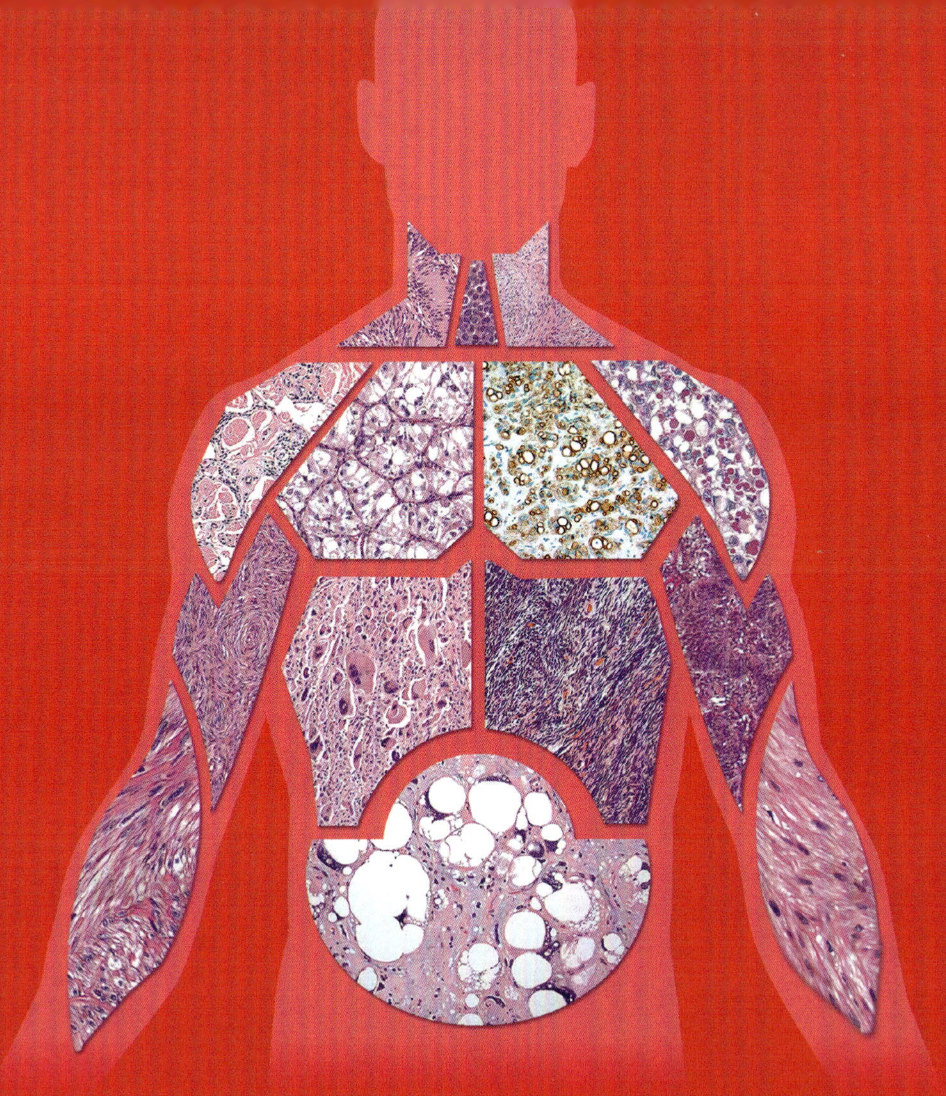

Diagnostic Pathology

Soft Tissue Tumors

Lindberg

ELSEVIER

THIRD EDITION

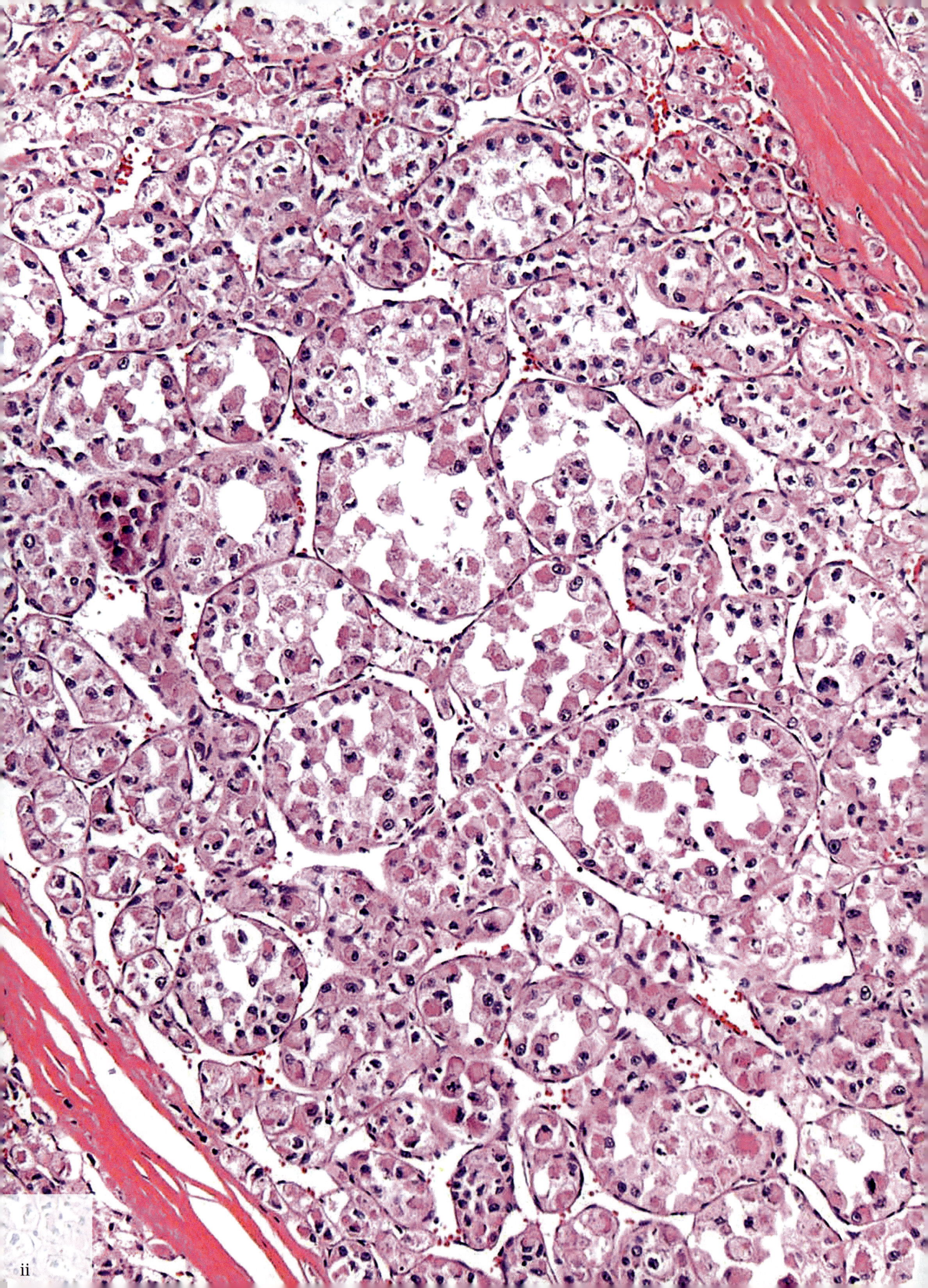

ii

Diagnostic Pathology

Soft Tissue Tumors

Third Edition

Matthew R. Lindberg, MD
Associate Professor of Pathology
University of Arkansas for Medical Sciences
Little Rock, Arkansas

DIAGNOSTIC PATHOLOGY: SOFT TISSUE TUMORS, THIRD EDITION

ISBN: 978-0-323-66110-2

Library of Congress Control Number: 2019931071

Cover Designer: Tom M. Olson, BA
Printed in Canada by Friesens, Altona, Manitoba, Canada

Last digit is the print number: 9 8 7 6 5 4 3 2 1

ELSEVIER

1600 John F. Kennedy Blvd.
Ste 1800
Philadelphia, PA 19103-2899

Dedication

To my wonderful wife, Rani, for her love, support, and infinite patience during the course of putting together this book. Also, to the excellent team of editors and coauthors with whom I have been very privileged to work. Many, many thanks for your hard work and high standards.

MRL

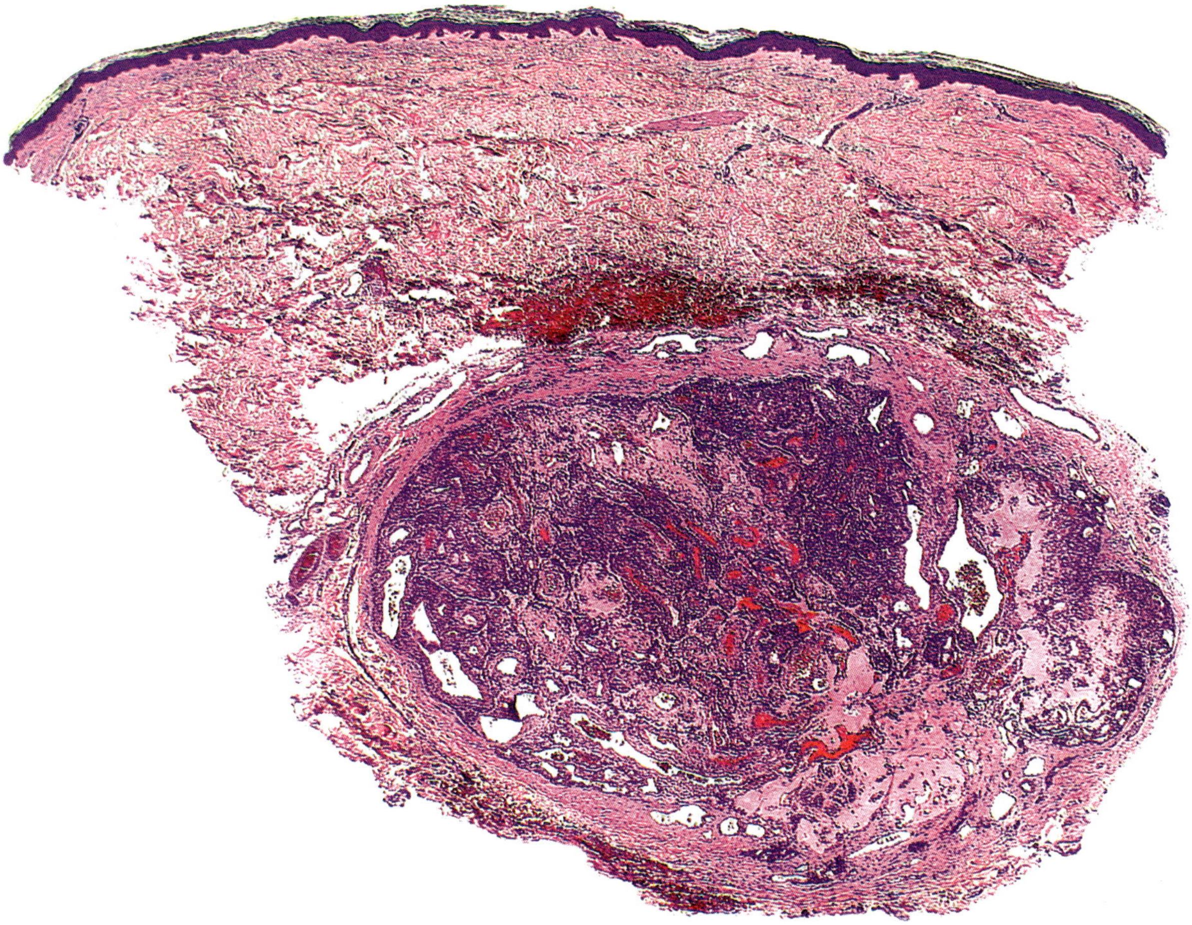

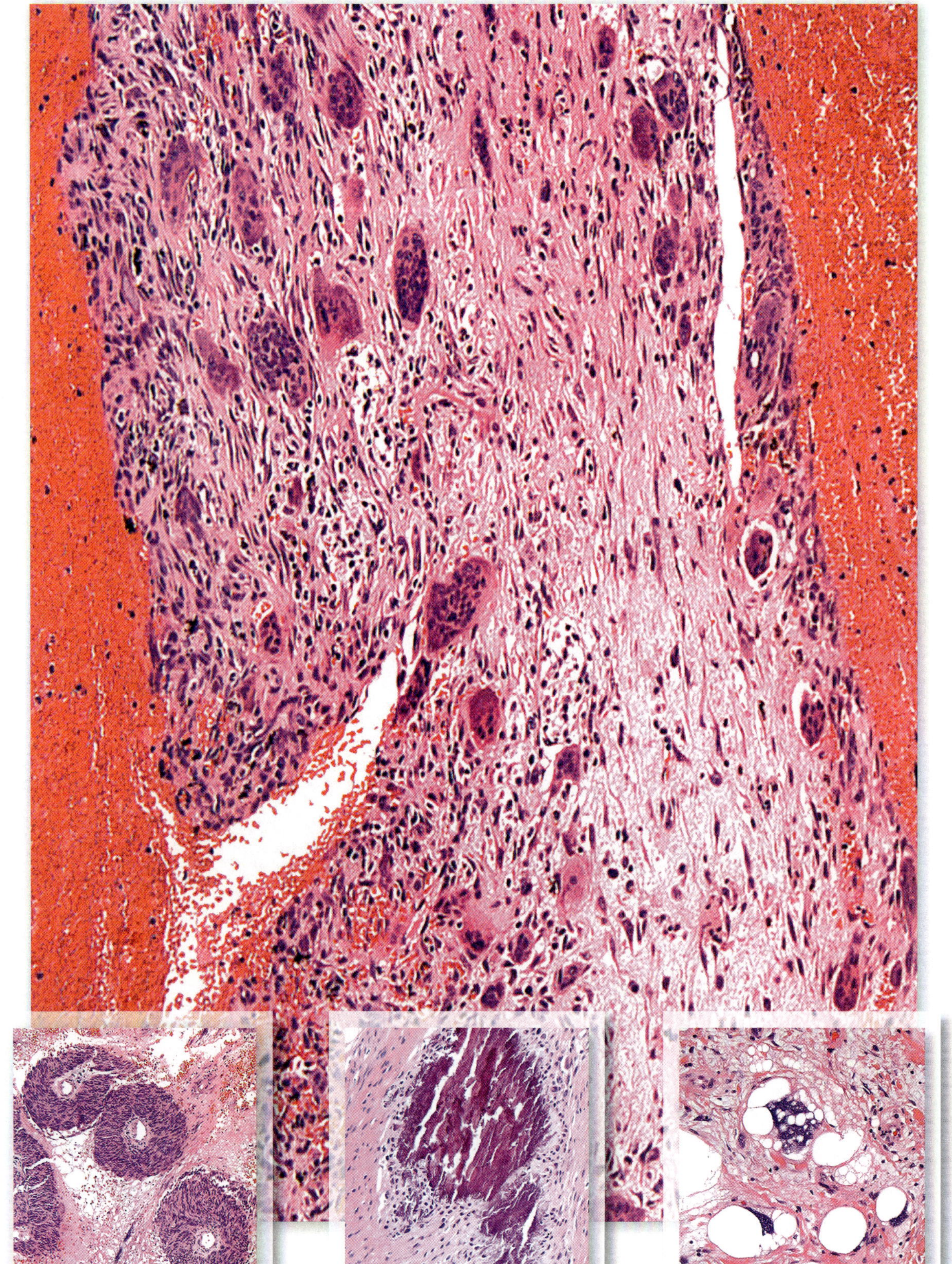

Contributing Authors

David Cassarino, MD, PhD
Dermatopathologist
Staff Pathologist
Los Angeles Permanente Medical Center
Los Angeles, California

Jerad M. Gardner, MD
Associate Professor of Pathology and Dermatology
Dermatopathology Fellowship Program Director
University of Arkansas for Medical Sciences
Little Rock, Arkansas

David Lucas, MD
Professor and Director of Anatomic Pathology
University of Michigan
Ann Arbor, Michigan

Charles Matthew Quick, MD
Associate Professor of Pathology
University of Arkansas for Medical Sciences
Little Rock, Arkansas

Kandi Stallings-Archer, MD
Assistant Professor of Pathology
University of Arkansas for Medical Sciences
Little Rock, Arkansas

Additional Contributing Authors

Jessica M. Comstock, MD

Cyril Fisher, MD, DSc, FRCPath

Jonathan B. McHugh, MD

L. Jeffrey Medeiros, MD

Thomas Mentzel, MD

Elizabeth A. Montgomery, MD

Amitabh Srivastava, MD

Lester D. R. Thompson, MD

Khin Thway, MD, FRCPath

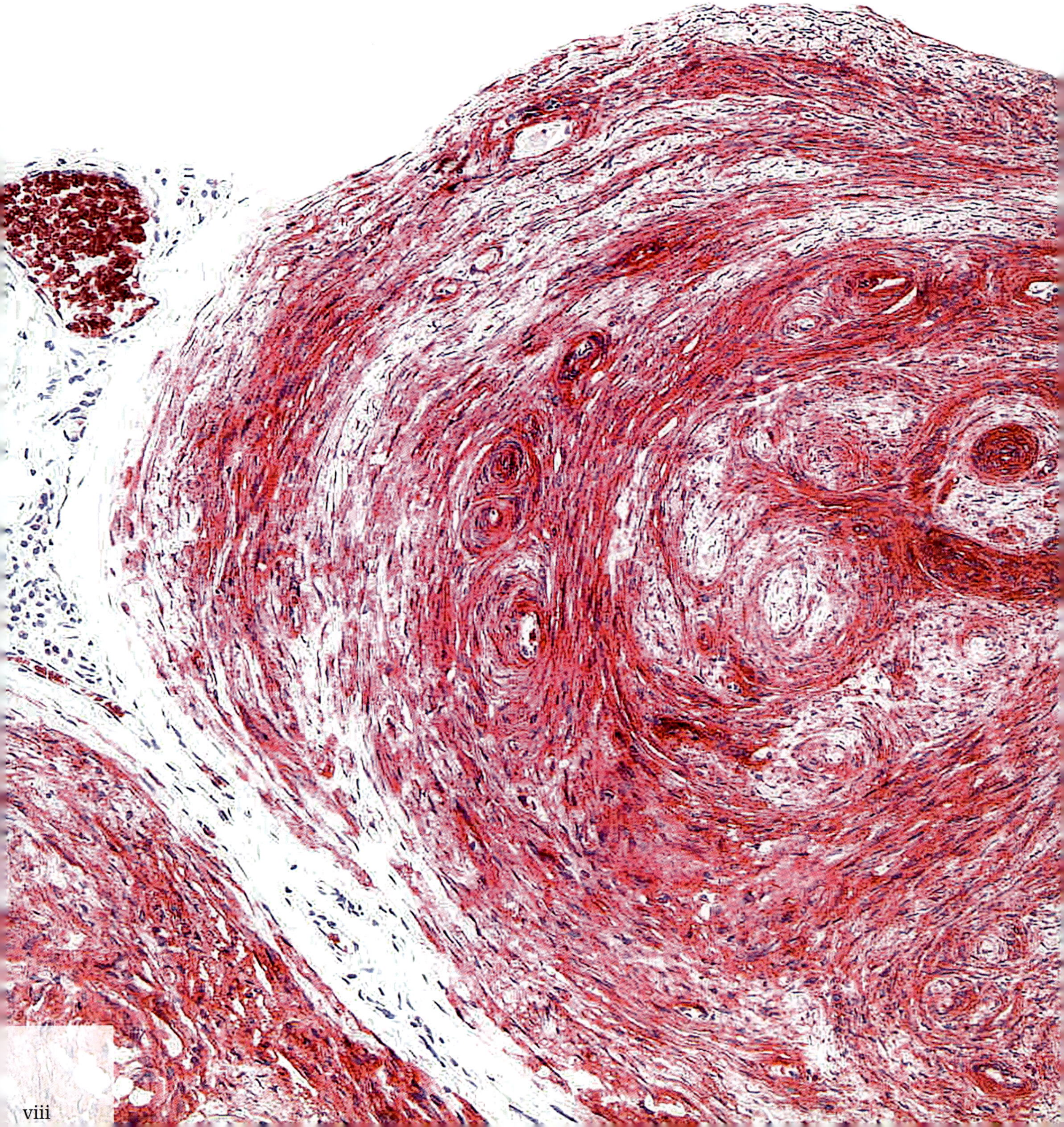

Preface

The field of soft tissue pathology continues to grow and change, with new diagnostic entities, immunohistochemical antibodies, and molecular tests introduced seemingly every month. The 3rd edition of *Diagnostic Pathology: Soft Tissue Tumors* strives to incorporate this new knowledge in the form of new chapters, updated text, and additional high-quality histologic images.

Since the publication of the 2nd edition, several new entities have been described in the scientific literature, including atypical spindle cell lipomatous tumor, superficial CD34-positive fibroblastic tumor, and *BCOR*-rearranged sarcoma. Chapters dedicated to each of these entities (as well as others) have been added in this new edition. Existing chapters devoted entirely to immunohistochemistry and molecular testing have also been updated to reflect recent discoveries in this span, and many individual chapters have seen a variety of text and gallery improvements. In particular, several galleries have been modified by swapping in new images that better reflect the extensive morphologic spectrum of soft tissue pathology.

As before, the 3 innovative "Approach to Diagnosis" chapters are still included in this new edition. Using a combination of clinical information, overall histologic pattern, and specific histologic findings, these chapters can aid the struggling pathologist in developing a thoughtful differential diagnosis for even some of the more challenging or unusual soft tissue cases. I hope you find these unique additions helpful in your own practice, both now and for many years to come.

Lastly, as always, owners of *Diagnostic Pathology: Soft Tissue Tumors*, 3rd edition, receive online access to all information and images contained in this text, plus much more. Enjoy!

Matthew R. Lindberg, MD
Associate Professor of Pathology
University of Arkansas for Medical Sciences
Little Rock, Arkansas

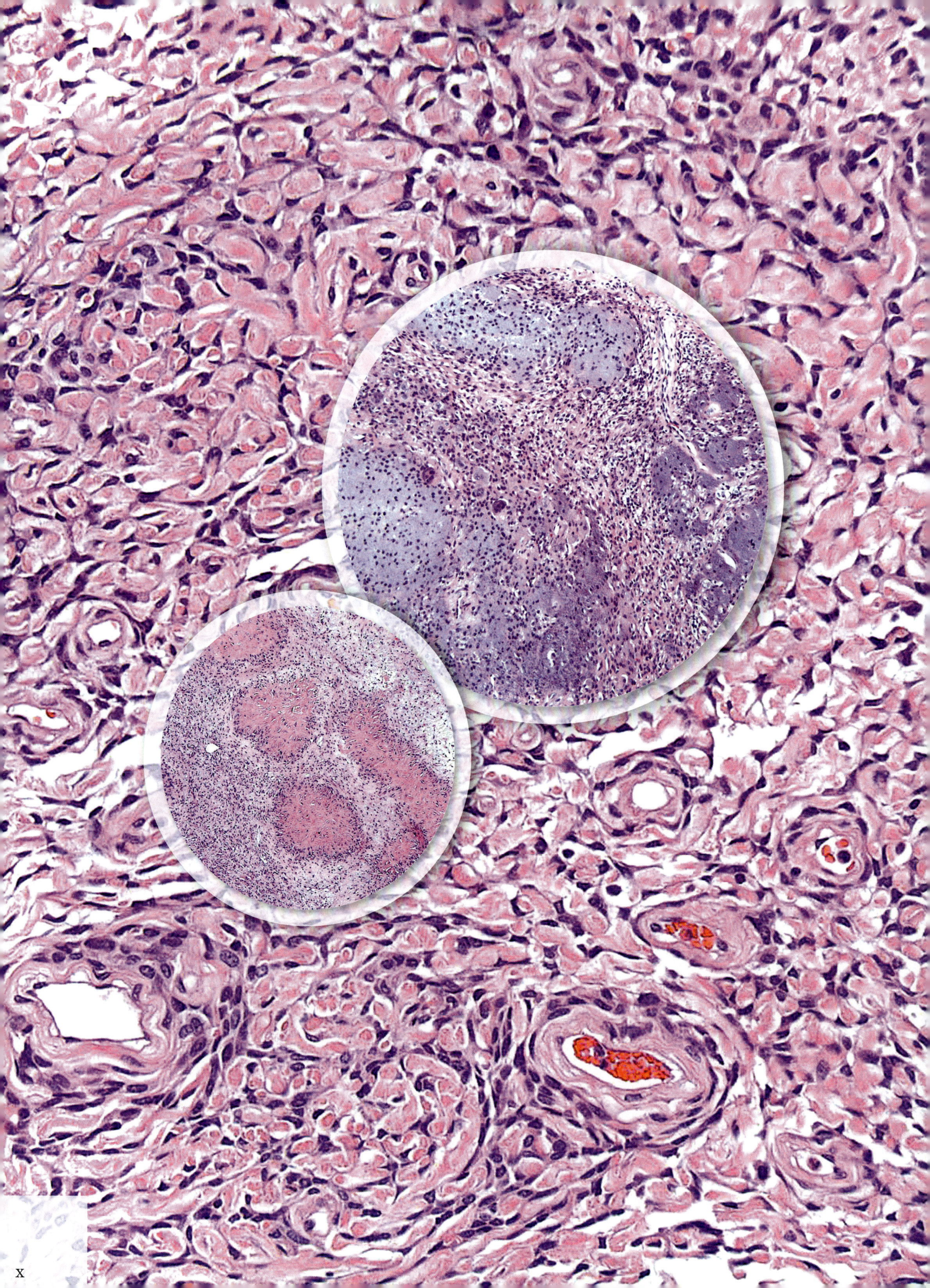

Acknowledgments

Lead Editor

Joshua Reynolds, PhD

Text Editors

Arthur G. Gelsinger, MA
Rebecca L. Bluth, BA
Nina I. Bennett, BA
Terry W. Ferrell, MS
Megg Morin, BA

Image Editors

Jeffrey J. Marmorstone, BS
Lisa A. M. Steadman, BS

Illustrations

Richard Coombs, MS
Lane R. Bennion, MS
Laura C. Wissler, MA

Art Direction and Design

Tom M. Olson, BA

Production Coordinators

Emily C. Fassett, BA
John Pecorelli, BS

ELSEVIER

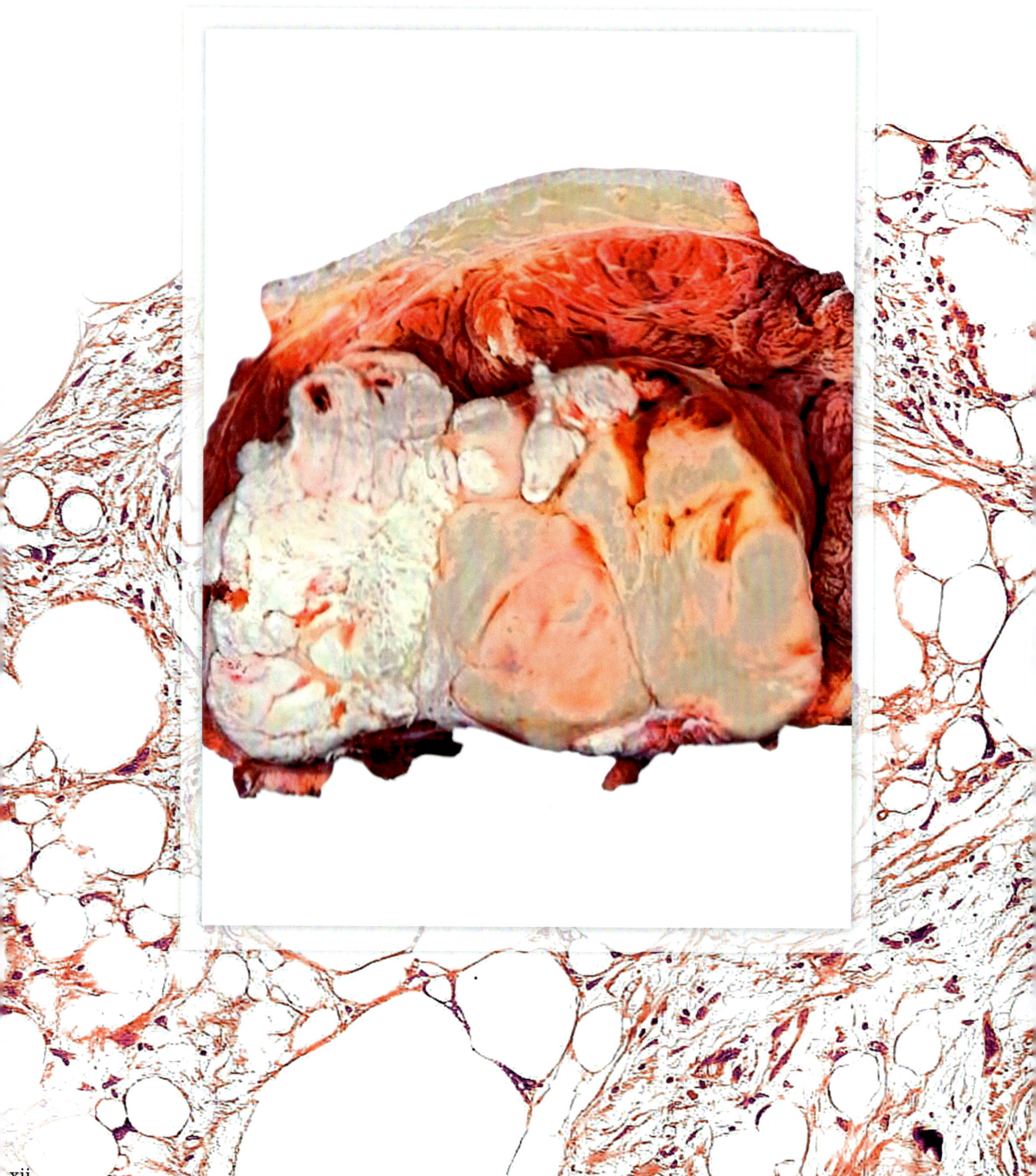

Sections

SECTION 1: Soft Tissue Introduction

SECTION 2: Diagnostic Approach to Soft Tissue Tumors

SECTION 3: Tumors of Adipose Tissue

SECTION 4: Fibroblastic/Myofibroblastic Lesions

SECTION 5: Pediatric Fibroblastic/Myofibroblastic Tumors

SECTION 6: Fibrohistiocytic, Histiocytic, and Dendritic Cell Tumors

SECTION 7: Smooth Muscle Tumors

SECTION 8: Pericytic (Perivascular) Tumors

SECTION 9: Tumors of Skeletal Muscle

SECTION 10: Vascular Tumors (Including Lymphatics)

SECTION 11: Chondroosseous Tumors

SECTION 12: Peripheral Nerve Sheath Tumors

SECTION 13: Genital Stromal Tumors

SECTION 14: Tumors of Mesothelial Cells

SECTION 15: Hematopoietic Tumors in Soft Tissue

SECTION 16: Tumors of Uncertain Differentiation

SECTION 17: Undifferentiated/Unclassified Sarcomas

SECTION 18: Mesenchymal Tumors of Gastrointestinal Tract

SECTION 19: Other Entities

TABLE OF CONTENTS

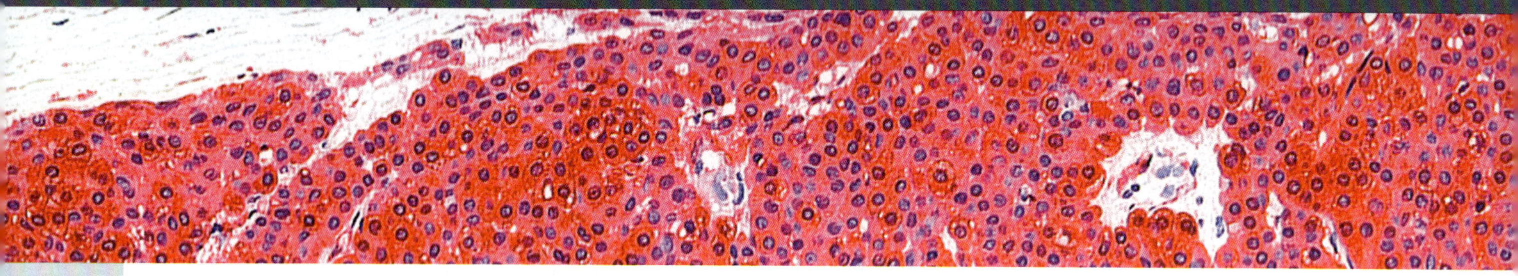

SECTION 1: SOFT TISSUE INTRODUCTION

INTRODUCTION AND OVERVIEW

4 **Gross Examination**
Matthew R. Lindberg, MD

6 **Grading and Staging**
Matthew R. Lindberg, MD

ANCILLARY TECHNIQUES

12 **Soft Tissue Immunohistochemistry**
Matthew R. Lindberg, MD

18 **Molecular Features of Soft Tissue Tumors**
Matthew R. Lindberg, MD

SECTION 2: DIAGNOSTIC APPROACH TO SOFT TISSUE TUMORS

OVERVIEW

22 **Biopsy and Resection of Soft Tissue Tumors**
Matthew R. Lindberg, MD

CLINICAL APPROACH

26 **Age- and Location-Based Approach to Diagnosis**
Matthew R. Lindberg, MD

HISTOLOGIC APPROACH

28 **Pattern-Based Approach to Diagnosis**
Matthew R. Lindberg, MD

36 **Feature-Based Approach to Diagnosis**
Matthew R. Lindberg, MD

SECTION 3: TUMORS OF ADIPOSE TISSUE

BENIGN

46 **Lipoma**
Matthew R. Lindberg, MD

52 **Lipomatosis of Nerve**
Jerad M. Gardner, MD

54 **Synovial Lipomatosis**
Matthew R. Lindberg, MD

56 **Angiolipoma**
Jerad M. Gardner, MD

60 **Spindle Cell/Pleomorphic Lipoma**
Matthew R. Lindberg, MD

66 **Chondroid Lipoma**
Matthew R. Lindberg, MD

70 **Myolipoma**
Jerad M. Gardner, MD

74 **Hibernoma**
Matthew R. Lindberg, MD

78 **Myelolipoma**
Matthew R. Lindberg, MD

80 **Lipoblastoma**
Matthew R. Lindberg, MD

84 **Atypical Spindle Cell Lipomatous Tumor**
Matthew R. Lindberg, MD

INTERMEDIATE, LOCALLY AGGRESSIVE

88 **Atypical Lipomatous Tumor/Well-Differentiated Liposarcoma**
Matthew R. Lindberg, MD

MALIGNANT

94 **Dedifferentiated Liposarcoma**
Matthew R. Lindberg, MD

100 **Myxoid Liposarcoma**
Matthew R. Lindberg, MD

106 **Pleomorphic Liposarcoma**
Matthew R. Lindberg, MD

SECTION 4: FIBROBLASTIC/MYOFIBROBLASTIC LESIONS

BENIGN

114 **Nodular Fasciitis**
Matthew R. Lindberg, MD

120 **Proliferative Fasciitis/Myositis**
Matthew R. Lindberg, MD

124 **Ischemic Fasciitis**
Matthew R. Lindberg, MD

126 **Myositis Ossificans**
Matthew R. Lindberg, MD

130 **Fibroosseous Pseudotumor of Digit**
David Lucas, MD and Elizabeth A. Montgomery, MD

134 **Fibroma of Tendon Sheath**
David Lucas, MD

140 **Desmoplastic Fibroblastoma**
David Cassarino, MD, PhD and Khin Thway, MD, FRCPath

142 **Elastofibroma**
Matthew R. Lindberg, MD

144 **Angiofibroma of Soft Tissue**
Matthew R. Lindberg, MD

148 **Mammary-Type Myofibroblastoma**
Matthew R. Lindberg, MD

152 **Intranodal Palisaded Myofibroblastoma**
Matthew R. Lindberg, MD

TABLE OF CONTENTS

156 **Pleomorphic Fibroma**
David Cassarino, MD, PhD

158 **Dermatomyofibroma**
David Cassarino, MD, PhD

160 **Storiform Collagenoma**
David Cassarino, MD, PhD

162 **Keloid**
David Cassarino, MD, PhD

164 **Nuchal-Type Fibroma**
Matthew R. Lindberg, MD

INTERMEDIATE (LOCALLY AGGRESSIVE)

166 **Palmar/Plantar Fibromatosis**
Matthew R. Lindberg, MD

168 **Desmoid-Type Fibromatosis**
Matthew R. Lindberg, MD

INTERMEDIATE (RARELY METASTASIZING)

174 **Dermatofibrosarcoma Protuberans**
Matthew R. Lindberg, MD

184 **Solitary Fibrous Tumor**
Matthew R. Lindberg, MD

192 **Low-Grade Myofibroblastic Sarcoma**
Matthew R. Lindberg, MD

196 **Inflammatory Myofibroblastic Tumor**
Matthew R. Lindberg, MD

202 **Myxoinflammatory Fibroblastic Sarcoma**
Matthew R. Lindberg, MD

210 **Superficial CD34(+) Fibroblastic Tumor**
Matthew R. Lindberg, MD

MALIGNANT

214 **Adult-Type Fibrosarcoma**
Jerad M. Gardner, MD

216 **Myxofibrosarcoma**
Matthew R. Lindberg, MD

222 **Low-Grade Fibromyxoid Sarcoma**
Matthew R. Lindberg, MD

232 **Sclerosing Epithelioid Fibrosarcoma**
Matthew R. Lindberg, MD

SECTION 5: PEDIATRIC FIBROBLASTIC/MYOFIBROBLASTIC TUMORS

BENIGN

240 **Fibrous Hamartoma of Infancy**
Matthew R. Lindberg, MD

244 **Calcifying Aponeurotic Fibroma**
Matthew R. Lindberg, MD

248 **Calcifying Fibrous Tumor**
Kandi Stallings-Archer, MD and Elizabeth A. Montgomery, MD

250 **Inclusion Body Fibromatosis**
Matthew R. Lindberg, MD

252 **Hyaline Fibromatosis Syndrome**
Kandi Stallings-Archer, MD, Elizabeth A. Montgomery, MD, and Cyril Fisher, MD, DSc, FRCPath

254 **Fibromatosis Colli**
Kandi Stallings-Archer, MD and Cyril Fisher, MD, DSc, FRCPath

256 **Gardner Fibroma**
Jerad M. Gardner, MD

INTERMEDIATE (LOCALLY AGGRESSIVE)

258 **Lipofibromatosis**
Kandi Stallings-Archer, MD and Elizabeth A. Montgomery, MD

260 **Giant Cell Fibroblastoma**
Matthew R. Lindberg, MD

INTERMEDIATE (RARELY METASTASIZING)

264 **Infantile Fibrosarcoma**
Matthew R. Lindberg, MD

SECTION 6: FIBROHISTIOCYTIC, HISTIOCYTIC, AND DENDRITIC CELL TUMORS

BENIGN

270 **Dermatofibroma and Fibrous Histiocytoma**
David Cassarino, MD, PhD

276 **Deep Benign Fibrous Histiocytoma**
Matthew R. Lindberg, MD

278 **Localized-Type Tenosynovial Giant Cell Tumor**
David Lucas, MD

284 **Diffuse-Type Tenosynovial Giant Cell Tumor**
David Lucas, MD

290 **Cellular Neurothekeoma**
Jerad M. Gardner, MD and Cyril Fisher, MD, DSc, FRCPath

294 **Xanthomas**
Matthew R. Lindberg, MD

298 **Solitary (Juvenile) Xanthogranuloma**
David Cassarino, MD, PhD and Elizabeth A. Montgomery, MD

300 **Reticulohistiocytoma**
David Cassarino, MD, PhD

304 **Deep Granuloma Annulare**
Jerad M. Gardner, MD

306 **Rheumatoid Nodule**
Jerad M. Gardner, MD

308 **Langerhans Cell Histiocytosis**
Matthew R. Lindberg, MD

310 **Extranodal Rosai-Dorfman Disease**
Matthew R. Lindberg, MD

314 **Crystal-Storing Histiocytosis**
Matthew R. Lindberg, MD and Elizabeth A. Montgomery, MD

INTERMEDIATE (RARELY METASTASIZING)

316 **Plexiform Fibrohistiocytic Tumor**
Matthew R. Lindberg, MD

320 **Giant Cell Tumor of Soft Tissue**
David Lucas, MD

TABLE OF CONTENTS

MALIGNANT

324 **Histiocytic Sarcoma**
Matthew R. Lindberg, MD

326 **Follicular Dendritic Cell Sarcoma**
Matthew R. Lindberg, MD

328 **Interdigitating Dendritic Cell Sarcoma**
Matthew R. Lindberg, MD, L. Jeffrey Medeiros, MD, and Cyril Fisher, MD, DSc, FRCPath

SECTION 7: SMOOTH MUSCLE TUMORS

BENIGN

332 **Smooth Muscle Hamartoma**
Jerad M. Gardner, MD

334 **Superficial Leiomyoma**
Jerad M. Gardner, MD and Jonathan B. McHugh, MD

338 **Deep Leiomyoma**
Matthew R. Lindberg, MD

INTERMEDIATE

342 **Epstein-Barr Virus-Associated Smooth Muscle Tumor**
David Lucas, MD

MALIGNANT

344 **Leiomyosarcoma**
Matthew R. Lindberg, MD

SECTION 8: PERICYTIC (PERIVASCULAR) TUMORS

BENIGN

352 **Glomus Tumors (and Variants)**
Thomas Mentzel, MD and Matthew R. Lindberg, MD

358 **Myopericytoma**
Matthew R. Lindberg, MD and Thomas Mentzel, MD

362 **Myofibroma and Myofibromatosis**
Matthew R. Lindberg, MD

366 **Angioleiomyoma**
Matthew R. Lindberg, MD

SECTION 9: TUMORS OF SKELETAL MUSCLE

BENIGN

370 **Focal Myositis**
Matthew R. Lindberg, MD and Cyril Fisher, MD, DSc, FRCPath

372 **Adult Rhabdomyoma**
Matthew R. Lindberg, MD

374 **Fetal Rhabdomyoma**
Matthew R. Lindberg, MD

376 **Genital Rhabdomyoma**
Matthew R. Lindberg, MD

378 **Cardiac Rhabdomyoma**
Matthew R. Lindberg, MD

MALIGNANT

380 **Embryonal Rhabdomyosarcoma**
Matthew R. Lindberg, MD

386 **Alveolar Rhabdomyosarcoma**
Matthew R. Lindberg, MD

392 **Spindle Cell Rhabdomyosarcoma**
Matthew R. Lindberg, MD

396 **Sclerosing Rhabdomyosarcoma**
Matthew R. Lindberg, MD

400 **Pleomorphic Rhabdomyosarcoma**
Jerad M. Gardner, MD

404 **Epithelioid Rhabdomyosarcoma**
Matthew R. Lindberg, MD

SECTION 10: VASCULAR TUMORS (INCLUDING LYMPHATICS)

BENIGN

408 **Papillary Endothelial Hyperplasia**
David Cassarino, MD, PhD and Amitabh Srivastava, MD

410 **Bacillary Angiomatosis**
David Cassarino, MD, PhD

412 **Congenital Hemangioma**
Kandi Stallings-Archer, MD

416 **Infantile Hemangioma**
Kandi Stallings-Archer, MD

420 **Lobular Capillary Hemangioma**
Matthew R. Lindberg, MD

422 **Epithelioid Hemangioma**
Matthew R. Lindberg, MD

426 **Spindle Cell Hemangioma**
Jerad M. Gardner, MD

430 **Intramuscular Hemangioma**
Matthew R. Lindberg, MD and Jonathan B. McHugh, MD

434 **Hobnail Hemangioma**
David Cassarino, MD, PhD

436 **Acquired Tufted Angioma**
David Cassarino, MD, PhD

438 **Microvenular Hemangioma**
David Cassarino, MD, PhD

440 **Sinusoidal Hemangioma**
David Cassarino, MD, PhD

442 **Glomeruloid Hemangioma**
David Cassarino, MD, PhD

444 **Angiomatosis**
David Lucas, MD

446 **Lymphangioma**
David Cassarino, MD, PhD

450 **Massive Localized Lymphedema**
Matthew R. Lindberg, MD

452 **Atypical Vascular Lesion**
David Lucas, MD

INTERMEDIATE (LOCALLY AGGRESSIVE)

454 **Kaposiform Hemangioendothelioma**
David Lucas, MD

TABLE OF CONTENTS

INTERMEDIATE (RARELY METASTASIZING)

456 **Papillary Intralymphatic Angioendothelioma**
David Cassarino, MD, PhD
458 **Retiform Hemangioendothelioma**
David Cassarino, MD, PhD
460 **Composite Hemangioendothelioma**
David Lucas, MD
462 **Pseudomyogenic Hemangioendothelioma**
Matthew R. Lindberg, MD

MALIGNANT

466 **Epithelioid Hemangioendothelioma**
Matthew R. Lindberg, MD and Thomas Mentzel, MD
470 **Angiosarcoma**
Matthew R. Lindberg, MD
476 **Kaposi Sarcoma**
Jerad M. Gardner, MD and Thomas Mentzel, MD

SECTION 11: CHONDROOSSEOUS TUMORS

BENIGN

486 **Soft Tissue Chondroma**
David Lucas, MD
492 **Synovial Chondromatosis**
David Lucas, MD

MALIGNANT

496 **Extraskeletal Osteosarcoma**
David Lucas, MD
500 **Extraskeletal Mesenchymal Chondrosarcoma**
David Lucas, MD

SECTION 12: PERIPHERAL NERVE SHEATH TUMORS

BENIGN

506 **Solitary Circumscribed Neuroma**
Jerad M. Gardner, MD
508 **Schwannoma**
Matthew R. Lindberg, MD
522 **Neurofibroma**
Matthew R. Lindberg, MD
530 **Perineurioma**
Matthew R. Lindberg, MD
536 **Hybrid Nerve Sheath Tumor**
Matthew R. Lindberg, MD
540 **Granular Cell Tumor**
Matthew R. Lindberg, MD
546 **Dermal Nerve Sheath Myxoma**
David Lucas, MD
550 **Ganglioneuroma**
Matthew R. Lindberg, MD
554 **Neuromuscular Choristoma**
David Lucas, MD

INTERMEDIATE

556 **Melanotic Schwannoma**
Matthew R. Lindberg, MD

MALIGNANT

558 **Malignant Peripheral Nerve Sheath Tumor**
Matthew R. Lindberg, MD
566 **Epithelioid Malignant Peripheral Nerve Sheath Tumor**
Matthew R. Lindberg, MD
570 **Ectomesenchymoma**
Matthew R. Lindberg, MD and Cyril Fisher, MD, DSc, FRCPath

SECTION 13: GENITAL STROMAL TUMORS

574 **Fibroepithelial Stromal Polyp**
Matthew R. Lindberg, MD
576 **Angiomyofibroblastoma**
Matthew R. Lindberg, MD
580 **Cellular Angiofibroma**
Matthew R. Lindberg, MD
584 **Deep (Aggressive) Angiomyxoma**
Matthew R. Lindberg, MD

SECTION 14: TUMORS OF MESOTHELIAL CELLS

BENIGN

590 **Adenomatoid Tumor**
Matthew R. Lindberg, MD
592 **Multicystic Peritoneal Mesothelioma**
Matthew R. Lindberg, MD
594 **Well-Differentiated Papillary Mesothelioma**
David Lucas, MD and Cyril Fisher, MD, DSc, FRCPath

MALIGNANT

598 **Malignant Mesothelioma**
Matthew R. Lindberg, MD and Cyril Fisher, MD, DSc, FRCPath

SECTION 15: HEMATOPOIETIC TUMORS IN SOFT TISSUE

606 **Solitary Extramedullary Plasmacytoma**
Matthew R. Lindberg, MD
608 **Myeloid Sarcoma**
Matthew R. Lindberg, MD
610 **Lymphoma of Soft Tissue**
Matthew R. Lindberg, MD and Khin Thway, MD, FRCPath

SECTION 16: TUMORS OF UNCERTAIN DIFFERENTIATION

BENIGN

614 **Intramuscular Myxoma**
Matthew R. Lindberg, MD

TABLE OF CONTENTS

618 **Juxtaarticular Myxoma**
Matthew R. Lindberg, MD and Khin Thway, MD, FRCPath

620 **Superficial Angiomyxoma**
Jerad M. Gardner, MD

624 **Acral Fibromyxoma**
Matthew R. Lindberg, MD

626 **Pleomorphic Hyalinizing Angiectatic Tumor**
Matthew R. Lindberg, MD and Cyril Fisher, MD, DSc, FRCPath

630 **Aneurysmal Bone Cyst of Soft Tissue**
Matthew R. Lindberg, MD

632 **Ectopic Hamartomatous Thymoma**
Matthew R. Lindberg, MD

INTERMEDIATE (LOCALLY AGGRESSIVE)

634 **Hemosiderotic Fibrolipomatous Tumor**
Matthew R. Lindberg, MD

INTERMEDIATE (RARELY METASTASIZING)

636 **Atypical Fibroxanthoma**
David Cassarino, MD, PhD

642 **Angiomatoid Fibrous Histiocytoma**
Matthew R. Lindberg, MD

650 **Ossifying Fibromyxoid Tumor**
Matthew R. Lindberg, MD

656 **Myoepithelioma of Soft Tissue**
Matthew R. Lindberg, MD

664 **Phosphaturic Mesenchymal Tumor**
Matthew R. Lindberg, MD

MALIGNANT

666 **Synovial Sarcoma**
Matthew R. Lindberg, MD

678 **Epithelioid Sarcoma**
Matthew R. Lindberg, MD

684 **Alveolar Soft Part Sarcoma**
Matthew R. Lindberg, MD

688 **Clear Cell Sarcoma**
Jerad M. Gardner, MD

692 **Perivascular Epithelioid Cell Tumor (PEComa)**
Matthew R. Lindberg, MD

700 **Desmoplastic Small Round Cell Tumor**
Matthew R. Lindberg, MD

706 **Extraskeletal Ewing Sarcoma**
Kandi Stallings-Archer, MD and Cyril Fisher, MD, DSc, FRCPath

712 **Extraskeletal Myxoid Chondrosarcoma**
David Lucas, MD

716 **Extrarenal Rhabdoid Tumor**
Matthew R. Lindberg, MD

720 **Intimal Sarcoma**
Jerad M. Gardner, MD

SECTION 17: UNDIFFERENTIATED/UNCLASSIFIED SARCOMAS

724 **Undifferentiated Pleomorphic Sarcoma**
Matthew R. Lindberg, MD

728 **Undifferentiated Round Cell Sarcoma With *CIC-DUX4* Translocation**
David Lucas, MD

734 ***BCOR-CCNB3* Fusion-Positive Sarcoma**
David Lucas, MD

SECTION 18: MESENCHYMAL TUMORS OF GASTROINTESTINAL TRACT

740 **Benign Neural Gastrointestinal Polyps**
Matthew R. Lindberg, MD

744 **Gastrointestinal Stromal Tumor**
Matthew R. Lindberg, MD

760 **Gastrointestinal Schwannoma**
Matthew R. Lindberg, MD

762 **Gastrointestinal Smooth Muscle Neoplasms**
Matthew R. Lindberg, MD

766 **Inflammatory Fibroid Polyp**
Matthew R. Lindberg, MD

770 **Gangliocytic Paraganglioma**
Matthew R. Lindberg, MD

772 **Plexiform Fibromyxoma**
Matthew R. Lindberg, MD

776 **Malignant Gastrointestinal Neuroectodermal Tumor**
Matthew R. Lindberg, MD

SECTION 19: OTHER ENTITIES

BENIGN

782 **Amyloidoma**
Matthew R. Lindberg, MD

784 **Ganglion Cyst**
Matthew R. Lindberg, MD

786 **Tumoral Calcinosis**
Matthew R. Lindberg, MD

788 **Idiopathic Tumefactive Fibroinflammatory Lesions**
Matthew R. Lindberg, MD

792 **Cardiac Myxoma**
Matthew R. Lindberg, MD

796 **Cardiac Fibroma**
Matthew R. Lindberg, MD

798 **Congenital Granular Cell Epulis**
Matthew R. Lindberg, MD

800 **Nasopharyngeal Angiofibroma**
Matthew R. Lindberg, MD, Lester D. R. Thompson, MD, and Cyril Fisher, MD, DSc, FRCPath

804 **Sinonasal Glomangiopericytoma**
Matthew R. Lindberg, MD and Jonathan B. McHugh, MD

810 **Ectopic Meningioma**
Matthew R. Lindberg, MD

812 **Glial Heterotopia**
Matthew R. Lindberg, MD

INTERMEDIATE

814 **Paraganglioma**
Matthew R. Lindberg, MD

822 **Peripheral Hemangioblastoma**
Matthew R. Lindberg, MD

824 **Melanotic Neuroectodermal Tumor of Infancy**
Matthew R. Lindberg, MD

TABLE OF CONTENTS

826 **Ependymoma of Soft Tissue**
Matthew R. Lindberg, MD

MALIGNANT

828 **Metastatic Tumors to Soft Tissue Sites**
Matthew R. Lindberg, MD

832 **Neuroblastoma and Ganglioneuroblastoma**
Kandi Stallings-Archer, MD, Jessica M. Comstock, MD, and Cyril Fisher, MD, DSc, FRCPath

842 **Extraaxial Soft Tissue Chordoma**
Jerad M. Gardner, MD

844 **Undifferentiated Embryonal Sarcoma of Liver**
Matthew R. Lindberg, MD

846 **Primary Pulmonary Myxoid Sarcoma**
David Lucas, MD

850 **Biphenotypic Sinonasal Sarcoma**
Matthew R. Lindberg, MD

854 **Spindle Epithelial Tumor With Thymus-Like Differentiation**
Matthew R. Lindberg, MD

856 **Low-Grade Endometrial Stromal Sarcoma**
Charles Matthew Quick, MD and Khin Thway, MD, FRCPath

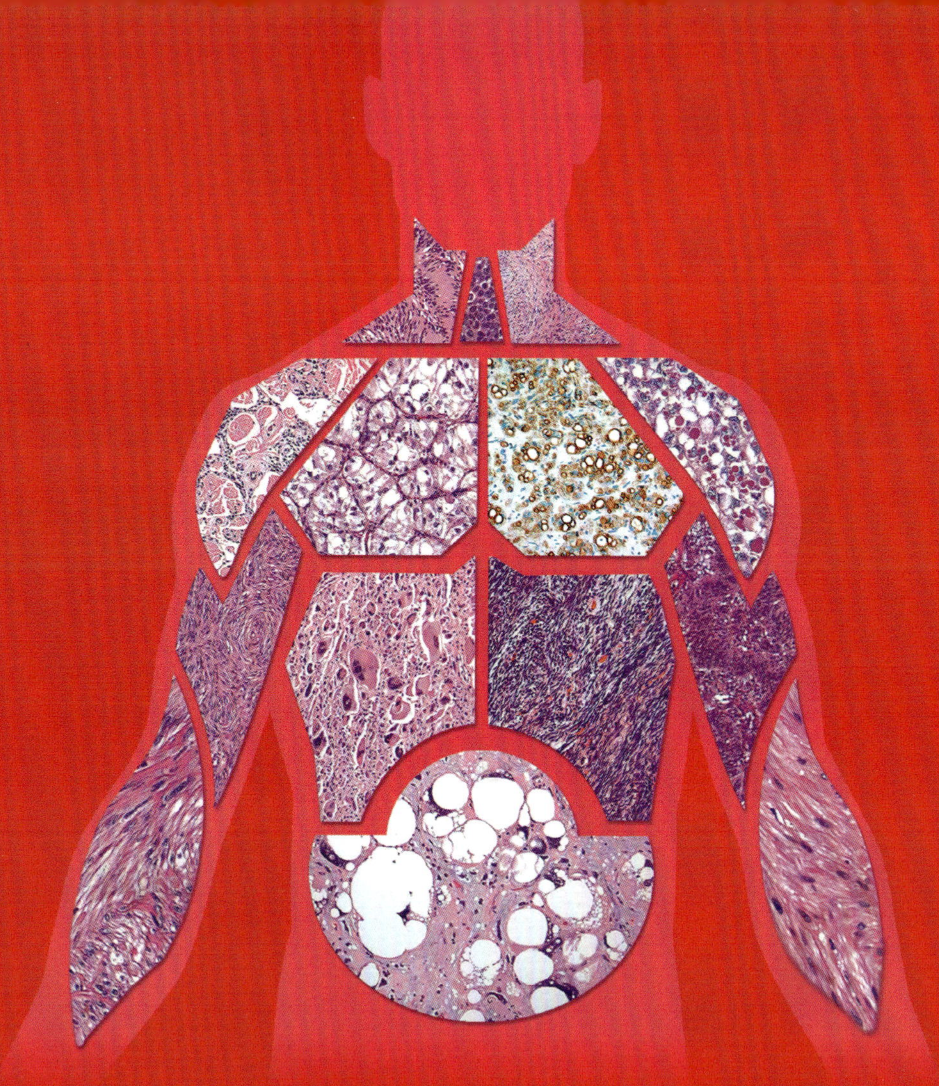

Diagnostic Pathology

Soft Tissue Tumors

Lindberg

ELSEVIER

THIRD EDITION

SECTION 1
Soft Tissue Introduction

Introduction and Overview

Gross Examination 4

Grading and Staging 6

Ancillary Techniques

Soft Tissue Immunohistochemistry 12

Molecular Features of Soft Tissue Tumors 18

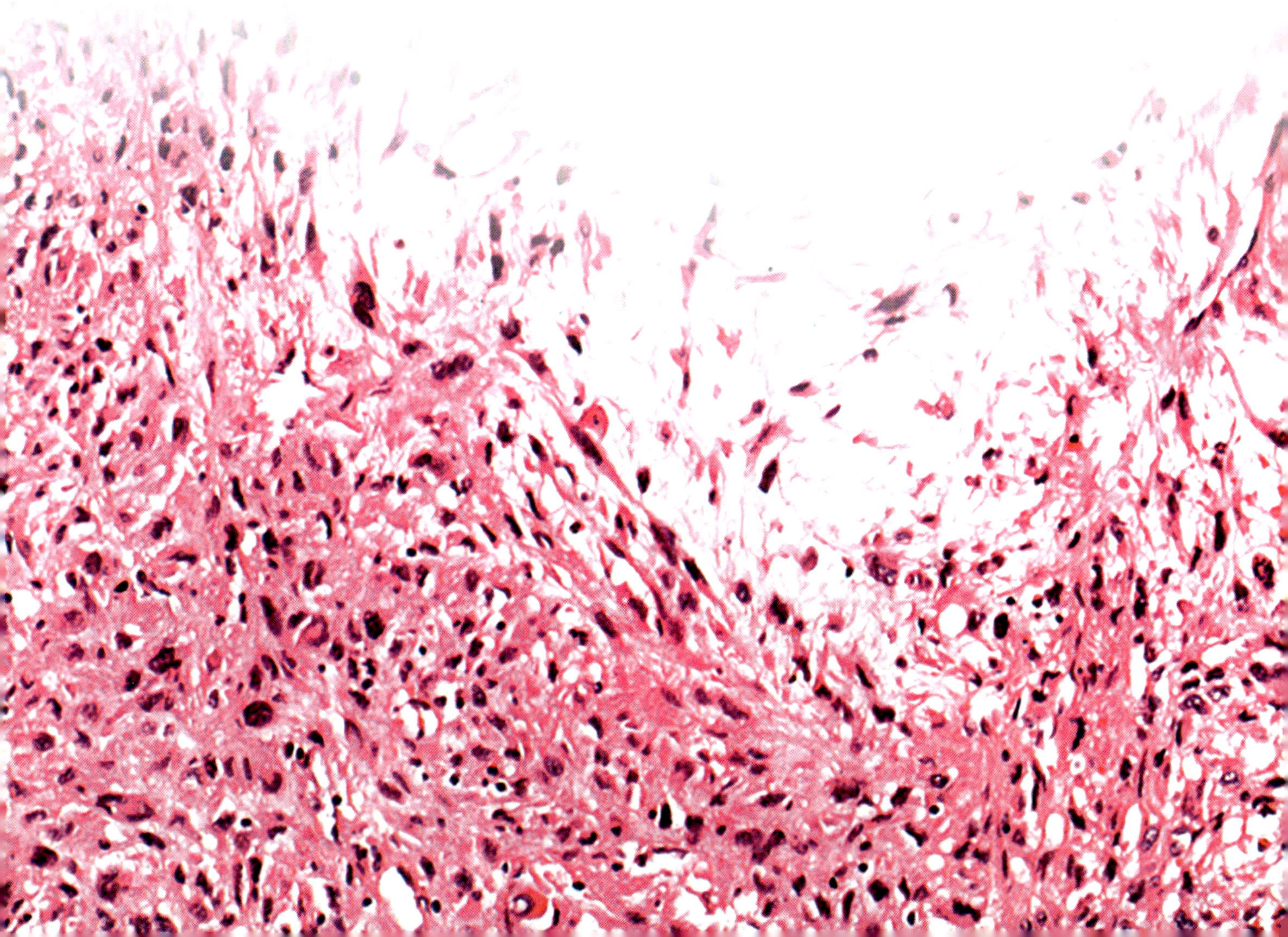

INTRODUCTION

Overview

- Thorough but focused gross examination is vital component of overall evaluation and diagnostic work-up of soft tissue tumors
- Common errors (e.g., undersampling, inappropriate sampling, not inking margins) can severely hamper or preclude accurate diagnosis, pathologic staging, and subsequent clinical planning
- Review of patient clinical history and information prior to gross examination is strongly recommended

CLINICAL FINDINGS

History

- Review any available clinical notes or operative report
  - Note age of patient and clinical presentation of tumor
  - Note if patient has prior history of tumor in same anatomic location, nearby, or elsewhere
- Determine whether tumor has been previously biopsied or treated or if there is established diagnosis

Imaging

- Review any pertinent radiographs, CT, or MR scans
  - Determine if tumor is homogeneous or heterogeneous
  - Identify any notable structures involved (e.g., large nerve trunk)
  - Determine whether radiologist favors benign or malignant process
- Note anatomic location (e.g., thigh, neck, retroperitoneum, finger)
- Note tissue plane (i.e., superficial/subcutaneous vs. deep/intramuscular)

GROSSING PROCEDURE

External Examination

- Specimen should be weighed and measured in 3 dimensions
- Describe external appearance and shape of mass
- Note any orientation provided by surgeon (e.g., stitches, strip of overlying skin, large nerves)
  - Skin is often excised to remove previous biopsy tract with rest of specimen
- Ink peripheral margins of specimen
  - Oriented tumors often require inking with up to 6 different colors
  - Unoriented tumors may be inked in 1 color

Sectioning and Internal Evaluation

- Serially section ("bread loaf") mass in 1-cm thick sections, perpendicular to long axis of specimen
- Lay out all slabs of tumor and examine cut surfaces
- Describe appearance of cut surface and note areas of different coloration &/or texture
  - Common colors: Tan, white, gray, red, brown
  - Common textures: Firm/fibrous, fleshy, gelatinous/glistening, fatty
- Note any areas of hemorrhage &/or necrosis
  - Quantify necrosis (none, ≤ 50%, or > 50%)
  - Highly necrotic tumors should be placed in formalin to fix and to minimize fragmentation
- Take representative fresh tissue for possible ancillary techniques or treatment protocols (may be snap frozen)

Sampling

- Standard approach is to take 1 section per cm of greatest tumor dimension (margin sections counted separately)
  - e.g., 16-cm tumor gets 16 blocks with 1 tissue piece in each or 8 blocks with 2 tissue pieces in each
  - Fewer sections may be submitted for large tumors with diffuse homogeneous appearance
- Inked margins, specifically close (< 2 cm) margins, should be sampled with perpendicular sections
- Sections should be taken from all distinctive areas (e.g., fibrous, gelatinous, fleshy, etc.)
  - Sections taken at interface between different areas can provide very useful histologic information
- Obviously necrotic areas should be minimally sampled
  - These areas often represent high-grade morphologies and are generally less useful diagnostically

External Examination

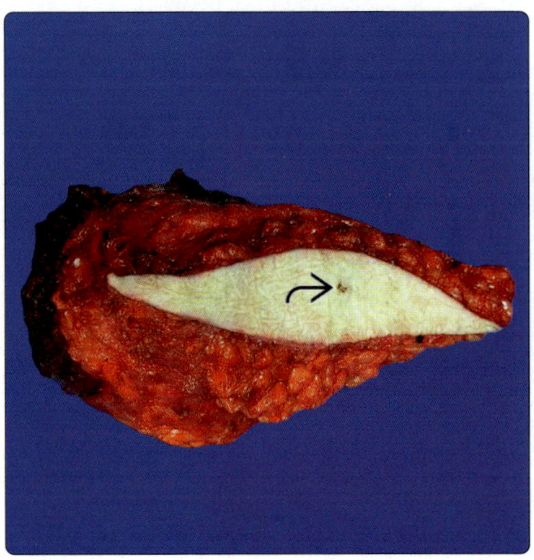

Specimen Inking

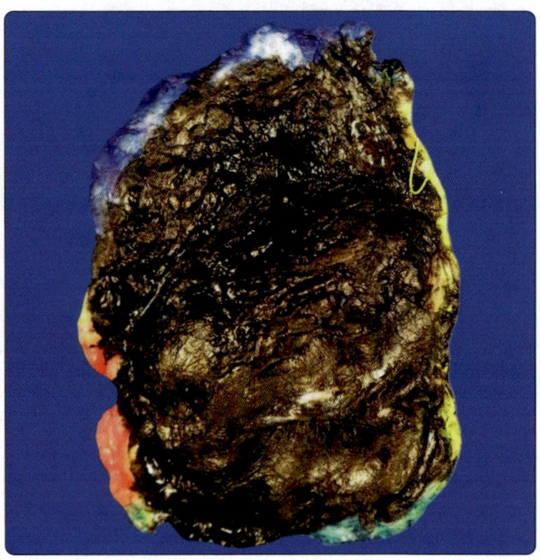

(Left) *The gross appearance of a soft tissue tumor specimen varies depending on the type of surgery, but many tumors (especially sarcomas) are removed with at least a thin rim of surrounding soft tissue. If the tumor has been previously sampled by core biopsy, the biopsy tract* ➩ *and skin strip are often removed as well.* **(Right)** *Although known benign soft tissue tumors are often excised without orientation by the surgeon, sarcomas often arrive oriented by stitches and require inking, as depicted, for satisfactory margin evaluation.*

Serial Sectioning

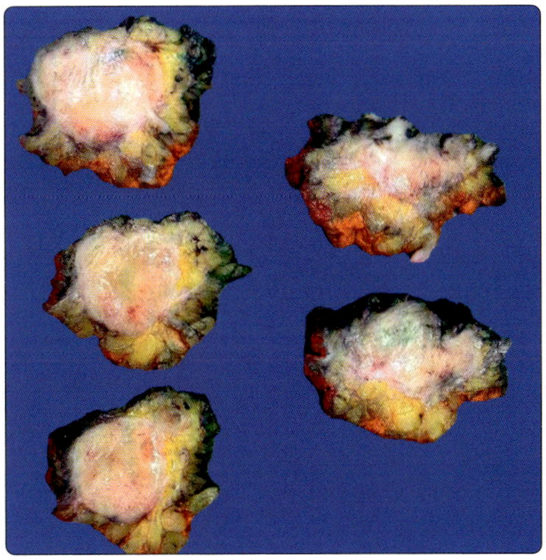

Evaluation of Cut Surface

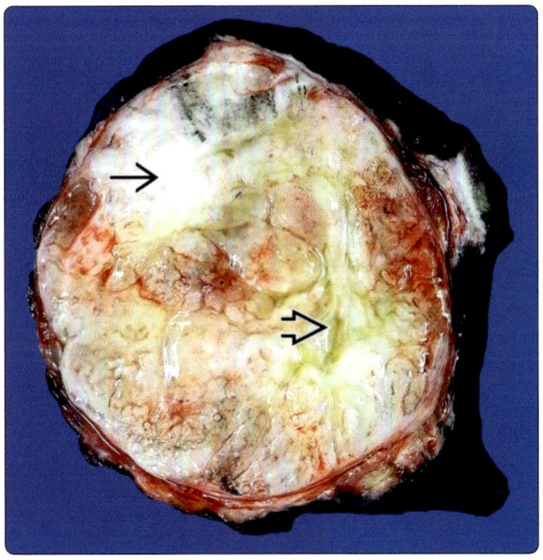

(Left) *After external examination and inking of the soft tissue tumor specimen, it should be serially sectioned in ~ 1-cm slices. After all sections are laid out, the margins should be assessed and sampled, and the appearance of the cut surfaces should be evaluated with any variations noted.* **(Right)** *The cut surface of a soft tissue tumor may show a variety of appearances (e.g., fibrous ⇨, fleshy, fatty, gelatinous ⇨), and all distinctive areas should be noted and sampled. Transition areas should be particularly targeted.*

Evaluation of Cut Surface

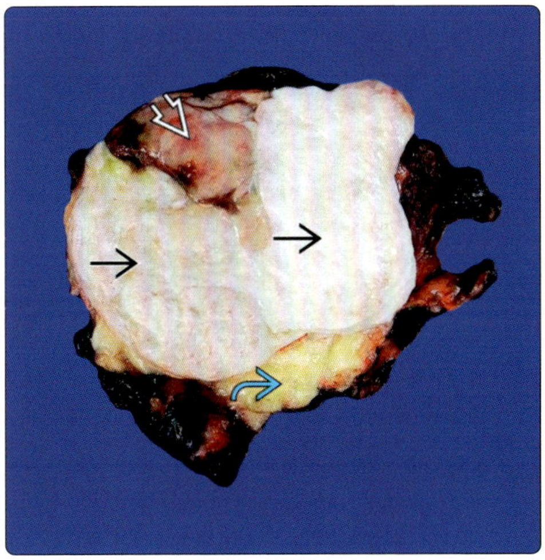

Documentation of Necrosis

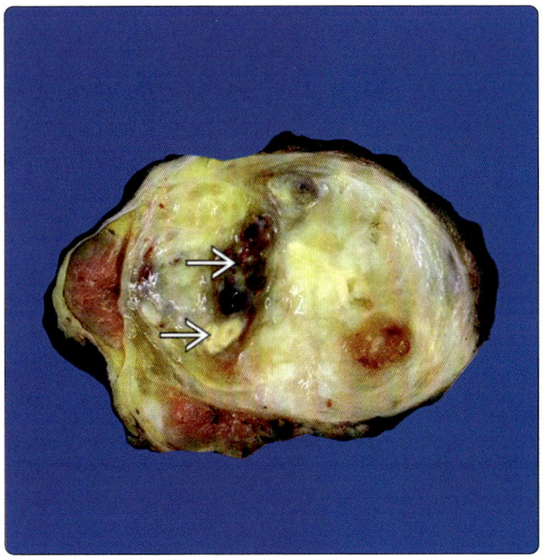

(Left) *Gross photo of a dedifferentiated liposarcoma shows a mixture of fibrous ⇨ and fleshy ➡ areas representing the high-grade component. The minimal, well-differentiated component ⇨ may be easily mistaken for normal fat and ignored.* **(Right)** *It is important to assess and document the amount of necrosis ➡ present during gross examination, as it may be useful in subsequent grading of the tumor. Of note, sometimes nonnecrotic, degenerative, edematous, or myxoid areas may be mistaken for necrosis grossly.*

Large Homogeneous Tumors

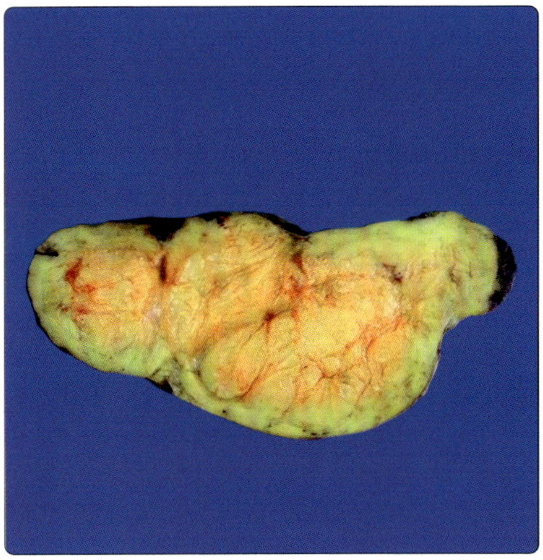

En Bloc Radical Resection Specimen

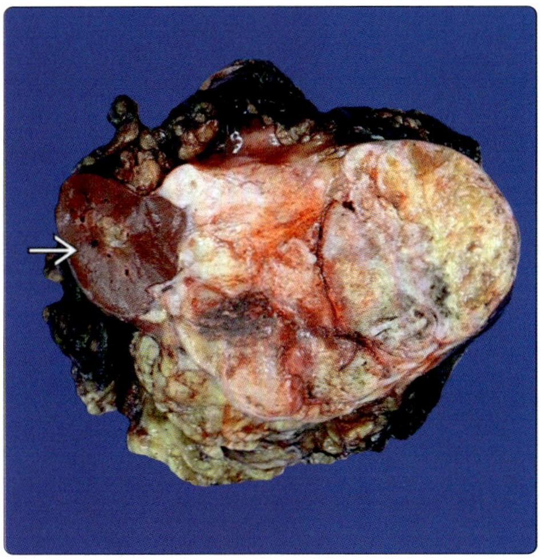

(Left) *Some larger soft tissue tumors show a similar homogeneous cut surface on all gross slices without areas of variation, as is seen in this gross photo of a lipoma. The "1 section per cm" rule may be relaxed in this situation.* **(Right)** *Soft tissue tumors that arise in body cavities (particularly the retroperitoneum) can grow to incredible sizes and may require radical surgical resection and debulking. This gross photo shows a dedifferentiated liposarcoma with renal ➡ involvement.*

GRADING AND STAGING SYSTEMS

Grading System

- French FNCLCC system most commonly utilized

Staging System

- TNM system (AJCC Cancer Staging Manual, 8th edition)

HISTOLOGIC FEATURES EVALUATED IN GRADING (FNCLCC)

Method

- Assign following 3 independent scores based upon particular histologic parameters
  - Differentiation
  - Mitotic rate
  - Necrosis
- 3 independent scores are totaled to determine histologic grade of sarcoma

Degree of Cellular Differentiation

- Score 1: Sarcomas closely resembling normal, adult mesenchymal tissue
  - Well-differentiated examples of liposarcoma (LPS)
  - Leiomyosarcoma
  - Malignant peripheral nerve sheath tumor (MPNST)
  - Others
- Score 2: Sarcoma for which histologic typing is certain
  - Myxofibrosarcoma
  - Myxoid LPS (excluding cellular/round cell)
  - Conventional leiomyosarcoma
  - MPNST
  - Others
- Score 3: Embryonal or undifferentiated sarcomas, synovial sarcoma, or sarcoma of uncertain type
  - Dedifferentiated LPS
  - Pleomorphic LPS
  - High-grade myxoid LPS (formerly round cell LPS)
  - Most rhabdomyosarcoma
  - Ewing sarcoma
  - Mesenchymal chondrosarcoma
  - Extraskeletal osteosarcoma
  - Pleomorphic leiomyosarcoma
  - Pleomorphic MPNST
  - Undifferentiated pleomorphic sarcoma

Mitotic Rate (Mitoses per 10 HPF)

- Score 1: 0-9
- Score 2: 10-19
- Score 3: > 19
  - Count total number in 10 successive HPF (40x objective) in most mitotically active areas
  - Avoid ulcerated, necrotic, or hypocellular areas

Percentage of Microscopic Tumor Necrosis

- Score 0: No necrosis
- Score 1: Necrosis < 50% total tumor volume
- Score 2: Necrosis ≥ 50% total tumor volume
  - Tumor necrosis should be evaluated at macroscopic and microscopic levels

Overall Histologic Grade

- Summation of 3 individual scores indicates grade
  - Grade 1 (low grade): Total score 2 or 3
  - Grade 2 (intermediate grade): Total score 4 or 5
  - Grade 3 (high grade): Total score 6, 7, or 8

Limitations

- Grading schemata apply best to fully excised specimens that have not been preoperatively treated with neoadjuvant therapies
  - Only minimum grade can be applied to limited (biopsy) sample
  - Sarcomas treated preoperatively with chemotherapy &/or radiation cannot be accurately graded
- For some sarcomas, grade is automatically defined by histologic subtype
  - Always grade 1 (low grade)
    - Well-differentiated LPS
    - Conventional dermatofibrosarcoma protuberans
    - Infantile fibrosarcoma
  - Always grade 3 (high grade)
    - Ewing sarcoma
    - High-grade myxoid LPS (formerly round cell LPS)
    - Pleomorphic LPS
    - Dedifferentiated LPS
    - Extraskeletal osteosarcoma
    - Mesenchymal chondrosarcoma
    - Desmoplastic small round cell tumor
    - Extrarenal rhabdoid tumor
  - Not formally graded but often managed as high grade
    - Alveolar soft part sarcoma
    - Clear cell sarcoma
    - Epithelioid sarcoma
    - Extraskeletal myxoid chondrosarcoma
    - Angiosarcoma
    - Embryonal and alveolar rhabdomyosarcoma

Additional Considerations

- Some mesenchymal neoplasms have unique criteria for histologic grading (or risk assessment) and do not routinely utilize FNCLCC system
  - Epithelioid hemangioendothelioma
  - Gastrointestinal stromal tumor
  - Solitary fibrous tumor
  - Ossifying fibromyxoid tumor
  - PEComa

Soft Tissue Sarcoma Staging (TNM System) for Trunk and Extremities

Pathologic Staging Category	Description
Primary Tumor (T)	
TX	Primary tumor cannot be assessed
T0	No evidence of primary tumor
T1	Tumor ≤ 5 cm in greatest dimension
T2	Tumor > 5 cm and ≤ 10 cm in greatest dimension
T3	Tumor > 10 cm and ≤ 15 cm in greatest dimension
T4	Tumor > 15 cm in greatest dimension
Regional Lymph Nodes (N)	
N0	No regional lymph node metastasis
N1	Regional lymph node metastasis
Distant Metastasis (M)	
M1	Distant metastasis [specify site(s), if known]

All tables adapted from 8th edition AJCC Staging Forms (2018). Nx designation not used for soft tissue tumors.

Soft Tissue Sarcoma Staging (TNM System) for Retroperitoneum

Pathologic Staging Category	Description
Primary Tumor (T)	
TX	Primary tumor cannot be assessed
T0	No evidence of primary tumor
T1	Tumor ≤ 5 cm in greatest dimension
T2	Tumor > 5 cm and ≤ 10 cm in greatest dimension
T3	Tumor > 10 cm and ≤ 15 cm in greatest dimension
T4	Tumor > 15 cm in greatest dimension
Regional Lymph Nodes (N)	
N0	No regional lymph node metastasis
N1	Regional lymph node metastasis
Distant Metastasis (M)	
M1	Distant metastasis [specify site(s), if known]

Soft Tissue Sarcoma Staging (TNM System) for Orbit

Pathologic Staging Category	Description
Primary Tumor (T)	
TX	Primary tumor cannot be assessed
T0	No evidence of primary tumor
T1	Tumor ≤ 2 cm in greatest dimension
T2	Tumor > 2 cm in greatest dimension without invasion of bony walls or globe
T3	Tumor of any size with invasion of bony walls
T4	Tumor of any size with invasion of globe or periorbital structures, including eyelid, conjunctiva, temporal fossa, nasal cavity, paranasal sinuses, &/or central nervous system
Regional Lymph Nodes (N)	
N0	No regional lymph node metastasis
N1	Regional lymph node metastasis
Distant Metastasis (M)	
M1	Distant metastasis [specify site(s), if known]

Soft Tissue Sarcoma Staging (TNM System) for Abdomen and Thoracic Organs

Pathologic Staging Category	Description
Primary Tumor (T)	
TX	Primary tumor cannot be assessed
T1	Tumor is organ confined
T2	Tumor extension into tissue beyond organ
T2a	Tumor invades serosa or visceral peritoneum
T2b	Tumor extends beyond serosa (mesentery)
T3	Tumor invades another organ
T4	Multifocal involvement
T4a	Multifocal (2 sites)
T4b	Multifocal (3-5 sites)
T4c	Multifocal (> 5 sites)
Regional Lymph Nodes (N)	
N0	No regional lymph node metastasis
N1	Regional lymph node metastasis
Distant Metastasis (M)	
M1	Distant metastasis [specify site(s), if known]

All tables adapted from 8th edition AJCC Staging Forms (2017).

Soft Tissue Sarcoma Staging (pTNM System) for Head and Neck

Pathologic Staging Category	Description
Primary Tumor (T)	
TX	Primary tumor cannot be assessed
T1	Tumor ≤ 2 cm
T2	Tumor > 2 to ≤ 4 cm
T3	Tumor > 4 cm
T4	Tumor with invasion of adjoining structures
T4a	Tumor with orbital invasion, skull base/dural invasion, invasion of central compartment viscera, involvement of facial skeleton, or invasion of pterygoid muscles
T4b	Tumor with brain parenchymal invasion, carotid artery encasement, prevertebral muscle invasion, or central nervous system involvement via perineural spread
Regional Lymph Nodes (N)	
N0	No regional lymph node metastasis
N1	Regional lymph node metastasis
Distant Metastasis (M)	
M1	Distant metastasis [specify site(s), if known]

Additional Descriptors (pTNM system)

Descriptor	Meaning
Prefix	
y	Tumor is being staged post therapy (i.e., neoadjuvant chemotherapy, radiation therapy, or both chemotherapy and radiation)
r	Tumor is recurrent (must follow documented disease-free interval)
Suffix	
m	Multiple primary tumors involving single site

Example: ypT3(m)N0 in pathologic stage T3 sarcoma, multifocal, treated with neoadjuvant therapy prior to resection.

Anatomic Stage/Prognostic Groups (Trunk and Extremities)

Stage	Tumor	Node	Metastasis	Grade (G)
Stage IA	T1	N0	M0	G1 or GX (low grade)
Stage IB	T2	N0	M0	G1 or GX (low grade)
	T3	N0	M0	G1 or GX (low grade)
	T4	N0	M0	G1 or GX (low grade)
Stage II	T1	N0	M0	G2 or G3 (high grade)
Stage IIIA	T2	N0	M0	G2 or G3 (high grade)
Stage IIIB	T3	N0	M0	G2 or G3 (high grade)
	T4	N0	M0	G2 or G3 (high grade)
Stage IV	Any T	N1	M0	Any G
	Any T	Any N	M1	Any G

All tables adapted from 8th edition AJCC Staging Forms (2017). GX: Grade cannot be assessed; M0: No distant metastasis.

Anatomic Stage/Prognostic Groups (Retroperitoneum)

Stage	Tumor	Node	Metastasis	Grade (G)
Stage IA	T1	N0	M0	G1 or GX (low grade)
Stage IB	T2	N0	M0	G1 or GX (low grade)
	T3	N0	M0	G1 or GX (low grade)
	T4	N0	M0	G1 or GX (low grade)
Stage II	T1	N0	M0	G2 or G3 (high grade)
Stage IIIA	T2	N0	M0	G2 or G3 (high grade)
Stage IIIB	T3	N0	M0	G2 or G3 (high grade)
	T4	N0	M0	G2 or G3 (high grade)
Stage IV	Any T	N1	M0	Any G
	Any T	Any N	M1	Any G

No formal stage groupings exist for head and neck, orbit, abdominal visceral organs, and thoracic visceral organ sites.

(Left) *Axial graphic of the thigh shows a T1 soft tissue sarcoma →. By definition, these tumors are ≤ 5 cm in greatest dimension. The previous "a" and "b" designations used to denote superficial (T1a) and deep localization (T1b) are no longer utilized.* (Right) *Axial graphic of the thigh shows a T1 soft tissue sarcoma → measuring < 5 cm. Though once designated "pT1b" in previous staging schema due to its deep/subfascial involvement, this tumor would now be staged purely as T1.*

T1 (TNM Staging)

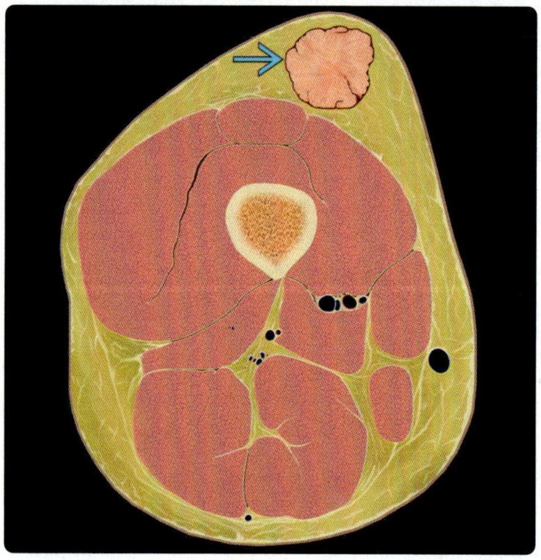

T1 (TNM Staging)

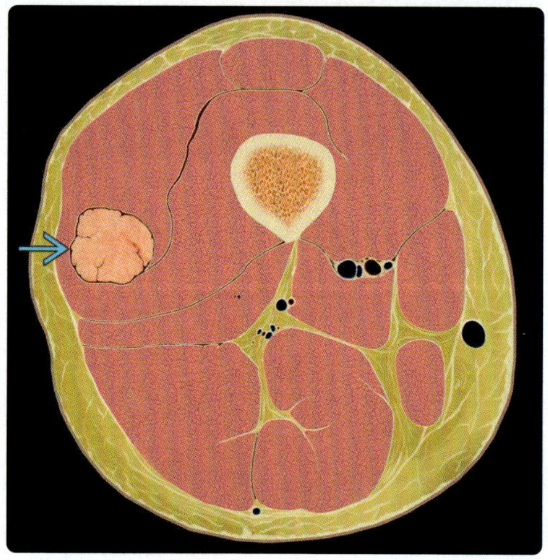

(Left) *Axial graphic of the thigh shows a T2 soft tissue sarcoma →. By definition, these tumors measure 5-10 cm in greatest dimension. Localization above or below the fascia is no longer taken into account.* (Right) *Axial graphic of the thigh shows a T3 soft tissue sarcoma →. By definition, these tumors measure 10-15 cm in greatest dimension. Although the tumor arises in the muscle, it does not affect the staging designation.*

T2 (TNM Staging)

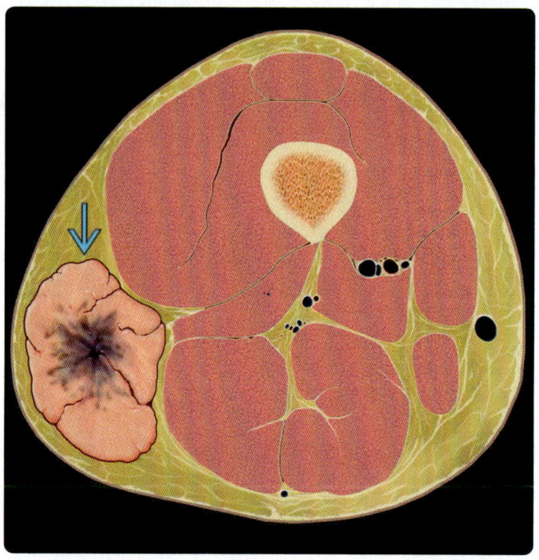

T3 (TNM Staging)

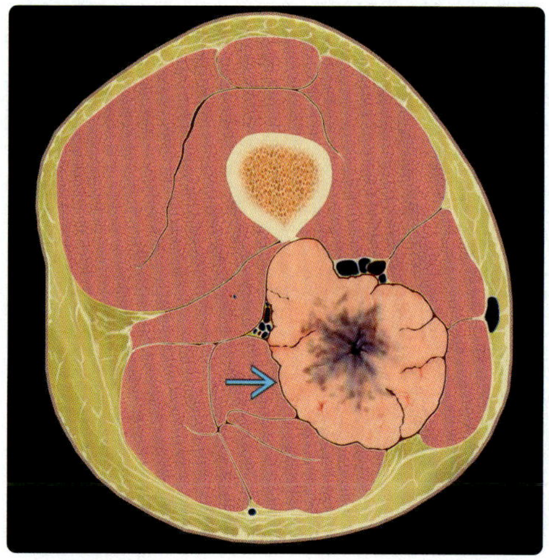

(Left) *Axial graphic of the thigh shows a T4 soft tissue sarcoma →. By definition, these tumors measure > 15 cm in greatest dimension.* (Right) *Axial graphic and MR show an anatomic stage IA soft tissue sarcoma → of the extremity. By definition, the tumor is < 5 cm, histologically low grade, and no metastases (nodal or distant) are present. If this tumor were > 5 cm, it would be grouped as IB.*

T4 (TNM Staging)

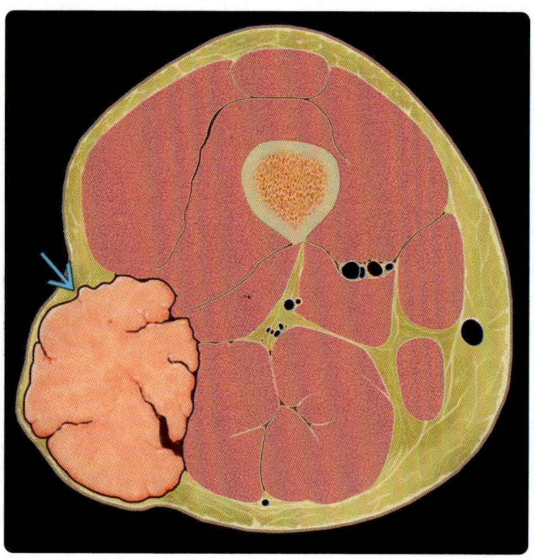

Anatomic/Prognosis Stage IA Group

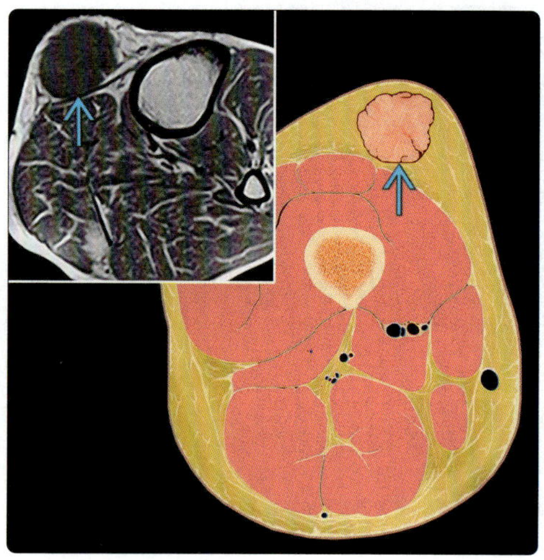

Anatomic/Prognosis Stage II Group

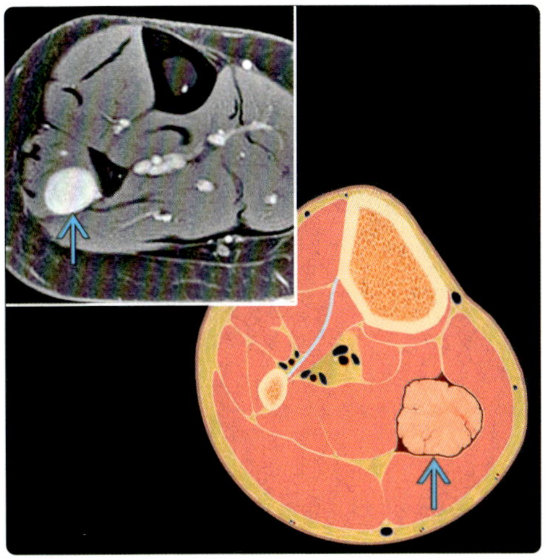

Anatomic/Prognosis Stage IIIB Group

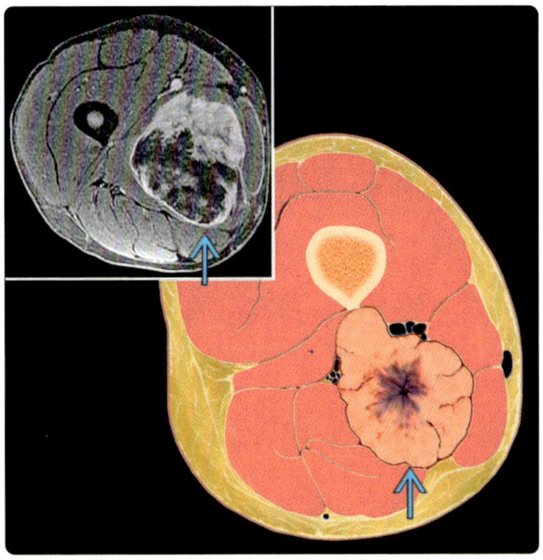

(Left) *Axial graphic and MR of the extremity show a stage II soft tissue sarcoma. These lesions are G2 or G3 (high grade) and all measure < 5 cm in greatest dimension. No metastases are present.* **(Right)** *Axial graphic and MR of the extremity show a stage IIIB soft tissue sarcoma. These tumors are G2 or G3 (high grade), and all measure > 10 cm in greatest dimension. No nodal metastases are present. If this same tumor measured between 5-10 cm, it would be grouped as IIIA.*

Anatomic/Prognosis Stage IV Group

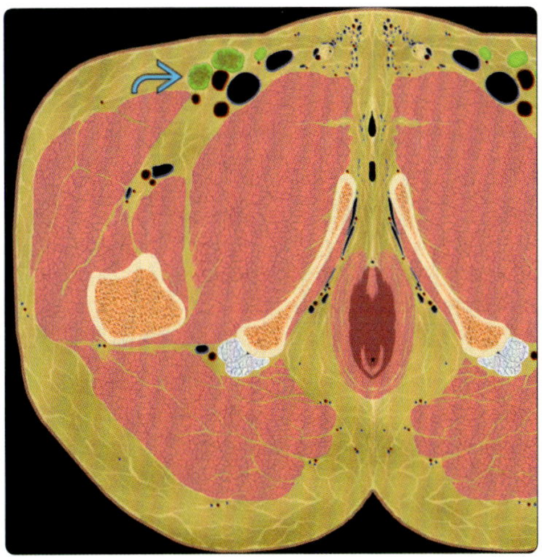

Anatomic/Prognosis Stage III Group

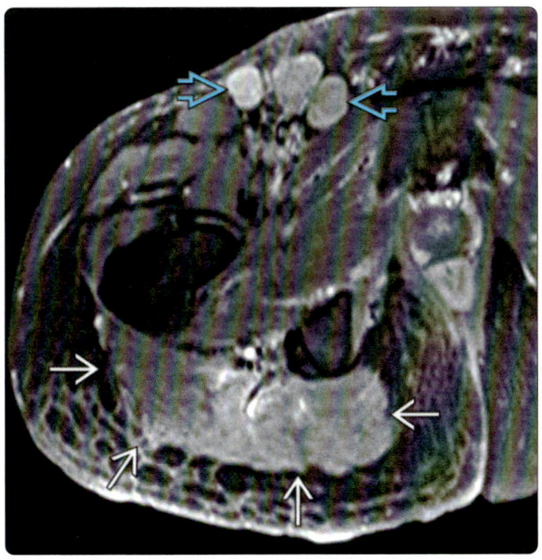

(Left) *Axial graphic through the low pelvis shows inguinal adenopathy. The presence of involved lymph nodes, though uncommon in sarcoma, makes this stage IV disease. The primary tumor can be any size or histologic grade.* **(Right)** *Axial MR with contrast shows an abnormal gluteus maximus muscle, which was infiltrated with tumor. Note the prominent inguinal adenopathy, making this a stage IV sarcoma.*

Anatomic/Prognosis Stage IV Group

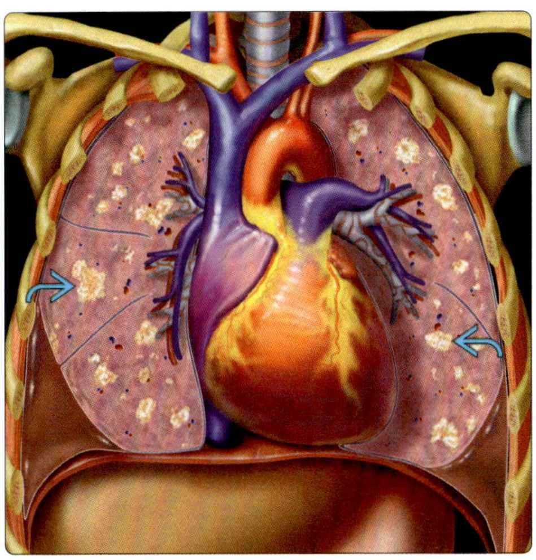

Anatomic/Prognosis Stage IV Group

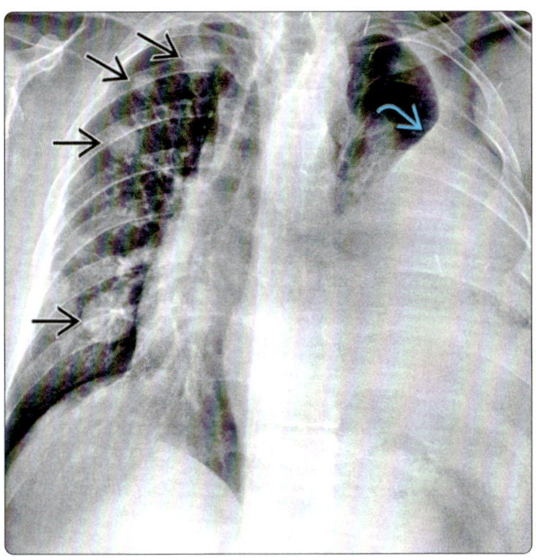

(Left) *Coronal graphic through the lungs demonstrates multiple bilateral pulmonary metastases from a soft tissue sarcoma. The presence of distant metastases makes this stage IV disease. In this setting, the size and histologic grade of the primary tumor are irrelevant.* **(Right)** *This chest radiograph in a patient with a malignant nerve sheath tumor shows multiple pulmonary metastases and a large malignant effusion filling the left hemithorax.*

Commonly Used Antibodies in Soft Tissue Pathology

Antibody Name	Main Diagnostic Utility	Specific Notes or Caveats
ALK1	Inflammatory myofibroblastic tumor (IMT), epithelioid fibrous histiocytoma, angiomatoid fibrous histiocytoma	50-60% of IMTs; occasionally seen in other tumors, including rhabdomyosarcoma and neuroblastoma
β-catenin	Nuclear expression in fibromatosis (50-75% of cases)	Nuclear expression occasionally seen in other tumors, limiting specificity; cytoplasmic expression nonspecific
Brachyury	Chordoma	Nuclear expression specific for notochordal origin
Caldesmon	Smooth muscle neoplasms, glomus, perivascular epithelioid cell tumor (PEComa)	Similar to desmin; can also be expressed in GIST
Calponin	Smooth muscle neoplasms, myoepithelioma; myofibroblastic lesions	Relatively nonspecific; better markers available
Calretinin	Malignant mesothelioma	Also common in synovial sarcoma and schwannoma
CD163	Histiocytic proliferations	Truly histiocyte specific; superior to CD68
CD21	Follicular dendritic cell sarcoma	Absent in interdigitating dendritic cell sarcoma
CD31	Vascular lesions (endothelial marker)	Pitfall: Weak granular expression in histiocytes
CD34	Dermatofibrosarcoma protuberans, solitary fibrous tumor (SFT), spindle cell lipoma, cellular angiofibroma, mammary-type myofibroblastoma, vascular lesions, epithelioid sarcoma	Always use in conjunction with morphology; diffuse expression is usually significant; weak &/or focal expression is often nonspecific
CD45	Hematolymphoid proliferations (including lymphoma)	Can be negative in lymphoblastic lymphomas
CD56	Limited applications due to lack of specificity	Usually negative in Ewing sarcoma and lymphoblastic lymphomas but expressed in many other small round blue cell tumors, including poorly differentiated synovial sarcoma; nonspecific in spindle cell lesions.
CD68	Histiocytic proliferations, fibrous histiocytomas, granular cell tumor	Lacks specificity (lysosome specific instead of histiocyte specific); CD163 is superior
CD99	Ewing sarcoma (strong, diffuse membranous expression)	Caveat: Many other small round blue cell tumors may show patchy, focal, &/or weak expression; always negative in neuroblastoma
CD117 (C-kit)	Gastrointestinal stromal tumor (GIST)	Highest specificity in GI tract; can also be seen in clear cell sarcoma, melanoma, PEComa, Kaposi sarcoma
CDK4	Atypical lipomatous tumor/well-differentiated liposarcoma, dedifferentiated liposarcoma	Nuclear expression; negative in lipoma and most other pleomorphic sarcomas; best utilized in conjunction with MDM2
Claudin-1	Perineurioma	May be seen focally in low-grade fibromyxoid sarcoma
Clusterin	Follicular dendritic cell sarcoma	Absent in interdigitating dendritic cell sarcoma
D2-40 (podoplanin)	Lymphatic lesions; malignant mesothelioma	Lacks specificity for lymphatic endothelium
Desmin	Myogenic tumors, angiomatoid fibrous histiocytoma, desmoplastic small round cell tumor (DSRCT), angiomyofibroblastoma	Good screening marker for myogenic differentiation; can be focally expressed in myofibroblastic tumors
DOG1	GIST	Helpful second-line marker in GISTs that are CD117(-)
EMA	Perineurioma, synovial sarcoma, epithelioid sarcoma, myoepithelioma, ectopic meningioma	Limited utility due to nonspecificity; can also be seen in low-grade fibromyxoid sarcoma
ERG	Vascular neoplasms	Nuclear expression; more specific than FLI-1
ER and PR	Angiomyofibroblastoma, cellular angiofibroma, aggressive (deep) angiomyxoma, deep smooth muscle neoplasms	Expressed in mammary/gynecologic carcinomas
FLI-1	Vascular tumors, Ewing sarcoma	Nuclear expression; similar to but less specific than ERG; may also be expressed in lymphocytes, lymphoblastic lymphoma, and other tumors
Factor XIII	Fibrous histiocytoma (dermatofibroma)	Stains intralesional histiocytes; limited utility as better markers are available
FOSB	Pseudomyogenic hemangioendothelioma, epithelioid hemangioma	Nuclear expression
GFAP	Myoepithelioma, schwannoma, soft tissue ependymoma, gastrointestinal schwannoma	Limited utility due to better markers available
GLUT1	Infantile hemangioma, perineurioma	Negative in congenital hemangioma, kaposiform

Commonly Used Antibodies in Soft Tissue Pathology (Continued)

Antibody Name	Main Diagnostic Utility	Specific Notes or Caveats
		hemangioendothelioma, and vascular malformations
H3K27me3	Malignant peripheral nerve sheath tumor (MPNST)	Only loss of nuclear expression counts
HHV8 (LANA)	Kaposi sarcoma	Highly useful; nuclear expression
HMB-45	Melanoma, PEComa, clear cell sarcoma, melanotic schwannoma	Can be negative or focally positive; often best used in panel of melanocytic markers
INI1 (SMARCB1)	Epithelioid sarcoma, malignant extrarenal rhabdoid tumor	Only loss of nuclear expression counts; subset of epithelioid MPNST, malignant myoepithelioma, and extraskeletal myxoid chondrosarcoma show loss
Keratins	Evidence of epithelial differentiation (epithelioid sarcoma, synovial sarcoma, DSRCT, myoepithelioma, others)	Caveat: Must always exclude carcinoma; can also be expressed in some epithelioid vascular tumors
MDM2	Atypical lipomatous tumor/well-differentiated liposarcoma, dedifferentiated liposarcoma	Nuclear expression; negative in lipoma and most other pleomorphic sarcomas
Melan-A (MART-1)	Melanoma, PEComa, clear cell sarcoma, melanotic schwannoma	Can be negative; best used in panel of melanocytic markers; may also be focally expressed in epithelioid GIST
MiTF	Melanoma, PEComa, cellular neurothekeoma, clear cell sarcoma	Nuclear expression; also expressed in granular cell tumor; occasionally positive in histiocytes
MUC4	Low-grade fibromyxoid sarcoma, sclerosing epithelioid fibrosarcoma	Also seen in subset of ossifying fibromyxoid tumor
Muscle-specific actin (HHF-35)	Myogenic tumors, PEComa	Similar to desmin
MyoD1	Rhabdomyoma, rhabdomyosarcomas, rhabdomyoblastic elements	Only nuclear expression should be considered positive
Myogenin (Myf4)	Rhabdomyoma, rhabdomyosarcomas, rhabdomyoblastic elements	Only nuclear expression should be considered positive
NB84	Neuroblastoma	Not entirely specific; occasionally seen focally in Ewing sarcoma and several other small round blue cell tumors
Retinoblastoma (Rb) protein	Spindle cell lipoma, cellular angiofibroma, mammary-type myofibroblastoma, atypical spindle cell lipomatous tumor	Only loss of nuclear expression is significant
S100 protein	Schwannoma, neurofibroma, hybrid nerve sheath tumor, MPNST, melanoma, myoepithelioma, ossifying fibromyxoid tumor, extranodal Rosai-Dorfman disease, others	Always use in conjunction with morphology and panel of other immunostains
SATB2	Extraskeletal osteosarcoma	Nuclear expression; expressed in any osteoblastic cell (not specific for osteosarcoma)
Smooth muscle actin	Smooth muscle, myofibroblasts, glomus, PEComa	Pattern of expression helpful (diffuse cytoplasmic vs. wispy submembranous)
SOX10	Melanoma, peripheral nerve sheath tumors, MPNST, myoepithelioma	Nuclear expression; shows very similar sensitivity, specificity, and tissue distribution to S100 protein; does not mark histiocytes; notable for expression in basal-type breast carcinoma
STAT6	SFT	Nuclear expression; appears highly specific for SFT
Synaptophysin	Paraganglioma, neuroblastoma	Can be expressed in some cases of extraskeletal myxoid chondrosarcoma and alveolar rhabdomyosarcoma
TdT	Lymphoblastic lymphoma	Assists in diagnosis of CD45(-) lymphoblastic lymphomas
TFE3	Alveolar soft part sarcoma, granular cell tumor	Also expressed in subsets of PEComa and epithelioid hemangioendothelioma
TLE1	Synovial sarcoma	Strong, diffuse nuclear expression; focal &/or weak expression is nonspecific
Vimentin	Generally not helpful in most situations (widespread expression)	Extremely nonspecific overall but may be useful as marker of antigen preservation
WT1	Mesothelioma, desmoplastic small round cell tumor, adenomatoid tumor, *CIC-DUX4* sarcoma	Nuclear expression; for DSRCT, antibodies recognizing carboxy-terminus must be utilized

Immunohistochemical Panel for Selected Spindle Cell Tumors in Soft Tissue

Tumor	Keratin	S100 Protein	SMA	Desmin	CD34	Other Markers
Cellular angiofibroma	-	-	-	-	+++	Loss of nuclear Rb protein expression
Dermatofibrosarcoma protuberans (DFSP)	-	-	-	-	+++	CD34 expression decreased or absent in fibrosarcomatous DFSP
Fibromatosis	-	-	+/-	-	-	Nuclear β-catenin expression in majority of tumors
Inflammatory myofibroblastic tumor	+/-	-	+++	+/-	-	ALK1(+) in over 50% of cases
Leiomyosarcoma	-	-	+++	+/-	-	Caldesmon (+); occasional focal keratin (+)
Low-grade myofibroblastic sarcoma	-	-	+/-	+/-	-	Nuclear atypia, desmin (+), and absence of nuclear β-catenin favors this diagnosis over fibromatosis
Low-grade fibromyxoid sarcoma	-	-	+/-	-	-	MUC4 most specific marker; focal EMA expression common
Malignant peripheral nerve sheath tumor (MPNST)	-	+/-	-	-	+/-	S100(+) and SOX10(+) usually focal or patchy; desmin expression seen in rhabdomyoblastic elements; loss of nuclear H3L27me3 expression also seen
Mammary-type myofibroblastoma	-	-	-	+++	+++	Loss of nuclear Rb protein expression
Neurofibroma	-	+++	-	-	+++	Contains mixture of S100(+) Schwann cells, CD34(+) stromal cells, and EMA/claudin-1 (+) perineurial cells
Nodular fasciitis	-	-	+++	-	-	Rare focal desmin (+)
Perivascular epithelioid cell tumor (PEComa)	-	-	+++	+/-	-	Myomelanocytic immunophenotype with additional variable expression of HMB-45, melan-A, &/or MITF
Perineurioma	-	-	-	-	+/-	EMA(+), claudin-1 (+), GLUT1(+)
Schwannoma	-	+++	-	-	+/-	CD34 expression usually subcapsular; focal keratin (+) in retroperitoneal schwannomas
Solitary fibrous tumor	-	-	-	-	+++	Nuclear STAT6(+) is highly specific
Spindle cell lipoma	-	-	-	-	+++	Loss of nuclear Rb protein expression
Spindle cell rhabdomyosarcoma	-	-	+/-	+++	-	Myogenin (+), MYOD1(+)
Synovial sarcoma	+++	+/-	-	-	-	TLE1(+); also expresses CD56 and calretinin

(+++) = typically positive; (+/-) = variably positive or negative; (-) = typically negative.

Immunohistochemical Panel for Selected Highly Pleomorphic Soft Tissue Tumors

Tumor	Keratin	S100 Protein	SMA	Desmin	Myogenin	MDM2/ CDK4	Notes
Dedifferentiated liposarcoma	-	-	+/-	-	-	+++	Most common in retroperitoneum
Malignant perivascular epithelioid cell tumor (PEComa)	-	-	+++	+/-	-	-	Variable melanocytic marker expression
Pleomorphic leiomyosarcoma	-	-	+++	+/-	-	-	Should show morphologic features of smooth muscle differentiation
Melanoma	-	+++	-	-	-	-	Also SOX10(+); variable melanocytic markers
Pleomorphic rhabdomyosarcoma	-	-	+/-	+++	+++	+/-	Myogenin (+) often focal
Sarcomatoid carcinoma	+++	-	+/-	-	-	-	p63(+) and p40(+) in squamous cell carcinoma
Undifferentiated pleomorphic sarcoma	-	-	+/-	-	-	-	Diagnosis of exclusion

(+++) = typically positive; (+/-) = variably positive or negative; (-) = typically negative.

Immunohistochemical Panel for Large, Epithelioid Cell Tumors in Soft Tissue

Tumor	Keratin	S100 Protein	SMA	Desmin	CD34	HMB-45	INI1	TFE3	Notes
Alveolar soft part sarcoma	-	-	+/-	+/-	-	-	Retained	+++	May show significant nuclear pleomorphism
Epithelioid angiosarcoma	+/-	-	-	-	+++	-	Retained	-	Also positive for CD31 and ERG
Epithelioid hemangio-endothelioma	+/-	-	-	-	+++	-	Retained	Subset	Also positive for CD31 and ERG
Epithelioid malignant peripheral nerve sheath tumor (MPNST)	-	+++	-	-	-	-	Lost (50%)	-	Mosaic (patchy) loss of nuclear INI1 expression
Epithelioid sarcoma	+++	-	-	-	+/-	-	Lost	-	Negative for p63 and CD31
Extrarenal rhabdoid tumor	+++	-	-	-	-	-	Lost	-	May also appear as small round blue cell tumor
Granular cell tumor	-	+++	-	-	-	-	Retained	+++	Prominent granular cytoplasm
Melanoma	-	+++	-	-	-	+++	Retained	-	Other melanocytic markers (melan-A, MITF, tyrosinase)
Myoepithelioma	+++	+++	+/-	+/-	-	-	Retained	-	Also expresses calponin; variable GFAP, p63
Perivascular epithelioid cell tumor (PEComa)	-	-	+++	+/-	-	+++	Retained	Subset	Can also express caldesmon, melan-A, MITF
Poorly differentiated carcinoma	+++	-	-	-	-	-	Retained	-	p63 for squamous cell carcinoma; various markers for adenocarcinoma (TTF-1, pax-8, Hep-Par1, etc.)

(+++) = typically positive; (+/-) = variably positive or negative; (-) = typically negative.

Immunohistochemical Panel for Selected Small Round Blue Cell Tumors

Tumor	Keratin	CD99	NB84	CD45	Desmin	Myogenin	Synaptophysin	Other Markers
Alveolar rhabdomyosarcoma	+/-	-	-	-	+++	+++	+/-	Also MyoD1(+)
Desmoplastic small round cell tumor	+++	+/-	+/-	-	+++ (dot)	-	+/-	WT1(+) if antibody recognizes carboxy-terminus
Ewing sarcoma	+/-	+++	+/-	-	-	-	+/-	FLI-1(+); notably CD56(-)
Extrarenal rhabdoid tumor	+++	+/-	-	-	-	-	+/-	Characteristic loss of nuclear INI1
Lymphoma	-	+/-	-	+++	-	-	-	TdT(+) to help exclude CD45(-) lymphoblastic lymphomas
Melanoma	-	-	-	-	-	-	-	S100(+), SOX10(+); variable melanocytic
Neuroblastoma	-	-	+++	-	-	-	+++	Notable CD99 negativity
Poorly differentiated synovial sarcoma	+/-	+++	-	-	-	-	-	TLE1(+); also commonly expresses CD56
Small cell neuroendocrine carcinoma	+++	-	-	-	-	-	+++	TTF-1(+)

(+++) = typically positive; (+/-) = variably positive or negative; (-) = typically negative.

Immunohistochemical Panel for Spindle Cell Tumors in GI Tract

Tumor	Keratin	S100 Protein	CD117 (C-kit)	DOG1	CD34	SMA	Desmin	Notes
Desmoid fibromatosis	-	-	-	-	-	+/-	-	Nuclear β-catenin (+) in majority; extrinsic to GI tract
Ganglioneuroma	-	+++	-	-	-	-	-	Contains ganglion cells
Gastrointestinal stromal tumor (GIST)	-	-	+++	+++	+++	+/-	-	Most common overall
Granular cell tumor	-	+++	-	-	–	-	-	Prominent granular cytoplasm; also epithelioid/polygonal tumor cells
Hybrid nerve sheath tumor	-	+++	-	–	+/-	-	-	Also expresses perineurial markers (e.g., EMA, claudin-1)
Inflammatory fibroid polyp	-	-	-	-	+++	-	-	Submucosal
Inflammatory myofibroblastic tumor	+/-	-	-	-	-	+++	+/-	ALK1(+) in majority; typically extrinsic to GI tract
Kaposi sarcoma	-	-	+/-	-	+++	-	-	Also HHV8(+), CD31(+), and ERG
Leiomyoma	-	-	-	-	-	+++	+++	More common than GIST in esophagus
Leiomyosarcoma	-	-	-	-	-	+++	+/-	Often pleomorphic
Perineurioma (polyp)	-	-	-	-	+/-	-	-	EMA(+), claudin-1 (+)
Plexiform fibromyxoma	-	-	-	-	-	+++	-	Arises in gastric antrum; conspicuous plexiform growth
Schwannoma	-	+++	-	-	-	-	-	Peripheral lymphoid cuff
Solitary fibrous tumor	-	-	-	-	+++	-	-	Nuclear STAT6(+)

(+++) = typically positive; (+/-) = variably positive or negative; (-) = typically negative.

Immunohistochemical Panel for Epithelioid Tumors in GI Tract

Tumor	Keratin	S100 Protein	CD117 (C-kit)	DOG1	SMA	HMB45	Notes
Epithelioid gastrointestinal stromal tumor (GIST)	-	-	+++	+++	-	-	Also CD34(+); occasionally CD117 can be negative; rare focal melan-A; some tumors are pleomorphic and resemble carcinoma or melanoma
Glomus tumor	-	-	-	-	+++	-	Can resemble epithelioid GIST
Malignant gastrointestinal neuroectodermal tumor	-	+++	-	-	-	-	Variable expression of synaptophysin, NB84, CD56; negative for CD99 and melan-A
Melanoma	-	+++	+/-	-	-	+++	Also expresses other melanocytic markers
Perivascular epithelioid cell tumor (PEComa)	-	-	+/-	-	+++	+++	Can also express caldesmon, melan-A, MITF
Poorly differentiated carcinoma	+++	-	-	-	-	-	Should always be excluded clinically, histologically, &/or immunohistochemically
Poorly differentiated synovial sarcoma	+/-	-	-	-	-	-	Strong diffuse nuclear TLE1 expression; molecular analysis in difficult cases
SDH-deficient GIST	-	-	+++	+++	-	-	Loss of cytoplasmic SDHB protein expression diagnostic (subset also shows loss of SDHA protein)

(+++) = typically positive; (+/-) = variably positive or negative; (-) = typically negative.

Selected Soft Tissue Tumors With Prominent CD34 Expression

Tumor	Helpful Clues to Diagnosis
Acral fibromyxoma	Location (hands or feet, often subungual); generally bland spindle cells within myxoid to fibrous stroma; loss of nuclear Rb expression
Angiosarcoma	Location (scalp, breast, etc.); evidence of vasoformation with infiltrative or dissecting growth; CD31(+), ERG(+)
Atypical spindle cell lipomatous tumor	Loose fascicles of bland spindle cells in myxoid to fibrous stroma; variable number of mono- and multivacuolated lipoblasts with atypical nuclei; loss of nuclear Rb expression; negative for MDM2/CDK4
Cellular angiofibroma	Usually genital region; hyalinized vessels; neural-like cytomorphology; desmin (-); loss of nuclear Rb expression
Deep benign fibrous histiocytoma	Well circumscribed, often with fibrous capsule; storiform growth pattern; admixed chronic inflammatory infiltrate common; ectatic vasculature
Dermatofibrosarcoma protuberans	Dermal/subcutaneous tumor; prominent storiform growth pattern; honeycomb-like fat infiltration; contains *COL1A1-PDGFB* fusion
Elastofibroma	Location (infrascapular deep soft tissue); affects older/elderly women; contains abnormal coarse, fragmented, beaded elastic fibers
Epithelioid hemangioendothelioma	Characteristic myxohyaline matrix; angiocentricity; blister cells; CD31(+); ERG(+)
Epithelioid hemangioma	Location (head, distal extremities); abundant lymphocytes and eosinophils; vasoformation present; CD31(+); CD34(+)
Epithelioid sarcoma	Location (distal extremity in classic type); nests of eosinophilic epithelioid cells, often with central necrosis; keratin (+); loss of nuclear INI1 expression
Fibrous hamartoma of infancy	Affect infants; organoid growth pattern with 3 distinct components; diffuse CD34 expression only in collagenized pseudoangiomatous (or neurofibroma-like) areas
Gastrointestinal stromal tumor	Arises in muscularis propria of GI tract or rarely omentum/mesentery; CD117(+), DOG1(+)
Giant cell fibroblastoma	Common in children; often on trunk; irregular clefts lined by multinucleated cells; may contain areas of DFSP; CD31(-); contains *COL1A1-PDGFB* fusion
Hemosiderotic fibrolipomatous tumor	Location (often distal lower extremity); adult women; abundant mature adipose tissue and hemosiderin; *TGFBR3* &/or *MGEA3* rearrangements
Kaposiform hemangioendothelioma	Occurs in children; associated with clinical Kasabach-Merritt syndrome; cannonball growth pattern with glomeruloid structures
Kaposi sarcoma	Hemorrhage common; clinical scenario (e.g., AIDS); lymph node involvement; HHV8(+); CD31(+)
Mammary-type myofibroblastoma	Genital region or extremities; features coarse collagen bundles; vasculature usually not prominent; additionally desmin (+); loss of nuclear Rb expression
Myeloid sarcoma	Clinical context (acute myeloid leukemia); myeloperoxidase (+); negative for vascular markers
Neurofibroma	Often cutaneous or originating from deeper nerve; admixed CD34(+) stromal cells with S100(+) Schwann cells
Perineurioma	Low-grade cytology; whorling growth; usually EMA(+), claudin-1 (+)
Pleomorphic hyalinizing angiectatic tumor	Location (often distal lower extremity); characteristic hyalinized/fibrin-lined vasculature; pleomorphic nuclei with pseudoinclusions; hemosiderin
Solitary fibrous tumor	Prominent ectatic staghorn vasculature; conspicuous stromal collagen; "patternless" architectural pattern; nuclear STAT6(+)
Spindle cell/pleomorphic lipoma	Classic distribution (neck, back, shoulders); adipose tissue component usually conspicuous, but not always; floret cells in pleomorphic lipoma; desmin (-); loss of nuclear Rb expression
Superficial CD34(+) fibroblastic tumor	Prominent nuclear pleomorphism, often bizarre; macronucleoli; patchy keratin (+)

**Rarely, prominent CD34(+) reported in various other tumors, including dedifferentiated liposarcoma, retroperitoneal leiomyosarcoma, myxofibrosarcoma, and myxoinflammatory fibroblastic sarcoma.*

Diagnostically Useful Molecular and Cytogenetic Findings

Histologic Classification	Key Abnormality	Comment
Acral fibromyxoma	Loss of 13q12 (*RB1*)	Similar to spindle cell lipoma and related lesions
Alveolar rhabdomyosarcoma	t(2;13)(q35;q14) with *PAX3-FOXO1* fusion	Most common (60% of cases)
	t(1;13)(p36;q14) with *PAX7-FOXO1* fusion	
Alveolar soft part sarcoma	der(17)t(X;17)(p11;q25) with *ASPSCR1-TFE3* fusion	Same gene fusion present in subset of distinctive pediatric renal cell carcinoma
Aneurysmal bone cyst of soft tissue	17p13 rearrangements	Involves *USP6* gene
Angiofibroma of soft tissue	t(5;8)(p15;q13) with *AHRR-NCOA2* fusion	
Angiosarcoma	Amplification of 8q24 (*MYC*)	Characteristic of tumors arising in association with radiation or lymphedema
Atypical spindle cell lipomatous tumor	Loss of 13q14 (*RB1*)	Similar to spindle cell lipoma, cellular angiofibroma, mammary-type myofibroblastoma, acral fibromyxoma
Atypical lipomatous tumor	Ring form of chromosome 12; amplification of *MDM2, CDK4, CPM*	Same tumor as well-differentiated liposarcoma
Angiomatoid fibrous histiocytoma	t (2;22)(q33;q12) with *EWSR1-CREB1* fusion t(12;22)(q13;q12) with *EWSR1-ATF1* fusion	t(2;22) most common (90% of cases); also present in clear cell sarcoma and malignant gastrointestinal neuroectodermal tumor
	t(12;16)(q13;p11) with *FUS-ATF1* fusion	Uncommon variant
Cellular angiofibroma	Loss of 13q14 (*RB1*)	Same abnormality in mammary-type myofibroblastoma and spindle cell/pleomorphic lipoma
Chondroid lipoma	t(11;16)(q13;p13) with *C11orf95-MKL2* fusion	
Clear cell sarcoma	t(12;22)(q13;q12) with *EWSR1-ATF1* fusion t(2;22)(q33;q12) with *EWSR1-CREB1* fusion	t(12;22) most common (90% of cases); also present in angiomatoid fibrous histiocytoma and malignant gastrointestinal neuroectodermal tumor
Dedifferentiated liposarcoma	Ring form of chromosome 12, amplification of *MDM2, CDK4, CPM* by FISH analysis	Also present in atypical lipomatous tumor/well-differentiated liposarcoma
Deep aggressive angiomyxoma	Rearrangements of 12q14.3	Involves *HMGA2*
Dermatofibrosarcoma protuberans (DFSP)	t(17;22)(q21;q13) with *COL1A1-PDGFB* fusion	Also present in giant cell fibroblastoma
	Novel *PDGFD* fusion with *COL6A3* or *EMILIN2*	Uncommon
Desmoid-type fibromatosis	*CTNNB1* (β-catenin gene) mutations in sporadic lesions	*APC* mutations in tumors arising within setting of Gardner syndrome
Desmoplastic fibroblastoma	11q12 rearrangements	Recurrent t(2;11)(q31;q12) reported
Desmoplastic small round cell tumor	t(11;22)(p13;q12) with *EWSR1-WT1* fusion	
Epithelioid hemangioendothelioma	t(1;3)(p36.3;q23-25) with *WWTR1-CAMTA1* fusion	Nearly all cases
	t(x;11)(p11;q22) with *YAP1-TFE3* fusion	Minor subset
Epithelioid hemangioma	*FOS* rearrangements (14q24.3)	
Epithelioid fibrous histiocytoma	2p23 (*ALK* gene) rearrangements	Most cases
Epithelioid sarcoma	22q11-12 abnormalities	Inactivation of *SMARCB1* (a.k.a. *INI1* or *SNF5*)
Ewing sarcoma	t(11;22)(q24;q12) with *EWSR1-FLI1* fusion	Most common (85% of cases)
	t(21;22)(q22;q12) with *EWSR1-ERG* t(2;22)(q33;q12) with *EWSR1-FEV* t(7;22)(p22;q12) with *EWSR1-ETV1* t(17;22)(q21;q12) with *EWSR1-ETV4* Very rare fusions involving *FUS*	Variants
Extrarenal rhabdoid tumor	Deletion of 22q11.2	Inactivation of *SMARCB1* (a.k.a. *INI1* or *SNF5*)

Diagnostically Useful Molecular and Cytogenetic Findings (Continued)

Histologic Classification	Key Abnormality	Comment
Extraskeletal myxoid chondrosarcoma	t(9;22)(q22;q12) with *EWSR1-NR4A3* fusion	Most common
	t(9;17) with *TAF15-NR4A3* t(9;15) with *TCF12-NR4A3* t(9;3) with *TFG-NR4A3*	All variant translocations associated with more aggressive course (high-grade morphology, rhabdoid cells)
Gastrointestinal stromal tumor	*KIT, PDGFRA* mutations	Rare: Mutations in SDH subunit genes (usually *SDHB*) or *NF1*
Giant cell fibroblastoma	t(17;22)(q21;q13) with *COL1A1-PDGFB* fusion	Also present in DFSP
Hemosiderotic fibrolipomatous tumor	t(1;10)(p22;q24) with *TGFBR3-MGEA5* fusion	
Hibernoma	11q13 rearrangements	
Infantile fibrosarcoma	t(12;15)(p13;q26) with *ETV6-NTRK3* fusion	Identical aberration seen in cellular mesoblastic nephroma of kidney
Inflammatory myofibroblastic tumor	2p23 rearrangements	Results in *ALK* gene fusion
Intramuscular myxoma	*GNAS* gene mutations	
Intranodal palisaded myofibroblastoma	*CTNNB1* (β-catenin gene) mutations	
Lipoblastoma	8q11-13 rearrangements	Involves *PLAG1*
Low-grade fibromyxoid sarcoma	t(7;16)(q33;p11) with *FUS-CREB3L2*	Most common (65-70% of cases); also present in some cases of sclerosing epithelioid fibrosarcoma
	t(11;16)(p11;p11) with *FUS-CREB3L1*	Rare
Mammary-type myofibroblastoma	Loss of 13q14 (*RB1*)	Same as spindle cell/pleomorphic lipoma and cellular angiofibroma
Myoepithelioma of soft tissue	t(6;22)(p12;q12) with *EWSR1-POU5F1* fusion t(1;22)(q23;q12) with *EWSR1-PBX1* fusion	50% of cases
	t(19;22)(q13;q12) with *EWSR1-ZNF444* fusion	Rare
Myxoid liposarcoma	t(12;16)(q13;p11) with *FUS-DDIT3* fusion	Most common (95% of cases)
	t(12;22)(q13;q12) with *EWSR1-DDIT3* fusion	Rare
Malignant gastrointestinal neuroectodermal tumor	t(2;22)(q33;q12) with *EWSR1-CREB1* fusion t(12;22)(q13;q12) with *EWSR1-ATF1* fusion	Also seen in clear cell sarcoma and angiomatoid fibrous histiocytoma
Myxoinflammatory fibroblastic sarcoma	t(1;10)(p22;q24) with *TGFBR3-MGEA5* fusion	Controversial; also present in hemosiderotic fibrolipomatous tumor and pleomorphic hyalinizing angiectatic tumor
Nodular fasciitis	t(17;22)(p13;q13) with *MYH9-USP6* fusion	
Ossifying fibromyxoid tumor	6p21 rearrangements	Involves *PHF1*
PEComa	Deletion of 16p	Loss of *TSC2*
	TFE3 rearrangements	Minor subset of cases
Pleomorphic hyalinizing angiectatic tumor	t(1;10)(p22;q24) with *TGFBR3-MGEA5* fusion	Also found hemosiderotic fibrolipomatous tumor
Pseudomyogenic (epithelioid sarcoma-like) hemangioendothelioma	t(7;19)(q22;q13) with *SERPINE1-FOSB* fusion	
Solitary fibrous tumor	12q13 aberrations with *NAB2-STAT6* fusion	Intrachromosomal rearrangement
Spindle cell/pleomorphic lipoma	Loss of 13q14 (*RB1*)	Also present in myofibroblastoma and cellular angiofibroma
Synovial sarcoma	t(X;18)(p11;q11) involving *SS18* (SYT) gene	Fusions between *SS18* and *SSX1* (most common), *SSX2*, or *SSX4* (rare)
BCOR-CCNB3 fusion-positive sarcoma	X chromosome (paracentric inversion)	Other fusions described (*BCOR-MAML3*)
Tenosynovial giant cell tumor	t(1;2)(2p;13q) with *CSF1-COL6A3* fusion	Both localized and diffuse forms
CIC-DUX4 translocation sarcoma	t(4;19)(q35;q13.1) t(10;19)(q26;3q13)	Both translocations result in *CIC-DUX4* fusion
Well-differentiated liposarcoma	Ring form of chromosome 12; amplification of *MDM2, CDK4, CPM*	Same tumor as atypical lipomatous tumor

SECTION 2

Diagnostic Approach to Soft Tissue Tumors

Overview

Biopsy and Resection of Soft Tissue Tumors 22

Clinical Approach

Age- and Location-Based Approach to Diagnosis 26

Histologic Approach

Pattern-Based Approach to Diagnosis 28
Feature-Based Approach to Diagnosis 36

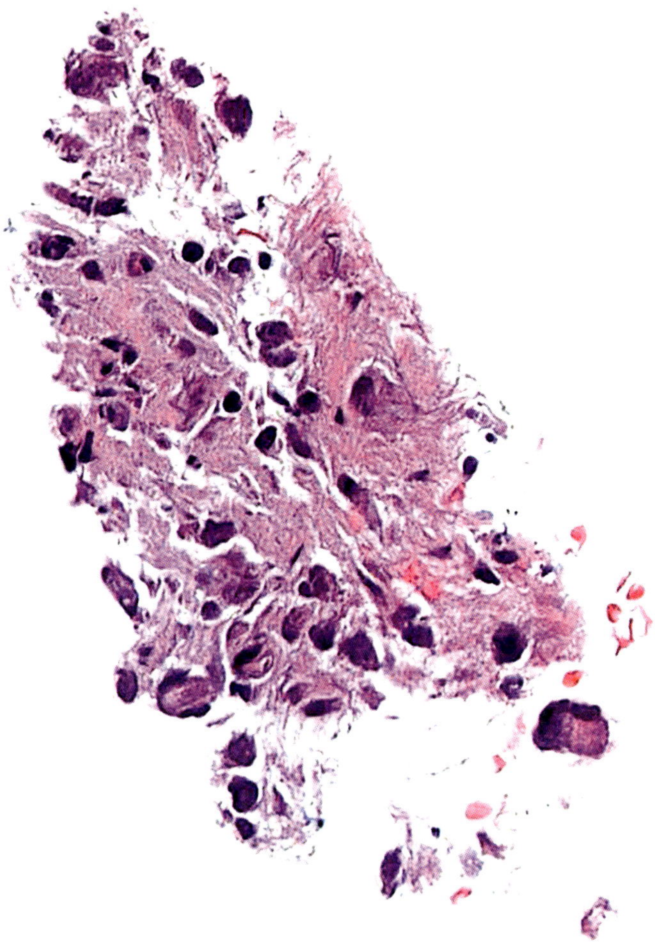

OVERVIEW

General Points

- Variety of diagnostic procedures are currently available to surgeons and clinicians to evaluate soft tissue tumors
  - Initial tumor tissue sampling may or may not be sought, depending on overall impression of tumor biologic potential derived from synthesis of clinical features and imaging characteristics
    - Tumors that appear likely benign are often surgically excised without sampling or followed clinically
    - Tumors that appear likely malignant or potentially malignant are usually sampled preoperatively
      - With increasing frequency, soft tissue tumors are sampled initially by core needle biopsy, fine-needle aspiration (FNA), or limited biopsy due to minimal morbidity to patient
      - Nondiagnostic results may reflex into larger open surgical biopsy with intraoperative frozen section evaluation or even outright resection, depending on clinical impression of tumor biology
      - Successful diagnosis usually leads to local excision, wide resection with margins, or preoperative adjuvant chemotherapy &/or radiation
- Smaller specimens are generally more challenging to evaluate due to sampling problems and issues related to immunohistochemistry
  - Underdiagnosis often poses greater risk than overdiagnosis
  - Misclassification is possible if several different tumors share morphologic overlap

Types of Specimens

- Core needle biopsy
  - Very small sample of tumor/lesion
  - Popular due to minimal risk of morbidity to patient
  - May be done in outpatient setting for superficial lesions or under CT guidance for deep or visceral lesions
- FNA
  - Very small sample of tumor/lesion
  - Aspiration allows for immediate evaluation of sampling adequacy (success or failure of attaining diagnostic tissue) with added benefit of cell block for histologic and immunohistochemical evaluation
  - Popular due to minimal risk of morbidity to patient
- Open surgical biopsy
  - Small sample of tumor/lesion but generally contains more intact tissue than core needle biopsy or FNA
  - Tissue may be sent for intraoperative frozen section consultation or just permanent sectioning
  - Smaller risk of underdiagnosis or misdiagnosis compared to needle biopsy and FNA
- Local excision
  - Entire tumor available for histologic evaluation
  - Surgical focus is on removal of tumor and not achieving rim of uninvolved soft tissue
  - Standard approach for benign, superficial tumors that are not believed to be locally aggressive
- Resection with margins
  - Includes wide resection and radical resection
    - Radical resection often contains extensive normal tissue or, in cases of intraabdominal, intrathoracic, or retroperitoneal tumors, may contain organs involved by tumor
  - Entire tumor available for histologic evaluation
  - Standard approach for locally aggressive benign tumors (e.g., fibromatosis), deep (subfascial) tumors, and sarcomas
  - May be performed following chemotherapy &/or radiation to improve resectability and decrease potential morbidity

BIOPSY SPECIMENS

General Histologic Approach

- Ensure that lesional tissue is present
- Evaluate histologic growth pattern and architecture in conjunction with cytologic features of tumor cells
  - Looks for histologic clues that suggest specific differentiation (e.g., lipoblasts)
- Assess mitotic activity and presence or absence of necrosis

Core Needle Biopsy

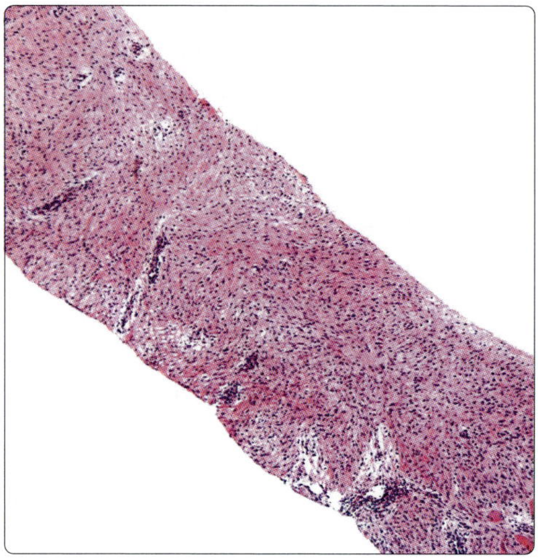

Fine-Needle Aspiration

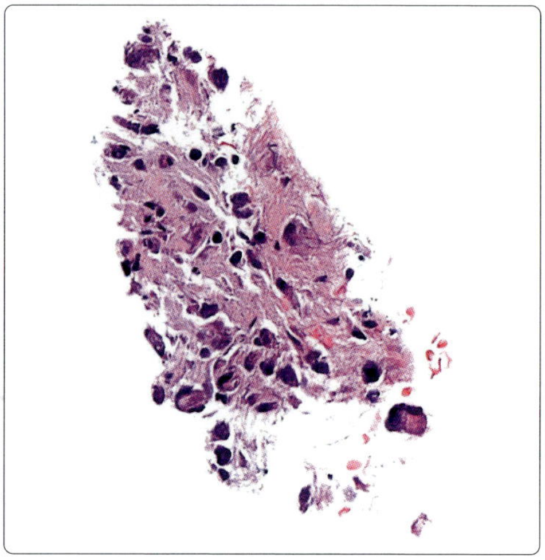

(Left) *Collecting tissue by core needle biopsy has become popular due to both the ease of performance and minimal morbidity to the patient as compared with open surgical biopsy. Despite the limited tissue sample, a diagnosis is often possible with careful histologic evaluation and judicious use of ancillary techniques.* **(Right)** *Cell block collected from a fine-needle aspiration (FNA) can also be used for diagnosis. However, tissue is often heavily fragmented and scant, as depicted.*

- Utilize ancillary studies (e.g., immunohistochemistry, molecular analysis) as needed
- If constellation of features is classic for particular tumor, diagnosis can be made
- If clear diagnosis cannot be made, determine whether tumor appears benign, low-grade malignant, or high-grade malignant
  - Even in absence of clear diagnosis, this information is helpful to guide surgical/clinical planning

Caveats

- Always exclude carcinoma, melanoma, lymphoma, and mesothelioma before committing to mesenchymal diagnosis
- At times, actual tumor does not get sampled
  - Some tumors may incite prominent peripheral host fibroblastic or inflammatory reaction that is inadvertently sampled
  - Normal subcutaneous fat adjacent to tumor may be sampled and mistaken for lipomatous tumor
- Be wary of sampling issues related to biopsy evaluation
  - Tumors that appear low grade on biopsy may contain higher grade areas upon resection
    - Particularly important in tumors of adipocytic and neural origin
  - Tumors that appear as nonspecific high-grade pleomorphic sarcomas on biopsy often can be more specifically classified on resection
    - e.g., dedifferentiated liposarcoma, pleomorphic liposarcoma, extraskeletal osteosarcoma
    - Diagnosis "undifferentiated pleomorphic sarcoma" should not be made on biopsy, as it is diagnosis of exclusion
- Awareness of particular idiosyncrasies of soft tissue pathology is very important
  - Sarcomas may appear paradoxically bland and therefore benign
    - e.g., low-grade fibromyxoid sarcoma, myxoid liposarcoma, myxoid synovial sarcoma
  - Benign tumors may show histologic features that suggest malignancy
    - e.g., nodular fasciitis, proliferative fasciitis/myositis, cellular schwannoma
- Only commit to clear diagnosis on biopsy if it is well supported
  - In general, conservative diagnosis on biopsy better serves patient

Reporting

- Every effort should be taken to establish clear diagnosis (and histologic grade, if applicable) on biopsy
  - Modern ancillary techniques are making this much easier for pathologists
  - Margin status cannot be evaluated
- If clear diagnosis cannot be established, descriptive diagnosis can help guide surgical/clinical planning
  - e.g., benign fibroblastic lesion
  - e.g., low-grade myxoid neoplasm, favor benign
  - e.g., high-grade pleomorphic sarcoma, not further classified
- Descriptive comment is highly recommended in many cases to discuss differential diagnosis options
  - e.g., "Although these findings are suggestive of a low-grade neoplasm, such as an intramuscular myxoma, a low-grade sarcoma, such as low-grade fibromyxoid sarcoma or low-grade myxofibrosarcoma, cannot be excluded in this limited sample."
  - e.g., "Although the histologic features are consistent with a neurofibroma, given the large size of the lesion clinically, the possibility of an unsampled malignant component cannot be excluded in this limited sample."

RESECTION SPECIMENS

General Histologic Approach

- Surgical removal without neoadjuvant therapy
  - If tumor has been sampled previously, review original biopsy (if available) and confirm diagnosis and adequacy of sampling
    - If diagnosis is established or confirmed, assure accuracy of histologic grade (if applicable)
      - Tumors diagnosed as "low grade" on biopsy may contain higher grade areas in resection specimen
    - Ancillary techniques (e.g., immunohistochemistry, molecular analysis) may be utilized as needed
  - If tumor has not been sampled previously, evaluate all histologic sections of tumor to establish diagnosis
    - Ancillary techniques may be utilized as needed
  - Evaluate margin status (mainly sarcomas and locally aggressive benign tumors)
- Surgical removal following neoadjuvant therapy
  - If tumor has been sampled previously, review original biopsy (if available) and confirm diagnosis
  - Determine whether diagnosis can be established or confirmed on resection (may not be possible due to treatment effect)
    - Overall histologic picture depends heavily upon biologic response of tumor to therapy
      - Tumors may be extensively necrotic, inflamed, &/or fibrotic/hyalinized
      - Tumor cells may become markedly pleomorphic and atypical, including bizarre cytomorphologies
  - Document approximate percentage of residual tumor viability
  - Evaluate margin status

Caveats

- Despite all efforts, small percentage of soft tissue tumors defy classification after resection
  - Distinction between benign, low-grade malignant, and high-grade malignant should be goal in these cases
  - Always ensure carcinoma, melanoma, lymphoma, and mesothelioma have been excluded before committing to soft tissue diagnosis
- Care is warranted when attempting to classify soft tissue tumor treated preoperatively with chemotherapy/radiation
  - Tumors that are usually cytologically monomorphic may appear pleomorphic following therapy
  - Cytoplasmic vacuolizations may be prominent, mimicking lipoblastic differentiation
  - Ancillary techniques are unreliable following chemotherapy/radiation and should not be utilized

Reporting

- Surgical pathology reports for soft tissue resections should contain tumor diagnosis, histologic grade (if applicable), and margin status (if appropriate)
  - Additional staging information (e.g., size) can be included as checklist
- For tumors that cannot be definitively classified after all options are exhausted, descriptive diagnosis can be utilized
  - e.g., low-grade myxoid sarcoma, not otherwise specified (NOS)
  - e.g., epithelioid malignant mesenchymal neoplasm, favor high-grade sarcoma
- For tumors treated with neoadjuvant therapy prior to resection
  - High-grade sarcoma with extensive therapy effect (20% tumor viability)

SPECIAL TOPICS

Intraoperative Frozen Section Consultation for Diagnosis

- May be requested by surgeon in certain scenarios
  - Tumor has not been sampled previously
  - To confirm previous biopsy diagnosis
  - Tumor was sampled previously by biopsy but no specific diagnosis was attained
  - Tumor with previous benign or low-grade biopsy diagnosis, and there is clinical concern for unsampled, higher grade component
- Intraoperative diagnosis or confirmation of diagnosis can be sought to confirm surgical/clinical treatment plan
  - Variability exists between individual surgeons
    - May continue with resection plans for benign or low-grade malignancies
    - May halt further surgery and administer neoadjuvant therapy if high-grade malignancy
- In many instances, specific soft tissue diagnosis cannot be made by frozen section evaluation
  - Most helpful information pathologist can provide: Whether tumor appears benign, low-grade malignant, or high-grade malignant
    - Exercise caution when calling soft tissue tumor "benign" on frozen section
      - Use of term "low grade" recommended over "benign," unless benignity is absolutely certain
      - Some low-grade sarcomas can be easily mistaken for benign tumors on frozen section, which can lead to inappropriately conservative treatment
  - If diagnosis cannot be made on frozen section, and alternative descriptive interpretation cannot be comfortably provided by pathologist, it is appropriate to document presence of satisfactory lesional tissue and defer to evaluation of permanent sections
  - Examples of appropriate frozen section interpretations
    - Low-grade spindle cell proliferation
    - High-grade sarcoma
    - Spindle cell sarcoma, favor low grade
    - Tumor present, defer to permanents
    - Malignant neoplasm, defer to permanents

Evaluation by Ancillary Testing

- Immunohistochemistry
  - Wide array of antibodies available today has made it easier for pathologists to make confident soft tissue diagnoses on limited tissue samples
  - It is recommended that every attempt be made to establish diagnosis or limited differential by routine histology
  - When needed, limited screening panel of immunohistochemical stains is helpful for supporting (or excluding) diagnoses
    - Specific screening panels vary depending on pathologist's comfort level with soft tissue pathology
  - Common 5-stain screening panel: Keratin, S100 protein, SMA, desmin, CD34
    - Provides reasonably broad coverage
    - Can be modified with additional stains as necessary depending upon histologic/clinical context
  - Recommendations and caveats
    - Always confirm that external and internal controls are functioning properly
    - Examine entire slide and all tissue fragments
    - Know what constitutes positive staining for each antibody (e.g., nuclear, cytoplasmic, membranous expression)
    - If stain appears positive, confirm that actual cells of interest are staining
    - Important: On very limited tissue sample, negative staining for particular antibody may not reflect status of entire tumor
      - e.g., myogenin expression in embryonal rhabdomyosarcoma can be patchy and focal
- Molecular analysis
  - Representative paraffin tissue block can be used for variety of sophisticated testing (e.g., FISH, RT-PCR)

Expert Consultation

- Pathologists who are experienced in evaluation of soft tissue tumors may be consulted to review case
- Common reasons
  - Primary pathologist is uncomfortable with &/or has limited experience in soft tissue pathology
  - Surgeon, primary care provider, or patient may request 2nd opinion
    - Histologic diagnosis is at odds with clinical impression
    - Diagnosis of very rare or unusual tumor is rendered
  - Newer immunohistochemical antibodies or molecular tests are not readily available to primary pathologist
- Sending 1 or more paraffin tissue blocks along with slides for ancillary testing can be helpful
  - Ideal blocks contain well-processed tissue and minimal to no necrosis
    - Blocks containing areas of lower grade histology are more likely to show diagnostically useful antigen expression than blocks containing predominantly high-grade pleomorphic morphology
- Inclusion of recent clinical history, imaging reports, and surgical notes can also provide useful information

High-Grade Pleomorphic Sarcoma

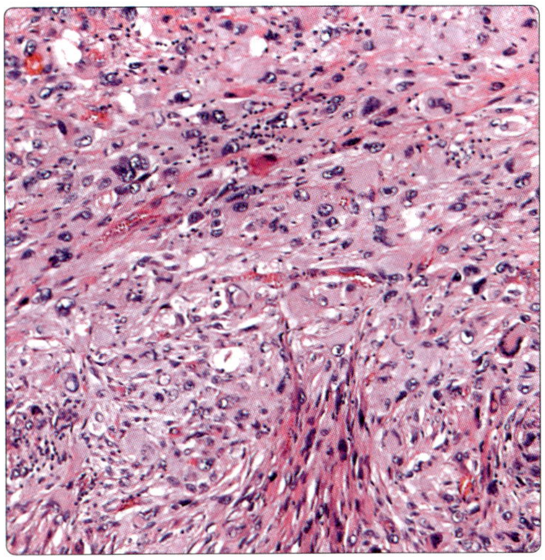

Well-Differentiated Adipocytic Neoplasms

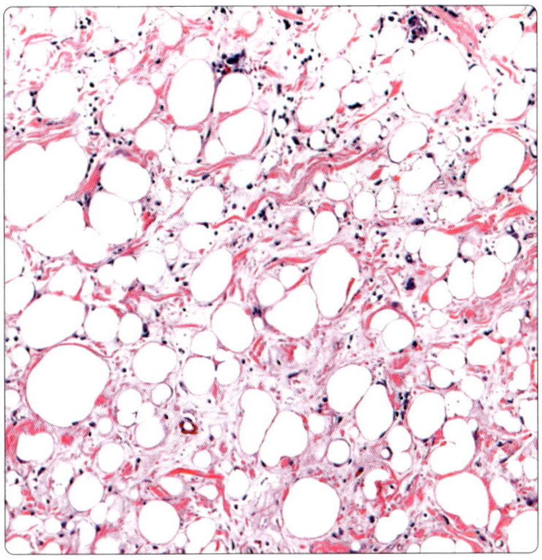

(Left) *On core needle biopsy, it may be difficult to distinguish one high grade pleomorphic sarcoma from another, particularly if discriminatory immunohistochemical stains or molecular tests are not available to the pathologist. Fortunately, in many cases, designation of "high-grade sarcoma" is often sufficient.* **(Right)** *Care should be taken in classifying well-differentiated adipocytic neoplasms on limited biopsy, as atypical lipomatous tumor/well-differentiated liposarcoma can contain large areas resembling conventional lipoma.*

Low-Grade Spindle Cell Neoplasm

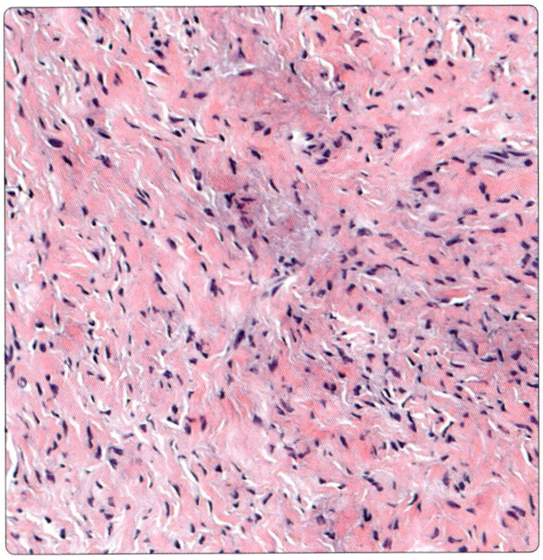

Deceptively Bland Sarcoma

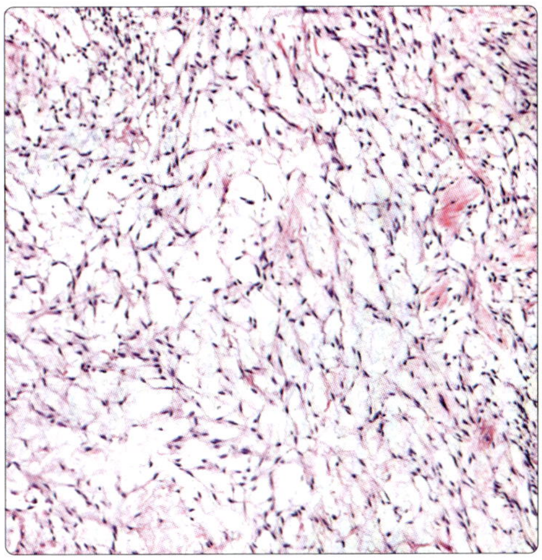

(Left) *Classification of low-grade spindle cell neoplasms on limited biopsy can be challenging without ancillary tests mainly because some low-grade sarcomas can closely resemble benign entities morphologically. This H&E shows a core biopsy specimen of a low-grade fibromyxoid sarcoma mimicking a benign neural or fibroblastic neoplasm.* **(Right)** *This H&E depicts a largely myxoid synovial sarcoma. On a limited biopsy specimen, this tumor could easily be mistaken for a benign or low-grade process.*

Posttherapy Changes

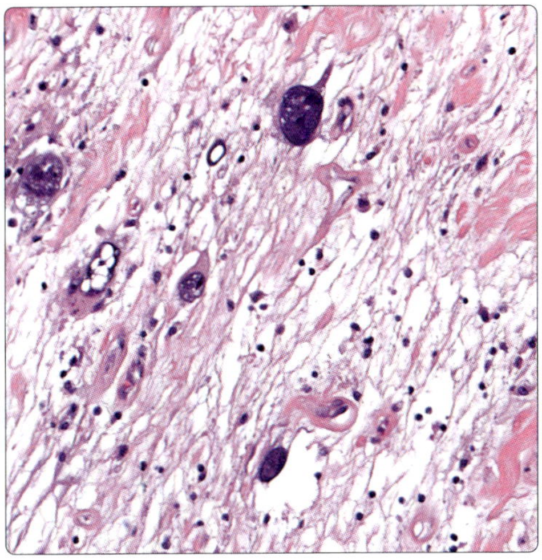

Immunohistochemistry

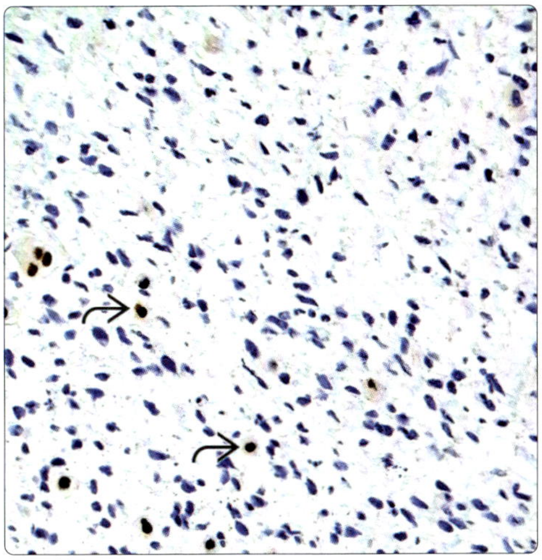

(Left) *If a specific diagnosis is not established prior to neoadjuvant therapy, definitive classification of a soft tissue sarcoma may not be possible due to therapy-related histologic changes, including bizarre nuclear atypia, stromal fibrosis, and edema. IHC and molecular analysis are also largely unhelpful in this setting.* **(Right)** *Care must always be taken with IHC performed on limited tissue. One pitfall is focal tumor antigen expression ➔ (e.g., myogenin, shown) that is not present on biopsy.*

Age- and Location-Based Approach to Diagnosis

DIRECTIONS

How to Use These Guides

- The following guides are neither comprehensive nor perfect and are meant to serve only as a starting point for working up a suspected mesenchymal neoplasm
- Includes entities that are most commonly or classically associated with particular clinical and histologic findings

Specific Directions for This Guide

- For each site and associated age range listed below, a selection of most commonly or characteristically associated diagnoses are provided
- Compile an assortment of potential diagnoses from the guide using age of patient and provided tumor site from your particular case
- Compare this selection to those created from the other 2 approach chapters in this section
- Overlapping diagnoses derived from these 3 distinct approaches are highest yield and should be your focus
- Once high-yield diagnoses have been identified, specific entity chapters should be directly consulted for detailed information and image galleries
    - In particular, the Differential Diagnosis sections should be fully utilized to broaden search and increase chances of securing the correct diagnosis

Important Caveat

- Always exclude carcinoma, melanoma, lymphoma, and mesothelioma before committing to a mesenchymal diagnosis

AGE-BASED APPROACH

Infancy (< 3 Years Old)

- Fibrous hamartoma of infancy
- Inclusion body fibromatosis
- Infantile fibrosarcoma
- Lipoblastoma
- Lipofibromatosis
- Myofibroma

Infants, Children, or Adolescents (< 20 Years Old)

- Angiomatosis
- Calcifying aponeurotic fibroma
- Dabska tumor (infants and children)
- Embryonal rhabdomyosarcoma
- Extrarenal rhabdoid tumor (infants and children)
- Fibromatosis
- Gardner fibroma
- Giant cell fibroblastoma
- Kaposiform hemangioendothelioma (infants and children)

Adolescents to Young Adults (~ 10 to 35 Years Old)

- Alveolar rhabdomyosarcoma
- Alveolar soft part sarcoma
- Angiomatoid fibrous histiocytoma
- Desmoplastic small round cell tumor (and children)
- Epithelioid sarcoma (classic type)
- Fibromatosis
- Inflammatory myofibroblastic tumor
- Low-grade fibromyxoid sarcoma
- Myxoid liposarcoma
- Plexiform fibrohistiocytic tumor
- Synovial sarcoma

Young to Middle-Aged Adults (~ 20 to 50 Years Old)

- Clear cell sarcoma
- Dermatofibrosarcoma protuberans
- Epithelioid hemangioendothelioma
- Epithelioid sarcoma (proximal type)
- Fibroma of tendon sheath
- Fibromatosis
- Hibernoma
- Leiomyosarcoma
- Low-grade myofibroblastic sarcoma
- Myositis ossificans
- Myxoinflammatory fibroblastic sarcoma
- Nodular fasciitis
- Pseudomyogenic hemangioendothelioma
- Tenosynovial giant cell tumor (both localized and diffuse types)

Inclusion Body Fibromatosis

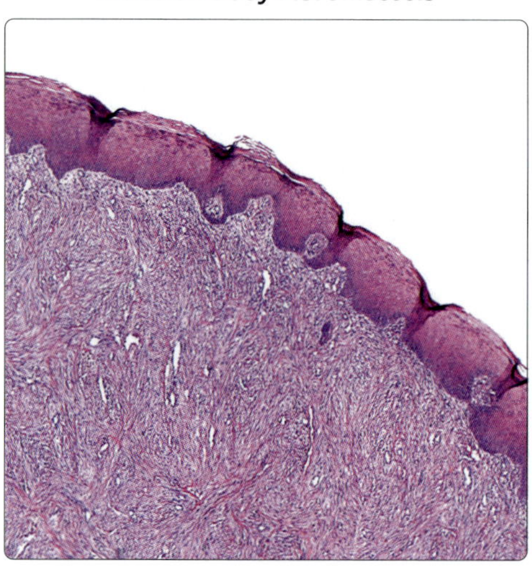

Dedifferentiated Liposarcoma

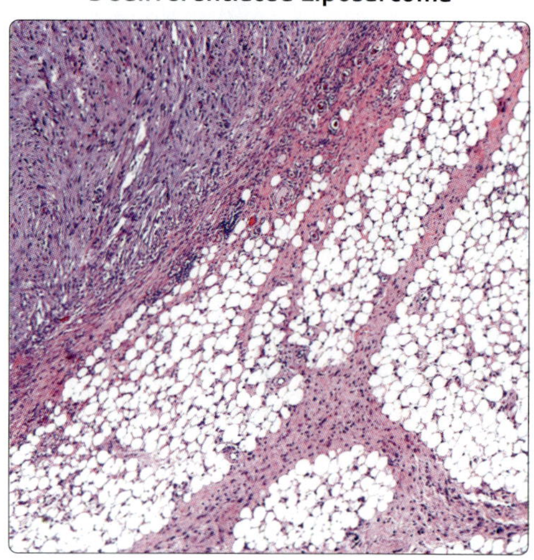

(Left) *Some mesenchymal neoplasms show a striking predilection for very specific age groups and very specific anatomic locations. For example, inclusion body fibromatosis (a.k.a. infantile digital fibromatosis) most frequently arises in the digits of infants.* **(Right)** *Dedifferentiated liposarcoma is the most common pleomorphic sarcoma of the retroperitoneum and should always be at the top of the differential diagnosis for retroperitoneal tumors in older adults.*

Middle-Aged to Older Adults (~ 40 to 65 Years Old)

- Atypical lipomatous tumor/well-differentiated liposarcoma
- Dedifferentiated liposarcoma
- Desmoplastic fibroblastoma
- Extraskeletal myxoid chondrosarcoma
- Extraskeletal osteosarcoma
- Hemosiderotic fibrolipomatous tumor
- Intramuscular myxoma
- Mammary-type myofibroblastoma
- Ossifying fibromyxoid tumor
- Proliferative fasciitis/myositis
- Sclerosing epithelioid fibrosarcoma
- Spindle cell/pleomorphic lipoma

Older and Elderly Adults (> 50 Years Old)

- Atypical fibroxanthoma
- Elastofibroma
- Ischemic fasciitis
- Myxofibrosarcoma
- Pleomorphic liposarcoma
- Pleomorphic rhabdomyosarcoma
- Undifferentiated pleomorphic sarcoma

LOCATION-BASED APPROACH

Distal Extremities

- Calcifying aponeurotic fibroma
- Clear cell sarcoma
- Epithelioid sarcoma (classic type)
- Fibromatosis
- Hemosiderotic fibrolipomatous tumor
- Lipofibromatosis
- Palmar/plantar fibromatosis
- Pleomorphic hyalinizing angiectatic tumor

Fingers and Toes

- Acral fibromyxoma
- Dermal nerve sheath myxoma
- Epithelioid hemangioma
- Fibroma of tendon sheath
- Glomus tumor
- Inclusion body fibromatosis
- Localized-type tenosynovial giant cell tumor
- Myxoinflammatory fibroblastic sarcoma
- Soft tissue chondroma

Genital Region and Groin

- Angiomyofibroblastoma
- Cellular angiofibroma
- Deep (aggressive) angiomyxoma
- Genital rhabdomyoma
- Intranodal palisaded myofibroblastoma
- Mammary-type myofibroblastoma
- Spindle cell rhabdomyosarcoma (paratesticular)

Mesentery/Omentum/Peritoneum

- Desmoid fibromatosis
- Desmoplastic small round cell tumor
- Gastrointestinal stromal tumor
- Inflammatory myofibroblastic tumor

Head and Neck

- Alveolar soft part sarcoma (infants and children)
- Atypical fibromyxoma
- Cellular neurothekeoma
- Ectopic meningioma
- Embryonal rhabdomyosarcoma
- Epithelioid hemangioma
- Paraganglioma
- Rhabdomyoma (adult and fetal types)
- Solitary circumscribed neuroma
- Spindle cell rhabdomyosarcoma

Retroperitoneum

- Dedifferentiated liposarcoma
- Desmoid fibromatosis
- Extrarenal rhabdoid tumor
- Ganglioneuroma
- Inflammatory myofibroblastic tumor
- Leiomyosarcoma
- PEComa
- Schwannoma (cellular variant)
- Well-differentiated liposarcoma

Trunk, Shoulders, and Back

- Dermatofibrosarcoma protuberans
- Desmoid fibromatosis
- Elastofibroma
- Lipoblastoma
- Proliferative myositis
- Spindle cell/pleomorphic lipoma

GASTROINTESTINAL MESENCHYMAL TUMORS (MOST COMMON BY LOCATION)

Esophagus

- Leiomyoma (mural)
- Granular cell tumor

Stomach

- Gastrointestinal stromal tumor
- Inflammatory fibroid polyp
- Schwannoma

Small Bowel

- Gastrointestinal stromal tumor
- Inflammatory fibroid polyp

Colorectum

- Leiomyoma (polyp; nonmural)
- Gastrointestinal stromal tumor

MESENCHYMAL TUMORS INVOLVING LYMPH NODES (MOST COMMON)

Metastasis

- Epithelioid sarcoma
- Clear cell sarcoma
- Rhabdomyosarcomas

Nodal Primary

- Kaposi sarcoma
- Intranodal palisaded myofibroblastoma

DIRECTIONS

How to Use These Guides

- These guides are neither comprehensive nor perfect and are meant to serve only as starting point for working up suspected mesenchymal neoplasm
- They include entities that are most commonly or classically associated with particular histologic patterns in soft tissue

Specific Directions for This Guide

- Following list of histologic patterns has been generated using combination of cell types (spindle or epithelioid), cytologic features (monomorphism vs. pleomorphism), and various stromal characteristics (e.g., myxoid, prominent vasculature)
- For each histologic pattern listed below, selection of more commonly or characteristically associated diagnoses are provided
- Compile assortment of potential diagnoses from each guide using main histologic pattern(s) from your particular case
- Compare this selection to those created from other 2 approach chapters
- Overlapping diagnoses derived from these 3 distinct approaches are highest yield and should be your focus
- Once high-yield diagnoses have been identified, specific entity chapters should be directly consulted for detailed information and image galleries
  - In particular, differential diagnosis sections should be fully utilized to broaden search and increase chances of securing correct diagnosis

Important Caveats

- Always exclude carcinoma, melanoma, lymphoma, and mesothelioma before committing to mesenchymal diagnosis
- Always exclude gastrointestinal stromal tumor when tumor arises within abdominal cavity or pelvis
  - Can demonstrate almost any morphologic pattern

MONOMORPHIC SPINDLE CELL PATTERNS

Monomorphic Spindle Cells Arranged in Sheets

- Angiomatoid fibrous histiocytoma
- Infantile fibrosarcoma
- Solitary fibrous tumor
- Synovial sarcoma

Monomorphic Spindle Cells Featuring Hyper- and Hypocellular Areas

- Low-grade fibromyxoid sarcoma
- Malignant peripheral nerve sheath tumor (MPNST)
- Schwannoma
- Solitary fibrous tumor
- Synovial sarcoma

Monomorphic Spindle Cells Arranged in Bundles or Fascicles

- Angioleiomyoma
- Deep leiomyoma
- Fibromatosis
- Fibrous hamartoma of infancy
- Inclusion body fibromatosis
- Infantile fibrosarcoma
- Kaposi sarcoma
- Leiomyosarcoma
- Lipofibromatosis
- Mammary-type myofibroblastoma
- Plexiform fibrohistiocytic tumor
- Schwannoma
- Solitary circumscribed neuroma

Monomorphic Spindle Cells Arranged in Cellular Herringbone Fascicles

- Adult-type fibrosarcoma
- Fibrosarcomatous dermatofibrosarcoma protuberans (DFSP)
- Infantile fibrosarcoma
- MPNST
- Spindle cell rhabdomyosarcoma

Monomorphic Spindle Cells: Sheets

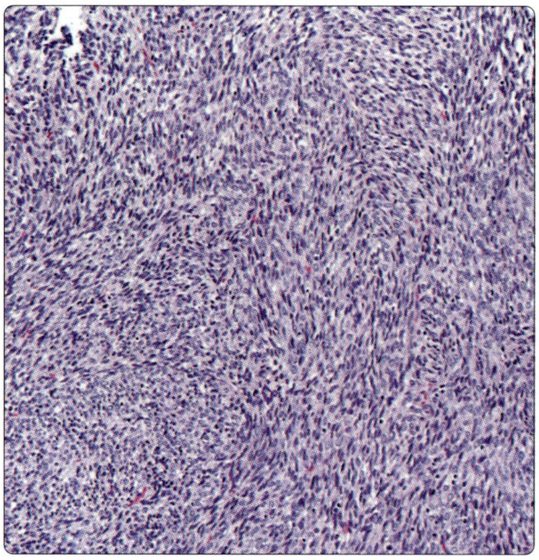

Monomorphic Spindle Cells: Sheets (Syncytia)

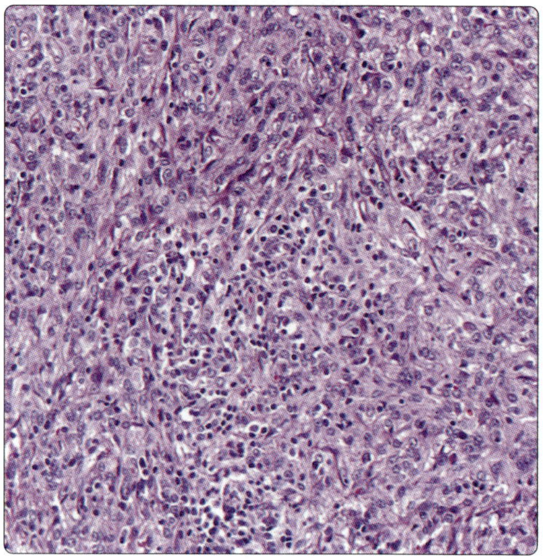

(Left) *A sheet-like pattern tends to feature diffuse growth of spindle cells without obvious directional orientation, however, areas of bundled or fascicular growth are not uncommon. This pattern is common in synovial sarcoma (shown) and solitary fibrous tumor.* **(Right)** *Sheets of spindled cells can also have a syncytial appearance in which cytoplasmic borders are inconspicuous, and independent cell nuclei appear to share the same cytoplasm. This appearance is common in angiomatoid fibrous histiocytoma.*

- Synovial sarcoma

Monomorphic Spindle Cells Arranged in Storiform or Whorled Architecture

- Deep benign fibrous histiocytoma
- Dermatofibroma (fibrous histiocytoma)
- Dermatofibrosarcoma protuberans
- Follicular dendritic cell sarcoma
- Hybrid nerve sheath tumor
- Inclusion body fibromatosis
- Low-grade fibromyxoid sarcoma
- Low-grade myofibroblastic sarcoma
- Nodular fasciitis
- Perineurioma

Monomorphic Spindle Cells Arranged in Multinodular or Plexiform Architecture

- Granular cell tumor
- Plexiform fibrohistiocytic tumor
- Plexiform neurofibroma
- Plexiform schwannoma
- Solitary circumscribed neuroma

Monomorphic Spindle Cells Arranged in Reticular or Microcystic Pattern

- Extraskeletal myxoid chondrosarcoma
- Myoepithelioma
- Perineurioma (variant)
- Schwannoma (variant)

Monomorphic Spindle Cells Within Myxoid Stroma

- Acral fibromyxoma
- Deep (aggressive) angiomyxoma
- Dermal nerve sheath myxoma
- Dermatofibrosarcoma protuberans (myxoid type)
- Desmoid fibromatosis
- Embryonal rhabdomyosarcoma
- Hybrid nerve sheath tumor
- Inflammatory myofibroblastic tumor
- Intramuscular myxoma
- Leiomyosarcoma (variant)
- Low-grade fibromyxoid sarcoma
- Myxoid liposarcoma
- Neurofibroma
- Nodular fasciitis
- Perineurioma
- Proliferative fasciitis/myositis
- Synovial sarcoma
- Spindle cell lipoma

Monomorphic Spindle Cells Within Collagenous, Hyalinized, or Sclerotic Stroma

- Acral fibromyxoma
- Calcifying fibrous tumor
- Cellular angiofibroma
- Desmoplastic fibroblastoma
- Elastofibroma
- Fibroma of tendon sheath
- Fibromatosis
- Inflammatory myofibroblastic tumor
- Low-grade fibromyxoid sarcoma
- Low-grade myofibroblastic sarcoma
- Neurofibroma
- Nodular fasciitis
- Perineurioma
- Sclerosing rhabdomyosarcoma
- Solitary fibrous tumor

Monomorphic Spindle Cells Amidst Prominent Stromal Vasculature

- Angiofibroma of soft tissue
- Angioleiomyoma
- Deep (aggressive) angiomyxoma
- Dermatofibrosarcoma protuberans (myxoid type)
- Low-grade fibromyxoid sarcoma
- Myopericytoma
- Myxoid liposarcoma
- Schwannoma
- Solitary fibrous tumor

Monomorphic Spindle Cells Associated With Mature Adipose Tissue

- Angiomyofibroblastoma
- Cellular angiofibroma
- Elastofibroma
- Fibrous hamartoma of infancy
- Hemosiderotic fibrolipomatous tumor
- Lipoblastoma
- Lipofibromatosis
- Mammary-type myofibroblastoma
- Myolipoma
- Solitary fibrous tumor (variant)
- Spindle cell lipoma

PLEOMORPHIC SPINDLE CELL PATTERNS

Pleomorphic Spindle Cells Arranged in Sheets

- Angiosarcoma
- Dedifferentiated liposarcoma
- Extraskeletal osteosarcoma
- Pleomorphic liposarcoma
- Pleomorphic rhabdomyosarcoma
- Superficial CD34(+) fibroblastic tumor
- Undifferentiated pleomorphic sarcoma

Pleomorphic Spindle Cells Arranged in Fascicles

- Dedifferentiated liposarcoma
- Leiomyosarcoma
- MPNST
- Pleomorphic rhabdomyosarcoma
- Undifferentiated pleomorphic sarcoma

Pleomorphic Spindle Cells Within Myxoid Stroma

- Ancient schwannoma
- Atypical neurofibroma
- Dedifferentiated liposarcoma
- Embryonal rhabdomyosarcoma (anaplastic)
- Giant cell fibroblastoma
- MPNST
- Myxofibrosarcoma
- Myxoinflammatory fibroblastic sarcoma
- Well-differentiated liposarcoma (variant)

Pleomorphic Spindle Cells Within Collagenous, Hyalinized, or Sclerotic Stroma

- Atypical lipomatous tumor/well-differentiated liposarcoma
- Giant cell fibroblastoma
- Myxoinflammatory fibroblastic sarcoma
- Undifferentiated pleomorphic sarcoma

Pleomorphic Spindle Cells Arranged in Storiform Architecture

- Dedifferentiated liposarcoma
- Myxofibrosarcoma (high grade)
- Pleomorphic liposarcoma
- Undifferentiated pleomorphic sarcoma

Pleomorphic Spindle Cell Amidst Prominent Stromal Vasculature

- Myxofibrosarcoma
- Pleomorphic hyalinizing angiectatic tumor
- Solitary fibrous tumor (malignant)
- Undifferentiated pleomorphic sarcoma

EPITHELIOID CELL PATTERNS

Epithelioid Cells Arranged in Nests or Lobules

- Alveolar rhabdomyosarcoma
- Alveolar soft part sarcoma
- Cellular neurothekeoma
- Clear cell sarcoma
- Desmoplastic small round cell tumor
- Epithelioid MPNST
- Epithelioid sarcoma (classic type)
- Glomus tumor
- Granular cell tumor
- Myoepithelioma of soft tissue
- Paraganglioma
- Perivascular epithelioid cell tumor (PEComa)

Epithelioid Cells Arranged in Cords or Trabeculae

- Ossifying fibromyxoid tumor
- Mammary-type myofibroblastoma (epithelioid variant)
- Myoepithelioma of soft tissue
- Sclerosing epithelioid fibrosarcoma

Epithelioid Cells Arranged in Sheets (Abundant Cytoplasm)

- Adult rhabdomyoma
- Alveolar soft part sarcoma
- Epithelioid angiosarcoma
- Epithelioid sarcoma (proximal type)
- Extrarenal rhabdoid tumor
- Tenosynovial giant cell tumor (both types)

Epithelioid Cells Arranged in Sheets (Minimal/Scant Cytoplasm)

- Alveolar rhabdomyosarcoma
- Ewing sarcoma
- Extrarenal rhabdoid tumor
- Extraskeletal mesenchymal chondrosarcoma
- Infantile fibrosarcoma
- Neuroblastoma
- Synovial sarcoma (poorly differentiated)

Epithelioid Cells Within Myxoid Stroma

- Epithelioid hemangioendothelioma
- Epithelioid MPNST
- Extraskeletal myxoid chondrosarcoma
- Glomus tumor
- Myoepithelioma of soft tissue
- Myxofibrosarcoma (variant)
- Soft tissue chondroma (variant)

Epithelioid Cells Within Collagenous, Hyalinized, or Sclerotic Stroma

- Desmoplastic small round cell tumor
- Epithelioid sarcoma
- Myoepithelioma of soft tissue
- Perineurioma (variant)
- Sclerosing epithelioid fibrosarcoma
- Tenosynovial giant cell tumor (both types)

Epithelioid Cells Associated With Prominent Stromal Vasculature

- Alveolar soft part sarcoma
- Angiomyofibroblastoma
- Glomus tumor
- Paraganglioma
- PEComa
- Cellular solitary fibrous tumor (formerly hemangiopericytoma)

Epithelioid Cells Associated With Adipose Tissue

- Angiomyofibroblastoma
- Chondroid lipoma
- Hibernoma

OTHER PATTERNS

Mixed Epithelioid and Spindle Cells

- Angiomyofibroblastoma
- Epithelioid sarcoma
- Leiomyoma
- Malignant mesothelioma (biphasic)
- Myoepithelioma of soft tissue
- PEComa
- Plexiform fibrohistiocytic tumor
- Schwannoma
- Synovial sarcoma (biphasic)

Checkerboard Skeletal Muscle Pattern

- Intramuscular hemangioma
- Intramuscular lipoma
- Intramuscular myxoma
- Low-grade myofibroblastic sarcoma
- Proliferative myositis

Nuclear Palisading

- Dermatofibroma (fibrous histiocytoma)
- Leiomyoma
- Leiomyosarcoma
- MPNST
- Schwannoma
- Synovial sarcoma

Monomorphic Spindle Cells: Hypocellular and Hypercellular Areas

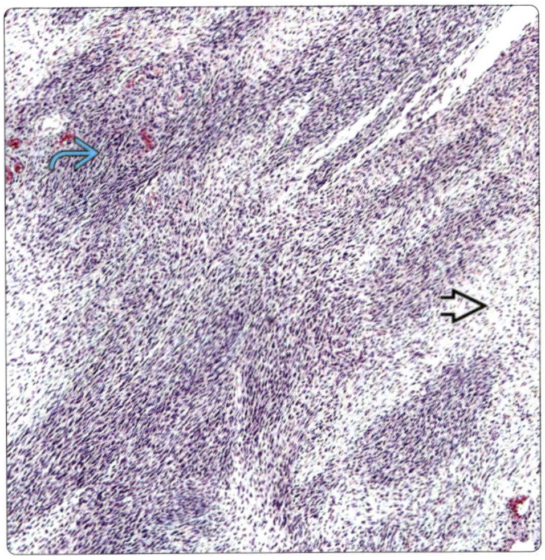

Monomorphic Spindle Cells: Bundles or Fascicles

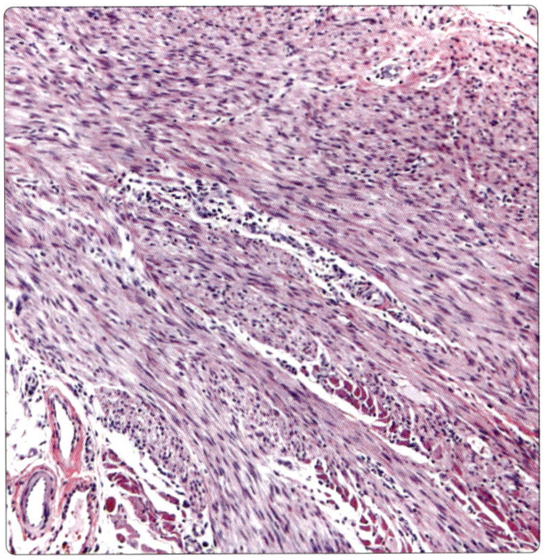

(Left) *A mixed light and dark pattern due to alternating areas of low and high cellularity is often best appreciated at low magnification. This pattern is commonly seen in schwannoma and MPNST.* **(Right)** *Classic bundled or fascicular growth features cells oriented in parallel groups. Directionality is more conspicuous than is usually seen in the sheet-like pattern, and bundles/fascicles may intersect or be organized in different directions. This image shows fibrous hamartoma of infancy.*

Monomorphic Spindle Cells: Cellular Herringbone Fascicles

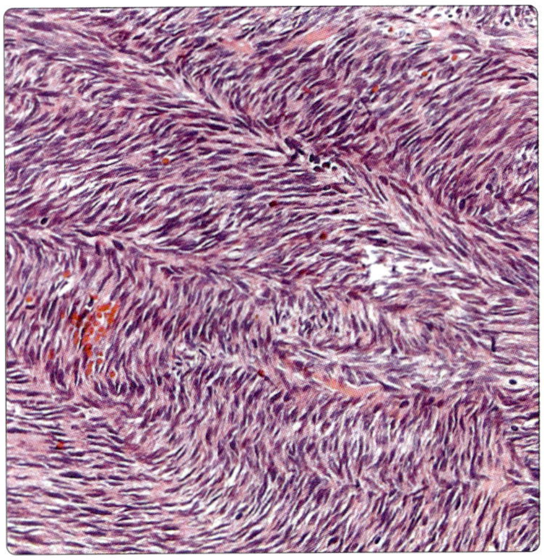

Monomorphic Spindle Cells: Storiform or Whorled Architecture

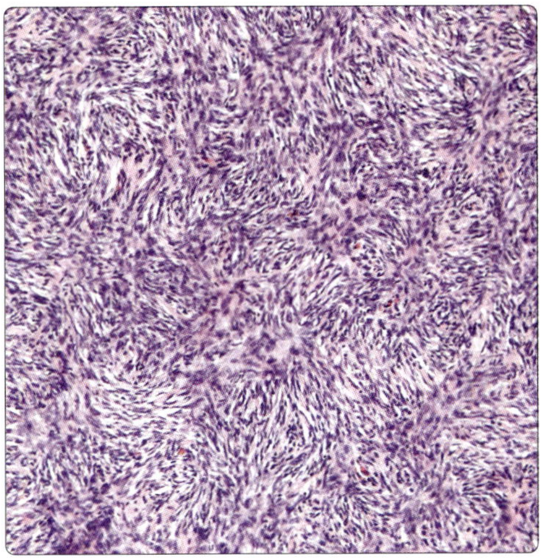

(Left) *A herringbone pattern is created when spindle cells within adjacent fascicles are oriented in roughly the same direction yet appear to slope away from each other. This orientation results in a wide V-shaped or chevron morphology.* **(Right)** *A storiform pattern is manifested by spindled cells that appear to radiate outward from a central point, often with a vague swirling or whorling, similar to a pinwheel. This pattern is most closely associated with DFSP but may be seen in a variety of other tumors.*

Monomorphic Spindle Cells: Multinodular or Plexiform Architecture

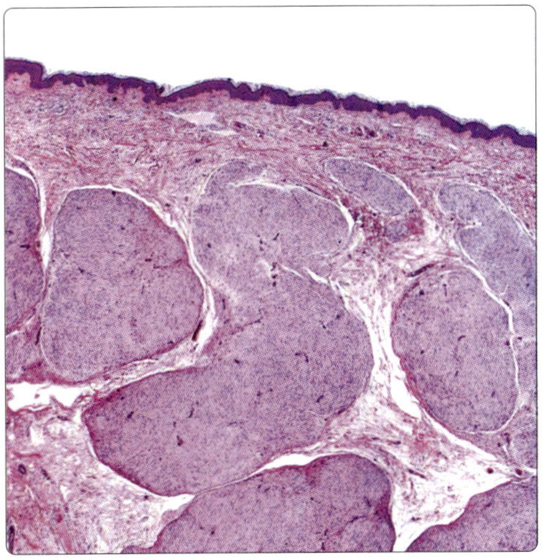

Monomorphic Spindle Cells: Reticular or Microcystic Pattern

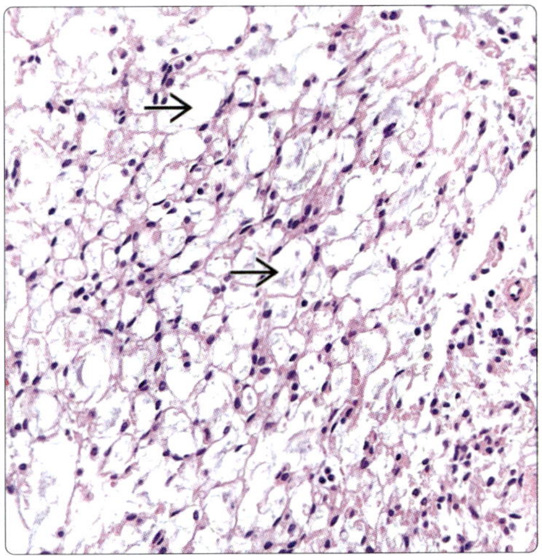

(Left) *Plexiform growth is characterized by discrete globular &/or serpiginous nodules of tumor cells. It tends to be most common in neural tumors, including plexiform neurofibroma and plexiform schwannoma (shown).* **(Right)** *A reticular pattern is created by thin spindled or stellate cells arranged such that cytoplasmic extensions appear to interconnect in a net-like or sieve-like fashion. Acellular microcystic spaces in between cells are also seen.*

(Left) *Myxoid stroma is very common in soft tissue tumors, particularly spindled lesions that are cytologically monomorphic. This pattern is inherent to some tumors (e.g., intramuscular myxoma) but is often seen in variants of other tumors (e.g., spindle cell lipoma, DFSP).* **(Right)** *Some tumors, such as myxoid liposarcoma (shown) or low-grade fibromyxoid sarcoma, may feature areas of increased cellularity. However, significant nuclear pleomorphism is absent.*

Monomorphic Spindle Cells: Myxoid Stroma

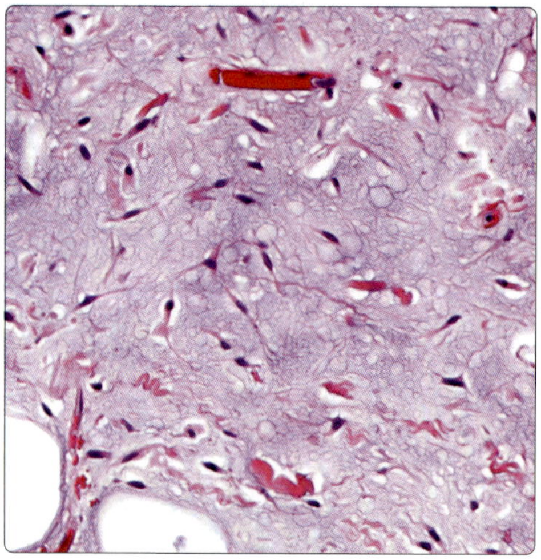

Monomorphic Spindle Cells: Myxoid Stroma (Cellular)

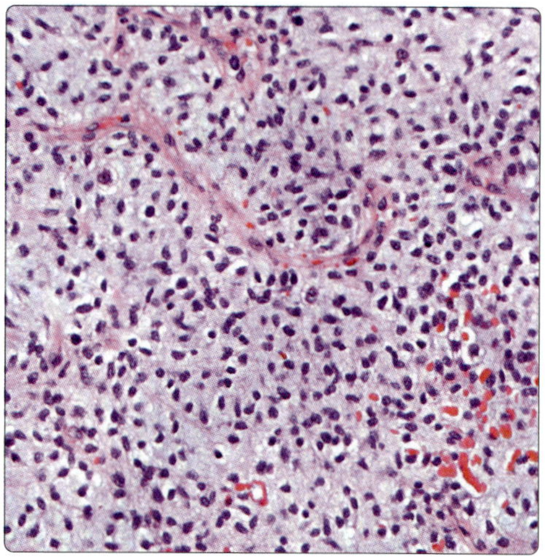

(Left) *Some monomorphic spindle cell tumors characteristically feature a conspicuous collagenous stroma that may or may not show prominent hyalinization or dense sclerosis. Tumor cells may show fascicular, storiform, or haphazard arrangements.* **(Right)** *Large, dilated or ectatic blood vessels* ⇒ *are relatively common as a focal finding in soft tissue tumors. Although these vessels are not usually prominent, some tumors (particularly solitary fibrous tumor) are notable exceptions.*

Monomorphic Spindle Cells: Collagenous, Hyalinized, Sclerotic Stroma

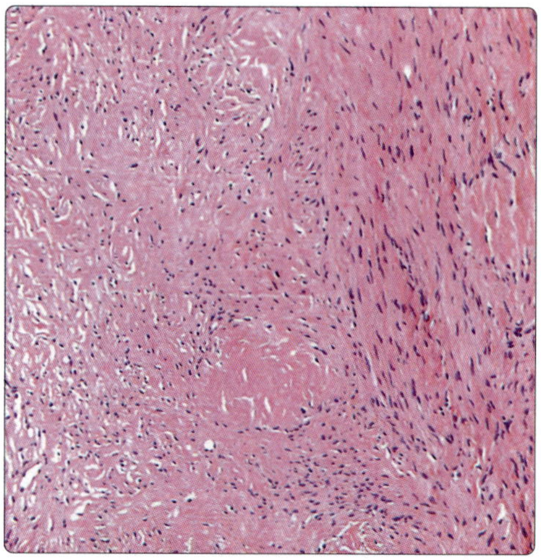

Monomorphic Spindle Cells: Prominent Stromal Vasculature (Large)

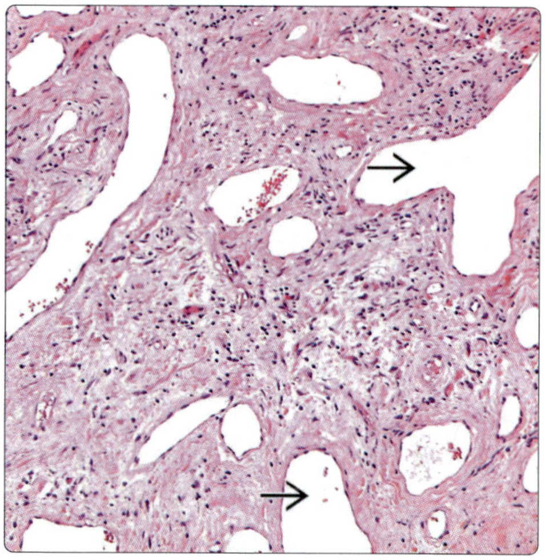

(Left) *Smaller capillary vascular channels* ⇒ *are conspicuous in some lesions, perhaps most notably myxoid liposarcoma.* **(Right)** *Although mature adipose tissue may be present in a tumor as a result of infiltration, some lesions feature fat as a true component of the tumor. Examples include spindle cell lipoma and mammary-type myofibroblastoma.*

Monomorphic Spindle Cells: Prominent Stromal Vasculature (Small)

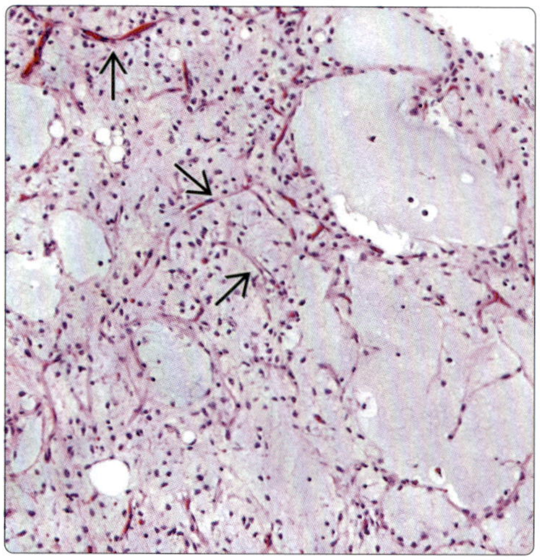

Monomorphic Spindle Cells: Adipose Tissue Component

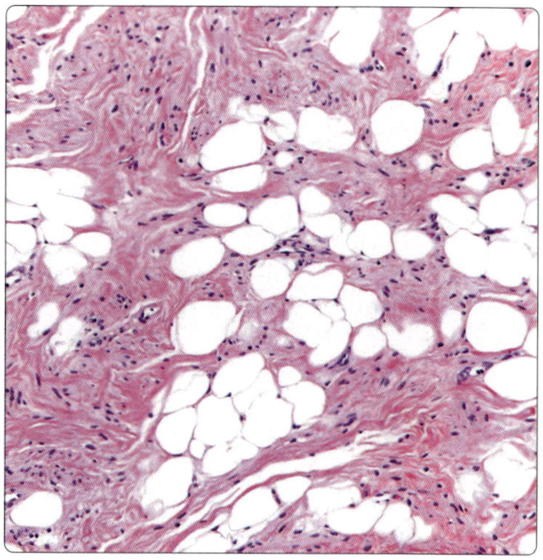

Pleomorphic Spindle Cells: Sheets

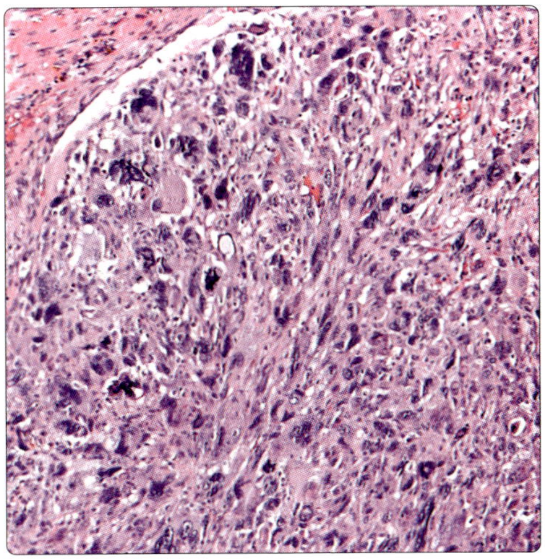

Pleomorphic Spindle Cells: Bundles and Fascicles

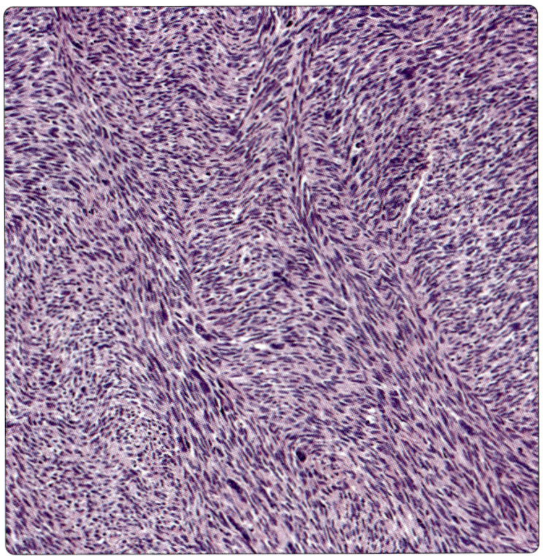

(Left) *Diffuse, cellular sheets of highly pleomorphic cells are typical of many high-grade sarcomas, including undifferentiated pleomorphic sarcoma, dedifferentiated liposarcoma, and high-grade myxofibrosarcoma.* **(Right)** *Fascicular and bundled growth patterns can also be present in pleomorphic spindle cell neoplasms, particularly leiomyosarcoma and MPNST. Pleomorphic cells within a herringbone growth pattern is often MPNST.*

Pleomorphic Spindle Cells: Myxoid Stroma

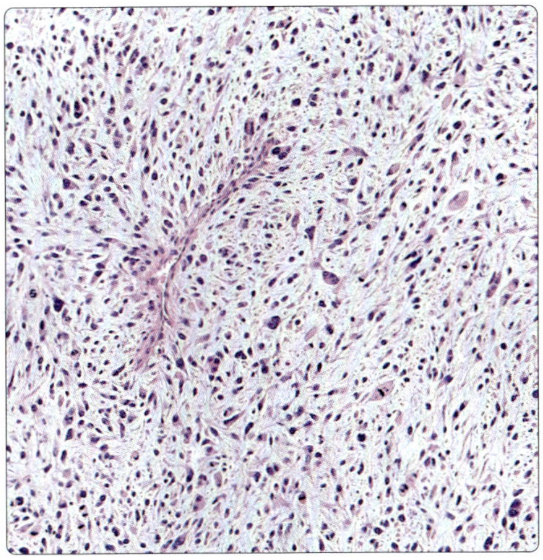

Pleomorphic Spindle Cells: Collagenous, Hyalinized, or Sclerotic Matrix

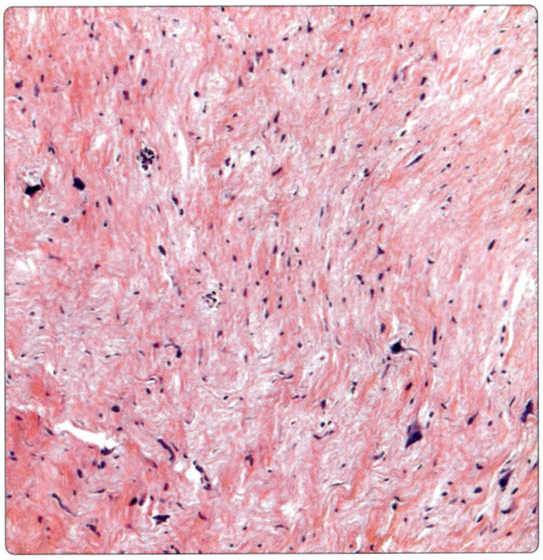

(Left) *Significant pleomorphism within a prominent myxoid stroma is most frequently associated with myxofibrosarcoma; however, it can also be seen in dedifferentiated and pleomorphic types of liposarcoma.* **(Right)** *Pleomorphism within a prominent collagenous matrix is often associated with various high-grade sarcomas; however, it can also be the pattern of sclerosing well-differentiated liposarcoma (shown).*

Pleomorphic Spindle Cells: Storiform or Whorled Architecture

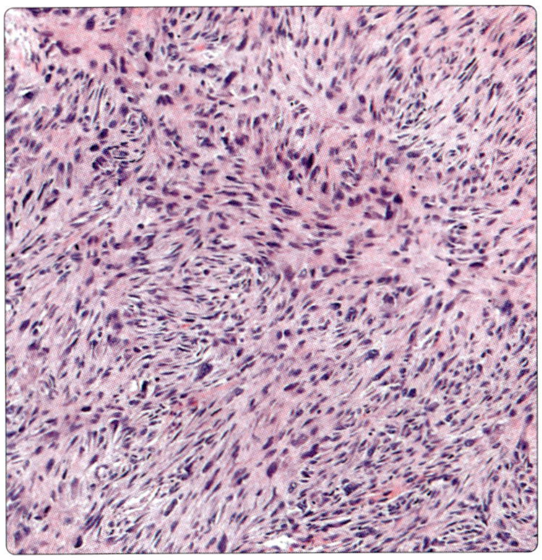

Pleomorphic Spindle Cells: Prominent Stromal Vessels

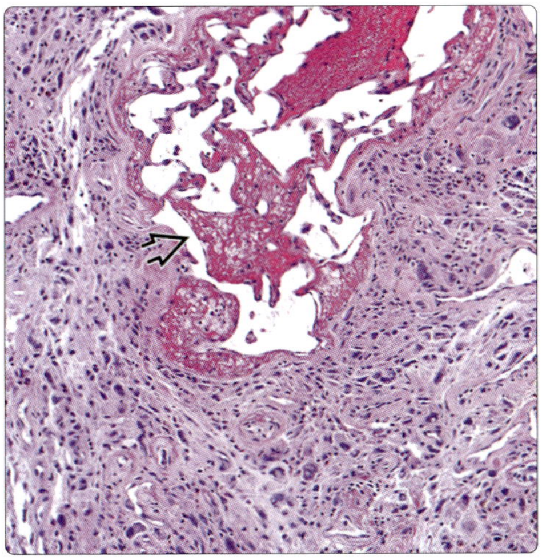

(Left) *The pattern of pleomorphic spindle cells arranged in whorls or storiform arrays is rather nonspecific and can be seen in a variety of often morphologically similar high-grade sarcomas.* **(Right)** *A prominent nonneoplastic stromal vasculature ⇒ is a feature of some pleomorphic spindle cell neoplasms, including both low-grade (e.g., pleomorphic hyalinizing angiectatic tumor, shown) and higher grade (e.g., myxofibrosarcoma) tumors.*

(Left) *Nested or lobular patterns are common in epithelioid neoplasms. Some tumors, such as alveolar soft part sarcoma (shown), may also show a central loss of cellular cohesion* ➔ *imparting a pseudoalveolar appearance.* **(Right)** *Distinct, linear arrangements of epithelioid cells may be seen within a myxoid, fibromyxoid, or fibrous stroma. Myoepithelioma and ossifying fibromyxoid tumor (shown) are examples.*

Epithelioid Cells: Nests or Lobules

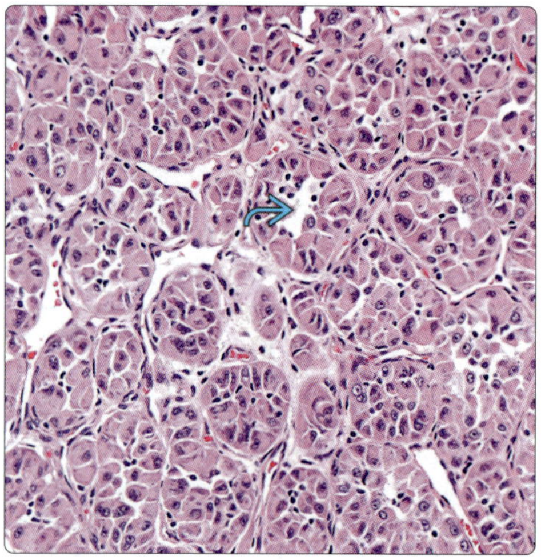

Epithelioid Cells: Cords or Trabeculae

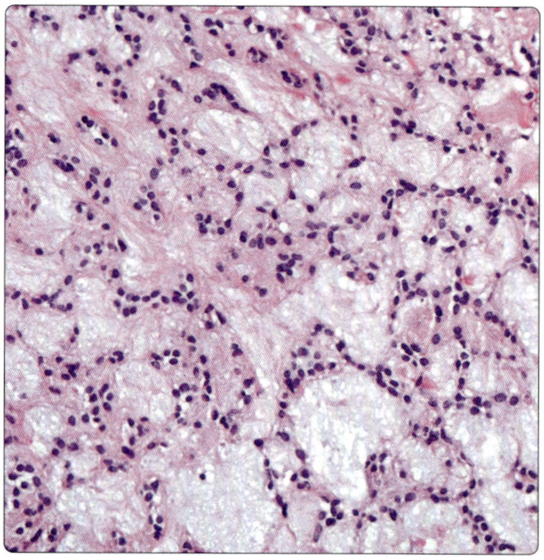

(Left) *Tumors that show a diffuse sheet-like arrangement of epithelioid cells are often high grade and feature marked cytologic atypia and mitotic activity. This morphology can closely mimic carcinoma or melanoma.* **(Right)** *Tumors with sheets of smaller epithelioid cells with minimal cytoplasm appear very blue or basophilic due to increased cell density. These neoplasms are often referred to as small, round, blue cell tumors. Immunohistochemistry is often necessary for diagnosis.*

Epithelioid Cells: Sheets (Abundant Cytoplasm)

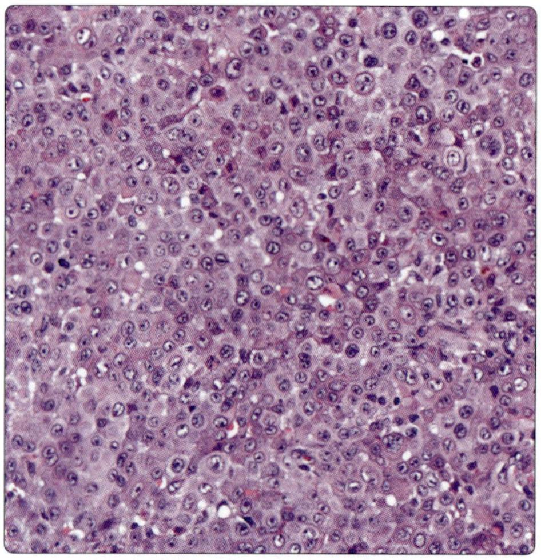

Epithelioid Cells: Sheets (Minimal/Scant Cytoplasm)

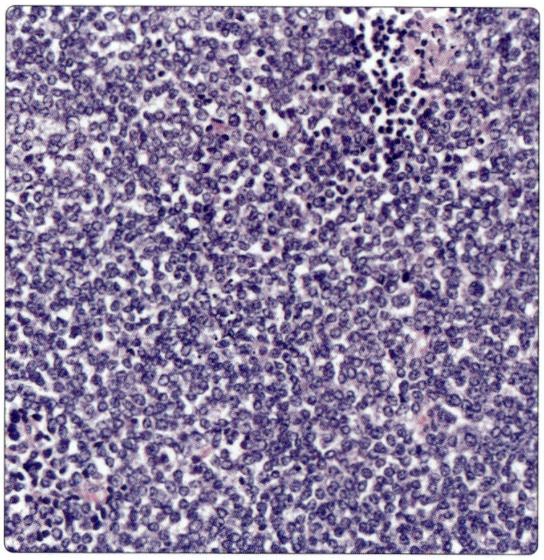

(Left) *The pattern of epithelioid cells within a myxoid stroma is distinctive but not generally common. Examples of tumors include myoepithelioma, extraskeletal myxoid chondrosarcoma, and epithelioid MPNST.* **(Right)** *Epithelioid cells within a collagenous stroma should always lead to consideration of sclerosing epithelioid fibrosarcoma (shown), however, this pattern can also be seen in myoepithelioma, epithelioid sarcoma, and others.*

Epithelioid Cells: Myxoid Stroma

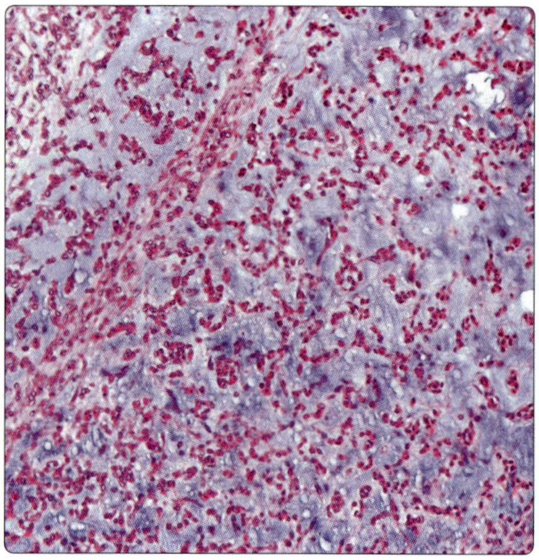

Epithelioid Cells: Collagenous, Hyalinized, or Sclerotic Stroma

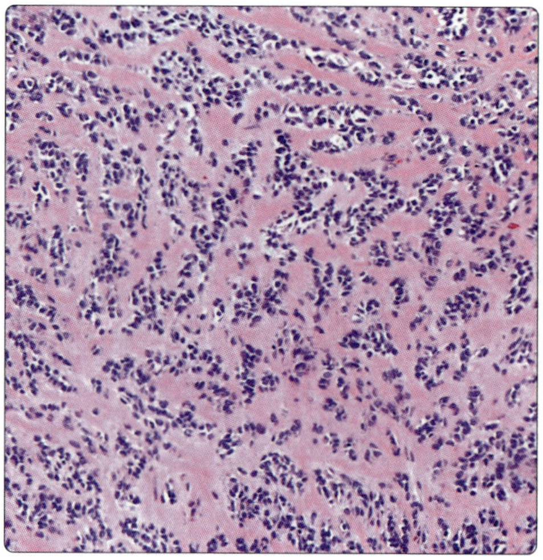

Epithelioid Cells: Prominent Stromal Vasculature

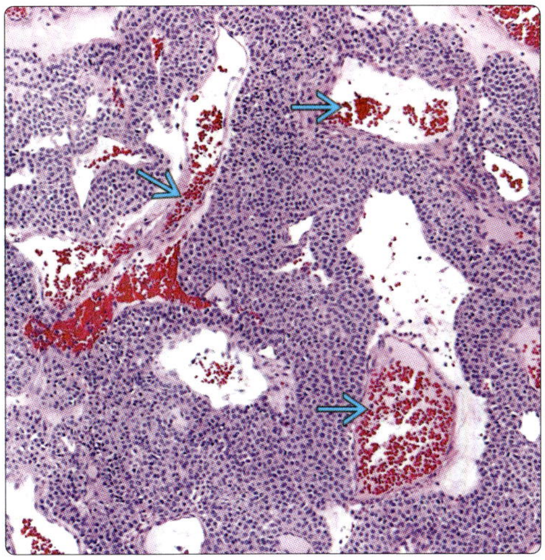

Epithelioid Cells: Adipose Tissue Component

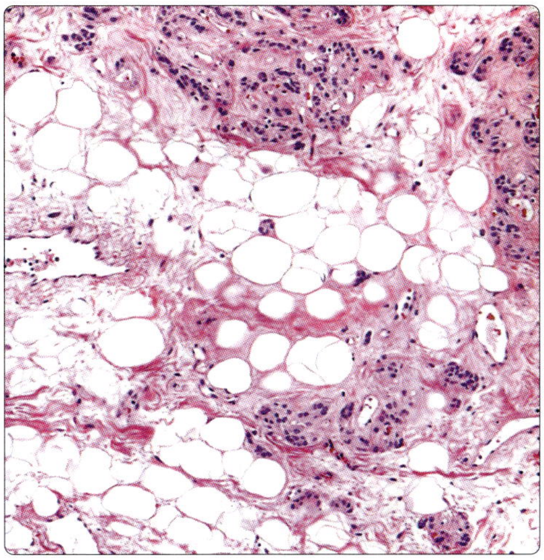

(Left) *Sheets or nests of epithelioid cells arranged around a prominent vasculature* → *(either small or larger vessels) are classically associated with glomus tumor but can also be seen in cellular solitary fibrous tumor (previously hemangiopericytoma) and others.* **(Right)** *Adipose tissue can be an integral part of some epithelioid soft tissue tumors but is generally uncommon. Examples include angiomyofibroblastoma (shown) and chondroid lipoma.*

Mixed Spindle and Epithelioid Cells

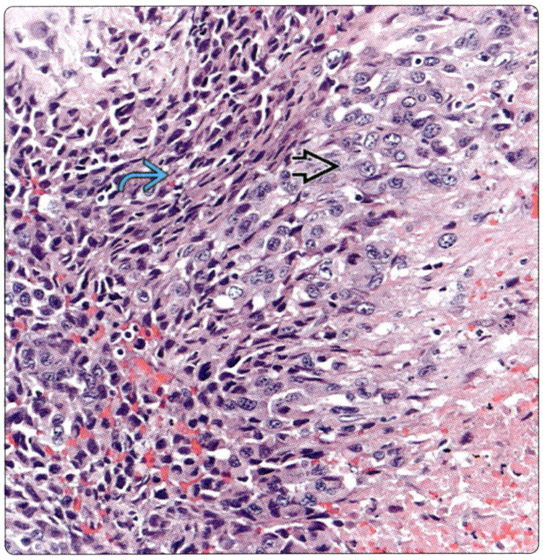

Spindle and Epithelioid Cells

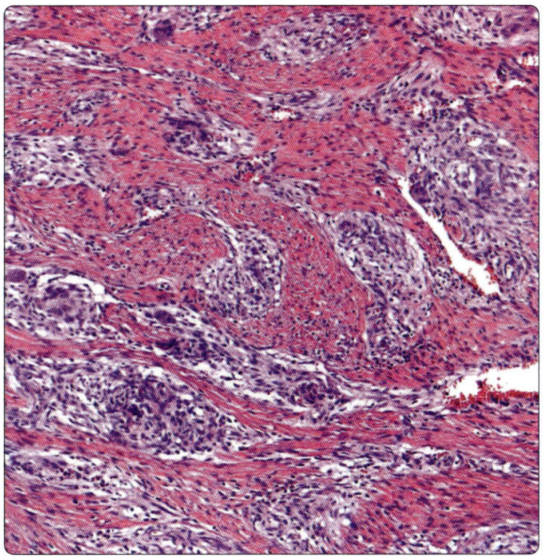

(Left) *Some soft tissue tumors feature a mixture of spindled* ↗ *and epithelioid* ⇨ *tumor cells, either as discrete components or closely admixed. Examples include synovial sarcoma and epithelioid sarcoma (shown).* **(Right)** *Plexiform fibrohistiocytic tumor is a neoplasm that may feature predominantly spindled cells in bundles/fascicles, predominantly epithelioid cells in nests, or a mixture of the 2 patterns (shown).*

Checkerboard Skeletal Muscle Pattern

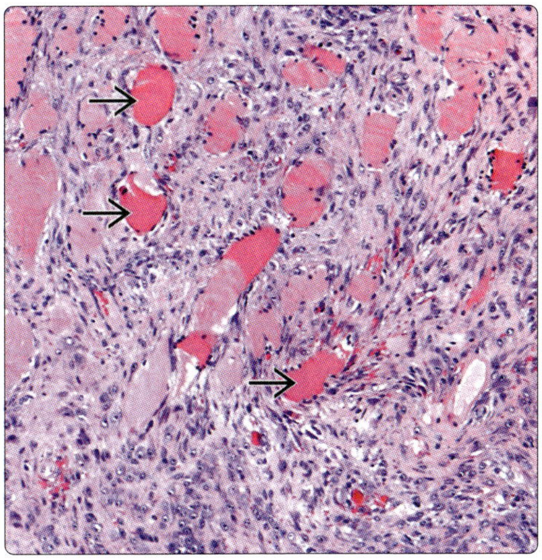

Nuclear Palisading

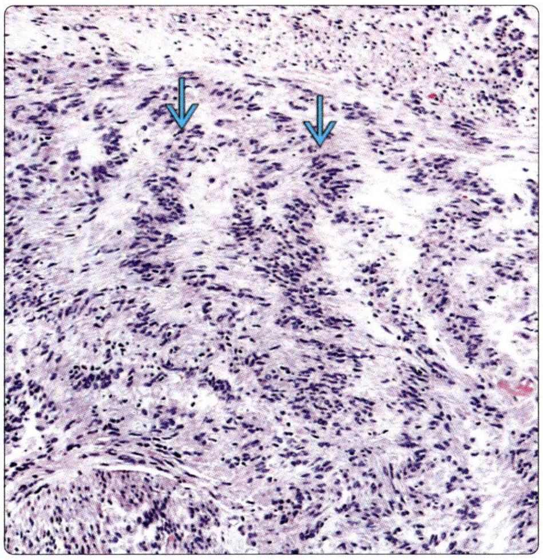

(Left) *Although any intramuscular neoplasm can show infiltration of normal skeletal muscle, some tumors characteristically feature cells growing between fibers* →*, imparting a checkerboard pattern. Examples include proliferative myositis and low-grade myofibroblastic sarcoma.* **(Right)** *Linear rows of nuclei (or cells)* → *typify a palisading pattern, as shown. Although classically associated with neural tumors, this pattern can also be seen in nonneural tumors including leiomyoma, GIST, and synovial sarcoma.*

DIRECTIONS

How to Use These Guides

- These guides are neither comprehensive nor perfect and are meant to serve only as starting point for working up suspected mesenchymal neoplasm
- They include entities that are most commonly or classically associated with particular clinical and histologic findings

Specific Directions for This Guide

- This list contains variety of distinctive histologic features ranging from unique nuclear and cellular morphologies to specific stromal components
  - Each listed feature is more commonly or characteristically associated with some soft tissue tumors and not others
- For each histologic feature listed below, selection of most commonly or characteristically associated diagnoses are provided
- Compile assortment of potential diagnoses from guide using particular feature(s) from your particular case
  - Compare this selection to those created from other 2 approach chapters
  - Overlapping diagnoses derived from these 3 distinct approaches are highest yield and should be your primary focus
- Once high-yield diagnoses have been identified, chapters on specific entities should be directly consulted for detailed information and image galleries
  - In particular, differential diagnosis sections should be fully utilized to broaden search and increase chances of securing correct diagnosis

Important Caveat

- Always exclude carcinoma, melanoma, lymphoma, and mesothelioma before committing to mesenchymal diagnosis
- Always consider GIST for tumors in abdomen, pelvis, and retroperitoneum

CYTOLOGIC FEATURES

Clear Cells

- Alveolar soft-part sarcoma
- Clear cell sarcoma
- Desmoplastic small round cell tumor
- Ewing sarcoma
- Myoepithelioma
- Myoepithelial carcinoma
- PEComa
- Sclerosing epithelioid fibrosarcoma

Granular Cells

- Adult rhabdomyoma
- Alveolar soft-part sarcoma
- Chondroid lipoma
- Congenital granular cell epulis
- Extranodal Rosai-Dorfman disease
- Granular cell tumor
- Hibernoma
- Leiomyoma
- PEComa

Hobnail Cells

- Epithelioid hemangioma
- Hobnail hemangioma
- Papillary intralymphatic angioendothelioma (Dabska)
- Retiform hemangioendothelioma

Rhabdoid Cells

- Angiomatoid fibrous histiocytoma
- Desmoplastic small round cell tumor
- Epithelioid malignant peripheral nerve sheath tumors (MPNST)
- Epithelioid sarcoma
- Extrarenal rhabdoid tumor
- Extraskeletal myxoid chondrosarcoma
- Myoepithelial carcinoma
- Pseudomyogenic hemangioendothelioma
- Synovial sarcoma (poorly differentiated)

(Left) *Soft tissue tumors featuring cells with clear cytoplasm include myoepithelioma, PEComa, and alveolar soft-part sarcoma (shown), among others. Unlike epithelial neoplasms, clear cell change in mesenchymal tumors is usually focal or patchy and rarely diffuse.* **(Right)** *Cells with prominent granular, eosinophilic cytoplasm are most commonly associated with granular cell tumor but can also be seen in congenital granular cell epulis (shown), PEComa, hibernoma, and adult rhabdomyoma.*

Clear Cells

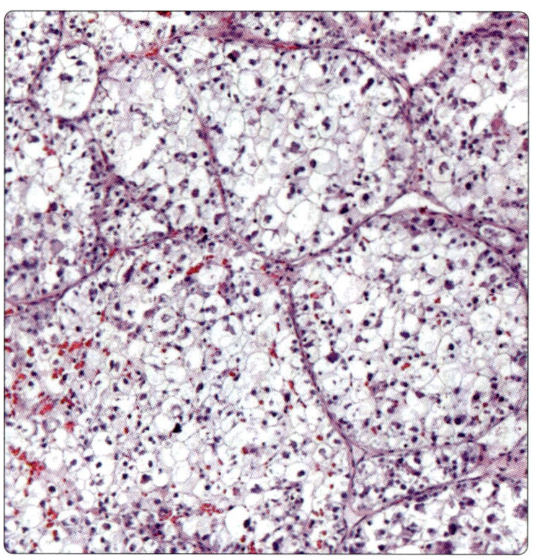

Granular Cells

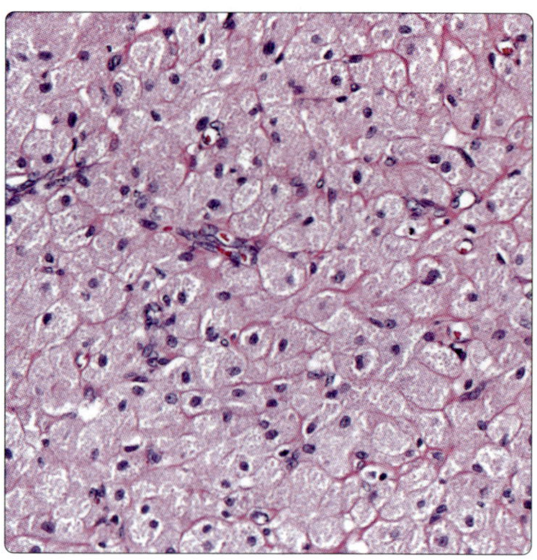

Rhabdomyoblastic Elements

- Dedifferentiated liposarcoma
- MPNST (a.k.a. malignant Triton tumor)
- Rhabdomyosarcomas

Paranuclear Vacuoles

- Intranodal palisaded myofibroblastoma
- Leiomyoma
- Leiomyosarcoma

Vacuolated Cells (Nonlipoblast)

- Chondroid lipoma
- Epithelioid hemangioma
- Epithelioid hemangioendothelioma
- Hibernoma
- Myoepithelioma (parachordoma)
- Myxofibrosarcoma
- Myxoinflammatory fibroblastic sarcoma
- Spindle cell hemangioma
- Peripheral hemangioblastoma

INFLAMMATORY COMPONENT

Prominent Eosinophils

- Epithelioid hemangioma
- Inflammatory myofibroblastic tumor
- Myxoinflammatory fibroblastic sarcoma
- Solitary (juvenile) xanthogranuloma

Prominent Foamy Histiocytes

- Schwannoma
- Dermatofibroma (fibrous histiocytoma)
- Tenosynovial giant cell tumor (both types)

Prominent Lymphocytes

- Angiomatoid fibrous histiocytoma (peripheral cuff)
- Cellular schwannoma (peripheral cuff)
- Dendritic cell sarcomas
- Epithelioid hemangioma (peripheral cuff)
- EBV-associated smooth muscle tumor
- Extranodal Rosai-Dorfman disease
- Inflammatory myofibroblastic tumor
- Kaposi sarcoma
- Retiform hemangioendothelioma

Prominent Mast Cells

- Acral fibromyxoma
- Cellular angiofibroma
- Mammary-type myofibroblastoma
- Pleomorphic hyalinizing angiectatic tumor
- Solitary fibrous tumor
- Spindle cell lipoma
- Synovial sarcoma

Prominent Mixed Inflammation

- Dedifferentiated liposarcoma
- Leiomyosarcoma (inflammatory variant)
- Myxoinflammatory fibroblastic sarcoma
- Well-differentiated liposarcoma (inflammatory variant)
- Superficial CD34-positive fibroblastic tumor

Prominent Neutrophils

- Dedifferentiated liposarcoma (rare)
- Myxoinflammatory fibroblastic sarcoma
- Pseudomyogenic hemangioendothelioma
- Superficial angiomyxoma

Prominent Plasma Cells

- Extranodal Rosai-Dorfman disease
- Inflammatory myofibroblastic tumor
- Kaposi sarcoma

MULTINUCLEATED CELLS

Entrapped Atrophic Skeletal Muscle Fibers

- Desmoid fibromatosis
- Intramuscular hemangioma
- Intramuscular lipoma

Floret-Like Tumor Cells

- Atypical lipomatous tumor/well-differentiated liposarcoma
- Giant cell fibroblastoma
- Myxofibrosarcoma
- Pleomorphic lipoma

Various Multinucleated Giant Cells

- Alveolar rhabdomyosarcoma
- Calcifying aponeurotic fibroma
- Clear cell sarcoma
- Dermatofibroma (fibrous histiocytoma)
- Extraskeletal osteosarcoma
- Giant cell tumor of soft tissue
- Myxoinflammatory fibroblastic sarcoma
- Nodular fasciitis (including intravascular variant)
- PEComa
- Phosphaturic mesenchymal tumor
- Plexiform fibrohistiocytic tumor
- Tenosynovial giant cell tumor (both types)
- Soft tissue chondroma (chondroblastoma-like variant)
- Solitary (juvenile) xanthogranuloma
- Undifferentiated pleomorphic sarcoma

NUCLEAR FEATURES

Grooves

- Soft tissue chondroma (chondroblastoma-like variant)
- Spindle cell lipoma
- Tenosynovial giant cell tumor (both types)

Prominent Nucleoli

- Alveolar soft-part sarcoma
- Clear cell sarcoma
- Dendritic cell sarcomas
- Epithelioid angiosarcoma
- Epithelioid sarcoma (proximal type)
- Epithelioid MPNST
- Extrarenal rhabdoid tumor
- Inflammatory myofibroblastic tumor
- Myoepithelial carcinoma
- Myxoinflammatory fibroblastic sarcoma
- Proliferative fasciitis/myositis
- Superficial CD34-positive fibroblastic tumor

Pseudoinclusions

- Pleomorphic hyalinizing angiectatic tumor
- Paraganglioma
- Superficial CD34-positive fibroblastic tumor

Smudgy Nuclei

- Ancient schwannoma
- Atypical lipomatous tumor/well-differentiated liposarcoma
- Atypical neurofibroma
- Inflammatory myofibroblastic tumor
- Ischemic fasciitis
- Massive localized lymphedema
- Myxoinflammatory fibroblastic sarcoma

STROMAL FINDINGS

Blood-Filled Spaces

- Aneurysmal bone cyst of soft tissue
- Aneurysmal dermatofibroma (fibrous histiocytoma)
- Angiomatoid fibrous histiocytoma
- Giant cell tumor of soft tissue

Calcification

- Calcifying aponeurotic fibroma
- Calcifying fibrous pseudotumor
- Leiomyoma
- Melanotic schwannoma
- Phosphaturic mesenchymal tumor ("grungy" calcification)
- Synovial sarcoma

Cleft-Like Spaces

- Fibroma of tendon sheath
- Fibrous hamartoma of infancy
- Giant cell fibroblastoma
- Sclerosing rhabdomyosarcoma
- Solitary circumscribed neuroma
- Spindle cell lipoma (angiomatous variant)
- Tenosynovial giant cell tumor, diffuse type

Extravasated Red Blood Cells

- Intranodal palisaded myofibroblastoma
- Kaposi sarcoma
- Nodular fasciitis

Keloidal Collagen

- Desmoid fibromatosis
- Keloid
- Nodular fasciitis
- Solitary fibrous tumor

Peripheral Bone Formation

- Aneurysmal bone cyst of soft tissue
- Myositis ossificans
- Ossifying fibromyxoid tumor

Pigment (Various)

- Aneurysmal dermatofibroma (fibrous histiocytoma)
- Angiomatoid fibrous histiocytoma
- Dermatofibrosarcoma protuberans (Bednar type)
- Giant cell tumor of soft tissue
- Hemosiderotic fibrolipomatous tumor
- Melanotic schwannoma
- Myxoinflammatory fibroblastic sarcoma
- Pleomorphic hyalinizing angiectatic tumor
- Schwannoma
- Tenosynovial giant cell tumor (both types)

Stromal Microcystic Spaces

- Lipoblastoma
- Myxoid liposarcoma
- Nodular fasciitis

STRUCTURES

Nodular Eosinophilic Structures

- Intranodal palisaded myofibroblastoma
- Low-grade fibromyxoid sarcoma
- Schwannoma (neuroblastoma-like variant)

True Epithelial Elements

- Ectopic hamartomatous thymoma
- Myoepithelioma (mixed tumor)
- Synovial sarcoma (biphasic)

VASCULATURE

Curvilinear Vessels

- Myxofibrosarcoma
- Low-grade fibromyxoid sarcoma

Ectatic Staghorn Vasculature

- Deep benign fibrous histiocytoma
- Infantile fibrosarcoma
- Glomus tumor
- Leiomyosarcoma
- Myopericytoma/myofibroma
- Paraganglioma
- Solitary fibrous tumor
- Synovial sarcoma

Perivascular Cellularity

- Low-grade fibromyxoid sarcoma
- Myxofibrosarcoma
- MPNST

Perivascular Hyalinization

- Cellular angiofibroma
- PEComa
- Pleomorphic hyalinizing angiectatic tumor
- Schwannoma
- Solitary fibrous tumor

Perivascular Tumor Cell Viability

- Ewing sarcoma
- Gastrointestinal stromal tumor
- MPNST

Plexiform Capillary Vasculature

- Atypical spindle cell lipomatous tumor
- Lipoblastoma
- Myxoid liposarcoma
- Superficial angiomyxoma
- Well-differentiated liposarcoma (myxoid variant)

Hobnail Cells

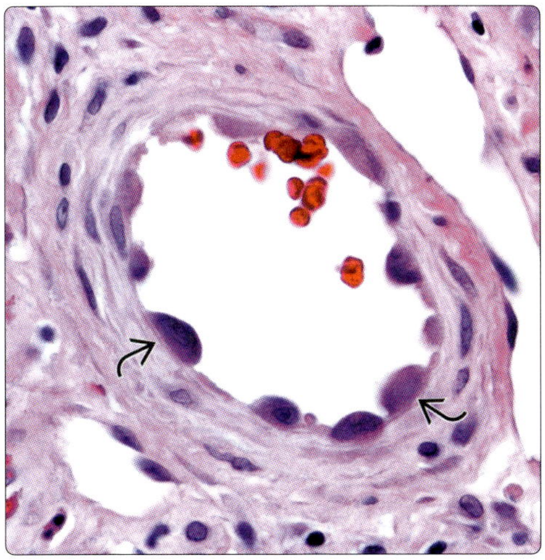

Rhabdoid Cells

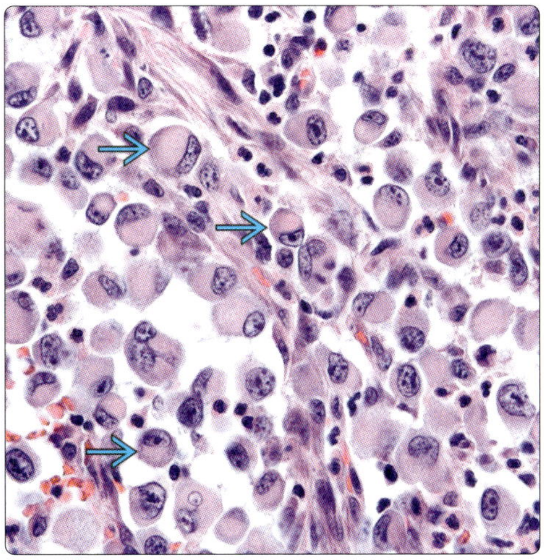

(Left) *Hobnail cells are plump endothelial cells that project independently into a vascular lumen (also referred to as matchstick or tombstone cells).* **(Right)** *Rhabdoid cells feature a large, eosinophilic, and often glassy intracytoplasmic inclusion with an eccentrically located nucleus. Nucleoli are often prominent. Although classically associated with extrarenal rhabdoid tumors, these cells are now known to be featured in a variety of other high-grade sarcomas, including epithelioid sarcoma.*

Paranuclear Vacuoles

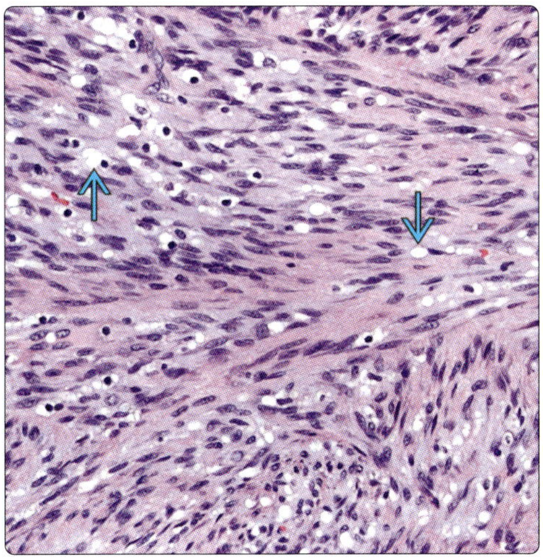

Vacuolated Cells

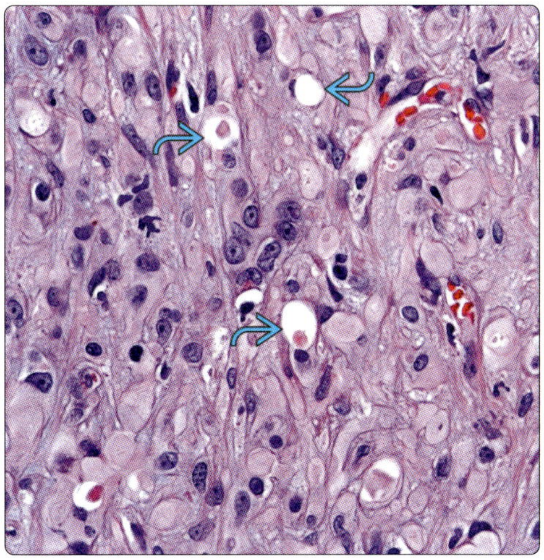

(Left) *Small, clear paranuclear vacuoles can be seen in smooth muscle neoplasms, particularly leiomyoma and leiomyosarcoma, but also gastrointestinal stromal tumor and intranodal palisaded myofibroblastoma.* **(Right)** *Vacuolated tumor cells may feature 1, several, or numerous intracytoplasmic vacuoles. A single vacuole (if any at all) is most typical of vascular tumors, such as epithelioid hemangioendothelioma (shown), epithelioid hemangioma, or spindle cell hemangioma.*

Multivacuolated Cells

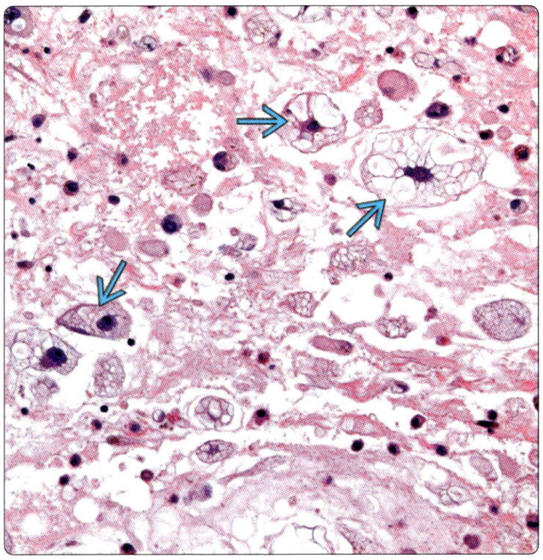

Brown Fat Cells

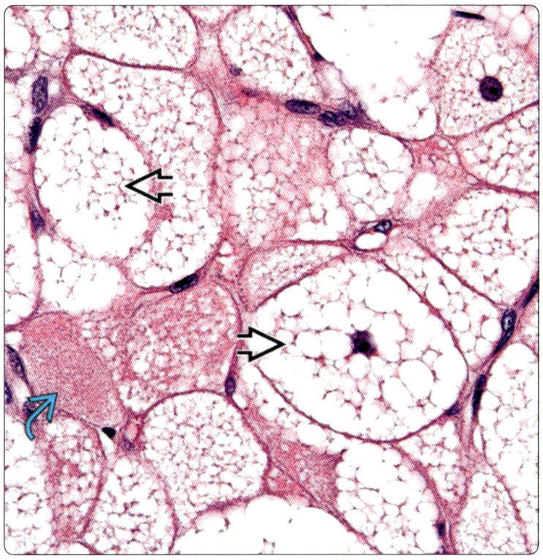

(Left) *Multivacuolated tumor cells often resemble true lipoblastic cells and may be referred to as pseudolipoblasts. Unlike true lipoblasts, however, the cytoplasm contains mucin instead of lipid.* **(Right)** *Brown fat cells are characteristically hypervacuolated, as depicted. In hibernomas, these cells are often associated with other cells featuring finely granular eosinophilic cytoplasm. Hibernoma-like cells may also be occasionally seen in myxoid liposarcoma or lipoblastoma.*

(Left) *A mild lymphocytic infiltrate is common in soft tissue tumors and is entirely nonspecific. A prominent infiltrate is a common finding in some entities, such as inflammatory myofibroblastic tumor (IMT) and the dendritic cell sarcomas.* **(Right)** *Several tumors are well known to feature a conspicuous, patchy lymphoid cuff, including angiomatoid fibrous histiocytoma, cellular forms of schwannoma, and epithelioid hemangioma. Consideration of lymphoma or a nodal metastasis is possible when this cuff is prominent.*

Prominent Lymphocytic Infiltrate

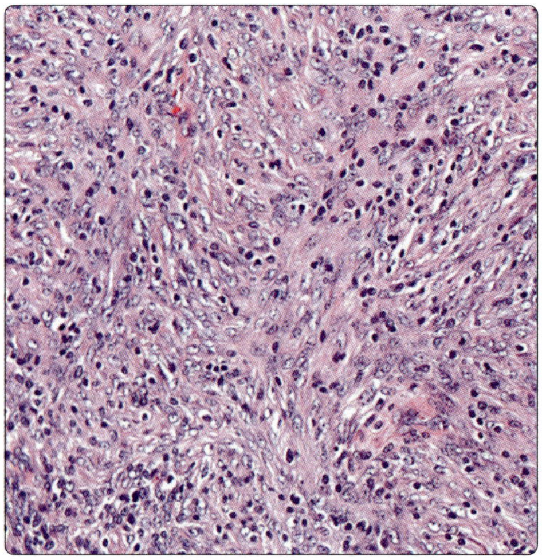

Lymphocytic Cuff

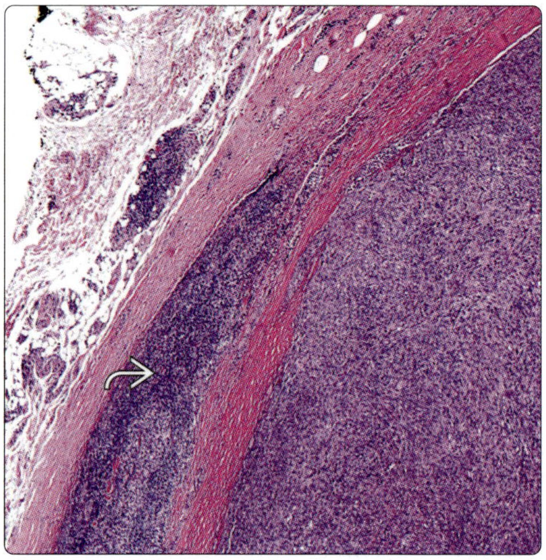

(Left) *A prominent neutrophilic infiltrate is generally uncommon in soft tissue tumors; however, it can be a striking finding in a few entities, particularly pseudomyogenic (epithelioid sarcoma-like) hemangioendothelioma.* **(Right)** *A prominent infiltrate of plasma cells is a common and classic finding in IMT but can be seen in other tumors, including extranodal Rosai-Dorfman disease.*

Neutrophilic Infiltrate

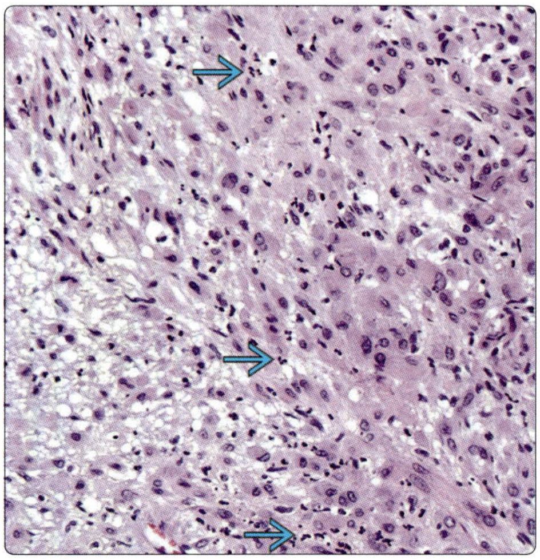

Prominent Plasma Cell Infiltrate

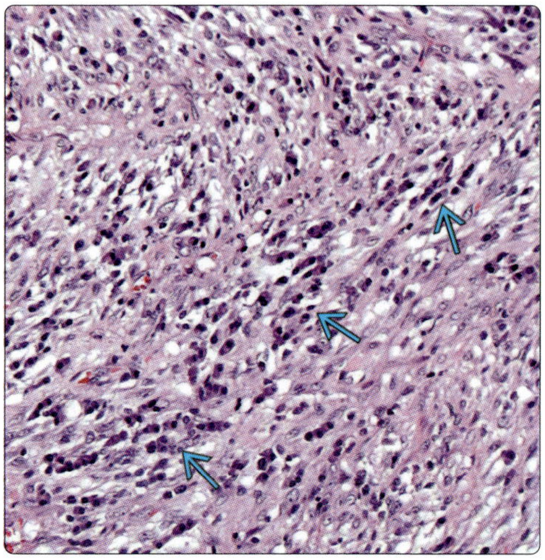

(Left) *Entrapped benign skeletal myocytes are a relatively common finding in intramuscular hemangioma and intramuscular lipoma. Note the grape-like clustering of small nuclei and dark eosinophilic cytoplasm.* **(Right)** *Floret-like tumor cells with hyperchromatic nuclei arranged radially around the periphery of part of the cell are best recognized as a feature of pleomorphic lipoma; however, they can also be seen in some sarcomas, including well-differentiated liposarcoma and myxofibrosarcoma (shown).*

Entrapped Skeletal Muscle Cells

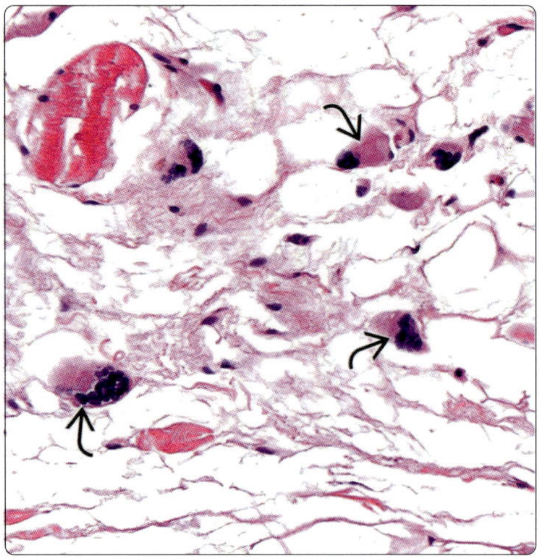

Floret-Like Multinucleated Cells

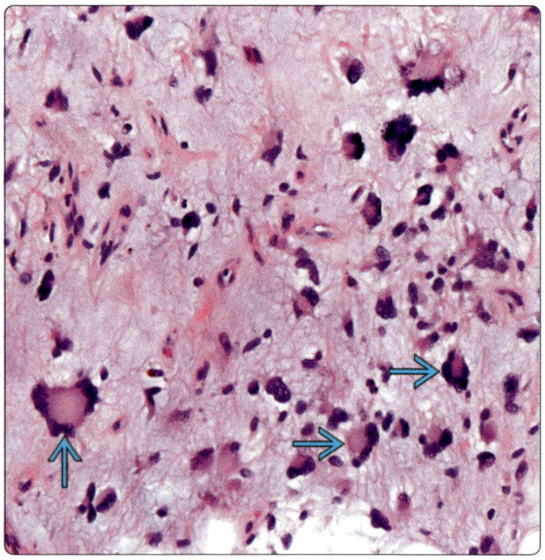

Osteoclast-Like Giant Cells

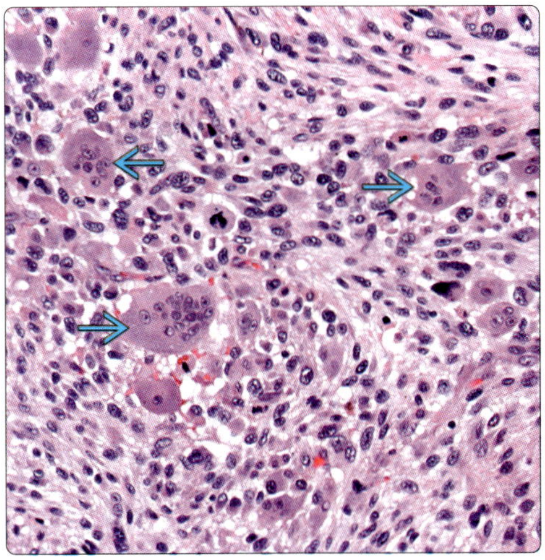

Wreath-Like Giant Cells

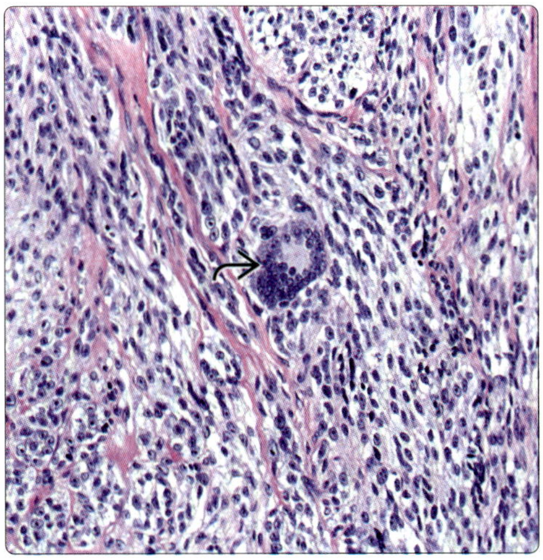

(Left) *Osteoclast-like multinucleated giant cells are seen in a variety of soft tissue neoplasms, both benign and malignant, and feature a variable number of uniform nuclei arranged randomly within the cytoplasm.* **(Right)** *Some tumors feature multinucleated giant cells with nuclei arranged peripherally in a wreath-like arrangement. This type of giant cell morphology is more commonly associated with clear cell sarcoma and alveolar rhabdomyosarcoma.*

Nuclear Grooves

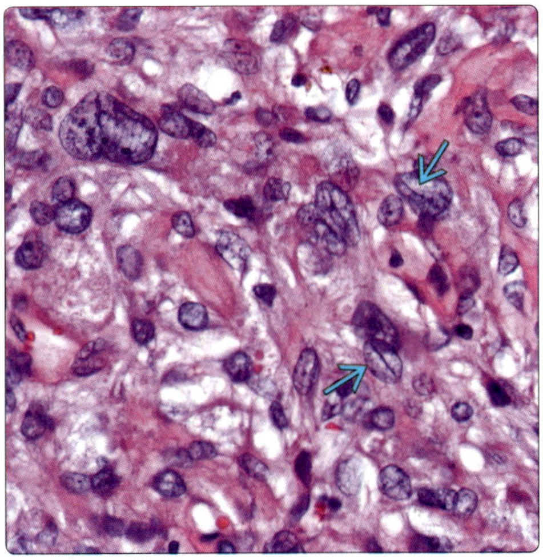

Prominent Nucleoli

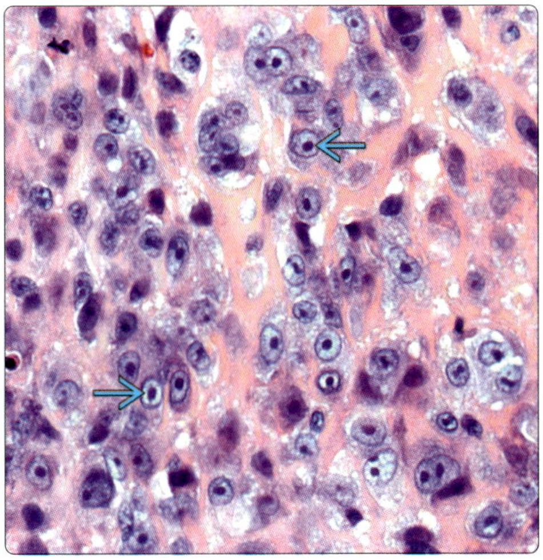

(Left) *Nuclear grooves or clefts are rarely striking but can be seen upon close cytologic inspection in some tumors, including spindle cell lipoma, tenosynovial giant cell tumors, and angiomatoid fibrous histiocytoma (shown).* **(Right)** *Prominent nucleoli are generally nonspecific; however, diffusely prominent uniform nucleoli are more characteristic of some entities, including clear cell sarcoma and epithelioid MPNST. Ganglion cell-like myofibroblasts in proliferative fasciitis/myositis also feature prominent nucleoli.*

Macronucleoli

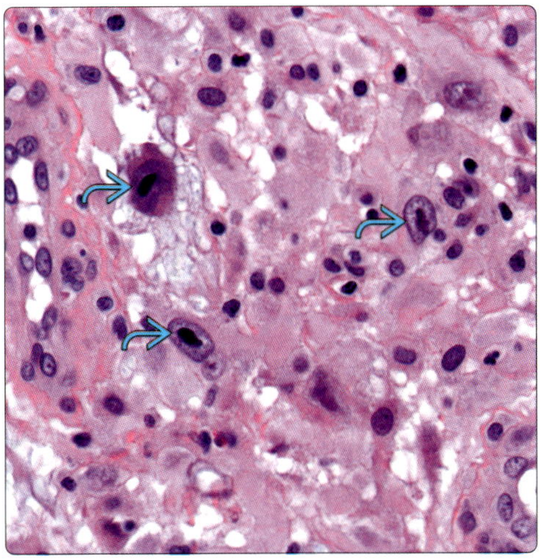

Nuclear Pseudoinclusions

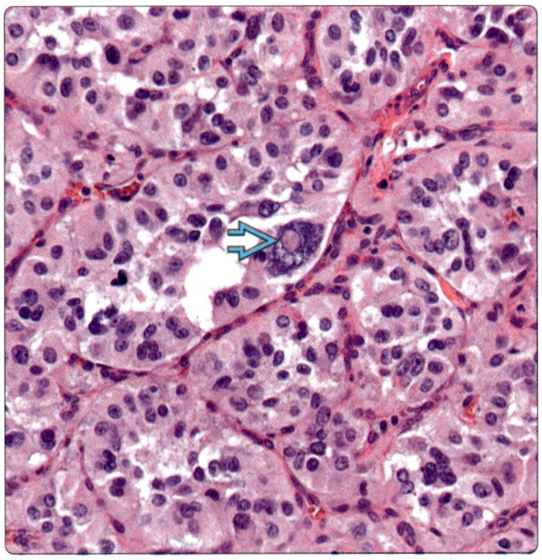

(Left) *A small group of mesenchymal neoplasms are well known to feature prominent basophilic or eosinophilic macronucleoli (reminiscent of viral infection), including myxoinflammatory fibroblastic sarcoma.* **(Right)** *Nuclear pseudoinclusions, or intranuclear cytoplasmic invaginations, are often conspicuous in some tumors, including pleomorphic hyalinizing angiectatic tumor, superficial CD34-positive fibroblastic tumor, and paraganglioma, and they may be eosinophilic or pale/clear.*

(Left) *Enlarged, poorly defined hyperchromatic nuclei* → *with smudgy chromatin can be seen in tumors, such as atypical lipomatous tumor (well-differentiated liposarcoma) and some forms of IMT (shown) and likely represent degenerative changes. This finding can also be seen in some benign neural and smooth muscle tumors.* **(Right)** *Cleft-like spaces are commonly seen in fibroma of the tendon sheath (shown) and solitary circumscribed neuroma and may represent thin vessels* ⇨ *or artifactual spaces.*

Smudgy Nuclei

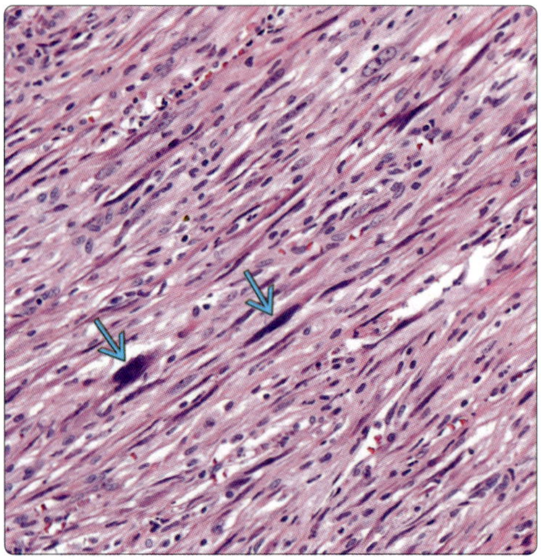

Cleft-Like Spaces

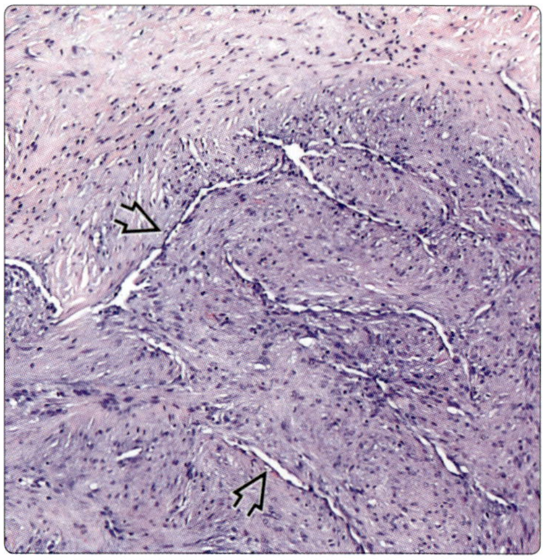

(Left) *Some tumors can feature irregular cleft-like spaces* → *lined by hyperchromatic mono- or multinucleated cells, including giant cell fibroblastoma (shown) and fibrous hamartoma of infancy. These areas can resemble a vascular neoplasm.* **(Right)** *Thick, brightly eosinophilic, and glassy collagen fibers or bundles* → *can be seen in lesions other than keloids, including nodular fasciitis, desmoid fibromatosis (shown), and solitary fibrous tumor.*

Pseudovascular Cleft-Like Spaces

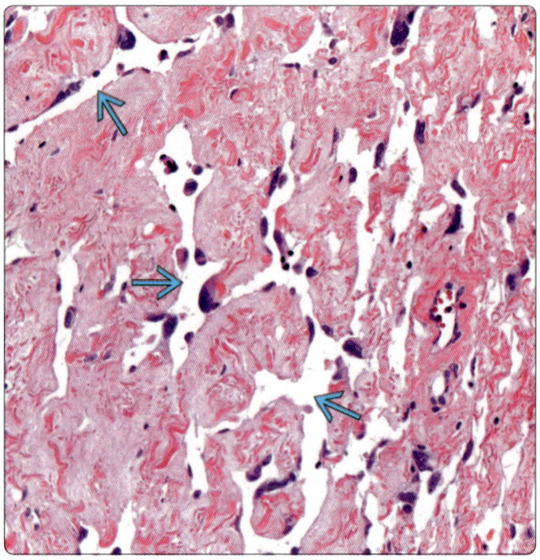

Keloidal Collagen

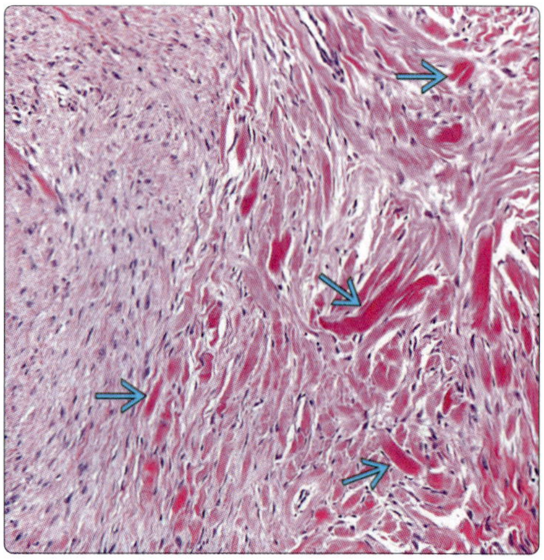

(Left) *Discrete microcystic spaces* → *are most characteristic of myxoid liposarcoma (shown) but can also be seen much less commonly in myxoid areas of some tumors, such as lipoblastoma. This finding is also common in nodular fasciitis; however, the spaces are irregular, resembling torn tissue paper.* **(Right)** *Nodular eosinophilic structures* → *are most typically associated with morphologic variants of low-grade fibromyxoid sarcoma and schwannoma but can very rarely be seen in other tumors.*

Stromal Microcystic Spaces

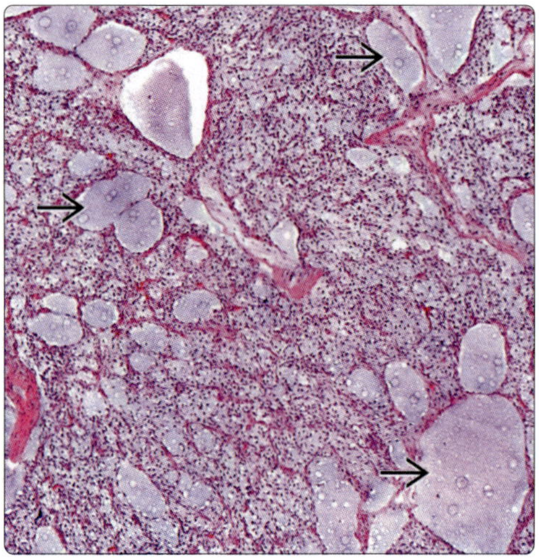

Nodular Eosinophilic Structures

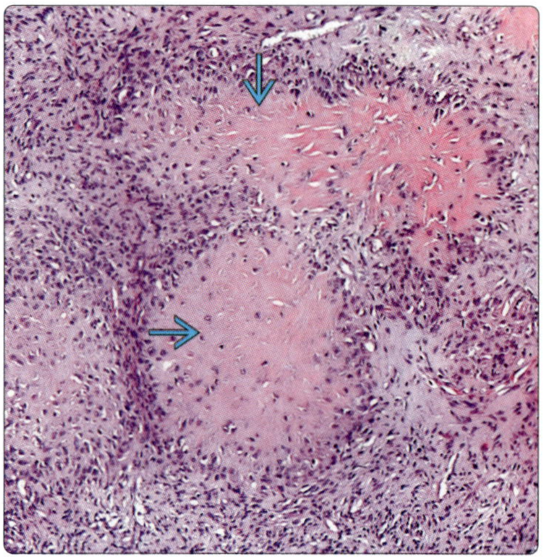

Prominent Ectatic, Staghorn Vasculature

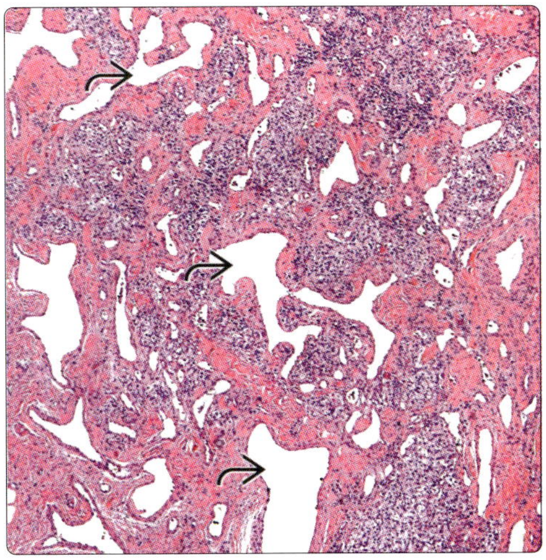

Curvilinear Vasculature

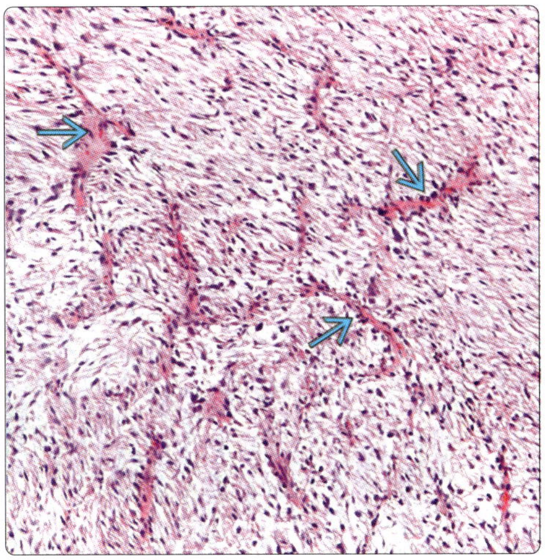

(Left) *Scattered, irregularly shaped and dilated vascular spaces ↪ (a.k.a. staghorn or hemangiopericytoma-like vessels) can be prominent in some tumors, the most well known of which is solitary fibrous tumor.* **(Right)** *Thin-walled capillary blood vessels ➔ lined by inflammatory cells and tumor cells and arranged in linear and curving arrays (curvilinear) are a characteristic feature of myxofibrosarcoma but can also be seen in myxoid regions of low-grade fibromyxoid sarcoma (LGFMS).*

Perivascular Cellularity

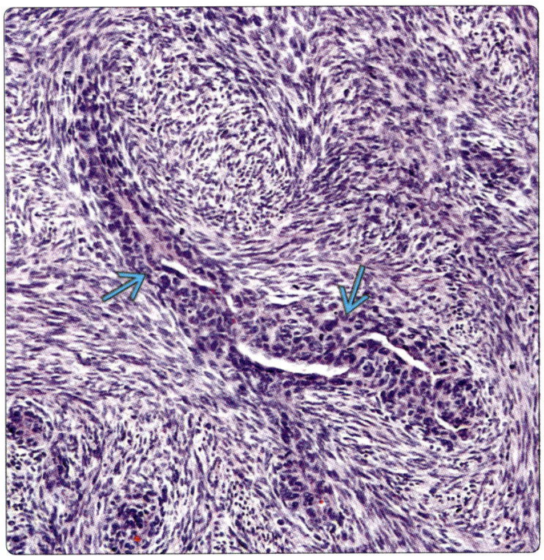

Perivascular Hyalinization

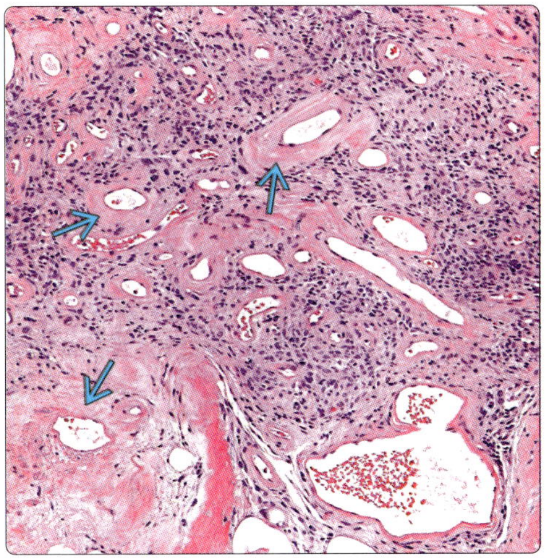

(Left) *Some tumors characteristically show an increase in tumor cell density ➔ around stromal blood vessels, as depicted in this case of MPNST. Other tumors include myxofibrosarcoma and LGFMS.* **(Right)** *Stromal vessels lined or rimmed by dense, acellular collagen ➔ or fibrin are seen in tumors, such as schwannoma, solitary fibrous tumor, and cellular angiofibroma and represent degenerative changes.*

Perivascular Tumor Cell Viability

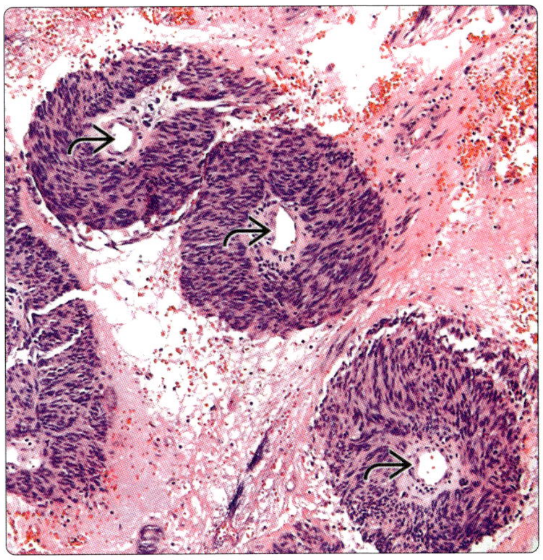

Plexiform Capillary Vasculature

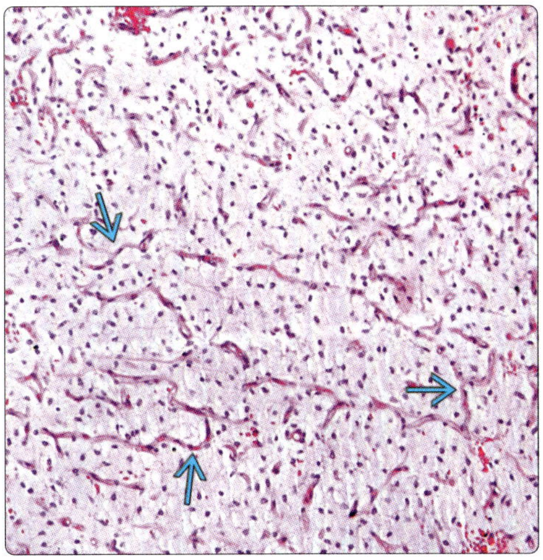

(Left) *In the setting of extensive geographic necrosis (and less commonly extensive degenerative changes), some tumors can show retained cell viability only around stromal vessels ↪, creating a distinctive peritheliomatous appearance, as depicted in this case of GIST. This finding can also be seen in MPNST.* **(Right)** *A delicate ramifying, arborizing, or plexiform capillary vasculature ➔ is characteristic of myxoid liposarcoma (shown) but can also be seen in myxoid areas of lipoblastoma or well-differentiated liposarcoma.*

SECTION 3

Tumors of Adipose Tissue

Benign

Lipoma 46
Lipomatosis of Nerve 52
Synovial Lipomatosis 54
Angiolipoma 56
Spindle Cell/Pleomorphic Lipoma 60
Chondroid Lipoma 66
Myolipoma 70
Hibernoma 74
Myelolipoma 78
Lipoblastoma 80
Atypical Spindle Cell Lipomatous Tumor 84

Intermediate, Locally Aggressive

Atypical Lipomatous Tumor/Well-Differentiated Liposarcoma 88

Malignant

Dedifferentiated Liposarcoma 94
Myxoid Liposarcoma 100
Pleomorphic Liposarcoma 106

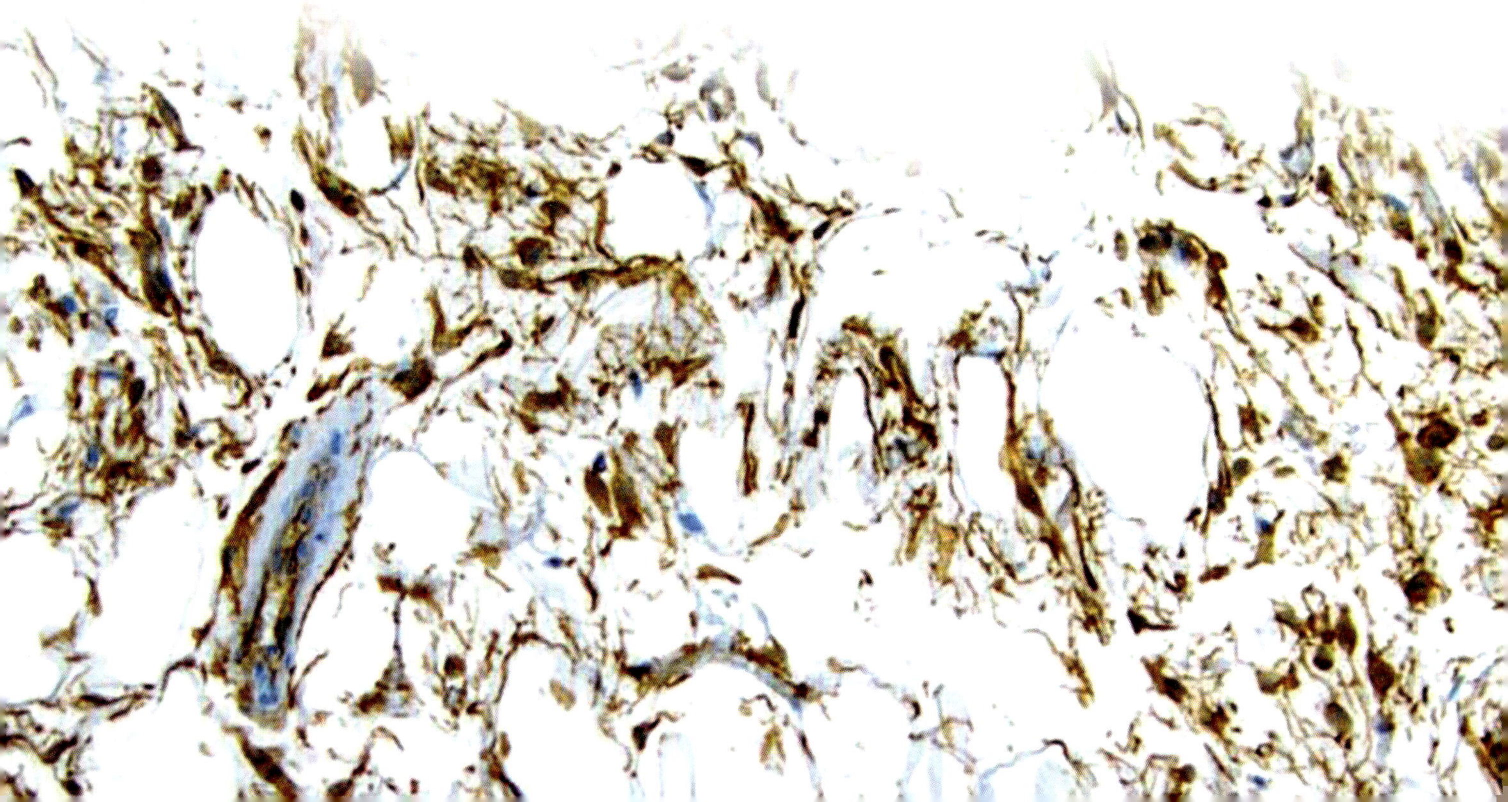

Lipoma

KEY FACTS

TERMINOLOGY
- Benign neoplasm of mature adipocytes (white fat)

CLINICAL ISSUES
- Very common (most common soft tissue tumor overall)
- Superficial lipomas are most common in upper back, shoulder, neck, and abdomen
  - Rarely may be multiple
- Surgical excision is generally curative
  - Intramuscular lipoma can recur (15% rate)
- Lipomatosis
  - Diffuse &/or regional overgrowth of mature adipose tissue

MACROSCOPIC
- Well circumscribed, often lobulated with thin capsule
- Yellow, greasy cut surface with very thin to no fibrous septa

MICROSCOPIC
- Lobules and sheets of mature adipocytes with minimal size variation and no nuclear atypia
- May show fat necrosis, myxoid changes, or other degenerative features
- Variants: Fibrolipoma, myxolipoma, intramuscular lipoma, lipoma with osseous or cartilaginous metaplasia

ANCILLARY TESTS
- Aberrations involving locus at 12q13-15 are most common
- No amplification of MDM2

TOP DIFFERENTIAL DIAGNOSES
- Atypical lipomatous tumor/well-differentiated liposarcoma
- Spindle cell lipoma
- Lipomatosis of nerve
- Myxoid liposarcoma
- Hibernoma (lipoma-like variant)

(Left) *A lipoma is surrounded by a thin, delicate, and transparent capsule ➡ and is often highly lobulated. It is also often taken out by the surgeon piecemeal.* **(Right)** *The cut surface of a lipoma is yellow, homogeneous, and greasy. Note the thin, delicate fibrous septa ➡, which separate the tumor into lobules. Some variants may show myxoid areas or small foci of hemorrhage.*

Lipoma

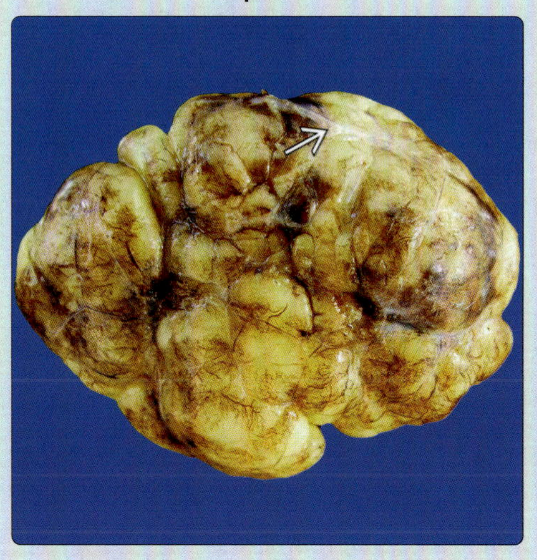

LIpoma, Cut Surface

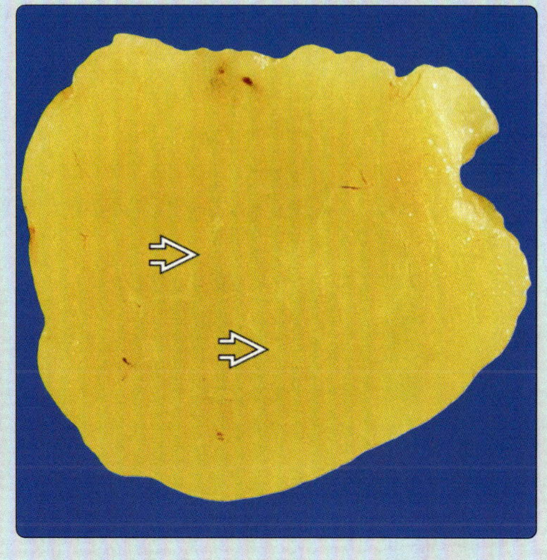

(Left) *A conventional lipoma is composed of lobules and sheets of mature adipocytes (white fat). Small to medium-sized vessels ➡ are often scattered in the background but are usually not prominent.* **(Right)** *The mature adipocytes of a lipoma usually vary little in size from one another. Thin fibrous septa ➡ are commonly seen separating the lobules; however, thicker, more fibrotic septa may be present along with fat necrosis in traumatized tumors.*

Mature Adipose Tissue

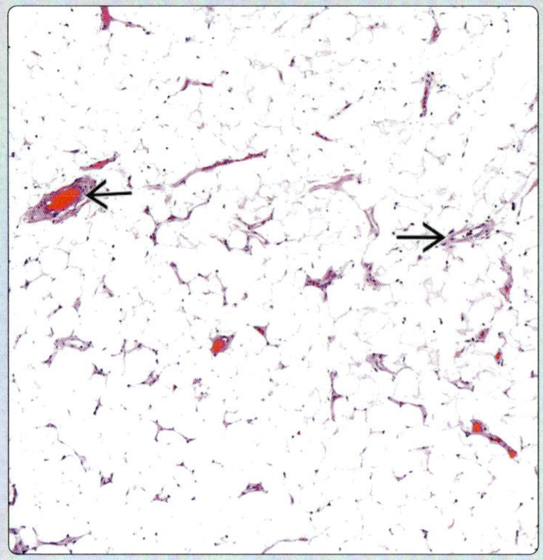

Mature Adipose Tissue

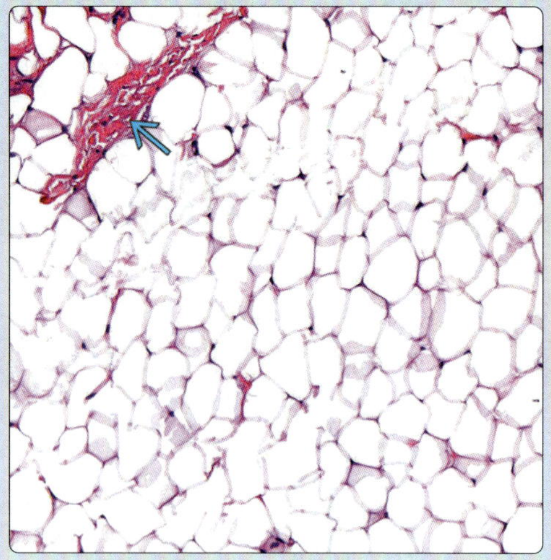

TERMINOLOGY

Definitions

- Benign neoplasm of mature adipocytes (white fat)

CLINICAL ISSUES

Epidemiology

- Incidence
  - Very common (most common soft tissue tumor overall)
  - More common in obese people
- Age
  - Wide range (40-60 years most common)
  - Rare < 20 years

Site

- Superficial lipomas are most common in upper back, shoulder, neck, and abdomen
  - Rare in hands, feet, lower legs, and face
- Deep lipomas may arise in deep soft tissues as well as thorax, mediastinum, pelvis, and, rarely, retroperitoneum
  - May also occur near bone (periosteal/parosteal lipoma)
- Intramuscular lipoma is most common within large muscles of thigh, upper arm, and shoulder
- Mature adipose tissue proliferation within synovium of large joint (synovial lipoma or lipoma arborescens) may clinically simulate diffuse-type tenosynovial giant cell tumor/pigmented villonodular synovitis

Presentation

- Painless mass
  - Larger lesions may be painful
- May be multiple (5% of cases)
  - Range in number from several to hundreds
  - Predilection for upper arm, shoulder, and back in older men
  - May be hereditary in 30% of cases (familial multiple lipomas)
  - Multiple lipomas can occur in various syndromes, including Cowden, Proteus, and Fröhlich

Treatment

- Surgical excision is curative

Prognosis

- Recurrences are rare
- Higher recurrence rate in intramuscular lipoma (15%)

Clinical Variants

- Lipomatosis
  - Diffuse &/or regional overgrowth of mature adipose tissue
    - Not same as multiple discrete lipomas
  - Subtypes: Diffuse, symmetric, pelvic, steroid, and HIV-associated lipodystrophy
  - Adipose tissue often appears poorly marginated, resulting in tendency toward recurrence
  - Significant growth may lead to obstruction of regional structures (larynx, ureter, bowel, etc.)
  - Cytologically and morphologically similar to conventional lipoma, except may show infiltration of muscle or regional structures

MACROSCOPIC

General Features

- Well circumscribed, often lobulated
- Thin, delicate capsule
- Yellow, greasy cut surface
- Myxoid change, focal hemorrhages, bone, or cartilage may be evident
- Infiltrative margins may be present in intramuscular cases

Size

- Usually 2-10 cm
- Deep and intramuscular lipomas are often larger

MICROSCOPIC

Histologic Features

- Lobules and sheets of mature adipocytes
  - In small samples, adipocytes are often indistinguishable from normal, nonlesional fat
- Minimal variation in adipocyte size
- Bland nuclei are small and often peripherally flattened
  - May appear absent
  - May show small intranuclear vacuoles (Lochkern change)
- Small to medium-sized vessels sparsely distributed throughout tumor
  - May be more prominent in atrophic lipomas
- Thin, discontinuous fibrous bands with collagen may be present, particularly in larger lesions
- Degenerative changes, including foci of fat necrosis, myxoid change, or hemorrhage, are not uncommon
  - Fat necrosis may be extensive in some cases
- Ischemic changes, infarction, and cystic degeneration may be present, particularly in traumatized lipomas

Morphologic Variants

- Fibrolipoma
  - Contains variably prominent fibrous tissue and septa with abundant collagen
  - Extensively fibrous examples ("sclerotic lipoma") have predilection for hands and scalp of young men
- Myxolipoma
  - Prominent/diffuse stromal myxoid change in otherwise conventional lipoma
  - May also show prominent vascular component (so-called angiomyxolipoma)
- Lipoma with cartilaginous metaplasia (chondrolipoma)
  - Additional component of mature cartilage
- Lipoma with osseous metaplasia (osteolipoma)
  - Additional component of mature bone
- Intramuscular lipoma
  - Often much larger than subcutaneous forms
  - Variable amounts of admixed mature skeletal muscle fibers, most prominent at periphery
    - Imparts checkerboard appearance at low magnification
    - Often infiltrative margins
  - Atrophic skeletal muscle fibers, if present, often mimic atypical stromal cells ("smudge cells") of atypical lipomatous tumor (ALT)/well-differentiated liposarcoma

ANCILLARY TESTS

Immunohistochemistry

- Mature adipocytes express S100 protein
- MDM2(-), CDK4(-)

Genetic Testing

- Majority of lipomas have abnormal karyotype
  - Aberrations involving 12q13-15 (most cases)
    - t(3;12)(q27-28;q13-15) most common translocation
  - Also aberrations involving 6p21-23, 13q11-12, and 12q22-24
- No amplification of *MDM2*

DIFFERENTIAL DIAGNOSIS

Atypical Lipomatous Tumor/Well-Differentiated Liposarcoma

- Often larger and more deeply seated than lipoma but may occur in subcutaneous tissue (ALT)
- Contain variably thickened fibrous septa containing atypical stromal cells ("smudge cells")
  - Atypical stromal cells may be extremely focal
- Lipoblasts may or may not be present and are not required for diagnosis
- May arise intramuscularly and show similar myoinfiltrative checkerboard pattern as in intramuscular lipoma
- MDM2(+) and CDK4(+) by IHC
- *MDM2* amplification by FISH
- In retroperitoneum, well-differentiated liposarcoma is far more common than lipoma

Spindle Cell Lipoma

- Predilection for upper arms, shoulders, and posterior neck
- Classically contains "ropey" collagen and population of bland, spindled fibroblastic cells
- Myxoid stroma is common and may be extensive
- Mast cells common
- CD34(+) spindle cells
- Loss of nuclear Rb expression by IHC

Myxoid Liposarcoma

- Plexiform chicken wire capillary vascular pattern
- Variable numbers of early lipoblasts and maturing adipocytes
- Generally more cellular than myxolipoma
- *DDIT3* rearrangements

Hibernoma

- Often occurs in younger patients than conventional lipoma
- Most common in thigh but can occur in variety of sites
- Contains multivacuolated "brown fat" cells
  - May be very focal (lipoma-like hibernoma)
- Karyotypic aberrations involving 11q13-21

Lipomatosis of Nerve

- Children and young adults
- Predominantly affects hand, wrist, forearm
- May be associated with macrodactyly
- Mature adipose tissue infiltrating around and between nerve branches and along perineurium

Diffuse-Type Neurofibroma

- Infiltrative growth within connective and adipose tissues
- Neural element may be sparse compared to adipocytic component
- S100(+) spindle cells
- Often show pseudomeissnerian bodies

Intramuscular Hemangioma

- May contain abundant mature adipose tissue, mimicking intramuscular lipoma
- Most patients < 30 years of age
- Contains prominent benign capillary or large vessel vascular component
- Significant recurrence rate (~ 50%)

Chondroid Lipoma

- Contains regions of myxoid or sclerotic lipoblastic differentiation that superficially resemble cartilage
- Lacks mature cartilage and contains numerous lipoblasts
- May contain large zones of relatively unremarkable-appearing mature adipose tissue

DIAGNOSTIC CHECKLIST

Pathologic Interpretation Pearls

- Most examples are clinically superficial/subcutaneous
- Homogeneous, yellow cut surface and lacking prominent, thick fibrous septations
- Adipocytes are mature and nuclei lack enlargement, irregularity, and hyperchromasia
- Fat necrosis and atrophic skeletal muscle fibers may mimic atypical stromal cells of well-differentiated liposarcoma/ALT

SELECTED REFERENCES

1. Michal M et al: Dysplastic lipoma: a distinctive atypical lipomatous neoplasm with anisocytosis, focal nuclear atypia, p53 overexpression, and a lack of mdm2 gene amplification by FISH; a report of 66 cases demonstrating occasional multifocality and a rare association with retinoblastoma. Am J Surg Pathol. 42(11):1530-40, 2018
2. Stojanov IJ et al: Lipomas of the oral cavity: utility of MDM2 and CDK4 in avoiding overdiagnosis as atypical lipomatous tumor. Head Neck Pathol. ePub, 2018
3. Agaimy A: Anisometric cell lipoma: Insight from a case series and review of the literature on adipocytic neoplasms in survivors of retinoblastoma suggest a role for RB1 loss and possible relationship to fat-predominant ("fat-only") spindle cell lipoma. Ann Diagn Pathol. 29:52-56, 2017
4. Manor E et al: Oral lipoma: analysis of 58 new cases and review of the literature. Ann Diagn Pathol. 15(4):257-61, 2011
5. Macarenco RS et al: Retroperitoneal lipomatous tumors without cytologic atypia: are they lipomas? A clinicopathologic and molecular study of 19 cases. Am J Surg Pathol. 33(10):1470-6, 2009
6. Sakurai H et al: Intrathoracic lipomas: their clinicopathological behaviors are not as straightforward as expected. Ann Thorac Surg. 86(1):261-5, 2008
7. Laskin WB et al: Sclerotic (fibroma-like) lipoma: a distinctive lipoma variant with a predilection for the distal extremities. Am J Dermatopathol. 28(4):308-16, 2006
8. Gaskin CM et al: Lipomas, lipoma variants, and well-differentiated liposarcomas (atypical lipomas): results of MRI evaluations of 126 consecutive fatty masses. AJR Am J Roentgenol. 182(3):733-9, 2004
9. Tardío JC et al: Angiomyxolipoma (vascular myxolipoma) of subcutaneous tissue. Am J Dermatopathol. 26(3):222-4, 2004
10. Willén H et al: Comparison of chromosomal patterns with clinical features in 165 lipomas: a report of the CHAMP study group. Cancer Genet Cytogenet. 102(1):46-9, 1998
11. Zelger BG et al: Sclerotic lipoma: lipomas simulating sclerotic fibroma. Histopathology. 31(2):174-81, 1997
12. Fletcher CD et al: Intramuscular and intermuscular lipoma: neglected diagnoses. Histopathology. 12(3):275-87, 1988

Mature Adipocytes

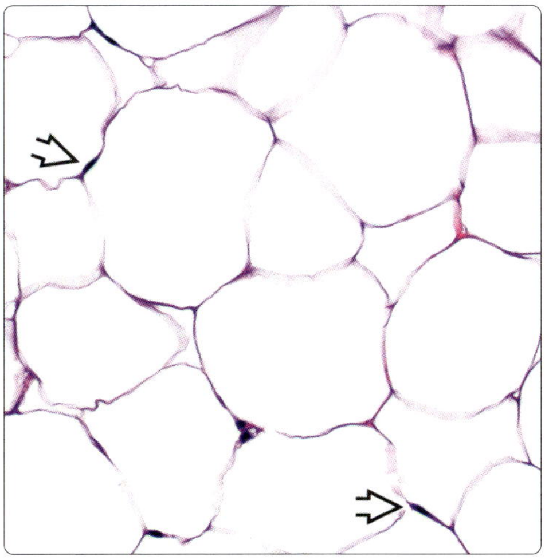

Lochkern Nuclear Change

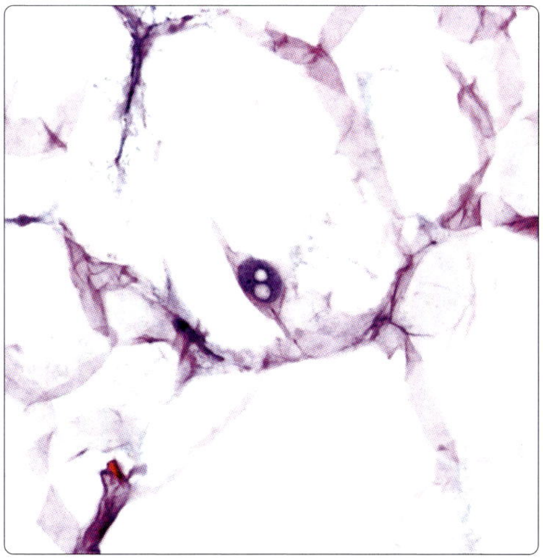

(Left) *A lipoma is composed entirely of mature white fat. The adipocyte nucleus ➲ is bland, small, and typically compressed against the periphery of the cell by the large fat vacuole. Of note, most adipocytes appear to lack a nucleus as a result of 2D tissue sectioning.* **(Right)** *Adipocytes showing nuclear vacuolization (or Lochkern change) is relatively common and may be mistaken for multivacuolated lipoblasts. The vacuoles (usually 1 or 2) are not external to the nucleus as would be seen in lipoblasts.*

Stromal Myxoid Change

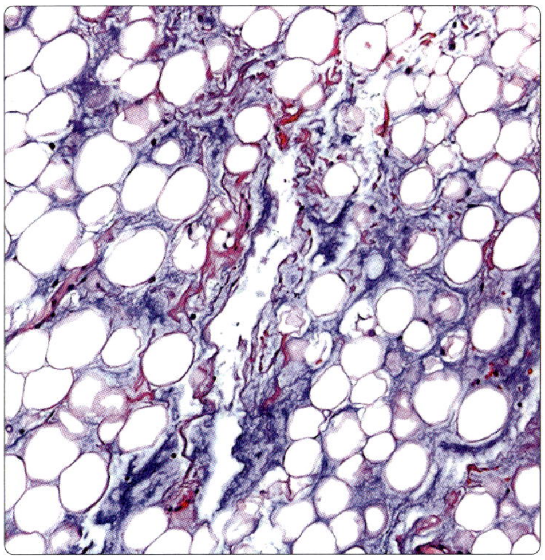

Fat Necrosis

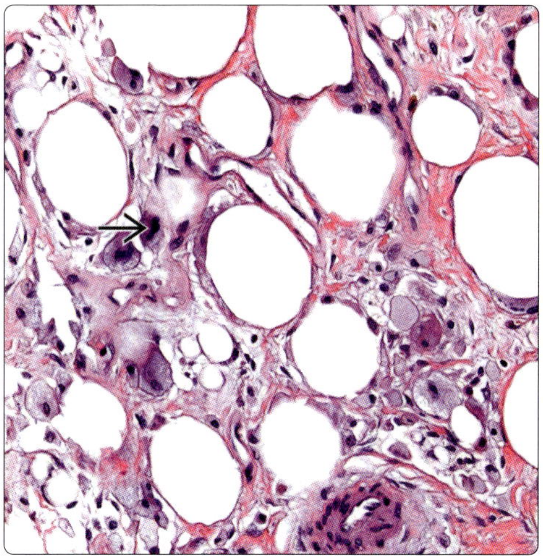

(Left) *Focal stromal myxoid change is a common finding in lipomas, particularly ones that have been traumatized. Fat necrosis is often present elsewhere.* **(Right)** *Fat necrosis is represented by foamy histiocytes surrounding and reacting to damaged adipocytes. Not uncommonly, the histiocytes are multinucleated, and the apparent hyperchromasia caused by nuclear overlap ➲ may raise concern for an atypical lipomatous tumor/well-differentiated liposarcoma.*

Focal Fat Necrosis

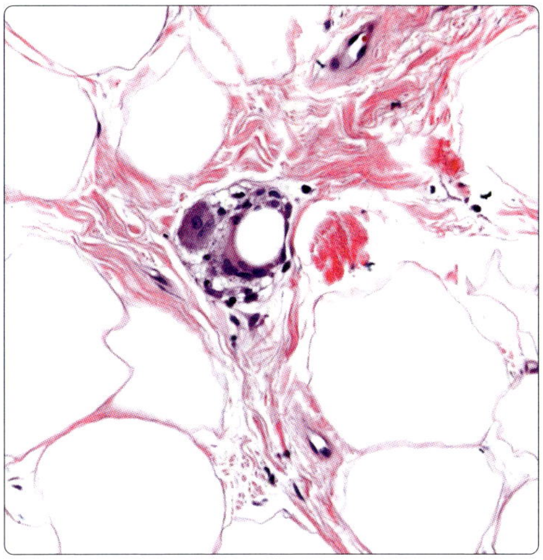

Fibrolipoma

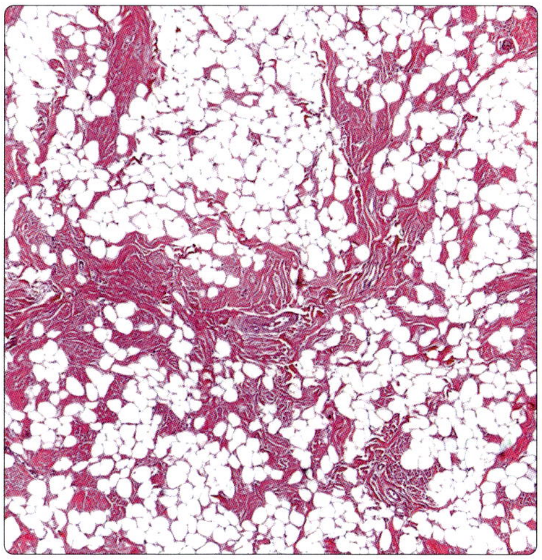

(Left) *Fat necrosis presents in a wide variety of histologic patterns, and the constituent histiocytes are commonly misidentified as lipoblasts or atypical cells indicative of an atypical lipomatous tumor/well-differentiated liposarcoma, particularly when focal and isolated.* **(Right)** *A lipoma containing abundant fibrous tissue and collagen is appropriately designated as a fibrolipoma. Examples with extensive fibrosis have been referred to as sclerotic lipomas.*

(Left) *Fibrolipomas often contain an abundance of collagen in the form of apparent septa or ill-defined aggregates. The exact amount of collagen varies from one case to the next.* **(Right)** *Some cases of fibrolipoma show well-demarcated bundles of collagen* ➩ *cut in cross section. This morphology may be easily confused with the smooth muscle bundles of a myolipoma when diffuse or even neural elements when focal.*

Abundant Collagen

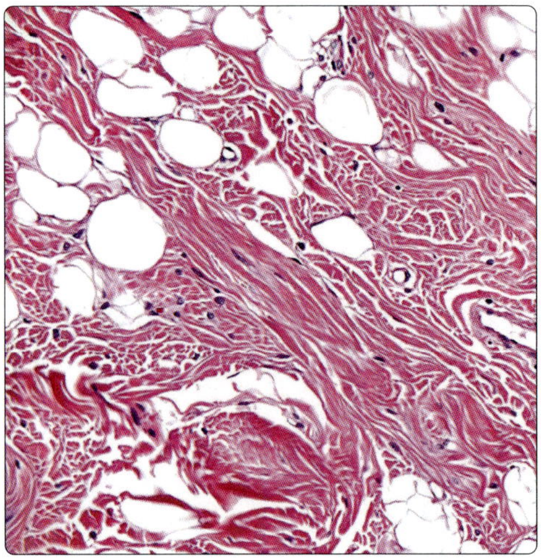

Bundles of Collagen

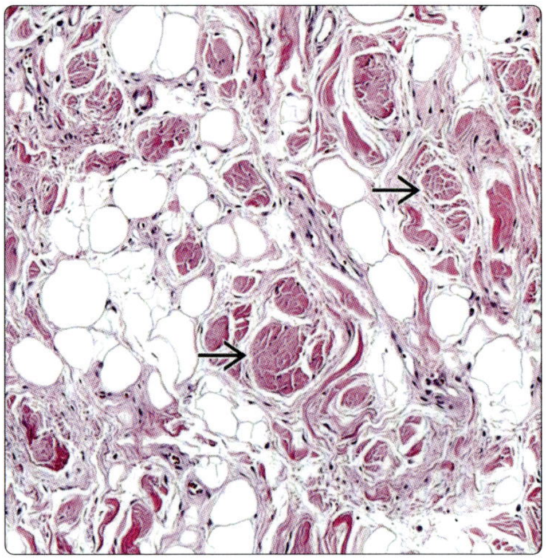

(Left) *This example of an otherwise conventional fibrolipoma contains foci of thickened collagen bundles similar to what is seen in spindle cell lipoma. The distinction in such cases is largely academic.* **(Right)** *A lipoma that demonstrates extensive and diffuse stromal myxoid change is appropriately classified as a myxolipoma. If a component of bland spindle cells is also present, a diagnosis of spindle cell lipoma is more appropriate.*

Fibrolipoma

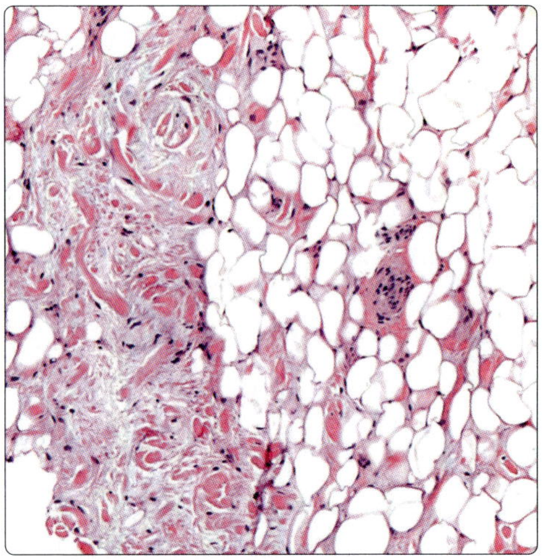

Stromal Myxoid Change

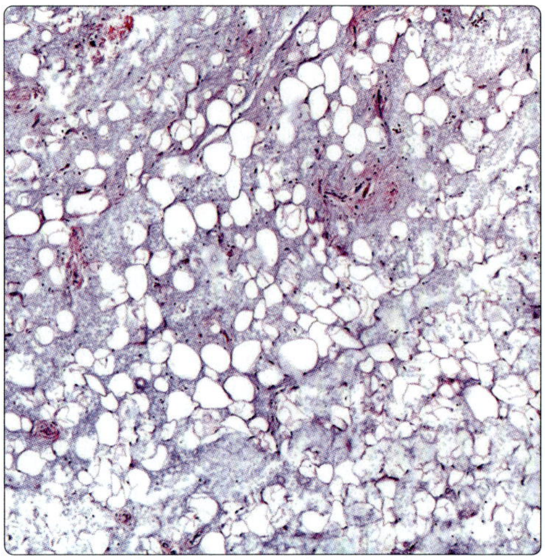

(Left) *Compared to a myxoid spindle cell lipoma, myxolipoma lacks a component of bland spindle cells as well as "ropey" collagen. The myxoid stroma is largely acellular. Although not seen in this H&E, prominent vessels may also be seen (so-called angiomyxolipoma).* **(Right)** *Metaplastic bone formation in a lipoma may be focal or extensive and is often first evident at the time of gross examination.*

Myxolipoma

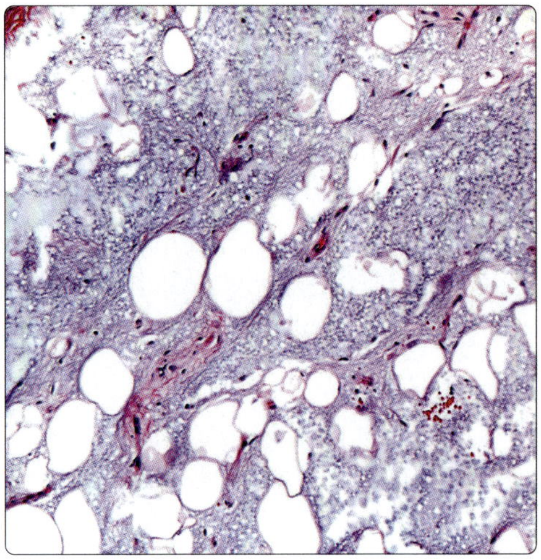

Osseous Metaplasia

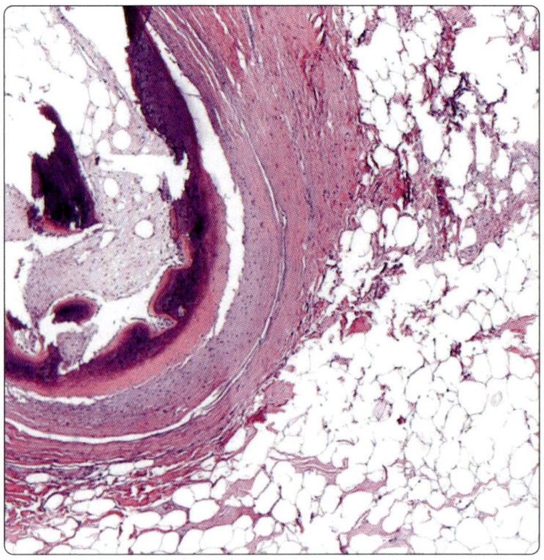

Cartilaginous Metaplasia

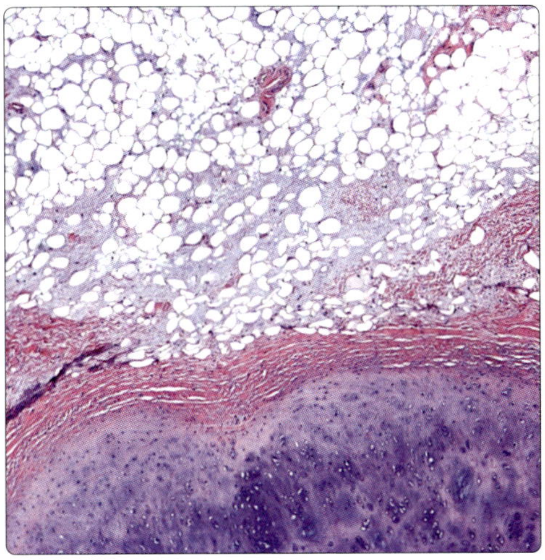

Intramuscular Lipoma

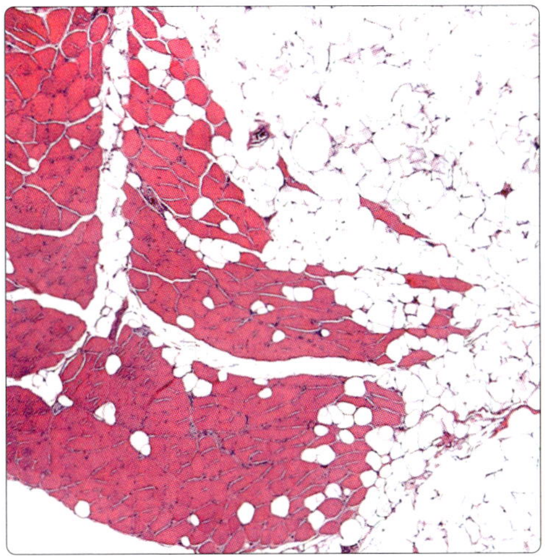

(Left) *Cartilaginous metaplasia in a lipoma may be isolated or associated with foci of metaplastic bone. Not uncommonly, the background adipose tissue shows increased fibrosis and collagen or myxoid stromal change.* **(Right)** *Intramuscular or intermuscular lipomas typically show bundles of mature skeletal muscle intermixed to some degree with the elements of mature adipose tissue.*

Checkerboard Pattern

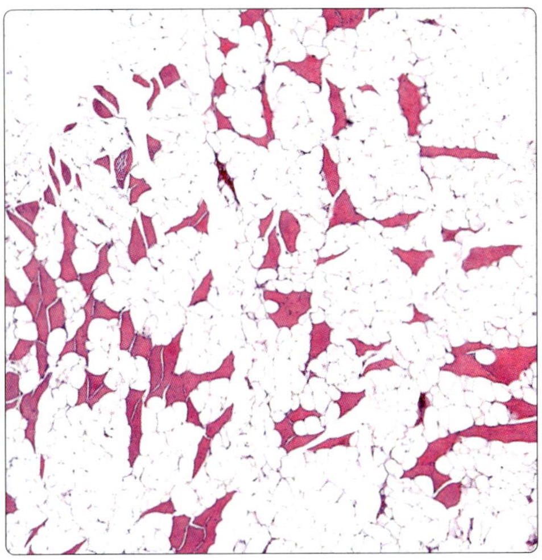

Mature Skeletal Muscle

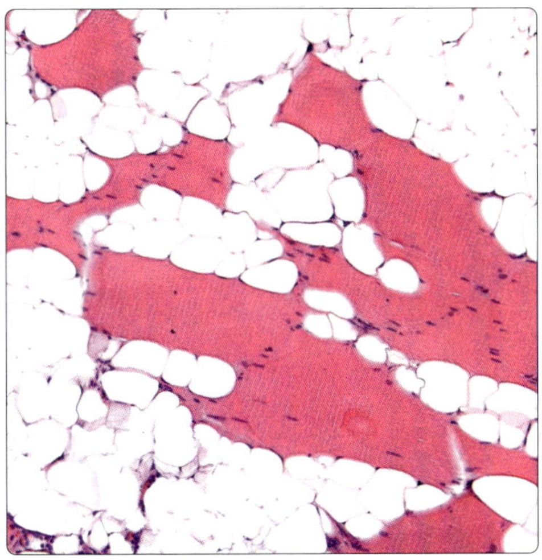

(Left) *The adipose tissue component of intramuscular lipoma is often highly intermixed with the skeletal muscle bundles and demonstrates the classic alternating checkerboard appearance.* **(Right)** *The skeletal muscle bundles in an intramuscular lipoma are composed of mature myocytes. They may be present focally in some tumors and extensively in others.*

Atrophic Skeletal Muscle

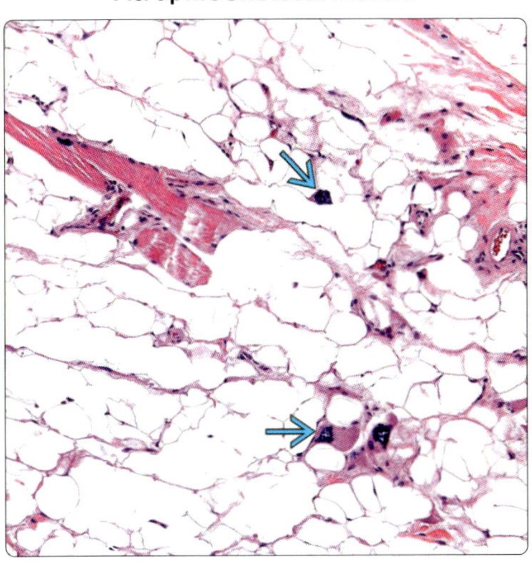

Atrophic Myocytes

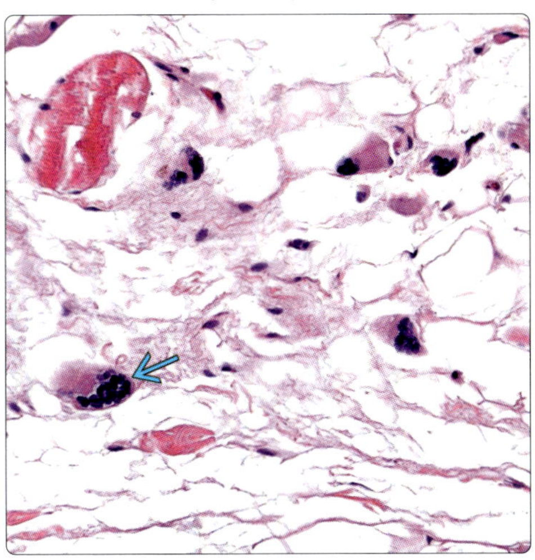

(Left) *Atrophic skeletal muscle fibers* → *are commonly identified in cases of intramuscular lipoma, although the extent of this finding may be very focal. This finding is not specific to lipomas and may be seen in other intramuscular tumors.* **(Right)** *Atrophic myocytes characteristically contain bright pink cytoplasm and numerous small, overlapping nuclei in a cluster of grapes configuration* →*. It is important to not confuse these cells with atypical stromal cells ("smudge cells") of liposarcoma.*

Lipomatosis of Nerve

KEY FACTS

TERMINOLOGY

- Increased fibrofatty tissue infiltrating and surrounding nerves
- Synonym: Fibrolipomatous hamartoma of nerve

CLINICAL ISSUES

- Predominantly in children, often congenital
    - Some in young adults up to 30 years; rare in older adults
- Median nerve and digital branches most common (80%)
    - Symptoms often similar to compression neuropathy or carpal tunnel syndrome
- Slowly progressive swelling/mass of palm (if median nerve affected)
- Macrodactyly present in 30%
- Biopsy not needed if classic MR findings
    - Complete excision usually contraindicated because of potential nerve damage
- Good prognosis when conservatively managed

IMAGING

- Coaxial cable-like (axial view) and spaghetti-like (coronal view) appearances due to linear nerve bundles encased in fat

MACROSCOPIC

- Sausage-shaped mass
- Yellow-white fibroadipose tissue surrounds and distends nerve

MICROSCOPIC

- Mature adipose and fibrous tissue infiltrate nerve
    - Individual nerve bundles separated and encased by fat
- Marked epineurial and perineurial fibrous thickening
- Concentric hyperplasia of perineurium

TOP DIFFERENTIAL DIAGNOSES

- Lipoma of nerve
- Neuroma

Nerve Surrounded by Fat and Fibrosis

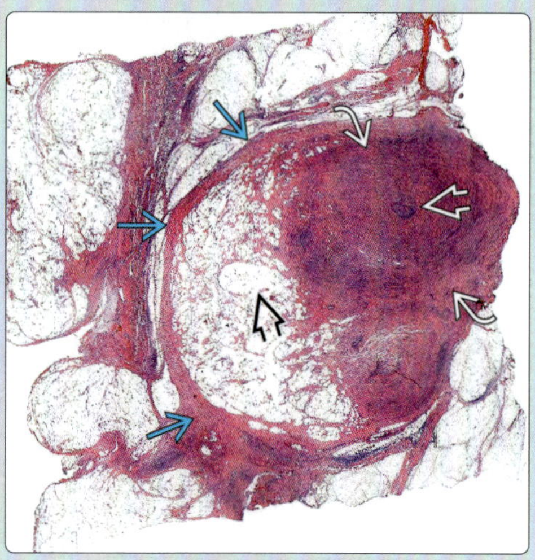

Perineurial Hyperplasia

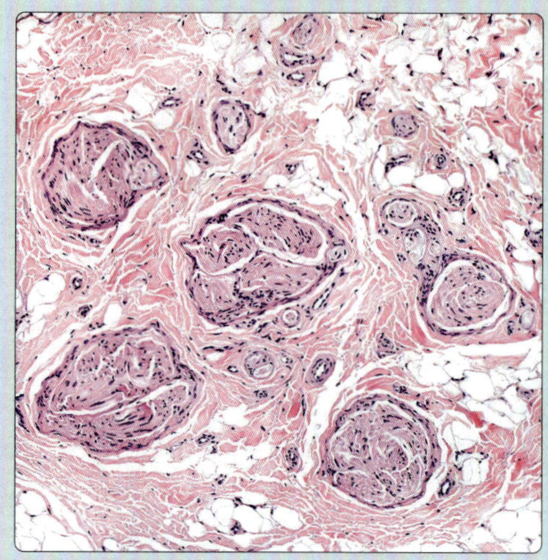

(Left) *In this H&E of lipomatosis of nerve (fibrolipomatous hamartoma), a small, solitary nerve bundle is surrounded by concentric layers of dense fibrosis, mature adipose tissue, and a thick layer of epineurial fibrosis.* **(Right)** *At higher magnification, nerve bundles with perineurial hyperplasia are separated from one another by fibrous tissue and mature fat.*

Frequent Involvement of Median Nerve

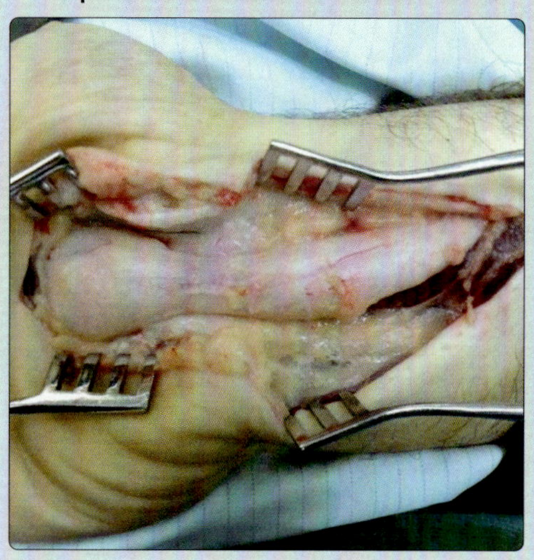

Appearance on Axial MR

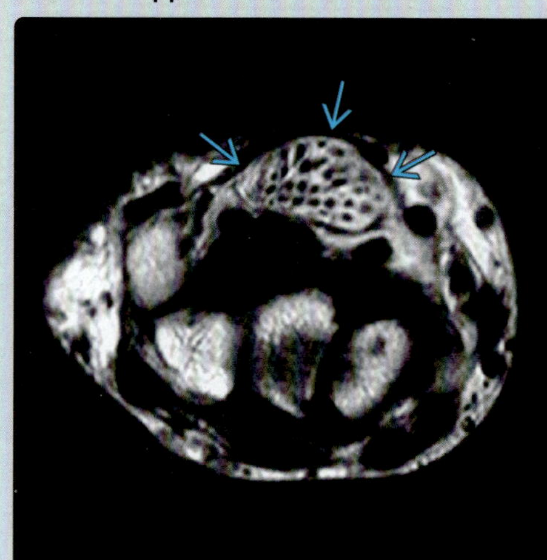

(Left) *In this gross photograph of lipomatosis of nerve, the median nerve is markedly enlarged and distended by pale yellow-white adipose tissue. (Courtesy T. Al-Jabri, MD.)* **(Right)** *The median nerve is massively enlarged on this axial T1 MR and has an appearance likened to a cross section of a coaxial cable. Multiple individual nerve bundles (dark) are divided from one another by intervening fibroadipose tissue (light). (Courtesy Dr. A, Lawson, Radiopaedia.org.)*

Lipomatosis of Nerve

TERMINOLOGY

Synonyms

- Fibrolipomatous hamartoma of nerve
- Neural fibrolipoma, neurolipomatosis
- Fatty infiltration of median nerve

Definitions

- Increased fibrofatty tissue infiltrating and surrounding nerves

CLINICAL ISSUES

Epidemiology

- Age
  - Predominantly in children, often congenital
  - Some in young adults up to 30 years; rare in older adults

Site

- Median nerve and digital branches most common (80%)
  - Affects palmar surface of hand, wrist, forearm, digits
- Rarely ulnar, radial, sciatic, peroneal, or cranial nerve; any nerve can be involved
- Vast majority are unilateral

Presentation

- Slowly progressive swelling/mass of palm (if median nerve affected)
- Paresthesia and dysesthesia
  - Symptoms often similar to compression neuropathy or carpal tunnel syndrome
- Macrodactyly (digital gigantism, macrodystrophia lipomatosa) in 30%
  - Can be congenital and progressive
  - Increased growth of bone and soft tissue of affected digit

Treatment

- Biopsy not needed if MR findings are classic
- Complete excision usually contraindicated because of potential nerve damage
- Surgical decompression (e.g., carpal tunnel release) or debulking may reduce symptoms
- For macrodactyly, may remove deformed digit

Prognosis

- Good prognosis when conservatively managed

IMAGING

MR Findings

- Fusiform enlargement of affected nerve segment
- Coaxial cable-like (axial view) and spaghetti-like (coronal view) appearances due to linear nerve bundles encased in fat

MACROSCOPIC

General Features

- Sausage-shaped mass
- Yellow-white fibroadipose tissue surrounds and distends nerve

Size

- Variable, up to 10 cm length of nerve may be involved

MICROSCOPIC

Histologic Features

- Mature adipose and fibrous tissue infiltrate nerve
  - Individual nerve bundles separated and encased by fat
- Marked epineurial and perineurial fibrous thickening
- Concentric hyperplasia of perineurium
- Nerves can become atrophic in longstanding cases
- Rare metaplastic bone formation

DIFFERENTIAL DIAGNOSIS

Lipoma of Nerve

- Circumscribed and confined within nerve
- Fat does not entrap and separate individual nerve bundles

Neuroma

- Increased number of nerve bundles, disorganized and tangled together
- Minimal fatty component

Lipomatosis

- Histologically similar; clinical information is key to distinction
- May have secondary nerve involvement but primarily lesion of skin/subcutis or muscle

Neurofibromatosis Type 1

- Also may cause macrodactyly
- Expanded nerve in neurofibromatosis type 1 (NF1) may grossly resemble lipomatosis of nerve
  - Histologically easy to distinguish by typical features of neurofibroma and lack of fat
- Other distinct clinical features of NF1 not usually seen in lipomatosis of nerve

SELECTED REFERENCES

1. Prasad NK et al: A new pattern of lipomatosis of nerve: case report. J Neurosurg. 126(3):933-7, 2017
2. Chiaradia G et al: Precalcaneal congenital fibrolipomatous hamartoma: report of 2 cases. J Pediatr Surg. 46(3):e11-2, 2011
3. Al-Jabri T et al: Lipofibromatous hamartoma of the median nerve. J Orthop Surg Res. 5:71, 2010
4. Chiang CL et al: MRI diagnosis of fibrolipomatous hamartoma of the median nerve and associated macrodystrophia lipomatosa. J Chin Med Assoc. 73(9):499-502, 2010
5. Flann S et al: Precalcaneal congenital fibrolipomatous hamartoma. Clin Exp Dermatol. 34(4):495-6, 2009
6. Bisceglia M et al: Neural lipofibromatous hamartoma: a report of two cases and review of the literature. Adv Anat Pathol. 14(1):46-52, 2007
7. Jain TP et al: Fibrolipomatous hamartoma of median nerve. Australas Radiol. 51 Spec No.:B98-B100, 2007
8. Razzaghi A et al: Lipofibromatous hamartoma: review of early diagnosis and treatment. Can J Surg. 48(5):394-9, 2005
9. Al-Qattan MM: Lipofibromatous hamartoma of the median nerve and its associated conditions. J Hand Surg [Br]. 26(4):368-72, 2001
10. Marom EM et al: Fibrolipomatous hamartoma: pathognomonic on MR imaging. Skeletal Radiol. 28(5):260-4, 1999
11. Berti E et al: Fibrolipomatous hamartoma of a cranial nerve. Histopathology. 24(4):391-2, 1994
12. Amadio PC et al: Lipofibromatous hamartoma of nerve. J Hand Surg [Am]. 13(1):67-75, 1988
13. Silverman TA et al: Fibrolipomatous hamartoma of nerve. A clinicopathologic analysis of 26 cases. Am J Surg Pathol. 9(1):7-14, 1985

Synovial Lipomatosis

KEY FACTS

TERMINOLOGY

- Benign, likely reactive, subsynovial proliferation of mature adipose tissue
  - May arise independently or in association with chronic joint disease
- Synonyms: Lipoma arborescens, synovial lipoma

CLINICAL ISSUES

- Wide age range
- Knee most common site
- Pain and swelling of affected joint
  - Secondary synovial lipomatosis arises in setting of joint disease, most commonly osteoarthritis
- Treatment: Arthroscopic or open synovectomy
- Benign
- Low risk of local recurrence
- Untreated lesions can lead to degenerative changes within affected joint

IMAGING

- Effusion
- Synovial hypertrophy with villous projections showing signal intensity of normal fat

MACROSCOPIC

- Yellow, fatty-appearing tissue

MICROSCOPIC

- Proliferation of mature adipose tissue beneath synovial membrane
- Synovium characteristically shows villous appearance
- Variable chronic inflammatory cell infiltrate

TOP DIFFERENTIAL DIAGNOSES

- Diffuse-type tenosynovial giant cell tumor
- Atypical lipomatous tumor
- Hoffa disease
- Rheumatoid arthritis

Synovial Lipomatosis

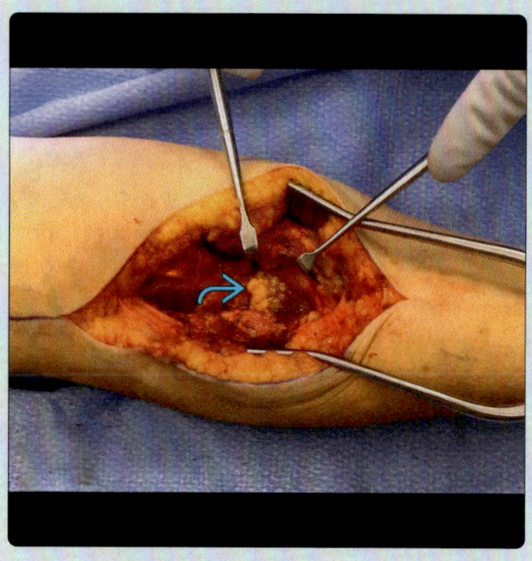

Villous Appearance

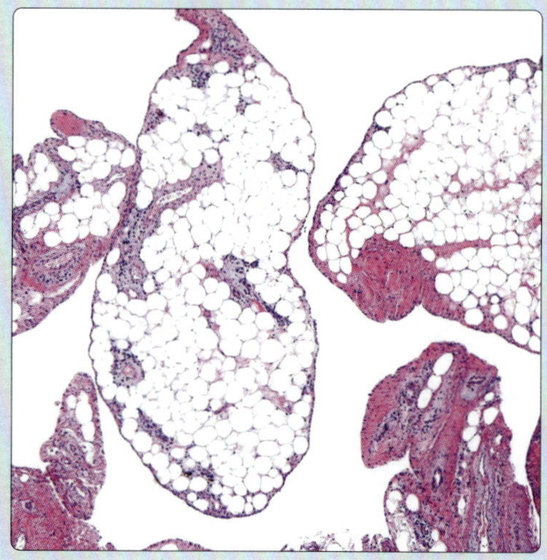

(Left) *Synovial lipomatosis, a.k.a. synovial lipoma or lipoma arborescens, is a benign proliferation of subsynovial adipose tissue. Grossly and intraoperatively, the lesion appears as yellow, fatty tissue, often with a villiform external contour. (Courtesy R. Nicholas, MD.)* **(Right)** *At low magnification, synovial lipomatosis shows abundant mature adipose tissue filling the subsynovial connective tissue. A villiform synovial architecture is often conspicuous.*

Subsynovial Mature Adipose Tissue

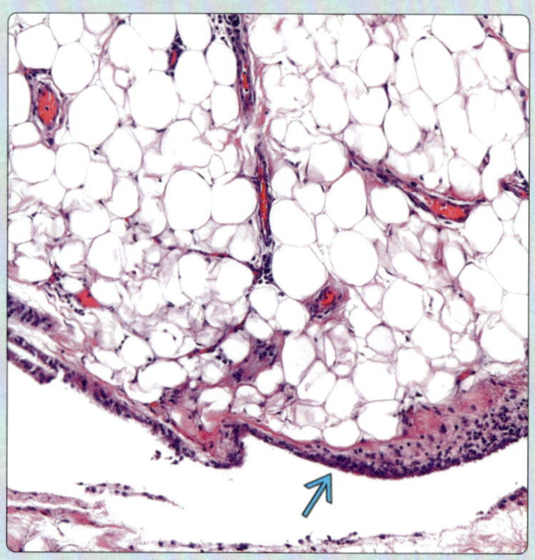

Mature Adipose Tissue

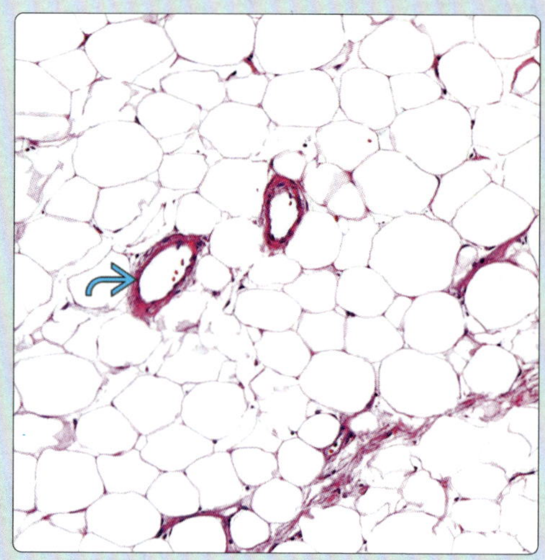

(Left) *The adipose tissue present in synovial lipomatosis is mature and devoid of atypia. A variable chronic inflammatory infiltrate is present in many cases. The overlying synovium may be unremarkable, hyperplastic, or inflamed.* **(Right)** *The mature adipose tissue of synovial lipomatosis is indistinguishable from conventional lipoma at high magnification. Small blood vessels are common as well.*

Synovial Lipomatosis

TERMINOLOGY

Synonyms

- Synovial lipoma
- Lipoma arborescens
- Villous lipomatous proliferation of synovial membrane

Definitions

- Benign, likely reactive, subsynovial proliferation of mature adipose tissue
  - May arise independently or in association with chronic joint disease

CLINICAL ISSUES

Epidemiology

- Incidence
  - Rare
- Age
  - Wide range
    - Rare in children and adolescents
- Sex
  - Male predominance

Site

- Knee most common
- Other sites
  - Ankle
  - Wrist
  - Elbow
  - Hip
- Occasionally bilateral

Presentation

- Pain and swelling of affected joint
- Secondary synovial lipomatosis arises in setting of joint disease, most commonly osteoarthritis
  - Associated with joint disease, most commonly osteoarthritis

Treatment

- Arthroscopic or open synovectomy

Prognosis

- Benign
- Untreated lesions can lead to degenerative changes within affected joint
- Low risk of local recurrence

IMAGING

MR Findings

- Effusion
- Synovial hypertrophy with villous projections showing signal intensity of normal fat

MACROSCOPIC

General Features

- Yellow, fatty-appearing tissue

MICROSCOPIC

Histologic Features

- Proliferation of mature adipose tissue beneath synovial membrane
- Synovium characteristically shows villous appearance
  - May show reactive hyperplasia
- Generally lacks hemorrhage and hemosiderin pigment
- Variable chronic inflammatory cell infiltrate

DIFFERENTIAL DIAGNOSIS

Diffuse-Type Tenosynovial Giant Cell Tumor

- Villonodular proliferation of epithelioid cells
- Sheet-like growth common
- Hemosiderin and foamy macrophages
- Fat typically absent

Atypical Lipomatous Tumor/Well-Differentiated Liposarcoma

- Large, lobular, expansile mass
- Rarely presents as intraarticular disease
- Combined MDM2(+) and CDK4(+) by immunohistochemistry
- MDM2 amplification
- Atypical stromal fibroblasts ("smudge cells")

Hoffa Disease

- Affects knee
- Hypertrophy of infrapatellar fat pad, related to prior trauma

Rheumatoid Arthritis

- Positive serologies for antirheumatoid factor
- Prominent lymphoplasmacytic synovial and subsynovial infiltrate

SELECTED REFERENCES

1. Kim S et al: An intra-articular synovial lipoma of the hip, possibly causing osteoarthritis: a case report and review of the literature. Skeletal Radiol. 47(5):717-721, 2018
2. Kulkarni HG et al: Lipoma arborescens - eyes see what mind knows! J Orthop Case Rep. 7(5):59-62, 2017
3. Tsifountoudis I et al: Lipoma arborescens of the knee: report of three cases and review of the literature. Case Rep Med. 2017:3569512, 2017
4. Miladore N et al: Synovial lipomatosis: a rare cause of knee pain in an adolescent female. World J Orthop. 6(3):369-73, 2015
5. Sailhan F et al: Bilateral lipoma arborescens of the knee: a case report. J Bone Joint Surg Am. 93(2):195-8, 2011
6. Chae EY et al: Lipoma arborescens of the glenohumeral joint causing bone erosion: MRI features with gadolinium enhancement. Skeletal Radiol. 38(8):815-8, 2009
7. Martín S et al: Diagnostic imaging of lipoma arborescens. Skeletal Radiol. 27(6):325-9, 1998
8. Soler T et al: Lipoma arborescens of the knee: MR characteristics in 13 joints. J Comput Assist Tomogr. 22(4):605-9, 1998

Angiolipoma

KEY FACTS

TERMINOLOGY

- Benign tumor consisting of mature adipocytes and thin-walled blood vessels with intraluminal fibrin thrombi

ETIOLOGY/PATHOGENESIS

- Majority are sporadic; rare familial cases

CLINICAL ISSUES

- Commonly in young adults
  - Male predominance
- Forearm, trunk, and upper arm most common sites
- Painful tender subcutaneous nodules
  - Often multiple
- Treatment: Simple surgical excision
- Excellent prognosis
  - Local recurrence very rare
  - No risk of malignant transformation

MACROSCOPIC

- Circumscribed, yellow-red nodule
- Typically < 2 cm in size

MICROSCOPIC

- Admixture of mature adipocytes and capillary-sized blood vessels
  - Hallmark: Fibrin thrombi within vessels
- Vascularity often more prominent in periphery
- No nuclear atypia in adipocytic or endothelial components
- Morphologic variant: Cellular angiolipoma

TOP DIFFERENTIAL DIAGNOSES

- Lipoma
- Intramuscular hemangioma
- Kaposi sarcoma
- Spindle cell hemangioma
- Angiomyolipoma (PEComa family)

Angiolipoma

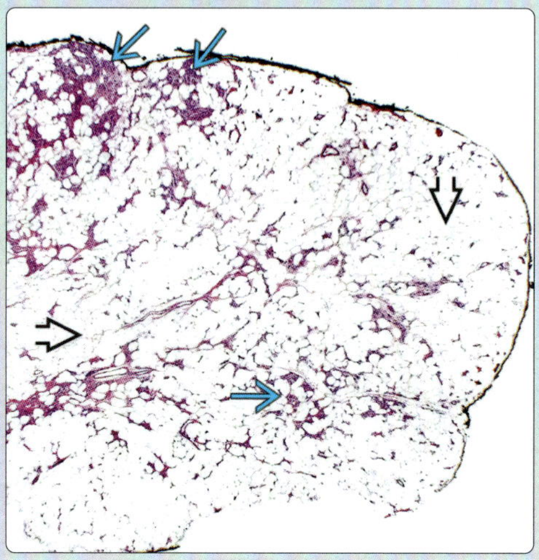

Abundant Adipose Tissue

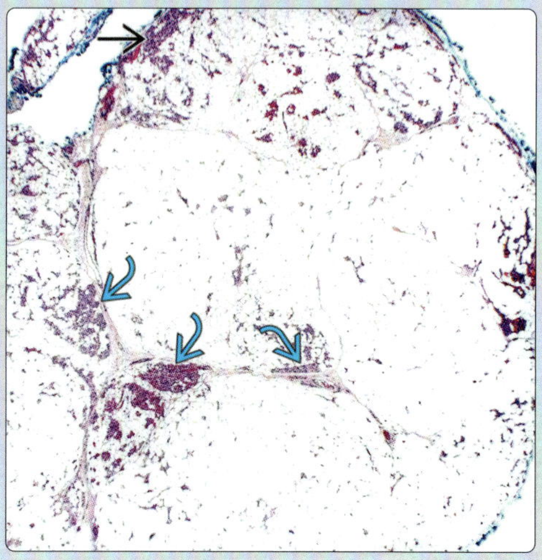

(Left) *Angiolipoma is composed of both vascular → and mature adipocytic ⇨ components admixed together in varying proportions. They are often small circumscribed lesions, as seen here.* **(Right)** *This angiolipoma is predominantly composed of adipose tissue. The focal vascular component is present as clusters of small vessels near the periphery → and near the thin fibrous septa ↗.*

Peripheral Vascular Component

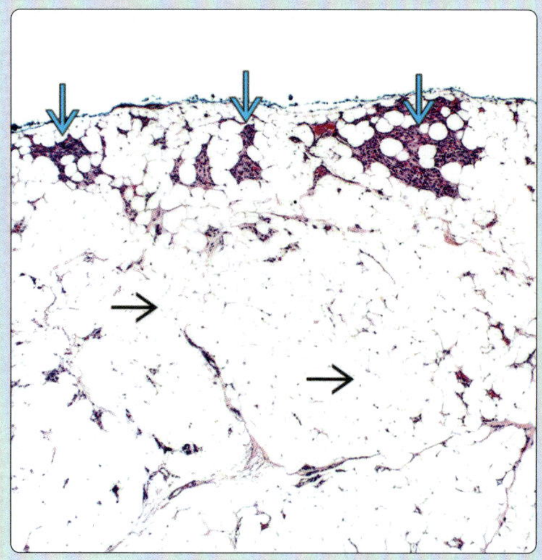

Characteristic Fibrin Thrombi

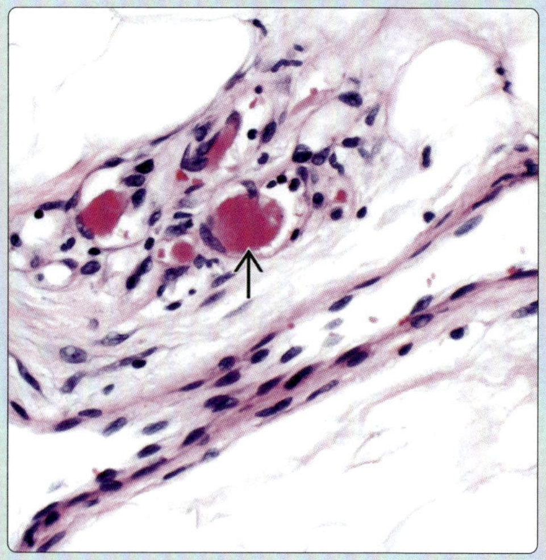

(Left) *The focal vascular component of angiolipoma is present as clusters of small vessels near the periphery of the mass →. The remainder of the lesion is composed of mature adipocytes →.* **(Right)** *Bright pink fibrin thrombi → are present in small clustered capillary vessels. This is the hallmark feature of angiolipoma.*

TERMINOLOGY

Definitions

- Benign tumor composed of mature adipocytes and clustered small blood vessels with intraluminal fibrin thrombi

ETIOLOGY/PATHOGENESIS

Unknown

- Majority are sporadic
- Rare familial predilection (5%)

CLINICAL ISSUES

Epidemiology

- Age
  - Most common in young adults
  - Rare in children or in adults > 50 years
- Sex
  - Male predominance

Site

- Forearm, trunk, and upper arm most common sites
- Rare on scalp or face

Presentation

- Painful subcutaneous nodule, often multiple (in 2/3 of cases)

Treatment

- Simple surgical excision

Prognosis

- Excellent: Benign
  - Very low risk of local recurrence
  - No known risk of malignant transformation

MACROSCOPIC

Gross Features

- Well circumscribed
- Yellow-red nodules
- Typically < 2 cm in size

MICROSCOPIC

Histologic Features

- 2 components present in varying proportions
  - Mature adipocytes
  - Clustered capillary-sized vessels with fibrin thrombi
    - Vascularity often more prominent in periphery
- No nuclear atypia in adipocytic or endothelial components

Morphologic Variant

- Cellular angiolipoma
  - Vascular component predominates

ANCILLARY TESTS

Immunohistochemistry

- Immunostains not useful for diagnosis

DIFFERENTIAL DIAGNOSIS

Lipoma

- Mass composed of mature adipose tissue
  - May have increased single vessels but lacks clustered vessels and fibrin thrombi
- Lipomas possess various translocations of chromosome 12q or 6p
- Fat-predominant angiolipoma may mimic lipoma
  - Even 1 cluster of small vessels with microthrombi is diagnostic of angiolipoma

Intramuscular Hemangioma

- Previously known as "infiltrating angiolipoma"
- Large infiltrative lesion in deep muscle (not in subcutis)
- Often has adipose tissue and large thick-walled vessels
  - Lacks clustered small vessels with luminal thrombi
  - May have organizing thrombi in large vessels

Kaposi Sarcoma

- More spindled and fascicular endothelial proliferation
- Blood-filled slit-like spaces and extravasated RBCs
- Plasma cells almost always present
- PAS(+) hyaline globules, but no fibrin thrombi
- HHV8(+) endothelial cells

Angiomyolipoma (PEComa Family)

- Spindle cells with pale/granular pink cytoplasm
- HMB-45 &/or MART-1(+) plus smooth muscle actin &/or desmin (+)
- Vessels are large caliber and thick walled
- Vanishingly rare in subcutis or peripheral soft tissue

Spindle Cell Hemangioma

- Painful multiple subcutaneous nodules in extremities
- Unlike cellular angiolipoma, spindle cell hemangioma has:
  - Large, cavernous vascular spaces
  - Cellular zones of spindled and epithelioid endothelial cells and clustered endothelial vacuoles resembling miniature adipocytes
  - Large calcified thrombi (phleboliths), but lacks clustered small vessels with luminal thrombi

DIAGNOSTIC CHECKLIST

Pathologic Interpretation Pearls

- Mature adipocytes
- Clusters of capillary-sized vessels
- Fibrin microthrombi in vessels

SELECTED REFERENCES

1. Hofvander J et al: Frequent low-level mutations of protein kinase D2 in angiolipoma. J Pathol. 241(5):578-82, 2017
2. Sheng W et al: Cellular angiolipoma: a clinicopathological and immunohistochemical study of 12 cases. Am J Dermatopathol. 35(2):220-5, 2013
3. Sciot R et al: Cytogenetic analysis of subcutaneous angiolipoma: further evidence supporting its difference from ordinary pure lipomas: a report of the CHAMP Study Group. Am J Surg Pathol. 21(4):441-4, 1997
4. Fletcher CD et al: Correlation between clinicopathological features and karyotype in lipomatous tumors. A report of 178 cases from the Chromosomes and Morphology (CHAMP) Collaborative Study Group. Am J Pathol. 148(2):623-30, 1996
5. Hunt SJ et al: Cellular angiolipoma. Am J Surg Pathol. 14(1):75-81, 1990

(Left) *Fibrin thrombi within capillary lumina are pink and amorphous.* **(Right)** *The capillaries in angiolipoma often have a lobular arrangement and may appear reminiscent of a hemangioma in some cases; however, pink fibrin thrombi are present in many of the lumina in angiolipoma.*

Fibrin Thrombi

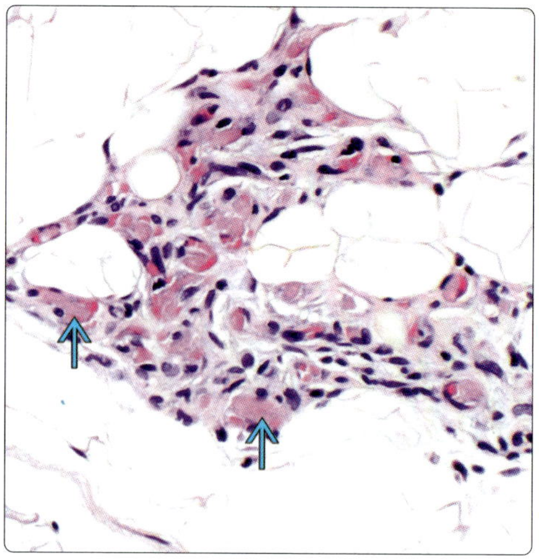

Abundant Fibrin Thrombi

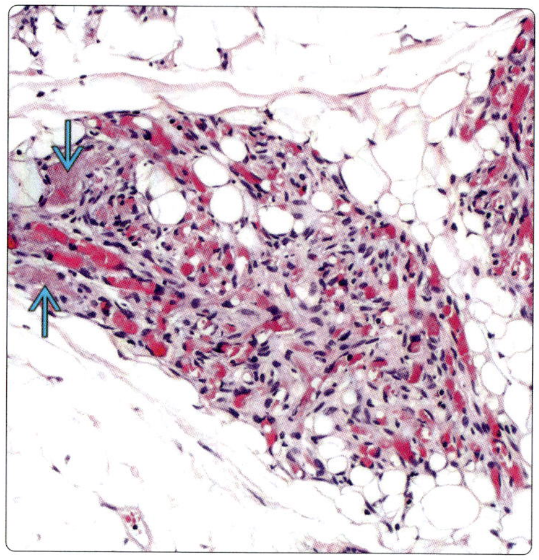

(Left) *More cellular vascular areas are admixed with mature adipose tissue in this angiolipoma. The vascularity is still enhanced at the peripheral aspect of the mass.* **(Right)** *Spindled endothelial cells and pericytes appear to infiltrate into mature adipose tissue. This more cellular and spindled pattern can mimic Kaposi sarcoma; however, note the characteristic fibrin thrombi.*

Moderate Cellularity

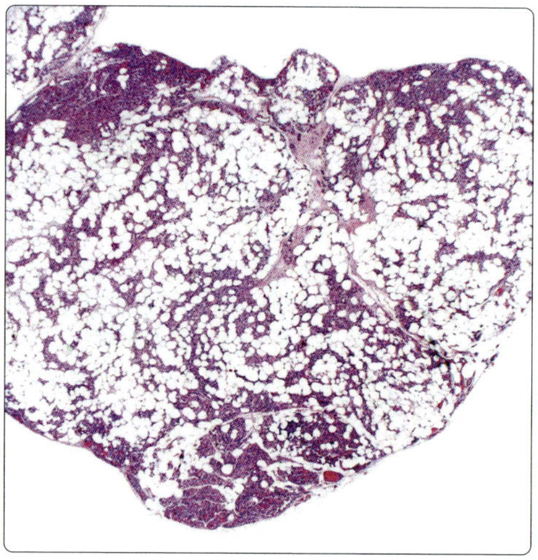

Kaposi-Like Cellularity

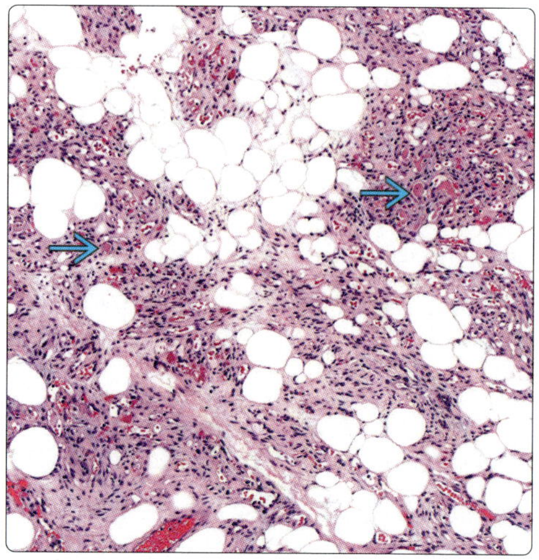

(Left) *Capillary lumina with bland endothelial cells can be appreciated at high power in the cellular zones. Fibrin thrombi are present, unlike in Kaposi sarcoma.* **(Right)** *Angiolipoma may have spindled cellular foci, but there are still small well-formed vessels. The spindled cells are endothelial and pericytic (perivascular modified smooth muscle cells). Both cell types are bland and lack nuclear atypia or significant mitotic activity in angiolipoma.*

Fibrin Thrombi

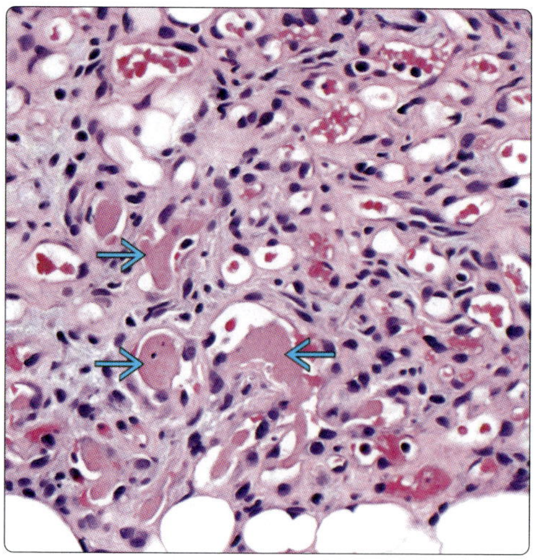

Focal Spindled Morphology

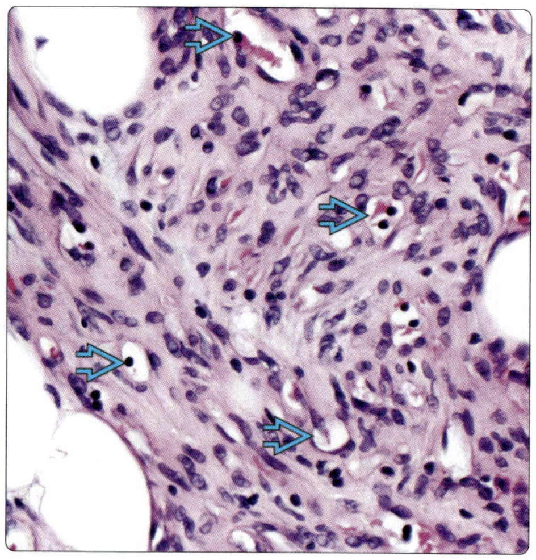

Cellular Angiolipoma

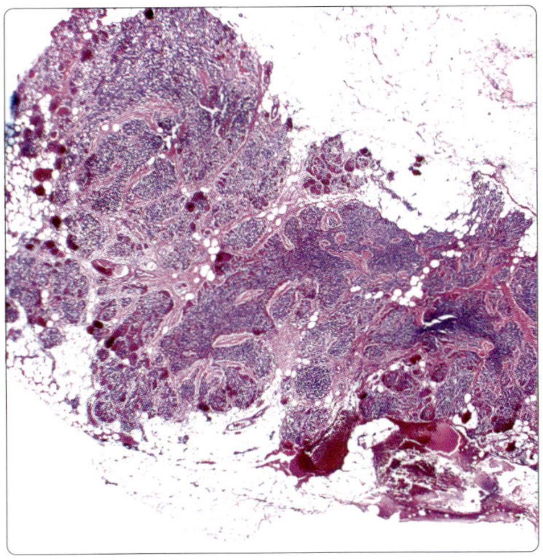

Lobular Arrangement

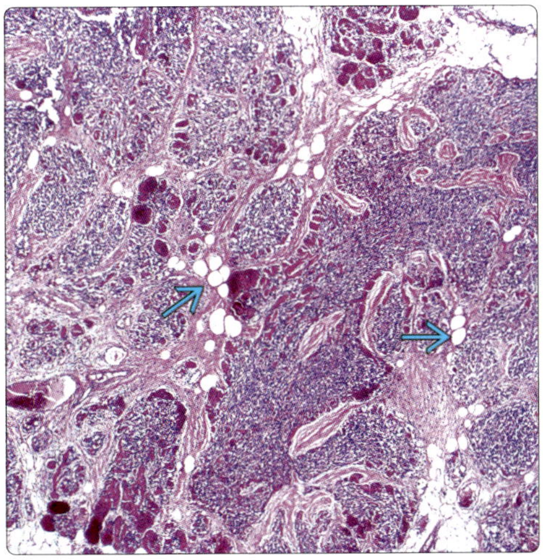

(Left) *The cellular variant of angiolipoma is composed almost entirely of densely packed small blood vessels. There is very little adipose component within the mass.* **(Right)** *There is often a lobular arrangement of vessels in cellular angiolipoma. Focal adipocytes* ➙ *appear to be entrapped between the vascular lobules, which may give a false impression of aggressive infiltrative growth.*

Tightly Packed Capillary Channels

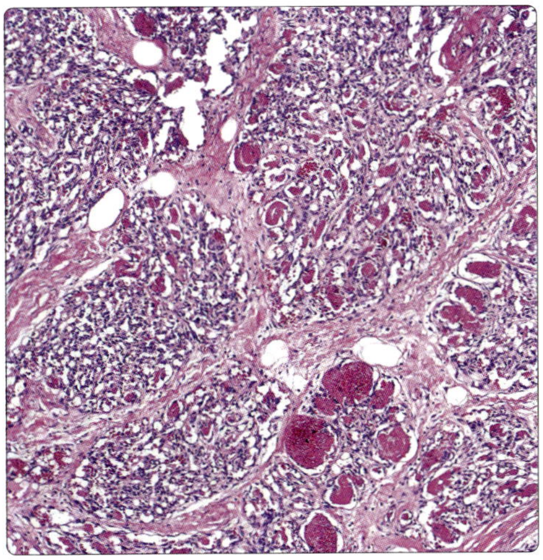

Numerous Thrombi

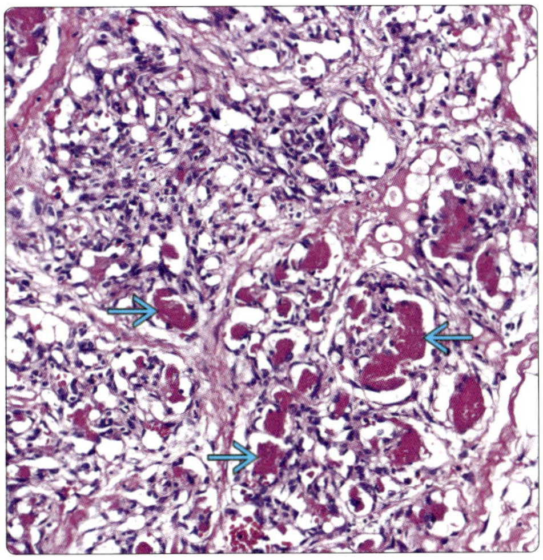

(Left) *Vascular zones in cellular angiolipoma are composed of tightly packed, well-formed small vessels.* **(Right)** *Numerous fibrin thrombi* ➙ *are present within the lumina of the vessels, helping to establish the diagnosis of angiolipoma.*

Well-Formed Vessels

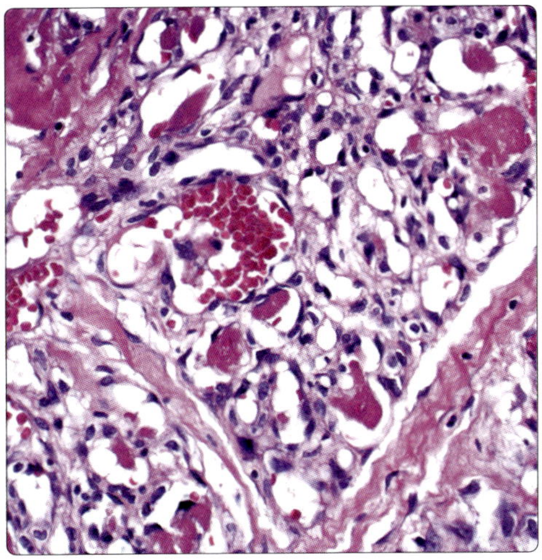

Bland Cytology

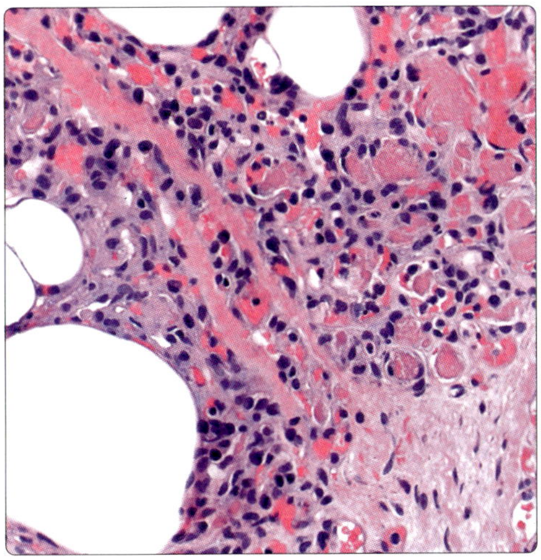

(Left) *The vessels in a cellular angiolipoma are well formed and lined by bland endothelial cells.* **(Right)** *The endothelial cells here are bland and uniform. The presence of intraluminal fibrin thrombi in cellular angiolipoma is helpful in distinguishing it from Kaposi sarcoma.*

Spindle Cell/Pleomorphic Lipoma

KEY FACTS

CLASSIFICATION

- Benign adipocytic tumor with variable admixture of spindle cells, "ropey" collagen, mature adipose tissue, and multinucleate tumor giant cells
- Spindle cell lipoma and pleomorphic lipoma (PL) are morphologic variations of same neoplasm

CLINICAL ISSUES

- Most common in older (> 50 years) men
- Most arise in shoulder, posterior neck, or back
    - Tumors in women more likely to arise in atypical locations
- Treatment: Conservative surgical excision only
- Benign; excellent prognosis

MACROSCOPIC

- Well-circumscribed subcutaneous (or less commonly dermal) mass
- Yellow-tan cut surface with variable gray-white &/or myxoid foci

MICROSCOPIC

- Variable admixture of bland spindle cells, "ropey" collagen, mature adipose tissue, myxoid stroma, and mast cells
    - PL contains multinucleated tumor cells
- Morphologic variants: Fat free, fat poor, angiomatous

ANCILLARY TESTS

- CD34(+); loss of nuclear retinoblastoma expression
- Molecular: Deletion of *RB1* (13q14)

TOP DIFFERENTIAL DIAGNOSES

- Atypical lipomatous tumor
- Neurofibroma
- Cellular angiofibroma
- Mammary-type myofibroblastoma
- Atypical spindle cell lipomatous tumor
- Solitary fibrous tumor

(Left) *Like conventional lipomas, spindle cell (SCL) and pleomorphic lipomas (PL) have a homogeneous, yellow cut surface. Both tumors also often show subtle, gray-white foci ⮕ that are firm in consistency and correlate histologically with spindle cell areas containing "ropey" collagenous matrix.* **(Right)** *At low power, SCL is composed of a mixture of adipose tissue and a variable myxoid to collagenous stroma containing bland spindle cells.*

Spindle Cell Lipoma

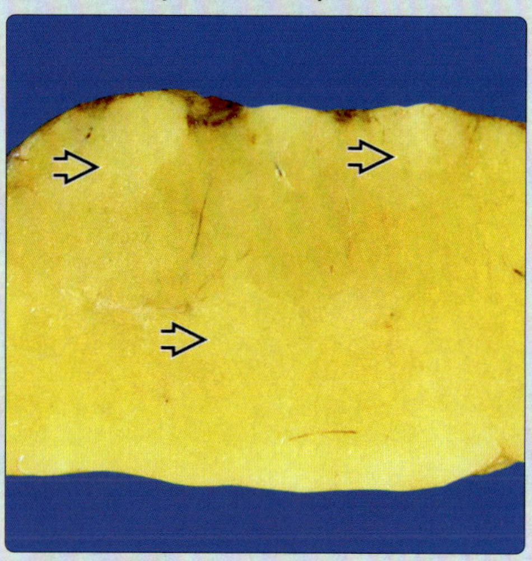

Spindle Cell Lipoma

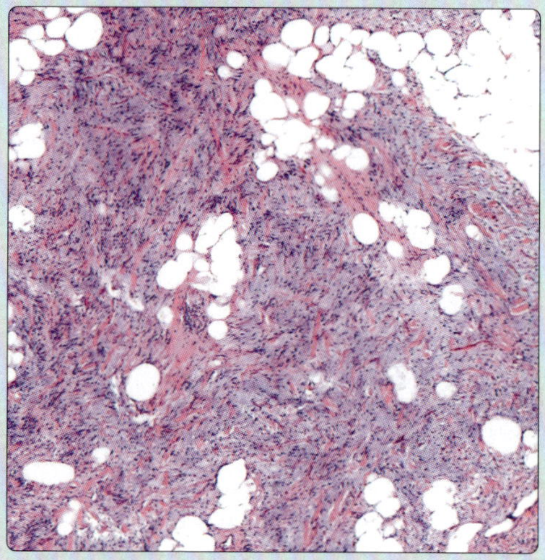

(Left) *Blocky bundles and strips of collagen ("ropey" collagen) are a consistent finding in SCL/PL and a helpful diagnostic feature. Mast cells ⮕ are also very commonly identified.* **(Right)** *The lesional cells of SCL are cytologically bland and show bipolar or stellate cytoplasmic processes. Nuclear grooves may be identified in some cases ⮕. Mitoses are rare.*

"Ropey" Collagen and Mast Cells

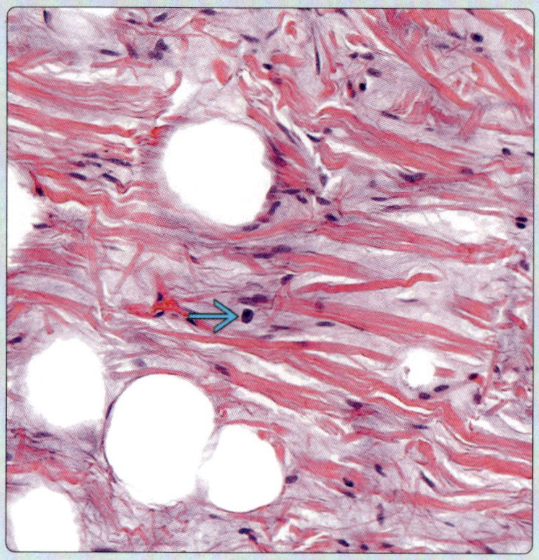

Bland Spindle Cells

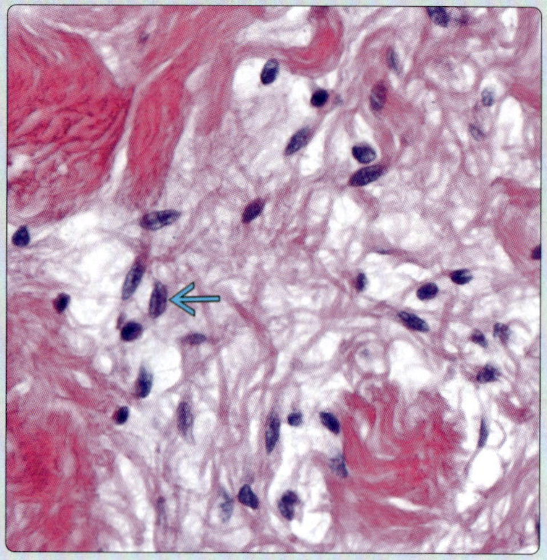

TERMINOLOGY

Abbreviations

- Spindle cell lipoma (SCL)
- Pleomorphic lipoma (PL)

Definitions

- Benign adipocytic tumor with variable admixture of spindle cells, "ropey" collagen, and mature adipose tissue
  - PL additionally contains multinucleated tumor giant cells
- SCL and PL are considered morphologic variations on same entity

CLINICAL ISSUES

Epidemiology

- Age
  - Typically in older age group (> 50 years)
  - Very rare < 20 years
- Sex
  - Strong male predilection
    - Dermal SCL appears to be more common in women

Site

- Most occur superficially in subcutaneous tissue or dermis
  - Exceptionally rare in deep soft tissues
- Shoulder, posterior neck, and back most common (80% of cases)
  - Atypical locations: Face, oral cavity, trunk, extremities
    - In women, SCL more likely to arise in these locations

Presentation

- Very similar to conventional lipoma
  - Painless, slow-growing mass
  - Often present for long duration
- Rarely arise in multiple sites (synchronous or metachronous)
  - May be familial

Treatment

- Conservative surgical excision

Prognosis

- Benign; excellent prognosis
- Local recurrence is very rare
- Atypical findings in SCL/PL, such as lipoblasts and very rare abnormal mitoses, do not appear to affect behavior

MACROSCOPIC

General Features

- Well circumscribed
  - Dermal tumors usually less circumscribed
- Yellow-tan cut surface
- Subtle, gray-white foci correlate with spindle cell foci
- May show focal myxoid areas or be extensively gelatinous
- Very rare multinodular, plexiform growth pattern

Size

- Usually 3-5 cm (rarely > 10 cm)

MICROSCOPIC

Histologic Features

- SCL and PL exist as 2 ends of single morphologic spectrum
  - Some tumors show morphology of SCL exclusively and some show morphology of PL exclusively
  - Tumors demonstrating intermixed features or discrete areas of both SCL and PL are common
- SCL
  - Variable admixture of 3 components
    - Uniform, bland spindle cell proliferation
      - Bipolar to stellate cytoplasmic projections
      - May cluster together akin to "schools of fish" or show nuclear palisading
      - May show nuclear grooves
      - Mitotic figures rare to absent
    - Mature adipocytes
    - Bundles of "ropey" collagen fibers
  - Myxoid stroma is common and may be extensive
  - Mast cells are very common and nearly constant finding
- PL
  - Characterized by variable numbers of multinucleated giant cells with dense eosinophilic cytoplasm and peripherally arranged nuclei (floret cells)
    - Also cells with "smudgy" nuclei &/or nuclear pseudoinclusions
  - Bland spindled cells, "ropey" collagen, mast cells, and adipose tissue also usually present
  - Mitotic figures rare to absent (may be atypical)
  - May contain lipoblasts

Morphologic Variants

- Fat-free or fat-poor SCL
  - Minimal to no mature adipose tissue component
  - May show abundant collagen, abundant myxoid stroma, or predominantly spindle cells
  - Fat-free and fat-poor forms of PL also exist
- Pseudoangiomatoid SCL
  - Also described as angiomatous SCL
  - Contains prominent slit-like to ectatic cleavage spaces (sometimes lined by endothelial cells)
  - Nodules or lobules of tumor may appear to float in empty space
  - May also show prominent myxoid stroma or minimal mature adipose tissue
  - Can be combined with fat-free or fat-poor morphology

ANCILLARY TESTS

Immunohistochemistry

- Strong, diffuse CD34(+) in spindled or multinucleated cells
- Loss of nuclear retinoblastoma (Rb) expression
- Generally S100 protein, smooth muscle actin, and desmin (-)
  - Rare cases with S100(+) or desmin (+) spindle cells

Molecular Genetics

- Characteristic deletion (monoallelic or biallelic) of *RB1* on 13q14
  - Identical deletion present in mammary-type myofibroblastoma and cellular angiofibroma
- No *MDM2* amplification

DIFFERENTIAL DIAGNOSIS

Atypical Lipomatous Tumor/Well-Differentiated Liposarcoma

- Usually large tumors
- Commonly arise in deep locations [especially retroperitoneum in well-differentiated liposarcoma (WDLPS)]
- "Ropey" collagen bundles and mast cells are not typical features
- MDM2(+), CDK4(+) by IHC
  - Rare cases of SCL show focal expression
- Amplification of *MDM2* by FISH in most cases

Neurofibroma

- Presence of bland spindle cells with intermixed adipose tissue in SCL may suggest diffuse-type neurofibroma
- "Ropey" collagen bundles in myxoid background in SCL may suggest plexiform neurofibroma
- S100(+) in most spindle cells
- CD34(+) component of admixed fibroblastic cells

Cellular Angiofibroma

- Most cases occur in lower external genital tract in women
  - May also occur in men in same general region
- Can show morphologic overlap with SCL
  - Hyalinized vessels common in cellular angiofibroma
- Strong CD34(+)
- Loss of nuclear Rb expression
- Deletion of *RB1* on 13q14

Mammary-Type Myofibroblastoma

- Histologically identical to myofibroblastoma of breast
- Short fascicles of monomorphic spindle cells in collagenous stroma
- Can show morphologic overlap with SCL
  - Thickened, coarse collagen bundles are characteristic feature of myofibroblastoma
- Strong CD34(+), desmin (+)
- Loss of nuclear Rb expression
- Deletion of *RB1* on 13q14

Atypical Spindle Cell Lipomatous Tumor

- Predilection for upper and lower extremities
- Nearly 1/2 of cases arise in deep soft tissue
- Nuclear hyperchromasia and lipoblasts common
- Generally lacks "ropey" collagen bundles

Solitary Fibrous Tumor

- Prominent ectatic "staghorn" vascular network in most cases
- "Ropey" collagen bundles are not feature
- Diffusely CD34(+) in vast majority of cases
- May also show intratumoral adipose tissue (lipomatous solitary fibrous tumor)

Myxoid Liposarcoma

- Usually affects younger age group than SCL/PL
- Often strikingly lobular growth pattern
- Usually shows prominent delicate plexiform capillary vascular pattern
- Uni- and multivacuolated lipoblasts are common
- May contain cellular ("round cell") foci
- CD34(-)
- Characteristic t(12;16) in most cases

Dermatofibrosarcoma Protuberans

- Usually occurs in younger individuals than SCL/PL
- Monomorphic spindle cells arranged in broad or tight storiform pattern
- May be focally or extensively myxoid
- Prominent infiltration of peripheral adipose tissue or skeletal muscle (honeycomb infiltration)
- Mast cells uncommon
- Diffuse CD34(+) in vast majority of cases
- t(17;22) with *COL1A1-PDGFB* fusion

Giant Cell Fibroblastoma

- Most common in children < 6 years
- Multinucleated stromal giant cells lining pseudovascular spaces/clefts
  - Tumors with inconspicuous pseudovascular spaces can resemble PL
- CD34(+)
- t(17;22) with *COL1A1-PDGFB* fusion

SELECTED REFERENCES

1. McCarthy AJ et al: Tumours composed of fat are no longer a simple diagnosis: an overview of fatty tumours with a spindle cell component. J Clin Pathol. 71(6):483-92, 2018
2. Creytens D et al: "Atypical" pleomorphic lipomatous tumor: a clinicopathologic, immunohistochemical and molecular study of 21 cases, emphasizing its relationship to atypical spindle cell lipomatous tumor and suggesting a morphologic spectrum (atypical spindle cell/pleomorphic lipomatous tumor). Am J Surg Pathol. 41(11):1443-1455, 2017
3. Ko JS et al: Spindle cell lipomas in women: a report of 53 cases. Am J Surg Pathol. 41(9):1267-1274, 2017
4. Mariño-Enriquez A et al: Atypical spindle cell lipomatous tumor: clinicopathologic characterization of 232 cases demonstrating a morphologic spectrum. Am J Surg Pathol. 41(2):234-244, 2017
5. Michal M et al: Lipoblasts in spindle cell and pleomorphic lipomas: a close scrutiny. Hum Pathol. 65:140-6, 2017
6. Ud Din N et al: Spindle cell lipomas arising at atypical locations. Am J Clin Pathol. 146(4):487-95, 2016
7. Cheah A et al: Spindle cell/pleomorphic lipomas of the face: an under-recognized diagnosis. Histopathology. 66(3):430-7, 2015
8. Creytens D et al: Atypical spindle cell lipoma: a clinicopathologic, immunohistochemical, and molecular study emphasizing its relationship to classical spindle cell lipoma. Virchows Arch. 465(1):97-108, 2014
9. Chen BJ et al: Loss of retinoblastoma protein expression in spindle cell/pleomorphic lipomas and cytogenetically related tumors: an immunohistochemical study with diagnostic implications. Am J Surg Pathol. 36(8):1119-28, 2012
10. Wood L et al: Cutaneous CD34+ spindle cell neoplasms: Histopathologic features distinguish spindle cell lipoma, solitary fibrous tumor, and dermatofibrosarcoma protuberans. Am J Dermatopathol. 32(8):764-8, 2010
11. Sachdeva MP et al: Low-fat and fat-free pleomorphic lipomas: a diagnostic challenge. Am J Dermatopathol. 31(5):423-6, 2009
12. Billings SD et al: Diagnostically challenging spindle cell lipomas: a report of 34 "low-fat" and "fat-free" variants. Am J Dermatopathol. 29(5):437-42, 2007
13. Fanburg-Smith JC et al: Multiple spindle cell lipomas: a report of 7 familial and 11 nonfamilial cases. Am J Surg Pathol. 22(1):40-8, 1998
14. Hawley IC et al: Spindle cell lipoma--a pseudoangiomatous variant. Histopathology. 24(6):565-9, 1994
15. Shmookler BM et al: Pleomorphic lipoma: a benign tumor simulating liposarcoma. A clinicopathologic analysis of 48 cases. Cancer. 47(1):126-33, 1981
16. Enzinger FM et al: Spindle cell lipoma. Cancer. 36(5):1852-9, 1975

"Ropey" Collagen

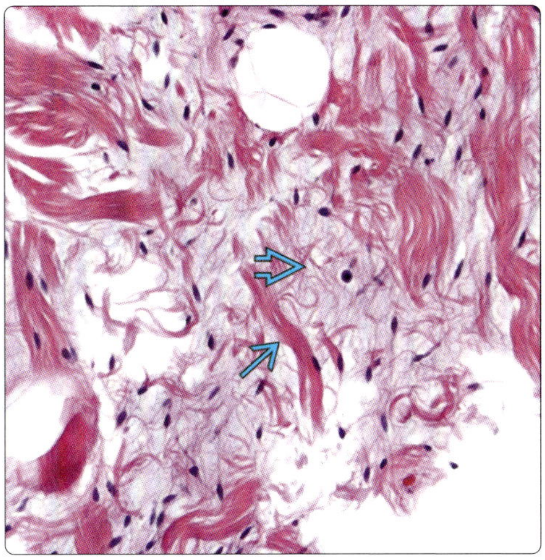

Thick Collagen Bundles

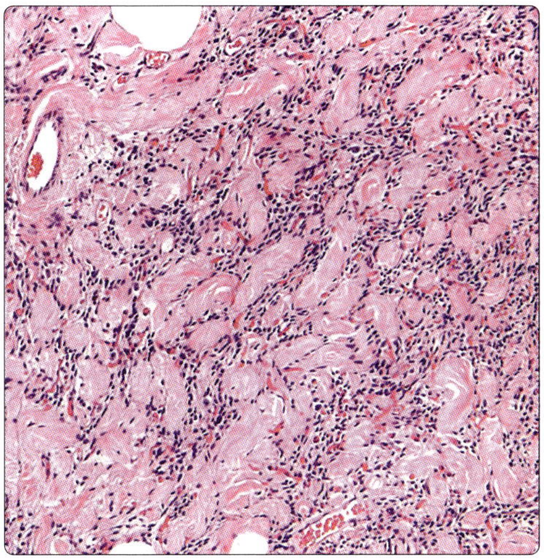

(Left) *The characteristic "ropey" collagen bundles ⇨ of SCL/PL vary widely in extent and distribution. Thin, wispy fibers ⇨ are often present as well and may be the predominant form of collagen in some cases.* **(Right)** *In some cases of SCL, the collagen fibers have a thickened and organized appearance, reminiscent of mammary-type myofibroblastoma, a tumor that appears to be histogenetically related to SCL.*

Prominent Collagen

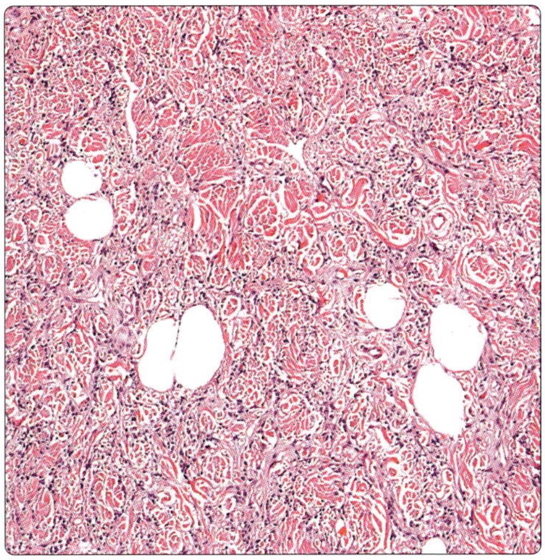

Haphazard Components

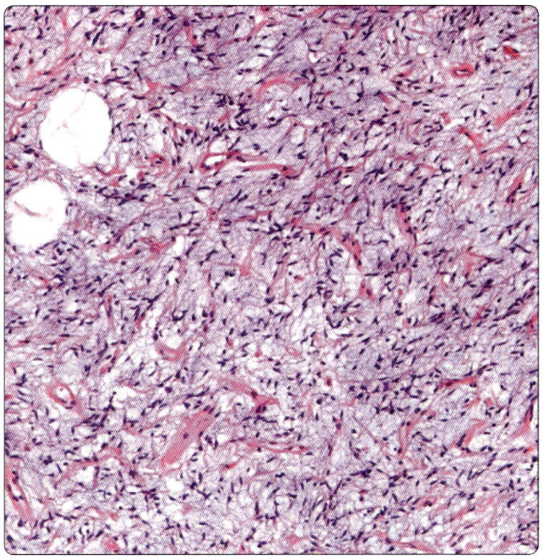

(Left) *Some cases of SCL show prominent stromal collagen, such as in this example where the "ropey" fibers are densely packed in together.* **(Right)** *Many cases of SCL show a haphazard, disorganized distribution of bipolar and stellate spindle cells with "ropey" or wispy collagen. This morphology may lead to consideration of a peripheral nerve sheath tumor like neurofibroma.*

Myxoid Stroma

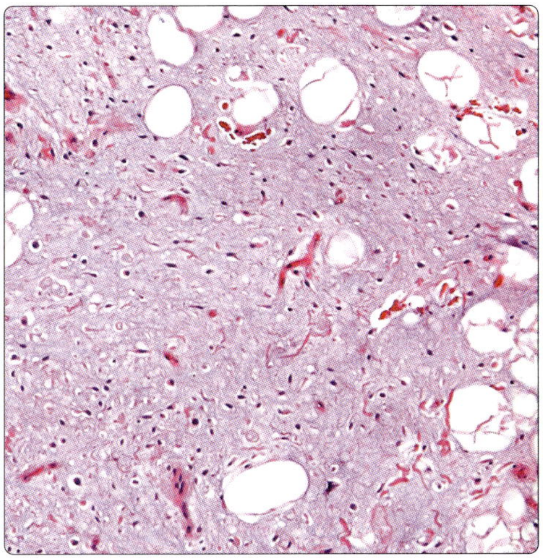

Myxoid Spindle Cell Lipoma

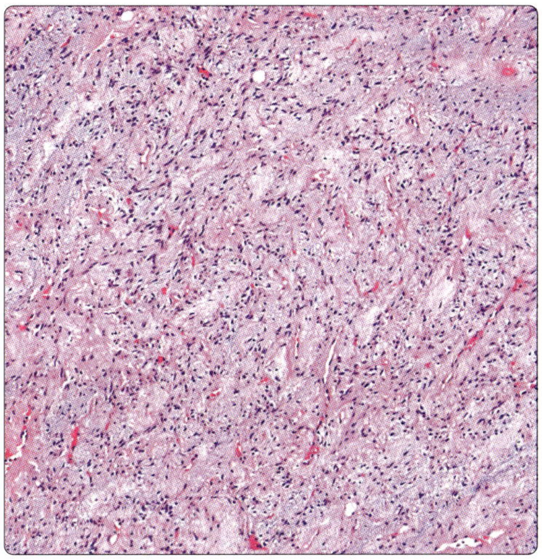

(Left) *SCL may show a markedly abundant myxoid stroma and overall striking hypocellularity that is suggestive of a myxoma or myxolipoma. Identification of a discrete component of scattered bland spindle cells is helpful, as are foci of "ropey" collagen.* **(Right)** *This case of myxoid SCL showed a relative paucity of adipocytes. This variant has been described as "fat poor" or "fat free."*

(Left) *Nuclear palisading is not an uncommon finding in myxoid SCL, but it is usually not extensive. Many cases, however, show small clusters or linear arrangements of tumor cells, akin to schools of fish.* **(Right)** *In some cases of SCL, there is little to no mature adipose tissue. These cases can be very challenging to diagnose; however, the characteristic spindle cells and collagen bundles are helpful clues, as is possibly the clinical presentation.*

Nuclear Palisading

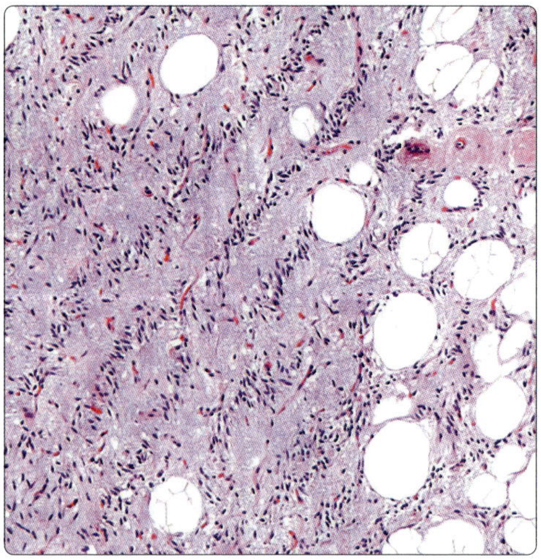

Fat-Free and Fat-Poor Variant

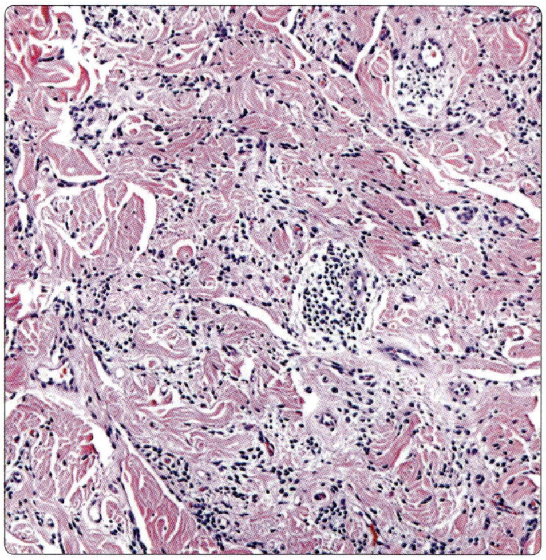

(Left) *The cellularity of fat-poor and fat-free SCL may be strikingly increased in some cases, resulting in the lesion looking nothing like an adipocytic tumor.* **(Right)** *Despite the cellularity, the cytologic features of this fat-free variant of SCL are not worrisome for malignancy, and mitotic figures are inconspicuous or absent. Note the mast cell →.*

Fat-Free Variant

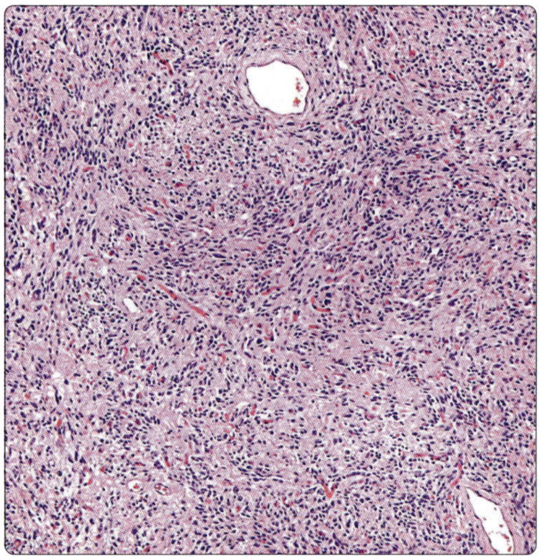

Fat-Free Variant

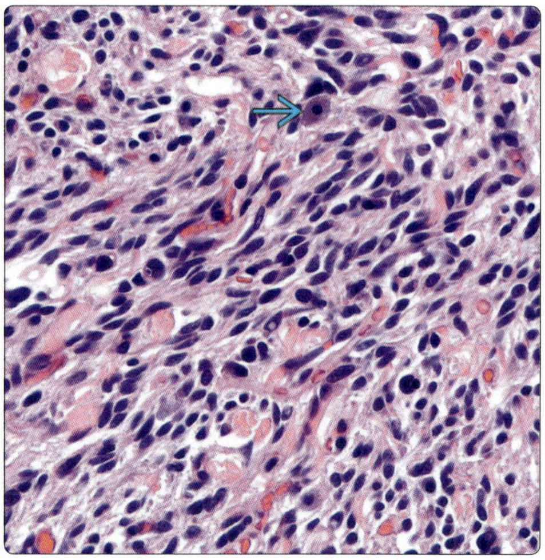

(Left) *The unusual pseudoangiomatoid variant of SCL demonstrates slit-like to markedly dilated cleavage spaces associated with the otherwise characteristic features of SCL.* **(Right)** *Some cases of the pseudoangiomatoid SCL variant show nodules of tumor "floating" in relatively empty spaces, as depicted. Red blood cells may also be seen in these spaces. This particular example was highly myxoid as well.*

Pseudoangiomatoid Variant

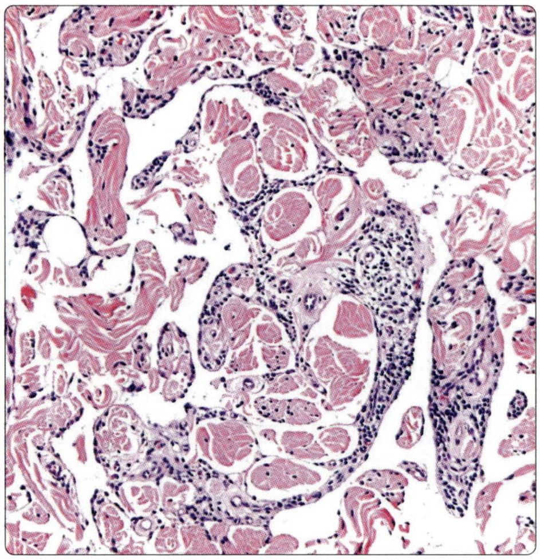

Pseudoangiomatoid Spindle Cell Lipoma

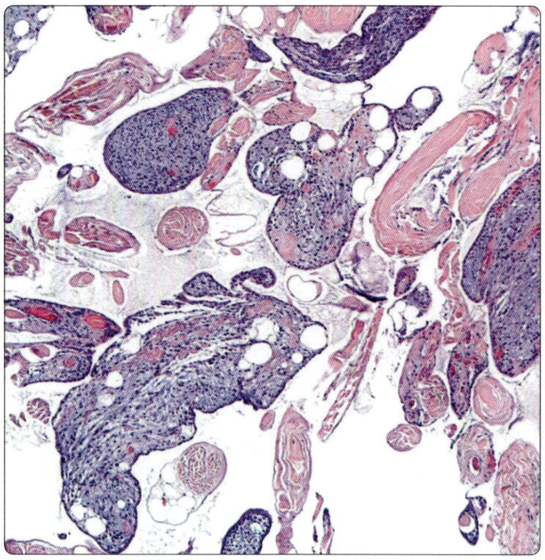

Endothelial Lining

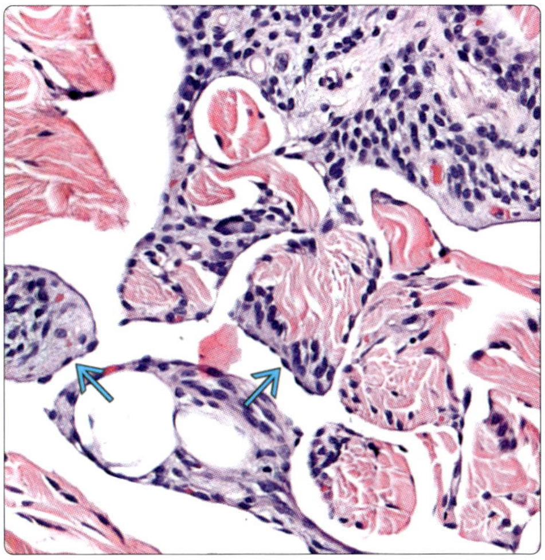

Pleomorphic Lipoma

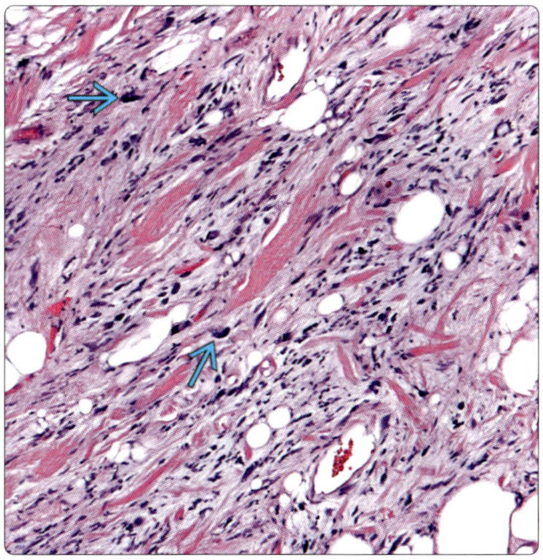

(Left) *A conspicuous endothelial lining ➔ can sometimes be identified in pseudoangiomatoid SCL, suggesting that "angiomatous" might be a better term. A CD31 immunostain will highlight the endothelial cells.* **(Right)** *PL is essentially the same neoplasm as SCL. Accordingly, many features of SCL are often present in PL, including bland spindle cells and "ropey" collagen bundles. Notably, there is also a variably prominent population of multinucleated tumor giant cells termed floret cells ➔.*

Pleomorphic Lipoma

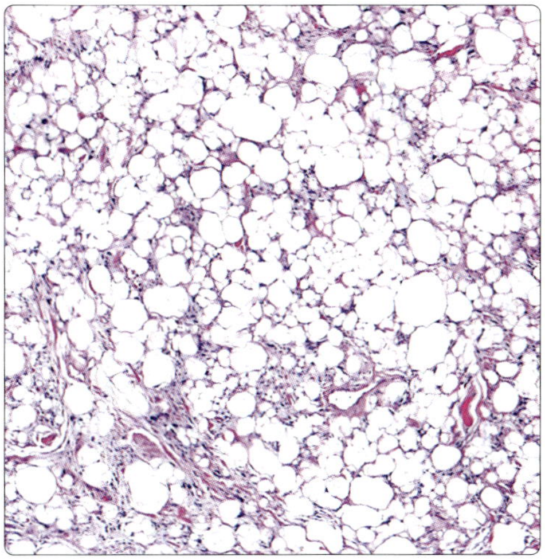

Floret Tumor Cells

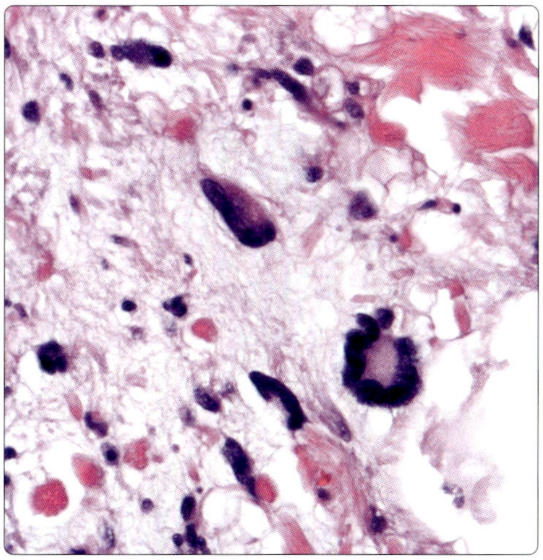

(Left) *Some cases of PL are mostly adipocytic with scattered foci of myxoid stroma containing the diagnostic findings. Examples such as these may at first resemble a myxolipoma or liposarcoma. Occasional cases of PL are fat poor or fat free.* **(Right)** *The floret cell defines the morphology of PL. These cells have eosinophilic cytoplasm and contain multiple hyperchromatic nuclei often arranged in a peripheral distribution, resembling that of a floral arrangement.*

Rare Multivacuolated Lipoblasts

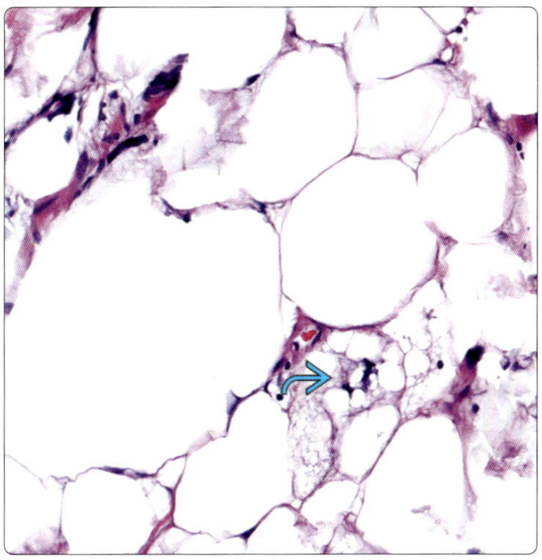

Diffuse CD34 Expression

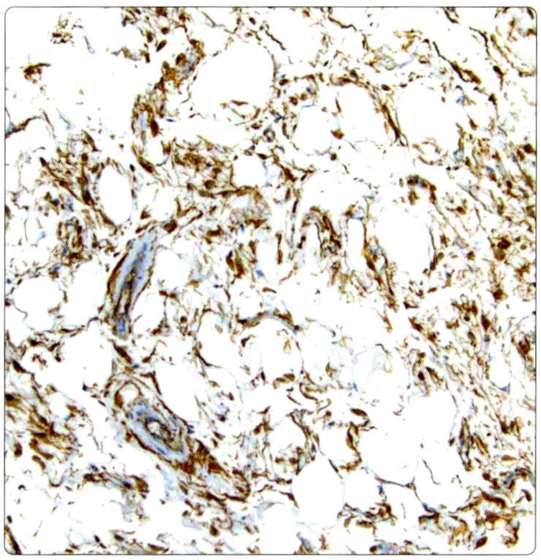

(Left) *Multivacuolated lipoblasts ⮳ may be rarely encountered in otherwise typical cases of PL. Similarly, a scattered atypical mitotic figure may also rarely be identified. Neither of these findings appears to alter the usual benign clinical course of these neoplasms.* **(Right)** *CD34 expression is strong, diffuse, and consistent in both SCL and PL and stains both the spindle cells and the multinucleated floret cells. S100 protein is expressed in adipocytes but is generally negative in the lesional cells.*

Chondroid Lipoma

KEY FACTS

TERMINOLOGY

- Benign mesenchymal neoplasm composed of lipoblastic cells and mature adipocytes within myxochondroid matrix

CLINICAL ISSUES

- Very rare
- Adults (20-40 years most common)
- Strong female predilection (4:1)
- Slow-growing, painless mass
- Most common in proximal limbs and limb girdles
  - Also trunk, head and neck
- Occurs in both superficial and deep tissues
- Simple complete excision is curative

MICROSCOPIC

- Well circumscribed, often encapsulated
- Nests, sheets, and cords of uni- and multivacuolated round cells
  - Some nonvacuolated tumor cells have granular eosinophilic cytoplasm
  - Classic multivacuolated lipoblasts common
- Myxochondroid to hyalinized matrix
- Variable mature adipose tissue component
- Interspersed thick- and thin-walled vessels with variable hemorrhage and hemosiderin deposition

ANCILLARY TESTS

- Variable S100 protein (+) in lipoblast-like cells
- Characteristic chromosomal translocation
  - t(11;16)(q13;p12-13) with *C11orf95-MKL2* fusion

TOP DIFFERENTIAL DIAGNOSES

- Soft tissue chondroma
- Atypical lipomatous tumor/well-differentiated liposarcoma
- Myxoid liposarcoma
- Extraskeletal myxoid chondrosarcoma
- Myoepithelioma of soft tissue

Chondroid Lipoma

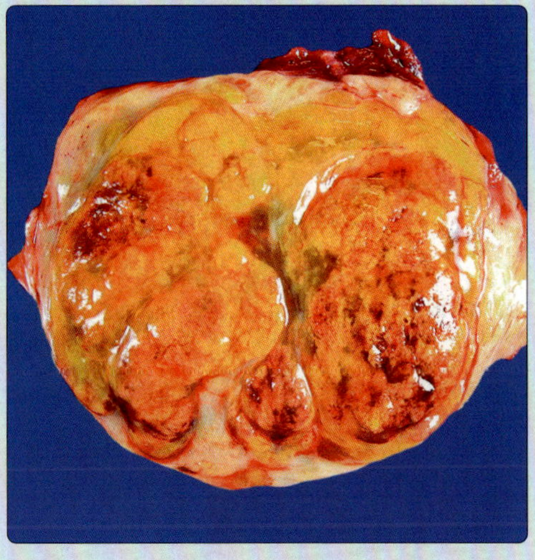

Sharp Circumscription

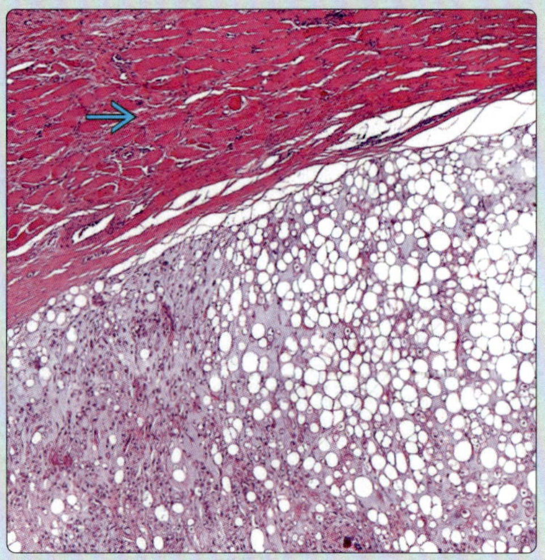

(Left) *Chondroid lipoma is classically a very well-circumscribed lesion with a multilobulated and yellow to tan cut surface. As in other forms of lipoma, foci of hemorrhage may be identified.* **(Right)** *Chondroid lipoma is usually sharply delineated from adjacent tissues and may or may not be encapsulated. It can occur in both superficial and deep soft tissues, the latter evidenced in this case by the presence of surrounding mature skeletal muscle ➔.*

Multilobulated Growth

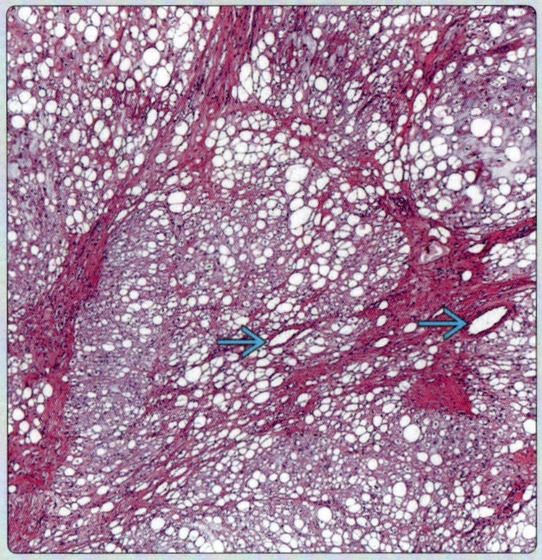

Classic Appearance

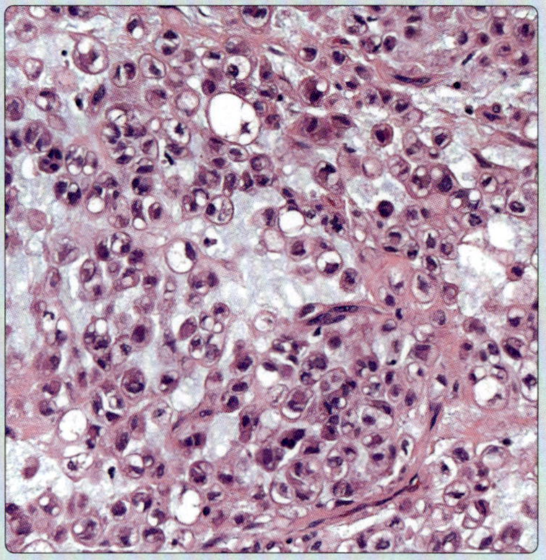

(Left) *Most cases of chondroid lipoma show a multilobulated growth pattern with each lobule delineated by a thin or thick fibrous septa. Dilated blood vessels ➔ are also abundant and conspicuous in this tumor.* **(Right)** *The classic image of chondroid lipoma shows a mixture of rounded eosinophilic cells with 1 to several intracytoplasmic vacuoles deposited in a myxochondroid matrix. Some cells, however, are not vacuolated.*

TERMINOLOGY

Definitions

- Benign mesenchymal neoplasm composed of lipoblastic cells and mature adipocytes within myxochondroid matrix

CLINICAL ISSUES

Epidemiology

- Incidence
  - Very rare
- Age
  - Adults (20-40 years most common)
- Sex
  - Strong female predilection (4:1)

Site

- Predominantly proximal limbs and limb girdles
- Also trunk, head and neck (particularly oral cavity)
- Occurs in both superficial and deep soft tissue

Presentation

- Painless, slowly enlarging mass
  - History of recent enlargement in 1/2 of cases

Treatment

- Simple complete excision

Prognosis

- Benign
- Does not recur or metastasize

MACROSCOPIC

General Features

- Well circumscribed and frequently encapsulated
- Tan-yellow cut surface; occasionally with hemorrhagic foci

Size

- 1.5-11.0 cm (median: 4.0 cm)

MICROSCOPIC

Histologic Features

- Well circumscribed
- Often lobulated with fibrous septa
- Nests, sheets, and cords of uni- and multivacuolated epithelioid cells
  - Cells may appear to be in lacunar spaces (chondrocyte-like)
  - Some nonvacuolated tumor cells have granular eosinophilic cytoplasm
  - No significant nuclear atypia or mitotic activity
- Classic multivacuolated lipoblasts common
- Myxochondroid matrix
  - May be hyalinized
- Variable mature adipose tissue component
- Interspersed thick- and thin-walled vessels with variable hemorrhage and hemosiderin deposition
- Can show fibrosis, calcification, metaplastic bone

ANCILLARY TESTS

Immunohistochemistry

- Variable S100 protein (+) in lipoblast-like cells
- Rarely focal keratin (+)
- Smooth muscle actin, HMB-45, EMA (-)

Genetic Testing

- Characteristic chromosomal translocation
  - t(11;16)(q13;p12-13) with *C11orf95-MKL2* fusion
- No amplification of *MDM2* or *CDK4*

DIFFERENTIAL DIAGNOSIS

Soft Tissue Chondroma

- Occurs in fingers, toes, hands, feet
- Contains true hyaline cartilage
- Lacks adipocytic component

Atypical Lipomatous Tumor/Well-Differentiated Liposarcoma

- Often large, slowly growing
- Lobules of atypical fat separated by thick fibrous septa containing atypical "smudgy" stromal cells
- Multivacuolated lipoblasts may be few, absent, or numerous
- May show prominent myxoid stroma
- *MDM2* amplification

Myxoid Liposarcoma

- Bland spindle cell component
- Plexiform capillary vascular pattern (staghorn vessels)
- Cellular (round cell) myxoid liposarcoma has larger, ovoid cells with monomorphic nuclei
- Characteristic t(12;16) translocation involving *FUS* and *DDIT3*

Extraskeletal Myxoid Chondrosarcoma

- Often larger, slowly growing, and infiltrative
- Anastomosing cords of spindled to stellate cells in prominent myxoid stroma
- No adipose tissue or lipoblasts
- Characteristic translocations involving *NR4A3*

Myoepithelioma of Soft Tissue

- Lacks lipoblasts
- Most cases show diffuse keratin (+) &/or S100 protein (+)
- Variable expression of SMA, EMA, calponin, GFAP, desmin

SELECTED REFERENCES

1. Flucke U et al: Presence of C11orf95-MKL2 fusion is a consistent finding in chondroid lipomas: a study of eight cases. Histopathology. 62(6):925-30, 2013
2. Thway K et al: Chondroid lipoma: an update and review. Ann Diagn Pathol. 16(3):230-4, 2012
3. de Vreeze RS et al: Delineation of chondroid lipoma: an immunohistochemical and molecular biological analysis. Sarcoma. 2011:638403, 2011
4. Ballaux F et al: Chondroid lipoma is characterized by t(11;16)(q13;p12-13). Virchows Arch. 444(2):208-10, 2004
5. Kindblom LG et al: Chondroid lipoma: an ultrastructural and immunohistochemical analysis with further observations regarding its differentiation. Hum Pathol. 26(7):706-15, 1995
6. Meis JM et al: Chondroid lipoma. A unique tumor simulating liposarcoma and myxoid chondrosarcoma. Am J Surg Pathol. 17(11):1103-12, 1993

Chondroid Lipoma

(Left) *The constituent cell of chondroid lipoma is small and round, contains abundant eosinophilic cytoplasm, and has a small, bland nucleus with irregular contours. Focal enlargement* → *may be seen, but significant nuclear pleomorphism is not typically a feature.* **(Right)** *Chondroid lipoma resembles a cartilaginous tumor in part due to the presence of cells* → *with cytoplasmic vacuoles surrounding the nucleus that create a compressed peripheral rim of eosinophilic cytoplasm, simulating a chondrocyte within a lacuna.*

Eosinophilic Cells

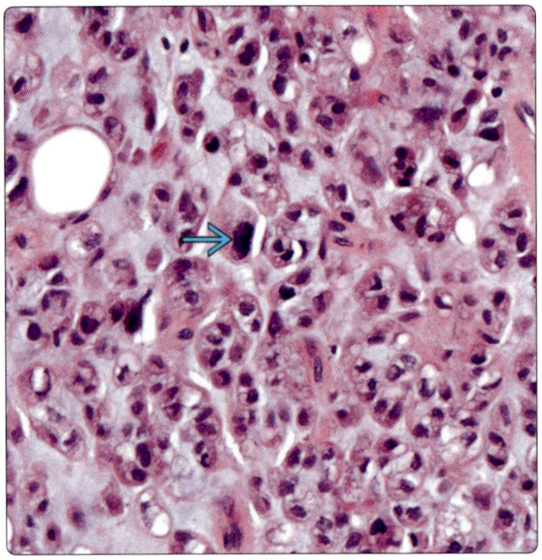

Chondroid Morphology

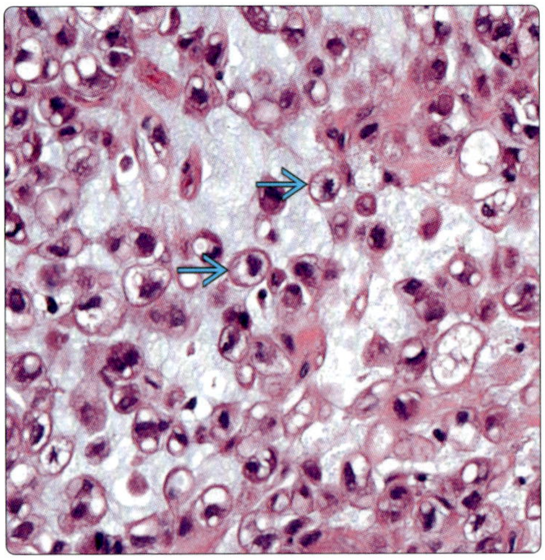

(Left) *Most cells of chondroid lipoma contain at least 1 cytoplasmic vacuole. In the cells that contain only 1* →*, the nucleus may be compressed at the periphery, reminiscent of a signet ring cell. When prominent, this morphology may be confused with carcinoma.* **(Right)** *Vague spindling of tumor cells is a rare and generally focal finding in chondroid lipoma and may lead to confusion with pleomorphic lipoma or even forms of liposarcoma.*

Univacuolated Cells

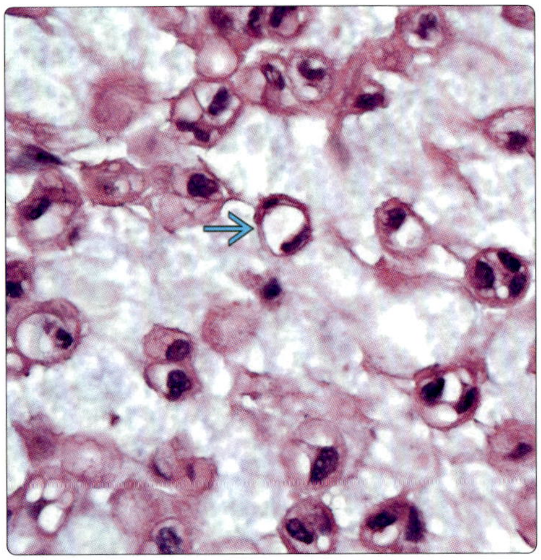

Rare Spindling of Tumor Cells

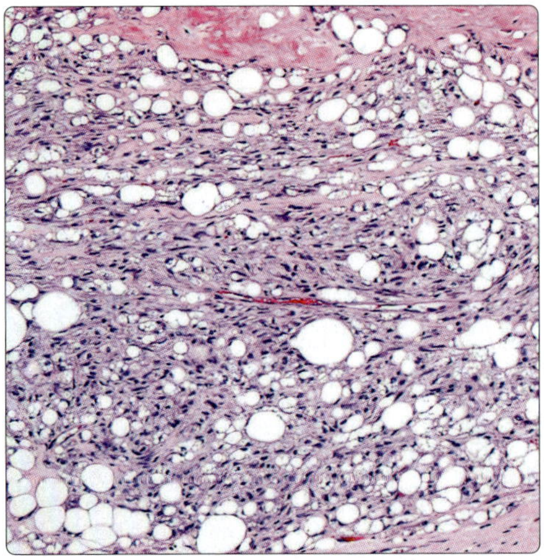

(Left) *Some of the multivacuolated tumor cells of chondroid lipoma are morphologically indistinguishable from the classic multivacuolated lipoblasts encountered in forms of liposarcoma. They vary in number from sparse to numerous but are usually quite abundant.* **(Right)** *A component of mature adipose tissue is almost always identified in chondroid lipoma, but the distribution varies from focal to extensive. In the latter setting, limited sampling may lead to diagnostic error.*

Multivacuolated Lipoblasts

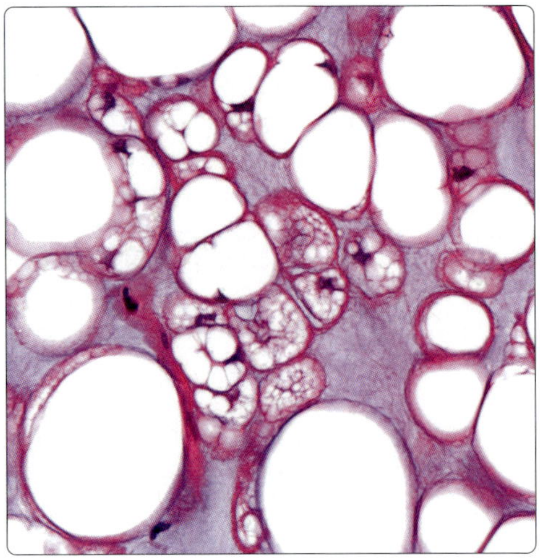

Mature Adipose Tissue

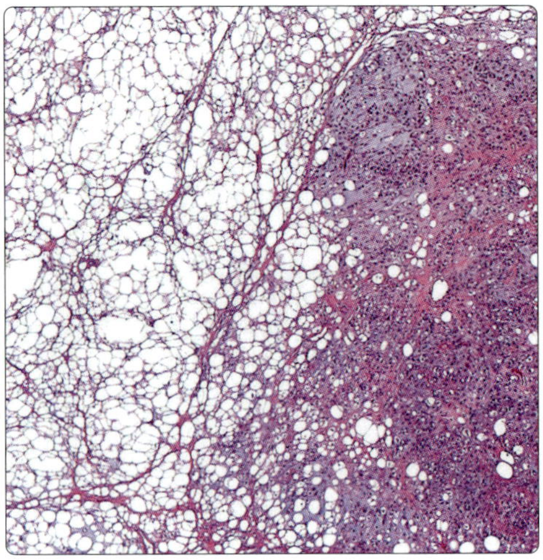

Mature Adipose Tissue

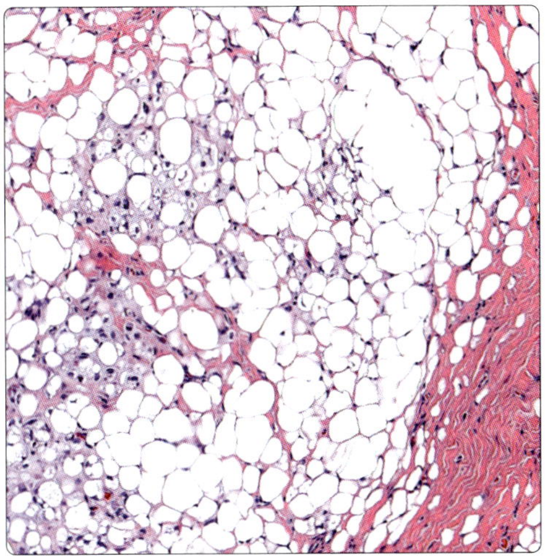

Myxoid Stroma

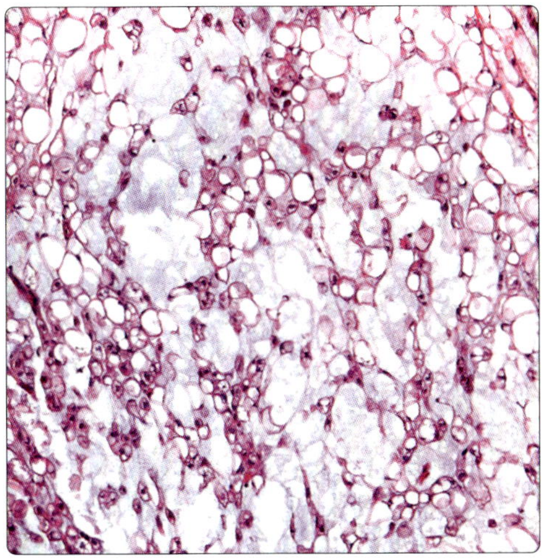

(Left) *In some cases of chondroid lipoma, the constituent tumor cells form small aggregates or nests within a background of abundant mature adipose tissue.* **(Right)** *Myxoid stroma is a common and relatively consistent feature of chondroid lipoma.*

Myxoid Stroma

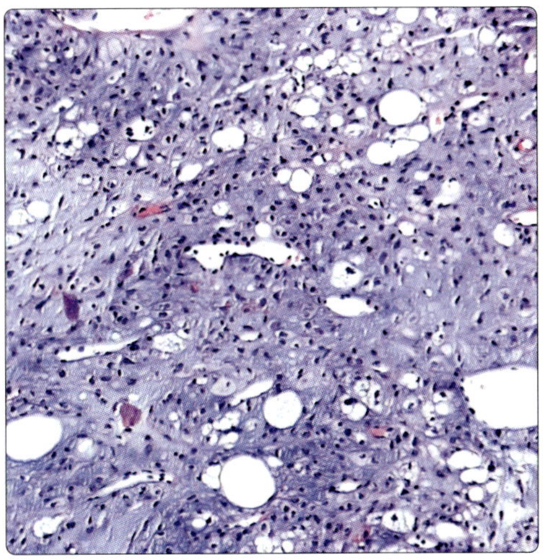

Hyalinized Stroma

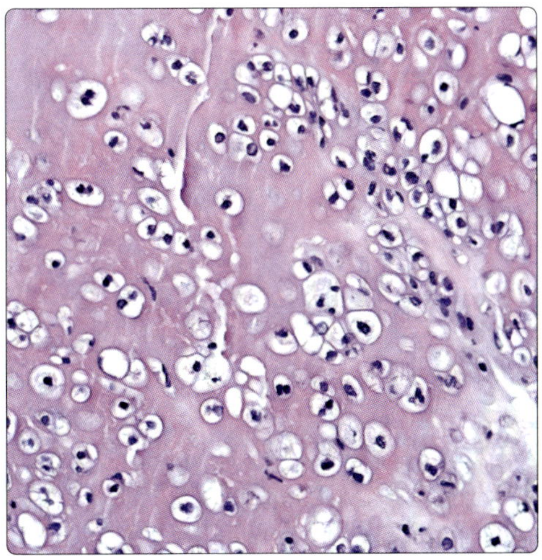

(Left) *In some heavily myxoid cases of chondroid lipoma, the overall appearance of scattered, small, bland tumor cells associated with adipose tissue and multivacuolated lipoblast-like cells may closely resemble a myxoid liposarcoma. However, chondroid lipoma does not demonstrate a delicate, plexiform vascular network.* **(Right)** *Foci of hyalinization are often intermingled with myxoid zones in chondroid lipoma; however, they are usually not prominent. In rare cases, the stroma is almost entirely hyalinized.*

Degenerative Changes

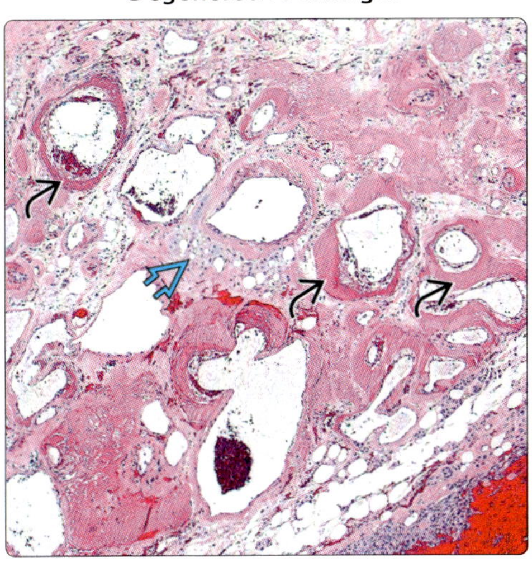

Conspicuous Vasculature

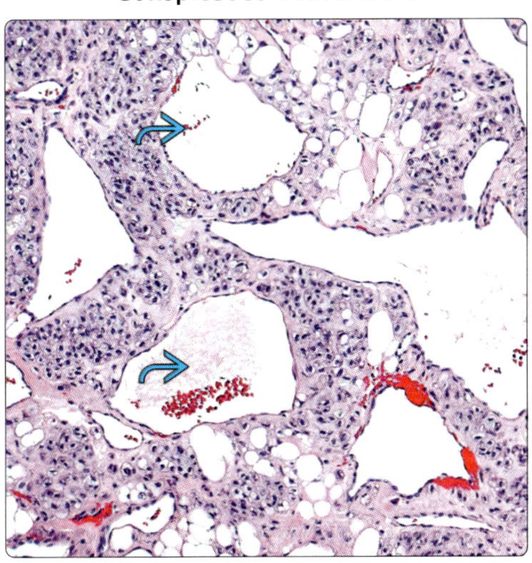

(Left) *This particular case of chondroid lipoma contained abundant degenerative changes, including prominent sclerosis, central ischemia, and perivascular hyalinization ↷. A small aggregate of tumor cells ⇨ can be identified at the center.* **(Right)** *Thin- to thick-walled dilated blood vessels ↷ are a common finding in chondroid lipoma and are often easily identified. They may be associated with stromal hemorrhage as well as hemosiderin deposition and fibrosis.*

Myolipoma

KEY FACTS

TERMINOLOGY

- Benign soft tissue neoplasm composed of mature adipose tissue & smooth muscle

CLINICAL ISSUES

- Adults; peak 5th-6th decades
- Female predilection
- Most occur in retroperitoneum, pelvis, inguinal region, & abdominal wall
- Excellent prognosis

MACROSCOPIC

- Intraabdominal tumors often large (mean: 10-15 cm)

MICROSCOPIC

- Mixture of mature adipose tissue & smooth muscle
  - Smooth muscle component is usually arranged in short fascicles
  - Adipose component consists of mature adipocytes
  - Muscle & fat evenly intermixed throughout tumor (sieve-like appearance)
  - Majority show smooth muscle predominance
- Scattered thin-walled vessels are often present but lack thick-walled muscular arteries
- Lack cytologic atypia
- Mitoses very rare or absent

ANCILLARY TESTS

- Smooth muscle markers (actins, desmin, calponin, H-caldesmon) (+) in spindle cell component
- Estrogen receptor (+) (86%) & HMGA2 (+) (60%)
- HMB-45, MART-1, CD34, & S100 protein (-)

TOP DIFFERENTIAL DIAGNOSES

- Angiomyolipoma (PEComa)
- Leiomyoma with fatty metaplasia/degeneration
- Dedifferentiated liposarcoma (with low-grade morphology)
- Spindle cell lipoma

Myolipoma

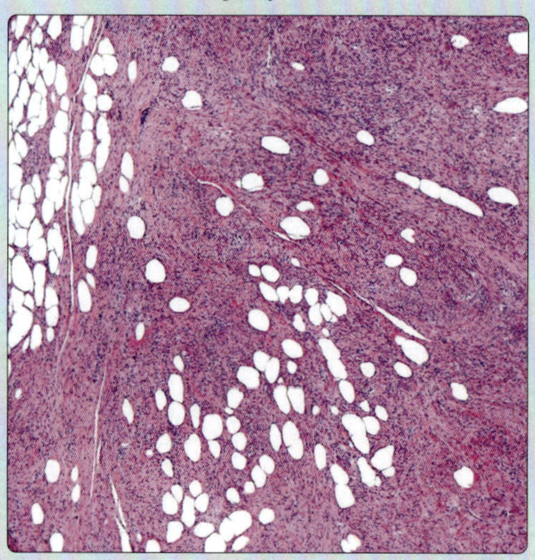

Sieve-Like Appearance

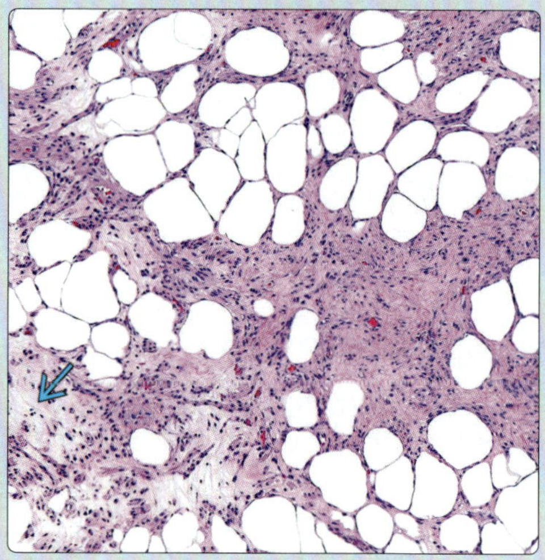

(Left) *Myolipoma is composed of an even admixture of smooth muscle and mature adipose tissue, imparting a sieve-like appearance. Most tumors have a predominance of smooth muscle, as demonstrated here in this example from the retroperitoneum.* **(Right)** *Eosinophilic smooth muscle cells intercalate between mature adipocytes in myolipoma. Hypocellular sclerotic and edematous areas are also present →. (Courtesy T. Bocklage, MD and R. Berry, MD.)*

Vague Fascicle Formation

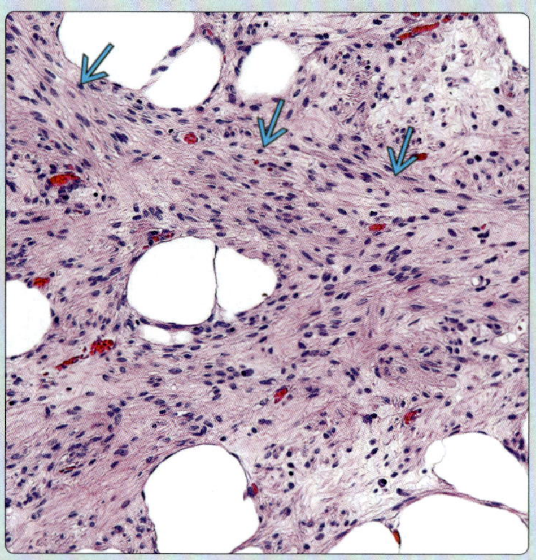

Desmin Expression

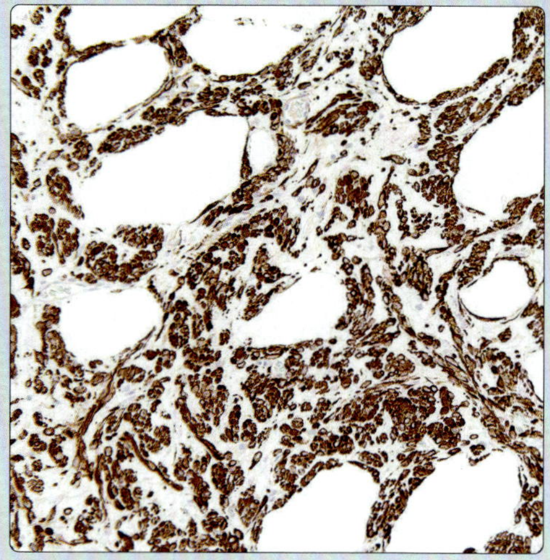

(Left) *Vague fascicle formation → by smooth muscle cells is often seen in myolipoma. Note also the component of mature adipose tissue. (Courtesy T. Bocklage, MD and R. Berry, MD.)* **(Right)** *The smooth muscle component of myolipoma displays strong, diffuse desmin expression. (Courtesy T. Bocklage, MD and R. Berry, MD.)*

TERMINOLOGY

Synonyms

- Extrauterine lipoleiomyoma

Definitions

- Benign soft tissue neoplasm composed of mature adipose tissue & smooth muscle

CLINICAL ISSUES

Epidemiology

- Incidence
  - Rare
- Age
  - Adults; peak in 5th-6th decades
- Sex
  - Female predilection

Site

- Most occur in retroperitoneum, pelvis, inguinal canal, & abdominal wall
- Less often occurs in extremities (subcutaneous or deep)

Presentation

- Painless mass
- May be incidentally discovered if deep

Treatment

- Complete surgical excision is treatment of choice

Prognosis

- Excellent prognosis
- Very low risk of recurrence after complete excision
- No metastatic potential

MACROSCOPIC

General Features

- Circumscribed & typically encapsulated
- Yellow to tan-white depending on relative amounts of fat & muscle
- More white-gray, firm, & whorled cut surface if muscle component predominates

Size

- Intraabdominal tumors often large (mean: 10-15 cm)
  - Usually much smaller when superficially located

MICROSCOPIC

Histologic Features

- Mixture of variable amounts of mature adipose tissue & smooth muscle
  - Majority show smooth muscle predominance
  - Muscle & fat evenly intermixed throughout tumor (sieve-like appearance)
- Smooth muscle component composed of elongated spindle cells with abundant eosinophilic fibrillary cytoplasm
  - Usually arranged in short intersecting fascicles
  - May have paranuclear vacuoles
  - Lack cytologic atypia
  - Mitoses very rare or absent
- Adipose component consists of mature adipocytes
  - No lipoblasts or floret-type giant cells
- Background sclerosis or chronic inflammation may be prominent
- Lacks thick-walled muscular arteries; scattered thin-walled vessels often present
- Similar appearance to uterine lipoleiomyoma but unrelated
- Rare unusual features may be present focally
  - Hypercellular fascicles, degenerative nuclear atypia, round cell morphology, hemosiderin deposition, metaplastic bone/cartilage, eosinophil infiltrates

ANCILLARY TESTS

Immunohistochemistry

- Smooth muscle markers (actins, desmin, calponin, H-caldesmon) (+) in spindle cell component
- Estrogen receptor (+) (86%) & HMGA2(+) (60%)
- HMB-45, MART-1, CD34, & S100 protein (-)
- MDM2 & CDK4 (-)

In Situ Hybridization

- Rearrangements of *HMGA2* gene
  - Also seen in conventional lipomas & uterine leiomyomas

DIFFERENTIAL DIAGNOSIS

Angiomyolipoma (PEComa)

- Granular or clear plump/epithelioid smooth muscle cells spin off of thick-walled muscular vessels
- Express HMB-45 &/or MART-1 with actin &/or desmin

Leiomyoma With Fatty Metaplasia/Degeneration

- Focal rather than uniform (sieve-like) distribution of fat throughout muscle component of tumor
- Fatty degeneration common in uterine leiomyomas, seen in subset of subcutaneous leiomyomas

Dedifferentiated Liposarcoma (Low-Grade Morphology)

- Can have myogenic differentiation & thus mimic myolipoma
- Diagnostic, large, hyperchromatic, atypical spindle cells present in adipocytic component
- Spindle cell component displays atypia & mitotic activity
- Often HMGA2 (+) (like myolipoma)
- *MDM2* & *CDK4* amplification by FISH (unlike myolipoma)

Spindle Cell Lipoma

- Exceedingly rare in retroperitoneum & pelvis
- May also have sieve-like admixture of fat & spindle cells
  - Spindle cells are not smooth muscle by H&E & IHC
    - No eosinophilic fibrillary cytoplasm or paranuclear vacuoles
    - Myoid markers usually (-)

SELECTED REFERENCES

1. Fukushima M et al: Myolipoma of soft tissue: clinicopathologic analysis of 34 cases. Am J Surg Pathol. 41(2):153-160, 2017
2. Panagopoulos I et al: Fusion of the HMGA2 and C9orf92 genes in myolipoma with t(9;12)(p22;q14). Diagn Pathol. 11:22, 2016
3. Michal M: Retroperitoneal myolipoma. A tumour mimicking retroperitoneal angiomyolipoma and liposarcoma with myosarcomatous differentiation. Histopathology. 25(1):86-8, 1994
4. Meis JM et al: Myolipoma of soft tissue. Am J Surg Pathol. 15(2):121-5, 1991

(Left) *Some myolipomas, such as this pelvic tumor, have a predominance of mature adipose tissue. The smooth muscle component intercalates between mature adipocytes.* **(Right)** *In some areas, the myogenic component of myolipoma may predominate. Bland smooth muscle cells are arranged into long fascicles similar to a leiomyoma. There is no atypia, and mitotic activity is minimal. Scattered mast cells are present in this case ➡. (Courtesy T. Bocklage, MD and R. Berry, MD.)*

Fat Predominant Tumors

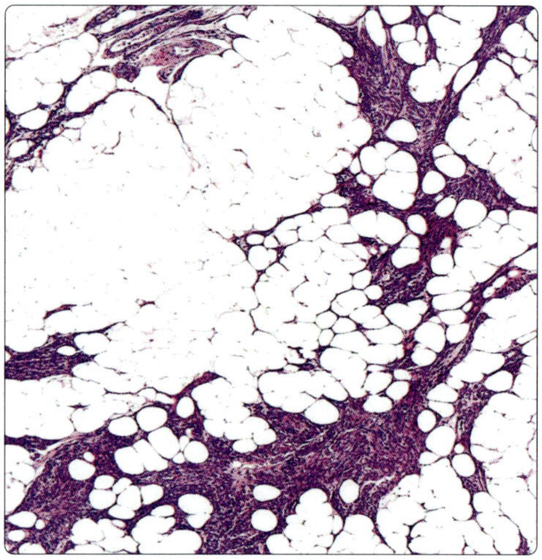

Smooth Muscle Predominant Tumors

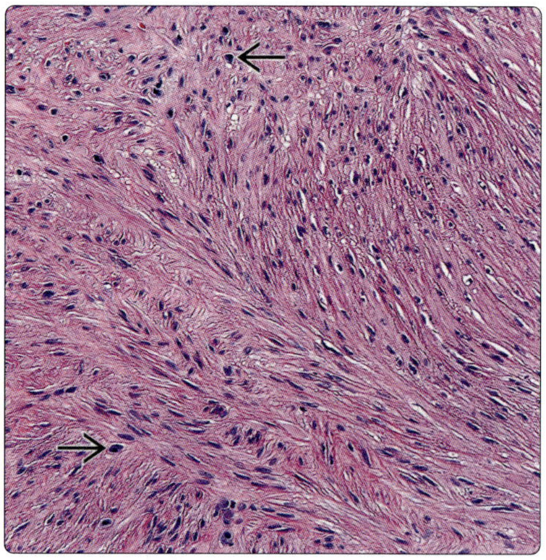

(Left) *At low power, myolipoma has a well-circumscribed border ➡ and lacks a capsule. Smooth muscle may predominate at the periphery, as depicted, with the bulk of the tumor interior composed of fat.* **(Right)** *Mature adipocytes are evenly distributed in a sieve-like pattern throughout the pink smooth muscle component of myolipoma. Hypocellular edematous areas are also present ➡. (Courtesy T. Bocklage, MD and R. Berry, MD.)*

Myolipoma

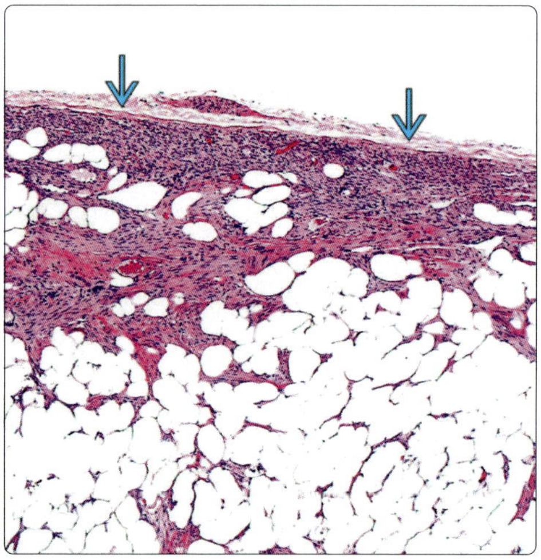

Hypocellular Edematous Areas

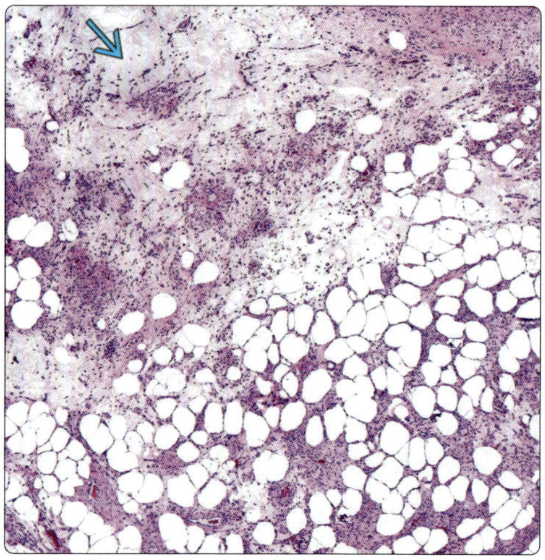

(Left) *Smooth muscle cells with intervening edema ➡ are seen on this H&E. (Courtesy T. Bocklage, MD and R. Berry, MD.)* **(Right)** *Dilated, thin-walled vessels ➡ are typical of myolipoma, but medium-sized muscular arteries, as would be seen in angiomyolipoma (PEComa), are not present.*

Edematous Foci

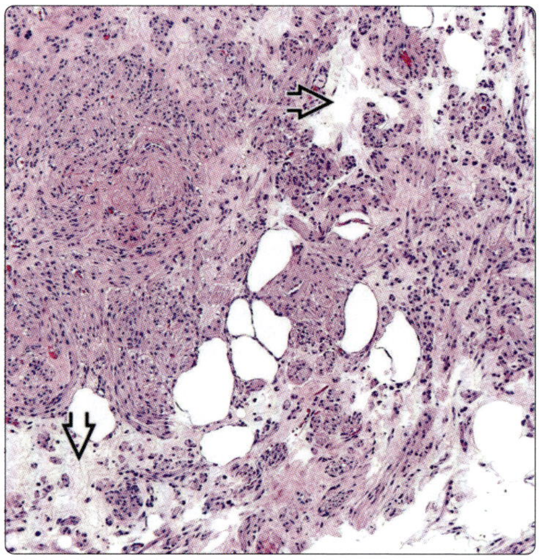

Thin-Walled Vessels

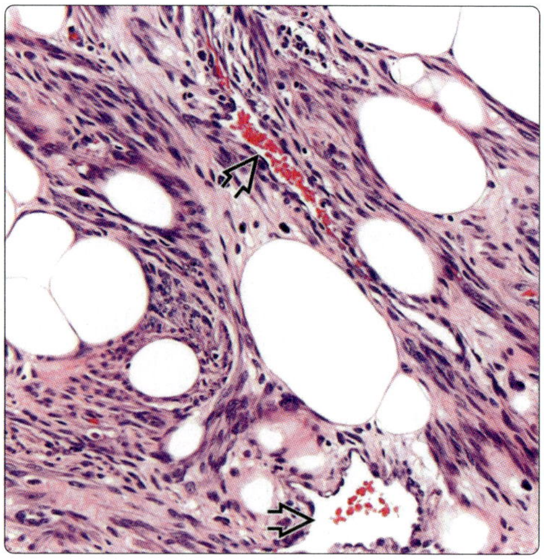

Foci of Sclerosis

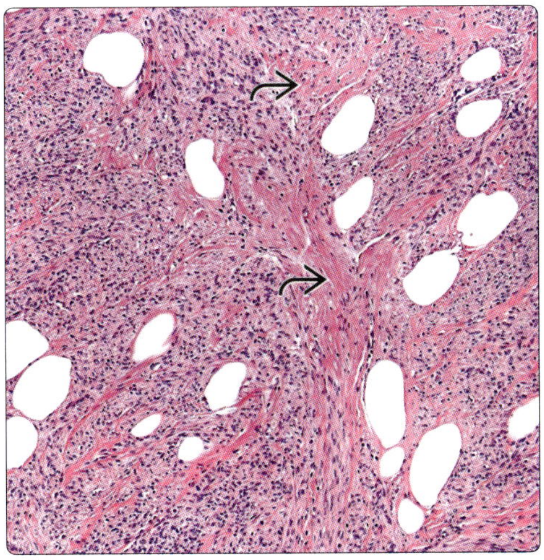

Foci of Sclerosis

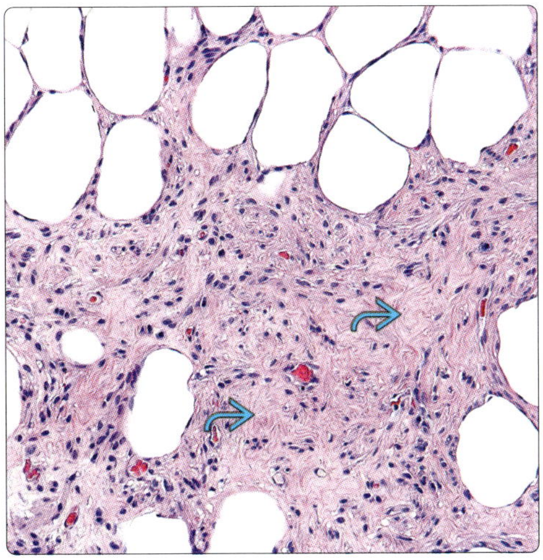

(Left) *Intermediate-power H&E shows evenly dispersed adipose tissue and short fascicles of smooth muscle, the typical appearance of myolipoma. Focal areas of sclerosis can be seen.* **(Right)** *The smooth muscle cells and mature adipocytes that comprise myolipoma lack atypia and mitotic activity. Background sclerosis may be present. (Courtesy T. Bocklage, MD and R. Berry, MD.)*

Fascicle Formation

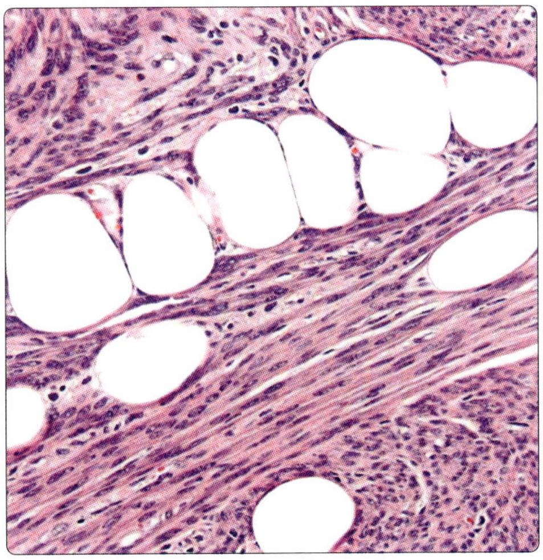

Focal Round Cell Morphology

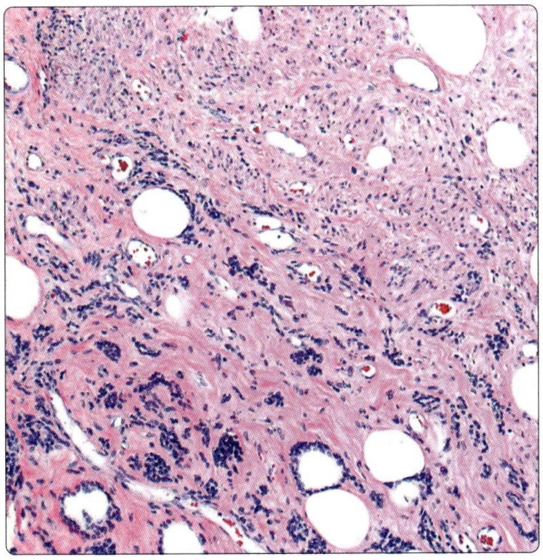

(Left) *Short fascicles of elongated spindle cells with oval, cytologically bland nuclei and abundant eosinophilic fibrillary cytoplasm are seen in myolipoma, similar to leiomyoma.* **(Right)** *Rare cases of myolipoma contain foci of tumor cells featuring a small round cell morphology (bottom left) rather than the usual spindling. These cells are cytologically banal, and the finding is of no clinical or prognostic significance.*

Minimal Atypia and Mitotic Activity

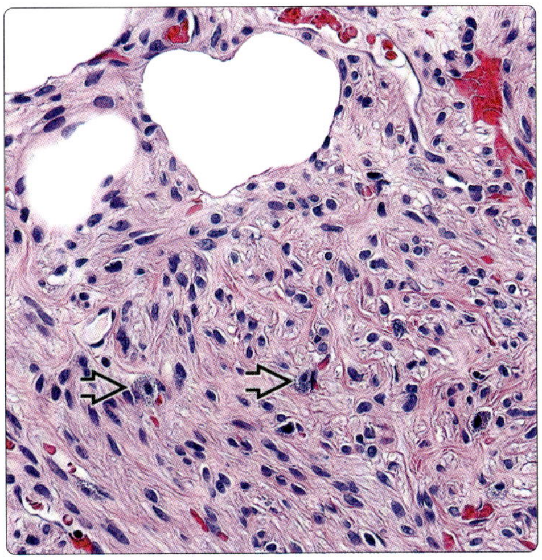

Sclerotic and Edematous Areas

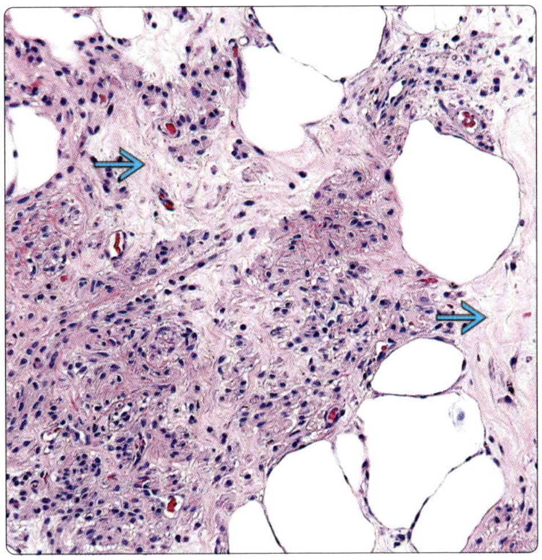

(Left) *The smooth muscle cells of myolipoma lack atypia and significant mitotic activity. Mast cells are also present on this H&E. (Courtesy T. Bocklage, MD and R. Berry, MD.)* **(Right)** *Hypocellular areas of sclerosis and edema may be present in myolipoma, as depicted. (Courtesy T. Bocklage, MD and R. Berry, MD.)*

Hibernoma

KEY FACTS

TERMINOLOGY

- Benign lipomatous tumor composed of lobules of cells resembling brown fat

CLINICAL ISSUES

- Age: 20-40 years most common
- Painless, slow-growing mass
- Most common in thigh, upper trunk, & neck
    - Subcutaneous (most common) or intramuscular
- Treatment: Simple surgical excision
- Benign; very rare recurrences

MACROSCOPIC

- Circumscribed, lobulated lesion
- Tan-yellow to yellow-brown, greasy cut surface
- Mean size: 9.3 cm

MICROSCOPIC

- Lobulated tumor composed of mixture of cell types in varying proportions
    - Polygonal cells with granular eosinophilic cytoplasm, multivacuolated cells, univacuolated adipocytes
- Small, bland, central nuclei ± nucleoli
- Stromal vessels are common & may be prominent
- Morphologic variants: Lipoma-like, myxoid, spindle cell

ANCILLARY TESTS

- Variable S100 protein (+)
- Molecular: Rearrangements of 11q13-21

TOP DIFFERENTIAL DIAGNOSES

- Normal brown fat
- Lipoblastoma
- Atypical lipomatous tumor/well-differentiated liposarcoma

Hibernoma

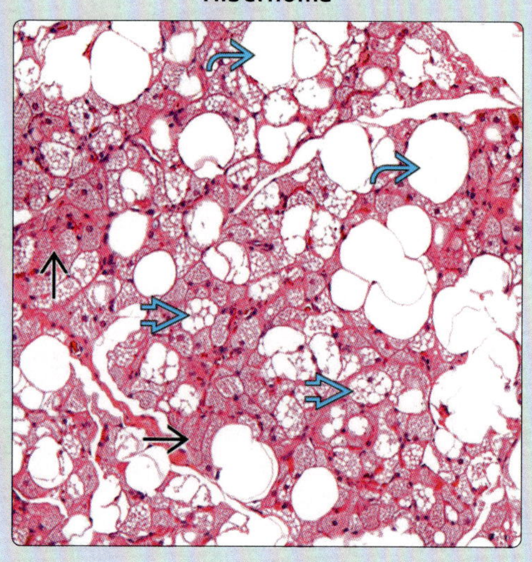

Multivacuolated Cells

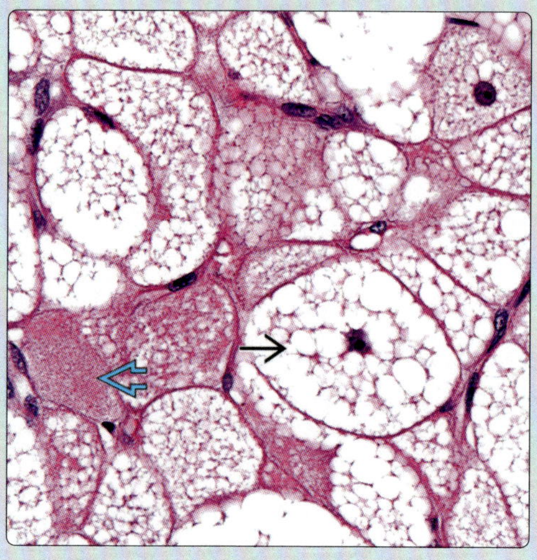

(Left) *Hibernoma is a benign lipomatous neoplasm composed of cells resembling brown fat. This classic case shows a mixture of granular eosinophilic cells →, multivacuolated cells →, & scattered univacuolated mature adipocytes →.* **(Right)** *The multivacuolated cells → usually contain innumerable lipid droplets & resemble multivacuolated lipoblasts, however, the latter have enlarged, hyperchromatic, & scalloped nuclei. The eosinophilic cells → get their coloration from numerous mitochondria.*

Prominent Vacuoles

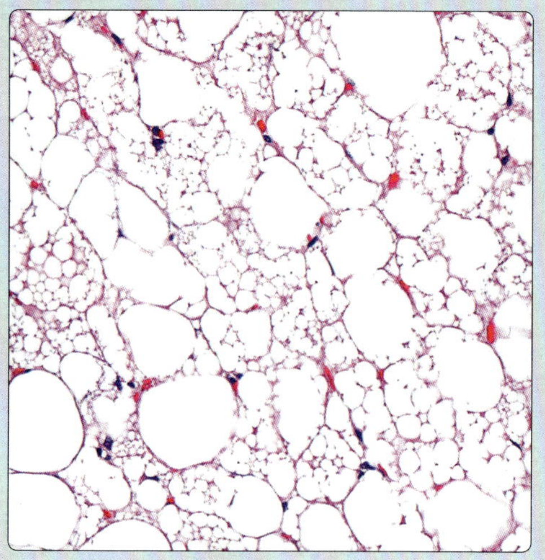

Lipoma-Like Hibernoma

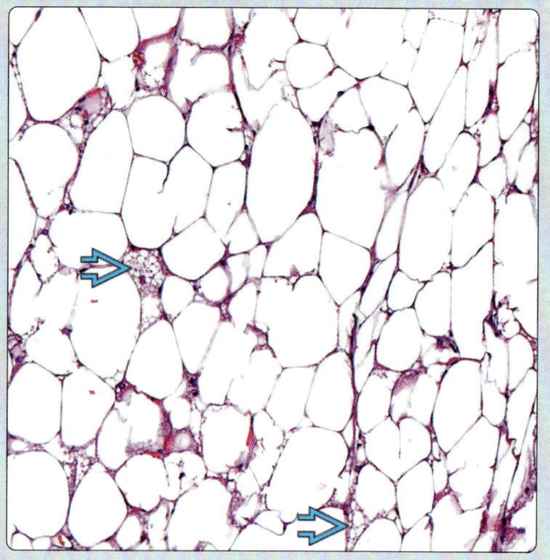

(Left) *Multivacuolated cells can be prominent & diffuse in some cases of hibernoma. Such cases often resemble the multivacuolated lipoblasts of atypical lipomatous tumor/well-differentiated liposarcoma. Enlarged, scalloped nuclei are absent in hibernoma, however.* **(Right)** *Occasional cases of hibernoma show predominantly univacuolated white fat cells with only scattered multivacuolated → & eosinophilic granular cells. These tumors may be easily misclassified as conventional lipoma.*

TERMINOLOGY

Synonyms

- Fetal lipoma
- Lipoma of embryonic fat

Definitions

- Benign lipomatous tumor composed of lobules of cells resembling brown fat

CLINICAL ISSUES

Epidemiology

- Age
  - 20-40 years most common
  - Rare in children & elderly > 60 years

Site

- Subcutaneous (most common) or intramuscular
- Most common in thigh
  - Also neck, arm, trunk, back, shoulder, & retroperitoneum
    - Rarely breast, kidney, or mediastinum

Presentation

- Painless, slow-growing mass

Treatment

- Simple surgical excision

Prognosis

- Benign
- Recurrences are very rare

MACROSCOPIC

General Features

- Circumscribed, lobulated lesions
- Tan-yellow to yellow-brown, greasy cut surface

Size

- Range: 1-24 cm (mean: 9.3 cm)

MICROSCOPIC

Histologic Features

- Lobulated tumor composed of mixture of cell types in varying proportions
  - Polygonal cells with granular eosinophilic cytoplasm
  - Multivacuolated cells with numerous lipid droplets
  - Univacuolated adipocytes
- Medium-sized stromal vessels are common & may be prominent
- Small, bland, central nuclei ± nucleoli
- Mitotic figures are rare

Morphologic Variants

- Lipoma-like
  - Mostly univacuolated adipocytes
  - Eosinophilic granular & multivacuolated cells are sparse
  - Most common in thigh
- Myxoid
  - Predominantly occurs in male patients
    - In head & neck
  - Constituent cells separated by acellular myxoid stroma
- Spindle cell
  - Hybrid features of hibernoma & spindle cell lipoma
    - Hibernoma cells, thick collagen bundles, mast cells, mature fat
  - Rare
    - Found in posterior neck or scalp

ANCILLARY TESTS

Immunohistochemistry

- Variable S100 protein (+)
- Spindle cell variant is often CD34(+)
- UCP1(+) in brown fat cells

Molecular Genetics

- Rearrangements of 11q13-21 common & characteristic
- Concomitant deletions of tumor suppressor genes *AIP* & *MEN1*

DIFFERENTIAL DIAGNOSIS

Normal Brown Fat

- More abundant in children & young adults than older adults
- Usually found in neck, axilla, mediastinum, & paraspinal regions
- No discrete mass lesion

Lipoblastoma

- May contain brown fat cells
- Usually occurs in infants (< 3 years of age)
- Prominent lobularity with myxoid stroma & lipoblasts
- *PLAG1* gene rearrangements

Atypical Lipomatous Tumor/Well-Differentiated Liposarcoma

- Atypical "smudge" cells in thickened fibrous septa
- True lipoblasts with hyperchromatic scalloped nuclei may be present
- MDM2 amplification by FISH

Granular Cell Tumor

- Diffuse cytoplasmic granularity
- No multivacuolated cells
- Diffuse S100 protein (+)

Myxoid Liposarcoma

- Delicate, plexiform vascular pattern; lipoblasts common
- Hibernoma-like cells uncommon
- Characteristic t(12;16) or t(12;22)

SELECTED REFERENCES

1. Greenbaum A et al: Hibernoma: diagnostic and surgical considerations of a rare benign tumour. BMJ Case Rep. 2016, 2016
2. Vassos N et al: Deep-seated huge hibernoma of soft tissue: a rare differential diagnosis of atypical lipomatous tumor/well differentiated liposarcoma. Int J Clin Exp Pathol. 6(10):2178-84, 2013
3. Manieri M et al: Morphological and immunohistochemical features of brown adipocytes and preadipocytes in a case of human hibernoma. Nutr Metab Cardiovasc Dis. Oct;20(8):567-74, 2010
4. Chirieac LR et al: Characterization of the myxoid variant of hibernoma. Ann Diagn Pathol. 10(2):104-6, 2006
5. Furlong MA et al: The morphologic spectrum of hibernoma: a clinicopathologic study of 170 cases. Am J Surg Pathol. 25(6):809-14, 2001

(Left) *Hibernoma with sheets of eosinophilic cells can resemble granular cell tumor or even oncocytoma. Intracytoplasmic material resembling mucin can also be seen focally in some cases.* **(Right)** *Hibernoma often has a lobulated appearance at low magnification. These tumors are highly vascular as well, as evidenced by the prominent large blood vessels seen in most cases. Small lymphoid aggregates may be present as well.*

Prominent Eosinophilic Cells

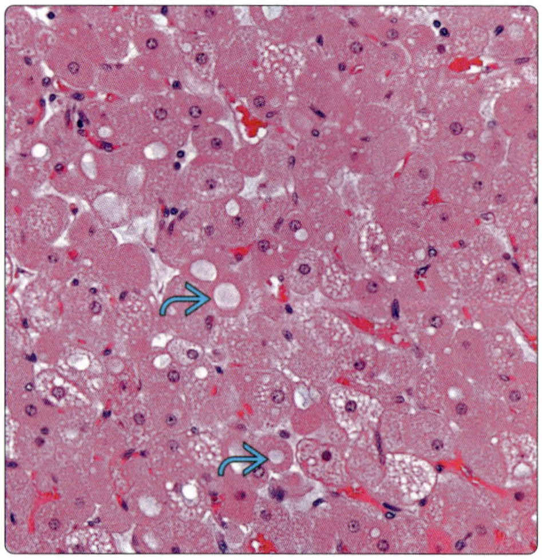

Vasculature

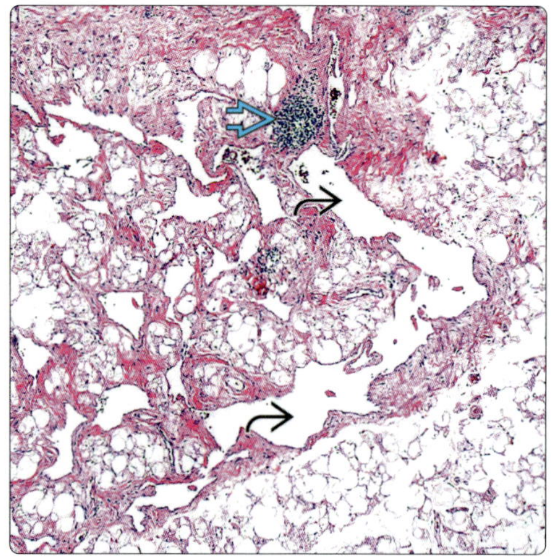

(Left) *Hibernoma can show areas with apparent hypervascularity, producing the appearance of cell clusters floating within clear spaces. In some cases, an endothelial lining can be appreciated.* **(Right)** *A rare variant of hibernoma features myxoid stromal change that may be diffuse. Scattered multivacuolated cells & mature adipocytes can be identified. Identification of other more typical areas of hibernoma is helpful.*

Angiomatous Pattern

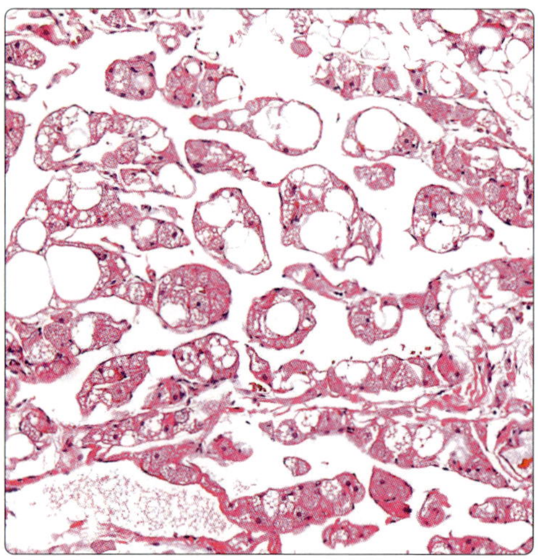

Myxoid Hibernoma

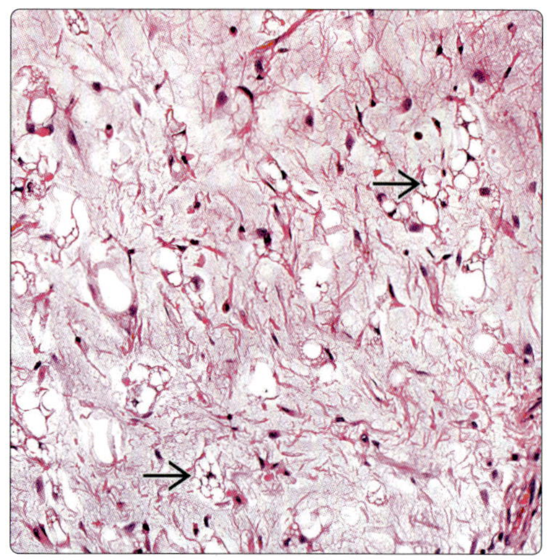

(Left) *In some cases of myxoid hibernoma, the stroma is less blue & myxoid & more pale & edematous. Note the scattered tumor cells.* **(Right)** *Hybrid tumors with features of hibernoma & spindle cell lipoma have been described, & most arise in the posterior neck & shoulder region. As expected, the spindle cells in such lesions are often CD34(+).*

Myxoedematous Stroma

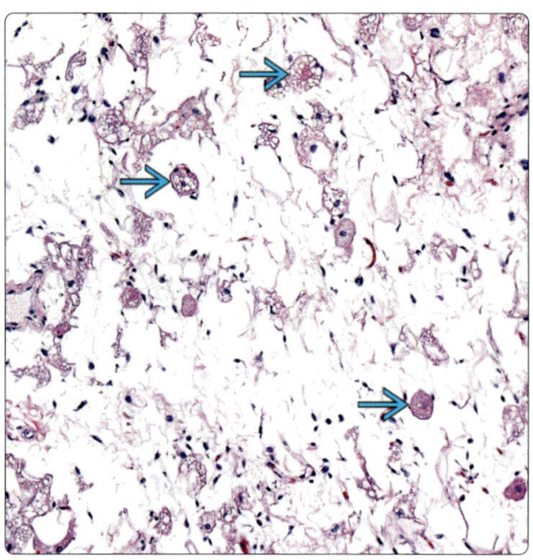

Spindle Cells in Hibernoma

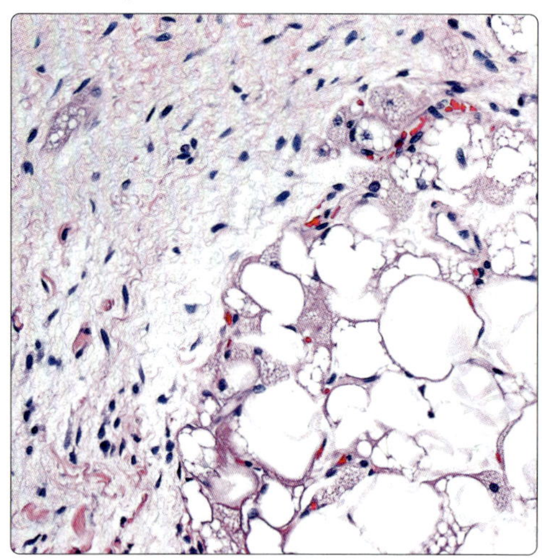

Skeletal Muscle

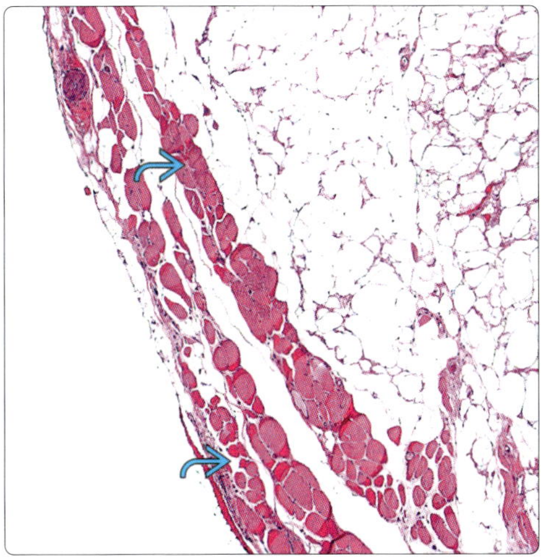

Cluster Morphology

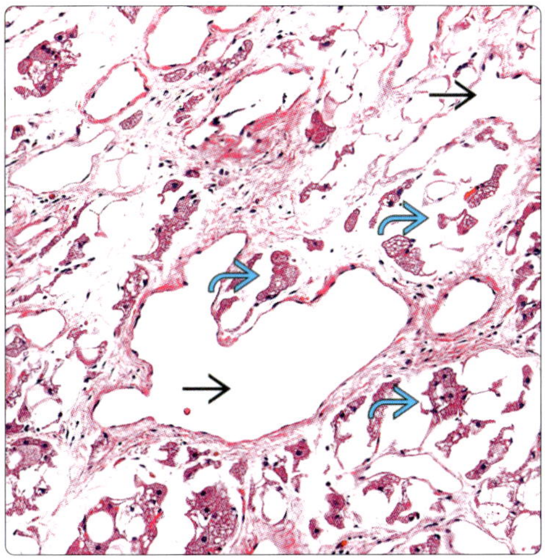

(Left) *Most cases of hibernoma arise within the subcutaneous fat of the extremity or neck, however, occasional tumors are more deeply located & may involve skeletal muscle* ↪. **(Right)** *In some cases, clusters of hibernoma cells* ↪ *may retract from each other, resembling a pattern often seen in mucinous epithelial tumors. Note the gaping vascular spaces* →, *a common feature of hibernoma.*

Frozen Section of Hibernoma

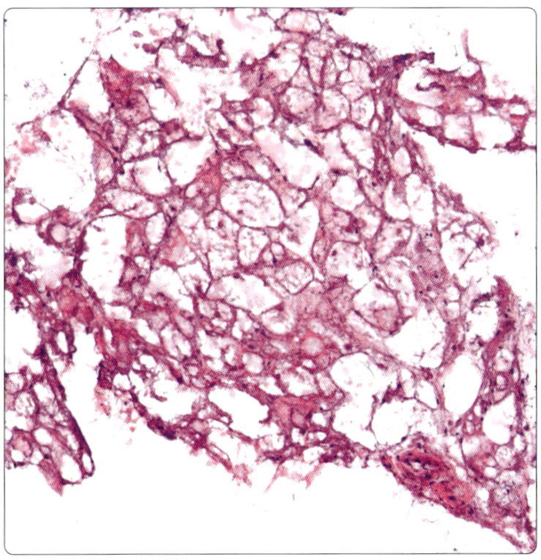

Infarcted Hibernoma

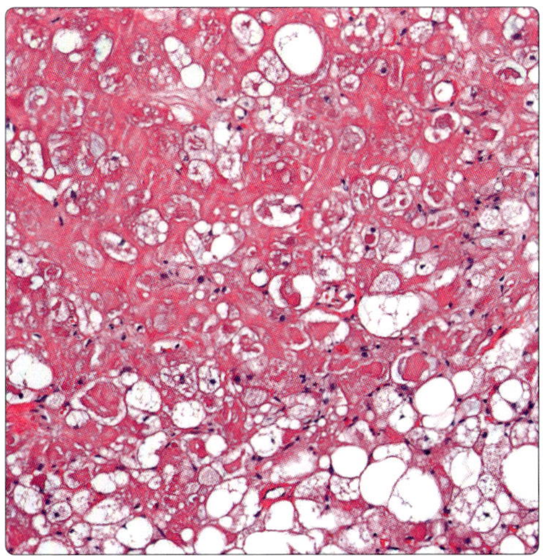

(Left) *Unlike white fat, which is very difficult to freeze & section adequately, brown fat cells with abundant mitochondria can often be visualized on frozen section, making a preliminary diagnosis possible.* **(Right)** *This case of a large hibernoma showed a centralized zone of infarction. In some of the interface areas, the dense eosinophilic appearance is somewhat reminiscent of hyalinized zones in chondroid lipoma.*

Focal Calcification

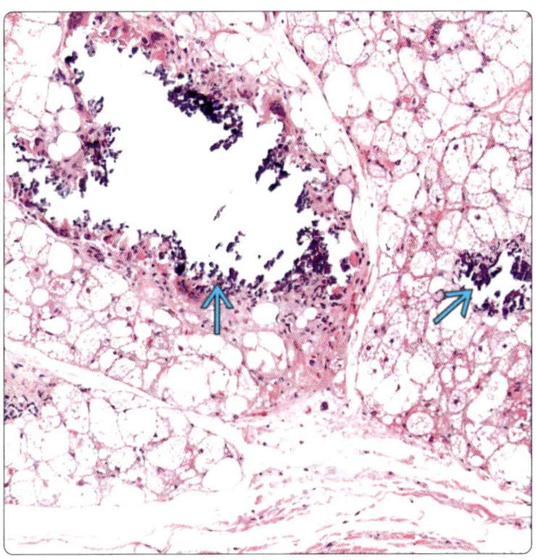

Mitochondria

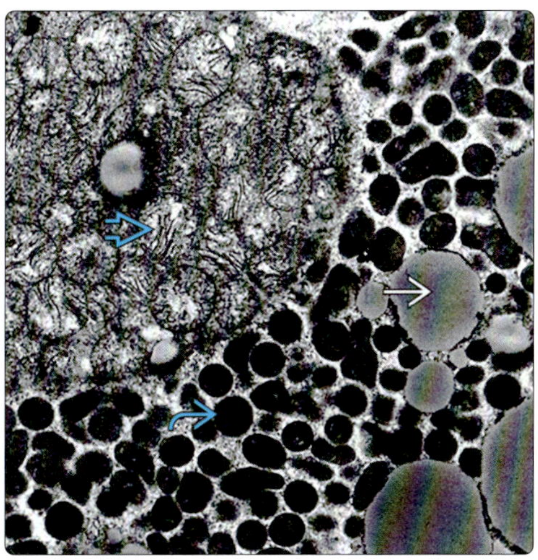

(Left) *As in other fatty tumors, calcification* → *may be present in hibernoma, particularly in the setting of local trauma, but it is rare. Fat necrosis & a multinucleated giant cell reaction can also rarely be seen.* **(Right)** *Electron micrograph of hibernoma shows numerous tightly packed mitochondria displaying transverse cristae* ⇨. *There are also small electron-dense lysosomes* ↪ & *lipid droplets* ➡.

Myelolipoma

KEY FACTS

TERMINOLOGY
- Benign, likely neoplastic proliferation composed of mature fat and hematopoietic tissues

ETIOLOGY/PATHOGENESIS
- Most are idiopathic
- Some associated with various endocrine neoplasms or hyperhormonal states

CLINICAL ISSUES
- Older adults, usually > 40 years
- Most common in adrenal gland
  - Extraadrenal locations rare
- Most are incidental findings and asymptomatic
- Treatment: Surgical excision or clinically follow
- Benign; overall excellent prognosis

MACROSCOPIC
- Well-circumscribed nodule
- Yellow-tan cut surface with red-gray areas
- Most are < 5 cm but may be larger

MICROSCOPIC
- Sharply circumscribed, often with rim of adrenal cortex
- Mature adipose tissue without atypia or lipoblasts
- Mature bone marrow hematopoietic elements
  - All 3 cell lines (myeloid, erythroid, megakaryocytic) represented
- Rare findings: Metaplastic bone, myxoid change

TOP DIFFERENTIAL DIAGNOSES
- Extramedullary hemopoiesis
- Conventional lipoma
- Well-differentiated liposarcoma
- Myeloid sarcoma (granulocytic sarcoma)
- Adrenocortical adenoma

Myelolipoma

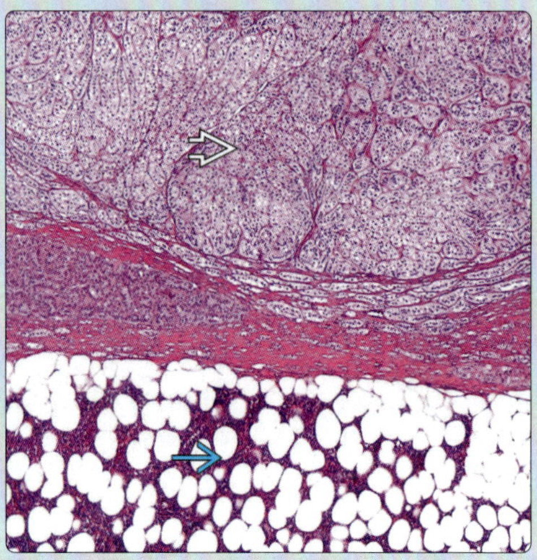

Hematopoietic Elements and Fat

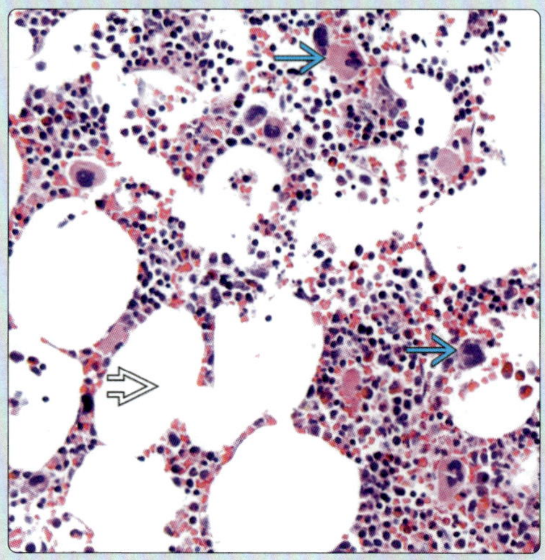

(Left) *Myelolipoma is a benign tumor that usually arises in the adrenal gland and rarely in other sites. There is a sharp demarcation between the adrenal cortex and the underlying lesion. The cortex is often thinned; however, this patient had adrenocortical hyperplasia, which may be seen in some cases.* **(Right)** *The hematopoietic component of myelolipoma consists of all 3 cell lines (erythroid, myeloid, and megakaryocytic). Note the admixed mature adipocytes.*

Mature Adipose Tissue

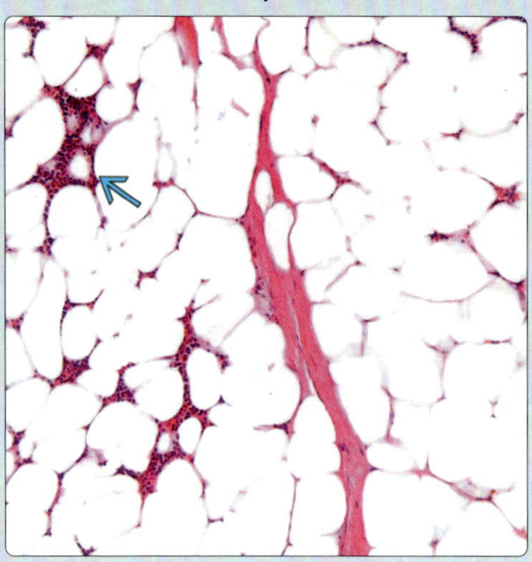

Rare Metaplastic Bone

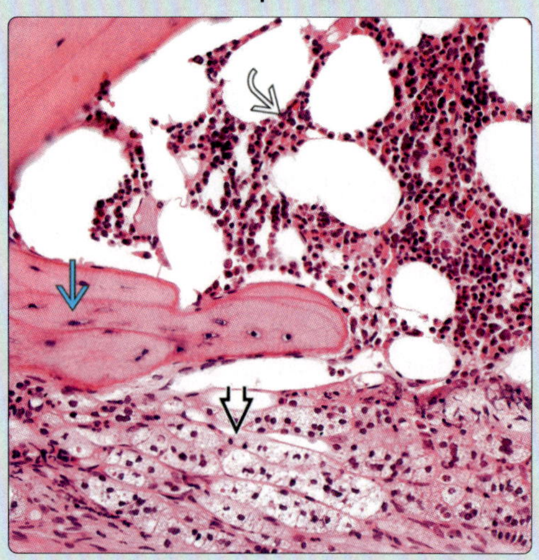

(Left) *The mature adipose tissue component often predominates in myelolipoma, and no atypical adipocytic/stromal nuclei or lipoblasts are present. In some cases, the hematopoietic elements may be sparse and easily overlooked.* **(Right)** *Metaplastic bone is an unusual finding in adrenal myelolipoma. Note peripheral adrenal cortical tissue, mature bone, and fatty hematopoietic lesional tissue.*

Myelolipoma

TERMINOLOGY

Definitions

- Benign, likely neoplastic proliferation composed of mature fat and hematopoietic tissues

ETIOLOGY/PATHOGENESIS

Idiopathic

- Most cases

Associated Conditions

- Hormonally active endocrine neoplasms
  - Adrenocortical adenoma, adrenocortical carcinoma, pheochromocytoma
- Hypercortisolic or hyperaldosteronic states
  - Adrenal cortical hyperplasia, Conn syndrome, 21-hydroxylase deficiency
- Obesity

CLINICAL ISSUES

Epidemiology

- Incidence
  - Rare
- Age
  - Older adults, usually > 40 years
- Sex
  - M = F

Site

- Most common in adrenal gland
- Extraadrenal locations rare
  - Retroperitoneum, presacral region, mediastinum, others

Presentation

- Most are incidental findings and asymptomatic
- Large lesions may cause abdominal symptoms
  - Massive acute hemorrhage in rare cases

Treatment

- Surgical excision is curative
- Small lesions may be followed without surgery

Prognosis

- Benign
- Excellent prognosis
  - Very rare spontaneous rupture and hemorrhage reported

IMAGING

Radiographic Findings

- Circumscribed lucent mass, often in adrenal gland

MACROSCOPIC

General Features

- Well-circumscribed nodule
- Yellow-tan cut surface with red-gray areas

Size

- Usually small, and most are < 5 cm
- Rare examples are large (giant myelolipoma)

MICROSCOPIC

Histologic Features

- Sharply circumscribed, often with rim of adrenal cortex
- Mature adipose tissue without atypia or lipoblasts
- Mature bone marrow hematopoietic elements
  - May be extensive or sparse
  - All 3 cell lines (myeloid, erythroid, megakaryocytic) represented
  - Lymphoid foci may be present
- Rare findings: Metaplastic bone, myxoid change

ANCILLARY TESTS

Molecular Genetics

- Reports of t(3;21)(q25;p11) translocation
- Nonrandom X chromosome inactivation

DIFFERENTIAL DIAGNOSIS

Extramedullary Hemopoiesis

- Typically arises in patients with myeloproliferative disease or severe anemia
- Multiple deposits common
- Often associated with splenomegaly

Conventional Lipoma

- Encapsulated
- Lacks bone marrow elements

Well-Differentiated Liposarcoma

- Lacks myeloid elements
- Variably thickened fibrous septa containing enlarged, hyperchromatic stromal cells
- May contain lipoblasts

Myeloid Sarcoma

- Generally lacks fatty component
- Sheets of primitive myeloid cells
- Usually occurs in association with acute leukemia

Adrenocortical Adenoma

- Expansile proliferation of adrenocortical cells
- Lacks adipose tissue and bone marrow elements

SELECTED REFERENCES

1. Decmann Á et al: Adrenal myelolipoma: a comprehensive review. Endocrine. 59(1):7-15, 2018
2. Littrell LA et al: Extra-adrenal myelolipoma and extramedullary hematopoiesis: imaging features of two similar benign fat-containing presacral masses that may mimic liposarcoma. Eur J Radiol. 93:185-194, 2017
3. Shi Q et al: Primary mediastinal myelolipoma: a case report and literature review. J Thorac Dis. 9(3):E219-E225, 2017
4. Ramirez M et al: Adrenal myelolipoma: to operate or not? A case report and review of the literature. Int J Surg Case Rep. 5(8):494-496, 2014
5. Suárez-Peñaranda JM et al: Unusual forms of adrenal and extra-adrenal myelolipomas. Int J Surg Pathol. 22(5):473-477, 2014
6. Goltz JP et al: [Ruptured giant myelolipoma of the adrenal gland with acute retroperitoneal hemorrhage.] Rofo. 181(5):485-7, 2009
7. Bishop E et al: Adrenal myelolipomas show nonrandom X-chromosome inactivation in hematopoietic elements and fat: support for a clonal origin of myelolipomas. Am J Surg Pathol. 30(7):838-43, 2006
8. Chang KC et al: Adrenal myelolipoma with translocation (3;21)(q25;p11). Cancer Genet Cytogenet. 134(1):77-80, 2002
9. Sanders R et al: Clinical spectrum of adrenal myelolipoma: analysis of 8 tumors in 7 patients. J Urol. 153(6):1791-3, 1995

Lipoblastoma

KEY FACTS

TERMINOLOGY

- Well-circumscribed, benign, lobular lipomatous neoplasm with resemblance to fetal adipose tissue
  - Deep tumors with infiltrative borders may be designated "diffuse lipoblastoma" or "lipoblastomatosis"

CLINICAL ISSUES

- Majority occur in first 3 years of life
- 2:1 male predominance
- Trunk and extremities most common
  - May involve mediastinum, retroperitoneum, viscera
- Treatment: Complete surgical excision
- Benign; excellent prognosis
- Local recurrence likely related to incomplete excision

MACROSCOPIC

- Pale tan-yellow, variably gelatinous cut surface
- Usually 2-6 cm

MICROSCOPIC

- Most are well circumscribed and lobular
- Lobules of immature adipocytes in various states of development, separated by fibrous septa
  - Spindle/stellate cells, univacuolated and multivacuolated lipoblasts
- Myxoid stromal change is common
- Delicate capillary vasculature often present
- Recurrent tumors often show evidence of maturation (lipoma-like)

ANCILLARY TESTS

- Molecular: Rearrangement of 8q11-13 (*PLAG1*)

TOP DIFFERENTIAL DIAGNOSES

- Myxoid liposarcoma
- Lipoma
- Lipoblastoma-like tumor of vulva

Lipoblastoma

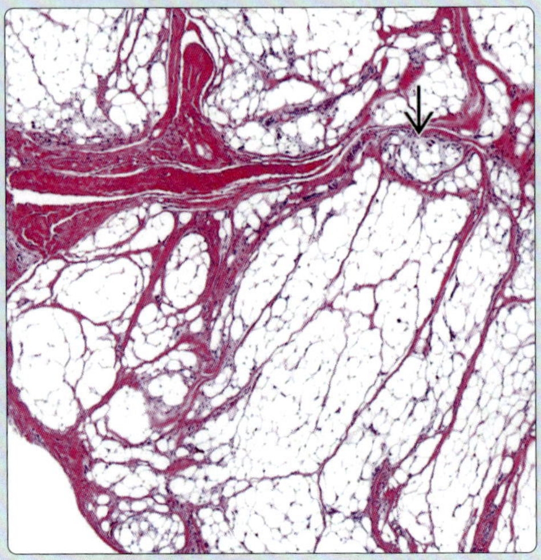

Fibrous Septa

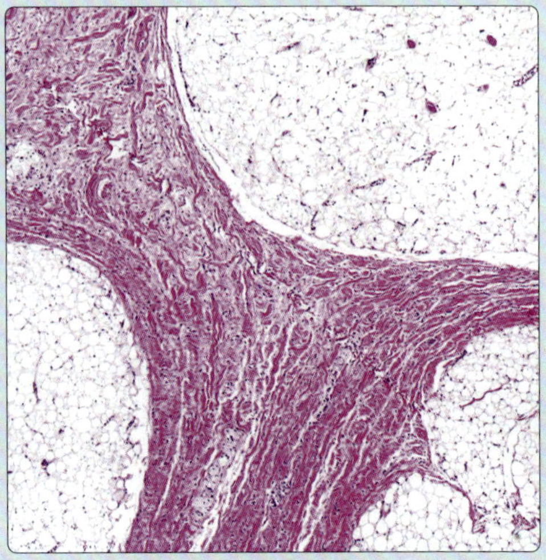

(Left) *Lipoblastoma is a benign adipocytic neoplasm that is most commonly identified in the first 3 years of life. At low magnification, it is characterized by a prominent lobularity imparted by extensive fibrous septation. Foci of myxoid change* ➙ *are also evident.* **(Right)** *In some cases of lipoblastoma, the fibrous septa are very thick, although the overall lobularity is retained. Rarely, the fibrous tissue may predominate over the fat component, suggesting a fibroblastic process.*

Immature Fat

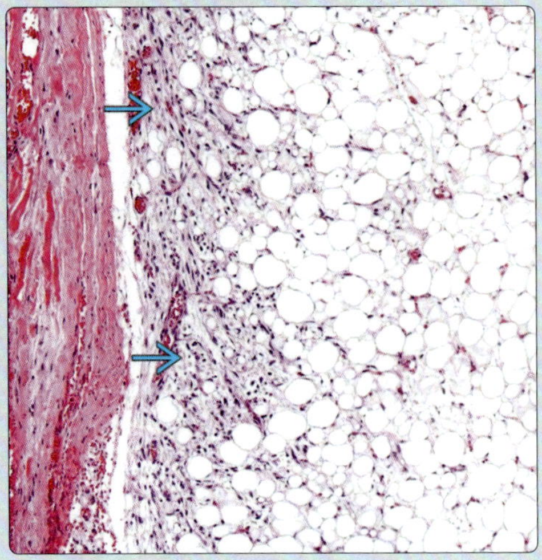

Immature Fat

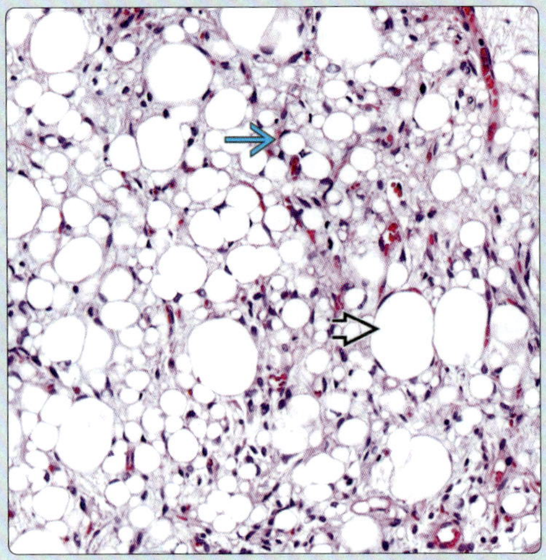

(Left) *The presence of immature fat is definitional for lipoblastoma and is characterized by lipoblasts in various stages of development. The more primitive foci often show myxoid stroma and are most common at the periphery of the lobules* ➙. **(Right)** *Lipocytes are seen in all stages of development, including spindled preadipocytes, small signet ring-like univacuolated lipoblasts* ➙*, multivacuolated lipoblasts, and large mature-appearing adipocytes* ➙.

TERMINOLOGY

Synonyms

- Fetal lipoma; embryonic lipoma

Definitions

- Well-circumscribed, benign, lobular lipomatous neoplasm with resemblance to fetal adipose tissue
  - Deep tumors with infiltrative borders may be designated "diffuse lipoblastoma" or "lipoblastomatosis"

CLINICAL ISSUES

Epidemiology

- Age
  - Majority occur in first 3 years of life
    - Rare in older children and adolescents
    - Very rare in adults
- Sex
  - 2:1 male predominance

Site

- Most frequent in trunk and extremities
  - Subcutaneous tissue (most common)
  - Deep/intramuscular (diffuse lipoblastoma/lipoblastomatosis)
- May also arise in head/neck region, mediastinum, retroperitoneum, mesentery, visceral organs

Presentation

- Painless, slow- or rapidly growing mass
- Subset of patients have central nervous system disorders
  - e.g., developmental delays, seizures, autism, congenital malformations

Treatment

- Complete surgical excision

Prognosis

- Benign; excellent outcome
- Local recurrences not uncommon, particularly in diffuse, infiltrative forms
  - Likely related to incomplete excision

MACROSCOPIC

General Features

- Pale tan-yellow cut surface with variable myxoid or gelatinous quality

Size

- Usually 2-6 cm
  - Rare cases > 10 cm

MICROSCOPIC

Histologic Features

- Most are lobular and well circumscribed
- Lobules of immature adipocytes separated by variably thickened fibrous septa
  - Immature adipocytes
    - Spindled or stellate cells (preadipocytes), small signet ring-like univacuolated lipoblasts, multivacuolated lipoblasts
  - Mature adipocytes may be seen, particularly near center of lobules
  - No significant nuclear atypia
  - Mitoses rare to absent
- Myxoid stromal change is common and may be focal or extensive
  - Stromal mucin pools may be seen
- Delicate capillary vasculature often present
  - Often conspicuous and plexiform in myxoid areas
- Rare findings: Collagen deposition, hibernoma-like cells, chondroid metaplasia, extramedullary hematopoiesis, multinucleated cells
- Diffuse lipoblastoma (lipoblastomatosis)
  - Deep variant with infiltrative growth with less pronounced lobular pattern
  - Entrapped skeletal muscle may be seen
- Recurrent tumors often show evidence of maturation
  - Increased proportion of mature adipose tissue; may be indistinguishable from lipoma or fibrolipoma

ANCILLARY TESTS

Molecular Genetics

- Rearrangement of 8q11-13 involving *PLAG1* gene common
  - Fusion partner genes include *HAS2, COL1A2, RAD51B, COL3A1, RAB2A*

DIFFERENTIAL DIAGNOSIS

Myxoid Liposarcoma

- Rare in first 10 years of life
- More likely to arise in deep soft tissue
- Lobular but generally less septated than lipoblastoma
- Hypercellular or "round cell" areas with nuclear atypia in some cases
- Characterized by t(12;16) or t(16;22) with *DDIT3* rearrangements
- Lacks rearrangements of *PLAG1* (8q11-13)

Lipoma

- Occurs in older patient population than lipoblastoma
- Lacks lipoblasts and myxoid stroma with plexiform capillary vasculature

Lipoblastoma-Like Tumor of Vulva

- Rare; recently described
- Affects adults; arises in vulva or groin
- Loss of nuclear Rb expression (often in mosaic pattern)
- Almost all reported cases lack *PLAG1* rearrangement

SELECTED REFERENCES

1. Abdul-Ghafar J et al: Lipoblastoma: a clinicopathologic review of 23 cases from a major tertiary care center plus detailed review of literature. BMC Res Notes. 11(1):42, 2018
2. Schoolmeester JK et al: Lipoblastoma-like tumor of the vulva: a clinicopathologic, immunohistochemical, fluorescence in situ hybridization and genomic copy number profiling study of seven cases. Mod Pathol. ePub, 2018
3. Kok KY et al: Lipoblastoma: clinical features, treatment, and outcome. World J Surg. 34(7):1517-22, 2010
4. Coffin CM et al: Lipoblastoma (LPB): a clinicopathologic and immunohistochemical analysis of 59 cases. Am J Surg Pathol. 33(11):1705-12, 2009
5. Collins MH et al: Lipoblastoma/lipoblastomatosis: a clinicopathologic study of 25 tumors. Am J Surg Pathol. 21(10):1131-7, 1997

Gross Appearance

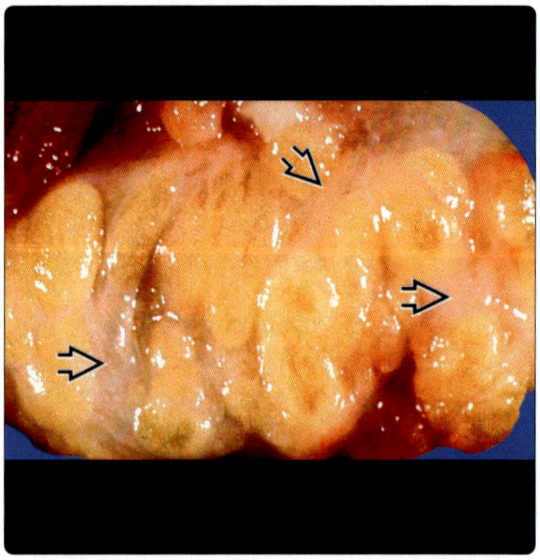

Capillary Vasculature

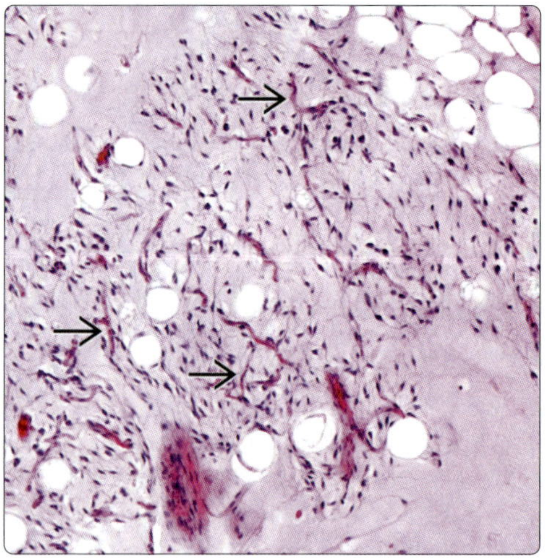

(Left) *Lipoblastomas have a glistening, pale yellow, lobular appearance with interlobular fibrous septation, which may also be apparent on gross examination.* **(Right)** *Lipoblastoma contains a variably prominent, delicate, branching capillary vascular network very similar to that seen in myxoid liposarcoma. Note the presence of conspicuous bland, spindled preadipocytes, also reminiscent of myxoid liposarcoma.*

Delicate Capillary Vasculature

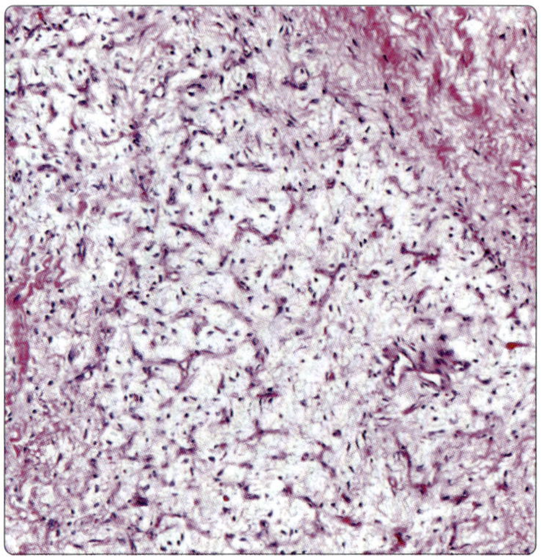

Maturing Fat

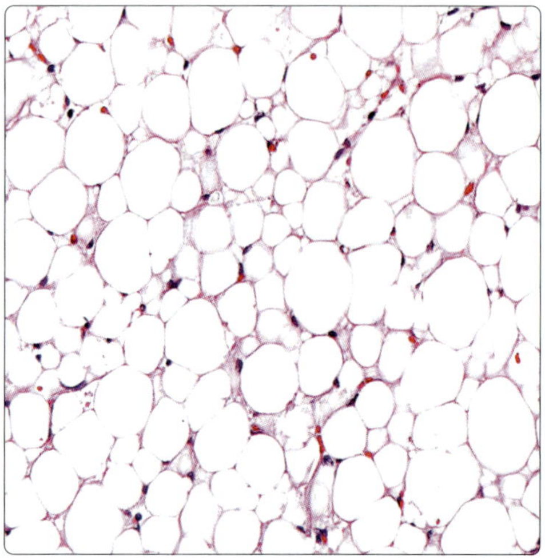

(Left) *The capillary network of lipoblastoma is usually most prominent in areas of myxoid change and may occasionally be striking.* **(Right)** *In most cases of lipoblastoma, the adipocytes near the center of a lobule are more mature than those at the periphery. Note, however, the variation in size, a feature not generally seen in conventional lipoma.*

Cellular Foci

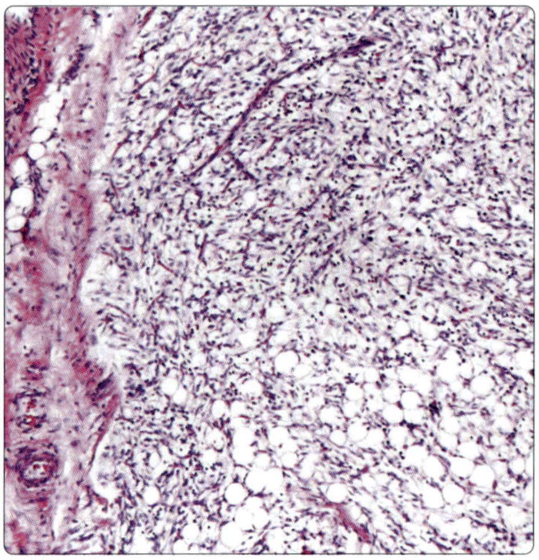

Cellular Foci

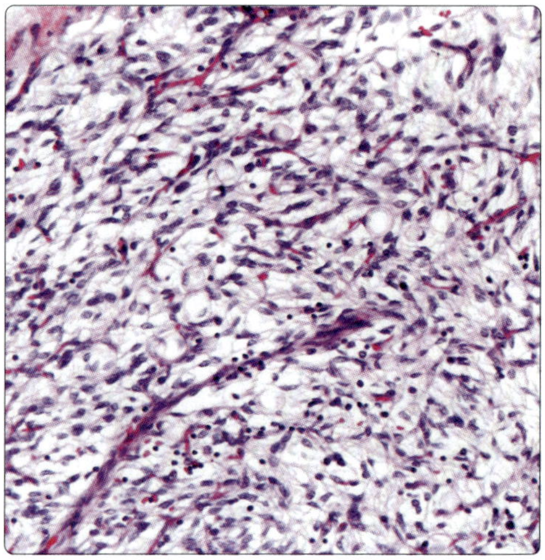

(Left) *Rare cases of lipoblastoma may show an increase in lobule cellularity, raising concerns for myxoid liposarcoma; however, more conventional morphology is often seen in other fields. FISH analysis may be helpful in difficult cases.* **(Right)** *Cellular foci in lipoblastoma are characterized by a proliferation of very bland, uniform spindled cells associated with delicate capillaries. The very young age of the patient is often a major clue to avoiding a misdiagnosis of myxoid liposarcoma in these cases.*

Myxoid Stroma

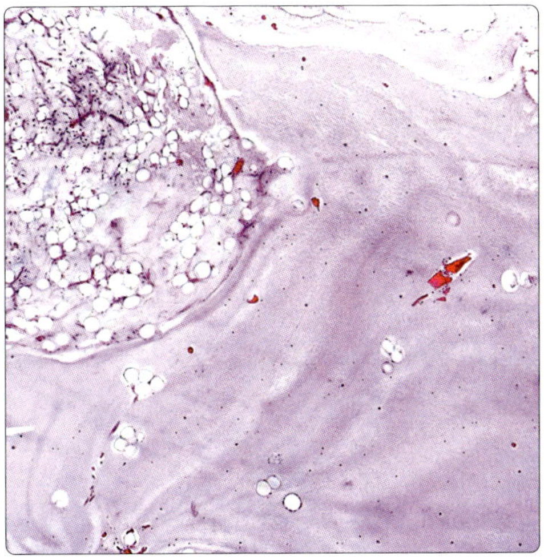

Stromal Mucin Pools

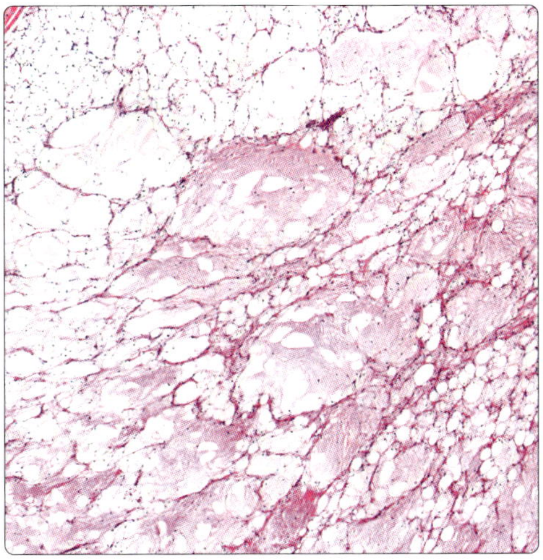

(Left) *Occasionally, lipoblastoma may show extensive myxoid stromal change, as depicted. A more conventional area can be seen in the upper left.* **(Right)** *Stromal mucin pools are present in some cases of lipoblastoma and are morphologically reminiscent of pulmonary edema in the lung. In general, however, this feature is more commonly identified in myxoid liposarcoma than lipoblastoma.*

Multivacuolated Cells

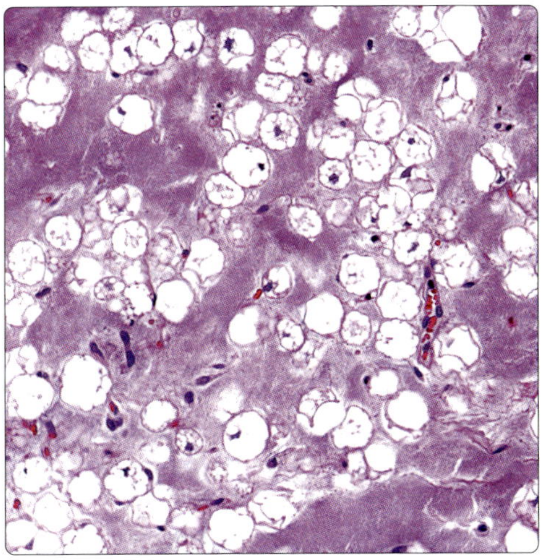

Diffuse Lipoblastoma

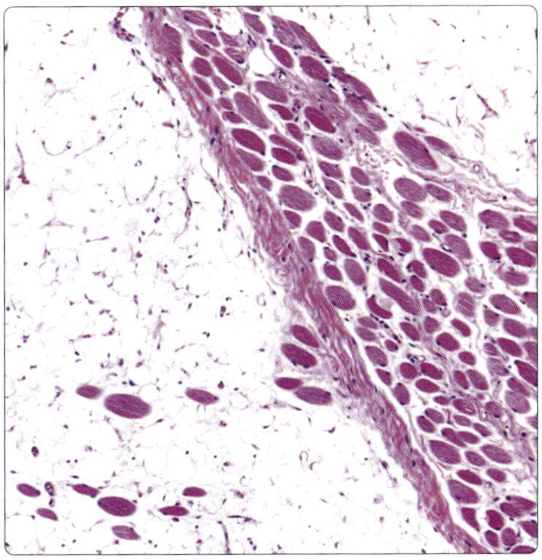

(Left) *Multivacuolated lipoblasts, similar to what can be seen in myxoid liposarcoma and atypical lipomatous tumor, can also be seen in lipoblastoma.* **(Right)** *Diffuse lipoblastoma (or lipoblastomatosis) is almost indistinguishable histologically from solitary lipoblastoma; however, the former is less lobular, more infiltrative, and more likely to involve muscle (shown). It is also more likely to be incompletely excised and recur.*

Maturing Lipoblastoma

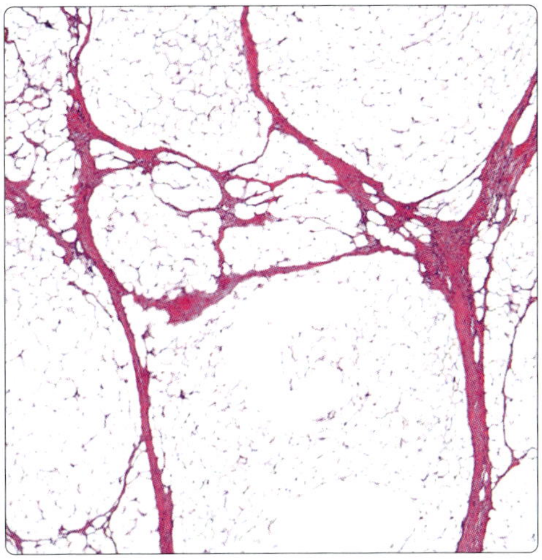

Maturing Lipoblastoma

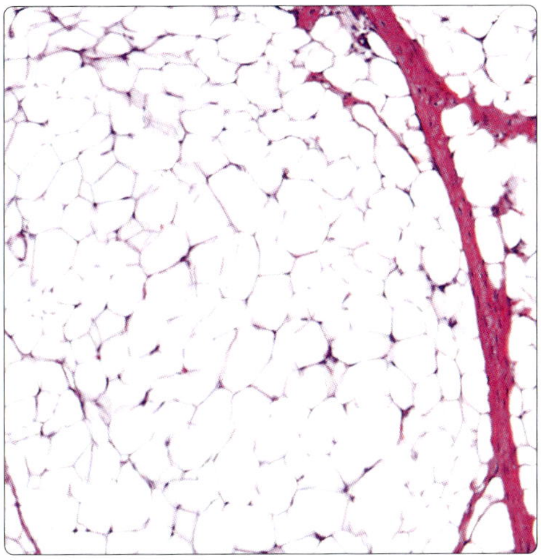

(Left) *Fat maturation has been well documented in recurrent cases of lipoblastoma, as evidenced by the presence of mostly mature adipose tissue with minimal to no primitive fat or myxoid component. Note the prominent lobularity and fibrous septa.* **(Right)** *This area of a recurrent lipoblastoma with maturation is indistinguishable from conventional lipoma at high magnification.*

Atypical Spindle Cell Lipomatous Tumor

KEY FACTS

TERMINOLOGY

- Low-grade atypical spindle cell neoplasm with adipocytic differentiation
- Synonyms: Spindle cell liposarcoma, fibrosarcoma-like lipomatous neoplasm, atypical spindle cell lipoma

CLINICAL ISSUES

- Wide age range (mean: 54 years)
- Slowly growing mass or swelling
- Majority arise in limbs and limb girdles
  - Also head/neck, trunk, genital region
- May arise in superficial or deep soft tissue
- Treatment: Complete surgical excision
- Low risk of local recurrence (~ 10%)
- No reports of malignant progression

MACROSCOPIC

- Median size: 5 cm

MICROSCOPIC

- Vaguely lobular, unencapsulated lesion, often with ill-defined or infiltrative peripheral border
- Relatively uniform spindle cell proliferation
  - Variable nuclear atypia and hyperchromasia
- Mature adipocytic component ± lipoblasts
  - Uni-, bi-, and multivacuolated lipoblasts frequent
- Myxoid to collagenous stroma
- Mitoses rare; no necrosis

ANCILLARY TESTS

- Variable CD34 and S100 protein expression
- Loss of nuclear Rb expression in 50%
- No *MDM2* amplification

TOP DIFFERENTIAL DIAGNOSES

- Spindle cell lipoma
- Atypical lipomatous tumor
- Mammary-type myofibroblastoma

Atypical Spindle Cell Lipomatous Tumor

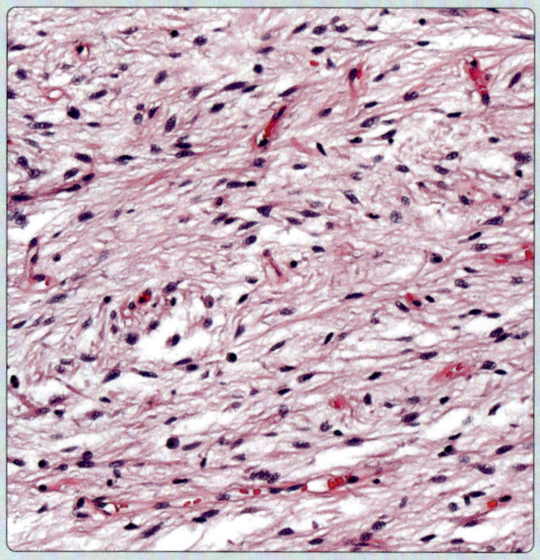

Adipocytic Component

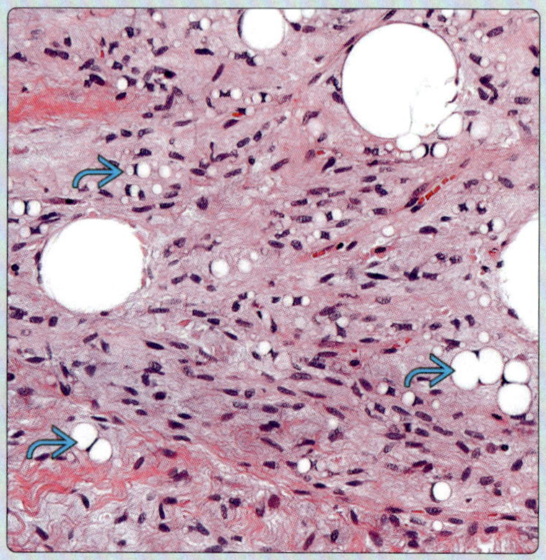

(Left) *Atypical spindle cell lipomatous tumor (ASCLT) is an unusual low-grade adipocytic neoplasm composed of variably atypical spindle cells and lipoblasts within a collagenous to myxoid stroma. It has also been described as "spindle cell liposarcoma" and "fibrosarcoma-like lipomatous neoplasm."* **(Right)** *Adipocytic differentiation is a consistent feature of ASCLT and takes the form of mature adipocytes ± lipoblasts.*

Lipoblast Cytomorphology

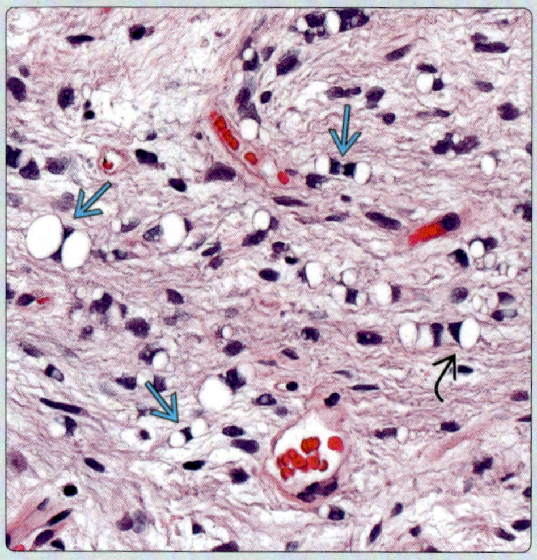

Absence of MDM2 Nuclear Expression

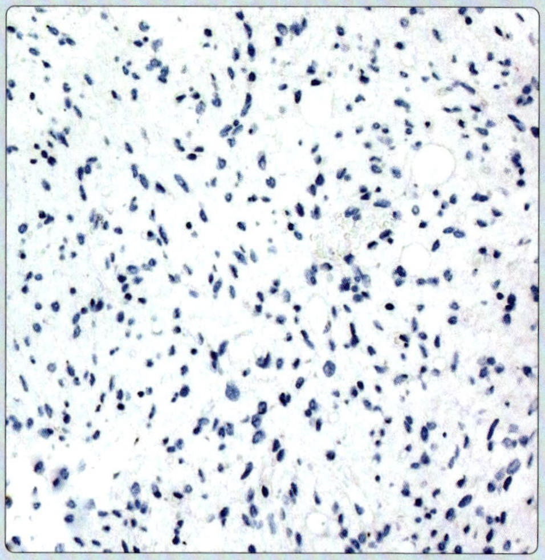

(Left) *Univacuolated and bivacuolated lipoblasts are a common finding in ASCLT and display cytomorphologies that can resemble either an ice cream cone or hourglass, respectively.* **(Right)** *Unlike atypical lipomatous tumor/well-differentiated liposarcoma, ASCLT does not show MDM2 gene amplification nor does it show coexpression of MDM2 and CDK4 by immunohistochemistry. This is a helpful distinguishing feature of the tumor.*

TERMINOLOGY

Abbreviations

- Atypical spindle cell lipomatous tumor (ASCLT)

Synonyms

- Spindle cell liposarcoma
- Fibrosarcoma-like lipomatous neoplasm
- Atypical spindle cell lipoma

Definitions

- Low-grade atypical spindle cell neoplasm with adipocytic differentiation

CLINICAL ISSUES

Epidemiology

- Age
  - Wide range (mean: 54 years)
- Sex
  - Male predominance

Site

- Majority arise in limbs and limb girdles
  - Mostly commonly hands, feet, thigh
- May arise in superficial or deep soft tissue
- Also head/neck, trunk, genital region
- Rarely mediastinum, retroperitoneum, other

Presentation

- Slowly growing mass or swelling
- May be present for years

Treatment

- Complete surgical excision

Prognosis

- Low risk of local recurrence (~ 10%)
- No reports of malignant progression

MACROSCOPIC

Size

- Wide range (0.5-28.0 cm)
  - Median: 5.0 cm

MICROSCOPIC

Histologic Features

- Vaguely lobular, unencapsulated lesion, often with ill-defined peripheral border
  - Infiltration of adjacent tissue common
- Wide range in cellularity (often low to moderate)
- Relatively uniform spindle cell proliferation
  - Variable nuclear atypia and hyperchromasia
  - May show bizarre, hyperchromatic, multinucleated cells
    - Floret-like cells can resemble those of pleomorphic lipoma
    - Some cases referred to in literature as "atypical pleomorphic lipomatous tumor"
- Adipocytic component
  - Variably sized, mature adipocytes
  - Uni-, bi-, &/or multivacuolated lipoblasts frequent
- Myxoid to collagenous stroma
  - Wispy collagen may be seen, but "ropey" bundles rare
- Mitoses rare; necrosis absent

ANCILLARY TESTS

Immunohistochemistry

- Variable CD34(+) in majority of cases
- Spindle cells may be S100(+) &/or focally desmin (+)
- Loss of nuclear Rb expression in 50%
- MDM2/CDK4 coexpression (-)

Molecular Genetics

- Heterozygous deletion of *RB1* in subset of cases
- No amplification of *MDM2*

DIFFERENTIAL DIAGNOSIS

Spindle Cell/Pleomorphic Lipoma

- Absence of infiltrative growth
- Most are subcutaneous, affecting neck, back, or shoulders
- Spindle cell component lacks nuclear atypia
- Characteristic "ropey" collagen bundles

Atypical Lipomatous Tumor/Well-Differentiated Liposarcoma

- Retroperitoneum common site
- Lacks well-developed spindle cell component
- MDM2/CDK4 overexpression by IHC
- *MDM2* amplification

Dedifferentiated Liposarcoma (Low Grade)

- Retroperitoneum common site
- Higher grade zones often present
- MDM2/CDK4 overexpression by IHC
- *MDM2* amplification

Mammary-Type Myofibroblastoma

- Well-circumscribed lesions
- Usually CD34(+) and desmin (+)
- Mature adipose tissue, if present, lacks lipoblasts

Dermatofibrosarcoma Protuberans

- Conspicuous storiform growth pattern common
- "Honeycomb" infiltration of subcutaneous fat
- t(17;22) with *COL1A1-PDGFB* fusion

SELECTED REFERENCES

1. Creytens D et al: "Atypical" pleomorphic lipomatous tumor: a clinicopathologic, immunohistochemical and molecular study of 21 cases, emphasizing its relationship to atypical spindle cell lipomatous tumor and suggesting a morphologic spectrum (atypical spindle cell/pleomorphic lipomatous tumor). Am J Surg Pathol. 41(11):1443-1455, 2017
2. Mariño-Enriquez A et al: Atypical spindle cell lipomatous tumor: clinicopathologic characterization of 232 cases demonstrating a morphologic spectrum. Am J Surg Pathol. 41(2):234-244, 2017
3. Creytens D et al: Atypical spindle cell lipoma: a clinicopathologic, immunohistochemical, and molecular study emphasizing its relationship to classical spindle cell lipoma. Virchows Arch. 465(1):97-108, 2014
4. Deyrup AT et al: Fibrosarcoma-like lipomatous neoplasm: a reappraisal of so-called spindle cell liposarcoma defining a unique lipomatous tumor unrelated to other liposarcomas. Am J Surg Pathol. 37(9):1373-8, 2013
5. Mentzel T et al: Well-differentiated spindle cell liposarcoma ('atypical spindle cell lipomatous tumor') does not belong to the spectrum of atypical lipomatous tumor but has a close relationship to spindle cell lipoma: clinicopathologic, immunohistochemical, and molecular analysis of six cases. Mod Pathol. 23(5):729-36, 2010

(Left) *At low power, ASCLT often shows a vaguely lobular growth pattern with most cases demonstrating an ill-defined peripheral margin (often infiltrative). However, a minority of cases are well circumscribed, as depicted.* **(Right)** *This case of ASCLT arose in the quadriceps muscle and showed obvious infiltration of adjacent skeletal muscle ➙. FISH analysis was negative for MDM2 gene amplification.*

Peripheral Border

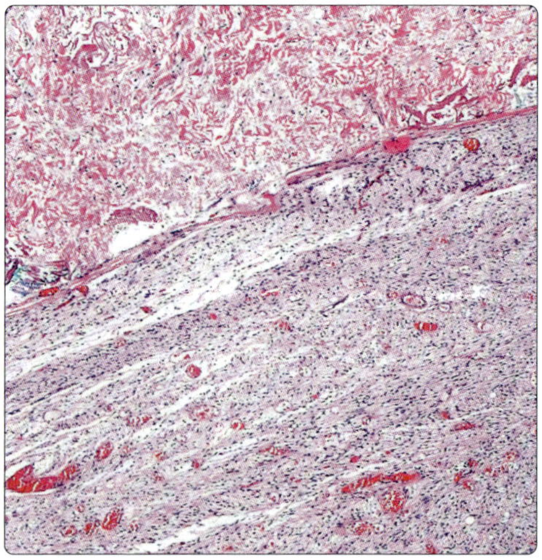

Infiltrative Periphery

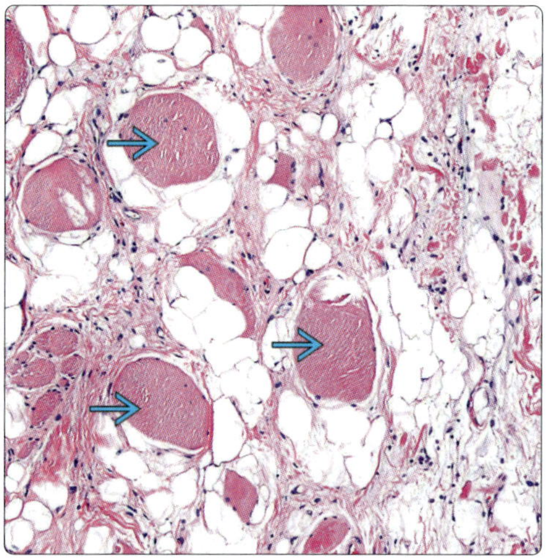

(Left) *Cellularity is variable in ASCLT with most cases falling on the low end of the spectrum. Some cases can show areas of moderate to high cellularity and architectural organization, mimicking low-grade dedifferentiated liposarcoma.* **(Right)** *Stromal myxoid change is common in ASCLT. Note the minimal to mild nuclear atypia in the spindled tumor cells and also the univacuolated lipoblasts ➙.*

Variation in Cellularity

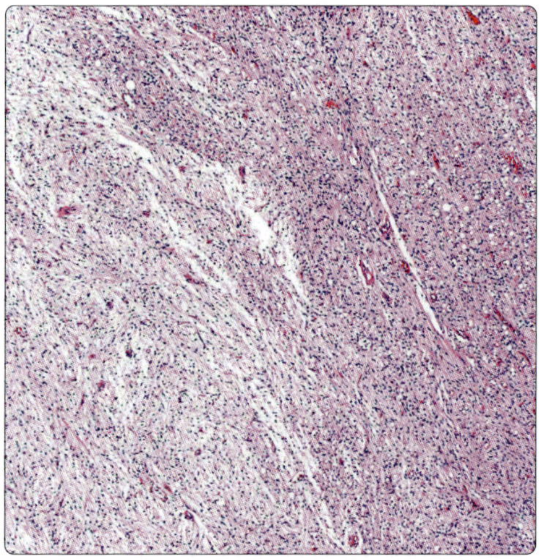

Myxoid Stroma

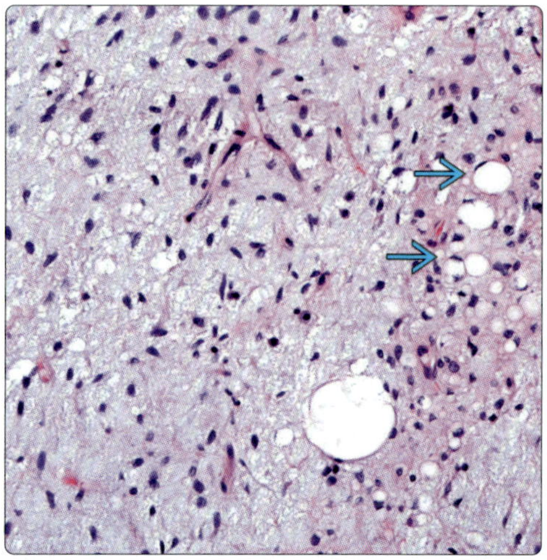

(Left) *Stromal collagen can be prominent in ASCLT, as depicted. Delicate wisps or bundles of collagen fibers can be seen in some cases, creating morphologic overlap with spindle cell lipoma.* **(Right)** *Mitotic figures ➙ are generally challenging to find in ASCLT and may be completely absent in histologic sections. Coagulative tumor necrosis is never seen.*

Collagenous Stroma

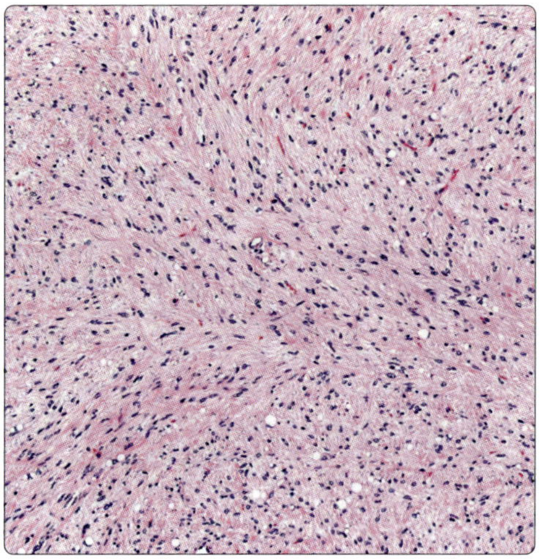

Sparse to Absent Mitotic Activity

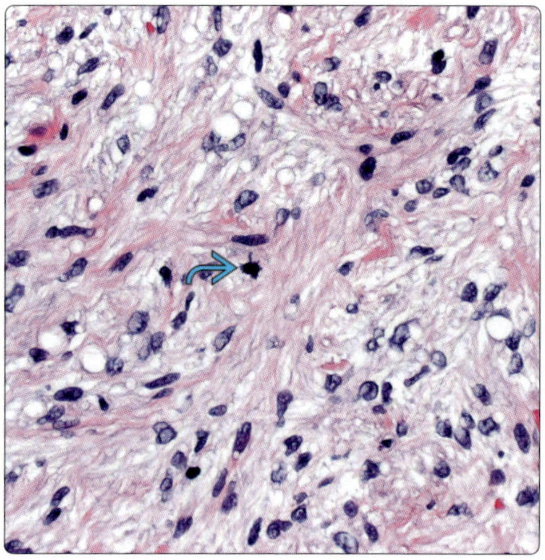

Delicate Capillary Vasculature

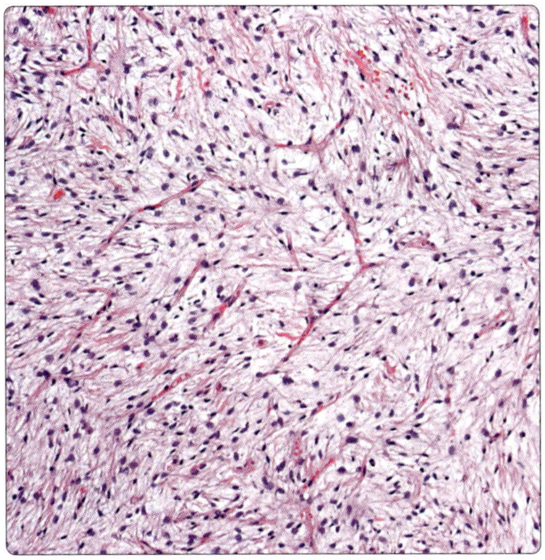

Lipoblastic Differentiation

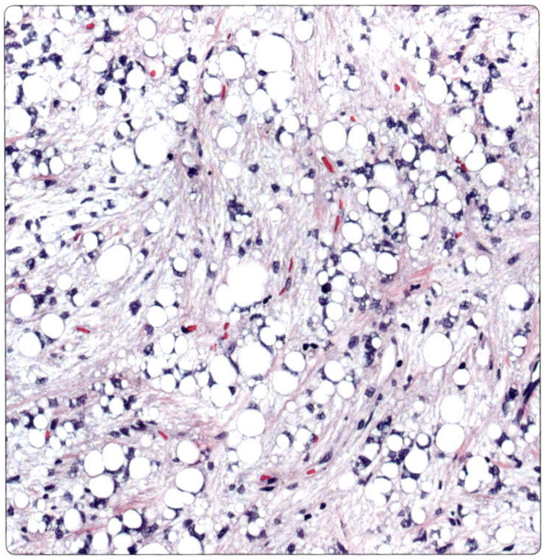

(Left) *Some cases of ASCLT may show a delicate, arborizing capillary network similar to myxoid liposarcoma. This finding, if present, is generally focal and not as extensive as that typically seen in myxoid liposarcoma.* **(Right)** *Although the number of lipoblasts varies widely from one case to the next, they may be a prominent finding in ASCLT, as depicted in this hematoxylin and eosin.*

Mature Adipose Tissue

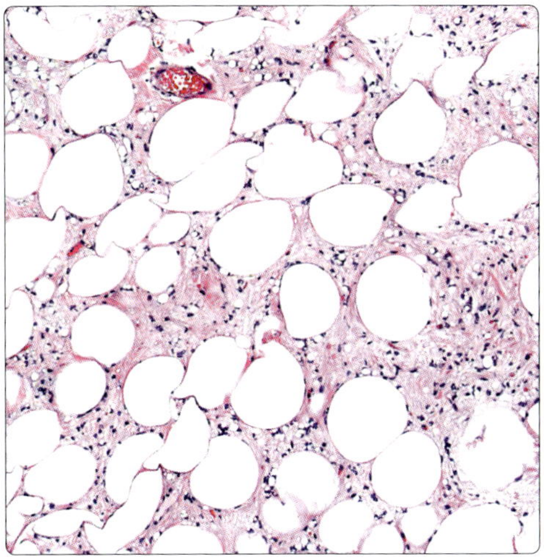

Cellular, Nonlipogenic Areas

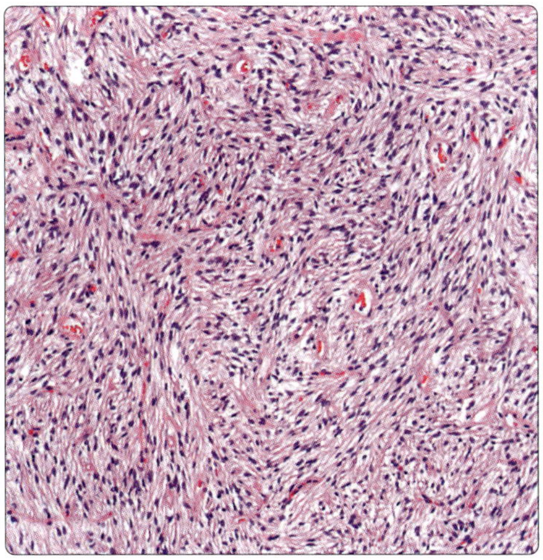

(Left) *Mature adipose tissue is a common feature of ASCLT, and the adipocytes often show variation in size. Hematoxylin and eosin also shows scattered univacuolated lipoblasts between the larger mature adipocytes.* **(Right)** *In some cases of ASCLT, there may be a decrease or absence of lipogenic tissue associated with an increase in cellularity. This finding may lead to consideration of dedifferentiation; however, MDM2 gene amplification is absent as is coexpression of MDM2 and CDK4 by immunohistochemistry.*

S100 Protein Expression

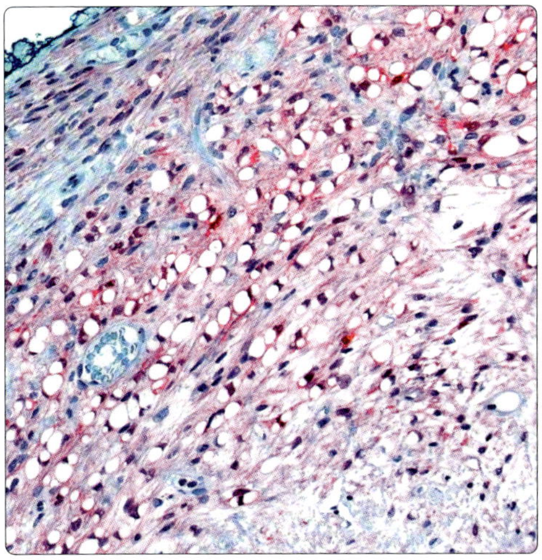

Atypical Pleomorphic Lipomatous Tumor

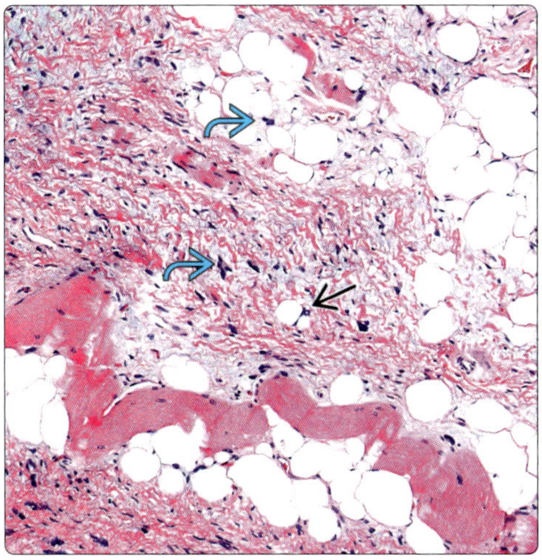

(Left) *Expression of S100 is common in ASCLT and can show positivity in both lesional spindle cells and lipoblasts (red chromogen here).* **(Right)** *Cases of ASCLT may also show bizarre, hyperchromatic, multinucleated, floret-like cells ↗, reminiscent of pleomorphic lipoma. These tumors have been recently described in the literature as "atypical pleomorphic lipomatous tumor" and appear to be histogenetically related to ASCLT. Note also the multivacuolated lipoblast →.*

Atypical Lipomatous Tumor/Well-Differentiated Liposarcoma

KEY FACTS

TERMINOLOGY

- Locally aggressive mesenchymal neoplasm composed of atypical adipocytes and demonstrating at least focal nuclear atypia in adipocytes &/or stromal cells

CLINICAL ISSUES

- Most common form of liposarcoma (40-45% of cases)
- Most occur in middle-aged to elderly adults
- Extremities, retroperitoneum, abdominal cavity, paratesticular region, mediastinum
- Treatment: Complete surgical excision with negative margins
- Anatomic site is most important prognostic factor
  - Low risk of recurrence and dedifferentiation in extremities
  - More significant risk of recurrence/dedifferentiation in body cavities
- No metastatic potential

MICROSCOPIC

- Sheets and lobules of relatively mature adipocytes of varying sizes
- Thickened, irregular fibrous bands or septa common
- Stromal &/or adipocyte nuclear atypia characteristic
- Lipoblasts vary in number and may be absent
- Rarely may show prominent myxoid stroma
- Other subtypes: Sclerosing, inflammatory, myxoid

ANCILLARY TESTS

- Overexpression of nuclear MDM2 and CDK4 by IHC
- Molecular: *MDM2* amplification
- Supernumerary ring and giant marker chromosomes

TOP DIFFERENTIAL DIAGNOSES

- Lipoma
- Pleomorphic lipoma
- Atypical spindle cell lipomatous tumor
- Dedifferentiated liposarcoma

Atypical Lipomatous Tumor

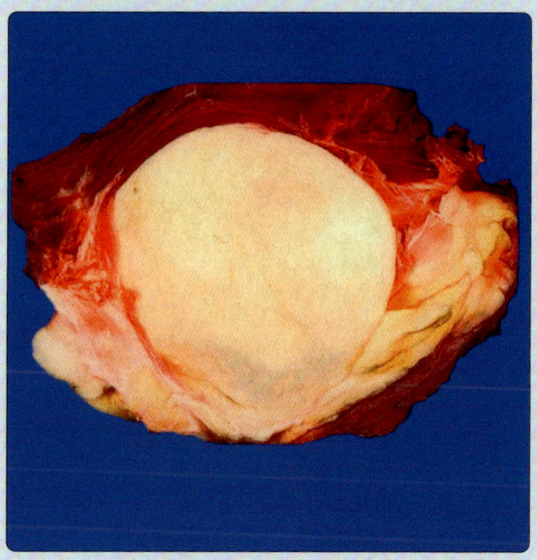

Atypical Lipomatous Tumor

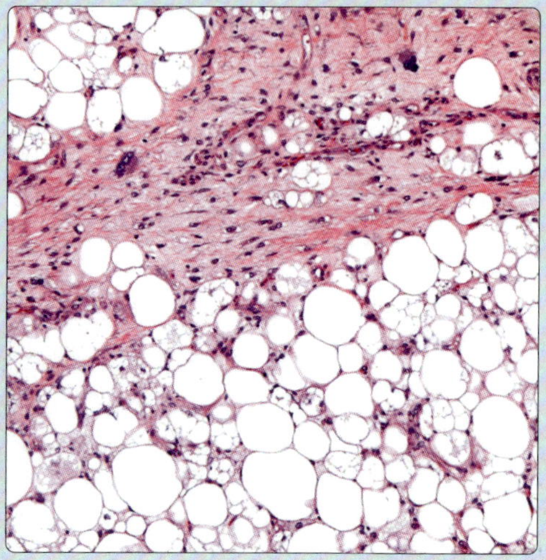

(Left) *Atypical lipomatous tumor (ALT) is generally well circumscribed and often shows a variable tan to yellow, firm to fatty cut surface. Well-differentiated liposarcoma (WDLPS) is an alternate term for the same entity.* **(Right)** *This image shows the classic morphologic appearance of ALT: Thickened fibrous bands containing atypical stromal cells and lobules of adipose tissue containing variable numbers of multivacuolated lipoblasts.*

Thickened Fibrous Bands

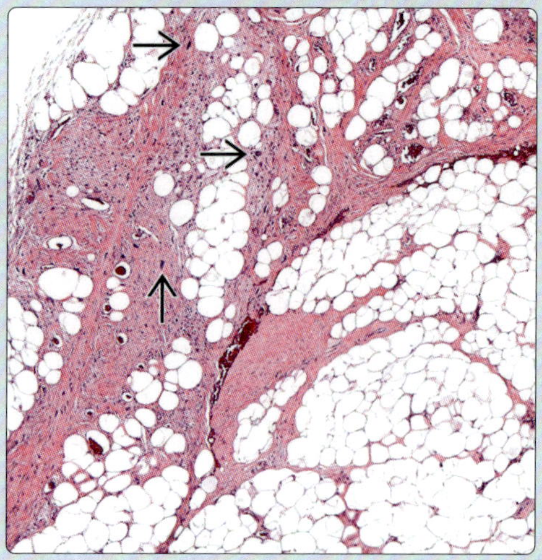

Fibrosis With Atypical Stromal Cells

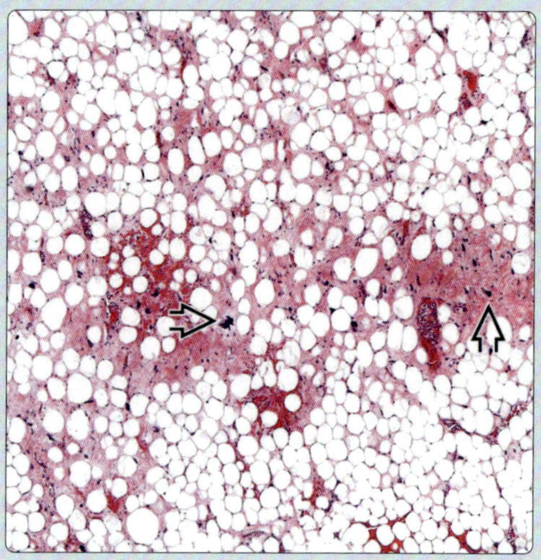

(Left) *Most cases of ALT/WDLPS characteristically show irregular expansion of fibrous septa/bands between lobules of adipocytes; however, in some cases they may be sparse. Atypical stromal cell nuclei → can often be appreciated from low power.* **(Right)** *Fibrosis in ALT/WDLPS may be seen within the adipocytic lobules as patchy splotches or irregular deposits, as depicted. Note the atypical stromal cell nuclei ⇒.*

TERMINOLOGY

Abbreviations

- Atypical lipomatous tumor (ALT)
- Well-differentiated liposarcoma (WDLPS)

Synonyms

- Atypical lipoma (obsolete)

Definitions

- Locally aggressive mesenchymal neoplasm composed of atypical adipocytes and demonstrating at least focal nuclear atypia in adipocytes &/or stromal cells
  - Histologic subtypes: Adipocytic (lipoma-like), sclerosing, inflammatory, myxoid
    - Spindle cell liposarcoma is now considered to be distinct from ALT/WDLPS
      - Described in literature as "atypical spindle cell lipomatous tumor" or "fibrosarcoma-like lipomatous neoplasm"
- Terms "atypical lipomatous tumor" and "well-differentiated liposarcoma" are synonyms for same neoplasm
  - "Well-differentiated liposarcoma" is best utilized only for tumors occurring within body cavities (retroperitoneum, mediastinum, abdominopelvic sites) or paratesticular region
    - Due to significant morbidity in these sites; also, increased risk of dedifferentiation

CLINICAL ISSUES

Epidemiology

- Incidence
  - Most common form of liposarcoma (40-45% of cases)
- Age
  - Most occur in middle-aged to elderly adults
  - Extremely rare in childhood

Site

- Overall, most frequently arise in deep soft tissues of extremities
  - May also arise in subcutaneous tissue and very rarely in skin
- Also common in retroperitoneum, abdominal cavity, paratesticular region, mediastinum
- Less frequent in head/neck area
- Subtype site predilections
  - Sclerosing subtype most common in retroperitoneum and spermatic cord
  - Inflammatory subtype most common in retroperitoneum

Presentation

- Slow-growing, painless, deep-seated mass
- Retroperitoneal tumors may only be discovered after attaining significant growth (> 20 cm)

Treatment

- Complete surgical excision with negative margins
- Surgical debulking for large, multifocal retroperitoneal/intraabdominal tumors
  - May require partial or complete resection of intraabdominal organs

Prognosis

- Anatomic site of occurrence is most important prognostic factor
  - Tumors in surgically amenable locations (e.g., extremities)
    - Recur only rarely after complete excision with clearly negative margins
  - Intraabdominal, retroperitoneal, mediastinal, or paratesticular tumors
    - Often recur locally and may cause significant morbidity and lead to death
      - Long-term mortality rate in retroperitoneal WDLPS up to 80%
- Risk of dedifferentiation
  - Very rare in extremities (< 2%)
  - Much higher in retroperitoneum (> 20%)
    - May arise de novo or in recurrences
- No metastatic potential for ALT/WDLPS unless dedifferentiation is present

MACROSCOPIC

General Features

- Well-circumscribed, lobular
- Variable yellow, fatty to tan-gray cut surface
- Thickened fibrous bands may be evident grossly
- Fat necrosis may be seen in larger tumors

Sections to Be Submitted

- Sampling very important in well-differentiated tumors
- 1 section submitted per cm of greatest linear dimension
- Focus sampling on firm or tan-gray areas

Size

- Wide size range (usually > 5 cm)
  - May grow to enormous sizes (> 20 cm), particularly in retroperitoneum and abdominal cavity

MICROSCOPIC

Histologic Features

- Sheets and lobules of relatively well-differentiated adipocytes
  - Adipocytes show significant variation in size and shape
    - Usually show at least focal nuclear hyperchromasia and atypia
- Variably prominent, thickened, irregular fibrous bands or septa
  - Often contain atypical, nonlipogenic fibroblastic cells
    - 1 or several enlarged, hyperchromatic nuclei
    - Variable amphophilic to eosinophilic cytoplasm
    - May show indistinct nuclear &/or cytoplasmic membranes ("smudge cells")
    - May show floret-like morphology
- Lipoblasts may be seen but are not essential for diagnosis (as they may be absent)
  - Usually multivacuolated
  - Hyperchromatic nuclei that are compressed and indented/scalloped by vacuoles
  - Significant nuclear pleomorphism/atypia absent
- Atypical cells may be present within walls of larger stromal blood vessels

- Prominent stromal collagenization/hyalinization in some tumors (sclerosing subtype)
  - Minimal adipocytic component
  - Atypical stromal cells often frequent
  - Chronic inflammatory infiltrate may be seen
- Dense stromal chronic inflammatory infiltrate in some tumors (inflammatory subtype)
  - Mainly lymphocytes, plasma cells
  - Scattered atypical stromal cells and lipoblasts
  - Often edematous stroma
- Myxoid stromal changes in some cases
  - May be prominent and extensive
- Heterologous differentiation rare
  - Bone, cartilage, smooth muscle, or skeletal muscle

ANCILLARY TESTS

Immunohistochemistry

- S100 protein (+) in adipocytes and lipoblasts
- Nuclear MDM2(+) and CDK4(+) in majority
  - Pitfall: Nuclear expression in reactive histiocytes (fat necrosis)
- Nuclear Rb expression intact

Cytogenetics

- Characteristic supernumerary ring and giant marker chromosomes
  - Contain amplified sequences originating from 12q14-15 region

Molecular Genetics

- *MDM2* amplification
  - Also, *CDK4*, *CPM*, *HMGA2*, *FRS2*, and *YEATS4* frequently coamplified
  - Can be detected by FISH, PCR, array CGH

DIFFERENTIAL DIAGNOSIS

Lipoma

- Most are smaller than ALT/WDLPS, but some can grow to very large sizes
- Lacks atypical stromal cells with irregular, hyperchromatic, pleomorphic nuclei
- Usually lacks significant variation in size and shape of adipocytes
- Generally no lipoblasts
- Negative for MDM2 and CDK4 by IHC
- No amplification of *MDM2*

Pleomorphic Lipoma

- Usually small lesions, often subcutaneous
- Variable number of floret-like cells
- Ropey collagen and scattered mast cells common
- Loss of nuclear Rb expression by IHC
- No *MDM2* amplification

Atypical Spindle Cell Lipomatous Tumor

- Previously known as spindle cell liposarcoma
- Bland spindle cells within fibrous to myxoid stroma
- Variable adipocytic differentiation, often with univacuolar lipoblasts
- Negative for MDM2 and CDK4 by IHC
- Loss of nuclear Rb expression by IHC in over 50% of cases
- No amplification of *MDM2*

Dedifferentiated Liposarcoma

- Cellular, usually nonlipogenic sarcoma with wide morphologic spectrum
  - Component of WDLPS may be present
- Positive for MDM2, CDK4 by IHC
- Shows *MDM2* amplification

Hibernoma

- Variably prominent component of brown fat
- Enlarged atypical stromal cells rare
- No *MDM2* amplification

Idiopathic Retroperitoneal Fibrosis

- Often bilateral, with impingement of ureters and subsequent hydronephrosis
- Lacks atypical stromal cells of WDLPS
- No *MDM2* amplification

Massive Localized Lymphedema

- Large superficial pseudotumor in morbidly obese patients
- Often show retention but expansion of overall architecture of subcutaneous tissue
- Reactive fibroblast nuclei may simulate atypical stromal cells of ALT/WDLPS
- No *MDM2* amplification

Myxoid Liposarcoma

- Prominent arborizing "chicken-wire" capillary vasculature; stromal mucin cysts common
- Lacks atypical stromal cells of ALT/WDLPS
- Characteristic t(12;16) in most cases, with *DDIT3* fusion

SELECTED REFERENCES

1. Kammerer-Jacquet SF et al: Differential diagnosis of atypical lipomatous tumor/well-differentiated liposarcoma and dedifferentiated liposarcoma: utility of p16 in combination with MDM2 and CDK4 immunohistochemistry. Hum Pathol. 59:34-40, 2017
2. Mariño-Enriquez A et al: Atypical spindle cell lipomatous tumor: clinicopathologic characterization of 232 cases demonstrating a morphologic spectrum. Am J Surg Pathol. 41(2):234-44, 2017
3. Dei Tos AP: Liposarcomas: diagnostic pitfalls and new insights. Histopathology. 64(1):38-52, 2014
4. Deyrup AT et al: Fibrosarcoma-like lipomatous neoplasm: a reappraisal of so-called spindle cell liposarcoma defining a unique lipomatous tumor unrelated to other liposarcomas. Am J Surg Pathol. 37(9):1373-8, 2013
5. Sioletic S et al: Well-differentiated and dedifferentiated liposarcomas with prominent myxoid stroma: analysis of 56 cases. Histopathology. 62(2):287-93, 2013
6. Piperi E et al: Well-differentiated liposarcoma/atypical lipomatous tumor of the oral cavity: report of three cases and review of the literature. Head Neck Pathol. 6(3):354-63, 2012
7. Aleixo PB et al: Can MDM2 and CDK4 make the diagnosis of well differentiated/dedifferentiated liposarcoma? An immunohistochemical study on 129 soft tissue tumours. J Clin Pathol. 62(12):1127-35, 2009
8. Evans HL: Atypical lipomatous tumor, its variants, and its combined forms: a study of 61 cases, with a minimum follow-up of 10 years. Am J Surg Pathol. 31(1):1-14, 2007
9. Sirvent N et al: Detection of MDM2-CDK4 amplification by fluorescence in situ hybridization in 200 paraffin-embedded tumor samples: utility in diagnosing adipocytic lesions and comparison with immunohistochemistry and real-time PCR. Am J Surg Pathol. 31(10):1476-89, 2007
10. Binh MB et al: MDM2 and CDK4 immunostainings are useful adjuncts in diagnosing well-differentiated and dedifferentiated liposarcoma subtypes: a comparative analysis of 559 soft tissue neoplasms with genetic data. Am J Surg Pathol. 29(10):1340-7, 2005

Atypical Stromal Cells

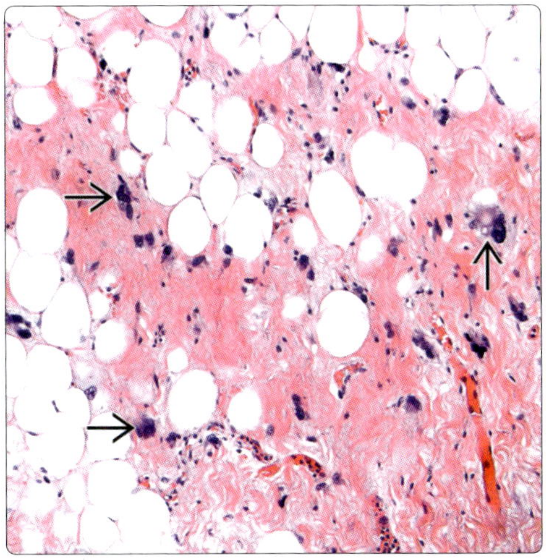

Floret-Like Cells

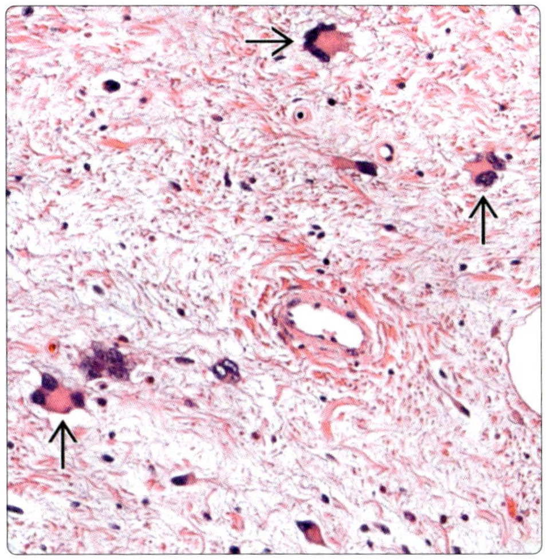

(Left) *Atypical stromal cells* ⇒ *are a key finding in ALT/WDLPS but vary widely in number and distribution from case to case. The nuclei are characteristically enlarged, irregular, and hyperchromatic and sometimes show a "smudgy" quality. These cells are usually most easily identified within the fibrous areas of ALT/WDLPS.* **(Right)** *Frequently, the atypical stromal cells of ALT/WDLPS show a floret-like morphology* ⇒ *similar to the cells seen in pleomorphic lipoma and some other tumors.*

Atypical Adipocyte Nuclei

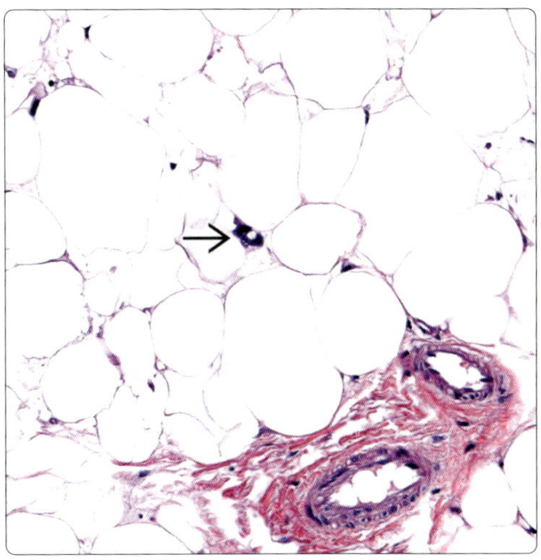

Fat Necrosis

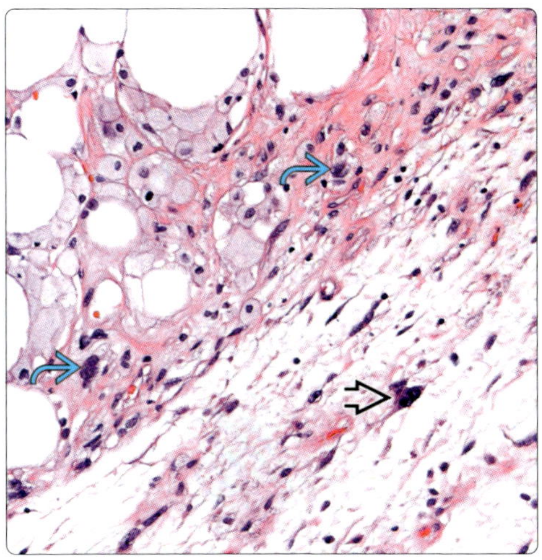

(Left) *Atypical adipocytic nuclei* ⇒ *may also be seen in ALT/WDLPS. The enlargement and hyperchromasia distinguish them from benign nuclei with vacuolated Lochkern change.* **(Right)** *Fat necrosis (particularly overlapping histiocyte nuclei* ↪*) in a lipoma may lead to the overcalling of nuclear atypia and a subsequent misdiagnosis of ALT/WDLPS. However, true ALT/WDLPS can also contain fat necrosis. Note the true atypical stromal cell* ⇒ *within the adjacent fibrous band, which helps support the diagnosis.*

Occasional Vascular Changes

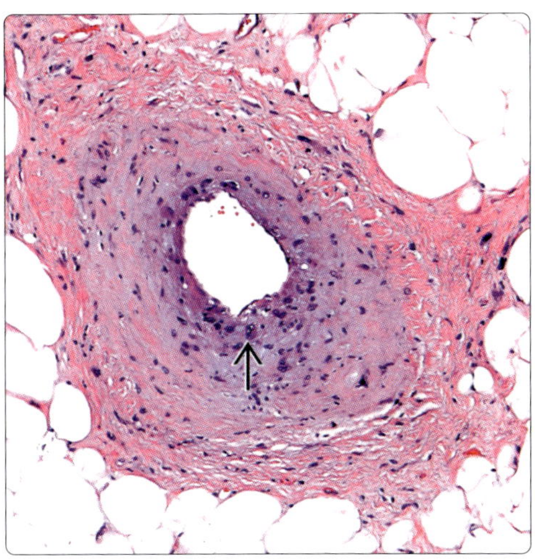

Atrophic Skeletal Muscle Fibers

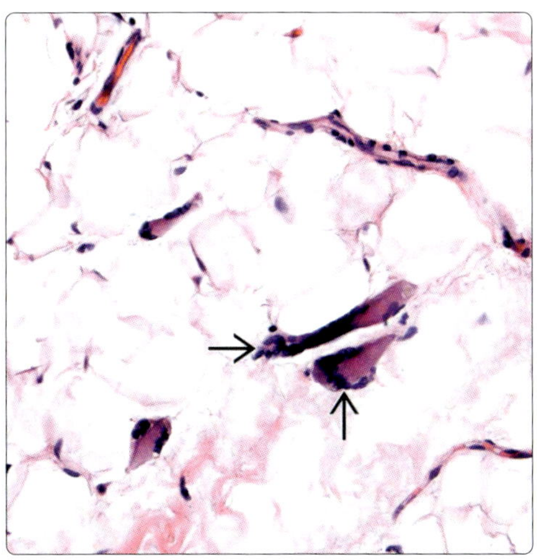

(Left) *Rare cases of ALT/WDLPS show atypical cells* ⇒ *within the muscular walls of stromal vessels. These cases also frequently contain a component of heterologous smooth muscle (so-called lipoleiomyosarcoma).* **(Right)** *Intramuscular adipocytic tumors may contain foci of atrophic skeletal muscle fibers, which should not be confused with true atypical cells of ALT/WDLPS. These cells* ⇒ *often show dense eosinophilic cytoplasm and clustering/overlapping of numerous small rounded nuclei.*

(Left) *Multivacuolated lipoblasts are a common but numerically variable finding in ALT/WDLPS; however, they can be absent in some cases and are therefore not required to make the diagnosis. They are identified by multiple intracytoplasmic fat vacuoles that compress and indent/scallop the hyperchromatic adipocyte nuclei* →. **(Right)** *The fibrous septa or bands of ALT/WDLPS may be quite cellular, as depicted, and should not be taken as evidence of dedifferentiation.*

Multivacuolated Lipoblasts

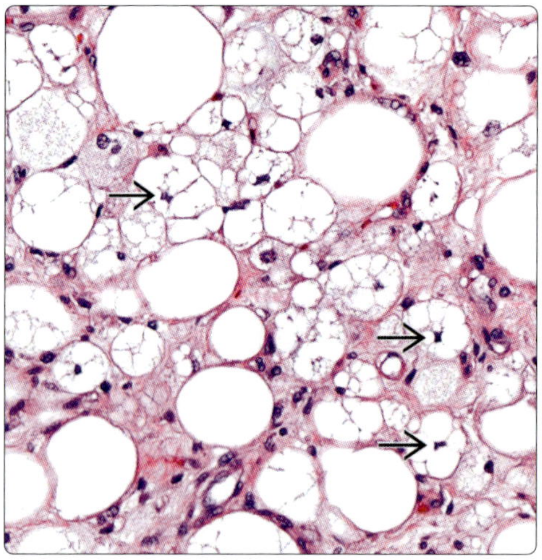

Cellular Fibrous Bands

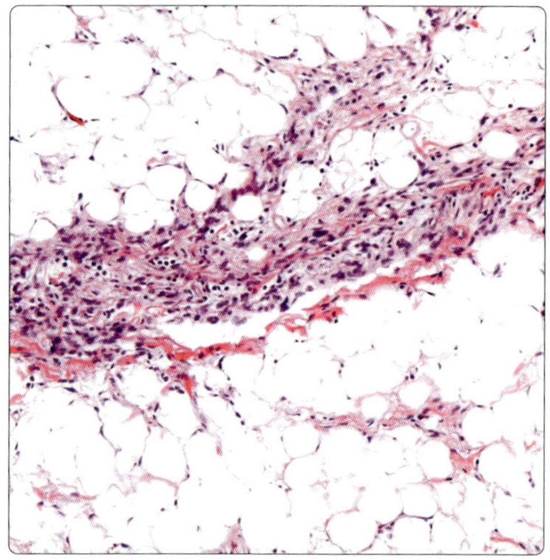

(Left) *In some cases of ALT/WDLPS, stromal fibrosis is more extensive and diffuse. Note the variation in size of the adipocytes in ALT/WDLPS, another common finding in this tumor.* **(Right)** *Examples of ALT/WDLPS with extensive stromal fibrosis and collagen that contain a minimal lipogenic component are sometimes referred to as the sclerosing type. Note the hypocellularity that, along with the essentially absent mitotic activity, distinguishes this morphology from true dedifferentiation.*

Fibrosis

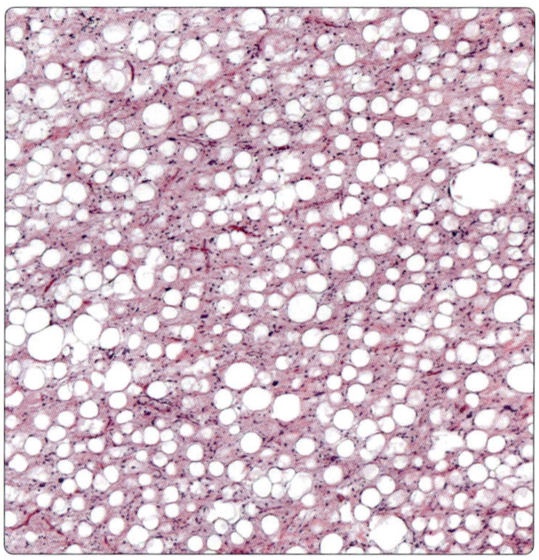

Sclerosing Subtype

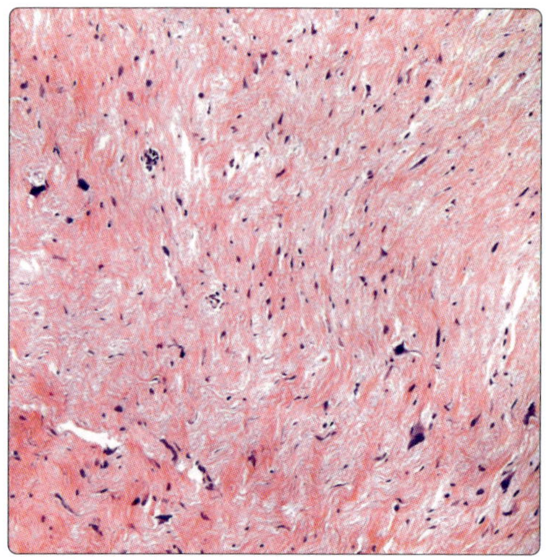

(Left) *Thickened or even "ropey" collagen bundles are a rare finding in ALT/WDLPS and are more suggestive of spindle cell or pleomorphic lipoma. However, in large tumors, MDM2 (or related) testing should be performed to aid in the diagnosis.* **(Right)** *Myxoid stroma is seen in a subset of ALT/WDLPS and may lead to serious consideration of other myxoid neoplasms, including myxoid liposarcoma. Other more conventional areas and features of ALT/WDLPS are usually present. Molecular techniques can also be utilized.*

Rare Thickened Collagen Bundles

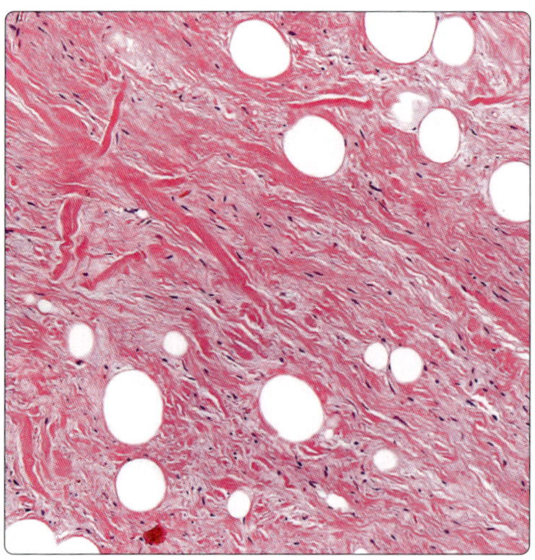

Myxoid Stroma

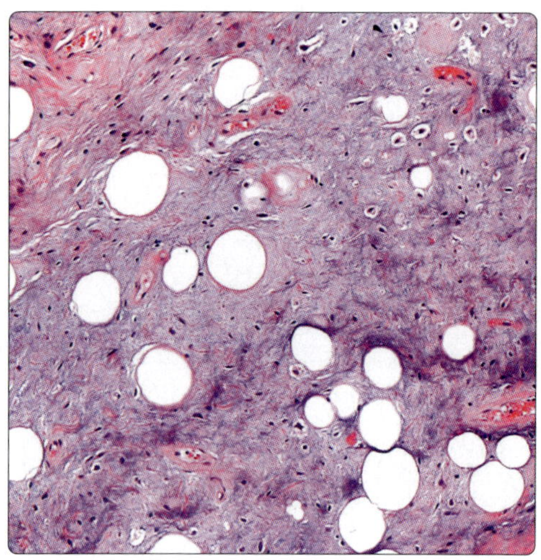

Rare Arborizing Capillary Vasculature

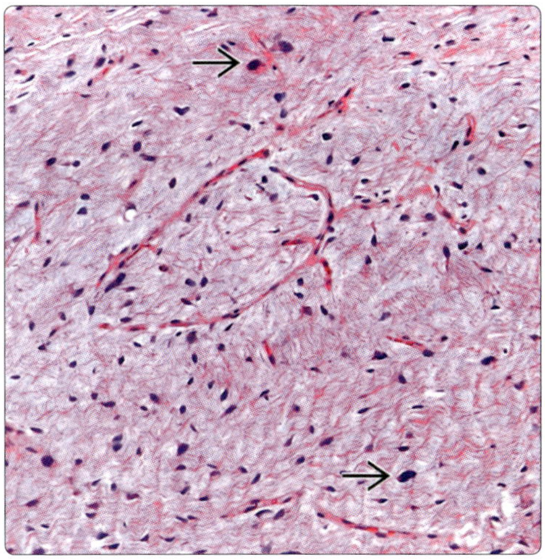

Chronic Inflammation

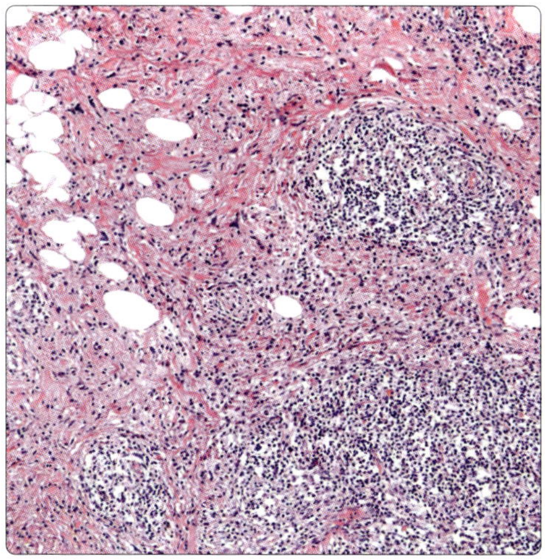

(Left) *An arborizing capillary vasculature, similar to that seen in myxoid liposarcoma, may be seen rarely in ALT/WDLPS. Note the hyperchromatic atypical stromal cells* →. **(Right)** *Lymphoid aggregates or collections of chronic inflammatory cells may be seen in ALT/WDLPS. Rarely, this chronic inflammatory component is very prominent (inflammatory-type ALT/WDLPS).*

Inflammatory Subtype

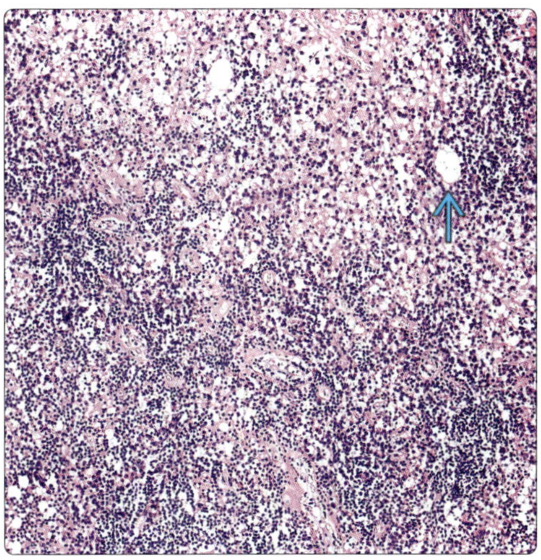

Rare Brown Fat Component

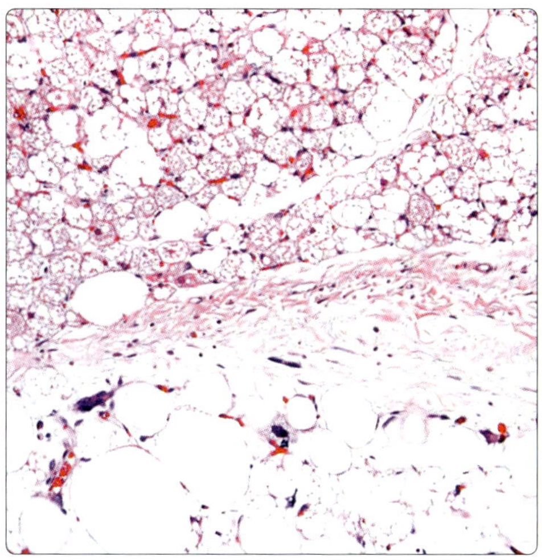

(Left) *The inflammatory subtype of ALT/WDLPS shows a prominent chronic inflammatory infiltrate and only scattered atypical stromal cells &/or multivacuolated lipoblasts* →. **(Right)** *A component of brown fat (top of image) is a rare finding in ALT/WDLPS but may lead to misdiagnosis as hibernoma. Molecular testing can be helpful in such cases.*

CT Scan

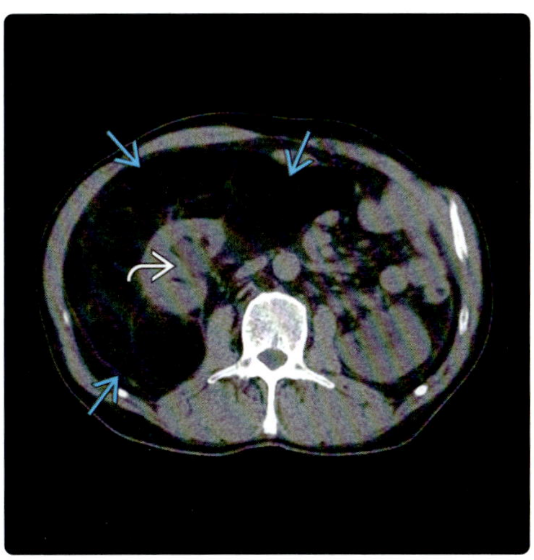

MDM2 Amplification

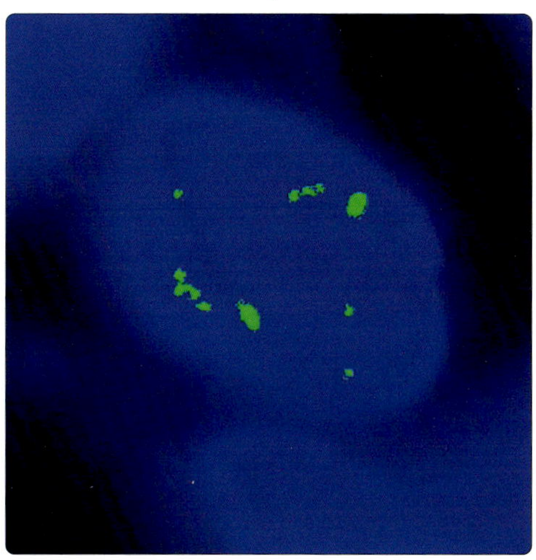

(Left) *This abdominal CT scan shows a large, well-differentiated liposarcoma* → *surrounding and almost encasing the right kidney* ➔. *Despite its size, no dedifferentiated component was identified histologically.* **(Right)** *In situ hybridization FISH analysis shows MDM2 amplification, a characteristic feature of ALT/WDLPS (and also dedifferentiated liposarcoma). Note numerous green signals in an analyzed tumor cell nucleus.*

Dedifferentiated Liposarcoma

KEY FACTS

TERMINOLOGY

- Malignant, generally nonlipogenic sarcoma of variable histologic grade often arising in association with identifiable component of atypical lipomatous tumor (ALT)/well-differentiated liposarcoma (WDLPS)

CLINICAL ISSUES

- Dedifferentiation occurs in up to 10% of ALT/WDLPS
  - Vast majority (90%) arise de novo
- Middle-aged to elderly adults
- Most common in retroperitoneum/abdominal cavity
  - Also spermatic cord, trunk, extremities, head/neck
- Treatment: Complete surgical resection with negative margins
- Anatomic location is most important prognostic factor
- Local recurrence in ~ 40% of cases
- Distant metastases observed in 15-20% of cases

MACROSCOPIC

- Well-demarcated, large mass with variable cut surface
- Important to sample thoroughly

MICROSCOPIC

- Classic appearance shows abrupt or gradual transition from ALT/WDLPS to nonlipogenic, cellular sarcoma
- Nonlipogenic component shows broad morphologic spectrum (often high grade)
- Mitotic rate > 5 per 10 HPF

ANCILLARY TESTS

- Diffuse nuclear MDM2(+) and CDK4(+)
- Molecular: Overexpression of *MDM2*

TOP DIFFERENTIAL DIAGNOSES

- Undifferentiated pleomorphic sarcoma
- Myxofibrosarcoma
- Pleomorphic liposarcoma

(Left) *The cut surface of dedifferentiated liposarcoma (DDLPS) varies in appearance depending upon the exact composition of the tumor. Lipogenic ➔ and nonlipogenic ⇨ (dedifferentiated) components are often readily distinguished from one another by differences in color and consistency.* **(Right)** *DDLPS may appear entirely or almost entirely composed of fibrous or fleshy nonlipogenic sarcoma ⇨. Sampling of peripheral fatty tissue ➔ to detect a minor lipogenic component is important.*

Dedifferentiated Liposarcoma

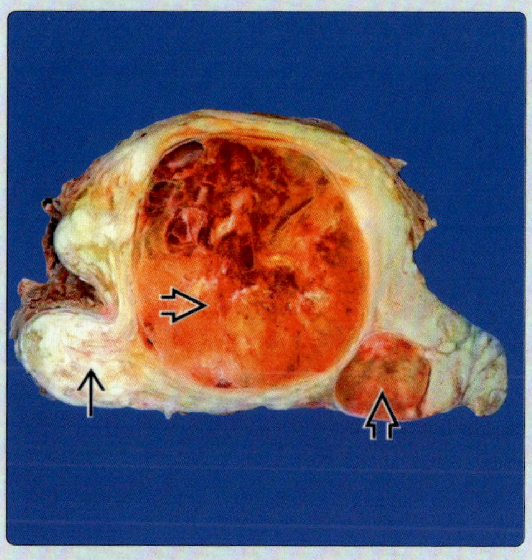

Dedifferentiated Liposarcoma

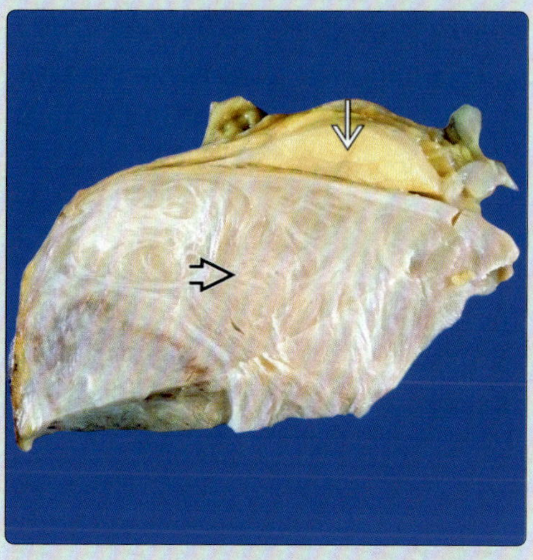

(Left) *This classic example of DDLPS shows a transition from a well-differentiated liposarcoma component (right) to a nonlipogenic sarcoma component (left). This transition may appear abrupt, as shown, with a sharp demarcation between the 2 components.* **(Right)** *The transitional interface in classic DDLPS may be more gradual and less abrupt, as depicted, with atypical fat cells admixed with otherwise nonlipogenic sarcoma.*

Abrupt Transition

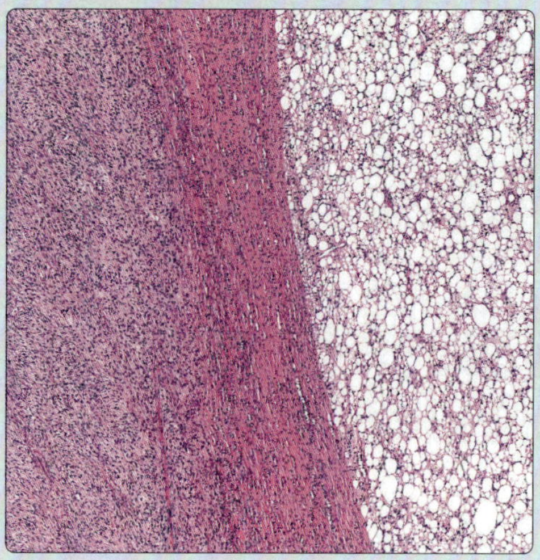

Gradual Transition

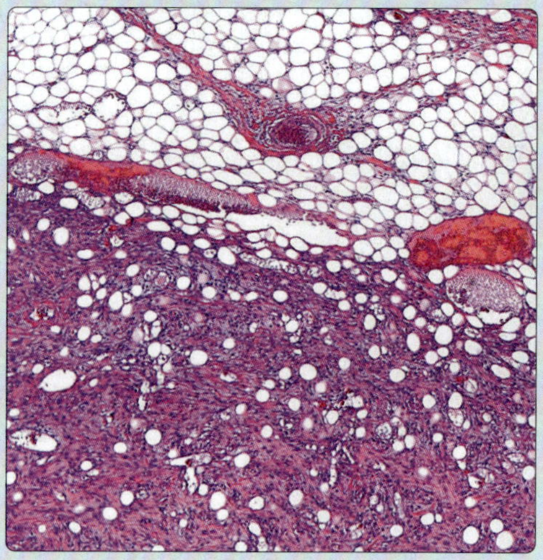

TERMINOLOGY

Abbreviations

- Dedifferentiated liposarcoma (DDLPS)

Definitions

- Malignant, generally nonlipogenic sarcoma of variable histologic grade often arising in association with identifiable component of atypical lipomatous tumor (ALT)/well-differentiated liposarcoma (WDLPS)

CLINICAL ISSUES

Epidemiology

- Incidence
  - Relatively common form of liposarcoma
  - Vast majority (90%) arise de novo
    - Minority develop in local recurrences of ALT/WDLPS
  - Dedifferentiation occurs in up to 10% of ALT/WDLPS
    - Probably represents time-dependent phenomenon
- Age
  - Middle-aged to elderly adults

Site

- Most common in retroperitoneum and abdominal cavity
- Also spermatic cord, trunk, extremities, head/neck region
- Most tumors arise in deep soft tissue
  - Rarely subcutaneous

Presentation

- Large, painless mass
- May be incidentally discovered in retroperitoneum
- In limbs, may present as longstanding mass that exhibits recent increase in size

Treatment

- Complete surgical resection with negative margins
- Surgical debulking for large, multifocal retroperitoneal/intraabdominal tumors
  - May require partial or complete resection of intraabdominal organs

Prognosis

- Anatomic location is most important prognostic factor
  - Retroperitoneal/intraabdominal tumors exhibit worst clinical behavior
- Local recurrence in ~ 40% of cases
  - Nearly all retroperitoneal tumors recur with long-term follow-up
- Distant metastases observed in 15-20% of cases
  - Less frequent than typically seen in other adult-type pleomorphic sarcomas
- Overall mortality 25-30% at 5-year follow-up
  - Likely higher rate with long-term follow-up
- Amount &/or histologic grade of dedifferentiated component generally shows no prognostic importance
  - However, in retroperitoneal tumors, high-grade morphology has been associated with decreased survival
- Presence of myogenic (especially rhabdomyoblastic) differentiation in retroperitoneal tumors has been associated with significantly decreased survival rates
- Epithelioid morphology (particularly when prominent) portends more aggressive clinical course

MACROSCOPIC

General Features

- Well demarcated, large, uni- or multinodular
- Dedifferentiated areas are often tan-gray-white with firm or fleshy cut surface
- Well-differentiated components, if present, are yellow and fatty
- Hemorrhage &/or necrosis common

Sections to Be Submitted

- Sections of both dedifferentiated and well-differentiated components must be sampled thoroughly
  - 1 section per cm of greatest linear tumor dimension
- If well-differentiated component is not obvious, sampling of peripheral adipose tissue is important

Size

- Often large (> 5 cm)
  - Retroperitoneal/intraabdominal tumors may be enormous

MICROSCOPIC

Histologic Features

- Classic appearance is transition from ALT/WDLPS to (usually) nonlipogenic, cellular sarcoma
  - ALT/WDLPS may be adipocytic (lipoma-like), sclerosing, or inflammatory subtypes
  - Transition may be abrupt or gradual
  - Component of ALT/WDLPS may be focal or absent
- Nonlipogenic sarcoma component shows very broad morphologic spectrum and may be high or low histologic grade
  - Many tumors show mixture of patterns
  - Cellular, pleomorphic morphology
    - Resembles undifferentiated pleomorphic sarcoma and other adult-type pleomorphic sarcomas
  - Prominent myxoid stroma morphology
    - Usually resembles intermediate- to high-grade myxofibrosarcoma
      - Pleomorphic, multinucleated tumor cells and curvilinear stromal vasculature
    - Rare focal areas may resemble myxoid liposarcoma
  - Fascicular spindle cell morphology
    - Variable nuclear atypia and pleomorphism
      - May appear low grade and resemble fibromatosis
    - Variable hyalinized stroma
  - Storiform, meningothelial-like morphology
    - Resembles neural proliferation or dermatofibrosarcoma protuberans
    - May be associated with metaplastic bone formation
  - Inflammatory morphology
    - Abundant neutrophilic infiltrate
    - Also plasma cells, lymphoid infiltrate
  - Epithelioid morphology
    - Diffuse, sheet-like growth
    - Rhabdoid cells may be apparent; rare acinar-like epithelial structures

- Often resemble carcinoma, melanoma, mesothelioma, or other sarcomas with epithelioid morphology
- Some areas may be indistinguishable from alveolar rhabdomyosarcoma
  - Identical immunophenotype as well (desmin, myogenin)
- Rare homologous lipoblastic morphology
  - Contains lipoblasts or pleomorphic lipoblasts
    - Occurring throughout lesion or in aggregates away from interface with ALT/WDLPS component
  - Can closely resemble pleomorphic liposarcoma
- Hemangiopericytoma-like vasculature may be prominent in rare cases
- Mitotic rate > 5 per 10 HPF
- Necrosis common
- Heterologous differentiation present in up to 10% of cases
  - Myogenic (rhabdomyoblastic, leiomyomatous), osteosarcoma, chondrosarcoma

ANCILLARY TESTS

Immunohistochemistry

- Diffuse nuclear MDM2(+) and CDK4(+) in majority
- Variable SMA, desmin, CD34
- Intact nuclear INI1 expression
- Nuclear H3K27me3 expression usually intact
  - Rarely lost, often in tumors with heterologous elements
- Heterologous elements in nonlipogenic areas can be highlighted by pertinent markers
  - e.g., desmin (+), myogenin (+) in rhabdomyoblastic elements
- Generally keratin and S100 protein (-)
  - Rare cases feature anomalous keratin expression (usually focal or patchy)
    - Often seen in epithelioid DDLPS

Molecular Genetics

- Similar to changes seen in ALT/WDLPS
  - Supernumerary ring and giant marker chromosomes
  - Amplified sequences originating from 12q13-15 region
    - Overexpression of *MDM2*, *CDK4*, &/or *HMGA2* detectable by FISH
- Rare *DDIT3* gene amplification
  - May be associated with myxoid liposarcoma-like morphology &/or homologous lipoblastic differentiation

DIFFERENTIAL DIAGNOSIS

Undifferentiated Pleomorphic Sarcoma

- Very rare in retroperitoneum
  - Most retroperitoneal tumors with undifferentiated pleomorphic sarcoma morphology are actually DDLPS
- Lacks component of ALT/WDLPS
- Generally less morphologically heterogeneous than DDLPS
- No *MDM2* amplification

Myxofibrosarcoma

- Very rare in retroperitoneum/abdomen
- Lacks component of ALT/WDLPS
- No *MDM2* amplification

Pleomorphic Liposarcoma

- May arise in retroperitoneum
- Lacks component of ALT/WDLPS
- No *MDM2* amplification

Well-Differentiated Liposarcoma

- May contain cellular areas, but mitotic activity is low to absent
- Lacks overtly fibrous or fleshy appearance grossly

Atypical Spindle Cell Lipomatous Tumor

- Lacks significant cytologic atypia
- Mitotic figures scarce or absent
- No *MDM2* amplification

Myxoid Liposarcoma

- Very rare in retroperitoneum/abdomen
- Lacks component of ALT/WDLPS
- No *MDM2* amplification
- Characteristic t(12;16)

Malignant Peripheral Nerve Sheath Tumor

- Fascicles of spindle cells with tapering nuclei; rarely markedly pleomorphic
- Characteristic perivascular cellularity in many cases
- May show origin from benign peripheral nerve sheath tumor (e.g., neurofibroma)
- May contain heterologous elements
- No *MDM2* amplification

Leiomyosarcoma

- Diffuse smooth muscle cytology (eosinophilic cytoplasm, cigar-shaped nuclei, etc.)
- Diffuse SMA(+)
- Variable desmin (+), caldesmon (+)
- No *MDM2* amplification

SELECTED REFERENCES

1. Agaimy A et al: Dedifferentiated liposarcoma composed predominantly of rhabdoid/epithelioid cells: a frequently misdiagnosed highly aggressive variant. Hum Pathol. 77:20-7, 2018
2. Makise N et al: Dedifferentiated liposarcoma with epithelioid/epithelial features. Am J Surg Pathol. 41(11):1523-31, 2017
3. Thway K et al: Dedifferentiated liposarcoma: updates on morphology, genetics, and therapeutic strategies. Adv Anat Pathol. 23(1):30-40, 2016
4. Gronchi A et al: Myogenic differentiation and histologic grading are major prognostic determinants in retroperitoneal liposarcoma. Am J Surg Pathol. 39(3):383-93, 2015
5. Liau JY et al: Dedifferentiated liposarcoma with homologous lipoblastic differentiation: expanding the spectrum to include low-grade tumours. Histopathology. 62(5):702-10, 2013
6. Ghadimi MP et al: Diagnosis, management, and outcome of patients with dedifferentiated liposarcoma systemic metastasis. Ann Surg Oncol. 18(13):3762-70, 2011
7. Thway K et al: Dedifferentiated liposarcoma with meningothelial-like whorls, metaplastic bone formation, and CDK4, MDM2, and p16 expression: a morphologic and immunohistochemical study. Am J Surg Pathol. 35(3):356-63, 2011
8. Lucas DR et al: Dedifferentiated liposarcoma with inflammatory myofibroblastic tumor-like features. Am J Surg Pathol. 34(6):844-51, 2010
9. Mariño-Enríquez A et al: Dedifferentiated liposarcoma with "homologous" lipoblastic (pleomorphic liposarcoma-like) differentiation: clinicopathologic and molecular analysis of a series suggesting revised diagnostic criteria. Am J Surg Pathol. 34(8):1122-31, 2010
10. Sirvent N et al: Detection of MDM2-CDK4 amplification by fluorescence in situ hybridization in 200 paraffin-embedded tumor samples: utility in diagnosing adipocytic lesions and comparison with immunohistochemistry and real-time PCR. Am J Surg Pathol. 31(10):1476-89, 2007

Pleomorphic Morphology

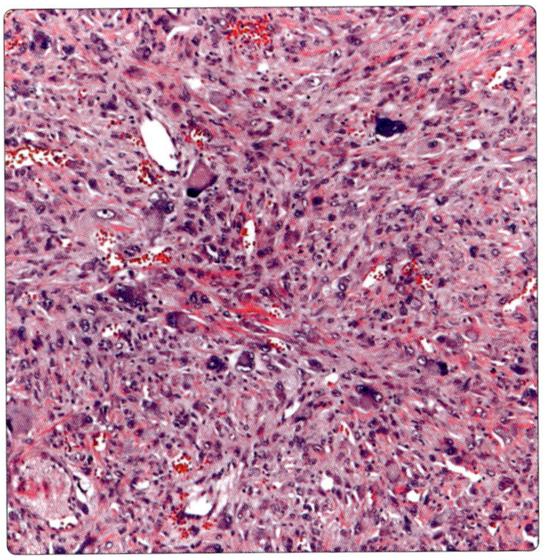

Myxofibrosarcoma-Like Morphology

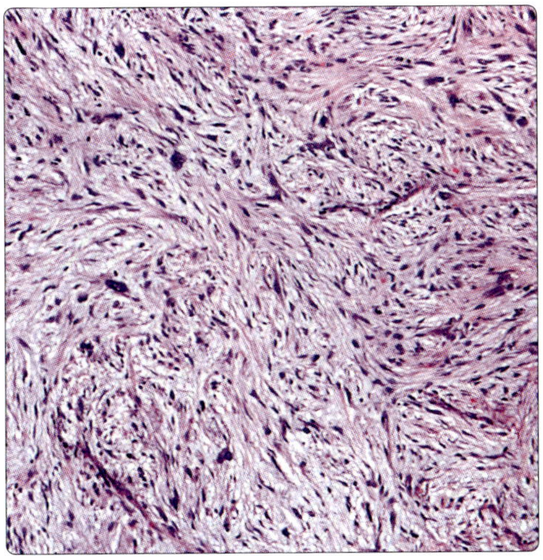

(Left) *A common morphologic appearance in DDLPS is that of a high-grade, cellular pleomorphic sarcoma. Out of context, this morphology is indistinguishable from that of an undifferentiated pleomorphic sarcoma.* **(Right)** *A prominent myxoid morphology with distinct stromal vessels is common in DDLPS and may closely simulate myxofibrosarcoma; however, the latter is very rare in the retroperitoneum in contrast to DDLPS.*

Low-Grade Myxoid Morphology

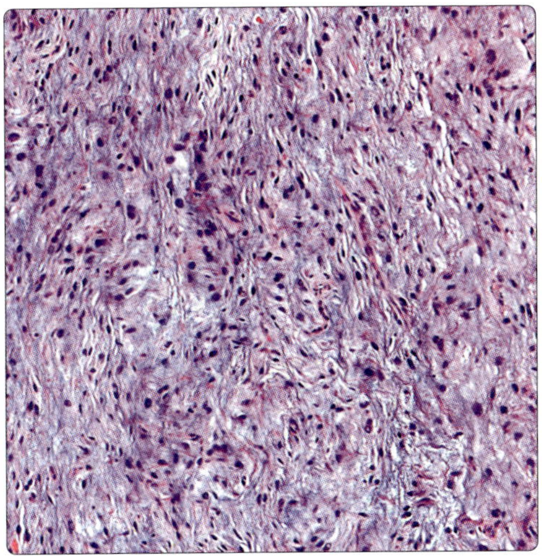

Spindled Morphology

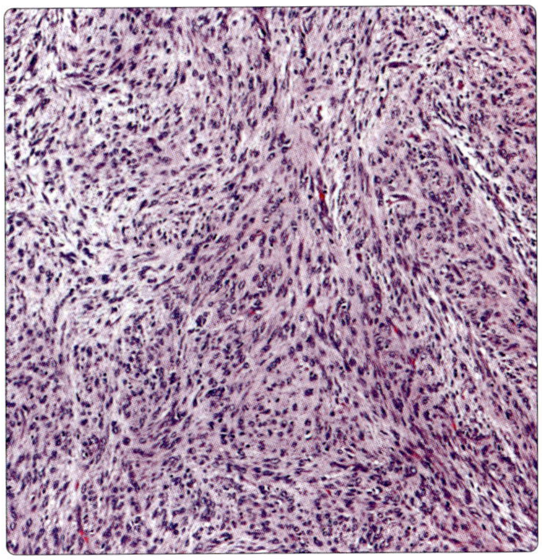

(Left) *Some myxoid nonlipogenic areas of DDLPS are cytologically low grade and may lead to consideration of other myxoid tumors, such as myxoid liposarcoma or low-grade fibromyxoid sarcoma. Identification of more conventional, higher grade areas is useful.* **(Right)** *Tumor cells may be spindled and loosely fascicular in DDLPS. This morphology may lead to consideration of other diagnoses, including leiomyosarcoma and malignant peripheral nerve sheath tumor.*

Fascicular Morphology

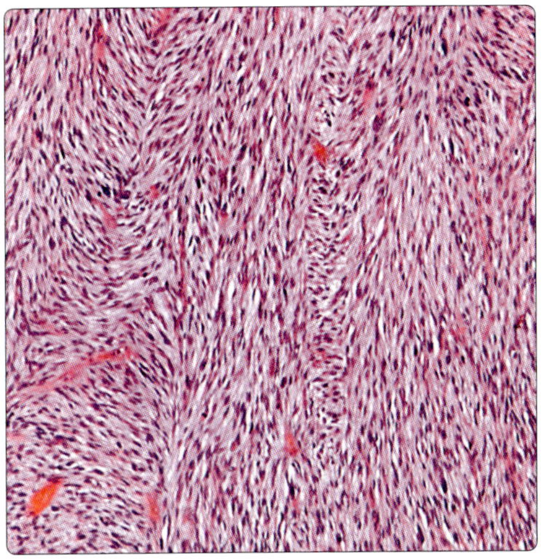

Low-Grade Fascicular Morphology

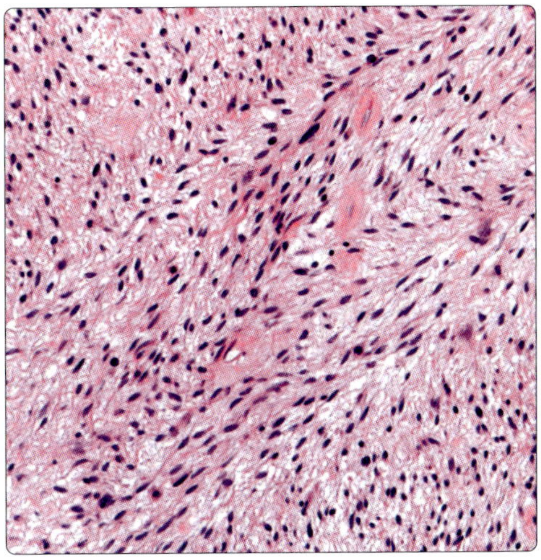

(Left) *Fascicular growth may be well developed in DDLPS and show a herringbone architecture, as shown, leading to consideration of entities like leiomyosarcoma and fibrosarcoma.* **(Right)** *Spindled, fascicular areas in DDLPS may be cytologically low grade, imparting an appearance suggestive of fibromatosis or a variety of low-grade sarcomas.*

Sclerotic Matrix

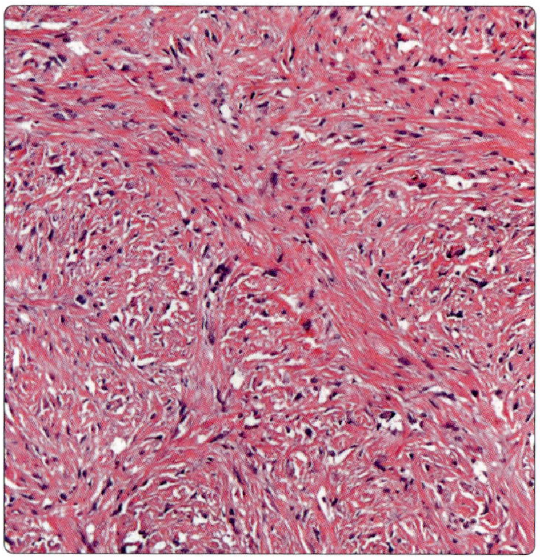

Storiform Morphology

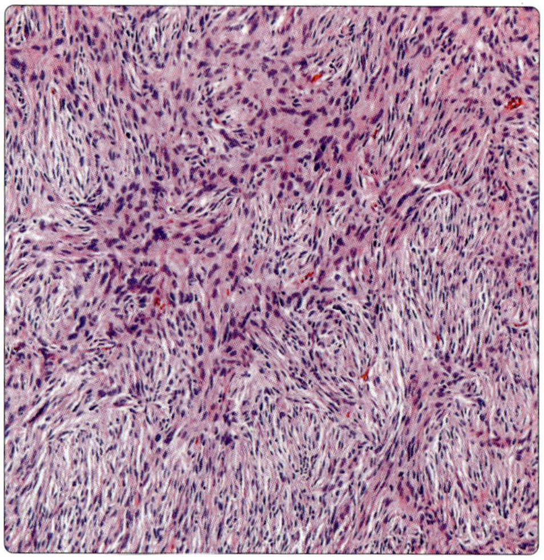

(Left) *Some cases of DDLPS may contain focal or prominent regions of hyalinized/sclerotic matrix. The overall fascicular growth, presence of mitoses, and lack of fat help distinguish this pattern from sclerosing ALT/WDLPS.* **(Right)** *A storiform growth pattern is not uncommon in DDLPS and may superficially resemble tumors such as dermatofibrosarcoma protuberans, perineurioma, or follicular dendritic cell sarcoma.*

Whorled Morphology

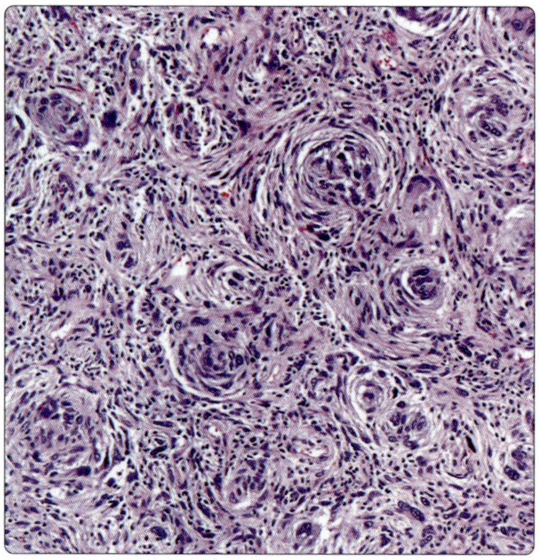

Inflammatory Component

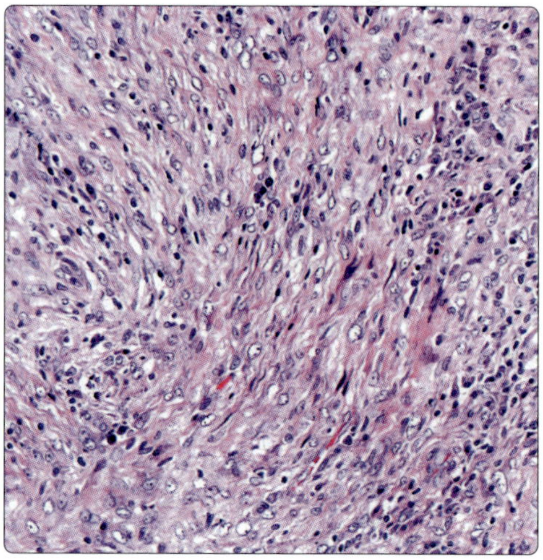

(Left) *A peculiar, meningothelial-like whorling growth may be seen in rare cases of DDLPS. This pattern has been associated with metaplastic bone formation in some cases.* **(Right)** *A chronic inflammatory component may be seen in DDLPS and often consists of plasma cells and lymphocytes. In conjunction with a fascicular morphology, this finding may suggest inflammatory myofibroblastic tumor.*

Abundant Neutrophils

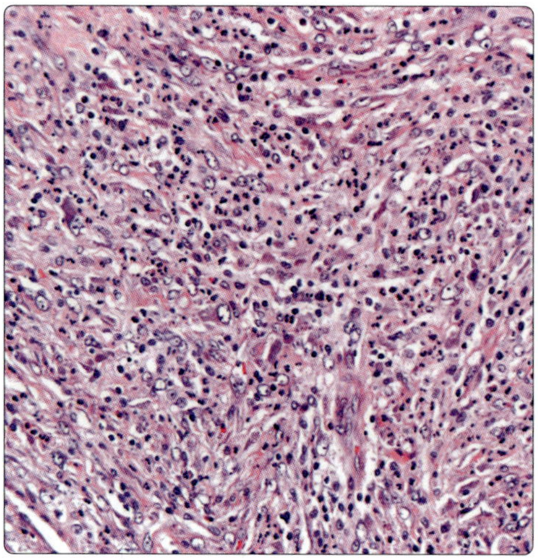

Epithelioid Morphology

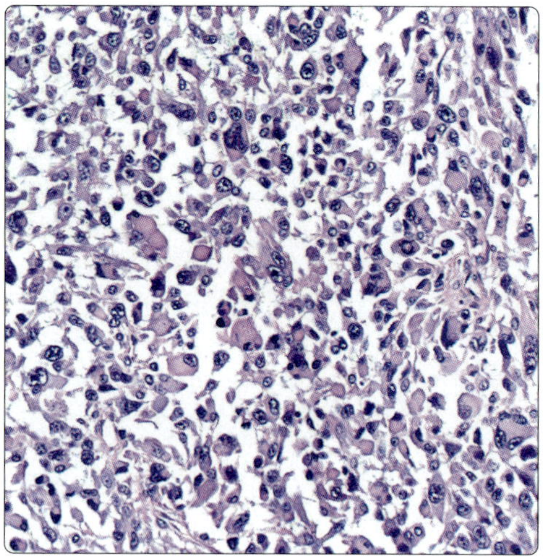

(Left) *Occasional cases of DDLPS show a prominent neutrophilic infiltrate and may not be readily identifiable as a liposarcoma. This finding is most frequently seen in the retroperitoneum. Detection of MDM2/CDK4 overexpression or amplification can be very helpful.* **(Right)** *An epithelioid morphology in DDLPS, though rare, is well described and can mimic carcinoma, melanoma, and other sarcomas with an epithelioid appearance. Rhabdoid change, as seen in this H&E, is also possible.*

Heterologous Elements

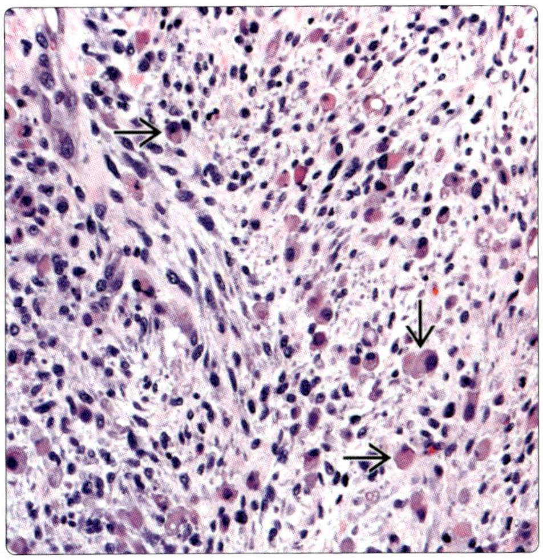

Rhabdomyosarcoma-Like Areas

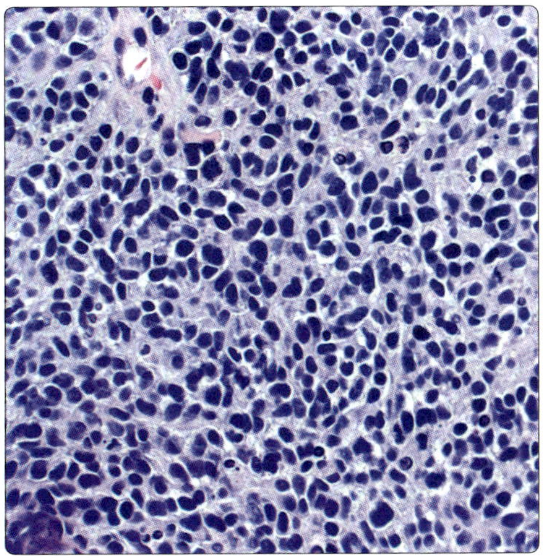

(Left) *Heterologous differentiation is seen in up to 10% of cases of DDLPS. Rhabdomyoblasts* ⇨ *are one of many types of elements and may be highlighted with desmin and myogenin immunostains.* **(Right)** *Rare cases of DDLPS can show epithelioid areas that closely resemble alveolar rhabdomyosarcoma (ARMS), including cytoplasmic clearing and scattered rhabdomyoblasts. Further, IHC staining supports rhabdomyoblastic differentiation.*

Myogenin

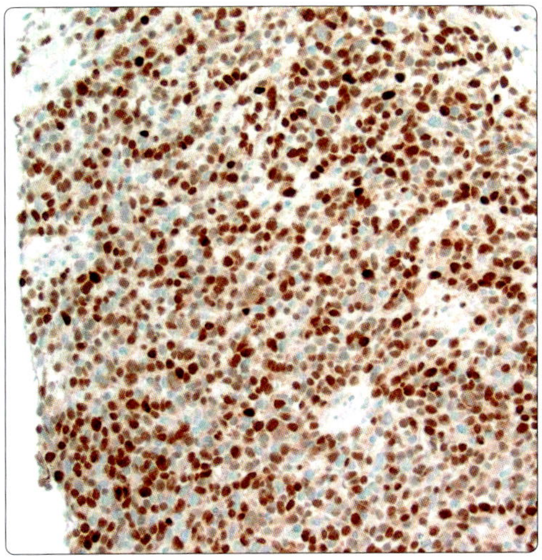

Heterologous Elements

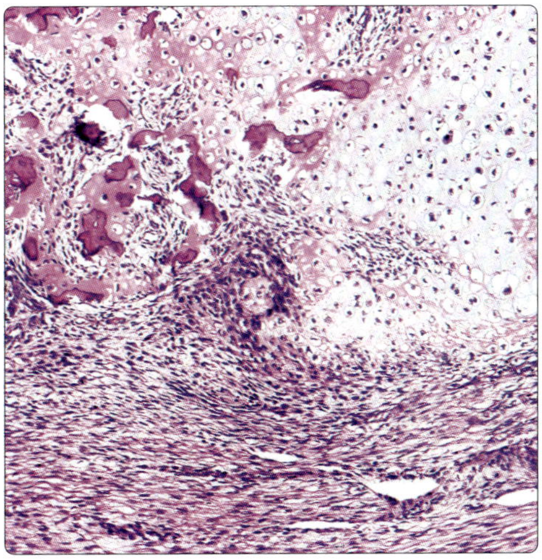

(Left) *Epithelioid DDLPS with areas resembling ARMS show diffuse myogenin expression, similar to actual ARMS. Demonstration of classic WDLPS zones or MDM2 gene amplification is often required to make the diagnosis of DDLPS.* **(Right)** *Heterologous osteosarcoma &/or chondrosarcoma may be seen in some cases of DDLPS, as shown. Additional types of elements include leiomyosarcoma and, rarely, angiosarcoma.*

Homologous Lipoblastic Differentiation

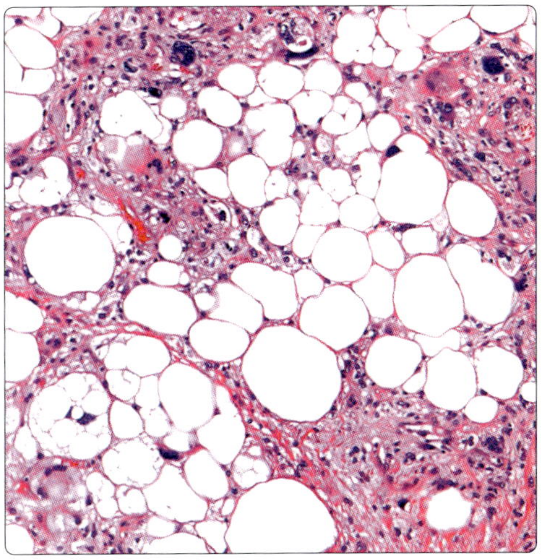

Unusual Morphologies

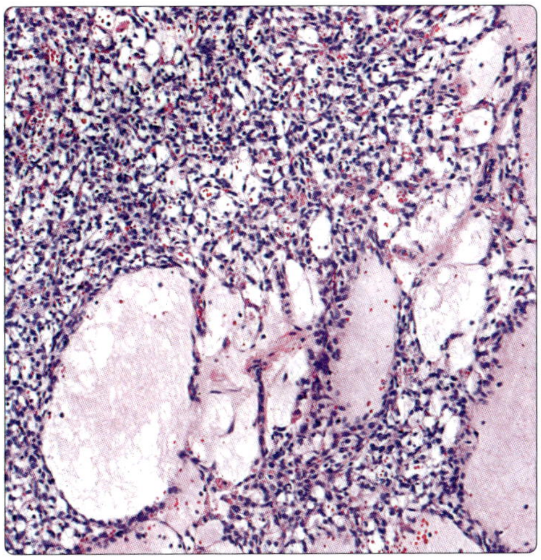

(Left) *Rare cases of DDLPS contain lipoblastic differentiation within the high-grade dedifferentiated component and is considered by some as homologous differentiation. The morphology often closely resembles pleomorphic liposarcoma.* **(Right)** *A variety of unusual morphologies can be noted in DDLPS, including ones that resemble cellular myxoid liposarcoma or even hemangioblastoma. This case (shown) features microcysts and abundant cytoplasmic eosinophilic globules.*

Myxoid Liposarcoma

KEY FACTS

TERMINOLOGY

- Malignant neoplasm composed of primitive nonlipogenic mesenchymal cells and variable number of lipoblasts set in prominent myxoid stroma with characteristic branching capillary vasculature

CLINICAL ISSUES

- Accounts for ~ 30-35% of all liposarcomas
- Most occur in young to middle-aged adults
- Usually arise in deep soft tissue of extremities
- Treatment: Complete surgical resection with negative margins
- Local recurrence in ~ 30% of cases
- Metastatic risk varies by histologic grade (< 10% up to 60%)
  - Presence of hypercellular (round cell) areas is most important histologic predictor of outcome

MACROSCOPIC

- Usually large (median 10-12 cm)

MICROSCOPIC

- Typically shows lobular growth pattern
- Abundant myxoid stroma
- Characteristic delicate, arborizing capillary vasculature
- Small spindled, stellate, and ovoid nonlipogenic tumor cells
- Uni-, bi-, and multivacuolated lipoblasts frequently present
- Mitoses generally scarce
- Progression to hypercellular or round cell areas may be present

ANCILLARY TESTS

- Molecular: Characteristic t(12;16) with *FUS-DDIT3* fusion

TOP DIFFERENTIAL DIAGNOSES

- Atypical lipomatous tumor/well-differentiated liposarcoma
- Myxofibrosarcoma
- Lipoblastoma
- Low-grade fibromyxoid sarcoma
- Intramuscular myxoma

Myxoid Liposarcoma

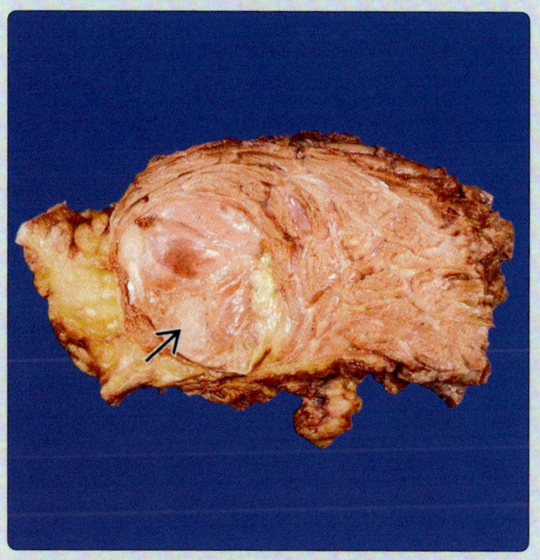

Lobular Growth

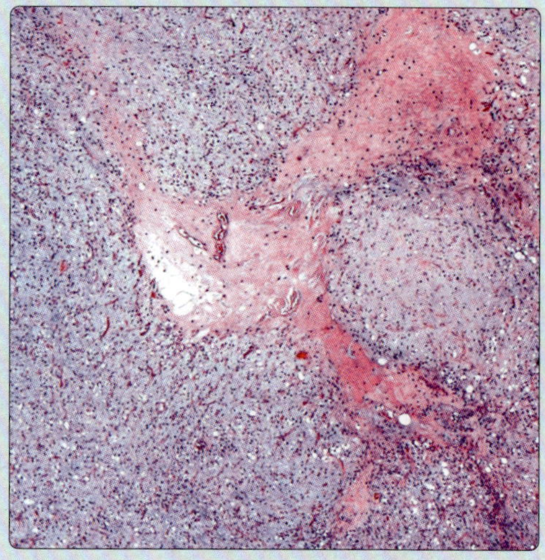

(Left) *Grossly, myxoid liposarcoma (MLPS) typically shows a glistening, gelatinous cut surface; however, more cellular, high-grade areas often appear more firm and gray-white ⇒. Thorough sampling of this neoplasm is critical for proper histologic grading.* **(Right)** *Lobular growth is a typical feature of MLPS, and lobules may be separated by hypocellular, pink fibrous zones. Although not shown in this image, an increase in cellularity may be present at the periphery of these lobules.*

Abundant Myxoid Stroma

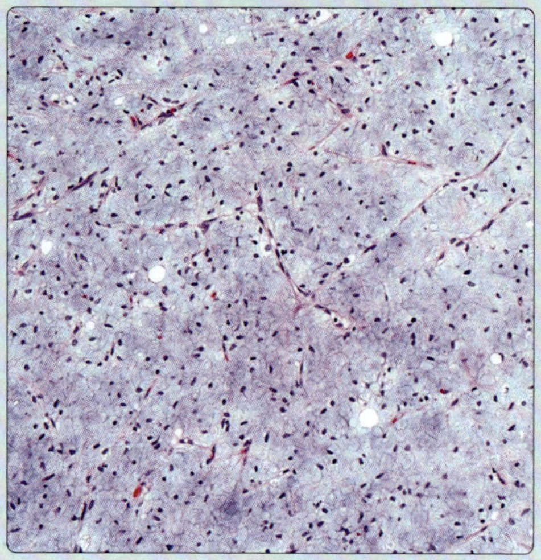

Bland Cytologic Features

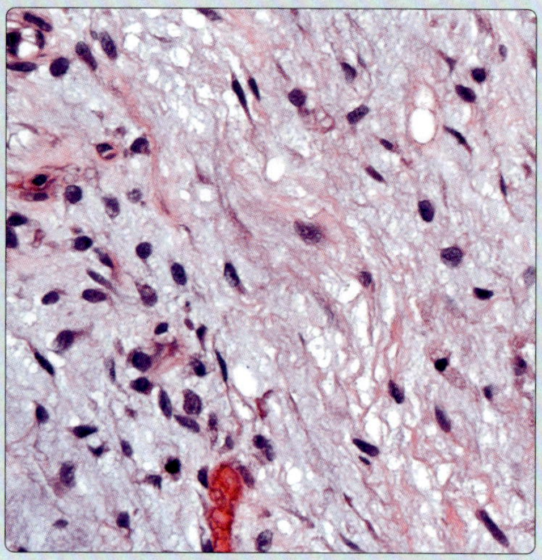

(Left) *Myxoid liposarcoma is characterized in most cases by an abundant myxoid stroma, particularly in low-grade areas; however, this stroma becomes less conspicuous in hypercellular, higher grade areas.* **(Right)** *The lesional cells of MLPS are spindled, stellate, or ovoid and usually contain small, bland nuclei. Mitoses are often scarce. With very rare exceptions, nuclear pleomorphism is not a feature of MLPS and should prompt consideration of other diagnoses.*

TERMINOLOGY

Abbreviations

- Myxoid liposarcoma (MLPS)

Synonyms

- Round cell liposarcoma (high-grade MLPS)

Definitions

- Malignant neoplasm composed of primitive nonlipogenic mesenchymal cells and variable number of lipoblasts set in prominent myxoid stroma with characteristic branching capillary vasculature
  - Use of term "round cell liposarcoma" no longer advocated (2013 WHO classification)
    - Current recommendation: High-grade MLPS

CLINICAL ISSUES

Epidemiology

- Incidence
  - Accounts for ~ 30-35% of all liposarcomas
  - Represents 5-10% of all sarcomas in adults
  - Most common form of liposarcoma in children and adolescents
- Age
  - Most occur in young to middle-aged adults (usually 20-50 years)
  - Rare in children

Site

- Deep soft tissue of extremities
  - Majority of cases arise within musculature of thigh
  - Rarely in subcutaneous tissue
- Exceptionally rare in retroperitoneum and body cavities
  - More likely to be primary well-differentiated liposarcoma or metastatic MLPS from somatic soft tissue site

Presentation

- Painless, slow-growing, deep-seated mass
- May present with synchronous or metachronous multifocal disease
  - Likely represent hematogenous soft tissue metastases rather than distinctly separate tumors

Treatment

- Complete surgical resection with negative margins
- Radiotherapy may reduce risk of local recurrence
- Trabectedin may be effective in treating metastatic MLPS

Prognosis

- Local recurrence in ~ 30% of cases
- Most frequent sites of metastasis include other soft tissue sites, bone, retroperitoneum, lungs
  - Metastatic risk varies by histologic grade
    - Low-grade tumors have < 10% risk
    - Higher-grade tumors have significantly increased risk (40-60%)
- Presence of hypercellular (round cell) areas is most important histologic predictor of outcome
  - > 5% hypercellularity is associated with unfavorable outcome (considered high grade)
    - Some studies recommend cutoff of 25% to consider high grade
- Other adverse prognostic factors: Age (> 45 years), presence of coagulative necrosis, p53 overexpression, *TP53* and *CDKN2A* mutations
- Overall mortality rate 25-40%

MACROSCOPIC

General Features

- Well circumscribed, multinodular
- Homogeneous, gelatinous cut surface in low-grade lesions
- Higher grade lesions are often tan-white and firm or fleshy
- Macroscopic evidence of necrosis uncommon

Size

- Usually large (median 10-12 cm)

Sections to Be Submitted

- Thorough sampling is necessary to adequately estimate percentage of hypercellular or round cell component, if present

MICROSCOPIC

Histologic Features

- Typically shows lobular growth pattern
  - Often increased cellularity at periphery of lobules
- Characteristic abundant myxoid stroma
  - May show areas of mucin pooling (pulmonary edema-like pattern)
- Characteristic delicate, arborizing capillary vasculature (chicken-wire pattern)
- Small spindled, stellate, and ovoid nonlipogenic tumor cells with scant cytoplasm
  - Bland nuclei with fine chromatin and inconspicuous nucleoli
    - General absence of nuclear pleomorphism
      - Exception: Very rare multinucleated cells
  - Mitoses generally scarce
- Uni-, bi-, and multivacuolated lipoblasts frequently present
  - Vary widely in number from case to case; may be sparse
  - Often most numerous at periphery of lobules or around stromal blood vessels
  - Some are highly vacuolated with eosinophilic, granular cytoplasm (hibernoma-like cells)
- Other findings: Interstitial hemorrhage, mature adipose tissue, stromal hyalinization (often following radiotherapy), rare foci of cartilaginous differentiation
- Progression to hypercellular or round cell areas
  - Nests or solid sheets of back-to-back &/or overlapping cells
    - Nuclei often larger and more hyperchromatic; may show more conspicuous nucleoli
    - Mitoses and apoptotic cells more frequent
  - Characteristic arborizing vasculature less conspicuous but present
  - Lipoblasts and stromal mucin pools may be present
  - Percentage of reportable hypercellular/round cell component varies from 5% to > 80%
  - Round cell areas may rarely show corded growth in hyalinized matrix

ANCILLARY TESTS

Immunohistochemistry

- Best utilized to exclude other entities
- Variable S100 protein (+)
  - May highlight lipoblasts or show focal expression in round cell areas
- Negative for keratin, CD34, SMA, desmin
- Usually negative for MDM2 and CDK4 (rare focal nuclear expression)

Molecular Genetics

- Characteristic recurrent t(12;16)(q13;p11) involving *DDIT3* (*CHOP*) and *FUS* genes
  - Vast majority of cases (90-95%)
- Infrequent variant t(12;22)(q13;q12) involving *DDIT3* and *EWSR1*
- Also, activating *PIK3CA* mutations or homozygous loss of *PTEN* in some tumors
- *TP53* mutations in 1/3 of cases, independent of histologic grade

DIFFERENTIAL DIAGNOSIS

Atypical Lipomatous Tumor/Well-Differentiated Liposarcoma

- May contain focal to extensive zones of myxoid stromal change
- Contains scattered enlarged, hyperchromatic stromal cells (including floret-like cells)
- Variably thickened fibrous bands
- Absence of delicate, arborizing vasculature in most cases
- Most show MDM2(+) and CDK4(+) by immunohistochemistry
- *MDM2* amplification
- Lacks *DDIT3* fusions

Myxofibrosarcoma

- Generally affects older age group than MLPS
- Nuclear pleomorphism and atypia are characteristic
- Lacks true lipoblasts
  - May contain pseudolipoblasts (vacuolated fibroblastic tumor cells containing mucin)
- Elongated curvilinear vessels of myxofibrosarcoma are different from delicate arborizing vasculature of MLPS
- Lacks *DDIT3* fusions

Lipoblastoma

- Most common in infancy and early childhood
- *PLAG1* rearrangements
- Lacks molecular signature of MLPS

Intramuscular Myxoma

- Often smaller, well-circumscribed tumors
- Lacks lipoblasts and arborizing capillary vascular pattern of MLPS
- Lacks *DDIT3* fusions

Low-Grade Fibromyxoid Sarcoma

- Bland fibrous zones punctuated by more cellular and vascularized myxoid nodules
- Lacks delicate arborizing capillary channels of MLPS
- Lacks lipoblasts
- Characteristic t(7;16) with *FUS-CREB3L2* fusion

Lipoblastoma-Like Tumor of Vulva

- Rare; only affect vulva
- Striking lobularity
- Loss of nuclear Rb expression by IHC
- Lacks *DDIT3* fusions

Extraskeletal Myxoid Chondrosarcoma

- Small spindled, stellate, or round eosinophilic tumor cells arranged in clusters and cords
- Lacks lipoblasts and arborizing capillary vascular pattern
- Variable S100 protein (+) in minority of cases
- Characteristic *NR4A3* gene arrangements

Dermatofibrosarcoma Protuberans (Myxoid Variant)

- Infiltrative dermal/subcutaneous neoplasm
- Diffuse infiltration of preexisting structures and adjacent soft tissue (honeycomb pattern)
- Lacks lipoblasts
- Vascular network and absence of nuclear pleomorphism may somewhat resemble that of MLPS
- Diffuse CD34(+) expression
- Characteristic *COL1A1-PDGFB* gene fusion

Synovial Sarcoma (Poorly Differentiated)

- May resemble hypercellular round cell areas of MLPS
- Often shows areas of cellular fascicular growth
- Lacks lipoblasts and arborizing capillary vasculature of MLPS
- Variable keratin (+) &/or EMA(+), often focal
- Diffuse nuclear TLE1 expression by immunohistochemistry
- Characteristic t(X;18) involving *SS18* (*SYT*)

Ewing Sarcoma

- Lacks lipoblasts and arborizing capillary vascular pattern of MLPS
- Usually strong, membranous CD99(+)
- Most contain *EWSR1* translocation
  - No rearrangement of *DDIT3* (*CHOP*)

SELECTED REFERENCES

1. Chowdhry V et al: Myxoid liposarcoma: treatment outcomes from chemotherapy and radiation therapy. Sarcoma. 2018:8029157, 2018
2. Muratori F et al: Myxoid liposarcoma: prognostic factors and metastatic pattern in a series of 148 patients treated at a single institution. Int J Surg Oncol. 2018:8928706, 2018
3. Bekers EM et al: Myxoid liposarcoma of the foot: a study of 8 cases. Ann Diagn Pathol. 25:37-41, 2016
4. Iwasaki H et al: Extensive lipoma-like changes of myxoid liposarcoma: morphologic, immunohistochemical, and molecular cytogenetic analyses. Virchows Arch. 466(4):453-64, 2015
5. Hoffman A et al: Localized and metastatic myxoid/round cell liposarcoma: clinical and molecular observations. Cancer. 119(10):1868-77, 2013
6. Gronchi A et al: Phase II clinical trial of neoadjuvant trabectedin in patients with advanced localized myxoid liposarcoma. Ann Oncol. 23(3):771-6, 2012
7. Moreau LC et al: Myxoid\round cell liposarcoma (MRCLS) revisited: an analysis of 418 primarily managed cases. Ann Surg Oncol. 19(4):1081-8, 2012
8. de Vreeze R et al: Multifocal myxoid liposarcoma–metastasis or second primary tumor?: a molecular biological analysis. J Mol Diagn. 12(2):238-43, 2010
9. ten Heuvel SE et al: Clinicopathologic prognostic factors in myxoid liposarcoma: a retrospective study of 49 patients with long-term follow-up. Ann Surg Oncol. 14(1):222-9, 2007
10. Orvieto E et al: Myxoid and round cell liposarcoma: a spectrum of myxoid adipocytic neoplasia. Semin Diagn Pathol. 18(4):267-73, 2001

Arborizing Capillary Vasculature

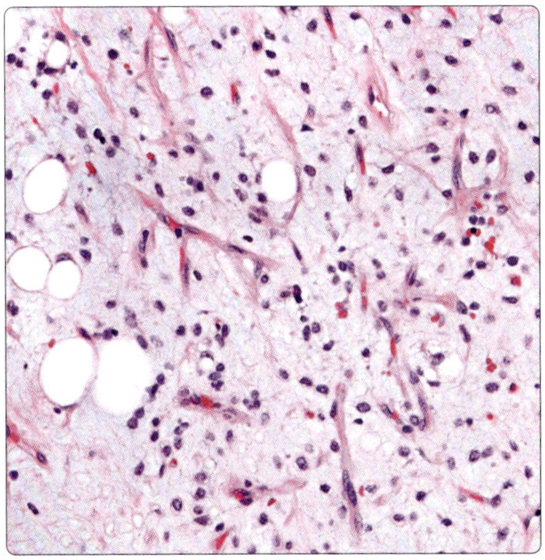

Arborizing Capillary Vasculature

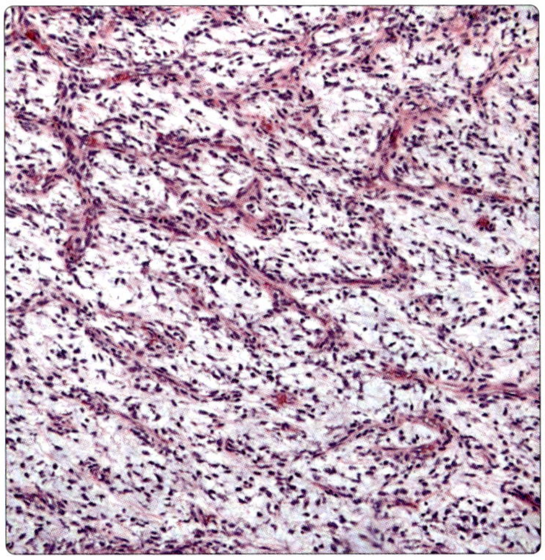

(Left) *The stromal vascular network of MLPS is highly characteristic and composed of delicate, arborizing or ramifying, thin-walled capillary channels. This pattern may be referred to as chicken-wire or crow's feet.* **(Right)** *Rarely, in some areas the arborizing vasculature of MLPS may appear more prominent secondary to increased perivascular cell density and may raise the possibility of myxofibrosarcoma or low-grade fibromyxoid sarcoma.*

Lipoblasts

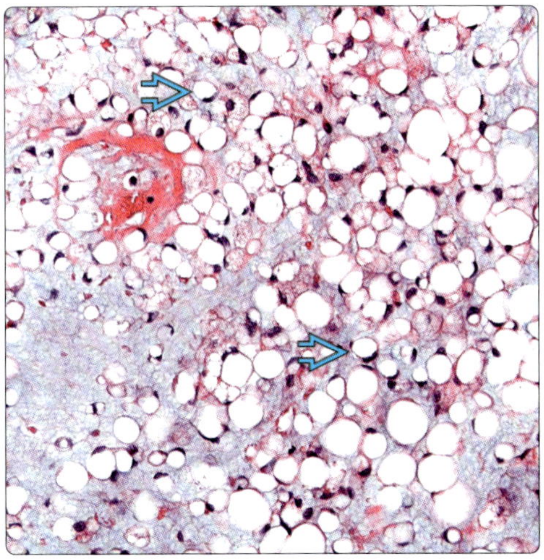

Sparse Lipoblasts

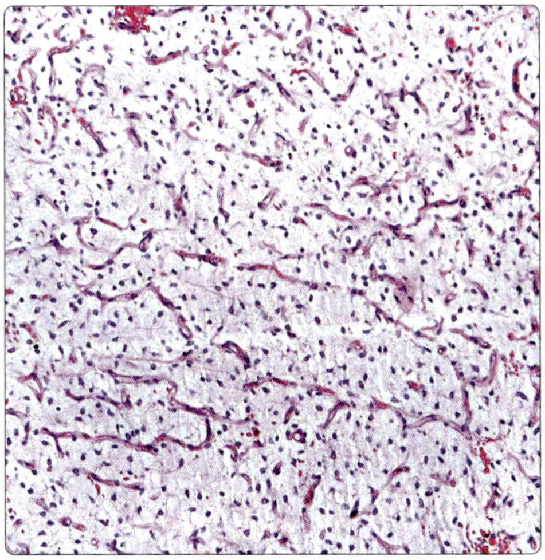

(Left) *Lipoblasts are a common finding in MLPS and are often univacuolated (resembling signet-ring cells) or bivacuolated. Multivacuolated forms are also seen. Lipoblasts vary widely in number and distribution and show a tendency to cluster around stromal blood vessels.* **(Right)** *This image of MLPS was taken from a case that showed a nicely developed "chicken-wire" vasculature but a relatively low number of lipoblasts. In a limited biopsy, absence of lipoblasts should never exclude the possibility of MLPS.*

Rare Multinucleated Cells

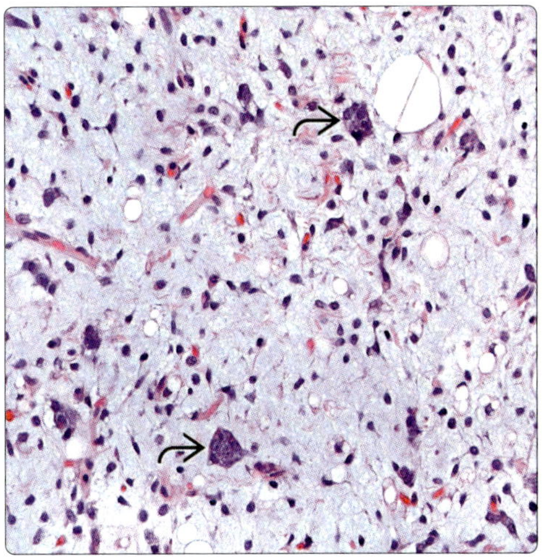

Hibernoma-Like Cells

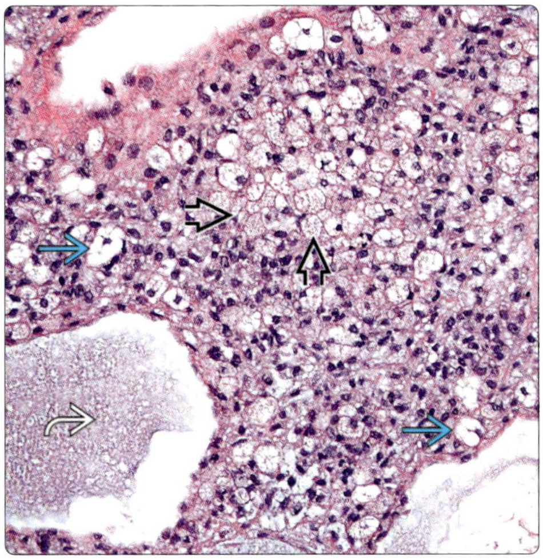

(Left) *Very rare cases of MLPS may show scattered cells with nuclear pleomorphism or multinucleation. This finding does not appear to affect prognosis.* **(Right)** *Some cases of MLPS contain highly vacuolated lipogenic cells with eosinophilic, granular cytoplasm. These cells resemble those of hibernoma. More characteristic lipoblasts and stromal mucin pools are also seen.*

(Left) *The formation of stromal mucin pools* → *is a relatively common finding in MLPS and has been described as a pulmonary edema-like or lymphangioma-like pattern. The size of the pools vary from small to quite large.* **(Right)** *Rare cases of MLPS show confluence of mucin pools and formation of large cystic structures, which may be so large as to be apparent at the time of gross examination.*

Stromal Mucin Pools

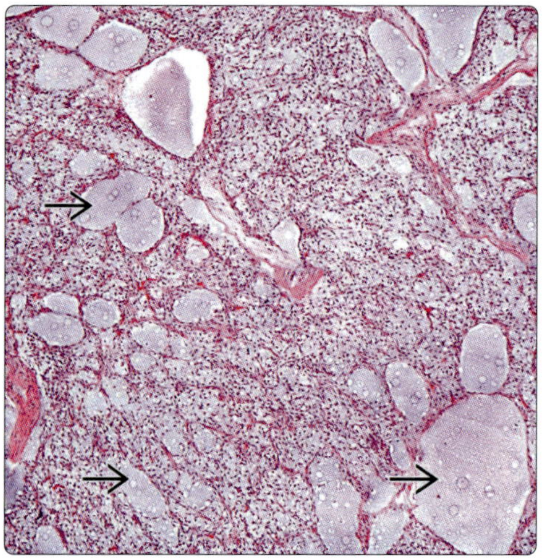

Stromal Mucin Pools

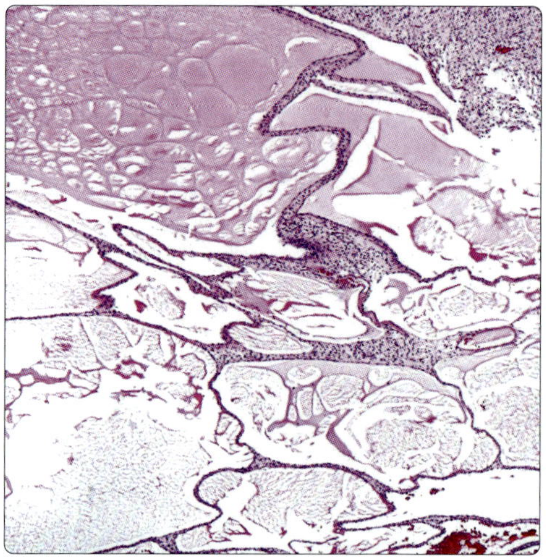

(Left) *Small, scattered foci of mature adipose tissue are not uncommon in MLPS; however, a dominant component of mature fat, as depicted, is much less frequent and may lead to underdiagnosis as a myxolipoma or spindle cell lipoma.* **(Right)** *Stromal hyalinization is often present in cases of MLPS treated preoperatively with radiation; however, it can be seen in untreated tumors as well, albeit less frequently. Note the intact capillary vasculature* ⇨ *and scattered lipoblasts* →.

Mature Adipose Tissue

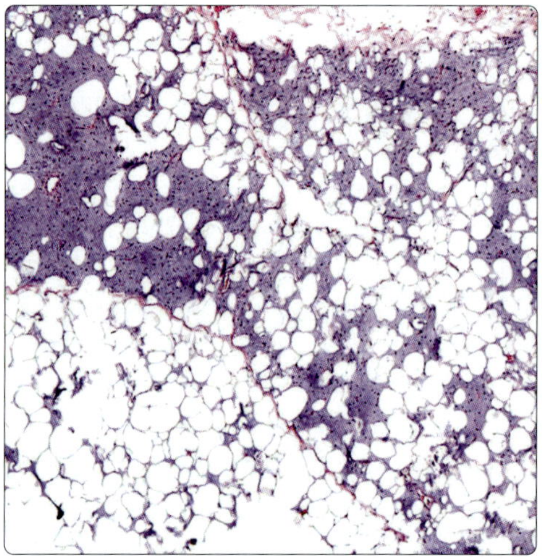

Stromal Hyalinization

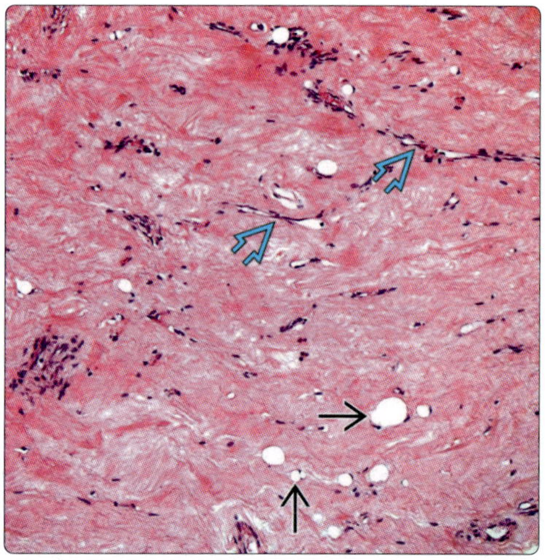

(Left) *S100 protein expression is generally limited to lipoblasts and adipocytes in MLPS and is not seen in lesional spindled/ovoid cells. However, focal expression may be seen in hypercellular round cell areas.* **(Right)** *Low-grade MLPS is generally hypocellular; however, a modest increase in cellularity is not uncommon. Note that, unlike prognostically significant hypercellular or round cell areas, the nuclei in these transitional areas do not show marked crowding or overlapping.*

S100 Protein Expression

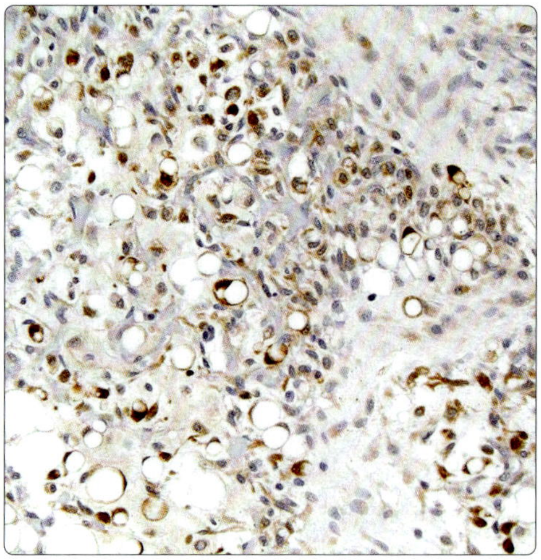

Transitional Areas

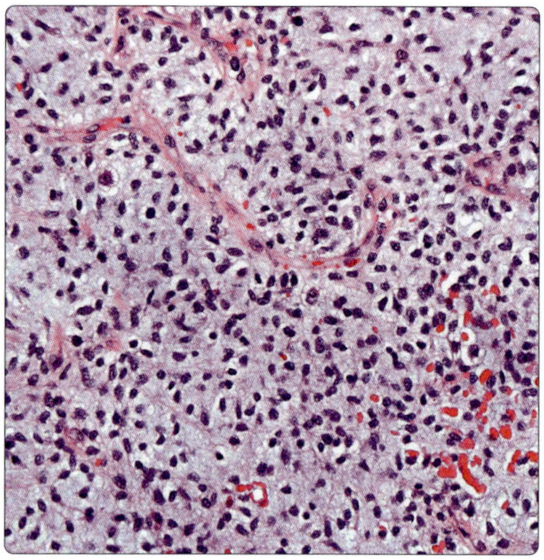

Hypercellularity

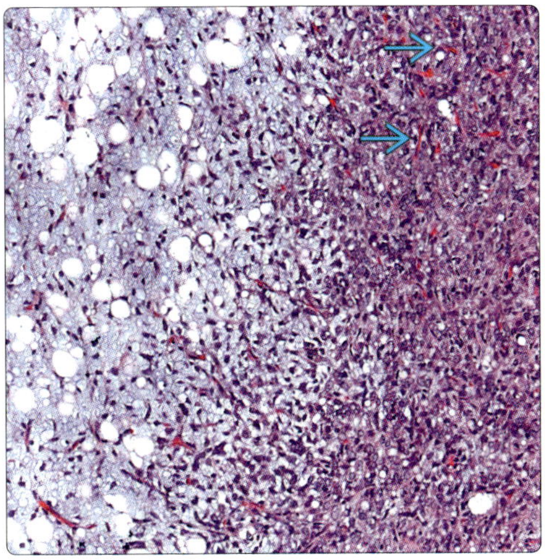

Hypercellularity

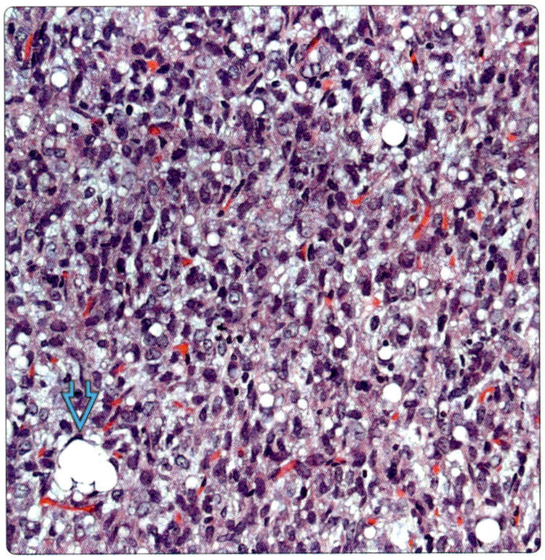

(Left) *Quantification of hypercellularity in MLPS is critical for histologic grading and prognostication. Hypercellular areas show dense crowding of cells and nuclei with limited or no myxoid stroma. Note that the arborizing capillary vasculature* → *is still present and identifiable but much less conspicuous.* **(Right)** *Lipoblasts* ⇒ *may be seen in hypercellular areas of MLPS but are much less frequent compared to lower grade areas. Note that significant nuclear pleomorphism is not a feature of high-grade MLPS.*

Cytology of Hypercellular Areas

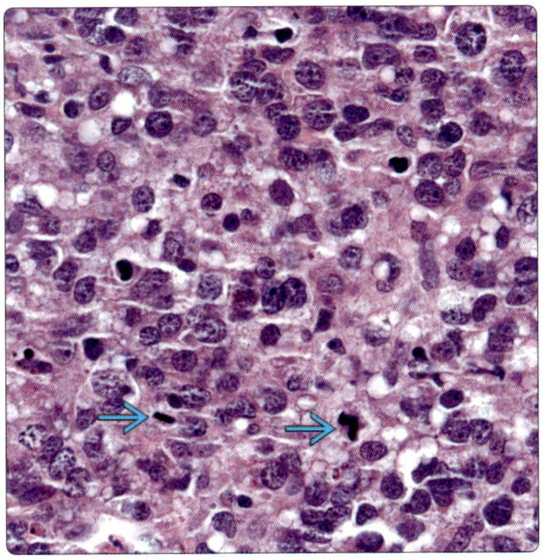

Mucin Pools in Hypercellular Areas

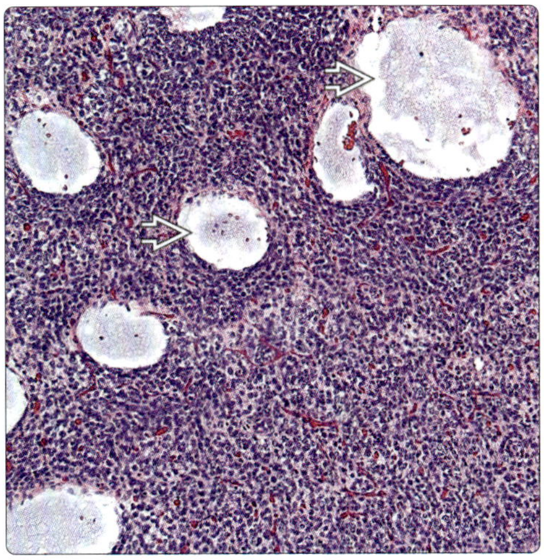

(Left) *Although still lacking significant pleomorphism, the nuclei in high-grade areas of MLPS are often rounder and show greater atypia and more conspicuous nucleoli than those in lower grade areas. Mitoses* → *are also more frequent in these areas.* **(Right)** *Similar to conventional low-grade areas of MLPS, high-grade areas may also show formation of stromal mucin pools* ➡*. Along with scattered lipoblasts, this finding can be a helpful clue to the diagnosis in diffusely hypercellular or round cell tumors.*

Round Cell Morphology

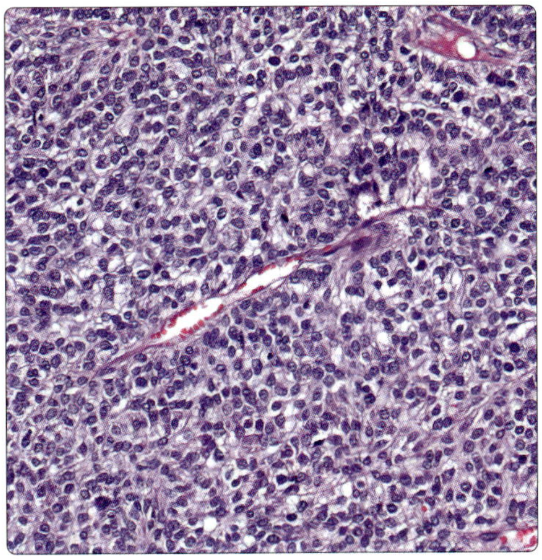

Round Cell Variations

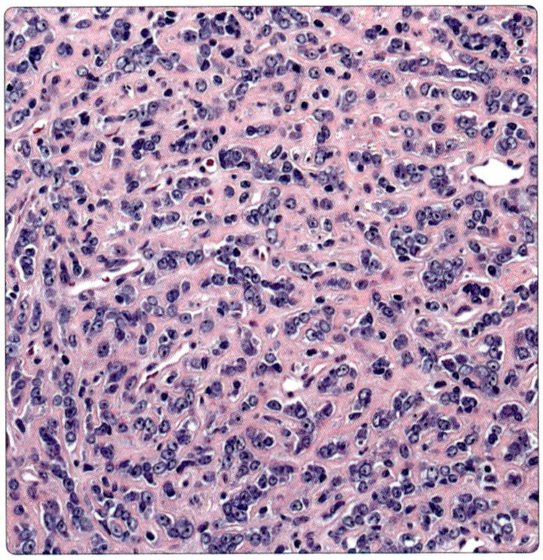

(Left) *Hypercellular areas in high-grade MLPS may show a prominent round cell morphology, as shown, and out of context can be easily confused with a variety of other round cell sarcomas and nonmesenchymal neoplasms. Ancillary studies are often helpful in making the diagnosis.* **(Right)** *Rare cases of high-grade MLPS may contain areas of round cells embedded in a sclerotic or hyalinized stroma, often forming short cords.*

Pleomorphic Liposarcoma

KEY FACTS

TERMINOLOGY

- High-grade, pleomorphic sarcoma demonstrating evidence of lipoblastic differentiation in absence of component of well-differentiated liposarcoma or another line of differentiation

CLINICAL ISSUES

- Least common variant of liposarcoma (5% of cases)
- Most common in patients > 50 years
- Deep soft tissues of extremities (75% of cases)
- Also trunk, retroperitoneum, other sites
- Treatment: Complete surgical resection with negative margins
- Aggressive sarcoma with poor prognosis
    - Metastases in 30-50% of cases

MACROSCOPIC

- Usually large (median size: 8-10 cm)

MICROSCOPIC

- Lipoblasts (often pleomorphic) are characteristic and requisite finding
    - Vary widely in number and distribution
- Multiple morphologic patterns in varying proportions
    - Cellular pleomorphic sarcoma (most common), myxofibrosarcoma-like, epithelioid
- Mitoses and necrosis common in all patterns

ANCILLARY TESTS

- MDM2 and CDK4 (-)
- Molecular: Complex, nonspecific karyotypes

TOP DIFFERENTIAL DIAGNOSES

- Undifferentiated pleomorphic sarcoma
- Dedifferentiated liposarcoma
- Myxofibrosarcoma
- Poorly differentiated carcinoma

(Left) *A gross photograph of a pleomorphic liposarcoma (PLPS) shows an intramuscular, partly necrotic neoplasm with tan and gray-white, firm cut surfaces. Most examples are large with a median size of 8-10 cm.* **(Right)** *This typical example of PLPS shows a variable number of lipoblasts and pleomorphic lipoblasts ⇨ scattered within a background of cellular, pleomorphic sarcoma. The number of pleomorphic lipoblasts vary considerably in number and distribution from case to case.*

Pleomorphic Liposarcoma

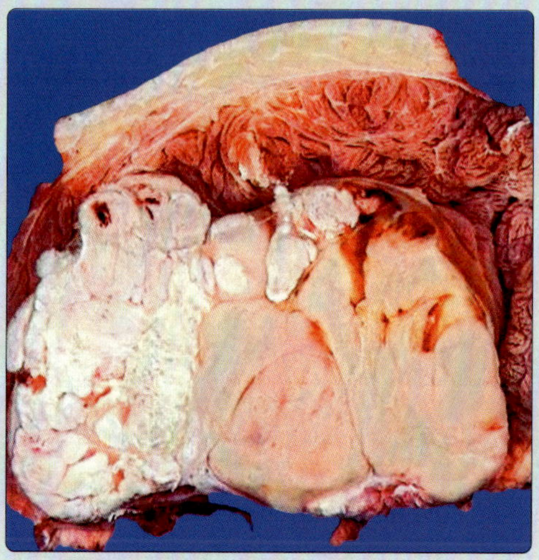

Pleomorphic Liposarcoma

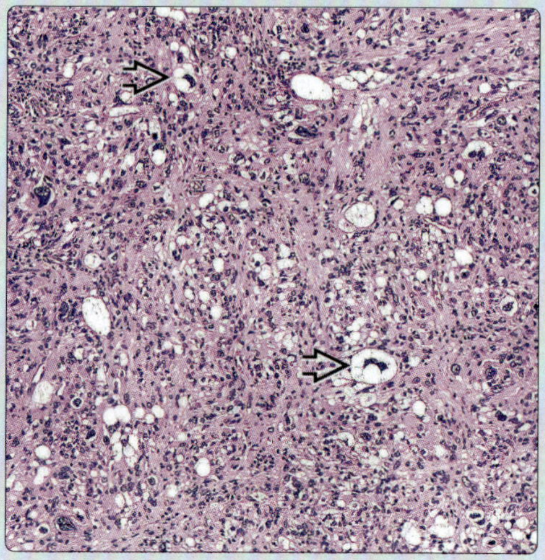

(Left) *Pleomorphic lipoblasts are similar to conventional multivacuolated lipoblasts, except that the nuclei are much larger, hyperchromatic, and pleomorphic than what is typically seen in lower grade liposarcomas. Note that some pleomorphic lipoblasts can show bizarre nuclear atypia.* **(Right)** *Mitotic figures are often numerous in PLPS, and atypical forms ⇨ are quite common.*

Pleomorphic Lipoblasts

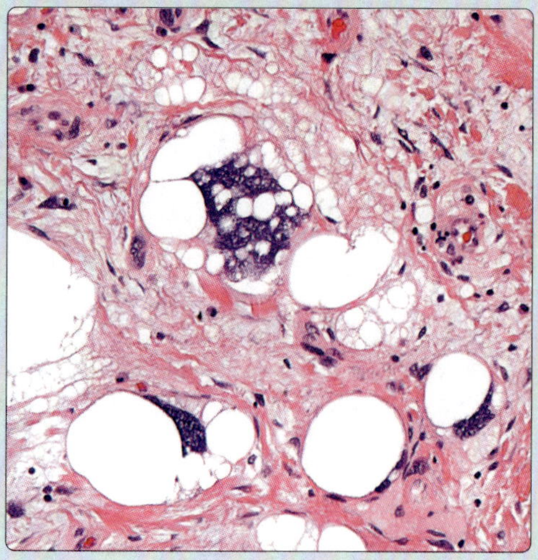

Atypical Mitotic Figures

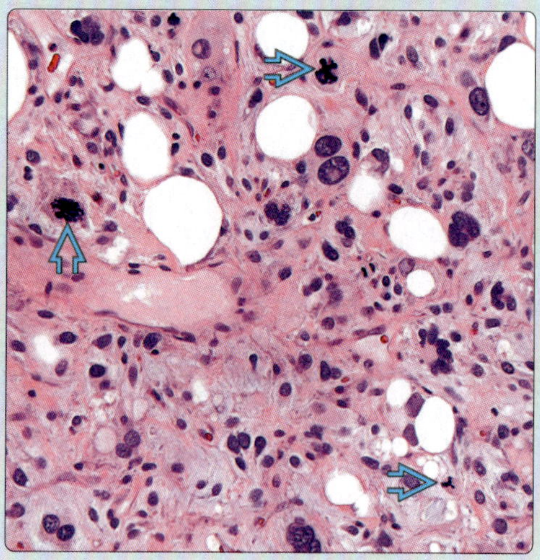

TERMINOLOGY

Abbreviations

- Pleomorphic liposarcoma (PLPS)

Definitions

- High-grade, pleomorphic sarcoma demonstrating evidence of lipoblastic differentiation in absence of component of well-differentiated liposarcoma or another line of differentiation

CLINICAL ISSUES

Epidemiology

- Incidence
  - Rare
    - Least common variant of liposarcoma (5% of cases)
- Age
  - Most common in patients > 50 years
- Sex
  - Slight male predominance

Site

- Deep soft tissues of extremities (75% of cases), most commonly thigh
  - Less commonly arise in subcutaneous tissue
  - Purely dermal lesions rare
- Trunk and retroperitoneum less commonly involved
- Rare sites include mediastinum, paratesticular region, scalp, abdominal/pelvic cavities

Presentation

- Enlarging, firm, painless mass
- Often short preoperative history

Treatment

- Complete surgical resection with negative margins
- Postoperative radiotherapy may be given for large, incompletely excised neoplasms

Prognosis

- Aggressive malignant neoplasm
  - Local recurrence common
  - Metastases in 30-50% of cases
    - Most commonly to lungs
  - Overall 5-year survival: ~ 50-60%
- Adverse prognostic factors
  - Age (> 60 years), nonextremity location, size (> 10 cm), mitotic rate (> 10 per 10 HPF), and deeply situated tumors

MACROSCOPIC

General Features

- Well defined and multinodular or irregular and infiltrative
- Tan-white-yellow cut surface with myxoid &/or necrotic foci

Size

- Usually large (median size: 8-10 cm)

Sections to Be Submitted

- Thorough gross sampling is critical for accurate classification of PLPS
  - Lipoblastic differentiation may be very focal

MICROSCOPIC

Histologic Features

- Infiltrative periphery
- Lipoblasts (often pleomorphic) are characteristic and requisite finding
  - Enlarged, hyperchromatic nuclei scalloped by cytoplasmic vacuoles
    - Nuclear atypia may be extreme in some lipoblasts
  - Vary widely in number from sparse and scattered to abundant and sheet-like
- Multiple morphologic patterns in varying proportions
  - Cellular pleomorphic sarcoma (most common)
    - Pleomorphic spindled, round, and polygonal cells
      - Sheets, short fascicles, storiform arrays
    - Severe nuclear atypia, multinucleation common
    - Numerous mitoses, including atypical forms
    - Intra- and extracellular eosinophilic droplets (represent lysosomal structures) may be noted
  - Myxofibrosarcoma-like morphology
    - Myxoid stroma containing prominent stromal vasculature
    - Pleomorphic tumor cell nuclei, including multinucleated floret-like cells
    - Scattered pleomorphic lipoblasts
    - Rare cystic and microcystic stromal changes
  - Epithelioid morphology
    - Solid, cohesive sheets of epithelioid cells with clear to eosinophilic cytoplasm
      - Can resemble clear cell renal cell carcinoma or adrenocortical carcinoma
    - Pleomorphic lipoblasts scattered singly or in aggregates
  - Coagulative necrosis common in all patterns

ANCILLARY TESTS

Immunohistochemistry

- Lipoblasts often S100 protein (+)
- Loss of nuclear Rb protein (by IHC) reported in one series
- Epithelioid variant may show focal keratin (+) or EMA(+)
- MDM2 and CDK4 (-)

Molecular Genetics

- Complex, nonspecific chromosomal abnormalities
- Loss of *RB1* in few reported cases

DIFFERENTIAL DIAGNOSIS

Dedifferentiated Liposarcoma

- Much more common in retroperitoneum than PLPS
- Cellular, nonlipogenic sarcoma with range of morphologic appearances
  - Pleomorphic lipoblasts rare (only seen in "homologous" dedifferentiation)
- Most cases contain component of well-differentiated liposarcoma
  - Presence of this component essentially precludes diagnosis of PLPS
- MDM2 and CDK4 (+) by IHC
- *MDM2* amplification by FISH

Undifferentiated Pleomorphic Sarcoma

- Usually cellular, high-grade, pleomorphic morphology
  - Can show significant morphologic overlap with PLPS
- No evidence of lipoblastic differentiation
  - Thorough gross sampling critical for correct classification

Myxofibrosarcoma

- More common in subcutaneous than deep tissue
- Multinodular growth
- No true lipoblastic component
  - But may contain fibroblastic "pseudolipoblasts"
- Can show significant morphologic overlap with PLPS
  - However, myxofibrosarcoma lacks lipoblastic differentiation

Atypical Lipomatous Tumor/Well-Differentiated Liposarcoma

- Sheets and lobules of low-grade, atypical adipocytes separated by thickened fibrous septa containing atypical, hyperchromatic stromal cells
- Lacks component of cellular, nonlipogenic pleomorphic sarcoma
- Lacks pleomorphic lipoblasts
- Mitotic activity generally low
- MDM2 and CDK4 (+) by IHC
- *MDM2* amplification by FISH

Silicone Granuloma

- Morphologic appearance may mimic sheets of lipoblasts
- History of silicone injection or implants present
- No atypical mitoses or coagulative necrosis

Myxoid Liposarcoma

- Young to middle-aged adults
- Fine, chicken-wire arborizing capillary vasculature
- Generally lacks degree of nuclear pleomorphism seen in PLPS
- Lacks pleomorphic lipoblasts
- t(12;16) or t(12;22)

Poorly Differentiated Carcinoma

- Renal cell and adrenocortical carcinomas are most common types on differential of epithelioid PLPS
- No evidence of lipoblastic differentiation
- More than focal expression of keratin, EMA, and other epithelial markers

Metastatic Malignant Melanoma

- No evidence of lipoblastic differentiation
- S100 protein (+) in tumor cells
- Expression of melanocytic markers

SELECTED REFERENCES

1. Creytens D et al: "Atypical" pleomorphic lipomatous tumor: a clinicopathologic, immunohistochemical and molecular study of 21 cases, emphasizing its relationship to atypical spindle cell lipomatous tumor and suggesting a morphologic spectrum (atypical spindle cell/pleomorphic lipomatous tumor). Am J Surg Pathol. 41(11):1443-55, 2017
2. Ramírez-Bellver JL et al: Primary dermal pleomorphic liposarcoma: utility of adipophilin and MDM2/CDK4 immunostainings. J Cutan Pathol. 44(3):283-8, 2017
3. Mariño-Enríquez A et al: Dedifferentiated liposarcoma and pleomorphic liposarcoma: a comparative study of cytomorphology and MDM2/CDK4 expression on fine-needle aspiration. Cancer Cytopathol. 122(2):128-37, 2014
4. Al-Zaid T et al: Dermal pleomorphic liposarcoma resembling pleomorphic fibroma: report of a case and review of the literature. J Cutan Pathol. 40(8):734-9, 2013
5. Wang L et al: Pleomorphic liposarcoma: a clinicopathological, immunohistochemical and molecular cytogenetic study of 32 additional cases. Pathol Int. 63(11):523-31, 2013
6. Gardner JM et al: Cutaneous and subcutaneous pleomorphic liposarcoma: a clinicopathologic study of 29 cases with evaluation of MDM2 gene amplification in 26. Am J Surg Pathol. 36(7):1047-51, 2012
7. Ghadimi MP et al: Pleomorphic liposarcoma: clinical observations and molecular variables. Cancer. 117(23):5359-69, 2011
8. Mariño-Enríquez A et al: Dedifferentiated liposarcoma with "homologous" lipoblastic (pleomorphic liposarcoma-like) differentiation: clinicopathologic and molecular analysis of a series suggesting revised diagnostic criteria. Am J Surg Pathol. 34(8):1122-31, 2010
9. Fiore M et al: Myxoid/round cell and pleomorphic liposarcomas: prognostic factors and survival in a series of patients treated at a single institution. Cancer. 109(12):2522-31, 2007
10. Singer S et al: Gene expression profiling of liposarcoma identifies distinct biological types/subtypes and potential therapeutic targets in well-differentiated and dedifferentiated liposarcoma. Cancer Res. 67(14):6626-36, 2007
11. Idbaih A et al: Myxoid malignant fibrous histiocytoma and pleomorphic liposarcoma share very similar genomic imbalances. Lab Invest. 85(2):176-81, 2005
12. Hornick JL et al: Pleomorphic liposarcoma: clinicopathologic analysis of 57 cases. Am J Surg Pathol. 28(10):1257-67, 2004
13. Panoussopoulos D et al: Focal divergent chondrosarcomatous differentiation in a primary pleomorphic liposarcoma and expression of transforming growth factor beta. Int J Surg Pathol. 12(1):79-85, 2004
14. Val-Bernal JF et al: Primary purely intradermal pleomorphic liposarcoma. J Cutan Pathol. 30(8):516-20, 2003
15. Gebhard S et al: Pleomorphic liposarcoma: clinicopathologic, immunohistochemical, and follow-up analysis of 63 cases: a study from the French Federation of Cancer Centers Sarcoma Group. Am J Surg Pathol. 26(5):601-16, 2002
16. Huang HY et al: Epithelioid variant of pleomorphic liposarcoma: a comparative immunohistochemical and ultrastructural analysis of six cases with emphasis on overlapping features with epithelial malignancies. Ultrastruct Pathol. 26(5):299-308, 2002
17. Cai YC et al: Primary liposarcoma of the orbit: a clinicopathologic study of seven cases. Ann Diagn Pathol. 5(5):255-66, 2001
18. Downes KA et al: Pleomorphic liposarcoma: a clinicopathologic analysis of 19 cases. Mod Pathol. 14(3):179-84, 2001
19. Meis-Kindblom JM et al: Cytogenetic and molecular genetic analyses of liposarcoma and its soft tissue simulators: recognition of new variants and differential diagnosis. Virchows Arch. 439(2):141-51, 2001
20. Oliveira AM et al: Pleomorphic liposarcoma. Semin Diagn Pathol. 18(4):274-85, 2001
21. Dei Tos AP: Liposarcoma: new entities and evolving concepts. Ann Diagn Pathol. 4(4):252-66, 2000
22. Miettinen M et al: Epithelioid variant of pleomorphic liposarcoma: a study of 12 cases of a distinctive variant of high-grade liposarcoma. Mod Pathol. 12(7):722-8, 1999
23. Dei Tos AP et al: Primary liposarcoma of the skin: a rare neoplasm with unusual high grade features. Am J Dermatopathol. 20(4):332-8, 1998
24. Mertens F et al: Cytogenetic analysis of 46 pleomorphic soft tissue sarcomas and correlation with morphologic and clinical features: a report of the CHAMP Study Group. Chromosomes and MorPhology. Genes Chromosomes Cancer. 22(1):16-25, 1998
25. Schneider-Stock R et al: No correlation of c-myc overexpression and p53 mutations in liposarcomas. Virchows Arch. 433(4):315-21, 1998
26. Zagars GK et al: Liposarcoma: outcome and prognostic factors following conservation surgery and radiation therapy. Int J Radiat Oncol Biol Phys. 36(2):311-9, 1996
27. Klimstra DS et al: Liposarcoma of the anterior mediastinum and thymus. A clinicopathologic study of 28 cases. Am J Surg Pathol. 19(7):782-91, 1995
28. Azumi N et al: Atypical and malignant neoplasms showing lipomatous differentiation. A study of 111 cases. Am J Surg Pathol. 11(3):161-83, 1987
29. Weiss LM et al: Ultrastructural distinctions between adult pleomorphic rhabdomyosarcomas, pleomorphic liposarcomas, and pleomorphic malignant fibrous histiocytomas. Hum Pathol. 15(11):1025-33, 1984

Cellular Pleomorphic Sarcoma Morphology

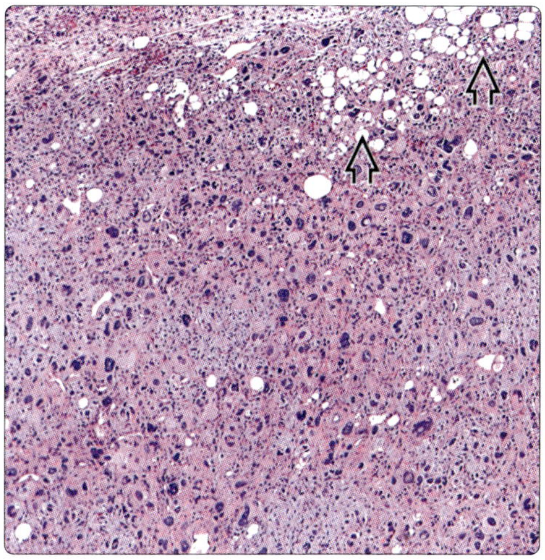

Marked Nuclear Pleomorphism

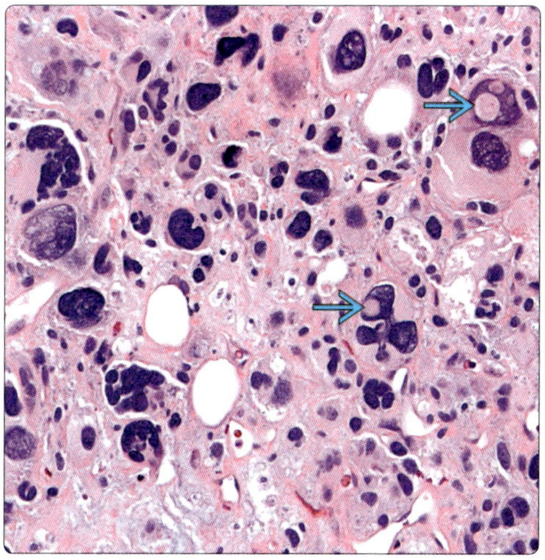

(Left) *The most common morphologic pattern in PLPS is that of a high-grade, cellular pleomorphic sarcoma. Scattered areas of definite lipoblastic differentiation* ⇨ *are required to distinguish PLPS from other pleomorphic sarcomas.* **(Right)** *Nuclear pleomorphism is often characteristically severe in PLPS with numerous bizarre and highly multinucleated forms. Nuclear pseudoinclusions* → *are also common.*

Eosinophilic Globules

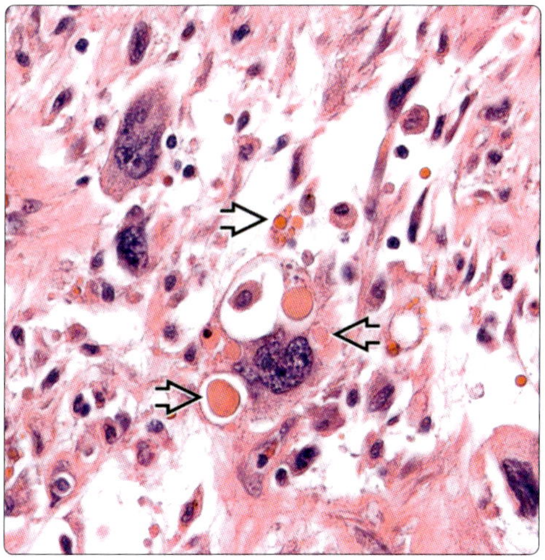

Abundant Globules

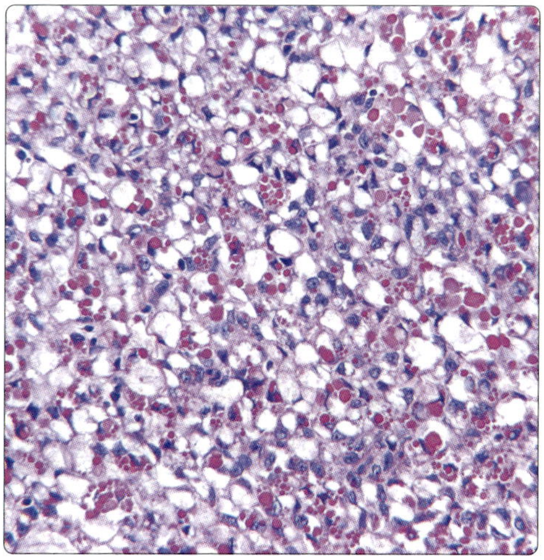

(Left) *Intracellular or extracellular eosinophilic globules* ⇨ *are a feature of some cases of PLPS but may be focal. This finding is not pathognomonic of PLPS, however, and can be seen in other tumors.* **(Right)** *This example of PLPS shows diffuse cytoplasmic eosinophilic globules, creating a striking morphologic appearance.*

Spindled Morphology

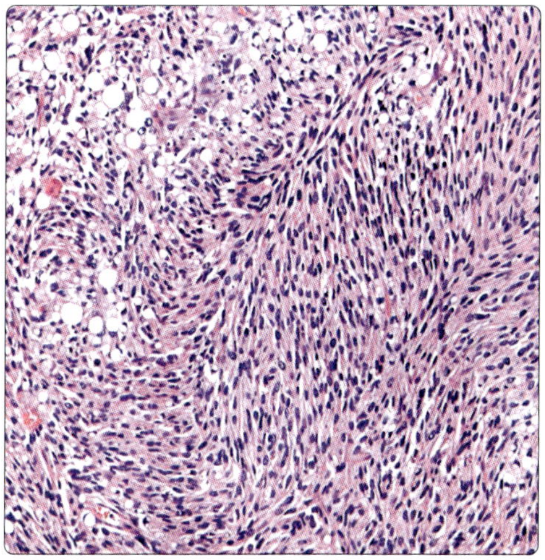

Spindled Morphology

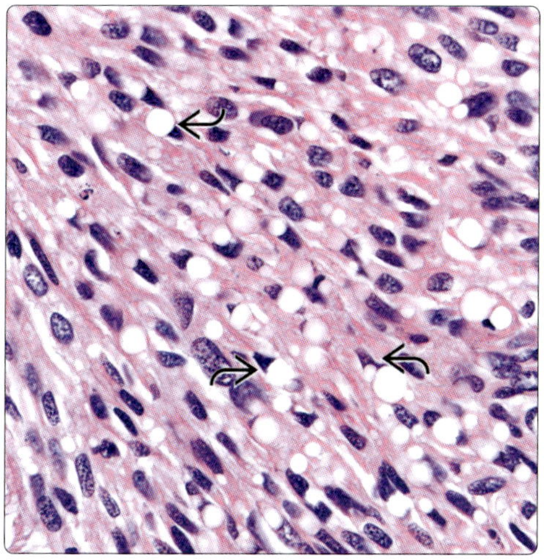

(Left) *As is the case with other pleomorphic sarcomas, PLPS may show areas that are more spindled and fascicular and less pleomorphic; however, this morphology is usually not prominent. A more conventional pleomorphic morphology was seen in most other fields in the depicted case. Note the focus of lipoblastic differentiation (upper left).* **(Right)** *There are numerous small, lipid-laden vacuoles in this H&E of PLPS, many of which indent or scallop the adjacent nuclei* ↶*.*

(Left) *Coagulative tumor necrosis is a common finding in PLPS and may appear as small pockets or geographic zones. Note the prominent nuclear pleomorphism in this H&E.* **(Right)** *In some cases of PLPS, the tumor is predominantly composed of or contains large sheets made up of almost entirely lipoblasts and pleomorphic lipoblasts. Note the atypical mitotic figure.*

Coagulative Necrosis

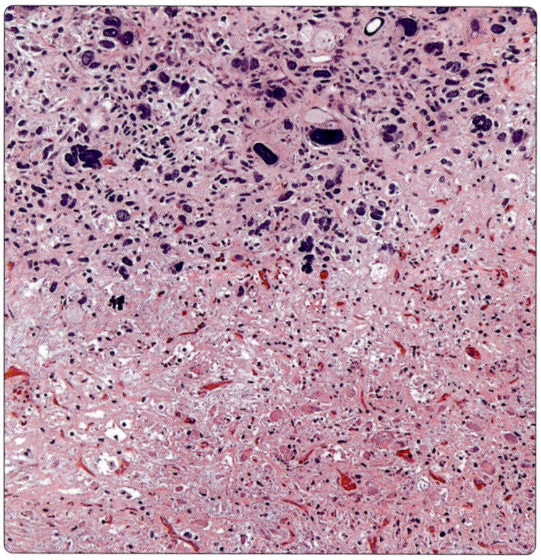

Sheets of Lipoblasts

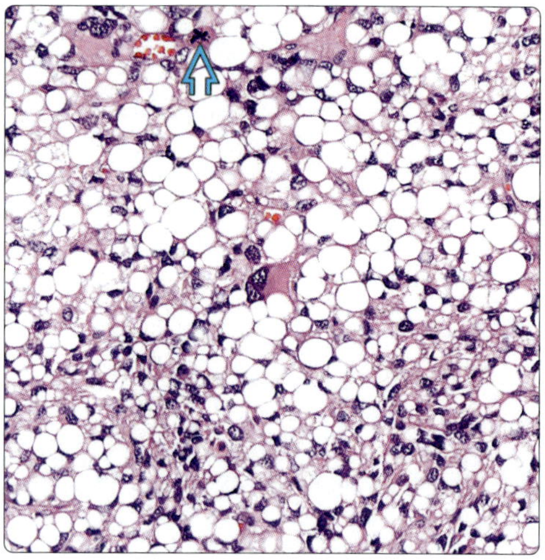

(Left) *This case of PLPS shows extensive lipoblastic differentiation and marked variation in the size of the lipoblasts. Note the focally severe nuclear atypia.* **(Right)** *This case of PLPS contains extensive lipoblastic differentiation and shows numerous highly pleomorphic lipoblasts with marked nuclear atypia.*

Sheets of Lipoblasts

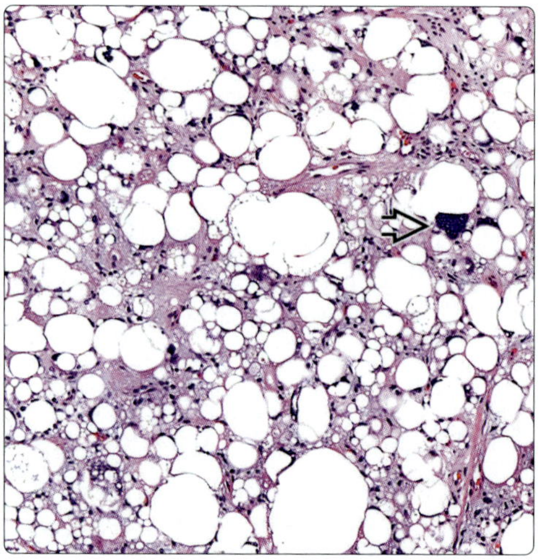

Sheets of Pleomorphic Lipoblasts

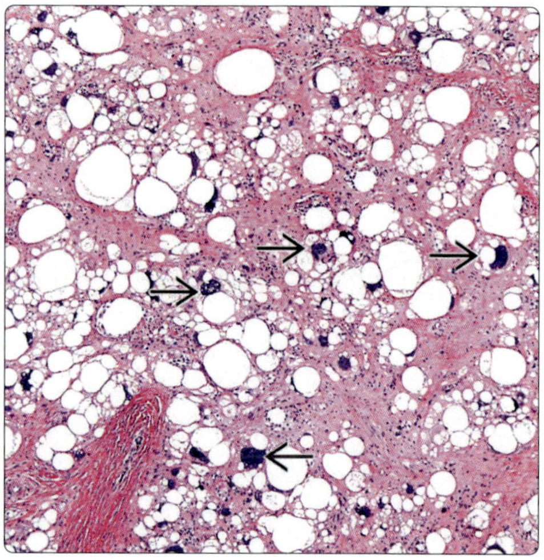

(Left) *Another common pattern in PLPS is that of prominent myxoid stroma containing conspicuous, thin-walled curvilinear blood vessels and scattered pleomorphic cells, reminiscent of intermediate- to high-grade myxofibrosarcoma.* **(Right)** *In some cases, the myxofibrosarcoma-like pattern of PLPS may be histologically indistinguishable from true myxofibrosarcoma. Identification of true lipoblastic differentiation clarifies the issue.*

Myxofibrosarcoma-Like Pattern

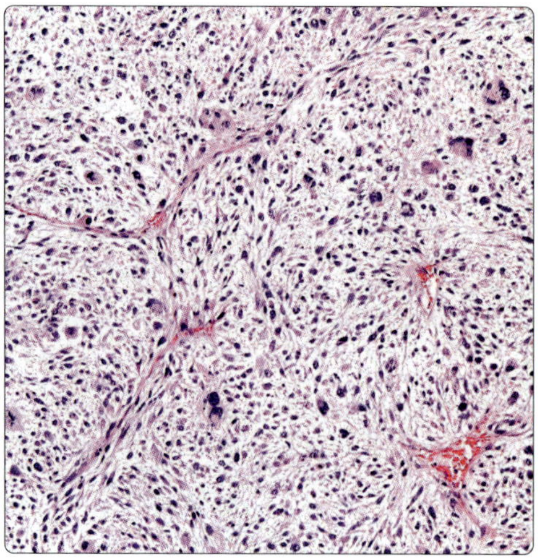

Myxofibrosarcoma-Like Pattern

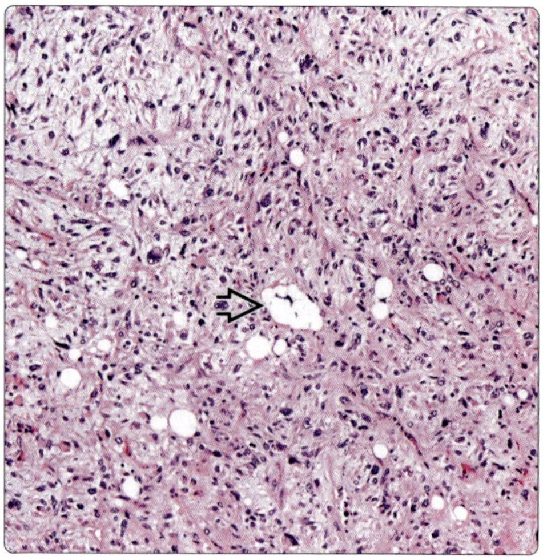

Myxofibrosarcoma-Like Pattern

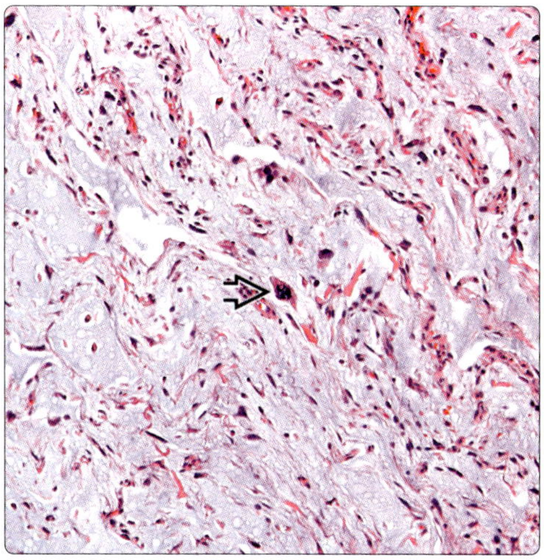

Cystic and Microcystic Changes

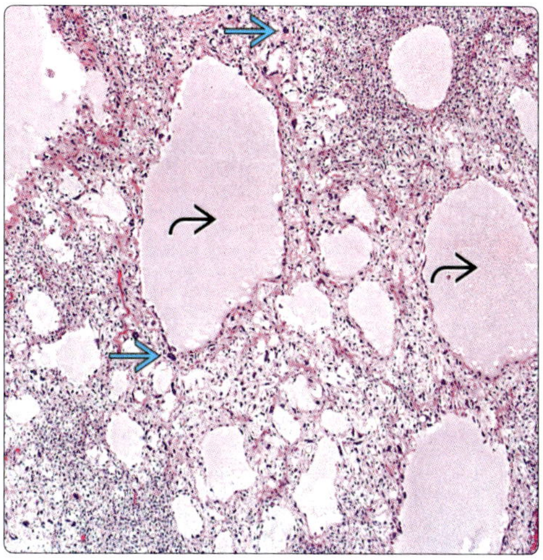

(Left) *Areas resembling low-grade myxofibrosarcoma are uncommon in PLPS and are usually associated with morphologically higher grade areas. Note the atypical mitotic figure.* **(Right)** *Stromal cystic changes, similar to what is often in myxoid liposarcoma, are occasionally seen in PLPS. Note the nuclear atypia identifiable even at low power.*

Epithelioid Morphology

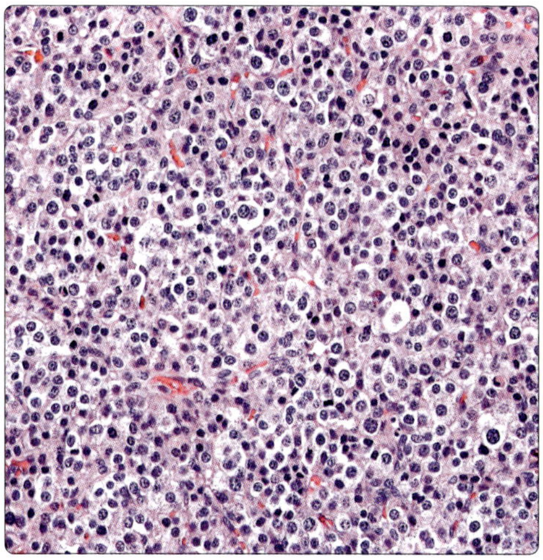

Epithelioid Morphology

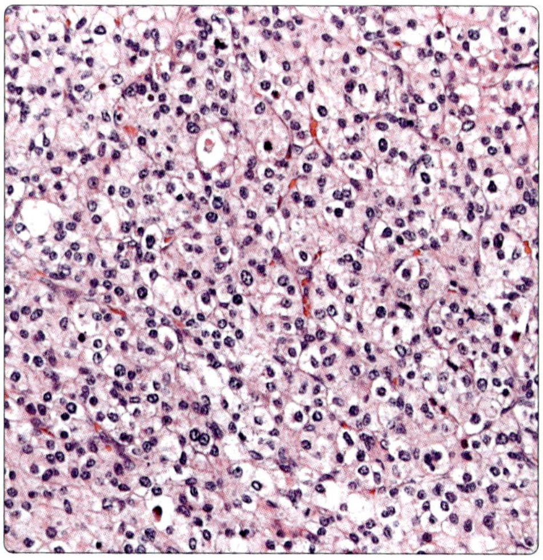

(Left) *An epithelioid morphology may be seen in occasional cases of PLPS but is the least common variant pattern overall. These tumors show diffuse, variably cohesive sheets and lobules of rounded cells, simulating an epithelial neoplasm.* **(Right)** *The tumor cells in epithelioid PLPS can show granular, eosinophilic to clear or foamy-appearing cytoplasm, morphologically suggesting a carcinoma, e.g., clear cell renal cell carcinoma or adrenocortical carcinoma. This confusion is most likely in retroperitoneal tumors, given the regional anatomy.*

Epithelioid Morphology

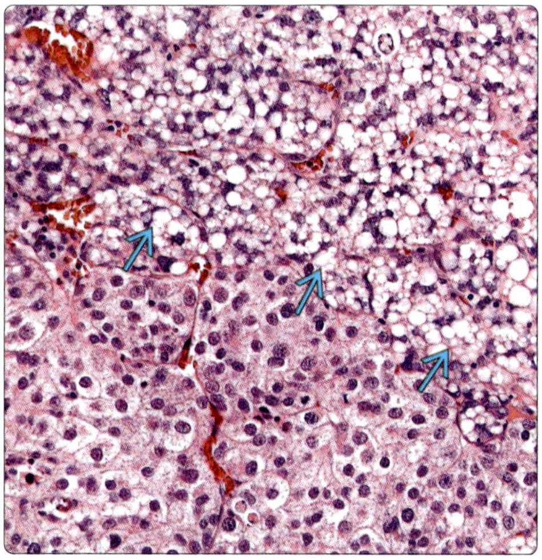

Unusual Epithelioid Cells

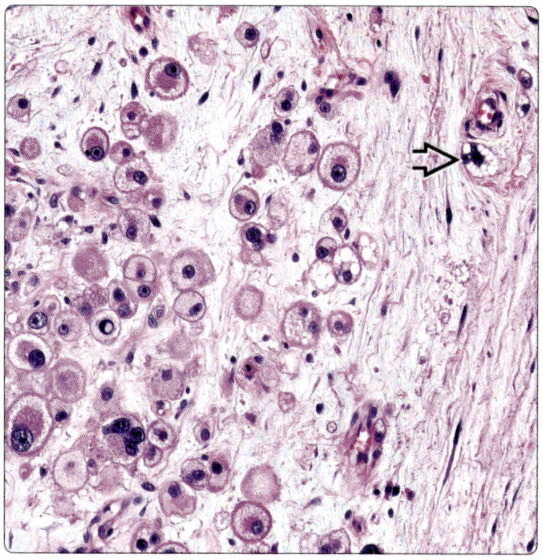

(Left) *The epithelioid cytomorphology and apparent lobular or nested growth of this variant of PLPS can lead to confusion with a poorly differentiated carcinoma, such as renal cell carcinoma. Lipoblastic differentiation and IHC help make the distinction.* **(Right)** *This unusual case of epithelioid PLPS shows atypical epithelioid tumor cells with abundant pale eosinophilic, granular, and xanthomatous cytoplasm. Note the pleomorphic lipoblast.*

SECTION 4

Fibroblastic/Myofibroblastic Lesions

Benign

Nodular Fasciitis 114
Proliferative Fasciitis/Myositis 120
Ischemic Fasciitis 124
Myositis Ossificans 126
Fibroosseous Pseudotumor of Digit 130
Fibroma of Tendon Sheath 134
Desmoplastic Fibroblastoma 140
Elastofibroma 142
Angiofibroma of Soft Tissue 144
Mammary-Type Myofibroblastoma 148
Intranodal Palisaded Myofibroblastoma 152
Pleomorphic Fibroma 156
Dermatomyofibroma 158
Storiform Collagenoma 160
Keloid 162
Nuchal-Type Fibroma 164

Intermediate (Locally Aggressive)

Palmar/Plantar Fibromatosis 166
Desmoid-Type Fibromatosis 168

Intermediate (Rarely Metastasizing)

Dermatofibrosarcoma Protuberans 174
Solitary Fibrous Tumor 184
Low-Grade Myofibroblastic Sarcoma 192
Inflammatory Myofibroblastic Tumor 196
Myxoinflammatory Fibroblastic Sarcoma 202
Superficial CD34(+) Fibroblastic Tumor 210

Malignant

Adult-Type Fibrosarcoma 214
Myxofibrosarcoma 216
Low-Grade Fibromyxoid Sarcoma 222
Sclerosing Epithelioid Fibrosarcoma 232

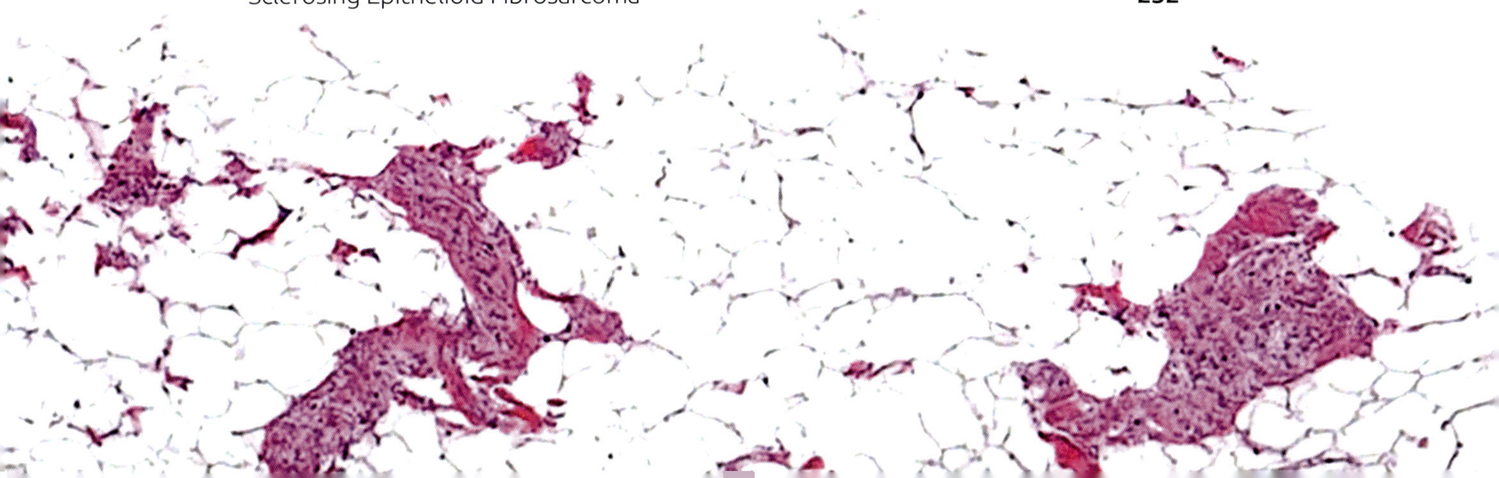

Nodular Fasciitis

KEY FACTS

TERMINOLOGY

- Self-limited, benign fibroblastic/myofibroblastic neoplasm characterized in most cases by *USP6-MYH9* gene fusion
  - Variants: Intravascular fasciitis, cranial fasciitis

CLINICAL ISSUES

- Wide range (most common: 20-40 years)
- Most common in extremities (particularly forearm), trunk, and head and neck
- Usually in subcutaneous tissue
- Small tumor with rapid growth characteristic
- Treatment: Conservative surgical excision
- Excellent prognosis; local recurrence very rare

MACROSCOPIC

- Usually small (average: 2-3 cm)

MICROSCOPIC

- Plump, spindled fibroblasts and myofibroblasts
  - No nuclear hyperchromasia or pleomorphism
  - Variable mitotic rate; may be numerous
- Variable short fascicular and loose storiform growth patterns
  - Overall cellularity varies widely
  - Loose, myxoid matrix is common; may be collagenous
- Extravasated erythrocytes, stromal lymphocytes, and osteoclast-like giant cells common

ANCILLARY TESTS

- Molecular: *USP6* gene rearrangement in most cases
  - *USP6-MYH9* fusion most common

TOP DIFFERENTIAL DIAGNOSES

- Desmoid fibromatosis
- Inflammatory myofibroblastic tumor
- Proliferative fasciitis/myositis
- Leiomyosarcoma
- Pseudosarcomatous myofibroblastic proliferation

(Left) *Nodular fasciitis is a benign self-limited myofibroblastic neoplasm that most commonly affects young to middle-aged adults. Although usually small (< 2-3 cm), most cases show rapid growth, raising clinical concerns for malignancy.* **(Right)** *Most cases of nodular fasciitis arise in the superficial soft tissues and are well to moderately circumscribed; however, limited peripheral soft tissue infiltration may be present ➡. Occasional cases are entirely intramuscular.*

Nodular Fasciitis

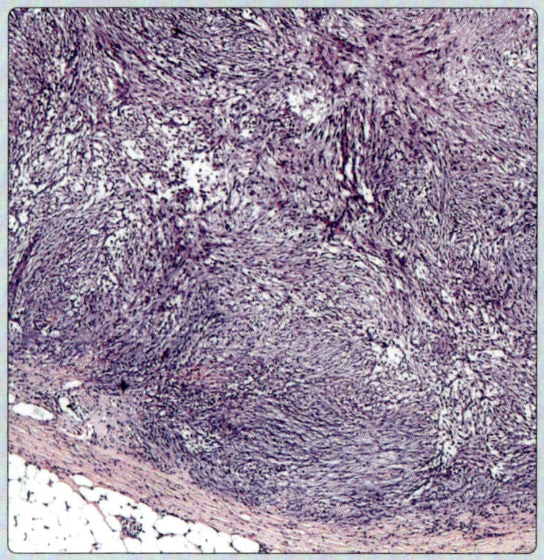

Nodular Fasciitis

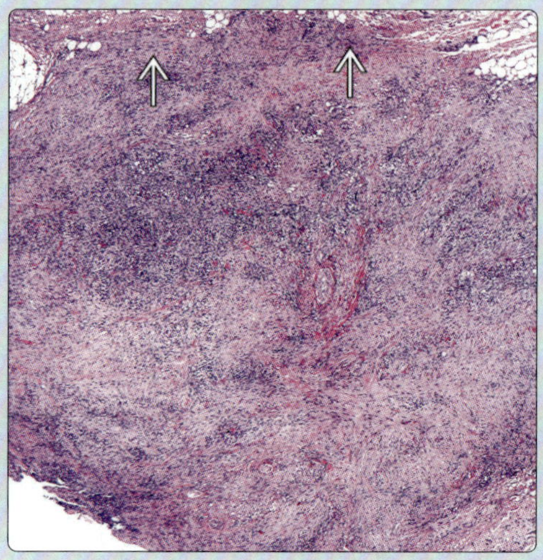

(Left) *A loose, myxoid stroma is common in nodular fasciitis, particularly in lesions that are excised early. Tumor cells are characteristically arranged loosely in a haphazard fashion, reminiscent of tissue culture growth.* **(Right)** *Tumor cells in nodular fasciitis are cytologically myofibroblastic with vesicular nuclei and 1 or 2 tiny nucleoli. Nuclear hyperchromasia and pleomorphism are not present.*

Myxoid Stroma

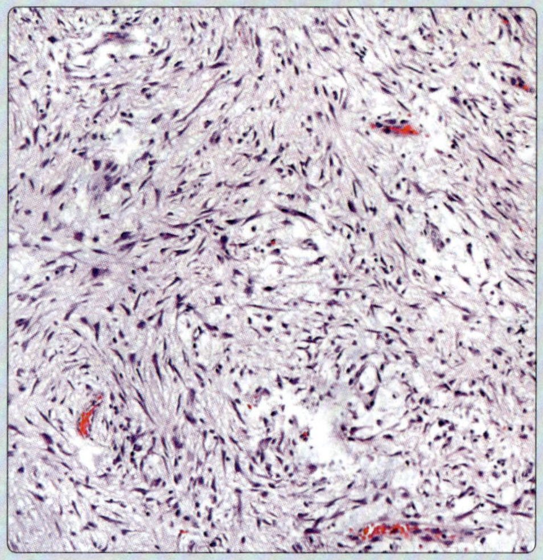

Cytologic Features

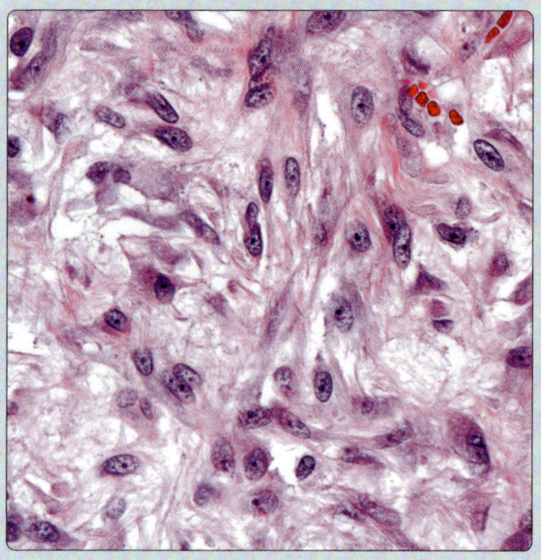

TERMINOLOGY

Synonyms

- Pseudosarcomatous fasciitis

Definitions

- Self-limited, benign fibroblastic/myofibroblastic neoplasm characterized in most cases by recurrent *USP6-MYH9* gene fusion
    - May arise from small or medium-sized vessels (intravascular fasciitis)
    - May arise in scalp in infants and involve underlying skull (cranial fasciitis)

ETIOLOGY/PATHOGENESIS

Trauma

- History of local trauma may be reported in minority (~ 15%) of cases of nodular fasciitis
- Birth trauma has been associated with development of cranial fasciitis

CLINICAL ISSUES

Epidemiology

- Incidence
    - Relatively common
- Age
    - Wide range (most common: 20-40 years)
    - Cranial fasciitis usually arises in infants
- Sex
    - Cranial fasciitis shows male predilection
    - M = F in other forms

Site

- Most arise in subcutaneous tissue
    - Minority arise entirely within skeletal muscle
    - Rarely in skin (intradermal fasciitis)
- Most common in extremities (particularly forearm), trunk, and head and neck
- Rare in distal/acral extremities, joints, other sites
- Cranial fasciitis arises in periosteum of skull and involves adjacent soft tissue of scalp; may extend inward and involves meninges

Presentation

- Usually small, tender or nontender nodule or mass
- Rapid growth (several weeks to a few months) characteristic

Treatment

- Conservative surgical excision

Prognosis

- Excellent
    - Local recurrence very rare
    - Can show spontaneous regression
- Does not metastasize or show malignant transformation

MACROSCOPIC

General Features

- Well marginated but unencapsulated
    - May rarely appear infiltrative
- Variable fibrous to myxoid cut surface

Size

- Usually small (average: 2-3 cm)
    - Very rarely > 5 cm

MICROSCOPIC

Histologic Features

- Usually well-demarcated peripheral border, but focal infiltration common
    - Often shows limited peripheral extension along fibrous septa between fat in subcutis or between skeletal muscle fibers in deeper lesions
- Plump, spindled fibroblasts and myofibroblasts
    - Eosinophilic cytoplasm and vesicular nuclei with 1 or 2 distinct nucleoli
    - Resemble cells in granulation tissue or tissue culture
    - No nuclear hyperchromasia or pleomorphism
    - Variable mitotic rate
        - Mitoses may be numerous
        - No atypical forms
- Variable short fascicular and loose storiform growth patterns
    - Overall cellularity varies widely both within and between cases
        - May be alarmingly hypercellular
- Loose, myxoid matrix is common and often abundant
    - More cellular areas may show loose, dyscohesive foci
    - Older lesions are often less myxoid and more collagenous and hypocellular
        - May contain thickened, keloidal collagen fibers
- Extravasated erythrocytes and lymphocytes are frequent finding
    - Also histiocytes, scattered or in small aggregates
- Osteoclast-like giant cells are not uncommon
- Frank intratumoral hemorrhage or cystic change is rare
- Rare metaplastic bone formation (ossifying fasciitis or fasciitis ossificans)
    - No zonal maturation in these lesions
- Necrosis rare (usually focal and centralized)
- Cranial fasciitis shows similar morphology to conventional nodular fasciitis
    - May be more myxoid and show metaplastic bone formation

Morphologic Variants

- Intravascular fasciitis
    - Arises from small to medium-sized vessels, often veins
        - Can be partly or entirely intravascular
            - May show multinodular or plexiform growth in latter
    - Often more solid than conventional nodular fasciitis
    - Osteoclast-like giant cells are often abundant

ANCILLARY TESTS

Immunohistochemistry

- SMA(+), often diffuse
- Rare desmin (+), usually focal
- Negative for keratin, S100 protein, CD34, nuclear β-catenin

- CD68(+) in intralesional histiocytes

Molecular Genetics

- Recurrent *USP6* gene rearrangement (17p13) in majority of tumors
  - *USP6-MYH9* fusion most common (60-80% of cases)
  - Many other fusion partners identified, including *RRBP1*, *COL6A2*, *CTNNB1*
  - *USP6* rearrangement also reported in aneurysmal bone cyst, myositis ossificans, fibroosseous pseudotumor of digit, and cellular fibroma of tendon sheath

DIFFERENTIAL DIAGNOSIS

Desmoid Fibromatosis

- Larger, infiltrative lesions
- Long, sweeping fascicles of fibroblasts/myofibroblasts
- Evenly distributed stromal collagen
- Some myxoid areas may resemble nodular fasciitis
- Nuclear β-catenin expression in 70% of cases

Inflammatory Myofibroblastic Tumor

- Chronic inflammatory component (particularly plasma cells)
- Usually larger size than nodular fasciitis
- ALK(+) in 50% of cases
- Lacks *USP6* rearrangements

Proliferative Fasciitis/Myositis

- Histologically similar to nodular fasciitis
- Contains large, ganglion cell-like myofibroblasts
- Lacks *USP6* rearrangement

Leiomyosarcoma

- Often larger tumors
- Intersected fascicles of eosinophilic cells with elongated, blunted nuclei
- Nuclear pleomorphism and hyperchromasia common
- SMA(+), desmin (+), caldesmon (+)

Pseudosarcomatous Myofibroblastic Proliferation

- Histologically similar to nodular fasciitis
- Usually arises in mucosal sites, particularly bladder
- May be associated with prior trauma or surgery
- Keratin (+) common; also, SMA(+)
- Lack *USP6* rearrangements

Dermatofibroma (Fibrous Histiocytoma)

- Most are small dermal lesions
- Generally lacks plump myofibroblastic cells
- Mixed chronic inflammatory component (lymphocytes, plasma cells, foamy histiocytes) common
- Usually SMA(-)

Neurofibroma

- Small, hyperchromatic, wavy or buckled nuclei
- May have history of neurofibromatosis type 1
- S100 protein (+)
- SMA(-)

Fibroma of Tendon Sheath

- Occurs predominantly in acral locations (particularly finger)
- Cellular tumors can show overlap with nodular fasciitis
- Peripheral slit-like vessels common

Undifferentiated Pleomorphic Sarcoma

- Usually large, deep tumors
- Most common in older adults and elderly
- Overtly malignant cytologic atypia
- Atypical mitotic figures and coagulative necrosis

Angiomatoid Fibrous Histiocytoma

- Multinodular, often with peripheral lymphocytic cuff
- Centralized hemorrhagic foci common
- Variable desmin (+)
- *EWSR1* gene translocation

Desmoplastic Fibroblastoma (Collagenous Fibroma)

- Usually very well circumscribed and markedly hypocellular
  - Spindled to stellate cells

Myositis Ossificans

- Presence of zonal maturation
  - Centralized fasciitis-like areas transitioning to mature bone at periphery
- Also features *USP6* rearrangement

Soft Tissue Aneurysmal Bone Cyst

- Features large, dilated, blood-filled spaces
- Peripheral rim of metaplastic bone
- Also features *USP6* rearrangement

Low-Grade Myofibroblastic Sarcoma

- Usually highly infiltrative
- Enlarged, hyperchromatic nuclei present, at least focally
- SMA(+), often patchy; variable desmin (+)

Kaposi Sarcoma

- Typically found in immunocompromised patients (especially AIDS patients)
- CD31(+), CD34(+), HHV8(+)

Myofibroma

- Most common in infants and children
- Myoid nodules with variably prominent hemangiopericytoma-like vascular component

SELECTED REFERENCES

1. Erber R et al: Misses and near misses in diagnosing nodular fasciitis and morphologically related reactive myofibroblastic proliferations: experience of a referral center with emphasis on frequency of USP6 gene rearrangements. Virchows Arch. 473(3):351-60, 2018
2. Patel NR et al: USP6 activation in nodular fasciitis by promoter-swapping gene fusions. Mod Pathol. 30(11):1577-88, 2017
3. Kumar E et al: Cutaneous nodular fasciitis with genetic analysis: a case series. J Cutan Pathol. 43(12):1143-9, 2016
4. Shin C et al: USP6 gene rearrangement in nodular fasciitis and histological mimics. Histopathology. 69(5):784-91, 2016
5. Oliveira AM et al: USP6-induced neoplasms: the biologic spectrum of aneurysmal bone cyst and nodular fasciitis. Hum Pathol. 45(1):1-11, 2014
6. Chi AC et al: Intravascular fasciitis: report of an intraoral case and review of the literature. Head Neck Pathol. 6(1):140-5, 2012
7. Erickson-Johnson MR et al: Nodular fasciitis: a novel model of transient neoplasia induced by MYH9-USP6 gene fusion. Lab Invest. 91(10):1427-33, 2011
8. de Feraudy S et al: Intradermal nodular fasciitis: a rare lesion analyzed in a series of 24 cases. Am J Surg Pathol. 34(9):1377-81, 2010
9. Weinreb I et al: Nodular fasciitis of the head and neck region: a clinicopathologic description in a series of 30 cases. J Cutan Pathol. 36(11):1168-73, 2009
10. Hornick JL et al: Intraarticular nodular fasciitis–a rare lesion: clinicopathologic analysis of a series. Am J Surg Pathol. 30(2):237-41, 2006

Cytologic Features

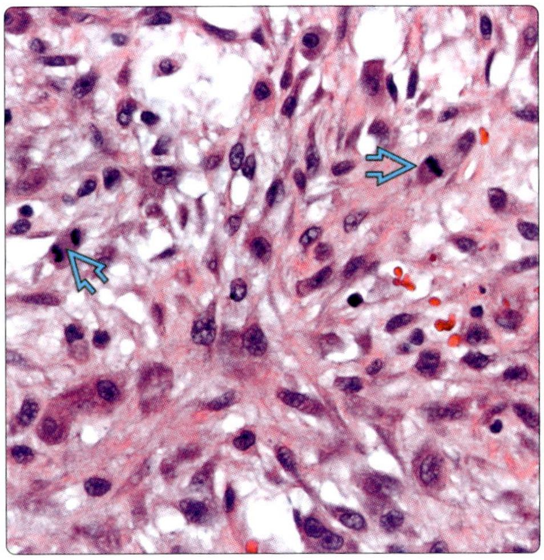

Stromal Dyscohesion

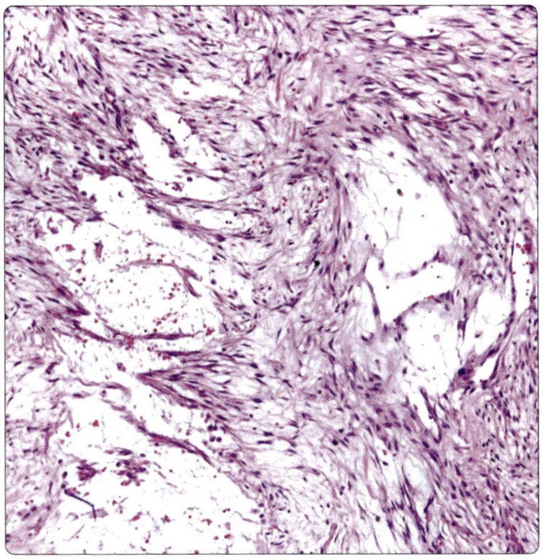

(Left) *Mitotic figures ➡ are very common in nodular fasciitis and naturally align with the frequent rapid growth seen clinically. In some cases, mitoses are so numerous that a sarcoma is considered (or misdiagnosed). However, importantly, abnormal mitoses are not seen.* **(Right)** *Stromal "tears" or dyscohesive foci are a common finding in nodular fasciitis, as depicted. These areas may be focal or abundant.*

Extravasated Blood Cells

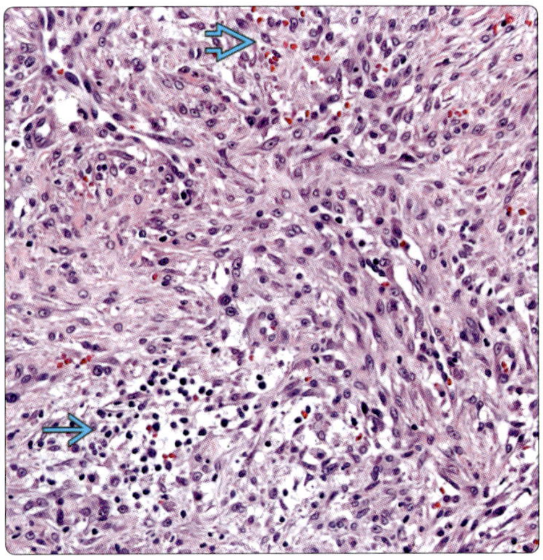

Osteoclast-Like Giant Cells

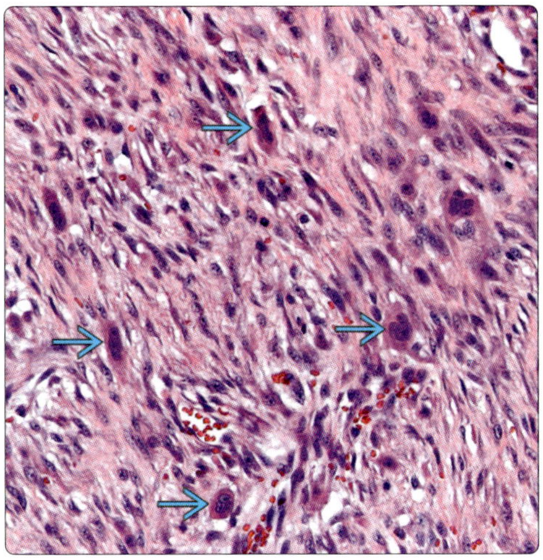

(Left) *Extravasated erythrocytes ➡ and chronic inflammatory cells (particularly lymphocytes ➡) are relatively common in nodular fasciitis. Scattered plasma cells may also be seen in some tumors; however, they are generally inconspicuous.* **(Right)** *Multinucleated osteoclast-like giant cells ➡ are a frequent finding in nodular fasciitis. They may be identified singly or in small clusters. Overlapping nuclei in these cells may be mistaken for nuclear pleomorphism.*

Stromal Collagen

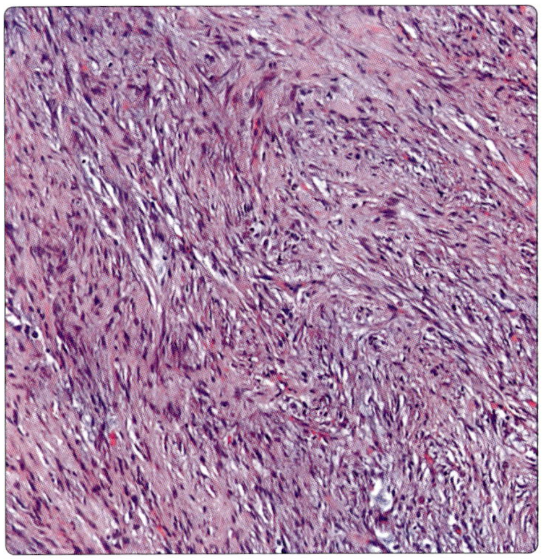

Storiform Growth

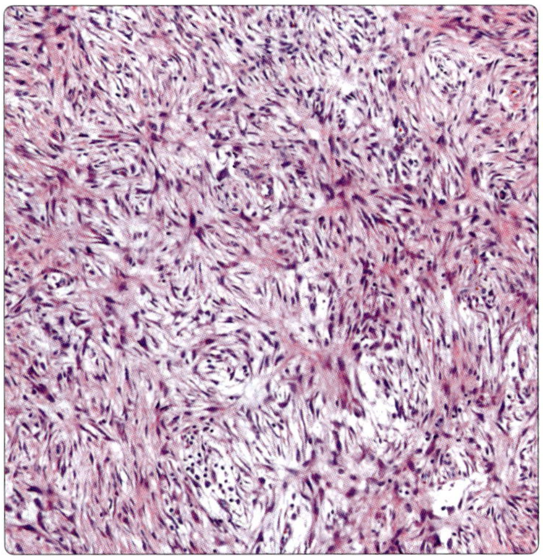

(Left) *As nodular fasciitis progresses, the amount of myxoid stroma often decreases and stromal collagen increases. The lesional cells, in turn, start to appear less haphazard and somewhat more organized.* **(Right)** *A storiform growth pattern may be seen in some cases of nodular fasciitis, as depicted.*

(Left) *Older lesions of nodular fasciitis often show a greater degree of stromal collagen and subsequent hyalinization. Cellularity is variable in these cases, and myxoid zones may or may not be present.* **(Right)** *Focal keloidal collagen is not uncommon in nodular fasciitis, as depicted in this image. In rare cases, it may be a prominent finding.*

Stromal Hyalinization

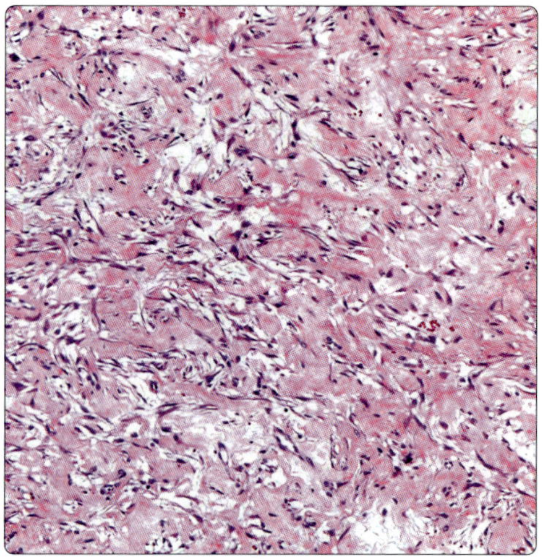

Keloidal Collagen

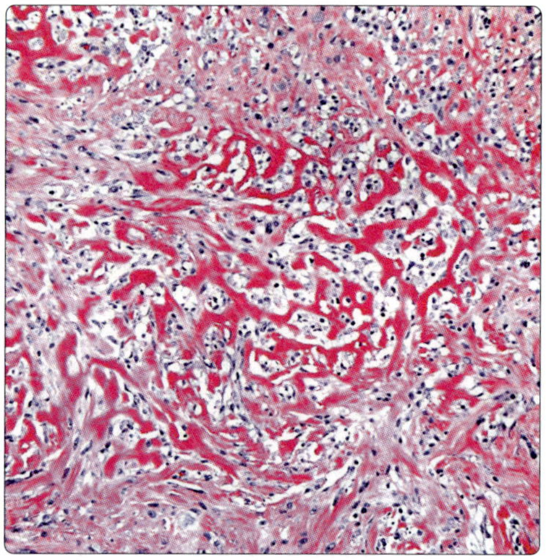

(Left) *Foci or zones of increased cellularity and organization ➙ are not uncommon in nodular fasciitis and can easily lead to consideration (or misdiagnosis) of sarcoma. Mitotic figures are usually frequent as well, further increasing the risk of overdiagnosis.* **(Right)** *Nodular fasciitis may show areas of striking cellularity. Short linear or curved fascicles or bundles are common findings in these areas. Mitoses are common, but never abnormal.*

Increased Cellularity

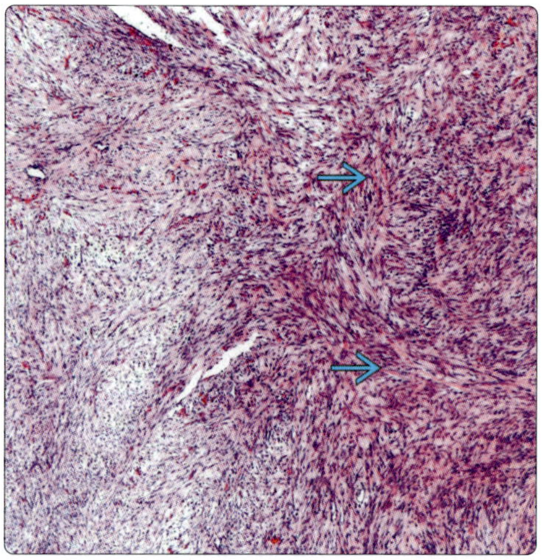

Cellular Areas

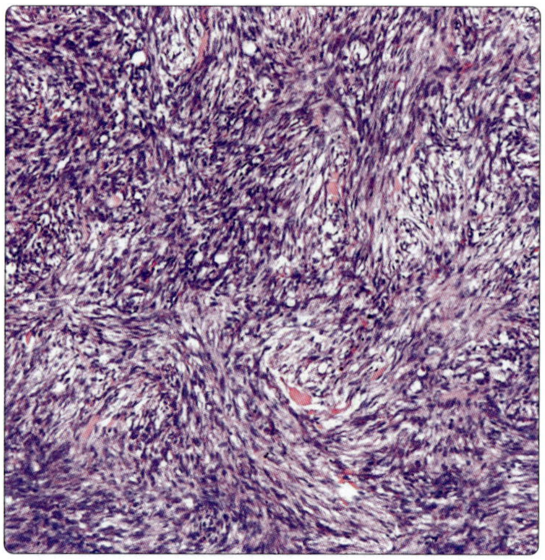

(Left) *Areas of increased stromal collagen and architectural organization in nodular fasciitis, as shown in this image, may lead to consideration of fibromatosis or a low-grade myofibroblastic sarcoma.* **(Right)** *A minority of cases of nodular fasciitis arise entirely within muscle ➪, as depicted. Care must be taken not to misidentify entrapped atrophic skeletal muscle fibers ➙ as pleomorphic hyperchromatic tumor cells.*

Cellular Areas

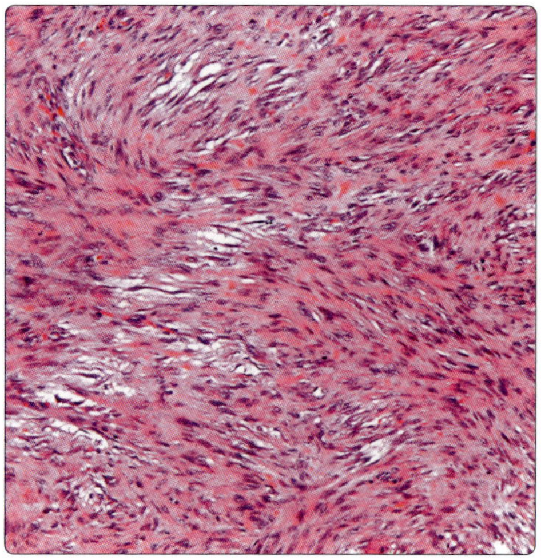

Origin in Muscle

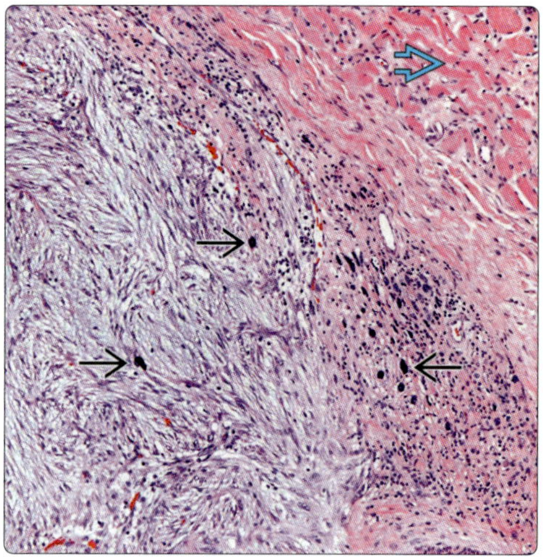

Peripheral Extension

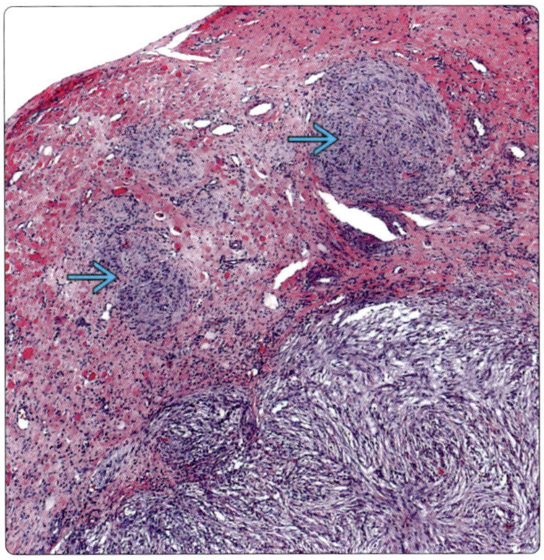

Intravascular Fasciitis

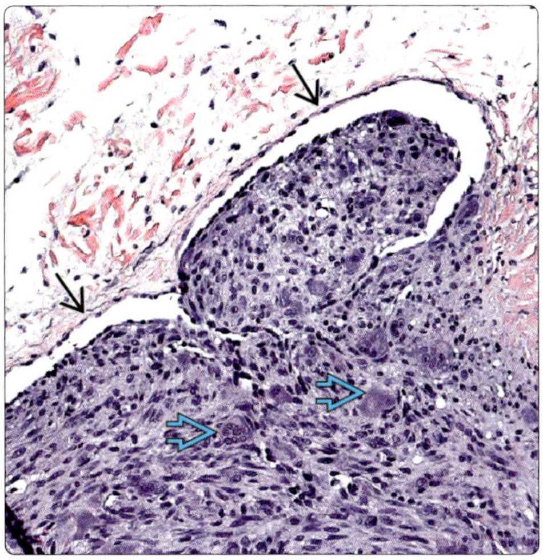

(Left) *Some cases of nodular fasciitis, particularly those that arise within skeletal muscle, can show a nodular morphology → at the periphery of the tumor, which may lead to consideration of a malignant, invasive process.* **(Right)** *Nodular fasciitis may grow partially or entirely within a vessel and is recognized by the term intravascular fasciitis. Note the protrusion into an endothelial-lined space →. Of note, osteoclast-like giant cells → are often more prominent in this variant.*

Intravascular Growth

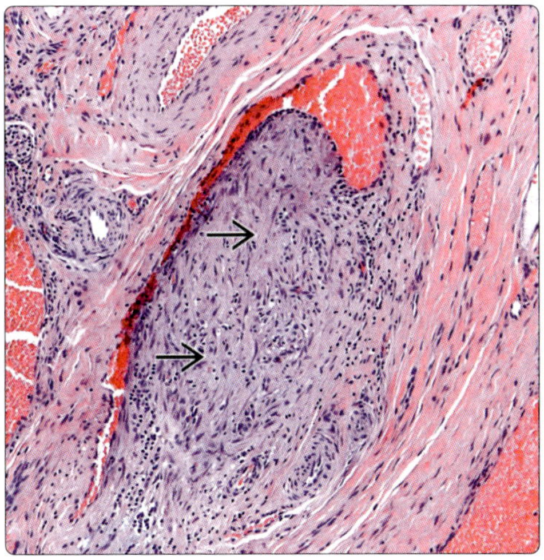

Fibrous or Myxoid Stroma

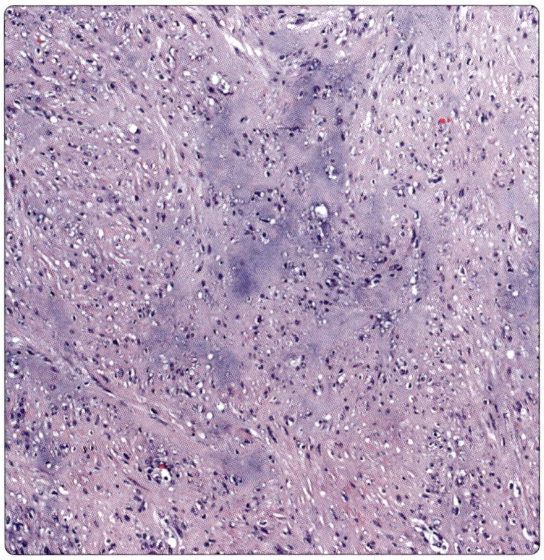

(Left) *Intravascular growth → may be identified within vessels located around the periphery of the tumor in some cases, as seen here. The main lesion had otherwise typical features of nodular fasciitis.* **(Right)** *Intravascular fasciitis closely resembles conventional nodular fasciitis morphologically and can feature a fibrous or myxoid stroma. Cellularity can also vary.*

Intravascular Fasciitis, Trichrome Stain

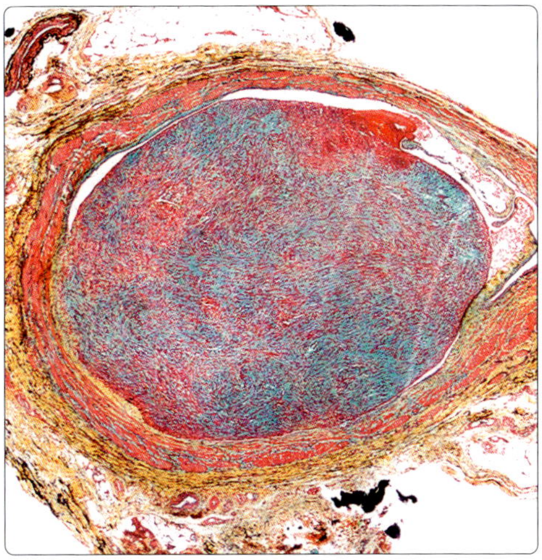

SMA Expression

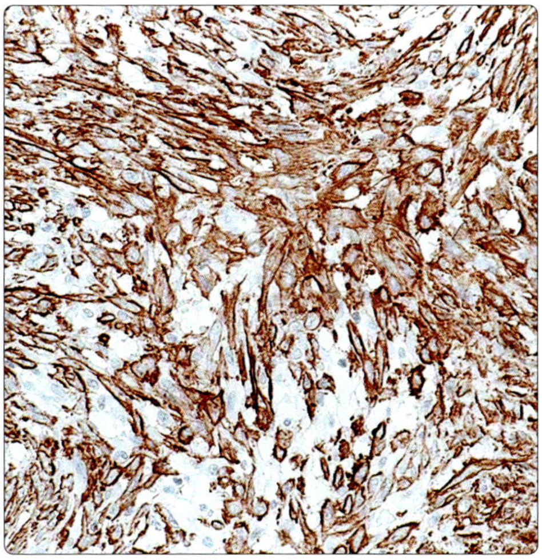

(Left) *A trichrome stain shows an entirely intravascular example of intravascular fasciitis. Despite the occlusive growth, this does not usually result in any functional impairment, and the lesion presents as a mass clinically. Veins or arteries can be involved, and the lesional tissue sometimes extends through the vessel wall.* **(Right)** *Strong staining with smooth muscle actin (SMA) is common in nodular fasciitis, and expression is often peripheral and submembranous as seen in other myofibroblastic lesions.*

Proliferative Fasciitis/Myositis

KEY FACTS

TERMINOLOGY

- Pseudosarcomatous myofibroblastic proliferation featuring ganglion-like cells and occurring in subcutaneous tissue (proliferative fasciitis) or intramuscularly (proliferative myositis)

CLINICAL ISSUES

- Middle-aged and older adults
  - Can arise in children (uncommon)
- Fasciitis: Subcutaneous tissue of upper extremity (particularly forearm), lower extremity, trunk
- Myositis: Muscles of trunk, shoulder, upper arm
- Rapidly growing, often tender mass
- Treatment: Simple excision
- Benign; local recurrence very rare

MACROSCOPIC

- Poorly circumscribed, elongated mass, usually < 4 cm

MICROSCOPIC

- Shows many morphologic features of nodular fasciitis
- Additional component of large ganglion-like fibroblasts (hallmark)
  - 1 or more nuclei, often eccentric with prominent macronucleoli
- Proliferative fasciitis in children is often more cellular and mitotically active
- Checkerboard growth pattern in proliferative myositis

ANCILLARY TESTS

- SMA(+)
- Desmin, keratin, S100 protein, myogenin (-)

TOP DIFFERENTIAL DIAGNOSES

- Nodular fasciitis
- Embryonal rhabdomyosarcoma
- Pleomorphic rhabdomyosarcoma
- Undifferentiated pleomorphic sarcoma

Proliferative Fasciitis

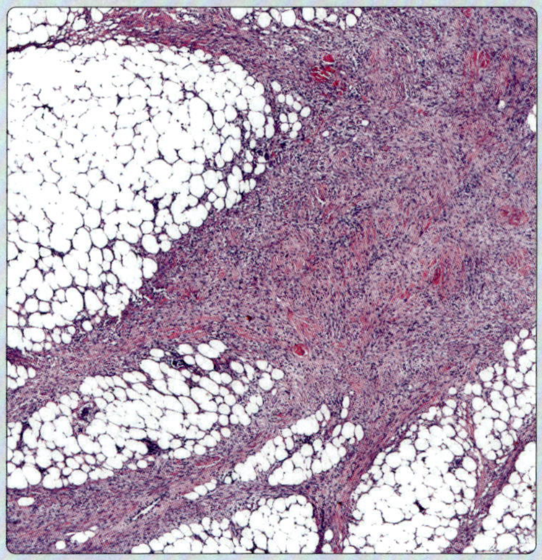

Proliferative Fasciitis

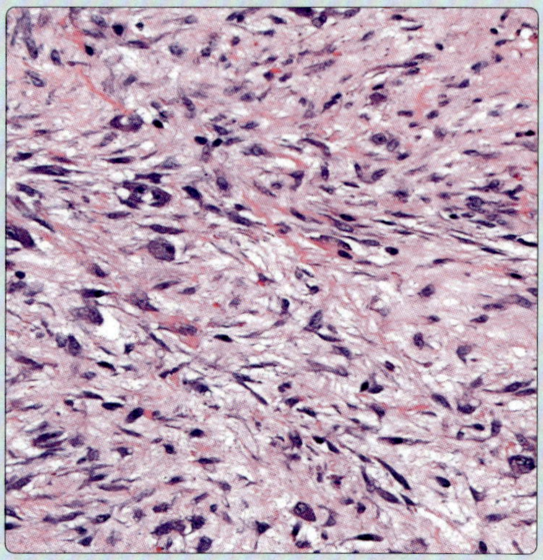

(Left) *Proliferative fasciitis usually presents clinically as a small but rapidly growing subcutaneous mass. At low magnification, it often tracks along fibrous connective tissue septa.* **(Right)** *Histologically, proliferative fasciitis (and myositis) shares many similarities with nodular fasciitis, including spindled to stellate myofibroblastic cells within a loose myxoid to collagenous stroma. Extravasated erythrocytes are common.*

Ganglion-Like Cells

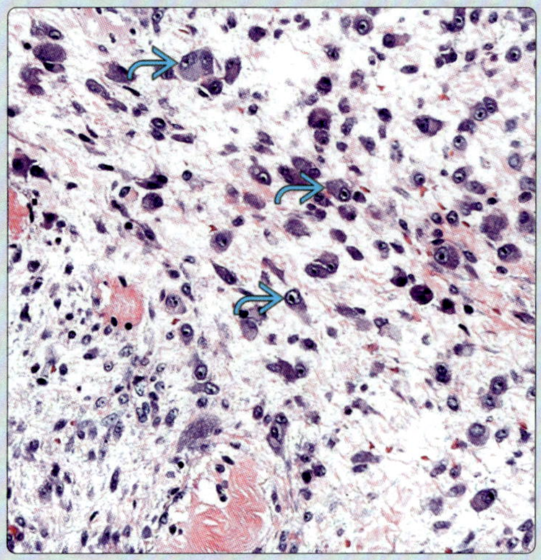

Ganglion-Like Cells

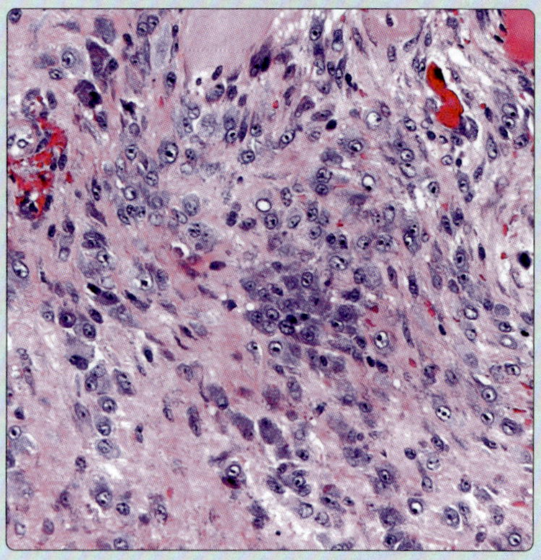

(Left) *The hallmark of proliferative fasciitis/myositis is the presence of enlarged epithelioid or polygonal cells* ➩ *with basophilic or amphophilic cytoplasm and large, eccentric vesicular nuclei with prominent macronucleoli. These cells resemble ganglion cells but are actually fibroblasts.* **(Right)** *Within any given case of proliferative fasciitis, the ganglion-like cells may be distributed singly, in loose clusters, or in aggregates. The actual density varies from microscopic field to field.*

TERMINOLOGY

Definitions

- Pseudosarcomatous myofibroblastic proliferation featuring ganglion-like cells and occurring in subcutaneous tissue (proliferative fasciitis) or intramuscularly (proliferative myositis)

CLINICAL ISSUES

Epidemiology

- Incidence
  - Rare
    - Less common than nodular fasciitis
- Age
  - Middle-aged and older adults
    - Can arise in children (uncommon)

Site

- Proliferative fasciitis
  - Subcutaneous tissue of upper extremity (particularly forearm), lower extremity, trunk
    - May also arise in dermis or involve underlying fascia
- Proliferative myositis
  - Muscles of trunk, shoulder, upper arm

Presentation

- Rapidly growing, often tender mass
- History of trauma reported in minority of cases

Treatment

- Simple excision

Prognosis

- Benign
- Usually no local recurrence, even with incomplete excision

MACROSCOPIC

General Features

- Poorly circumscribed, elongated mass
  - Childhood tumors are often well circumscribed and lobular

Size

- Usually < 4 cm

MICROSCOPIC

Histologic Features

- Similar morphologic features to nodular fasciitis
  - Plump, spindled, and stellate myofibroblasts in variably myxoid or collagenous stroma
    - Myxoid tumors often have loose tissue culture appearance
    - Vesicular nuclei with 1 or 2 small but conspicuous nucleoli
    - Mitotic activity often brisk; no atypical forms
  - Extravasated erythrocytes and stromal lymphocytic infiltrate common
  - Older lesions may have abundant hyalinized collagen
- Large ganglion-like fibroblasts (hallmark)
  - Epithelioid cells with abundant amphophilic or basophilic cytoplasm
  - Contain 1 or 2 vesicular nuclei, often eccentric with prominent macronucleoli
  - Can form large aggregates or loose clusters
- Proliferative fasciitis in children is often much more cellular and mitotically active
  - May have acute inflammation and foci of necrosis
- Checkerboard pattern of intramuscular growth in proliferative myositis
- Older lesions may show stromal hyalinization
- Focal metaplastic bone formation rare

ANCILLARY TESTS

Immunohistochemistry

- SMA(+)
- Desmin, keratin, S100 protein, myogenin, MYOD1 (-)

DIFFERENTIAL DIAGNOSIS

Nodular Fasciitis

- More common in younger adults
- Histologically similar to proliferative fasciitis/myositis
- Lacks ganglion-like cells
- Well circumscribed
- *USP6* gene rearrangements

Embryonal Rhabdomyosarcoma

- Usually involves genital region or head/neck of infants and young children
- Mucosal tumors often show enhanced cellularity beneath epithelium (cambium layer)
- Usually malignant cytologic features
- Desmin (+), myogenin (+)

Pleomorphic Rhabdomyosarcoma

- Usually large, intramuscular, and in older adults
- Markedly pleomorphic cells with numerous atypical mitoses and necrosis
- Desmin (+), myogenin (+)

Undifferentiated Pleomorphic Sarcoma

- Usually large, intramuscular, and in older adults
- Markedly pleomorphic cells with numerous atypical mitoses and necrosis

SELECTED REFERENCES

1. Wei N et al: Proliferative myositis in the right brachioradialis: a case report. Exp Ther Med. 13(5):2483-2485, 2017
2. Rosa G et al: A report of three cases of pediatric proliferative fasciitis. J Cutan Pathol. 41(9):720-3, 2014
3. Yamaga K et al: Proliferative fasciitis mimicking a sarcoma in a child: a case report. J Dermatol. 41(2):163-7, 2014
4. Satter EK et al: Intradermal proliferative fasciitis on the finger. Am J Dermatopathol. 37(3):246-8, 2013
5. Brooks JK et al: Intraoral proliferative myositis: case report and literature review. Head Neck. 29(4):416-20, 2007
6. Sasano H et al: Proliferative fasciitis of the forearm: case report with immunohistochemical, ultrastructural and DNA ploidy studies and a review of the literature. Pathol Int. 48(6):486-90, 1998
7. Meis JM et al: Proliferative fasciitis and myositis of childhood. Am J Surg Pathol. 16(4):364-72, 1992

Binucleation

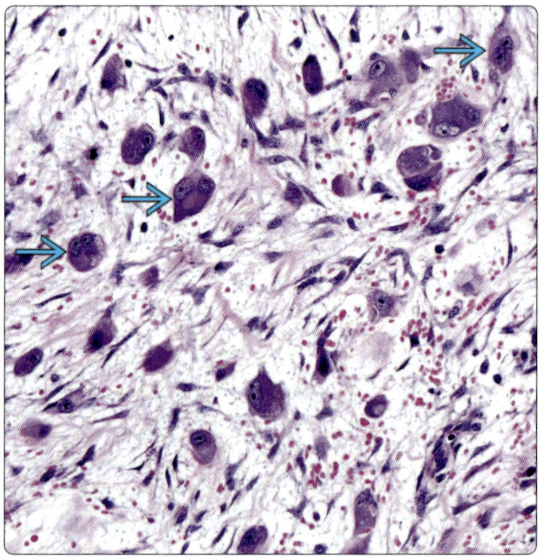

Pediatric Proliferative Fasciitis

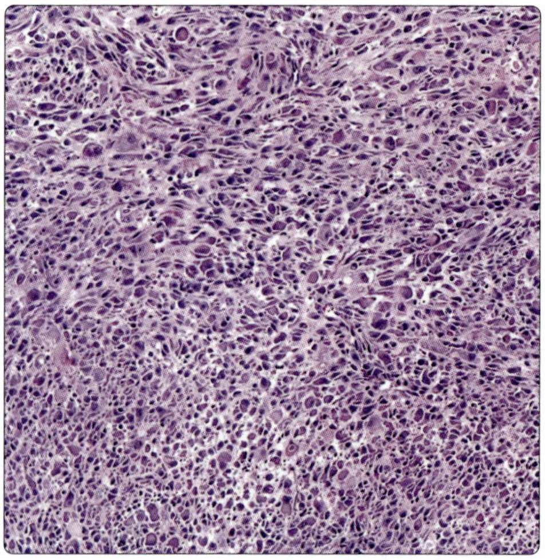

(Left) *Although most of the ganglion-like cells in proliferative fasciitis have single nuclei, some may be binucleated. This H&E shows several of these variant cells. Note also the loose myxoid stroma with extravasated erythrocytes.* **(Right)** *Pediatric proliferative fasciitis is often much more cellular and less myxoid than adult forms. This variant may naturally raise concerns for malignancy. A correct diagnosis can usually be derived from the clinical presentation and immunohistochemistry.*

Pediatric Proliferative Fasciitis

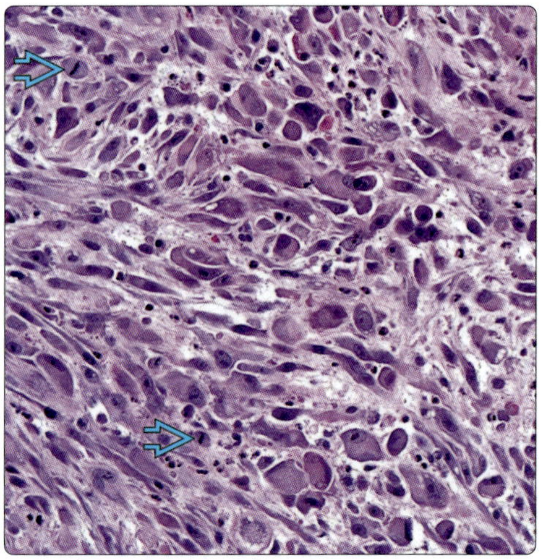

Pediatric Proliferative Fasciitis

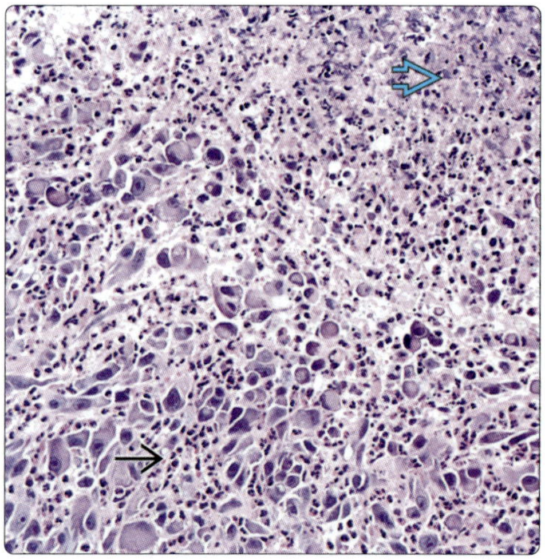

(Left) *Pediatric proliferative fasciitis is more likely to show increased mitotic activity than the typical adult form. Two mitotic figures are shown in this H&E. Importantly, mitoses are almost never atypical. If more than a rare atypical figure is identified, malignancy should be carefully excluded.* **(Right)** *Pediatric examples of proliferative fasciitis may also show pockets of acute inflammation as well as foci of necrosis.*

Stromal Hyalinization

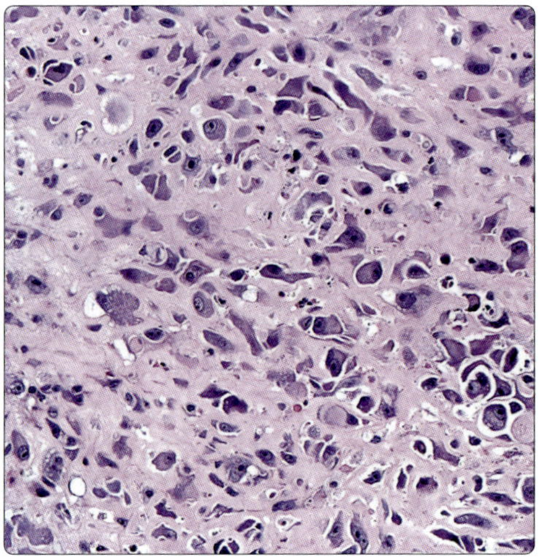

Proliferative Myositis

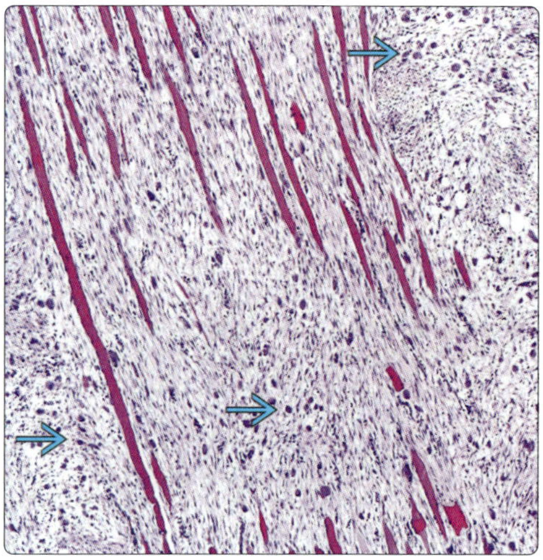

(Left) *Occasionally, older lesions may show stromal hyalinization. Together with the large, ganglion-like cells, this feature may mimic osteoid deposition and lead to misdiagnosis as osteosarcoma.* **(Right)** *Proliferative myositis is essentially the intramuscular counterpart to proliferative fasciitis. Characteristically, the proliferation splays out muscle fibers, imparting a highly infiltrative appearance. Ganglion-like cells can be seen even at low magnification.*

Proliferative Myositis

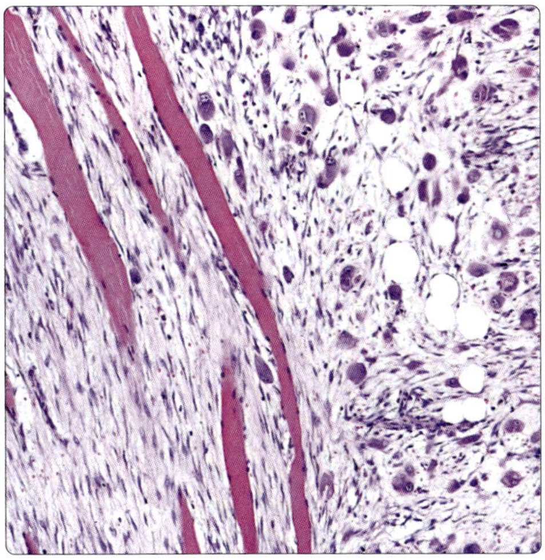

Checkerboard Pattern

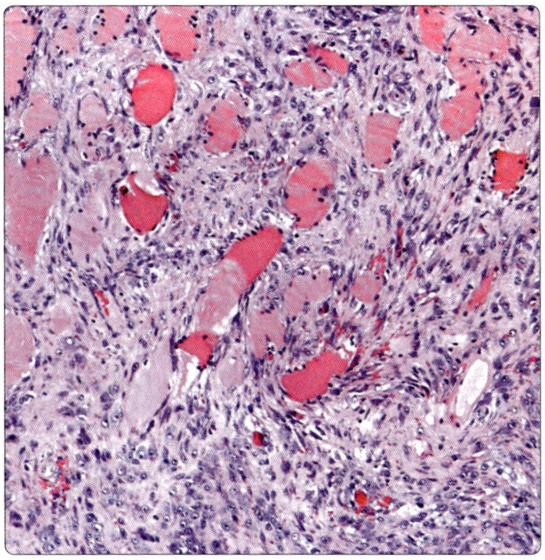

(Left) *Just as in proliferative fasciitis, proliferative myositis characteristically contains scattered ganglion-like cells with prominent nucleoli. The background stroma is loose and myxoid, similar to nodular fasciitis.* **(Right)** *When seen in cross section, the splayed muscle fibers appear to alternate with the lesional proliferation, imparting a checkerboard morphologic pattern.*

Spindled Morphology

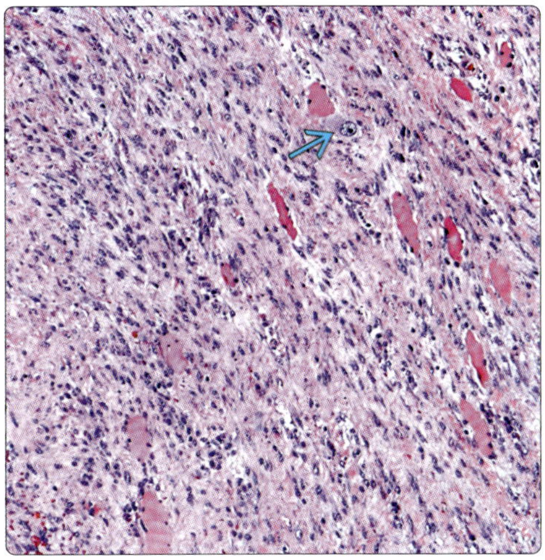

Rare Metaplastic Bone

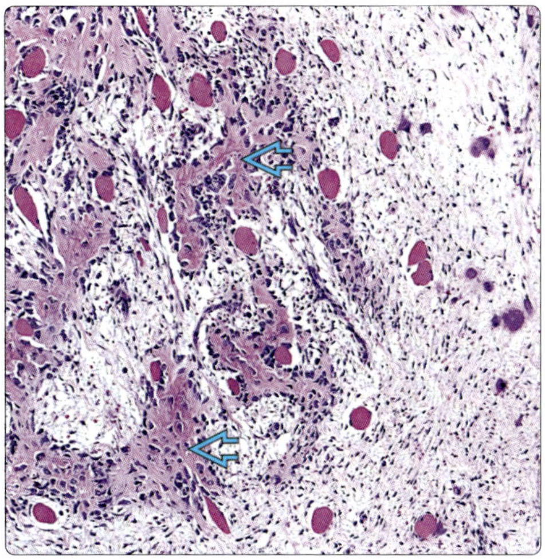

(Left) *In some areas of proliferative myositis, the lesional fibroblasts may adopt a subtle fascicular morphology, reminiscent of fibromatosis. Note, however, the presence of a ganglion-like cell →.* **(Right)** *Foci of metaplastic bone formation ⇨ may be seen in rare cases of proliferative myositis (or proliferative fasciitis). Note also the checkerboard pattern of muscle fibers.*

Cellular Foci

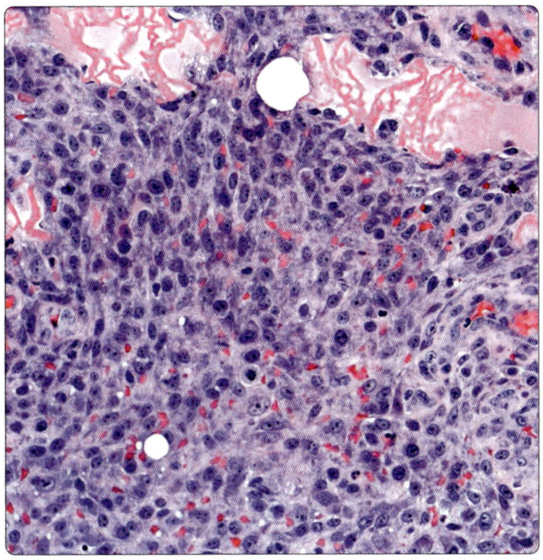

Fasciitis/Myositis Mimics

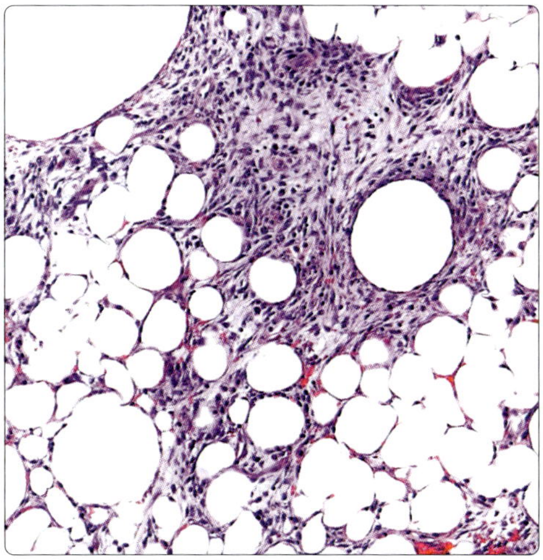

(Left) *Similar to proliferative fasciitis, the ganglion-like cells in proliferative myositis may show areas of increased cellular density.* **(Right)** *Reactive myofibroblastic proliferations, such as those seen in the setting of intraabdominal adhesions or incarcerated hernias, may closely mimic proliferative fasciitis histologically. However, there is often a prominent component of adipose tissue in reactive adhesions, and the clinical presentation is often very different from that of proliferative fasciitis.*

Ischemic Fasciitis

KEY FACTS

TERMINOLOGY

- Pseudosarcomatous proliferation composed of zones of fat and fibrinoid necrosis with ingrowth of capillaries, reactive fibroblasts, and myofibroblasts
- Synonym: Atypical decubital fibroplasia

CLINICAL ISSUES

- Peak incidence: 70-90 years of age
- Most common in soft tissues overlying bony prominences
  - Hip, shoulder, chest wall, back, sacrum
- Many patients are immobilized or debilitated
- Treatment: Simple surgical excision
- Benign
  - Local recurrences rare

MICROSCOPIC

- Characteristic zonal appearance
  - Central fibrinoid necrosis/degeneration
  - Vascularized granulation tissue typically surrounds necrotic foci
    - Thin-walled capillary channels lined by plump, reactive endothelial cells
    - Reactive fibroblasts often enlarged with amphophilic cytoplasm and variably prominent nucleoli
      - May resemble ganglion cells (ganglion cell-like myofibroblast)
  - Peripheral soft tissue shows variable myxoid change, fibrosis, fat necrosis
- Mitotic activity usually low but may be brisk
- Variable inflammatory infiltrate

TOP DIFFERENTIAL DIAGNOSES

- Proliferative fasciitis/myositis
- Nodular fasciitis
- Well-differentiated liposarcoma
- Myxofibrosarcoma (low grade)

Ischemic Fasciitis

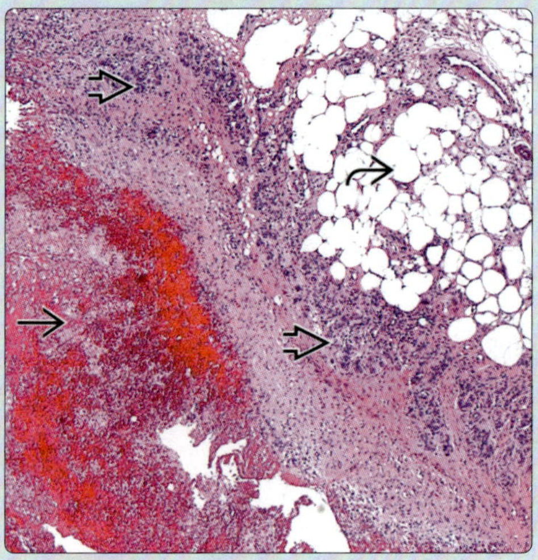

Vascularized Rim

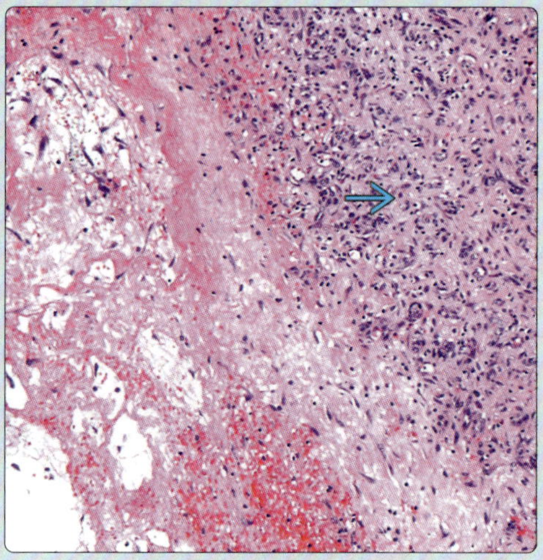

(Left) *Ischemic fasciitis (also referred to as atypical decubital fibroplasia) classically shows a zonal appearance with centralized fibrinoid necrosis, mantled by arcades of reactive capillaries admixed with reactive myofibroblasts and surrounding tissues. Adipose tissue often contains fat necrosis and may be partially infarcted.* **(Right)** *The vascularized granulation tissue-like rim shows small, reactive capillaries admixed with reactive myofibroblasts.*

Reactive Myofibroblasts

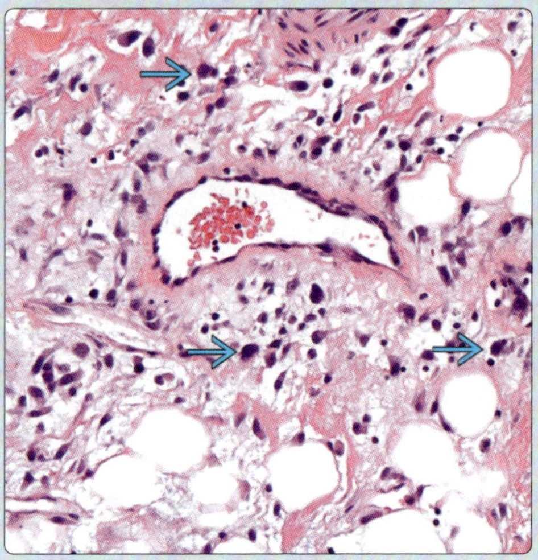

Reactive Myofibroblasts

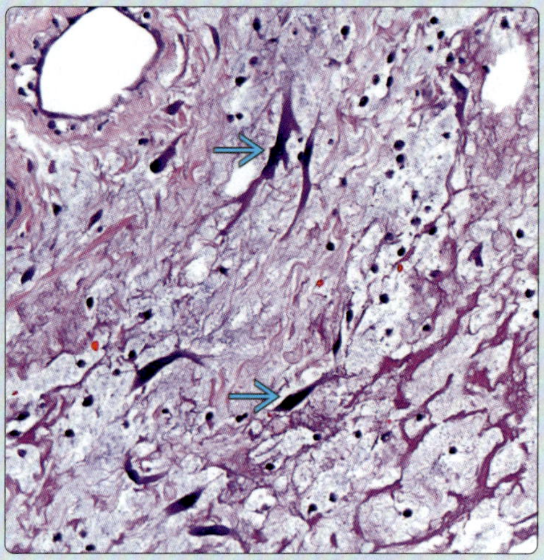

(Left) *The reactive myofibroblasts of ischemic fasciitis are often enlarged and contain basophilic to amphophilic cytoplasm. Nucleoli may be inconspicuous or prominent, the latter sometimes resembling ganglion cells. Mitoses vary in number, and rare atypical forms may be seen.* **(Right)** *In some cases of ischemic fasciitis, the myofibroblasts appear bipolar or stellate with hyperchromatic and "smudgy" degenerative nuclei, reminiscent of atypical lipomatous tumor/well-differentiated liposarcoma.*

TERMINOLOGY

Synonyms

- Atypical decubital fibroplasia

Definitions

- Pseudosarcomatous proliferation composed of zones of fat and fibrinoid necrosis with ingrowth of capillaries, reactive fibroblasts, and myofibroblasts

CLINICAL ISSUES

Epidemiology

- Age
    - Peak incidence: 70-90 years
        - Occasionally in younger adult patients
- Sex
    - Slight male predominance

Site

- Most common in soft tissues overlying bony prominences
    - Hip, shoulder, chest wall, back, and sacrum
- Usually deep subcutaneous tissue
    - May extend to involve dermis or underlying fascia/muscle

Presentation

- Painful or painless mass
    - Overlying skin usually not ulcerated
- Many patients are immobilized or debilitated
    - Some patients have history of local trauma (including previous surgical procedure) or chronic disease (e.g., osteoarthritis, COPD)

Treatment

- Simple surgical excision

Prognosis

- Benign
- Local recurrence is rare

MACROSCOPIC

General Features

- Ill-defined, tan-yellow mass with cut surface showing variable necrosis and hemorrhage

Size

- 1-10 cm

MICROSCOPIC

Histologic Features

- Vaguely lobular configuration and generally hypocellular
- Characteristic zonal appearance
    - Central fibrinoid necrosis/degeneration
        - May show pseudocyst formation &/or infarcted fat
    - Vascularized granulation tissue typically surrounds necrotic foci
        - Thin-walled capillary channels lined by plump, reactive endothelial cells
        - Reactive fibroblasts often enlarged with amphophilic cytoplasm and variably prominent nucleoli
            - May resemble ganglion cells (ganglion cell-like myofibroblast)
            - Nuclei may appear degenerative (hyperchromatic and "smudgy")
    - Peripheral soft tissue around lesion shows variable myxoid change, fibrosis, fat necrosis
- Mitotic activity usually low but may be brisk
    - Atypical mitoses rare
- Variable inflammatory infiltrate
    - Usually lymphocytes and plasma cells, occasionally neutrophils
- Other findings: Extravasated erythrocytes, hemosiderin, vascular hyalinization/thrombosis

ANCILLARY TESTS

Immunohistochemistry

- Variable SMA(+), desmin (+), CD34(+)
- Keratin (-), S100 protein (-)

DIFFERENTIAL DIAGNOSIS

Nodular Fasciitis/Proliferative Fasciitis/Proliferative Myositis

- Often occurs away from bony prominences
- Exuberant myofibroblastic proliferation with delicate vessels, extravasated erythrocytes, scattered lymphocytes
    - More evenly cellular than ischemic fasciitis
- Absence of zonal pattern with central fibrinoid necrosis
- Proliferative fasciitis/myositis: Randomly scattered or clustered myofibroblasts with eccentric nuclei and prominent nucleoli (ganglion cell-like myofibroblasts)

Well-Differentiated Liposarcoma

- Often large, deep tumors of extremities or in retroperitoneum
- Lobules of atypical fat separated by variably thickened fibrous septa containing hyperchromatic "smudgy" cells
- Multivacuolated lipoblasts may be present
- Absence of zonal pattern with central fibrinoid necrosis
- Minimal mitotic activity
- *MDM2* gene amplification

Myxofibrosarcoma (Low Grade)

- Absence of zonal pattern (central fibrinoid necrosis with surrounding reactive changes)
- Nuclear pleomorphism often present, at least focally

Epithelioid Sarcoma

- Large nests of eosinophilic epithelioid cells, often with central necrosis
    - Malignant cytologic features
- Keratin (+), EMA(+), loss of INI1

SELECTED REFERENCES

1. Yamada Y et al: HIF-1α, MDM2, CDK4, and p16 expression in ischemic fasciitis, focusing on its ischemic condition. Virchows Arch. 471(1):117-122, 2017
2. Lehmer LM et al: Ischemic fasciitis: enhanced diagnostic resolution through clinical, histopathologic and radiologic correlation in 17 cases. J Cutan Pathol. 43(9):740-8, 2016
3. Liegl B et al: Ischemic fasciitis: analysis of 44 cases indicating an inconsistent association with immobility or debilitation. Am J Surg Pathol. 32(10):1546-52, 2008

KEY FACTS

TERMINOLOGY

- Localized, self-limited, reactive fibroblastic lesion arising intramuscularly and featuring bone in varying stages of maturation
  - Biologically similar lesions occur in other specific sites (e.g., fibroosseous pseudotumor of digit, panniculitis ossificans)

ETIOLOGY/PATHOGENESIS

- Many cases are associated with history of localized trauma or injury

CLINICAL ISSUES

- Wide age range (most common around 30 years)
- 3:2 male predominance
- Skeletal muscle of thigh, buttock, elbow, shoulder most common sites
- Treatment: Simple surgical excision
- Benign; rare local recurrence

MACROSCOPIC

- Size range: 2-12 cm (mean: 5 cm)

MICROSCOPIC

- Well circumscribed
- Characteristic zonal appearance with peripheral maturation
  - Centralized proliferations of spindled fibroblasts and myofibroblasts
    - No nuclear atypia or atypical mitoses
  - Areas with woven bone formation and peripheral maturation

TOP DIFFERENTIAL DIAGNOSES

- Extraskeletal osteosarcoma
- Nodular fasciitis
- Aneurysmal bone cyst of soft tissue
- Ossifying fibromyxoid tumor

(Left) *Myositis ossificans (MO) is a reactive, self-limiting fibroblastic proliferation that features bone in various stages of maturation. It may be confused both clinically and histologically with a sarcoma.* **(Right)** *The presence of zonal maturation is a key feature of MO. Lesions tend to show gradual progression from loose or cellular fibroblastic zones → to areas containing immature woven bone formation ⇨ to more peripheral areas of remodeling and mature lamellar bone formation.*

Myositis Ossificans

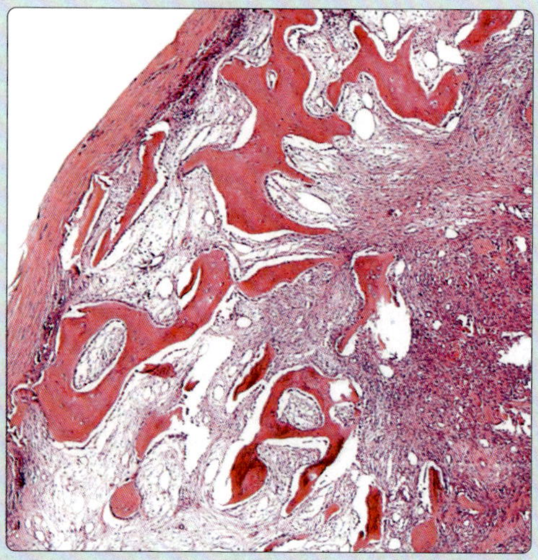

Zonal Maturation

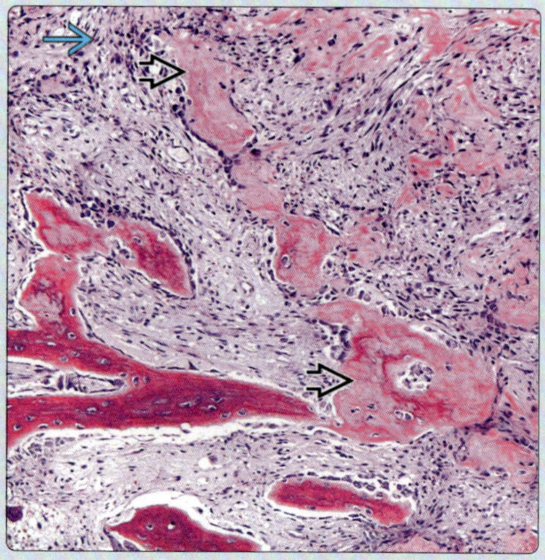

(Left) *The fibroblastic areas of MO are often centralized within the lesion and commonly resemble nodular fasciitis, as shown. The cellularity of these areas varies widely from loose and sparse to strikingly dense.* **(Right)** *Some fibroblastic areas in MO may be alarmingly cellular, usually in early lesions, and mitotic figures may be numerous. Importantly, nuclei are cytologically bland, and mitoses are not abnormal. Osteoclasts → are also a common finding.*

Nodular Fasciitis-Like Areas

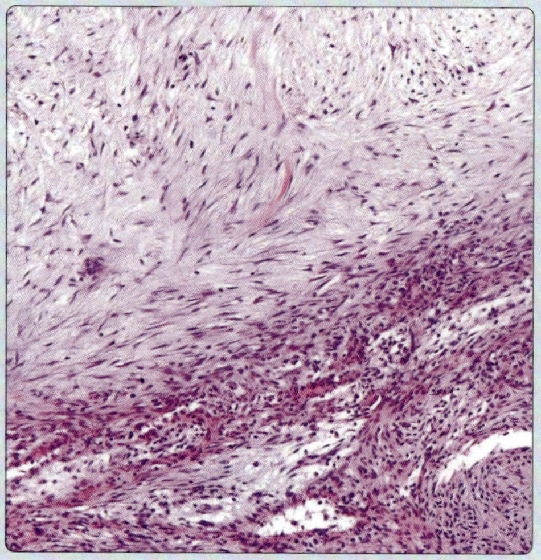

Cellular Foci

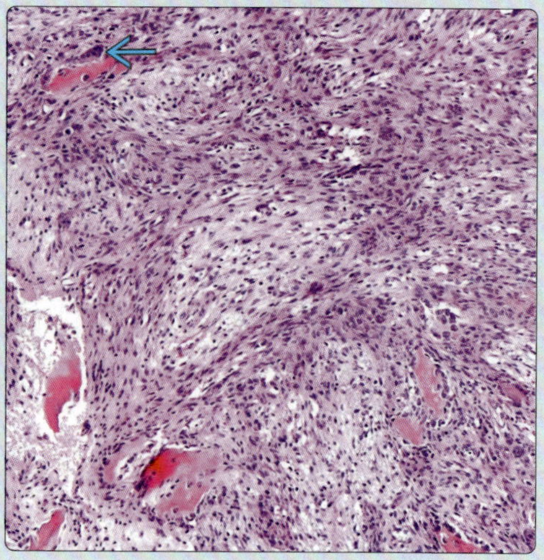

TERMINOLOGY

Abbreviations

- Myositis ossificans (MO)

Synonyms

- MO circumscripta/traumatica

Definitions

- Localized, self-limited, reactive fibroblastic lesion arising intramuscularly and featuring bone in varying stages of maturation
  - Biologically similar lesions occur in other specific sites
    - Fibroosseous pseudotumor of digits (fingers and toes)
    - Panniculitis ossificans (subcutaneous adipose tissue)
    - Also in fascia and mesentery

ETIOLOGY/PATHOGENESIS

Injury

- Many cases are associated with history of localized trauma or injury
  - Patients with MO are often physically active

CLINICAL ISSUES

Epidemiology

- Age
  - Wide age range (most common around 30 years)
- Sex
  - Male predominance

Site

- Arise intramuscularly in areas prone to local trauma
  - Thigh, buttock, elbow, shoulder most common

Presentation

- Rapidly growing, variably tender mass

Treatment

- Simple surgical excision

Prognosis

- Benign
  - Rare local recurrence
- Exceptionally rare reports of malignant transformation

IMAGING

CT Findings

- Early lesions: Soft tissue fullness
- 2-6 weeks later: Flocculent calcifications and eventual development of bony shell (eggshell-like)

MACROSCOPIC

Size

- 2-12 cm (mean: 5 cm)

MICROSCOPIC

Histologic Features

- Well circumscribed
- Characteristic zonal appearance with peripheral maturation
  - Centralized proliferations of spindled fibroblasts and myofibroblasts
    - Often closely resembles nodular fasciitis
    - Variably cellular and myxoid
    - Cells randomly oriented or in loose fascicles
    - Bland, vesicular nuclei ± small nucleoli
    - Mitoses may be numerous but never atypical
    - Vascularized stroma with extravasated erythrocytes, fibrin, and lymphocytes
    - Osteoclast-like giant cells are common
  - Peripheral portion with bone formation
    - Merges with cellular myofibroblastic portion
    - Irregular trabeculae of immature woven bone rimmed by osteoblasts
    - Maturation into well-developed trabeculae of lamellar bone at periphery of older lesions
      - Older lesions may be composed entirely of mature bone ± hematopoietic elements
    - Cartilage uncommon but may be seen
- Zonal appearance poorly developed in some lesions

ANCILLARY TESTS

In Situ Hybridization

- *USP6* gene rearrangements
  - Similar to nodular fasciitis and aneurysmal bone cyst

DIFFERENTIAL DIAGNOSIS

Extraskeletal Osteosarcoma

- Often large masses in older adults
- Marked cytologic atypia, atypical mitoses
- Lacks zonal maturation of MO
  - Random deposits of osteoid and bone associated with cytologically malignant cells

Nodular Fasciitis

- Most common in subcutaneous tissue
- Usually lacks prominent bone formation
- Early lesions of MO may be indistinguishable from nodular fasciitis

Aneurysmal Bone Cyst of Soft Tissue

- Large, centralized, cystic, hemorrhagic spaces
- Peripheral rim of bone common

Ossifying Fibromyxoid Tumor

- Uniform, generally rounded cells, often in lace-like pattern
- Incomplete, peripheral rim of mature bone in majority of cases
- Usually S100 protein (+); some desmin (+)
- *PHF1* gene rearrangements

SELECTED REFERENCES

1. Bekers EM et al: Myositis ossificans - another condition with USP6 rearrangement, providing evidence of a relationship with nodular fasciitis and aneurysmal bone cyst. Ann Diagn Pathol. 34:56-9, 2018
2. Sferopoulos NK et al: Myositis ossificans in children: a review. Eur J Orthop Surg Traumatol. 27(4):491-502, 2017
3. Sukov WR et al: Frequency of USP6 rearrangements in myositis ossificans, brown tumor, and cherubism: molecular cytogenetic evidence that a subset of "myositis ossificans-like lesions" are the early phases in the formation of soft-tissue aneurysmal bone cyst. Skeletal Radiol. 37(4):321-7, 2008

(Left) *CT through the left leg shows a partial rim of bone ➡ in this example of well-developed MO.* **(Right)** *This gross photo of MO shows a circumscribed but not encapsulated early lesion. There are foci of hemorrhage ➡ mainly in the center of the lesion with adjacent, firm, white-yellow tissue. Bone may be grossly obvious in older cases.*

Myositis Ossificans: CT Scan

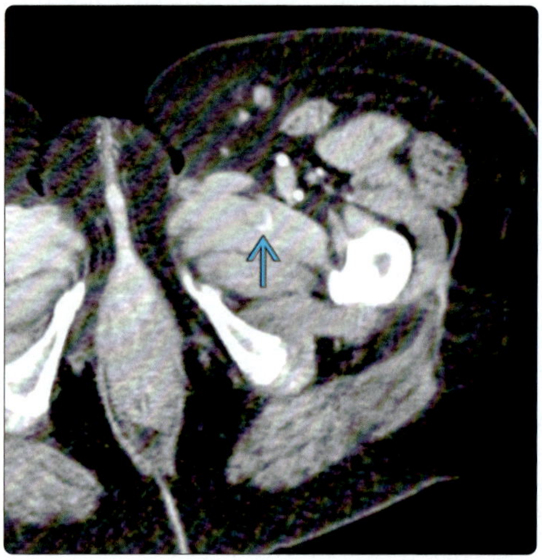

Gross Appearance

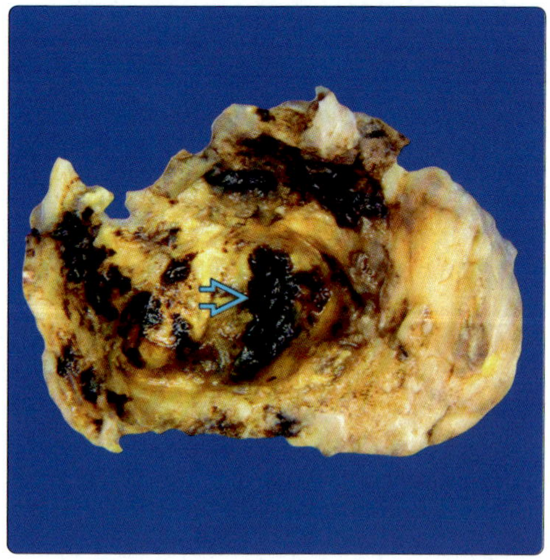

(Left) *The cytologic features of MO are similar to those of nodular fasciitis. The lesional fibroblastic/myofibroblastic cells are uniform and have bland nuclear features. Mitoses can be present (and numerous) but are not atypical.* **(Right)** *Evidence of zonal maturation is a key feature of MO. Woven bone formation with a conspicuous peripheral lining of osteoblasts ➡ is a typical finding.*

Cytologic Features

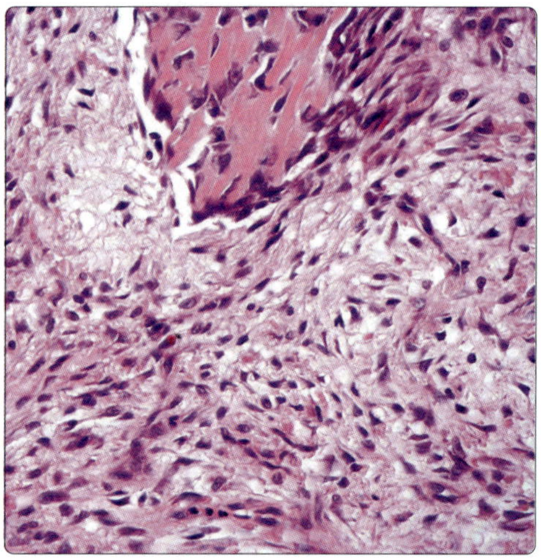

Zonal Maturation and Osteoblastic Rimming

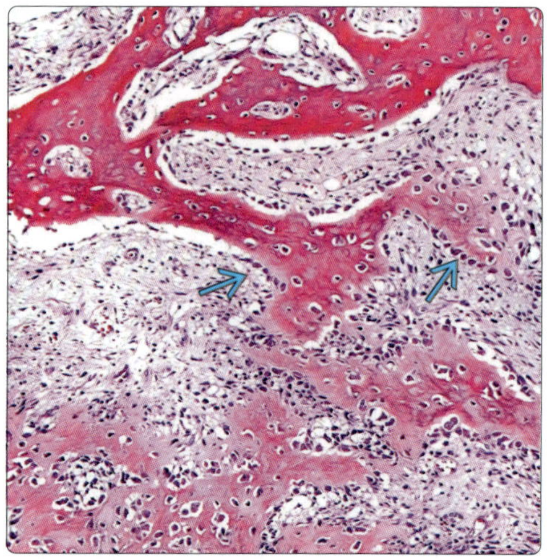

(Left) *Osteoclastic giant cells are commonly seen in MO, particularly in the centralized portion of early proliferative forms. In conjunction with the myofibroblastic cells and fibromyxoid stroma, the appearance is similar to nodular fasciitis.* **(Right)** *Extravasated red blood cells ➡ are common in the cellular, proliferative portion of MO and provide further morphologic similarity to nodular fasciitis.*

Osteoclastic Giant Cells

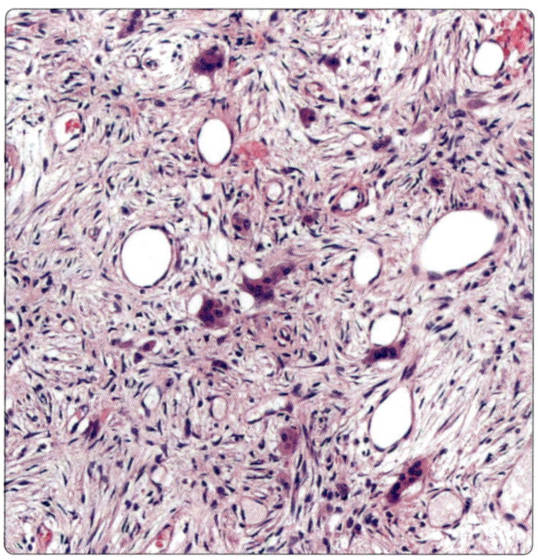

Extravasated Red Blood Cells

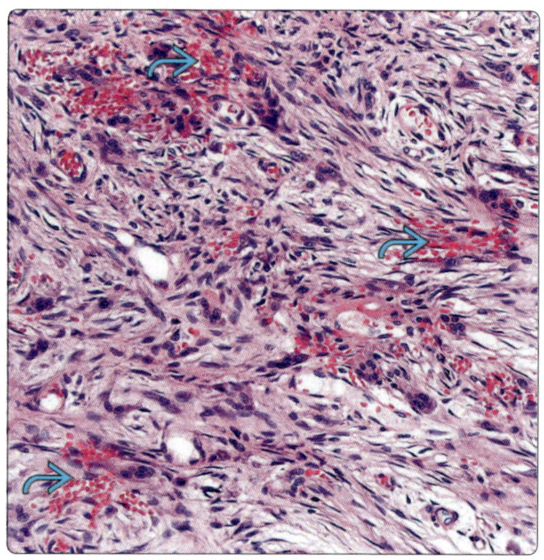

Cellular Proliferative Zones

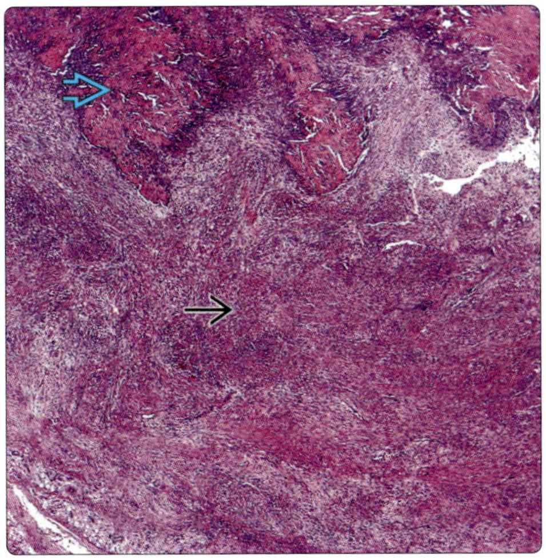

Osteoid Deposition and Immature Bone

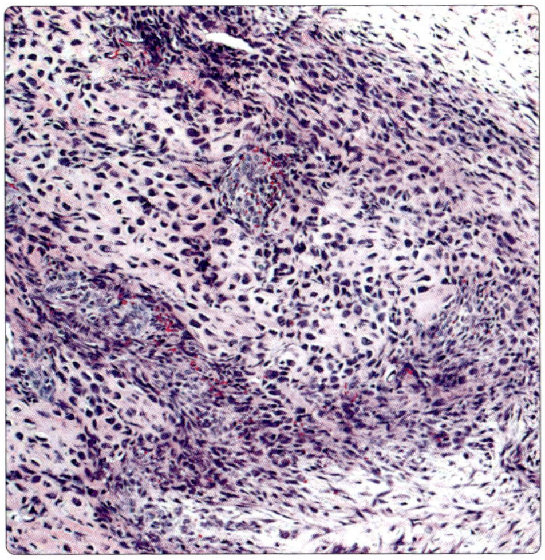

(Left) *MO is characterized by a zoned proliferation of myofibroblasts with a peripheral rim of woven bone . This example has a highly cellular central portion , which may be worrisome for sarcoma at low magnification.* **(Right)** *Foci of osteoid deposition with prominent osteoblasts in MO can be easily mistaken for a malignant process. The overall features of the lesion must be taken into account, including presence of zonal maturation and absence of malignant atypia.*

Primitive Trabecular Morphology

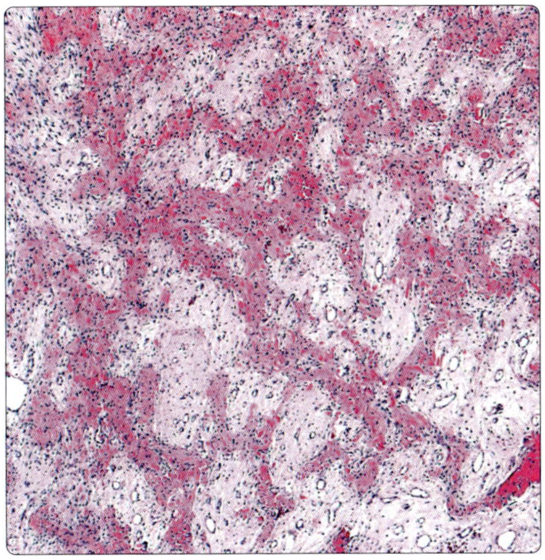

Vascularity

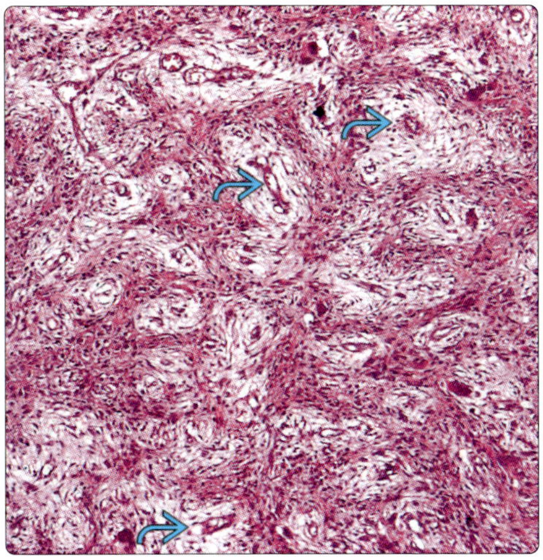

(Left) *Osteoid deposition and immature bone formation can form a ramifying, trabecular pattern in MO. Osteoblastic rimming is also common.* **(Right)** *The proliferative myofibroblastic zones of MO are often well vascularized, and myxoedematous change around the stromal vessels is not uncommon.*

Loose, Storiform Growth

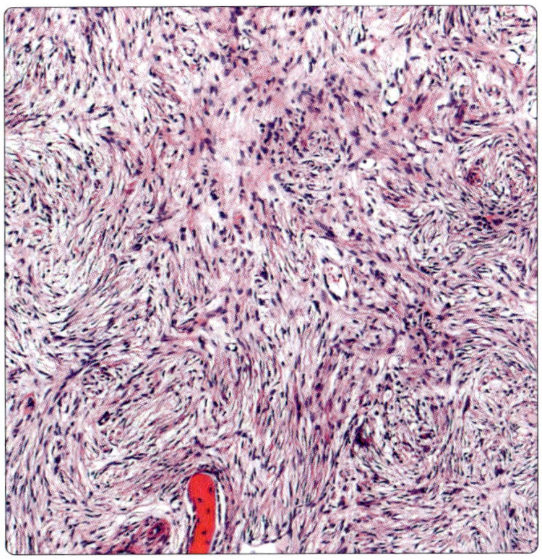

Mature Bone

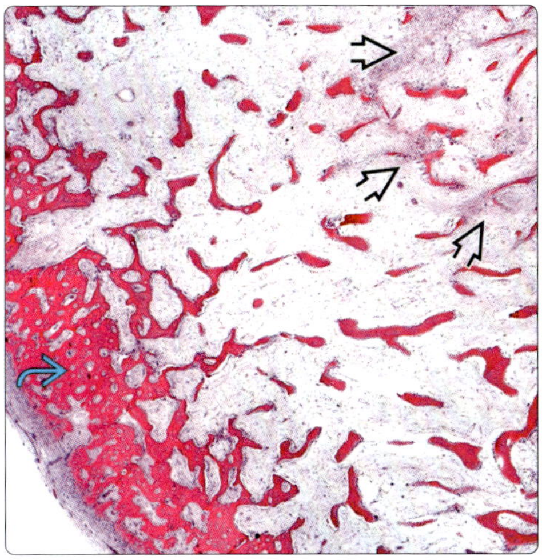

(Left) *Some cases of MO show a proliferative zone featuring bland myofibroblastic spindle cells in a storiform arrangement, as depicted here. Osteoclastic giant cells are not seen in this image.* **(Right)** *In the later stages of MO, mature bone is more prominent and well developed. A residual centralized and somewhat more cellular proliferative area is still identifiable in this image.*

Fibroosseous Pseudotumor of Digit

KEY FACTS

TERMINOLOGY

- Reactive-appearing, ossifying fibroblastic proliferation of soft tissue typically affecting digits of hands and feet
- Florid reactive periostitis

ETIOLOGY/PATHOGENESIS

- Clonal transient neoplasm with *USP6* rearrangement

CLINICAL ISSUES

- Fusiform swelling, often with erythema, pain, or ulceration
- Rapid onset; weeks to months
- Proximal phalanx of hand most common site
- Rarely occurs beyond acral extremities
- Benign, often self-limited
- Simple excision usually curative

IMAGING

- Early lesions characterized by ill-defined soft tissue density
- Older lesions with intralesional calcification
- Periosteal reaction common

MACROSCOPIC

- 0.5-5.6 cm; median: ~ 2.0 cm

MICROSCOPIC

- Fasciitis-like spindle cell proliferation with active ossification
- Myofibroblastic spindle and stellate cells with vesicular nuclei and amphophilic cytoplasm
- Ossification in various stages of maturation
- Peripheral zonal osseous maturation present in 50%
- Cartilage with endochondral ossification in some

TOP DIFFERENTIAL DIAGNOSES

- Extraskeletal osteosarcoma
- Myositis ossificans
- Fracture callus
- Bizarre parosteal osteochondromatous proliferation

Fibroosseous Pseudotumor

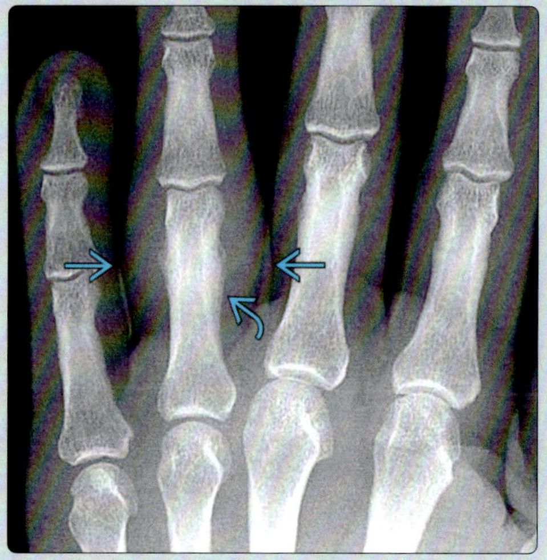

Low-Power Architecture

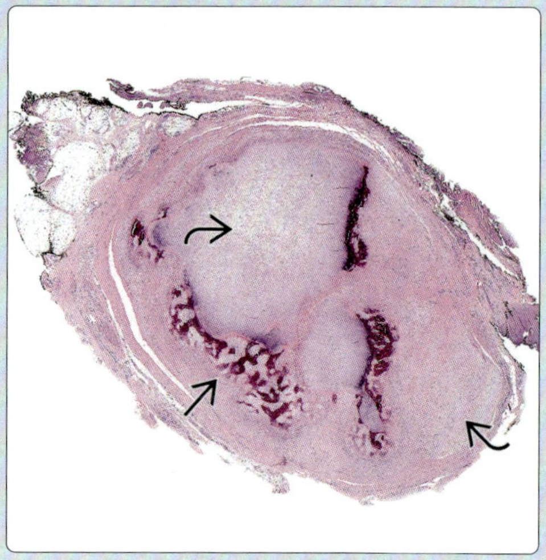

(Left) *Fibroosseous pseudotumor (FP) typically presents as fusiform swelling of a proximal phalanx of the hand. This radiograph depicts ill-defined soft tissue density and periosteal reaction. FP is also known as florid reactive periostitis.* **(Right)** *This scanning power micrograph depicts a circumscribed FP with lobular architecture, areas of bone formation, and loosely textured edematous, myxoid nodules. Bone formation in FP is usually distributed randomly as shown.*

Myofibroblasts and Reactive Bone

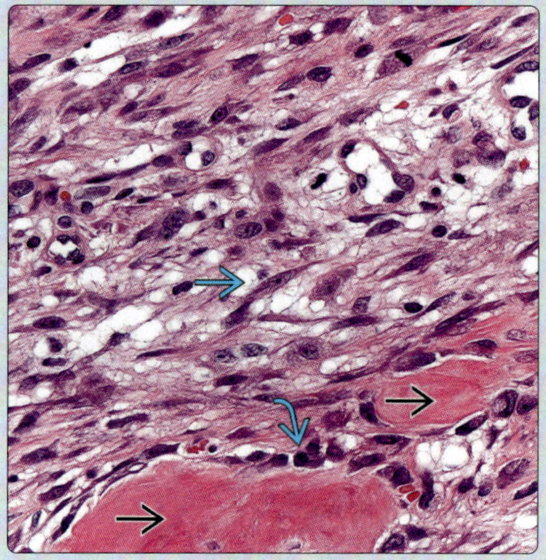

Osteoid and Woven Bone

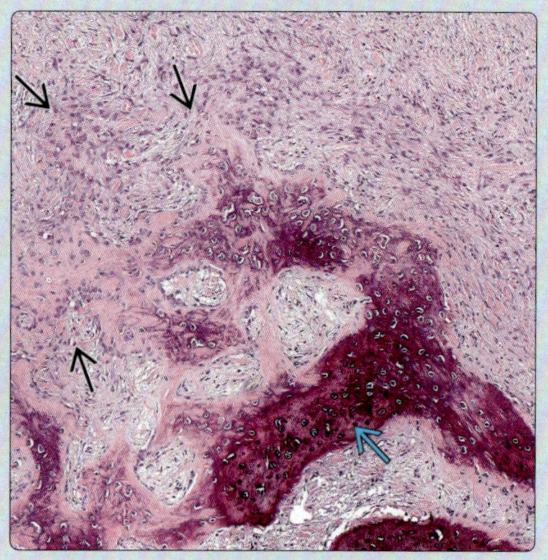

(Left) *FP consists of a fasciitis-like proliferation of spindle-shaped myofibroblasts with vesicular nuclei and abundant amphophilic cytoplasm admixed with reactive bone. The bone is rimmed by osteoblasts. FP is regarded as a reactive nonneoplastic process.* **(Right)** *Bone formation in FP typically shows a zonal pattern of maturation from osteoid to bone. In this example, eosinophilic osteoid undergoes progressive mineralization and transformation into trabeculae of woven bone.*

TERMINOLOGY

Abbreviations

- Fibroosseous pseudotumor (FP)

Synonyms

- Florid, reactive periostitis of tubular bones of hands and feet
- Fasciitis ossificans
- Parosteal fasciitis

Definitions

- Reactive-appearing, ossifying fibroblastic proliferation of soft tissue typically affecting digits of hands and feet

ETIOLOGY/PATHOGENESIS

Neoplastic

- Clonal transient neoplasm
- *USP6* rearrangement

CLINICAL ISSUES

Epidemiology

- Incidence
  - Rare; exact incidence unknown
- Age
  - 5-75 years; median: ~ 35 years
- Sex
  - Slight female predominance

Site

- Hands, feet
  - Proximal phalanx of hand most common site
  - Rarely occurs beyond acral extremities

Presentation

- Fusiform swelling, often with erythema, pain, or ulceration
- Rapid onset; weeks to months

Natural History

- Benign, often self-limited

Treatment

- Surgical approaches
  - Simple excision usually curative

IMAGING

General Features

- Early lesions characterized by ill-defined soft tissue density
- Older lesions with intralesional calcification
- Periosteal reaction common

MACROSCOPIC

Size

- 0.5-5.6 cm; median: ~ 2.0 cm

MICROSCOPIC

Histologic Features

- Fasciitis-like spindle cell proliferation with active ossification
- Cellular areas alternate with less cellular fibromyxoid areas in lobular pattern
- Ossification at various stages of maturation
  - Osteoid and wispy immature woven bone
  - Anastomosing trabeculae of woven bone rimmed by single layer of plump activated osteoblasts
  - Mature lamellar bone
- Geographic areas of collagenous matrix in some
- Cartilage with endochondral ossification in some

Cytologic Features

- Myofibroblastic spindle and stellate cells with vesicular nuclei and amphophilic cytoplasm

DIFFERENTIAL DIAGNOSIS

Extraskeletal Osteosarcoma

- Much larger tumor; very rare in digits
- Malignant cytoarchitectural features

Myositis Ossificans

- Larger tumor, involves skeletal muscle, proximal extremities, and trunk
- Well-defined peripheral zonal ossification

Fracture Callus

- Reactive proliferation of woven bone, granulation tissue, and reactive cartilage
- Radiographic evidence of fracture in most cases

Bizarre Parosteal Osteochondromatous Proliferation

- Tubular bones of hands and feet, adherent to periosteum
- Ossifying tumor with cartilage cap
- Spindle cell stroma, woven bone, and immature basophilic "blue" bone

Tenosynovial Giant Cell Tumor

- Common in fingers
- Polymorphous population of epithelioid cells, osteoclastic giant cells, macrophages, and xanthoma cells
- May have hyalinized collagenous matrix that mimics osteoid

Giant Cell Tumor of Soft Tissue

- Identical histology to giant cell tumor of bone
- Ovoid or spindled stromal cells and numerous osteoclastic giant cells
- Often has peripheral rim of bone

Ossifying Fibromyxoid Tumor

- Soft tissue tumor often with peripheral rim of bone
- Ovoid mesenchymal cells arranged in cords and clusters
- Usually S100 protein (+)
- Myxohyaline matrix

SELECTED REFERENCES

1. Flucke U et al: Fibro-osseous pseudotumor of digits - expanding the spectrum of clonal transient neoplasms harboring USP6 rearrangement. Ann Diagn Pathol. 35:53-5, 2018
2. Chaudhry IH et al: Fibro-osseous pseudotumor of the digit: a clinicopathological study of 17 cases. J Cutan Pathol. 37(3):323-9, 2010
3. Moosavi CA et al: Fibroosseous [corrected] pseudotumor of the digit: a clinicopathologic study of 43 new cases. Ann Diagn Pathol. 12(1):21-8, 2008
4. Dupree WB et al: Fibro-osseous pseudotumor of the digits. Cancer. 58(9):2103-9, 1986

(Left) *This medium-power micrograph depicts irregular interconnecting trabeculae of osteoid* → *within myxoid stromal background* →. *Spindle cells condense around the osteoid* ↪. **(Right)** *The bone in FP varies from immature woven bone* → *to mature lamellar bone. In this example, the bone arises within thick seams of pale osteoid matrix* →.

Interconnecting Trabeculae of Osteoid

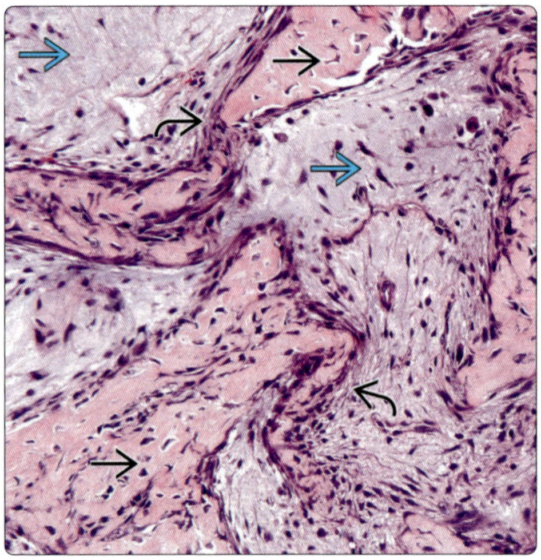

Immature Bone

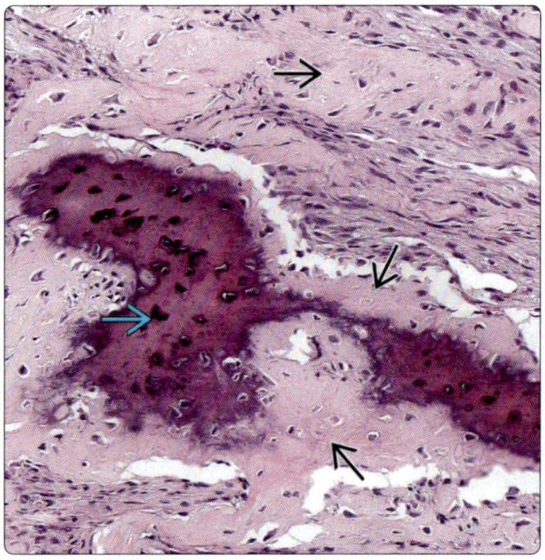

(Left) *FP typically contains a large amount of reactive-appearing bone as shown by a trabecula of immature woven bone* → *rimmed by a single-cell layer of plump activated osteoblasts with abundant basophilic granular cytoplasm and eccentric nuclei* ↪. **(Right)** *Large geographic sheets of collagenous matrix* → *in between spindle cell areas* ↪ *may be seen in FP as depicted in this low-power micrograph.*

Osteoblastic Rimming

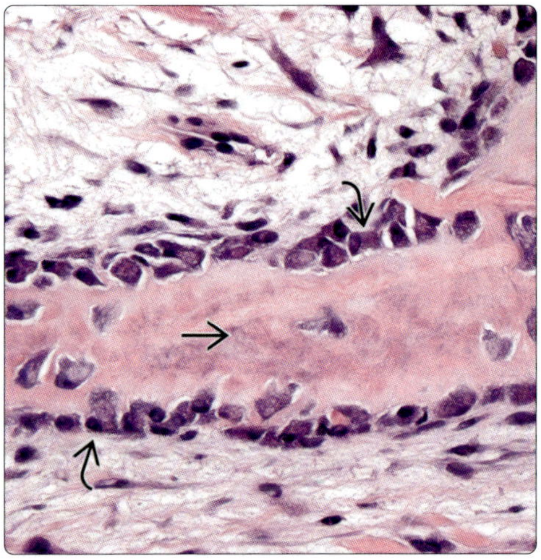

Geographic Area of Fibrous Matrix

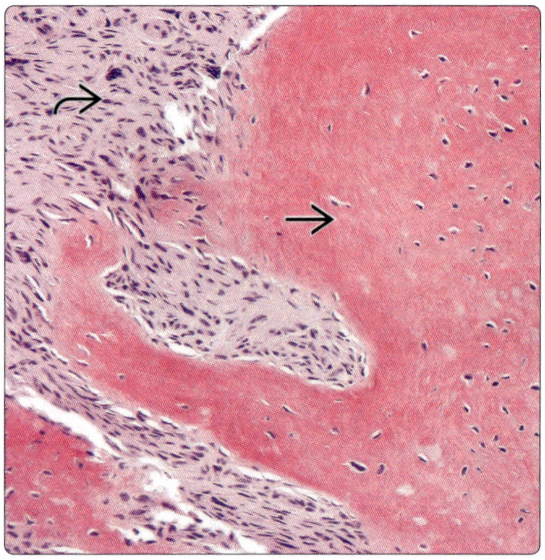

(Left) *The spindle cell component of FP typically resembles nodular fasciitis, consisting of fascicles of spindle-shaped myofibroblasts with brisk mitotic activity* → *and extravasated red blood cells* ↪. **(Right)** *This high-power micrograph illustrates the cytologic features of myofibroblasts in FP, consisting of plump spindle cells with abundant amphophilic cytoplasm* → *and vesicular nuclei with prominent solitary nucleoli* ↪.

Fasciitis-Like Histology

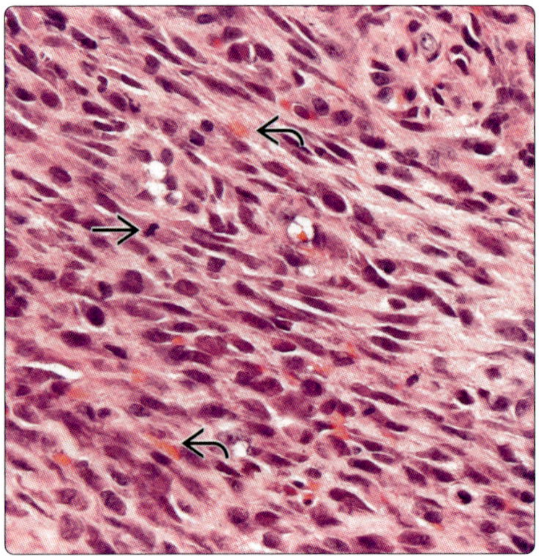

Myofibroblasts

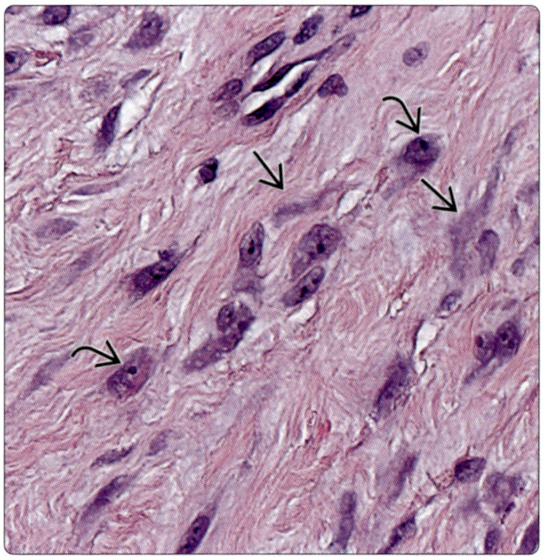

Fibroosseous Pseudotumor of Hand

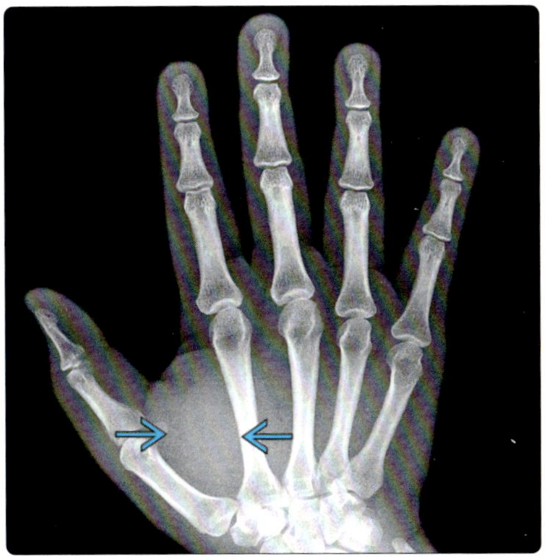

Hyalinized Collagen

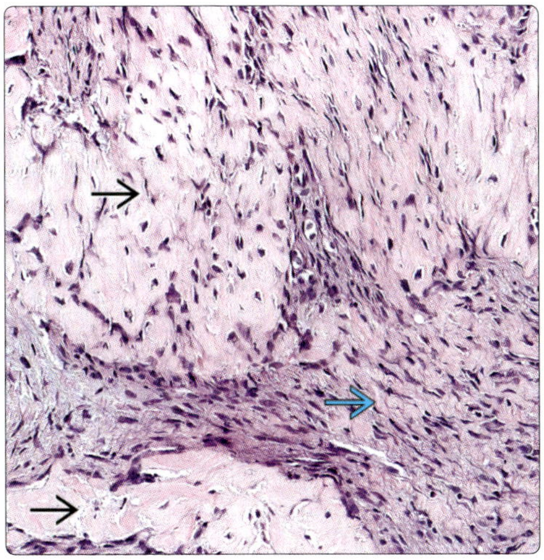

(Left) *Although the most common site is within a proximal phalanx of the hand, FP affects other sites such as the thenar compartment, depicted in this radiograph by an ill-defined soft tissue density ➔. Only rare examples have been reported outside the hands and feet.* **(Right)** *Geographic zones of densely hyalinized, pale eosinophilic collagen ➔ alternate with spindle cell areas ➔ as illustrated by this low-power micrograph.*

Myxoid Area

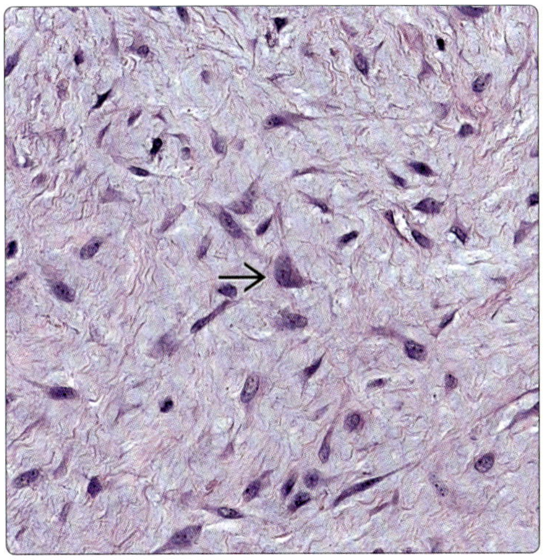

Osteoid and Myxoid Matrix

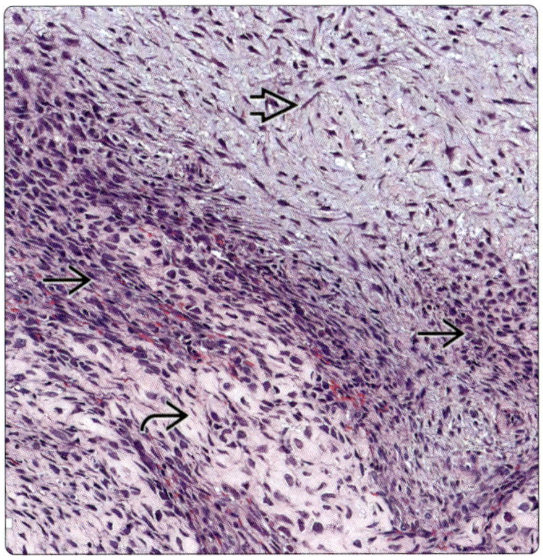

(Left) *Myxoid areas are common in FP, consisting of pale blue matrix containing myofibroblasts with plump, vesicular nuclei and abundant amphophilic cytoplasm often forming stellate-shaped cells ➔.* **(Right)** *Low-power micrograph depicts trabeculae of eosinophilic osteoid matrix ➔ surrounded by proliferating spindle cells and osteoblasts ➔ juxtaposed with a less cellular area containing abundant myxoid matrix ➔.*

Endochondral Ossification

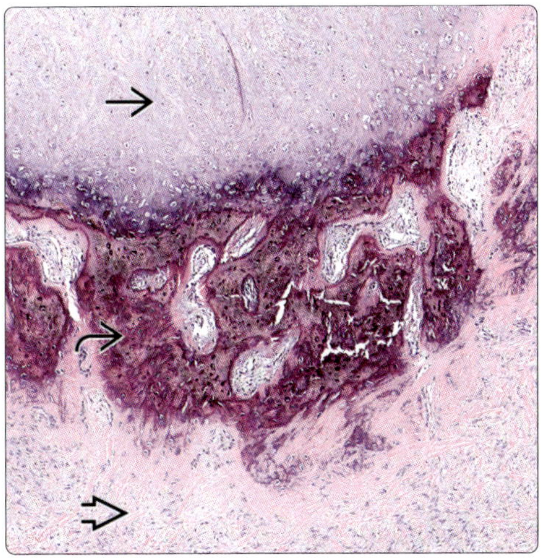

Fibrocartilage

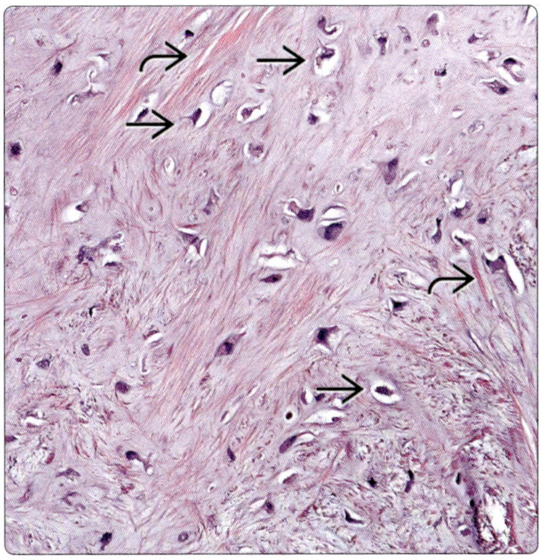

(Left) *Reactive endochondral ossification can sometimes be present in FP. In this example, fibrocartilage ➔ merges with woven bone ➔, which subsequently merges with a collagenous spindle cell area ➔, creating a distinctive zonal architecture.* **(Right)** *This high-power image depicts fibrocartilage within an FP consisting of chondrocytes in cleared-out lacunar spaces ➔ embedded within avascular, pale blue cartilaginous matrix containing bundles of eosinophilic collagen ➔.*

Fibroma of Tendon Sheath

KEY FACTS

TERMINOLOGY

- Benign fibrous nodule typically attached to tendon sheath

ETIOLOGY/PATHOGENESIS

- Generally regarded as reactive, nonneoplastic process
- Cellular fibroma of tendon sheath (FTS) has *USP6* fusions, indicating benign neoplasm related to nodular fasciitis

CLINICAL ISSUES

- Median age: 30 years
- Painless mass
- Slowly growing
- Hand (80%)
  - Finger most common site
- Intraarticular fibroma (rare)
  - Knee most common site
- Very low recurrence rate following complete excision

MACROSCOPIC

- Well circumscribed
- White-tan
- Uni- or multinodular
- Hard, rubbery, or gelatinous
- Median size: ~ 2.0 cm (range: 0.5-5.0 cm)

MICROSCOPIC

- Well demarcated
- Attached to tendon sheath or tendon
- Benign fibroblasts and myofibroblasts
- Slit-like vascular spaces
- Cellular nodular fasciitis-like areas

TOP DIFFERENTIAL DIAGNOSES

- Nodular fasciitis
- Superficial fibromatosis
- Localized tenosynovial giant cell tumor
- Desmoplastic fibroblastoma

Fibroma of Tendon Sheath

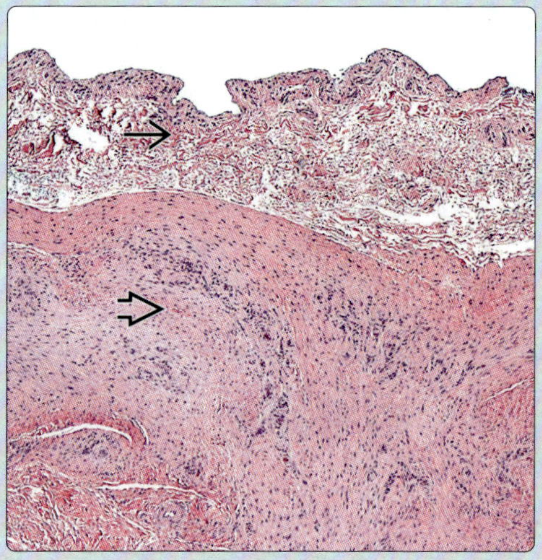

Slit-Like Blood Vessels

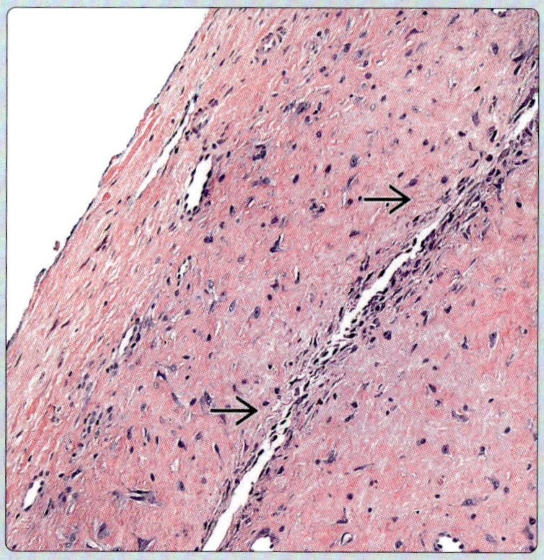

(Left) *Fibroma of tendon sheath (FTS) typically presents as a well-circumscribed soft tissue nodule, most of which occur in the finger. This micrograph depicts a circumscribed FTS ⇨ attached to a synovial-lined tendon sheath →.* **(Right)** *Long, slit-like blood vessels →, usually located at the periphery, is a characteristic feature of FTS. Note the dense collagenous stroma and wide distribution of plump spindle cells.*

Gross Photograph

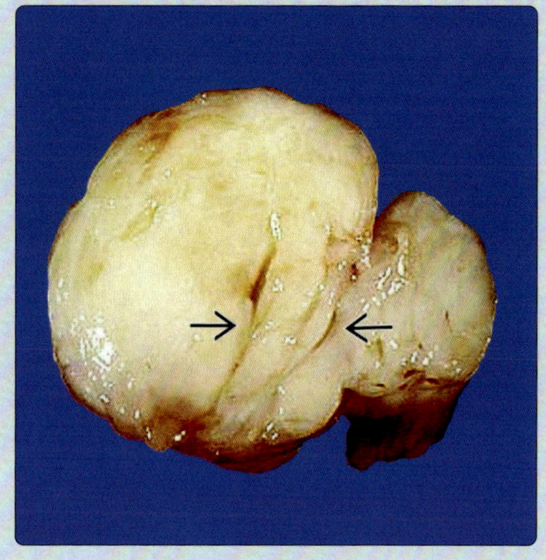

Multinodular

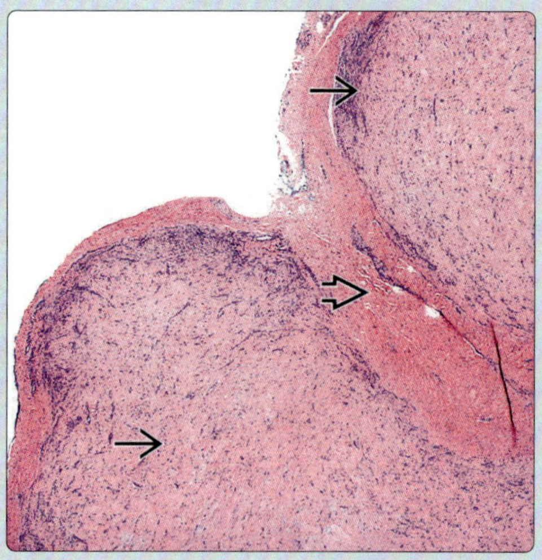

(Left) *Grossly, FTS presents as a well-circumscribed, white-tan nodule. It is often multinodular, as shown, and has a fibrous cut surface with clefts →. No intratumoral hemorrhage or hemosiderin pigment is evident, as would be present in tenosynovial giant cell tumor.* **(Right)** *Multinodular architecture is common in FTS, as depicted by spindle cell nodules → separated by a dense fibrous septum ⇨.*

TERMINOLOGY

Abbreviations

- Fibroma of tendon sheath (FTS)

Synonyms

- Tenosynovial fibroma
- Intraarticular fibroma

Definitions

- Benign fibrous nodule typically attached to tendon sheath

ETIOLOGY/PATHOGENESIS

Histogenesis

- Generally regarded as reactive, nonneoplastic process
- Cellular FTS has *USP6* fusions
    - Indicating benign neoplasm related to nodular fasciitis

CLINICAL ISSUES

Epidemiology

- Incidence
    - Uncommon, exact incidence unknown
- Age
    - Median: 30 years
        - Range: 5 months to 70 years
- Sex
    - Men outnumber women

Site

- Upper extremities
    - Hand (80%)
        - Finger most common site
            - Especially thumb and index and middle fingers
        - Palm
        - Wrist
    - Forearm
    - Biceps tendon
- Lower extremities
    - Anterior knee
    - Ankle
    - Foot
    - Toes
- Rare sites
    - Medial canthal tendon
    - Thigh
    - Shoulder
    - Back
    - Trunk
- Rare cases with multifocal involvement
- Intraarticular fibroma
    - Rare
    - Knee most common site
    - Less common sites
        - Ankle
        - Wrist
        - Acromioclavicular joint

Presentation

- Slowly growing
- Painless mass
- Uncommon findings
    - Nerve impingement
    - Carpal tunnel syndrome
    - Trigger finger
    - Bone erosion

Treatment

- Complete surgical excision

Prognosis

- Excellent
    - Low recurrence rate
        - Very low rate with good surgical technique and complete excision
        - Reexcision usually curative

IMAGING

MR Findings

- Focal nodular mass
- Variable signal
- No hemosiderin

MACROSCOPIC

General Features

- Well circumscribed
- Uni- or multinodular
- White-tan
- Hard, rubbery
- Some with gelatinous or cystic areas

Size

- Median: ~ 2.0 cm
    - Range: 0.5-5.0 cm

MICROSCOPIC

Histologic Features

- Well demarcated
- Attached to tendon sheath or portion of tendon
- Benign fibroblasts and myofibroblasts
    - Vesicular nucleus with single nucleolus
    - Abundant, finely granular, amphophilic cytoplasm
    - Bipolar and stellate forms
    - Low mitotic rate in most
- Variable fibrous to myxoid stroma
    - Some tumors with densely hyalinized, fibrous stroma
    - Some with myxoid matrix or cystic areas
- Slit-like vascular spaces
    - Characteristic feature of FTS
    - Most prevalent at periphery
    - Lined by flattened endothelial cells
- Cellular areas
    - Most prevalent at periphery
    - May resemble nodular fasciitis
    - Diffusely cellular tumors are termed cellular FTS
- Storiform areas in some tumors
- Rare tumors with cellular pleomorphism
    - May be referred to as pleomorphic FST
- Rare tumors with chondroid and osseous metaplasia

ANCILLARY TESTS

Immunohistochemistry

- SMA(+); may be focal
- Desmin (-)

Molecular Testing

- Cellular FTS shows *USP6* gene rearrangements
  - Suggest relationship to nodular fasciitis

DIFFERENTIAL DIAGNOSIS

Nodular Fasciitis

- Rare in fingers
- Usually arises from fascia
- Less circumscribed
- More cellular and mitotically active
- Cellular FTS often indistinguishable from nodular fasciitis
  - Appears be clonal neoplasm related to nodular fasciitis with alternate *USP6* fusions

Superficial Fibromatosis

- Arises from palmar or plantar fascia
- Infiltrates surrounding tissue
- Dupuytren contracture in palmar tumors
- Often nuclear β-catenin (+)
  - FTS is negative

Localized Tenosynovial Giant Cell Tumor

- Synonym: Giant cell tumor of tendon sheath
- Common in fingers
- Arises from tendon sheath
- Stromal cells with round to reniform, eccentric nuclei
- Osteoclastic giant cells
- Xanthoma cells
- Hemosiderin-laden macrophages
- Variable fibrosis
  - Markedly fibrotic tumors resemble FTS

Desmoplastic Fibroblastoma

- Synonym: Collagenous fibroma
- Rare in fingers
- Arises in subcutis or skeletal muscle
- Well circumscribed
- Larger size
- Stellate-shaped and bipolar myofibroblasts

Sclerosing Perineurioma

- Common in hands
- Well-demarcated nodule
- Whorling pattern
- Scant, ill-defined cytoplasm
- EMA(+), GLUT1(+)

Inclusion Body Fibromatosis

- Usually in hands and feet
- Dome-shaped dermal nodule
- 1st year of life
  - Very rare in adults
- Infiltrating fascicles in dermis
- Cytoplasmic spherical inclusions

Benign Fibrous Histiocytoma

- Rare in fingers
- Typically arises in dermis but can be more deeply seated
- Well-defined storiform pattern
- More cellular than FTS
- Plump spindle cells (fibrohistiocytic)
- Multinucleated giant cells common
- Infiltrative growth with entrapment of dermal collagen

SELECTED REFERENCES

1. Carter JM et al: USP6 genetic rearrangements in cellular fibroma of tendon sheath. Mod Pathol. 29(8):865-9, 2016
2. Al-Qattan MM: Fibroma of tendon sheath of the hand: a series of 20 patients with 23 tumours. J Hand Surg Eur Vol. 39(3):300-5, 2014
3. De Maeseneer M et al: Fibroma of the tendon sheath of the long head of the biceps tendon. Skeletal Radiol. 43(3):399-402, 2014
4. Glover M et al: Intra-articular fibroma of tendon sheath arising in the acromioclavicular joint. Skeletal Radiol. 43(5):681-6, 2014
5. Jacobs E et al: Fibroma of tendon sheath located within Kager's triangle. J Foot Ankle Surg. 53(2):208-11, 2014
6. Andrew N et al: Tendon sheath fibroma of the medial canthal tendon. Ophthal Plast Reconstr Surg. 29(1):e1-2, 2013
7. Nason GJ et al: Fibroma of the peroneus longus tendon sheath in a child: a case report. J Orthop Surg (Hong Kong). 21(3):387-90, 2013
8. Lucas DR: Tenosynovial giant cell tumor: case report and review. Arch Pathol Lab Med. 136(8):901-6, 2012
9. Moretti VM et al: Tendon sheath fibroma in the thigh. Orthopedics. 35(4):e607-9, 2012
10. Kosuge D et al: Flexor tendon fibroma as a cause of wrist triggering and carpal tunnel syndrome. J Hand Surg Eur Vol. 36(3):246-7, 2011
11. Park SY et al: Multiple fibromas of tendon sheath: unusual presentation. Ann Dermatol. 23 Suppl 1:S45-7, 2011
12. Moretti VM et al: Fibroma of tendon sheath in the knee: a report of three cases and literature review. Knee. 17(4):306-9, 2010
13. Ciatti R et al: Fibroma of tendon sheath located within the ankle joint capsule. J Orthop Traumatol. 10(3):147-50, 2009
14. Laskin WB, Miettinen M, Fetsch JF: Infantile digital fibroma/fibromatosis: a clinicopathologic and immunohistochemical study of 69 tumors from 57 patients with long-term follow-up. Am J Surg Pathol. 33(1):1-13, 2009
15. Gleason BC et al: Deep "benign" fibrous histiocytoma: clinicopathologic analysis of 69 cases of a rare tumor indicating occasional metastatic potential. Am J Surg Pathol. 32(3):354-62, 2008
16. Le Corroller T et al: Mineralized fibroma of the tendon sheath presenting as a bursitis. Skeletal Radiol. 37(12):1141-5, 2008
17. Carlson JW et al: Immunohistochemistry for beta-catenin in the differential diagnosis of spindle cell lesions: analysis of a series and review of the literature. Histopathology. 51(4):509-14, 2007
18. Fox MG et al: MR imaging of fibroma of the tendon sheath. AJR Am J Roentgenol. 180(5):1449-53, 2003
19. Varallo VM et al: Beta-catenin expression in Dupuytren's disease: potential role for cell-matrix interactions in modulating beta-catenin levels in vivo and in vitro. Oncogene. 22(24):3680-4, 2003
20. Dal Cin P et al: Translocation 2;11 in a fibroma of tendon sheath. Histopathology. 32(5):433-5, 1998
21. Evans HL: Desmoplastic fibroblastoma. A report of seven cases. Am J Surg Pathol. 19(9):1077-81, 1995
22. Lamovec J et al: Pleomorphic fibroma of tendon sheath. Am J Surg Pathol. 15(12):1202-5, 1991
23. Pulitzer DR et al: Fibroma of tendon sheath. A clinicopathologic study of 32 cases. Am J Surg Pathol. 13(6):472-9, 1989
24. Jablokow VR et al: Fibroma of tendon sheath. J Surg Oncol. 19(2):90-2, 1982
25. Chung EB et al: Fibroma of tendon sheath. Cancer. 44(5):1945-54, 1979

Fibroma of Tendon Sheath

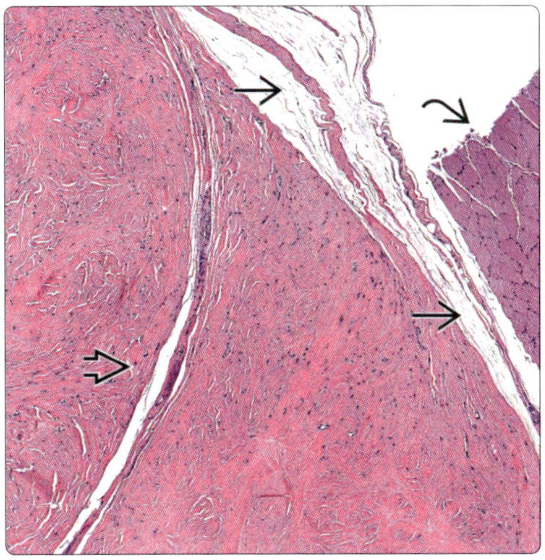

Fibroma of Tendon Sheath

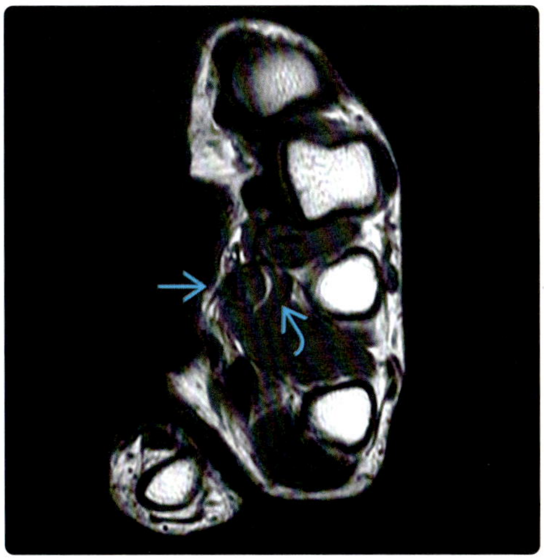

(Left) *Typical low-power appearance of FTS, depicting a hypocellular, collagenous tumor, which is sharply demarcated and attached to tenosynovium* →*, is shown. This tumor is traversed by a muscular vein with artifactual clefting* ⇨*. Note attached, uninvolved skeletal muscle at the edge* ↷*.* **(Right)** *T1 MR demonstrates a 1.6-cm, well-circumscribed FTS* → *within the flexor retinaculum of the hand, situated superficial to a flexor tendon* ↷*. The nodule is isointense with skeletal muscle.*

Tendon Attachment

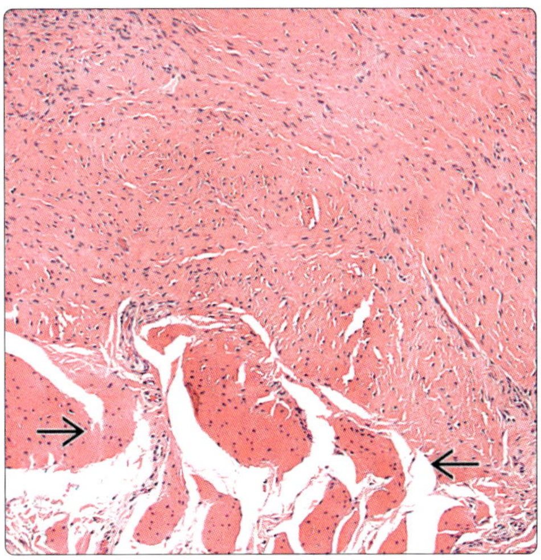

Multinodular Architecture

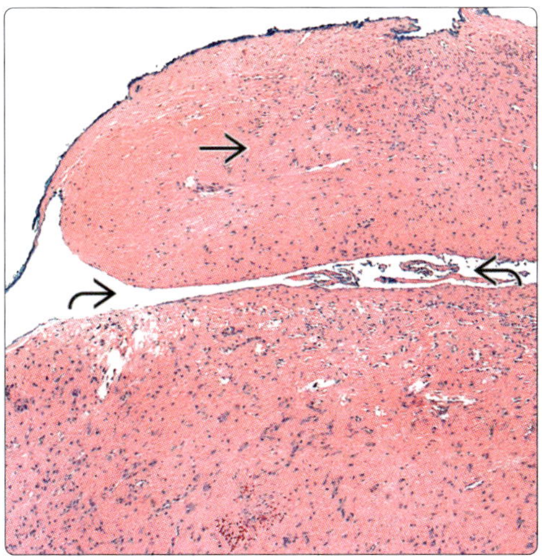

(Left) *In some cases, FTS has direct attachment to the tendon* →*. Note the lesional tissue at the top of the stain.* **(Right)** *This low-power micrograph depicts an FTS with a small, peripheral nodule* → *separated from the main lesion by a clefted space* ↷*. In some cases, these peripheral nodules may separate completely and become detached.*

Well-Circumscribed Nodule

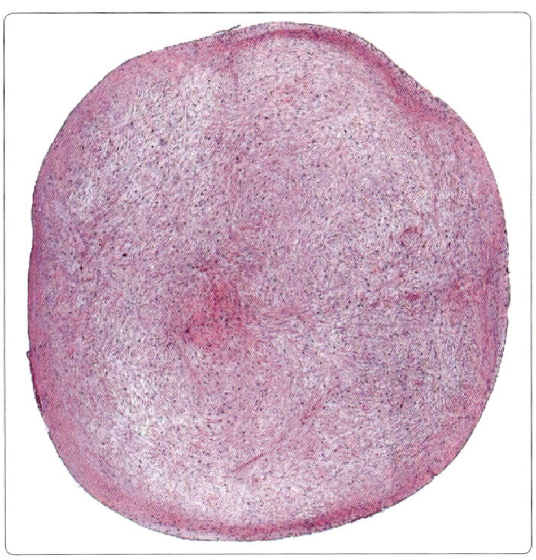

Multilobular Architecture

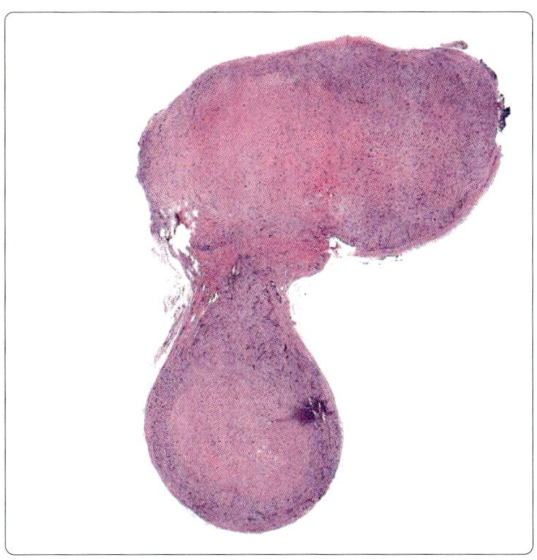

(Left) *FTS varies from 0.5-5.0 cm. Small tumors, such as this one, are uninodular and well circumscribed, as depicted. Despite the circumscription, marginal or incomplete excision may lead to local recurrence in some cases.* **(Right)** *Scanning power depicts a dumbbell-shaped FTS excised from a finger. Note the relatively smooth outer border of the lesion and lower cellularity at the centers of the nodules.*

(Left) *This hypocellular FTS has abundant, hyalinized, collagenous matrix associated with widely dispersed spindle cells and thin-walled, curvilinear blood vessels* →. *The spindled fibroblasts are devoid of nuclear atypia and mitotic activity.* **(Right)** *This FTS contains loosely textured fibrous stroma consisting of fibrillary collagen bundles within edematous matrix and a sparse population of uniform myofibroblasts.*

Hyalinized Matrix

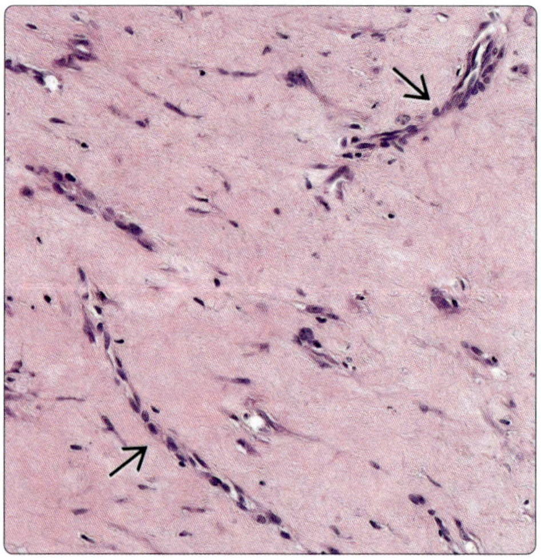

Loose Collagenous Stroma

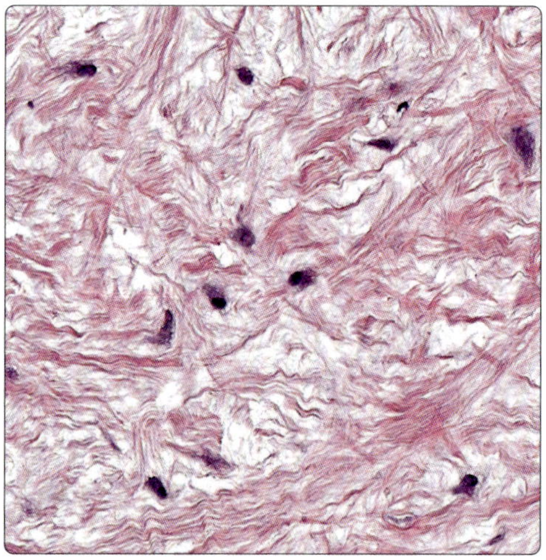

(Left) *FTS is often composed of dense, fibrous stroma consisting of mature collagen. Note the widely dispersed mature fibroblasts* →. *In some lesions, particularly older ones, stromal hyalinization may be diffuse.* **(Right)** *FTS frequently shows increased cellularity at the periphery* →, *while the center is hypocellular and more collagenous* ↪. *This zonation is often a useful clue to the diagnosis.*

Dense Collagenous Stroma

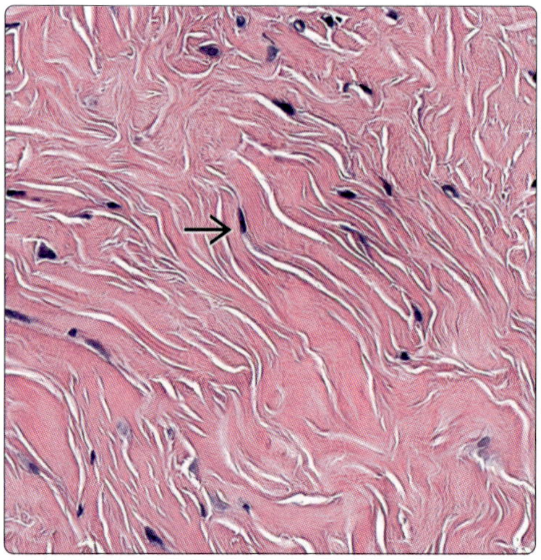

Peripheral Cellularity

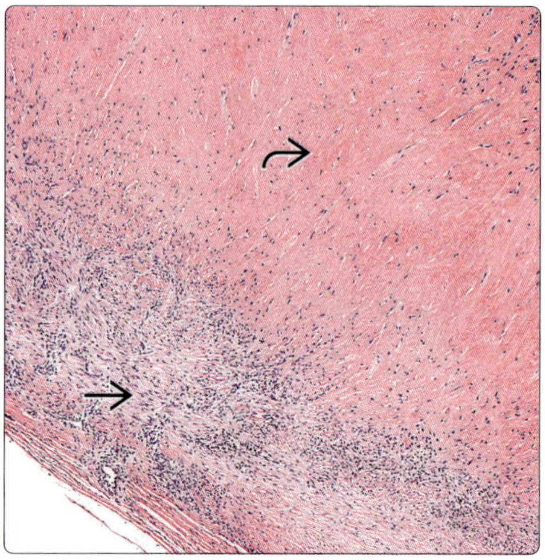

(Left) *FTS can be partially or exclusively composed of hypercellular areas containing fascicles and storiform arrays of plump myofibroblastic spindle cells, as depicted. This morphology resembles cellular foci in nodular fasciitis.* **(Right)** *Cellular zones in FTS may show a fascicular architecture, raising concerns for a sarcoma; however, the overall lesion is usually small and well circumscribed, and central hypocellularity is often present. Also, significant nuclear atypia is not seen.*

Cellular Fibroma of Tendon Sheath

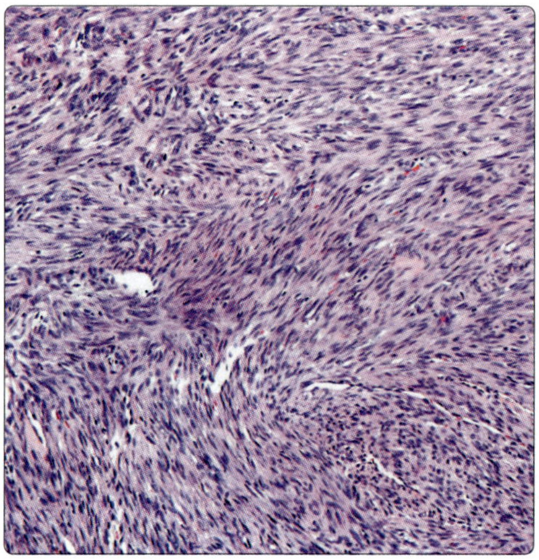

Cellular Fibroma of Tendon Sheath

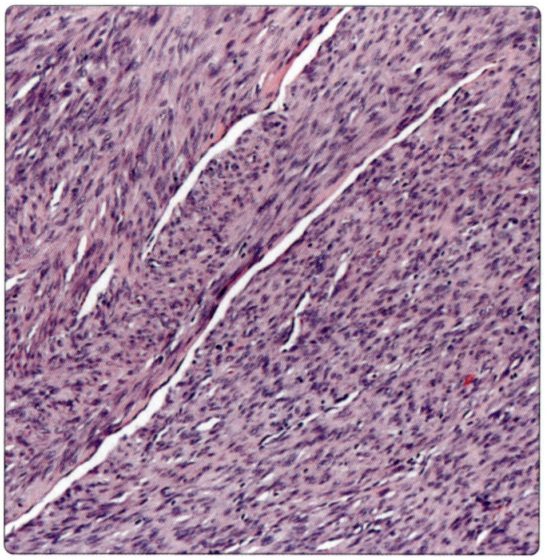

Resembling Nodular Fasciitis

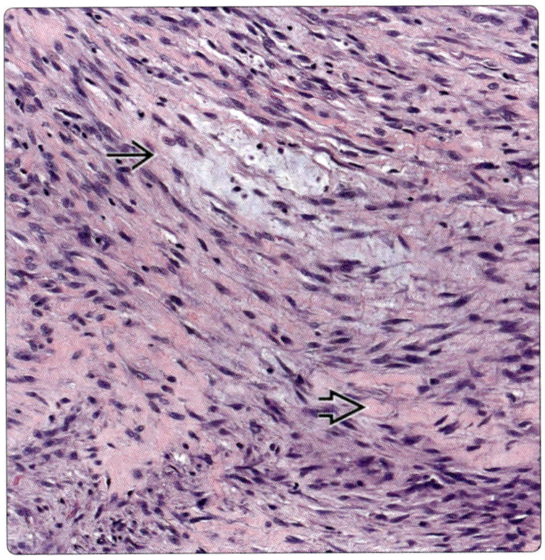

Cytological Features

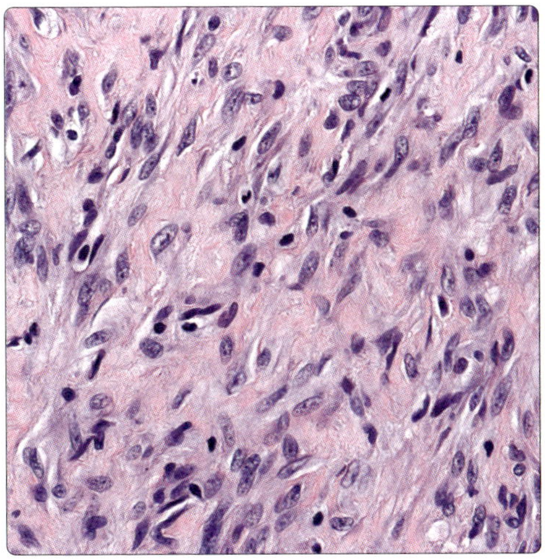

(Left) *Cellular areas of FTS can resemble nodular fasciitis, as depicted by loosely textured fascicles of myofibroblastic spindle cells, myxoid pools ➔, and keloidal collagen ➩.* **(Right)** *The proliferating cells in both conventional and cellular FTS consist of bland myofibroblasts with oval, vesicular nuclei containing single nucleoli and finely granular, amphophilic cytoplasm in bipolar and stellate configurations, as depicted.*

Cystic Degeneration

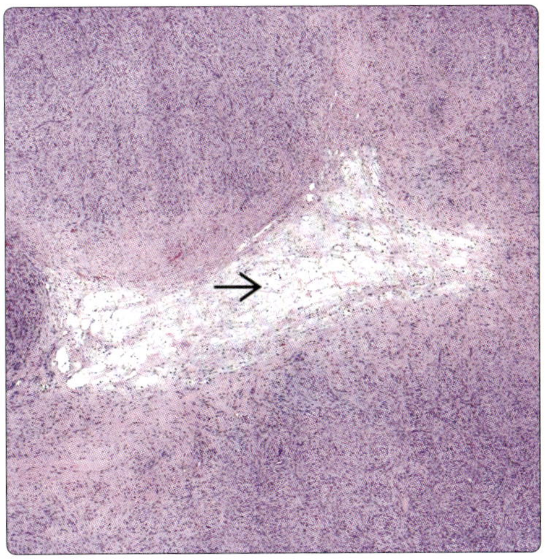

Myxoid Matrix

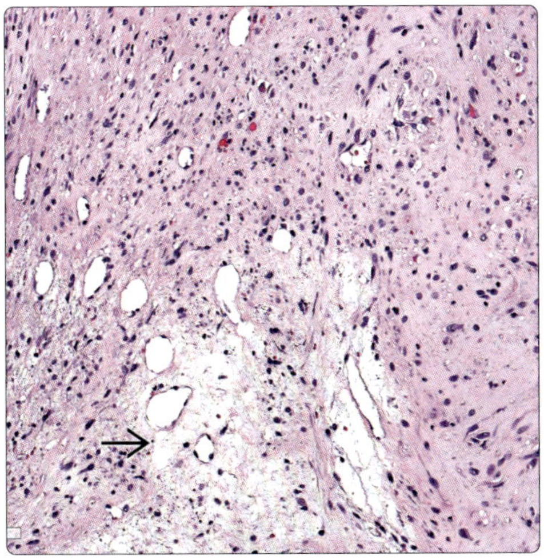

(Left) *Central cystic degeneration can be found in some FTS, as depicted by this stellate-shaped area of edematous myxoid matrix ➔. Other degenerative changes, such as metaplastic bone or cartilage, may be seen on occasion.* **(Right)** *Myxoid matrix consists of loosely textured areas of edematous mucoid material ➔. Cellularity in these areas is often low.*

Cellular Atypia

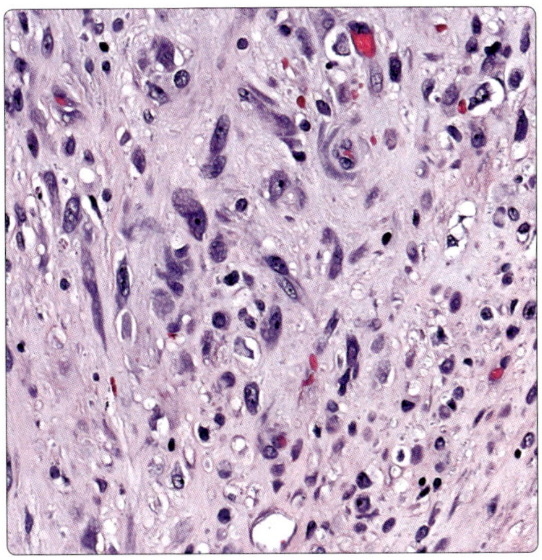

Intraarticular Fibroma

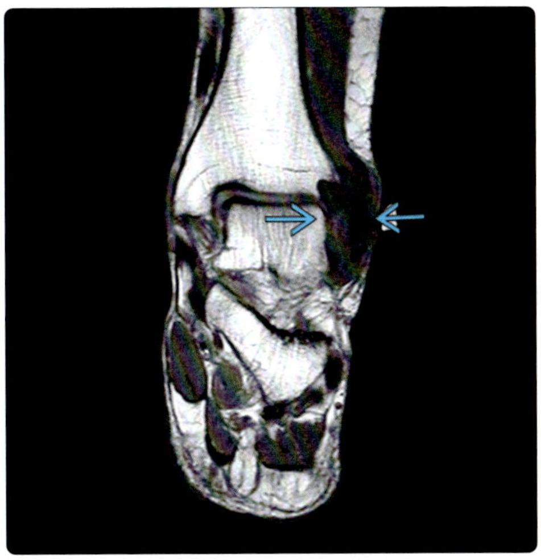

(Left) *This high-power H&E illustrates activated myofibroblasts with cellular and nuclear pleomorphism in a cellular FTS. Scattered, bizarre pleomorphic cells may rarely be a feature.* **(Right)** *Fibroma (of tendon sheath) can occasionally present as a purely intraarticular mass, as depicted by this T1 MR of a 3.4-cm mass ➔ in the anterior lateral ankle. The knee, however, is the most common site for intraarticular fibroma.*

Desmoplastic Fibroblastoma

KEY FACTS

TERMINOLOGY

- Rare, benign fibrous soft tissue neoplasm occurring mainly in adult males, consisting of paucicellular arrays of stellate and spindle-shaped fibroblasts
- a.k.a. collagenous fibroma

CLINICAL ISSUES

- Usually in older adults (5th-6th decades) as slow-growing, painless mass
- Male preponderance
- Most occur in subcutaneous tissue, but up to 25% involve skeletal muscle
- Most common in proximal extremity

MICROSCOPIC

- Generally well circumscribed, although may infiltrate adjacent soft tissues
- Characteristically hypocellular
- Patternless distribution of bland, spindled and stellate-shaped cells
- Hypovascular fibrous or fibromyxoid stroma
- Mitotic figures rare; no necrosis

ANCILLARY TESTS

- Variably SMA(+)
- CD34, desmin, S100 (-)
- Cytogenetics: Reciprocal translocation t(2;11)(q31;q12) reported in few cases

TOP DIFFERENTIAL DIAGNOSES

- Fibromatosis
- Neurofibroma
- Nodular fasciitis
- Elastofibroma
- Fibroma of tendon sheath
- Calcifying fibrous pseudotumor

Desmoplastic Fibroblastoma

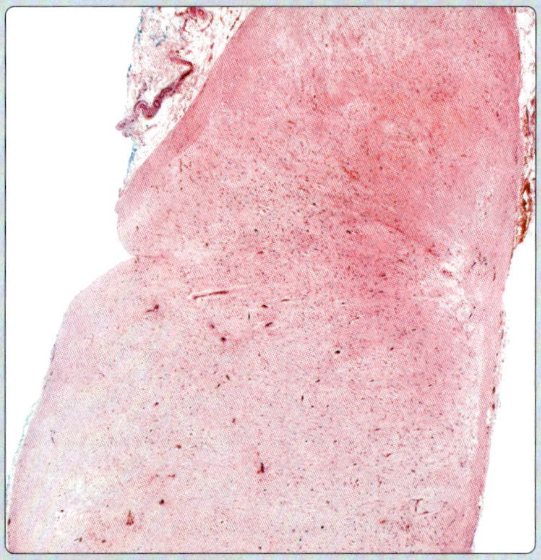

Desmoplastic Fibroblastoma at Higher Magnification

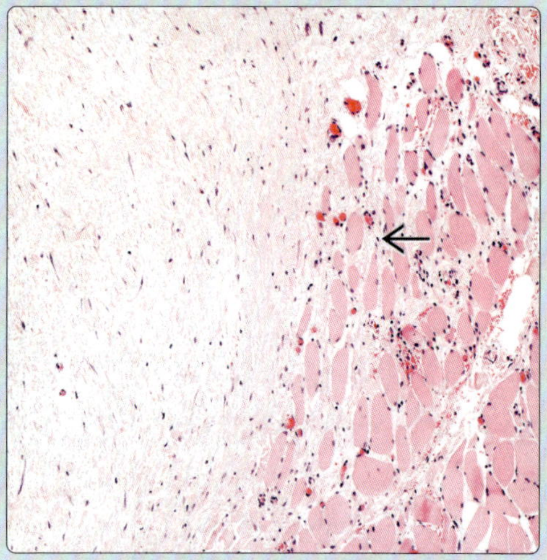

(Left) *Low-magnification examination of a desmoplastic fibroblastoma is shown. The lesion is a well-circumscribed, ovoid or fusiform mass. The characteristic hypocellularity is apparent at low power.* **(Right)** *Higher magnification of desmoplastic fibroblastoma is shown. Although the tumor is largely circumscribed, focal infiltration of surrounding soft tissue, including skeletal muscle in this case, may be seen ⇨.*

Myxoid Stroma in Desmoplastic Fibroblastoma

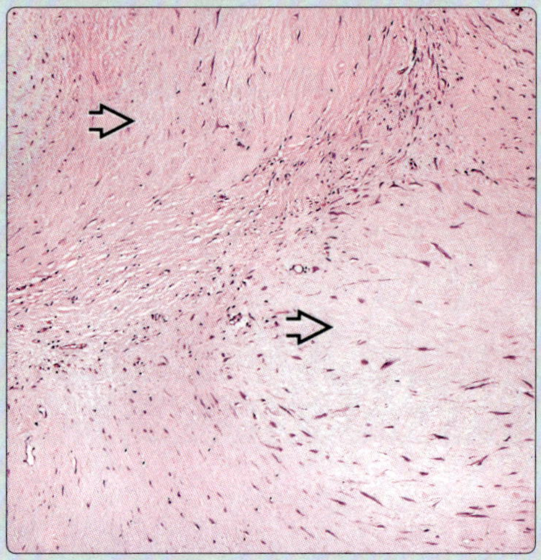

Spindled and Stellate Fibroblasts in Desmoplastic Fibroblastoma

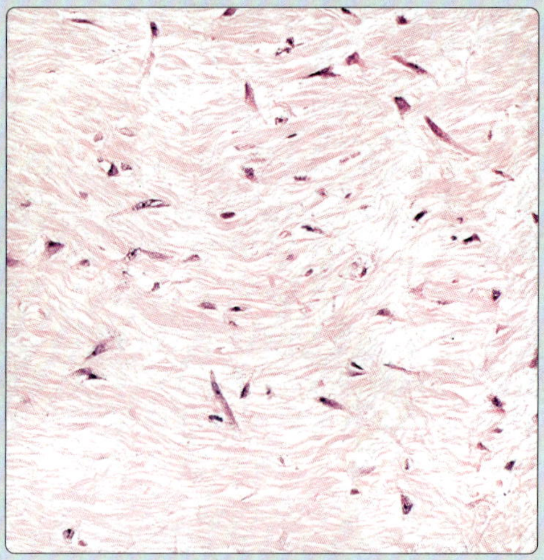

(Left) *H&E of desmoplastic fibroblastoma shows the sparsely cellular nature of the lesion. The stroma can be myxoid ⇨ in some cases. Although cells may be plump, no true atypia is seen, and mitotic figures are rare or absent.* **(Right)** *High magnification shows stroma that is densely collagenous and contains spindle and stellate fibroblasts in patternless distributions. Vessels are inconspicuous.*

TERMINOLOGY

Synonyms

- Collagenous fibroma

Definitions

- Rare, benign fibrous soft tissue neoplasm occurring mainly in adult males and consisting of paucicellular arrays of stellate and spindle fibroblasts

CLINICAL ISSUES

Epidemiology

- Age
  - All ages but particularly older adults (5th-6th decades)
- Sex
  - M > F

Site

- Most occur in subcutaneous tissue
  - Up to 25% involve skeletal muscle
- Most common in upper extremity (shoulder, upper arm, forearm) followed by lower extremity
- Rare in head and neck

Presentation

- Slow growing
- Painless mass

Treatment

- Simple complete excision but not necessary given benign behavior

Prognosis

- Benign; does not recur locally or metastasize

MACROSCOPIC

General Features

- Firm, circumscribed, lobulated mass
- White or gray cut surface
- No necrosis or hemorrhage

Size

- Often small (< 4 cm); range: 1.5-20.0 cm

MICROSCOPIC

Histologic Features

- Generally well circumscribed, although may infiltrate adjacent soft tissues
- Sparsely cellular
- Patternless proliferation of bland spindle or stellate cells
- Hypovascular fibrous or fibromyxoid stroma
- Mitotic figures very rare; no necrosis

ANCILLARY TESTS

Immunohistochemistry

- Variable SMA(+)
- CD34, desmin, S100 protein (-)
- Rare focal keratin expression

Genetic Testing

- Reciprocal translocation t(2;11)(q31;q12) reported in 2 cases
  - Same translocation has also been reported in 1 case of fibroma of tendon sheath
  - 11q12 breakpoint in 2 other cases

DIFFERENTIAL DIAGNOSIS

Fibromatosis

- More infiltrative and cellular
- Cells in loose fascicles
- Prominent vascular pattern and extravasated red blood cells

Neurofibroma

- Cell nuclei are usually angulated, wavy-appearing, or schwannian
- Strongly S100 protein (+)

Nodular Fasciitis (Late Stage)

- Foci of increased cellularity
- Chronic inflammation, extravasated red cells

Elastofibroma

- Typically located in subscapular region
- Fragmented elastic fibers

Fibroma of Tendon Sheath

- Peritendinous locations, particularly of hands

Calcifying Fibrous Pseudotumor

- Children and young adults
- Psammomatous calcifications
- Lymphoplasmacytic infiltrate

Low-Grade Fibromyxoid Sarcoma

- Often larger and more cellular; may show hyalinizing rosette formation
- MUC4(+)
- Characteristic translocations t(7;16) and t(11;16)

SELECTED REFERENCES

1. Vasconcelos AC et al: Oral bilateral collagenous fibroma: a previously unreported case and literature review. J Clin Exp Dent. 10(1):e96-e99, 2018
2. Hu SC et al: Dermal desmoplastic fibroblastoma presenting as a large sacral mass. Australas J Dermatol. 57(4):296-299, 2016
3. Tofuku Y et al: Case of collagenous fibroma (desmoplastic fibroblastoma) with vascular hyperplasia in the boundary area detected by Doppler sonography and histopathological examination. J Dermatol. 42(8):831-2, 2015
4. Nagaraja V et al: Desmoplastic fibroblastoma presenting as a parotid tumour: a case report and review of the literature. Head Neck Pathol. 7(3):285-90, 2013
5. Macchia G et al: FOSL1 as a candidate target gene for 11q12 rearrangements in desmoplastic fibroblastoma. Lab Invest. 92(5):735-43, 2012
6. Watanabe H et al: Desmoplastic fibroblastoma (collagenous fibroma). J Dermatol. 35(2):93-7, 2008
7. Bernal K et al: Translocation (2;11)(q31;q12) is recurrent in collagenous fibroma (desmoplastic fibroblastoma). Cancer Genet Cytogenet. 149(2):161-3, 2004
8. Miettinen M et al: Collagenous fibroma (desmoplastic fibroblastoma): a clinicopathologic analysis of 63 cases of a distinctive soft tissue lesion with stellate-shaped fibroblasts. Hum Pathol. 29(7):676-82, 1998
9. Evans HL: Desmoplastic fibroblastoma. A report of seven cases. Am J Surg Pathol. 19(9):1077-81, 1995

Elastofibroma

KEY FACTS

TERMINOLOGY

- Benign fibrous tumor containing abnormal elastic fibers within collagenous stroma admixed with variable component of mature adipose tissue

ETIOLOGY/PATHOGENESIS

- May be associated with repetitive physical labor

CLINICAL ISSUES

- Usually > 50 years
- Female predominance
- Most occur at inferior margin of scapula on chest wall
- Painless, slow-growing mass
- Treatment: Simple excision
- Benign

MACROSCOPIC

- Ill-defined, firm mass with admixed tan-white to yellow cut surface
- Usually 3-10 cm

MICROSCOPIC

- Infiltrative, ill-defined lesion
- Variable mixture of dense collagenous stroma and mature adipose tissue
- Numerous thickened and fragmented elastic fibers within collagenous stroma
    - Appear as beaded cords and individual rounded fragments of variable size

ANCILLARY TESTS

- Elastin stain highlights abnormal elastic fibers

TOP DIFFERENTIAL DIAGNOSES

- Desmoid fibromatosis
- Nuchal-type fibroma/Gardner fibroma
- Elastofibromatous change
- Fibrolipoma

Elastofibroma

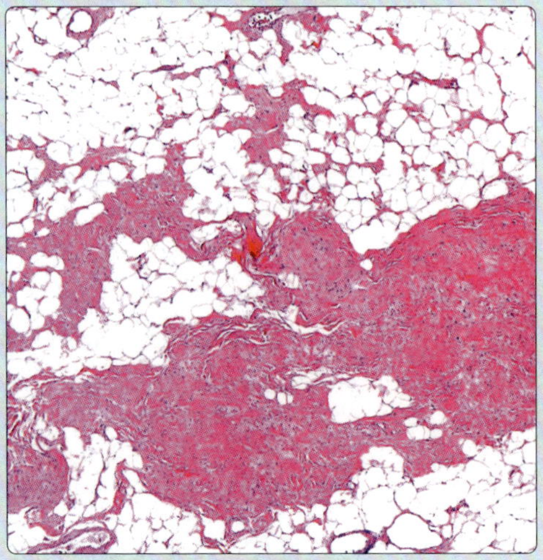

Dystrophic Elastic Fibers

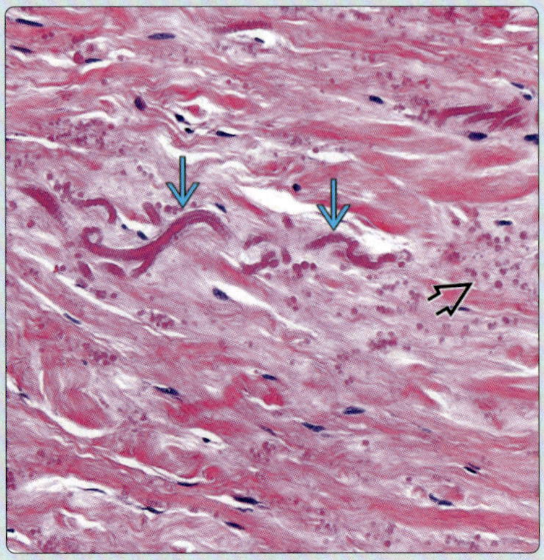

(Left) *Elastofibroma is a benign infiltrative lesion that classically occurs near the inferior border of the scapula and is composed of a variable admixture of densely collagenous tissue and mature fat.* **(Right)** *The characteristic finding in elastofibroma is the presence of enlarged fragments of abnormal elastic fibers arranged as irregular beaded cords → and solitary, rounded structures ⇒ of varying size.*

Elastic Fiber Special Stain

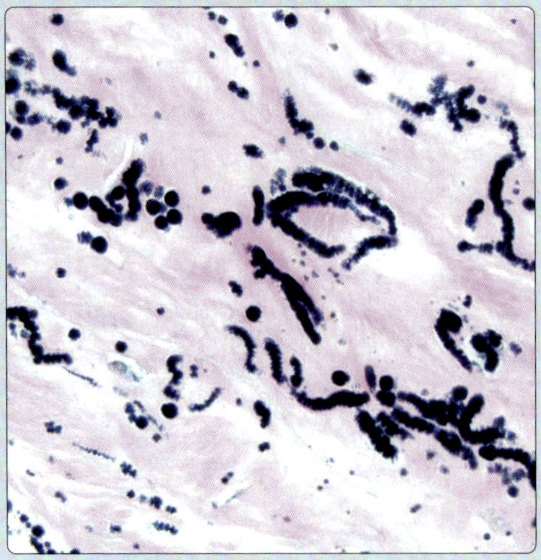

Edematous Stromal Change

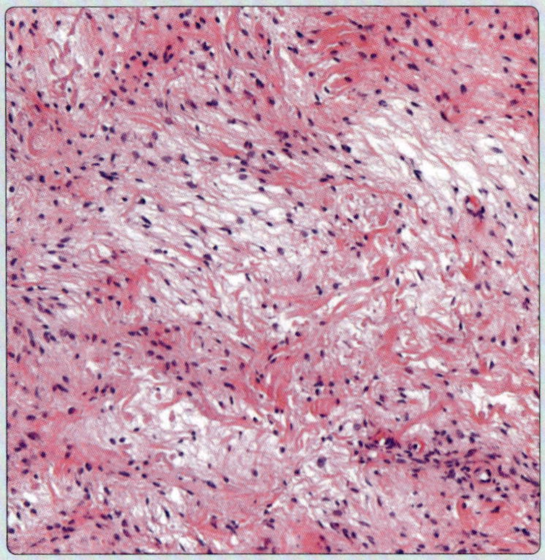

(Left) *Verhoeff van Gieson histochemical stain nicely highlights the abnormal elastic fibers in elastofibroma as dark, fragmented cords and spherules.* **(Right)** *The fibrous tissue in most cases of elastofibroma are densely collagenous, but occasional areas show loose, edematous change in which collagen bundles admix with dystrophic elastic fibers. Myxoid stromal change can be seen as well.*

TERMINOLOGY

Synonyms

- Elastofibroma dorsi

Definitions

- Benign fibrous tumor containing abnormal elastic fibers within collagenous stroma admixed with variable component of mature adipose tissue

ETIOLOGY/PATHOGENESIS

Environmental Exposure

- Some related to trauma or friction
  - Some cases reported in manual workers doing repetitive physical labor
  - Similar microscopic changes are found in 15% of autopsies of older patients
- Radiation therapy may play role in development

CLINICAL ISSUES

Epidemiology

- Incidence
  - Rare
  - Vast majority are sporadic; some familial
- Age
  - Most > 50 years
- Sex
  - Female predominance

Site

- Classically occur at inferior margin of scapula on chest wall
  - Deep to muscles of back
  - Can adhere to periosteum
- Also described in other soft tissue sites
- Visceral locations include oral cavity, stomach, rectum, omentum

Presentation

- Slow-growing, often painless mass
- Most are solitary; occasionally bilateral

Treatment

- Simple excision

Prognosis

- Benign
- Local recurrence is rare

MACROSCOPIC

General Features

- Ill-defined, firm mass with admixed tan-white to yellow cut surface
- Skeletal muscle infiltration or involvement of periosteum not uncommon

Size

- Usually 3-10 cm

MICROSCOPIC

Key Microscopic Features

- Infiltrative, ill-defined lesion
- Variable mixture of dense collagenous stroma with bland fibroblasts and mature adipose tissue
  - Stroma may be myxoid or edematous
- Numerous thickened and fragmented elastic fibers within collagenous stroma
  - Appear as beaded cords and individual rounded fragments of variable size
  - Elastic fibers may be sparse and subtle in areas
- May infiltrate and entrap skeletal muscle

ANCILLARY TESTS

Histochemistry

- Elastic special stains highlights abnormal elastic fibers

Molecular Genetics

- Nonrandom X chromosome inactivation or gains of Xq
- Recurrent chromosomal rearrangements in 1p and 7q

DIFFERENTIAL DIAGNOSIS

Desmoid Fibromatosis

- More cellular than elastofibroma
- Parallel-aligned sweeping fascicles of myofibroblasts
- Nuclear β-catenin (+) in many cases

Nuchal-Type Fibroma/Gardner Fibroma

- Different anatomic distribution from elastofibroma
- Predominantly dense collagen
- Absence of abnormal elastic fibers

Elastofibromatous Change

- Seen in gastrointestinal tract, usually colon or rectum
- Often centered about elastotic submucosal vessels
- May resemble amyloid; Congo red (-)

Fibrolipoma

- Different anatomic distribution from elastofibroma
- Lacks abnormal elastic fibers

Atypical Lipomatous Tumor/Well-Differentiated Liposarcoma

- Usually large tumors in extremity or retroperitoneum (well-differentiated liposarcoma)
- Atypical stromal cells and adipocyte atypia often present
- No abnormal elastic fibers

SELECTED REFERENCES

1. Deveci MA et al: Elastofibroma dorsi: Clinical evaluation of 61 cases and review of the literature. Acta Orthop Traumatol Turc. 51(1):7-11, 2017
2. Giannotti S et al: Elastofibroma dorsi: case series of a rare benign tumour of the back. Eur J Orthop Surg Traumatol. 23(6):643-5, 2013
3. Lococo F et al: Elastofibroma dorsi: clinicopathological analysis of 71 cases. Thorac Cardiovasc Surg. 61(3):215-22, 2013
4. Nishio J et al: Elastofibroma dorsi: diagnostic and therapeutic algorithm. J Shoulder Elbow Surg. 21(1):77-81, 2012
5. Vincent J et al: Elastofibroma: cytomorphologic, histologic, and radiologic findings in five cases. Diagn Cytopathol. 40 Suppl 2:E99-E103, 2012

Angiofibroma of Soft Tissue

KEY FACTS

TERMINOLOGY

- Low-grade fibrovascular neoplasm characterized by recurrent chromosomal translocation

CLINICAL ISSUES

- Occurs in superficial or deep soft tissues of extremities (lower limb most common)
- Slow-growing, painless mass
- Treatment: Simple conservative excision
- Benign; recurrence very rare

MACROSCOPIC

- Well circumscribed
- 1-12 cm (mean: 4.3 cm)

MICROSCOPIC

- Very well circumscribed, often with fibrous capsule
- Bland, uniform spindle cells in variably myxoid to collagenous stroma
- Very prominent and complex stromal vasculature
    - Vessels range from small and thin-walled to medium and large ectatic channels
- Stromal chronic inflammatory infiltrate common

ANCILLARY TESTS

- SMA, CD34, desmin usually (-) or at most focally positive
    - CD34 highlights prominent vascular network
- Negative for S100 protein, STAT6
- Molecular: Recurrent t(5;8) (p15;q13) translocation with *AHRR-NCOA2* gene fusion

TOP DIFFERENTIAL DIAGNOSES

- Low-grade fibromyxoid sarcoma
- Myxoid liposarcoma
- Solitary fibrous tumor
- Lobular capillary hemangioma (pyogenic granuloma)
- Myxofibrosarcoma (low grade)

Soft Tissue Angiofibroma

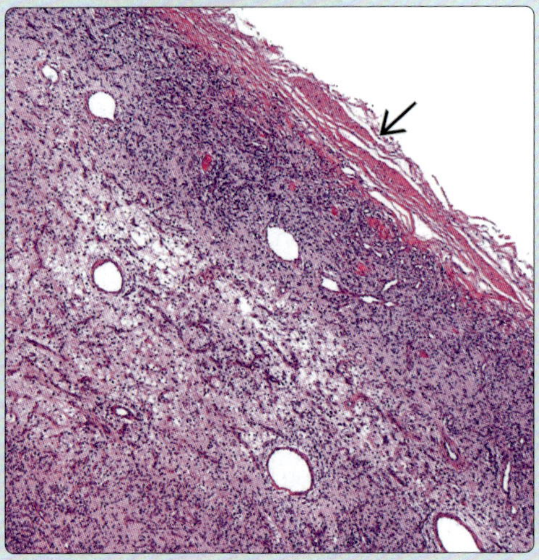

Soft Tissue Angiofibroma

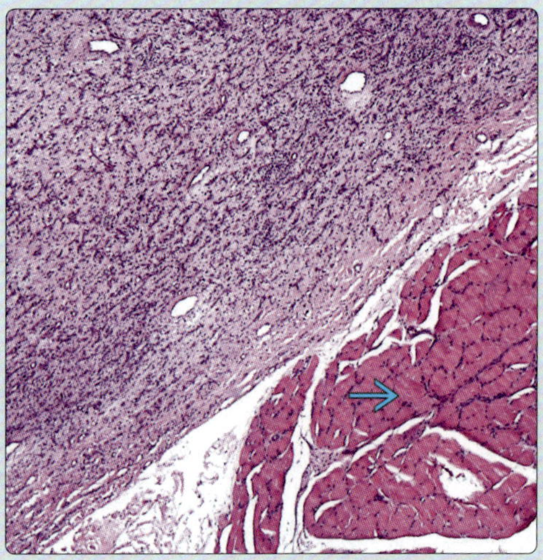

(Left) *Soft tissue angiofibroma (STA) is a benign fibrovascular neoplasm that most commonly occurs in the extremities, particularly the lower limbs. It is often well circumscribed, and > 1/2 of cases display a fibrous capsule ⇒ of varying thickness.* **(Right)** *STA appears to arise as often in deep soft tissues (subfascial or intramuscular ⇒) as it does in subcutaneous tissue. Note the sharp circumscription of the tumor, which is a feature of most, but not all, cases.*

Variable Cellularity

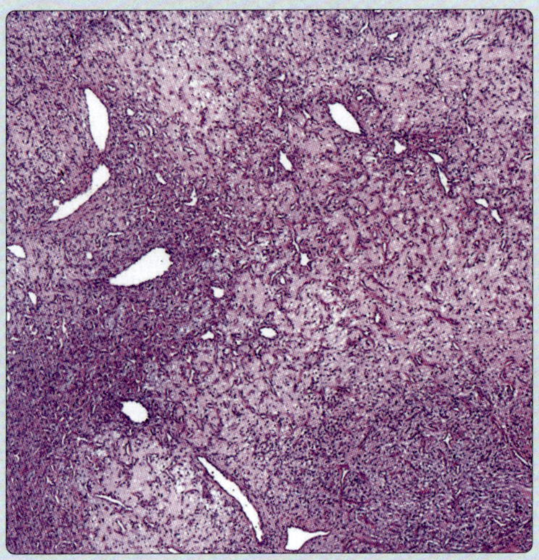

Prominent Vascular Network

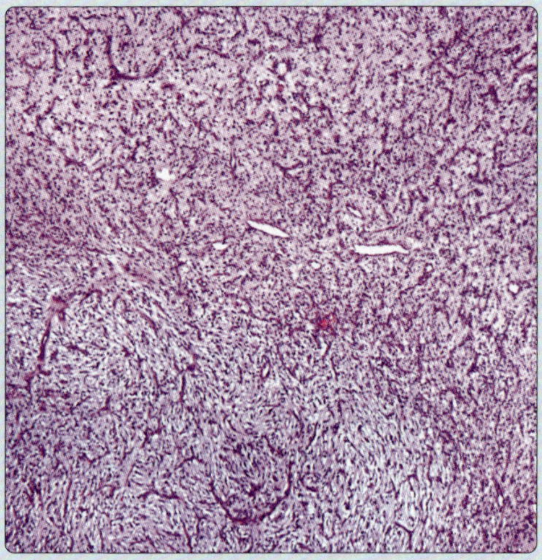

(Left) *At low magnification, STA often shows regional variation in cellularity (similar to solitary fibrous tumor), and the quality of the stroma varies from myxoid to collagenous. Note the prominent vascularity, a consistent feature of this tumor.* **(Right)** *Although the vessels vary widely in size in STA, the typical case shows numerous ramifying thin-walled vascular channels. This pattern is particularly striking in myxoid or edematous zones, as depicted.*

Angiofibroma of Soft Tissue

TERMINOLOGY

Definitions

- Low-grade fibroblastic neoplasm featuring prominent and complex stromal vasculature

CLINICAL ISSUES

Epidemiology

- Age
  - Wide range (median: 49 years)
- Sex
  - F:M (2:1)

Site

- Superficial or deep soft tissues of extremities (lower limb most common)
  - Also back, pelvis, chest wall, and abdominal wall

Presentation

- Slow-growing, painless mass

Treatment

- Simple conservative excision

Prognosis

- Benign
- Rarely recurs, even with incomplete excision

MACROSCOPIC

General Features

- Well circumscribed
- Firm, rubbery cut surface

Size

- 1-12 cm (mean: 4.3 cm)

MICROSCOPIC

Histologic Features

- Generally well circumscribed; ± fibrous capsule
- Cellularity varies widely
- Bland, uniform spindled to stellate cells in variably myxoid to collagenous stroma
  - Rare degenerative mild nuclear atypia
- Very prominent and complex stromal vasculature
  - Vessels range from small and thin-walled to medium and large ectatic "staghorn" channels
  - Variable perivascular hyalinization or fibrosis
- Stromal chronic inflammatory infiltrate common
- Extravasation of erythrocytes common
- Mitoses rare

ANCILLARY TESTS

Immunohistochemistry

- Focal EMA(+) in 1/2 of cases
- SMA, CD34, and desmin usually negative or at most focally positive
  - CD34 highlights prominent vascular network
- Estrogen receptor expression reported in 1 series
- Negative for S100 protein, CD31, MUC4, STAT6

Molecular Genetics

- Recurrent t(5;8) (p15;q13) translocation resulting in fusion of *AHRR* and *NCOA2* genes
  - *NCOA2* detectable by FISH

DIFFERENTIAL DIAGNOSIS

Low-Grade Fibromyxoid Sarcoma

- Large, deeply situated mass
- Alternating fibrous and myxoid zones
  - Prominent vascularity is seen only in myxoid zones
- MUC4(+)
- *FUS* gene fusions (*FUS-CREB3L2* most common)

Myxoid Liposarcoma

- Large, deeply situated mass
- Prominent myxoid stroma with delicate plexiform capillary vascular network
- Uni- and multivacuolated lipoblasts are common
- *DDIT3* gene fusions (*DDIT3-FUS* most common)

Solitary Fibrous Tumor

- Prominent branching ectatic "staghorn" vasculature
  - Usually lack abundant small vessels
- Diffuse CD34(+), STAT6(+)

Lobular Capillary Hemangioma (Pyogenic Granuloma)

- Usually arise in head and neck, particularly oral and nasal cavities
- Usually small (< 2.5 cm)
- Lobulated growth pattern with small capillaries arranged around larger "feeder" vessels

Myxofibrosarcoma (Low Grade)

- Very infiltrative myxoid neoplasm in superficial soft tissues of older adults
- Usually conspicuous nuclear hyperchromasia and pleomorphism
- Often shows thick-walled elongated curvilinear vessels with perivascular tumor cell accentuation

Deep Benign Fibrous Histiocytoma

- Vasculature may be prominent and contain branching &/or ectatic vessels
- Many cases contain stromal hyalinization, foamy histiocytes, &/or multinucleated giant cells
- CD34(+) in most cases

SELECTED REFERENCES

1. Bekers EM et al: Soft tissue angiofibroma: clinicopathologic, immunohistochemical and molecular analysis of 14 cases. Genes Chromosomes Cancer. 56(10):750-7, 2017
2. Yamada Y et al: Histological spectrum of angiofibroma of soft tissue: histological and genetic analysis of 13 cases. Histopathology. 69(3):459-69, 2016
3. Sugita S et al: Diagnostic utility of NCOA2 fluorescence in situ hybridization and STAT6 immunohistochemistry staining for soft tissue angiofibroma and morphologically similar fibrovascular tumors. Hum Pathol. 45(8):1588-96, 2014
4. Edgar MA et al: Soft tissue angiofibroma: report of 2 cases of a recently described tumor. Hum Pathol. 44(3):438-41, 2013
5. Mariño-Enríquez A et al: Angiofibroma of soft tissue: clinicopathologic characterization of a distinctive benign fibrovascular neoplasm in a series of 37 cases. Am J Surg Pathol. 36(4):500-8, 2012

(Left) *An extensive, branching vascular pattern is characteristic of STA but can also somewhat resemble the capillary network of myxoid liposarcoma; however, the vessels are more numerous and thicker walled in STA.* **(Right)** *The tumor cells of STA are bland, spindled, and uniform with inconspicuous cytoplasm. Rare degenerative nuclear changes may be seen, but significant nuclear atypia is not seen.*

Prominent Vascular Network

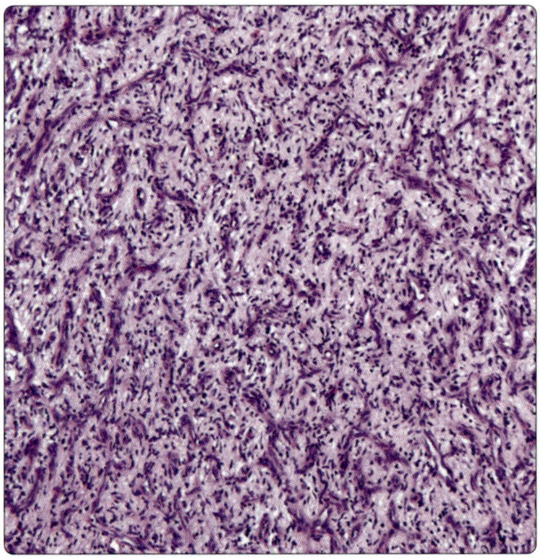

Bland Fibroblastic Spindle Cells

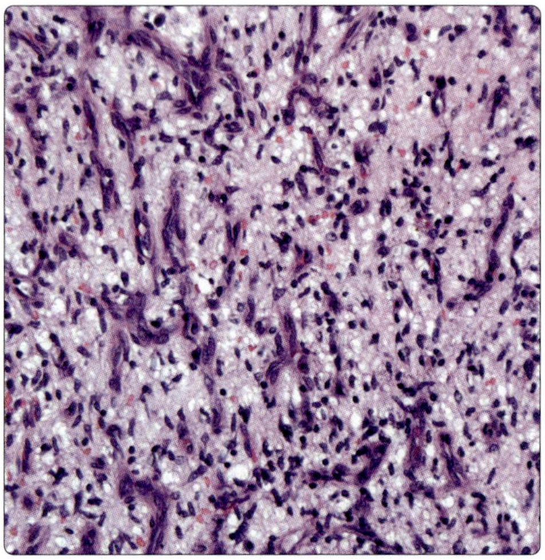

(Left) *Some areas of STA may show a moderate to marked increase in cellularity. Importantly, the lesional cells remain uniform and cytologically bland, and foci of more conventional morphology are often present.* **(Right)** *A variably brisk stromal infiltrate of chronic inflammatory cells, particularly lymphocytes, is a common finding in STA. Lymphocytes may also form small perivascular aggregates* ⇨.

Cellular Zones

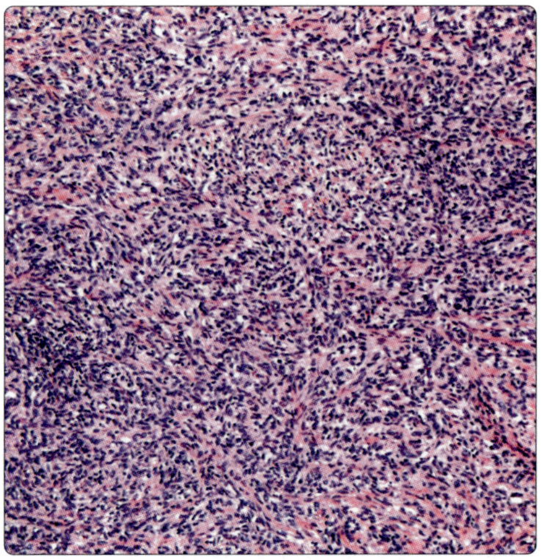

Chronic Inflammatory Infiltrate

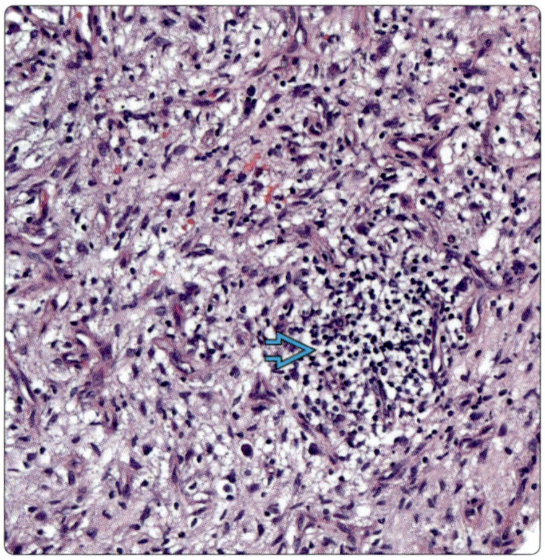

(Left) *In addition to lymphocytes, scattered mast cells* →*, plasma cells, and neutrophils may occasionally be present in STA.* **(Right)** *Soft tissue angiofibroma often contains variably prominent, fine or coarse stromal collagen* →*. In some cases, this collagenous stroma may be quite dominant.*

Chronic Inflammatory Infiltrate

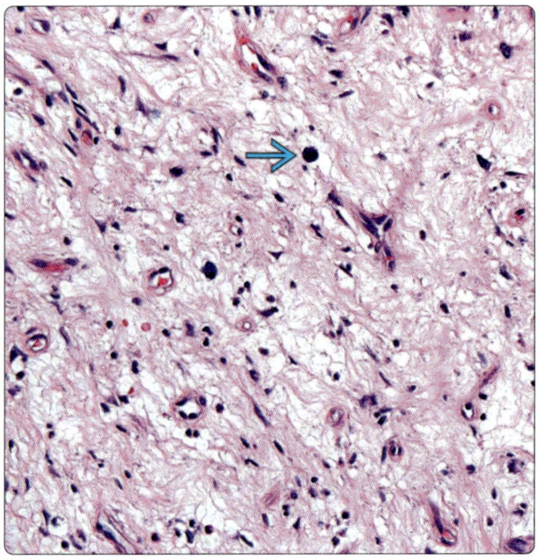

Stromal Collagen

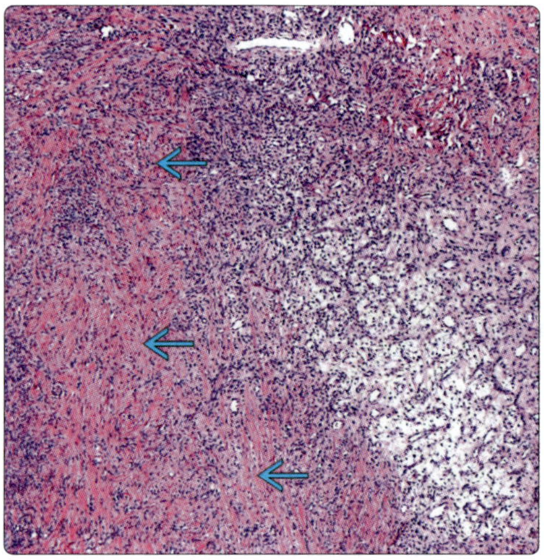

Collagenous Stroma

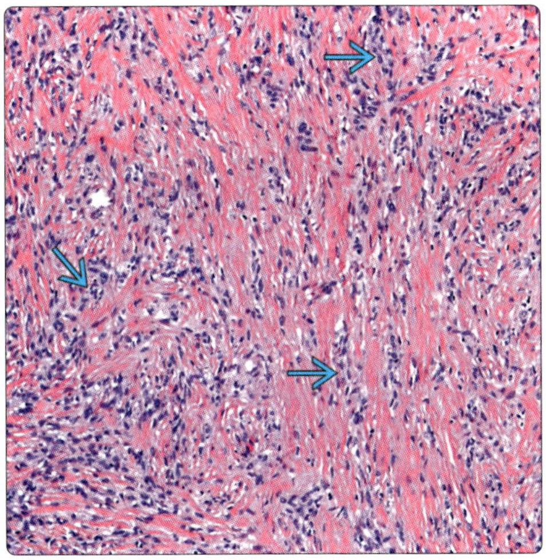

Coarse Collagen Bundles

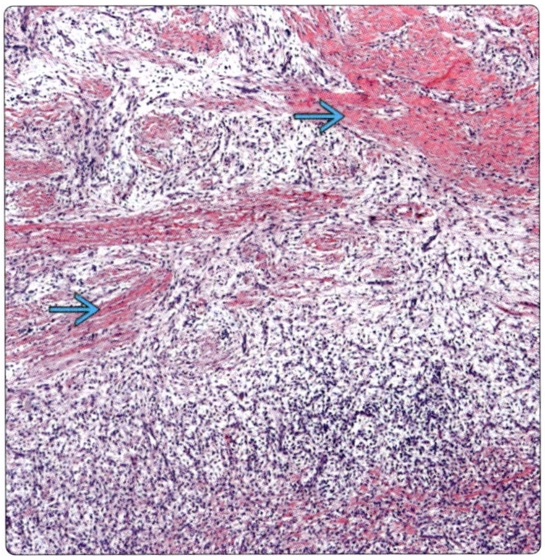

(Left) *In areas of STA that show prominent collagenous stroma, the characteristic vascular channels* ➡ *are present but are somewhat less conspicuous. The orientation of the collagen may also impart a fascicular morphologic appearance.* **(Right)** *In some areas of STA, the stromal collagen forms more discrete, coarse bundles* ➡*. The stroma in these areas is often myxoid and hypocellular.*

Perivascular Hyalinization

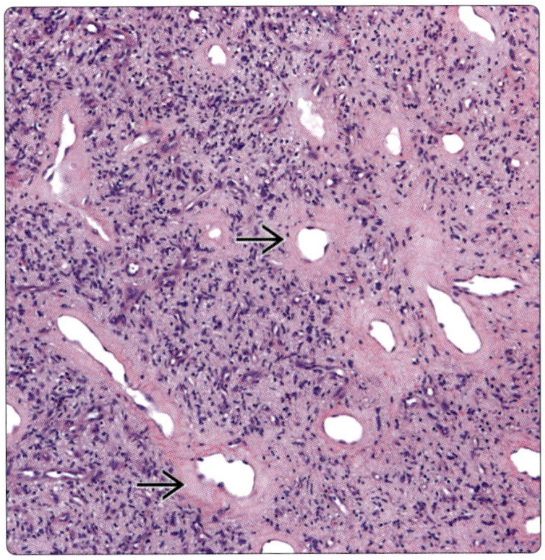

Ectatic "Staghorn" Vessels

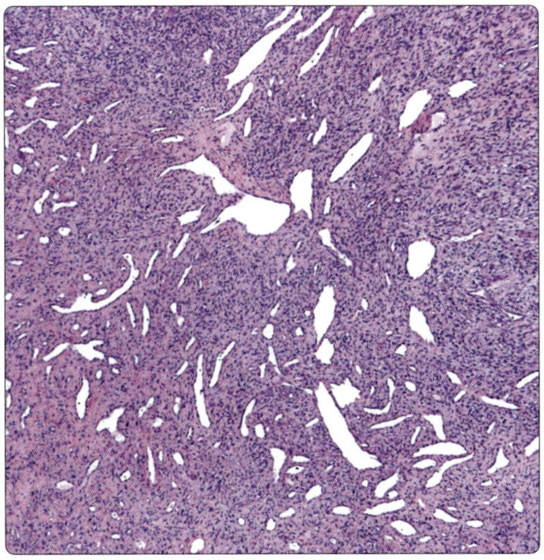

(Left) *Perivascular hyalinization* ➡ *(fibrosis or collagen deposition) is a common finding in STA but can also be a feature in several entities on the differential diagnosis.* **(Right)** *In addition to small and medium vessels, large ectatic channels are not uncommon in STA and may show an irregular "staghorn" morphology. When prominent, a diagnosis of solitary fibrous tumor may be entertained; however, STA is negative for STAT6 and CD34.*

Vascular Changes

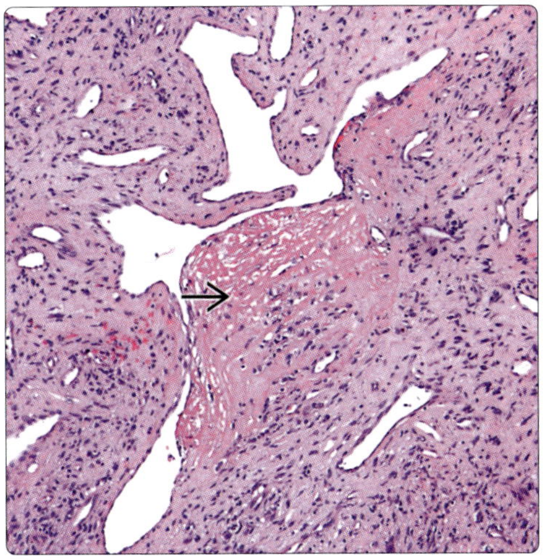

CD34 Immunostain

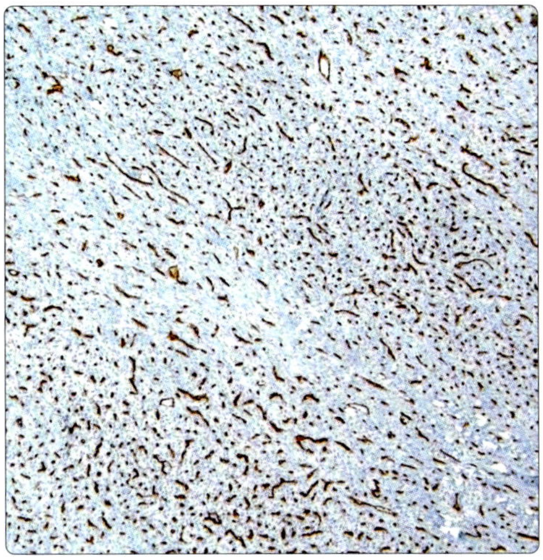

(Left) *Various changes may occur within the walls of the blood vessels in STA, including fibrinoid necrosis* ➡ *and focal thrombus formation.* **(Right)** *The lesional cells of STA are usually negative for SMA, desmin, and CD34, or at most are focally positive. Endothelial markers (such as CD31 and CD34) nicely highlight the prominent stromal vascular network, as depicted.*

Mammary-Type Myofibroblastoma

KEY FACTS

TERMINOLOGY

- Benign fibroblastic/myofibroblastic neoplasm featuring hyalinized bundles of stromal collagen and variable amounts of mature adipose tissue
  - Appears to form histogenetic continuum with spindle cell lipoma and cellular angiofibroma

CLINICAL ISSUES

- Affects 4th-7th decades (mean age: 55 years)
- Most arise in subcutaneous tissue of inguinal/groin or vulvovaginal region
- Slow-growing, often painless mass
- Treatment: Simple excision is usually curative
- Excellent prognosis

MACROSCOPIC

- Well circumscribed, unencapsulated
- Size range: 1-13 cm (median: 5.5 cm)

MICROSCOPIC

- Composed of variably sized fascicles of bland spindled cells
  - Tapered or ovoid banal nuclei and moderate eosinophilic cytoplasm
- Hyalinized bundles of stromal collagen are characteristic
- Variable mature adipose tissue component common
- Stromal vasculature is generally inconspicuous
- Morphologic variant: Epithelioid myofibroblastoma

ANCILLARY TESTS

- CD34(+), desmin (+)
- SMA(+) in 30% of cases
- Loss of nuclear retinoblastoma protein expression
- Molecular: Loss of 13q14 region characteristic

TOP DIFFERENTIAL DIAGNOSES

- Spindle cell lipoma
- Cellular angiofibroma
- Solitary fibrous tumor

Mammary-Type Myofibroblastoma

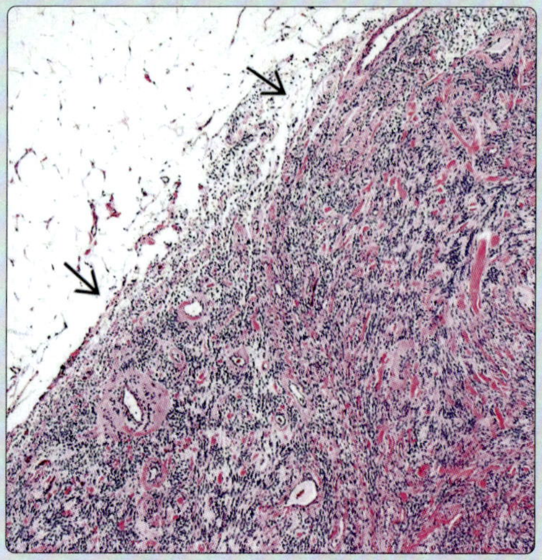

Mammary-Type Myofibroblastoma

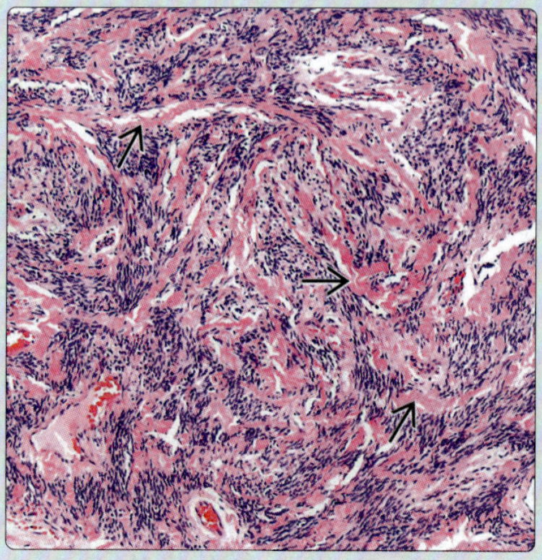

(Left) *Myofibroblastoma is a benign fibroblastic neoplasm of adults. Though originally described in the breast, it also occurs in extramammary soft tissue sites, particularly the inguinal and vulvovaginal regions. Most tumors are well circumscribed ⇒ but unencapsulated, as shown.* **(Right)** *The classic example of myofibroblastoma is composed of variably cellular and sized fascicles of cytologically bland spindle cells within a stroma containing coarse bundles of collagen ⇒.*

Bland Cytologic Features

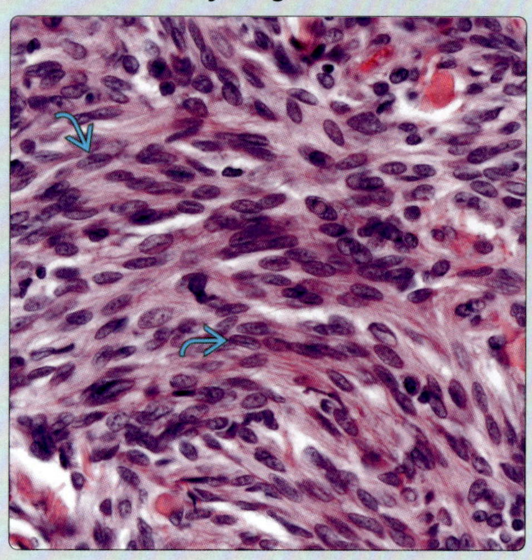

CD34 Expression

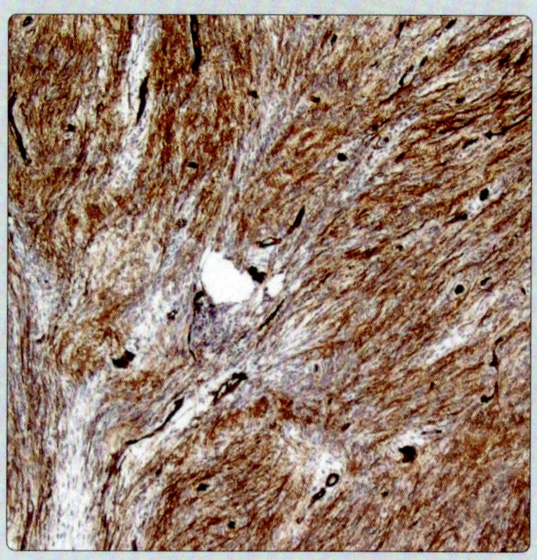

(Left) *The tumor cells of myofibroblastoma demonstrate ovoid to elongated bland nuclei, which often contain a small inconspicuous nucleolus. Nuclear grooves ⇗ may occasionally be seen. Mitotic activity is generally low.* **(Right)** *Diffuse CD34 expression is a characteristic feature of myofibroblastoma but can be seen in a variety of other mesenchymal neoplasms. In the rare negative cases, Rb IHC can be helpful (nuclear expression lost in myofibroblastoma).*

Mammary-Type Myofibroblastoma

TERMINOLOGY

Synonyms

- Soft tissue myofibroblastoma
- Extramammary myofibroblastoma

Definitions

- Benign fibroblastic/myofibroblastic neoplasm featuring hyalinized bundles of stromal collagen and variable amounts of mature adipose tissue
  - Histologically identical to myofibroblastoma of breast
- Appears to form histogenetic continuum with spindle cell lipoma and cellular angiofibroma

CLINICAL ISSUES

Epidemiology

- Age
  - Wide range (mean: 55 years)
- Sex
  - Slight male predominance

Site

- Most arise in subcutaneous tissue
- Inguinal/groin, vulvovaginal, scrotal regions most common extramammary sites
- Extremities (lower > upper) and trunk
- Retroperitoneum, abdominal cavity, head/neck, viscera uncommon
- Appears to occur more frequently along "milk line"
  - Line of potential breast tissue from axilla to inner groin

Presentation

- Slow-growing, often painless mass

Treatment

- Simple excision is usually curative

Prognosis

- Excellent
- No significant risk of recurrence
- Does not metastasize

MACROSCOPIC

General Features

- Circumscribed lesion
- Firm, tan, yellow, or white whorled cut surface

Size

- 1-13 cm diameter (median: 5.5 cm)

MICROSCOPIC

Histologic Features

- Well circumscribed, unencapsulated
- Composed of variably sized fascicles of bland spindled cells
  - Tapered or ovoid banal nuclei and moderate eosinophilic cytoplasm
    - Rare nuclear atypia ± multinucleation (degenerative changes)
  - May show focal epithelioid cytomorphology
  - Rare nuclear palisading (neurilemmoma-like)
  - Mitoses rare
- Hyalinized bundles of stromal collagen are characteristic
  - Some cases are paucicellular and show stromal sclerosis
- Variable mature adipose tissue component
- Stromal vasculature is generally inconspicuous
  - Lacks prominent perivascular hyalinization and large "staghorn" vessels
- Stromal myxoid change common
- Necrosis absent

Morphologic Variants

- Epithelioid myofibroblastoma
  - Composed predominantly of small, rounded or epithelioid tumor cells
  - Other features of myofibroblastoma often present

ANCILLARY TESTS

Immunohistochemistry

- CD34(+), desmin (+)
- SMA(+) in 30-40% of cases
- Loss of nuclear retinoblastoma (Rb) protein expression
  - Also seen in spindle cell lipoma and cellular angiofibroma
- Keratin, S100 protein, STAT6, myogenin, CD31 (-)

Molecular Genetics

- Loss of 13q14 region characteristic
  - Monoallelic deletion of *RB1* or *FOXO1* genes by FISH
  - Also seen in spindle cell lipoma and cellular angiofibroma

DIFFERENTIAL DIAGNOSIS

Spindle Cell Lipoma

- Most commonly arises in neck or back
- Frequent myxoid areas
- CD34(+); usually desmin (-)
- Loss of 13q14 and nuclear Rb protein expression

Cellular Angiofibroma

- Most common in genital/inguinal region
- Stromal vessels more conspicuous and often hyalinized
- CD34(+); desmin (-)
- Loss of 13q14 and nuclear Rb protein expression

Solitary Fibrous Tumor

- Characteristic prominent "staghorn" vasculature
- CD34(+), STAT6(+); desmin (-)
- Nuclear Rb protein expression intact
- Characteristic *NAB2-STAT6* gene fusion

SELECTED REFERENCES

1. McCarthy AJ et al: Tumours composed of fat are no longer a simple diagnosis: an overview of fatty tumours with a spindle cell component. J Clin Pathol. 71(6):483-92, 2018
2. Howitt BE et al: Mammary-type myofibroblastoma: clinicopathologic characterization in a series of 143 cases. Am J Surg Pathol. 40(3):361-7, 2016
3. Magro G et al: Mammary and vaginal myofibroblastomas are genetically related lesions: fluorescence in situ hybridization analysis shows deletion of 13q14 region. Hum Pathol. 43(11):1887-93, 2012
4. Flucke U et al: Cellular angiofibroma: analysis of 25 cases emphasizing its relationship to spindle cell lipoma and mammary-type myofibroblastoma. Mod Pathol. 24(1):82-9, 2011
5. McMenamin ME et al: Mammary-type myofibroblastoma of soft tissue: a tumor closely related to spindle cell lipoma. Am J Surg Pathol. 25(8):1022-9, 2001

(Left) *At low power, myofibroblastoma shows a clean border with the surrounding adipose tissue. No capsule is present. This particular case featured a myxoid and palisaded morphology.* **(Right)** *Nuclear palisading in myofibroblastoma is distinctive but rare. Unlike schwannoma, myofibroblastoma is S100 negative and often coexpresses CD34 and desmin.*

Scanning Magnification

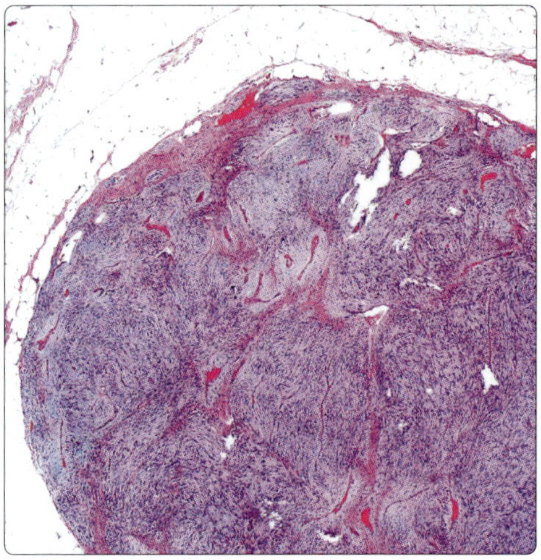

Nuclear Palisading

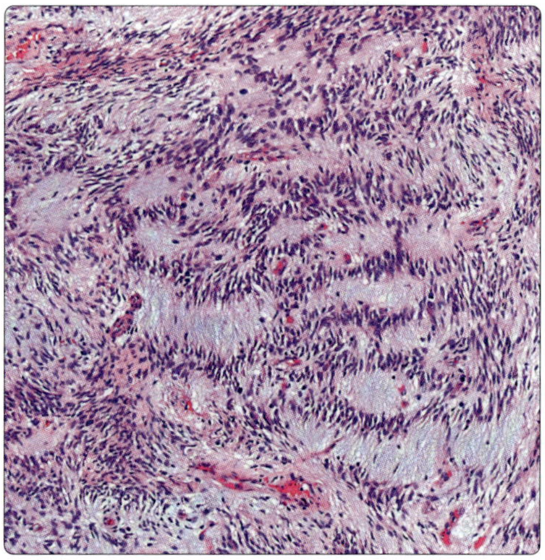

(Left) *Myofibroblastoma can also feature areas of increased cellularity (left) or stromal myxoid change (right). These variations may be focal or diffuse, depending on the individual lesion.* **(Right)** *Rare cases of myofibroblastoma show focal degenerative nuclear atypia, including multinucleation ⇨. The rest of the cells show the usual bland cytologic features.*

Cellular and Myxoid Variants

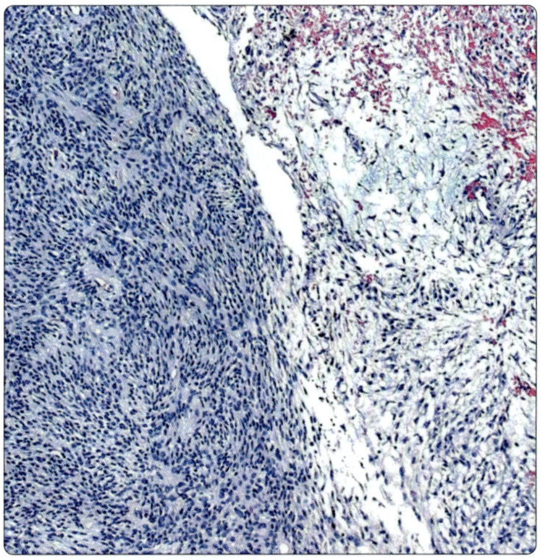

Rare Focal Atypia &/or Multinucleation

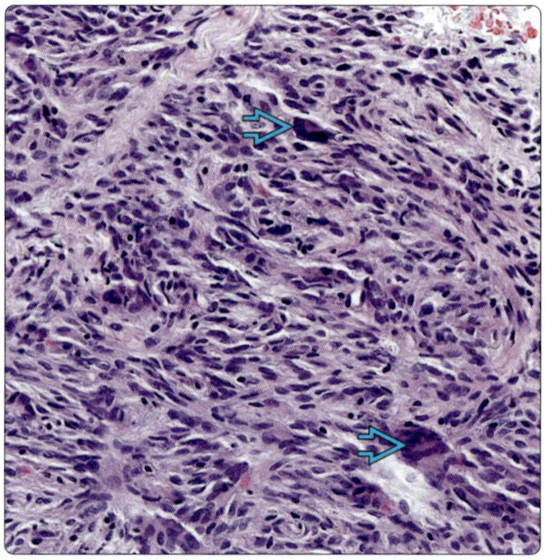

(Left) *Most cases of myofibroblastoma contain some degree of mature adipose tissue, as shown. In some cases it can be extensive, resembling a lipoma, though in other cases it can be focal. Note the presence of collagen bundles →, visible even at low power.* **(Right)** *Some cases of myofibroblastoma are extensively hyalinized and appear hypocellular, as shown in this image. Note the scattered mature adipocytes.*

Mature Adipose Tissue

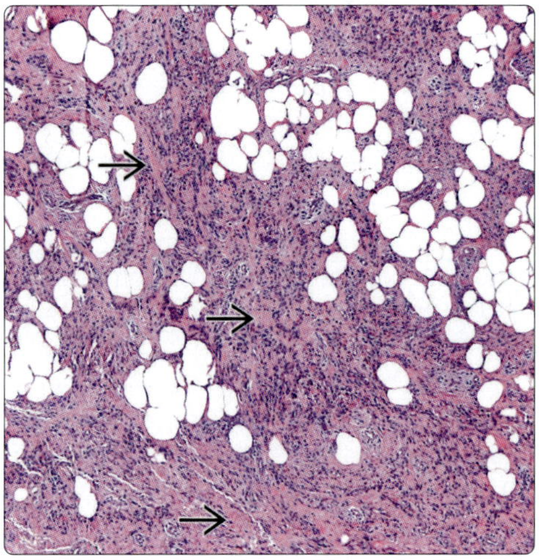

Prominent Stromal Hyalinization

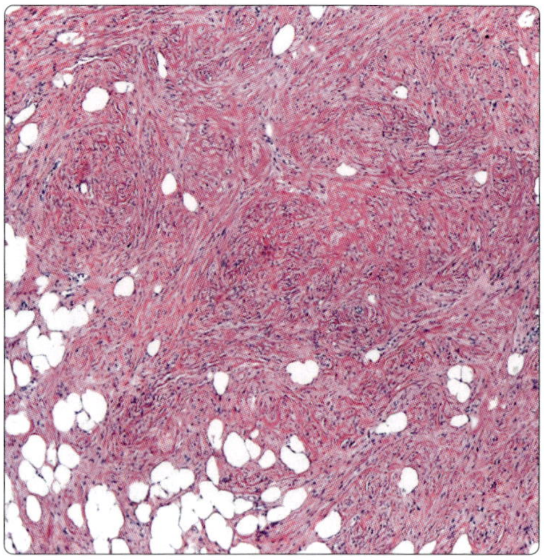

Prominent Stromal Hyalinization

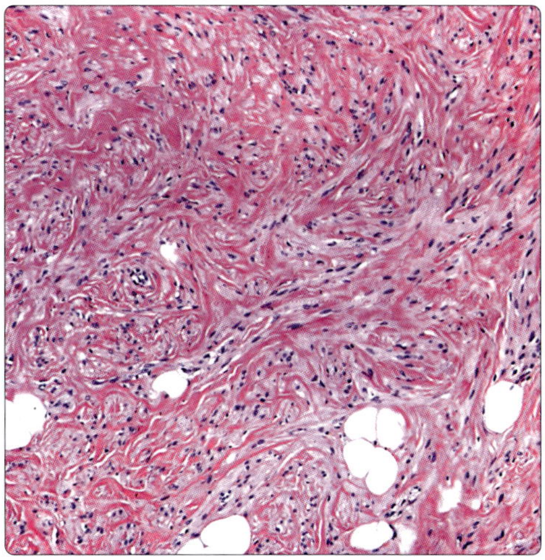

Desmin Expression

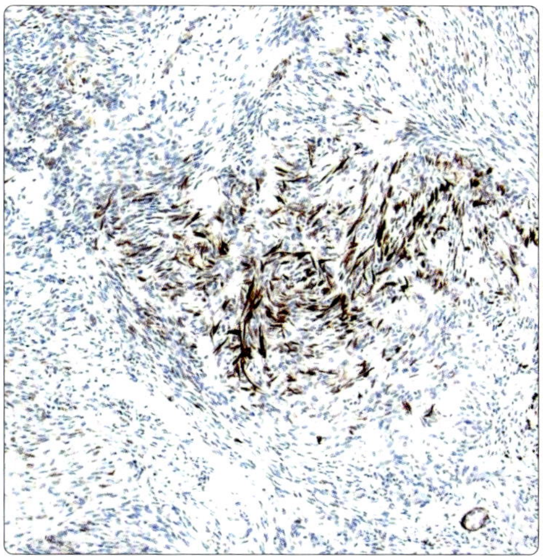

(Left) *The tumor cells in hyalinized cases of myofibroblastoma are cytologically similar to conventional cases. Given the prominent overall eosinophilia of the lesion, a smooth muscle tumor may be considered.* **(Right)** *Desmin is expressed in the majority of cases of myofibroblastoma and may be diffuse, patchy, or focal. In some tumors, desmin is negative.*

Smooth Muscle Actin Expression

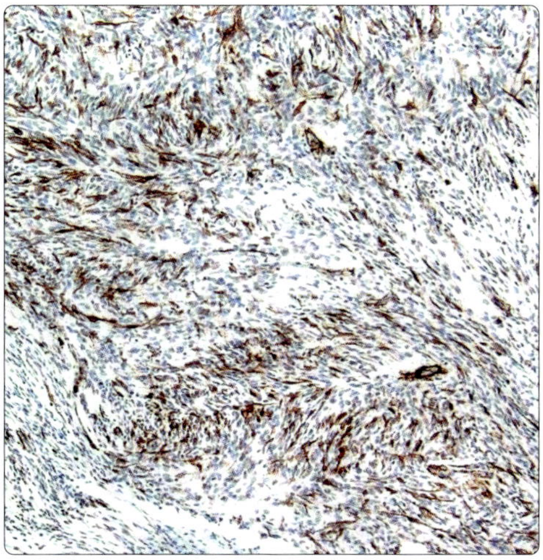

Epithelioid Variant

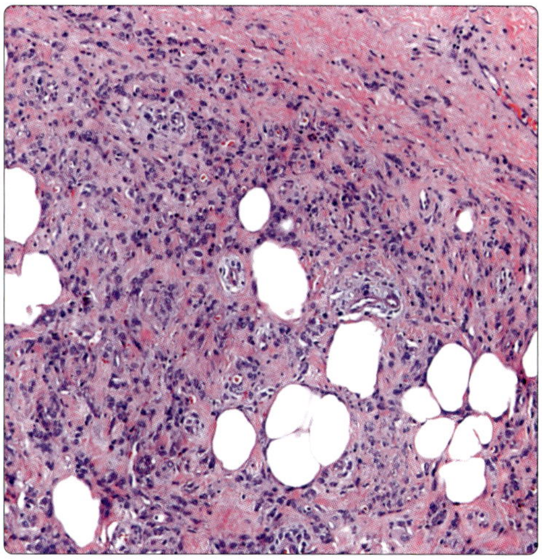

(Left) *Approximately 30-40% of myofibroblastomas show smooth muscle actin (SMA) expression, often in a patchy distribution. This finding can be used for diagnostic support in cases that are CD34(+) but desmin (-).* **(Right)** *Epithelioid cytomorphologic change is uncommon but well documented in mammary myofibroblastoma and may be focal or diffuse. This morphology may also be seen in extramammary soft tissue sites.*

Epithelioid Variant: Cytology

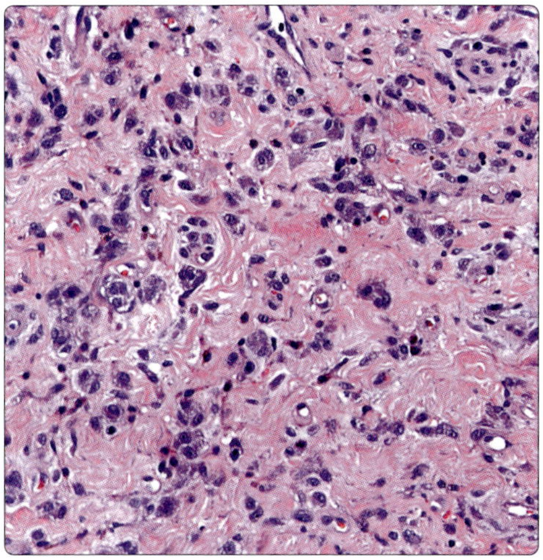

Epithelioid Variant: Growth Patterns

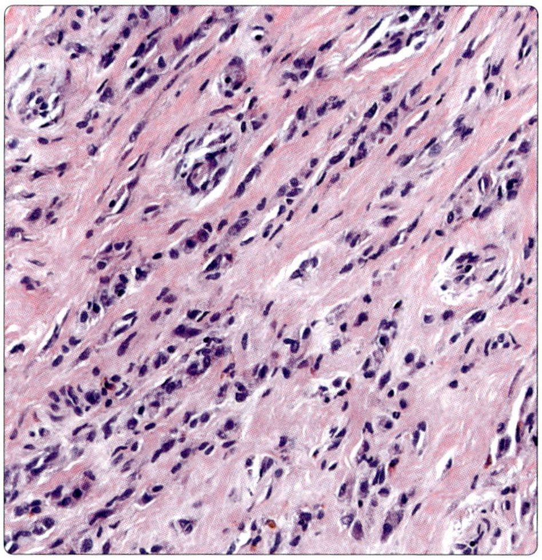

(Left) *The tumor cells of epithelioid myofibroblastoma are small and bland with indistinct eosinophilic cytoplasm. At lower magnification, they can mimic inflammatory cells (particularly plasma cells).* **(Right)** *Epithelioid myofibroblastoma shows a tendency to form cords or linear arrays of tumor cells, as depicted, mimicking infiltrating carcinoma. This is particularly problematic in mammary cases but can also be seen in extramammary sites.*

Intranodal Palisaded Myofibroblastoma

KEY FACTS

TERMINOLOGY

- Distinctive benign spindle cell tumor that occurs in lymph nodes, particularly within inguinal region

CLINICAL ISSUES

- Most common 45-55 years
- 2:1 male predominance
- Most arise in inguinal lymph nodes
- Slow-growing, usually painless mass
- Treatment: Simple surgical excision
- Benign; local recurrences rare

MACROSCOPIC

- Well circumscribed
- Usually < 5 cm in size

MICROSCOPIC

- Rim of compressed residual lymph node tissue at periphery
- Uniform, elongated spindled cells in variably cellular bundles, fascicles, and whorls
  - Nuclear palisading is common, particularly around hyalinized blood vessels
  - Perinuclear vacuolization common
- Bland, uniform nuclei
- Frequent stromal microhemorrhages
  - Hemosiderin pigment and extravasated erythrocytes
- Collagenous bodies are characteristic

ANCILLARY TESTS

- SMA(+)
- Negative for S100, desmin, CD31, CD34, keratin, HMB-45

TOP DIFFERENTIAL DIAGNOSES

- Schwannoma
- Kaposi sarcoma
- Desmoid fibromatosis
- Lymph node metastasis

Intranodal Palisaded Myofibroblastoma

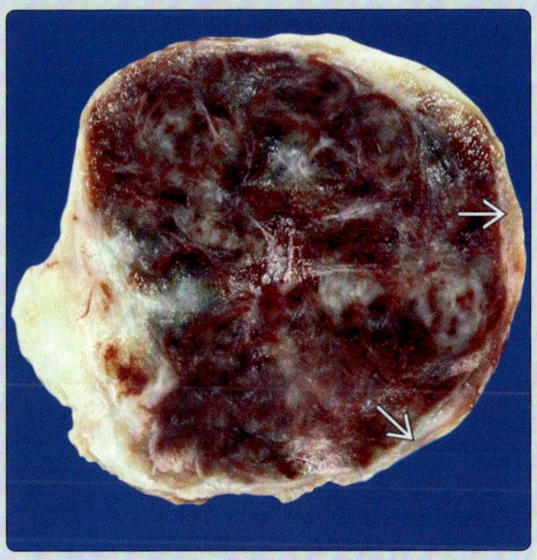

Resemblance to Involved Lymph Node

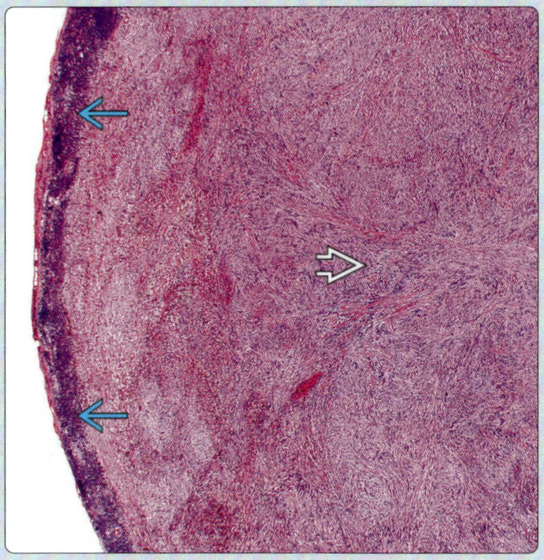

(Left) *Intranodal palisaded myofibroblastoma (IPM) is a distinctive benign spindle cell tumor that shows a strong predilection for inguinal lymph nodes. This tumor is well circumscribed, and compressed residual nodal tissue is usually seen at the periphery.* **(Right)** *A peripheral rim of compressed residual lymph node is usually easily identifiable histologically in IPM. The tumor arises centrally and is composed of fascicles and whorls of spindle cells.*

Fibrous Pseudocapsule

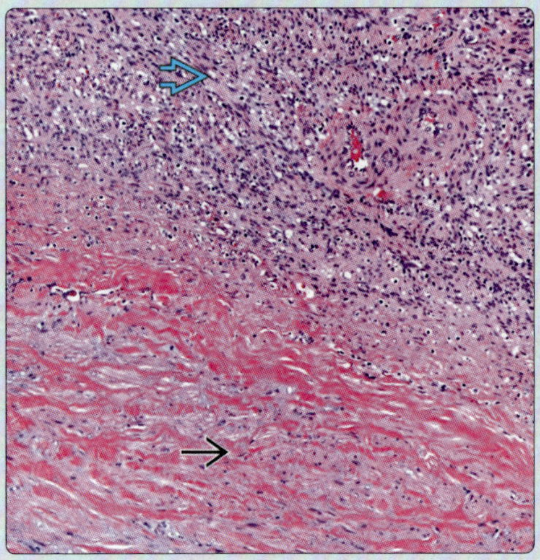

Nuclear Palisading

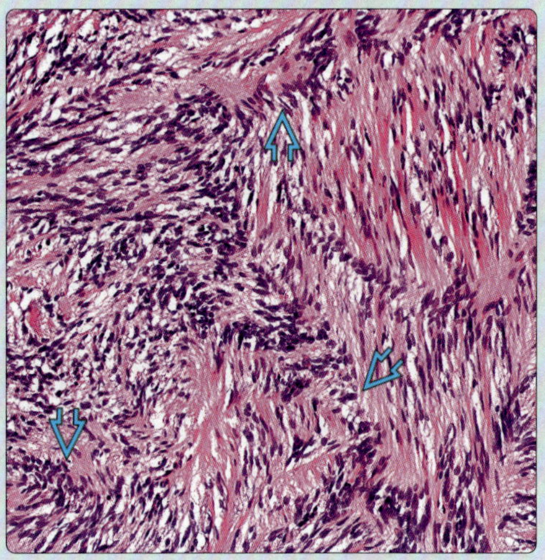

(Left) *Most cases of IPM demonstrate a fibrous or collagenous pseudocapsule at the interface between the tumor and the peripheral residual nodal tissue (not shown in this image).* **(Right)** *The lesional cells of IPM are uniform and spindled with eosinophilic cytoplasm and elongated, cytologically bland nuclei. Some degree of nuclear palisading is commonly present in these tumors.*

TERMINOLOGY

Synonyms

- Intranodal hemorrhagic spindle cell tumor with amianthoid fibers
- Solitary spindle cell tumor with myoid differentiation of lymph node

Definitions

- Distinctive benign spindle cell tumor that occurs in lymph nodes, particularly within inguinal region

CLINICAL ISSUES

Epidemiology

- Incidence
  - Rare
- Age
  - Most common 45-55 years
- Sex
  - 2:1 male predominance

Site

- Most arise in inguinal lymph nodes
- Rare cases reported in submandibular nodes, cervical nodes, and mediastinum

Presentation

- Slow-growing, usually painless mass
- Usually solitary; very rarely multicentric

Treatment

- Simple surgical excision

Prognosis

- Benign
- Local recurrence is very rare

MACROSCOPIC

General Features

- Well circumscribed, often with compressed residual nodal tissue at periphery
- Solid tan-red-brown cut surface

Size

- Usually < 5 cm

MICROSCOPIC

Histologic Features

- Rim of compressed residual lymph node tissue at periphery
  - Tumor is often separated from residual nodal tissue by fibrocollagenous pseudocapsule
- Uniform, elongated spindled cells in variably cellular bundles, fascicles, and whorls
  - Nuclear palisading is common, particularly around hyalinized blood vessels
  - Perinuclear artifactual clearing is common
  - Fascicles may be collagenized and resemble fibromatosis
  - Intracytoplasmic perinuclear pale eosinophilic globules have been reported
- Bland, uniform nuclei
  - Can show occasional intranuclear pseudoinclusions, nuclear grooves
  - Mitoses usually infrequent
- Finely collagenous to myxoedematous stroma with frequent microhemorrhages
  - Often associated with hemosiderin pigment and extravasated erythrocytes
  - Mild chronic inflammatory infiltrate may be present
- Collagenous bodies are characteristic findings
  - Variably sized bundles of acellular collagen, reminiscent of amianthoid fibers
  - Occasionally calcified
- Rare findings: Metaplastic bone, extramedullary hematopoiesis, focal "staghorn" vasculature

ANCILLARY TESTS

Immunohistochemistry

- SMA(+)
- Negative for S100 protein, desmin, CD31, CD34, keratin, HMB-45
- Nuclear β-catenin (+), cyclin-D1 (+)

Molecular Genetics

- *CTNNB1* gene mutations reported

DIFFERENTIAL DIAGNOSIS

Schwannoma

- Rare in lymph nodes
- S100 protein (+); negative for SMA

Kaposi Sarcoma

- Often associated with history of immunosuppression
- CD34(+), CD31(+), ERG(+), D2-40(+), HHV8(+)
- Negative for SMA

PEComa

- Can show dyscohesive, fascicular morphology with stromal hemorrhage
- Does not arise in lymph nodes
- SMA(+), HMB45(+), MART-1(+)

Desmoid Fibromatosis

- Does not arise in lymph nodes
- Lacks nuclear palisading and amianthoid-like collagen fibers

Lymph Node Metastasis

- Spindle cell carcinoma or spindle cell melanoma
- Clinical history of primary tumor
- Immunohistochemistry may be necessary

SELECTED REFERENCES

1. Agaimy A et al: CTNNB1 (β-catenin)-altered neoplasia: a review focusing on soft tissue neoplasms and parenchymal lesions of uncertain histogenesis. Adv Anat Pathol. 23(1):1-12, 2016
2. Bhullar JS et al: Intranodal palisaded myofibroblastoma: a review of the literature. Int J Surg Pathol. 21(4):337-41, 2013
3. Kandemir NO et al: Intranodal palisaded myofibroblastoma (intranodal hemorrhagic spindle cell tumor with amianthoid fibers): a case report and literature review. Diagn Pathol. 5:12, 2010
4. Nguyen T et al: Intranodal palisaded myofibroblastoma. Arch Pathol Lab Med. 131(2):306-10, 2007

Irregular Fascicular Growth

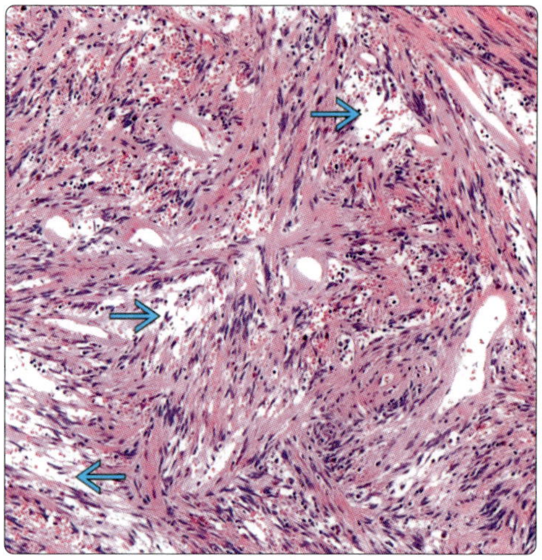

Cellularity

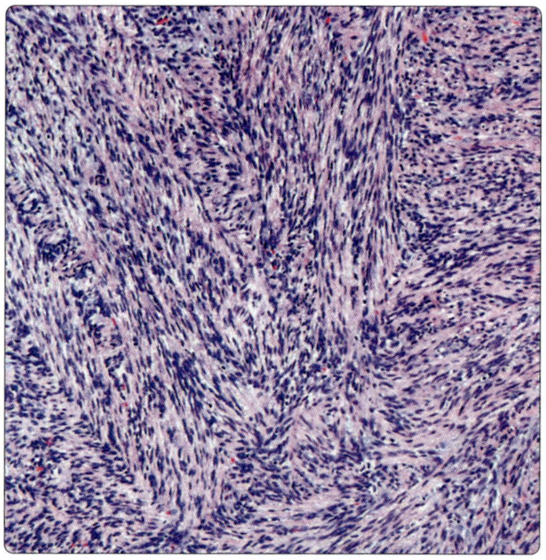

(Left) *A haphazard organization of spindled cells in fascicles is a common morphology in IPM. Note also the stromal and cellular dyscohesion* → *associated with hemorrhage, a prominent finding in some tumors.* **(Right)** *Fascicles of spindle cells vary in length, cellularity, and organization in IPM. Prominent, well-developed, and cellular fascicles, as seen here, may lead to consideration of a sarcoma.*

Fibromatosis-Like Morphology

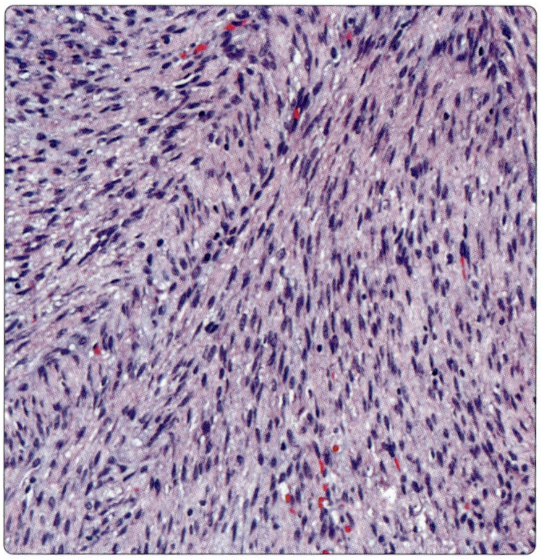

Bland Nuclear Cytology

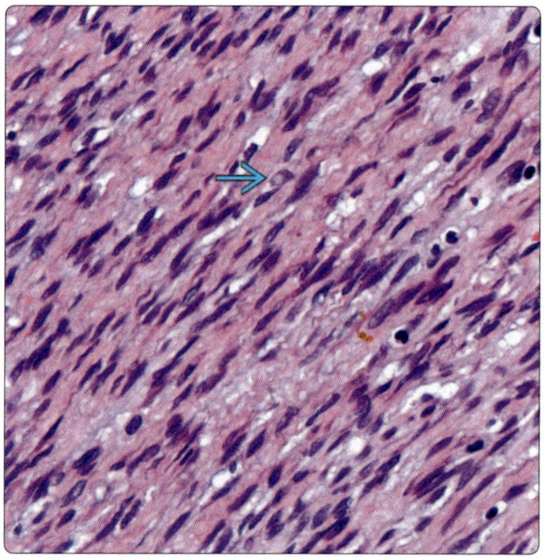

(Left) *In some cases of IPM, the fascicles are broad and show increased collagen deposition, imparting a similar morphologic appearance to fibromatosis.* **(Right)** *The lesional cell nuclei of IPM are elongated, uniform, and cytologically bland. The nuclei may also appear wavy (shown) and can occasionally show grooves or small, pale pseudoinclusions* →*.*

Artifactual Clearing

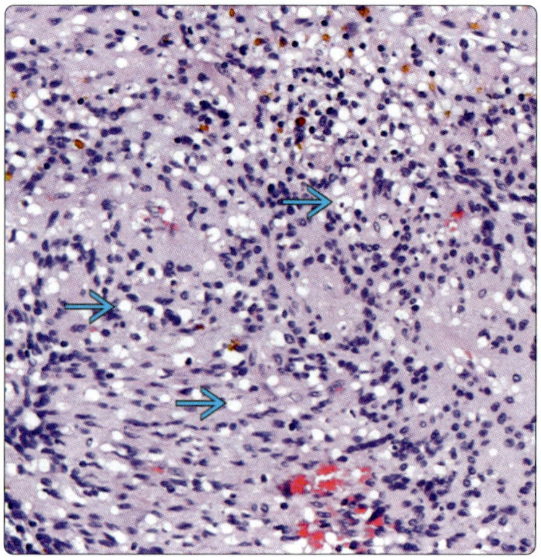

Extramedullary Hematopoiesis

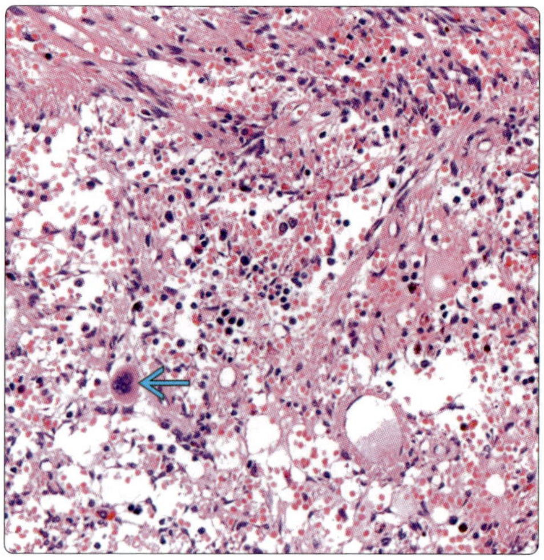

(Left) *Artifactual perinuclear clearing* → *is a relatively common finding in IPM but varies widely in distribution from case to case. This finding is similar to that seen in some spindled gastrointestinal stromal tumors.* **(Right)** *Extramedullary hematopoiesis is an uncommon but documented finding in IPM. Note the presence of a megakaryocyte* →*.*

Microhemorrhages

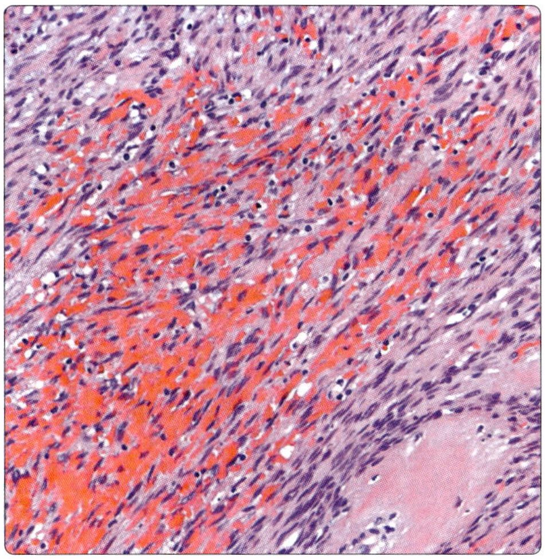

Perivascular Collagen

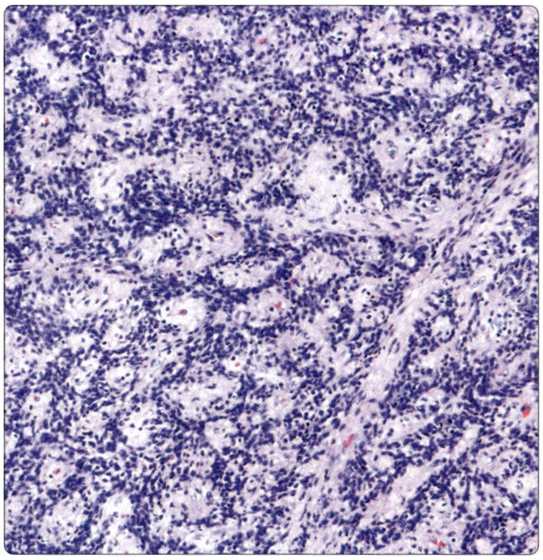

(Left) *Stromal microhemorrhages are common and characteristic of IPM, and associated extravasated erythrocytes and hemosiderin pigment are also seen. At times, this appearance of blood between elongated eosinophilic cells may closely simulate Kaposi sarcoma.* **(Right)** *Perivascular collagen deposition can be seen in IPM, and some cases show a diffuse lattice-like arrangement when vessel density increases.*

Perivascular Collagen

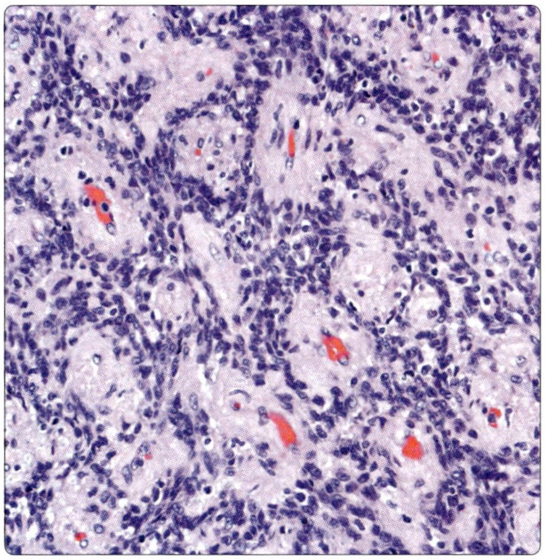

Collagenous Bodies

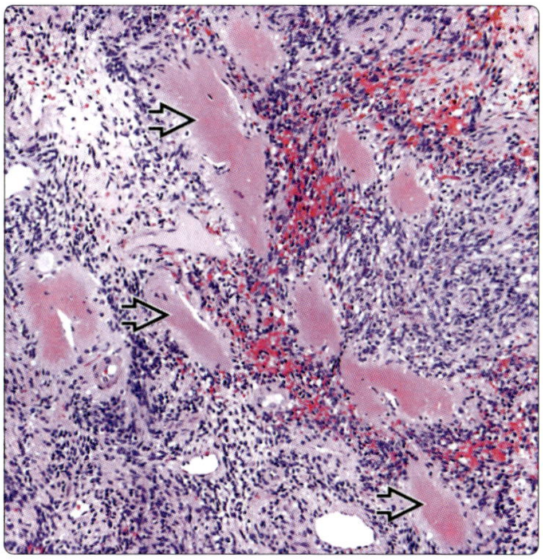

(Left) *This higher magnification view shows perivascular collagen deposition in IPM, as evidenced by hypocellular eosinophilic zones around centralized capillary channels.* **(Right)** *Dense collagenous bodies ⇨, resembling amianthoid fibers, are another characteristic finding seen in many cases of IPM. They may be focal and easily overlooked or numerous and dominate the histologic picture.*

Eosinophilic Collagen

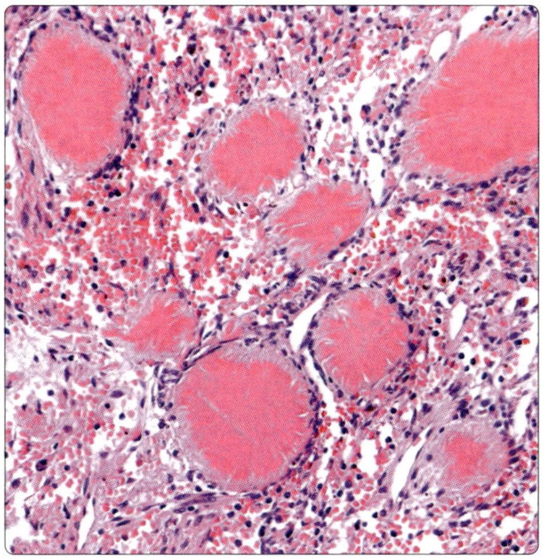

Myxoid Stromal Change

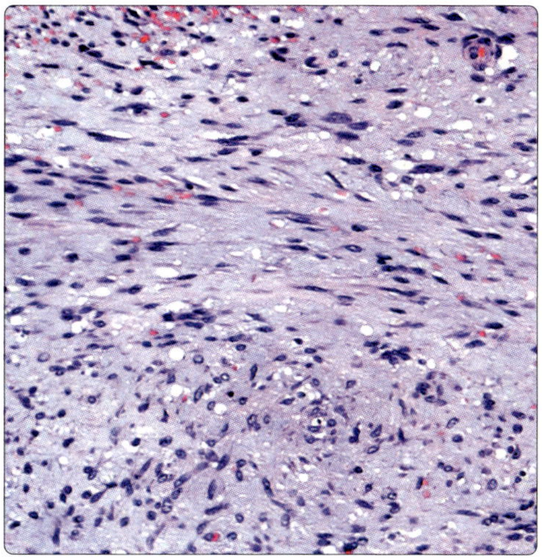

(Left) *The eosinophilic collagenous bodies in IPM typically show a denser centralized portion and a lighter or paler periphery. These bodies may also show calcification in rare cases.* **(Right)** *The stroma in IPM is usually finely collagenous but may also show myxoid or edematous change. Perinuclear vacuoles and extravasated erythrocytes are often prominent in these areas.*

Pleomorphic Fibroma

KEY FACTS

TERMINOLOGY

- Pleomorphic fibroma (PF)
- Benign, dermal-based neoplasm composed of pleomorphic-appearing myofibroblasts

ETIOLOGY/PATHOGENESIS

- Unknown; some cases may be related to ischemia, trauma, or degenerative changes

CLINICAL ISSUES

- Slow-growing skin nodule
- Usually dome-shaped or polypoid-appearing
- May show local recurrence if incompletely excised

MACROSCOPIC

- Size range: 0.4-1.6 cm

MICROSCOPIC

- Well-circumscribed, dome-shaped, or polypoid hypocellular proliferation of dermal spindle cells
- Lesional cells are predominantly spindle shaped with few larger stellate and multinucleated cells
- Mitotic figures are rare or absent
- Stroma typically is composed of hyalinized-appearing collagen fibers
- Cells show enlarged, hyperchromatic nuclei with small nucleoli and scant amounts of eosinophilic cytoplasm

ANCILLARY TESTS

- CD34(+), SMA(+), and vimentin (+)
- Variable FXIIIA(+)

TOP DIFFERENTIAL DIAGNOSES

- Atypical fibroxanthoma
- Dermatofibroma (fibrous histiocytoma)
- Fibrous papule (angiofibroma)
- Sclerotic fibroma

Pleomorphic Fibroma

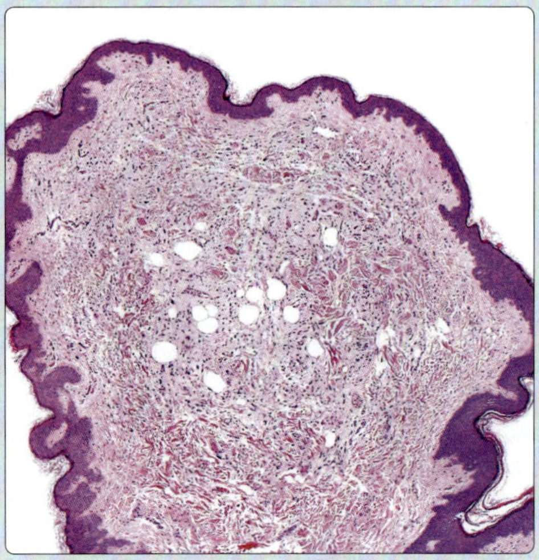

Superficial Multinucleated Cells

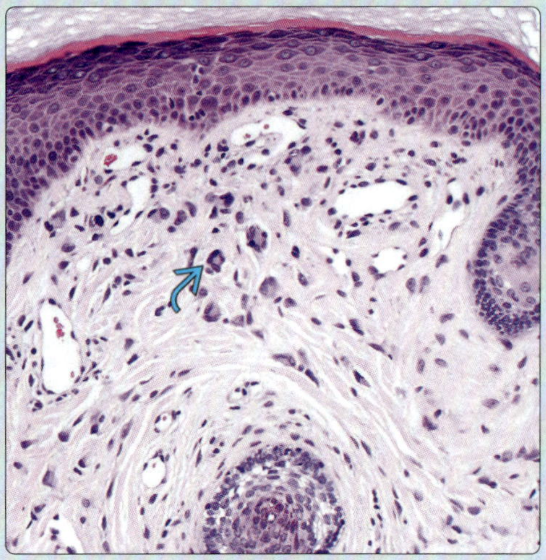

(Left) *Scanning magnification shows a polypoid (skin-tag-like) lesion with a fibromyxoid stroma. The lesion is usually solitary and occurs on the trunk, head and neck region, or extremities.* **(Right)** *Higher magnification shows multinucleated histiocytic cells in the superficial dermis with a background of fibrosis and telangiectasia.*

Cytologic Features

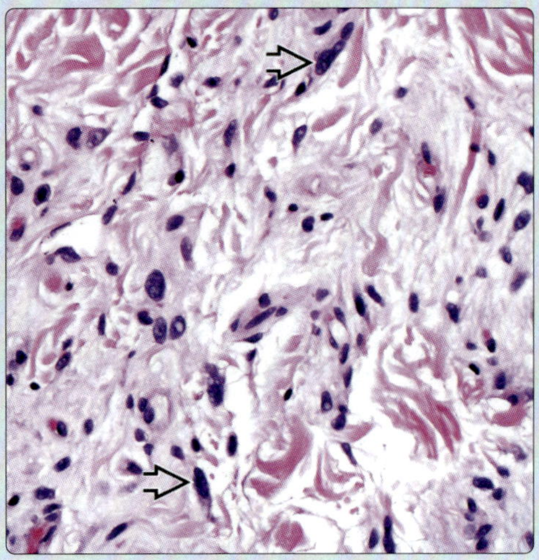

CD34 Expression

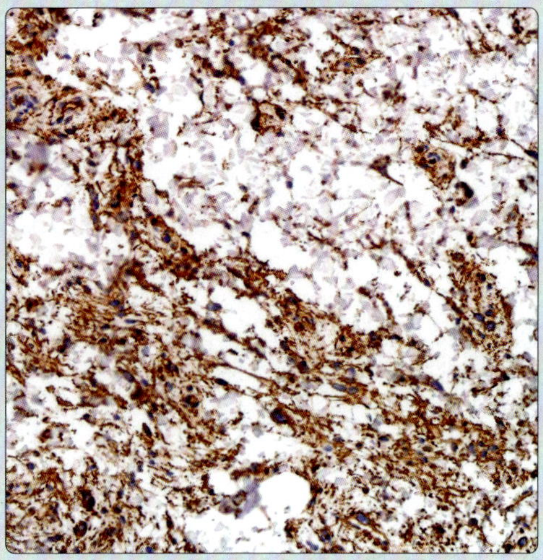

(Left) *High-power examination shows a population of enlarged, hyperchromatic-staining, spindled, stellate, and multinucleated cells set in a fibromyxoid stroma. No mitoses are seen.* **(Right)** *CD34 shows strong and diffuse staining of the spindled and multinucleated cells. This is in contrast to atypical fibroxanthoma and dermatofibroma (fibrous histiocytoma), which are often negative for this antigen.*

TERMINOLOGY

Abbreviations

- Pleomorphic fibroma (PF)

Definitions

- Benign, dermal-based neoplasm composed of pleomorphic-appearing myofibroblasts

ETIOLOGY/PATHOGENESIS

Unknown

- Some cases may be related to ischemia, trauma, or degenerative changes

CLINICAL ISSUES

Presentation

- Slow-growing skin papule or nodule
  - Usually dome-shaped or polypoid-appearing
  - Flesh colored and nonulcerated
- Typically occurs on trunk, extremities, or head and neck region

Treatment

- Complete conservative excision is curative

Prognosis

- Benign tumors with excellent prognosis
- May show local recurrence if incompletely excised

MACROSCOPIC

Size

- Range: 0.4-1.6 cm

MICROSCOPIC

Histologic Features

- Well-circumscribed, dome-shaped, or polypoid hypocellular proliferation of dermal spindle cells
- Lesional cells are predominantly spindle-shaped with scattered larger stellate and multinucleated cells
- Cells show enlarged, hyperchromatic nuclei with small nucleoli and scant amounts of eosinophilic cytoplasm
- Mitotic figures are rare or absent
  - No atypical mitoses should be seen
- Stroma typically composed of hyalinized-appearing collagen fibers
  - Some cases show overlapping features with sclerotic fibroma
    - i.e., these cases show storiforming of hyalinized collagen bundles with collagen clefts
- Myxoid areas may be present
  - Can be prominent/diffuse in some cases (myxoid PF)

ANCILLARY TESTS

Immunohistochemistry

- CD34(+), SMA(+), and vimentin (+)
- Variable FXIIIA(+), often weak
- Loss of Rb protein expression

DIFFERENTIAL DIAGNOSIS

Atypical Fibroxanthoma

- Highly cellular and atypical-appearing, dermal-based tumor associated with solar elastosis in head and neck region
- Mitotic figures are easily found in most cases, including atypical forms
- Typically CD34(-), and nonspecific markers (including CD68, CD10, and CD99) are usually (+)

Dermatofibroma (Fibrous Histiocytoma)

- Usually does not show degree of pleomorphism seen in PF, although rare cases may (i.e., atypical dermatofibroma or "dermatofibroma with monster cells")
- More typical dermatofibroma areas should be present at periphery of tumor
  - Collagen trapping, histiocytoid cells, and overlying epidermal hyperplasia are usually present
- Typically CD34(-), unlike PF

Fibrous Papule (Angiofibroma)

- Small, dome-shaped papule that shows dermal fibrosis and increased blood vessels with telangiectasia
- Scattered, enlarged, mildly pleomorphic-appearing fibroblasts may be present
- CD34(-), FXIIIA(+)

Sclerotic Fibroma

- Shows characteristic storiform pattern of thickened, hyalinized-appearing collagen bundles with clefts between them
- Some cases show overlapping features with PF with population of enlarged, pleomorphic-appearing spindled cells
  - Some authors believe that PF is variant of sclerotic fibroma, but this is not universally accepted

DIAGNOSTIC CHECKLIST

Pathologic Interpretation Pearls

- Hypocellular dermal proliferation of spindled, stellate, and multinucleated cells
- Cells appear pleomorphic and hyperchromatic but lack mitotic activity

SELECTED REFERENCES

1. Tashakori M et al: Pleomorphic fibroma of the skin with MDM2 immunoreactivity: a potential diagnostic pitfall. J Cutan Pathol. 45(1):59-62, 2018
2. Hinds B et al: Loss of retinoblastoma in pleomorphic fibroma: an immunohistochemical and genomic analysis. J Cutan Pathol. 44(8):665-71, 2017
3. Halteh P et al: Subungual pleomorphic fibroma: a case report and review of the literature. Dermatol Online J. 22(11), 2016
4. Al-Zaid T et al: Pleomorphic fibroma and dermal atypical lipomatous tumor: are they related? J Cutan Pathol. 40(4):379-84, 2013
5. Yadav Y et al: Cytomorphology of pleomorphic fibroma of skin: a diagnostic enigma. J Cytol. 30(1):71-3, 2013
6. Mahmood MN et al: Solitary sclerotic fibroma of skin: a possible link with pleomorphic fibroma with immunophenotypic expression for O13 (CD99) and CD34. J Cutan Pathol. 30(10):631-6, 2003
7. Pitt MA et al: Myxoid cutaneous pleomorphic fibroma. Histopathology. 25(3):300, 1994
8. Kamino H et al: Pleomorphic fibroma of the skin: a benign neoplasm with cytologic atypia. A clinicopathologic study of eight cases. Am J Surg Pathol. 13(2):107-13, 1989

Dermatomyofibroma

KEY FACTS

TERMINOLOGY

- a.k.a. plaque-like dermal fibromatosis
- Myofibroblastic tumor with features overlapping with dermatofibroma

ETIOLOGY/PATHOGENESIS

- May be related to trauma in some cases

CLINICAL ISSUES

- Rare, slow-growing plaque or nodule
  - Often red-brown in color
- Usually occurs in young adult females
- No malignant potential but may continue to enlarge if not completely removed

MACROSCOPIC

- Small, dermal-based nodule
- Usually 1-2 cm in size but occasionally much larger

MICROSCOPIC

- Dermal-based spindle cell proliferation
- Tumor is composed of broad fascicles of elongated monomorphic spindle cells oriented parallel to surface
  - Bland nuclei; palely eosinophilic cytoplasm
- Overlying epidermal hyperplasia often present
- Elastic fibers are typically increased in numbers and fragmented
- Mitotic figures are rare and not atypical

ANCILLARY TESTS

- Variable SMA(+)
- CD34(-), MSA(-), desmin (-), S100 protein (-), and FXIIIA(-)

TOP DIFFERENTIAL DIAGNOSES

- Dermatofibroma
- Superficial (palmar/plantar) fibromatosis
- Leiomyoma
- Hypertrophic scar

Scanning Magnification of Dermatomyofibroma

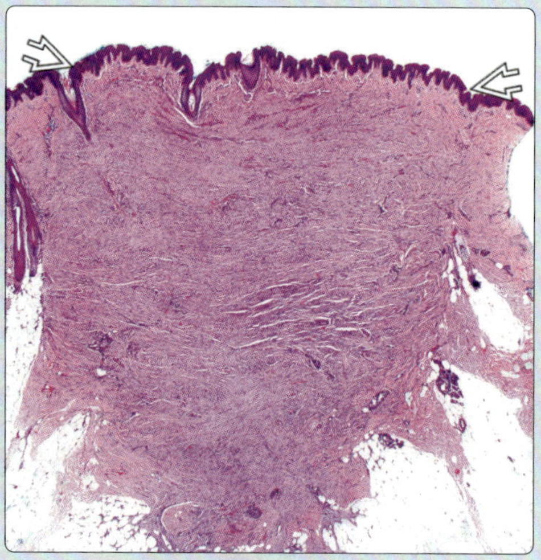

Higher Magnification of Dermatomyofibroma

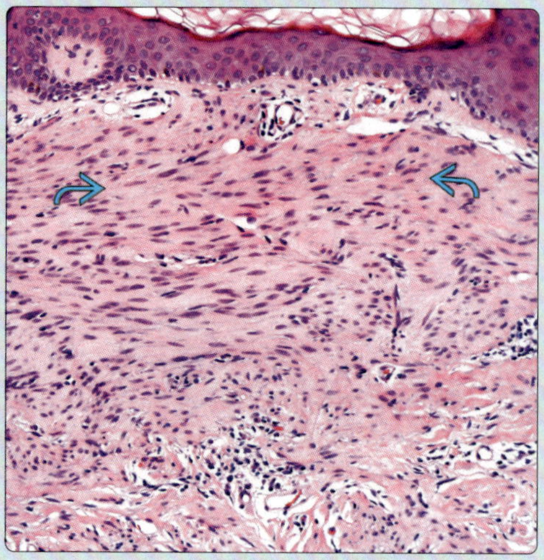

(Left) *Dermatomyofibroma is a dermal-based, plaque-like spindle proliferation with overlying epidermal hyperplasia ➔ and basilar pigmentation, similar to a dermatofibroma.* **(Right)** *Higher magnification shows the superficial portion of the spindle cell proliferation closely approaching the epidermis. Note the parallel arrangement and the prominent eosinophilic-staining cytoplasm of the spindled cells ➔.*

High Magnification of Dermatomyofibroma

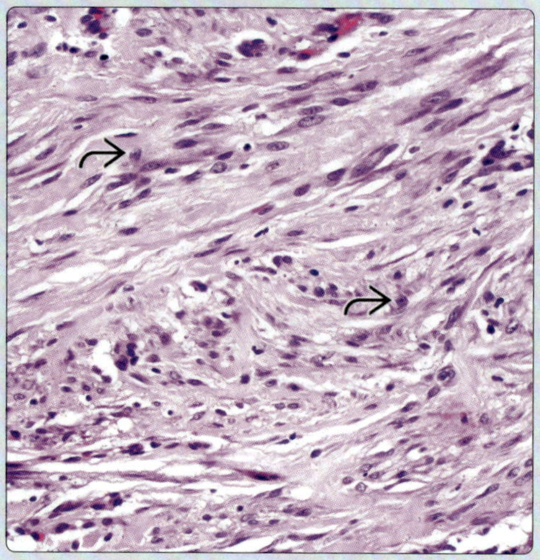

SMA Staining in Dermatomyofibroma

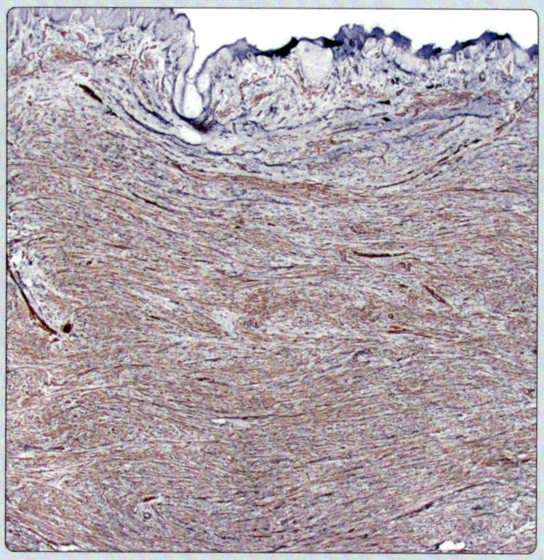

(Left) *High magnification shows the cytologic features of dermatomyofibroma. The lesion is composed of bland-appearing, elongated, eosinophilic-staining spindled cells with inconspicuous to small nucleoli ➔.* **(Right)** *SMA shows diffuse positivity in the spindle cells of dermatomyofibroma. Desmin is typically negative.*

TERMINOLOGY

Synonyms

- Plaque-like dermal fibromatosis

Definitions

- Myofibroblastic tumor with many features similar to dermatofibroma

ETIOLOGY/PATHOGENESIS

Unknown

- May be related to trauma in some cases

CLINICAL ISSUES

Epidemiology

- Incidence
  - Rare tumor
- Age
  - Usually occurs in young adults
- Sex
  - M:F = 1:8

Site

- Typically present in shoulder and axillary regions
  - Also present in trunk, head and neck

Presentation

- Slow-growing indurated plaque or nodule
  - Often red-brown in color
- Rarely may present as multiple lesions

Treatment

- Complete surgical excision is curative, but not necessary, given benign nature of these tumors

Prognosis

- Excellent
  - No malignant potential but may continue to enlarge if not completely removed
- Does not generally recur, even if incompletely excised

MACROSCOPIC

General Features

- Small, dermal-based nodule

Size

- Usually 1-2 cm in size but occasionally much larger

MICROSCOPIC

Histologic Features

- Dermal-based, plaque-like spindle cell proliferation
  - Usually located in reticular dermis but may show involvement of superficial subcutis
  - Adnexal structures are usually preserved
  - Often see overlying epidermal hyperplasia (similar to dermatofibroma)
- Tumor is composed of broad fascicles of elongated monomorphic spindle cells
  - Fascicles often run in parallel to epidermis
  - Nuclei bland and tapered
  - Uniform chromatin with small nucleoli
  - Palely eosinophilic cytoplasm, poorly delineated
- Foci of collagen trapping may be present but not as prominent as in dermatofibroma
- Mitotic figures are rare and not atypical
- Elastic fibers are typically increased in numbers and fragmented
  - Can highlight this with elastic stains

ANCILLARY TESTS

Immunohistochemistry

- Variable SMA(+)
- CD34(-), MSA(-), desmin (-), S100 protein (-), and FXIIIA(-)

DIFFERENTIAL DIAGNOSIS

Dermatofibroma

- Lacks parallel orientation and muscle differentiation
- Shows more prominent peripheral collagen trapping

Superficial (Palmar/Plantar) Fibromatosis

- Occurs in hands or feet
- Nodular growth, rather than plaque-like

Leiomyoma

- Shows more clear-cut smooth muscle differentiation with strong SMA, MSA, and desmin expression
- Fascicles of spindle cells not typically oriented parallel to epidermis

Hypertrophic Scar

- Dense proliferation of collagen with vertically oriented vessels
- Adnexal structures are lost as opposed to dermatomyofibroma

Dermatofibrosarcoma Protuberans

- Plaque-like variant of dermatofibrosarcoma protuberans can show histologic features similar to dermatomyofibroma
- Strong CD34(+), SMA(-)

SELECTED REFERENCES

1. Borucki R et al: Fluorescence microscopy for the evaluation of elastic tissue patterns within fibrous proliferations of the skin on hematoxylin-eosin-stained slides. J Am Acad Dermatol. ePub, 2018
2. Lima LAF et al: Multiple dermatomyofibromas. An Bras Dermatol. 93(2):268-270, 2018
3. Ma JE et al: Dermatomyofibromas arising in children: report of two new cases and review of the literature. Pediatr Dermatol. 34(3):347-351, 2017
4. Cano Martínez N et al: Dermatomyofibroma mimicking granuloma annulare. Dermatol Online J. 17(6):3, 2011
5. Gomez-Moyano E et al: Two cases of dermatomyofibroma (plaque-like dermal fibromatosis). Int J Dermatol. 49(8):914-7, 2010
6. Mentzel T et al: Dermatomyofibroma: clinicopathologic and immunohistochemical analysis of 56 cases and reappraisal of a rare and distinct cutaneous neoplasm. Am J Dermatopathol. 31(1):44-9, 2009
7. Mortimore RJ et al: Dermatomyofibroma: a report of two cases, one occurring in a child. Australas J Dermatol. 42(1):22-5, 2001
8. Mentzel T et al: Dermatomyofibroma: additional observations on a distinctive cutaneous myofibroblastic tumour with emphasis on differential diagnosis. Br J Dermatol. 129(1):69-73, 1993
9. Cooper PH: Dermatomyofibroma: a case of fibromatosis revisited. J Cutan Pathol. 19(2):81-2, 1992
10. Kamino H et al: Dermatomyofibroma. A benign cutaneous, plaque-like proliferation of fibroblasts and myofibroblasts in young adults. J Cutan Pathol. 19(2):85-93, 1992

Storiform Collagenoma

KEY FACTS

TERMINOLOGY

- Synonym: Sclerotic fibroma
- Benign, dermal-based fibroblastic proliferation

ETIOLOGY/PATHOGENESIS

- May be related to trauma
- Some cases may represent regressed dermatofibromas
- Multiple lesions are associated with Cowden syndrome, consistent with genetic influence

CLINICAL ISSUES

- May occur at any age, including infants and elderly
- Excellent prognosis; may locally recur but no metastatic potential
- Present most commonly on face, extremities, and trunk

MACROSCOPIC

- Typically 0.5-3.0 cm in size
- Dermal nodule with firm, yellow-tan surface

MICROSCOPIC

- Composed of thickened, hyalinized-appearing collagen bundles in storiform/whorled pattern
  - Prominent clefts often seen between collagen bundles
- Cells are typically small, bland, spindled to stellate fibroblasts
- Occasional cases may show large, bizarre-appearing cells (pleomorphic sclerotic fibroma)
  - These cells do not show infiltrative features or increased mitotic activity

ANCILLARY TESTS

- FXIIIA(+), vimentin (+), focal CD34(+)

TOP DIFFERENTIAL DIAGNOSES

- Dermatofibroma
- Pleomorphic fibroma
- Collagenous fibroma
- Acral fibrokeratoma (subungual and periungual fibroma)

(Left) *Scanning magnification view of sclerotic fibroma shows a dermal-based, symmetric-appearing nodular spindle cell proliferation with storiforming ➢ of collagen.* **(Right)** *Intermediate-power examination shows prominent areas of storiforming and clefting artifact between the collagen bundles ➢.*

Sclerotic Fibroma at Low Magnification

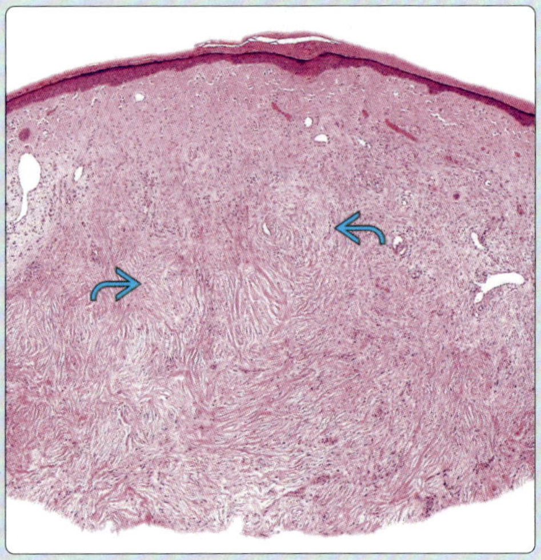

Intermediate Magnification of Sclerotic Fibroma

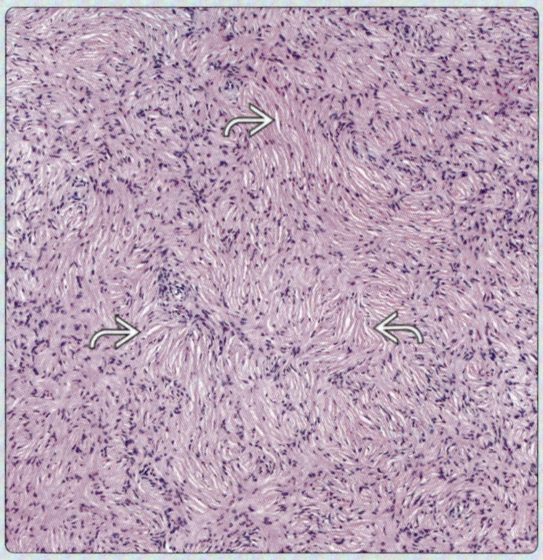

(Left) *High-power magnification shows spindled fibroblasts ➡ without nuclear atypia in a dense fibrous stroma with a few scattered small lymphocytes ➡.* **(Right)** *FXIIIA immunohistochemistry shows staining of scattered spindle cells ➡ in sclerotic fibroma (storiform collagenoma).*

Sclerotic Fibroma at High Magnification

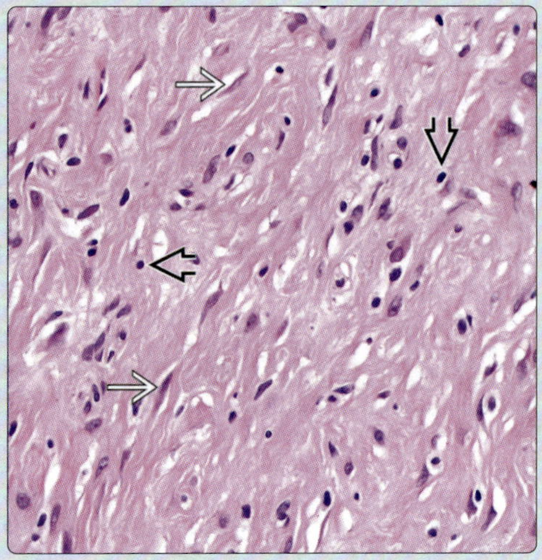

FXIIIA Expression

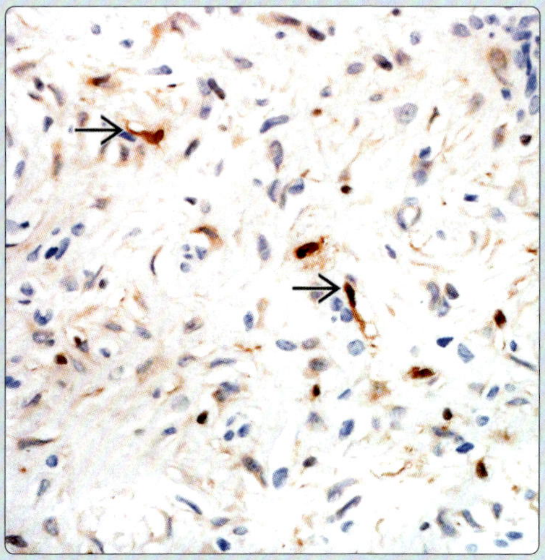

TERMINOLOGY

Synonyms

- Sclerotic fibroma

Definitions

- Benign, dermal-based fibroblastic proliferation with storiforming collagen

ETIOLOGY/PATHOGENESIS

Unknown

- May be related to trauma
- Some cases may represent regressed dermatofibromas
- Some cases are genetic
  - Multiple lesions are associated with Cowden syndrome (*PTEN* mutations, associated with multiple hamartomas and tricholemmomas)

CLINICAL ISSUES

Epidemiology

- Age
  - May occur at any age, including infants and elderly
- Sex
  - Occurs in both males and females

Site

- Present most commonly on face, extremities, and trunk

Presentation

- Slow-growing, flesh-colored papule or nodule

Treatment

- Complete conservative excision is curative

Prognosis

- Excellent; may locally recur but no metastatic potential

MACROSCOPIC

General Features

- Dermal nodule with firm, yellow-tan surface

Size

- Typically 0.5-3.0 cm

MICROSCOPIC

Histologic Features

- Circumscribed, unencapsulated dermal nodule
- Composed of thickened, hyalinized-appearing collagen bundles in storiform/whorled pattern
  - Prominent clefts often seen between collagen bundles (so-called plywood or fingerprint pattern)
- Cells are typically small, bland, spindled to stellate fibroblasts
- Occasional cases may show large, bizarre-appearing cells (pleomorphic sclerotic fibroma), similar to pleomorphic fibroma
  - These cells do not show infiltrative features or increased mitotic activity
- Pacinian collagenoma is rare variant with "onion-skin" mimicking pacinian corpuscle

ANCILLARY TESTS

Immunohistochemistry

- FXIIIA(+), vimentin (+), focal CD34(+)
- Ki-67 may highlight few scattered nuclei, but overall proliferative rate is low

DIFFERENTIAL DIAGNOSIS

Dermatofibroma

- Typically does not show prominent storiforming of collagen, although it may be focally present in rare cases
- Areas of conventional dermatofibroma with collagen trapping and histiocytic cells should be present
  - Some cases may show overlapping features, leading some investigators to believe that sclerotic fibromas are involuting dermatofibromas

Pleomorphic Fibroma

- Clinically resembles skin tag
- Pleomorphic cells are more prominent, and storiforming pattern of collagen should be absent

Collagenous Fibroma

- Usually subcutaneous tumors with only rare dermal involvement
- Densely collagenous or fibromyxoid stroma; lacks prominent storiforming of collagen

Acral Fibrokeratoma (Subungual and Periungual Fibroma)

- Usually shows overlying hyperkeratosis and acanthosis
- Proliferation of thick collagen bundles, often vertically oriented

DIAGNOSTIC CHECKLIST

Pathologic Interpretation Pearls

- Dermal nodule of thickened, hyalinized-appearing collagen bundles in storiform/whorled pattern

SELECTED REFERENCES

1. Ebadian M et al: Dermoscopy of a solitary storiform collagenoma. Dermatol Pract Concept. 8(2):120-122, 2018
2. Shi KY et al: Late-stage nodular erythema elevatum diutinum mimicking sclerotic fibroma. J Cutan Pathol. 45(1):94-96, 2018
3. Kieselova K et al: Multiple sclerotic fibromas of the skin: an important clue for the diagnosis of Cowden syndrome. BMJ Case Rep. 2017, 2017
4. Val-Bernal JF et al: Sclerotic fibroma (storiform collagenoma)-like stroma in a fibroadenoma of axillary accessory breast tissue. J Cutan Pathol. 39(8):798-802, 2012
5. Nakashima K et al: Solitary sclerotic fibroma of the skin: morphological characterization of the 'plywood-like pattern'. J Cutan Pathol. 35 Suppl 1:74-9, 2008
6. González-Vela MC et al: Sclerotic fibroma-like dermatofibroma: an uncommon distinctive variant of dermatofibroma. Histol Histopathol. 20(3):801-6, 2005
7. Chen TM et al: Pleomorphic sclerotic fibroma: a case report and literature review. Am J Dermatopathol. 24(1):54-8, 2002
8. Martín-López R et al: Pleomorphic sclerotic fibroma. Dermatology. 198(1):69-72, 1999
9. Pujol RM et al: Solitary sclerotic fibroma of the skin: a sclerotic dermatofibroma? Am J Dermatopathol. 18(6):620-4, 1996
10. Requena L et al: Multiple sclerotic fibromas of the skin. A cutaneous marker of Cowden's disease. J Cutan Pathol. 19(4):346-51, 1992
11. Rapini RP et al: Sclerotic fibromas of the skin. J Am Acad Dermatol. 20(2 Pt 1):266-71, 1989

Keloid

KEY FACTS

TERMINOLOGY

- Synonym: Scar with keloidal collagen
- Reactive/reparative proliferation with prominent thickened and hyalinized, eosinophilic-staining bundles of collagen extending beyond original biopsy/wound site

CLINICAL ISSUES

- Scar that grows beyond original biopsy/wound site
- Often erythematous, pruritic lesions with predilection for earlobe in black patients
- Most common in patients < 30 years
- Typically follows ear piercing or other trauma by a few months
- Direct injection of steroids is often 1st-line treatment
- Complete excision, accompanied by concurrent steroid injections or radiotherapy to decrease risk of recurrence
- Persistence and recurrence are common, but there is no risk of malignancy

MACROSCOPIC

- Large, nodular, dermal-based lesion with firm, white cut surface

MICROSCOPIC

- Dense proliferation of thickened, hyalinized-appearing collagen bundles in dermis
- Decreased vessels compared to conventional and hypertrophic scars
- Increased numbers of stromal fibroblasts, lymphocytes, and mast cells are usually present
- May be background of conventional or hypertrophic scar with smaller collagen bundles and perpendicular vessels

TOP DIFFERENTIAL DIAGNOSES

- Hypertrophic scar
- Desmoplastic melanoma
- Nodular fasciitis

Keloid

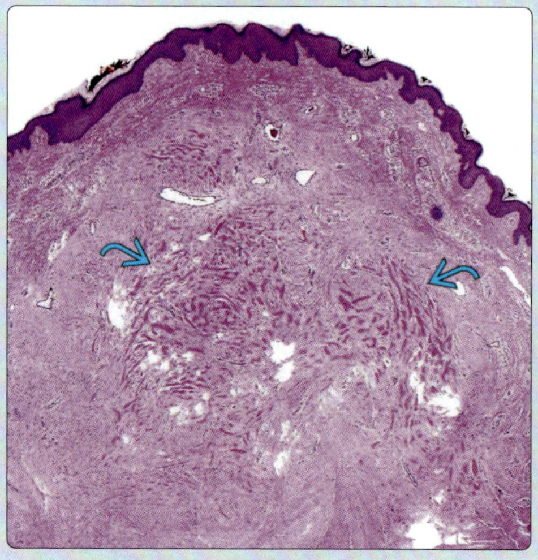

Low Magnification

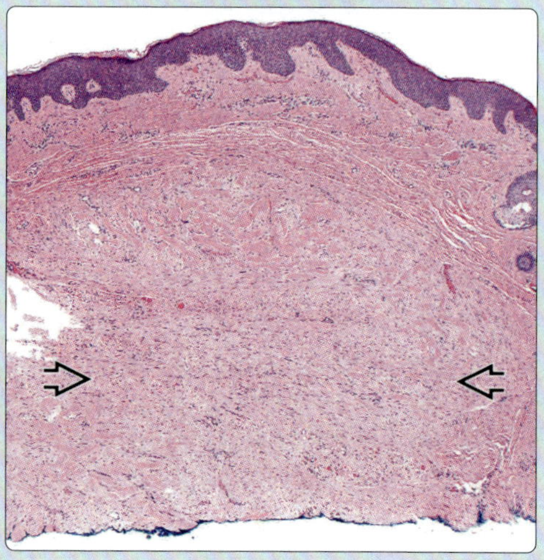

(Left) *This keloid forms a polypoid skin lesion and displays dense dermal collagen, especially in the center of the lesion. Note the mild epidermal hyperplasia. Commonly, the epidermis overlying a keloidal scar is atrophic-appearing.* **(Right)** *Keloids usually are dome-shaped or polypoid skin lesions, which show dense, thickened dermal collagen bundles, often with areas of hypertrophic scar. Note the overlying irregular epidermal hyperplasia in this example.*

Dense Dermal Scarring

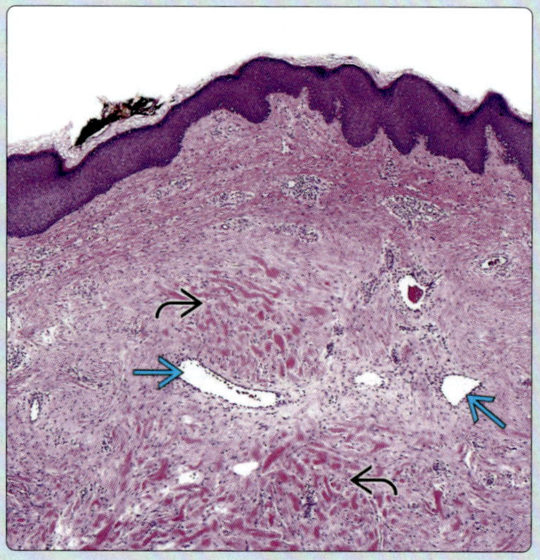

Ectatic Vessels

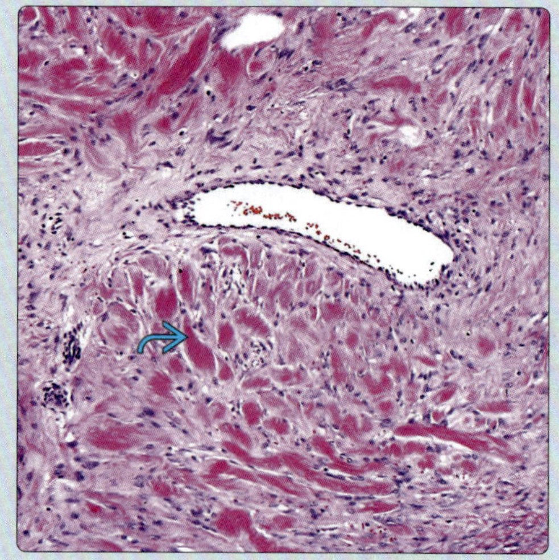

(Left) *Intermediate magnification shows the superficial aspects of a keloid. Note the dermal scarring with telangiectasia and prominent thickened, hyalinized-appearing collagen bundles.* **(Right)** *Higher magnification of the superficial portion of a keloid shows telangiectatic vessels surrounded by hyalinized, eosinophilic-staining collagen bundles.*

TERMINOLOGY

Synonyms

- Scar with keloidal collagen

Definitions

- Reactive/reparative proliferation with prominent thickened and hyalinized, eosinophilic-staining bundles of collagen extending beyond original biopsy/wound site

ETIOLOGY/PATHOGENESIS

Unknown, Possibly Genetic

- Fibroblasts from keloids show decreased apoptosis
- Many cytokines implicated in stimulating fibroblasts, including TNF-α, TGF-β1, IL-1α, IL-1β, IL-6, IL-15

CLINICAL ISSUES

Epidemiology

- Age
  - Most common in patients < 30 years
- Ethnicity
  - More common in black patients; least common in white patients

Site

- Earlobe is most common site
  - Typically follows ear piercing or other trauma by a few months

Presentation

- Mass lesion most common
- Scar that grows beyond confines of original wound
- Often erythematous, pruritic lesions with predilection for earlobe in black patients
- Potentially disfiguring

Treatment

- Surgical approaches
  - Complete excision, accompanied by concurrent steroid injections or radiotherapy to decrease risk of recurrence
- Drugs
  - Direct injection of steroids is often 1st-line treatment

Prognosis

- Persistence and recurrence are common, but there is no risk of malignancy

MACROSCOPIC

General Features

- Large, nodular, dermal-based lesion with firm, white cut surface

MICROSCOPIC

Histologic Features

- Dense proliferation of thickened, hyalinized collagen bundles in dermis
- May be background of conventional or hypertrophic scar with smaller collagen bundles and perpendicular vessels
- Decreased vessels compared to conventional and hypertrophic scars
  - Superficial telangiectatic vessels often present
  - Associated with mild, chronic inflammation
- Overlying epidermis may show atrophy or acanthosis
- Increased fibroblasts, lymphocytes, and mast cells are usually present

DIFFERENTIAL DIAGNOSIS

Hypertrophic Scar

- Lacks characteristic hyalinized collagen bundles of keloid
- Has more small, perpendicularly oriented vessels; lacks telangiectasia
- Overlapping cases often seen; may be diagnosed as hypertrophic scar with keloidal collagen
- Clinically not as elevated as keloid

Desmoplastic Melanoma

- Unlikely but rarely may enter differential diagnosis if no history of trauma or previous biopsy/surgery
- Reexcision specimens of desmoplastic melanoma may show keloidal collagen
- Usually S100(+)
  - Pitfall: Increased numbers of S100(+) dermal dendritic cells may be seen in scars
    - Should not show spindled morphology of desmoplastic melanoma cells

Nodular Fasciitis

- May rarely show focal keloidal collagen
- Background shows classic features of nodular fasciitis with loose, tissue culture appearance, mucin, and vessels
- Zonation with cellular, myxoid, and more fibrous areas

DIAGNOSTIC CHECKLIST

Pathologic Interpretation Pearls

- Nodular, elevated lesion compared to adjacent skin
- Thickened, hyalinized, eosinophilic collagen bundles
- Often see background of hypertrophic scar

SELECTED REFERENCES

1. Chen ZY et al: The mechanisms of β-catenin on keloid fibroblast cells proliferation and apoptosis. Eur Rev Med Pharmacol Sci. 22(4):888-95, 2018
2. Lee HJ et al: Recent understandings of biology, prophylaxis and treatment strategies for hypertrophic scars and keloids. Int J Mol Sci. 19(3):E711, 2018
3. Zhong L et al: Identification and integrated analysis of microRNA expression profiles in keloid. J Cosmet Dermatol. 17(5):917-24, 2018
4. Shi C et al: The pivotal role of inflammation in scar/keloid formation after acne. Dermatoendocrinol. 9(1):e1448327, 2017
5. Halim AS et al: Keloid scarring: understanding the genetic basis, advances, and prospects. Arch Plast Surg. 39(3):184-9, 2012
6. Iqbal SA et al: Identification of fibrocytes from mesenchymal stem cells in keloid tissue: a potential source of abnormal fibroblasts in keloid scarring. Arch Dermatol Res. 304(8):665-71, 2012
7. Shih B et al: Comparative genomic hybridisation analysis of keloid tissue in Caucasians suggests possible involvement of HLA-DRB5 in disease pathogenesis. Arch Dermatol Res. 304(3):241-9, 2012
8. Zhang G et al: Analyses of CDC2L1 gene mutations in keloid tissue. Clin Exp Dermatol. 37(3):277-83, 2012
9. Gauglitz GG et al: Hypertrophic scarring and keloids: pathomechanisms and current and emerging treatment strategies. Mol Med. 17(1-2):113-25, 2011
10. Wolfram D et al: Hypertrophic scars and keloids–a review of their pathophysiology, risk factors, and therapeutic management. Dermatol Surg. 35(2):171-81, 2009
11. Butler PD et al: Current progress in keloid research and treatment. J Am Coll Surg. 206(4):731-41, 2008
12. Köse O et al: Keloids and hypertrophic scars: are they two different sides of the same coin? Dermatol Surg. 34(3):336-46, 2008

Nuchal-Type Fibroma

KEY FACTS

TERMINOLOGY

- Benign pseudotumor composed of abundant collagen and showing predilection for posterior neck

ETIOLOGY/PATHOGENESIS

- Up to 1/2 of patients with nuchal-type fibroma also have diabetes

CLINICAL ISSUES

- Most common in young to middle-aged adults (20-50 years)
  - Rare in children
  - Strong male predominance
- Posterior neck region most common
  - Infrequently arises in upper back area, extremities, face
- Treatment: Simple surgical excision
- Local recurrence common

MACROSCOPIC

- Poorly delineated, firm mass
- Mean size: 3 cm

MICROSCOPIC

- Poorly circumscribed, unencapsulated
- Arises in dermis and subcutaneous tissue
- Abundant haphazardly arranged thickened collagen bundles
  - Elastic fibers present but often scant
- Markedly hypocellular, with scant admixed bland spindle cells
- Entrapment of mature adipose tissue, nerve twigs, and cutaneous adnexal structures

TOP DIFFERENTIAL DIAGNOSES

- Gardner fibroma
- Nuchal fibrocartilaginous pseudotumor
- Elastofibroma
- Fibrolipoma
- Solitary fibrous tumor

Nuchal-Type Fibroma

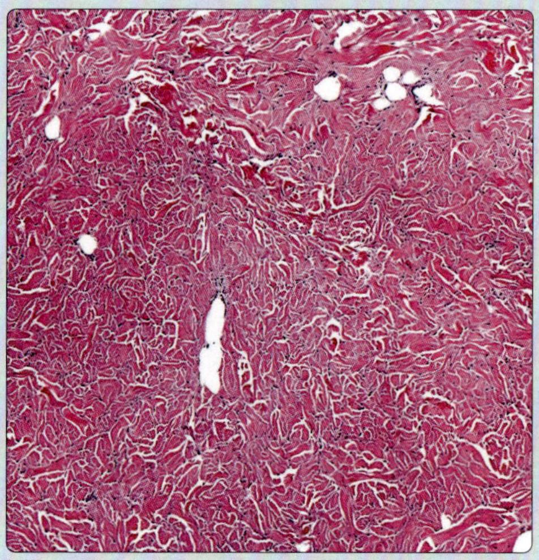

Poor Margination

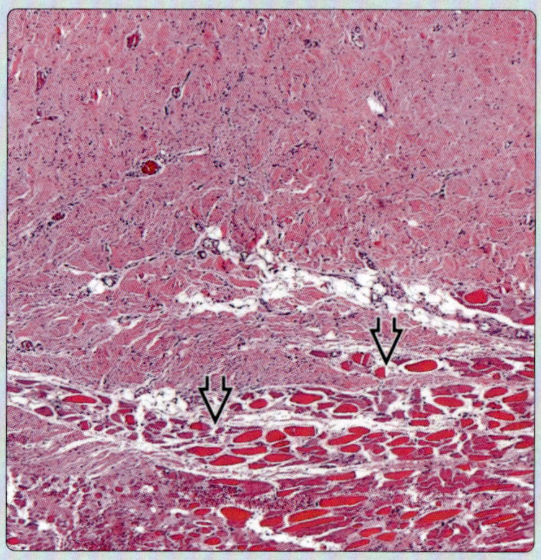

(Left) *Nuchal-type fibroma (NTF) is a benign pseudotumor of young to middle-aged adults that shows a predilection for the posterior neck. At low power, it appears as a paucicellular lesion composed predominantly of abundant thick collagen bundles.* **(Right)** *Most cases of NTF are poorly marginated and often show an irregular or infiltrative interface with the surrounding dermis, subcutaneous fat, and underlying skeletal muscle ⇨.*

Abundant Thick Collagen Bundles

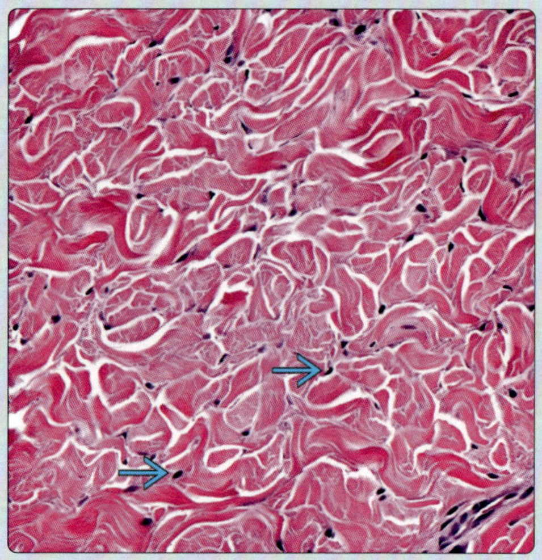

Entrapment of Adipose Tissue, Vessels, and Nerves

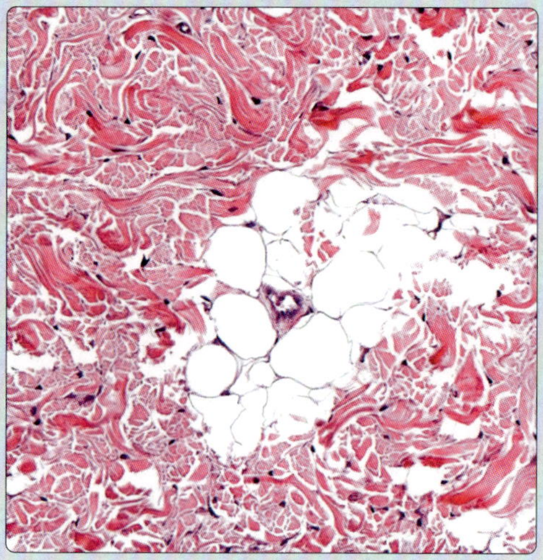

(Left) *Hypocellularity is the rule in NTF, and the lesion is composed of thick bundles of collagen with scattered bland fibroblastic spindle cells (often only identifiable by their nuclei ➡).* **(Right)** *Entrapment of normal structures and tissue is a frequent finding in NTF. This image shows mature adipose tissue (most common), but blood vessels and nerve twigs are also seen with some regularity.*

Nuchal-Type Fibroma

TERMINOLOGY

Abbreviations

- Nuchal-type fibroma (NTF)

Synonyms

- Nuchal fibroma
- Collagenosis nuchae

Definitions

- Benign pseudotumor composed of abundant collagen and showing predilection for posterior neck

ETIOLOGY/PATHOGENESIS

Disease Association

- Up to 1/2 of patients with NTF also have diabetes
  - NTF histologically resembles scleroderma-like process seen in this disease

CLINICAL ISSUES

Epidemiology

- Incidence
  - Rare
- Age
  - Most commonly 20-50 years
  - Rare in children
- Sex
  - Strong male predominance

Site

- Posterior neck region most common
- Infrequently arises in upper back area
- Rare cases described in extremities and face

Presentation

- Solitary, painless mass
  - Rarely multifocal

Treatment

- Simple surgical excision

Prognosis

- Excellent
- Local recurrence common
- No metastasis or malignant transformation

MACROSCOPIC

General Features

- Poorly delineated, firm mass
- White-gray cut surface

Size

- Mean: 3 cm

MICROSCOPIC

Histologic Features

- Poorly circumscribed, unencapsulated
- Arises in dermis and subcutaneous tissue
  - Often superficially involves underlying skeletal muscle
- Abundant haphazardly arranged thickened collagen bundles
  - Bundles may appear to intersect
  - Elastic fibers present but often scant
- Markedly hypocellular, with scant admixed bland spindle cells
- Entrapment of mature adipose tissue, nerve twigs, and cutaneous adnexal structures

ANCILLARY TESTS

Immunohistochemistry

- CD34(+) in spindle cells
- Negative for SMA, desmin, and nuclear β-catenin

DIFFERENTIAL DIAGNOSIS

Gardner Fibroma

- Mainly affects children (< 10 years)
- Most associated with familial adenomatous polyposis/Gardner syndrome
- Nuclear β-catenin (+)

Nuchal Fibrocartilaginous Pseudotumor

- History of trauma often present
- Arises in nuchal ligament but involves surrounding soft tissues
- Fibrocartilaginous composition

Elastofibroma

- Predominantly arises near inferior border of scapula
- Contains dystrophic, "beaded" elastic fibers

Fibrolipoma

- Well-circumscribed lesion
- Abundant mature adipose tissue component
- Fibrocollagenous bands or septa

Solitary Fibrous Tumor

- Prominent ectatic "staghorn" vasculature
- More cellular than NTF
- Striking, diffuse CD34(+)

SELECTED REFERENCES

1. Gong Y et al: Nuchal-type fibroma of the shoulder: a case report and review of the literature. Oncol Lett. 11(6):4152-4, 2016
2. Kim DH et al: Multiple nuchal-type fibromas on the scalp: a case report. Ann Dermatol. 27(2):194-6, 2015
3. LeBlanc KG Jr et al: Multiple nuchal fibromas in a 2-year-old without Gardner syndrome. Pediatr Dermatol. 28(6):695-6, 2011
4. Samadi DS et al: Nuchal fibroma: a clinicopathological review. Ann Otol Rhinol Laryngol. 109(1):52-5, 2000
5. Laskin WB et al: Nuchal fibrocartilaginous pseudotumor: a clinicopathologic study of five cases and review of the literature. Mod Pathol. 12(7):663-8, 1999
6. Michal M et al: Nuchal-type fibroma: a clinicopathologic study of 52 cases. Cancer. 85(1):156-63, 1999
7. O'Connell JX et al: Nuchal fibrocartilaginous pseudotumor: a distinctive soft-tissue lesion associated with prior neck injury. Am J Surg Pathol. 21(7):836-40, 1997
8. Balachandran K et al: Nuchal fibroma. A clinicopathological study of nine cases. Am J Surg Pathol. 19(3):313-7, 1995

Palmar/Plantar Fibromatosis

KEY FACTS

TERMINOLOGY

- Locally infiltrative but nonmetastasizing fibroblastic proliferation arising from aponeurosis of hand or foot
  - Similar proliferations may occur on knuckles (knuckle pads) or penile shaft (Peyronie disease)
- Synonyms
  - Palmar fibromatosis: Dupuytren contracture
  - Plantar fibromatosis: Ledderhose disease

CLINICAL ISSUES

- Palmar: Palm of hand in middle-aged to older adults
- Plantar: Plantar aponeurosis in children to young adults
- Solitary or multiple firm nodules
- Treatment
  - Complete surgical excision of involved aponeurosis/fascia, if possible
  - Collagenase clostridium histolyticum injections are effective alternative
- Benign, but significant rate of local recurrence

MACROSCOPIC

- Usually < 3 cm

MICROSCOPIC

- Nodules of uniform, elongated, spindled fibroblasts in long, "sweeping" fascicles
  - Cellularity varies with age of lesion
- Variably collagenous stroma with compressed, thin-walled stromal vessels

ANCILLARY TESTS

- SMA(+), desmin (variable)
- Keratin (-), S100(-), CD34(-)

TOP DIFFERENTIAL DIAGNOSES

- Desmoid fibromatosis
- Leiomyoma
- Synovial sarcoma (monophasic)
- Malignant peripheral nerve sheath tumor

Palmar Fibromatosis

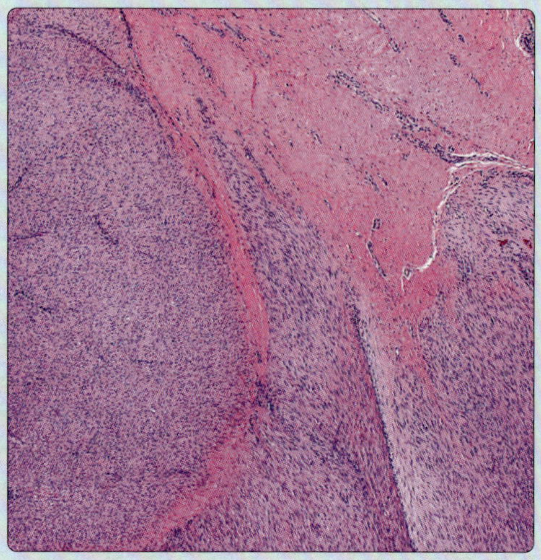

Bland Cytology

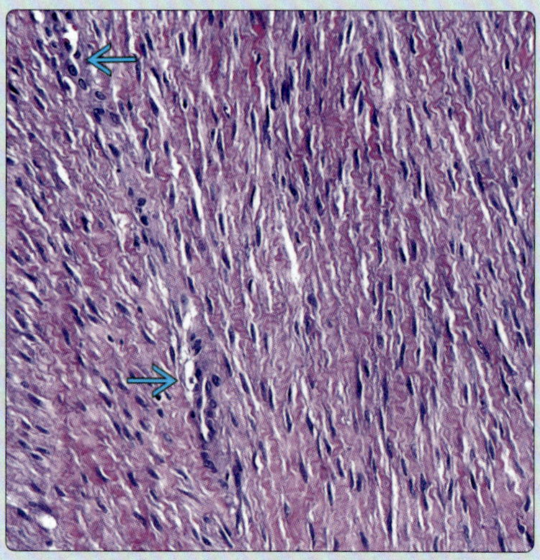

(Left) *Superficial fibromatosis is characterized by nodules and fascicles of uniform fibroblasts with a collagenous stroma. It most commonly arises in the palm of the hand or plantar aspect of the foot. Origin from fascia or aponeurosis may be histologically evident.* **(Right)** *All forms of superficial fibromatosis show uniformly bland, spindled fibroblastic cells with small nuclei. The cells are often plumper in earlier lesions, and older lesions contain more abundant collagen. Compressed vascular spaces ➡ are also common.*

Epithelioid Morphology

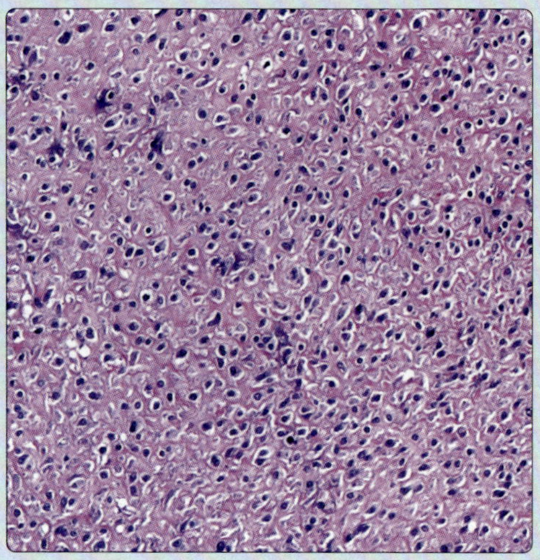

Plantar Fibromatosis

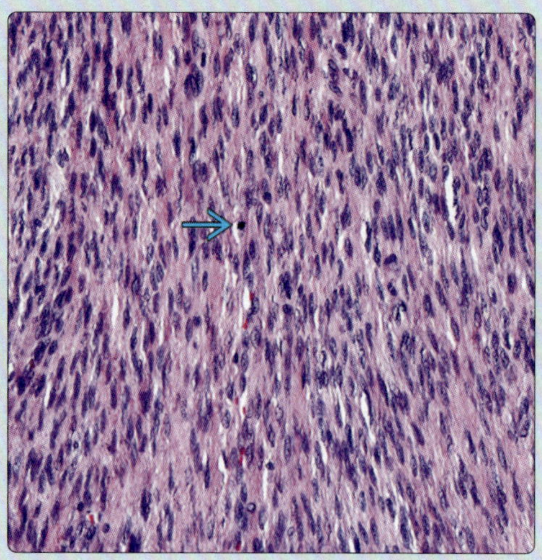

(Left) *It is important to note that the spindled fascicles of fibromatosis may appear epithelioid when viewed in cross section. Perinuclear clearing is often also evident in this morphology.* **(Right)** *Some cases of superficial fibromatosis may show alarming hypercellularity, particularly when in the foot (plantar). Mitoses ➡ may be present in any form of fibromatosis but are never atypical.*

TERMINOLOGY

Synonyms

- Aggressive fibromatosis
- Desmoid tumor
- Musculoaponeurotic fibromatosis

Definitions

- Intermediate (locally aggressive) but nonmetastasizing myofibroblastic neoplasm that is characterized by infiltrative growth and tendency toward local recurrence

CLINICAL ISSUES

Epidemiology

- Incidence
  - Less common than superficial (palmar/plantar) fibromatosis
  - Most are sporadic; 10% familial
- Age
  - Wide range (most common in young to middle-aged adults)
- Sex
  - Female predominance
    - Puberty to 40 years of age
  - Male = female
    - Later adulthood
    - Pediatric population

Site

- Extraabdominal
  - Shoulder, chest wall, back, thigh, head/neck
  - Anterior abdominal wall
- Intraabdominal
  - Mesentery, retroperitoneum, pelvis
- Very rare in hands and feet

Presentation

- Usually large, painless, slow-growing mass
- Abdominal wall fibromatosis classically occurs in pregnant women or within year following childbirth
- Intraabdominal fibromatosis
  - Asymptomatic, vague abdominal pain or symptoms related to adjacent organ involvement (small bowel, ureter, bladder, etc.)
  - ~ 50% of cases associated with prior trauma or surgical procedure
  - Mesenteric fibromatosis can occur within setting of familial adenomatous polyposis (FAP), Gardner syndrome
- May rarely arise in surgical scar (cicatricial fibromatosis)

Treatment

- Symptomatic tumors
  - Surgical excision with preservation of function
    - Reexcision of recurrences
    - Radiation, chemotherapy, hormone therapy ± NSAIDs for unresectable lesions
- Asymptomatic tumors may be followed clinically or treated medically to stabilize

Prognosis

- Benign; does not metastasize
- Prone to local recurrence
  - Higher risk associated with younger age, mesenteric or head/neck location, and particularly FAP/Gardner syndrome
- Rare deaths due to compromise of local vital structures

MACROSCOPIC

General Features

- Poorly circumscribed, firm
- Tan-white, gritty, fibrous or gelatinous cut surface

Size

- Variable range (usually 5-10 cm)
  - Intraabdominal tumors often > 10 cm

MICROSCOPIC

Histologic Features

- Majority of cases show infiltration of adjacent adipose tissue or skeletal muscle
- Uniform, spindled to stellate cells in long, "sweeping" fascicles or loose, vague storiform arrays
  - Small vesicular nuclei with 1 or several tiny nucleoli
  - Mitotic activity varies
  - Absence of nuclear pleomorphism and atypical mitotic figures
- Collagenous stroma
  - May appear sparse in cellular areas or abundant in hyalinized lesions
    - Some cases with keloidal collagen fibers
    - Heavily hyalinized tumors may show vague nodular growth
  - Occasional extensive myxoid or edematous stromal changes
    - Most common in mesenteric and pelvic tumors
    - Often associated with microhemorrhages and extravasated erythrocytes
- Small to medium-sized stromal blood vessels
  - Often show perivascular edema
  - Ectatic, thin-walled, staghorn or hemangiopericytoma-like vessels with perivascular hyalinization can be seen in intraabdominal tumors
- Metaplastic ossification or calcification rare

ANCILLARY TESTS

Immunohistochemistry

- SMA(+), MSA(+), focal desmin (+)
- CD34, h-caldesmon, S100 protein, CD117, STAT6 (-)
- Nuclear β-catenin (+) in ~ 75% of cases

Molecular Genetics

- Somatic mutations in β-catenin *CTNNB1* gene on 3p21 (sporadic tumors)
- Inactivating germline mutations in *APC* gene on 5q21-q22 (tumors in FAP/Gardner syndrome)

DIFFERENTIAL DIAGNOSIS

Low-Grade Myofibroblastic Sarcoma

- Highly infiltrative
- Most arise in head/neck or extremities
- Displays at least focal nuclear atypia
- Nuclear β-catenin (-)

Low-Grade Dedifferentiated Liposarcoma

- Most common in retroperitoneum
- May feature component of well-differentiated liposarcoma
- MDM2 (+) and CDK4 (+) by IHC
- *MDM2* amplification by FISH

Fibrous Scar

- Site of previous trauma or surgical procedure
  - Caveat: Rare cases of fibromatosis arise in scar tissue
- Usually lacks infiltrative growth pattern
- Nuclear β-catenin (-)

Sclerosing Mesenteritis/Idiopathic Retroperitoneal Fibrosis

- Middle-aged to older adults
- Prominent chronic inflammatory component (particularly plasma cells), often with fat necrosis
- Less cellular and fascicular than fibromatosis
- Nuclear β-catenin (-)

Nodular Fasciitis

- May show morphologic overlap with highly myxoid fibromatosis
- Small, rapidly growing, well-circumscribed lesion
- Usually lacks long, "sweeping" fascicles
- Nuclear β-catenin (-)

Proliferative Fasciitis/Myositis

- Features enlarged, ganglion cell-like myofibroblasts
- Fasciitis background can mimic myxoid fibromatosis

Low-Grade Fibromyxoid Sarcoma

- Hypocellular collagenous zones with myxoid foci
- Usually lacks long, "sweeping" fascicles
- MUC4(+), rare focal SMA(+)
- *FUS* gene translocations

Gastrointestinal Stromal Tumor (Spindle Cell Type)

- Arises from muscularis propria of gastrointestinal tract
- Usually lacks long, "sweeping" fascicles
- CD117(+), DOG1(+), CD34(+)
- *KIT* or *PDGFRA* mutation

Inflammatory Myofibroblastic Tumor

- Mesentery common location in pediatric age group
- Usually abundant inflammatory cells (plasma cells, lymphocytes)
- ALK(+) or *ALK* gene rearrangments in 50%
- SMA(+), nuclear β-catenin (-)

Leiomyoma

- Well circumscribed, expansile
- Smooth muscle cytologic features
- SMA(+), desmin (+)
- Nuclear β-catenin (-)

Deep (Aggressive) Angiomyxoma

- May show morphologic overlap with highly myxoid pelvic desmoids
- Lacks fascicular growth seen in fibromatosis
- Desmin (+), CD34 (variable); nuclear β-catenin (-)

SELECTED REFERENCES

1. Bekers EM et al: Multifocal occurrence of extra-abdominal desmoid type fibromatosis - a rare manifestation. A clinicopathological study of 6 sporadic cases and 1 hereditary case. Ann Diagn Pathol. 35:38-41, 2018
2. Koike H et al: Is immunohistochemical staining for β-catenin the definitive pathological diagnostic tool for desmoid-type fibromatosis?: a multi-institutional study. Hum Pathol. ePub, 2018
3. Agaimy A et al: CTNNB1 (β-Catenin)-altered neoplasia: a review focusing on soft tissue neoplasms and parenchymal lesions of uncertain histogenesis. Adv Anat Pathol. 23(1):1-12, 2016
4. Carter JM et al: CTNNB1 mutations and estrogen receptor expression in neuromuscular choristoma and its associated fibromatosis. Am J Surg Pathol. 40(10):1368-74, 2016
5. Huss S et al: β-catenin (CTNNB1) mutations and clinicopathological features of mesenteric desmoid-type fibromatosis. Histopathology. 62(2):294-304, 2013
6. Barak S et al: Immunoreactivity for calretinin and keratins in desmoid fibromatosis and other myofibroblastic tumors: a diagnostic pitfall. Am J Surg Pathol. 36(9):1404-9, 2012
7. Bertani E et al: Recurrence and prognostic factors in patients with aggressive fibromatosis. The role of radical surgery and its limitations. World J Surg Oncol. 10:184, 2012
8. Bo N et al: Analysis of β-catenin expression and exon 3 mutations in pediatric sporadic aggressive fibromatosis. Pediatr Dev Pathol. 15(3):173-8, 2012
9. Cates JM et al: Morphologic and immunophenotypic analysis of desmoid-type fibromatosis after radiation therapy. Hum Pathol. 43(9):1418-24, 2012
10. Cates JM et al: Signal transduction pathway analysis in fibromatosis: receptor and nonreceptor tyrosine kinases. Hum Pathol. 43(10):1711-8, 2012
11. Dumont AG et al: A nonrandom association of gastrointestinal stromal tumor (GIST) and desmoid tumor (deep fibromatosis): case series of 28 patients. Ann Oncol. 23(5):1335-40, 2012
12. Kim T et al: Prevalence of the CTNNB1 mutation genotype in surgically resected fibromatosis of the breast. Histopathology. 60(2):347-56, 2012
13. Romero S et al: Role of tumor-associated macrophages and angiogenesis in desmoid-type fibromatosis. Virchows Arch. 461(2):117-22, 2012
14. Wang B et al: Infantile intracranial aggressive fibromatosis: report of two cases with a review of the literature. Pediatr Neurosurg. 48(3):181-6, 2012
15. Grabellus F et al: The prevalence of the c-kit exon 10 variant, M541L, in aggressive fibromatosis does not differ from the general population. J Clin Pathol. 64(11):1021-4, 2011
16. de Camargo VP et al: Clinical outcomes of systemic therapy for patients with deep fibromatosis (desmoid tumor). Cancer. 116(9):2258-65, 2010
17. Lacroix-Triki M et al: β-catenin/Wnt signalling pathway in fibromatosis, metaplastic carcinomas and phyllodes tumours of the breast. Mod Pathol. 23(11):1438-48, 2010
18. Lips DJ et al: The role of APC and beta-catenin in the aetiology of aggressive fibromatosis (desmoid tumors). Eur J Surg Oncol. 35(1):3-10, 2009
19. Lazar AJ et al: Specific mutations in the beta-catenin gene (CTNNB1) correlate with local recurrence in sporadic desmoid tumors. Am J Pathol. 173(5):1518-27, 2008
20. Deyrup AT et al: Estrogen receptor-beta expression in extraabdominal fibromatoses: an analysis of 40 cases. Cancer. 106(1):208-13, 2006
21. Heinrich MC et al: Clinical and molecular studies of the effect of imatinib on advanced aggressive fibromatosis (desmoid tumor). J Clin Oncol. 24(7):1195-203, 2006
22. Bhattacharya B et al: Nuclear beta-catenin expression distinguishes deep fibromatosis from other benign and malignant fibroblastic and myofibroblastic lesions. Am J Surg Pathol. 29(5):653-9, 2005
23. Montgomery E et al: Beta-catenin immunohistochemistry separates mesenteric fibromatosis from gastrointestinal stromal tumor and sclerosing mesenteritis. Am J Surg Pathol. 26(10):1296-301, 2002
24. Montgomery E et al: Superficial fibromatoses are genetically distinct from deep fibromatoses. Mod Pathol. 14(7):695-701, 2001
25. Burke AP et al: Intra-abdominal fibromatosis. A pathologic analysis of 130 tumors with comparison of clinical subgroups. Am J Surg Pathol. 14(4):335-41, 1990
26. Burke AP et al: Mesenteric fibromatosis. A follow-up study. Arch Pathol Lab Med. 114(8):832-5, 1990

Characteristic Vasculature

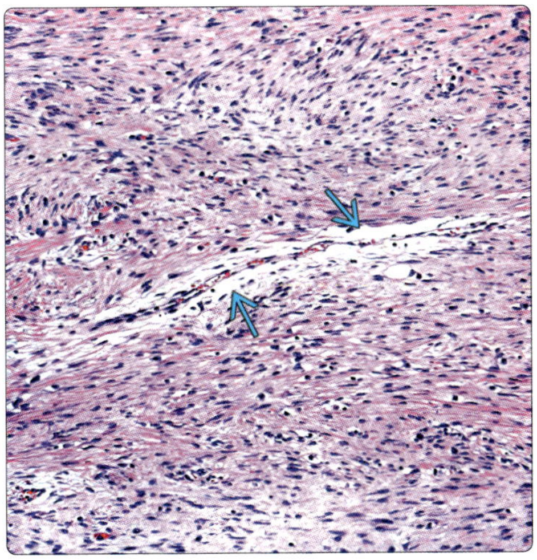

Haphazard Cellular Arrangement

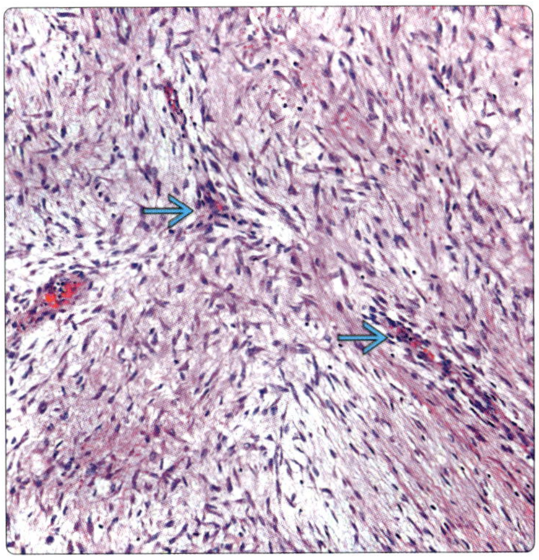

(Left) *The stromal blood vessels of fibromatosis are often elongated and compressed between lesional fascicles. It is common to see a slight rim of perivascular clearing (edema ➔) that may contain scattered chronic inflammatory cells.* **(Right)** *In some foci of desmoid fibromatosis, the cellular organization is less fascicular and storiform and more haphazard. This appearance is more common in myxedematous areas. Note the characteristic vessels ➔ with mild perivascular edema.*

Stromal Myxoid Change

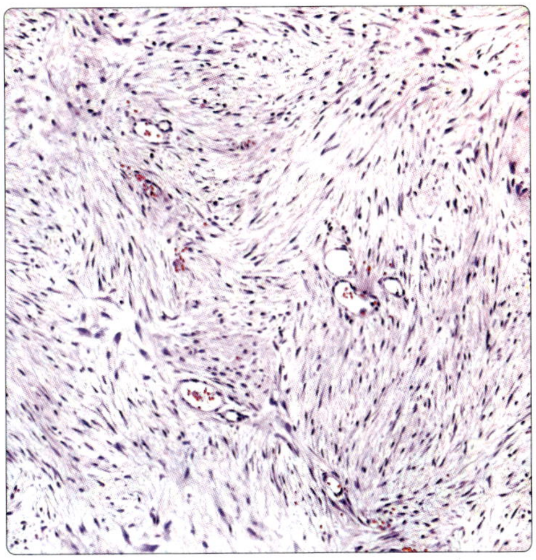

Fasciitis-Like Morphology

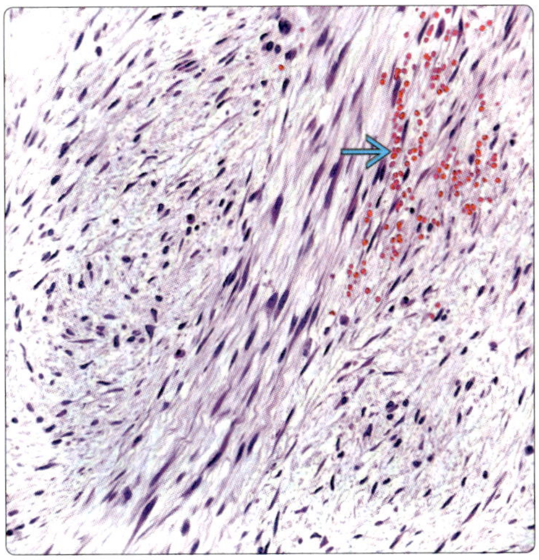

(Left) *Myxoid or edematous stromal change is not uncommon in desmoid fibromatosis and varies from focal to diffuse. This change is particularly common in mesenteric lesions.* **(Right)** *Extensive myxoid stromal change and a loose arrangement of lesional cells may impart an appearance similar to nodular fasciitis or inflammatory myofibroblastic tumor. Extravasated erythrocytes ➔ further add to the morphologic overlap.*

Stellate Cells

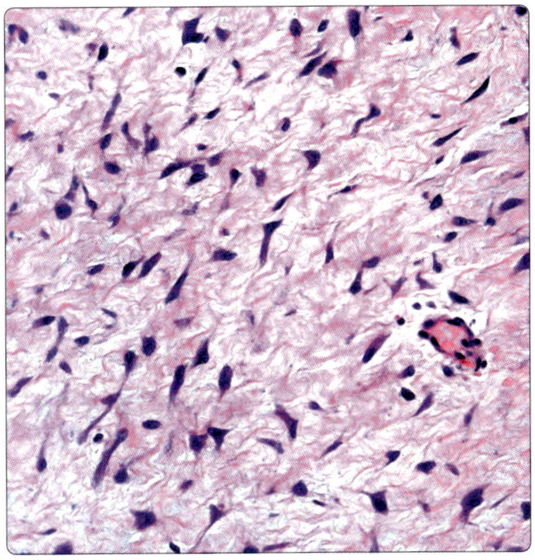

Myxocollagenous Stroma

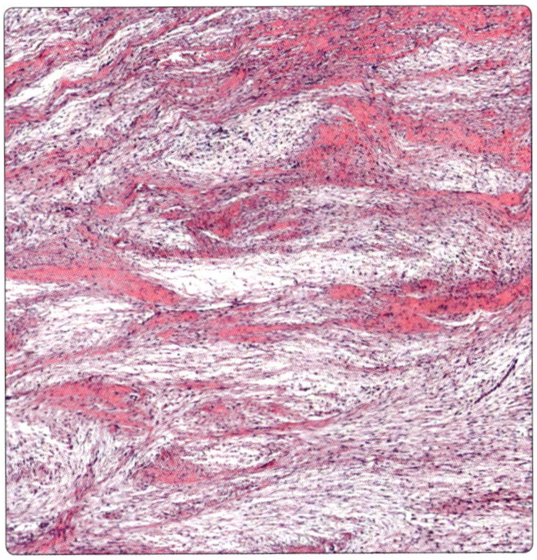

(Left) *In some myxedematous cases of desmoid fibromatosis, the lesional cells appear stellate as well as spindled. In hypocellular examples, this morphology may resemble desmoplastic fibroblastoma.* **(Right)** *Occasional cases of desmoid fibromatosis show alternating or swirling collagenous and myxedematous layers. This low-power appearance may raise concerns for low-grade fibromyxoid sarcoma.*

Epithelioid Cytomorphology

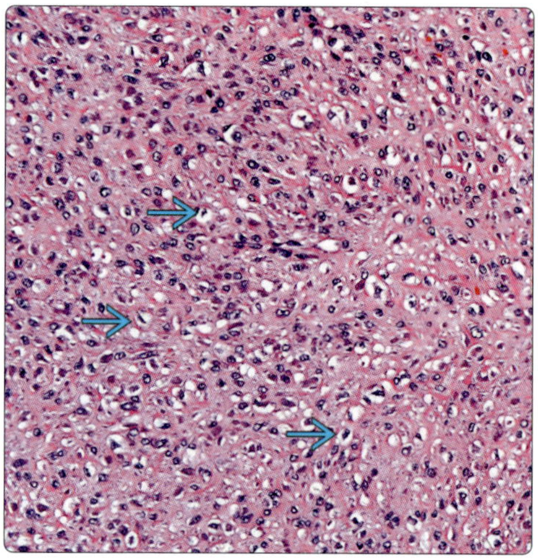

Large, Ectatic Blood Vessels

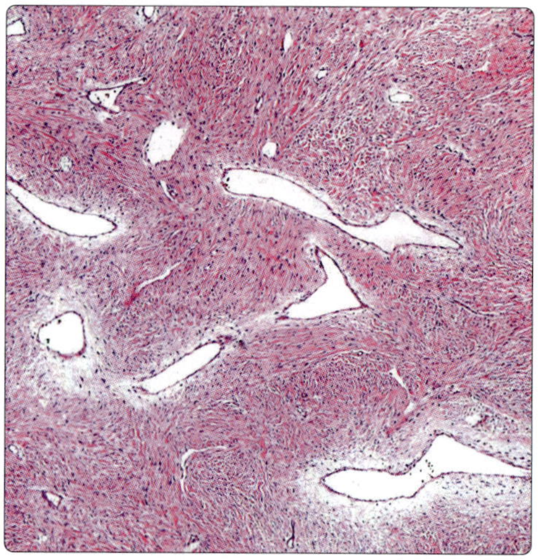

(Left) *Similar to superficial forms of fibromatosis, in desmoid tumors, an epithelioid morphology may be apparent if spindled fascicles are cut and viewed in cross section. A perinuclear rim of clearing* → *is often also seen in many of the cells.* **(Right)** *Dilated staghorn or hemangiopericytoma-like stromal vessels with perivascular hyalinization may be seen in desmoid fibromatosis, particularly intraabdominal tumors. This finding may be quite prominent in some cases.*

Sclerotic Stroma

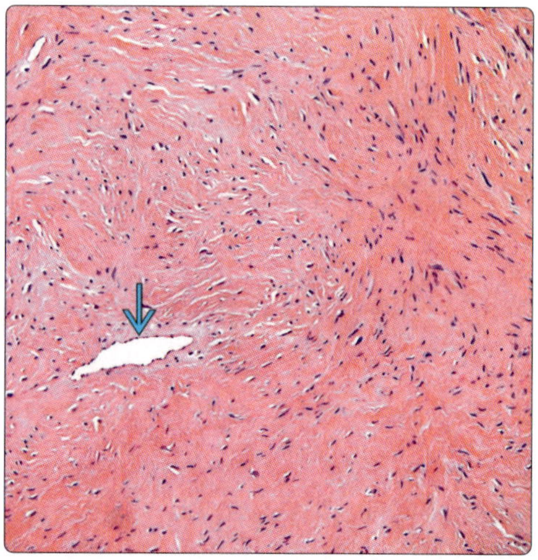

Vague Nodular Growth

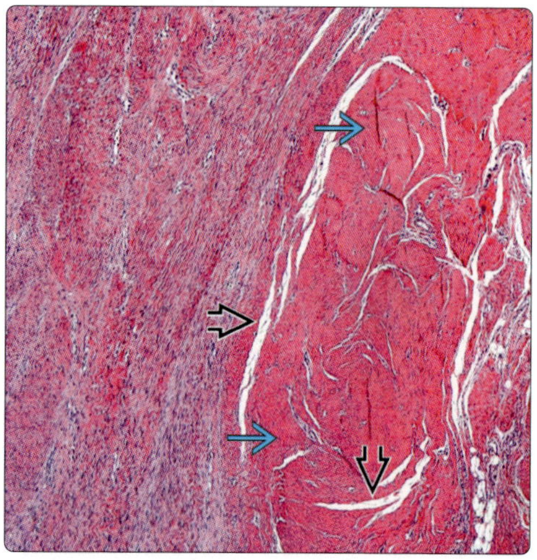

(Left) *Extensive stromal hyalinization or sclerosis may be seen in desmoid fibromatosis. These cases are often very hypocellular. Note the dilated blood vessel* →. **(Right)** *In addition to characteristic "streaming" fascicular growth, some cases of desmoid fibromatosis show formation of vague nodules* →. *The nodules are often highly collagenous and hypocellular and may show artifactual clefting* ⇨.

Keloidal Collagen

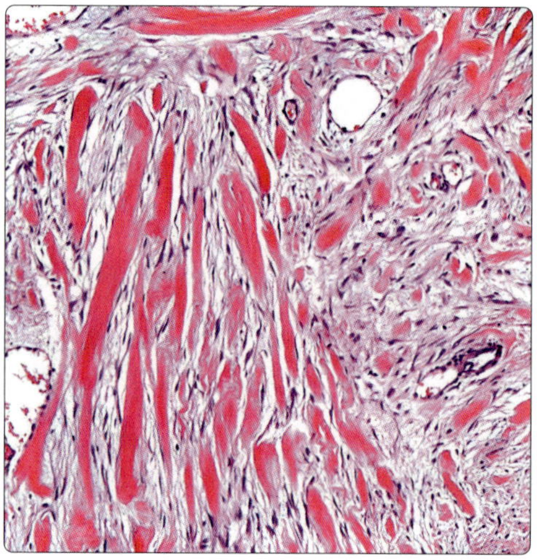

Stromal Microhemorrhage

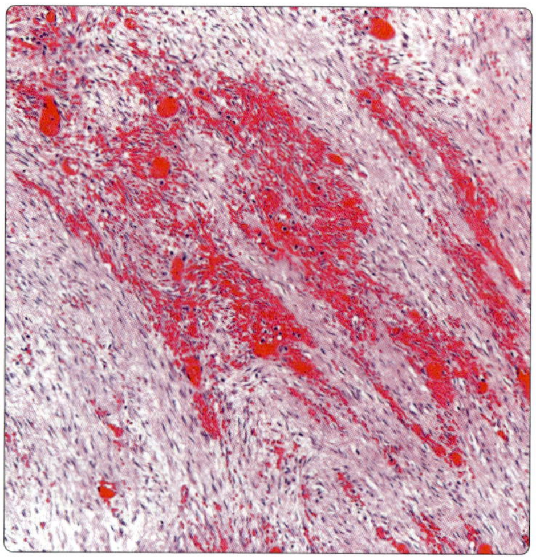

(Left) *Thick, glassy bundles of keloidal collagen are seen in some cases of desmoid fibromatosis. This finding is particularly common in intraabdominal tumors.* **(Right)** *Stromal microhemorrhages are a variable finding in desmoid fibromatosis. They are often focal and associated with myxoid stromal change but rarely may be somewhat prominent.*

Metaplastic Bone Formation

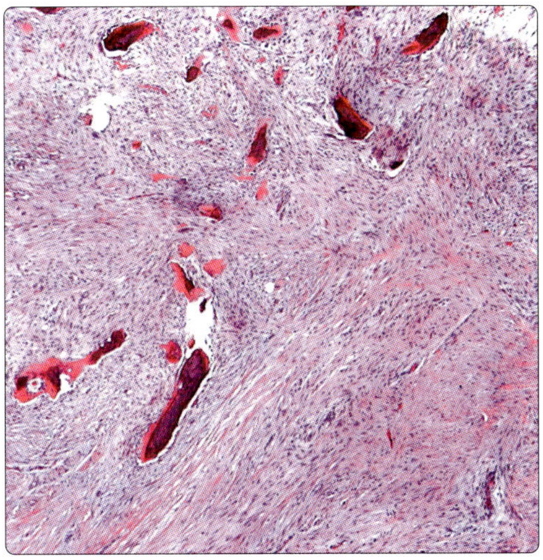

Infiltrative Growth

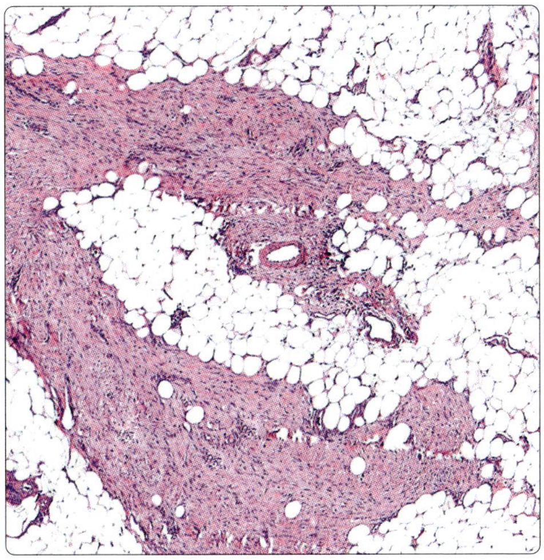

(Left) *Rare cases of desmoid fibromatosis contain focal stromal calcification or formation of metaplastic bone.* **(Right)** *Desmoid fibromatosis is generally a highly infiltrative and locally aggressive neoplasm. Depending upon the exact location of the tumor, infiltration of fat or muscle is often easily identified at the periphery.*

Infiltration of Fat and Skeletal Muscle

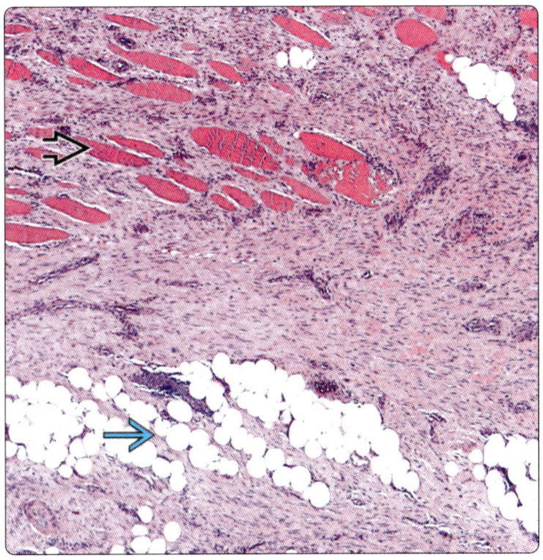

Entrapped Myocytes

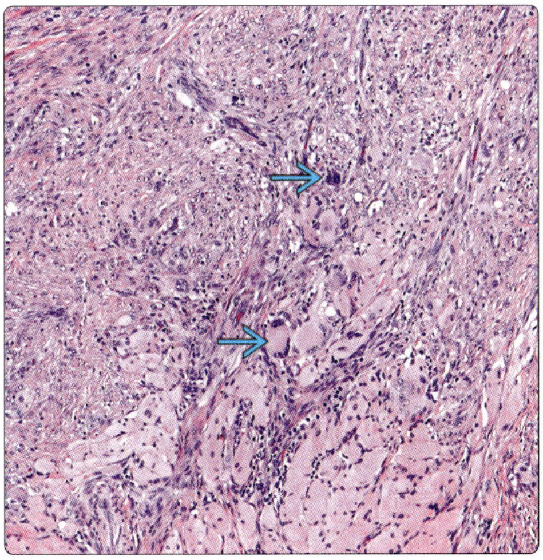

(Left) *H&E shows a desmoid tumor with extensive infiltration of both adipose tissue ➡ and skeletal muscle ➡. Note the checkerboard pattern of myoinfiltration in this case, a finding similar to what is usually seen in proliferative myositis.* **(Right)** *In intramuscular tumors, entrapped atrophic or regenerative skeletal muscle fibers may show compressed nuclei and mimic pleomorphic fibroblastic nuclei ➡. This phenomenon is similar to what can be seen in other intramuscular neoplasms.*

Wispy SMA Expression

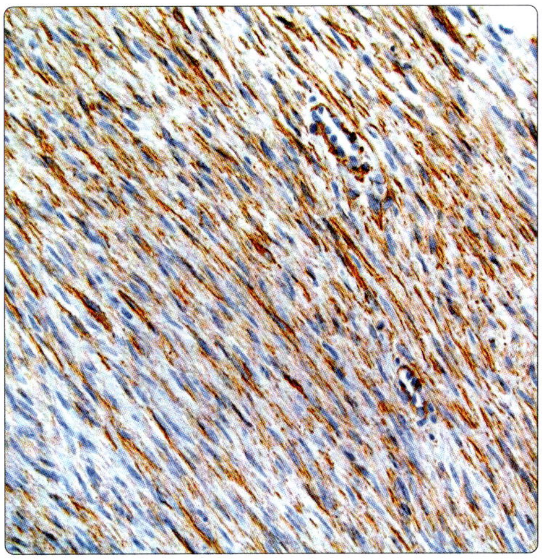

Nuclear β-Catenin Expression

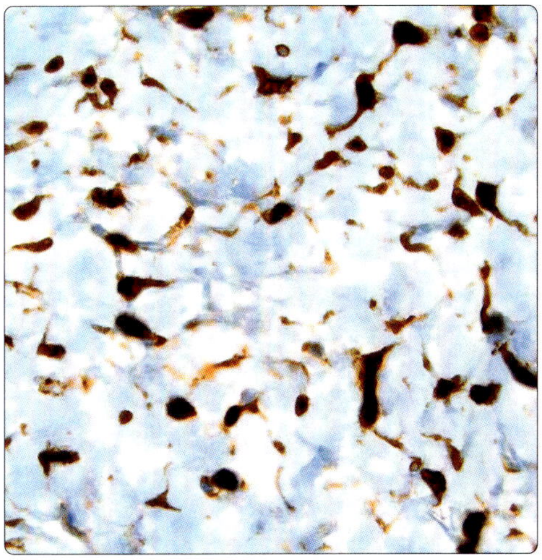

(Left) *SMA expression is common in desmoid fibromatosis and classically manifests as fine, "wispy" cytoplasmic positivity. This is in contrast to leiomyoma, which shows strong, diffuse cytoplasmic expression.* **(Right)** *Abnormal nuclear localization of β-catenin is seen in ~ 70% of cases of desmoid fibromatosis. Cytoplasmic expression is commonly seen in a variety of other tumors and is entirely nonspecific. Only nuclear expression counts in supporting the diagnosis.*

Dermatofibrosarcoma Protuberans

KEY FACTS

TERMINOLOGY

- Locally aggressive, low-grade, superficial fibroblastic sarcoma characterized in most cases by *COL1A1-PDGFB* gene fusion
  - May show progression to higher grade neoplasm with increased metastatic risk [fibrosarcomatous dermatofibrosarcoma protuberans (DFSP)]

CLINICAL ISSUES

- Young to middle-aged adults
- Most common in trunk and proximal extremities
- Persistent, slow-growing, plaque-like or protuberant nodular/multinodular cutaneous mass
- Treatment: Complete surgical excision with widely negative (2-3 cm) margins
- Local recurrences common (up to 50% of cases)
- Metastases extremely rare (< 0.5%)
  - 10-15% risk in tumors with fibrosarcomatous changes

MICROSCOPIC

- Diffuse infiltration of dermis and subcutis
  - Honeycomb pattern of fat infiltration
- Uniform spindled cells characteristically arranged in storiform or whorled growth pattern
- Variable myxoid stromal change
- Fibrosarcomatous DFSP
  - More cellular zones with fascicular growth
  - Increased cytologic atypia and mitotic activity

ANCILLARY TESTS

- Diffuse CD34(+)
- *COL1A1-PDGFB* fusion in most cases
  - Subset with *PDGFD* rearrangements

TOP DIFFERENTIAL DIAGNOSES

- Dermatofibroma (fibrous histiocytoma)
- Perineurioma
- Deep benign fibrous histiocytoma

(Left) *Dermatofibrosarcoma protuberans (DFSP) is a distinctive, superficial, low-grade sarcoma with a tendency toward local recurrence. It is characterized clinically by an exophytic, plaque-like or multinodular growth in most cases.* **(Right)** *At low magnification, DFSP often shows diffuse dermal and subcutaneous involvement with characteristic infiltration of subcutaneous fat ➡ by neoplastic cells that grow along fibrous septa ⇨.*

Dermatofibrosarcoma Protuberans

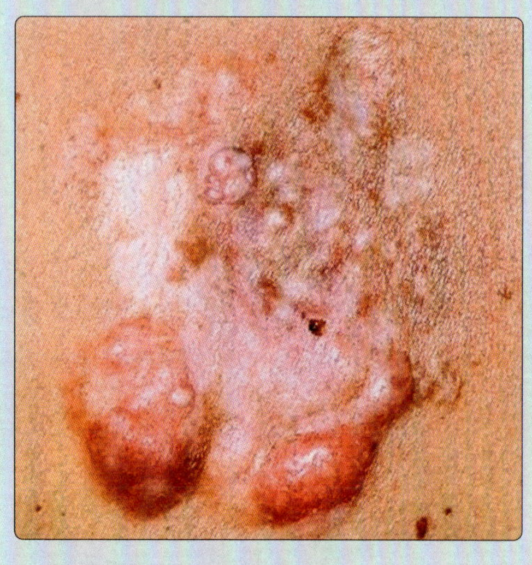

Infiltrative Growth Patterns

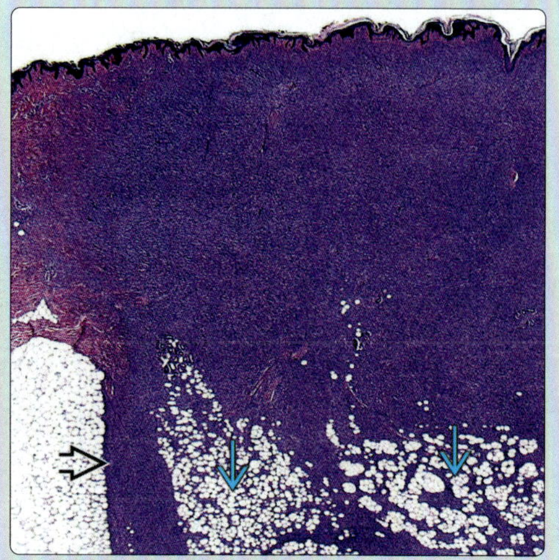

(Left) *Some cases of DFSP are more clearly nodular and multinodular, as depicted; however, infiltrative properties are still readily apparent as evidenced by infiltration of subcutaneous fat ➡.* **(Right)** *A tight storiform or pinwheel growth pattern (tumor cells radiating or spiraling out from a common center) is highly characteristic of DFSP, although not pathognomonic.*

Nodular Pattern

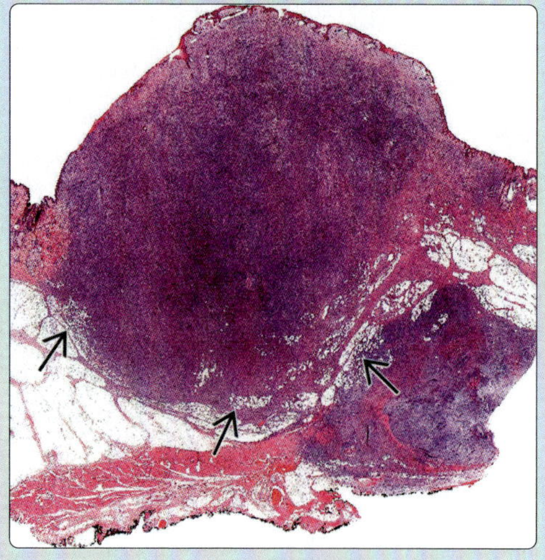

Storiform Architecture

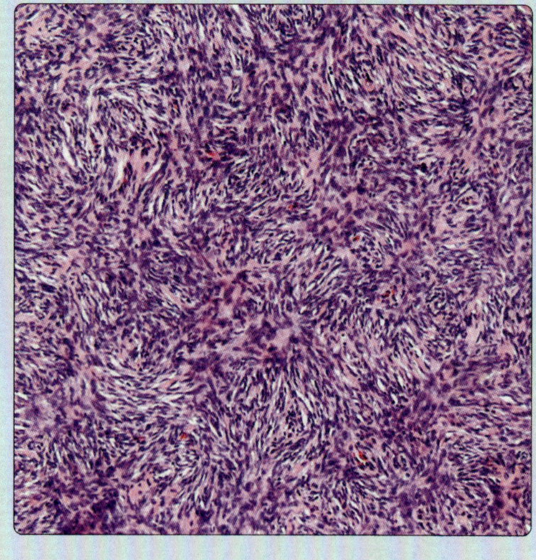

TERMINOLOGY

Abbreviations

- Dermatofibrosarcoma protuberans (DFSP)

Definitions

- Locally aggressive, low-grade, superficial fibroblastic sarcoma characterized in most cases by *COL1A1-PDGFB* gene fusion
  - May show progression to higher grade neoplasm with increased metastatic risk fibrosarcomatous DFSP

CLINICAL ISSUES

Epidemiology

- Incidence
  - Overall rare (< 1% of all sarcomas)
    - However, most common dermal sarcoma
- Age
  - Most common in young to middle-aged adults
    - May also occur in children (including congenitally) or elderly
- Sex
  - Slight male predominance

Site

- Most common in trunk (chest, back, shoulder, abdominal wall) and proximal extremities
- Also head/neck and distal extremities
- Rare in genital areas

Presentation

- Persistent, slow-growing, protuberant, nodular or multinodular cutaneous mass
  - Can show rapid growth within setting of fibrosarcomatous transformation
  - Rapid growth also seen in pregnancy
- Early lesions may appear flat and plaque-like

Treatment

- Complete surgical excision with widely negative margins
  - 2- to 3-cm margins recommended
  - Mohs surgery can significantly reduce local recurrence with less tissue loss
- Radiotherapy may be used for margin-positive, unresectable disease
- Treatment with imatinib and other tyrosine kinase inhibitors in advanced, fibrosarcomatous, and metastatic cases

Prognosis

- Local recurrences common (up to 50% of cases) if not completely excised
  - Can recur multiple times
- Metastases extremely rare (< 0.5%)
- Tumors with fibrosarcomatous progression
  - Similar recurrence risk as conventional DFSP
  - Distant metastases in 10-15%

MACROSCOPIC

General Features

- Indurated dermal plaque with nodularities
  - Multiple protuberances are often seen in recurrent cases
- Firm, gray-white cut surface
- Usually no tumor necrosis
- Rare tumors arise in subcutaneous tissue

Size

- Wide size range (average: 5 cm)
  - May grow to considerable sizes

MICROSCOPIC

Histologic Features

- Dermal-based, ill-defined proliferation
  - Diffuse infiltration of dermis and subcutis
    - Infiltration along fibrous connective tissue septa and into subcutaneous fat (honeycomb pattern)
    - Deeply growing or recurrent tumors may superficially infiltrate underlying fascia and skeletal muscle
    - Tumor cells encase, but do not destroy, cutaneous adnexal structures
    - Rare cases grow in linear, plaque-like fashion with less infiltration (atrophic DFSP or plaque-like DFSP)
  - Overlying skin is uninvolved
    - Uninvolved subepithelial layer of dermis (grenz zone) may or may not be present
  - Rare cases are confined to subcutaneous tissue with no dermal involvement
- Uniform spindled cells characteristically arranged in storiform or whorled growth pattern
  - Plump or elongated wavy nuclei
    - Minimal to mild nuclear atypia
    - Mitoses usually sparse (or < 5 mitoses per 10 HFP)
- Collagenous stroma containing small blood vessels
  - Rare cases show prominent vasculature
  - Myointimal proliferation may be seen in some vessels
    - When prominent and occlusive, appear as small nodules or "myoid balls"
- Variable myxoid stromal change
  - Rarely may be extensive (myxoid DFSP)
    - More nodular growth with accentuation of stromal vasculature
    - Prominent storiform growth often lost
    - Can mimic other low-grade myxoid neoplasms (especially neural)
- May contain scattered pigmented melanocytic cells
  - Described as pigmented DFSP or Bednar tumor
- Rare findings: Granular cytoplasmic change, bundled or braided growth pattern
- May show areas of giant cell fibroblastoma (GCFB) morphology
  - Pure DFSP may recur as pure GCFB and vice versa

Fibrosarcomatous Transformation

- Represents morphologic form of progression to higher grade tumor
  - Often intermediate grade; rarely high grade
- More frequently occurs de novo; rarely in local recurrence
  - May arise in any form or variant of DFSP
- Abrupt or gradual transformation from areas of conventional DFSP morphology to zones showing more cellular and fascicular architecture

- Herringbone pattern common
- Increased cytologic atypia and mitotic activity (> 5 per 10 HPF)
- Often nodular, expansile growth rather than infiltrative
- May show myxoid change or contain pigmented dendritic cells
- Necrosis may be present
- Rare high-grade pleomorphic morphology

ANCILLARY TESTS

Immunohistochemistry

- Diffuse CD34(+)
  - Often lost or decreased in areas of fibrosarcomatous transformation
- Negative for S100 protein, keratin, SMA, desmin
  - Myoid bundles are SMA(+)

Molecular Genetics

- Characteristic t(17;22)(q22;q13) leading to *COL1A1-PDGFB* fusion product
  - Identical rearrangement seen in GCFB
- Subset of *PDGFB*-fusion negative tumors contain *PDGFD* rearrangements
  - *COL6A3-PDGFD* and *EMILIN2-PDGFD* fusions reported

DIFFERENTIAL DIAGNOSIS

Dermatofibroma (Fibrous Histiocytoma)

- Particularly cellular and aneurysmal variants
- Often polymorphous cellular infiltrate
- Lacks diffuse honeycomb-like fat infiltration
- Lacks diffuse CD34 expression (peripheral positivity in some cellular variants)
- Lacks *COL1A1-PDGFB* fusion

Perineurioma

- Elongated tumor cells with thin, elongated cytoplasmic processes
- Lacks highly infiltrative growth of DFSP
- EMA(+), claudin-1 (+), GLUT-1(+)
- CD34(+) in many cases (focal to extensive)
- Lacks *COL1A1-PDGFB* fusion

Deep Benign Fibrous Histiocytoma

- Chronic inflammatory component
- Ectatic "staghorn" vasculature common
- Variable nuclear pleomorphism
- Lacks *COL1A1-PDGFB* fusion

Diffuse Neurofibroma

- Lacks prominent storiform pattern
- Presence of Meissner-like corpuscles is common
- S100 protein (+)
- Patchy to focal CD34(+)
- Lacks *COL1A1-PDGFB* fusion

Plaque-Like CD34(+) Dermal Fibroma

- Benign, superficial, plaque-like proliferation with medallion-like clinical appearance
- Tumor contains dilated venules and spares adnexal structures
- Lacks *COL1A1-PDGFB* fusion

Dermatomyofibroma

- Superficial, plaque-like dermal neoplasms
- Elongated spindled cells with myofibroblastic features
  - Cells oriented parallel to surface; no prominent storiform growth
- Increased number of small elastic fibers
- CD34(+), usually focal

Solitary Fibrous Tumor

- Predominantly arise in subcutaneous and deep soft tissues
- Generally well circumscribed and lacks infiltrative border with surrounding tissue
- Ectatic "staghorn" vasculature common
- CD34(+); STAT6(+)

Spindle Cell (Desmoplastic) Melanoma

- Often in actinically damaged skin in elderly patients
- Often associated with lentigo maligna
- Homogeneous expression of S100 protein

SELECTED REFERENCES

1. Dadone-Montaudié B et al: Alternative PDGFD rearrangements in dermatofibrosarcomas protuberans without PDGFB fusions. Mod Pathol. ePub, 2018
2. Dickson BC et al: Dermatofibrosarcoma protuberans with a novel COL6A3-PDGFD fusion gene and apparent predilection for breast. Genes Chromosomes Cancer. 57(9):437-45, 2018
3. Shah KK et al: Dermatofibrosarcoma protuberans of distal extremities and acral sites: a clinicopathologic analysis of 27 cases. Am J Surg Pathol. 42(3):413-9, 2018
4. Llombart B et al: Subcutaneous dermatofibrosarcoma protuberans, a rare subtype with predilection for the head: a retrospective series of 18 cases. J Am Acad Dermatol. 77(3):503-11.e1, 2017
5. Zhang Z et al: Application of COL1A1-PDGFB fusion gene detection by fluorescence in situ hybridization in biopsy tissue of dermatofibrosarcoma protuberans. J Dermatol. 44(7):798-802, 2017
6. Cesinaro AM et al: An unusual presentation of dermatofibrosarcoma protuberans with pleomorphic sarcomatous transformation: potential pitfall and diagnostic strategy. J Cutan Pathol. 43(7):589-93, 2016
7. Thway K et al: Dermatofibrosarcoma protuberans: pathology, genetics, and potential therapeutic strategies. Ann Diagn Pathol. 25:64-71, 2016
8. Santos-Briz A et al: Braided pattern in a dermatofibrosarcoma protuberans: a potential mimicker of neural neoplasms. Am J Dermatopathol. 36(11):920-4, 2014
9. Serra-Guillén C et al: Mohs micrographic surgery in dermatofibrosarcoma protuberans allows tumour clearance with smaller margins and greater preservation of healthy tissue compared with conventional surgery: a study of 74 primary cases. Br J Dermatol. ePub, 2014
10. Llombart B et al: Dermatofibrosarcoma protuberans: a comprehensive review and update on diagnosis and management. Semin Diagn Pathol. 30(1):13-28, 2013
11. Llombart B et al: Dermatofibrosarcoma protuberans: a clinicopathological, immunohistochemical, genetic (COL1A1-PDGFB), and therapeutic study of low-grade versus high-grade (fibrosarcomatous) tumors. J Am Acad Dermatol. 65(3):564-75, 2011
12. Llombart B et al: Dermatofibrosarcoma protuberans: clinical, pathological, and genetic (COL1A1-PDGFB) study with therapeutic implications. Histopathology. 54(7):860-72, 2009
13. Bague S et al: Dermatofibrosarcoma protuberans presenting as a subcutaneous mass: a clinicopathological study of 15 cases with exclusive or near-exclusive subcutaneous involvement. Am J Dermatopathol. 30(4):327-32, 2008
14. Reimann JD et al: Myxoid dermatofibrosarcoma protuberans: a rare variant analyzed in a series of 23 cases. Am J Surg Pathol. 31(9):1371-7, 2007
15. Terrier-Lacombe MJ et al: Dermatofibrosarcoma protuberans, giant cell fibroblastoma, and hybrid lesions in children: clinicopathologic comparative analysis of 28 cases with molecular data--a study from the French Federation of Cancer Centers Sarcoma Group. Am J Surg Pathol. 27(1):27-39, 2003

Uniform Cytologic Features

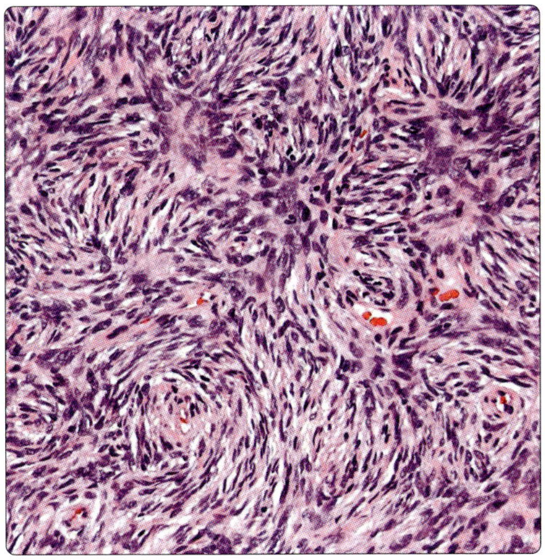

Cellular Storiform Pattern

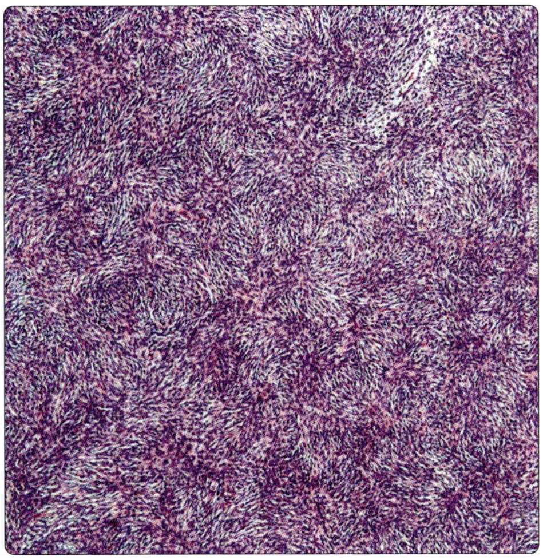

(Left) *All cases of DFSP are composed of uniform spindle cells with minimal to no nuclear atypia. Nuclei can appear wavy and suggest neural origin. Mitotic activity varies from sparse to no more than 5 figures per 10 HPF.* **(Right)** *Although many cases of DFSP show more than a single architectural pattern, some cases display only a repetitive, tight storiform growth pattern throughout the lesion, as depicted.*

Interstitial Collagen

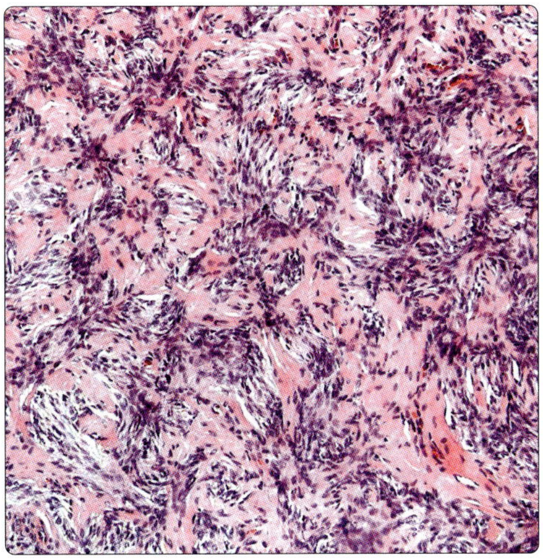

Interstitial Collagen

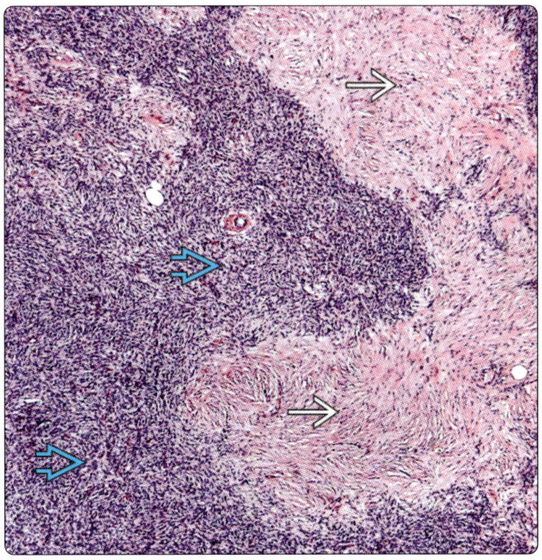

(Left) *The amount of interstitial collagen varies widely in DFSP. Some cases appear to have very little, and in others, like the case shown here, the collagen is more prominent. Note the underlying storiform architecture.* **(Right)** *More heavily collagenized areas ➡ may occasionally appear to interdigitate with more typical cellular areas ⇨ in DFSP.*

Subcutaneous Septal Growth

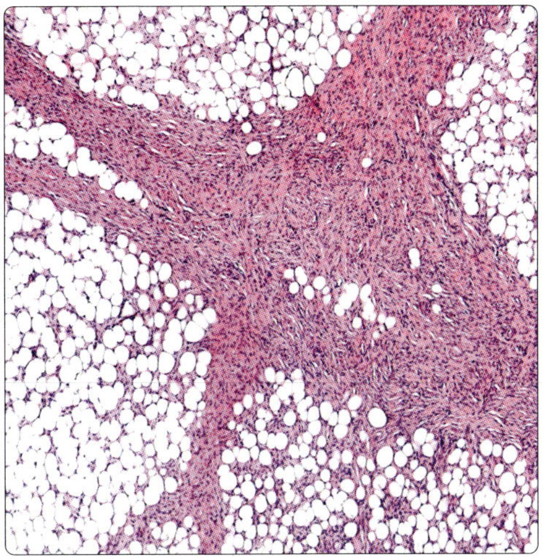

Honeycomb Fat Infiltration

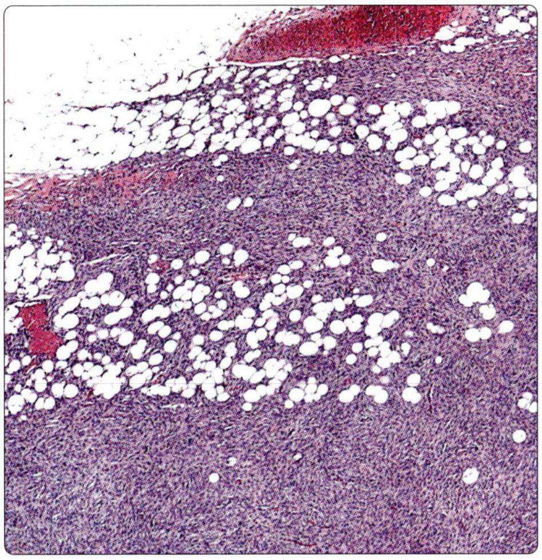

(Left) *Tumor cells in DFSP characteristically infiltrate along subcutaneous fibroconnective septa, as shown, and then out into the adipose tissue. Infiltration of adipose tissue is a nearly constant feature of this tumor.* **(Right)** *The tumor cells in DFSP not only grow around lobules of adipose tissue but also through them, usually with entrapment of single adipocytes. This overall appearance has been likened to a honeycomb pattern.*

(Left) *Fat infiltration may be impressively extensive in some cases of DFSP and may lead to confusion with diffuse-type neurofibroma, particularly on small biopsy.* **(Right)** *In some cases of DFSP, lobules of entrapped fat may contain many small atrophic adipocytes, closely simulating lipoblastic differentiation. Coupled with myxoid stroma, this finding may lead to confusion with myxoid liposarcoma.*

Fat Infiltration

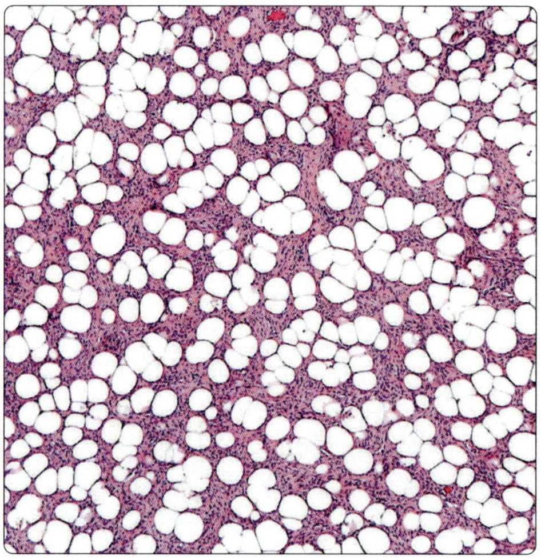

Pseudolipoblastic Entrapped Fat

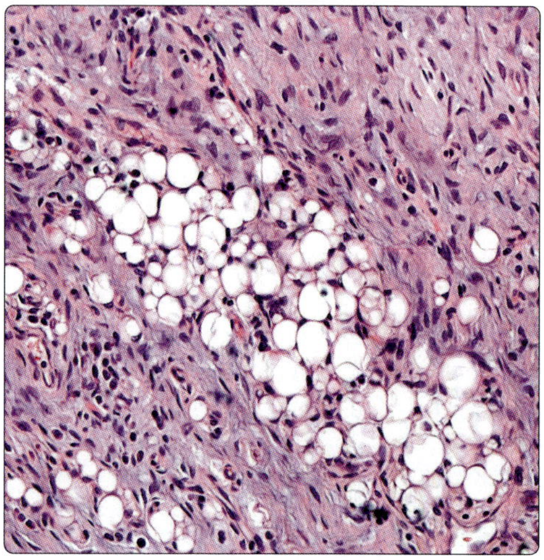

(Left) *Although a honeycomb pattern of fat infiltration is characteristic of DFSP, it is important to note that a similar pattern of skeletal muscle infiltration ➡ may be seen in deeply extending or recurrent tumors.* **(Right)** *As a testimony to its highly infiltrative nature, the tumor cells of DFSP are also commonly identified growing around and entrapping normal structures, such as nerve twigs ➡ and cutaneous adnexal structures (e.g., eccrine ducts) (not shown).*

Skeletal Muscle Infiltration

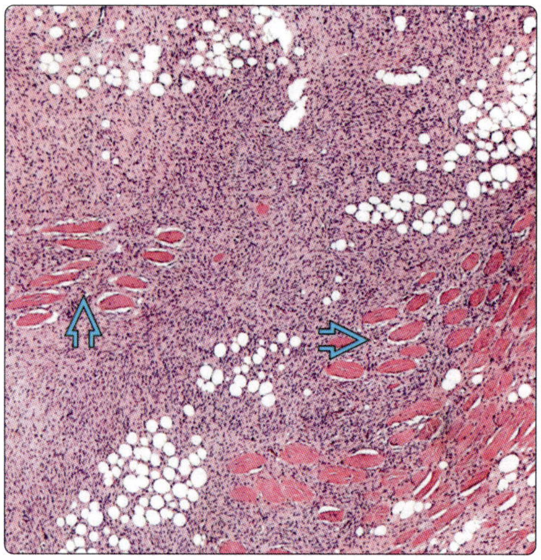

Entrapment of Normal Structures

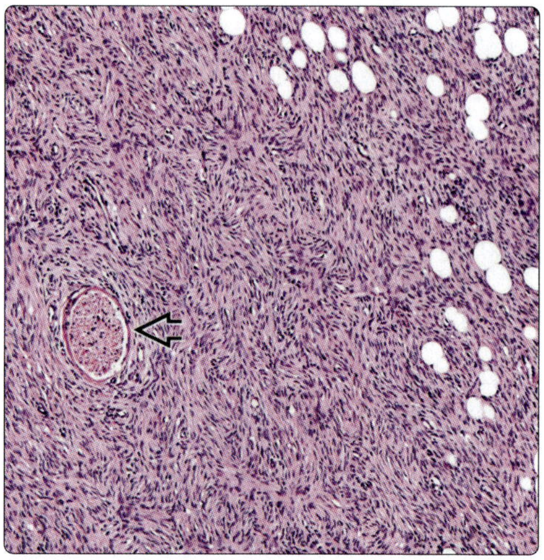

(Left) *Most cases of DFSP show a thin layer of uninvolved dermis ➡ (grenz zone) beneath the epidermis. In some cases, however, the tumor may appear to directly contact the surface.* **(Right)** *Infiltration of dermal collagen is not uncommon in DFSP and may lead to misdiagnosis as dermatofibroma (fibrous histiocytoma). More typical features of DFSP are usually present.*

Grenz Zone

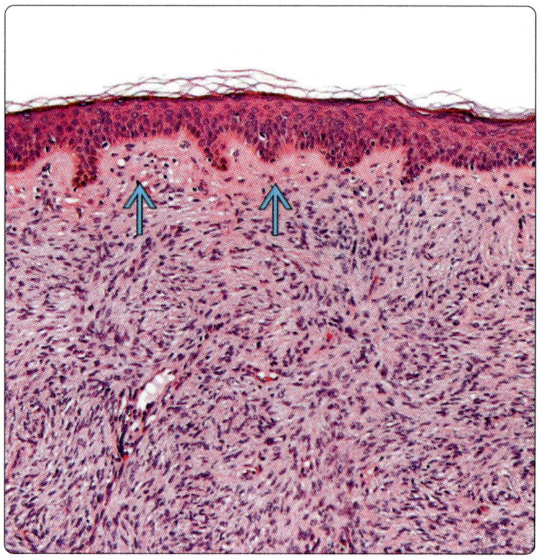

Infiltration of Dermal Collagen

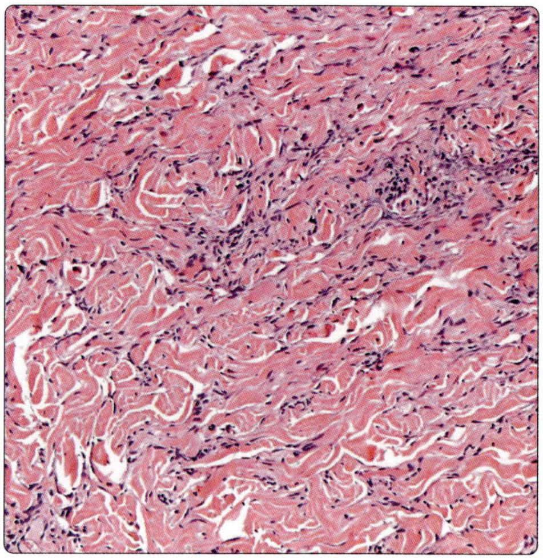

Less Prominent Storiform Growth

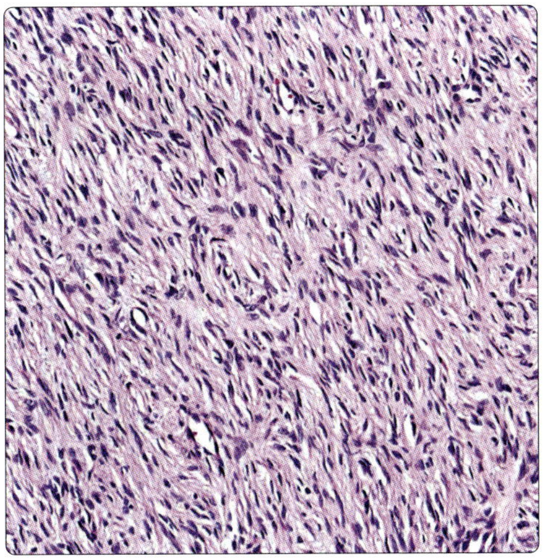

Rare Nuclear Palisading

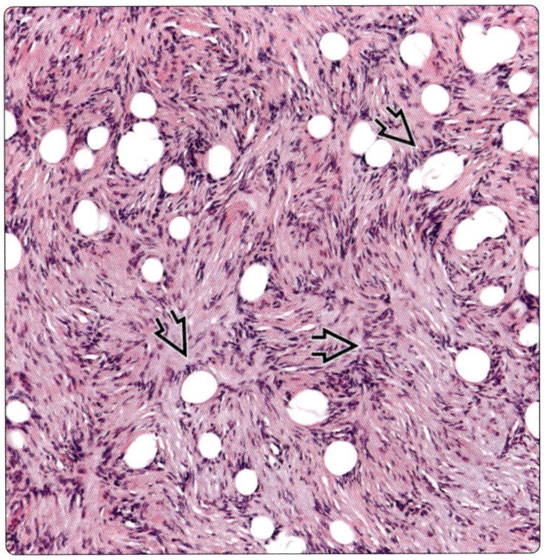

(Left) *Not uncommonly, storiform growth is less prominent in some areas of DFSP, and tumor cells may show a curly or lamellar growth. This finding is particularly common in the superficial (dermal) portion of the tumor.* **(Right)** *Nuclei appear to focally palisade ⇨ in this image of a collagenized DFSP. Nuclear palisading, however, is not a typical feature of DFSP and should lead to consideration of other entities first.*

Rare Bundled or Braided Growth

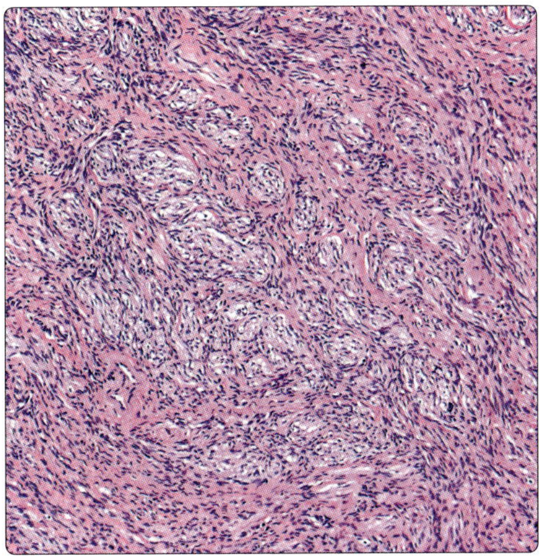

Rare Prominent Stromal Hyalinization

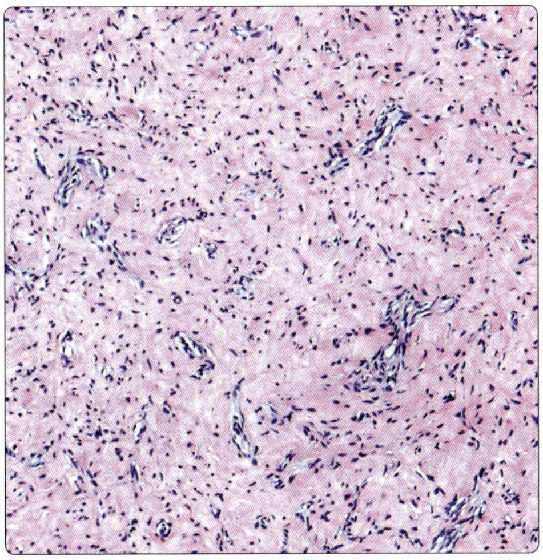

(Left) *A rare morphologic pattern in DFSP is that of intersecting or interwoven small bundles, cords, and nodules of tumor cells. This pattern may impart a neural appearance.* **(Right)** *In rare cases of DFSP, stromal collagenization or hyalinization is prominent and may leave little clue to the diagnosis; however, areas of more conventional morphology are usually present.*

Myoid Nodules

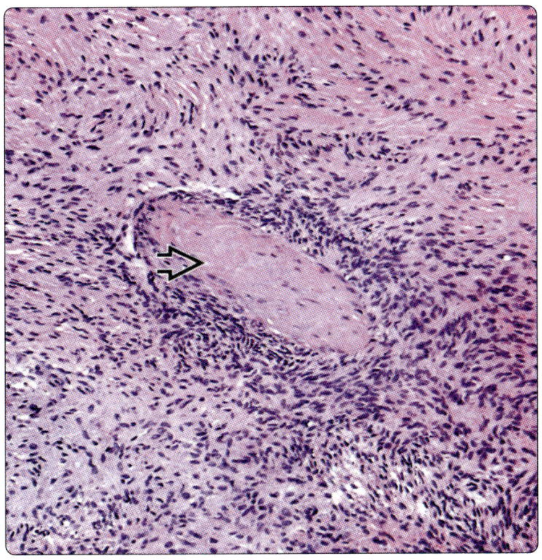

CD34 Expression

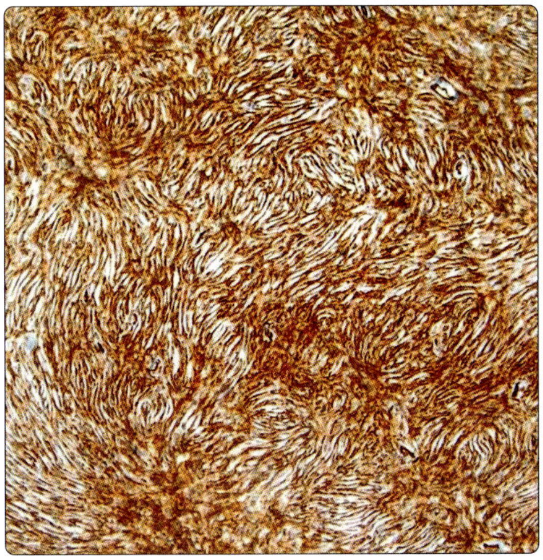

(Left) *Small, localized myoid nodules ⇨ are an unusual feature seen in some cases of DFSP. These structures likely represent a nonneoplastic myointimal proliferation within stromal vessels.* **(Right)** *CD34 expression is characteristically strong and diffuse in most cases of DFSP, making it a sensitive and useful marker for supporting the diagnosis. It lacks specificity, however, and can be expressed in a variety of spindled mesenchymal neoplasms, including neurofibroma and perineurioma.*

(Left) *Myxoid stromal change may be seen in DFSP. Although not uncommon as a focal finding, rare cases are predominantly or entirely myxoid.* **(Right)** *Although the characteristic storiform pattern of DFSP may be retained in myxoid variants, it is more often than not less well developed or lost completely. Stromal vessels often become more prominent and may lead to confusion with other tumors, such as myxofibrosarcoma.*

Myxoid Stroma

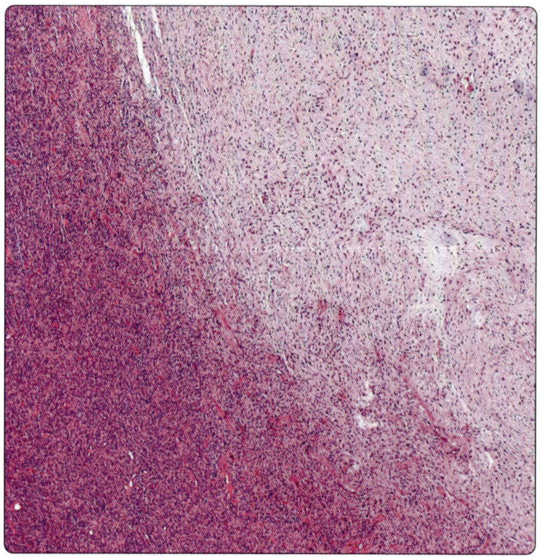

Myxoid Dermatofibrosarcoma Protuberans

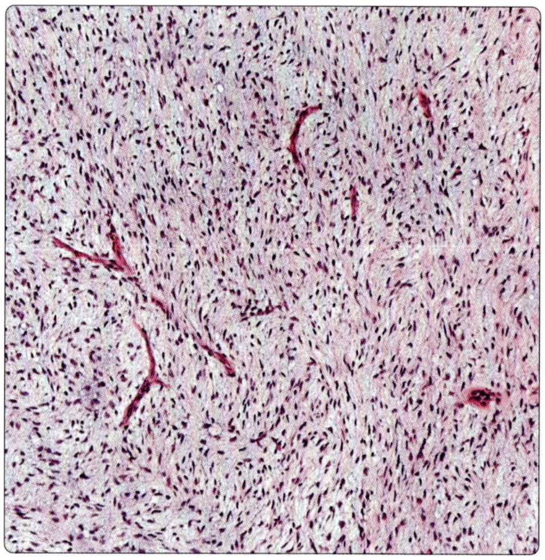

(Left) *This example of myxoid DFSP shows complete loss of storiform growth and prominent stromal blood vessels. Many nuclei also appear thin and wavy. A variety of other myxoid mesenchymal neoplasms must be considered with this morphologic appearance.* **(Right)** *Myxoid DFSP may show an interconnecting, reticulated or sieve-like morphology, similar to the microcystic/reticular variant of schwannoma. Note that pseudocystic or pseudovascular spaces may also be present.*

Myxoid Dermatofibrosarcoma Protuberans

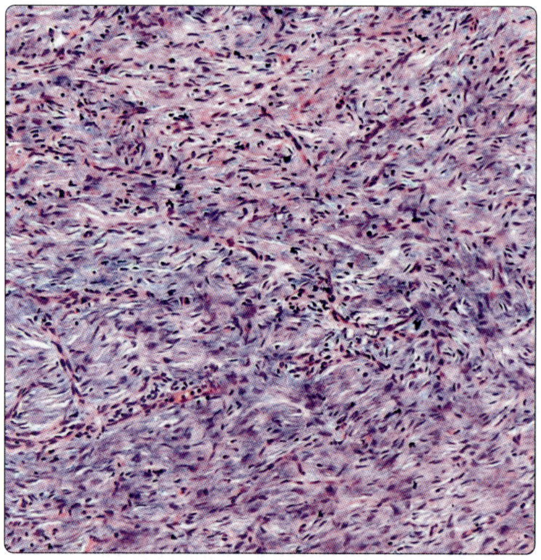

Reticulated Morphology

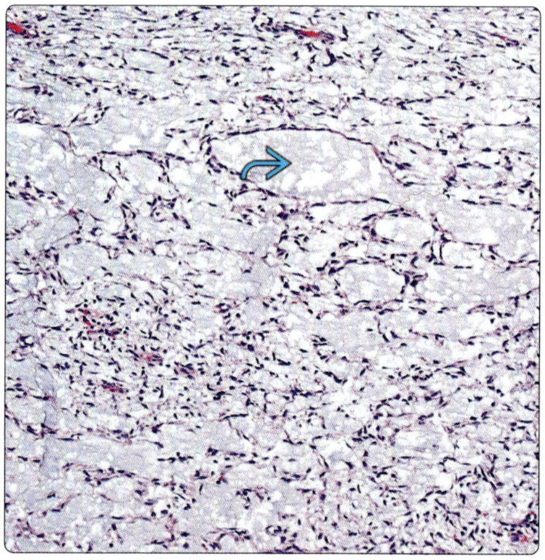

(Left) *Occasional cases of otherwise conventional DFSP may contain scattered dendritic cells containing melanin pigment. A stellate appearance to these cells is not uncommon. This variant is also known as a Bednar tumor. Rarely, these cells may also be seen in fibrosarcomatous transformation in DFSP.* **(Right)** *Rare cases of DFSP show a plaque-like growth with less conspicuous infiltration of subcutaneous adipose tissue. These neoplasms are easily misdiagnosed as benign mesenchymal neoplasms.*

Pigmented Dermatofibrosarcoma Protuberans (Bednar Tumor)

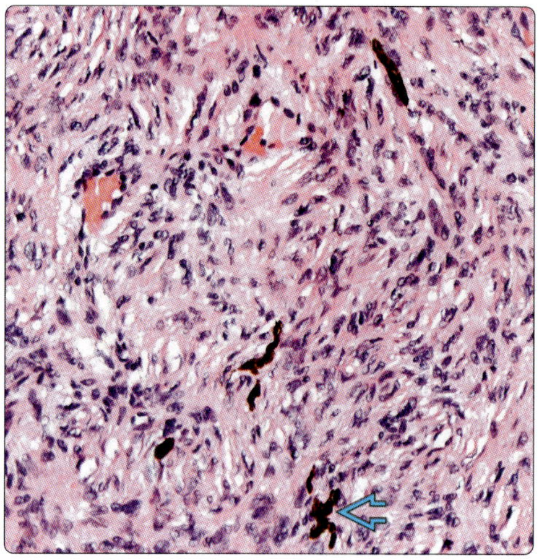

Plaque-Like or Atrophic Dermatofibrosarcoma Protuberans

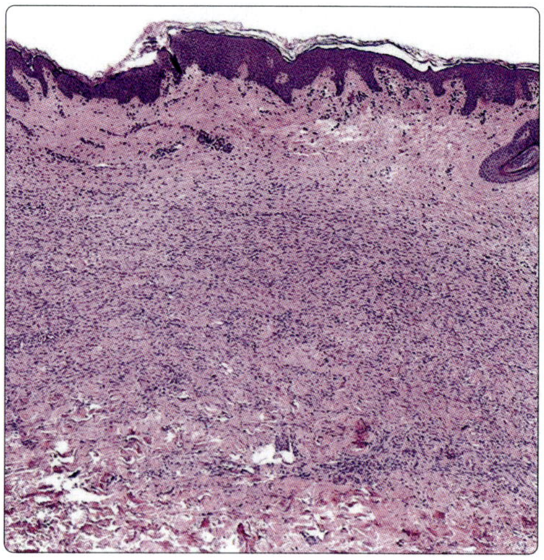

Giant Cell Fibroblastoma Morphology

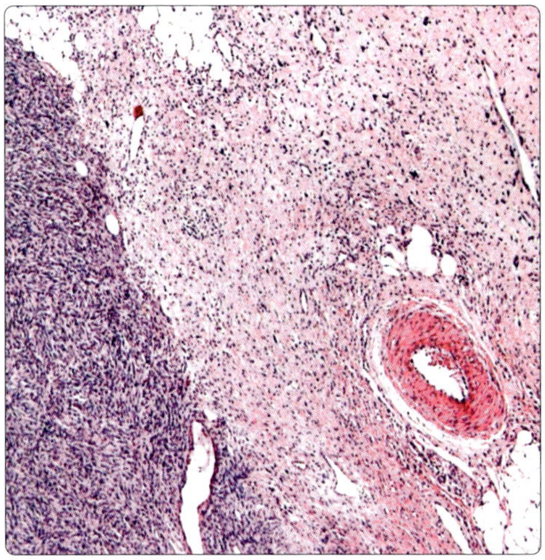

Giant Cell Fibroblastoma

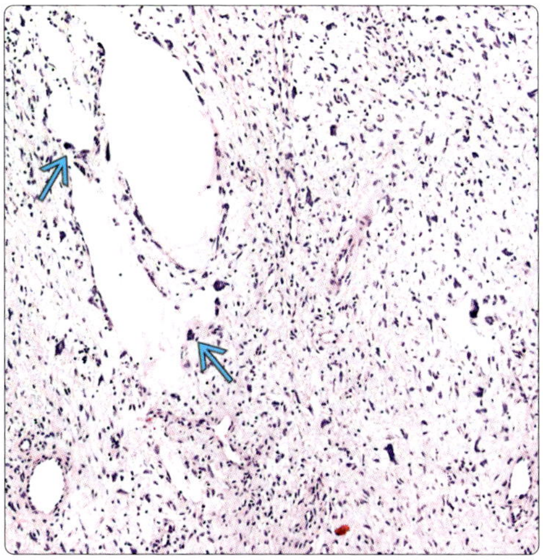

(Left) *Foci of giant cell fibroblastoma (right) may occur in otherwise conventional DFSP (far left). Of note, DFSP may recur in some patients as pure giant cell fibroblastoma and vice versa.* **(Right)** *Giant cell fibroblastoma characteristically contains hyperchromatic, multinucleated tumor cells within a hyalinized to myxoid stroma. The cells often line stromal clefts ⇒, imparting a pseudovascular appearance.*

Recurrent Myxoid Dermatofibrosarcoma Protuberans With Areas of Giant Cell Fibroblastoma

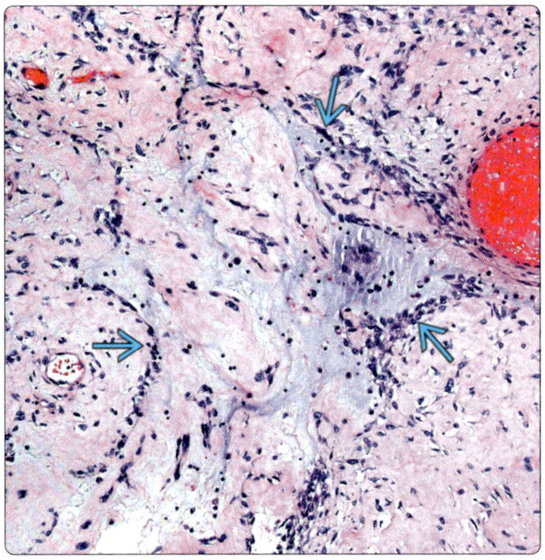

Fibrosarcomatous Dermatofibrosarcoma Protuberans

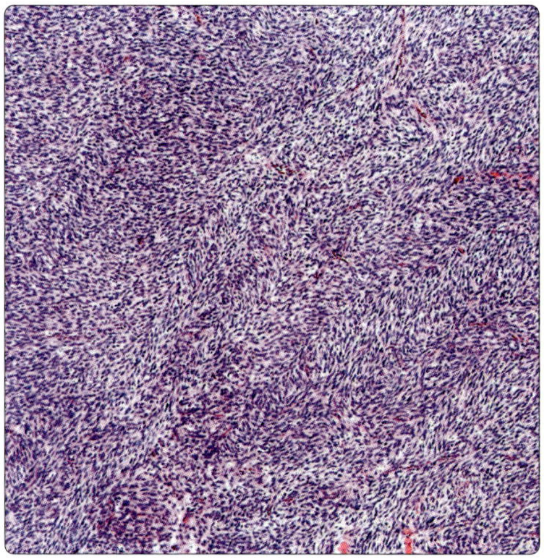

(Left) *This case of recurrent DFSP not only showed diffuse myxoid stromal changes but also foci resembling giant cell fibroblastoma. Note the vague pseudovascular spaces lined by tumor cells ⇒.* **(Right)** *Fibrosarcomatous dermatofibrosarcoma protuberans (FS-DFSP) is most easily recognized by a prominent cellular, fascicular growth pattern rather than a tight storiform pattern. This finding represents transition from a low-grade to a higher grade (usually intermediate) neoplasm.*

Fibrosarcomatous Dermatofibrosarcoma Protuberans

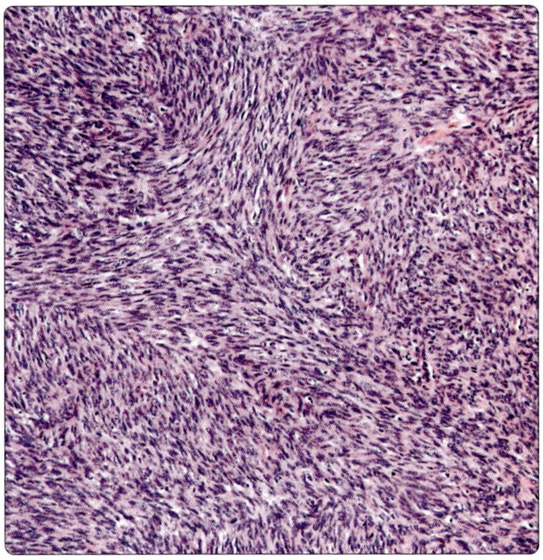

Herringbone Architecture

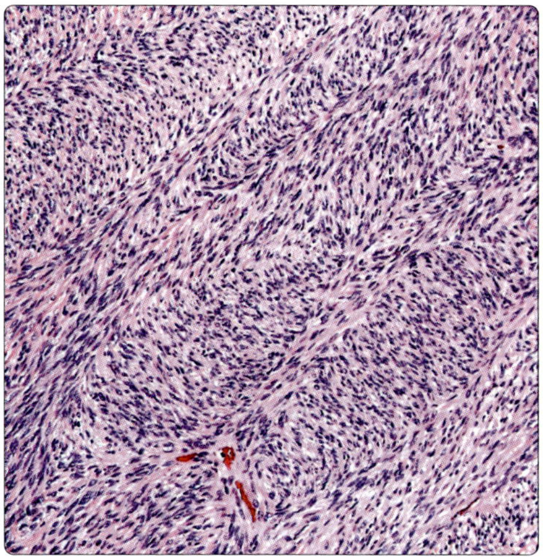

(Left) *Fascicular growth is well developed in FS-DFSP and is usually easily distinguished from conventional low-grade DFSP. Fibrosarcomatous transformation may be seen de novo (most common) or in recurrences.* **(Right)** *A well-developed herringbone architecture is a common finding in FS-DFSP and may lead to consideration of other entities, such as synovial sarcoma, malignant peripheral nerve sheath tumor (MPNST), and adult-type fibrosarcoma.*

(Left) *In contrast to conventional DFSP, FS-DFSP often shows a leading edge that is more expansile and "pushing" than frankly infiltrative. However, more typical infiltrative growth can also be seen.* **(Right)** *As in all forms of DFSP, tumor cell nuclei in FS-DFSP can appear thin and wavy. Combined with a fascicular growth pattern, this finding may lead to confusion with MPNST.*

Expansile Growth

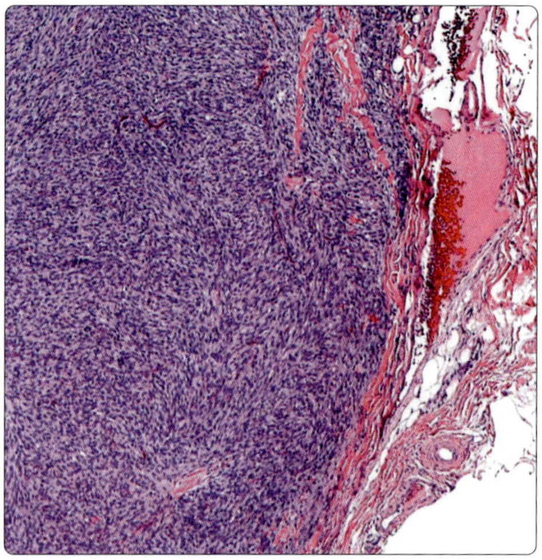

Neural-Like Morphology

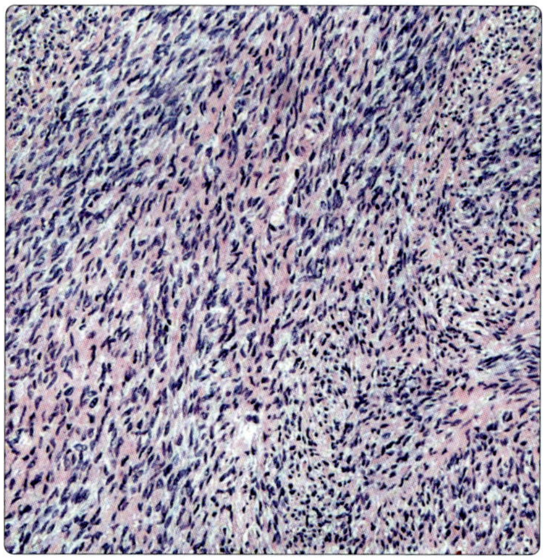

(Left) *Similar to low-grade DFSP, the tumor cells in FS-DFSP are relatively uniform; however, nuclei show greater atypia. Very rare cases show an undifferentiated pleomorphic sarcoma-like morphology.* **(Right)** *Compared to low-grade DFSP, the mitotic rate in FS-DFSP is usually higher than 5 figures per 10 HPF. Note the 3 mitoses ➩ in this image.*

Uniform Cytologic Features

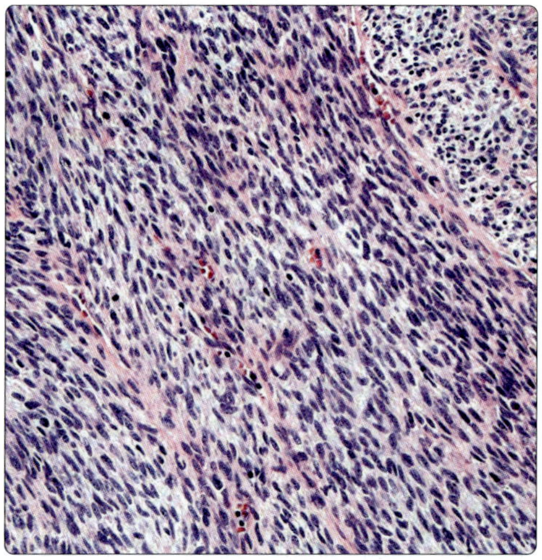

Increased Mitotic Rate

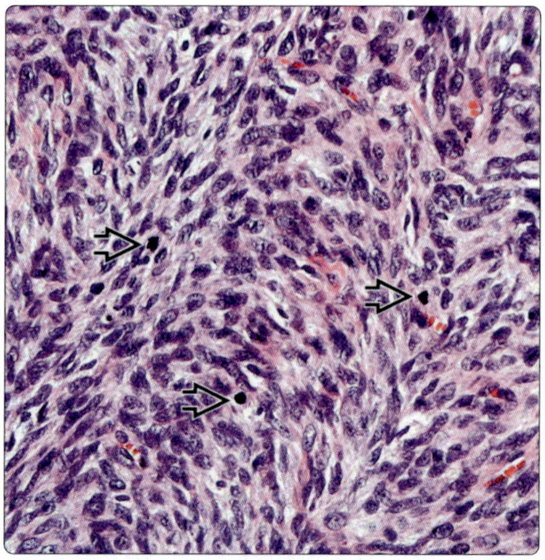

(Left) *Given its prominent fascicular growth, some areas of FS-DFSP may appear to show a round cell morphology when fascicles are viewed in cross section.* **(Right)** *As in conventional DFSP, FS-DFSP may also show increased stromal collagenization. Note the otherwise prominent fascicular growth.*

Round Cell Morphology

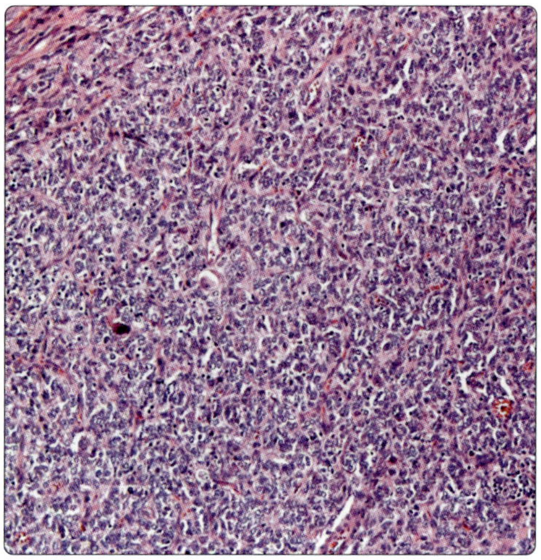

Stromal Collagenization in Fibrosarcomatous Dermatofibrosarcoma Protuberans

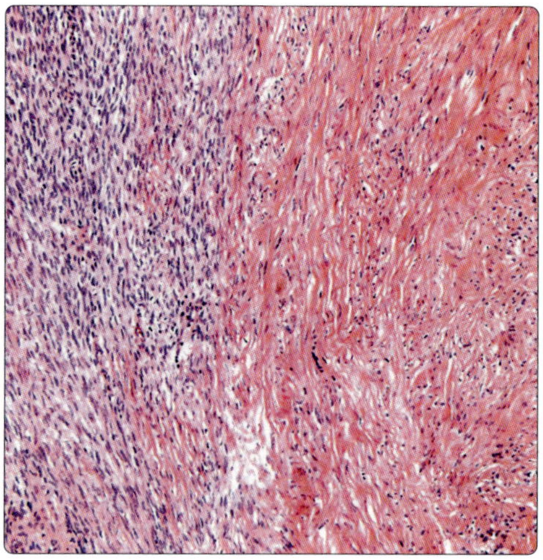

Stromal Collagenization in Fibrosarcomatous Dermatofibrosarcoma Protuberans

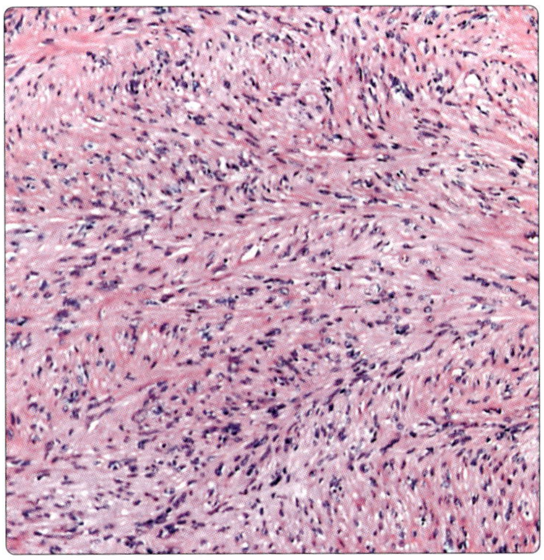

Myoid Nodules in Fibrosarcomatous Dermatofibrosarcoma Protuberans

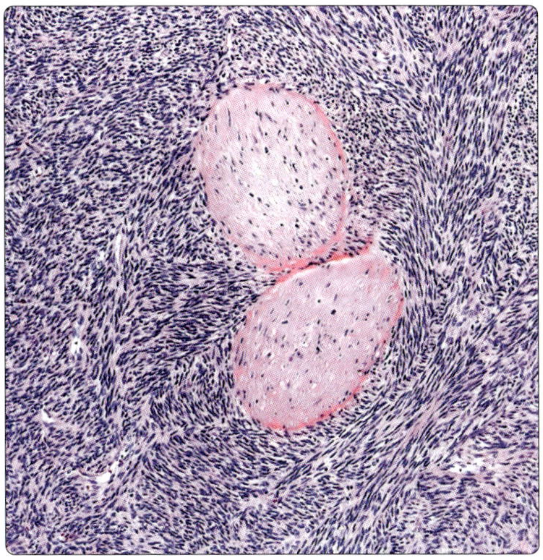

(Left) *Increased stromal collagen in conjunction with prominent fascicular growth in FS-DFSP may lead to confusion with leiomyosarcoma or low-grade myofibroblastic sarcoma.* **(Right)** *Myoid nodules may be seen in both conventional, low-grade DFSP and FS-DFSP; however, they are more common in the latter setting, as depicted.*

Myxoid Change in Fibrosarcomatous Dermatofibrosarcoma Protuberans

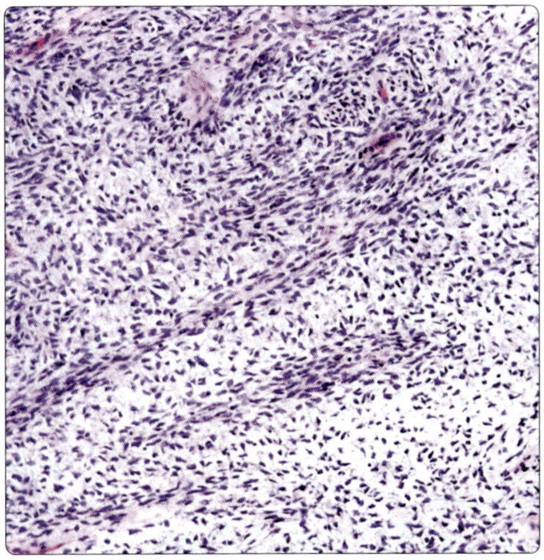

Rare Compartmentalized Pattern

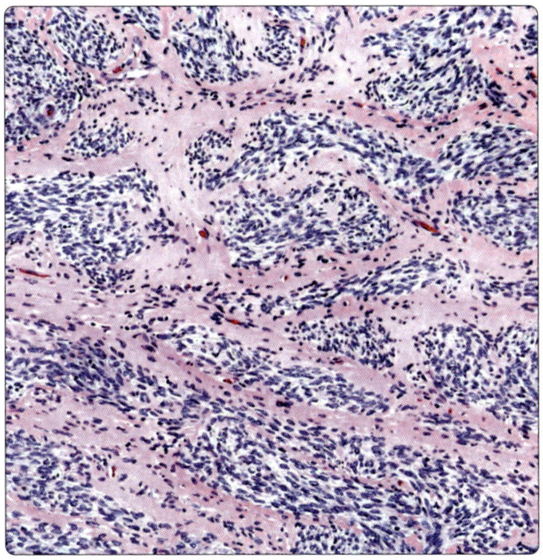

(Left) *Myxoid stromal change may be seen in FS-DFSP. In contrast to the myxoid variant of conventional DFSP, myxoid FS-DFSP usually retains its characteristic fascicular growth.* **(Right)** *This unusual case of FS-DFSP contained foci showing an interwoven, bundled or braided growth pattern similar to what has been reported in low-grade DFSP. Most of the tumor, however, showed more typical features of FS-DFSP.*

CD34 Expression Decreased or Lost

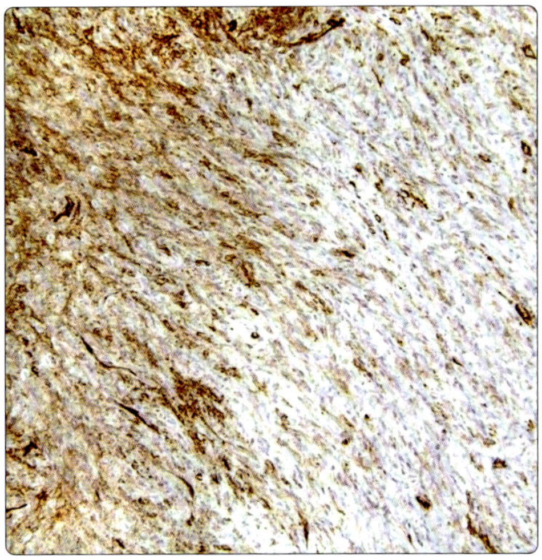

COL1A1-PDGFB **Fusion by FISH**

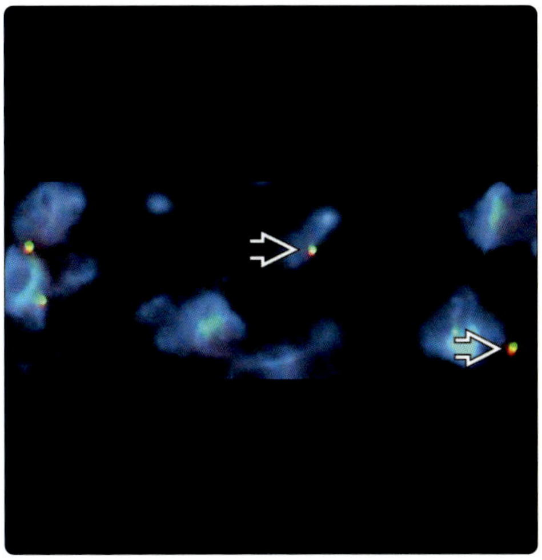

(Left) *In contrast to low-grade DFSP and its variants, FS-DFSP characteristically shows lost or diminished expression of CD34. This loss can often be demonstrated nicely in transition areas with low-grade areas (upper left). Rare cases of FS-DFSP retain strong expression of this antigen.* **(Right)** *FISH analysis of DFSP shows the characteristic 17;22 translocation with fusion of the COL1A1 and PDGFB genes. The red and green signals colocalize, resulting in a yellow signal* ➡*.*

Solitary Fibrous Tumor

KEY FACTS

TERMINOLOGY
- Fibroblastic mesenchymal neoplasm often featuring prominent branching staghorn vascular pattern
  - Includes tumors once classified as soft tissue hemangiopericytoma and giant cell angiofibroma

CLINICAL ISSUES
- Usually adults (range: 20-70 years)
- Can arise virtually anywhere (somatic or visceral)
  - Subcutaneous or deep soft tissue
- Treatment: Complete surgical resection
- Most are benign (85-90%)
- Combination of patient age, tumor size, mitotic activity, and necrosis is predictive of metastatic risk (Demicco et al)

MICROSCOPIC
- Classic variably cellular patternless pattern
- Uniform, spindled to ovoid fibroblastic cells
- Characteristic prominent staghorn vascular pattern
- Fibrous stroma often with abundant collagen
- Stromal myxoid change in some cases and may be diffuse
- Mitotic activity low (usually < 3 figures per 10 HPF)
- Malignant and dedifferentiated forms occur
- Variants: Lipomatous ("fat forming")

ANCILLARY TESTS
- Strong, diffuse CD34(+) and nuclear STAT6(+)
- Usually keratin, S100, desmin, CD117, CD31 (-)
- Molecular: Characteristic *NAB2-STAT6* fusion

TOP DIFFERENTIAL DIAGNOSES
- Deep benign fibrous histiocytoma
- Spindle cell lipoma
- Cellular angiofibroma
- Dermatofibrosarcoma protuberans
- Angiofibroma of soft tissue
- Synovial sarcoma (monophasic)

Solitary Fibrous Tumor

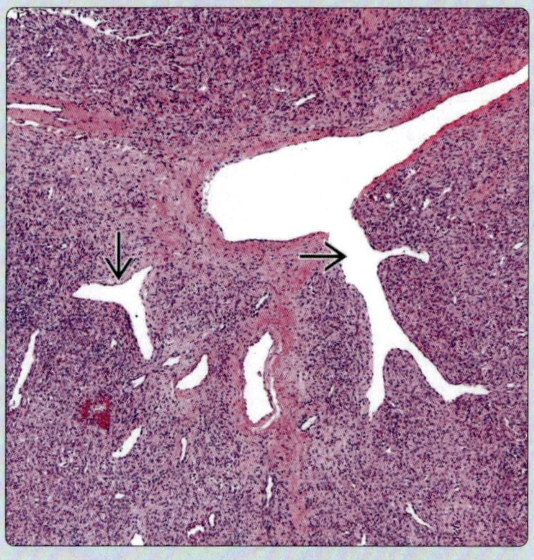

Bland Fibroblastic Cells

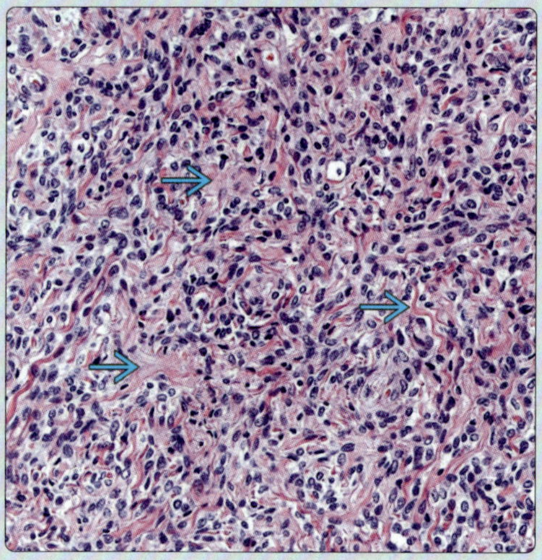

(Left) *Low-power view of a solitary fibrous tumor (SFT) shows areas of varying cellularity and a prominent vascularized stroma that classically features ectatic and irregularly shaped vessels →. These vessels are often described as staghorn, given their antler-like shapes.* **(Right)** *The lesional cells of SFT are spindled to ovoid, contain bland, relatively uniform nuclei, and are often arranged in a patternless pattern. A collagenous stroma → is characteristic, but its prominence varies by regional cellularity.*

CD34 Expression

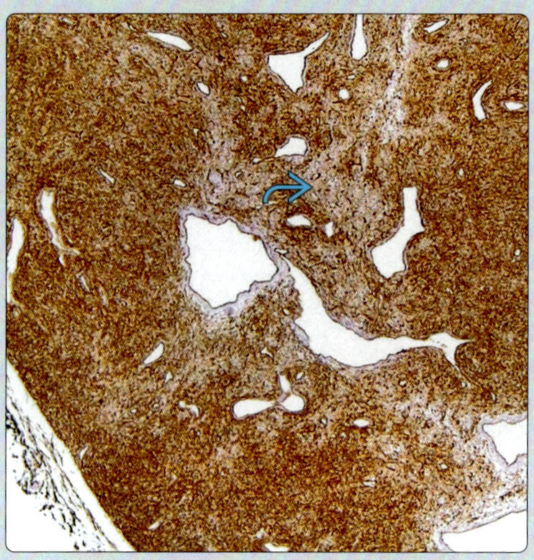

STAT6 Expression

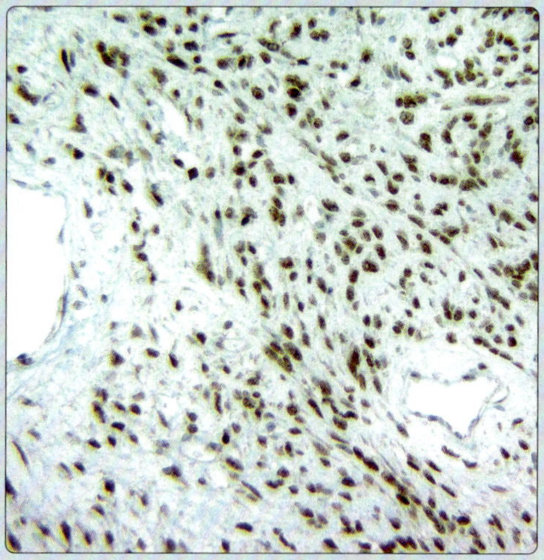

(Left) *CD34 expression is present in the vast majority of cases of SFT and is typically strong and diffuse, although there are often small foci of decreased or absent expression →. Rare cases are negative for this antigen.* **(Right)** *Diffuse nuclear expression of STAT6 is characteristic of SFT and is seen is the vast majority of cases. With the exception of rare cases of dedifferentiated liposarcoma, most entities on the differential diagnosis of SFT are negative.*

Solitary Fibrous Tumor

TERMINOLOGY

Abbreviations

- Solitary fibrous tumor (SFT)

Synonyms

- Hemangiopericytoma
- Giant cell angiofibroma (giant cell-rich variant of SFT)
- Localized fibrous mesothelioma (obsolete)

Definitions

- Fibroblastic mesenchymal neoplasm often featuring prominent branching staghorn vascular pattern
  - Includes tumors once classified as soft tissue hemangiopericytoma

CLINICAL ISSUES

Epidemiology

- Age
  - Usually adults (range: 20-70 years)
  - Occasionally in children and adolescents
- Sex
  - M = F
    - Slight male predominance in lipomatous SFT
    - Strong female predominance in superficial SFT

Site

- Pleura, thoracic cavity
- Extrathoracic sites
  - Extremities
  - Head and neck, including orbit and intracranial sites
  - Abdominal cavity, pelvis, retroperitoneum
  - Visceral organs
- However, may occur at almost any site

Presentation

- Slow-growing, often painless mass
- May arise in subcutaneous or deep soft tissue
  - Rare tumors are dermal/cutaneous
- Larger tumors may be associated with paraneoplastic hypoglycemia due to production of IGF2

Treatment

- Complete surgical resection with negative margins
- Combination of radiation therapy and chemotherapy may be utilized in malignant SFT

Prognosis

- Most are benign (85-90%)
- Minority behave aggressively
  - Recurrences and distant metastases
- Updated risk stratification model (Demicco et al)
  - Based on patient age, tumor size, mitotic activity, and necrosis
  - Scoring
    - Age: 0 if < 55 years; 1 if ≥ 50 years
    - Tumor size: 0 if < 5 cm; 1 if 5 to < 10 cm; 2 if 10 to < 15 cm; 3 if ≥ 15 cm
    - Mitotic activity: 0 if < 1 mitosis/10 HPF; 1 if 1-3 mitoses/10 HPF; 2 if ≥ 4 mitoses/10 HPF
    - Necrosis: 0 if < 10%, 1 if ≥ 10%
  - Total score
    - Low risk: 0-3
    - Intermediate risk: 4-5
    - High risk: 6-7
  - Metastatic risk (5 years): 10% (intermediate-risk group) and 73% (high-risk group)
    - No metastasis seen in low-risk group (in 2017 study)
- Activating mutations in telomerase reverse transcriptase gene (*TERT*) associated with adverse outcome
  - Strongly associated with older patient age, large tumor size, and higher risk classifications

MACROSCOPIC

General Features

- Lobulated, circumscribed mass
  - Histologically malignant tumors may be locally infiltrative
- Firm, gray-white or brown cut surface
- Occasional cystic degeneration or hemorrhage

Size

- Range: 1-20 cm (most 5-10 cm)

MICROSCOPIC

Histologic Features

- Classic patternless pattern showing field-to-field variations in cellularity and general absence of defined architectural organization
  - Spindled to ovoid fibroblastic cells with scanty cytoplasm and small, uniform, vesicular nuclei
    - Isolated degenerative nuclear atypia occasionally present
    - Mitotic activity low (usually < 3 figures per 10 HPF)
    - Rare rounded or epithelioid cytomorphology
  - Some tumors are diffusely cellular
    - Cellular SFT once classified as classic hemangiopericytoma
  - Cells often appear randomly arranged (patternless pattern)
    - Tumors can show areas of more defined storiform, trabecular, or loose fascicular growth
  - Characteristic prominent vascular pattern
    - Branching or staghorn-shaped vessels
    - Perivascular hyalinization common
  - Varying component of fibrous stroma (often abundant)
    - Frequent dense, keloid-like hyalinization
    - Densely hyalinized stroma may show cracking artifact
    - Distinctive collagen fibers may appear thick, irregular, or nodular
  - Stromal myxoid change in some cases and may be diffuse
  - Mast cells common
  - Occasional multinucleated stromal giant cells
    - May be abundant and line pseudovascular spaces
      - Originally described as distinct entity: Giant cell angiofibroma
- Atypical or potentially malignant features in SFT
  - Hypercellularity, nuclear pleomorphism, infiltrative margins, necrosis
  - > 4 mitoses per 10 HPF
    - One of better indicators of prognosis

- Dedifferentiated SFT
  - Abrupt transition from conventional low-grade SFT to areas of high-grade sarcoma
    - High-grade areas may contain heterologous elements

Morphologic Variant

- Lipomatous ("fat-forming") SFT
  - Conventional or cellular SFT admixed with variable amount of mature fat
  - Synonym: Lipomatous hemangiopericytoma
  - Rare histologically malignant forms
    - May contain lipoblasts or areas resembling well-differentiated liposarcoma

ANCILLARY TESTS

Immunohistochemistry

- Strong CD34(+), often diffuse (but can be patchy)
  - Rare, benign-appearing tumors (-)
  - May also be decreased or lost in malignant/dedifferentiated SFT
- Strong, diffuse nuclear STAT6(+)
- Diffuse TLE1(+) in rare subset (pitfall)
- Retained nuclear Rb protein expression
- Focal EMA(+) or SMA(+) in up to 40%
- Nuclear β-catenin (+) in minor subset
- Generally keratin, S100 protein, desmin, CD117, DOG1, CD31 (-)

Molecular Genetics

- Recurrent intrachromosomal rearrangement (12q) resulting in *NAB2-STAT6* fusion
  - Detectable by RT-PCR (difficult by FISH)

DIFFERENTIAL DIAGNOSIS

Deep Benign Fibrous Histiocytoma

- Well-developed storiform growth pattern common
- Uniform cellularity
- Foamy macrophages &/or giant cells in 50% of cases
- Variable CD34; STAT6(-)

Spindle Cell Lipoma

- Can show morphologic overlap with lipomatous SFT
- Most common in back, neck, shoulder
- Staghorn vasculature rare
- Loss of nuclear Rb protein expression
- STAT6(-)

Cellular Angiofibroma

- Can show morphologic overlap with SFT
- Most common in vulvovaginal/inguinal regions
- Vessels often smaller than in SFT and show hyalinization/fibrosis
- Loss of nuclear Rb protein expression
- STAT6(-)

Dermatofibrosarcoma Protuberans

- Dermal component
- Infiltrative growth and well-developed storiform pattern
- Staghorn vascular pattern absent
- STAT6(-)
- Characteristic t(17;22) with *COL1A1-PDGFB* fusion

Angiofibroma of Soft Tissue

- Can show marked morphologic overlap with SFT
- Prominent thin- to thick-walled stromal vasculature
- CD34 and STAT6 (-)
- t(5;8) with *AHRR-NCOA2* gene fusion

Synovial Sarcoma (Monophasic)

- Usually hypercellular spindle cell neoplasm with variable fascicular growth
- Prominent staghorn vascular pattern uncommon
- Focal cytokeratin (+) &/or EMA(+) expression
- Diffuse TLE1 (+) characteristic (but also rarely seen in SFT)
- STAT6 and CD34 (-)
- Characteristic t(X;18) with *SS18* (SYT) rearrangement

Myopericytoma

- Conspicuous perivascular growth or arrangement
- SMA(+); CD34 and STAT6 (-)

Gastrointestinal Stromal Tumor

- Arises from wall of GI tract, mesentery, or omentum
- Staghorn vasculature may be present
- CD117(+) and DOG1(+) in most cases; also CD34(+)
- Most show *KIT* or *PDGFRA* oncogenic mutations

Dedifferentiated Liposarcoma

- High-grade pleomorphic morphology in many cases
- Rare cases with SFT-like morphology
  - May also show STAT6(+)
- MDM2(+) and CDK4(+) by IHC
- *MDM2* amplification

SELECTED REFERENCES

1. Feasel P et al: Superficial solitary fibrous tumor: a series of 26 cases. Am J Surg Pathol. 42(6):778-785, 2018
2. Lin Y et al: Telomerase promoter mutations and copy number alterations in solitary fibrous tumours. J Clin Pathol. 71(9):832-839, 2018
3. Olson NJ et al: Dedifferentiated solitary fibrous tumor: a concise review. Arch Pathol Lab Med. 142(6):761-766, 2018
4. Demicco EG et al: Risk assessment in solitary fibrous tumors: validation and refinement of a risk stratification model. Mod Pathol. 30(10):1433-1442, 2017
5. Kouba E et al: Solitary fibrous tumour of the genitourinary tract: a clinicopathological study of 11 cases and their association with the NAB2-STAT6 fusion gene. J Clin Pathol. 70(6):508-514, 2017
6. Smith SC et al: Solitary fibrous tumors of the head and neck: a multi-institutional clinicopathologic study. Am J Surg Pathol. 41(12):1642-56, 2017
7. Yang EJ et al: Solitary fibrous tumour of the female genital tract: a clinicopathological analysis of 25 cases. Histopathology. 72(5):749-759, 2017
8. Bahrami A et al: TERT promoter mutations and prognosis in solitary fibrous tumor. Mod Pathol. 29(12):1511-1522, 2016
9. Doyle LA et al: Nuclear expression of STAT6 distinguishes solitary fibrous tumor from histologic mimics. Mod Pathol. 27(3):390-5, 2014
10. Koelsche C et al: Nuclear relocation of STAT6 reliably predicts NAB2-STAT6 fusion for the diagnosis of solitary fibrous tumour. Histopathology. 65(5):613-22, 2014
11. Demicco EG et al: Solitary fibrous tumor: a clinicopathological study of 110 cases and proposed risk assessment model. Mod Pathol. 25(9):1298-306, 2012
12. Lee JC et al: Malignant fat-forming solitary fibrous tumor (so-called "lipomatous hemangiopericytoma"): clinicopathologic analysis of 14 cases. Am J Surg Pathol. 35(8):1177-85, 2011
13. Mosquera JM et al: Expanding the spectrum of malignant progression in solitary fibrous tumors: a study of 8 cases with a discrete anaplastic component–is this dedifferentiated SFT? Am J Surg Pathol. 33(9):1314-21, 2009
14. Guillou L et al: Lipomatous hemangiopericytoma: a fat-containing variant of solitary fibrous tumor? Clinicopathologic, immunohistochemical, and ultrastructural analysis of a series in favor of a unifying concept. Hum Pathol. 31(9):1108-15, 2000

Variable Cellularity

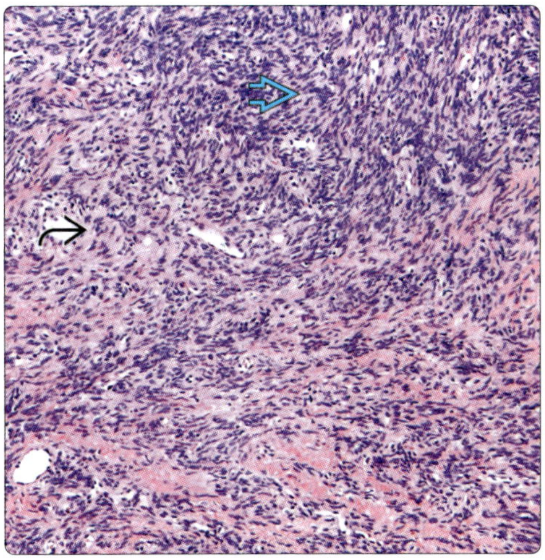

Stromal Collagen

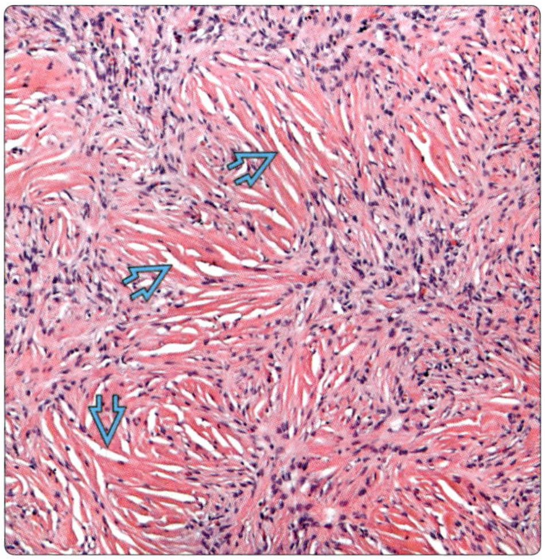

(Left) *Variations in cellularity are common in SFT, as seen in this H&E showing areas of both high → and low cell density →. Note also the absence of any defined cytoarchitectural pattern.* **(Right)** *Stromal collagen is generally more prominent in less cellular regions of SFT, as depicted. Note the artifactual clefts or "cracks" → present in the more densely collagenized foci.*

Bland Cytologic Features

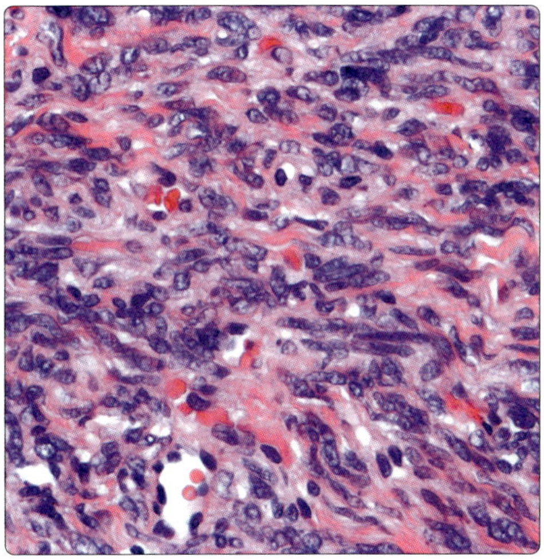

Vascular Hyalinization

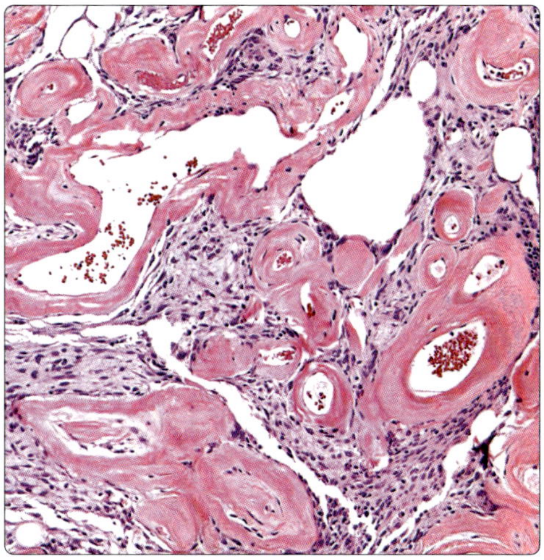

(Left) *The nuclei of SFT are small, vesicular, and relatively uniform. Nucleoli, if present, are small and inconspicuous. Mitotic activity is low and usually does not exceed 3 mitoses per 10 HPF.* **(Right)** *Ectatic staghorn vessels are characteristic of SFT but are not specific for the diagnosis. Perivascular hyalinization or fibrosis may also be seen and in some cases can be striking, as in this H&E.*

Cystic Hyalinized Vessels

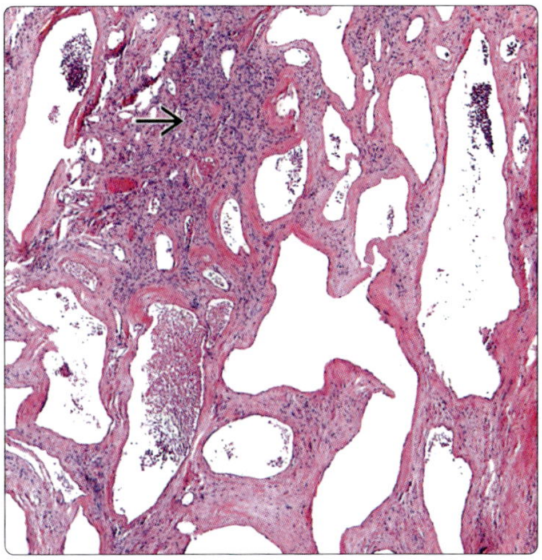

Focal Marked Vascularity

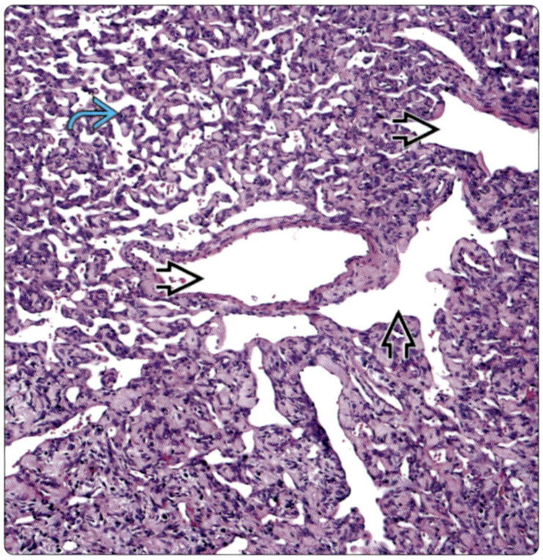

(Left) *This unusual case of SFT shows areas containing large, cystically dilated blood vessels. Hypervascular examples, such as this, may be embolized prior to surgery. Note the focus → of more typical SFT.* **(Right)** *This otherwise conventional case of SFT contains several discrete, centrally located foci featuring a more complex anastomosing vasculature →, as depicted. Note the more characteristic larger staghorn vessels →.*

(Left) *SFT may contain varying amounts of mature adipose tissue, as depicted, and has been referred to as the lipomatous or "fat-forming" variant of SFT. Cases containing abundant fat may be confused with a true lipomatous neoplasm.* **(Right)** *Some cases of SFT may feature both diffuse hyalinized stroma and abundant mature adipose tissue. In conjunction with CD34 expression, misdiagnosis as spindle cell lipoma, cellular angiofibroma, or myofibroblastoma is possible.*

Lipomatous ("Fat-Forming") Solitary Fibrous Tumor

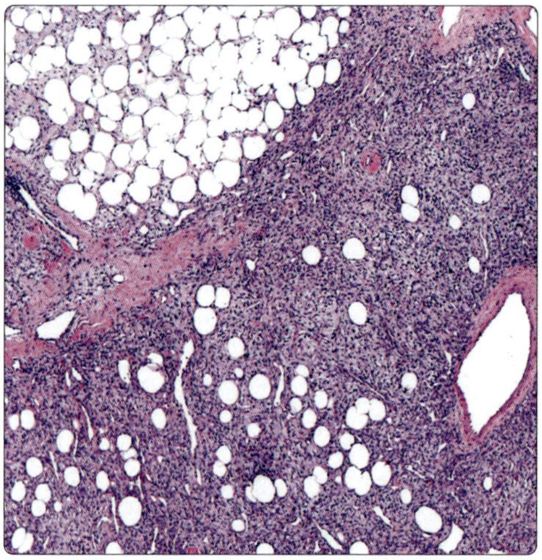

Hyalinized Lipomatous Solitary Fibrous Tumor

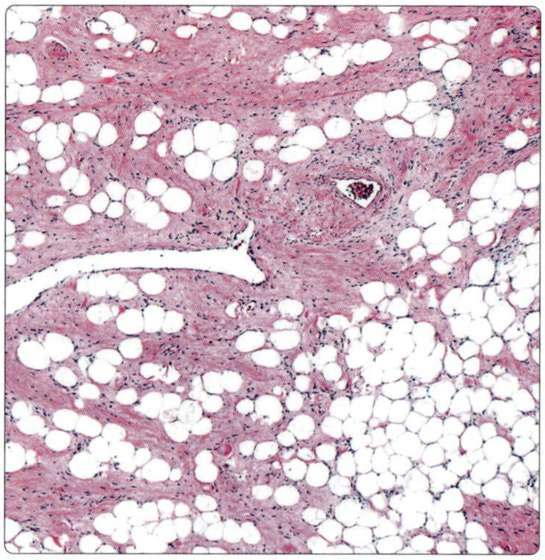

(Left) *Myxoid stromal change is not uncommon in SFT but is often focal when present. Rare tumors are predominantly myxoid and can be challenging to distinguish from other low-grade myxoid neoplasms. A prominent staghorn vasculature can be a helpful clue.* **(Right)** *H&E shows marked hypocellularity within a myxoid area of SFT. Note the dilated vessels.*

Myxoid Solitary Fibrous Tumor

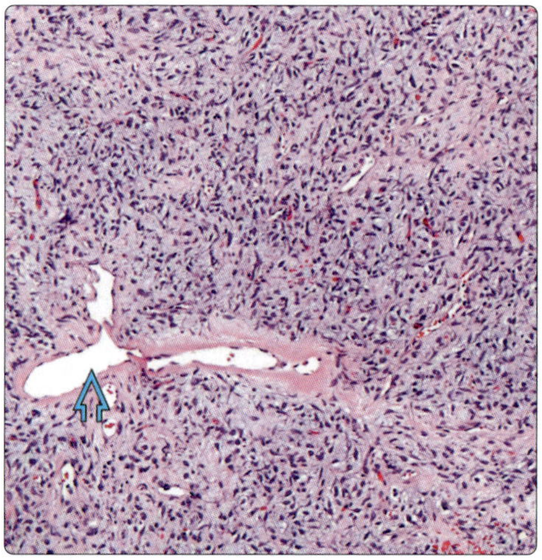

Myxoid Solitary Fibrous Tumor

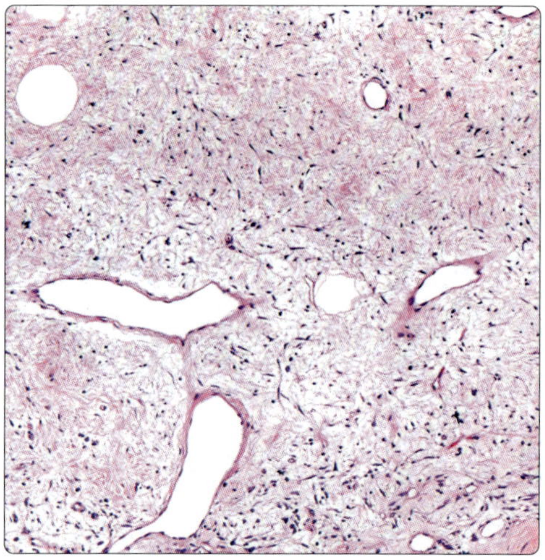

(Left) *This case of myxoid SFT contains diffuse mature adipose tissue, resembling myxoid liposarcoma; however, DDIT3 FISH is negative, and STAT6 immunohistochemistry is diffusely positive.* **(Right)** *Myxoid areas of SFT may also contain the characteristic prominent vasculature seen in more conventional, nonmyxoid areas.*

Myxoid Lipomatous Solitary Fibrous Tumor

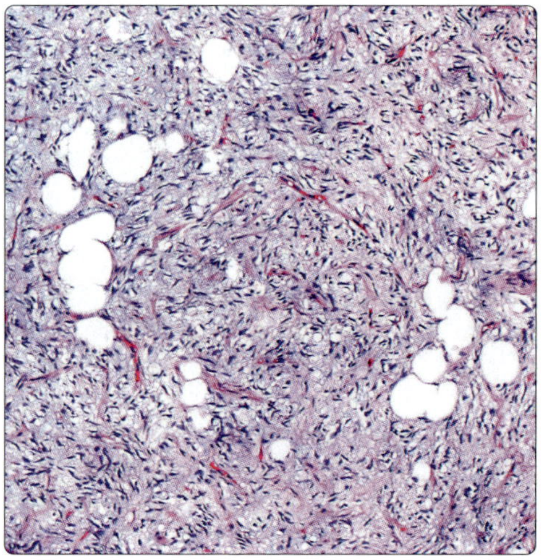

Myxoid Solitary Fibrous Tumor Vasculature

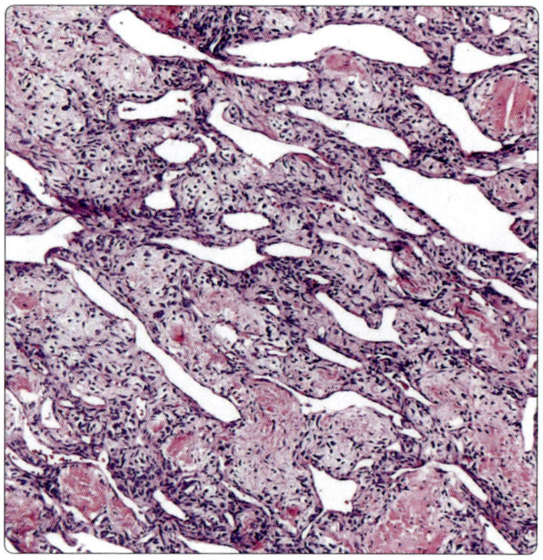

Prominent Stromal Collagen

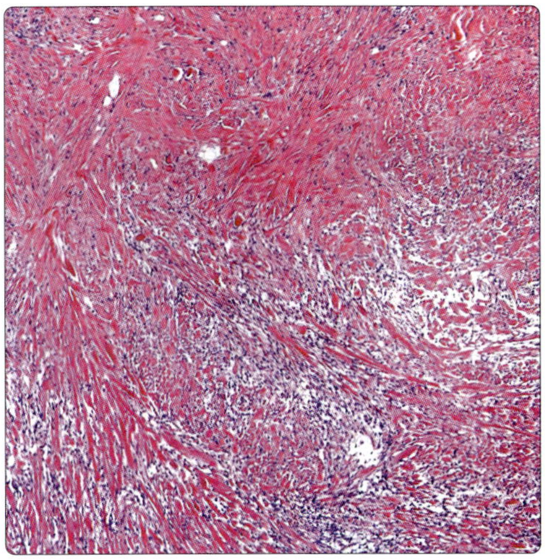

Keloidal Collagen Fibers

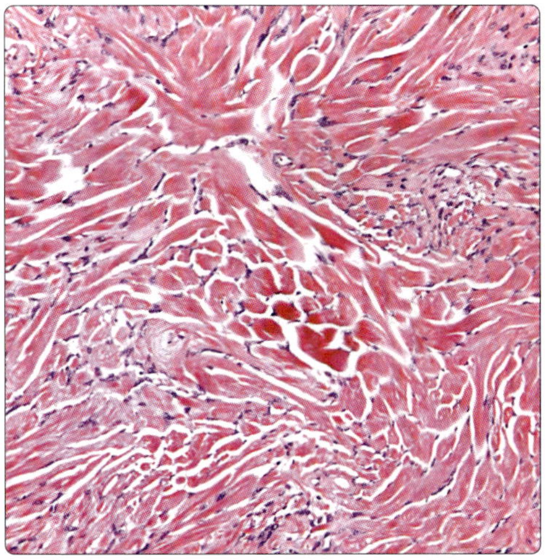

(Left) *This case of SFT shows prominent thickened collagen fibers arranged haphazardly. Dilated vascular channels are not evident in this particular field but were more conspicuous elsewhere in the tumor.* **(Right)** *Thick, glassy collagen bundles similar to those seen in keloids can be present in SFT. Note the prominent "cracking" artifact (clear slits and spaces) between collagen bundles.*

Hyalinized Solitary Fibrous Tumor

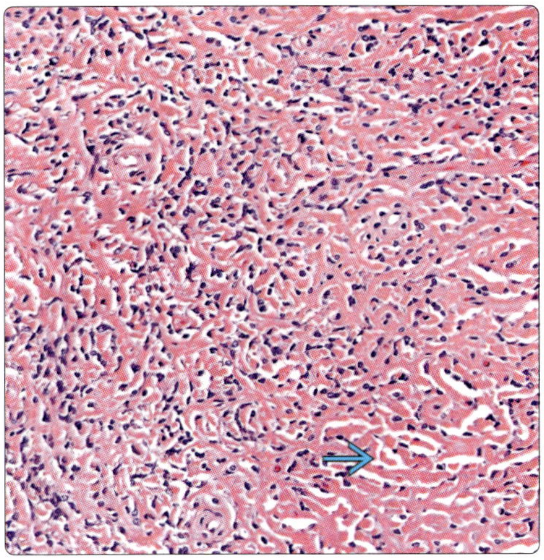

Hypocellular, Hyalinized Solitary Fibrous Tumor

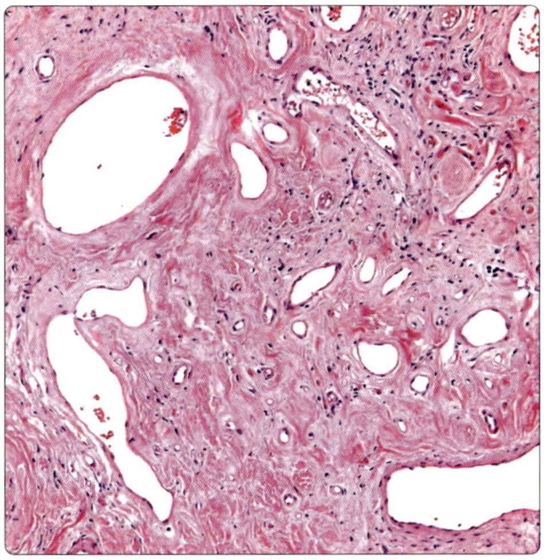

(Left) *H&E shows a hyalinized/sclerotic region of SFT in which the cells are arranged randomly rather than in linear cords. Artifactual clefting ⇨ or "cracking" is also conspicuous.* **(Right)** *H&E shows a longstanding case of SFT featuring prominent stromal sclerosing and marked hypocellularity. Note the various gaping vessels.*

Striking Collagen Production

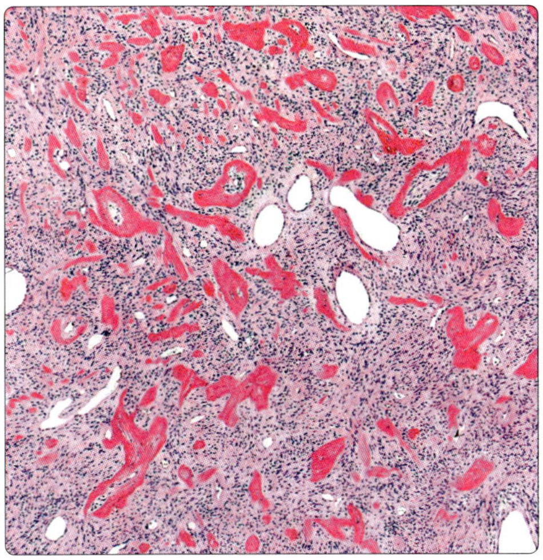

Architectural Patterns

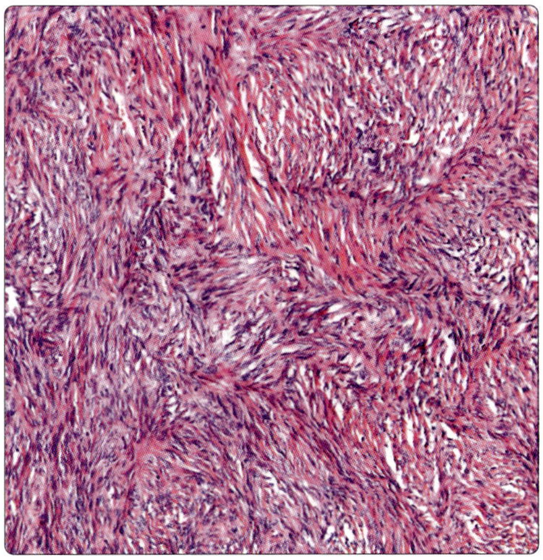

(Left) *This example of SFT features large, irregular bundles of eosinophilic, keloidal-like collagen, imparting a striking low-power appearance.* **(Right)** *Although tumor cells are classically arranged in a relatively random or haphazard fashion in most cases of SFT, it is not uncommon to find areas showing more defined architectures, including storiform arrays, short bundles, or loose fascicles.*

(Left) *Mast cells* → *are a common, but nonspecific finding in SFT. They are often more prominent in hypocellular regions with loose edematous or myxoid stroma.* **(Right)** *Focal cystic change can be present in some cases of SFT, as depicted, and may be quite prominent in rare cases. Associated hemorrhage may or may not be present.*

Mast Cells

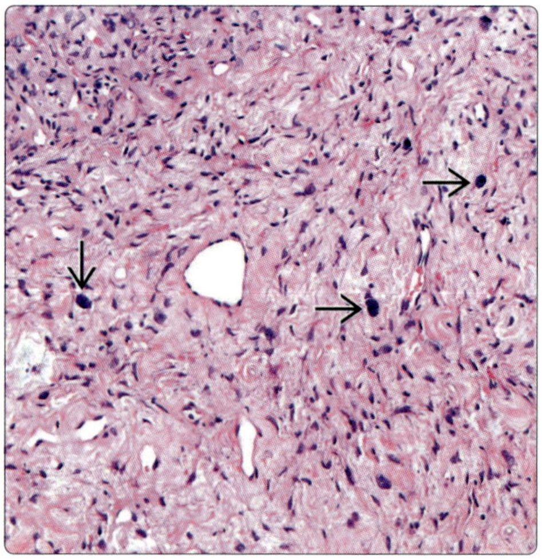

Cystic Change

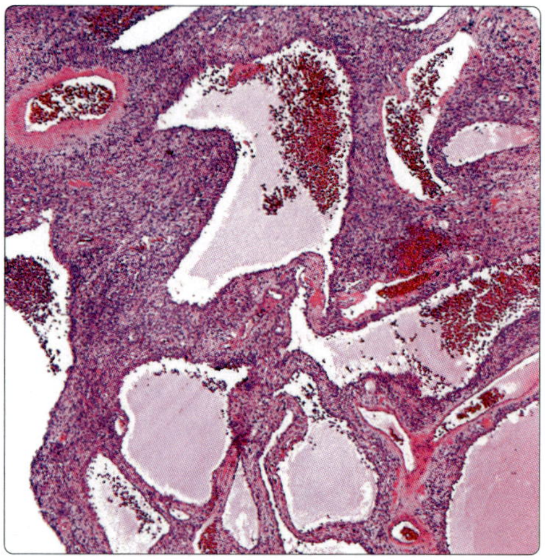

(Left) *Most cases of SFT contain areas of varying cellularity; however, some tumors show predominantly increased cellularity and can resemble synovial sarcoma or malignant peripheral nerve sheath tumor.* **(Right)** *Cellular examples of SFT with a more ovoid or rounded cytomorphology and prominent vasculature, as depicted, represent tumors that were formerly classified as classic hemangiopericytoma.*

Cellular Solitary Fibrous Tumor

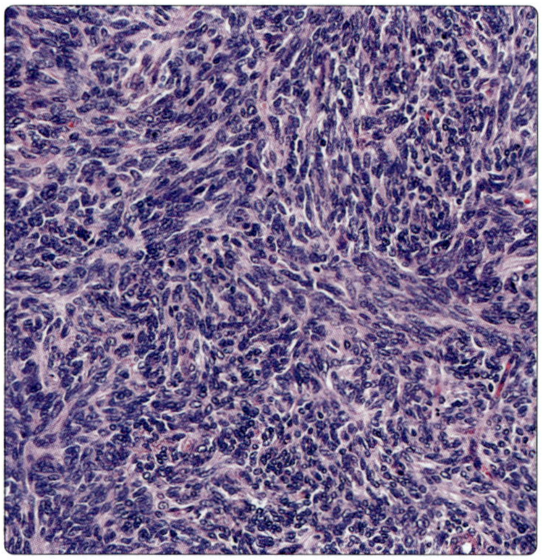

Cellular Solitary Fibrous Tumor

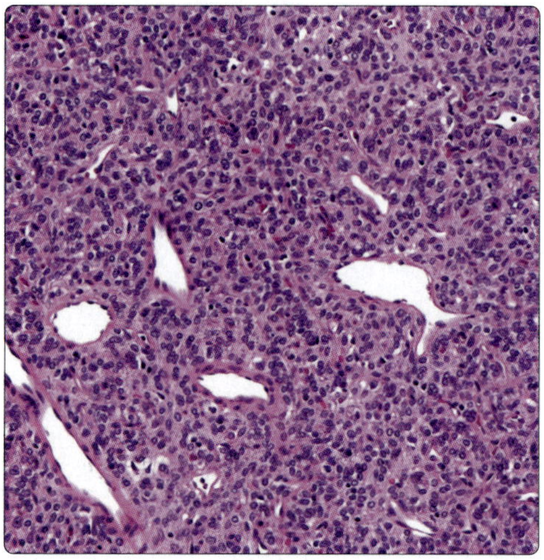

(Left) *The lesional cells of SFT are relatively uniform and usually show no more than mild pleomorphism. Some cases, however, contain cells featuring multiple enlarged nuclei* →. **(Right)** *In some cases of SFT, multinucleated stromal giant cells* ⇒ *are more abundant and can be seen lining pseudovascular spaces* →. *Tumors with this morphology were formerly classified as giant cell angiofibroma but are now recognized as a form of SFT. Areas of more conventional morphology are almost always present.*

Multinucleated Stromal Giant Cells

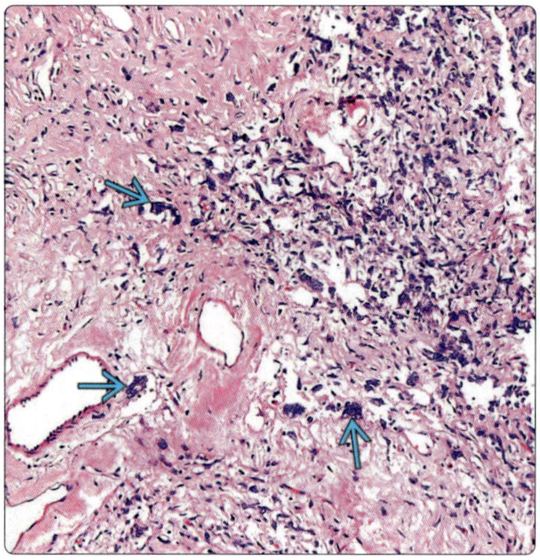

Giant Cell Angiofibroma Morphology

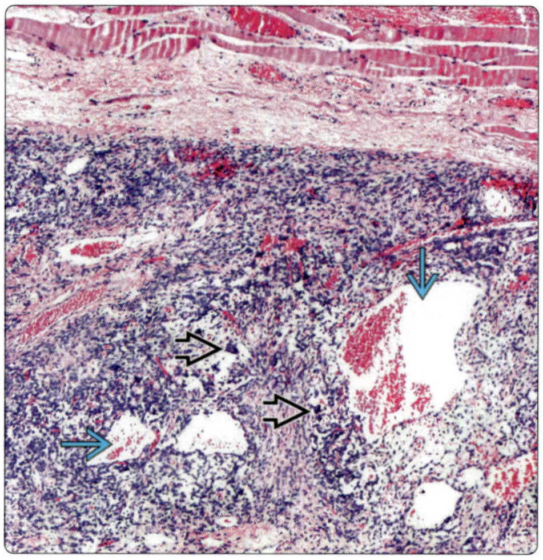

Osteoclast-Like Giant Cells

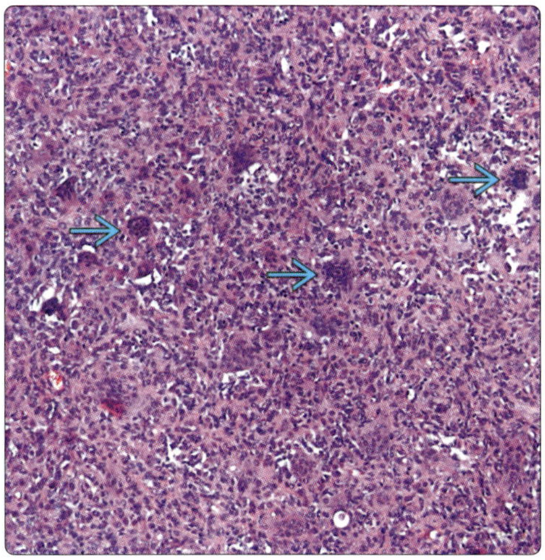

Malignant Solitary Fibrous Tumor

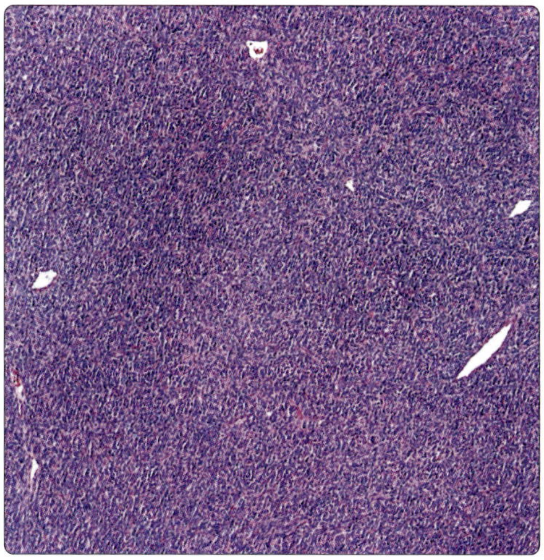

(Left) *Osteoclast-like giant cells* *are a rare finding in SFT and are distinct from the multinucleated stromal giant cells that line pseudovascular spaces in tumors with a giant cell angiofibroma morphology.* **(Right)** *Histologically malignant forms of SFT do occur but are uncommon. They are often characterized by a variable combination of hypercellularity (shown), nuclear pleomorphism, elevated mitotic activity, invasive growth, and necrosis.*

Malignant Solitary Fibrous Tumor: Elevated Mitotic Rate

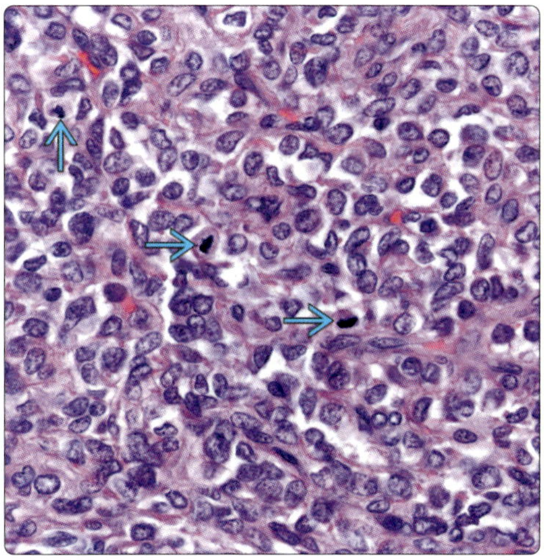

Malignant Solitary Fibrous Tumor: Fascicular Growth

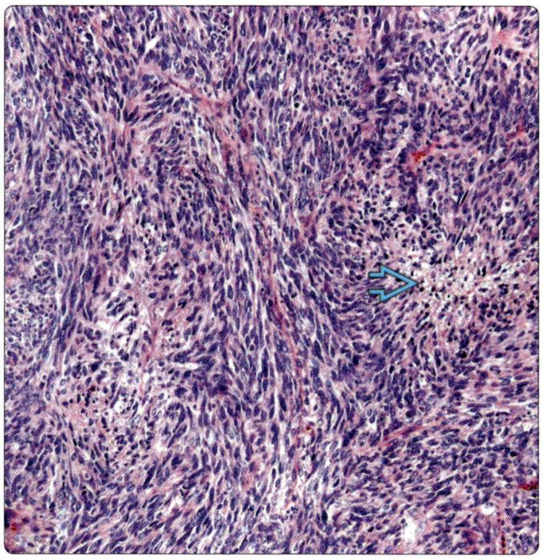

(Left) *Mitotic activity* *appears to be the best prognostic indicator of behavior in SFT, and the rate in malignant tumors often exceeds 4 mitoses per 10 HPF. As a point of practice, the mitotic rate should be assessed on all cases of cellular SFT, even in cases without nuclear pleomorphism.* **(Right)** *Malignant SFT can show a more prominently fascicular growth pattern, as depicted, resembling other spindle cell sarcomas. A small focus of tumor necrosis* *is also evident in this H&E.*

Malignant Solitary Fibrous Tumor: Pleomorphism

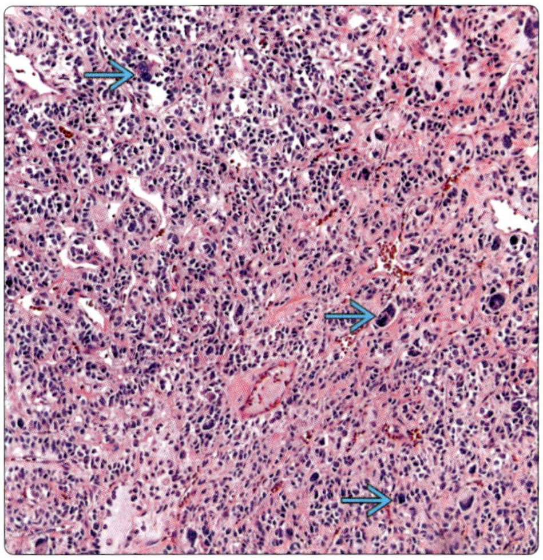

Malignant Solitary Fibrous Tumor: Loss of CD34

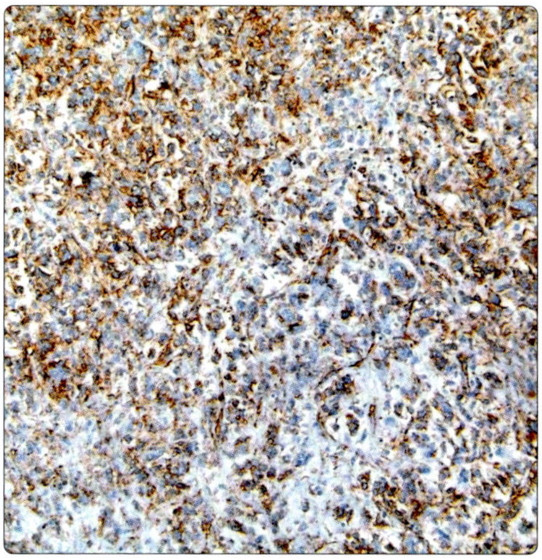

(Left) *In some cases, malignant SFT may feature prominent nuclear pleomorphism and atypia* *. Note that the overall background architecture and vasculature somewhat resembles conventional SFT.* **(Right)** *CD34 expression is highly variable in malignant SFT and may be patchy, decreased, or absent. Demonstration of nuclear STAT6 expression can be very helpful in CD34(-) cases.*

Low-Grade Myofibroblastic Sarcoma

KEY FACTS

TERMINOLOGY

- Atypical, infiltrative spindle cell neoplasm with morphologic, immunohistochemical, &/or ultrastructural evidence of myofibroblastic differentiation
- Synonym: Myofibrosarcoma

CLINICAL ISSUES

- Occurs predominantly in adult patients
- Frequently occurs in head and neck region
  - Also extremities, trunk, groin, abdomen/pelvis, other sites
- Treatment: Complete surgical excision
- Local recurrence is common
- Metastases are rare

MACROSCOPIC

- Well-circumscribed or ill-defined firm mass
- Variable size range, often < 5 cm

MICROSCOPIC

- Often diffusely infiltrative growth
- Fascicles or storiform arrays of spindled cells
  - Pale eosinophilic cytoplasm and indistinct borders
  - Elongated, fusiform, vesicular nuclei with variable nucleoli
    - Mild to moderate atypia present at least focally
- Prominent stromal collagen
- Mitotic rate often low (< 5 mitoses per 10 HPF)

ANCILLARY TESTS

- Variable SMA(+) &/or desmin (+)
- H-caldesmon, CD34, keratin, EMA, S100, myogenin (-)

TOP DIFFERENTIAL DIAGNOSES

- Desmoid fibromatosis
- Leiomyosarcoma
- Spindle cell rhabdomyosarcoma

Low-Grade Myofibroblastic Sarcoma

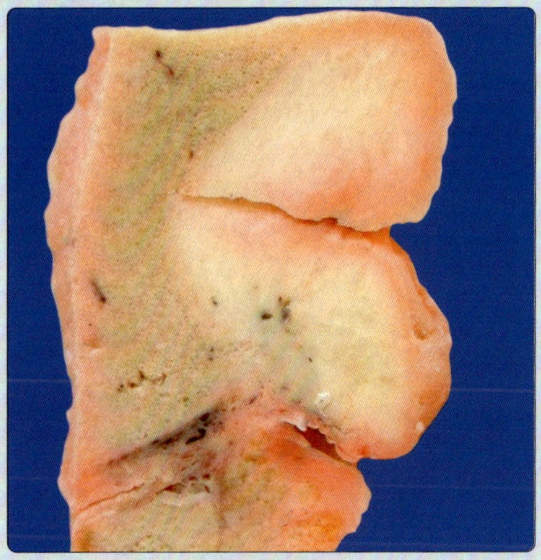

Low-Grade Myofibroblastic Sarcoma

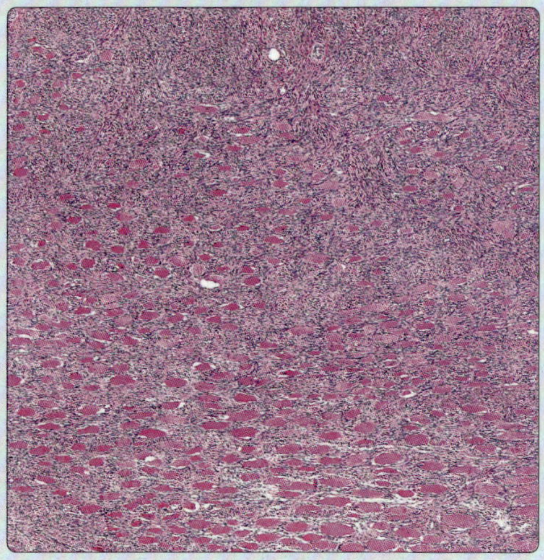

(Left) *Gross photograph shows a low-grade myofibroblastic sarcoma (LGMS) arising in the testis. The cut surface of this tumor usually appears tan-white-gray and fibrous on cut section.* **(Right)** *LGMS (a.k.a. myofibrosarcoma) is characterized in most cases by diffuse infiltration of preexisting structures and normal tissue, as seen in this H&E involving skeletal muscle.*

Infiltrative Growth

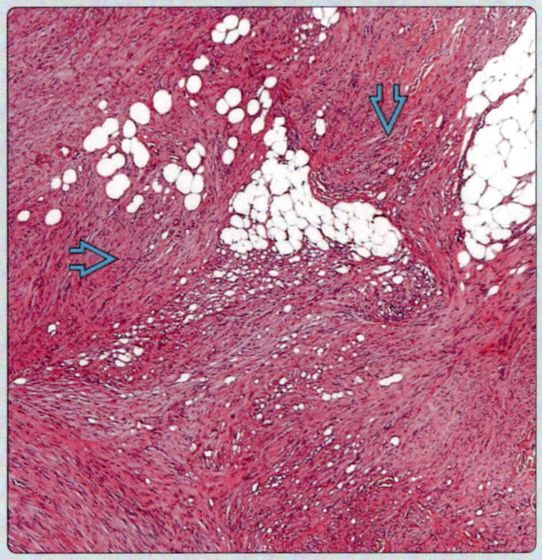

Infiltrative Growth

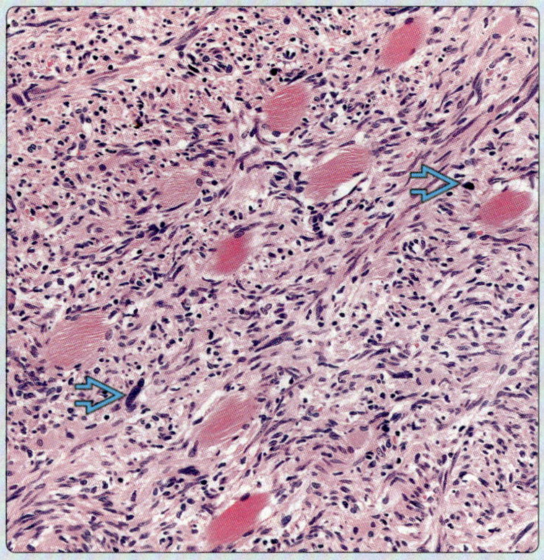

(Left) *Cases of LGMS that arise in subcutaneous tissue often show extensive infiltration of adipose tissue by fascicles of tumor cells →, as shown in this H&E.* **(Right)** *Infiltration of skeletal muscle fibers in LGMS often shows a checkerboard pattern with tumor cell growth around individual fibers. Also note the scattered hyperchromatic nuclei →, another characteristic feature of LGMS.*

Low-Grade Myofibroblastic Sarcoma

TERMINOLOGY

Abbreviations

- Low-grade myofibroblastic sarcoma (LGMS)

Synonyms

- Myofibrosarcoma

Definitions

- Atypical, infiltrative spindle cell neoplasm with morphologic, immunohistochemical, &/or ultrastructural evidence of myofibroblastic differentiation

CLINICAL ISSUES

Epidemiology

- Incidence
  - Rare
    - May be more common due to lack of well-defined diagnostic criteria
- Age
  - Occurs predominantly in adult patients
  - Children are rarely affected
- Sex
  - Slight male predominance

Site

- Occurs frequently in head and neck region
  - Particularly tongue and oral cavity
- Also extremities, trunk, groin, abdomen/pelvis, other sites
- May arise in subcutaneous or deep soft tissues
  - Very rare dermal origin

Presentation

- Slow-growing, painless mass

Treatment

- Complete surgical excision

Prognosis

- Local recurrence is common
  - May recur repeatedly
- Metastases are rare
  - Often after prolonged time interval

MACROSCOPIC

General Features

- Well-circumscribed or ill-defined firm mass
- Pale gray-white, fibrous cut surface

Size

- Variable, often < 5 cm
  - Some cases may grow to > 10 cm

MICROSCOPIC

Histologic Features

- Often highly infiltrative growth
  - Tumor cells may grow diffusely between individual preexisting cells and structures
    - Checkerboard pattern of infiltration within skeletal muscle
- Fascicles or storiform arrays of spindled cells
  - Often cellular or hypercellular; rarely hypocellular
  - Spindled cells show pale eosinophilic cytoplasm and indistinct borders
  - Elongated, fusiform, vesicular nuclei with variable nucleoli
    - May show nuclear indentations
    - Mild to moderate atypia present at least focally
      - □ Enlargement, hyperchromasia
    - Rare cases contain cells with marked nuclear pleomorphism
- Prominent stromal collagen
  - May show hyalinization or keloidal collagen
- Stroma may contain increased number of thin-walled capillaries
- Mitotic rate is often low (< 5 mitoses per 10 HPF)
- Tumor necrosis uncommon
- May progress to higher grade morphology

ANCILLARY TESTS

Immunohistochemistry

- Variable SMA(+) &/or desmin (+)
  - Diffuse desmin (+) may be seen in subset
- H-caldesmon, CD34, keratin, EMA, S100 protein, myogenin (-)
- Nuclear β-catenin (+) in subset

DIFFERENTIAL DIAGNOSIS

Desmoid Fibromatosis

- Shows infiltrative growth but lacks diffuse growth through and around preexisting structures
- Lacks cytologic atypia
- Desmin usually (-)

Leiomyosarcoma

- Cells with brightly eosinophilic cytoplasm and distinct cell borders
- Elongated, blunted, cigar-shaped nuclei
- Usually diffuse cytoplasmic SMA(+), h-caldesmon (+)

Spindle Cell Rhabdomyosarcoma

- Clinical and morphologic overlap with LGMS
- Contains scattered rhabdomyoblasts
- Desmin (+); focal myogenin (+)

Inflammatory Myofibroblastic Tumor

- Prominent inflammatory infiltrate (lymphocytes, plasma cells)
- Myxoid stroma common
- ALK(+) in 50% of cases

SELECTED REFERENCES

1. Taweevisit M et al: Distinctive features of low-grade myofibroblastic sarcoma on aspiration cytology: a case report. Cytopathology. 73(4): 634-44, 2018
2. Cai C et al: In myofibroblastic sarcomas of the head and neck, mitotic activity and necrosis define grade: a case study and literature review. Virchows Arch. 463(6):827-36, 2013
3. Fisher C: Myofibrosarcoma. Virchows Arch. 445(3):215-23, 2004
4. Montgomery E et al: Myofibrosarcoma: a clinicopathologic study. Am J Surg Pathol. 25(2):219-28, 2001
5. Mentzel T et al: Low-grade myofibroblastic sarcoma: analysis of 18 cases in the spectrum of myofibroblastic tumors. Am J Surg Pathol. 22(10):1228-38, 1998

(Left) *LGMS is composed of fascicles and storiform arrays of spindled myofibroblastic cells with ill-defined, pale eosinophilic cytoplasm. Scattered hyperchromatic nuclei are frequently identified* ⇨. **(Right)** *The nuclei of LGMS are cytologically myofibroblastic with vesicular chromatin and a small eosinophilic nucleolus. They may appear elongated and tapering or plump with irregular/notched contours.*

Nuclear Atypia

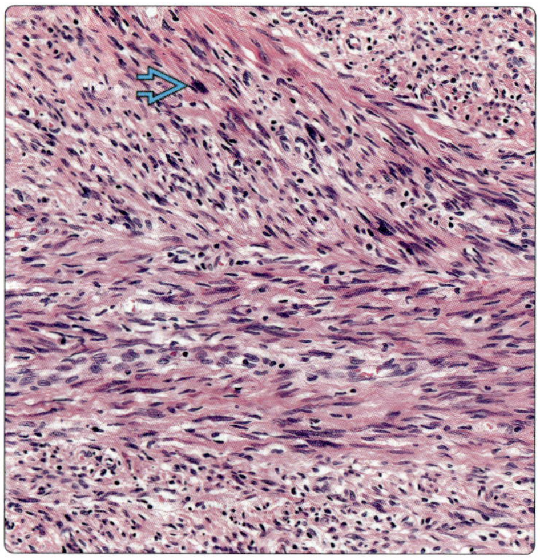

Cytologic Features

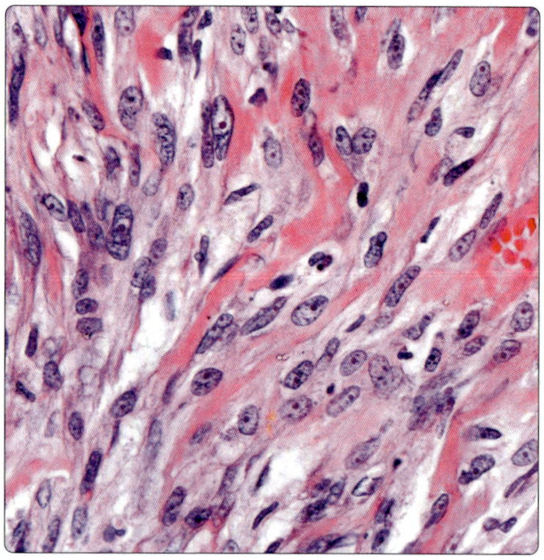

(Left) *Stromal collagen is a consistent feature of LGMS and is often abundant.* **(Right)** *In some cases of LGMS, the stromal collagen is more conspicuously bundled and thicker and may even appear keloidal. This morphologic appearance may be retained in the rare event of metastasis.*

Stromal Collagen

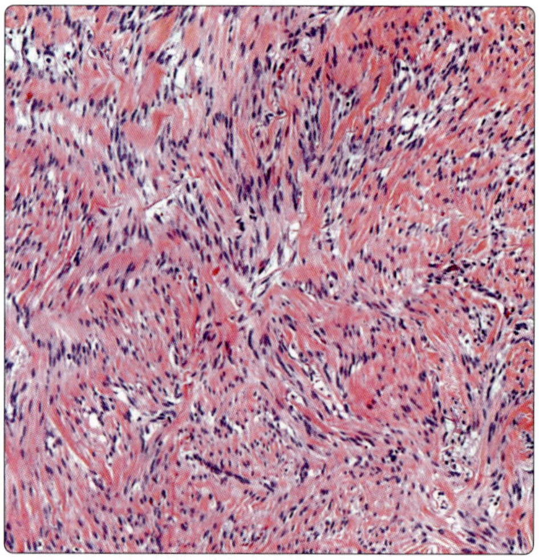

Stromal Collagen

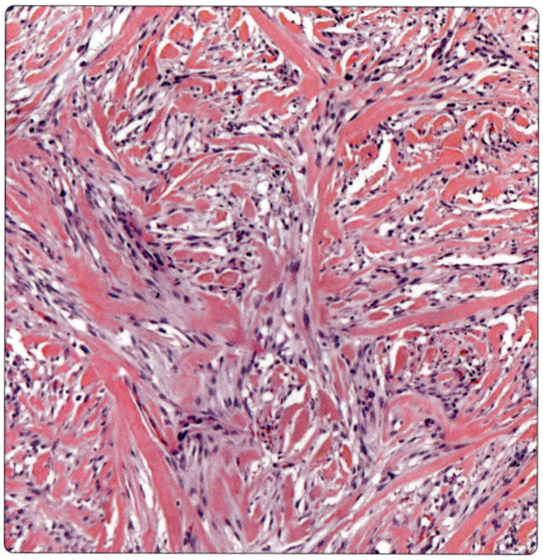

(Left) *Some areas of LGMS may show a streaming, fascicular growth similar to fibromatosis. Importantly, nuclear atypia/hyperchromasia is a feature of LGMS and not fibromatosis, and the former typically shows a greater degree of soft tissue infiltration.* **(Right)** *A fascicular growth pattern is common in LGMS and may show focal herringbone architecture, as depicted. Note the abundant stromal collagen.*

Fibromatosis-Like Morphology

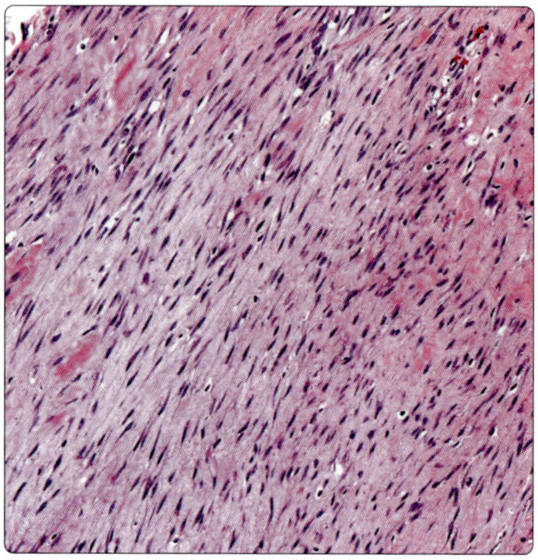

Fascicular Growth

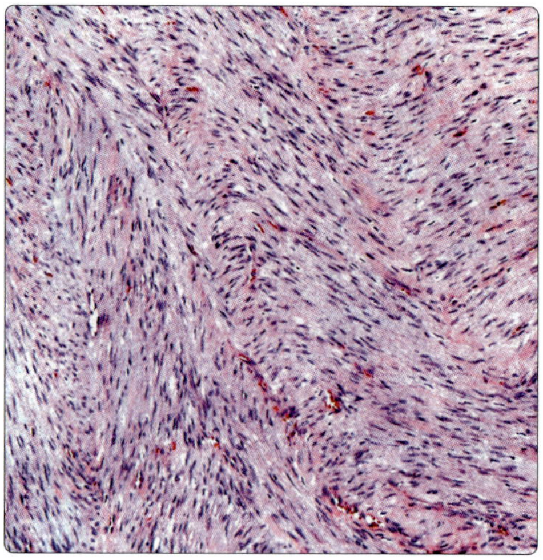

Rare Hypercellular Areas

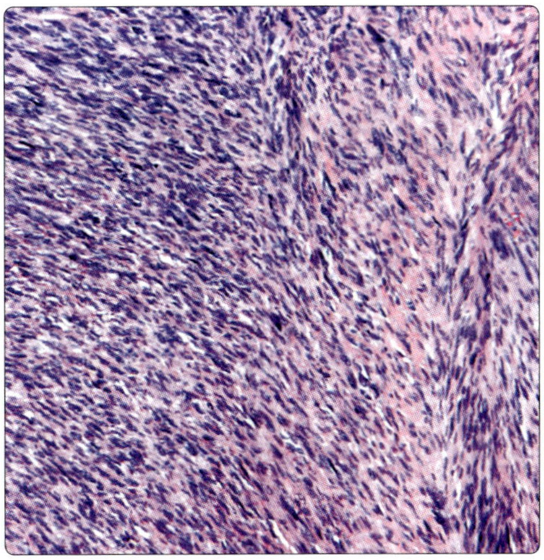

Fasciitis-Like Areas

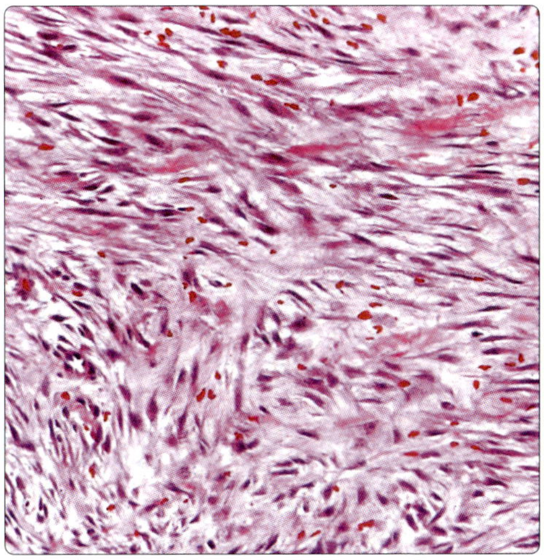

(Left) *Hypercellular areas may be found in LGMS but are generally very rare. Other entities, such as synovial sarcoma, adult-type fibrosarcoma, and leiomyosarcoma, must be carefully excluded.* **(Right)** *Myxoid and loosely arranged architecture may be seen focally in LGMS and may raise the possibility of nodular fasciitis or inflammatory myofibroblastic tumor. Infiltrative growth, nuclear atypia, and lack of a prominent chronic inflammatory cell component favor LGMS.*

Hypocellular Areas

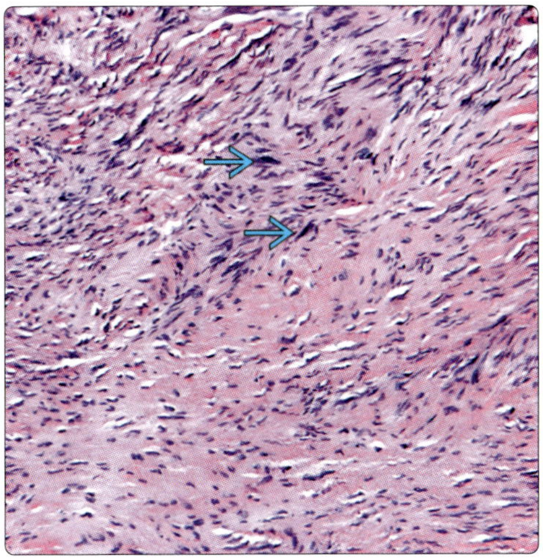

Stromal Hyalinization

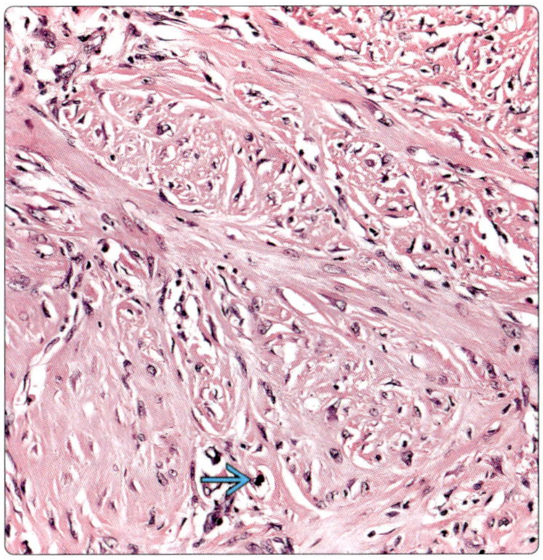

(Left) *Areas showing marked stromal hyalinization are not uncommon in LGMS; however, tumors with diffuse hyalinization are rare. Note the scattered hyperchromatic nuclei ➡ in this H&E.* **(Right)** *This example of LGMS is hypocellular and shows abundant stromal hyalinization. Scattered mitotic figures are also present ➡.*

Higher Grade Morphology

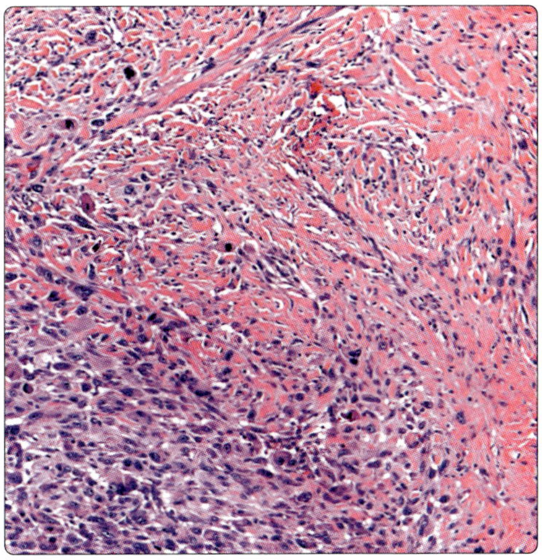

Rare Metastases

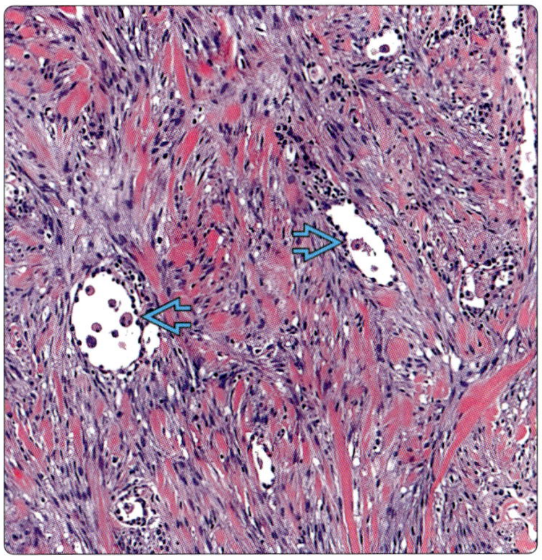

(Left) *Rare cases of LGMS may show areas of transition to a higher grade sarcoma; however, this is more likely to be seen in recurrences. Primary tumors with high-grade features are probably best classified as undifferentiated pleomorphic sarcoma.* **(Right)** *H&E shows a lung metastasis in a 45-year-old woman with LGMS of the hip diagnosed 3-4 years prior. The tumor is cytologically low grade and shows abundant collagen production, similar to the original. Note the entrapped alveolar spaces ⇨.*

Inflammatory Myofibroblastic Tumor

KEY FACTS

TERMINOLOGY

- Myofibroblastic spindle cell neoplasm of predominantly children and young adults that classically features mixed chronic inflammatory infiltrate

CLINICAL ISSUES

- Most common in children and young adults
- Abdominopelvic region (mesentery, omentum, retroperitoneum) common
  - Also lung, bladder, female genital tract, CNS, others
- Treatment: Complete surgical resection
- Prognosis variable but generally good
  - Up to 35% may recur and < 5% metastasize
  - Usually intraabdominal or retroperitoneal tumors
  - Distinctive intraabdominal morphologic variant, epithelioid inflammatory myofibroblastic sarcoma (EIMS), shows aggressive course

MICROSCOPIC

- Spindled or stellate myofibroblastic cells
- Main histologic patterns: Myxoid, fascicular, sclerosing
- Inflammatory cell infiltrate common

ANCILLARY TESTS

- SMA(+), variable desmin (+)
- Cytoplasmic ALK(+) in 50-60%
- Molecular: Rearrangement of 2p23 (*ALK*) in ~ 50% of cases
  - *ALK-RANBP2* rearrangement identified in EIMS variant
  - Other gene fusions reported in subset of *ALK*-negative inflammatory myofibroblastic tumor (IMT) (e.g., *ROS1*)

TOP DIFFERENTIAL DIAGNOSES

- Nodular fasciitis
- Desmoid fibromatosis
- Leiomyosarcoma
- IgG4-related sclerosing disease

(Left) *Inflammatory myofibroblastic tumor (IMT) is a myofibroblastic neoplasm of intermediate biologic potential that most frequently occurs in children and young adults. A variably cellular myxoid morphology is common in these tumors.* **(Right)** *The cells of IMT are typically spindled or stellate and show eosinophilic to amphophilic cytoplasm. Extravasated erythrocytes may be seen. Heavily myxoid tumors may resemble nodular fasciitis or a reactive process.*

Inflammatory Myofibroblastic Tumor

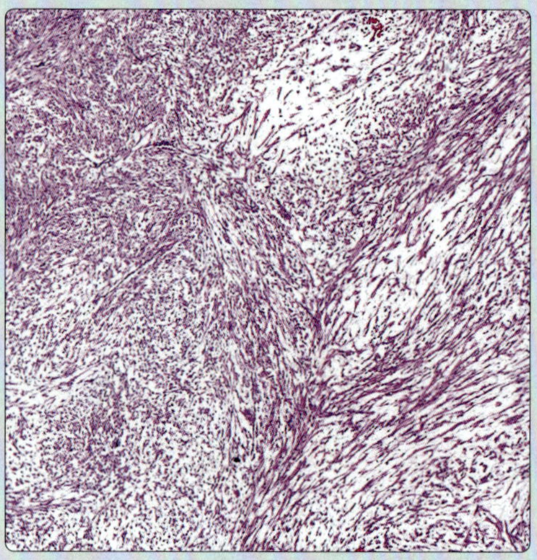

Myxoid Stroma

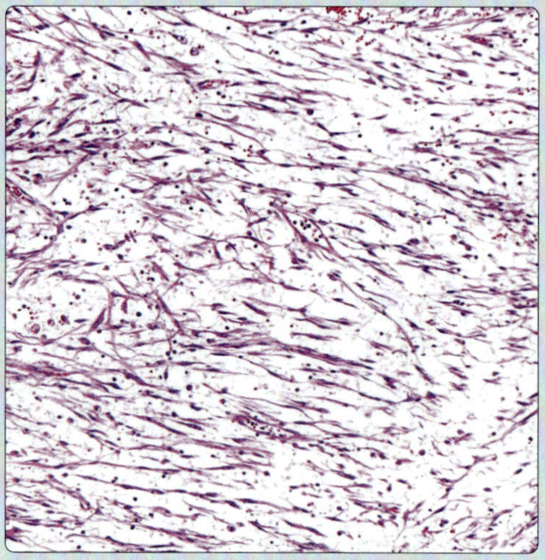

(Left) *Cytologically, the lesional cells of IMT show vesicular nucleoli with 1 or 2 conspicuous nucleoli. In some cases, the nucleoli may be larger and more prominent. The mitotic rate varies but is often low.* **(Right)** *Cytoplasmic ALK expression is identified in ~ 50% of cases of IMT and may be patchy or extensive. This expression roughly correlates with the presence of an ALK gene arrangement.*

Cytologic Features

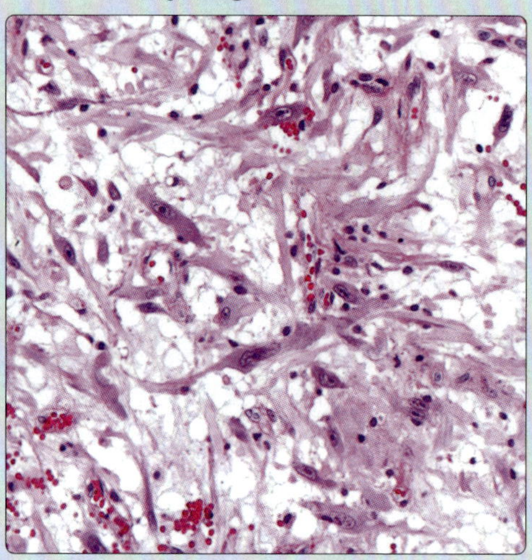

ALK Expression

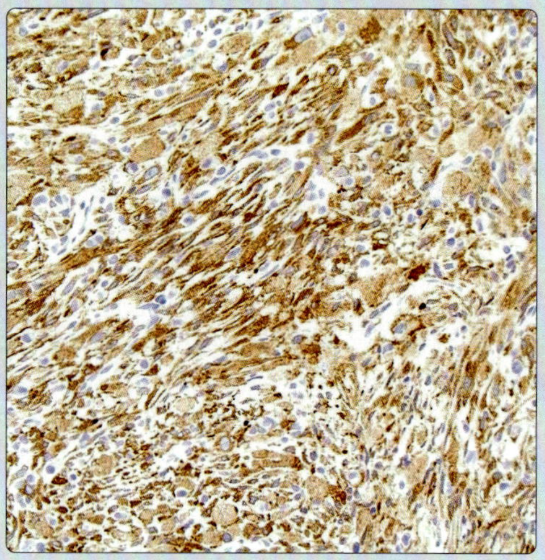

TERMINOLOGY

Abbreviations

- Inflammatory myofibroblastic tumor (IMT)

Synonyms

- Inflammatory myofibroblastic sarcoma
- Inflammatory fibrosarcoma
- Inflammatory pseudotumor
- Plasma cell granuloma

Definitions

- Myofibroblastic spindle cell neoplasm of predominantly children and young adults that classically features mixed chronic inflammatory infiltrate

CLINICAL ISSUES

Epidemiology

- Incidence
  - Rare
- Age
  - Wide range (most common in children and young adults)
- Sex
  - Slight female predominance

Site

- Abdominopelvic region (mesentery, omentum, retroperitoneum) most common
- Many other sites including head/neck, lung, bladder, female genital tract, CNS
  - Peripheral soft tissue sites are rare

Presentation

- Site specific
  - Lung
    - Chest pain, dyspnea
  - Mesentery, omentum, uterus, gastrointestinal tract
    - Obstruction (often large tumors)
    - May have constitutional symptoms (e.g., fever, weight loss)
    - May show laboratory evidence of anemia, hypergammaglobulinemia, or elevated ESR
  - Soft tissue
    - Painless mass
  - Bladder
    - Hematuria

Treatment

- Complete surgical resection
  - Reexcision of recurrences
- Potential for targeted therapy with specific tyrosine kinase inhibitors provides rationale for routine molecular analysis of IMT

Prognosis

- Variable but generally good
- Up to 35% may recur and < 5% metastasize
  - Usually intraabdominal or retroperitoneal tumors
    - Distinctive intraabdominal variant, epithelioid inflammatory myofibroblastic sarcoma (EIMS), shows aggressive course
- Tumor size, mitotic rate, cellularity, nuclear atypia, and necrosis do not appear to correlate well with outcome in conventional IMT

MACROSCOPIC

General Features

- Often multilobulated
- Solid tan-white-pink firm cut surface

Size

- 1-20 cm (most < 10 cm)

MICROSCOPIC

Histologic Features

- Expansile or infiltrative peripheral border
- Myofibroblastic cells
  - Usually spindled, ovoid, or stellate
    - Rarely epithelioid
  - Vesicular nuclei with 1 or 2 conspicuous nucleoli
  - Occasional cells have enlarged nuclei with macronucleoli or "smudgy" chromatin
- 3 main histologic patterns
  - Spindle or stellate cells within prominent loose myxoid stroma
  - Compact spindle cells in fascicles or storiform arrays
  - Hypocellular, sclerotic matrix
- Inflammatory cells common but vary in number
  - Lymphocytes and plasma cells predominate
  - Variable numbers of neutrophils and eosinophils
  - Histiocytes
- Mitotic rate varies (often low)
- Necrosis is rare
- Occasional calcification and ossification

Morphologic Variants

- EIMS
  - Predominantly composed of rounded to epithelioid cells with prominent nucleoli
  - Often shows prominent myxoid stroma rich in inflammatory cells, particularly neutrophils or lymphocytes
  - Strong desmin (+) and ALK(+) in nuclear membrane staining pattern

ANCILLARY TESTS

Immunohistochemistry

- SMA(+), variable desmin (+)
- Cytoplasmic ALK(+) in 50-60% of cases
  - Positive expression roughly correlates with presence of *ALK* gene rearrangement
  - ALK expression is more common in younger patients
  - ROS1(+) in subset of ALK(-) tumors (if *ROS1* rearrangement is present)
- Subset shows focal keratin (+)
- Negative for S100 protein, myogenin, CD117, and EMA

Molecular Genetics

- Rearrangement of 2p23 (*ALK*) in ~ 50% of cases
  - Variety of partner genes including *ATIC, TPM3, TPM4, CLTC, RANBP2, EML4, IGFBP5, THBS1*

- *ALK-RANBP2* rearrangement identified in most reported cases of EIMS
- Subset of *ALK*-negative tumors harbor fusions involving *ROS1*, *RET*, *PDGFRB*, or *ETV6* and *NTRK3*

DIFFERENTIAL DIAGNOSIS

Nodular Fasciitis

- Most common in extremity
- Usually subcutaneous and < 3 cm in size
- Negative for ALK by IHC
- *MYH9-USP6* fusion

Desmoid Fibromatosis

- Usually in small bowel mesentery
- Fascicles of spindle cells with interspersed collagen and usually negligible inflammation
- Small-caliber vessels often with perivascular edema
- SMA(+)
- Negative for ALK by IHC
- Nuclear β-catenin (+) in majority

Leiomyosarcoma

- May have prominent inflammation or myxoid stroma
  - Myxoid leiomyosarcoma usually lacks lymphoplasmacytic infiltrate
- Deep soft tissues of older adults
- Foci of classic leiomyosarcoma morphology may be present
- Generally diffuse SMA(+); variable desmin (+)
- Negative for ALK by IHC

IgG4-Related Sclerosing Disease

- May closely resemble sclerosing pattern of IMT
- Obstructive phlebitis common
- Negative for ALK by IHC
- Ratio of IgG4(+) to IgG(+) plasma cells much higher than IMT

Well-Differentiated Liposarcoma

- May show prominent chronic inflammatory component
- More common in older adults
- Adipocytic differentiation often clearly present elsewhere

Dedifferentiated Liposarcoma

- Most common in older adults
- Nonlipogenic component may rarely resemble IMT
- Often occurs in retroperitoneum of older adults
- Most contain component of conventional well-differentiated liposarcoma
- Negative for ALK by IHC

Gastrointestinal Stromal Tumor

- May occur in abdomen/pelvis but outside tubular GI tract
- Monomorphic spindled &/or epithelioid cells
- May have stromal lymphocytes; plasma cells or eosinophils are rare
- CD34(+)
- CD117(+)
- DOG1(+)
- Negative for ALK by IHC
- *KIT* or *PDGFRA* mutations

Inflammatory Fibroid Polyp

- Bland spindle cells in loose edematous or myxoid stroma with eosinophils and lymphocytes
- Usually in submucosa of gastric antrum or duodenum; often polypoid
- CD34(+)
- Negative for ALK by IHC
- *PDGFRA* mutations

Anaplastic Large Cell Lymphoma

- May show morphologic overlap with EIMS
- Seldom spindled
- Expresses lymphoid markers
- CD30(+), ALK(+), similar to EIMS

SELECTED REFERENCES

1. Mohammad N et al: ALK is a specific diagnostic marker for inflammatory myofibroblastic tumor of the uterus. Am J Surg Pathol. 42(10):1353-9, 2018
2. Bennett JA et al: Inflammatory myofibroblastic tumor of the uterus: a clinicopathological, immunohistochemical, and molecular analysis of 13 cases highlighting their broad morphologic spectrum. Mod Pathol. 30(10):1489-503, 2017
3. Haimes JD et al: Uterine inflammatory myofibroblastic tumors frequently harbor ALK fusions with IGFBP5 and THBS1. Am J Surg Pathol. 41(6):773-80, 2017
4. Inamura K et al: A novel fusion of HNRNPA1-ALK in inflammatory myofibroblastic tumor of urinary bladder. Hum Pathol. 69:96-100, 2017
5. Lahlou G et al: Sinonasal inflammatory myofibroblastic tumor with anaplastic lymphoma kinase 1 rearrangement: case study and literature review. Head Neck Pathol. 11(2):131-8, 2017
6. Pickett JL et al: Inflammatory myofibroblastic tumors of the female genital tract are under-recognized: a low threshold for ALK immunohistochemistry is required. Am J Surg Pathol. 41(10):1433-42, 2017
7. Antonescu CR et al: Molecular characterization of inflammatory myofibroblastic tumors with frequent ALK and ROS1 gene fusions and rare novel RET rearrangement. Am J Surg Pathol. 39(7):957-67, 2015
8. Hornick JL et al: Expression of ROS1 predicts ROS1 gene rearrangement in inflammatory myofibroblastic tumors. Mod Pathol. 28(5):732-9, 2015
9. Lovly CM et al: Inflammatory myofibroblastic tumors harbor multiple potentially actionable kinase fusions. Cancer Discov. 4(8):889-95, 2014
10. Li J et al: Inflammatory myofibroblastic tumor with RANBP2 and ALK gene rearrangement: a report of two cases and literature review. Diagn Pathol. 8:147, 2013
11. Mariño-Enríquez A et al: Epithelioid inflammatory myofibroblastic sarcoma: an aggressive intra-abdominal variant of inflammatory myofibroblastic tumor with nuclear membrane or perinuclear ALK. Am J Surg Pathol. 35(1):135-44, 2011
12. Yamamoto H et al: Inflammatory myofibroblastic tumor versus IgG4-related sclerosing disease and inflammatory pseudotumor: a comparative clinicopathologic study. Am J Surg Pathol. 33(9):1330-40, 2009
13. Gleason BC et al: Inflammatory myofibroblastic tumours: where are we now? J Clin Pathol. 61(4):428-37, 2008
14. Coffin CM et al: Inflammatory myofibroblastic tumor: comparison of clinicopathologic, histologic, and immunohistochemical features including ALK expression in atypical and aggressive cases. Am J Surg Pathol. 31(4):509-20, 2007
15. Patel AS et al: RANBP2 and CLTC are involved in ALK rearrangements in inflammatory myofibroblastic tumors. Cancer Genet Cytogenet. 176(2):107-14, 2007
16. Cole B et al: Inflammatory myofibroblastic tumor with thrombocytosis and a unique chromosomal translocation with ALK rearrangement. Arch Pathol Lab Med. 130(7):1042-5, 2006
17. Montgomery EA et al: Inflammatory myofibroblastic tumors of the urinary tract: a clinicopathologic study of 46 cases, including a malignant example inflammatory fibrosarcoma and a subset associated with high-grade urothelial carcinoma. Am J Surg Pathol. 30(12):1502-12, 2006
18. Coffin CM et al: Inflammatory myofibroblastic tumor, inflammatory fibrosarcoma, and related lesions: an historical review with differential diagnostic considerations. Semin Diagn Pathol. 15(2):102-10, 1998
19. Coffin CM et al: Extrapulmonary inflammatory myofibroblastic tumor (inflammatory pseudotumor). A clinicopathologic and immunohistochemical study of 84 cases. Am J Surg Pathol. 19(8):859-72, 1995

Inflammatory Infiltrate

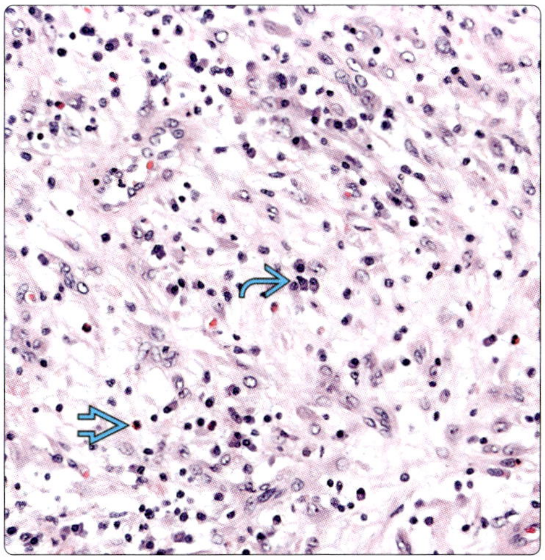

Plasma Cells

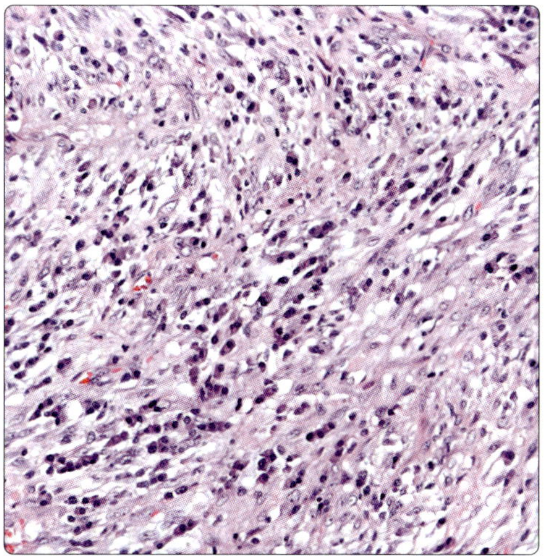

(Left) *A characteristic feature of IMT is the presence of a stromal inflammatory infiltrate. Lymphocytes and plasma cells are most common, but eosinophils and neutrophils may also be seen.* **(Right)** *A stromal inflammatory infiltrate is not specific for IMT and may be seen in a variety of other tumors; however, a prominent component of plasma cells is often considered more typical of IMT, as depicted. In some cases, the plasma cells may even form small aggregates.*

Fascicular Architecture

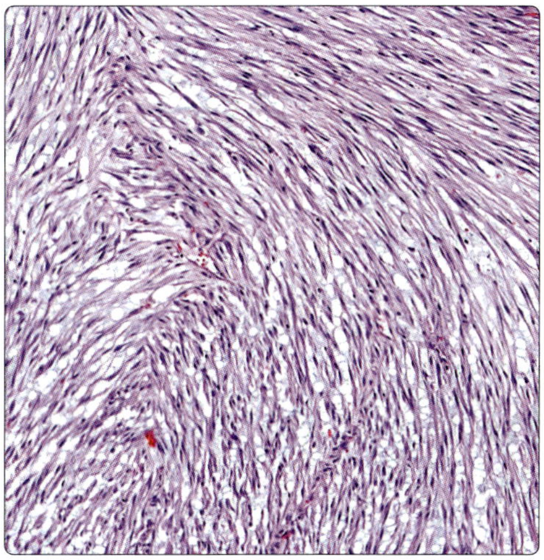

Fascicular Architecture

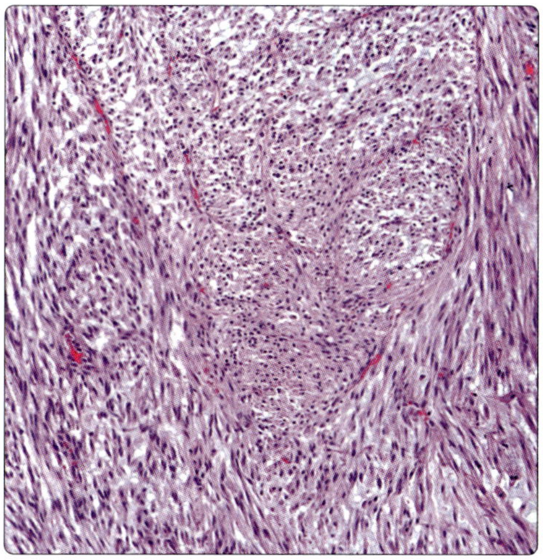

(Left) *In the more cellular areas of a myxoid IMT, the tumor cells often show a vague, subtle, or well-formed fascicular growth pattern.* **(Right)** *In some cellular examples of IMT, fascicular growth is more pronounced and may closely resemble a smooth muscle neoplasm, particularly leiomyosarcoma. These tumors can also be a challenge immunohistochemically, although strong cytoplasmic ALK expression would support IMT.*

Hemorrhage

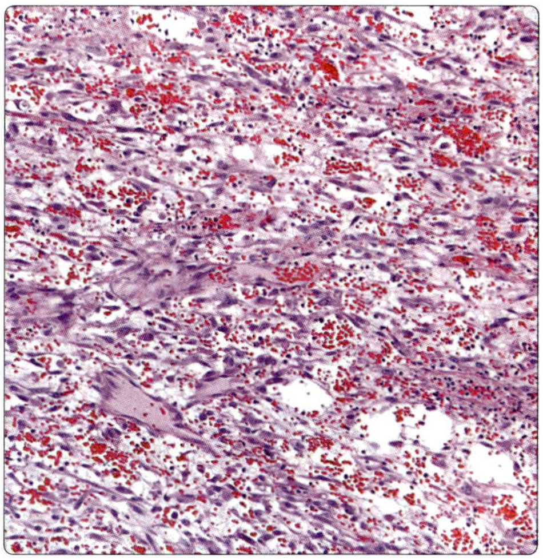

Cellular Fascicular Growth

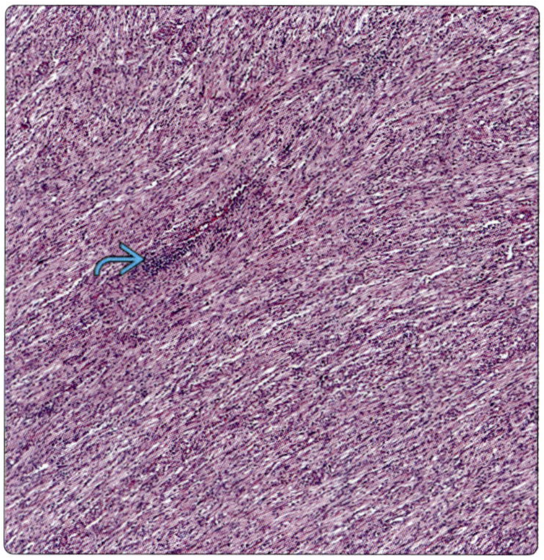

(Left) *Intratumoral hemorrhage may be seen in IMT, particularly myxoid tumors. When extensive, a vascular neoplasm may be considered.* **(Right)** *Another major morphologic pattern in IMT is solid, moderately cellular fascicular growth with prominent inflammatory cells. Scattered lymphoid aggregates may be present, occasionally with reactive germinal centers.*

Cytologic Features

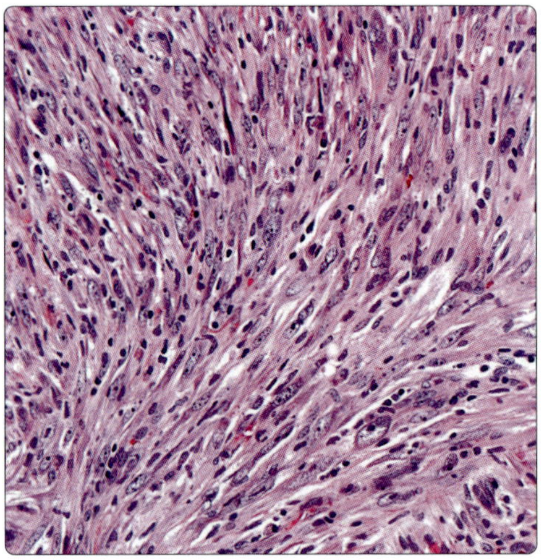

Macronucleoli

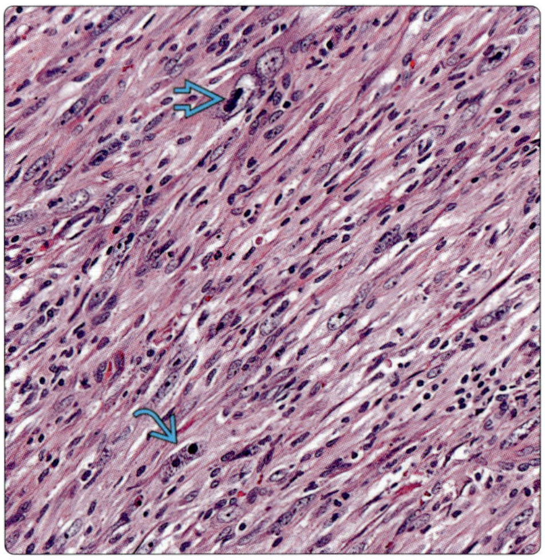

(Left) *The lesional cells of IMT show vesicular nucleoli with 1 or few conspicuous nucleoli. A conspicuous stromal inflammatory infiltrate is present.* **(Right)** *Some tumor cells in IMT contain enlarged nuclei with prominent basophilic or eosinophilic macronucleoli resembling Reed-Sternberg cells ➔ or viral infection ⇨. Although atypical, in isolation these cells do not appear to predict behavior.*

"Smudgy" Chromatin

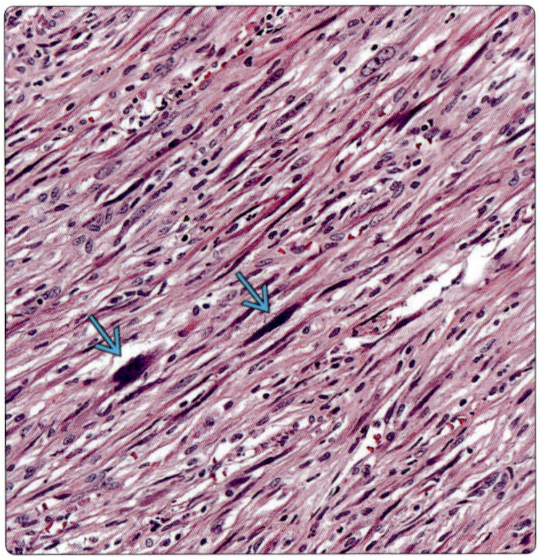

Occasional Herringbone Growth

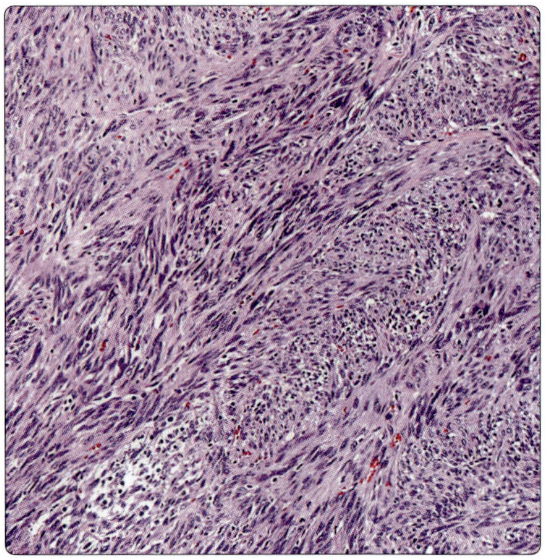

(Left) *Scattered tumor cells with hyperchromatic and "smudgy" chromatin ➔ are not uncommon in more cellular examples of IMT. In some cases, they may be more numerous.* **(Right)** *A focal herringbone fascicular growth pattern may be seen in cellular cases of IMT. This finding may lead to misclassification as a frank sarcoma.*

Vague Storiform Growth

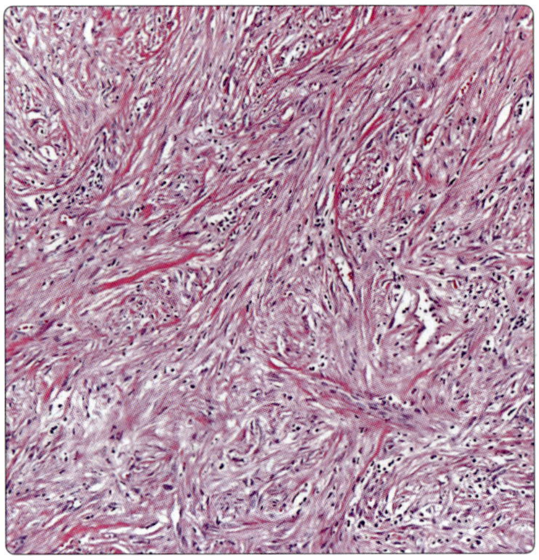

Hyalinized Stroma

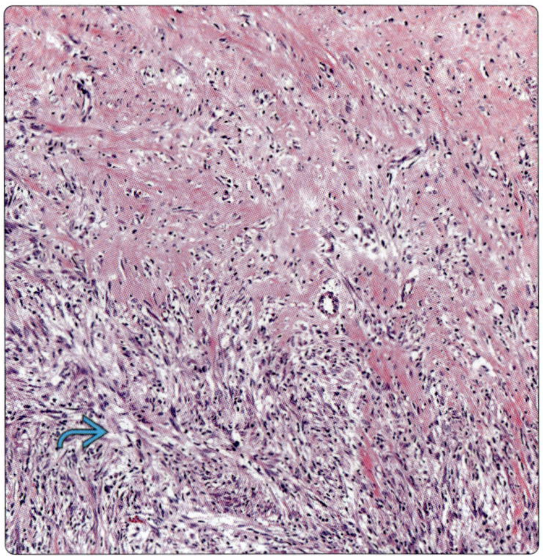

(Left) *A vague loose or tight storiform growth pattern may also be seen in IMT. This example also shows an increase in stromal collagen.* **(Right)** *Another major morphologic pattern in IMT is that of a prominent hyalinized or collagenous stroma with low cellularity. This pattern is often admixed with more cellular and morphologically typical areas ➔.*

Stromal Sclerosis

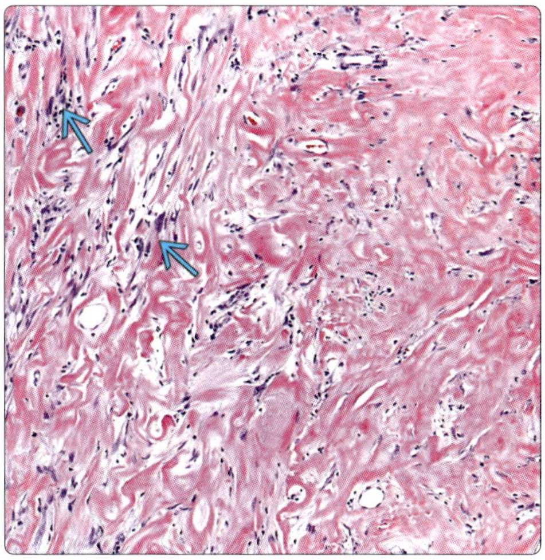

Stromal Sclerosis

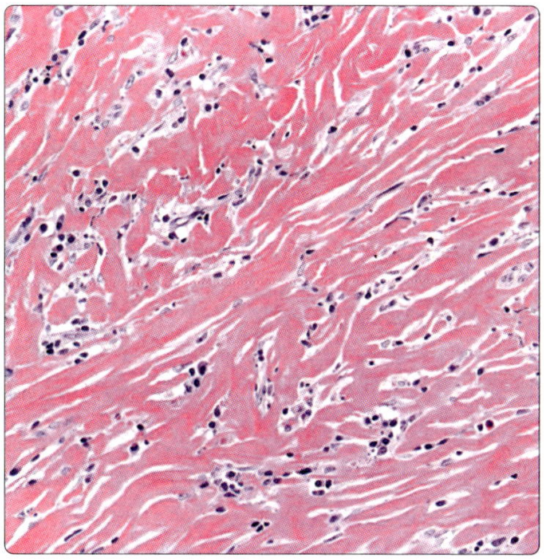

(Left) *In sclerotic areas of IMT, the lesional cells often form small clusters* → *within a prominent eosinophilic collagenized stroma. The characteristic inflammatory infiltrate is common in these zones.* **(Right)** *In this sclerotic focus of IMT, only stromal collagen and chronic inflammatory cells are conspicuous, and lesional cells are difficult to identify. This pattern may closely mimic IgG4-related sclerosing disease.*

Prominent Inflammation

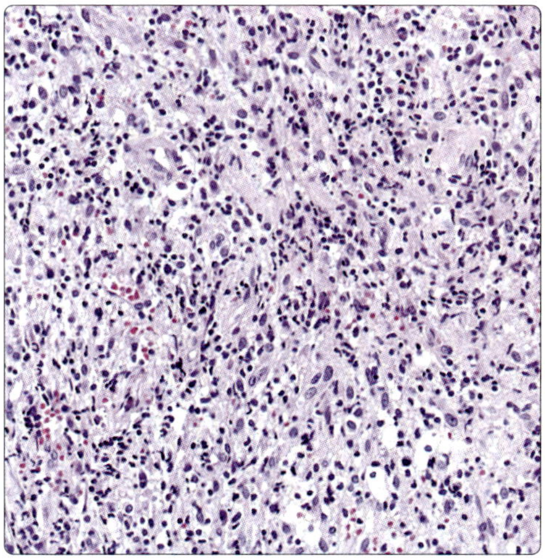

Rare Giant Cells

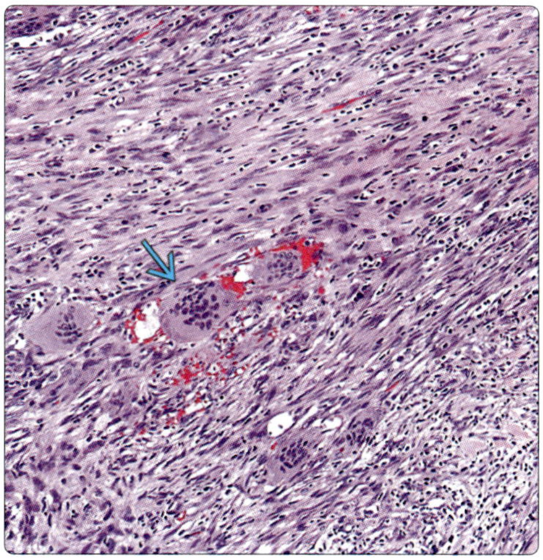

(Left) *In some cases of IMT, the stromal mixed inflammatory infiltrate is quite prominent, as depicted, and the neoplastic nature of the lesion may be overlooked.* **(Right)** *Osteoclast-like giant cells* → *are a rare finding in IMT and may be seen in association with focal calcification or metaplastic bone formation, which are also rare findings.*

Peripheral Changes

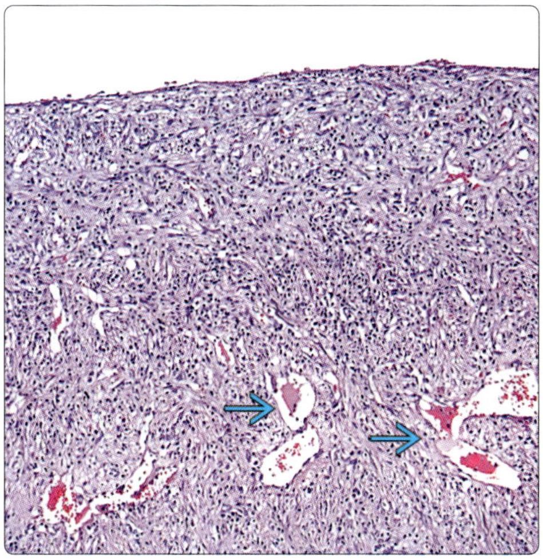

Epithelioid Morphology

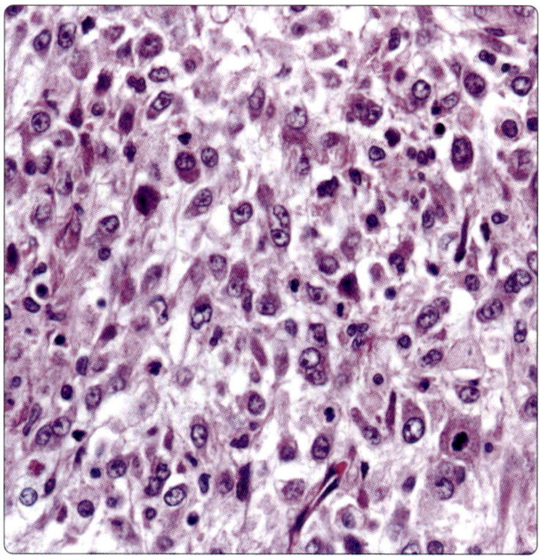

(Left) *The periphery of some expansile, intraabdominal IMTs may show ulceration, granulation tissue formation, or dilated congested blood vessels* →*, simulating a reactive process.* **(Right)** *An epithelioid morphology is occasionally seen in conventional IMT. When this morphology is diffuse, however, and the tumor arises in the abdominal cavity, the aggressive variant epithelioid inflammatory myofibroblastic sarcoma (EIMS) should be carefully excluded through molecular analysis.*

Myxoinflammatory Fibroblastic Sarcoma

KEY FACTS

TERMINOLOGY

- Distinctive locally aggressive and rarely metastasizing mesenchymal neoplasm of fibroblastic/myofibroblastic origin that shows predilection for distal (acral) extremities

CLINICAL ISSUES

- Slow-growing infiltrative mass in subcutaneous tissue of adults
- Predilection for distal (acral) extremities, particularly dorsal aspects of fingers and hand
- Treatment: Wide local excision with negative margins
- Local recurrence rate 30-50%
- Metastasis very rare
- Higher grade tumors have worse prognosis

MICROSCOPIC

- Poorly marginated, often multinodular tumor
- Variable mixture of hyalinized and myxoid zones merging with variably prominent inflammatory component
- Inflammatory component shows variable mixture of lymphocytes, plasma cells, neutrophils, and eosinophils
- Scattered enlarged epithelioid tumor cells with smudgy heterochromatin or enlarged/macronucleoli
- Pseudolipoblasts common in myxoid zones
- Low mitotic rate

ANCILLARY TESTS

- Nonspecific, variable expression of CD34, CD68, D2-40, CD117, EMA reported
- *BRAF* abnormalities identified in subset
- *TGFBR3* and *MGEA5* rearrangements rare in pure MIFS

TOP DIFFERENTIAL DIAGNOSES

- Myxofibrosarcoma
- Diffuse-type tenosynovial giant cell tumor
- Extranodal Hodgkin disease
- Hemosiderotic fibrolipomatous tumor
- Proliferative fasciitis

Multinodular Growth

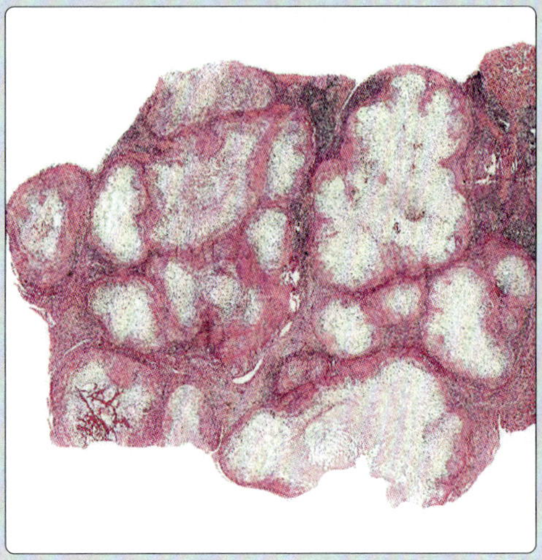

Stromal Variation

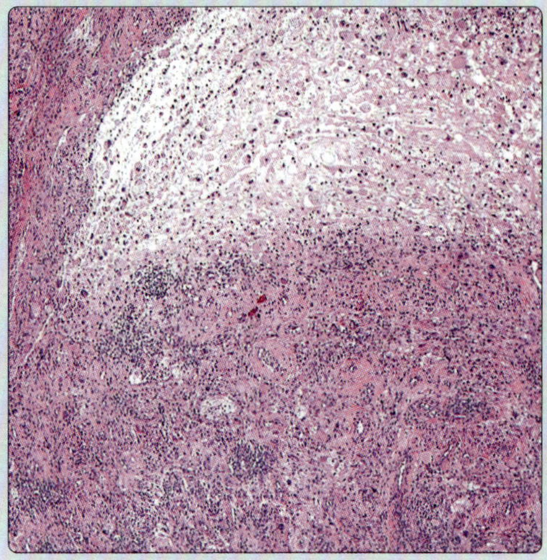

(Left) *At low magnification, myxoinflammatory fibroblastic sarcoma (MIFS) classically shows a multinodular growth pattern. This nodularity may be prominent and well delineated, as in this example, or subtle and more compartmentalized.* **(Right)** *MIFS typically shows a variable admixture of 3 morphologic zones: Myxoid, hyalinized, and inflammatory. The exact composition is highly variable, and some cases may show predominantly 1 type of zone.*

Conspicuous Inflammation

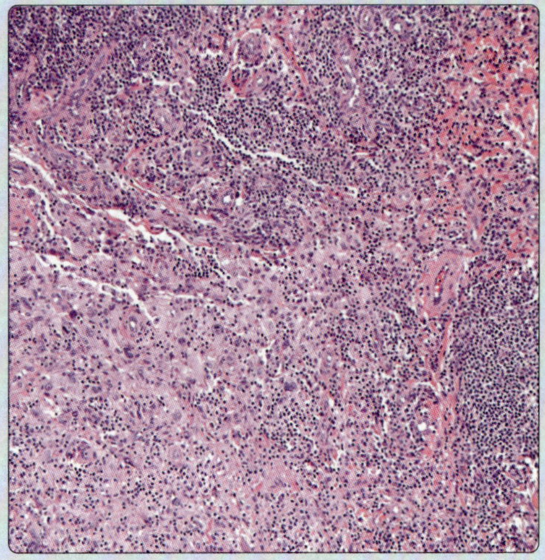

Viral Inclusion-Like Nucleoli

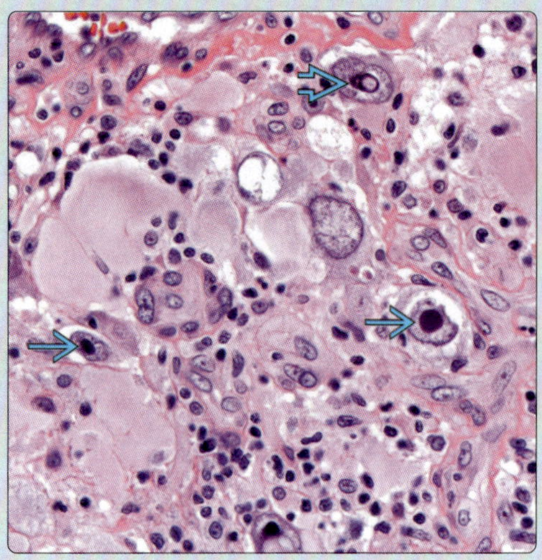

(Left) *A relatively consistent finding in MIFS is the presence of a conspicuous inflammatory infiltrate. This inflammation may be in the form of dense sheets of lymphocytes and plasma cells or appear as a scattered stromal infiltrate.* **(Right)** *The tumor cells in MIFS range from plump spindle cells to histiocytoid or epithelioid cells with enlarged basophilic or eosinophilic macronucleoli ➡. The latter are often reminiscent of virally infected nuclei. Intranuclear pseudoinclusions ➡ are also common.*

TERMINOLOGY

Abbreviations

- Myxoinflammatory fibroblastic sarcoma (MIFS)

Synonyms

- Acral myxoinflammatory fibroblastic sarcoma
- Atypical myxoinflammatory fibroblastic tumor
- Inflammatory myxohyaline tumor of distal extremities with virocyte or Reed-Sternberg-like cells

Definitions

- Distinctive locally aggressive and rarely metastasizing mesenchymal neoplasm of fibroblastic/myofibroblastic origin that shows predilection for distal (acral) extremities
- Recent evidence suggests that MIFS may not be related to hemosiderotic fibrolipomatous tumor (HFLT) or pleomorphic hyalinizing angiectatic tumor (PHAT)

CLINICAL ISSUES

Epidemiology

- Age
  - Adults (25-50 years most common)

Site

- Marked predilection for distal (acral) extremities, particularly dorsal aspects
  - Fingers and hand most common
  - Also wrist, forearm, toes, feet, ankles, lower leg
- Rare extraacral cases but increasingly reported
  - Higher grade tumors tend to arise in proximal locations

Presentation

- Slow-growing, painless, ill-defined mass
  - Usually subcutaneous
    - May involve dermis or invade underlying skeletal muscle
- May be mistaken clinically for ganglion cyst or lipoma

Treatment

- Wide local excision with negative margins
  - Amputation may be considered in distal lesions
- Indefinite clinical follow-up recommended
- Radiation therapy following excision may have role in reducing local recurrence

Prognosis

- Local recurrences common (30-50%)
  - Risk associated with adequacy of surgical excision
- Very low, but definite risk of metastasis
  - Most reported cases of metastatic MIFS in literature showed local recurrence before metastasis
- Tumors with high-grade or dedifferentiated morphology have worse prognosis
  - Metastasis in 50% of cases in one series (18 cases), including 7 deaths

MACROSCOPIC

General Features

- Usually multinodular, infiltrative, poorly circumscribed

Size

- 1-10 cm, usually 3-4 cm

MICROSCOPIC

Histologic Features

- Poorly marginated, multinodular
- Combination of myxoid and hyalinized zones merging with variably prominent inflammatory infiltrate
  - Exact composition varies from case to case
  - Zones may be separated by cleft-like spaces in more nodular tumors
- Inflammatory component shows variable mixture of lymphocytes, plasma cells, neutrophils, and eosinophils
  - Lymphoplasmacytic infiltrates can be dense and may show reactive germinal center formation
    - Can be prominent and extensive and mimic inflammatory pseudotumor, lymphoma, or reactive condition
  - Neutrophils may be prominent in myxoid areas
- Plump epithelioid to spindled cells with moderate to marked nuclear atypia
  - Epithelioid cells have eosinophilic cytoplasm and enlarged nucleoli
    - Basophilic or eosinophilic macronucleoli may resemble intranuclear viral inclusions
    - Some nuclei contain "smudgy" heterochromatin or show bizarre atypia
    - Occasional cells contain inflammatory cells in cytoplasm (emperipolesis)
  - Smaller epithelioid cells may appear ganglion-like and form clusters or larger aggregates
- Myxoid zones often contain unusual highly vacuolated cells that resemble lipoblasts (pseudolipoblasts)
- Generally low mitotic rate (usually ≤ 5 per 50 HPF)
- Multinucleated giant cells (including Touton forms) may be seen
- Unusual features
  - Branching or thick-walled arcuate curvilinear vessels
  - Cellular zones displaying solid, whorled, fascicular, or storiform patterns
  - Absence of large epithelioid cells with macronucleoli
- High-grade morphologic features
  - Variable combination of increased cellularity, marked nuclear atypia, high mitotic activity (> 10 per HPF), atypical mitoses, and necrosis
  - Dedifferentiation: Areas of conventional MIFS juxtaposed to undifferentiated pleomorphic sarcoma
- Rare tumors may contain areas resembling HFLT
  - Bland, spindled fibroblastic cells admixed with abundant adipose tissue with hemosiderin pigment
  - Recent evidence suggests that these tumors may actually represent HFLT with sarcomatous progression

ANCILLARY TESTS

Immunohistochemistry

- Nonspecific immunophenotype
  - Variable expression of CD34, CD68, D2-40, CD117, EMA
  - Rare cases show focal keratin expression
- Nuclear INI1 expression retained/intact

- Negative for desmin, clusterin
- Negative for CD15, CD30, CD45 in cells with inclusion-like macronucleoli

Molecular Genetics

- *BRAF* gene abnormalities recently described in subset of cases
  - *TOM1L2-BRAF* rearrangements in 5 cases; 1 case with *BRAF* amplification
  - Not yet reported in HFLT, PHAT, or so-called hybrid HFLT/MIFS
- Rearrangements of *TGFBR3* (1p22) and *MGEA5* (10q24) are rare in pure MIFS
  - These rearrangements mostly reported in cases of pure HFLT, hybrid HFLT/MIFS, and hybrid HFLT/PHAT
    - Recent data suggests that MIFS with *TGFBR3* or *MGEA5* rearrangements actually represents HFLT with sarcomatous progression

DIFFERENTIAL DIAGNOSIS

Myxofibrosarcoma

- Usually in superficial soft tissues of proximal extremities of older adults
- Often lobulated rather than infiltrative
- Myxoid stroma abundant in low- to intermediate-grade lesions
  - Curvilinear vascular network variably prominent
- No hyalinized zones
- Inflammatory cells comprise minor component
- Higher grade tumors show solid sheets of overtly malignant cells, often with numerous mitoses, including atypical forms

Diffuse-Type Tenosynovial Giant Cell Tumor

- a.k.a. pigmented villonodular synovitis
- Often localized to large joints, such as knee and hip
- Proliferation of uniform rounded histiocytoid cells in sheets and aggregates
- Background of hemosiderin, foamy histiocytes, and lymphoplasmacytic cells
- Myxoid stromal changes, pseudolipoblasts, and enlarged atypical cells with bizarre atypia not typical features of conventional diffuse-type tenosynovial giant cell tumor
- Often contains population of scattered desmin (+), dendritic-like cells

Extranodal Hodgkin Disease

- Patients usually have history of nodal disease
- Myxoid areas very unusual
- Inflammatory cells are mostly lymphoid
  - Neutrophils not common; eosinophils may be present
- Reed-Sternberg cells label with CD15 and CD30 and are lymphoid rather than fibroblastic

Hemosiderotic Fibrolipomatous Tumor

- Classically involves ankle and feet
- Mildly atypical spindle cells and hemosiderin in background of adipose tissue
- May show areas resembling MIFS
- Strongly CD34(+)
- t(1;10)(p22;q24) (*TGFBR3*; *MGEA5*)

Proliferative Fasciitis

- Small, often rapidly growing lesion on extremities of young adults
- Bland spindled to stellate myofibroblastic cells in loose myxoid to hyalinized stroma
- Contains variably prominent population of small ganglion cell-like myofibroblasts with prominent nucleoli
  - No bizarre nuclear atypia
- Mitotic figures are common; no atypical forms
- No pseudolipoblasts or prominent inflammatory component
- Variant occurring in childhood is highly cellular and may show necrosis and acute inflammation

Inflammatory Myofibroblastic Tumor

- Most commonly affects children and young adults
- Occurrence in extremity uncommon
- Variable loose myxoid to hyalinized stroma
- Intermingled chronic inflammatory infiltrate common, particularly plasma cells
- SMA(+), ALK(+) in most cases
- *ALK* gene rearrangements often detectable

Superficial CD34(+) Fibroblastic Tumor

- Rare, but increasingly reported
- Shows many overlapping histologic features with MIFS
- Generally more cellular than MIFS and lacks prominent myxoid and hyalinized zones
- Lacks t(1;10) and rearrangements of *TGFBR3* and *MGEA5*
- CD34(+); variable keratin (+)

SELECTED REFERENCES

1. Boland JM et al: Hemosiderotic fibrolipomatous tumor, pleomorphic hyalinizing angiectatic tumor, and myxoinflammatory fibroblastic sarcoma: related or not? Adv Anat Pathol. 24(5):268-77, 2017
2. Kao YC et al: Recurrent BRAF gene rearrangements in myxoinflammatory fibroblastic sarcomas, but not hemosiderotic fibrolipomatous tumors. Am J Surg Pathol. 41(11):1456-65, 2017
3. Lucas DR: Myxoinflammatory fibroblastic sarcoma: review and update. Arch Pathol Lab Med. 141(11):1503-7, 2017
4. Gaetke-Udager K et al: Myxoinflammatory fibroblastic sarcoma: spectrum of disease and imaging presentation. Skeletal Radiol. 45(3):347-56, 2016
5. Zreik RT et al: TGFBR3 and MGEA5 rearrangements are much more common in "hybrid" hemosiderotic fibrolipomatous tumor-myxoinflammatory fibroblastic sarcomas than in classical myxoinflammatory fibroblastic sarcomas: a morphological and fluorescence in situ hybridization study. Hum Pathol. 53:14-24, 2016
6. Michal M et al: High-grade myxoinflammatory fibroblastic sarcoma: a report of 23 cases. Ann Diagn Pathol. 19(3):157-63, 2015
7. Ieremia E et al: Myxoinflammatory fibroblastic sarcoma: morphologic and genetic updates. Arch Pathol Lab Med. 138(10):1406-11, 2014
8. Laskin WB et al: Myxoinflammatory fibroblastic sarcoma: a clinicopathologic analysis of 104 cases, with emphasis on predictors of outcome. Am J Surg Pathol. 38(1):1-12, 2014
9. Weiss VL et al: Myxoinflammatory fibroblastic sarcoma in children and adolescents: clinicopathologic aspects of a rare neoplasm. Pediatr Dev Pathol. 16(6):425-31, 2013
10. Jurcić V et al: Myxoinflammatory fibroblastic sarcoma: a tumor not restricted to acral sites. Ann Diagn Pathol. 6(5):272-80, 2002
11. Lambert I et al: Acral myxoinflammatory fibroblastic sarcoma with unique clonal chromosomal changes. Virchows Arch. 438(5):509-12, 2001
12. Meis-Kindblom JM et al: Acral myxoinflammatory fibroblastic sarcoma: a low-grade tumor of the hands and feet. Am J Surg Pathol. 22(8):911-24, 1998
13. Montgomery EA et al: Inflammatory myxohyaline tumor of distal extremities with virocyte or Reed-Sternberg-like cells: a distinctive lesion with features simulating inflammatory conditions, Hodgkin's disease, and various sarcomas. Mod Pathol. 11(4):384-91, 1998

Mixed Inflammatory Infiltrate

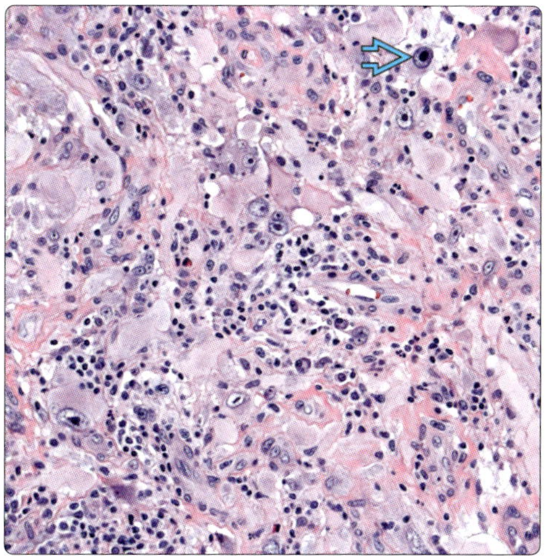

Large Ganglion-Like Cells

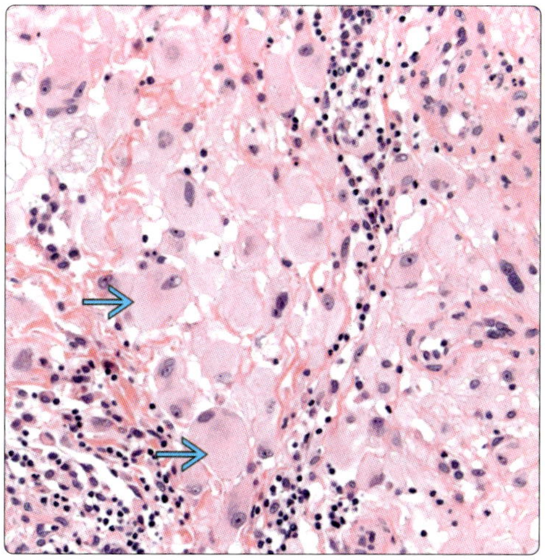

(Left) *The stromal inflammatory infiltrate is often composed of a mixture of cell types, including lymphocytes, plasma cells, eosinophils, and neutrophils. The exact composition varies, and some cases show a predominantly neutrophilic infiltrate. Note also the presence of macronucleoli ⇨.* **(Right)** *Enlarged epithelioid tumor cells → with abundant eosinophilic cytoplasm and eccentric nuclei may resemble ganglion cells, particularly when they form small aggregates or cluster in some tumors.*

Small Ganglion-Like Cells

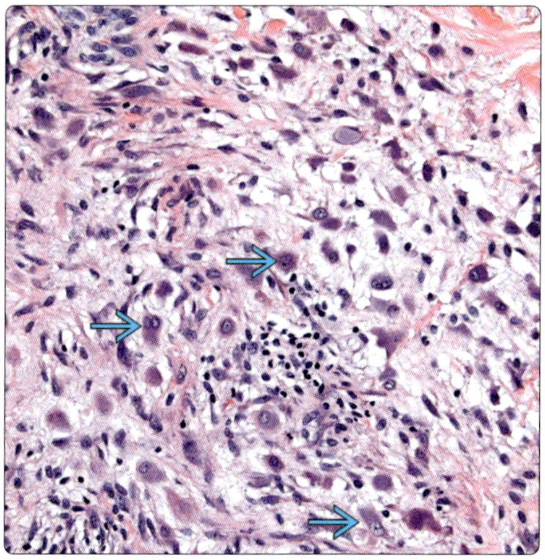

Sheets of Plump Tumor Cells

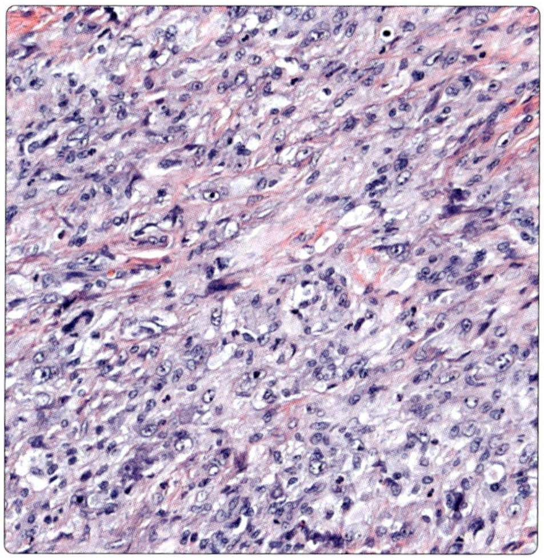

(Left) *Some of the tumor cells → in MIFS may resemble the ganglion cell-like myofibroblasts seen in proliferative fasciitis/myositis.* **(Right)** *In some cases of MIFS, sheets of plump spindled and epithelioid cells with conspicuous nucleoli, as depicted, may closely resemble cellular areas of a tenosynovial giant cell tumor. A more collagenized stroma may also be seen in these cases.*

Smudgy Heterochromatin

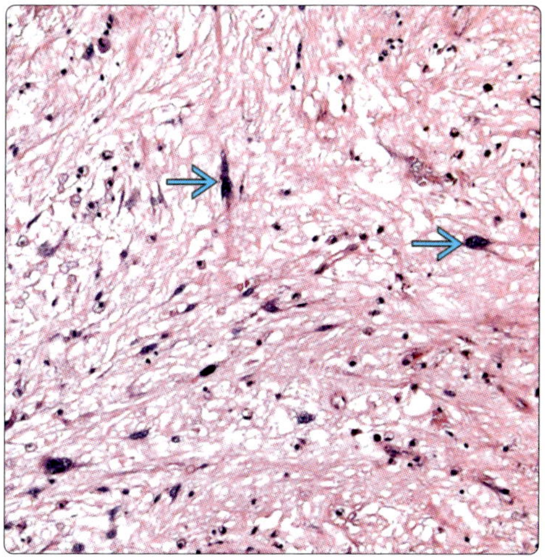

Low Mitotic Rate

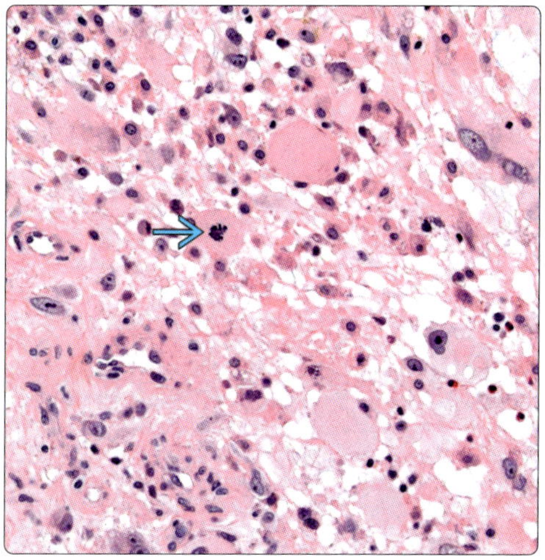

(Left) *Nuclear atypia in the form of irregular nuclear contours with smudgy heterochromatin is a common finding in MIFS. These cells → are similar in appearance to the atypical stromal cells of well-differentiated liposarcoma.* **(Right)** *Mitotic activity → in MIFS is often low (usually < 5 per 50 HPF) and may even be seemingly nonexistent. Rare atypical cases show a higher mitotic rate, and very rare cases can show atypical mitoses.*

(Left) *Myxoid areas are very common in MIFS and range from small foci to large zones. The tumor cells within these areas are often spindled and show mild to moderate nuclear atypia. These zones may also be quite paucicellular and resemble myxoma.* **(Right)** *Bizarre, enlarged tumor cells with extensive cytoplasmic vacuolization ⇒ are common in myxoid zones of MIFS and may be misconstrued as true lipoblasts. As a caveat, similar cells may also be seen in some cases of myxofibrosarcoma.*

Myxoid Zones

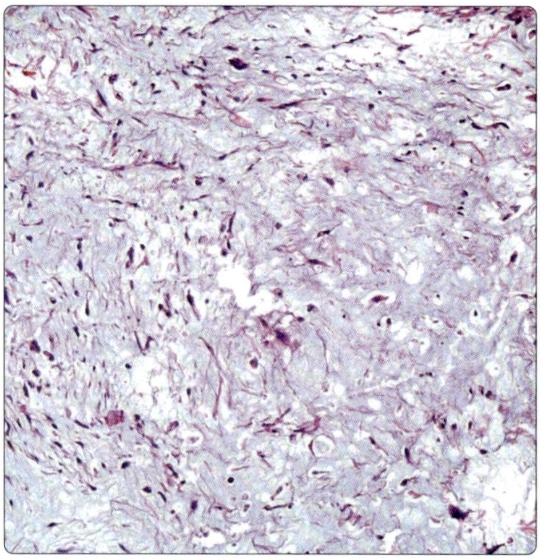

Pseudolipoblasts

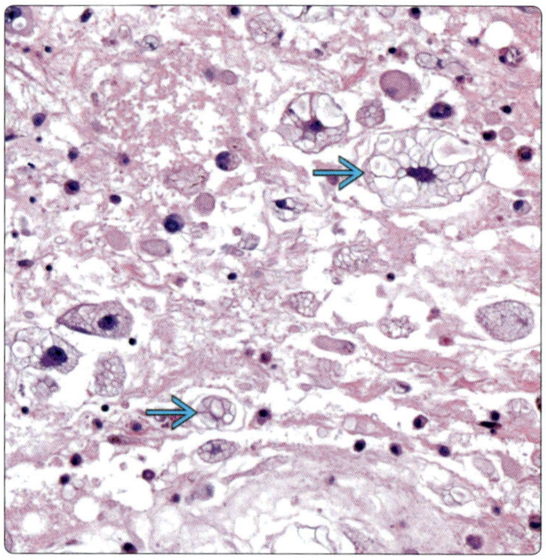

(Left) *Scattered large ganglion-like tumor cells may show emperipolesis of inflammatory cells, particularly neutrophils ⇒. In some cases, the cytoplasm may be packed with cells.* **(Right)** *Hyalinized zones in MIFS are often hypo- to modestly cellular and may show prominent sclerosis. The diagnosis may be challenging in rare cases that are predominantly sclerotic. Note the interface with a myxoid focus ⇒. In some cases, cleft-like spaces may separate these zones.*

Emperipolesis

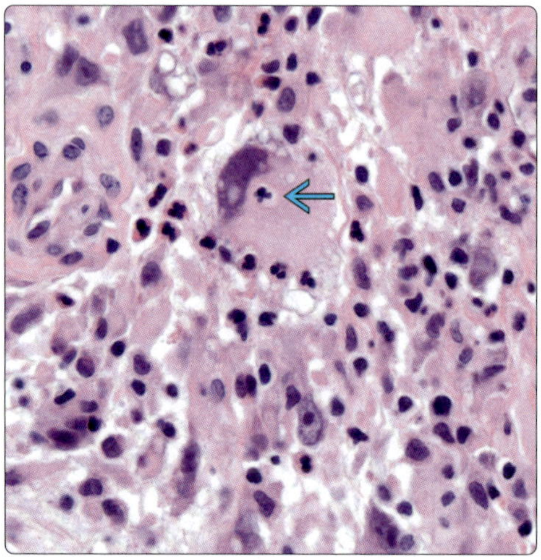

Hyalinized Zones

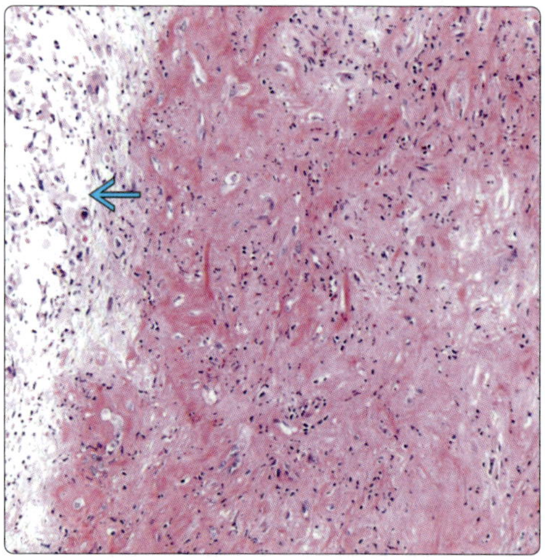

(Left) *The inflammatory zones in MIFS may be discrete and dense. In rare cases, this inflammation is so extensive that the neoplastic cells may be obscured, potentially leading to misdiagnosis as a reactive or infectious process.* **(Right)** *Occasionally, zones of dense lymphoplasmacytic inflammation will show reactive germinal center formation ➡. When located at the periphery of a tumor, this finding may mimic a lymph node metastasis.*

Inflammatory Zone

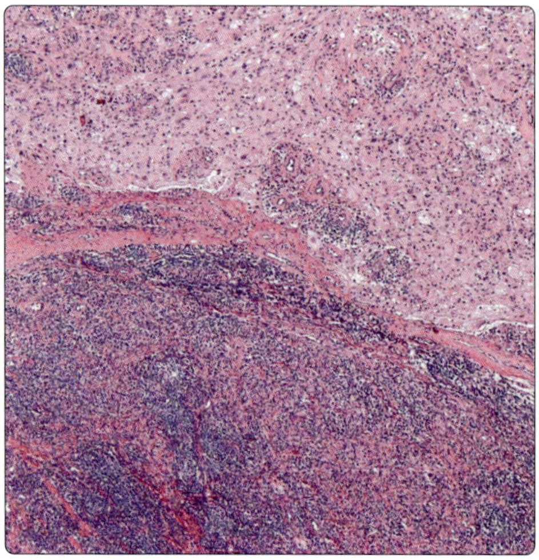

Germinal Center Formation

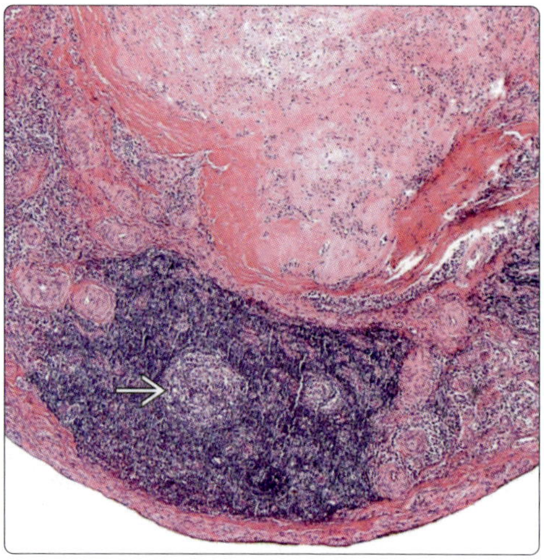

Reed-Sternberg-Like Cells

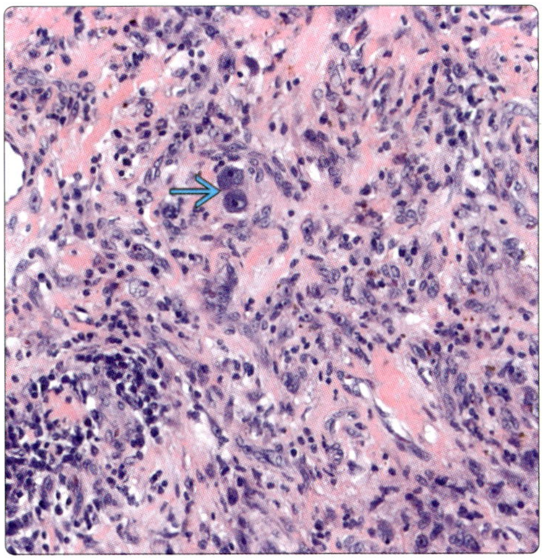

Multinucleated Giant Cells

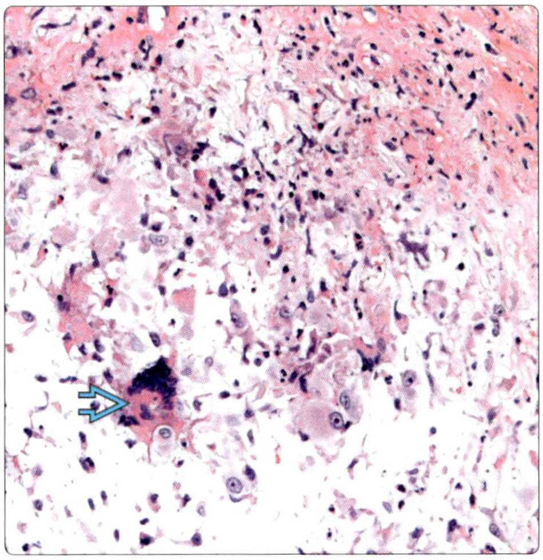

(Left) *Some atypical tumor cells in MIFS appear binucleated and are reminiscent of Reed-Sternberg cells. Within the setting of a predominantly inflammatory background, this finding may lead to confusion with Hodgkin lymphoma.* **(Right)** *Multinucleated giant cells are not infrequent in MIFS and may show a Touton-like morphology (similar to solitary/juvenile xanthogranuloma) or osteoclastic morphology. These cells may also show emperipolesis or engulfment of other cells.*

Arcuate Vasculature

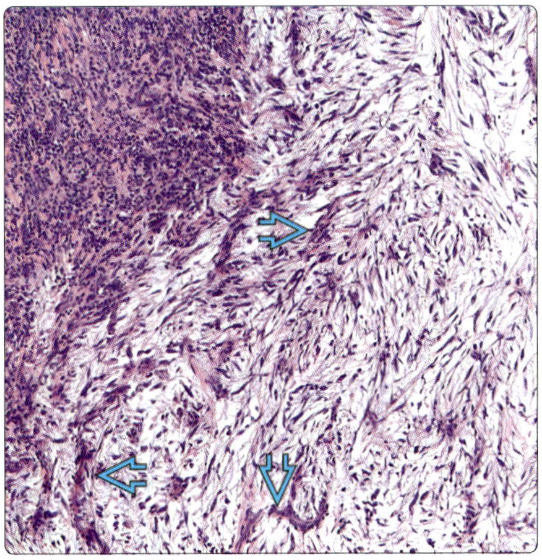

Rare Architectural Organization

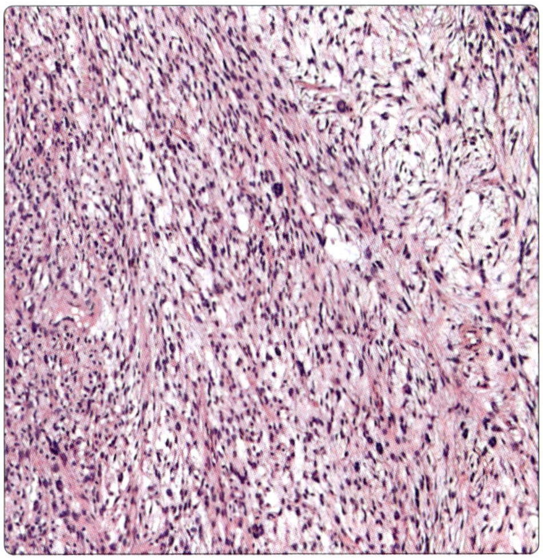

(Left) *A rare and unusual finding in MIFS is the presence of an arcuate or curvilinear vascular pattern. This vascularity is similar to what is often seen in myxofibrosarcoma and low-grade fibromyxoid sarcoma and may potentially lead to misdiagnosis if other clinical and histologic features are not taken into account.* **(Right)** *Very rare cases of MIFS may show focal architectures such as storiform, whorling, or fascicular growth patterns. Other more typical features of MIFS are often present elsewhere.*

Focal Necrosis

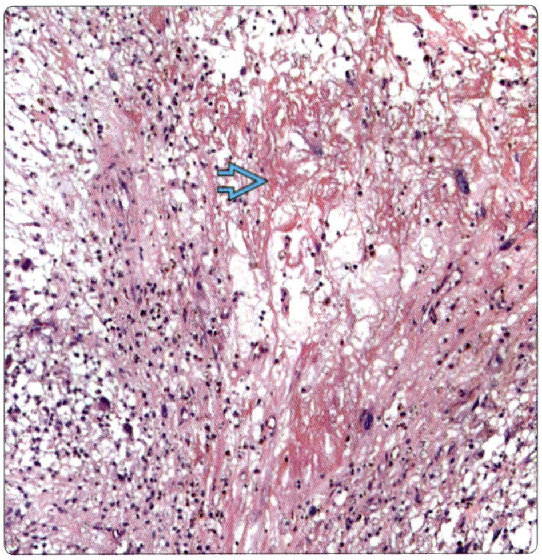

Hemosiderotic Fibrolipomatous Tumor-Like Areas

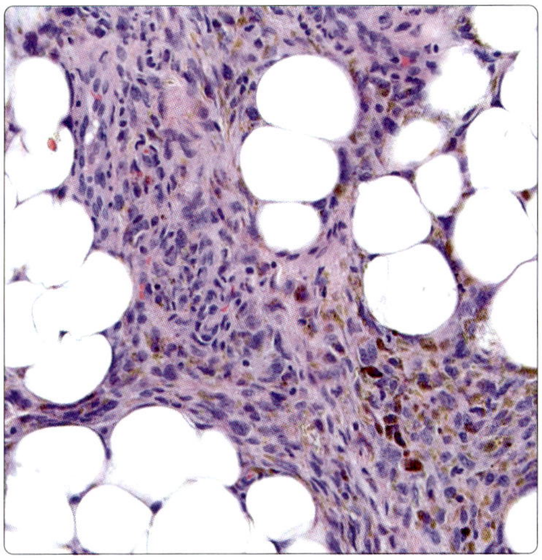

(Left) *Focal necrosis is rarely encountered in MIFS and can be fibrinoid or coagulative.* **(Right)** *Unusual tumors may show areas containing features of both MIFS and hemosiderotic fibrolipomatous tumor (HFLT), as depicted, and these tumors have been described as hybrid MIFS/HFLT. Recent studies have proposed that these tumors are actually HFLT with sarcomatous progression rather than a hybrid or variant of MIFS.*

(Left) *This MIFS is superficial and shows a myxoinflammatory expansion of the subcutaneous fat. Such neoplasms can also be associated with tendons and have an infiltrative appearance. A prominent lymphoid infiltrate is present throughout the neoplasm.* **(Right)** *This case of MIFS contained discrete areas of seemingly detached myxoid nodules separated from more cellular, inflammatory zones by cleft-like spaces.*

Superficial/Cutaneous Myxoinflammatory Fibroblastic Sarcoma

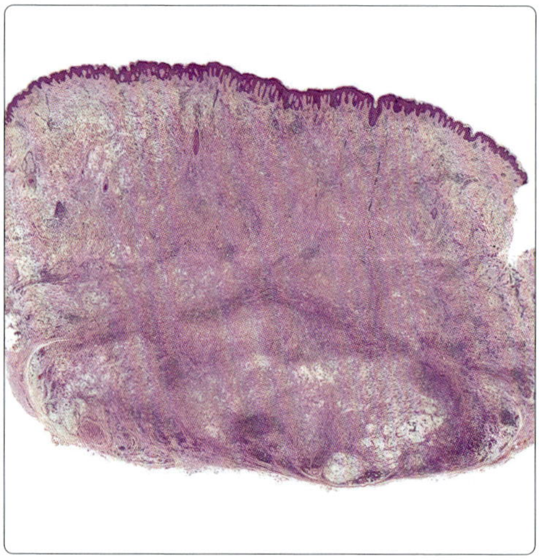

Cleft-Like Spaces

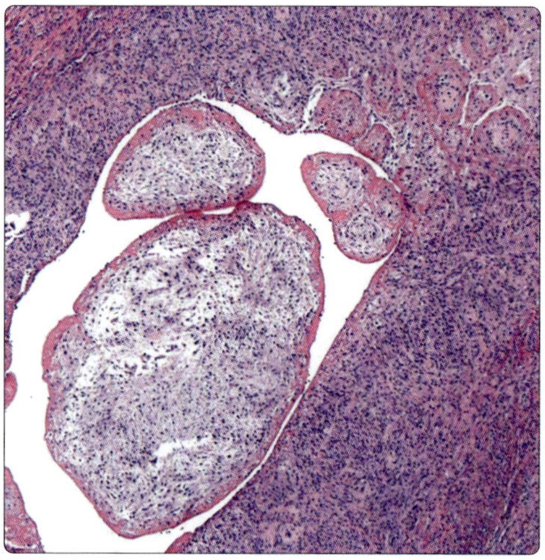

(Left) *MIFS most commonly arises superficially and demonstrates an infiltrative border with the surrounding tissue (in this case, mature fat).* **(Right)** *Given its strong tendency for infiltrative growth, MIFS can also show involvement/entrapment of normal structures such as vessels and nerves. A pacinian corpuscle ➔ is shown in this image.*

Infiltration of Fat

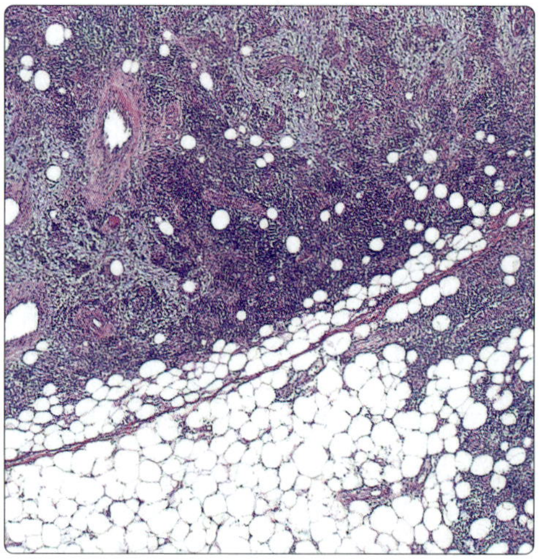

Infiltration of Dermal and Subcutaneous Structures

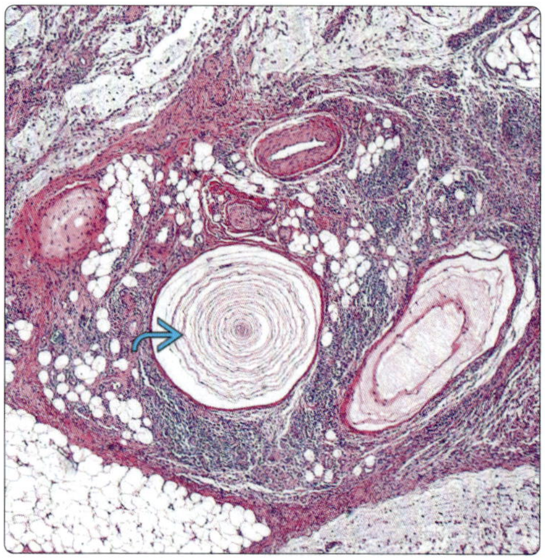

(Left) *This case of MIFS shows a massive chronic inflammatory infiltrate, raising concerns for Hodgkin lymphoma. Other, more conventional areas with typical features were identified in additional sections.* **(Right)** *Variable CD34 expression is not uncommon in MIFS and can be quite prominent in some cases, as depicted here.*

Prominent Chronic Inflammation

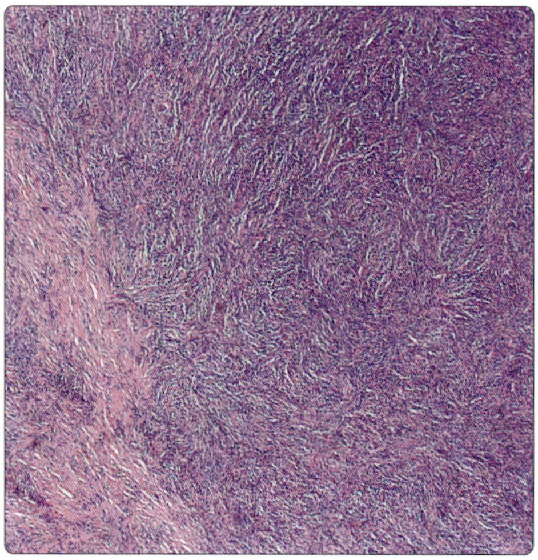

CD34 Expression

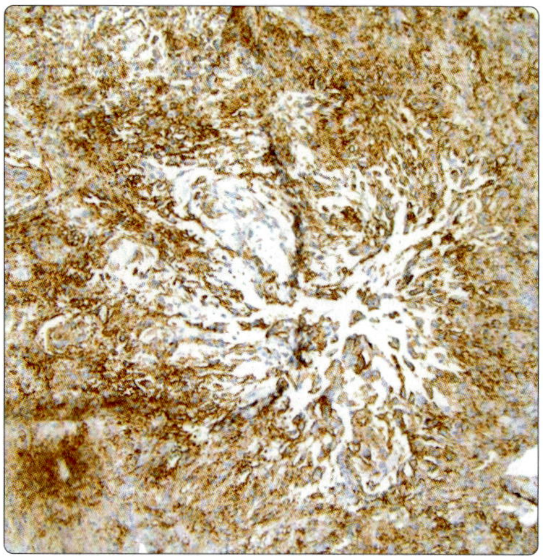

Eosinophils

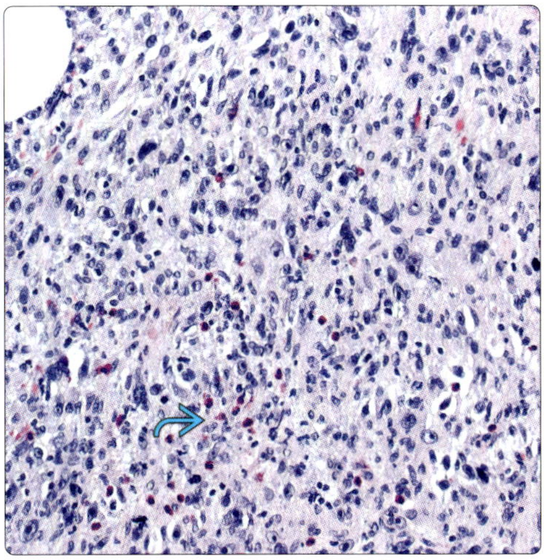

Cellular Zones

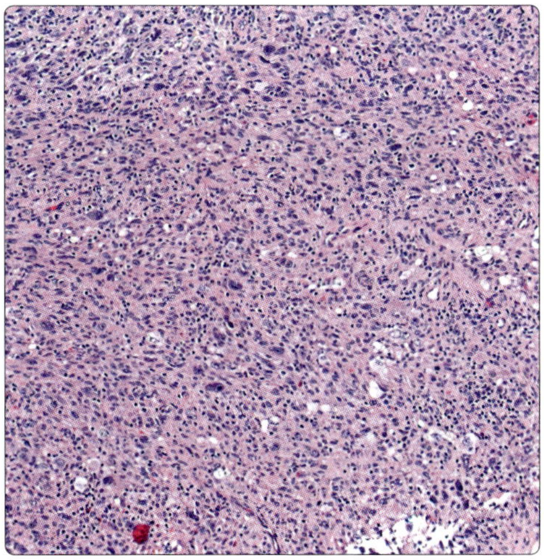

(Left) *Neutrophils are a relatively common finding in MIFS, but eosinophils → can also be conspicuous in some cases.* **(Right)** *Some cases of MIFS feature areas with increased cellularity and comparatively less myxoid, hyalinized, and inflammatory morphology. Despite the cellularity, mitotic activity is generally low, and characteristic virocyte-like macronucleoli can often be identified without trouble.*

Prominent Sclerotic and Inflammatory Zones

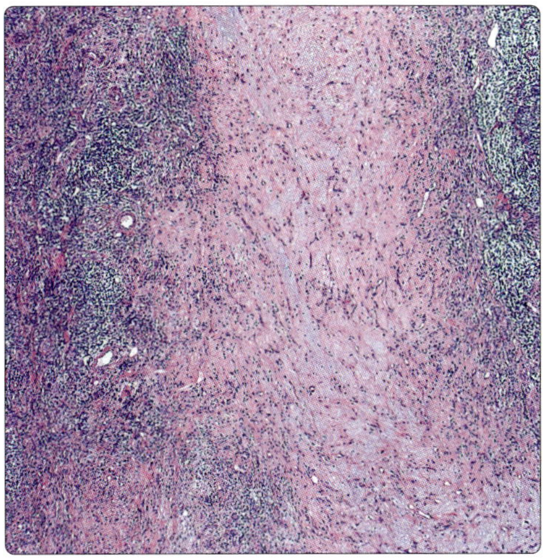

Sclerotic Matrix

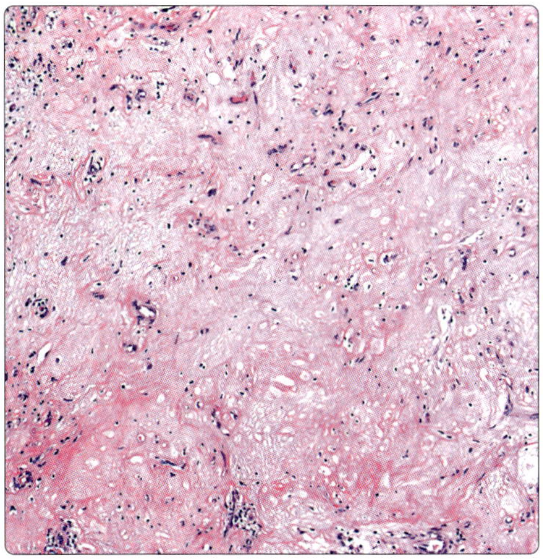

(Left) *The appearance of sclerotic and inflammatory zones in MIFS may lead to the mistaken impression of a nonneoplastic process.* **(Right)** *Sclerosing zones in MIFS can be markedly paucicellular, leading to confusion with a reactive process. This pitfall can cause particular problems on a small biopsy.*

Hypocellular Myxoid Zones

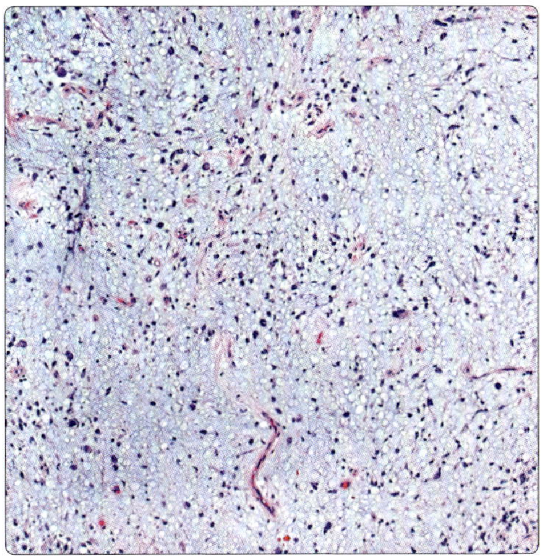

High-Grade Morphology

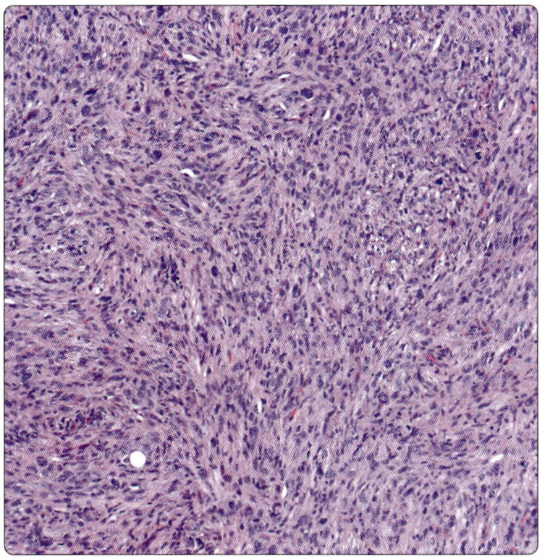

(Left) *This case of MIFS contained large myxoid zones with relatively small tumor cells and scattered inflammation. This pattern can mimic a low-grade myxofibrosarcoma; however, the 2 tumors often present differently clinically.* **(Right)** *Rare cases of MIFS contain high-grade features, including a mixture of marked atypia, cellularity, mitotic activity, &/or necrosis. Dedifferentiation (conventional MIFS adjacent to undifferentiated pleomorphic sarcoma) has also been reported.*

Superficial CD34(+) Fibroblastic Tumor

KEY FACTS

TERMINOLOGY

- Distinctive low-grade fibroblastic neoplasm arising in superficial soft tissues and featuring fascicular growth, prominent nuclear pleomorphism, and consistent CD34 expression

CLINICAL ISSUES

- Wide age range (median: 38 years)
- Solitary, slow-growing, painless mass or nodule arising in superficial soft tissues
- Lower extremity most common site
- Treatment: Complete surgical excision
- Generally indolent clinical course
  - No local recurrence or tumor-related deaths reported
  - Regional nodal metastases in 1 published case

MACROSCOPIC

- Mean size: 4.1 cm
- Well-circumscribed, firm mass

MICROSCOPIC

- Spindled to epithelioid cells arranged in fascicles or storiform arrays
  - Prominent eosinophilic cytoplasm, may be glassy
  - Characteristically striking nuclear pleomorphism
  - Prominent macronucleoli, also nuclear pseudoinclusions
- Mitotic figures rare to infrequent; no necrosis

ANCILLARY TESTS

- Strong, diffuse CD34(+)
- Patchy, focal cytokeratin (+) in majority of cases
- Retained nuclear INI1 expression
- Negative for *TGFBR3*, *MGEA5*, *PDGFB*, and *ALK* gene rearrangements

TOP DIFFERENTIAL DIAGNOSES

- Myxoinflammatory fibroblastic sarcoma
- Pleomorphic dermal sarcoma
- Epithelioid sarcoma

Superficial CD34(+) Fibroblastic Tumor

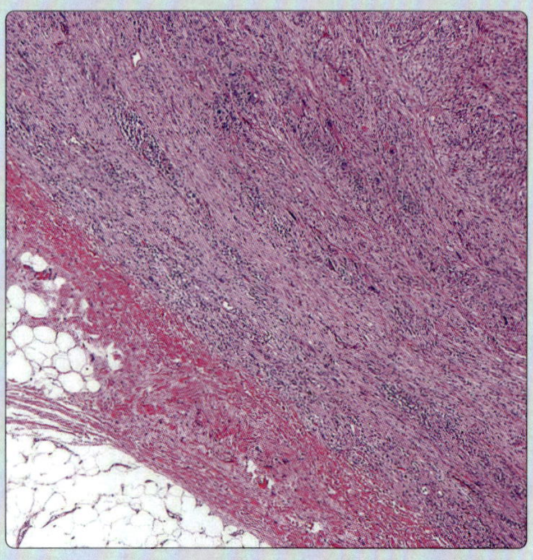

Prominent Nuclear Atypia

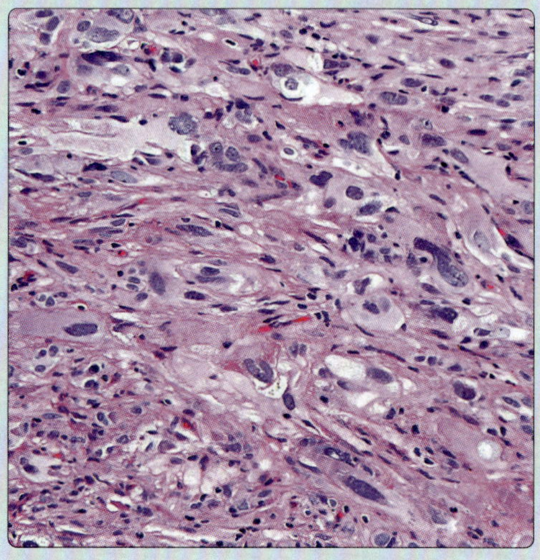

(Left) *Superficial CD34(+) fibroblastic tumor (SCD34FT) is a rare but distinctive mesenchymal neoplasm that arises in superficial soft tissue sites and is composed of variably pleomorphic spindle cells. It often shows a well-circumscribed peripheral border, as depicted.* **(Right)** *A characteristic feature of the tumor is striking nuclear atypia, often in the form of hyperchromasia, pleomorphism, and multinucleation. Bizarre atypia is also common, which can raise concerns for malignancy.*

Macronucleoli and Pseudoinclusions

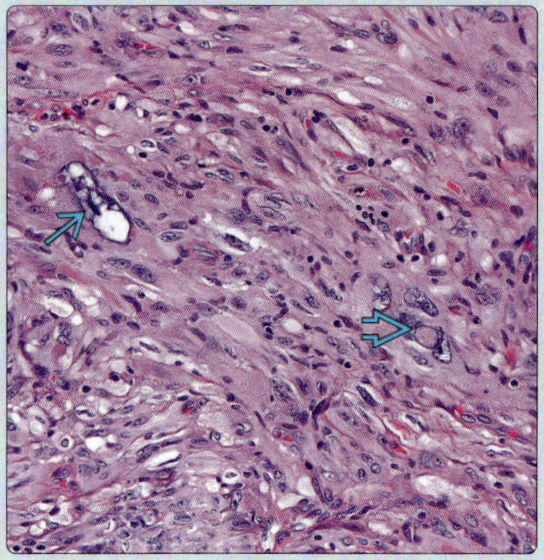

Strong CD34 Expression

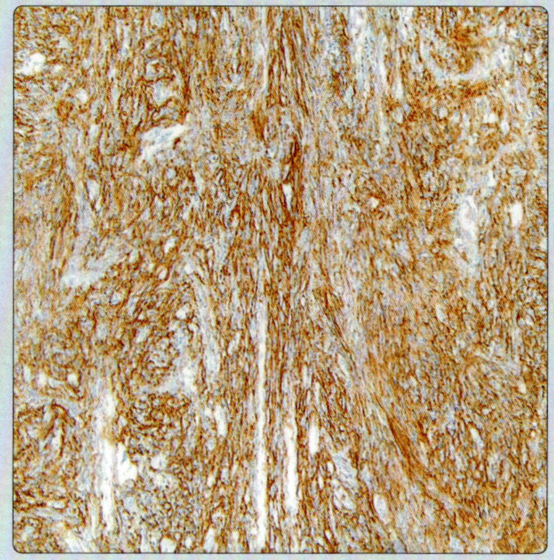

(Left) *Prominent basophilic or eosinophilic macronuclei ➙ can be seen in some of the larger cells. Intranuclear pseudoinclusions ⇨ are also common. Similar findings are seen in myxoinflammatory fibroblastic sarcoma, a neoplasm that does not appear to be related.* **(Right)** *All reported cases of SCD34FT have strong CD34 expression, usually in the majority of the tumor cells.*

TERMINOLOGY

Abbreviations

- Superficial CD34(+) fibroblastic tumor (SCD34FT)

Definitions

- Distinctive low-grade fibroblastic neoplasm arising in superficial soft tissues and featuring fascicular growth, prominent nuclear pleomorphism, and consistent CD34 expression

CLINICAL ISSUES

Epidemiology

- Incidence
  - Very rare (~ 35 cases reported in literature)
- Age
  - Wide range (median: 38 years)
  - No tumors reported < 18 years

Site

- Lower extremity most common
  - Thigh, buttock, lower leg, foot
- Also shoulder, upper arm, groin, others

Presentation

- Solitary, slow-growing, painless mass or nodule
  - Often present for > 1 year
- Arises in superficial soft tissues
  - Absent to minimal involvement of underlying muscle

Treatment

- Complete surgical excision

Prognosis

- Generally indolent clinical course
  - No local recurrence or tumor-related deaths reported thus far
  - Regional nodal metastases in 1 published case, occurring 7 years following incomplete excision

MACROSCOPIC

General Features

- Well-circumscribed, firm mass
- Tan/gray/yellow, fleshy cut surface

Size

- Mean: 4.1 cm (range: 1.5-10.0 cm)

MICROSCOPIC

Histologic Features

- Well demarcated but may show limited extension into adjacent adipose tissue
- Spindled to epithelioid cells arranged in fascicles or storiform arrays
  - Prominent eosinophilic cytoplasm, may be granular, fibrillar, or glassy
    - Large epithelioid or polygonal cells may appear ganglion-like
  - Characteristically striking nuclear atypia
    - Hyperchromatic, pleomorphic nuclei, often bizarre
    - Prominent macronucleoli common
    - Also nuclear pseudoinclusions
- Mild to moderate inflammatory cell infiltrate, particularly lymphocytes and mast cells
  - Occasional xanthoma cells
- Mitotic figures rare to infrequent
- Necrosis absent

ANCILLARY TESTS

Immunohistochemistry

- Strong, diffuse CD34(+)
- Patchy, focal cytokeratin (+) in majority of cases
- EMA, S100 protein, SMA, desmin, CD31, ERG, STAT6, HMB-45, Melan-A, ALK, and FLI-1 (-)
- Retained nuclear INI1 expression

In Situ Hybridization

- Negative for *TGFBR3*, *MGEA5*, *PDGFB*, and *ALK* gene rearrangements

DIFFERENTIAL DIAGNOSIS

Myxoinflammatory Fibroblastic Sarcoma

- Generally multinodular and poorly delineated
- Predilection for distal extremities
- Myxoid stroma common, also hyalinized and inflammatory zones

Pleomorphic Dermal Sarcoma

- Mitotic figures and necrosis are common
- CD34, keratin (-)
- Aggressive growth (can invade fascia, muscle)

Epithelioid Sarcoma

- Nodules of atypical epithelioid cells, ± central necrosis
- Spindle cell morphology in subset
- Diffuse cytokeratin (+); patchy CD34(+) in 50%
- Loss of nuclear INI1

Atypical Fibroxanthoma

- Dermal lesion, usually small
- Mitotic activity common, including atypical mitoses
- CD34, keratin (-)

Inflammatory Myofibroblastic Tumor

- Predilection for lung and abdominal cavity; rare in extremities
- SMA(+); subset are focally keratin (+)
- ALK expression in 50% of cases
- CD34(-)

SELECTED REFERENCES

1. Lao IW et al: Superficial CD34-positive fibroblastic tumour: a clinicopathological and immunohistochemical study of an additional series. Histopathology. 70(3):394-401, 2017
2. Sood N et al: Superficial CD34-positive fibroblastic tumor: a new entity; case report and review of literature. Indian J Pathol Microbiol. 60(3):377-380, 2017
3. Yamaga K et al: Detailed analysis of a superficial CD34-positive fibroblastic tumor: a case report and review of the literature. Oncol Lett. 14(3):3395-3400, 2017
4. Wada N et al: Superficial CD34-positive fibroblastic tumor: a new case from Japan. J Dermatol. 43(8):934-6, 2016
5. Carter JM et al: Superficial CD34-positive fibroblastic tumor: report of 18 cases of a distinctive low-grade mesenchymal neoplasm of intermediate (borderline) malignancy. Mod Pathol. 27(2):294-302, 2014

(Left) *Although all cases of SCD34FT are grossly well circumscribed, microscopic evidence of limited infiltration into adjacent adipose tissue is not uncommon.* **(Right)** *Similar to smooth muscle neoplasms, the tumor cells that comprise SCD34FT characteristically show prominent cytoplasmic eosinophilia. Morphologic architectures include fascicles, vague bundles, and storiform arrays.*

Limited Extension Into Adipose Tissue

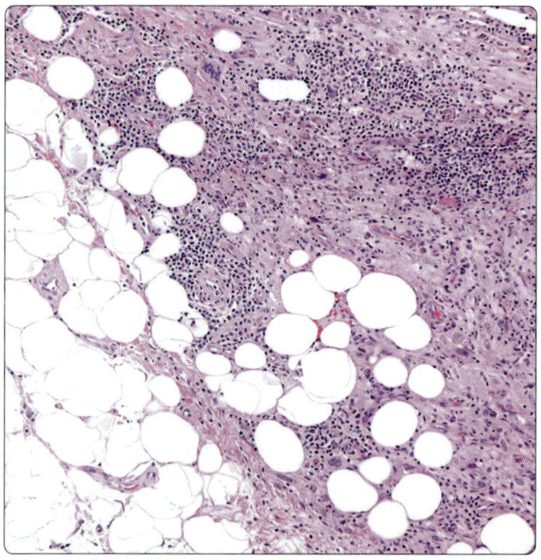

Cytoplasmic Eosinophilia

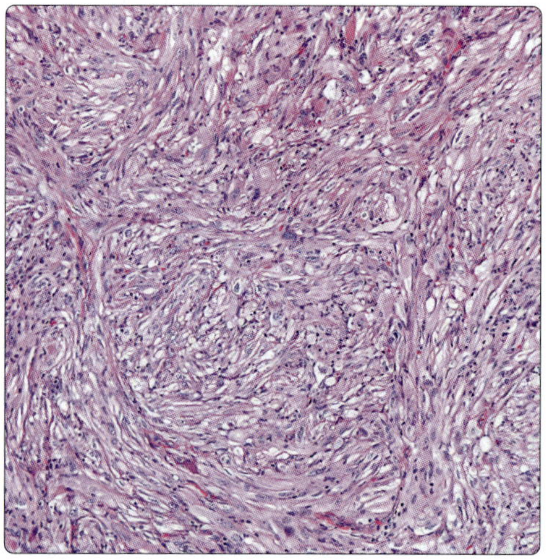

(Left) *Larger epithelioid or polygonal cells are a common finding in SCD34FT, similar to many cases of myxoinflammatory fibroblastic sarcoma.* **(Right)** *Tumor cell cytoplasm, though often eosinophilic, can also appear glassy, fibrillary, or granular in texture. A focal clear cell appearance is also possible. Similar findings can be seen in PEComa.*

Epithelioid or Polygonal Cells

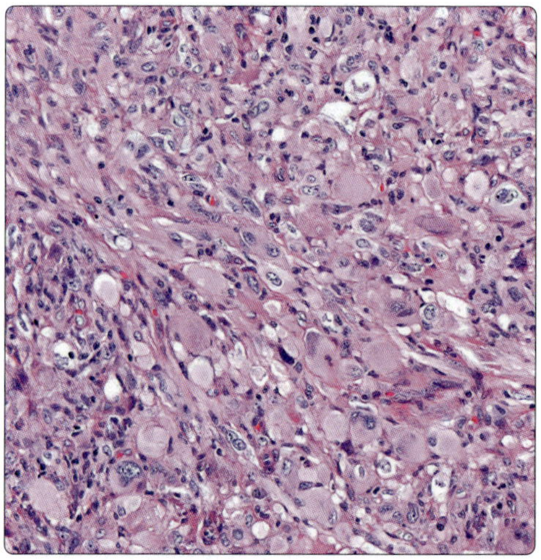

Glassy, Fibrillar, or Granular Cytoplasm

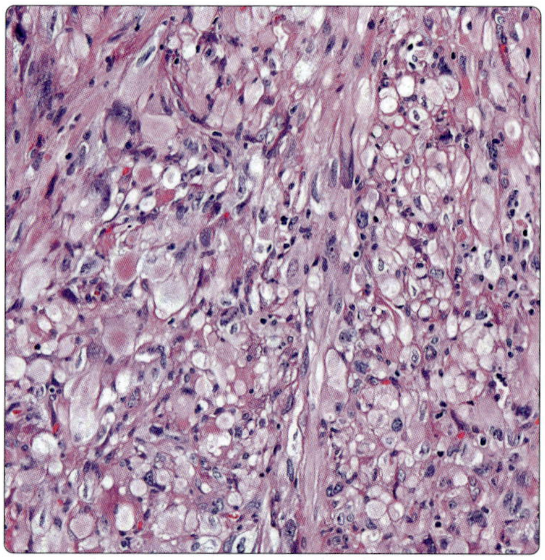

(Left) *An intratumoral infiltrate of chronic inflammatory cells is seen in most cases of SCD34FT. Lymphocytes are most common, but mast cells and histiocytes can also be present.* **(Right)** *Foamy histiocytes (xanthoma cells) → can be present focally in SCD34FT. Hemosiderin pigment may also be seen but is generally rare.*

Chronic Inflammatory Cells

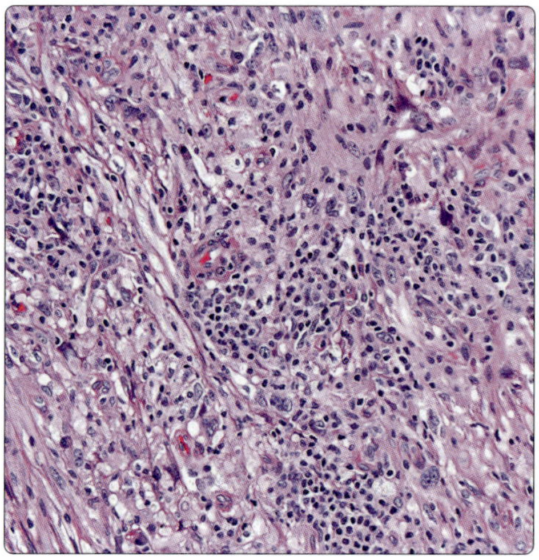

Xanthoma Cells

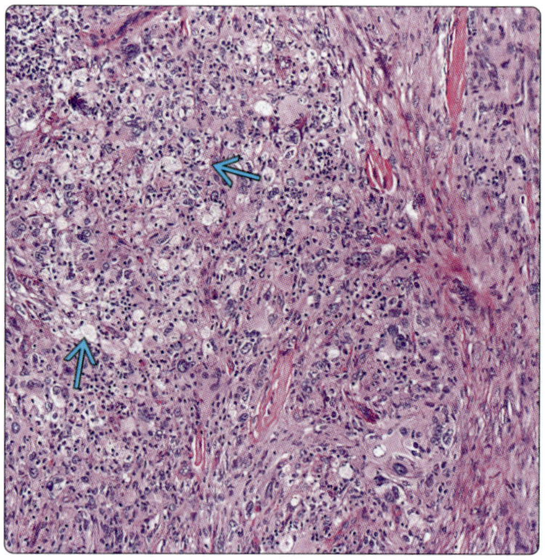

Focal Areas Lacking Atypia

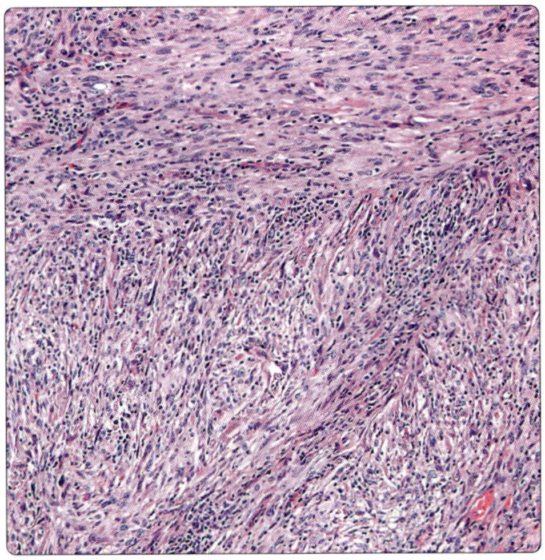

Rare Mitotic Figures

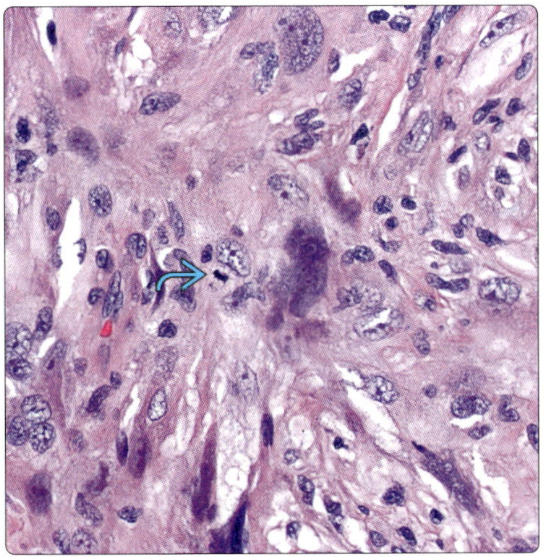

(Left) *Some regions lack the characteristic prominent nuclear atypia that characterizes SCD34FT, however, they do not tend to predominate.* **(Right)** *Mitotic figures are rare to absent in SCD34FT. This finding supports the notion that most of the nuclear atypia seen in this tumor is degenerative in nature.*

Glassy Epithelioid Cells

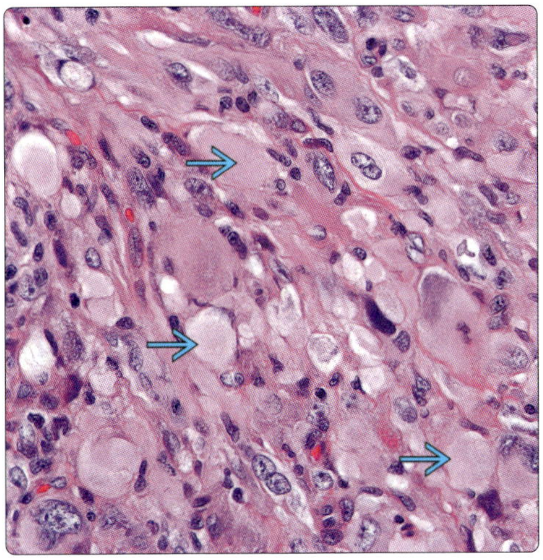

Nuclear Hyperchromasia

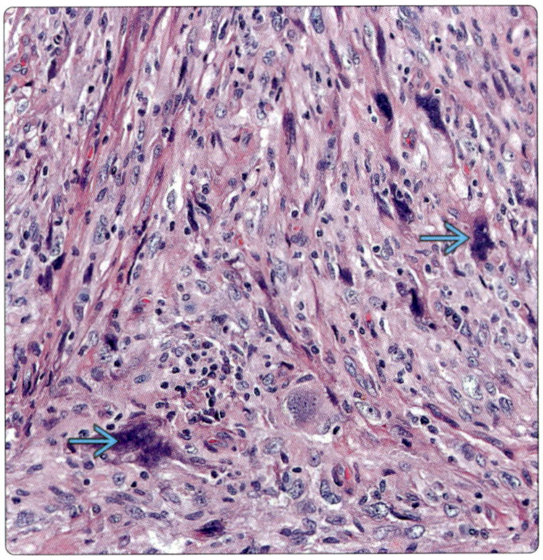

(Left) *This image shows epithelioid to polygonal tumor cells with smooth and glassy eosinophilic cytoplasm, a common finding in SCD34FT.* **(Right)** *Nuclear hyperchromasia, pleomorphism, and multinucleation can give some tumor cells a smudgy appearance, similar to cells seen in well-differentiated liposarcoma, myxoinflammatory fibroblastic sarcoma, and inflammatory myofibroblastic tumor.*

Collagen Fiber Entrapment

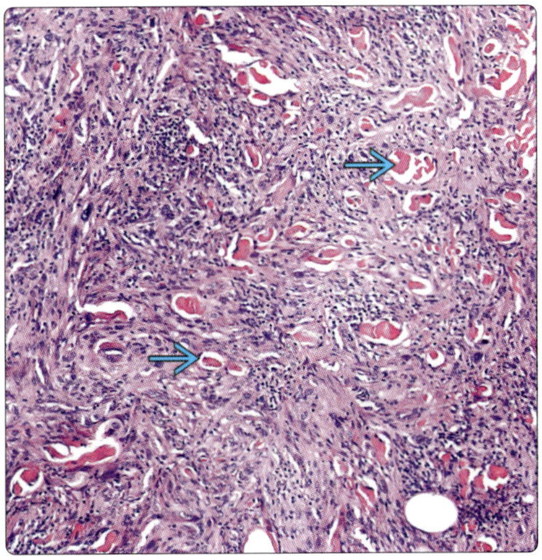

Focal to Patchy Keratin Expression

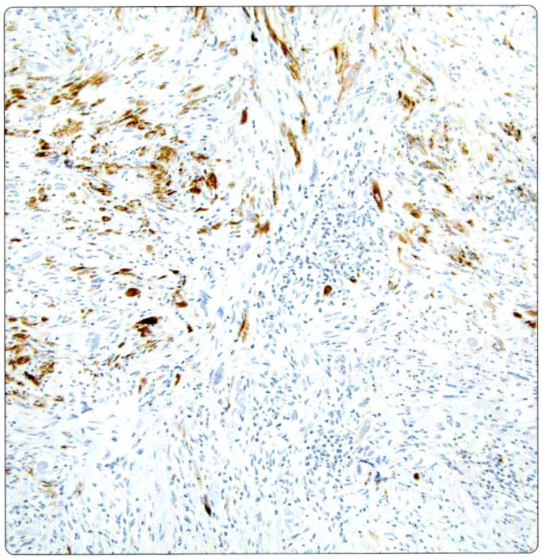

(Left) *Entrapment of dermal collagen fibers can be seen in the superficial aspects of SCD34FT, which may lead to diagnostic confusion with atypical fibrous histiocytoma (dermatofibroma).* **(Right)** *Keratin expression can be seen in up to 2/3 of cases of SCD34FT, however, this finding is characteristically focal or patchy.*

Adult-Type Fibrosarcoma

KEY FACTS

TERMINOLOGY

- Sarcoma composed of uniform spindle cells resembling fibroblasts
- Vast majority of tumors classified as fibrosarcoma in older literature now reclassified as other entities
- Currently, vanishingly rare entity; diagnosis of exclusion
- High-grade fibroblastic sarcomas with nuclear pleomorphism are currently classified as undifferentiated pleomorphic sarcoma rather than fibrosarcoma

CLINICAL ISSUES

- Most arise in deep soft tissues of extremities in adults
- Treatment: Wide surgical resection
- Limited prognostic data using modern, strict diagnostic criteria
- 50% overall mortality

MICROSCOPIC

- Uniform, hyperchromatic spindle cells in herringbone fascicles
- Lacks characteristic features of other defined entities

ANCILLARY TESTS

- Negative for keratins, EMA, S100 protein, desmin, most others
- Lacks molecular signatures of other defined sarcomas

TOP DIFFERENTIAL DIAGNOSES

- Undifferentiated pleomorphic sarcoma
- Synovial sarcoma
- Malignant peripheral nerve sheath tumor
- Fibrosarcomatous dermatofibrosarcoma protuberans
- Desmoid fibromatosis
- Cellular dermatofibroma
- Low-grade myofibroblastic sarcoma
- Leiomyosarcoma

Adult-Type Fibrosarcoma

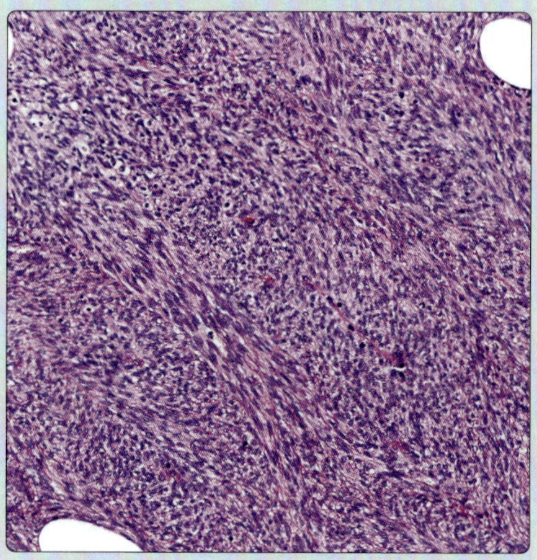

Fascicular Herringbone Pattern

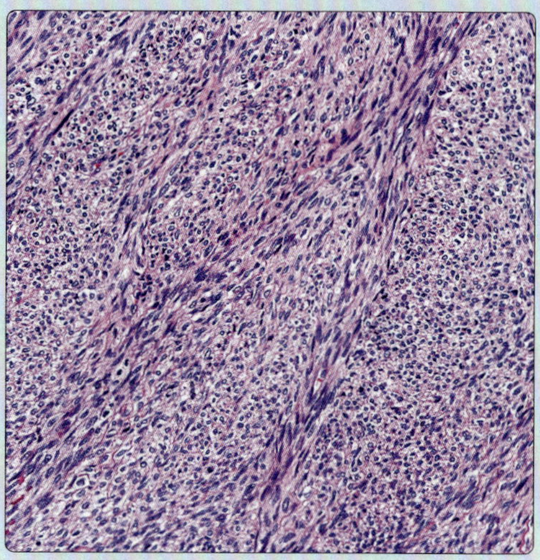

(Left) *The rare, adult-type fibrosarcoma should be diagnosed only after all morphologically similar entities have been rigorously excluded. All strictly defined cases demonstrate prominent fascicular growth by spindled tumor cells lacking significant nuclear pleomorphism. (Courtesy K. Fritchie, MD.)* **(Right)** *Relatively uniform spindle cells are arranged in prominent fascicles that intersect at acute angles, giving rise to the characteristic (but nonspecific) herringbone pattern. (Courtesy K. Fritchie, MD.)*

Mitoses

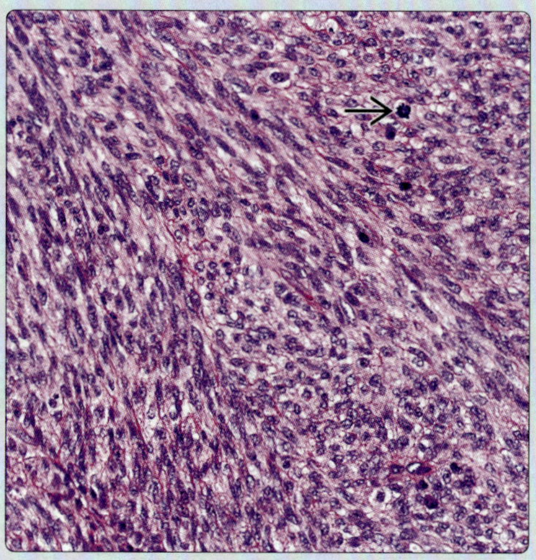

Intervening Collagen Fibers

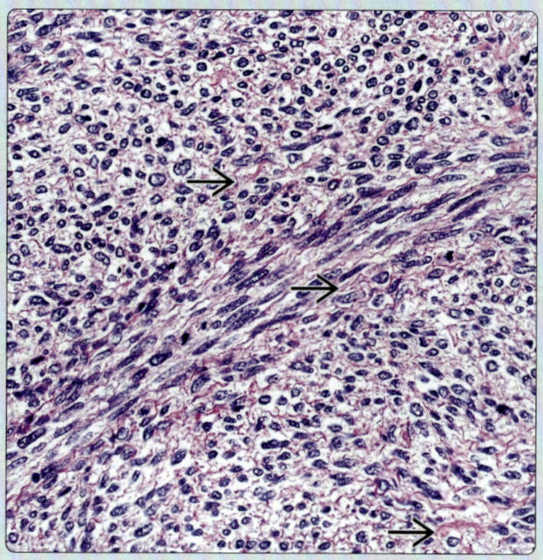

(Left) *Mitotic figures* → *are usually present in adult-type fibrosarcoma; however, the overall mitotic rate is variable. Importantly, the hyperchromatic tumor cells show no more than mild to moderate nuclear pleomorphism. (Courtesy K. Fritchie, MD.)* **(Right)** *Fine, wavy, pink collagen fibers* → *separate the hyperchromatic spindle cells from one another in adult-type fibrosarcoma. The amount of intervening collagen is variable, but it is usually less than that seen in desmoid fibromatosis. (Courtesy K. Fritchie, MD.)*

Adult-Type Fibrosarcoma

TERMINOLOGY

Definitions

- Sarcoma composed of uniform spindle cells resembling fibroblasts
  - Vast majority of tumors classified as fibrosarcoma in older literature now reclassified as other entities
  - Currently, vanishingly rare entity; diagnosis of exclusion
  - Diagnosis should only be made with extreme caution
- Lacks features of other distinct defined fibrosarcoma subtypes (e.g., myxofibrosarcoma, infantile fibrosarcoma, sclerosing epithelioid fibrosarcoma, etc.)
- High-grade fibroblastic sarcomas with nuclear pleomorphism are currently classified as undifferentiated pleomorphic sarcoma (UPS) rather than fibrosarcoma

CLINICAL ISSUES

Epidemiology

- Incidence
  - Very rare (if strictly defined)
- Age
  - Median age: 50 years

Presentation

- Usually deep mass of lower extremity but may occur anywhere
  - Rarely arise in subcutis; most apparent fibrosarcoma in skin or subcutis actually represent fibrosarcomatous transformation of dermatofibrosarcoma protuberans

Treatment

- Wide surgical resection

Prognosis

- Only 2 modern studies using strict diagnostic criteria
  - Most older series represent wide variety of sarcoma types (by current criteria); thus, unreliable data
- 50% mortality (low-grade tumors have better prognosis)

MACROSCOPIC

Size

- Median size: 6.5 cm (range: 2-17 cm)

MICROSCOPIC

Histologic Features

- Elongated, hyperchromatic, relatively uniform fusiform/spindle cells with little cytoplasm
  - Only mild-moderate pleomorphism allowed
  - If severe pleomorphism, classify as UPS, not fibrosarcoma
  - Variable mitotic rate, but mitoses present in most cases
- Fascicles, usually arranged in characteristic (but nonspecific) herringbone pattern
- Parallel collagen fibers between cells (variable)
- Hypocellular or myxoid areas may mimic fibromatosis
  - These are usually focal; other areas show more cellular zones typical of fibrosarcoma
- Lacks features of distinct, defined fibrosarcoma subtypes
  - Low-grade fibromyxoid sarcoma, sclerosing epithelioid fibrosarcoma, myxofibrosarcoma, infantile fibrosarcoma

ANCILLARY TESTS

Immunohistochemistry

- May express variable smooth muscle actin (SMA) (similar to other fibroblastic neoplasms)
- Most other markers negative: Keratins, EMA, S100 protein, desmin, CD34, etc.

Genetic Testing

- No known characteristic molecular abnormality
- Lacks molecular signatures that define other sarcomas

DIFFERENTIAL DIAGNOSIS

Undifferentiated Pleomorphic Sarcoma

- Sheets of markedly pleomorphic cells
- Severe nuclear atypia

Synovial Sarcoma

- Commonly has herringbone fascicular pattern
- Biphasic form also has glandular epithelial structures
- Monotonous spindle/ovoid nuclei; no pleomorphism
- Cytokeratin (+), EMA(+), diffuse nuclear TLE1(+)
- Characteristic t(X;18), *SS18-SSX1/2/4* gene fusion

Malignant Peripheral Nerve Sheath Tumor

- Commonly has herringbone fascicular pattern
- Perivascular cuffing by large atypical tumor cells
- Evidence of neural origin (clinical, cytologic, or IHC)
- Arises in: Nerve, neurofibroma, or patient with NF1
- Focal/patchy S100 or SOX10 (+) (50% are negative)
- Loss of nuclear H3K27me3 expression in majority

Fibrosarcomatous Dermatofibrosarcoma Protuberans

- Histologically identical to fibrosarcoma but arising from dermatofibrosarcoma protuberans
- CD34 expression may be lost in fibrosarcomatous zones
- Characteristic t(17;22), *COL1A1-PDGFB* gene fusion

Desmoid Fibromatosis

- Less cellular; broad sweeping fascicles, not herringbone

Cellular Dermatofibroma

- Majority in dermis/subcutis (unlike fibrosarcoma)
- Can have intersecting hypercellular fascicles with mitoses but also conventional dermatofibroma areas at periphery

Low-Grade Myofibroblastic Sarcoma

- Cells tend to have more cytoplasm than fibrosarcoma
- Multifocal SMA(+), sometimes focal desmin (+)

Leiomyosarcoma

- Abundant eosinophilic cytoplasm; diffuse SMA and desmin (+)
- Herringbone pattern uncommon

SELECTED REFERENCES

1. Bahrami A et al: Adult-type fibrosarcoma: a reevaluation of 163 putative cases diagnosed at a single institution over a 48-year period. Am J Surg Pathol. 34(10):1504-13, 2010
2. Hansen T et al: Low-grade fibrosarcoma–report on 39 not otherwise specified cases and comparison with defined low-grade fibrosarcoma types. Histopathology. 49(2):152-60, 2006

Myxofibrosarcoma

KEY FACTS

TERMINOLOGY

- Malignant fibroblastic neoplasm with cellular pleomorphism; variably prominent myxoid stroma; and prominent elongated, thin-walled stromal blood vessels
- Synonym: Myxoid malignant fibrous histiocytoma

CLINICAL ISSUES

- Most common sarcoma of elderly patients
- Most common in patients 50-70 years of age
- Most common in limbs and limb girdles
  - More often superficial than deep
  - Extremely rare in retroperitoneum and abdominal cavity
- Treatment: Complete surgical excision with negative margins
- Local, often repeated recurrences in up to 50-60% of cases, unrelated to histologic grade
- Metastatic potential and mortality rate are associated with histologic grade

MACROSCOPIC

- Often multinodular (particularly superficial tumors)

MICROSCOPIC

- Often multinodular growth with incomplete fibrous septa
- Myxoid stroma and characteristic elongated, curvilinear, thin-walled blood vessels
- Pseudolipoblasts may be seen
- Spectrum of cellularity, atypia, and proliferative activity reflected by 3 histologic grades (low, intermediate, high)
- Morphologic variant: Epithelioid myxofibrosarcoma (MFS)

TOP DIFFERENTIAL DIAGNOSES

- Low-grade fibromyxoid sarcoma
- Cellular myxoma
- Undifferentiated pleomorphic sarcoma
- Dedifferentiated liposarcoma
- Pleomorphic liposarcoma

(Left) *Unlike many sarcomas, myxofibrosarcoma (MFS) more often arises superficially in the subcutaneous tissue or dermis than in deep soft tissues locations, as shown in this photograph. Grossly, MFS is usually multinodular* ➡ *and demonstrates a variably gelatinous cut surface.* **(Right)** *Deep-seated (subfascial or intramuscular) cases of MFS may show the characteristic multinodular growth (shown) or more of a solitary nodular mass. Note the glistening, gelatinous cut surface.*

Myxofibrosarcoma

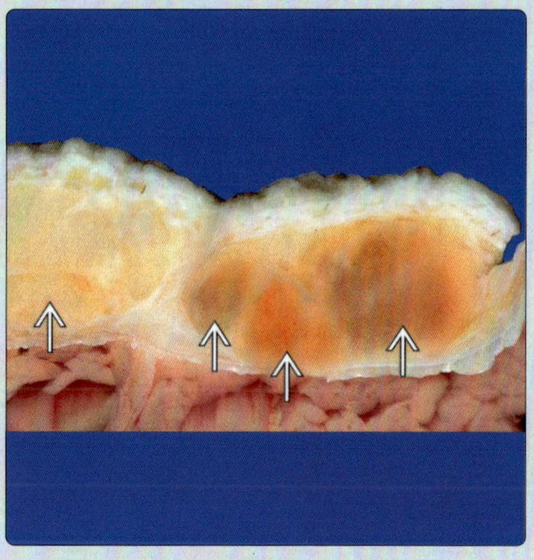

Myxofibrosarcoma

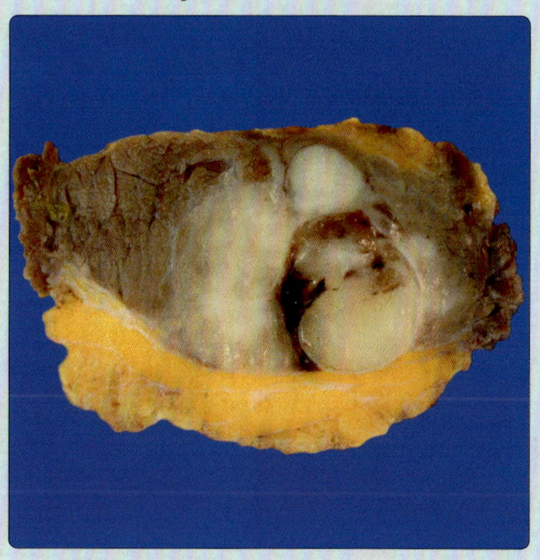

(Left) *MFS most commonly arises in the extremities of older/elderly adults. It is more likely to arise in the subcutaneous tissue, as depicted, than in skeletal muscle.* **(Right)** *A multinodular growth pattern with thin, variably incomplete fibrous septa is a feature of many cases of MFS. Note the infiltrated skeletal muscle* ➡ *in this deep-seated example.*

Superficial Tissues of Extremities

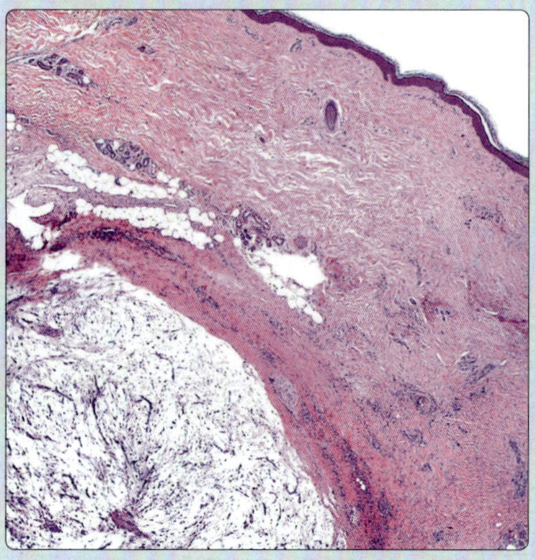

Multinodular With Fibrous Septa

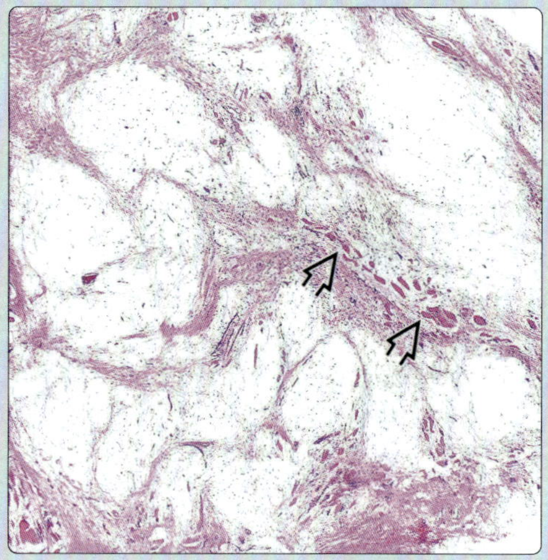

Myxofibrosarcoma

TERMINOLOGY

Abbreviations

- Myxofibrosarcoma (MFS)

Synonyms

- Myxoid malignant fibrous histiocytoma

Definitions

- Malignant fibroblastic neoplasm characterized by cellular pleomorphism; variably prominent myxoid stroma; and prominent elongated, thin-walled stromal blood vessels

CLINICAL ISSUES

Epidemiology

- Incidence
  - Relatively common
    - Most common sarcoma of elderly patients
- Age
  - Wide range but most common in patients 50-70 years
  - Exceptionally rare in patients < 20 years
- Sex
  - Slight male predominance

Site

- Most common in limbs and limb girdles
  - Lower extremity > upper extremity
  - Majority (65%) arise in superficial tissues (dermis/subcutaneous) vs. subfascial/intramuscular
- Also, rarely on trunk, head/neck region, and hands/feet
- Extremely rare in retroperitoneum and abdominal cavity

Presentation

- Slow-growing, painless mass

Treatment

- Complete surgical excision with negative margins
- Radiotherapy may decrease risk of local recurrence in some cases
- Chemotherapy has not been proven to be effective

Prognosis

- Local, often repeated recurrences in up to 50-60% of cases, unrelated to histologic grade
- Metastatic potential and mortality rate are associated with histologic grade
  - Low grade
    - Metastases very rare
    - May show tumor progression in subsequent recurrences and may acquire metastatic potential
  - Intermediate and high grade
    - Metastases in 20-35% of cases
  - Metastases to lungs, viscera, retroperitoneum, bone, regional lymph nodes
- Overall 5-year survival is 60-70%
  - Tumor size, histologic grade, and margin status are statistically significant predictors of survival
- Epithelioid variant of MFS appears to be more clinically aggressive
  - Local recurrence in 70% and metastases in 50%, even with relatively short follow-up period

MACROSCOPIC

General Features

- Often multinodular (particularly superficial tumors)
- Variably firm to gelatinous cut surfaces

Size

- Wide size range: 3 cm to > 10 cm

MICROSCOPIC

Histologic Features

- Often multinodular growth with incomplete fibrous septa
- Usually peripherally infiltrative
- Myxoid stroma is consistent but variable feature
- Conspicuous, elongated, curvilinear, thin-walled blood vessels are characteristic
  - Variation in number of these vessels from case to case
- Vacuolated fibroblastic cells containing mucin (pseudolipoblasts) are not uncommon
  - More common in lower grade tumors but may be seen in areas of high-grade examples
- Inflammatory cells may be present
- Spectrum of cellularity, cytologic atypia, and proliferative activity reflected by 3 histologic grades
  - Low-grade MFS
    - Hypocellular, prominently myxoid
    - Scattered, noncohesive, spindled to stellate cells with ill-defined eosinophilic cytoplasm and enlarged, hyperchromatic nuclei
    - Curvilinear vasculature often prominent
    - Mitoses infrequent
    - No tumor necrosis
  - Intermediate-grade MFS
    - More cellular and pleomorphic than low-grade tumors
      - Lacks solid/sheet-like areas of high-grade tumors
    - Mitoses more common than in low-grade tumors but are not numerous
    - Curvilinear vasculature often prominent
    - No tumor necrosis
  - High-grade MFS
    - Partly or predominantly composed of solid sheets and cellular fascicles of tumor cells
      - Often marked nuclear and cytologic pleomorphism
      - Bizarre, multinucleated tumor giant cells common
      - Mitotic figures, often atypical, and coagulative necrosis are common
    - At least focally, areas of lower grade MFS can be identified

Morphologic Variants

- Epithelioid MFS
  - Contains aggregates &/or cellular sheets of atypical epithelioid cells
    - Abundant eosinophilic cytoplasm
    - Round, vesicular nuclei with prominent nucleoli
      - Severe nuclear pleomorphism and atypia not uncommon
      - Frequent mitoses, often atypical
  - Other features or areas of conventional MFS present

ANCILLARY TESTS

Immunohistochemistry

- May show focal expression of SMA, MSA, CD34
  - Diffuse expression of CD34 more common in superficial tumors
- Desmin, keratins, S100 protein, CD163 (-)

Molecular Genetics

- Nondistinctive complex karyotypic abnormalities
  - Increasingly complex aberrations often seen in recurrent lesions

DIFFERENTIAL DIAGNOSIS

Low-Grade Fibromyxoid Sarcoma

- Usually affects younger age group than that of MFS
- More common in deep soft tissue sites than superficial
- Hypocellular fibrous zones alternating with more cellular myxoid areas
  - Whorling and swirling growth pattern of tumor cells
  - Arcades of blood vessels in myxoid areas are similar to those of MFS
  - Most cases lack significant nuclear atypia and pleomorphism
- *FUS* rearrangements (most commonly *FUS-CREB3L2*)

Cellular Myxoma (Superficial, Intramuscular, or Juxtaarticular)

- Absence of nuclear atypia and pleomorphism
- Lacks characteristic vasculature of MFS
- Activating mutations of *GNAS* gene in intramuscular myxoma

Neurofibroma

- Absence of significant nuclear pleomorphism in most cases
  - Atypical (degenerative) neurofibromas show disproportionately low mitotic rate for level of nuclear atypia
- Lacks characteristic vasculature of MFS
- Consistent S100 protein (+)

Myxoid Liposarcoma

- Usually affects younger age group than that of MFS
- More common in deep soft tissue sites than superficial
- Contains univacuolated and multivacuolated lipoblasts
- Delicate plexiform capillary vascular pattern
- No prominent cytologic atypia
- *DDIT3* rearrangements

Undifferentiated Pleomorphic Sarcoma

- Can be indistinguishable from cellular, solid, high-grade areas of MFS
- Lacks myxoid areas with curvilinear vasculature and other features of lower grade MFS
- Usually arises in deep soft tissue of extremities

Pleomorphic Liposarcoma

- Commonly contains areas that are essentially morphologically indistinguishable from MFS
- True lipoblastic differentiation (particularly pleomorphic lipoblasts) present

Dedifferentiated Liposarcoma

- Very common in retroperitoneum in contrast to MFS
- May contain areas that are essentially morphologically indistinguishable from MFS
- Component of well-differentiated liposarcoma is often present, at least focally
- MDM2(+), CDK4(+) by IHC
- *MDM2* amplification by FISH

Myxoinflammatory Fibroblastic Sarcoma

- Most frequently arises in subcutaneous tissues of distal extremities (hands, wrists, feet, and ankles)
  - Can rarely arise more proximally
- Spindled; polygonal; and bizarre, ganglion-like tumor cells with huge, inclusion-like nucleoli
- Characteristic prominent mixed inflammatory infiltrate in most cases

Malignant Peripheral Nerve Sheath Tumor

- Fascicular arrangement of spindle-shaped tumor cells common
- Often perivascular whorling or accentuation of tumor cells
  - Generally lacks characteristic vasculature of MFS
- Focal expression of S100 protein in 50% of cases
- May show evidence of origin from neurofibroma or nerve trunk
- Loss of h3k27me3 by IHC

Metastatic Carcinoma/Melanoma

- Can be difficult to distinguish morphologically from epithelioid MFS
- History of primary tumor may be present
- IHC helpful
  - Keratin (+) for carcinoma; S100 protein (+) for melanoma

SELECTED REFERENCES

1. Ma S et al: MET-overexpressing myxofibrosarcoma frequently exhibit polysomy of chromosome 7 but not MET amplification, especially in high-grade cases: clinical and pathological review of 30 myxofibrosarcoma cases. Diagn Pathol. 13(1):56, 2018
2. Heitzer E et al: Expanded molecular profiling of myxofibrosarcoma reveals potentially actionable targets. Mod Pathol. 30(12):1698-1709, 2017
3. Scoccianti G et al: Soft tissue myxofibrosarcoma: a clinico-pathological analysis of a series of 75 patients with emphasis on the epithelioid variant. J Surg Oncol. 114(1):50-5, 2016
4. Look Hong NJ et al: Prognostic factors and outcomes of patients with myxofibrosarcoma. Ann Surg Oncol. 20(1):80-6, 2013
5. Riouallon G et al: Superficial myxofibrosarcoma: assessment of recurrence risk according to the surgical margin following resection. A series of 21 patients. Orthop Traumatol Surg Res. 99(4):473-7, 2013
6. Smith SC et al: CD34-positive superficial myxofibrosarcoma: a potential diagnostic pitfall. J Cutan Pathol. 40(7):639-45, 2013
7. Olson MT et al: Myxofibrosarcoma: cytomorphologic findings and differential diagnosis on fine needle aspiration. Acta Cytol. 56(1):15-24, 2012
8. Sanfilippo R et al: Myxofibrosarcoma: prognostic factors and survival in a series of patients treated at a single institution. Ann Surg Oncol. 18(3):720-5, 2011
9. Nascimento AF et al: Epithelioid variant of myxofibrosarcoma: expanding the clinicomorphologic spectrum of myxofibrosarcoma in a series of 17 cases. Am J Surg Pathol. 31(1):99-105, 2007
10. Willems SM et al: Local recurrence of myxofibrosarcoma is associated with increase in tumour grade and cytogenetic aberrations, suggesting a multistep tumour progression model. Mod Pathol. 19(3):407-16, 2006
11. Mansoor A et al: Myxofibrosarcoma presenting in the skin: clinicopathological features and differential diagnosis with cutaneous myxoid neoplasms. Am J Dermatopathol. 25(4):281-6, 2003
12. Mentzel T et al: Myxofibrosarcoma. Clinicopathologic analysis of 75 cases with emphasis on the low-grade variant. Am J Surg Pathol. 20(4):391-405, 1996

Characteristic Stromal Vasculature

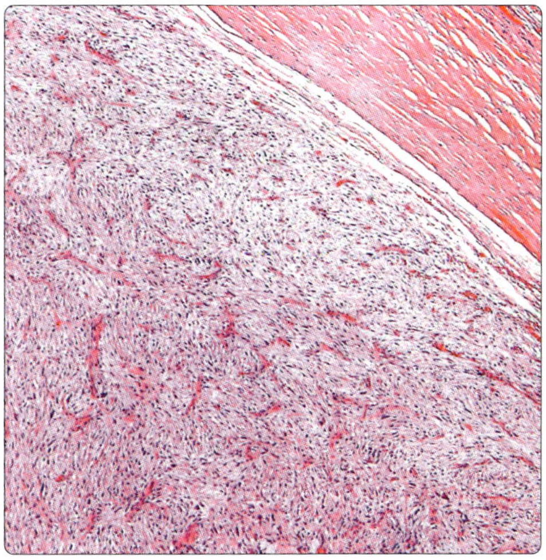

Elongated, Thin-Walled Vessels

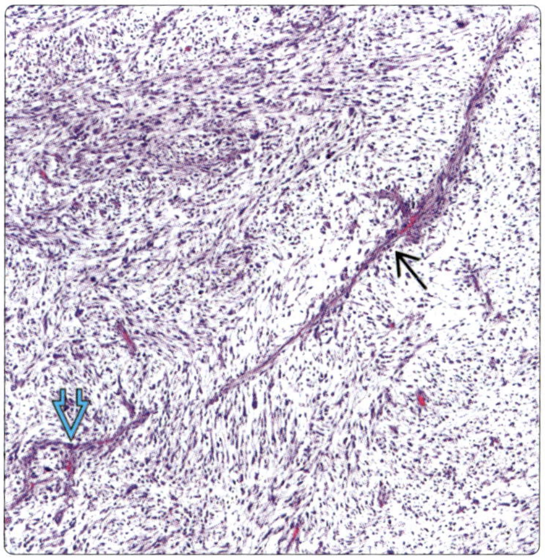

(Left) *A distinctive and characteristic feature of MFS is the presence of elongated, thin-walled stromal blood vessels in short arcs and linear arrays; however, in some cases, the vessels may not be prominent. Of note, this vascular pattern may be seen in other tumors, including low-grade fibromyxoid sarcoma.* **(Right)** *The characteristic blood vessels → in MFS are often referred to as curvilinear, given their frequent linear and short arcing appearance. Branching ⇨ is also a common finding.*

Perivascular Condensation

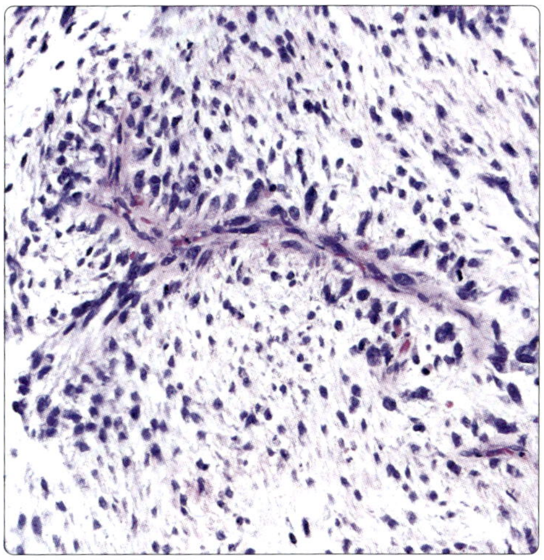

Nuclear Pleomorphism and Atypia

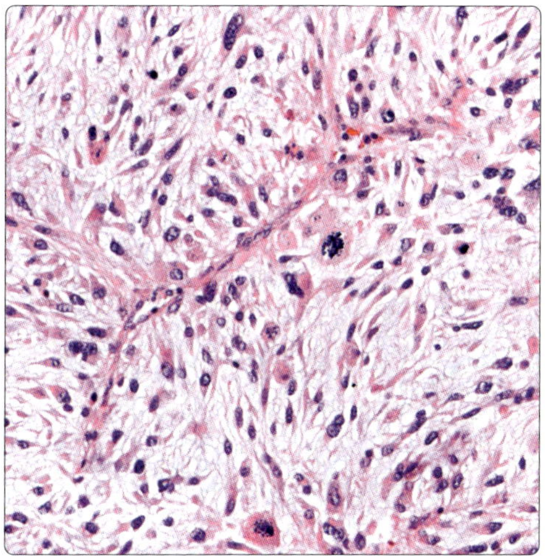

(Left) *An increase in tumor cell density around vessels is not uncommonly noted in MFS, as depicted. Chronic inflammatory cells may also congregate around these stromal vessels.* **(Right)** *The consistent presence of nuclear pleomorphism and atypia is one of the more important features of MFS. In low-grade examples, it may be one of the few clues that help distinguish MFS from morphologically similar myxoid neoplasms. Mitoses are also often conspicuous but vary with histologic grade.*

Nuclear Pleomorphism and Atypia

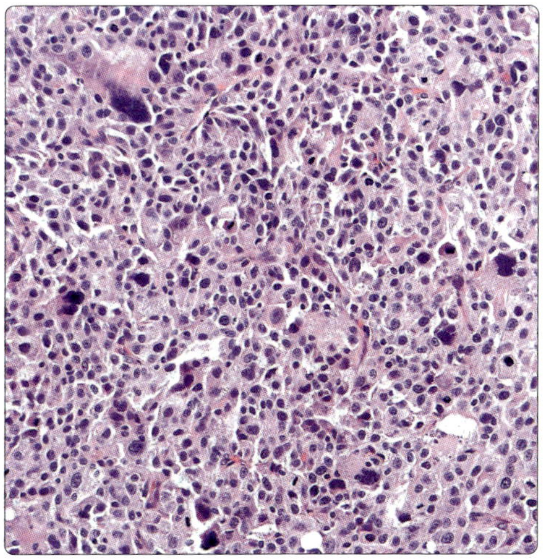

Multinucleated Tumor Cells

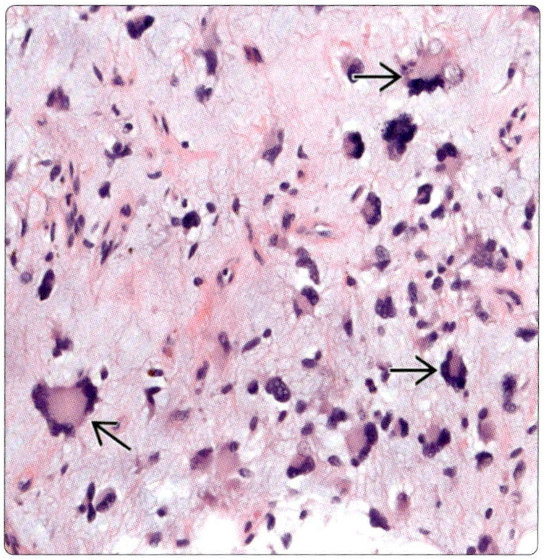

(Left) *Nuclear pleomorphism may be extreme in some cases of MFS, as shown. Such high-grade areas can be morphologically indistinguishable from undifferentiated pleomorphic sarcoma.* **(Right)** *Multinucleated tumor giant cells are commonly identified in MFS and often adopt a floret-like appearance → similar to what is seen in pleomorphic lipoma and well-differentiated liposarcoma. These cells often show densely eosinophilic cytoplasm and may even suggest myogenic differentiation.*

(Left) *The multinucleated tumor cells of MFS may also show a peripheral ring or wreath-like orientation of nuclei. The high-grade MFS depicted in this H&E shows numerous multinucleated cells within cellular nodules.* **(Right)** *Vacuolated fibroblastic tumor cells* ⇨ *distended with acid mucin are a common finding in MFS, particularly low- and intermediate-grade cases. These cells may erroneously suggest lipoblastic differentiation and are often described as pseudolipoblasts.*

Multinucleated Tumor Cells

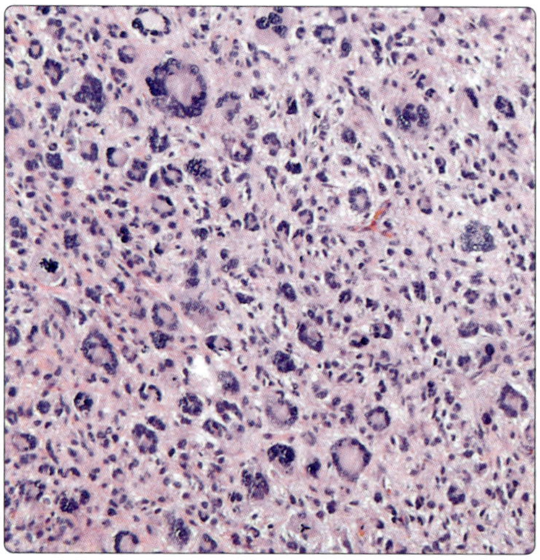

Pseudolipoblasts

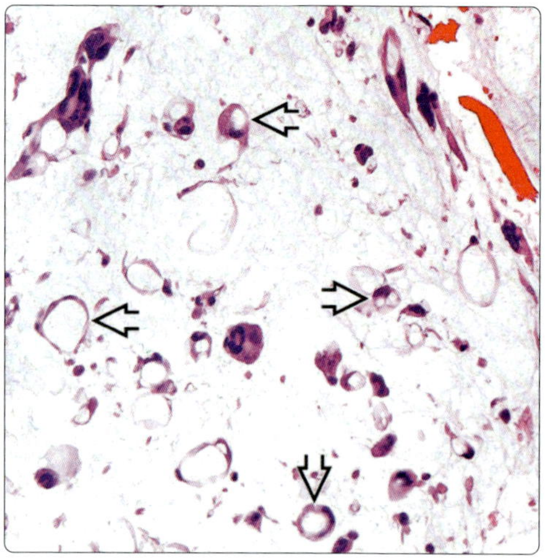

(Left) *The pseudolipoblasts of MFS contain cytoplasmic mucin instead of lipid and are not truly lipogenic. Histochemical stains can clarify the issue, but they are usually not necessary.* **(Right)** *Variable expression of CD34 may be seen in MFS, particularly superficial and cutaneous forms. Diffuse expression can lead to confusion with entities, such as pleomorphic lipoma and dermatofibrosarcoma protuberans.*

Pseudolipoblasts

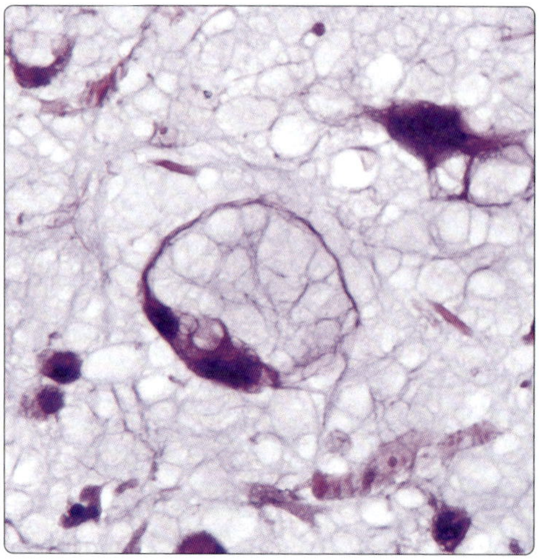

Variable CD34 Expression

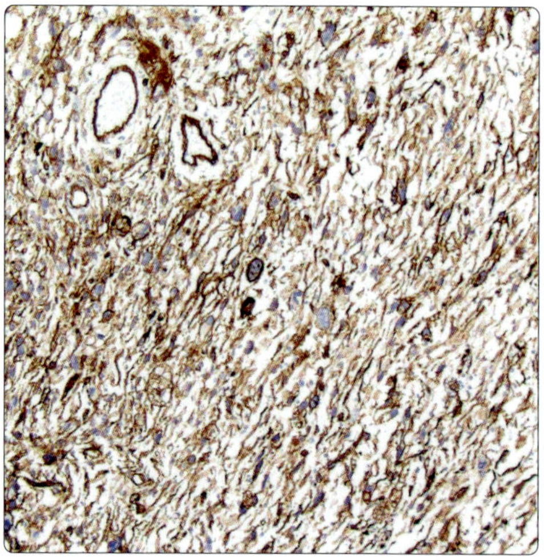

(Left) *The overall cellularity and level of atypia and mitotic activity vary depending on the histologic grade of MFS. Low-grade tumors are highly myxoid and of low cellularity and show scattered atypical hyperchromatic tumor cells with a low proliferation rate. Necrosis is absent.* **(Right)** *Some areas in low-grade MFS can be strikingly hypocellular and myxoid, and cytologic atypia can be focal. Other more conventional and atypical areas are often present; however, on small biopsy, these relatively banal zones can be treacherous.*

Low-Grade Myxofibrosarcoma

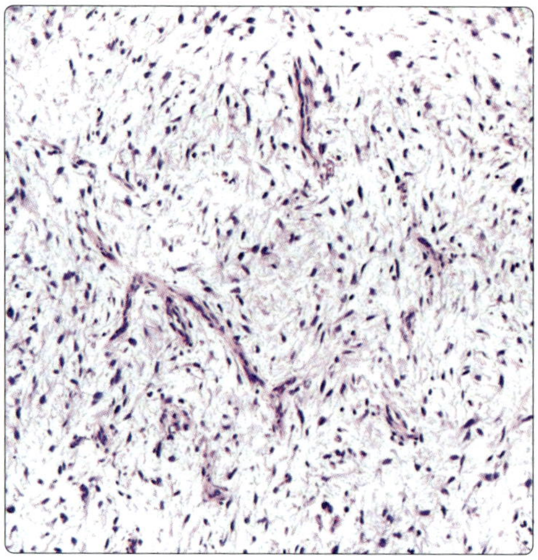

Low-Grade Myxofibrosarcoma

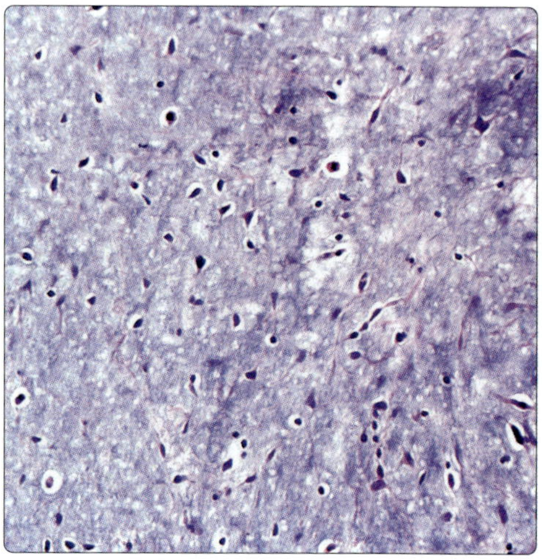

Intermediate-Grade Myxofibrosarcoma

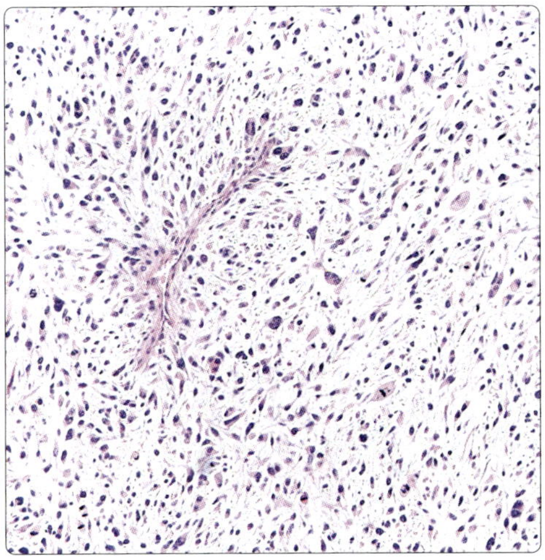

High-Grade Myxofibrosarcoma

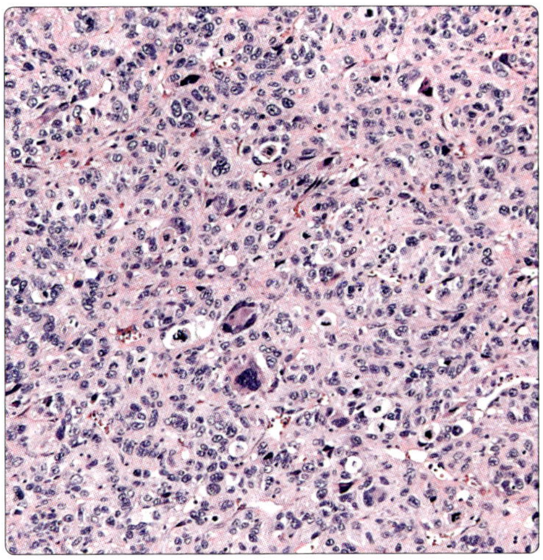

(Left) *Intermediate-grade MFS shows increased cellularity, nuclear pleomorphism, and mitotic activity compared to low-grade tumors; however, these features do not reach the severe degree seen in high-grade tumors.* **(Right)** *High-grade MFS contains cellular sheets and fascicles of highly pleomorphic tumor cells, essentially morphologically identical to other high-grade pleomorphic sarcomas. Mitoses, including atypical forms, and coagulative necrosis are also very common.*

Regional Variation in Histologic Grade

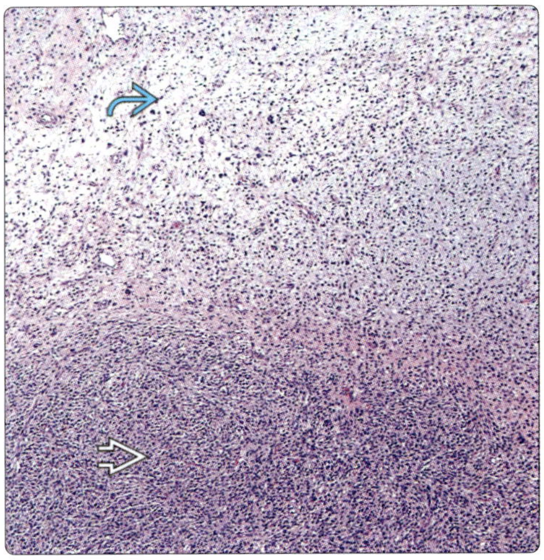

Epithelioid Variant

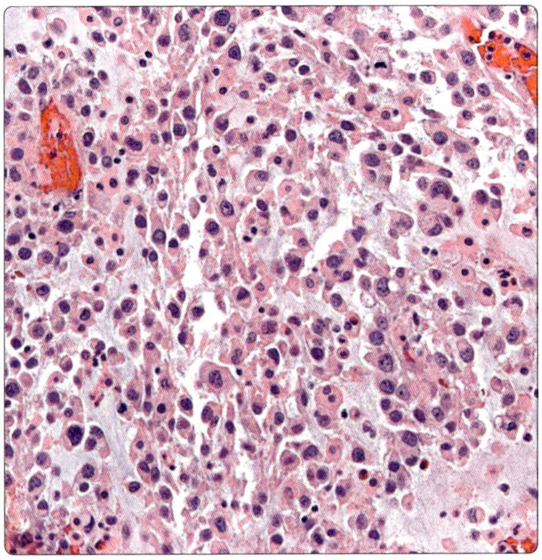

(Left) *In any given case of MFS, the histologic grade may vary from one field to the next, as evidenced at low magnification by the variation in cellularity and degree of myxoid stroma. Note the differences between high-grade ➔ and lower grade ➔ areas.* **(Right)** *The rare epithelioid variant of MFS contains areas of variably sized, rounded cells with abundant eosinophilic cytoplasm and vesicular nuclei with prominent nucleoli. Other areas showing features of conventional MFS are often present elsewhere.*

Epithelioid Variant

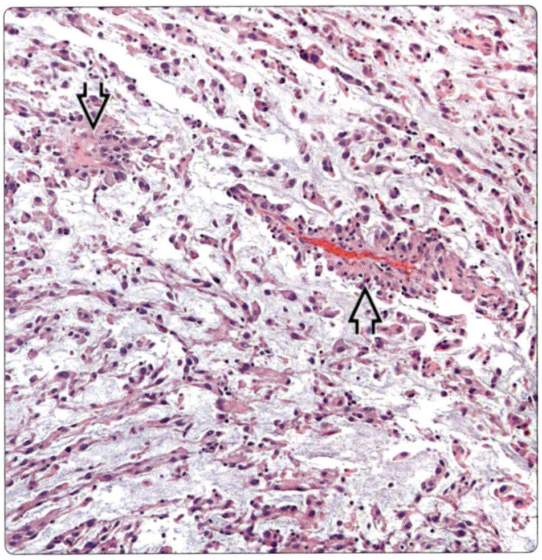

Epithelioid Variant

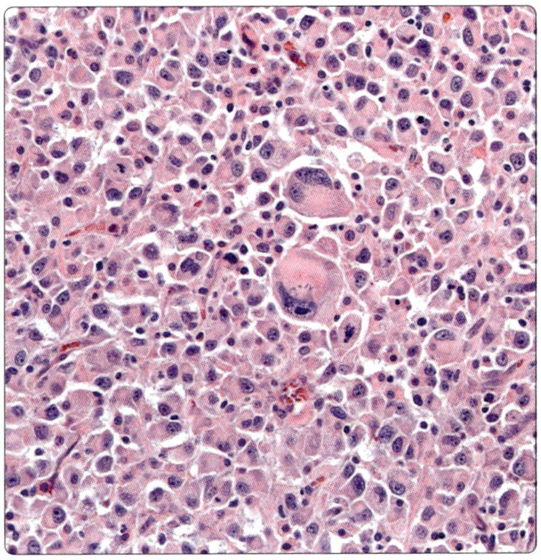

(Left) *The tumor cells in epithelioid MFS may be present singly or form architectures, including nests, aggregates, sheets, or linear cords. Increased perivascular tumor cell density ➔ can also be seen.* **(Right)** *In some areas of epithelioid MFS, the tumor cells form diffuse sheets and may closely resemble a poorly differentiated carcinoma or melanoma. IHC is very helpful in making the distinction.*

Low-Grade Fibromyxoid Sarcoma

KEY FACTS

TERMINOLOGY

- Deceptively bland, malignant fibroblastic neoplasm composed of spindle cells in variable collagenous to myxoid matrix and characterized in most cases by *FUS-CREB3L2* or *FUS-CREB3L1* fusion
- Synonym: Evans tumor

CLINICAL ISSUES

- Uncommon but incidence likely underestimated
- Most common in young adults
  - ~ 20% occur in patients < 18 years old
- Most common in proximal extremities and trunk
- Slow-growing, painless mass, often of long clinical duration
- Vast majority arise in deep soft tissue
- Treatment: Wide surgical excision
- Generally indolent clinical course
  - However, higher rates of recurrence and metastatic disease with longer clinical follow-up
- Indefinite, long-term follow-up is mandatory

MICROSCOPIC

- Classically shows combination of hypocellular fibrocollagenous and cellular myxoid zones
- Cytologically bland spindle cells with indistinct cytoplasm
- Short fascicular and whorling growth patterns characteristic
- Vasculature often prominent in myxoid zones
- Mitotic figures generally rare to absent
- Sclerosing epithelioid fibrosarcoma-like areas in some cases
- Morphologic variant with paucicellular collagen nodules

ANCILLARY TESTS

- Strong, diffuse MUC4(+) with cytoplasmic expression
- Molecular: t(7;16) with *FUS-CREB3L2* (75% of cases)

TOP DIFFERENTIAL DIAGNOSES

- Desmoid fibromatosis
- Perineurioma
- Intramuscular myxoma
- Myxofibrosarcoma

Low-Grade Fibromyxoid Sarcoma

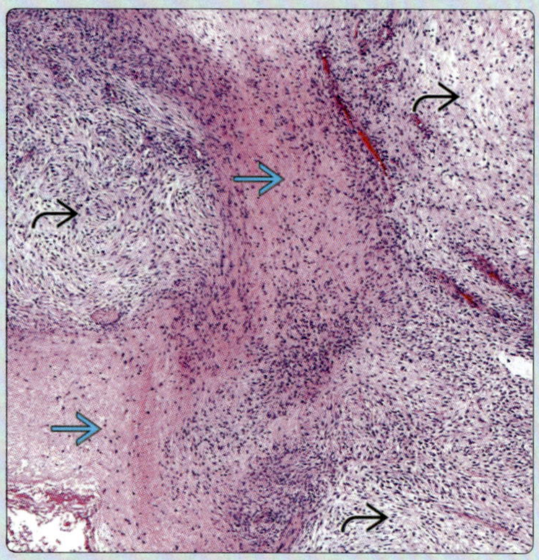

Fibrous Zones

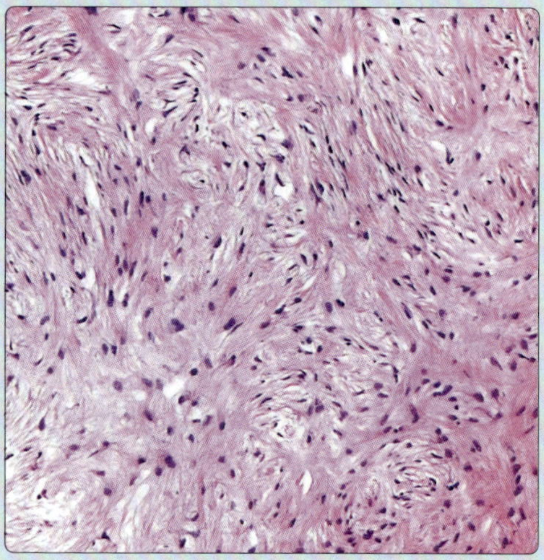

(Left) *Low-grade fibromyxoid sarcoma (LGFMS) is a malignant fibroblastic neoplasm that most commonly arises in the deep soft tissue of young adults. The classic low-power appearance is that of cellular myxoid zones admixed with hypocellular fibrocollagenous zones.* **(Right)** *The fibrous zones of LGFMS are often hypocellular and feature regular, cytologically banal spindle cells. Mitoses are rare. This deceptively bland appearance is a common reason for misdiagnosis as a benign neoplasm.*

Myxoid Zones

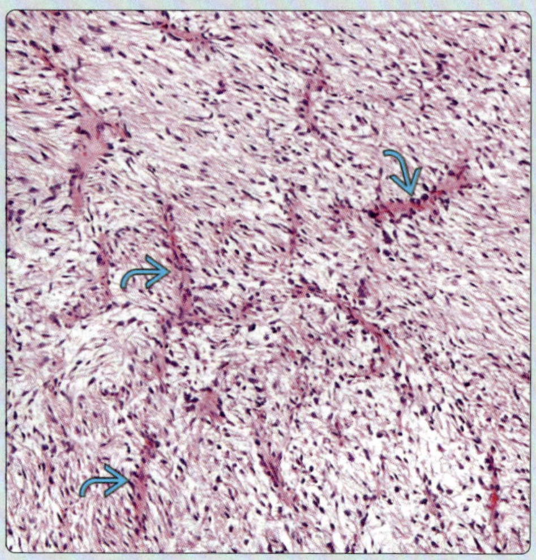

MUC4 Expression

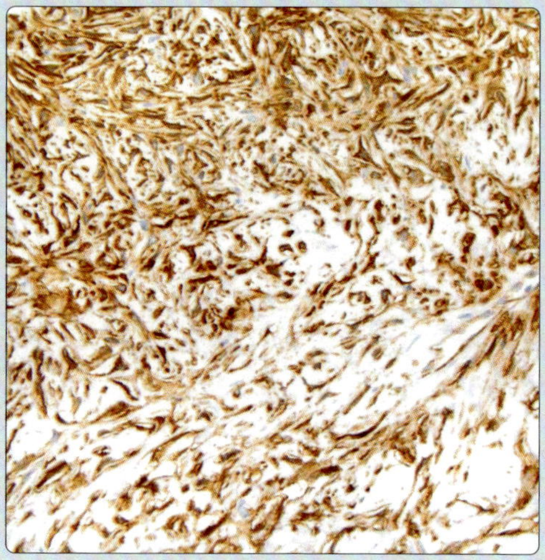

(Left) *The myxoid zones or nodules of LGFMS are generally more cellular than the fibrous zones and frequently show a variable prominent vascular network composed of arcades of thin-walled vessels. This vascularity may sometimes resemble that of myxofibrosarcoma.* **(Right)** *MUC4 is a highly sensitive and specific marker of LGFMS and is not seen in its morphologic mimics. Of note, MUC4 expression is also common in sclerosing epithelioid fibrosarcoma (SEF), a genetically related entity.*

TERMINOLOGY

Abbreviations

- Low-grade fibromyxoid sarcoma (LGFMS)

Synonyms

- Evans tumor
- Fibrosarcoma, fibromyxoid type
- Hyalinizing spindle cell tumor with giant rosettes (morphologic variant)

Definitions

- Deceptively bland, malignant fibroblastic neoplasm composed of spindle cells in variable collagenous to myxoid matrix and characterized in most cases by *FUS-CREB3L2* or *FUS-CREB3L1*
  - Appear to be genetically related to subset of sclerosing epithelioid fibrosarcoma (SEF)

CLINICAL ISSUES

Epidemiology

- Incidence
  - Once considered rare
    - Incidence likely underestimated and underreported in literature due to misclassification as other tumors
- Age
  - Young adults (typically in 4th decade) but wide age distribution
    - Significant proportion (~ 20%) occurs in patients < 18 years old

Site

- Most common in proximal extremities and trunk
- Rarely other locations, including viscera

Presentation

- Slow-growing, painless mass
  - Often of prolonged duration (> 1 year)
- Vast majority arise in deep soft tissue
- Rare tumors arise in subcutis or dermis
  - Superficial tumors more common in children

Treatment

- Wide surgical excision with negative margins
- Indefinite, long-term follow-up is mandatory to monitor for recurrences and late metastases

Prognosis

- Generally indolent clinical course
  - Low rates of local recurrence and metastatic disease in 1st few years after initial surgery
- Higher rates of recurrence and metastatic disease with longer clinical follow-up
  - Metastatic disease may occur many years after primary surgery (up to 45 years reported)
    - Most commonly to lung, pleura, and chest wall
  - In one recent study with long-term follow-up, death from disease occurred in 42% of patients with median interval to tumor-related death of 15 years
- Superficial tumors (subcutis or dermis) appear to have better overall outcome
  - Lower risk of local recurrence and as of yet, no reported cases of metastatic disease
- Generally, no correlation between histologic features or translocation status
  - Exception: "Dedifferentiated" LGFMS with undifferentiated round cells shows aggressive clinical course
- Exact behavior of LGFMS with areas resembling SEF (so-called hybrid LGFMS/SEF) is difficult to predict but appears to behave more like conventional LGFMS than pure SEF

MACROSCOPIC

General Features

- Well-defined mass
- White, fibrous cut surface, often with glistening areas
- Sometimes cystic foci but necrosis rare

Size

- Median: 5 cm (range: 1 cm to > 20 cm)

MICROSCOPIC

Histologic Features

- Well circumscribed but often shows microscopic infiltration of peripheral soft tissues
- Cytologically bland spindle cells with indistinct cytoplasm
  - Usually at most mild nuclear enlargement &/or hyperchromasia
  - Mitotic figures generally rare to absent
- Classically shows combination of fibrous and myxoid zones
  - Exact composition of given tumor is highly variable
    - Occasional cases are almost entirely fibrous or myxoid
  - Transitional interface may be gradual or abrupt (cannonball-like myxoid nodules)
  - Fibrous zones
    - Usually hypocellular with abundant fine, fibrillary or feathery stromal collagen
    - Short fascicular and whorling growth patterns characteristic
    - Scattered paucicellular collagen rosettes may be seen in subset of cases
  - Myxoid zones
    - More cellular than fibrous zones
    - Vasculature often prominent
      - Arcades of small blood vessels with variable perivascular sclerosis
      - Increased perivascular cellularity may be seen
- Necrosis rare (may be focal)
- Rare findings: Cystic degeneration, osseous metaplasia, staghorn blood vessels
- Minority of cases feature foci of increased cellularity, nuclear pleomorphism, mitoses, or epithelioid morphology
  - These findings are more common in recurrent and metastatic tumors
- Areas morphologically similar to or indistinguishable from SEF can be seen
  - Sheets, nests, and cords of small epithelioid cells with clear to eosinophilic cytoplasm within prominent sclerotic matrix
- Rare undifferentiated round cell component reported in recurrences ("dedifferentiated" LGFMS)

Morphologic Variants

- Hyalinizing spindle cell tumor with giant rosettes
  - Prominent paucicellular hyalinized nodules bordered by more rounded tumor cells
  - Background morphology similar to conventional LGFMS
  - No genetic, immunohistochemical, or behavioral differences in this variant
  - This term is no longer recommended

ANCILLARY TESTS

Immunohistochemistry

- Strong, diffuse MUC4(+) with cytoplasmic expression
- May show focal expression of EMA, CD34, SMA, p63, claudin-1
- Variable DOG1(+) reported in 5/10 cases in one series
- Desmin, S100 protein, keratin, p40, CD117 (-)
- Nuclear β-catenin expression absent

Molecular Genetics

- Characteristic chromosomal translocations
  - t(7;16)(q33;p11) is most common (75% of cases)
    - Results in *FUS-CREB3L2* fusion
  - t(11;16)(p11;p11)
    - Results in *FUS-CREB3L1* fusion
  - Very rare tumors reported with *EWSR1-CREB3L1* fusion

DIFFERENTIAL DIAGNOSIS

Desmoid Fibromatosis

- Infiltrative growth
- Characteristic sweeping fascicular pattern
- Nuclear β-catenin (+)
- MUC4(-)
- Lacks genetic features of LGFMS

Perineurioma

- Can show significant morphologic overlap with LGFMS
- Perivascular whorls and storiform arrays
- Myxoid areas lack prominent vasculature
- EMA(+), claudin-1 (+); variable CD34(+)
- MUC4(-)
- Lacks genetic features of LGFMS

Intramuscular Myxoma

- Paucicellular myxoid areas predominate
- Lacks prominent vasculature
- MUC4(-)
- Lacks genetic features of LGFMS

Myxofibrosarcoma

- Most common in superficial soft tissues of elderly patients
- Abundant myxoid stroma in lower grade tumors
- Prominent nuclear atypia and pleomorphism
- Can feature similar vasculature to LGFMS
- MUC4(-)
- Lacks genetic features of LGFMS

Sclerosing Epithelioid Fibrosarcoma

- Nests and cords of small epithelioid cells within prominent sclerotic matrix
- MUC4(+) in most cases
- May show pure SEF morphology or contain minor areas of conventional LGFMS
  - Clear point of distinction between classification as SEF vs. "hybrid LGFMS/SEF" is unclear
    - However, *EWSR1* and *CREB3L1* rearrangements appear to predominate in pure SEF
      - In contrast to predominately *FUS* and *CREB3L2* rearrangements in pure LGFMS and hybrid LGFMS/SEF

Myxoid Liposarcoma

- General absence of fibrous zones
- More delicate plexiform or arborizing capillary vasculature
- Often contains lipoblasts
- MUC4(-)
- Distinctive t(12;16) with *FUS-DDIT3* fusion in most cases

Hybrid Nerve Sheath Tumor

- Often resembles perineurioma
- Variable fibromyxoid matrix
- Contains Schwann cells and perineurial cells
  - S100 protein (+), EMA(+), claudin-1 (+)
- MUC4(-)
- Lacks genetic features of LGFMS

SELECTED REFERENCES

1. Swanson AA et al: Low-grade fibromyxoid sarcoma arising within the median nerve. Neuropathology. 38(3):309-14, 2018
2. Ud Din N et al: Abdominopelvic and retroperitoneal low-grade fibromyxoid sarcoma: a clinicopathologic study of 13 cases. Am J Clin Pathol. 149(2):128-34, 2018
3. Mohamed M et al: Low-grade fibromyxoid sarcoma: clinical, morphologic and genetic features. Ann Diagn Pathol. 28:60-7, 2017
4. Cowan ML et al: Low-grade fibromyxoid sarcoma of the head and neck: a clinicopathologic series and review of the literature. Head Neck Pathol. 10(2):161-6, 2016
5. Prieto-Granada C et al: A genetic dichotomy between pure sclerosing epithelioid fibrosarcoma (SEF) and hybrid SEF/low-grade fibromyxoid sarcoma: a pathologic and molecular study of 18 cases. Genes Chromosomes Cancer. 54(1):28-38, 2015
6. Thway K et al: Pediatric low-grade fibromyxoid sarcoma mimicking ossifying fibromyxoid tumor: adding to the diagnostic spectrum of soft tissue tumors with a bony shell. Hum Pathol. 46(3):461-6, 2015
7. Thway K et al: DOG1 expression in low-grade fibromyxoid sarcoma: a study of 11 cases, with molecular characterization. Int J Surg Pathol. 23(6):454-60, 2015
8. Lau PP et al: EWSR1-CREB3L1 gene fusion: a novel alternative molecular aberration of low-grade fibromyxoid sarcoma. Am J Surg Pathol. 37(5):734-8, 2013
9. Maretty-Nielsen K et al: Low-grade fibromyxoid sarcoma: incidence, treatment strategy of metastases, and clinical significance of the FUS gene. Sarcoma. 2013:256280, 2013
10. Doyle LA et al: MUC4 is a highly sensitive and specific marker for low-grade fibromyxoid sarcoma. Am J Surg Pathol. 35(5):733-41, 2011
11. Evans HL: Low-grade fibromyxoid sarcoma: a clinicopathologic study of 33 cases with long-term follow-up. Am J Surg Pathol. 35(10):1450-62, 2011
12. Rekhi B et al: Low-grade fibromyxoid sarcoma: a clinicopathologic study of 18 cases, including histopathologic relationship with sclerosing epithelioid fibrosarcoma in a subset of cases. Ann Diagn Pathol. 15(5):303-11, 2011
13. Guillou L et al: Translocation-positive low-grade fibromyxoid sarcoma: clinicopathologic and molecular analysis of a series expanding the morphologic spectrum and suggesting potential relationship to sclerosing epithelioid fibrosarcoma: a study from the French Sarcoma Group. Am J Surg Pathol. 31(9):1387-402, 2007
14. Billings SD et al: Superficial low-grade fibromyxoid sarcoma (Evans tumor): a clinicopathologic analysis of 19 cases with a unique observation in the pediatric population. Am J Surg Pathol. 29(2):204-10, 2005
15. Folpe AL et al: Low-grade fibromyxoid sarcoma and hyalinizing spindle cell tumor with giant rosettes: a clinicopathologic study of 73 cases supporting their identity and assessing the impact of high-grade areas. Am J Surg Pathol. 24(10):1353-60, 2000

Irregular Zonal Interface

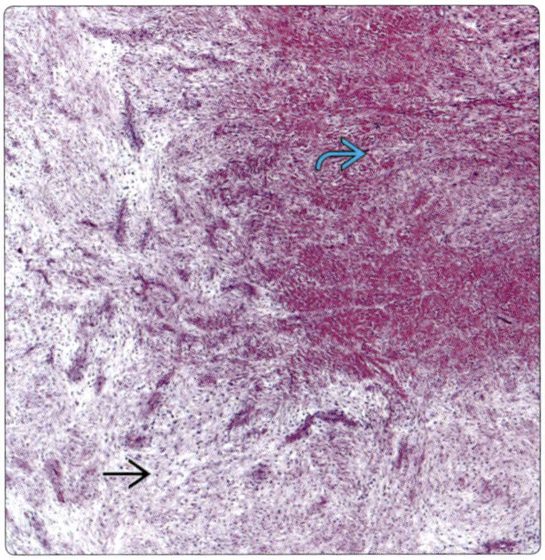

Abrupt Zonal Interface

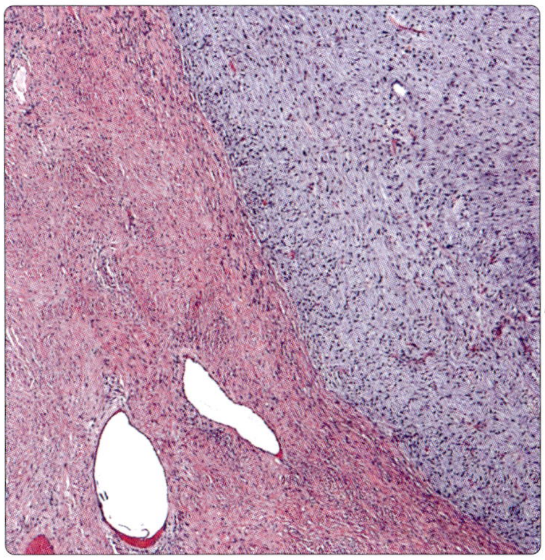

(Left) *In most cases of LGFMS, the fibrous ↪ and myxoid → zones are well delineated from one another, although the border/interface is often somewhat irregular, as depicted in this H&E.* **(Right)** *Occasionally, myxoid zones are very well demarcated in LGFMS and truly show an abrupt interface with the fibrous areas, as seen in this H&E.*

Gradual Zonal Interface

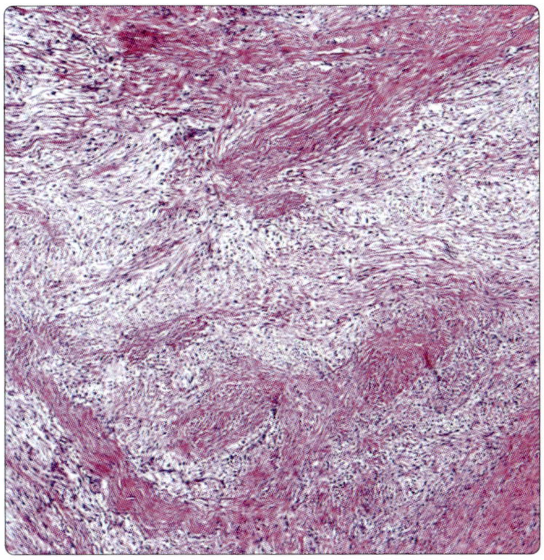

"Tigroid" Zonal Interface

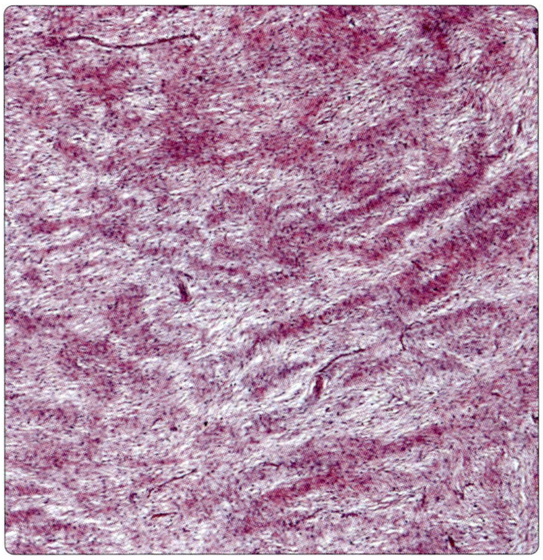

(Left) *Myxoid areas showing a more gradual transition to and from fibrous zones are also relatively common in LGFMS, as depicted in this H&E.* **(Right)** *Rare cases of LGFMS can show an unusual pattern of fibrous and myxoid zones alternating in rows. This striped morphology has been referred to as tigroid.*

Zonal Variations in Cellularity

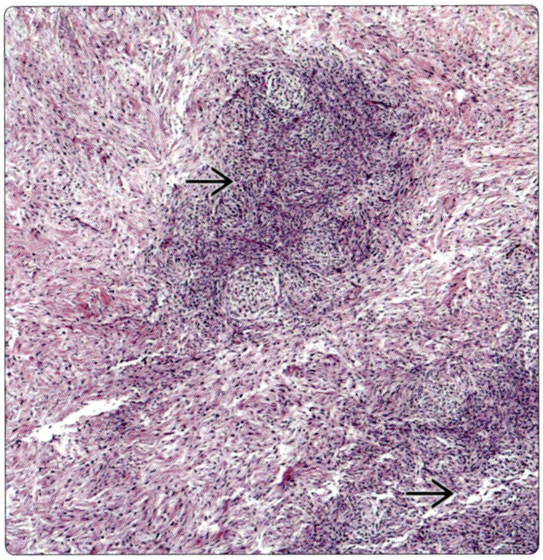

Hypocellular Myxoid Zones

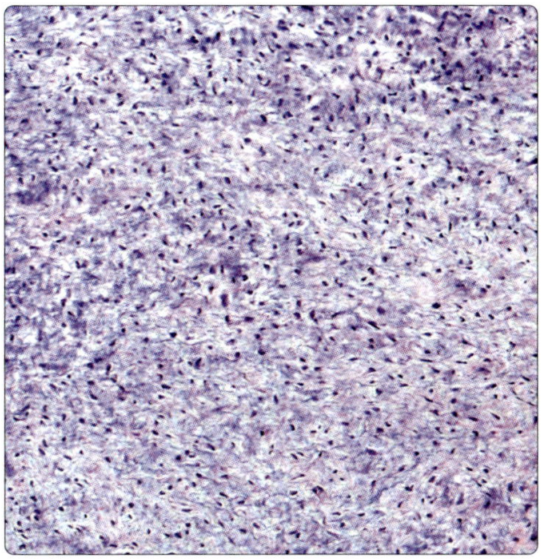

(Left) *The myxoid zones → of LGFMS are generally more cellular than the adjacent fibrous zones. This is in contrast to many other soft tissue tumors, wherein a myxoid matrix is often associated with a decrease in cellularity.* **(Right)** *Occasionally, a myxoid region in LGFMS is very hypocellular, as depicted. In conjunction with the bland spindled cells, these areas can resemble a benign tumor, such as myxoma or myxoid neurofibroma.*

Prominent Vasculature

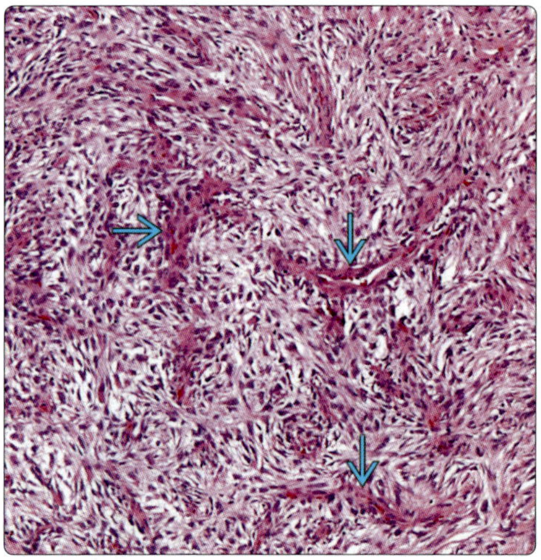

Prominent Vasculature

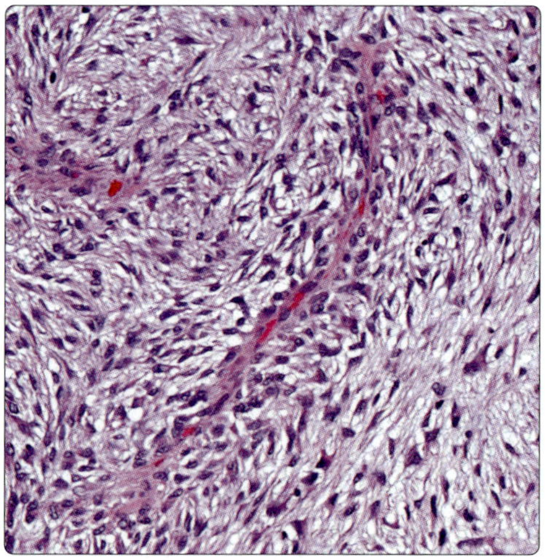

(Left) *A characteristic finding in many of the myxoid zones of LGFMS is an accentuated stromal vasculature composed of arcades of branching, thin-walled blood vessels* ➙*. A mild degree of perivascular sclerosis is also a frequent finding in some cases.* **(Right)** *An increase in cell density around blood vessels may be seen in LGFMS, as shown in this H&E. Note that the tumor cells show no more than mild atypia, unlike myxofibrosarcoma.*

Prominent Vasculature

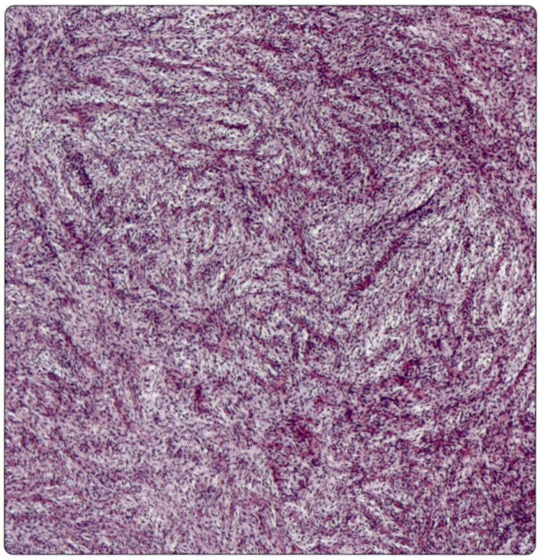

Prominent Vasculature

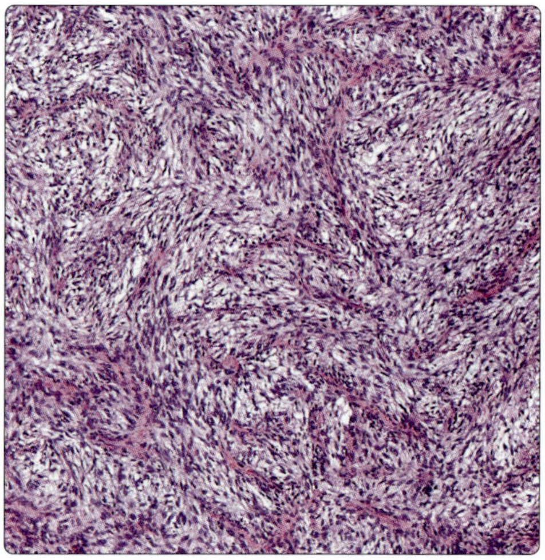

(Left) *The characteristic vasculature of LGFMS may be quite prominent and plexiform in some tumors, as depicted in this H&E. Although somewhat resembling the ramifying vascular pattern of myxoid liposarcoma, the fascicles and whorls of tumor cells are not features of that diagnosis.* **(Right)** *H&E shows increased cellularity in a highly vascular myxoid region of a case of LGFMS.*

Perivascular Sclerosis

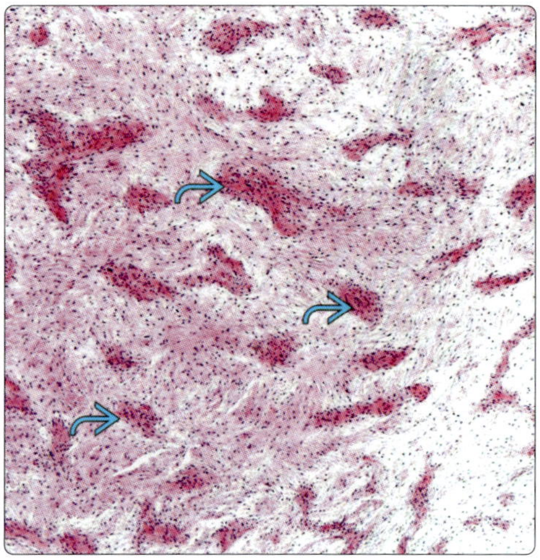

Perivascular Sclerosis

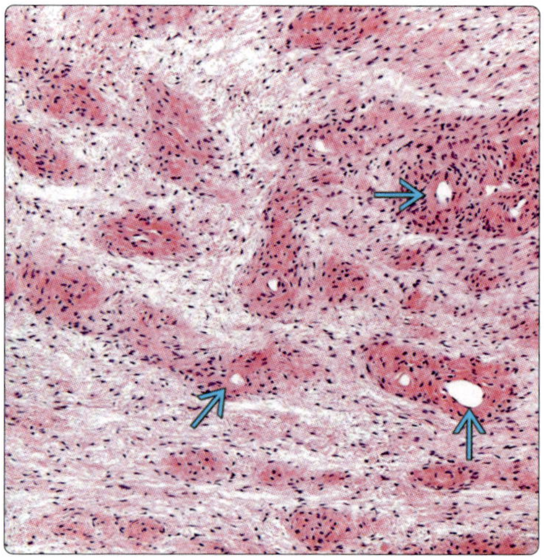

(Left) *A variable degree of perivascular hyalinization or sclerosis is not uncommon in LGFMS. This finding often imparts an eosinophilic accentuation* ➚ *to the individual blood vessels.* **(Right)** *Higher power H&E of LGFMS shows prominent perivascular sclerosis, as evidenced by eosinophilic collagen surrounding variably distinct vascular channels* ➙*.*

Cyst-Like Changes

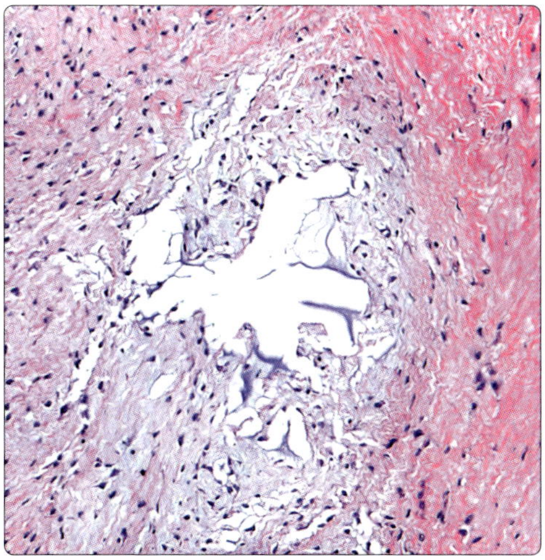

Cystic Degeneration

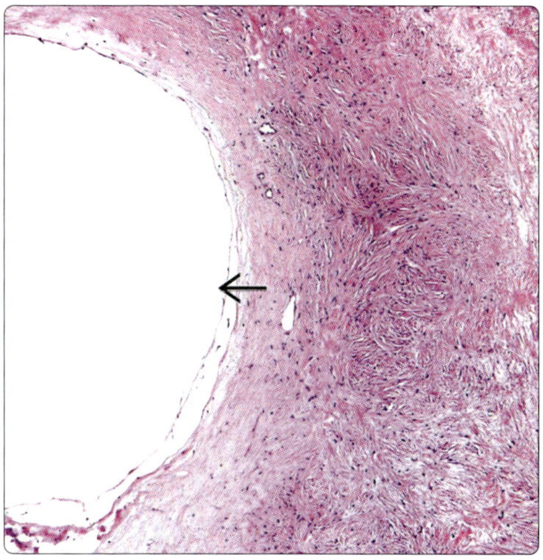

(Left) *Some myxoid foci in LGFMS can demonstrate a loose mucoid quality with cyst-like degeneration, similar to the stromal "holes" or "tears" seen in nodular fasciitis.* **(Right)** *Larger, degenerative cystic spaces ⇒ may be seen in some longstanding cases of LGFMS.*

Feathery Stromal Collagen

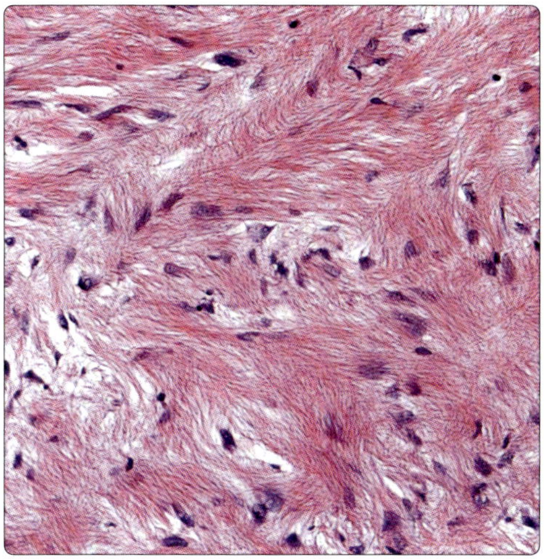

Haphazard Growth

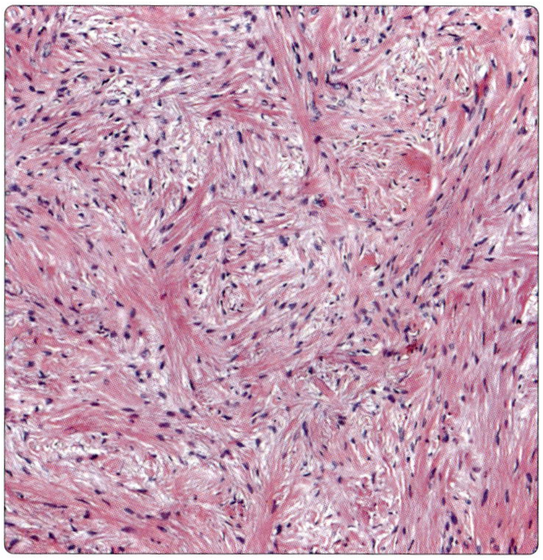

(Left) *The stromal collagen fibers of LGFMS often show a fine, fibrillary or feathery quality, as depicted in this H&E. Note the generally bland nuclei.* **(Right)** *A variety of architectural patterns may be seen in LGFMS, including fascicular, whorling, storiform, and random, haphazard growth. The latter pattern is featured in this case.*

Storiform Growth

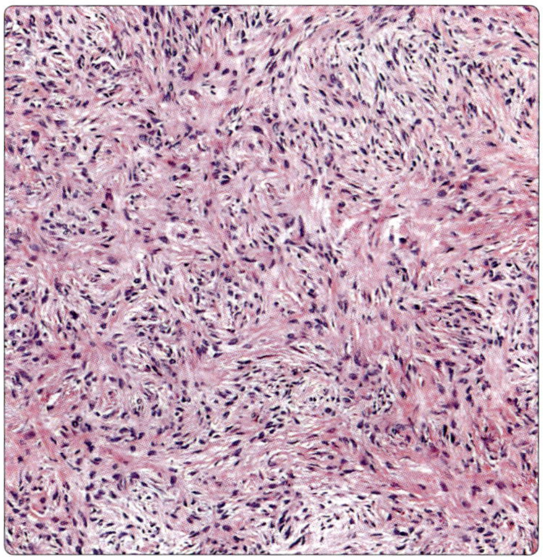

Hypocellular Fibrous Zone

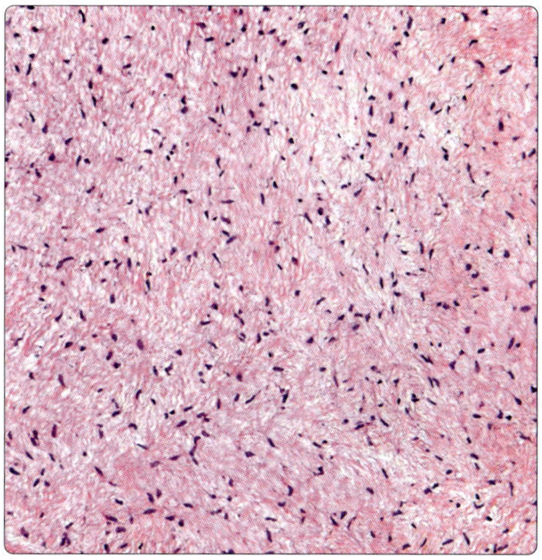

(Left) *H&E shows a loose storiform architectural pattern in a case of LGFMS.* **(Right)** *LGFMS shows hypocellular fibrous areas with haphazard cellular growth mimicking a nerve sheath tumor, such as neurofibroma. IHC is often helpful in this setting. Note the fine, fibrillary or feathery stromal collagen.*

(Left) *Collagen fibers may form more discrete bundles in LGFMS, as depicted in this H&E. This morphology can lead to serious consideration of neurofibroma. Note the scattered wavy nuclei →, further complicating the issue.* **(Right)** *Areas of increased cellularity are seen in a minor subset of cases of LGFMS, occurring both de novo and in recurrent/metastatic tumor (the latter being much more common).*

Discrete Collagen Fibers

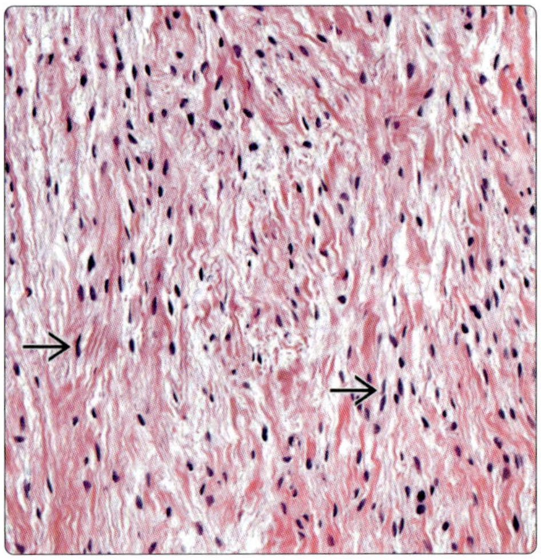

Increased Cellularity

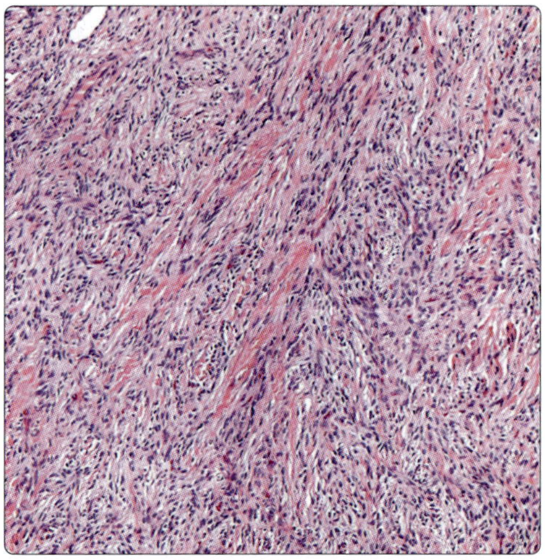

(Left) *Despite the finding of increased cellularity in this case of LGFMS, the tumor cells are regular and still relatively cytologically bland.* **(Right)** *Fascicular growth may be seen in LGFMS, particularly in cellular areas, as depicted in this H&E. Focal herringbone architecture can also be seen, similar to other types of fibrosarcoma.*

Cellular but Minimal Atypia

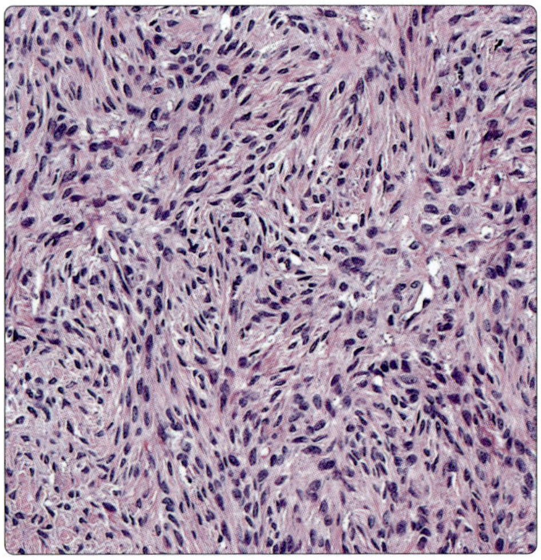

Fascicular Growth

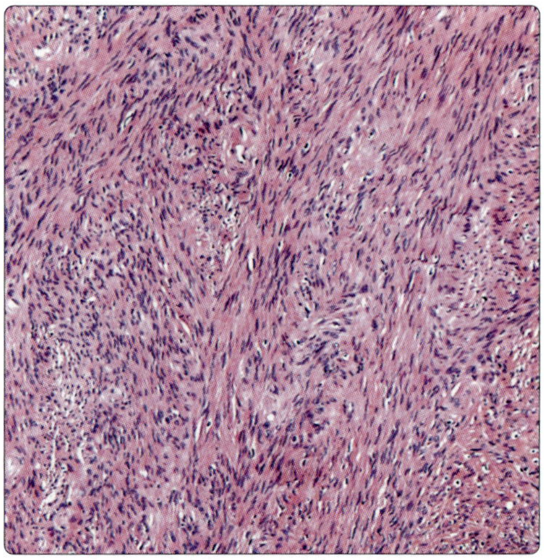

(Left) *The combination of fascicular growth and uniform, cytologically bland spindled cells in LGFMS can easily lead to consideration of fibromatosis, particularly on biopsy.* **(Right)** *Increased perivascular cellularity is not uncommon in myxoid zones of LGFMS; however, it can also be seen in fibrous areas, as shown in this H&E. Note the vessels →.*

Fascicular Growth

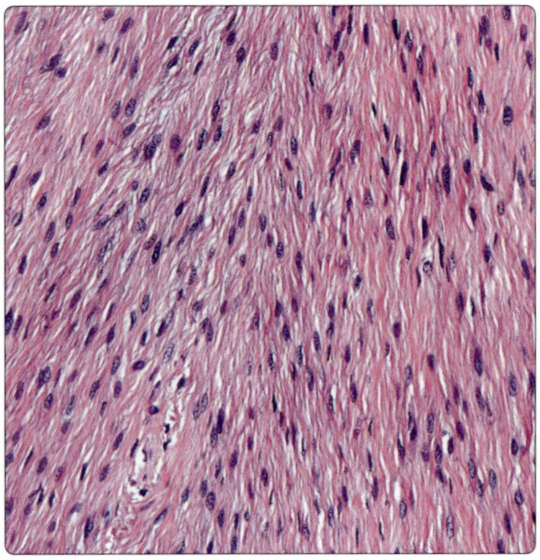

Perivascular Cellularity

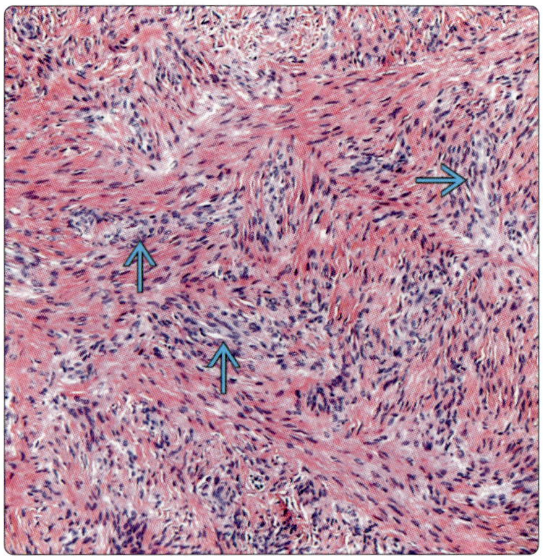

Perivascular Cellularity

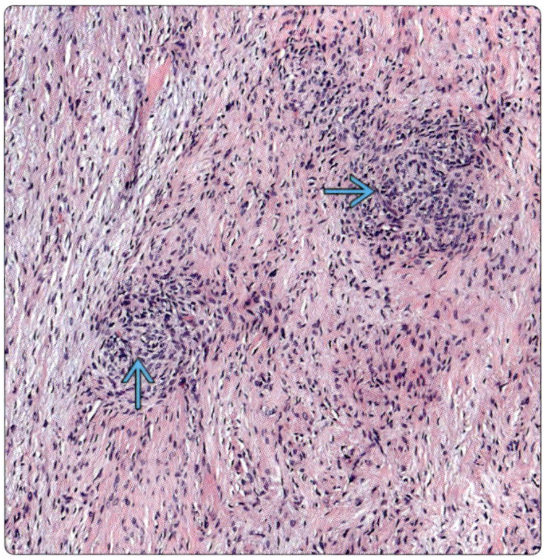

Focal Vague Palisaded Growth

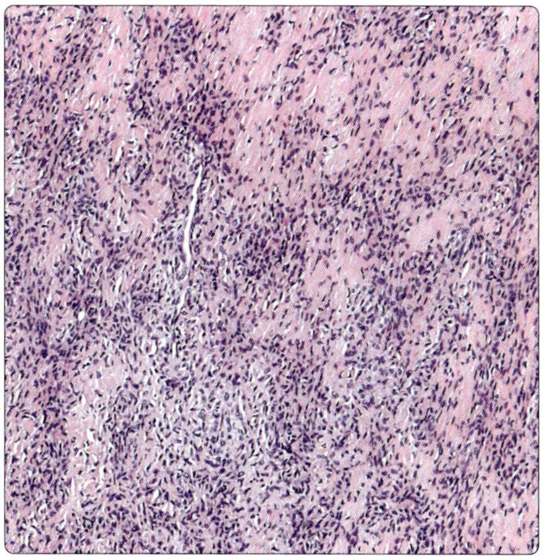

(Left) *In some cases of LGFMS, the increased perivascular cellularity is accentuated by a more epithelioid cytomorphology ➔ in the tumor cells. Occasionally, the vessels are inconspicuous, and the structures resemble loose epithelial nests.* **(Right)** *Focal vague palisading of tumor cells or nuclei is a rare finding in LGFMS, as depicted in this H&E.*

Stromal Hyalinization

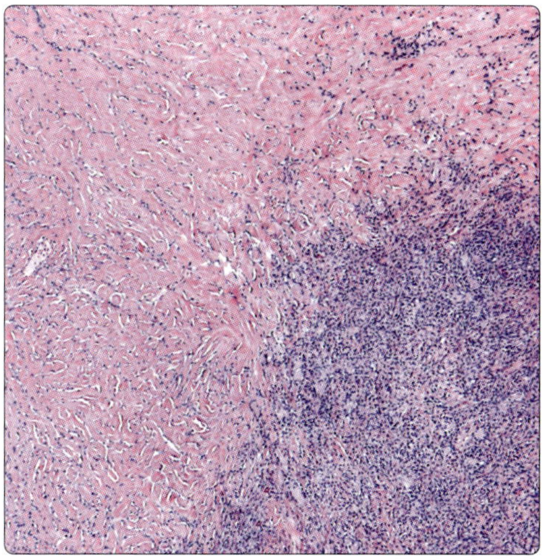

Stromal Hyalinization

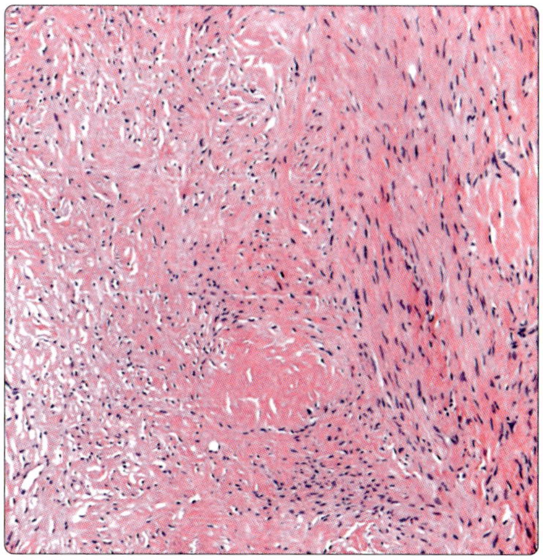

(Left) *Prominent hyalinization of a large fibrous area (upper left) is seen in this H&E of LGFMS. Note the more cellular myxoid region (lower right).* **(Right)** *Stromal hyalinization can be marked in LGFMS and may make for a challenging case if more conventional morphologic areas are not present. These areas can also closely resemble SEF.*

Metaplastic Bone Formation

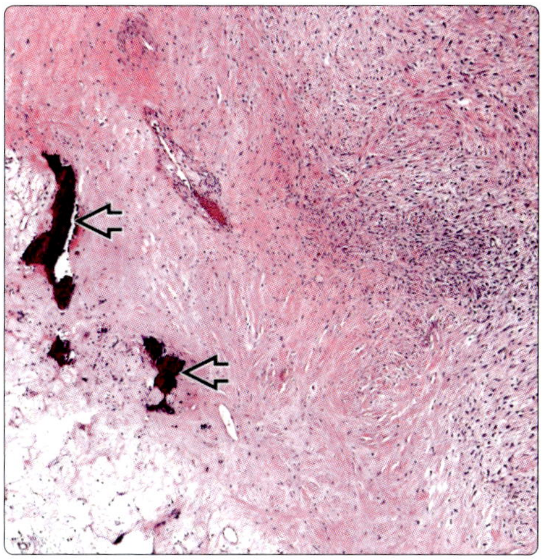

Rare Staghorn Blood Vessels

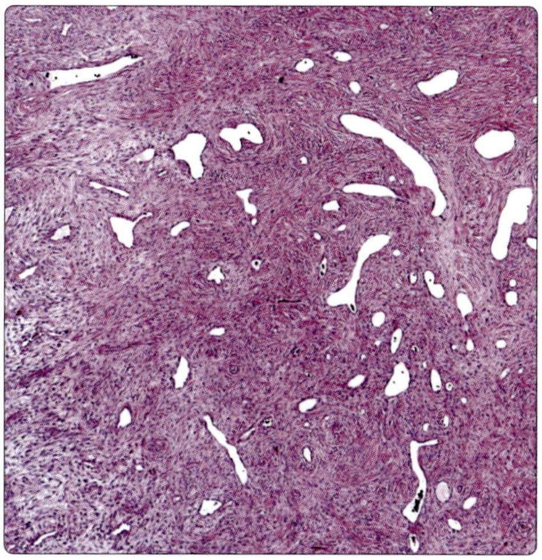

(Left) *Metaplastic bone formation ⇨ is an uncommon but well-documented finding in LGFMS.* **(Right)** *Larger ectatic or staghorn blood vessels are an uncommon finding in LGFMS. In rare cases, these vessels are quite prominent, as depicted in this H&E, and may lead to consideration of solitary fibrous tumor.*

(Left) *Up to 30% of cases of LGFMS feature unusual nodular structures composed of paucicellular collagen rimmed by plump tumor cells. These collagenous rosettes may range from focal and isolated to numerous and confluent.* **(Right)** *The tumor cells rimming the collagenous rosettes of LGFMS generally show a plumper and more epithelioid cytomorphology.*

Collagenous Rosettes

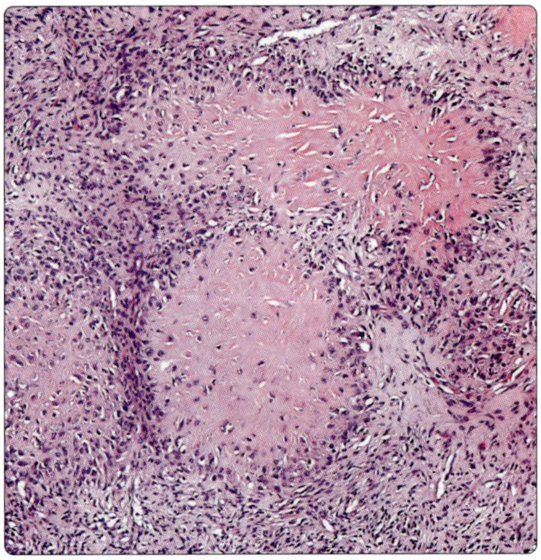

Epithelioid Perinodular Cells

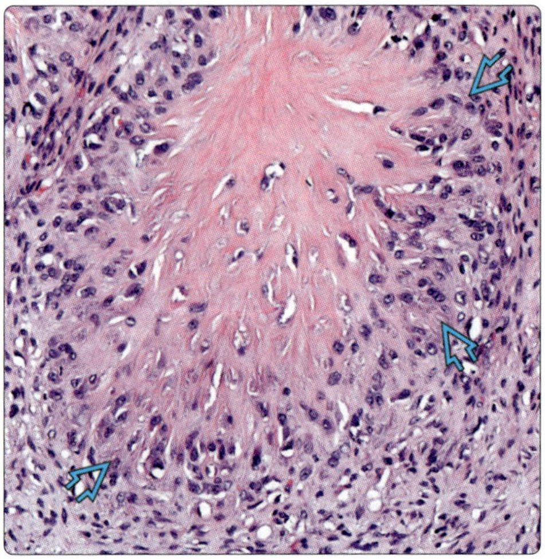

(Left) *In some cases of LGFMS with collagenous rosettes, the structures are only seen focally and can appear less distinctive than usual.* **(Right)** *The collagenous rosettes of LGFMS may be seen to encompass a central vessel and likely originate as nodules of perivascular hyalinization/sclerosis. Note the peripheral epithelioid fibroblastic tumor cells.*

Early Collagenous Rosettes

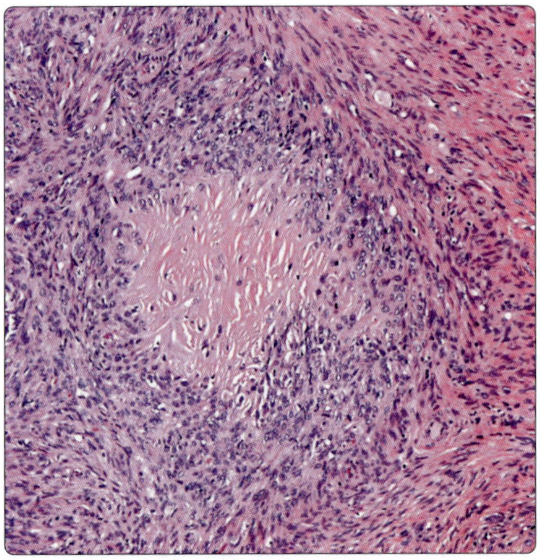

Perivascular Collagenous Rosettes

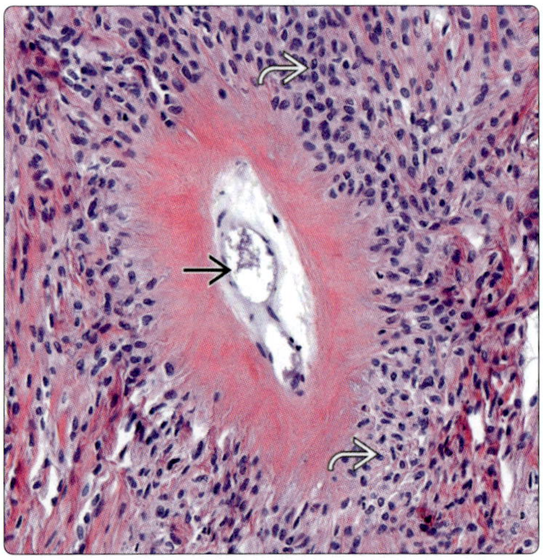

(Left) *Cases of LGFMS showing prominent collagenous rosettes, as depicted in this H&E, were previously classified as hyalinizing spindle cell tumor with giant rosettes (HSCTGR) before it become widely accepted as a morphologic variant of LGFMS.* **(Right)** *H&E shows a predominantly fibrocollagenous and hyalinized example of LGFMS (formerly HSCTGR). Note the numerous collagenous rosettes.*

Hyalinizing Spindle Cell Tumor With Giant Rosettes

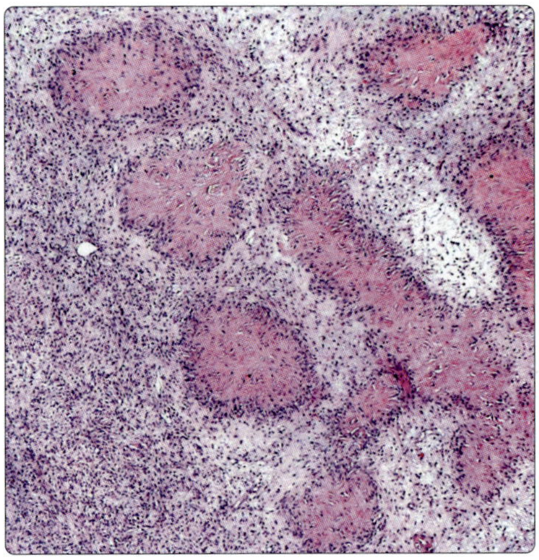

Hyalinizing Spindle Cell Tumor With Giant Rosettes

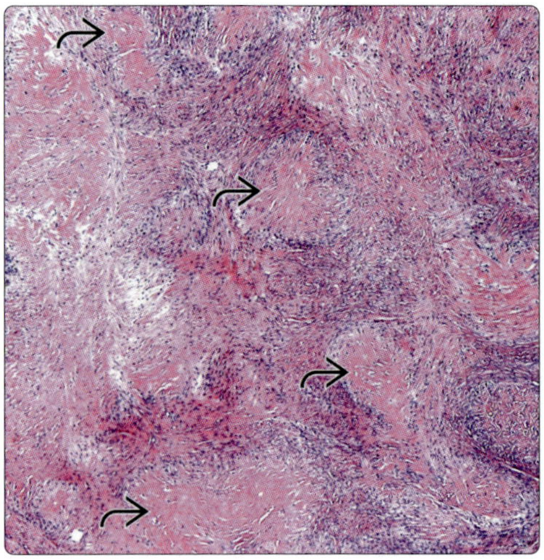

Infrequent Nuclear Atypia

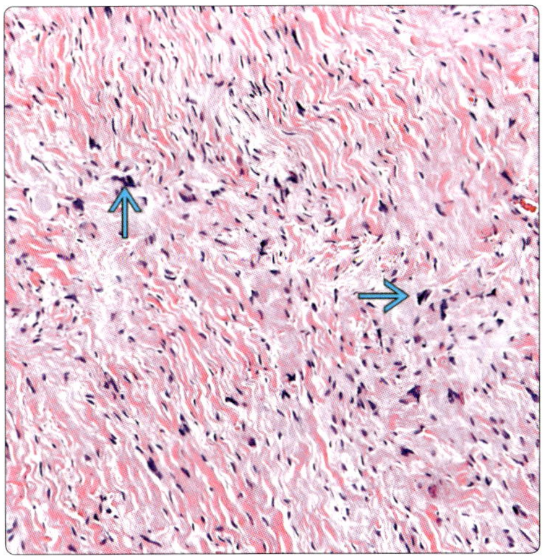

Epithelioid Cytomorphology

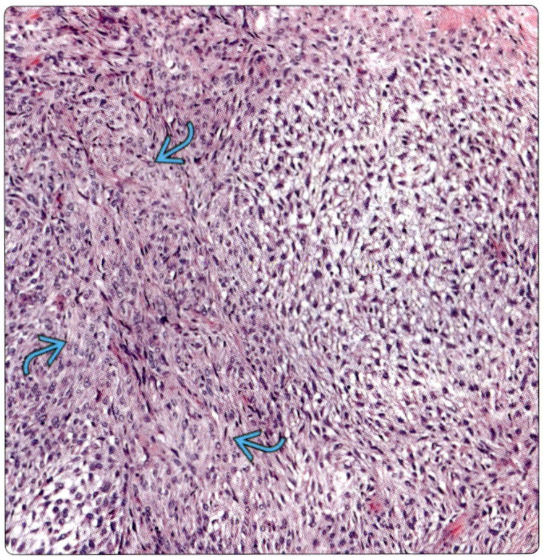

(Left) Nuclear atypia in the form of pleomorphism ➡ or multinucleation is an uncommon finding in LGFMS and is more likely to be present in recurrent or metastatic tumors. **(Right)** *Rare cases of LGFMS feature foci of plumper epithelioid cells ➡. Although not shown in this H&E, very rare cases of recurrent LGFMS may show "dedifferentiated" areas containing an anaplastic round cell component.*

Sclerosing Epithelioid Fibrosarcoma-Like Areas

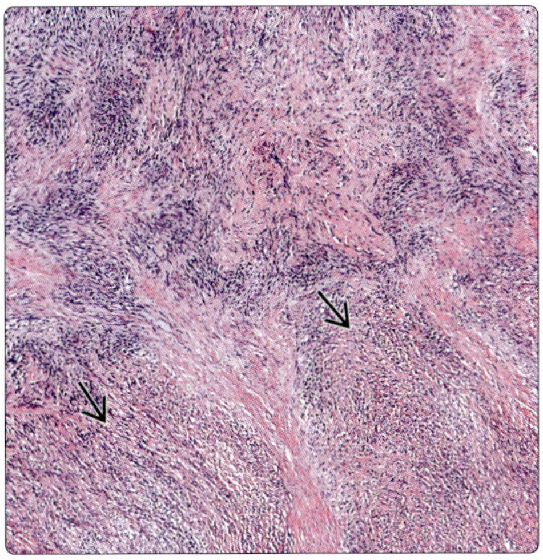

Sclerosing Epithelioid Fibrosarcoma-Like Areas

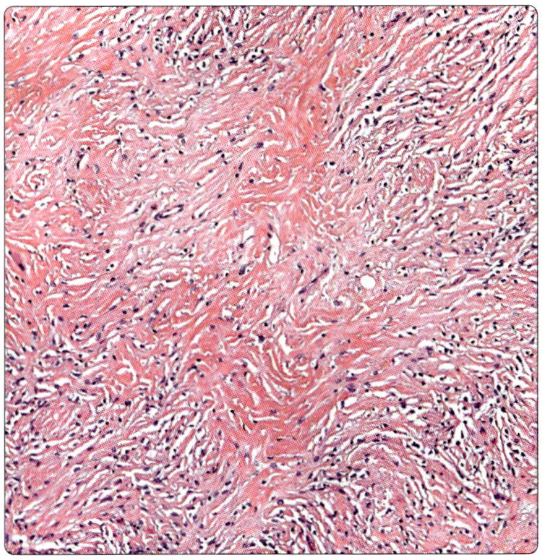

(Left) *Some cases of LGFMS may feature areas ➡ that are morphologically similar to or indistinguishable from SEF. Tumors featuring predominantly SEF morphology are probably better classified and followed as SEF, given its propensity for more aggressive behavior.* **(Right)** *Foci resembling SEF are characterized by small epithelioid tumor cells forming cords and nests within a prominent hyalinized or sclerotic matrix.*

Sclerosing Epithelioid Fibrosarcoma-Like Areas

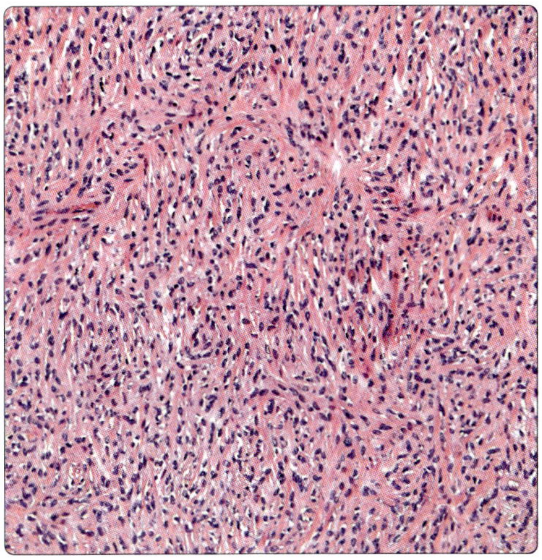

Sclerosing Epithelioid Fibrosarcoma-Like Areas

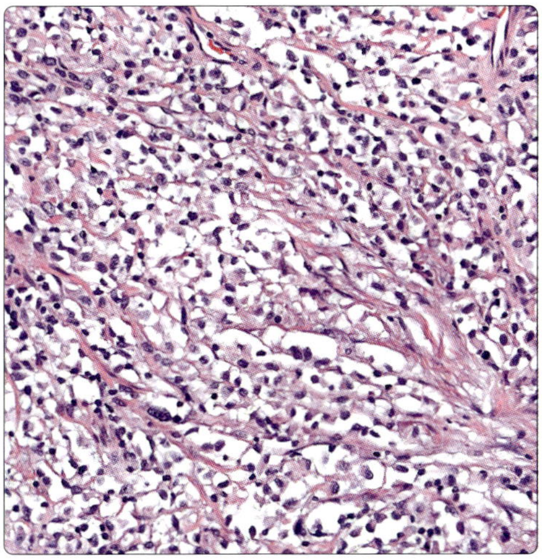

(Left) *A corded growth pattern is a common finding in SEF and may also be seen in SEF-like areas of LGFMS, as depicted.* **(Right)** *Clear cytoplasm is a common finding in tumor cells in SEF and SEF-like areas of LGFMS, as depicted. These areas may be completely indistinguishable from true "pure" SEF in a limited biopsy. Molecular analysis may assist in favoring diagnosis over the other.*

Sclerosing Epithelioid Fibrosarcoma

KEY FACTS

TERMINOLOGY

- Aggressive but deceptively bland sarcoma characterized by epithelioid tumor cells with prominent sclerotic matrix
  - Subset appears to be genetically related to low-grade fibromyxoid sarcoma (LGFMS)

CLINICAL ISSUES

- Most common in middle-aged to older adults
- Most common in limbs, limb girdles, trunk, neck
- Rarely in abdomen/pelvis, retroperitoneum, viscera, bone
- Solitary, deeply seated (intramuscular) mass
- Treatment: Wide surgical excision with negative margins
- Generally aggressive tumor with overall poor prognosis
  - Local recurrence in > 50% and metastasis in up to 80%

MICROSCOPIC

- Densely hyalinized, sclerotic matrix characteristic
- Nests, cords, and chains of small to medium-sized epithelioid cells
  - Clear to eosinophilic cytoplasm
  - Bland, ovoid, sometimes angulated, nuclei
- Mitotic rate low and necrosis uncommon
- Minor areas of conventional fibrosarcoma or LGFMS may be present

ANCILLARY TESTS

- MUC4(+) in majority
- SATB2, keratin, S100 protein, SMA, desmin (-)
- Molecular: Most cases show *EWSR1-CREB3L1* fusion

TOP DIFFERENTIAL DIAGNOSES

- Metastatic carcinoma
- LGFMS
- Sclerosing rhabdomyosarcoma
- Extraskeletal osteosarcoma

Sclerosing Epithelioid Fibrosarcoma

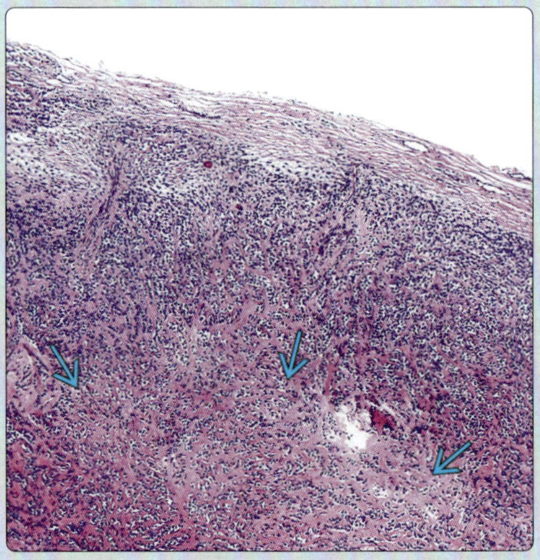

Prominent Hyalinized Matrix

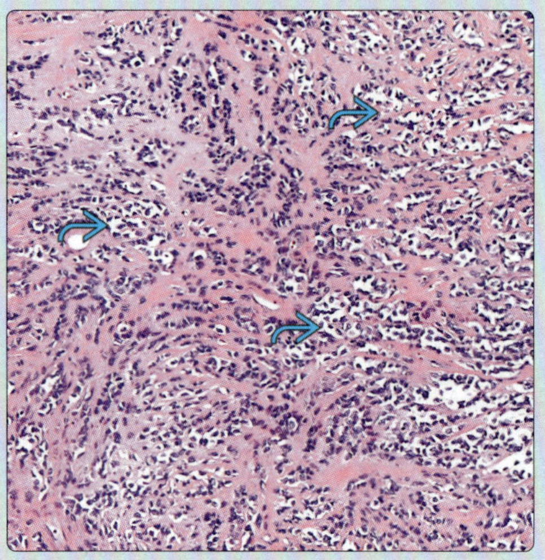

(Left) *Sclerosing epithelioid fibrosarcoma (SEF) is a clinically aggressive sarcoma that most commonly arises in the deep soft tissue of the extremities. The characteristic eosinophilic collagenous matrix is often evident at low power.* **(Right)** *A densely hyalinized or sclerotic matrix is a characteristic feature of SEF and may be strikingly abundant in areas. Lesional cells are small to medium sized and contain pale eosinophilic cytoplasm; however, a clear cell appearance is an extremely common finding in this tumor.*

Cytologic Features

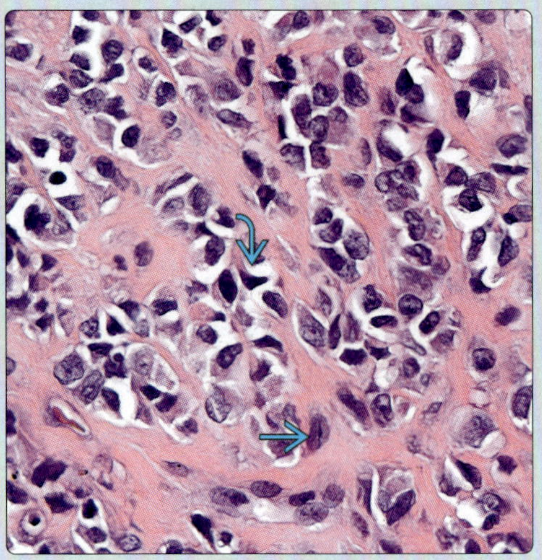

MUC4 Expression

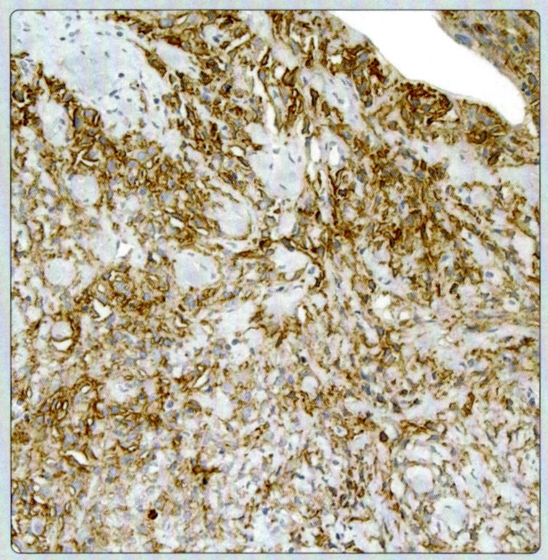

(Left) *The cells of SEF usually contain relatively bland, uniform, oval or angulated nuclei. Subtle nuclear grooves or folds may also be seen.* **(Right)** *MUC4 expression is seen in the majority of cases of SEF; however, it is also expressed in almost all cases of low-grade fibromyxoid sarcoma, which can show histologic and genetic overlap with SEF. MUC4 has also been reported in a minor subset of ossifying fibromyxoid tumor.*

TERMINOLOGY

Abbreviations

- Sclerosing epithelioid fibrosarcoma (SEF)

Definitions

- Aggressive but deceptively bland sarcoma characterized by epithelioid tumor cells with prominent sclerotic matrix
  - Subset appears to be genetically related to low-grade fibromyxoid sarcoma (LGFMS)

CLINICAL ISSUES

Epidemiology

- Age
  - Most common in middle-aged to older adults
    - Wide range reported
- Sex
  - M = F

Site

- Limbs and limb girdles most common
  - Lower > upper extremity
- Also trunk, neck
- May rarely arise in abdomen/pelvis, retroperitoneum, viscera, bone

Presentation

- Solitary, deeply seated (intramuscular) mass
  - May erode underlying bone
- Often painless but may be painful
- Metastatic disease may exist at time of presentation

Treatment

- Wide surgical excision with negative margins
  - Can require amputation especially when bone involved
- Chemotherapy or radiation therapy may be attempted to control recurrence and metastasis

Prognosis

- Generally aggressive tumor with overall poor prognosis
  - Local recurrence in > 50%
  - Metastasis in up to 80%
    - Most common to lung, pleura, bone, CNS
    - Metastases may occur many years after primary surgery
  - 5-year survival is 43-75%

MACROSCOPIC

General Features

- Circumscribed, nodular mass
- Often involves underlying periosteum
- Firm, gray-white cut surface
  - Can show calcification or ossification

Size

- Usually 5-10 cm in maximal dimension
  - Occasional tumors > 20 cm

MICROSCOPIC

Histologic Features

- Well-demarcated tumor but often microscopically infiltrative at periphery
- Prominent densely hyalinized, sclerotic matrix characteristic
  - Some areas may be largely paucicellular
  - Thin strands of collagen can resemble osteoid
  - Occasional myxoid foci
  - Calcification or metaplastic bone/cartilage may be seen
  - Rare cases are cellular without abundant hyalinization/sclerosis
- Nests, cords, and chains of small to medium-sized epithelioid cells
  - Clear to eosinophilic cytoplasm
  - Bland, ovoid, sometimes angulated, nuclei
    - Rare foci with prominent nuclear pleomorphism
  - Nests can appear to lose cohesion, imparting pseudoalveolar/pseudoacinar appearance
  - Generally low mitotic index
- Necrosis uncommon
- Focal staghorn vasculature pattern in some cases
- Other patterns of fibrosarcoma can coexist
  - Spindle cell fascicular areas, resembling conventional fibrosarcoma
  - Small areas resembling LGFMS (± collagenous rosettes)

ANCILLARY TESTS

Immunohistochemistry

- MUC4(+) in majority
- Focal EMA(+) in some cases
- SATB2, keratin, S100, SMA, desmin, CD34 (-)

Molecular Genetics

- *EWSR1-CREB3L1* fusion in most cases of pure SEF
  - *CREB3L2* and *CREB3L3* also reported
- Rare cases with *FUS-CREB3L2* fusion
  - In contrast to cases of pure LGFMS and "hybrid LGFMS/SEF" in which *FUS-CREB3L2* fusion clearly predominates

DIFFERENTIAL DIAGNOSIS

Metastatic Carcinoma

- Clinical evidence of primary tumor
- Cord-like growth in some breast carcinomas
- Densely sclerotic matrix generally uncommon
- Strong keratin (+), EMA(+)

Low-Grade Fibromyxoid Sarcoma

- Classic admixture of hypocellular fibrous zones and cellular myxoid zones
- May contain areas resembling SEF either in primary tumor (so-called hybrid LGFMS/SEF) or in recurrences
- LGFMS and "hybrid LGFMS/SEF" contain substantial component of tumor with LGFMS-type morphology
- Majority of cases characterized by t(7;16)(q33;p11) resulting in *FUS-CREB3L2* fusion
  - Includes pure LGFMS, "hybrid LGFMS/SEF," and LGFMS that recurs with areas resembling SEF

Sclerosing Lymphoma

- Relatively uniform cytology
- Expression of hematolymphoid immunohistochemical markers

Sclerosing Rhabdomyosarcoma

- May contain spindled fascicular component (spindle cell RMS)
- Occasional rhabdomyoblasts
- Dense hyaline or chondroid stroma with pseudovascular cellular growth pattern
- Variable desmin (+) and myogenin (+)
  - Desmin may show dot-like cytoplasmic expression
- Strong diffuse, nuclear MYOD1(+)
- MUC4(-)
- Lacks genetic features of SEF

Extraskeletal Osteosarcoma

- Sheets of variably pleomorphic spindled and polygonal tumor cells, often with significant nuclear atypia
- Mitoses common and often abnormal
- Variable degree of bone formation, often centralized
- MUC4(-)
- SATB2(+)

Ossifying Fibromyxoid Tumor

- Most arise in subcutaneous tissue
- Cytologically bland cells arranged in cords and trabeculae
  - Clear cytoplasm not generally feature of ossifying fibromyxoid tumor
- Stroma is often fibromyxoid but can show hyalinization
- S100 protein (+), variable desmin (+)
- Recurrent *PHF1* rearrangements

Alveolar Rhabdomyosarcoma

- Most common in adolescents and young adults
- Nests and sheets of cells in dense fibrous stroma
- Rhabdomyoblasts with eosinophilic cytoplasm
- Characteristic wreath-like multinucleated giant cells in some cases
- Strong diffuse desmin (+) and myogenin (+)
- *FOXO1* rearrangements

SELECTED REFERENCES

1. Chew W et al: Clinical characteristics and efficacy of chemotherapy in sclerosing epithelioid fibrosarcoma. Med Oncol. 35(11):138, 2018
2. Mok Y et al: Primary renal hybrid low-grade fibromyxoid sarcoma-sclerosing epithelioid fibrosarcoma: an unusual pediatric case with EWSR1-CREB3L1 fusion. Pediatr Dev Pathol. 1093526617754030, 2018
3. Arbajian E et al: In-depth genetic analysis of sclerosing epithelioid fibrosarcoma reveals recurrent genomic alterations and potential treatment targets. Clin Cancer Res. 23(23):7426-34, 2017
4. Dewaele B et al: A novel EWS-CREB3L3 gene fusion in a mesenteric sclerosing epithelioid fibrosarcoma. Genes Chromosomes Cancer. 56(9):695-9, 2017
5. Laliberte C et al: Sclerosing epithelioid fibrosarcoma of the jaw: late recurrence from a low grade fibromyxoid sarcoma. Head Neck Pathol. ePub, 2017
6. Argani P et al: Primary renal sclerosing epithelioid fibrosarcoma: report of 2 cases with EWSR1-CREB3L1 gene fusion. Am J Surg Pathol. 39(3):365-73, 2015
7. Prieto-Granada C et al: A genetic dichotomy between pure sclerosing epithelioid fibrosarcoma (SEF) and hybrid SEF/low-grade fibromyxoid sarcoma: a pathologic and molecular study of 18 cases. Genes Chromosomes Cancer. 54(1):28-38, 2015
8. Righi A et al: Sclerosing epithelioid fibrosarcoma of the thigh: report of two cases with synchronous bone metastases. Virchows Arch. 467(3):339-44, 2015
9. Arbajian E et al: Recurrent EWSR1-CREB3L1 gene fusions in sclerosing epithelioid fibrosarcoma. Am J Surg Pathol. 38(6):801-8, 2014
10. Folpe AL: Fibrosarcoma: a review and update. Histopathology. 64(1):12-25, 2014
11. Folpe AL: Selected topics in the pathology of epithelioid soft tissue tumors. Mod Pathol. 27 Suppl 1:S64-79, 2014
12. Stockman DL et al: Sclerosing epithelioid fibrosarcoma presenting as intraabdominal sarcomatosis with a novel EWSR1-CREB3L1 gene fusion. Hum Pathol. 45(10):2173-8, 2014
13. Wojcik JB et al: Primary sclerosing epithelioid fibrosarcoma of bone: analysis of a series. Am J Surg Pathol. 38(11):1538-44, 2014
14. Doyle LA et al: MUC4 is a sensitive and extremely useful marker for sclerosing epithelioid fibrosarcoma: association with FUS gene rearrangement. Am J Surg Pathol. 36(10):1444-51, 2012
15. Wang WL et al: FUS rearrangements are rare in 'pure' sclerosing epithelioid fibrosarcoma. Mod Pathol. 25(6):846-53, 2012
16. Rekhi B et al: Sclerosing epithelioid fibrosarcoma - a report of two cases with cytogenetic analysis of FUS gene rearrangement by FISH technique. Pathol Oncol Res. 17(1):145-8, 2011
17. Ossendorf C et al: Sclerosing epithelioid fibrosarcoma: case presentation and a systematic review. Clin Orthop Relat Res. 466(6):1485-91, 2008
18. Frattini JC et al: Sclerosing epithelioid fibrosarcoma of the cecum: a radiation-associated tumor in a previously unreported site. Arch Pathol Lab Med. 131(12):1825-8, 2007
19. Guillou L et al: Translocation-positive low-grade fibromyxoid sarcoma: clinicopathologic and molecular analysis of a series expanding the morphologic spectrum and suggesting potential relationship to sclerosing epithelioid fibrosarcoma: a study from the French Sarcoma Group. Am J Surg Pathol. 31(9):1387-402, 2007
20. Massier A et al: Sclerosing epithelioid fibrosarcoma of the pituitary. Endocr Pathol. 18(4):233-8, 2007
21. Battiata AP et al: Sclerosing epithelioid fibrosarcoma: a case report. Ann Otol Rhinol Laryngol. 114(2):87-9, 2005
22. Bhattacharya B et al: Nuclear beta-catenin expression distinguishes deep fibromatosis from other benign and malignant fibroblastic and myofibroblastic lesions. Am J Surg Pathol. 29(5):653-9, 2005
23. Chow LT et al: Primary sclerosing epithelioid fibrosarcoma of the sacrum: a case report and review of the literature. J Clin Pathol. 57(1):90-4, 2004
24. Hu WW et al: [Sclerosing epithelioid fibrosarcoma: a clinicopathologic study of eight cases] Zhonghua Bing Li Xue Za Zhi. 33(4):337-41, 2004
25. Ogose A et al: Sclerosing epithelioid fibrosarcoma with der(10)t(10;17)(p11;q11). Cancer Genet Cytogenet. 152(2):136-40, 2004
26. Watanabe K et al: Epithelioid fibrosarcoma of the ovary. Virchows Arch. 445(4):410-3, 2004
27. Genevay M et al: [Recent entities in soft tissue tumor pathology. Part 2] Ann Pathol. 23(2):135-48, 2003
28. Hindermann W et al: [Sclerosing epithelioid fibrosarcoma] Pathologe. 24(2):103-8, 2003
29. Abdulkader I et al: Sclerosing epithelioid fibrosarcoma primary of the bone. Int J Surg Pathol. 10(3):227-30, 2002
30. Jiao YF et al: Overexpression of MDM2 in a sclerosing epithelioid fibrosarcoma: genetic, immunohistochemical and ultrastructural study of a case. Pathol Int. 52(2):135-40, 2002
31. Antonescu CR et al: Sclerosing epithelioid fibrosarcoma: a study of 16 cases and confirmation of a clinicopathologically distinct tumor. Am J Surg Pathol. 25(6):699-709, 2001
32. Arya M et al: A rare tumour in the pelvis presenting with lower urinary symptoms: 'sclerosing epithelioid fibrosarcoma'. Eur J Surg Oncol. 27(1):121-2, 2001
33. Hanson IM et al: Evidence of nerve sheath differentiation and high grade morphology in sclerosing epithelioid fibrosarcoma. J Clin Pathol. 54(9):721-3, 2001
34. Bilsky MH et al: Sclerosing epithelioid fibrosarcomas involving the neuraxis: report of three cases. Neurosurgery. 47(4):956-9; discussion 959-60, 2000
35. Donner LR et al: Sclerosing epithelioid fibrosarcoma: a cytogenetic, immunohistochemical, and ultrastructural study of an unusual histological variant. Cancer Genet Cytogenet. 119(2):127-31, 2000
36. Eyden BP et al: Sclerosing epithelioid fibrosarcoma: a study of five cases emphasizing diagnostic criteria. Histopathology. 33(4):354-60, 1998
37. Gisselsson D et al: Amplification of 12q13 and 12q15 sequences in a sclerosing epithelioid fibrosarcoma. Cancer Genet Cytogenet. 107(2):102-6, 1998
38. Reid R et al: Sclerosing epithelioid fibrosarcoma. Histopathology. 28(5):451-5, 1996
39. Meis-Kindblom JM et al: Sclerosing epithelioid fibrosarcoma. A variant of fibrosarcoma simulating carcinoma. Am J Surg Pathol. 19(9):979-93, 1995

Circumscribed but Infiltrative

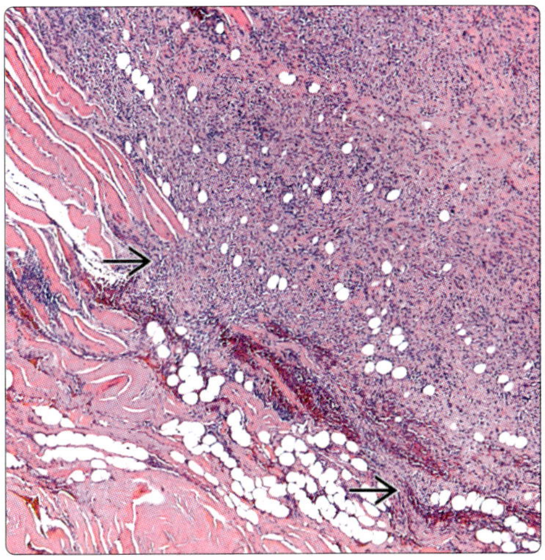

Corded Growth Pattern

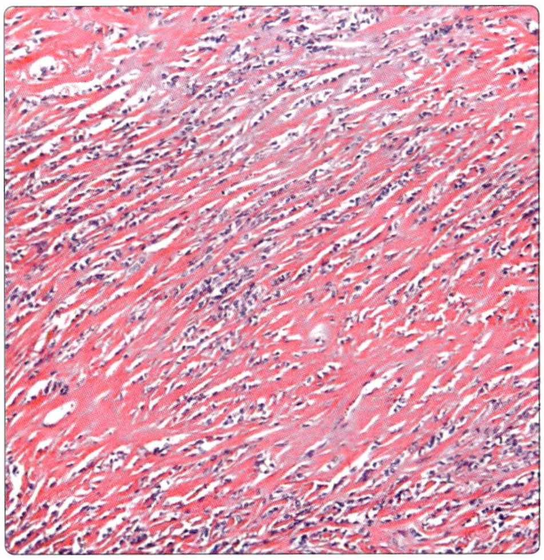

(Left) *The peripheral border of SEF is often well delineated, but microscopic evidence of infiltrative growth ⇒ can often be identified. Peritumoral foci of vascular invasion can also be seen (not shown).* **(Right)** *A linear corded growth pattern is a common feature of SEF, as depicted. Out of context, this architecture could easily be misconstrued as infiltrating carcinoma, particularly lobular carcinoma of the breast.*

Nests and Aggregates

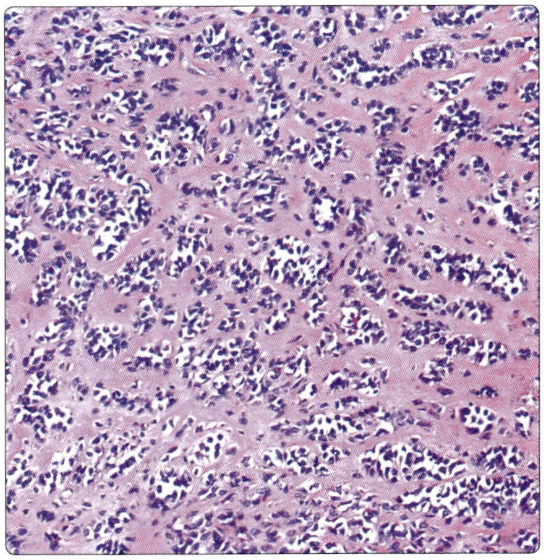

Pseudoalveolar Appearance

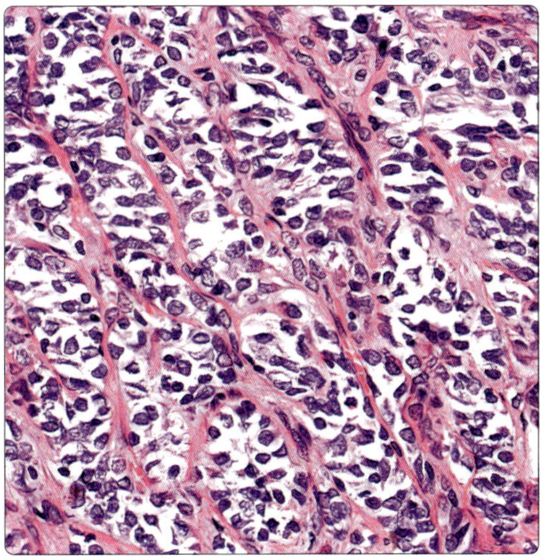

(Left) *Nests, clusters, and aggregates of tumor cells are a common finding in SEF. Note that although clear cells are frequently seen in most cases, in some areas they may not be well visualized.* **(Right)** *Nests of tumor cells in SEF can appear dyscohesive and may resemble alveolar or acinar structures, as shown in this H&E. Note also the prominent angulated nuclei.*

Polygonal Cells

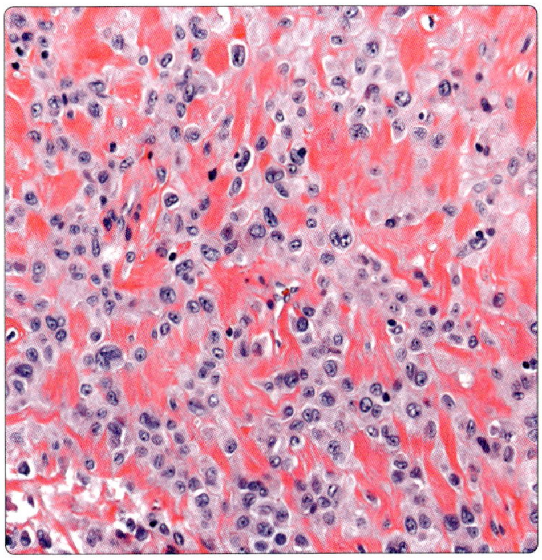

Deceptively Bland Appearance

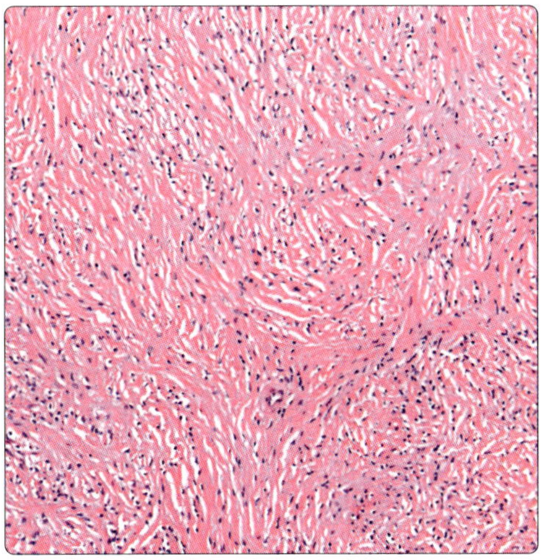

(Left) *In some cases of SEF, the tumor cells are more polygonal and may more closely resemble carcinoma, particularly with nested growth. Note the dense collagenous matrix.* **(Right)** *It is not uncommon for some areas of SEF to appear extremely bland, as depicted, which may easily lead to misdiagnosis as a benign neoplasm, particularly on limited biopsy.*

(Left) *The prominence of the fibrocollagenous matrix in SEF often varies from tumor to tumor and sometimes from field to field. Some cases may contain paucicellular areas with abundant matrix and striking cracking artifact, as shown here.* **(Right)** *Small areas demonstrating a spindled, fascicular appearance resembling low-grade fibrosarcoma are noted in some cases of SEF.*

Prominent Stromal Collagen

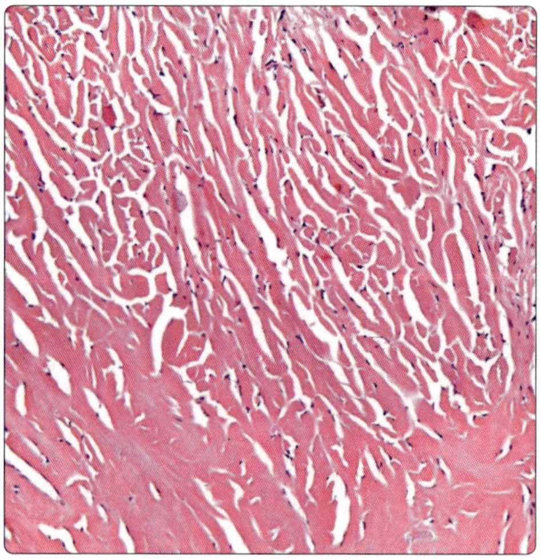

Spindled, Fibrosarcoma-Like Areas

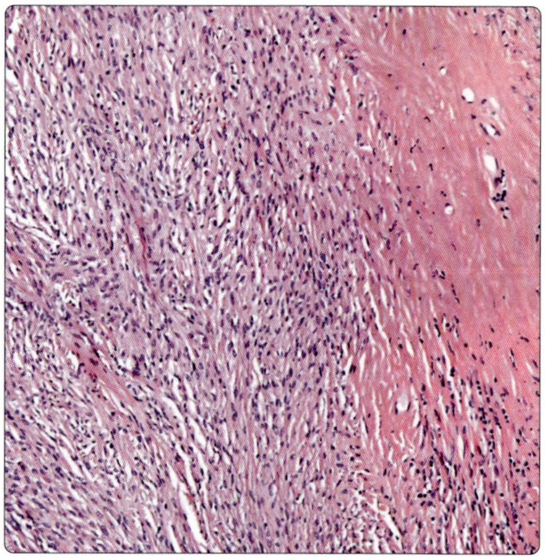

(Left) *This H&E shows an area of increased cellularity in SEF. Note that the collagenous matrix and clear cells are less prominent in this area.* **(Right)** *This H&E shows an area of SEF with markedly compressed cords and nests, resembling sheet-like growth; however, the intervening collagenous matrix ↷ can still be identified. Note also the relatively uniform, oval to angular nuclei.*

Cellular Areas

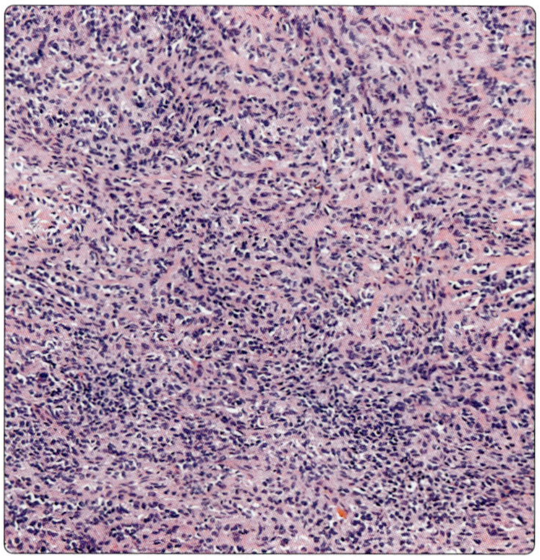

Cellular Areas

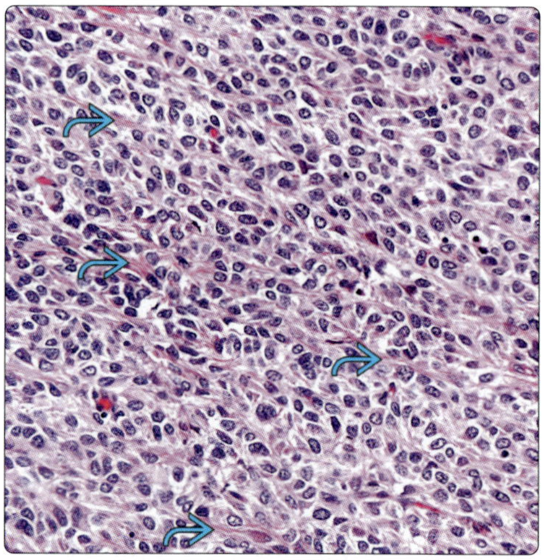

(Left) *Small tumor cells → with eccentric nuclei and eosinophilic cytoplasm may sometimes mimic plasma cells or even osteoblasts in SEF.* **(Right)** *Foci of increased nuclear pleomorphism and atypia may be seen in SEF but are generally uncommon. Necrosis is also uncommon in SEF but can be seen in larger tumors.*

Cytologic Pitfalls

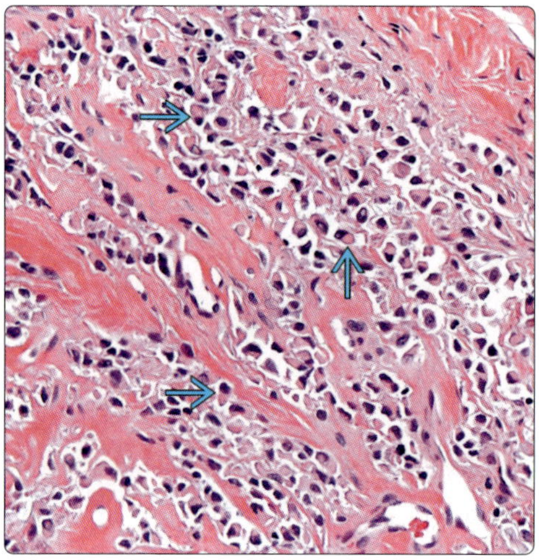

Focal Increased Pleomorphism

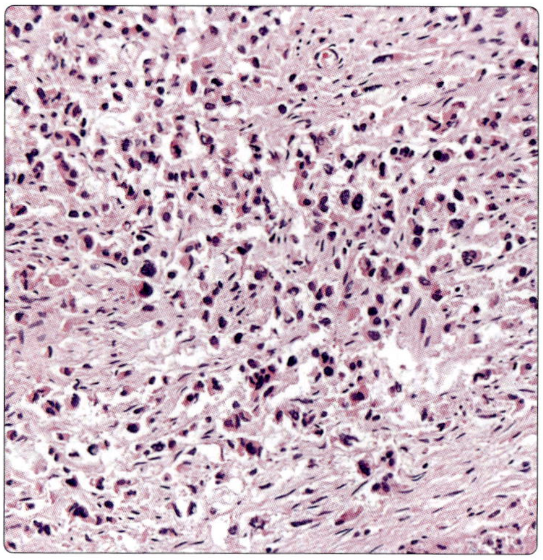

Metaplastic Bone or Cartilage

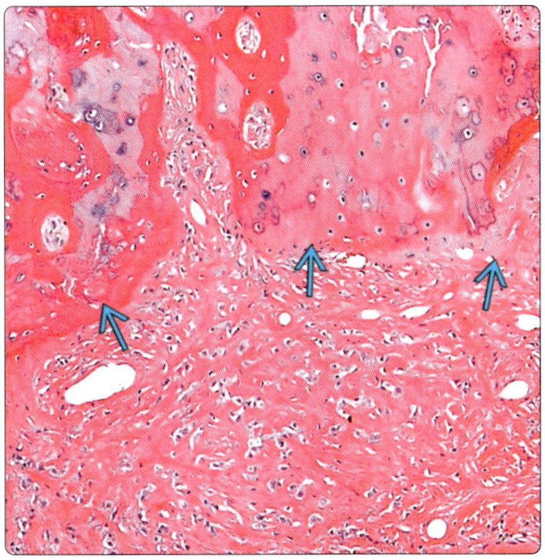

Focal Ectatic Staghorn Vasculature

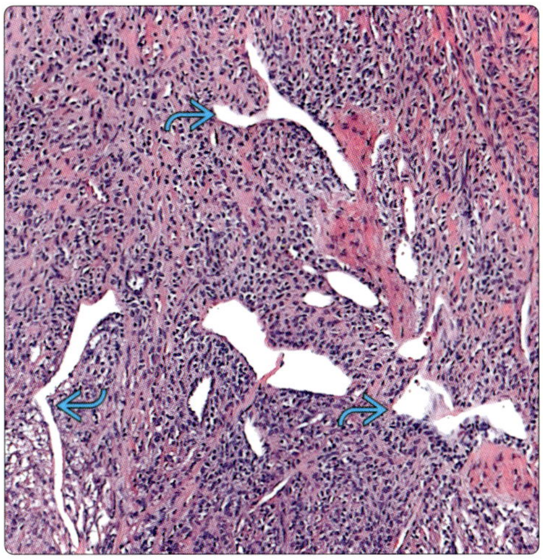

(Left) *Foci of metaplastic bone &/or cartilage can be seen in SEF. Bone formation may be extensive in some tumors and raise considerations of an extraskeletal osteosarcoma.* **(Right)** *Dilated staghorn-shaped blood vessels may be a focal finding in SEF, as depicted. This finding is very nonspecific and is seen in a wide variety of both benign and malignant soft tissue neoplasms.*

Focal Myxoid Change

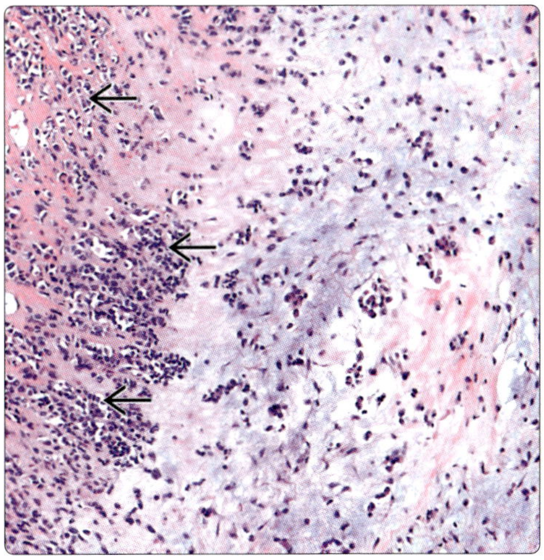

Myxoid Change

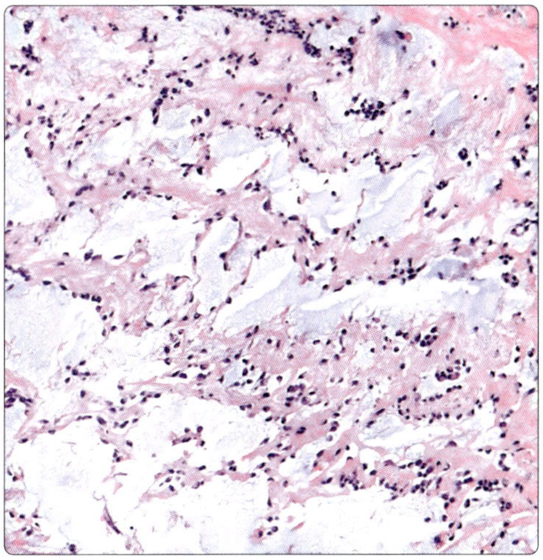

(Left) *Focal myxoid stromal change may be seen in SEF but is uncommon. Note the area of more conventional morphology featuring clear cells and a prominent hyalinized matrix.* **(Right)** *This case of a large SEF of the thigh predominantly features the characteristic sclerosing matrix but also shows several small myxoid foci, as depicted. Note the small epithelioid tumor cells that appear to line the cystic or cleft-like myxoid spaces.*

Low-Grade Fibromyxoid Sarcoma

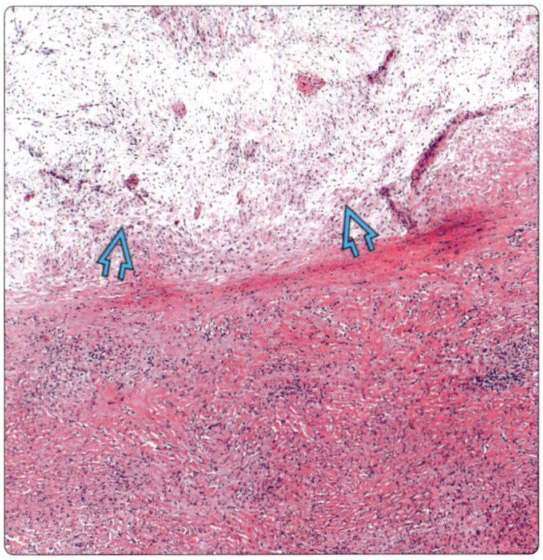

Lung Metastases

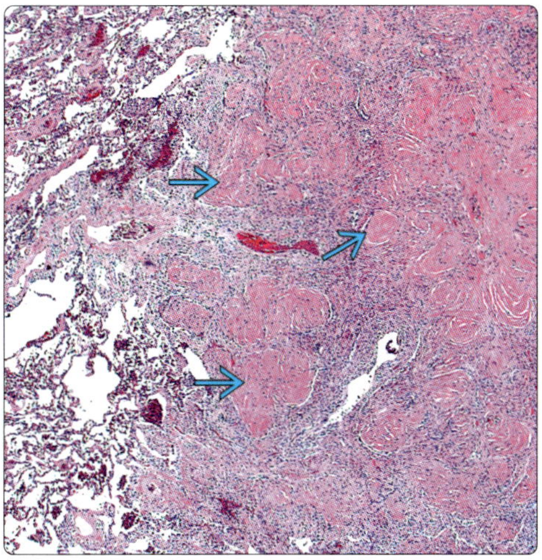

(Left) *Some cases of SEF contain minor areas with morphologic features of LGFMS. In light of current published reports, molecular analysis in these cases is more likely to show FUS/CREB3L2 than EWSR1/CREB3L1 rearrangements.* **(Right)** *Pulmonary metastases of SEF often feature nodular hyalinized deposits of hypocellular or acellular tumor filling alveolar spaces within the lesion. Note the normal lung tissue at the bottom left of the H&E.*

SECTION 5

Pediatric Fibroblastic/Myofibroblastic Tumors

Benign

Fibrous Hamartoma of Infancy 240
Calcifying Aponeurotic Fibroma 244
Calcifying Fibrous Tumor 248
Inclusion Body Fibromatosis 250
Hyaline Fibromatosis Syndrome 252
Fibromatosis Colli 254
Gardner Fibroma 256

Intermediate (Locally Aggressive)

Lipofibromatosis 258
Giant Cell Fibroblastoma 260

Intermediate (Rarely Metastasizing)

Infantile Fibrosarcoma 264

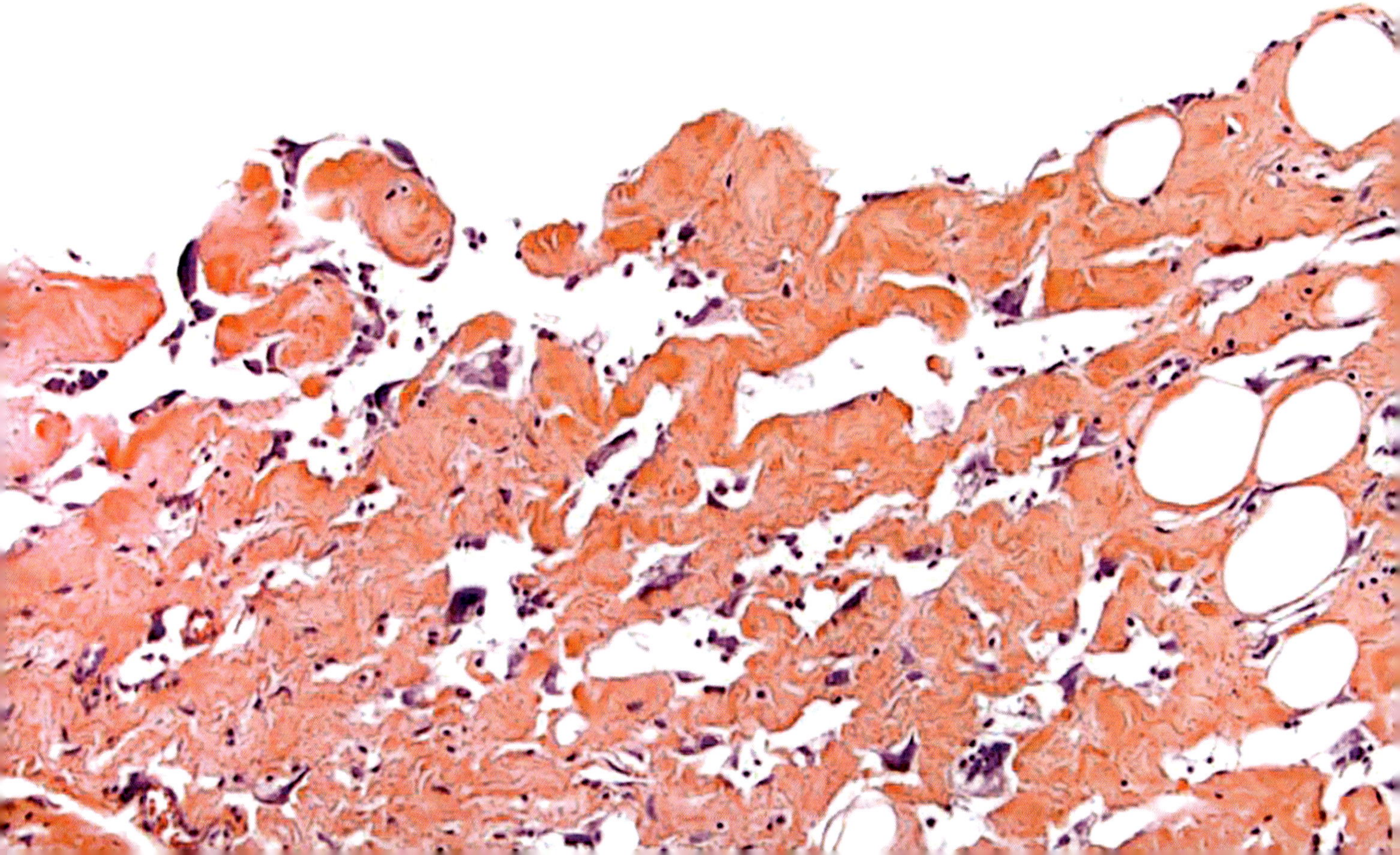

Fibrous Hamartoma of Infancy

KEY FACTS

TERMINOLOGY

- Benign superficial fibrous tumor with characteristic organoid pattern of 3 distinct components: Fibrous tissue, fat, primitive mesenchymal cells

CLINICAL ISSUES

- Infants and children up to 2 years
  - Up to 25% congenital
  - Male predilection
- Most common in deep dermis or subcutis of trunk, including axilla, upper back, and groin/perineum
- Slow-growing or rapidly enlarging, painless mass
- Treatment: Complete local excision
- Benign
- Up to 15% recur locally

MACROSCOPIC

- Soft, poorly defined mass
- Usually < 5 cm

MICROSCOPIC

- Classic organoid growth pattern
  - 3 distinct components in widely varying amounts
    - Fascicles and sheets of fibroblasts/myofibroblasts
    - Nests of immature mesenchymal cells in loose myxoid stroma
    - Mature adipose tissue
  - Also hypocellular areas with prominent stromal collagen

ANCILLARY TESTS

- SMA(+) in fibroblastic component
- CD34(+) in myxoid and collagenous/pseudovascular areas

TOP DIFFERENTIAL DIAGNOSES

- Lipofibromatosis
- Fibromatosis
- Giant cell fibroblastoma
- Lipofibromatosis-like neural tumor
- Lipoblastoma

Fibrous Hamartoma of Infancy

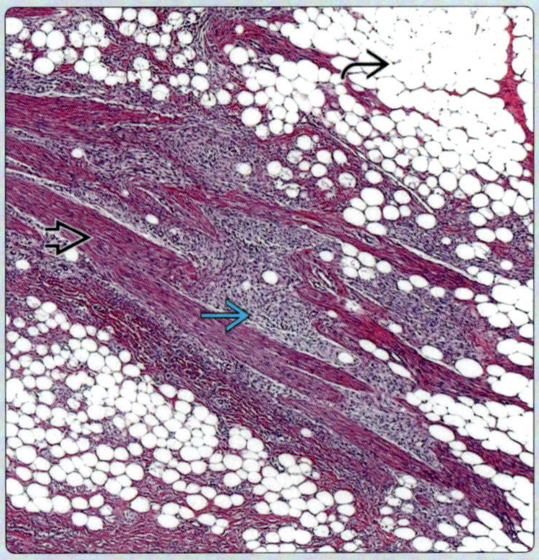

Fibroblastic Component

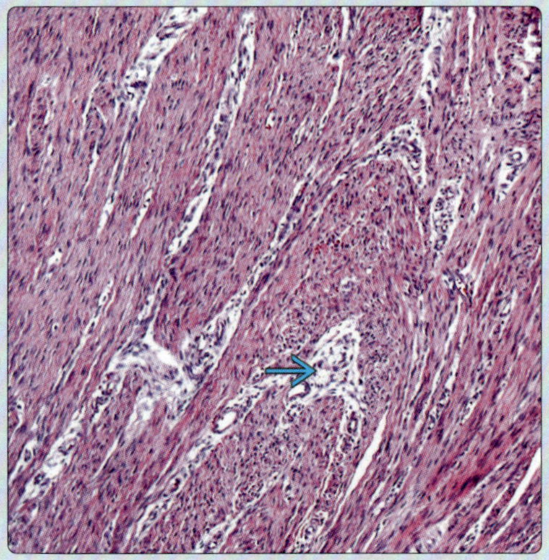

(Left) *Fibrous hamartoma of infancy (FHI) is a benign fibrous tumor that typically occurs in the 1st year of life and has a predilection for males. The usual case shows an irregular conglomeration of 3 main components: Immature mesenchymal zones →, fascicles of fibroblasts ⇨, and mature adipose tissue ↷.* **(Right)** *The fibroblastic portion of FHI is composed of irregular bands, fascicles, and sheets of bland spindled cells in a collagenous background. Note the small immature myxoid focus →.*

Immature Myxoid Mesenchymal Component

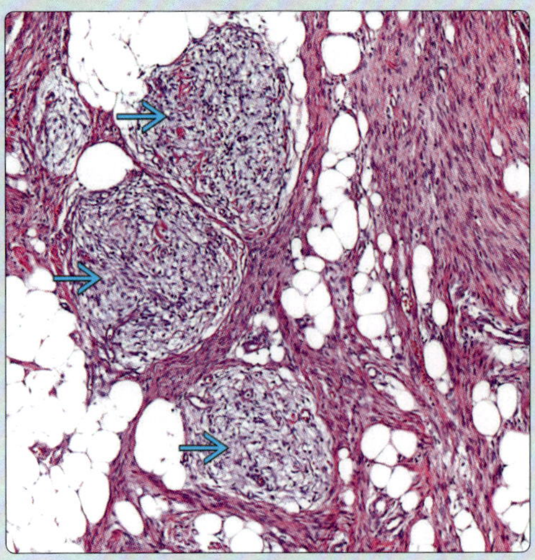

Collagenous Zones

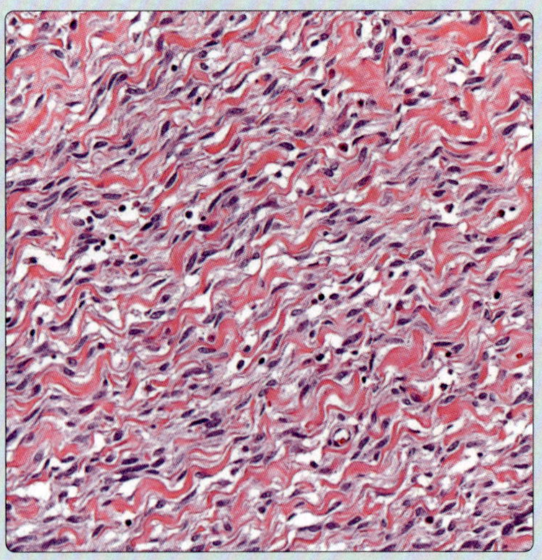

(Left) *The immature mesenchymal component of FHI is composed of bland spindled to ovoid cells within a basophilic myxoid matrix. These foci → are often small and scattered haphazardly, but rarely they may be large, confluent, or dominant.* **(Right)** *Approximately 1/2 of cases of FHI contain a highly collagenized zone with scattered blood vessels. These areas are often centrally located within the tumor and may somewhat resemble a neurofibroma.*

Fibrous Hamartoma of Infancy

TERMINOLOGY

Abbreviations

- Fibrous hamartoma of infancy (FHI)

Definitions

- Benign superficial fibrous tumor with characteristic organoid pattern of 3 distinct components: Fibrous tissue, fat, primitive mesenchymal cells

CLINICAL ISSUES

Epidemiology

- Age
  - Infants and children up to 2 years
    - Up to 25% congenital
  - Very rarely in older children
- Sex
  - Male predominance

Site

- Deep dermis or subcutis
- Most common in trunk, including axilla, upper back, and groin/perineum
  - Also extremities and many other reported sites
- Usually solitary

Presentation

- Slow-growing or rapidly enlarging painless mass
- May have overlying skin changes (e.g., altered pigmentation, hypertrichosis)
- No known syndromic or familial associations
  - Isolated reports of FHI occurring in setting of tuberous sclerosis or Williams syndrome

Treatment

- Complete local excision

Prognosis

- Benign
  - Has not been shown to spontaneously regress
- Up to 15% recur locally
  - Likely related to incomplete excision

MACROSCOPIC

General Features

- Soft, poorly defined mass
- Cut surface shows mixture of tan-white tissue and fat

Size

- Usually < 5 cm

MICROSCOPIC

Histologic Features

- Classic organoid growth pattern
  - 3 distinct components in widely variable proportions
    - Intersecting bands and sheets of mature fibroblasts/myofibroblasts
    - Nests of immature ovoid to spindled mesenchymal cells in loose basophilic, myxoid stroma
      - May contain subtle chronic inflammatory infiltrate
    - Mature adipose tissue
- Hypocellular areas with prominent stromal collagen also common
  - Can resemble vascular growth pattern (pseudoangiomatous) or neurofibroma
  - Often centrally located (may be maturation phenomenon)
- Mitotic figures rare to absent
- Exceptional cases reported with sarcomatous features
  - Undifferentiated spindled or round cell morphology
  - Hypercellularity with mitoses

ANCILLARY TESTS

Immunohistochemistry

- SMA(+) in fibroblastic component
  - Desmin rare
- CD34(+), CD31(-) in myxoid and collagenous/pseudovascular areas
- S100 protein (+) in mature adipose tissue only
- Absence of nuclear β-catenin expression

Molecular Genetics

- *EGFR* exon 20 insertion/duplication mutations
- No *PDGFB, PLAG1,* or *NTRK1* rearrangements

DIFFERENTIAL DIAGNOSIS

Lipofibromatosis

- Predilection for distal extremities
- Fascicles of fibroblasts infiltrating adipose tissue
- Absence of immature myxoid mesenchymal component and organoid growth pattern

Fibromatosis

- Adipose tissue not typically integral component
- Lacks organoid growth pattern and immature myxoid mesenchymal component
- Nuclear β-catenin (+) in majority

Giant Cell Fibroblastoma

- Irregular slit-like or ectatic pseudovascular spaces lined by multinucleated cells
- Lacks organoid growth pattern
- t(17;22) with *PDGFB-COL1A1* fusion

Lipofibromatosis-Like Neural Tumor

- Rare; recently described
- Affects older children and young adults
- Coexpression of CD34 and S100 protein
- *NTRK1* gene rearrangements

Lipoblastoma

- Prominent lobulated architecture
- Immature adipocytes (lipoblasts) in myxoid stroma
- Lacks organoid growth pattern

SELECTED REFERENCES

1. Al-Ibraheemi A et al: Fibrous hamartoma of infancy: a clinicopathologic study of 145 cases, including 2 with sarcomatous features. Mod Pathol. 30(4):474-85, 2017
2. Park JY et al: EGFR exon 20 insertion/duplication mutations characterize fibrous hamartoma of infancy. Am J Surg Pathol. 40(12):1713-8, 2016
3. Saab ST et al: Fibrous hamartoma of infancy: a clinicopathologic analysis of 60 cases. Am J Surg Pathol. 38(3):394-401, 2014

(Left) *This image shows an area of FHI that is composed of irregular, ramifying bands and fascicles of fibroblasts, admixed with mature adipose tissue, resembling lipofibromatosis. Immature mesenchymal foci were identified elsewhere.* **(Right)** *Fat is a predominant component in some cases of FHI. The fibroblastic component appears as thin ramifying fascicles infiltrating fat resembling lipofibromatosis; however, small immature mesenchymal foci are present* ➡.

Fat-Fibrous Pattern

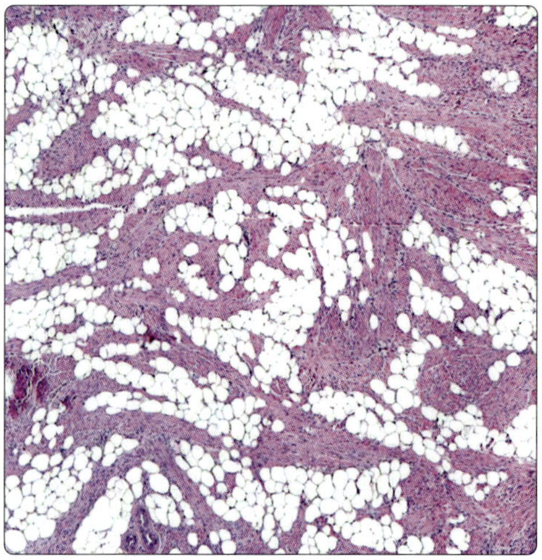

Fat-Predominant Pattern

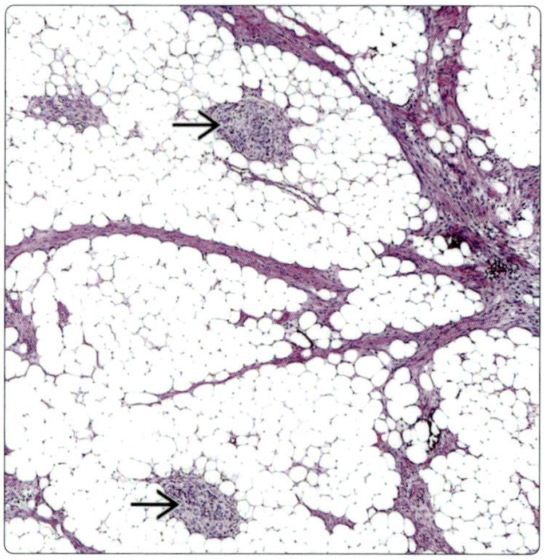

(Left) *In FHI with a fat-predominant morphology, identification of immature mesenchymal foci is diagnostic. In challenging cases, they may be small and widely scattered and thereby easily overlooked.* **(Right)** *The fibroblastic component of FHI is identified by sheets and fascicles of uniform spindled cells set in a collagenous background. Nuclear atypia is not present.*

Fat-Predominant Pattern

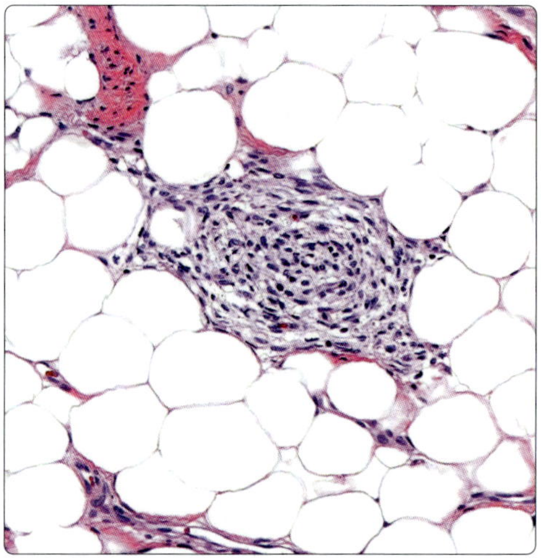

Fibroblastic Component

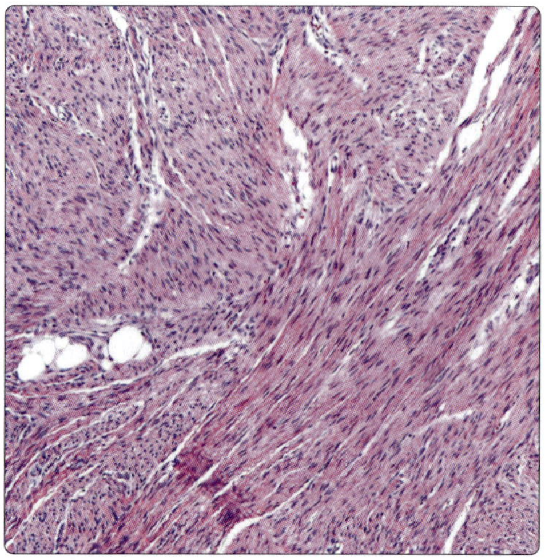

(Left) *The fibroblastic component may bear a striking resemblance to conventional fibromatosis, with long streaming fascicles of bland spindled cells in a collagenous background punctuated by blood vessels.* **(Right)** *The immature mesenchymal component of FHI is typically quite myxoid, but the cellularity varies. A subtle chronic inflammatory infiltrate may be seen in these foci. Note also the adipose* ➡ *and fibrous* ➡ *components.*

Fibroblastic Component

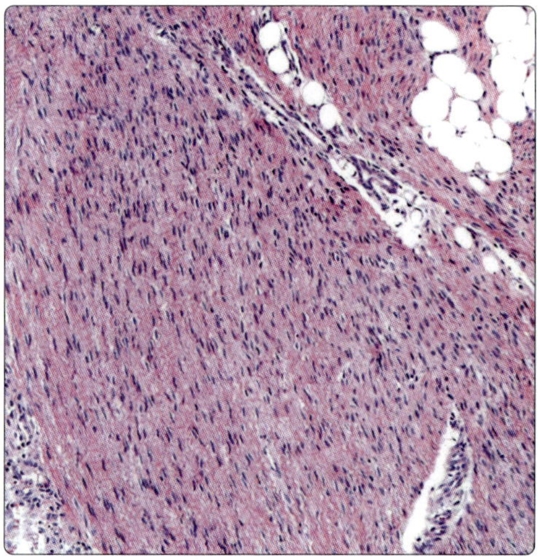

Immature Mesenchymal Component

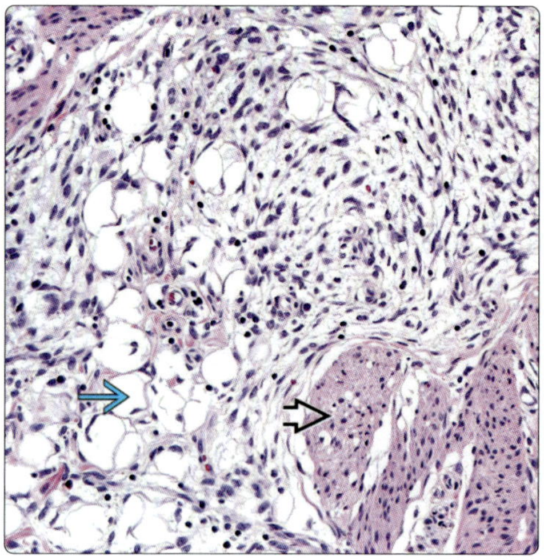

Immature Mesenchymal Component

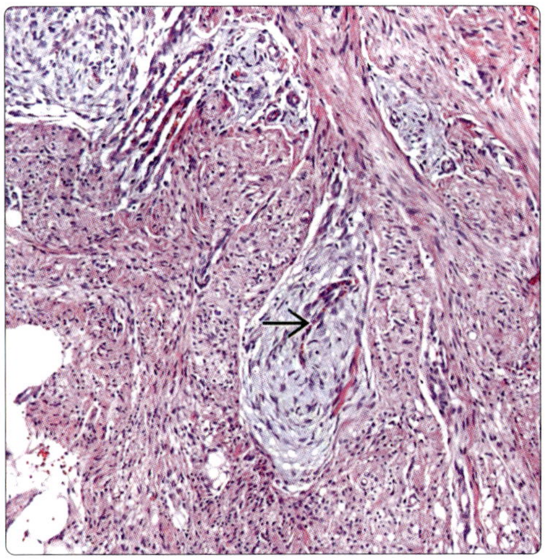

Immature Mesenchymal Component

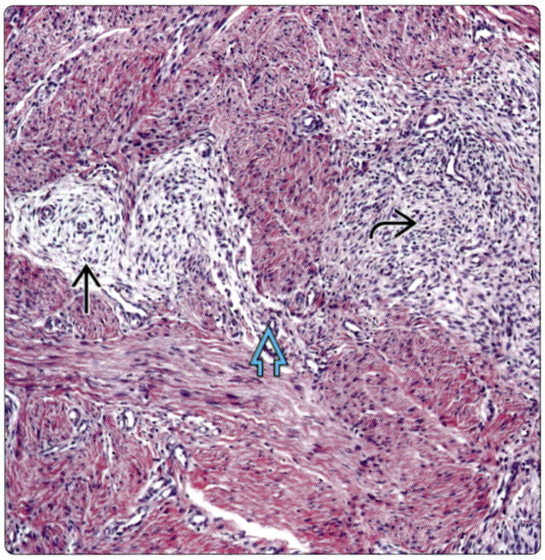

(Left) *This image shows immature myxoid foci within a prominent background of mature fibrous tissue. At times, these foci may appear to be organized around small veins or capillaries →.* **(Right)** *This image of FHI shows a typical immature mesenchymal focus → but with a progressive decrease in myxoid matrix ⇨ and apparent increase in cellularity ↪.*

Cellular Immature Mesenchymal Component

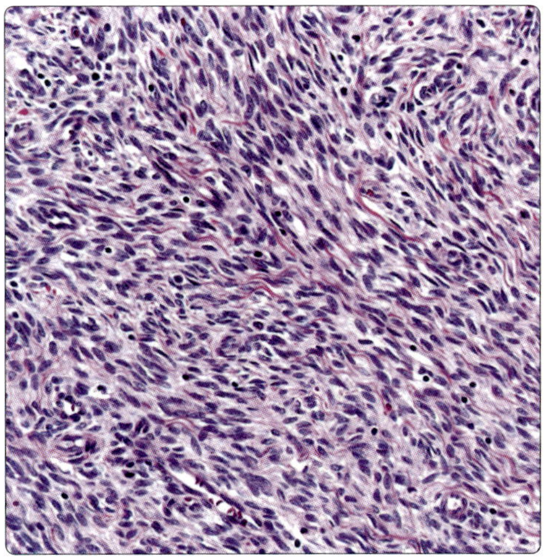

Collagenous Zones

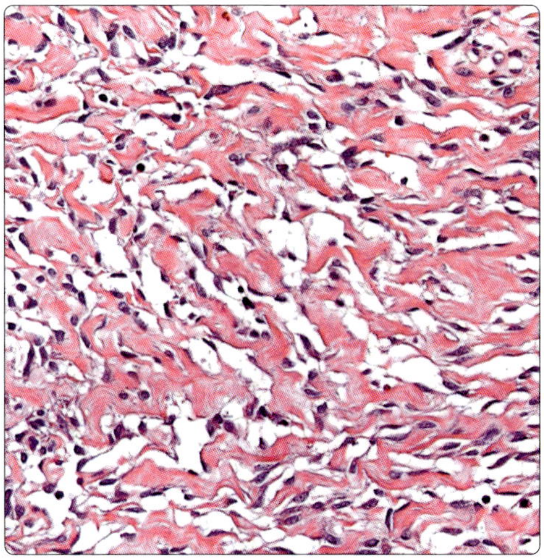

(Left) *Some immature foci may have comparatively little myxoid matrix and therefore appear more cellular than usual. Mitoses are absent.* **(Right)** *Vascular collagenized areas may be seen in a significant number of cases of FHI. Importantly, if a stromal separation artifact is present (shown), these zones may lead to misdiagnosis as a vascular lesion or giant cell fibroblastoma.*

Hyalinized Zones

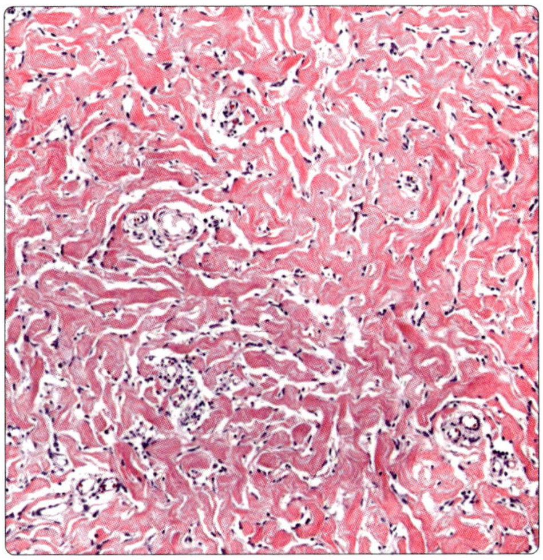

Collagenous/Hyalinized Zones

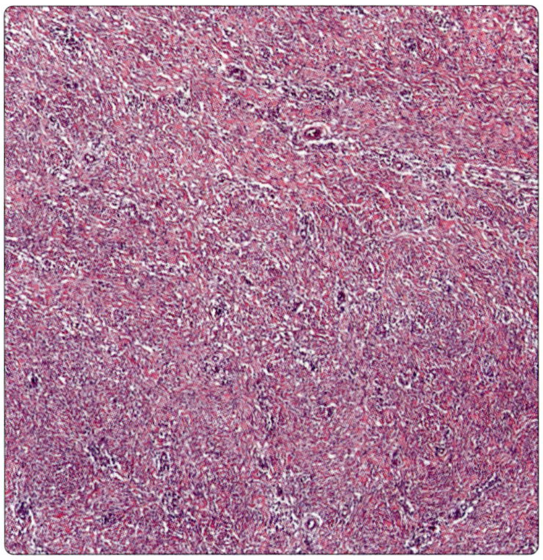

(Left) *In some cases of FHI, marked stromal hyalinization/sclerosis imparts a pseudovascular appearance similar to pseudoangiomatous stromal hyperplasia of the breast.* **(Right)** *Rare examples of FHI contain a large, centralized component of collagenous or hyalinized tissue. Foci of more conventional triphasic morphology are often seen at the periphery.*

Calcifying Aponeurotic Fibroma

KEY FACTS

TERMINOLOGY

- Distinctive, infiltrative fibroblastic lesion containing calcified &/or chondroid foci and typically arising in hands or feet of children

CLINICAL ISSUES

- Most common: 5-15 years
- 2:1 male predominance
- Fingers or palm of hand most common site
  - Also plantar foot, ankle, toes
- Painless, slow-growing mass
  - Arise in subcutaneous tissue or attached to aponeurosis/fascia
- Treatment: Complete but conservative excision for primary lesion and recurrences
  - ~ 40-50% recur locally

MACROSCOPIC

- Ill-defined, firm or rubbery, sometimes gritty cut surface
  - Older lesions tend to be more well circumscribed and calcified
- Usually < 3 cm in size

MICROSCOPIC

- Nodular growth with infiltration of surrounding tissue
- Spindled to ovoid fibroblasts without nuclear atypia in collagenous stroma
- Variable number of calcified or cartilaginous foci
  - Epithelioid cells may be arranged around these foci
  - Associated osteoclast-like giant cells may be present
- Mitoses uncommon
- Exact proportion of components generally varies with age

TOP DIFFERENTIAL DIAGNOSES

- Lipofibromatosis
- Monophasic synovial sarcoma
- Palmar and plantar fibromatosis
- Soft tissue chondroma

Calcifying Aponeurotic Fibroma

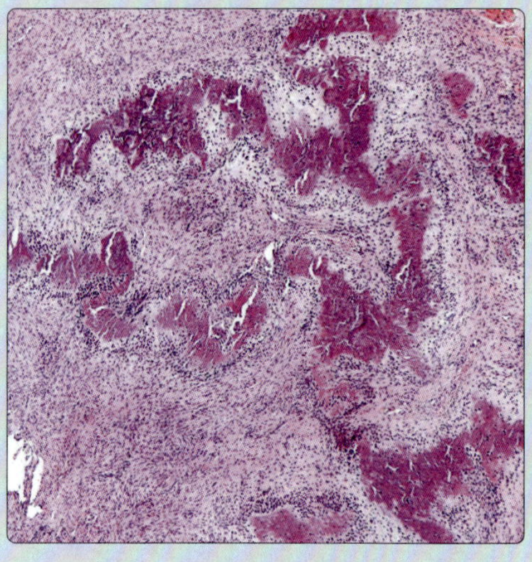

Calcified Foci

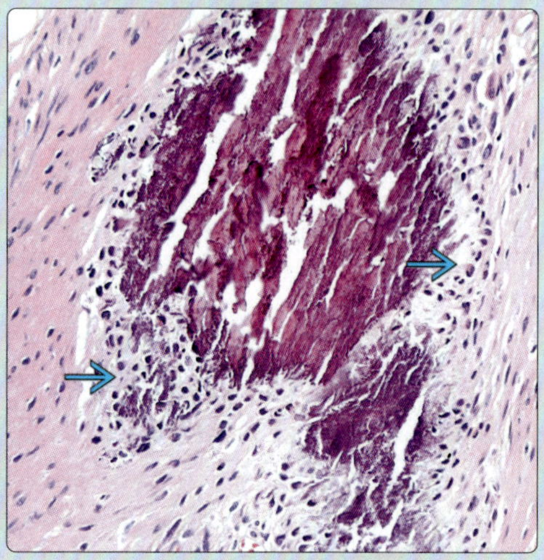

(Left) *Calcifying aponeurotic fibroma (CAF) is a rare fibroblastic lesion that most commonly occurs in the hands or feet of children. At low magnification, a classic example shows irregular calcified foci within a variably cellular proliferation of spindled fibroblasts.* **(Right)** *Calcifications in CAF are finely granular or coarse and chunky. The surrounding fibroblasts also typically adopt a more plump, epithelioid morphology* ➔ *and may radiate outward from the calcification.*

Osteoclast-Like Giant Cells

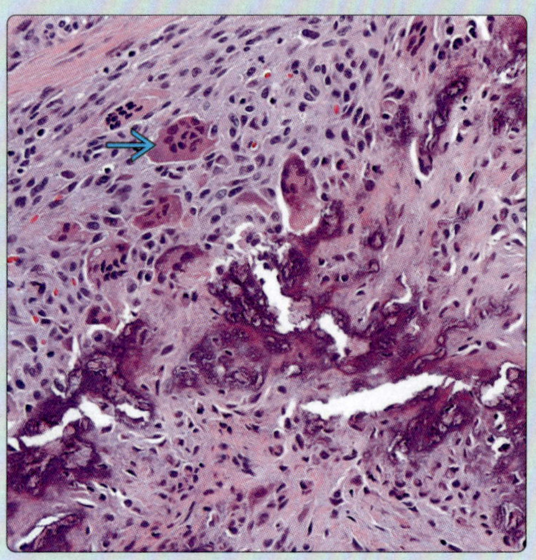

Spindle Cell Component

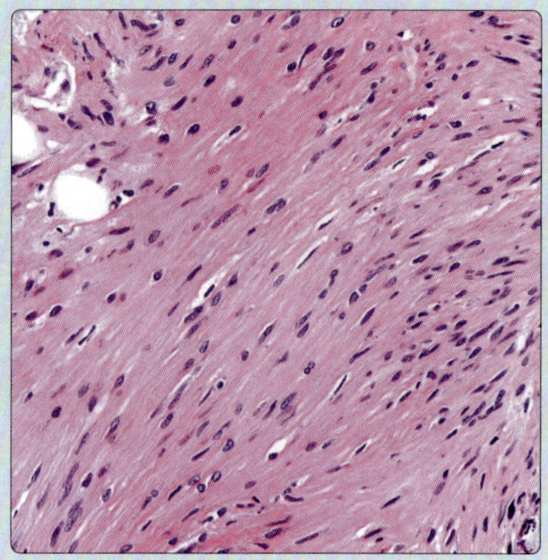

(Left) *Osteoclast-like giant cells* ➔ *are not uncommon in CAF and are most commonly identified in direct association with the calcified or cartilaginous foci.* **(Right)** *The fibromatosis-like spindled component of CAF varies in cellularity from area to area, but stromal collagen is generally prominent. Importantly, the fibroblastic cells are cytologically bland, and mitotic figures are generally scarce.*

TERMINOLOGY

Synonyms

- Juvenile aponeurotic fibroma
- Calcifying fibroma

Definitions

- Distinctive, infiltrative fibroblastic lesion containing calcified &/or chondroid foci and typically arising in hands or feet of children

CLINICAL ISSUES

Epidemiology

- Incidence
  - Rare
- Age
  - Most arise in children (most common: 5-15 years)
    - May occur in adults (often recurrence)
- Sex
  - 2:1 male predominance

Site

- Fingers or palm of hand most common
  - Subcutaneous tissue or attached to aponeurosis/fascia
- Also plantar foot, ankle, toes
- Very rarely other sites

Presentation

- Painless, slow-growing mass
- May be present for years

Treatment

- Complete, but conservative excision
  - Reexcision of recurrences

Prognosis

- Benign
  - Exceptionally rare case reports of malignant degeneration (controversial)
- ~ 40-50% recur locally

MACROSCOPIC

General Features

- Ill-defined, firm or rubbery, sometimes gritty cut surface
  - Older lesions tend to be more well circumscribed and calcified

Size

- Usually < 3 cm

MICROSCOPIC

Histologic Features

- Nodular growth with infiltration of surrounding tissue
- Spindled to ovoid fibroblasts without nuclear atypia in collagenous stroma
  - May be cellular with less stromal collagen
- Variable number of calcified and cartilaginous foci
  - Calcifications range from fine granules to large, chunky masses
  - Epithelioid chondrocyte-like cells may be arranged around these foci
  - Associated osteoclast-like giant cells may be present
  - Ossification rare
- Mitoses uncommon
- Overall appearance generally varies with age
  - Infants and young children often have predominant fibroblastic morphology with little to no calcification
  - Older lesions are generally more well circumscribed and contain more calcified/cartilaginous foci

DIFFERENTIAL DIAGNOSIS

Lipofibromatosis

- Usually involves proximal extremities or head and neck
- Fascicles of elongated fibroblasts, often diffusely infiltrative
- Calcification and osteoclast-like giant cells rare

Monophasic Synovial Sarcoma

- Large tumors, usually arising in deep soft tissue of extremities
- Often highly cellular
- Can be calcified, but calcified areas usually lack chondroid rim
- Focal expression of keratins or EMA in most cases
- *SS18 (SYT)* gene rearrangements

Palmar and Plantar Fibromatosis

- Uni- or multinodular, centered on fascia
- "Sweeping" cellular fascicles of fibroblasts with dense collagen
  - May show brisk mitotic activity
- Compressed or dilated stromal vessels common
- Usually lack calcification and cartilage formation

Soft Tissue Chondroma

- Sharply circumscribed nodular mass, most common in hand
- Usually affects older adults
- Chondroid differentiation is well developed
- Lack of prominent spindle cell fibromatosis-like component

SELECTED REFERENCES

1. Lee SM et al: Intraarticular calcifying aponeurotic fibroma of the wrist: mimicking gout or calcium pyrophosphate dihydrate deposition disease. Skeletal Radiol. 47(5):729-34, 2018
2. Corominas L et al: Calcifying aponeurotic fibroma in children: our experience and a literature review. J Pediatr Orthop B. 26(6):560-4, 2017
3. Shim SW et al: MRI features of calcifying aponeurotic fibroma in the upper arm: a case report and review of the literature. Skeletal Radiol. 45(8):1139-43, 2016
4. Kim OH et al: Calcifying aponeurotic fibroma: case report with radiographic and MR features. Korean J Radiol. 15(1):134-9, 2014
5. Giuffre JL et al: Recurrent calcifying aponeurotic fibroma of the thumb: case report. J Hand Surg Am. 36(1):110-5, 2011
6. Thakur JS et al: Calcifying (juvenile) aponeurotic fibroma of the scalp. Ear Nose Throat J. 90(10):E14-6, 2011
7. Kramer JM et al: Calcifying aponeurotic fibroma with bone islands exhibiting hematopoiesis: a case report and review of the literature. Oral Surg Oral Med Oral Pathol Oral Radiol Endod. 109(6):878-82, 2010
8. Fetsch JF et al: Calcifying aponeurotic fibroma: a clinicopathologic study of 22 cases arising in uncommon sites. Hum Pathol. 29(12):1504-10, 1998
9. Allen PW et al: Juvenile aponeurotic fibroma. Cancer. 26(4):857-67, 1970
10. Keasbey LE: Juvenile aponeurotic fibroma (calcifying fibroma); a distinctive tumor arising in the palms and soles of young children. Cancer. 6(2):338-46, 1953

(Left) *Most cases of CAF are histologically infiltrative into surrounding tissues, particularly those that occur in younger patients. Note the characteristic calcified foci →.* **(Right)** *In more infiltrative areas, CAF may show rays of fibroblastic fascicles extending into subcutaneous adipose tissue, closely resembling lipofibromatosis. The clinical presentation and presence of calcified foci are helpful in avoiding misdiagnosis.*

Infiltrative Growth

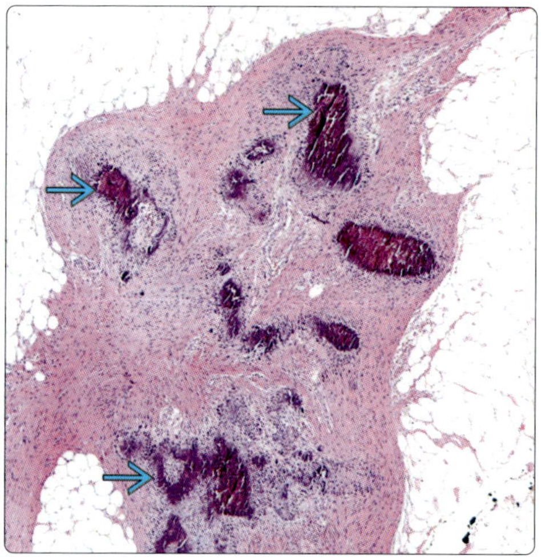

Infiltrative Growth

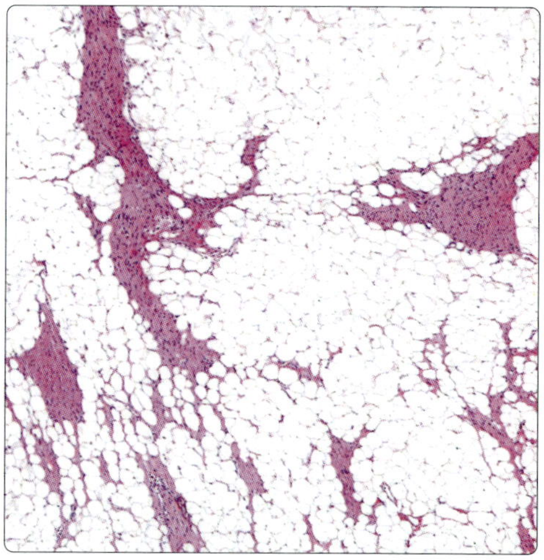

(Left) *The formation of true calcified or cartilaginous foci in CAF may be preceded by small aggregates of epithelioid fibroblastic or chondrocyte-like cells. This finding may be one of the only clues that distinguishes CAF from lipofibromatosis.* **(Right)** *Cartilage formation, as evidenced by the presence of chondrocytes within lacunae →, is common in CAF and may or may not be associated with calcification. Absence of calcification is more typical of early lesions in younger children.*

Noncalcified Foci

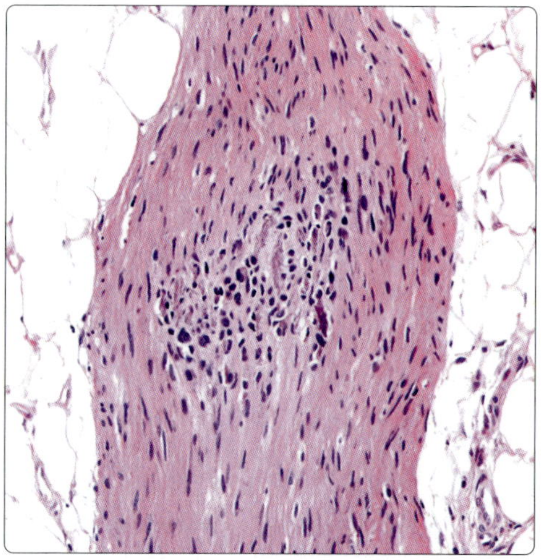

Cartilaginous Foci

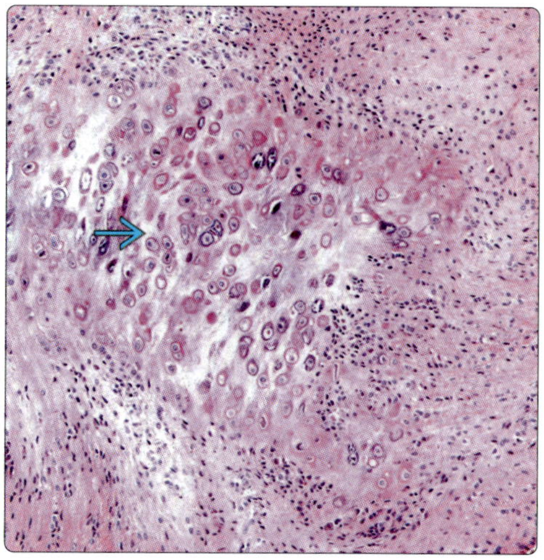

(Left) *Calcification may be extensive in some cases of CAF, particularly in established lesions and those that occur in older individuals. This feature may be readily apparent on gross examination and cut section.* **(Right)** *Some cases of CAF may show multiple hypocellular or myxoedematous nodules → with little or no evidence of cartilage formation ⇨.*

Extensive Calcification

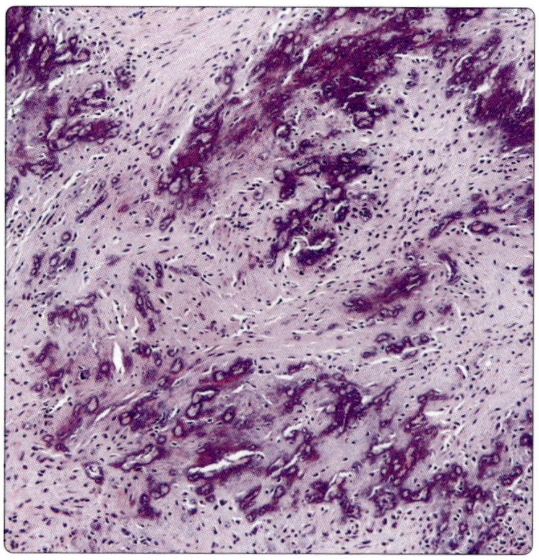

Immature Cartilaginous Nodules

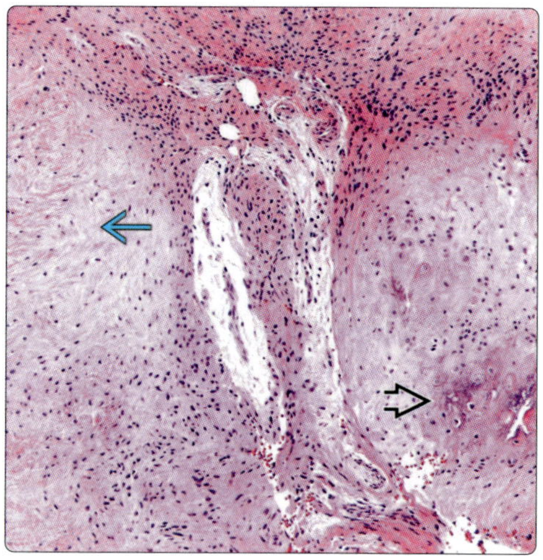

Osteoclast-Like Giant Cells

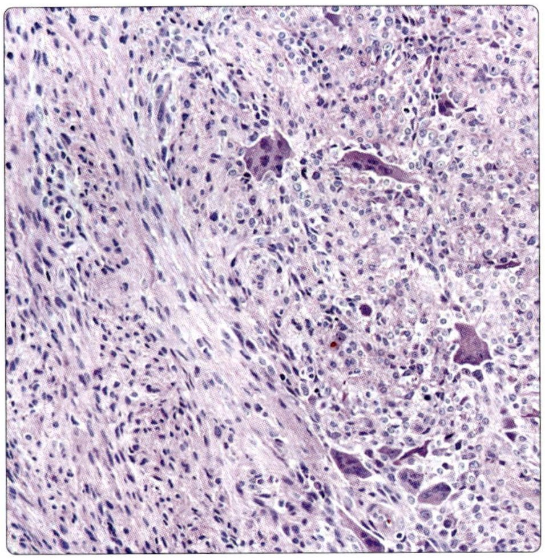

Fibroblastic Component

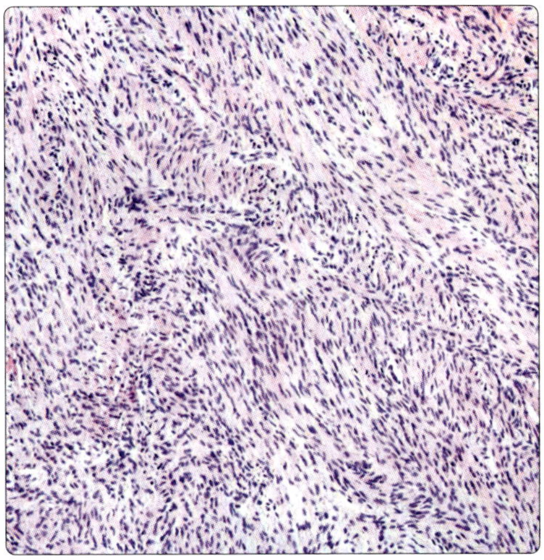

(Left) *Osteoclast-like giant cells, when present in CAF, are usually associated with the calcified or cartilaginous foci; however, rarely they may be isolated.* **(Right)** *The spindled fibroblastic component of CAF often shows varying degrees of cellularity, even within the same case. Some areas may be alarmingly cellular, but importantly, there is no nuclear atypia, and mitoses are rare.*

Fibroblastic Component

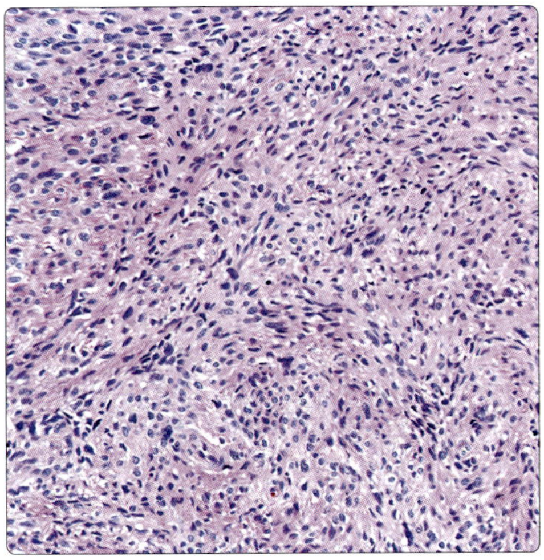

Rare Ossification

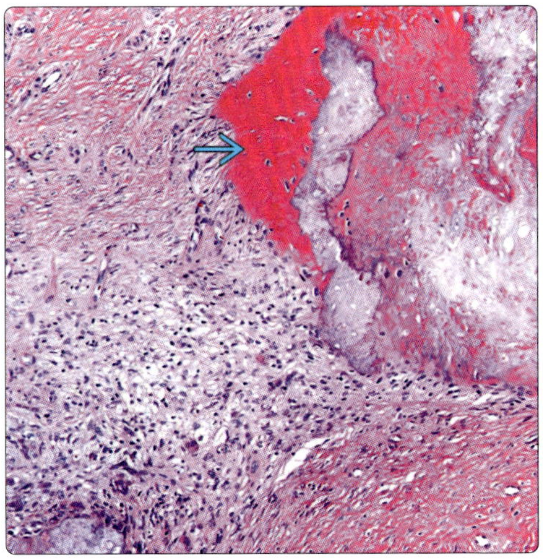

(Left) *Cellular fibroblastic regions in CAF may raise concerns for a possible sarcoma, such as synovial sarcoma or fibrosarcoma; however, the clinical presentation is generally different for these entities, and areas of more conventional morphology are often easily identified elsewhere.* **(Right)** *True bone formation → is a rare event in CAF. Hematopoiesis in these areas has also been reported.*

DDx: Lipofibromatosis

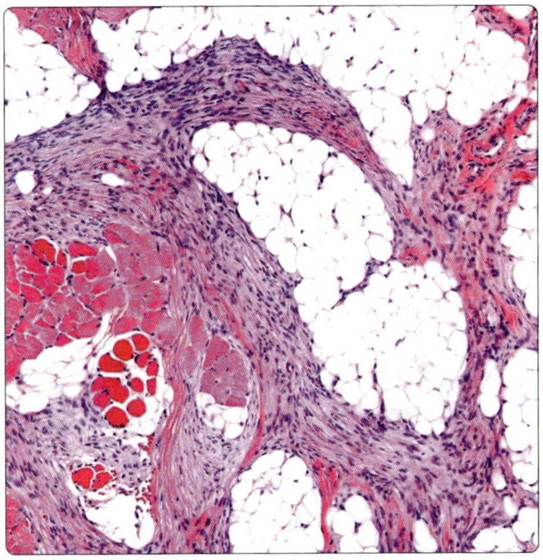

DDx: Soft Tissue Chondroma

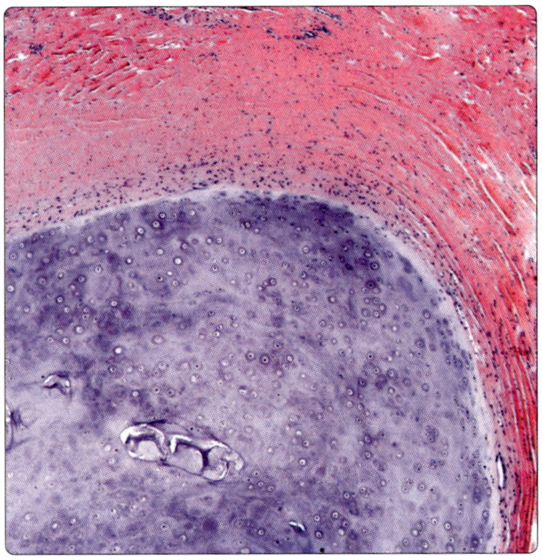

(Left) *Calcifying aponeurotic fibroma may closely resemble lipofibromatosis (shown), particularly in early lesions lacking calcification and cartilage formation; however, CAF is generally less infiltrative and rarely arises outside the hands and feet.* **(Right)** *In contrast to CAF, soft tissue chondroma occurs in older adults and usually shows very well-developed lobules of hyaline cartilage with or without myxoid change and calcification.*

Calcifying Fibrous Tumor

KEY FACTS

TERMINOLOGY

- Synonyms: Calcifying fibrous pseudotumor; childhood fibrous tumor with psammoma bodies

CLINICAL ISSUES

- Wide age range (12-83 years)
  - Soft tissue lesions more common < 20 years of age
  - Visceral lesions more common in adults
- Most common in subcutaneous and deep soft tissue of extremities, trunk, and head and neck
- Often asymptomatic; visceral lesions may produce site-dependent symptoms
- Treatment: Complete local excision
- Benign; excellent prognosis
- Rare local recurrence

MACROSCOPIC

- Well circumscribed and unencapsulated
- Firm, gray to white, gritty cut surfaces

MICROSCOPIC

- Hypocellular, fibrous lesion with bland spindled cells embedded in dense, hyalinized, collagenous stroma
- No atypia or mitotic activity
- Scattered psammomatous &/or dystrophic calcifications
- Variable lymphoplasmacytic infiltrate with lymphoid aggregates

ANCILLARY TESTS

- CD34(+), factor XIIIA(+)
- S100 protein, ALK1, keratin, CD117, DOG1, and STAT6 (-)

TOP DIFFERENTIAL DIAGNOSES

- Inflammatory myofibroblastic tumor
- Fibromatosis
- Synovial sarcoma
- Gastrointestinal stromal tumor
- Solitary fibrous tumor

Calcifying Fibrous Tumor

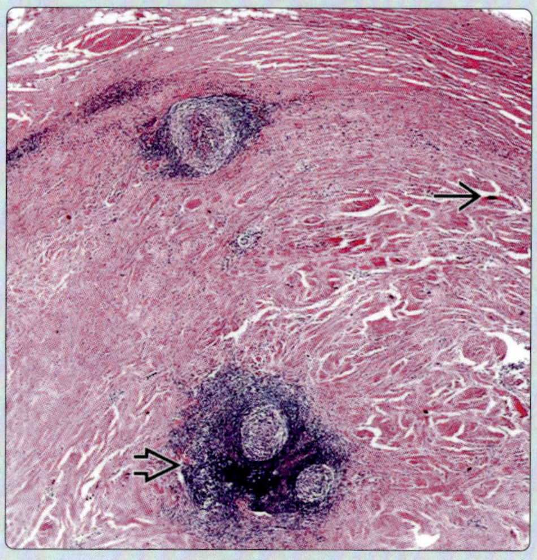

Calcifications

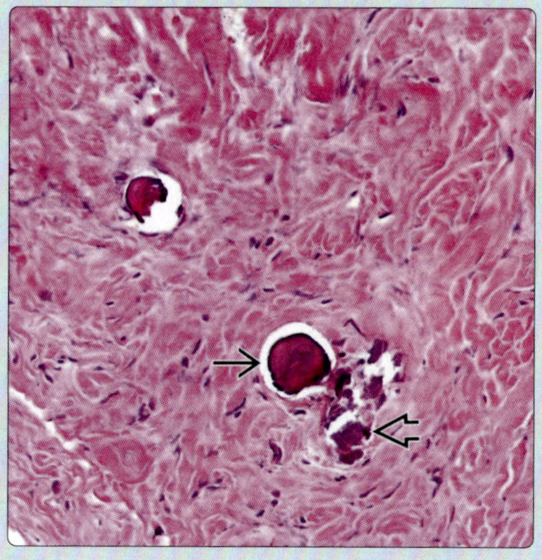

(Left) *A calcifying fibrous tumor (CFT) is a hypocellular lesion composed of hyalinized fibrous tissue with scattered calcifications* →*. Chronic inflammation with lymphoid aggregates is commonly seen* ⇨. **(Right)** *Although the presence of calcifications is the salient feature of CFT, they can be of variable size and prominence, ranging from scarce to extensive. The calcifications can be of the psammomatous type* → *or dystrophic type* ⇨*. The stroma is characteristically composed of hyalinized, collagenous tissue.*

Bland Fibroblasts

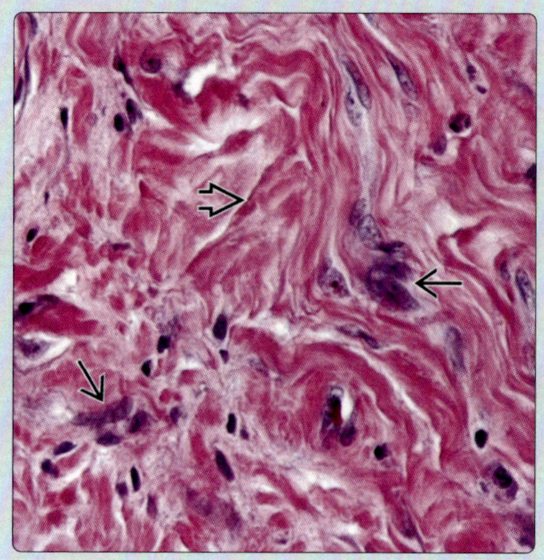

Lymphoplasmacytic Infiltrate

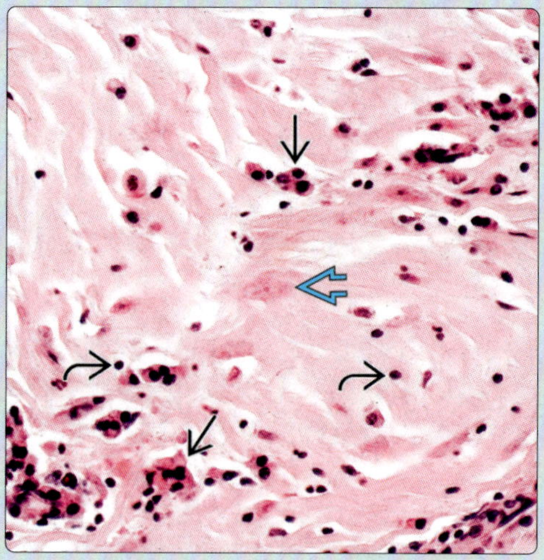

(Left) *The fibroblastic component of CFT is characterized by the presence of bland spindled cells* → *with ovoid/round nuclei, minimal cytologic atypia, and no mitotic activity. These cells are typically embedded in collagenous stroma* ⇨. **(Right)** *A variably prominent population of chronic inflammatory cells, including plasma cells* → *and lymphocytes* ↗ *(± lymphoid aggregates), is commonly seen in the background of CFT. Note the fibroblast nucleus* ⇨*.*

TERMINOLOGY

Abbreviations

- Calcifying fibrous tumor (CFT)

Synonyms

- Calcifying fibrous pseudotumor
- Childhood fibrous tumor with psammoma bodies

Definitions

- Rare benign fibroblastic lesion characterized by dense collagenization, psammomatous &/or dystrophic calcification, and variable lymphoplasmacytic infiltrate

ETIOLOGY/PATHOGENESIS

Neoplastic

- Favored to represent neoplastic rather than reactive process
- In past, postulated to represent sclerosing end-stage inflammatory myofibroblastic tumor (IMT)
  - Absence of ALK expression and chromosome 2 abnormalities in CFT, in contrast to IMT, suggests these are distinct entities
- Most are sporadic (rare reported occurrence of familial peritoneal multifocal lesion)
- Deleterious, heterozygotic de novo mutations in *ZNF717, CDC27,* and *FRG1* genes have been identified in pleural-based lesions

CLINICAL ISSUES

Presentation

- Wide age range
  - Soft tissue lesions more common in first 2 decades of life
  - Visceral lesions more common in adults (4th and 5th decades)
- No sex predilection
- Wide anatomical distribution
  - Most commonly occur in subcutaneous and deep soft tissues (extremities, trunk, head and neck, axilla, mediastinum, mesentery)
  - Pleural, peritoneal, and visceral lesions most commonly involving gastrointestinal tract
- Asymptomatic, painless soft tissue mass often discovered as incidental finding
  - Visceral lesions may produce site-dependent symptoms
- Most lesions are solitary with reported cases of multifocality (especially in pleura and peritoneum)
- Rare associations: Hyaline-type Castleman disease, IMT, and sclerosing angiomatoid nodular transformation of spleen

Treatment

- Complete local excision

Prognosis

- Benign; excellent prognosis
- Rare cases of nondestructive short- and long-term local recurrences ± complete local excision
- No reported malignant transformation

MACROSCOPIC

General Features

- Well circumscribed and unencapsulated
- Firm, gray to white, gritty cut surfaces
- Variable size (< 1 cm to > 10 cm in greatest dimension)

MICROSCOPIC

Histologic Features

- Well circumscribed and unencapsulated
- Hypocellular, fibrous lesion with bland spindled cells embedded in dense, hyalinized, collagenous stroma
- Scattered psammomatous &/or dystrophic calcifications
- Variable lymphoplasmacytic infiltrate with lymphoid aggregates
- No atypia or mitotic activity

ANCILLARY TESTS

Immunohistochemistry

- CD34(+), factor XIIIA(+)
- Rare cases with focal SMA(+) or desmin (+)
- S100 protein, ALK1, keratin, CD117, DOG1, and STAT6 (-)
- Absence of nuclear β-catenin staining

DIFFERENTIAL DIAGNOSIS

Inflammatory Myofibroblastic Tumor

- ALK1(+) in 40-60% of cases
- Chromosome 2p22-24 abnormalities often observed

Fibromatosis

- Cellular lesions with fascicular architecture
- Lacks prominent inflammation and calcifications
- Nuclear β-catenin (+), particularly in deep lesions

Synovial Sarcoma

- Highly cellular lesions that can be calcified
- Focal keratin (+) &/or EMA(+) in most cases
- Characteristic t(X;18) with *SS18* (SYT) translocations

Gastrointestinal Stromal Tumor

- Cellular lesions with minimal inflammation
- Lack hyalinized collagen and calcifications
- CD117(+), DOG1(+)

Solitary Fibrous Tumor

- Calcification and lymphoplasmacytic infiltrate not typically present
- CD34(+), STAT6(+)
- *NAB2-STAT6* gene fusion

SELECTED REFERENCES

1. Mehrad M et al: Whole exome sequencing identifies unique mutations and copy number losses in calcifying fibrous tumor of the pleura: report of three cases and review of the literature. Hum Pathol. 78:36-43, 2018
2. Pezhouh MK et al: Clinicopathologic study of calcifying fibrous tumor of the gastrointestinal tract: a case series. Hum Pathol. 62:199-205, 2017
3. Chorti A et al: Calcifying fibrous tumor: review of 157 patients reported in international literature. Medicine (Baltimore). 95(20):e3690, 2016
4. Valladolid G et al: Calcifying fibrous tumor of the small intestine associated with Castleman-like lymphadenopathy. J Gastrointest Surg. 18(6):1205-8, 2014

Inclusion Body Fibromatosis

KEY FACTS

TERMINOLOGY

- Synonym: Infantile digital fibromatosis
- Benign fascicular myofibroblastic proliferation containing eosinophilic intracytoplasmic inclusions that occur on digits of young children

CLINICAL ISSUES

- Majority occur in 1st year of life (1/3 congenital)
- Most arise on dorsal or lateral aspects of fingers or toes
- Rapidly growing, nontender, dome-shaped swelling
- Treatment: Observation ± conservative surgical excision
- Benign
- High rate of local recurrence (> 50% of cases)

MACROSCOPIC

- Most < 2 cm
- Usually covered by intact skin

MICROSCOPIC

- Overlying skin is often compressed/flattened with fewer/no rete ridges
  - Entrapped dermal adnexal structures common
- Fascicles, sheets, and whorls of uniform, bland, spindled fibroblasts
- Paranuclear intracytoplasmic eosinophilic spherical inclusions
  - Highlighted by Masson trichrome stain
  - Inclusions are less prominent in older lesions
- No necrosis

TOP DIFFERENTIAL DIAGNOSES

- Superficial/desmoid fibromatoses
- Pilar leiomyoma
- Perineurioma
- Calcifying aponeurotic fibroma

Inclusion Body Fibromatosis

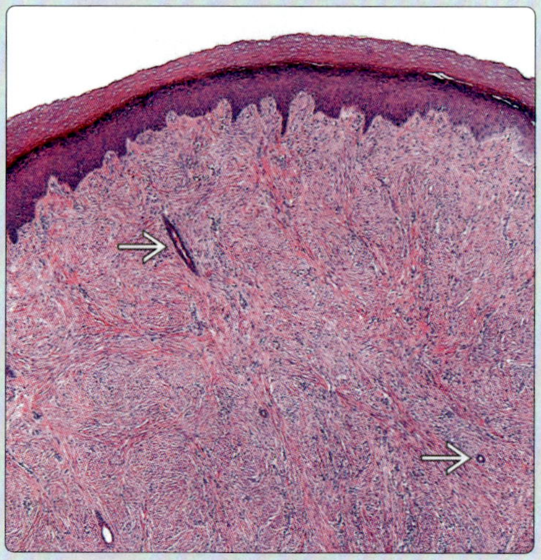

Irregular Fascicular Architecture

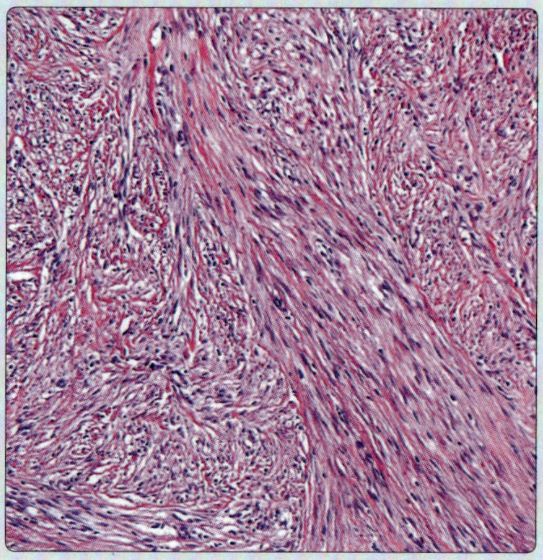

(Left) *Inclusion body fibromatosis (a.k.a. infantile digital fibromatosis) usually arises in the fingers or toes of infants and presents as a rapidly growing, dome-shaped mass with intact overlying skin. Note the entrapped adnexal structures* ➡. **(Right)** *The lesional cells of inclusion body fibromatosis are uniform and spindled and form a variety of patterns, including irregular fascicles, sheets, and whorls.*

Paranuclear Inclusions

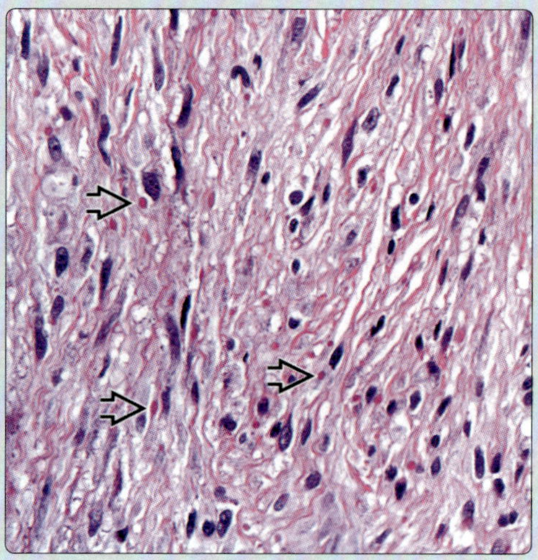

Paranuclear Inclusions (Trichrome)

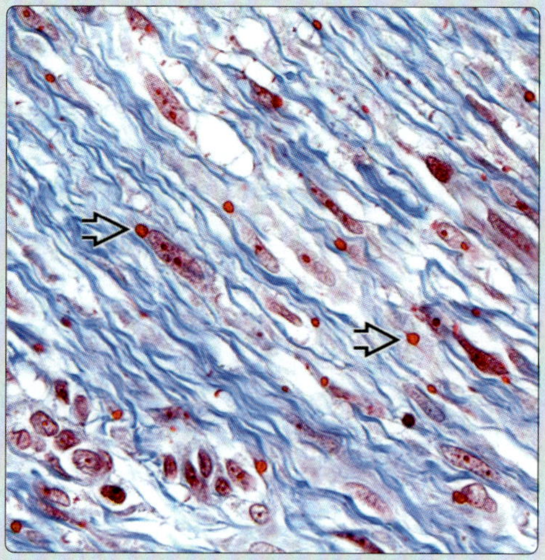

(Left) *A characteristic finding in inclusion body fibromatosis is the presence of intracytoplasmic eosinophilic inclusions, often situated alongside adjacent nuclei. These inclusions* ➡ *can be identified on routine H&E stain, as depicted.* **(Right)** *A trichome stain nicely highlights the characteristic inclusions* ➡ *of inclusion body fibromatosis. The number of inclusions varies from case to case but are generally less prominent in more mature lesions.*

Inclusion Body Fibromatosis

TERMINOLOGY

Synonyms

- Infantile digital fibromatosis
- Infantile digital fibroma
- Digital fibrous tumor of childhood

Definitions

- Benign fascicular myofibroblastic proliferation containing eosinophilic intracytoplasmic inclusions that occur on digits of young children

CLINICAL ISSUES

Epidemiology

- Incidence
  - Rare
- Age
  - Majority occur in 1st year of life
    - ~ 30% are congenital
  - Rarely seen in older children and adults

Site

- Dorsal or lateral aspects of fingers or toes
  - Thumb or big toe is only very rarely affected
- Very rare extradigital sites (i.e., arm, breast) have been reported
- Most cases are superficial (dermal/subcutaneous), but rare cases may involve periosteum or underlying bone

Presentation

- Rapidly growing, nontender, dome-shaped swelling
  - Rarely multiple

Treatment

- Complete but conservative surgical excision
  - Some authorities recommend observation after diagnosis, utilizing excision only for lesions that show continuing growth or functional impairment, or for cosmetic purposes
- Intralesional injections of fluorouracil or corticosteroids have been reported to induce regression in some cases

Prognosis

- Benign
- High rate of local recurrence (> 50% of cases)
  - Spontaneous regression reported in some cases

MACROSCOPIC

General Features

- Firm, ill-defined growth with gray-white cut surface
- Usually covered by intact skin

Size

- Usually < 2 cm

MICROSCOPIC

Histologic Features

- Overlying skin is often compressed/flattened with fewer/no rete ridges
  - Dermal adnexal structures often present and entrapped
- Fascicles, sheets, and whorls of uniform, bland, spindled fibroblasts
- Stomal collagen usually abundant
- Intracytoplasmic eosinophilic spherical inclusions
  - Often in perinuclear location
  - Highlighted by Masson trichrome stain
  - Inclusions are less prominent in older lesions
- Rare mitoses
- No necrosis

ANCILLARY TESTS

Immunohistochemistry

- SMA(+), calponin (+)
- Most cases desmin (-), CD34(-), β-catenin (-)
- S100 protein (-)

DIFFERENTIAL DIAGNOSIS

Superficial/Desmoid Fibromatoses

- Paranuclear cytoplasmic inclusions absent
- Superficial fibromatosis occurs in children but is rare in infants
- Desmoid fibromatosis occurs in older children/adults and in more proximal locations
  - Nuclear β-catenin expression in ~ 70%

Pilar Leiomyoma

- Rare in infants
- Discrete nodules and bundles of eosinophilic spindled cells
- Paranuclear cytoplasmic inclusions absent
- Diffuse cytoplasmic SMA(+), desmin (+)

Perineurioma

- Rare in infants
- Paranuclear cytoplasmic inclusions absent
- EMA(+), Claudin-1 (+), SMA(-), desmin (-)

Calcifying Aponeurotic Fibroma

- Usually contains at least focal calcification or cartilage formation
- Paranuclear cytoplasmic inclusions absent

Acral Fibromyxoma

- Occurs in adults
- Varying myxoid and collagenous stroma
- Paranuclear cytoplasmic inclusions absent
- CD34(+), SMA(-), desmin (-)

Epithelioid Sarcoma

- Often shows ulceration clinically
- Spindled morphology rare
- Keratin (+); loss of nuclear INI1

SELECTED REFERENCES

1. Marks E et al: Infantile digital fibroma: a rare fibromatosis. Arch Pathol Lab Med. 140(10):1153-6, 2016
2. Henderson H et al: Anti-calponin 1 antibodies highlight intracytoplasmic inclusions of infantile digital fibromatosis. Histopathology. 64(5):752-5, 2014
3. Spingardi O et al: Infantile digital fibromatosis: our experience and long-term results. Chir Main. 30(1):62-5, 2011
4. Laskin WB et al: Infantile digital fibroma/fibromatosis: a clinicopathologic and immunohistochemical study of 69 tumors from 57 patients with long-term follow-up. Am J Surg Pathol. 33(1):1-13, 2009

Hyaline Fibromatosis Syndrome

KEY FACTS

TERMINOLOGY

- Synonyms: Juvenile hyaline fibromatosis (JHF), infantile systemic hyalinosis (ISH), inherited systemic hyalinosis

ETIOLOGY/PATHOGENESIS

- Mutations in *ANTXR2* (CMG2) gene
- JHF and ISH represent allelic variations

CLINICAL ISSUES

- Autosomal recessive transmission
- Usually presents at < 5 years of age with development of new lesions throughout life
- Cutaneous and soft tissue lesions of head, neck, gingiva, and perianal areas
- Progressive joint contractures
- Mild phenotype presents later in childhood (JHF)
- Severe phenotype presents during infancy (ISH)
    - Visceral involvement, malnutrition, and protein-losing enteropathy
- High rate of local recurrence after surgical excision

MICROSCOPIC

- Bland, round to spindle cells embedded in homogeneous, hyalinized stroma
- PAS(+), diastase-resistant hyalinized stroma
    - May not be present in early lesions
- Pericellular clearing may impart chondroid-like appearance
- No significant pleomorphism, atypia, or mitoses

TOP DIFFERENTIAL DIAGNOSES

- Infantile myofibromatosis
- Fibrodysplasia (myositis) ossificans progressiva
- Lipoid proteinosis

Hyaline Fibromatosis Syndrome

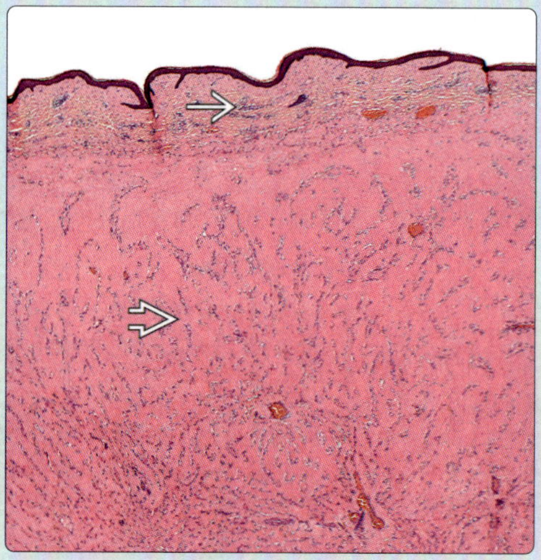

Variable Cellularity

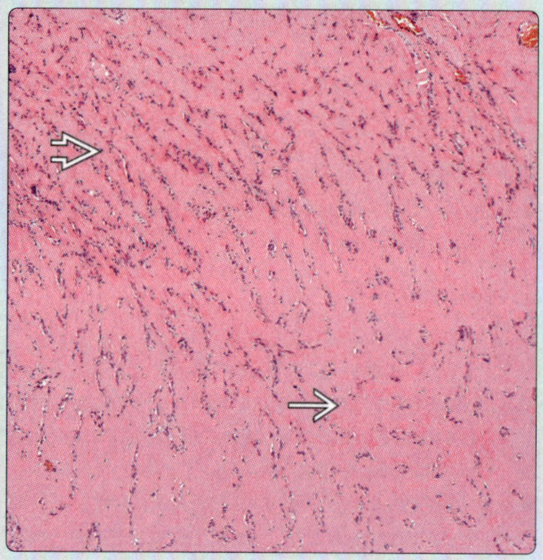

(Left) *Hyaline fibromatosis syndrome (juvenile hyaline fibromatosis) is characterized by well-defined dermal and subcutaneous hyalinization of the stroma ➡. Some lesions have a tumor-free (grenz) zone between the epidermis and lesional tissue ➡.* **(Right)** *The intratumoral cellularity in hyaline fibromatosis may be variable with some areas of sparse cellularity ➡ located adjacent to areas of increased cellularity. In more cellular areas, the cells may form cords that assume a vaguely parallel arrangement ➡.*

Hyalinized Matrix

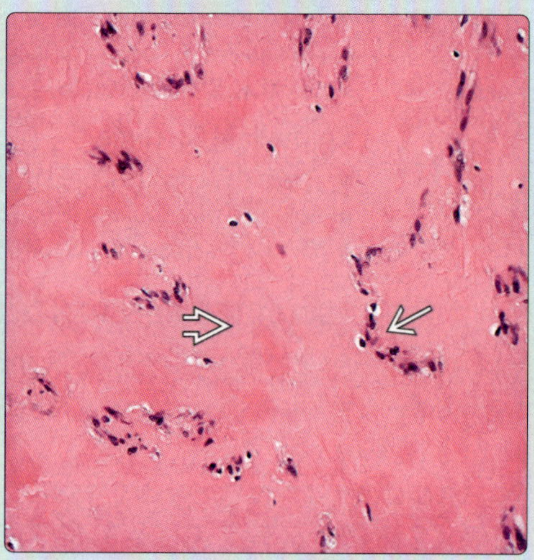

Cytologic Features

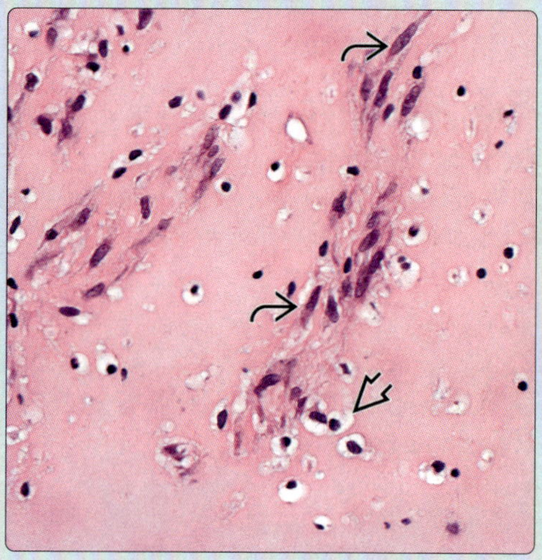

(Left) *The stroma is replaced by uniform, glassy, eosinophilic matrix imparting a hyalinized appearance ➡. This hyalinized material is strongly positive with PAS and diastase resistant. The embedded fibroblasts are small, uniform, and arranged in short curved cords ➡.* **(Right)** *The fibroblasts are variable in shape and may be spindled ➡ or round. The round cells often times exhibit pericellular clearing and resemble chondrocytes ➡. Note the absence of cytologic atypia and mitotic activity.*

TERMINOLOGY

Synonyms

- Juvenile hyaline fibromatosis (JHF)
- Infantile systemic hyalinosis (ISH)
- Inherited systemic hyalinosis

Definitions

- Rare autosomal recessive disorder characterized by hyaline deposition in skin, soft tissue, bones, and viscera

ETIOLOGY/PATHOGENESIS

Genetic Disorder

- Due to deleterious mutations in *ANTXR2* (CMG2) gene on chromosome 4q21
  - Results in abnormal biosynthesis of glycosaminoglycans and collagen and disruption of basement membrane formation
- JHF and ISH represent allelic variations
- Autosomal recessive transmission

CLINICAL ISSUES

Epidemiology

- Incidence
  - Very rare
  - Increased incidence in consanguineous populations
- Age
  - Usually presents at < 5 years with development of new lesions throughout life

Presentation

- Continuous phenotypic spectrum with variable levels of severity
- Skin and soft tissue manifestations
  - Multiple plaques and papulonodular skin lesions on scalp, face, neck, thorax, and perianal areas
  - Large superficial and deep soft tissue masses
- Extracutaneous manifestations
  - Gingival hyperplasia (most common)
  - Progressive joint contractures with severe limitation of joint mobility
  - Osteolytic bone lesions and generalized osteoporosis
  - Variable visceral involvement (bowel, spleen, thyroid, adrenal glands, heart, lung, and liver)
- Clinical variants
  - JHF characterized by milder clinical phenotype
    - Presents later in childhood
    - Skin, soft tissue, gingiva, and joint involvement
  - ISH characterized by severe clinical phenotype
    - Very early onset at birth or within first 6 months of life
    - Visceral involvement in addition to skin, soft tissue, and joint abnormalities
    - Chronic diarrhea and malnutrition due to protein-losing enteropathy

Treatment

- Surgical excision of skin, soft tissue, and gingival lesions for functional improvement or cosmetic purposes
- Intralesional steroid injections

Prognosis

- High rate of local recurrence after surgical excision
- Severe phenotype carries poor prognosis with death by 2 years of age
  - Death due to complications of protein-losing enteropathy, infection, or multiorgan failure
- Mild phenotype carries better prognosis with survival into adulthood

MACROSCOPIC

General Features

- Larger cutaneous lesions form soft tissue masses
- Poorly circumscribed with uniform, waxy, white cut surfaces

MICROSCOPIC

Histologic Features

- Poorly circumscribed proliferation of bland, round to spindled fibroblasts embedded in homogeneous, eosinophilic hyalinized stroma
- Pericellular clearing may impart chondroid-like appearance
- PAS(+), diastase-resistant hyalinized stroma
  - Degree of hyalinization increases with age of lesions and may not be present in early lesions
- No significant pleomorphism, atypia, or mitoses
- Displaces normal dermal components

DIFFERENTIAL DIAGNOSIS

Infantile Myofibromatosis

- Multiple lesions appearing in infancy
- May involve skin, soft tissue, bone, and viscera
- Biphasic pattern with central hemangiopericytoma-like zones and peripheral myoid nodules

Fibrodysplasia (Myositis) Ossificans Progressiva

- Rare and autosomal dominant
- Soft tissue ossification at multiple sites and skeletal abnormalities of digits and cervical spine
- Trauma (accidental or surgical) results in painful soft tissue lesions
- Mitotically active myofibroblasts and variable ossification depending on age of lesions

Lipoid Proteinosis

- Dermal pericapillary PAS(+), diastase-resistant hyaline deposits and prominent basement membrane thickening
  - Basement membrane thickening not seen in hyaline fibromatosis
- Due to mutations in *ECM1* gene (1q21)

SELECTED REFERENCES

1. Bürgi J et al: CMG2/ANTXR2 regulates extracellular collagen VI which accumulates in hyaline fibromatosis syndrome. Nat Commun. 8:15861, 2017
2. Haidar Z et al: Diagnosis implications of the whole genome sequencing in a large Lebanese family with hyaline fibromatosis syndrome. BMC Genet. 18(1):3, 2017
3. Kalgaonkar PS et al: Juvenile hyaline fibromatosis- a rare autosomal recessive disease. J Clin Diagn Res. 11(7):SD04-SD06, 2017
4. Rahvar M et al: Systemic hyalinosis with heterozygous CMG2 mutations: a case report and review of literature. Am J Dermatopathol. 38(5):e60-3, 2016

Fibromatosis Colli

KEY FACTS

TERMINOLOGY

- Sterno(cleido) mastoid (pseudo)tumor of infancy

ETIOLOGY/PATHOGENESIS

- Associated with birth trauma, forceps delivery, breech presentation, difficult labor, and primiparous birth

CLINICAL ISSUES

- Most common cause of neck mass in perinatal period
- Occurs in neonates and infants (presents within first 8 weeks of life)
- Painless, firm mass in middle to lower 1/3 of sternocleidomastoid muscle
  - Most commonly unilateral, right-sided mass
    - Rare reported bilateral cases
- 14-30% of cases are associated with congenital muscular torticollis (CMT)
- Primarily conservative management with physiotherapy and stretching exercises
- Most cases are self-limited with spontaneous regression by 4-8 months of age

MICROSCOPIC

- Fibroblastic infiltrate between skeletal muscle fibers producing fine, checkerboard-like pattern
- Muscle fibers swell followed by progressive degeneration and atrophy
- No significant nuclear hyperchromasia, pleomorphism, or mitotic activity

ANCILLARY TESTS

- Lesional cells are nuclear β-catenin (-)

TOP DIFFERENTIAL DIAGNOSES

- Nodular fasciitis
- Fibromatosis
- Focal myositis

Fibromatosis Colli

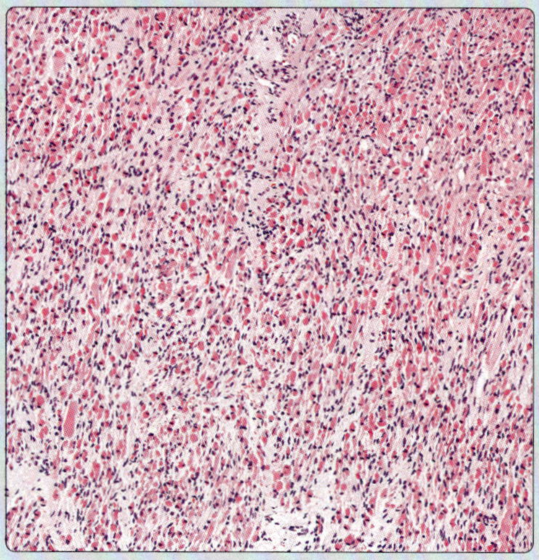

Degenerative Muscle

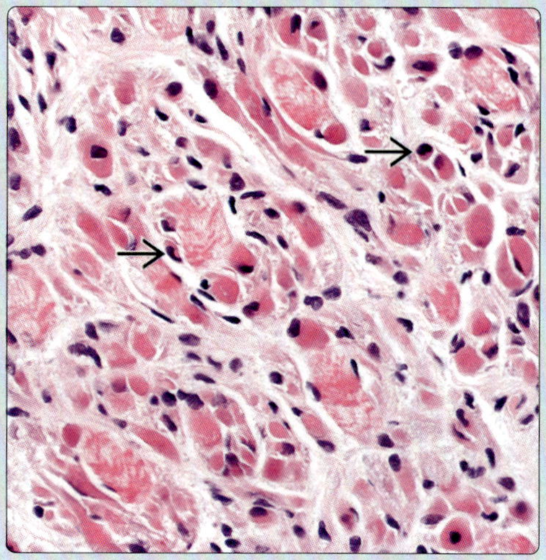

(Left) *Fibromatosis colli is characterized by intramuscular interstitial fibrosis. The proliferating fibroblasts infiltrate between and surround individual muscle fibers, imparting a fine, checkerboard-like pattern.* **(Right)** *The infiltrating fibroblasts dissect muscle fiber groups to surround individual myocytes. With time, the myocytes show degenerative and atrophic changes, including myocyte swelling and reduction in the size of myofibers ⇨.*

Early Stage

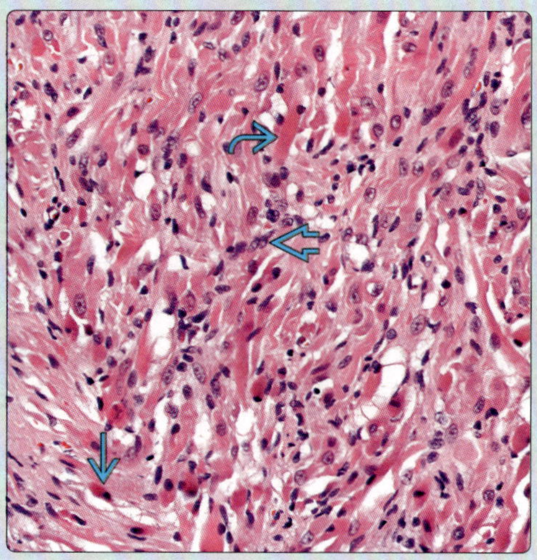

Late Stage

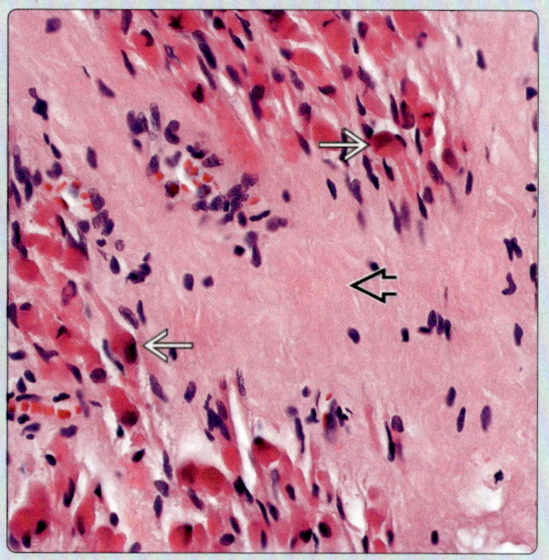

(Left) *Early-stage fibromatosis colli lesions show increased interstitial cellularity with bland fibroblasts ⇨ and scant inflammation. The myofibers show architectural disarray and progressive atrophic changes, including hypereosinophilia ⇗ and reduction in size ⇨. Fatty replacement of atrophied muscle is not a feature of this condition.* **(Right)** *In later stage lesions, the degree of cellularity decreases as muscle fibers become replaced by confluent areas of fibrosis ⇨. The surrounding muscle fibers are atrophic ➡.*

TERMINOLOGY

Synonyms

- Sterno(cleido) mastoid (pseudo)tumor of infancy

Definitions

- Benign fibrous proliferation involving sternocleidomastoid muscle (SCM) in infants

ETIOLOGY/PATHOGENESIS

Developmental Anomaly

- May be related to venous ischemia of muscle secondary to intrauterine malposition or birth trauma

Environmental Exposure

- Associated with birth trauma, forceps delivery, breech presentation, difficult labor, and primiparous birth

CLINICAL ISSUES

Epidemiology

- Incidence
  - Rare, 0.4% of live births
  - Most common cause of neck mass in perinatal period
- Age
  - Neonates and infants (presents within first 8 weeks of life)
- Sex
  - Slight male predominance (M:F = 1.3-2.3:1.0)

Site

- Intramuscular location within SCM
  - Most commonly involves middle and lower 1/3 of muscle
- Most commonly unilateral with rare reported bilateral cases
  - Predominantly right sided (75% of cases)

Presentation

- Painless, firm mass in body of SCM
  - Rare reported cases of trapezius muscle involvement
  - Initial growth phase over 1st several weeks, then stabilizes in size
- 14-30% of cases are associated with congenital muscular torticollis (CMT)
  - Prolonged torticollis may result in craniofacial asymmetry
- Associated with developmental dysplasia of hip in 2.4-10.0% of cases

Treatment

- Primarily conservative management with physiotherapy and stretching exercises
- Surgical management reserved for patients with persistence of disease after 1 year of age or those with craniofacial abnormalities

Prognosis

- Most cases are self-limited with spontaneous regression by 4-8 months of age
- If conservative therapy is initiated early, 80-90% of cases resolve permanently

IMAGING

Ultrasonographic Findings

- Initial modality of choice (sensitivity ~ 100%)
- Focal or diffuse fusiform enlargement within SCM
- Lesion displays synchronous mobility with SCM

MACROSCOPIC

General Features

- Firm, white, infiltrative lesion involving body of muscle
- Does not extend into adjacent soft tissue
- Average size: 2-3 cm in diameter

MICROSCOPIC

Histologic Features

- Fibroblastic infiltrate between skeletal muscle fibers producing fine, checkerboard-like pattern
- Increased cellularity during early proliferative phase
- Increased fibrosis in later stages
- Muscle fibers swell followed by progressive degeneration and atrophy
- No significant nuclear hyperchromasia, pleomorphism, or mitotic activity

ANCILLARY TESTS

Immunohistochemistry

- Infiltrating fibroblasts are SMA(+) in early stages
- Lesional cells are nuclear β-catenin (-)

DIFFERENTIAL DIAGNOSIS

Nodular Fasciitis

- Does not infiltrate between muscle bundles
- Myxoid and storiform patterns are common
- Admixed extravasated red blood cells, lymphocytes, and plasma cells are commonly seen

Fibromatosis

- Solitary or multiple masses
- Not confined to single muscle group as in fibromatosis colli
- May entrap muscle fibers at periphery but does not replace muscle
- Deep lesions exhibit nuclear β-catenin immunoreactivity

Focal Myositis

- Can occur at any age
- Gastrocnemius and vastus lateralis muscles are most common sites
- Intramuscular mass with interstitial mixed inflammatory infiltrate and dense fibrosis
- Degenerative and regenerative myopathic changes

SELECTED REFERENCES

1. Sargar KM et al: Pediatric fibroblastic and myofibroblastic tumors: a pictorial review. Radiographics. 36(4):1195-214, 2016
2. Adamoli P et al: Rapid spontaneous resolution of fibromatosis colli in a 3-week-old girl. Case Rep Otolaryngol. 2014:264940, 2014
3. Coffin CM et al: Fibroblastic and myofibroblastic tumors in children and adolescents. Pediatr Dev Pathol. 15(1 Suppl):127-80, 2012

Gardner Fibroma

KEY FACTS

TERMINOLOGY

- Uncommon fibrocollagenous lesion classically arising in paraspinal or back region of child
- Majority linked to familial adenomatous polyposis (FAP)/Gardner syndrome

CLINICAL ISSUES

- Majority (80%) arise in 1st decade of life
- Slight male predominance
- Back and paraspinal most common sites (60%)
    - Also head/neck, extremities, abdomen/chest
- Painless subcutaneous mass, occasionally multiple
- Treatment: Simple surgical excision
- Benign but may recur after incomplete excision
- Majority (70%) associated with FAP/Gardner syndrome
    - Nearly 20% of patients also have desmoid fibromatosis

MACROSCOPIC

- Poorly circumscribed subcutaneous mass
- Range 1 cm to > 10 cm (mean: 3-4 cm)

MICROSCOPIC

- Sheets of dense collagen bundles with intervening cleft/cracking artifact
- Sparse intermixed population of small bland fibroblastic spindle cells
- Variable amounts of entrapped fat, vessels, and nerves, especially at periphery

ANCILLARY TESTS

- Nuclear β-catenin (+) in majority

TOP DIFFERENTIAL DIAGNOSES

- Nuchal-type fibroma
- Nuchal fibrocartilaginous pseudotumor
- Fibrolipoma
- Elastofibroma
- Desmoid fibromatosis

(Left) *Gardner fibroma arises as a hypocellular densely collagenous mass in the subcutis. This case was from the scalp of a 5-year-old patient.* **(Right)** *Islands of adipocytes are often entrapped within the dense collagen of Gardner fibroma.*

Subcutaneous Mass

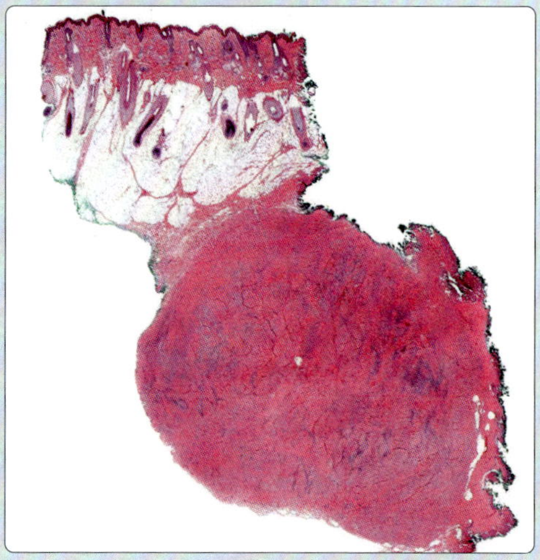

Entrapped Fat

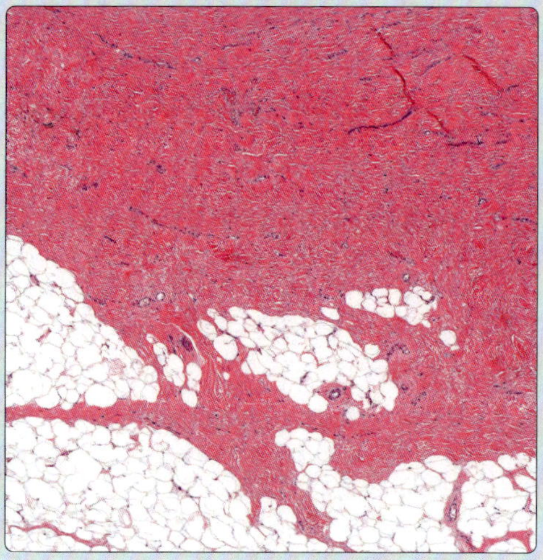

(Left) *Gardner fibroma is composed of sheets of dense collagen with sparsely scattered, bland, spindled fibroblasts.* **(Right)** *Scattered, small, spindled fibroblastic cells ➔ are present among the dense collagen bundles and are often only identifiable by their thin, bland nuclei. Cracking artifact ⇨ is clearly seen in this H&E. (Courtesy M. Edgar, MD.)*

Hypocellular Sheets of Dense Collagen

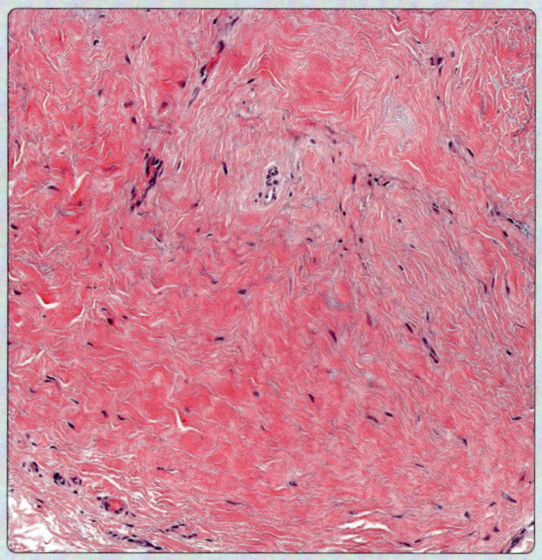

Artifactual Clefting

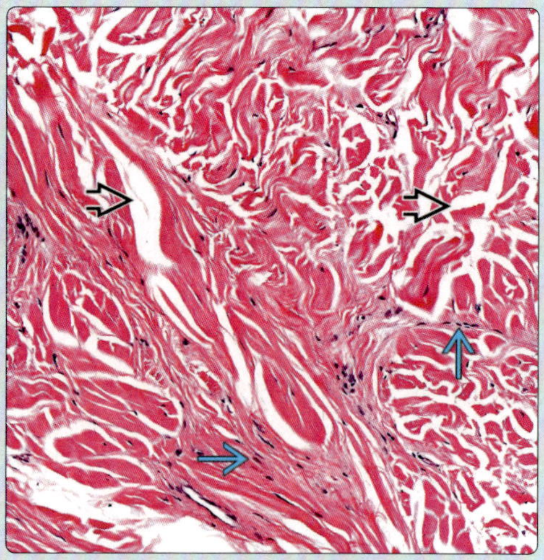

Gardner Fibroma

TERMINOLOGY

Synonyms

- Gardner-associated fibroma; desmoid precursor lesion

Definitions

- Uncommon fibrocollagenous lesion classically arising in paraspinal or back region of child
  - Majority linked to familial adenomatous polyposis (FAP)/Gardner syndrome
- Distinct entity from nuchal-type fibroma (despite very similar histologic features)
- Uncertain whether benign neoplasm or malformation

CLINICAL ISSUES

Epidemiology

- Age
  - Majority (80%) arise in 1st decade (mean age: 5 years)
    - Remainder in teens or young adults
- Sex
  - Slight male predominance

Site

- Back and paraspinal most common sites (60%)
- Also head/neck, extremities, abdomen/chest

Presentation

- Painless subcutaneous mass
- Usually solitary; multiple lesions in 15% of patients
  - Multiple lesions more likely in FAP
- Large/unresectable lesions more likely in FAP

Treatment

- Simple surgical excision
- Celecoxib has been used for large/unresectable cases

Prognosis

- Benign but may recur after incomplete excision
- May transform into desmoid fibromatosis
- 24% of desmoid fibromatosis have adjacent areas of Gardner fibroma (may be subtle)
- 70% are associated with FAP/Gardner syndrome
  - Nearly 20% of patients also have desmoid fibromatosis
  - Gardner fibroma may be sentinel event of FAP

MACROSCOPIC

General Features

- Poorly circumscribed subcutaneous mass
- Rubbery white to yellow cut surface

Size

- Range 1 cm to > 10 cm (mean: 3-4 cm)

MICROSCOPIC

Histologic Features

- Identical for sporadic vs. FAP-associated cases
- Sheets of dense collagen bundles with intervening cleft/cracking artifact
- Sparse intermixed small bland fibroblasts
- Variable amounts of entrapped fat, vessels, and nerves, especially at periphery
- Scattered mast cells may be present

ANCILLARY TESTS

Immunohistochemistry

- Immunostains usually not required for diagnosis
- Majority (+) for β-catenin (nuclear), CD34, cyclin-D1, myc
- Subset are β-catenin (-), particularly sporadic non-FAP cases

DIFFERENTIAL DIAGNOSIS

Nuchal-Type Fibroma

- Histologically very similar to Gardner fibroma
- Arises in young to middle-aged adults (not children)
- Lacks nuclear β-catenin (+)
- Uncommonly associated with FAP/Gardner syndrome
- Some have proliferation of small nerve bundles, unlike Gardner fibroma

Nuchal Fibrocartilaginous Pseudotumor

- Arises in specific site: Posterior neck at junction of nuchal ligament and deep cervical fascia
- Contains prominent cartilaginous tissue

Elastofibroma

- Arises beneath inferior tip of scapula; often bilateral
- Dense collagen admixed with mature adipose tissue
- Hallmark finding: Degenerated serrated elastic fibers with "petaloid globules" or "caterpillar bodies"

Desmoid Fibromatosis

- Usually large deep mass
- Long, broad, sweeping fascicles of bland fibroblastic cells
  - Much more cellular and fascicular than Gardner fibroma
- Infiltration and entrapment of skeletal muscle fibers

Fibrolipoma

- Circumscribed mass of mature adipose tissue with intervening fibrocollagenous septa
- Much more fat/less collagen than Gardner fibroma

Desmoplastic Fibroblastoma (Collagenous Fibroma)

- Dense sheets of collagen but usually more homogeneous
- Multinodular and well circumscribed; not infiltrative
- Has large stellate fibroblasts not seen in Gardner fibroma

DIAGNOSTIC CHECKLIST

Clinically Relevant Pathologic Features

- Raise possibility of FAP/Gardner syndrome; recommend consultation with genetic counselor for further work-up

SELECTED REFERENCES

1. Dahl NA et al: Gardner fibroma: clinical and histopathologic implications of germline APC mutation association. J Pediatr Hematol Oncol. 38(5):e154-7, 2016
2. Cates JM et al: Desmoid-type fibromatosis-associated Gardner fibromas: prevalence and impact on local recurrence. Cancer Lett. 353(2):176-81, 2014
3. Coffin CM et al: Gardner fibroma: a clinicopathologic and immunohistochemical analysis of 45 patients with 57 fibromas. Am J Surg Pathol. 31(3):410-6, 2007
4. Wehrli BM et al: Gardner-associated fibromas (GAF) in young patients: a distinct fibrous lesion that identifies unsuspected Gardner syndrome and risk for fibromatosis. Am J Surg Pathol. 25(5):645-51, 2001

Lipofibromatosis

KEY FACTS

TERMINOLOGY

- Infiltrating, fibrofatty soft tissue tumor of childhood with predilection for distal extremities
- Synonym: Infantile/juvenile fibromatosis, nondesmoid type (obsolete)

CLINICAL ISSUES

- Presents from birth to childhood
  - Majority present prior to 3 years of age
  - Male predominance
- Most commonly involves distal extremities (hands and feet)
- Painless, slow-growing, subcutaneous or deep soft tissue mass
- Treatment: Complete surgical resection
- Benign with high rate of local recurrence
- No reported cases of metastasis

MACROSCOPIC

- Poorly demarcated with tan to yellow, firm cut surfaces
- Most 1-3 cm

MICROSCOPIC

- Lobules of mature adipose tissue traversed by fascicles of bland, spindled fibroblasts
- Infiltrative growth pattern
- No nuclear pleomorphism
- Low to absent mitotic activity

TOP DIFFERENTIAL DIAGNOSES

- Fibrous hamartoma of infancy
- Lipomatosis of nerve
- Lipoblastoma
- Fibroblastic connective tissue nevus
- Lipofibromatosis-like neural tumor

Lipofibromatosis

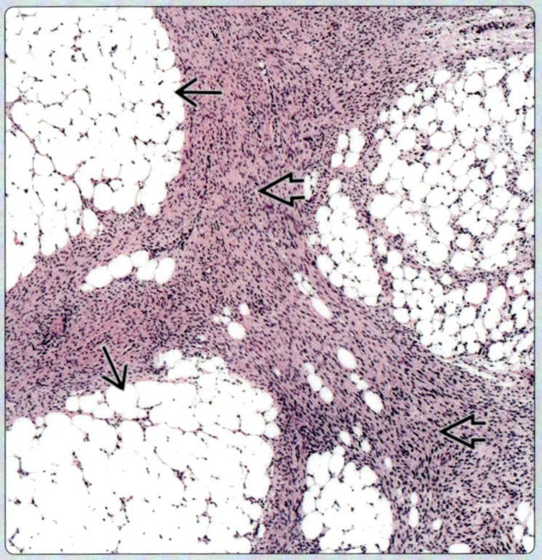

Adipocytes and Fibroblasts

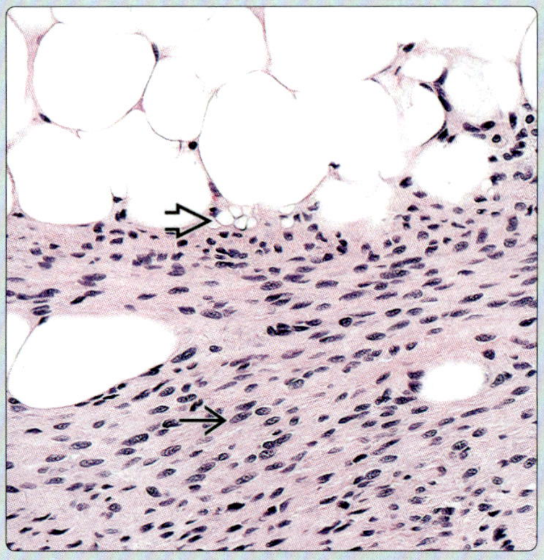

(Left) *Lipofibromatosis is a benign lesion characterized by alternating lobules of mature adipocytes* → *and fascicles of variably cellular but bland fibrous tissue* ⇨. **(Right)** *This lesion is composed of 2 cell types: Mature adipose tissue and fibroblasts. The fibroblasts are spindled in shape with ovoid nuclei, no cytologic atypia, and minimal mitotic activity* →. *Although the majority of adipocytes are mature, occasional univacuolated lipoblast-like cells* ⇨ *are encountered at the interface of adipose and fibrous tissue.*

Variable Proportions

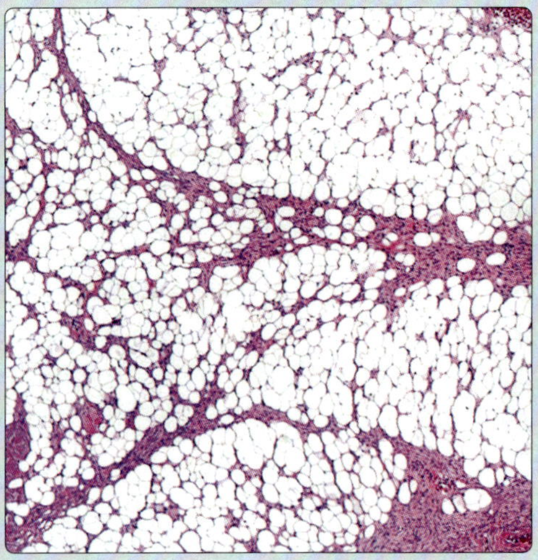

Infiltrative Growth Pattern

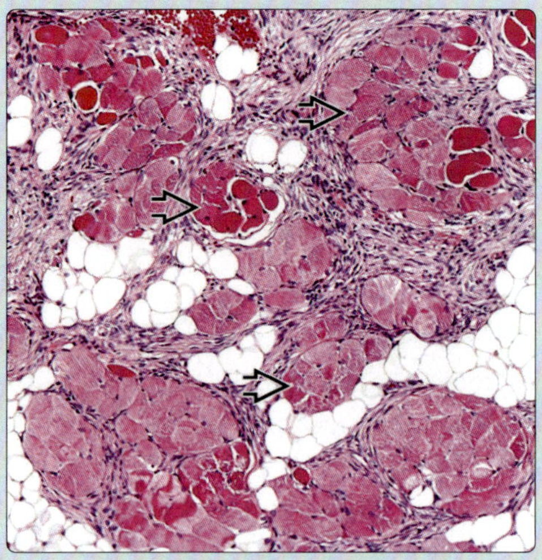

(Left) *The adipocytic and fibrous components of lipofibromatosis vary widely in proportion from tumor to tumor. Typically, the adipocytic component is abundant and comprises at least 50% of the lesion.* **(Right)** *Lipofibromatosis displays a tendency for infiltrative growth and can entrap muscle* ⇨*, nerves, and adnexal structures. As such, there is a high rate of local recurrence after excision.*

TERMINOLOGY

Synonyms

- Infantile/juvenile fibromatosis, nondesmoid type (former designation)

Definitions

- Infiltrating, fibrofatty soft tissue tumor of childhood with predilection for distal extremities

ETIOLOGY/PATHOGENESIS

Genetics

- Single reported case of balanced 3-way t(4;9;6) translocation
- Fibroblastic component demonstrates high expression of connective tissue growth factor (CCN2), which is encoded by gene located on chromosome 6q23.1

CLINICAL ISSUES

Epidemiology

- Presents from birth to childhood
  - Median age of presentation: 1 year
  - Majority of cases present prior to 3 years of age
- Tendency for male predominance (M:F = 2.7:1.0)

Site

- Most commonly involves distal extremities (hands and feet)
- Less common sites: Head, neck, orbit, jaw, back, chest wall, abdominal wall

Presentation

- Slow-growing, subcutaneous or deep soft tissue mass

Treatment

- Complete surgical resection

Prognosis

- Benign
- High rate of local recurrence due to infiltrative growth pattern
- Factors associated with recurrence
  - Congenital presentation, male sex, high mitotic activity, and incomplete excision

MACROSCOPIC

General Features

- Tan to yellow, firm cut surfaces
- Poorly demarcated with ill-defined margins

Size

- Most 1-3 cm (rarely > 5 cm)

MICROSCOPIC

Histologic Features

- Lobules of mature adipose tissue traversed by fascicles of bland, spindled fibroblasts
  - No nuclear pleomorphism
  - Low to absent mitotic activity
- Infiltrative growth pattern with entrapped muscle, nerves, and adnexal structures
- Vacuolated (lipoblast-like) cells at areas of interface between adipose and fibrous tissue
- Scattered pigmented cells (containing melanin) reported in rare cases

ANCILLARY TESTS

Immunohistochemistry

- Variable focal SMA(+), CD34(+), CD99(+)
- Nuclear β-catenin expression absent
- Fibroblasts/myofibroblasts (-) for S100, desmin, and ALK1

DIFFERENTIAL DIAGNOSIS

Fibrous Hamartoma of Infancy

- More commonly occurs in axillary fold, proximal extremities, and groin (rare in hands and feet)
- Classic organoid growth pattern with 3 distinct components in varying amounts
  - Mature adipose tissue
  - Fascicles and sheets of fibroblasts/myofibroblasts
  - Primitive mesenchymal cells in myxoid stroma

Lipomatosis of Nerve

- Typically affects median nerve and digital branches (80%)
- Associated with macrodactyly in 30% of cases
- Infiltration of perineurium and epineurium by adipose tissue

Lipoblastoma

- Admixture of mature and immature adipocytes
  - Adipocytes mature over time and become separated by prominent fibrous septa
- Lipoblasts prominent in early lesions
- Prominent plexiform vasculature within fat lobules
- Variable amounts of myxoid stroma
- *PLAG1* (8q11-13) gene rearrangements

Fibroblastic Connective Tissue Nevus

- Isolated plaque-like or nodular lesion on trunk, head and neck, and extremities of children
- Interlacing fascicles of spindled fibroblasts/myofibroblasts within reticular dermis and subcutis
- Entrapped adnexal structures and adipocytes

Lipofibromatosis-Like Neural Tumor

- Fascicles of spindle cells infiltrating adipocytes in subcutis
- May display mild cytologic atypia
- S100(+), CD34(+) and NTRK1(+)
- *NTRK1* gene rearrangements

SELECTED REFERENCES

1. Lao QY et al: [Lipofibromatosis: a clinicopathological analysis of eight cases.] Zhonghua Bing Li Xue Za Zhi. 47(3):186-191, 2018
2. Pennacchia I et al: Fibroblastic connective tissue nevus: clinicopathological and immunohistochemical study of 14 cases. J Cutan Pathol. 44(10):827-834, 2017
3. Agaram NP et al: Recurrent NTRK1 gene fusions define a novel subset of locally aggressive lipofibromatosis-like neural tumors. Am J Surg Pathol. 40(10):1407-16, 2016
4. Boos MD et al: Lipofibromatosis: an institutional and literature review of an uncommon entity. Pediatr Dermatol. 31(3):298-304, 2014

Giant Cell Fibroblastoma

KEY FACTS

TERMINOLOGY

- Locally aggressive fibroblastic neoplasm, predominantly of childhood and adolescence, that classically features multinucleated giant cells lining pseudovascular spaces
  - Histologically and genetically related to dermatofibrosarcoma protuberans (DFSP)

CLINICAL ISSUES

- Most arise in children (median: 6 years)
- 2:1 male predominance
- Most common in superficial soft tissues of trunk
- Superficial, often protuberant mass
  - May arise in site of previous DFSP excision
- Treatment: Wide surgical excision with margins
- Local recurrence in up to 50%
- No documented reports of metastasis in histologically pure giant cell fibroblastoma

MICROSCOPIC

- Infiltrative growth
- Hypocellular proliferation of bland spindled cells within myxoid to collagenous stroma
- Multinucleated giant cells in stroma and lining irregular pseudovascular spaces
- Mitoses rare; necrosis absent
- Minority of cases contain areas of conventional DFSP

ANCILLARY TESTS

- CD34(+) in spindled and multinucleated giant cells
- Molecular: Characteristic t(17;22) with *COL1A1-PDGFB* fusion

TOP DIFFERENTIAL DIAGNOSES

- DFSP
- Angiosarcoma
- Dermatofibroma (fibrous histiocytoma)
- Myxofibrosarcoma

(Left) *Giant cell fibroblastoma (GCFB) is a benign but locally aggressive fibroblastic neoplasm that most frequently arises on the trunk, usually in children. As shown on this H&E, GCFB ⇒ is a superficial lesion and arises in the dermis &/or subcutis.* **(Right)** *The classic histologic appearance of GCFB shows irregular, pseudovascular ("angiectoid") spaces lined by multinucleated giant cells within a variable collagenous to myxoid stroma. An initial impression of a vascular neoplasm like angiosarcoma is not uncommon.*

Giant Cell Fibroblastoma

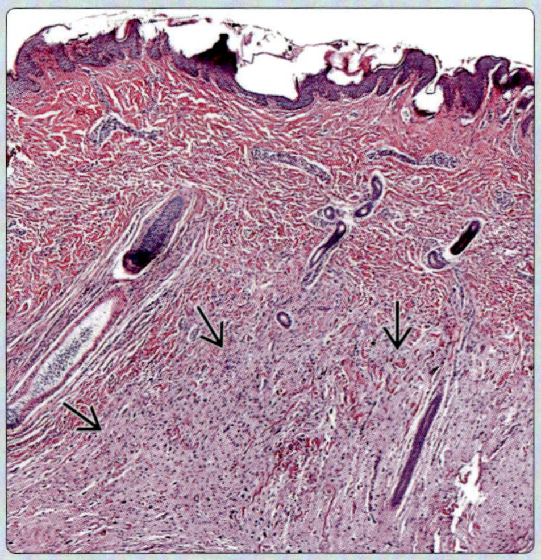

Giant Cell Fibroblastoma

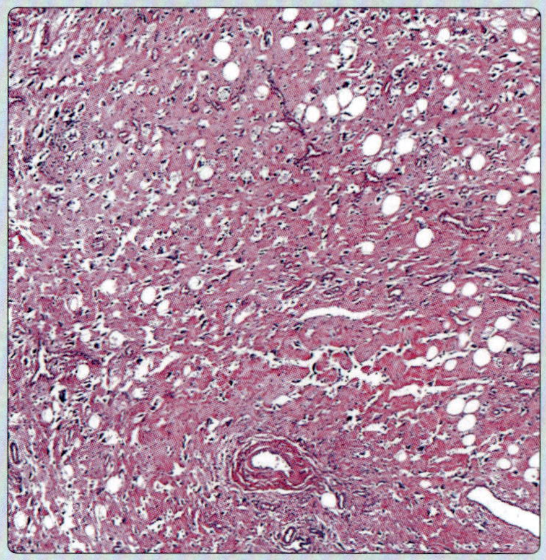

(Left) *Two types of stromal fibroblastic cells can be identified in GCFB: Mononuclear cells ⇒ with bland, wavy nuclei and multinucleated giant cells ⇒ with nuclei in a floret-like or centrally clustered arrangement. Mitotic activity is low to absent.* **(Right)** *Although not seen in every case, many examples of GCFB contain characteristic irregular pseudovascular spaces lined by mono- and multinucleated stromal cells. These spaces, when present, may be dilated and prominent, as depicted, or slit-like and prominent.*

Mono- and Multinucleated Stromal Cells

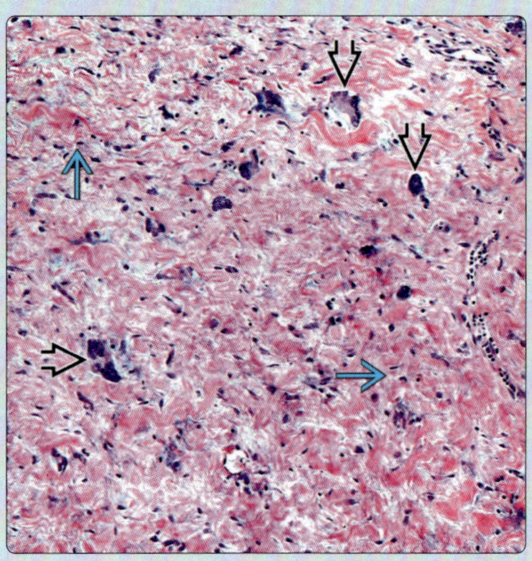

Irregular Pseudovascular Spaces

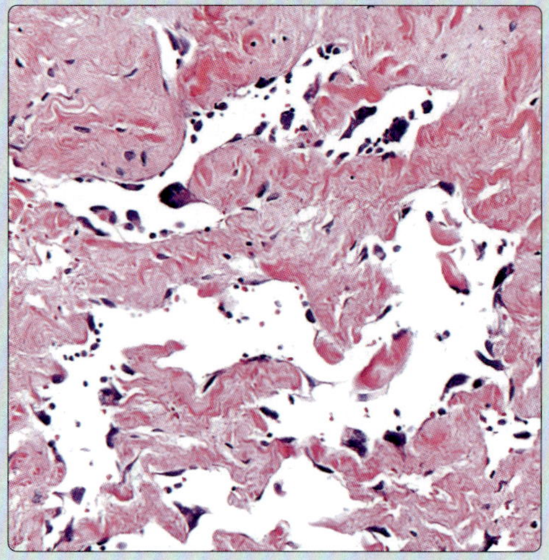

Giant Cell Fibroblastoma

TERMINOLOGY

Abbreviations

- Giant cell fibroblastoma (GCFB)

Definitions

- Locally aggressive fibroblastic neoplasm, predominantly of childhood and adolescence, that classically features multinucleated giant cells lining pseudovascular spaces
  - Histologically and genetically related to dermatofibrosarcoma protuberans (DFSP)

CLINICAL ISSUES

Epidemiology

- Incidence
  - Rare
- Age
  - Most arise in children (median: 6 years)
  - 75% occur before 20 years
  - Occasionally may occur in adults
- Sex
  - 2:1 male predominance

Site

- Arises in dermis &/or subcutaneous tissue
- Most common on trunk
- Infrequent on extremities, head/neck region

Presentation

- Superficial, often protuberant mass
  - May be polypoid
- Slow growing, often painless
- May arise in site of previous DFSP excision

Treatment

- Wide surgical excision with margins

Prognosis

- Local recurrence in up to 50%
  - Often related to marginal or incomplete excision
- No documented reports of metastasis in histologically pure GCFB
  - Hybrid GCFB/DFSP tumors behave more like DFSP

MACROSCOPIC

General Features

- Poorly defined, superficial lesion
- Tan-gray to yellow mucoid cut surface

Size

- Mean: 3.5 cm

MICROSCOPIC

Histologic Features

- Infiltrative growth
  - Adnexal structures entrapped but not destroyed
  - Often shows honeycomb pattern of fat infiltration
- Hypocellular proliferation of small spindled cell with bland, wavy nuclei within myxoid to collagenous stroma
  - Areas of increased cellularity can be seen
- Variable number of multinucleated giant cells in stroma
  - These cells also characteristically line irregular, cleft-like pseudovascular spaces
- Mitoses rare; necrosis absent
- Intralesional hemorrhage may be present
- Perivascular chronic inflammatory infiltrate not uncommon
- Minority of cases contain areas of conventional DFSP (hybrid DFSP/GCFB)
  - May be present in primary tumor or in recurrence
  - Rare pigmented cells, myoid nodules, or fibrosarcomatous change

ANCILLARY TESTS

Immunohistochemistry

- CD34(+) in spindled and multinucleated giant cells
- S100 protein, SMA, desmin, keratin (-)

Molecular Genetics

- Characteristic t(17;22) leading to *COL1A1-PDGFB* fusion protein

DIFFERENTIAL DIAGNOSIS

Dermatofibrosarcoma Protuberans

- Pure DFSP lacks multinucleated giant cells
- Well-developed storiform architecture in most cases
- DFSP can contain areas of GCFB

Angiosarcoma

- Very rare in pediatric age group
- Prominent nuclear atypia and mitoses
- CD31(+), CD34(+)

Dermatofibroma (Fibrous Histiocytoma)

- May contain multinucleated giant cells
- Lacks irregular pseudovascular spaces lined by multinucleated cells
- Generally CD34(-)
- Lacks *COL1A1-PDGFB* fusion

Pleomorphic Lipoma

- Well circumscribed, noninfiltrative
- Contains characteristic floret-like multinucleated cells
- Adipose tissue component often abundant
- Lacks *COL1A1-PDGFB* fusion

Myxofibrosarcoma

- Most common in older/elderly adults
- Usually prominent nuclear atypia and mitotic activity
- Occasionally shows CD34(+)

SELECTED REFERENCES

1. Shah KK et al: Dermatofibrosarcoma protuberans of distal extremities and acral sites: a clinicopathologic analysis of 27 cases. Am J Surg Pathol. 42(3):413-419, 2018
2. Macarenco RS et al: Genomic gains of COL1A1-PDFGB occur in the histologic evolution of giant cell fibroblastoma into dermatofibrosarcoma protuberans. Genes Chromosomes Cancer. 47(3):260-5, 2008
3. Jha P et al: Giant cell fibroblastoma: an update and addition of 86 new cases from the Armed Forces Institute of Pathology, in honor of Dr. Franz M. Enzinger. Ann Diagn Pathol. 11(2):81-8, 2007
4. Terrier-Lacombe MJ et al: Dermatofibrosarcoma protuberans, giant cell fibroblastoma, and hybrid lesions in children: clinicopathologic comparative analysis of 28 cases with molecular data–a study from the French Federation of Cancer Centers Sarcoma Group. Am J Surg Pathol. 27(1):27-39, 2003

(Left) *The pseudovascular spaces of GCFB may appear to be lined by either the mononuclear or multinucleated cells. Importantly, these cells are stromal rather than endothelial.* **(Right)** *The pseudovascular spaces can be prominent and sinusoidal in some cases of GCFB.*

Cells Lining Pseudovascular Spaces

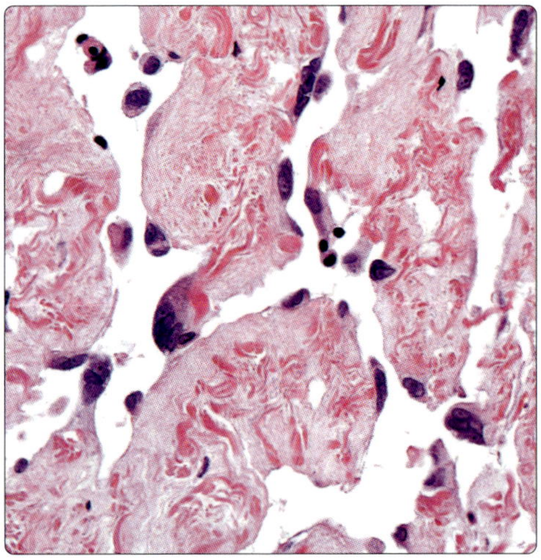

Prominent Pseudovascular Spaces

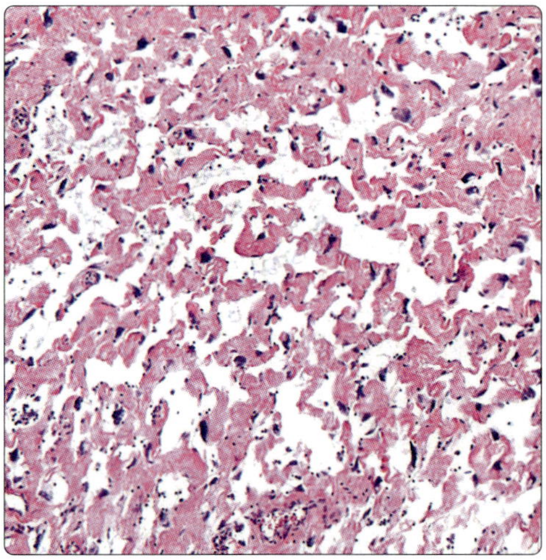

(Left) *When present, the pseudovascular spaces of GCFB may be small, slit-like, and less prominent, as shown on this H&E.* **(Right)** *GCFB is a highly infiltrative tumor and can display extension into both dermal connective tissues and subcutaneous fat. Cutaneous adnexal structures* ⇨*, if present, are often entrapped but spared.*

Inconspicuous Pseudovascular Spaces

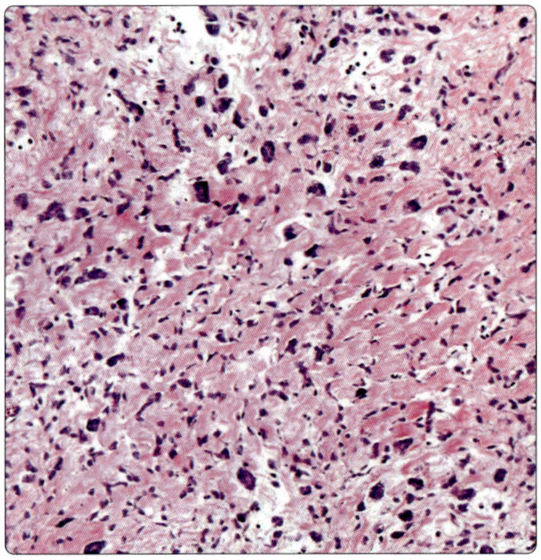

Adnexal Sparing

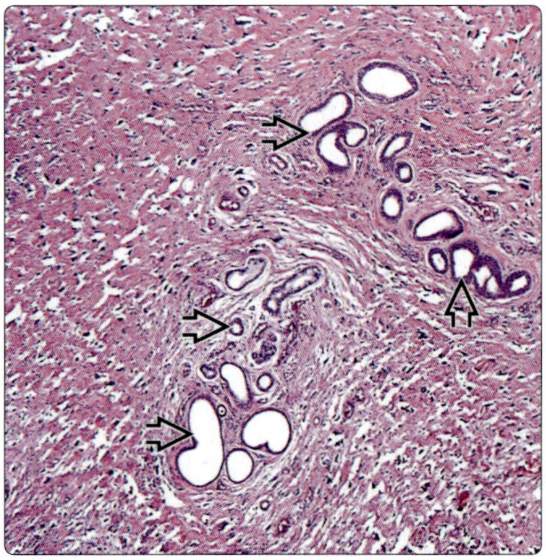

(Left) *Similar to the related dermatofibrosarcoma protuberans (DFSP), GCFB often shows a honeycomb pattern of infiltrative growth into subcutaneous adipose tissue.* **(Right)** *When multinucleated giant cells are prominent in GCFB, the honeycomb pattern of fat infiltration can lead to the mistaken impression of a pleomorphic lipoma or well-differentiated liposarcoma.*

"Honeycomb" Fat Infiltration

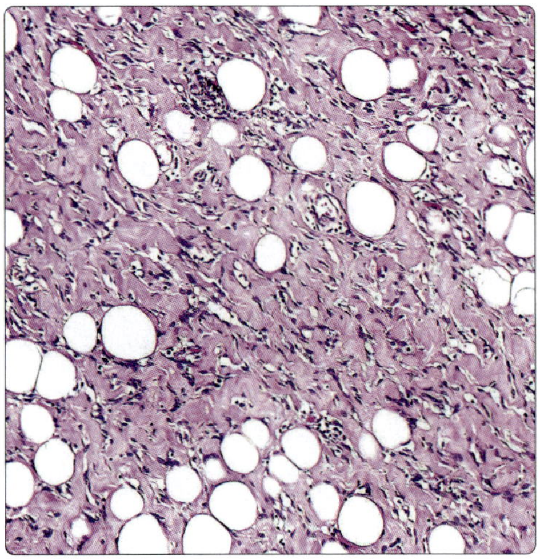

Mimicry of Lipomatous Neoplasm

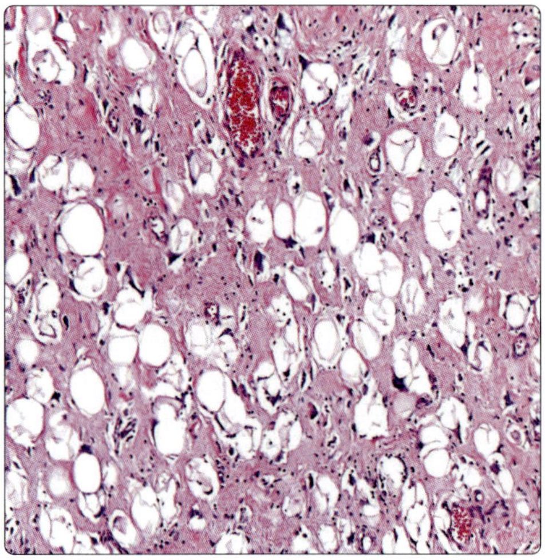

Parallel Cellular Orientation

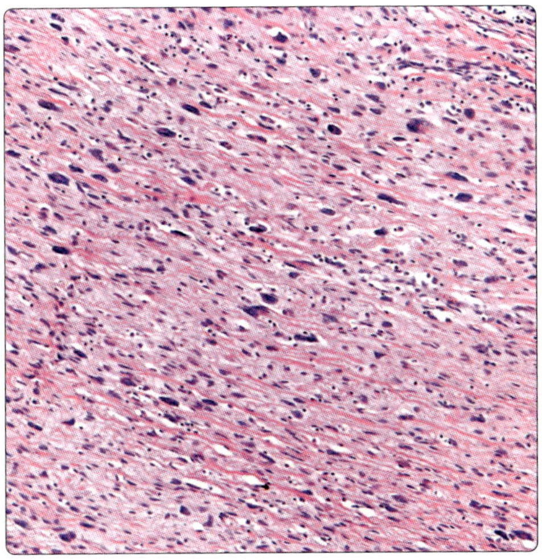

Increased Cellularity

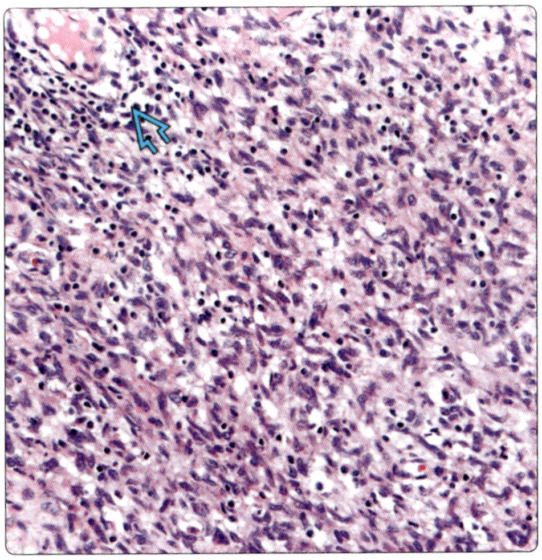

(Left) *The lesional cells of GCFB may show a more orderly but loose parallel arrangement, as depicted. A storiform growth pattern is absent, unless a component of DFSP is present.* **(Right)** *Most cases of GCFB are largely hypocellular; however, some areas can show increased cellularity, as seen on this H&E. This field lacks multinucleated cells. Also note the presence of a perivascular lymphoid infiltrate ⇨, a relatively common finding.*

Prominent Collagenous Stroma

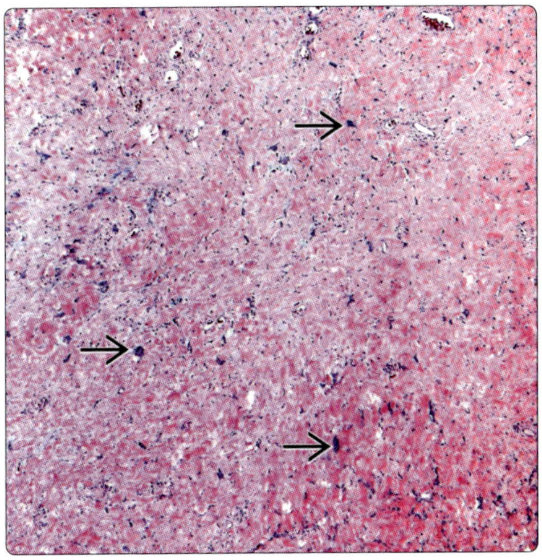

Prominent Myxoid Stroma

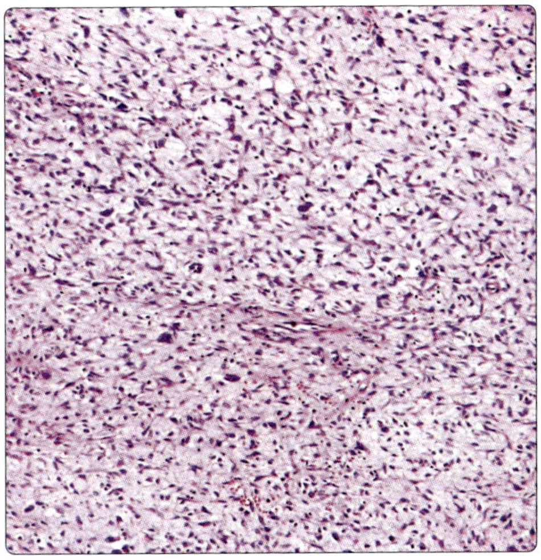

(Left) *Prominent collagenous stroma is a common finding in GCFB and may impart an overall hyalinized or sclerotic appearance to the lesion. Note the multinucleated cells → evident even at low power.* **(Right)** *Myxoid stroma is common in GCFB but varies in extent. The combination of a prominent myxoid stroma and multinucleated floret-like cells may lead to confusion with myxofibrosarcoma. The latter tumor, however, occurs in a much older age group than GCFB.*

Intralesional Hemorrhage

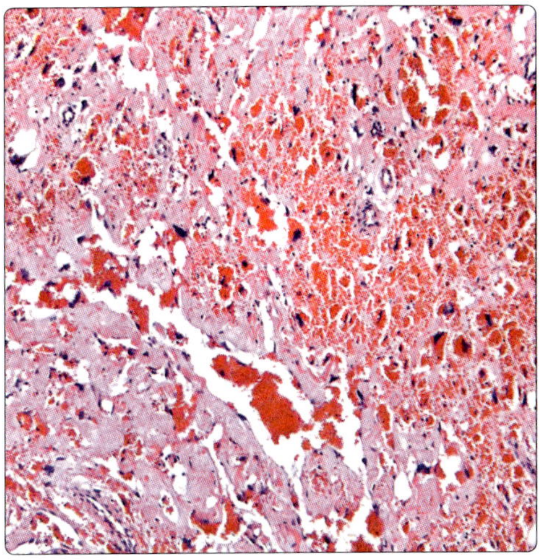

Areas of Conventional Dermatofibrosarcoma Protuberans

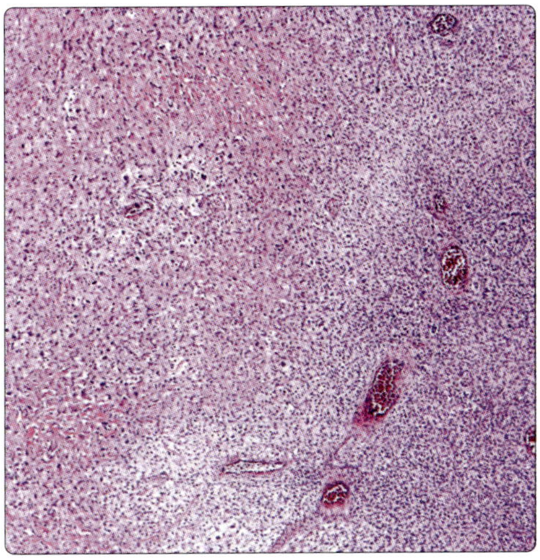

(Left) *Intralesional hemorrhage can be seen in a significant number of cases and, in conjunction with the irregular stromal clefts and spaces, can lead to misdiagnosis as angiosarcoma.* **(Right)** *Areas of DFSP morphology (bottom right) may be seen in some cases of GCFB (hybrid DFSP/GCFB). This component may be identified by a significant increase in cell density and an absence of multinucleated cells and pseudovascular spaces. Evidence of storiform growth is also supportive.*

Infantile Fibrosarcoma

KEY FACTS

TERMINOLOGY

- Synonym: Congenital fibrosarcoma
- Infiltrative, rarely metastasizing fibroblastic sarcoma of infancy associated with *ETV6-NTRK3* gene fusion

CLINICAL ISSUES

- Most arise in 1st year of life (often congenital)
- Superficial and deep soft tissues of distal extremities (most common site)
  - Also trunk and head/neck; rarely visceral sites
- Solitary, rapidly enlarging, often large mass
- Treatment: Complete surgical excision ± chemotherapy
- Overall favorable prognosis
  - Recurrence rate varies (5-50%); metastases are rare

MICROSCOPIC

- Infiltrative growth
- Sheets and intersecting or sweeping fascicles of monomorphic spindled to ovoid cells
  - May show primitive round cell morphology in some cases
  - Mitoses common and may be brisk
- Scattered foci of hemorrhage and necrosis common
- Other findings: Myxoid foci, hemangiopericytoma-like vasculature

ANCILLARY TESTS

- May show SMA(+) or CD34(+) but often focally
- Pan-TRK cytoplasmic positivity
- Desmin, myogenin, keratin, S100 protein (-)
- Molecular: Characteristic t(12;15)(p13;q25) producing *ETV6-NTRK3* gene fusion

TOP DIFFERENTIAL DIAGNOSES

- Lipofibromatosis
- Infantile myofibroma
- Fibrosarcomatous dermatofibrosarcoma protuberans
- Spindle cell rhabdomyosarcoma
- Synovial sarcoma

Infantile Fibrosarcoma

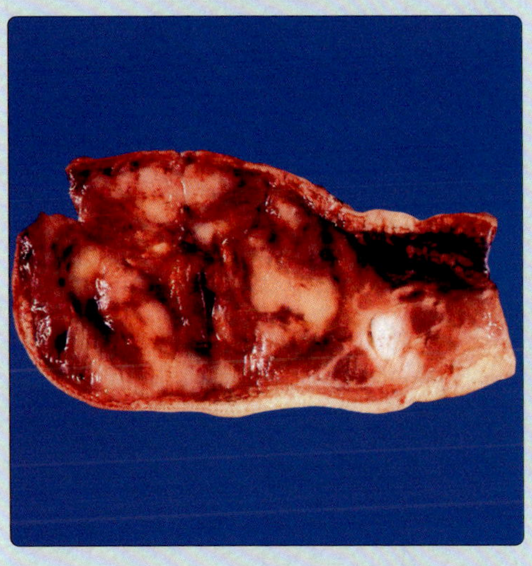

Infantile Fibrosarcoma

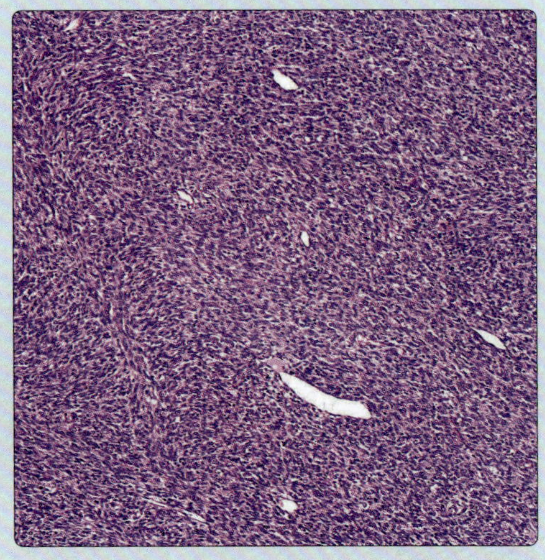

(Left) *Infantile fibrosarcoma (IFS) is a low- to intermediate-grade sarcoma that predominantly affects infants and is often present at birth. Grossly, IFS often forms a large, lobulated mass with a tan, fleshy cut surface and areas of hemorrhage and necrosis.* **(Right)** *Most cases of IFS are densely cellular and resemble adult-type fibrosarcoma; however, the degree of cellularity varies with the stromal collagen content. Significant nuclear pleomorphism is not a feature.*

Infiltration and Entrapment

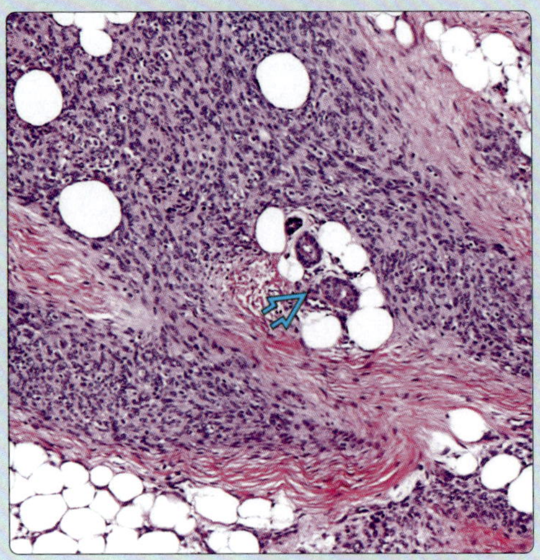

Uniform Cytology

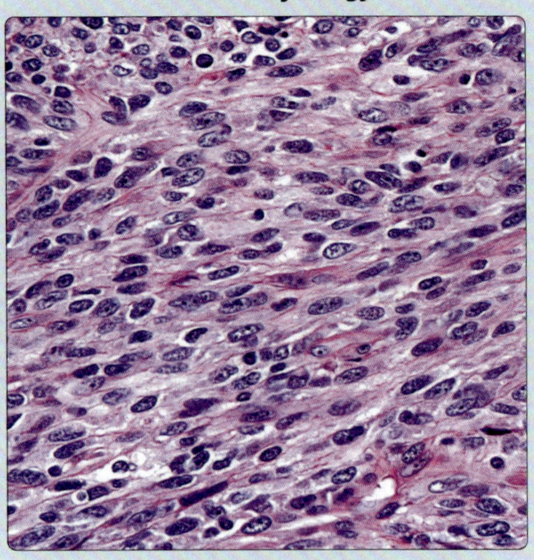

(Left) *IFS is generally an infiltrative neoplasm and grows through adipose tissue and around muscle bundles, nerves, and cutaneous adnexal structures ➲. Some highly fat-infiltrative tumors may resemble lipofibromatosis.* **(Right)** *Nuclei in IFS are atypical but relatively uniform and not pleomorphic. Nucleoli may or may not be identifiable. Mitotic activity is often conspicuous.*

TERMINOLOGY

Abbreviations

- Infantile fibrosarcoma (IFS)

Synonyms

- Congenital fibrosarcoma

Definitions

- Infiltrative, rarely metastasizing fibroblastic sarcoma of infancy associated with *ETV6-NTRK3* gene fusion

CLINICAL ISSUES

Epidemiology

- Age
  - Most arise in 1st year of life
    - Over 1/2 are congenital
      - May be detected and diagnosed antenatally

Site

- Superficial and deep soft tissues of distal extremities (most common)
- Also trunk and head/neck; rarely visceral sites

Presentation

- Solitary, rapidly enlarging, often large mass
- Overlying skin may be erythematous &/or ulcerated

Treatment

- Complete surgical excision with negative margins
- Preoperative chemotherapy also effective

Prognosis

- Overall indolent clinical course with favorable prognosis
  - Recurrence rate up to 50%; metastasis are rare
  - Mortality usually < 5%
    - Often related to local invasion of vital structures
- Spontaneous regression has been reported

MACROSCOPIC

General Features

- Poorly circumscribed, lobulated, tan-gray, firm or fleshy

Size

- Often large (reports up to 30 cm)

MICROSCOPIC

Histologic Features

- Irregular peripheral border
  - May show pseudocapsule formation
- Infiltrative growth
  - Entraps adipose tissue, muscle, nerves, cutaneous adnexal structures
- Sheets and intersecting or sweeping fascicles of monomorphic spindled to ovoid cells
  - May show herringbone architecture
  - Occasional vague storiform growth
- Immature spindled or ovoid cells
  - Tapered, relatively uniform nuclei with variable nucleoli
    - Lacks significant nuclear pleomorphism
  - May show primitive round cell morphology in some cases
  - Mitoses common and may be brisk
- Scattered foci of hemorrhage and necrosis common
- Variable stromal collagen formation
- Other findings
  - Chronic inflammatory infiltrate, myxoid foci, hemangiopericytoma-like vasculature, dystrophic calcification, extramedullary hematopoiesis
  - May contain areas reminiscent of myofibroma
- Postchemotherapy changes include diffuse fibrosis and hypocellular scar-like appearance

ANCILLARY TESTS

Immunohistochemistry

- Variable, often focal SMA(+), CD34(+)
- Desmin, myogenin, keratin, S100 protein (-)
- Pan-TRK(+)
  - Cytoplasmic expression sensitive but not specific for *NTRK3* fusion

Molecular Genetics

- Characteristic t(12;15)(p13;q25) with *ETV6-NTRK3* fusion
  - Also seen in cellular mesoblastic nephroma of kidney
- Rare *EML4-NTRK3* fusion also reported

DIFFERENTIAL DIAGNOSIS

Lipofibromatosis

- Less cellular than IFS; lower mitotic rate; no necrosis
- Pan-TRK(-)
- Lacks *ETV6-NTRK3* fusion

Myofibroma/Myofibromatosis

- Biphasic growth pattern in most cases
- Consistently SMA(+), often diffuse
- Lacks *ETV6-NTRK3* fusion

Synovial Sarcoma

- More common in teenagers and young adults
- Keratin (+), EMA(+), TLE-1(+)
- Characteristic t(X;18)(p11;q11) involving *SS18* (SYT)

Spindle Cell Rhabdomyosarcoma

- Arise predominantly in paratesticular location in kids
- Desmin (+), myogenin (+)
- Rearrangements of *NCOA2* or *VGLL2* in infantile cases

Fibrosarcomatous DFSP

- Usually affects older patients but may be congenital
- Diffuse CD34(+)
- Characteristic *COL1A1-PDGFB* gene fusion

Lipofibromatosis-Like Neural Tumor

- Spindled cells with variable cytologic atypia
- Diffuse S100 protein (+); pan-TRK cytoplasmic positivity
- *NTRK1* gene rearrangements

SELECTED REFERENCES

1. Church AJ et al: Recurrent EML4-NTRK3 fusions in infantile fibrosarcoma and congenital mesoblastic nephroma suggest a revised testing strategy. Mod Pathol. 31(3):463-473, 2018
2. Hung YP et al: Evaluation of pan-TRK immunohistochemistry in infantile fibrosarcoma, lipofibromatosis-like neural tumour and histological mimics. Histopathology. 73(4):634-644, 2018

(Left) *Although the rate is variable, mitotic figures ➡ are usually easily identified in IFS. In some cases, mitoses are numerous.* **(Right)** *Fascicular growth is a common feature of IFS and may be prominent. A herringbone architectural pattern may be seen focally in some cases. Others show more sheet-like growth or, rarely, a focal, vague storiform architecture.*

Mitoses Common

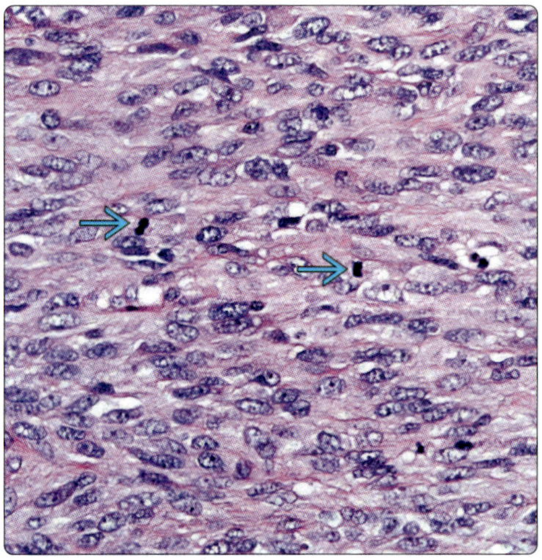

Fascicular Growth

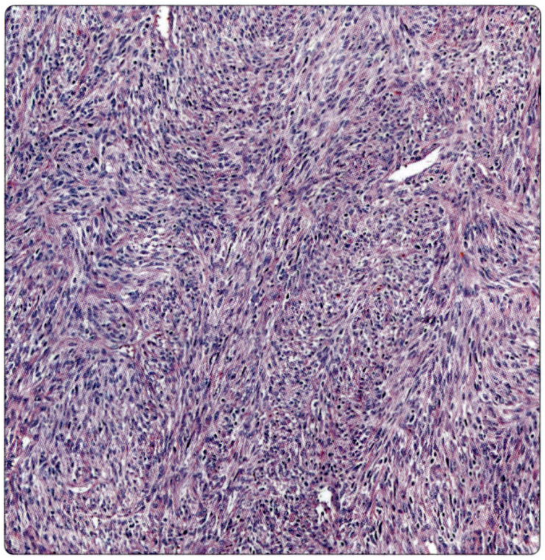

(Left) *When viewed in cross section, fascicles of spindled tumor cells often appear more rounded. Some tumors may show alternating spindled ➡ and round cell areas ⇨.* **(Right)** *Small, thin-walled vascular channels are a common finding in IFS but in some cases appear markedly dilated and irregular, imparting a staghorn appearance, similar to what is seen in a solitary fibrous tumor, among other neoplasms.*

Fascicular Growth

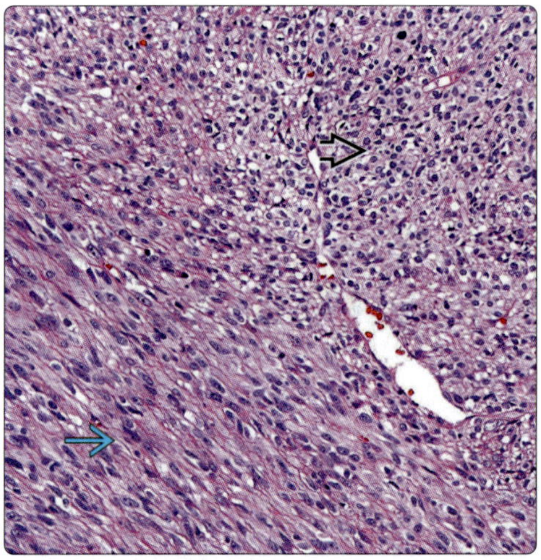

Thin-Walled Vasculature

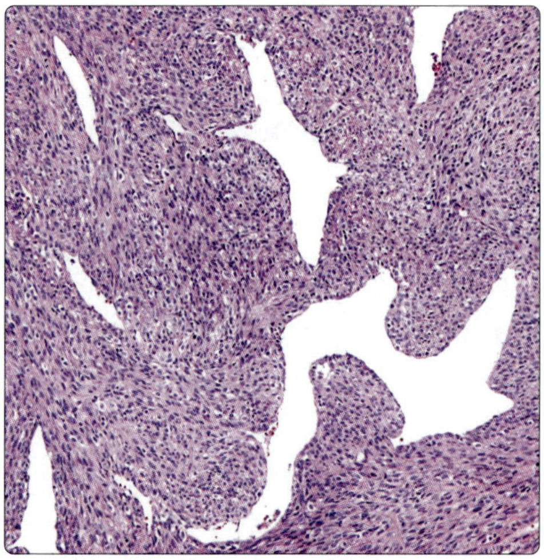

(Left) *A focally prominent ramifying hemangiopericytoma-like pattern composed of extensive irregular and ectatic vascular channels is depicted in this example of IFS. Most other fields demonstrated more conventional solid growth.* **(Right)** *Although not present in all tumors, some cases of IFS show perivascular edema or myxoid change, as depicted.*

Hemangiopericytoma-Like Vasculature

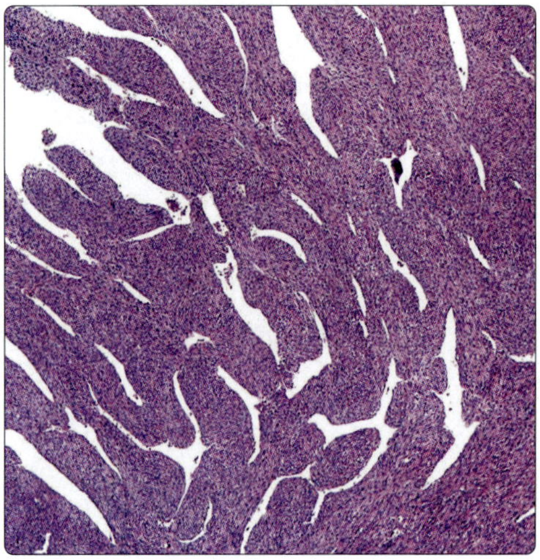

Perivascular Edema

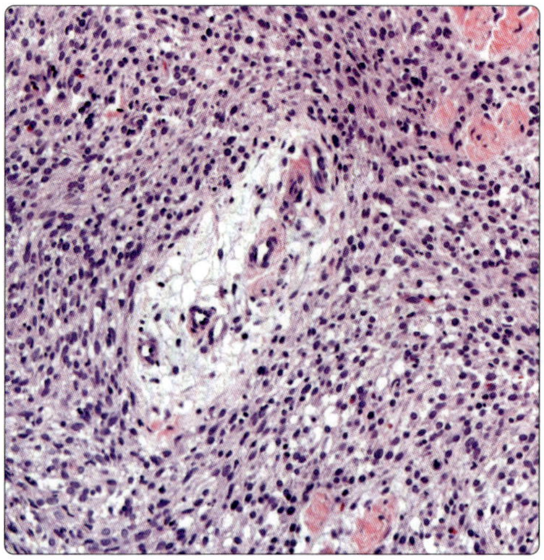

Necrosis

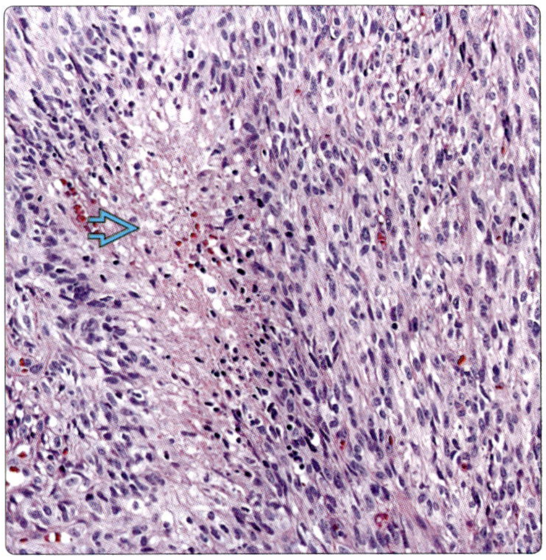

Chronic Inflammatory Infiltrate

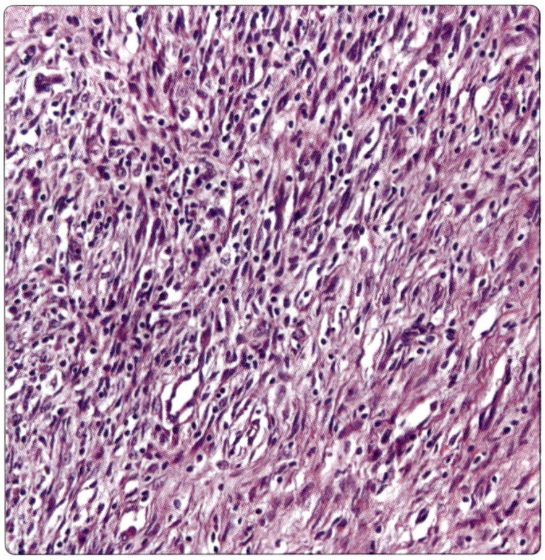

(Left) *Foci of tumor necrosis* ➡ *and hemorrhage are common in IFS and are often also identifiable at the time of gross examination. Occasional cases show widespread, zonal necrosis.* **(Right)** *A chronic inflammatory infiltrate, usually composed of lymphocytes, is a relatively common finding in IFS but varies in degree from brisk to very subtle.*

Immature Round Cell Morphology

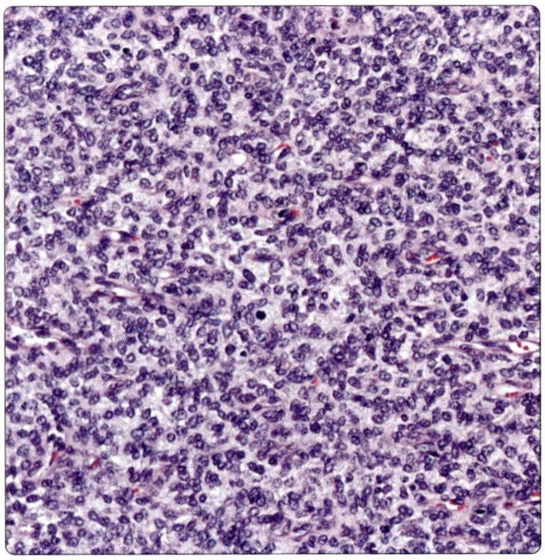

Cutaneous Extension

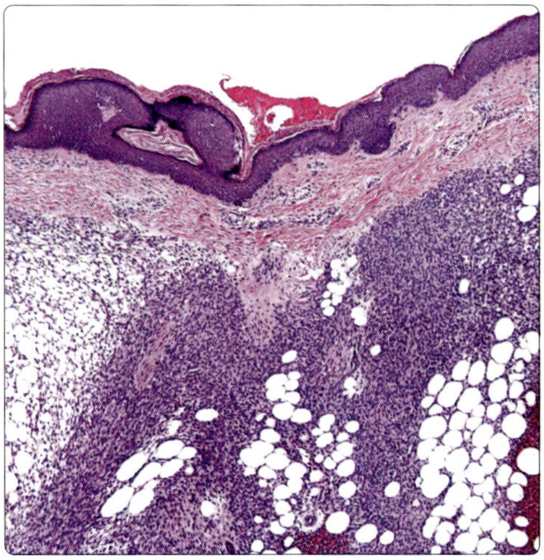

(Left) *In some cases of IFS, tumor cells adopt a cellular immature round cell morphology. Spindled areas are often present elsewhere but may be inconspicuous.* **(Right)** *Larger examples of IFS may show involvement of the overlying skin, and ulceration is not uncommon. Entrapment of adipose tissue and adnexal structures is typical, given the infiltrative nature of the tumor.*

Myxoid Change

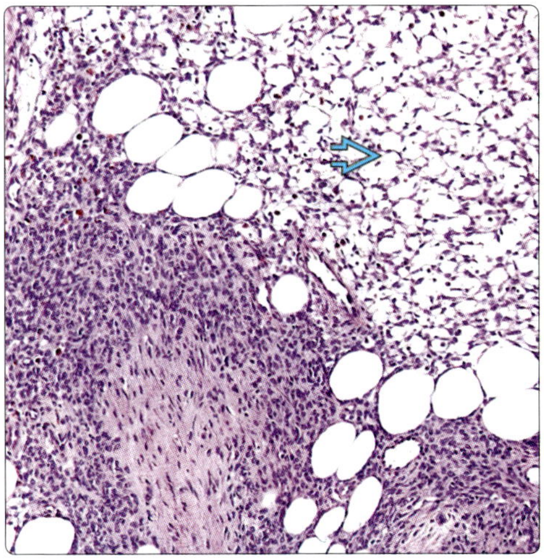

Cellular Mesoblastic Nephroma of Kidney

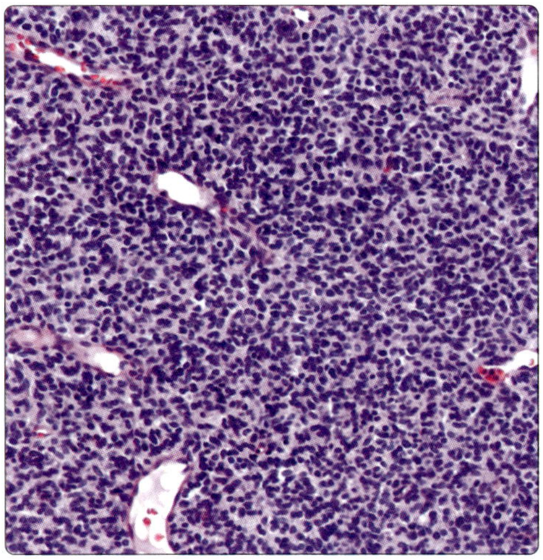

(Left) *Myxoid change* ➡ *may be seen focally in IFS. Note the more conventional spindled morphology (lower left).* **(Right)** *IFS is characterized by a distinctive chromosomal translocation, t(12;15)(p13;q25), resulting in ETV6-NTRK3 gene fusion. An identical translocation is present in cellular mesoblastic nephroma (shown), a renal neoplasm that shows histologic similarity to IFS.*

SECTION 6

Fibrohistiocytic, Histiocytic, and Dendritic Cell Tumors

Benign

Dermatofibroma and Fibrous Histiocytoma 270
Deep Benign Fibrous Histiocytoma 276
Localized-Type Tenosynovial Giant Cell Tumor 278
Diffuse-Type Tenosynovial Giant Cell Tumor 284
Cellular Neurothekeoma 290
Xanthomas 294
Solitary (Juvenile) Xanthogranuloma 298
Reticulohistiocytoma 300
Deep Granuloma Annulare 304
Rheumatoid Nodule 306
Langerhans Cell Histiocytosis 308
Extranodal Rosai-Dorfman Disease 310
Crystal-Storing Histiocytosis 314

Intermediate (Rarely Metastasizing)

Plexiform Fibrohistiocytic Tumor 316
Giant Cell Tumor of Soft Tissue 320

Malignant

Histiocytic Sarcoma 324
Follicular Dendritic Cell Sarcoma 326
Interdigitating Dendritic Cell Sarcoma 328

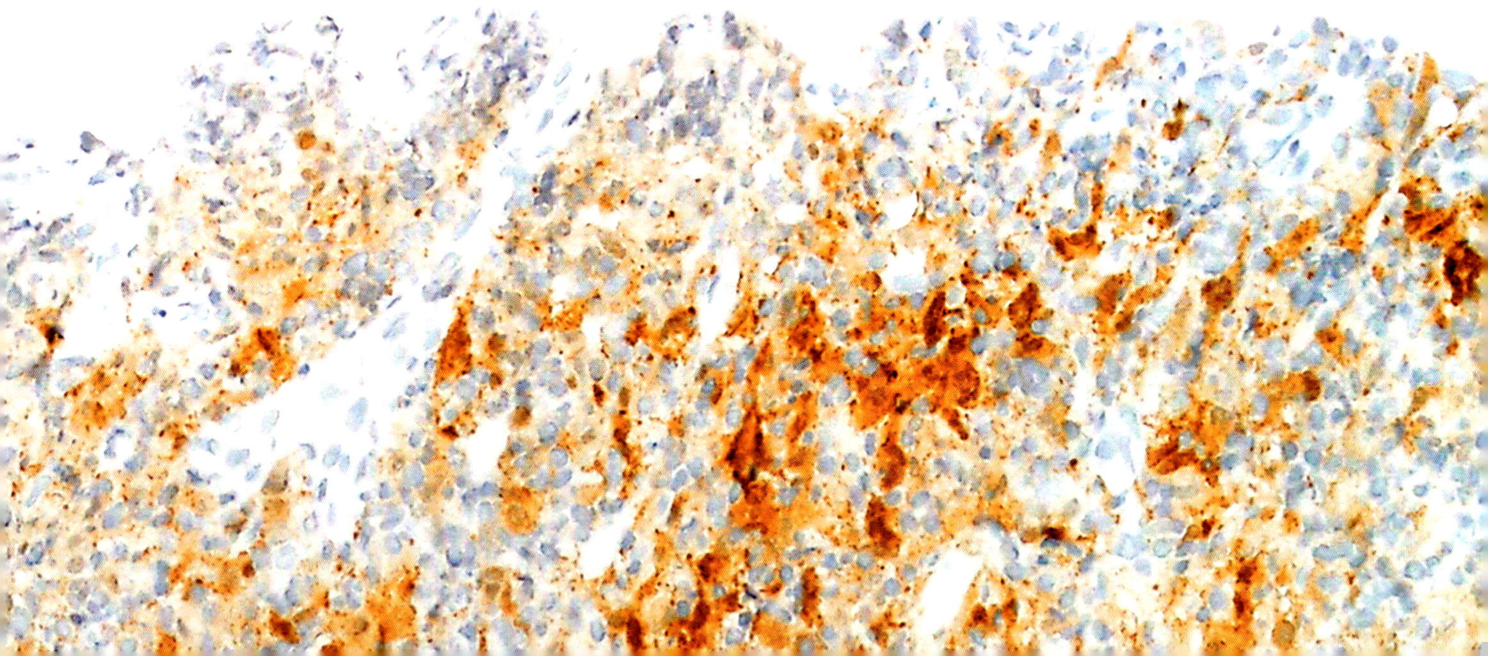

Dermatofibroma and Fibrous Histiocytoma

KEY FACTS

TERMINOLOGY

- Benign, limited proliferation of histiocytic and fibroblastic cells in dermis
- Terms dermatofibroma (DF) and fibrous histiocytoma (FH) are interchangeable

ETIOLOGY/PATHOGENESIS

- Evidence supports both neoplastic and reactive pathogenesis

CLINICAL ISSUES

- Affects all ages but most common in young adults
- Typically occur on distal extremities but may present at any cutaneous site
- Firm, isolated, flesh-colored, subcutaneous papule or nodule
- Excellent prognosis in vast majority of cases
  - Metastasis and death in very rare cases of cellular and atypical DF

MICROSCOPIC

- Dermal-based proliferation of typically bland, spindled to histiocytoid-appearing cells
  - Early lesions typically show more histiocytes and lymphocytes
- Characteristic collagen trapping at periphery
- Overlying epithelial basilar induction with hyperpigmentation
- Numerous morphologic variants

ANCILLARY TESTS

- FXIIIA(+), CD163(+), CD68(+), CD34(-)

TOP DIFFERENTIAL DIAGNOSES

- Dermatofibrosarcoma protuberans
- Atypical fibroxanthoma
- Basal cell carcinoma
- Angiosarcoma

Dermatofibroma

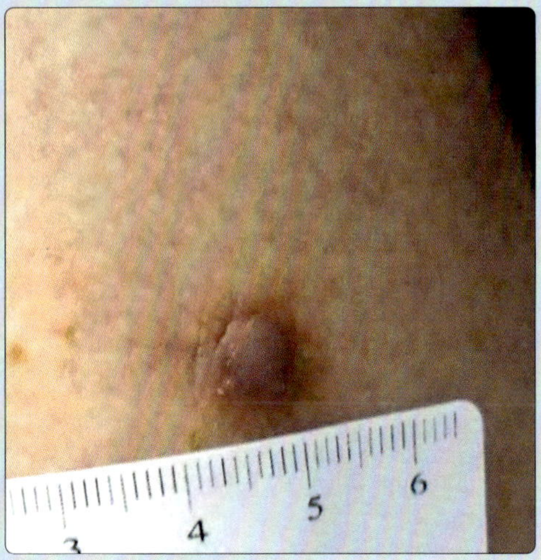

Dermal Spindle Cell Proliferation With Epidermal Hyperplasia

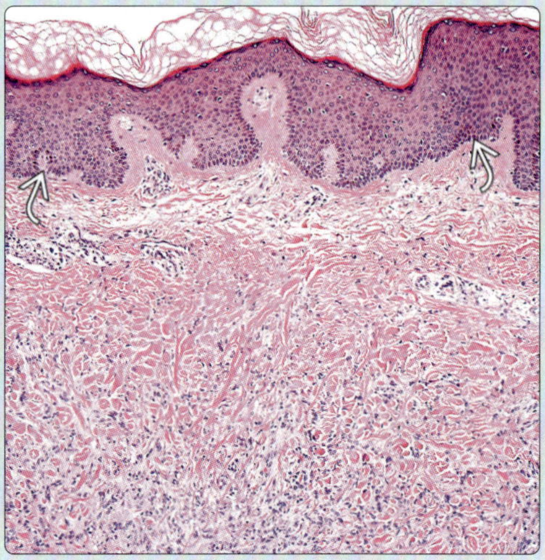

(Left) *This photograph shows the typical appearance of dermatofibroma (DF), occurring here on the lower leg of an adult patient, which is a common presentation of this tumor. Note the light reddish/brown appearance of the lesion.* **(Right)** *Classic DF shows a dermal-based proliferation of small, bland, spindled to histiocytic-appearing cells associated with a grenz zone. Note the overlying epidermal hyperplasia with basilar pigmentation* ➡.

Collagen Entrapment

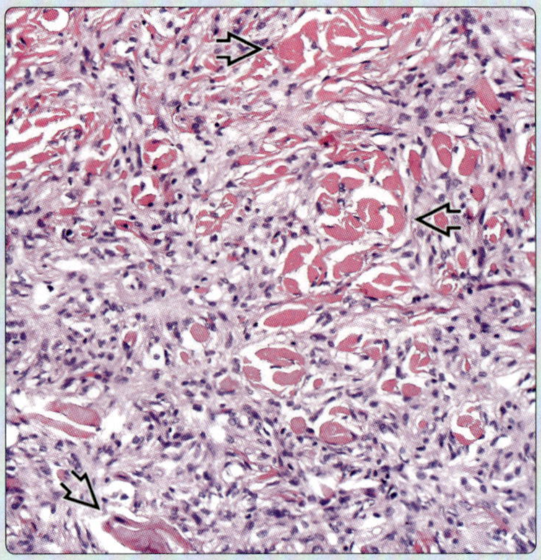

Hemosiderotic Dermatofibroma With Sclerosis

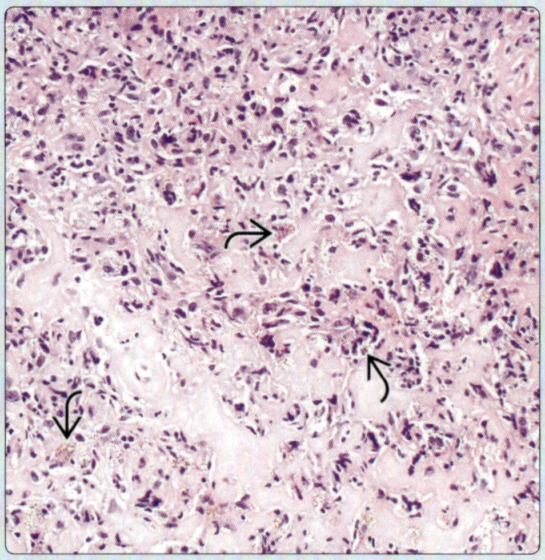

(Left) *Higher power examination of a classic DF shows a proliferation of bland, spindled to histiocytoid cells entrapping numerous hyalinized balls of collagen* ➡. **(Right)** *This is an example of a hemosiderotic (or sclerosing hemangioma) variant of DF with prominent stromal sclerosis and hemosiderin within many of the histiocytic cells* ➡.

TERMINOLOGY

Abbreviations

- Dermatofibroma (DF)
- Fibrous histiocytoma (FH)

Synonyms

- Cutaneous FH
- Sclerosing hemangioma

Definitions

- Common, benign, localized proliferation of fibroblastic and histiocytic cells in dermis
- DF and FH are interchangeable terms

ETIOLOGY/PATHOGENESIS

Unknown

- Evidence supports both reactive and neoplastic pathogenesis
  - Histiocytic population may be clonal; fibroblast/myofibroblastic population may be polyclonal (reactive)
- Tumor may be preceded by local trauma, including insect bite, in some cases
  - However, no inciting event identified in majority of cases

CLINICAL ISSUES

Epidemiology

- Incidence
  - Common tumors in most populations
- Age
  - All but most common in 4th and 5th decades
- Sex
  - Occur in male and female patients equally

Site

- Typically occur on distal extremities but may present at any cutaneous site

Presentation

- Firm, isolated, flesh-colored, subcutaneous papule or nodule
  - New DFs are typically pink (vascular); older DFs are brown (overlying epidermal hyperplasia with basilar pigmentation)
- Multiple DFs may occur in immunosuppressed populations
- Dimpling sign when in vivo DF is pinched by fingers

Treatment

- Complete excision is curative in most cases
- Reexcision &/or clinical follow-up of cellular, atypical, and aneurysmal variants may be prudent

Prognosis

- Excellent in vast majority of cases
  - Local recurrence potentially significant (up to 30%) with cellular variant
  - Very rare reports of metastasis and death from otherwise benign-appearing DF/FH
    - Most are cellular, aneurysmal, or atypical morphologic variants
    - Usually large and deep, cellular lesions

MACROSCOPIC

General Features

- Firm, circumscribed, but nonencapsulated, dermal-based tumor
- White to yellow cut surface
- Can have cystic changes and hemorrhage

MICROSCOPIC

Histologic Features

- Tumors are grossly circumscribed but microscopically have irregular, often jagged borders
- Dermal-based proliferation of typically bland, spindled to histiocytoid-appearing cells
  - Either spindled (fibroblastic) or histiocytoid cells may predominate
  - Early lesions typically show more histiocytes and lymphocytes
  - Established lesions show greater cellularity and spindled cells
  - Older lesions show more fibrosis
  - Spindled cells show elongated eosinophilic cytoplasmic processes
  - Histiocytic-type cells are larger, epithelioid-shaped, and have abundant, pale, vacuolated cytoplasm
  - Cytologic atypia and pleomorphism are usually minimal but can be present
- Collagen trapping at periphery
  - Spheres of intensely eosinophilic collagen (so-called collagen balls) separated by bands of pale fibrohistiocytic cells
- Grenz zone
  - Tumor often spares band of superficial papillary dermis
- Folliculosebaceous induction and basilar epidermal hyperplasia overlying DF
  - Can mimic basal cell carcinoma (BCC) if basilar induction is marked, especially in superficial shave biopsy
- Overlying epidermal hyperplasia with basilar hyperpigmentation is common, occasional melanocytic hyperplasia
  - So-called dirty feet or dirty sock sign
- Adjacent adnexal hyperplasia

Morphologic Variants

- Aneurysmal
  - Also described as hemosiderotic/sclerosing hemangioma variant of DF/FH
  - Pseudovascular spaces, hemosiderin, reactive spindled and epithelioid cells
    - May mimic vascular tumor, including Kaposi sarcoma and angiosarcoma
  - Aneurysmal DF can show mild cytologic atypia but lacks high-grade atypia, infiltrative features, and increased or atypical mitotic figures
- Cellular
  - Uncommon, often large, deeply penetrating tumors
    - May show overlapping features with atypical DF
    - Occasional mitoses and multinucleated cells are seen
    - Up to 12% of cases may show focal central necrosis

- Most likely subtype to recur (up to 30% in some studies)
- Epithelioid
  - Also described as epithelioid cell histiocytoma and may represent distinct tumor
  - Nodular to sheet-like, well-circumscribed proliferation of plump cells in papillary dermis
    - Often has associated epidermal collarette
- Atypical
  - Also described as pseudosarcomatous DF or DF with monster cells
  - Shows population of atypical cells with nuclear hyperchromasia and prominent nucleoli, often with abundant cytoplasm
    - Mitotic figures are sparse, usually not atypical in appearance
- Lipidized
  - Often large tumors, typically present in ankle region
  - Numerous large, foamy cells are present with few hemosiderin-containing cells
  - Stromal hyalinization is typically present, which may be wiry or keloidal in appearance
- Many other rare variants described, including granular cell, clear cell, histiocytic/xanthomatous, osteoclastic, myxoid, keloidal/scar-like, palisading, deep penetrating [may mimic dermatofibrosarcoma protuberans (DFSP)], and lichenoid

ANCILLARY TESTS

Immunohistochemistry

- FXIIIA, CD10, CD163, HMGA1/HMGA2, MMP-11 (+)
  - CD68(+) but may be weak; typically highlights histiocytic-appearing cells
  - Focal SMA(+); may indicate myofibroblastic differentiation
- Recent reports of ALK1 expression in epithelioid FH
- CD34 typically (-) but may show focal staining, especially at periphery of lesion (but should lack strong and diffuse staining typical of DFSP)
- S100, MART-1/Melan-A, HMB-45, CD31, cytokeratins, desmin, nestin (-)

DIFFERENTIAL DIAGNOSIS

Dermatofibrosarcoma Protuberans

- Shows deep, cellular, monotonous proliferation of spindled cells
- Typically extends deeply along septa of subcutaneous fat with honeycomb-like fat entrapment
- CD34(+), nestin (+), CD163(-), HMGA1/HMGA2(-), FXIIIA(±)

Basal Cell Carcinoma

- In superficial biopsies, BCC may be difficult to distinguish from benign follicular induction overlying DF
  - CK20 highlights Merkel cells in basal layer overlying DF; these cells are typically absent in BCC

Angiosarcoma

- May be considered in differential diagnosis with aneurysmal DF
- Infiltrative, dissecting growth pattern with endothelial atypia in most cases
- CD31, CD34 (+)

Kaposi Sarcoma

- Nodular/tumor stage Kaposi sarcoma shows atypical cellular spindle cell proliferation
- Slit-like vascular spaces and extravasated red blood cells are often present
  - CD31, HHV8 (+)

Atypical Fibroxanthoma

- Dermal nodule composed of highly atypical spindled and pleomorphic epithelioid cells
- Typically occurs in heavily sun-damaged skin (especially head and neck area) of elderly patients
  - Both atypical fibroxanthoma (AFX) and DF are positive for nonspecific markers, including CD68, CD10, and vimentin
  - FXIIIA may show greater positivity in DF

DIAGNOSTIC CHECKLIST

Clinically Relevant Pathologic Features

- Cellularity and atypia
- Tumor size (more aggressive cases typically large and deep)

Pathologic Interpretation Pearls

- "Collagen balls" classically seen
- Basilar epidermal induction with hyperpigmentation
- Occasional adnexal and melanocytic hyperplasia

SELECTED REFERENCES

1. Acar EM et al: Hemosiderotic dermatofibroma mimicking melanoma in a 12-year-old boy: a case report. Clin Case Rep. 6(6):1006-9, 2018
2. Felty CC et al: Epithelioid fibrous histiocytoma: a concise review. Am J Dermatopathol. ePub, 2018
3. Jedrych JJ et al: Aneurysmal fibrous histiocytomas with recurrent rearrangement of the PRKCD gene and LAMTOR1-PRKCD fusions. J Cutan Pathol. 45(12):966-8, 2018
4. Liu S et al: Giant aneurysmal benign fibrous histiocytoma (dermatofibroma). J Cutan Pathol. 45(10):774-6, 2018
5. Beatrous SV et al: Associated conditions in patients with multiple dermatofibromas: case reports and literature review. Dermatol Online J. 23(9), 2017
6. Romano RC et al: Fibrohistiocytic tumors. Clin Lab Med. 37(3):603-31, 2017
7. Jedrych J et al: Epithelioid cell histiocytoma of the skin with clonal ALK gene rearrangement resulting in VCL-ALK and SQSTM1-ALK gene fusions. Br J Dermatol. 172(5):1427-9, 2014
8. Doyle LA et al: Metastasizing "benign" cutaneous fibrous histiocytoma: a clinicopathologic analysis of 16 cases. Am J Surg Pathol. 37(4):484-95, 2013
9. Fernandez-Flores A et al: Mitosis in dermatofibroma: a worrisome histopathologic sign that does not necessarily equal recurrence. J Cutan Pathol. 35(9):839-42, 2008
10. Gleason BC et al: Deep "benign" fibrous histiocytoma: clinicopathologic analysis of 69 cases of a rare tumor indicating occasional metastatic potential. Am J Surg Pathol. 32(3):354-62, 2008
11. Mori T et al: Expression of nestin in dermatofibrosarcoma protuberans in comparison to dermatofibroma. J Dermatol. 35(7):419-25, 2008
12. Sachdev R et al: Expression of CD163 in dermatofibroma, cellular fibrous histiocytoma, and dermatofibrosarcoma protuberans: comparison with CD68, CD34, and Factor XIIIa. J Cutan Pathol. 33(5):353-60, 2006
13. Mahmoodi M et al: Anti-cytokeratin 20 staining of Merkel cells helps differentiate basaloid proliferations overlying dermatofibromas from basal cell carcinoma. J Cutan Pathol. 32(7):491-5, 2005
14. Hui P et al: Clonal analysis of cutaneous fibrous histiocytoma (dermatofibroma). J Cutan Pathol. 29(7):385-9, 2002
15. Kaddu S et al: Atypical fibrous histiocytoma of the skin: clinicopathologic analysis of 59 cases with evidence of infrequent metastasis. Am J Surg Pathol. 26(1):35-46, 2002
16. Chen TC et al: Dermatofibroma is a clonal proliferative disease. J Cutan Pathol. 27(1):36-9, 2000
17. Altman DA et al: Differential expression of factor XIIIa and CD34 in cutaneous mesenchymal tumors. J Cutan Pathol. 20(2):154-8, 1993

Hemosiderotic and Cellular Dermatofibroma

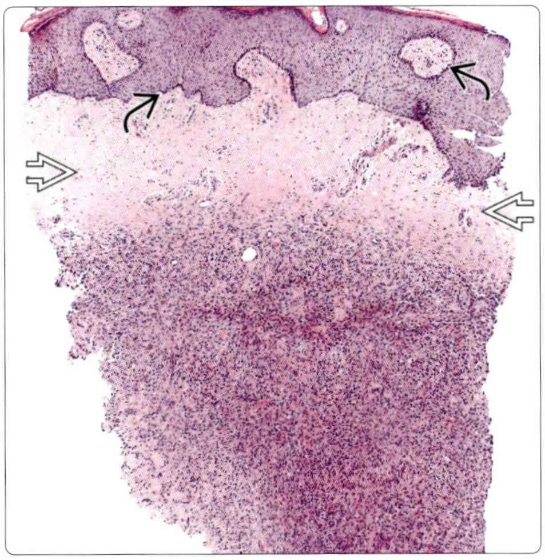

Hemosiderotic and Cellular Dermatofibroma

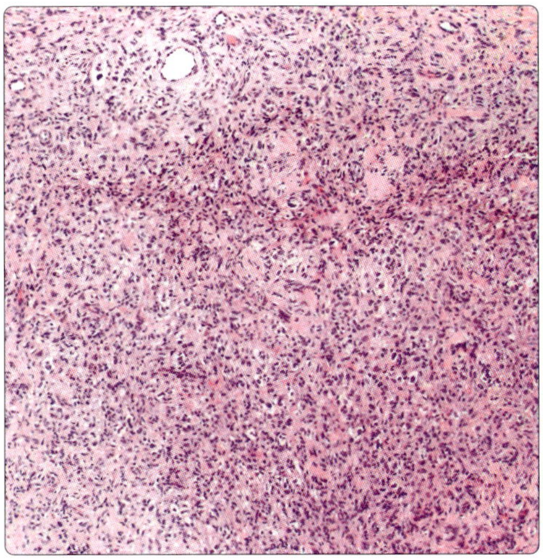

(Left) *This is an example of a hemosiderotic and cellular DF with a prominent grenz zone separating the lesion from the overlying epidermis. Note the marked epidermal acanthosis and basilar pigmentation also present.* **(Right)** *Intermediate magnification of the dermal tumor in the same patient shows a cellular proliferation of spindled and histiocytic cells associated with a sclerotic stroma.*

Aneurysmal Variant

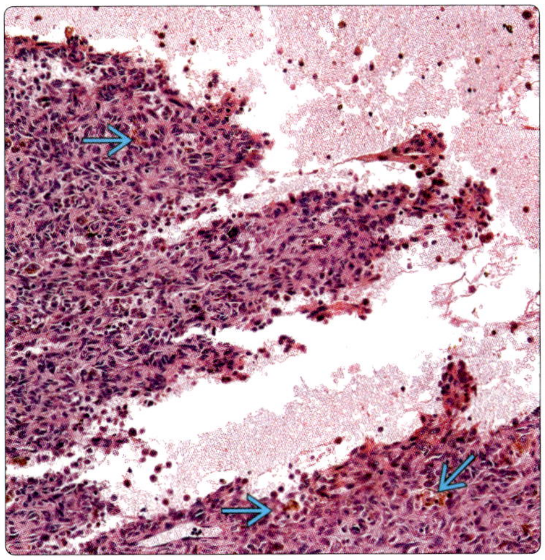

Hemosiderin-Laden Macrophages

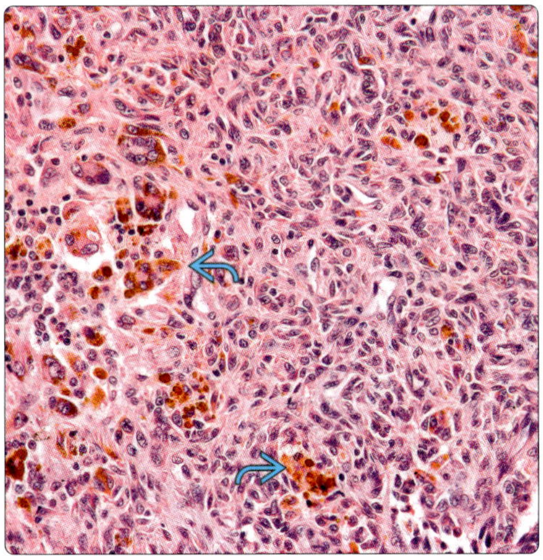

(Left) *An example of an aneurysmal fibrous histiocytoma shows large, irregular, blood-filled spaces and prominent hemosiderin deposition.* **(Right)** *Higher magnification of an aneurysmal fibrous histiocytoma shows numerous hemosiderin-laden multinucleated macrophages.*

Histiocytic Variant

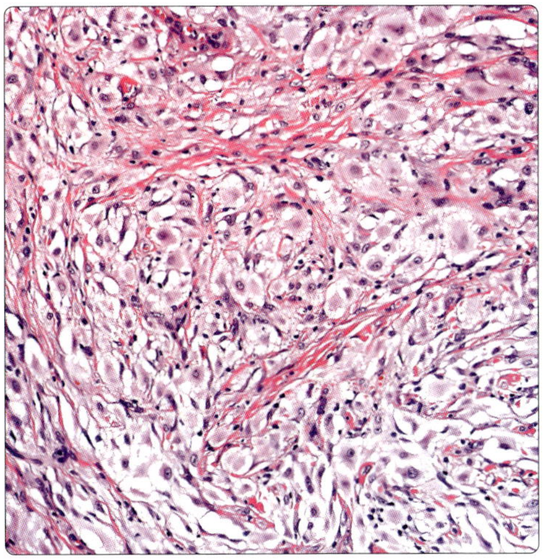

Histiocytic Variant

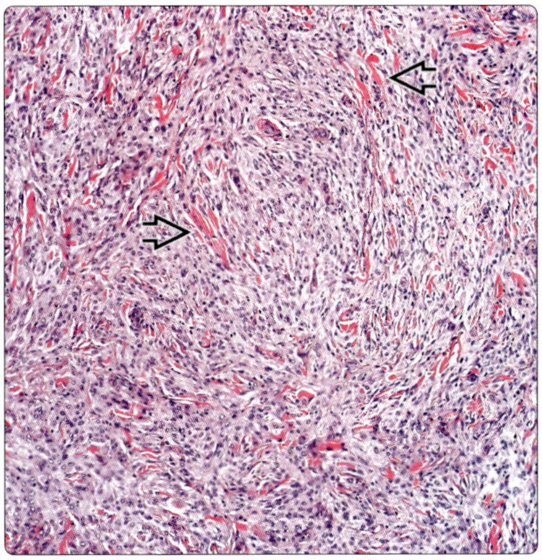

(Left) *High-power examination of histiocytic DF shows a proliferation of large, epithelioid-shaped cells with abundant, pale to vacuolated cytoplasm and bland-appearing nuclei.* **(Right)** *Histiocyte-predominant DF shows a proliferation of large, epithelioid-appearing cells with abundant, pale/vacuolated cytoplasm and scattered, small, entrapped collagen bundles.*

(Left) *Scanning magnification shows an otherwise typical-appearing DF with overlying epidermal hyperplasia and a small associated osteoma cutis ➙.* **(Right)** *Higher power view of scar-like DF shows dense and glassy-appearing bundles of keloidal collagen ➩.*

Incidental Osteoma Cutis in Dermatofibroma

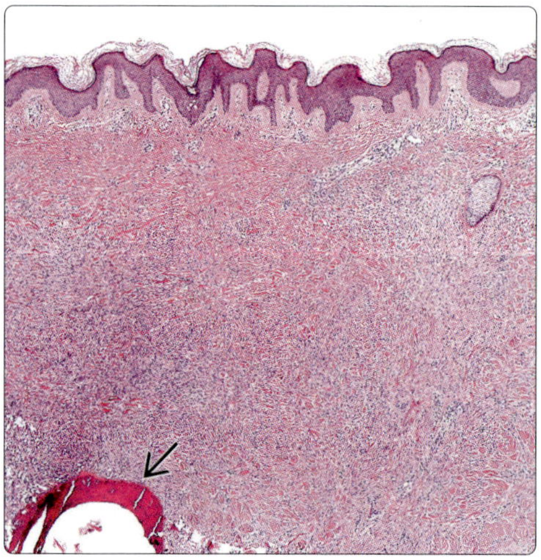

Scar-Like Dermatofibroma With Keloidal Collagen

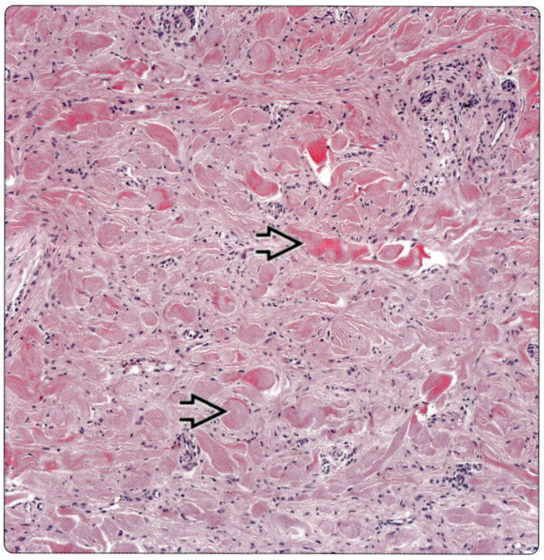

(Left) *Low-power view of an epithelioid cell histiocytoma (DF variant) shows a relatively cellular proliferation of histiocytic-appearing cells. These tumors often have an associated epidermal collarette, a feature not seen in conventional DFs.* **(Right)** *High-power view of an epithelioid cell histiocytoma shows a relatively cellular proliferation of small, bland, histiocytic-appearing cells. The stroma is vascular and fibrotic but does not show prominent collagen entrapment.*

Epithelioid Cell Histiocytoma

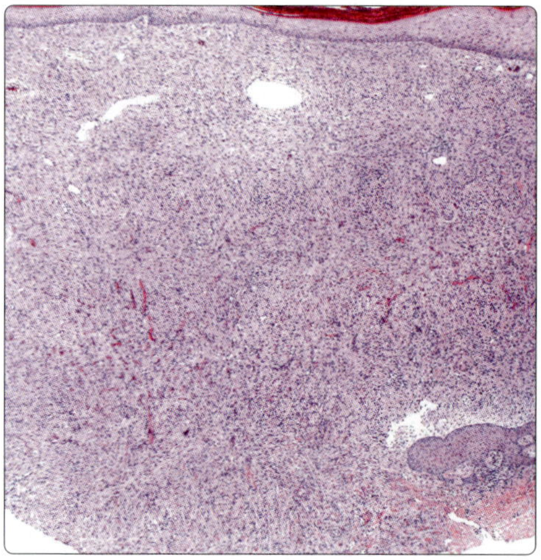

Epithelioid Cell Histiocytoma

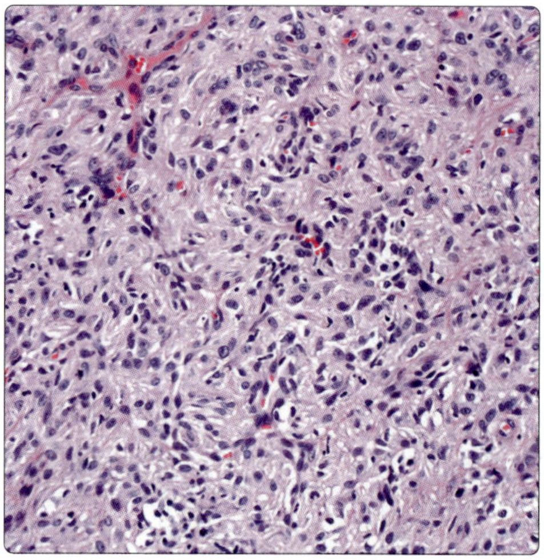

(Left) *Low-power view of a cellular DF shows a dense proliferation of spindled and histiocytic-appearing cells with nuclear hyperchromasia.* **(Right)** *Higher power view of a cellular DF with focal atypia (or so-called DF with monster cells) shows scattered, bizarre-appearing cells with enlarged, irregular, hyperchromatic-staining nuclei ➩.*

Cellular Variant

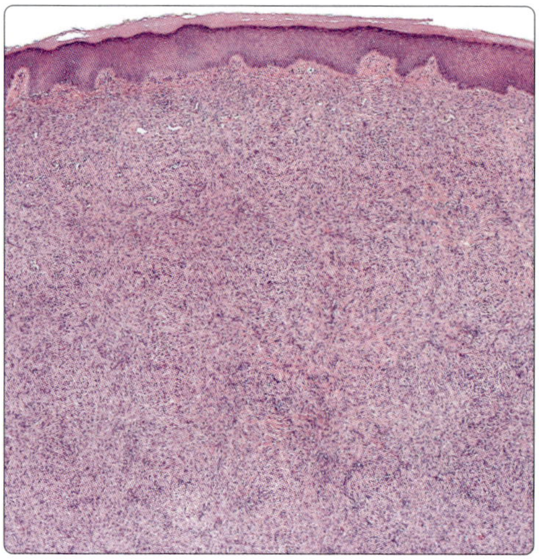

Cellular Variant With Atypia

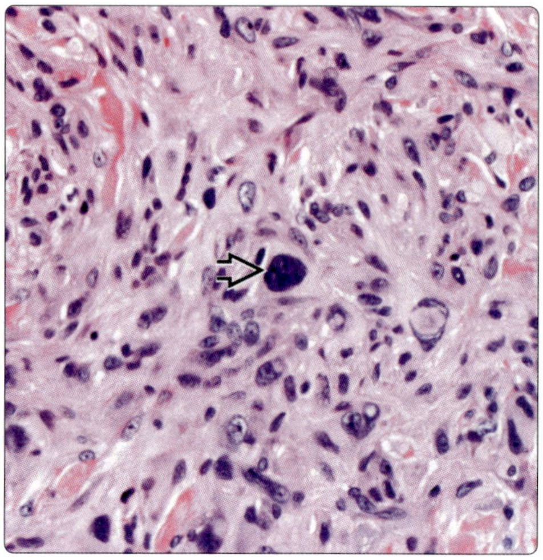

FXIIIA Expression

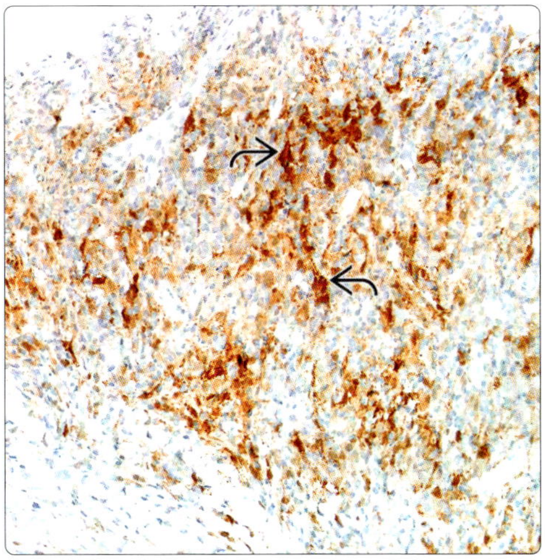

FXIIIA Expression

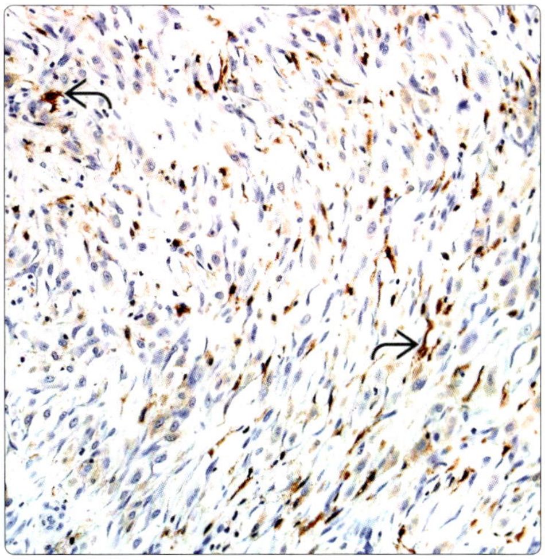

(Left) *Strongly positive FXIIIA staining of many of the spindled and dendritic-appearing tumor cells* ➲ *is seen in some cases of DF.* **(Right)** *Weakly positive FXIIIA stain in a biopsy shows weak/patchy staining of the tumoral spindled cells and stronger staining of scattered dermal dendritic cells* ➲.

CD163 Expression

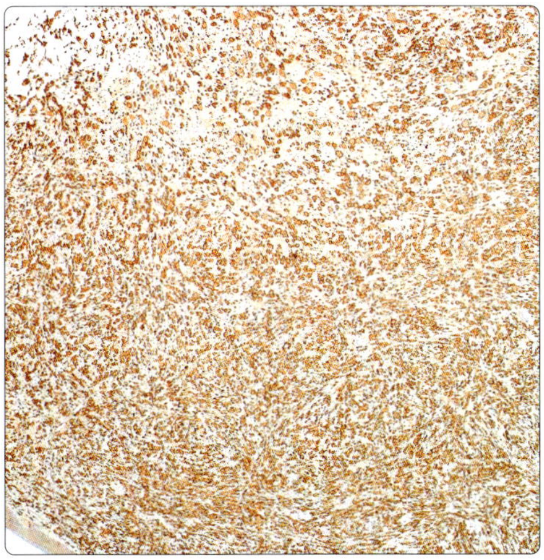

CD34 Staining

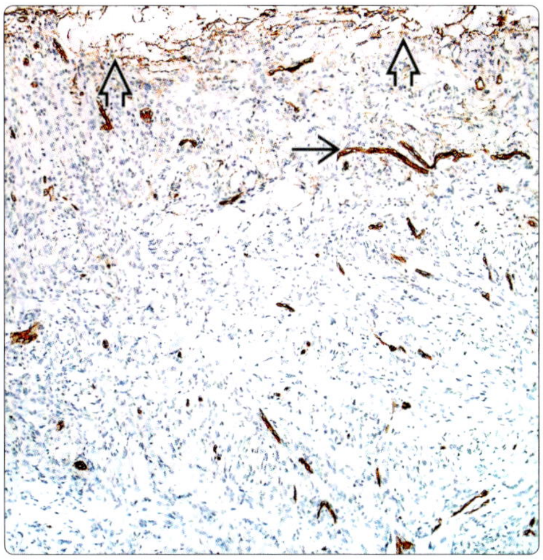

(Left) *CD163 IHC shows strong and diffuse staining in a cellular and histiocytic-type DF. CD163 is a more sensitive marker and usually shows stronger staining than FXIIIA.* **(Right)** *CD34 strongly highlights vessels* ➜ *and shows weak background staining of some of the peripheral dermis* ⇧ *but is negative within the tumoral cells.*

Differential Diagnosis: Dermatofibrosarcoma Protuberans

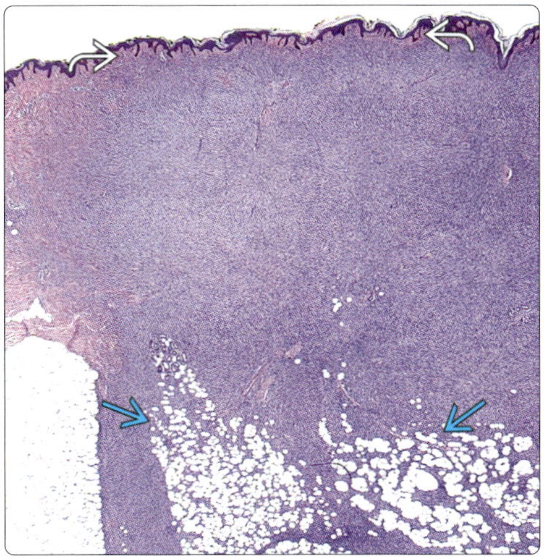

Higher Magnification of Dermatofibrosarcoma Protuberans

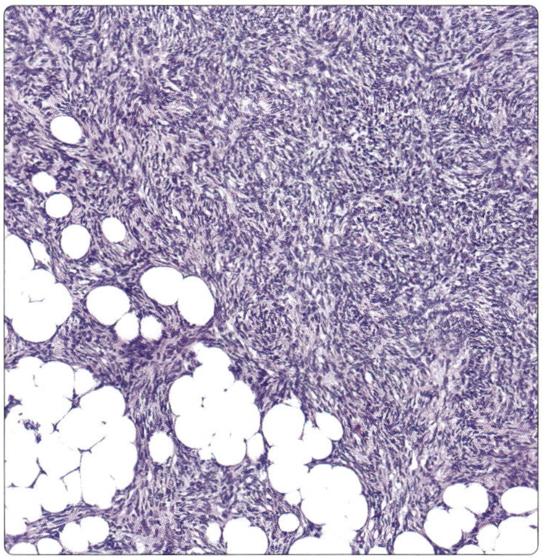

(Left) *Low magnification of a dermatofibrosarcoma protuberans (DFSP) shows a deep dermal and subcutaneous cellular spindle cell tumor with honeycombing fat entrapment* ➜. *The epidermis is separated from the tumor by a thin grenz zone* ➲. **(Right)** *Higher power examination of DFSP shows a cellular, deep dermal and subcutaneous spindle cell tumor with storiforming and honeycombing fat invasion.*

Deep Benign Fibrous Histiocytoma

KEY FACTS

TERMINOLOGY

- Distinctive variant of cutaneous fibrous histiocytoma (dermatofibroma) that occurs in subcutaneous tissue

CLINICAL ISSUES

- Wide age range (median: 40 years)
- Subcutaneous tissue of extremities most common site
  - Also head and neck, trunk
  - Rarely retroperitoneum, mediastinum, pelvis
- Slow-growing, often painless mass
- Treatment: Complete surgical excision
- Local recurrences common (~ 20%)
- Rare metastases and rarer tumor-associated deaths reported

MACROSCOPIC

- Size usually 2-3 cm (subcutaneous lesions)
  - Visceral lesions can be very large (up to 25 cm reported)

MICROSCOPIC

- Well circumscribed ± thin fibrous pseudocapsule
- Storiform &/or short fascicular growth patterns
- Plump, ovoid to spindle cells with indistinct cytoplasm
- Secondary chronic inflammatory component often present
- Large, branching "staghorn" vessels common
- Variable stromal hyalinization or myxoid change
- Mitotic activity varies (median: 3 per 10 HPF)

ANCILLARY TESTS

- CD34(+) in almost 1/2 of cases
- Desmin (-), EMA(-), STAT6(-)

TOP DIFFERENTIAL DIAGNOSES

- Dermatofibrosarcoma protuberans
- Solitary fibrous tumor
- Perineurioma
- Tenosynovial giant cell tumor, localized type

Deep Benign Fibrous Histiocytoma

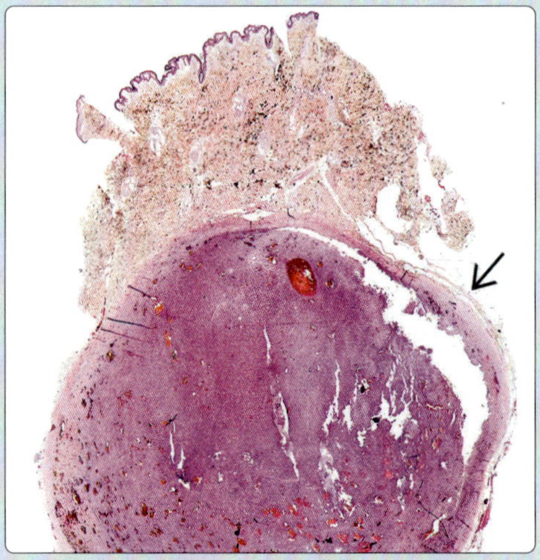

Chronic Inflammatory Component

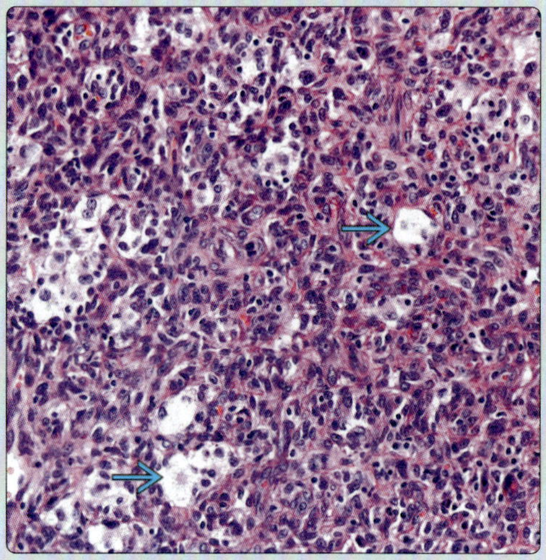

(Left) *Deep benign fibrous histiocytoma (BFH) is a distinct variant of cutaneous fibrous histiocytoma (dermatofibroma) that occurs in the subcutaneous tissue. Essentially, all cases are well circumscribed and many show a fibrous pseudocapsule ➡.* **(Right)** *The lesional cells of deep BFH are generally cytologically bland and similar to those seen in conventional cutaneous cases. Stromal chronic inflammatory cells, including lymphocytes and foamy histocytes ➡, are common.*

Hemangiopericytoma-Like Vasculature

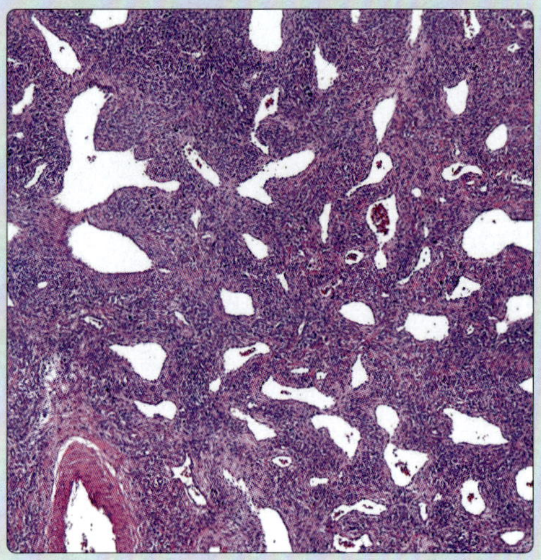

Stromal Changes

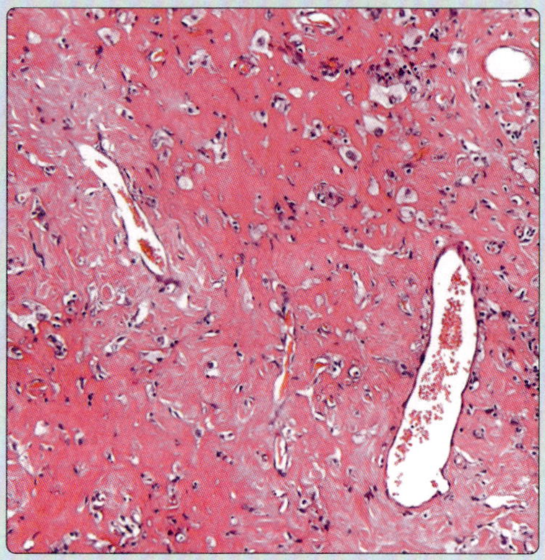

(Left) *A common finding in deep BFH, in contrast to cutaneous forms, is the presence of large, dilated, and branching "staghorn" hemangiopericytoma-like vasculature, which may be focal or numerous. When these vessels are prominent, a solitary fibrous tumor must be considered.* **(Right)** *Although most cases of deep BFH show a uniform, cellular storiform or short fascicular morphology, areas showing stromal hyalinization (shown) or myxoid changes are occasionally seen.*

TERMINOLOGY

Synonyms

- Deep penetrating dermatofibroma

Definitions

- Distinctive, well-circumscribed variant of cutaneous fibrous histiocytoma (dermatofibroma) occurring in subcutaneous tissue

CLINICAL ISSUES

Epidemiology

- Incidence
  - Rare
- Age
  - Wide range (median: 40 years)
- Sex
  - Slight male predominance

Site

- Subcutaneous tissue of extremities most common
- Head and neck, trunk
- Also rarely retroperitoneum, mediastinum, pelvis

Presentation

- Slow-growing, often painless mass

Treatment

- Complete surgical excision

Prognosis

- Local recurrences common (~ 20%)
- Rare metastases and rarer tumor-associated deaths reported
  - Currently no reliable features for predicting aggressive behavior
    - Local recurrence and presence of necrosis may increase risk (limited data)

MACROSCOPIC

General Features

- Well marginated and often encapsulated
- Yellow-tan, firm cut surface

Size

- Usually 2-3 cm (subcutaneous lesions)
- Visceral lesions can be very large (up to 25 cm reported)

MICROSCOPIC

Histologic Features

- Well circumscribed ± thin fibrous pseudocapsule
  - May focally extend into dermis, where conventional peripheral collagen trapping is present
- Storiform &/or short fascicular growth patterns
- Plump, ovoid to spindle cells with indistinct cytoplasm
  - Bland nuclei, vesicular chromatin, delicate nucleoli
- Secondary chronic inflammatory component often present
  - Lymphocytes, plasma cells, foamy histocytes, osteoclast-like giant cells
- Large, branching hemangiopericytoma-like "staghorn" vessels common
- Variable stromal hyalinization or myxoid change
- Variable hemorrhage and stromal hemosiderin (aneurysmal change)
- Rare scattered pleomorphic cells with prominent nuclear atypia
- Mitotic activity varies (median: 3 per 10 HPF)

ANCILLARY TESTS

Immunohistochemistry

- CD34(+) in almost 1/2 of cases
- Variable SMA(+)
- Desmin (-), EMA(-), STAT6(-)

DIFFERENTIAL DIAGNOSIS

Dermatofibrosarcoma Protuberans

- Superficial, usually localized to dermis
- Highly infiltrative growth pattern with entrapped skin appendages and "honeycomb" fat infiltration
- Uniform spindle cells in diffuse storiform growth pattern
- Negligible chronic inflammatory component, no giant cells
- Consistently CD34(+)
- t(17;22)(q22;q23) with *COL1A1-PDGFB* fusion

Solitary Fibrous Tumor

- Classic patternless pattern with regional variations in cellularity
- Prominent hemangiopericytoma-like vascular pattern
- Stromal collagen and hyalinization varies
- Minimal stromal chronic inflammation
- Consistently CD34(+)
- Nuclear STAT6(+)

Perineurioma

- Often show storiform or whorled growth
- Lack "staghorn" vessels and chronic inflammatory component
- EMA(+), claudin-1 (+)

Tenosynovial Giant Cell Tumor, Localized Type

- Most common on fingers/toes
- Composed of histiocytoid cells with variable hemosiderin, giant cells, and stromal sclerosis
- Lacks "staghorn" vessels
- CD34(-)

SELECTED REFERENCES

1. Puopolo A et al: Deep benign fibrous histiocytoma of the anterior mediastinum mimicking malignancy. Lung. 195(4):503-506, 2017
2. Kim SI et al: Deep penetrating fibrous histiocytoma: a case report and implications for surgical management. Am J Dermatopathol. 38(4):e49-51, 2016
3. Chung J et al: Deep penetrating benign fibrous histiocytoma of the foot associated with throbbing pain. Ann Dermatol. 23(Suppl 2):S239-42, 2011
4. Gleason BC et al: Deep "benign" fibrous histiocytoma: clinicopathologic analysis of 69 cases of a rare tumor indicating occasional metastatic potential. Am J Surg Pathol. 32(3):354-62, 2008
5. Fletcher CD: Benign fibrous histiocytoma of subcutaneous and deep soft tissue: a clinicopathologic analysis of 21 cases. Am J Surg Pathol. 14(9):801-9, 1990

Localized-Type Tenosynovial Giant Cell Tumor

KEY FACTS

TERMINOLOGY

- Localized-type tenosynovial giant cell tumor (L-TGCT)
- Giant cell tumor of tendon sheath, nodular tenosynovitis, localized pigmented villonodular synovitis (PVNS)
- Benign soft tissue tumor of synovial origin
- Arises from tendon sheath, intraarticular site, bursa

ETIOLOGY/PATHOGENESIS

- Balanced translocation involving 1p13 (*CSF1* gene)
  - CSF1 overexpression by neoplastic stromal cells
  - Autocrine activation of neoplastic cells via CSF1R
  - Recruitment and activation of macrophages and giant cells via CSF1R

CLINICAL ISSUES

- 2nd most common tumor of hand
- Any age; peak: 3rd-4th decades
- Digits (85%)
- Around large joints (10%)
- Benign but recurs locally (10-20%)
- Intraarticular tumors called localized PVNS

MACROSCOPIC

- Average size: 1.1 cm (range: 0.5-6.0 cm)

MICROSCOPIC

- Polymorphous population of epithelioid cells, macrophages, and osteoclast-like giant cells
- Well demarcated
- Multinodular with fibrous septa
- Stromal fibrosis
- Mitotic rate 1-20 per 10 HPF (average: 5 per 10 HPF)

TOP DIFFERENTIAL DIAGNOSES

- Diffuse-type TGCT (PVNS)
- Giant cell tumor of soft tissue
- Fibroma of tendon sheath
- Dermatofibroma

Localized-Type Tenosynovial Giant Cell Tumor

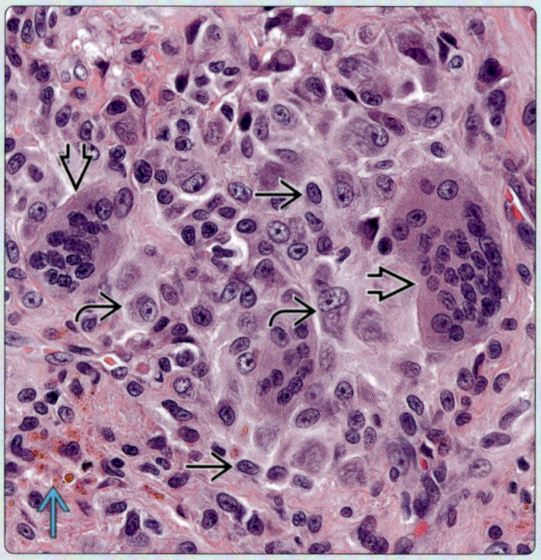

Clinical Presentation

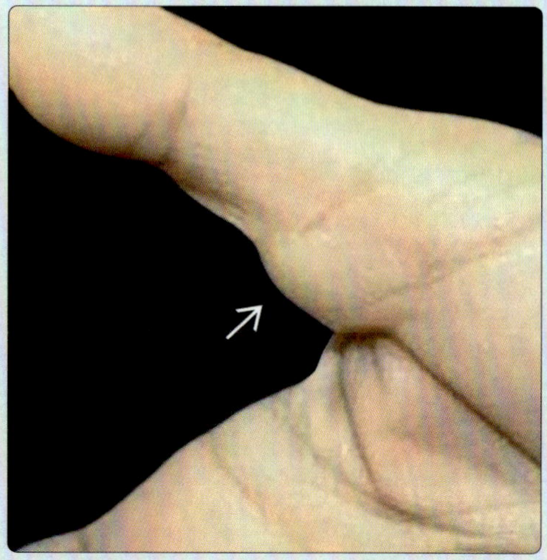

***(Left)** Localized-type tenosynovial giant cell tumor (L-TGCT) is composed of a polymorphous cell population, including large epithelioid cells with abundant eosinophilic cytoplasm and eccentric vesicular nuclei ⮫; mononuclear stromal cells with smaller, round or reniform nuclei ⇨; and osteoclast-like giant cells ⇨. Note the hemosiderin deposits ⇨. **(Right)** L-TGCT typically presents as a painless, slowly growing mass that arises from a tendon sheath, most often on the volar aspect of a finger, such as this thumb mass ➡.*

Gross Appearance

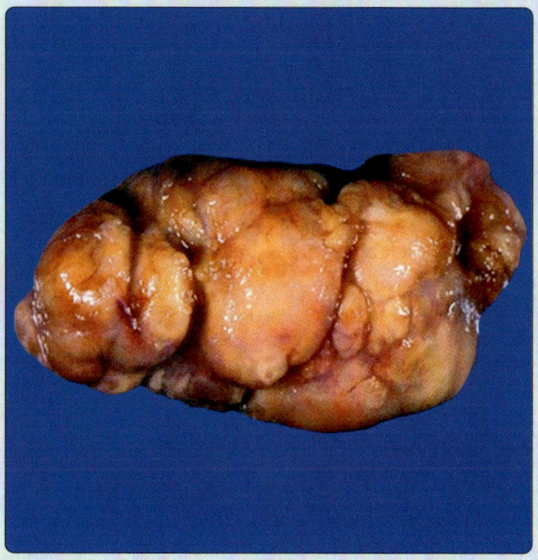

Lobular Architecture

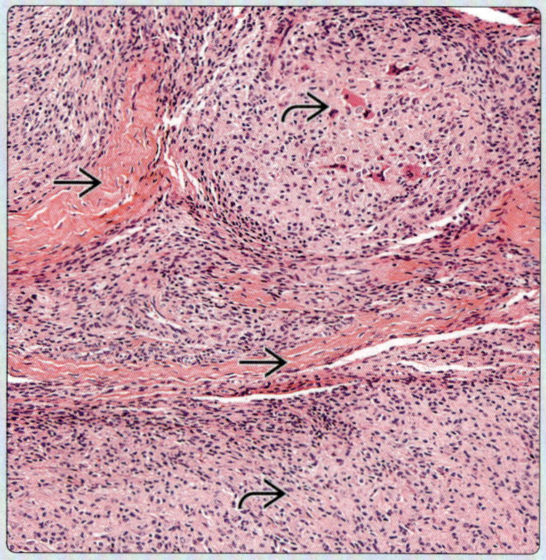

***(Left)** Grossly, L-TGCT is well demarcated, yellow to red-brown, and typically has a lobular configuration with surface clefting, as depicted. Average size is 1.1 cm, ranging from 0.5-6.0 cm. **(Right)** L-TGCT has a multinodular architecture, as illustrated by this low-power micrograph. Note the long, thick fibrous septa ⇨ that divide the tumor into nodules ⮫.*

Localized-Type Tenosynovial Giant Cell Tumor

TERMINOLOGY

Abbreviations

- Localized-type tenosynovial giant cell tumor (L-TGCT)

Synonyms

- Giant cell tumor of tendon sheath
- Nodular tenosynovitis
- Localized pigmented villonodular synovitis (PVNS)
  - Intraarticular forms

Definitions

- Benign soft tissue neoplasm of synovial origin
  - Polymorphous cell population
    - Large epithelioid cells
    - Macrophages
    - Osteoclast-like giant cells
  - Well circumscribed, noninvasive

ETIOLOGY/PATHOGENESIS

Histogenesis

- Neoplastic growth
  - Balanced translocation involving 1p13 (*CSF1* gene) in many tumors
    - *COL6A3-CSF1* fusion transcripts often present
    - CSF1 overexpression by neoplastic stromal cells
    - Autocrine activation of neoplastic cells via CSF1R
    - Recruitment and activation of intratumoral macrophages and osteoclasts via CSF1R
- Synoviocytic differentiation
  - Clusterin (+)

CLINICAL ISSUES

Epidemiology

- Incidence
  - 40 patients/1 million
    - 2nd most common tumor of hand
      - Ganglion cyst most common
- Age
  - Wide spectrum
    - Peak: 3rd-4th decades
- Sex
  - F > M: 2:1

Site

- Digits (85%)
  - Especially fingers (75%)
  - Tendon sheath
    - Usually volar
    - Often adjacent to interphalangeal joint
- Around large joints (10%)
  - Ankle
  - Knee
  - Wrist
  - Elbow
- Unusual sites
  - Scapular region
  - Brachial plexus
  - Spine
- Within bursae
- Intraarticular L-TGCT
  - Also called localized PVNS
  - Knee most common site
  - Complete excision usually curative

Presentation

- Painless mass
- Slowly growing
- Uncommon findings
  - Triggering
  - Carpal and ulnar tunnel syndromes
  - Multifocal cases

Treatment

- Complete local excision

Prognosis

- Benign but recurs locally (10-20%)
- Risk factors for recurrence
  - Degenerative joint disease
  - Distal phalanx
  - Interphalangeal joint of thumb
  - Osseous erosion

IMAGING

Radiographic Findings

- Soft tissue mass
- Cortical bony erosion (10%)
  - Rarely invades bone to mimic primary bone tumor

MR Findings

- Lobulated mass with low T1 and T2 signal

MACROSCOPIC

General Features

- Well circumscribed
- Partially encapsulated
- Multinodular configuration
  - Surface clefting
  - Sometimes grooved along tendon interface
- Variegated cut surface: Tan, red-brown, yellow

Size

- Average: 1.1 cm (range: 0.5-6.0 cm)
  - Large joint tumors often larger than digital tumors (average: 2.0 cm)

MICROSCOPIC

Histologic Features

- Well demarcated
- Multinodular with fibrous septa
- Stromal fibrosis
  - Can be extensive
  - Can mimic osteoid
- Hemosiderin deposits
- Dyscohesive areas render pseudoglandular appearance
- Cleft-like spaces lined by synoviocytes
- Distal tumors can invade dermis

Cytologic Features

- Polymorphous cell population
  - Large epithelioid cells
    - Abundant, eccentric, eosinophilic cytoplasm
      - Often contain hemosiderin pigment
    - Vesicular, round nuclei with prominent nucleoli
  - Histiocytes with pale cytoplasm and round or reniform nuclei
  - Osteoclast-like multinucleated giant cells
    - Can be sparse in some tumors
  - Xanthoma cells
  - Hemosiderin-laden macrophages
- Mitotic rate 1-20 per 10 HPF (average: 5 per 10 HPF)

ANCILLARY TESTS

Immunohistochemistry

- Epithelioid cells are clusterin (+)
- Histiocytes are CD68(+)
- Osteoclast-like giant cells are CD68(+), CD45(+), TRAP(+)
- Desmin (+) cells in 50% of tumors
  - Usually patchy

DIFFERENTIAL DIAGNOSIS

Diffuse-Type Tenosynovial Giant Cell Tumor (PVNS)

- Microscopically similar to L-TGCT
- Diffuse intraarticular tumors form villonodular masses
- Large joints; knee most common site
- Diffuse extraarticular tumors invade adjacent tissues

Giant Cell Tumor of Soft Tissue

- More uniform, less polymorphous mononuclear stromal cell population
- Osteoclast-like giant cell component prominent
- Less stromal fibrosis
- Often encased by shell of bone

Giant Cell Tumor of Bone

- Identical histology to giant cell tumor of soft tissue
- Primary osseous tumor but can invade soft tissue
- Immunohistochemically (+) for G34W-mutated site of histone H3.3
  - L-TGCT(-)

Fibroma of Tendon Sheath

- Lacks hemosiderin and multinucleated giant cells
- Peripheral, thin-walled vessels &/or clefts
- Usually occurs in fingers
- L-TGCT may show diffuse fibrosis mimicking fibroma of tendon sheath (FTS)

Dermatofibroma

- Rare in digits
- Lacks osteoclast-like giant cells
- L-TGCT can sometimes invade dermis

Plexiform Fibrohistiocytic Tumor

- Often has osteoclast-like giant cells
- Plexiform architecture but can be nodular
- Involves dermis and subcutis
- Rare in acral extremities
- Usually children and young adults

SELECTED REFERENCES

1. Ehrenstein V et al: Tenosynovial giant cell tumor: incidence, prevalence, patient characteristics, and recurrence. a registry-based cohort study in Denmark. J Rheumatol. 44(10):1476-83, 2017
2. Mastboom MJL et al: Higher incidence rates than previously known in tenosynovial giant cell tumors. Acta Orthop. 88(6):688-94, 2017
3. Beytemür O et al: Localized giant cell tenosynovial tumor seen in the knee joint. Case Rep Orthop. 2014:840243, 2014
4. Ding Y et al: Tenosynovial giant cell tumors lacking giant cells: report of diagnostic pitfalls. Ann Clin Lab Sci. 44(2):222-7, 2014
5. Palmerini E et al: Tenosynovial giant cell tumour/pigmented villonodular synovitis: outcome of 294 patients before the era of kinase inhibitors. Eur J Cancer. 51(2):210-7, 2014
6. Panagopoulos I et al: Novel CSF1-S100A10 fusion gene and CSF1 transcript identified by RNA sequencing in tenosynovial giant cell tumors. Int J Oncol. 44(5):1425-32, 2014
7. Ye JM et al: Tenosynovial giant cell tumour of brachial plexus. J Clin Neurosci. 21(6):1070-2, 2014
8. Yoshimoto T et al: Hepatoid tenosynovial giant cell tumor - a rare morphologic variant case report. Pathol Res Pract. 210(10):694-7, 2014
9. Atik E et al: Tenosynovial giant cell tumor in an unusual localization. Acta Orthop Traumatol Turc. 47(2):139-41, 2013
10. Di Grazia S et al: Giant cell tumor of tendon sheath: study of 64 cases and review of literature. G Chir. 34(5-6):149-52, 2013
11. Fukuda A et al: Tenosynovial giant cell tumor arising on the scapular region. Case Rep Dermatol. 5(3):267-71, 2013
12. Lanzinger WD et al: Giant cell tumor of the tendon sheath. J Hand Surg Am. 38(1):154-7; quiz 157, 2013
13. van der Heijden L et al: A multidisciplinary approach to giant cell tumors of tendon sheath and synovium–a critical appraisal of literature and treatment proposal. J Surg Oncol. 107(4):433-45, 2013
14. Ho CY et al: Giant cell tumor of tendon sheath: cytomorphologic and radiologic findings in 41 patients. Diagn Cytopathol. 40 Suppl 2:E94-8, 2012
15. Lucas DR: Tenosynovial giant cell tumor: case report and review. Arch Pathol Lab Med. 136(8):901-6, 2012
16. Okutan O et al: Tenosynovial giant cell tumor in the cervico-thoracic junction. Turk Neurosurg. 22(6):769-71, 2012
17. Kim HS et al: Localized tenosynovial giant cell tumor in both knee joints. Skeletal Radiol. 39(9):923-6, 2010
18. Boland JM et al: Clusterin is expressed in normal synoviocytes and in tenosynovial giant cell tumors of localized and diffuse types: diagnostic and histogenetic implications. Am J Surg Pathol. 33(8):1225-9, 2009
19. Darwish FM et al: Giant cell tumour of tendon sheath: experience with 52 cases. Singapore Med J. 49(11):879-82, 2008
20. Möller E et al: Molecular identification of COL6A3-CSF1 fusion transcripts in tenosynovial giant cell tumors. Genes Chromosomes Cancer. 47(1):21-5, 2008
21. Murphey MD et al: Pigmented villonodular synovitis: radiologic-pathologic correlation. Radiographics. 28(5):1493-518, 2008
22. Cupp JS et al: Translocation and expression of CSF1 in pigmented villonodular synovitis, tenosynovial giant cell tumor, rheumatoid arthritis and other reactive synovitides. Am J Surg Pathol. 31(6):970-6, 2007
23. Dines JS et al: Long-term follow-up of surgically treated localized pigmented villonodular synovitis of the knee. Arthroscopy. 23(9):930-7, 2007
24. Jafarian F et al: Plexiform fibrohistiocytic tumor in three children. Pediatr Dermatol. 23(1):7-12, 2006
25. West RB et al: A landscape effect in tenosynovial giant-cell tumor from activation of CSF1 expression by a translocation in a minority of tumor cells. Proc Natl Acad Sci U S A. 103(3):690-5, 2006
26. Nilsson M et al: Molecular cytogenetic mapping of recurrent chromosomal breakpoints in tenosynovial giant cell tumors. Virchows Arch. 441(5):475-80, 2002
27. Reilly KE et al: Recurrent giant cell tumors of the tendon sheath. J Hand Surg Am. 24(6):1298-302, 1999
28. Enzinger FM et al: Plexiform fibrohistiocytic tumor presenting in children and young adults. An analysis of 65 cases. Am J Surg Pathol. 12(11):818-26, 1988
29. Ushijima M et al: Giant cell tumor of the tendon sheath (nodular tenosynovitis). A study of 207 cases to compare the large joint group with the common digit group. Cancer. 57(4):875-84, 1986
30. Chung EB et al: Fibroma of tendon sheath. Cancer. 44(5):1945-54, 1979

Localized-Type Tenosynovial Giant Cell Tumor

Gross Cut Surface

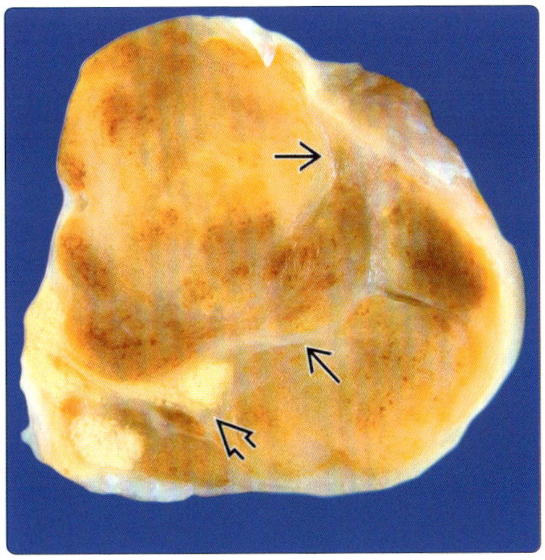

Radiographic Appearance

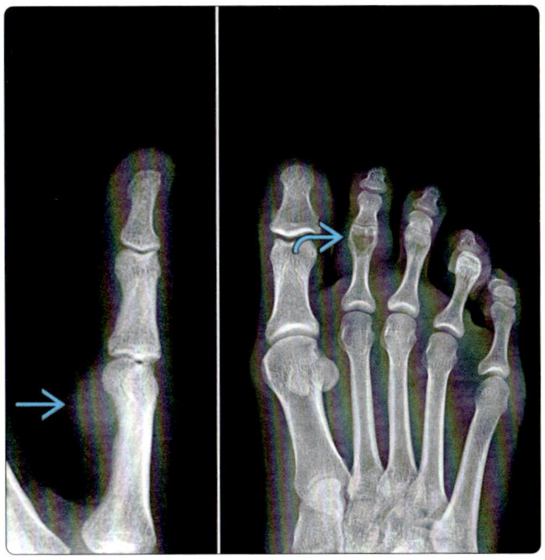

(Left) *L-TGCT is well circumscribed, encapsulated, and multinodular. Fibrous septa* → *divide it into nodules. The cut surface is variegated with gold, tan, red-brown, and yellow areas. Bright yellow areas* ⇨ *represent xanthoma cells.* **(Right)** *Radiographically, L-TGCT appears as a soft tissue density most often on the volar side of a finger* →*. Approximately 10% erode the bony cortex as shown. Rare tumors invade medullary bone, mimicking a primary bone tumor* ↗*, such as this 2nd toe tumor.*

Medium-Power View

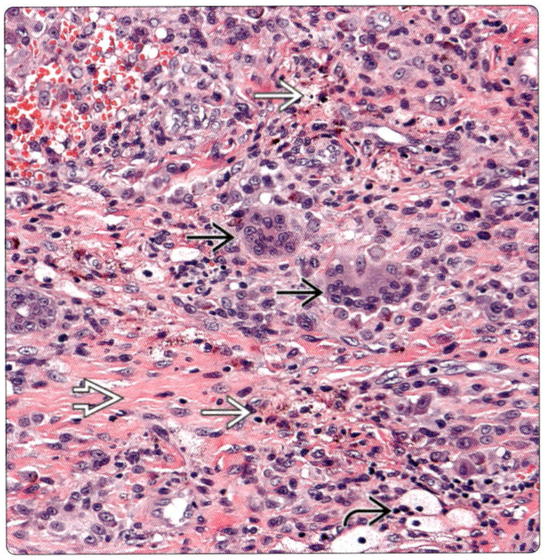

Polymorphous Cellular Population

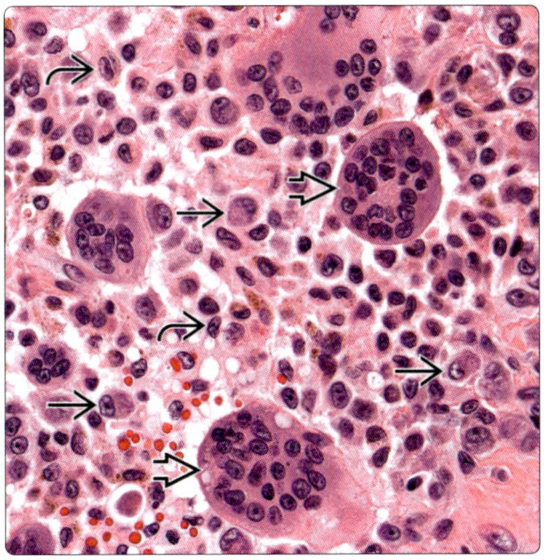

(Left) *L-TGCT has a mixture of mononuclear stromal cells, multinucleated giant cells* →*, and macrophages, including xanthoma cells* ↗*. Stromal fibrosis* ➡ *and hemosiderin deposits* ➡ *are very common.* **(Right)** *This high-power view depicts large epithelioid cells with eccentric nuclei* →*, (believed to be the neoplastic element), macrophages with smaller round to reniform nuclei* ↗*, and osteoclast-like giant cells* ⇨*.*

Xanthoma Cells

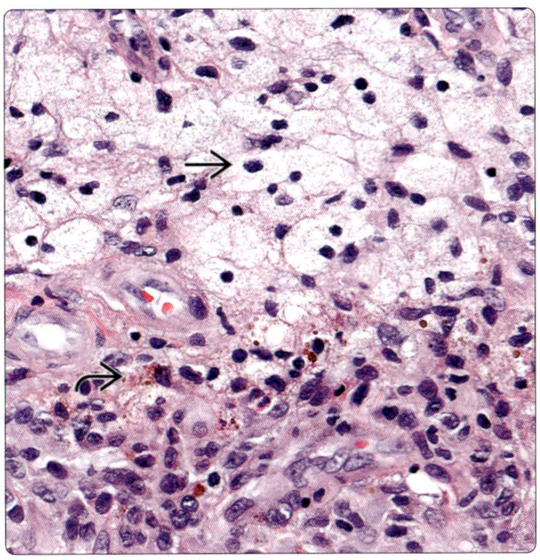

Hemosiderin Deposition

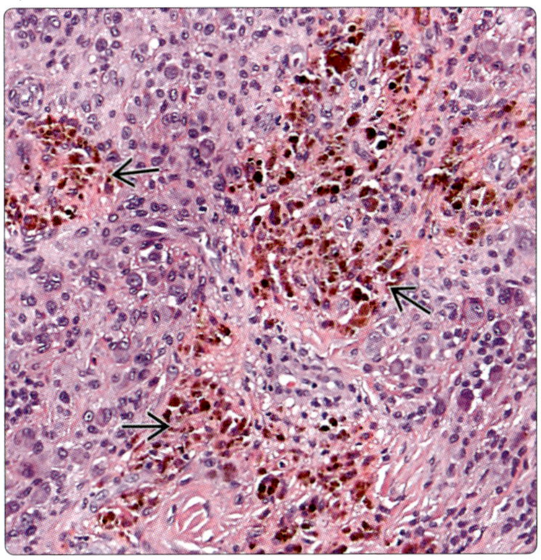

(Left) *Sheets and clusters of xanthoma cells are very common in L-TGCT. Xanthoma cells (foamy macrophages) have copious, finely vacuolated cytoplasm and small, central nuclei as depicted* →*. Hemosiderin-laden macrophages* ↗ *are also common.* **(Right)** *Some tumors have very extensive hemosiderin deposition, as depicted* →*.*

(Left) *Stromal fibrosis is usually present in L-TGCT but highly variable in its extent. In some tumors, fibrosis consists of lace-like, hyalinized collagen that resembles osteoid* ➡. **(Right)** *Occasionally, fibrosis can be very extensive, affecting large areas of a tumor. This low-power micrograph shows diffuse stromal fibrosis that entraps both mononuclear stromal cells and multinucleated giant cells* ➡.

Osteoid-Like Fibrosis

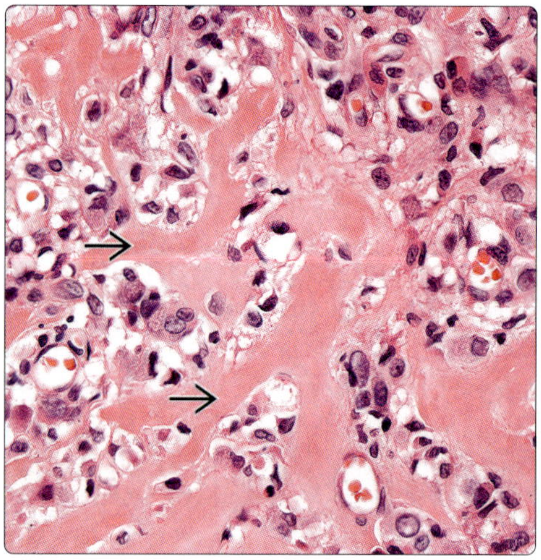

Stromal Fibrosis

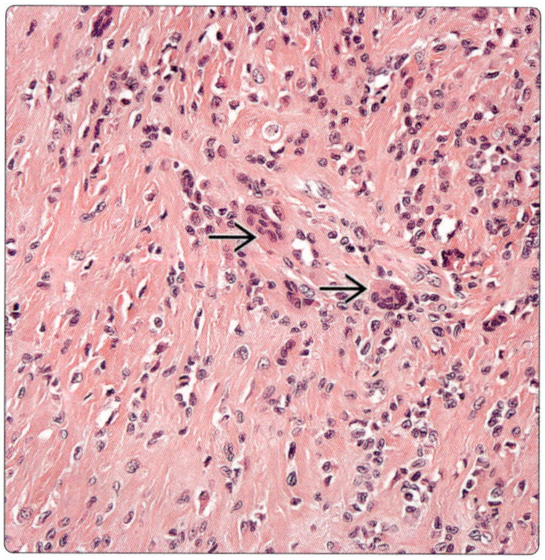

(Left) *Areas of cellular dyscohesion are not uncommon in L-TGCT. In some tumors, it can be so pronounced as to form cystic spaces* ➡, *creating a pseudoglandular pattern.* **(Right)** *Occasionally, L-TGCT can have very few giant cells as in this example, which consists of a uniform population of mononuclear stromal cells with round nuclei.*

Pseudoglandular Pattern

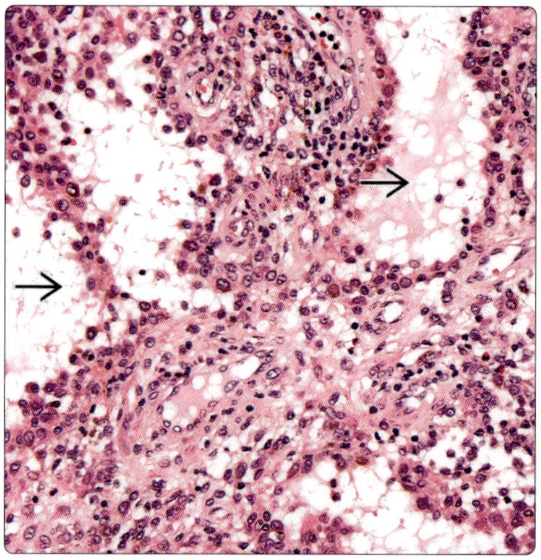

Localized-Type Tenosynovial Giant Cell Tumor Without Giant Cells

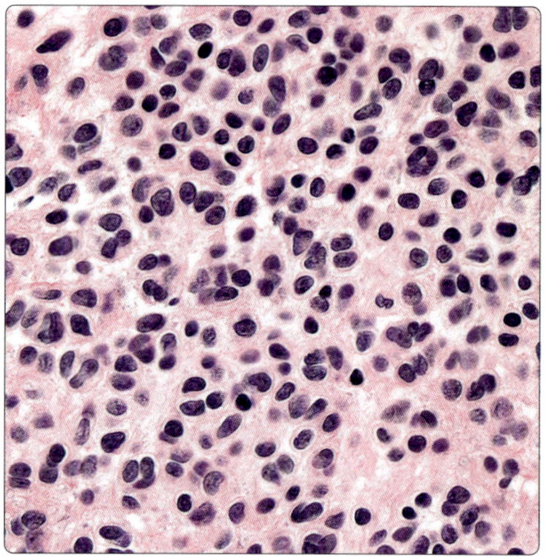

(Left) *Some L-TGCTs contain sheets of large epithelioid cells with abundant eosinophilic cytoplasm and eccentric vesicular nuclei. Note the intracytoplasmic hemosiderin deposits* ➡. **(Right)** *The large epithelioid cells are positive for clusterin* ➡, *indicating synoviocytic differentiation. By contrast, infiltrating macrophages and giant cells* ↪ *are negative.*

Epithelioid Cells

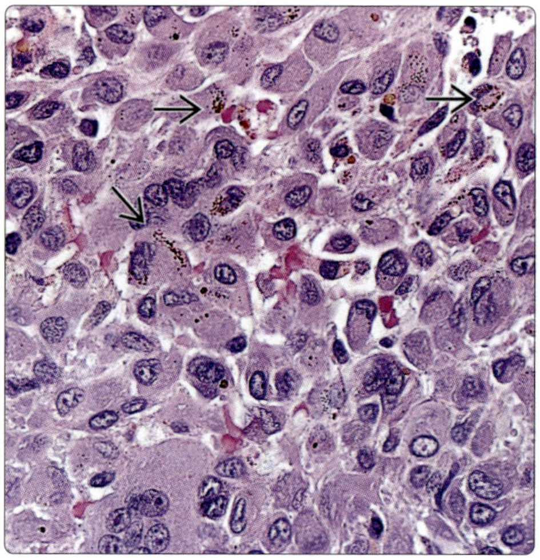

Clusterin Immunostain

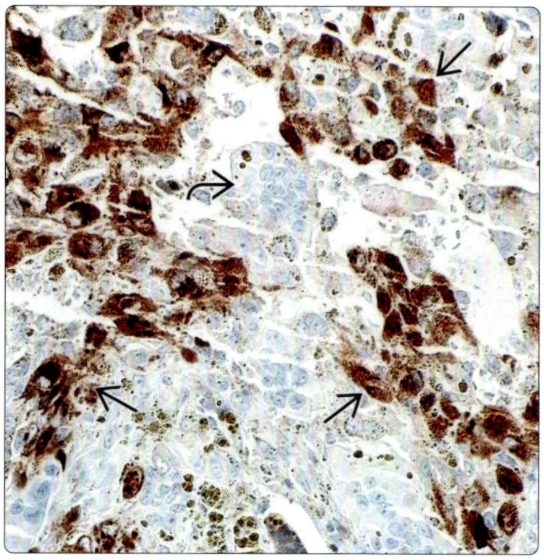

Brisk Mitotic Activity

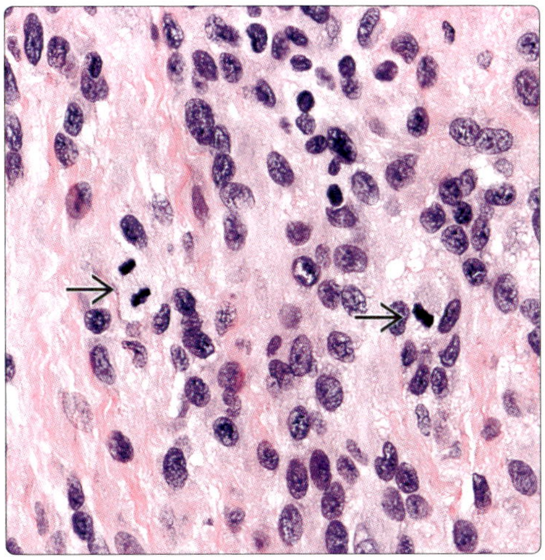

Giant Cells

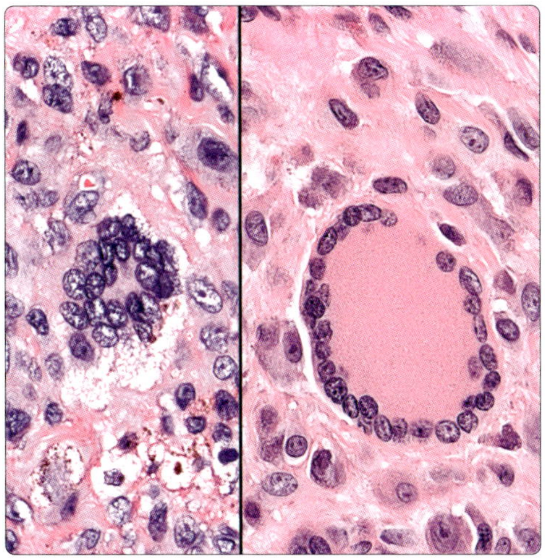

(Left) *Mitotic activity ranges from 1-20 mitoses per 10 HPF (average 5 per 10 HPF). Brisk mitotic activity, therefore, is not uncommon in these lesions, as evidenced by 2 mitotic figures in this single high-power field ➩.* **(Right)** *Although osteoclast-like multinucleated giant cells are most common, occasionally, L-TGCT can have Touton-like (left) or Langhans-type (right) giant cells.*

Skin Involvement

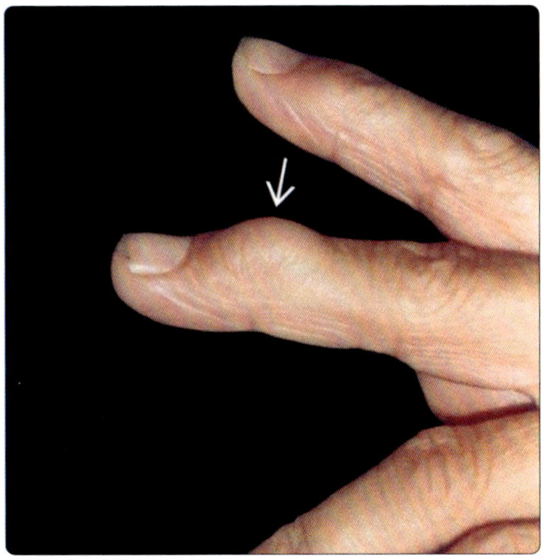

Skin Involvement

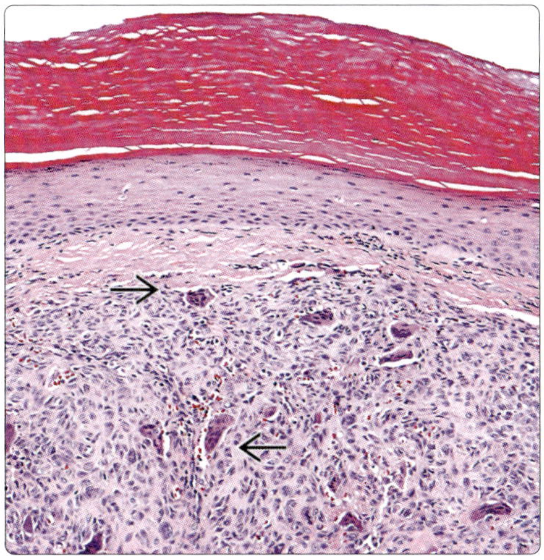

(Left) *In a distal acral location, L-TGCT can adhere to and invade the overlying skin, as depicted ➡ by this tumor of the middle finger.* **(Right)** *In this example of L-TGCT, the tumor invades the dermis, mimicking a dermatofibroma. Unlike L-TGCT, however, dermatofibroma does not contain osteoclast-like giant cells ➩.*

Intraarticular Localized-Type Tenosynovial Giant Cell Tumor (Localized PVNS)

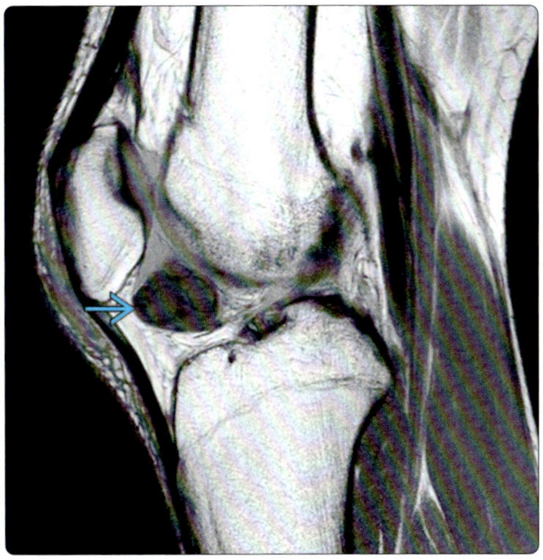

Intraarticular Localized-Type Tenosynovial Giant Cell Tumor (Localized PVNS)

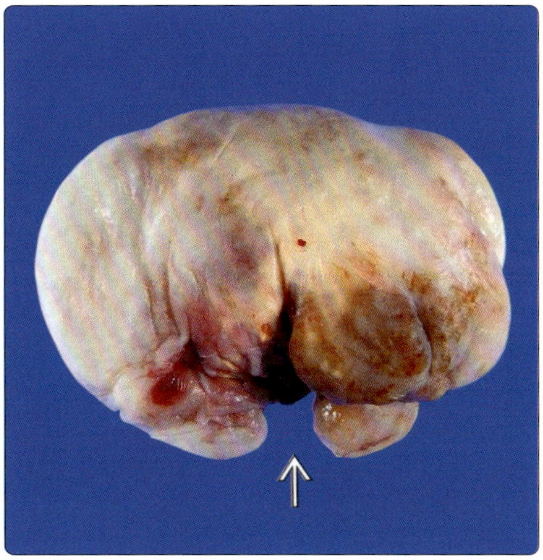

(Left) *Localized intraarticular TGCT [or localized pigmented villonodular synovitis (PVNS)] forms a well-demarcated tumor within the joint space. The knee is the most common site, as depicted in this MR ➩.* **(Right)** *Grossly, intraarticular tumors are well circumscribed and form pedunculated or sessile polypoid masses attached to the synovial surface by a stalk ➡ (inverted here). Unlike diffuse-type TGCT, localized intraarticular tumors rarely recur following complete excision and have an excellent prognosis.*

Diffuse-Type Tenosynovial Giant Cell Tumor

KEY FACTS

TERMINOLOGY

- Diffuse-type tenosynovial giant cell tumor (D-TGCT)
- Synonym: Pigmented villonodular synovitis (PVNS)
- Generally benign, locally aggressive neoplastic proliferation of synovial origin
  - Intra- or extraarticular

ETIOLOGY/PATHOGENESIS

- Balanced translocation involving 1p13 (*CSF1*)

CLINICAL ISSUES

- Average age: 35 years; range: 1st-7th decades
- Knee (75-80%)
- High recurrence rate (15-55%)

IMAGING

- Low signal on T1 and T2, enhancement with contrast
- MR signal voids secondary to hemosiderin

MACROSCOPIC

- Most of synovial surface affected
- Villous, nodular, or villonodular
- Large, usually > 5 cm

MICROSCOPIC

- Thin, delicate villi and broad papillary structures
- Solid cellular areas with multinodular architecture
- Heterogeneous cell population
  - Large epithelioid cells
  - Osteoclastic giant cells
  - Macrophages/xanthoma cells
- Hemosiderin, fibrosis

TOP DIFFERENTIAL DIAGNOSES

- Localized tenosynovial giant cell tumor
- Hemarthrosis
- Chondroblastoma of craniofacial bones
- Giant cell tumor of soft tissue

Diffuse-Type Tenosynovial Giant Cell Tumor

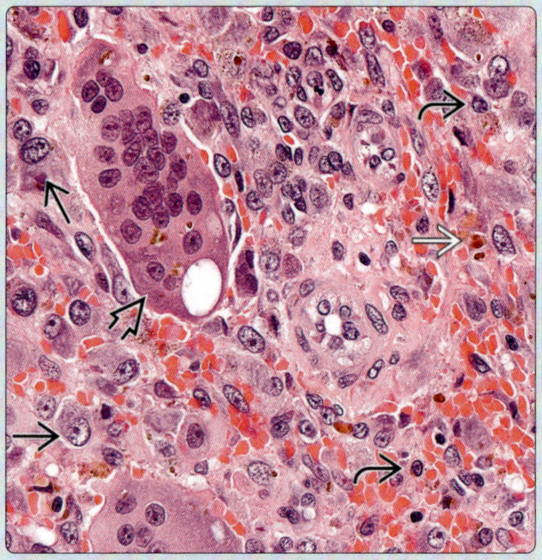

Villonodular Architecture

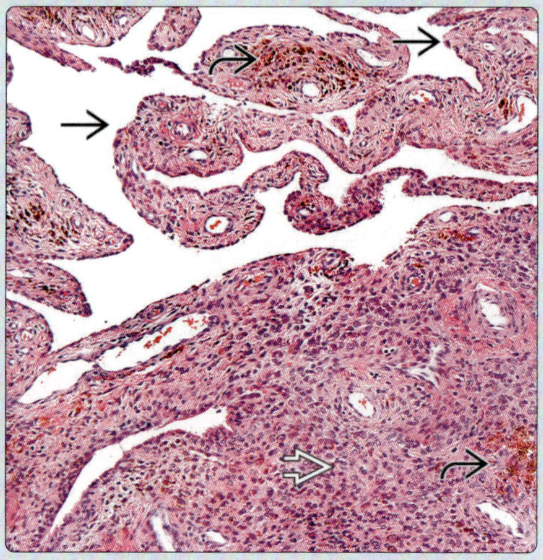

(Left) *D-TGCT typically has a mix of large eosinophilic cells with eccentric vesicular nuclei ⇨, smaller stromal cells and macrophages with oval to reniform nuclei →, and osteoclast-like giant cells ↪. Note the presence of stromal hemorrhage and hemosiderin deposits ➡.* **(Right)** *D-TGCT has a villonodular architecture composed of elongated villi →, solid cellular areas ⇨ containing a heterogeneous population of mononuclear stromal cells and multinucleated giant cells, and hemosiderin deposits ↪.*

Gross Appearance

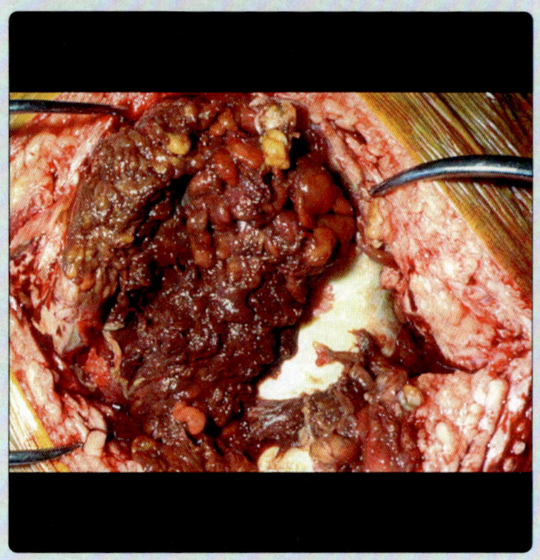

MR of Knee Tumor

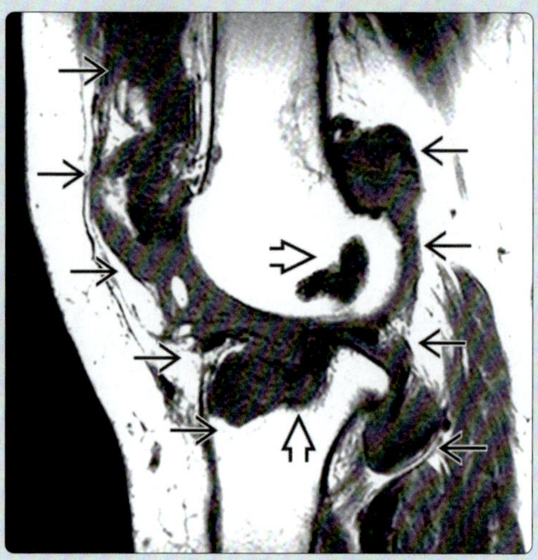

(Left) *D-TGCT (or pigmented villonodular synovitis) usually presents as a large, intraarticular mass. 75-80% occur in the knee. It diffusely covers most of the synovial surface, has a villonodular appearance, and is red-brown.* **(Right)** *Sagittal T1 MR of the knee depicts an advanced, locally destructive D-TGCT forming a large mass involving both anterior and posterior synovium →, which erodes into the distal femur and proximal tibia ⇨. On MR, D-TGCT shows low signal on T1 and T2 and enhances with contrast.*

TERMINOLOGY

Abbreviations

- Diffuse-type tenosynovial giant cell tumor (D-TGCT)

Synonyms

- Pigmented villonodular synovitis (PVNS)
- Diffuse-type giant cell tumor
- Giant cell tumor of tendon sheath, diffuse type

Definitions

- Generally benign but locally aggressive neoplastic proliferation of synovial origin
  - Intraarticular tumors within large joints
  - Extraarticular invasive tumors of tendon sheath, bursa, or soft tissue origin

ETIOLOGY/PATHOGENESIS

Neoplastic Proliferation

- Balanced translocation involving 1p13 (*CSF1*) in most tumors
  - Most often fused with 2q35 (*COL6A3*), promoter
  - Overexpression of CSF1 by neoplastic cells
  - Autocrine activation via CSFR1
  - Paracrine inflammatory cell recruitment and activation via CSFR1
- Trisomy 5 or 7 in some tumors

CLINICAL ISSUES

Epidemiology

- Incidence
  - Rare, annual incidence 4-8 patients/1 million
- Age
  - Wide range (1st-7th decades)
    - Average: 35 years
- Sex
  - Women slightly outnumber men

Site

- Intraarticular
  - Knee (75-80%)
  - Hip (15%)
  - Ankle, elbow, shoulder, temporal mandibular joint, spine
- Extraarticular
  - Knee region most common
  - Foot, wrist, inguina, elbow region, digits

Presentation

- Painful mass
- Long duration of symptoms (years)
- Hemorrhagic joint effusion
- Decreased range of motion

Treatment

- Surgical approaches
  - Wide local excision
  - Total synovectomy
  - Prosthetic joint replacement
  - Amputation in advanced cases
- Drugs
  - Tyrosine kinase inhibitors (e.g., CSFR1 inhibitor or imatinib) for relapsing or uncontrolled tumors
- Radiation
  - May improve local control

Prognosis

- Locally aggressive
  - High recurrence rate (15-55%)
  - Multiple relapses common
  - Very rare tumors progress to malignancy
    - Often radiation associated
  - Very rare histologically benign tumors metastasize

IMAGING

General Features

- Ill-defined periarticular soft tissue mass
- Bone erosions
- Subchondral cysts

MR Findings

- Low signal on T1 and T2
- Enhancement with contrast
- MR signal voids secondary to hemosiderin ("blooming")

MACROSCOPIC

General Features

- Diffusely covers most of synovial surface
- Villous, nodular, or villonodular
  - Heterogeneous synovial projections
    - Thin villi, thick papillae, nodules
- Firm to sponge-like
- Variegated cut surface
  - Red-brown, tan, yellow
- Poorly demarcated from adjacent soft tissue
- Extraarticular tumors form multinodular masses

Size

- Large, usually > 5 cm

MICROSCOPIC

Histologic Features

- Elongated villi
  - Vary from thin, delicate villi to broad papillary structures
  - Lined by 1 to few layers of synoviocytes
- Solid cellular areas
  - Multinodular architecture
  - Fibrous septa surround nodules
  - Stromal fibrosis
    - Varies from minimal to extensive
    - Irregular, hyalinized collagen mimics osteoid
  - Hemosiderin deposits usually abundant

Cytologic Features

- Heterogeneous cell population
  - Large epithelioid cells
    - Abundant eosinophilic cytoplasm
      - ▫ Often contain hemosiderin pigment
    - Vesicular, round to oval, eccentric nuclei with prominent nucleoli

- Macrophages with smaller, oval or reniform nuclei
  - Xanthoma cells
  - Hemosiderin-laden macrophages
- Osteoclast-like giant cells
  - Usually abundant
- Synoviocytes line villi and cleft-like spaces
- Frequent mitotic figures
- Homogenous mononuclear cell population in some tumors
  - Large areas may be devoid of giant cells

Diffuse-Type Tenosynovial Giant Cell Tumor of Temporal Mandibular Joint

- Distinctive microscopic features
- Sheets of large epithelioid cells
- Chondroid metaplasia
- Can invade temporal bone
- May be mistaken for chondroblastoma of craniofacial bones

ANCILLARY TESTS

Immunohistochemistry

- Large epithelioid cells clusterin (+)
  - Indicates synovial differentiation
- Often desmin (+)
  - Usually patchy but sometimes diffuse
- Macrophages CD163(+)
- Osteoclastic giant cell CD68(+), CD45(+), TRAP(+)
- G34W mutated site of histone H3.3 (-)
  - Giant cell tumor of bone (+)

DIFFERENTIAL DIAGNOSIS

Localized Tenosynovial Giant Cell Tumor

- Well circumscribed and encapsulated
- Lacks villi
- Otherwise identical microscopic features
- Localized to digits (85%)
- Intraarticular tumors (usually knee)
  - Localized PVNS

Hemarthrosis

- Villiform synovial hyperplasia with hemosiderosis
- Lacks solid cellular areas
- History of repetitive hemarthrosis
  - Trauma or hemophilia

Malignant Tenosynovial Giant Cell Tumor

- Malignant cytoarchitectural features
  - Pleomorphic spindle cells
  - Epithelioid cells with prominent nucleoli
  - High mitotic rate and necrosis
  - Often with past history of radiation therapy

Chondroblastoma

- D-TGCT of temporal mandibular joint can invade temporal bone mimicking primary bone tumor
  - Large epithelioid cells
  - Zones of chondroid matrix
  - Dystrophic chicken-wire calcification
  - Closely resembles chondroblastoma of craniofacial bones
    - Many reported cases of chondroblastoma in temporal bone probably represent D-TGCT with chondroid metaplasia

Giant Cell Tumor of Soft Tissue

- Identical histology to giant cell tumor of bone
  - Uniform mononuclear stromal cells
  - Numerous evenly distributed giant cells
  - Metaplastic bone may be present
- Less heterogeneous cell population
- Less stromal fibrosis

SELECTED REFERENCES

1. Ehrenstein V et al: Tenosynovial giant cell tumor: incidence, prevalence, patient characteristics, and recurrence. a registry-based cohort study in Denmark. J Rheumatol. 44(10):1476-83, 2017
2. Lüke J et al: H3F3A mutation in giant cell tumour of the bone is detected by immunohistochemistry using a monoclonal antibody against the G34W mutated site of the histone H3.3 variant. Histopathology. 71(1):125-33, 2017
3. Mastboom MJL et al: Higher incidence rates than previously known in tenosynovial giant cell tumors. Acta Orthop. 88(6):688-94, 2017
4. Staals EL et al: Diffuse-type tenosynovial giant cell tumour: current treatment concepts and future perspectives. Eur J Cancer. 63:34-40, 2016
5. Righi A et al: Metastasizing tenosynovial giant cell tumour, diffuse type/pigmented villonodular synovitis. Clin Sarcoma Res. 5:15, 2015
6. Asano N et al: Multiple metastases from histologically benign intraarticular diffuse-type tenosynovial giant cell tumor: a case report. Hum Pathol. 45(11):2355-8, 2014
7. Ding Y et al: Tenosynovial giant cell tumors lacking giant cells: report of diagnostic pitfalls. Ann Clin Lab Sci. 44(2):222-7, 2014
8. Pina S et al: Recurrent temporal bone tenosynovial giant cell tumor with chondroid metaplasia: the use of imaging to assess recurrence. Neuroradiol J. 27(1):97-101, 2014
9. Wang K et al: Primary diffuse-type tenosynovial giant cell tumor of the spine: a report of 3 cases and systemic review of the literature. Turk Neurosurg. 24(5):804-13, 2014
10. Yoshimoto T et al: Hepatoid tenosynovial giant cell tumor - a rare morphologic variant case report. Pathol Res Pract. 210(10):694-7, 2014
11. Fisher M et al: Chondroid tenosynovial giant cell tumor of the temporal bone. Otol Neurotol. 34(6):e49-50, 2013
12. Lucas DR: Tenosynovial giant cell tumor: case report and review. Arch Pathol Lab Med. 136(8):901-6, 2012
13. van der Heijden L et al: The management of diffuse-type giant cell tumour (pigmented villonodular synovitis) and giant cell tumour of tendon sheath (nodular tenosynovitis). J Bone Joint Surg Br. 94(7):882-8, 2012
14. Hoch BL et al: Chondroid tenosynovial giant cell tumor: a clinicopathological and immunohistochemical analysis of 5 new cases. Int J Surg Pathol. 19(2):180-7, 2011
15. Yoon HJ et al: Malignant pigmented villonodular synovitis of the temporomandibular joint with lung metastasis: a case report and review of the literature. Oral Surg Oral Med Oral Pathol Oral Radiol Endod. 111(5):e30-6, 2011
16. Boland JM et al: Clusterin is expressed in normal synoviocytes and in tenosynovial giant cell tumors of localized and diffuse types: diagnostic and histogenetic implications. Am J Surg Pathol. 33(8):1225-9, 2009
17. Blay JY et al: Complete response to imatinib in relapsing pigmented villonodular synovitis/tenosynovial giant cell tumor (PVNS/TGCT). Ann Oncol. 19(4):821-2, 2008
18. Oda Y et al: Pigmented villonodular synovitis with chondroid metaplasia, resembling chondroblastoma of the bone: a report of three cases. Mod Pathol. 20(5):545-51, 2007
19. West RB et al: A landscape effect in tenosynovial giant-cell tumor from activation of CSF1 expression by a translocation in a minority of tumor cells. Proc Natl Acad Sci U S A. 103(3):690-5, 2006
20. Nilsson M et al: Molecular cytogenetic mapping of recurrent chromosomal breakpoints in tenosynovial giant cell tumors. Virchows Arch. 441(5):475-80, 2002
21. Bertoni F et al: Malignant giant cell tumor of the tendon sheaths and joints (malignant pigmented villonodular synovitis). Am J Surg Pathol 21(2):153-63, 1997
22. Fletcher JA et al: Trisomy 5 and trisomy 7 are nonrandom aberrations in pigmented villonodular synovitis: confirmation of trisomy 7 in uncultured cells. Genes Chromosomes Cancer. 4(3):264-6, 1992
23. Bertoni F et al: Chondroblastoma of the skull and facial bones. Am J Clin Pathol. 88(1):1-9, 1987

Villous Architecture

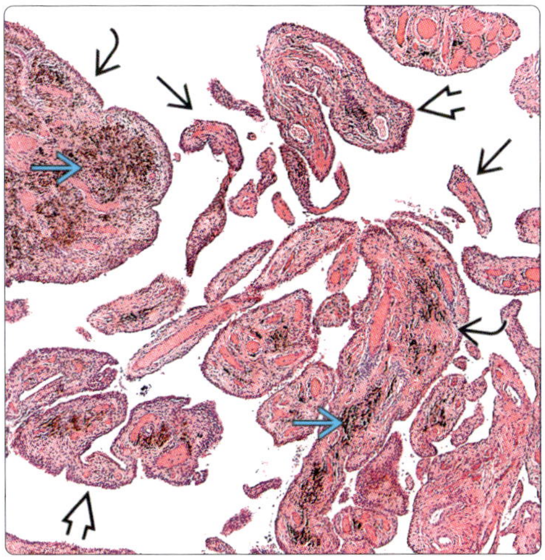

Nodular Architecture

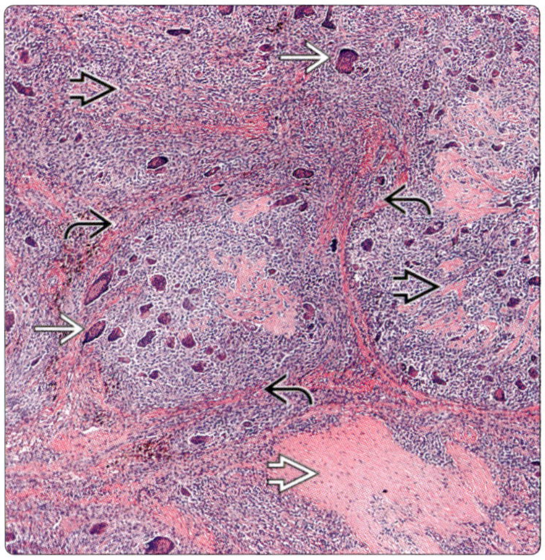

(Left) *Intraarticular D-TGCT (pigmented villonodular synovitis) forms long villous processes that extend into the joint space. They vary from thin and delicate ⇨ to broad ⇨ and are lined by plump synoviocytes ⇨. Hemosiderin is often abundant in the villi ⇨.* **(Right)** *In the solid areas, D-TGCT has a multinodular architecture composed of cellular areas ⇨ separated by fibrous septa ⇨. Giant cells ⇨ and zones of stromal fibrosis ⇨ are also seen.*

Slit-Like Clefts

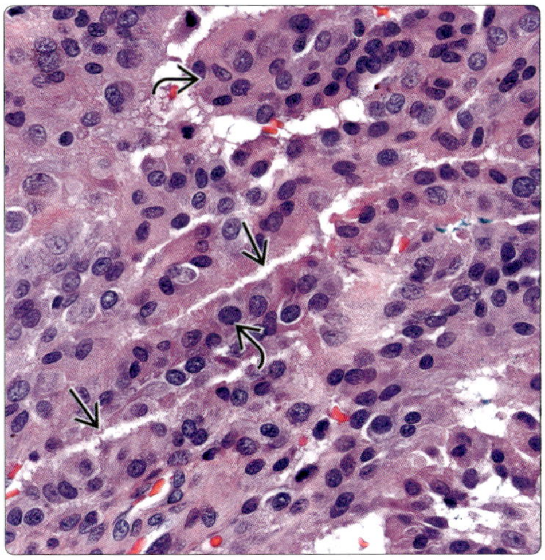

Gross Appearance

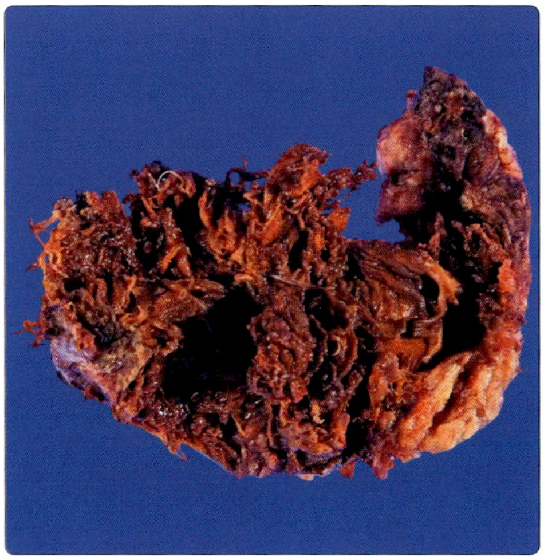

(Left) *Slit-like, clefted areas lined by synoviocytes are common in D-TGCT. This micrograph depicts linear clear spaces ⇨ rimmed by plump synoviocytes with abundant eosinophilic cytoplasm and rounded nuclei ⇨.* **(Right)** *D-TGCT broadly involves the synovial membrane and has a very distinctive gross appearance consisting of villiform papillary fronds that extend into the joint cavity. It is usually red-brown, secondary to congestion and hemosiderosis.*

Gross Appearance

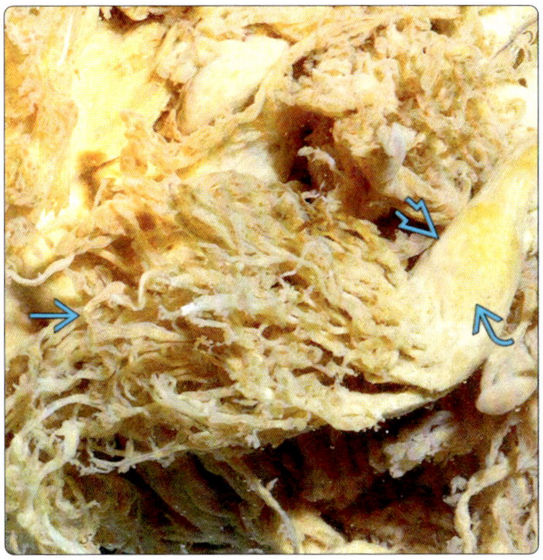

Erosion of Bone and Cartilage

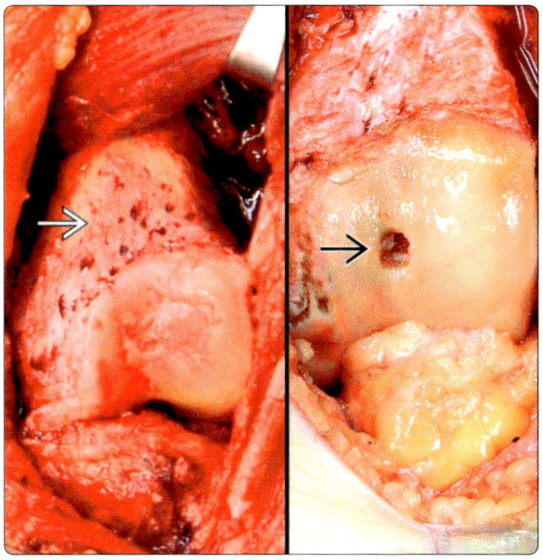

(Left) *This close-up photograph depicts long, delicate villi ⇨ emanating from a broad papillary stalk ⇨ resembling a sea anemone. The yellow coloration ⇨ is due to sheets of xanthoma cells.* **(Right)** *Intraoperative postsynovectomy photographs from 2 patients with D-TGCT of the knee illustrate multiple surface bone erosions ⇨ and penetration of the articular cartilage ⇨.*

Epithelioid Cells and Macrophages

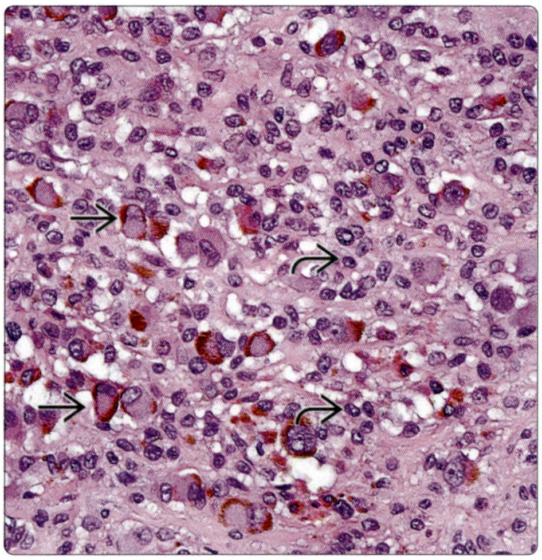

Dyscohesive Pattern

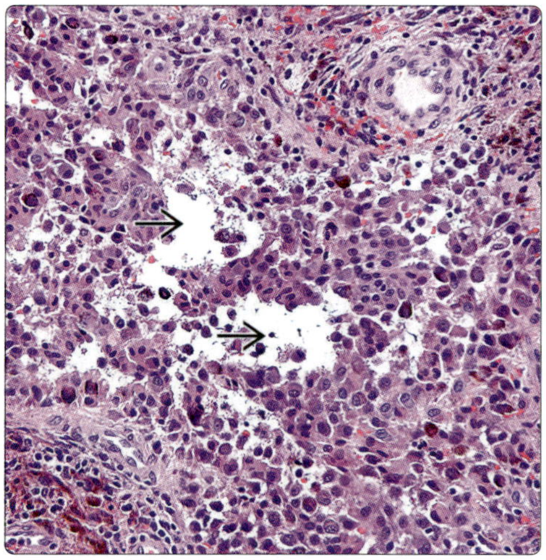

(Left) *This micrograph depicts a mix of large epithelioid cells (many with hemosiderin-laden cytoplasm) ➡ and smaller mononuclear inflammatory cells ↪. Inflammatory cells are recruited into the milieu by CSF1, a potent inflammatory cytokine, produced by the neoplastic cells.* **(Right)** *In areas, the cells become dyscohesive and form irregular cystic spaces ➡, creating a pseudoalveolar pattern, a common finding in D-TGCT.*

Diffuse-Type Tenosynovial Giant Cell Tumor Without Giant Cells

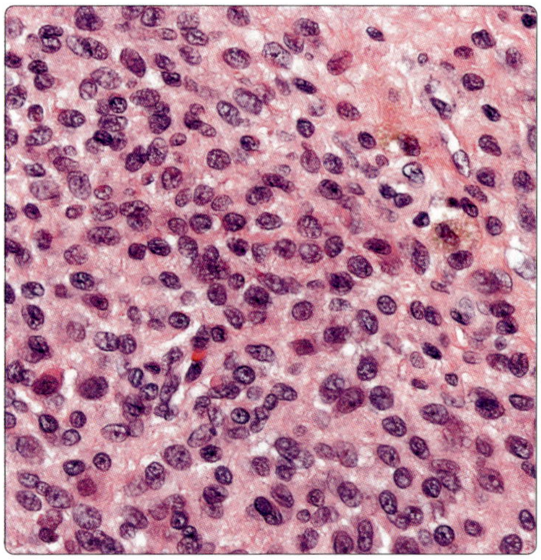

Osteoid-Like Fibrosis

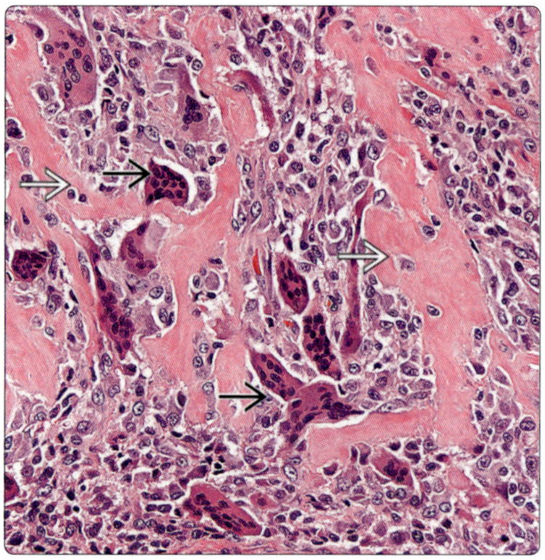

(Left) *Large zones containing uniform, mononuclear cells with few or no giant cells may be present. This H&E depicts a monotonous population of histiocytoid stromal cells with uniform, round to oval nuclei and abundant eosinophilic cytoplasm.* **(Right)** *Stromal fibrosis and hyalinization are common in D-TGCT. Hyalinized collagen can form irregular branching structures that mimic an osteoid ➡. Numerous osteoclast-like giant cells are present ➡, further adding to this mimicry.*

Xanthoma Cells and Hemosiderin Pigment

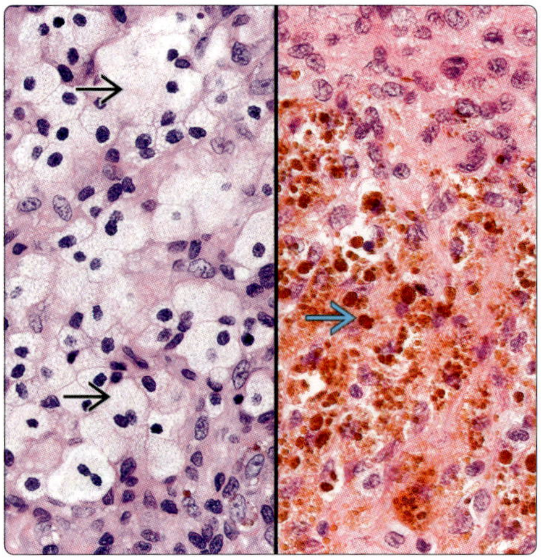

Clusterin

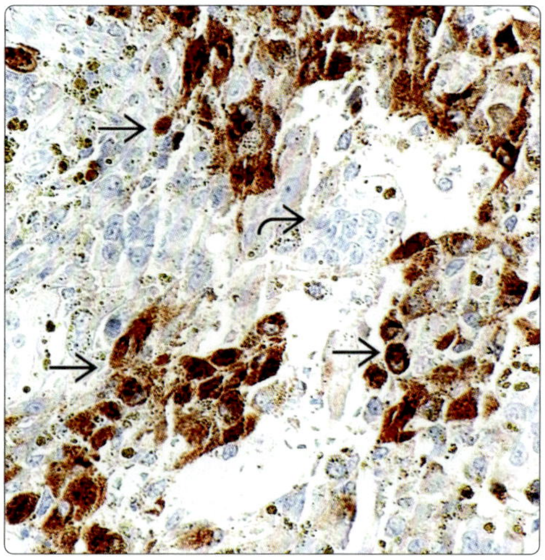

(Left) *Clusters of xanthoma cells (foamy macrophages) ➡ are common. They have abundant, vacuolated, lipid-filled cytoplasm, which imparts a yellow color to the gross tissue. Hemosiderin deposits secondary to remote hemorrhage are common and can be abundant as illustrated ➡.* **(Right)** *The large epithelioid cells in D-TGCT are positive for clusterin ➡, indicative of synovial differentiation. By contrast, the osteoclast-like giant cells ↪ and macrophages are negative.*

Extraarticular Diffuse-Type Tenosynovial Giant Cell Tumor

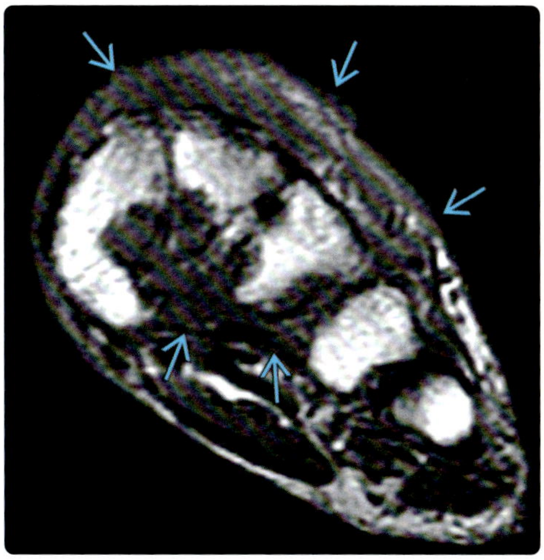

Invasive Growth in Extraarticular Tumor

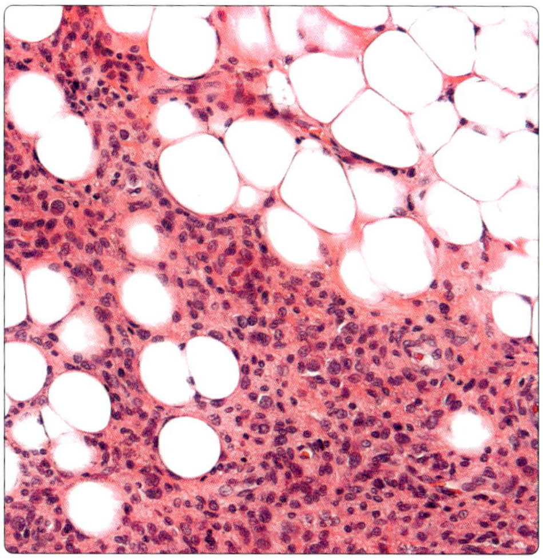

(Left) *Extraarticular D-TGCT presents as an invasive soft tissue tumor arising from a tendon sheath, bursa, or soft tissue. This T1-weighted MR depicts a low-signal mass that diffusely infiltrates between metatarsals to involve both deep and superficial compartments of the foot* →. **(Right)** *Unlike localized-type TCGT, which is usually encased by a pseudocapsule, D-TGCT invades adjacent tissues as illustrated by infiltration and entrapment of adipose tissue.*

Temporal Mandibular Joint Tumor

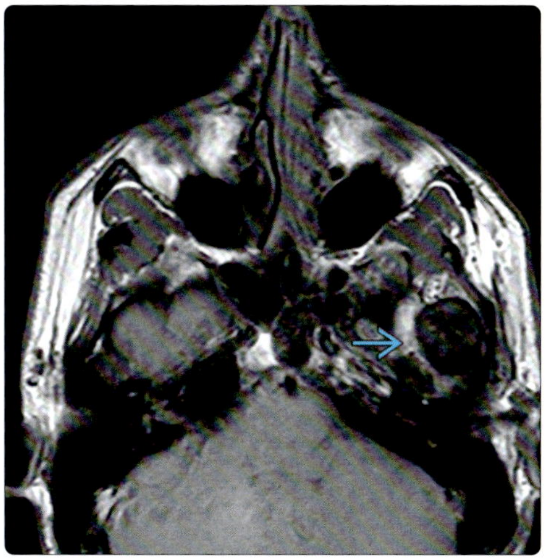

Epithelioid Cells in Temporal Mandibular Joint Tumor

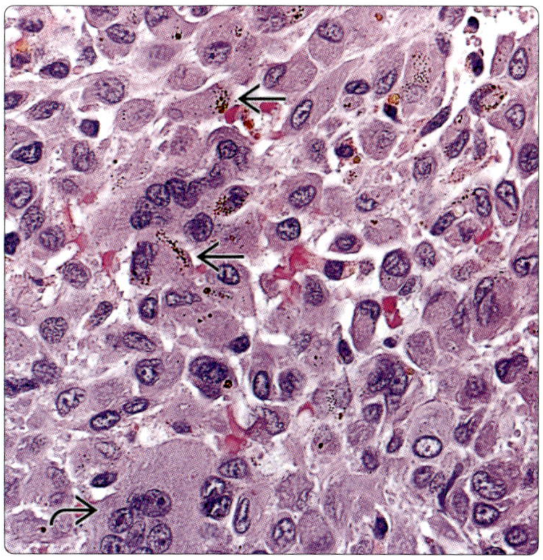

(Left) *D-TGCT can arise in the temporal mandibular joint (TMJ) as depicted in this TI MR of recurrent tumor* →. *In this location, it may invade into the temporal bone to mimic a primary bone tumor.* **(Right)** *TMJ tumors have distinctive histologic features characterized by sheets of large epithelioid cells with abundant eosinophilic cytoplasm, eccentric nuclei, and hemosiderin pigmentation* →. *Note the single osteoclast-like giant cell* ↪.

Chondroid Metaplasia

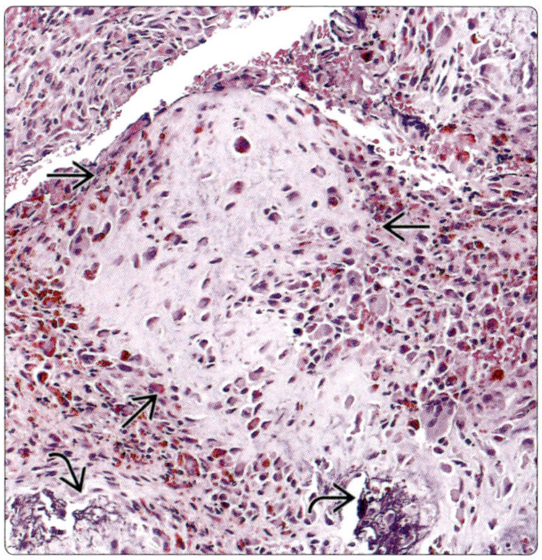

Malignant Tenosynovial Giant Cell Tumor

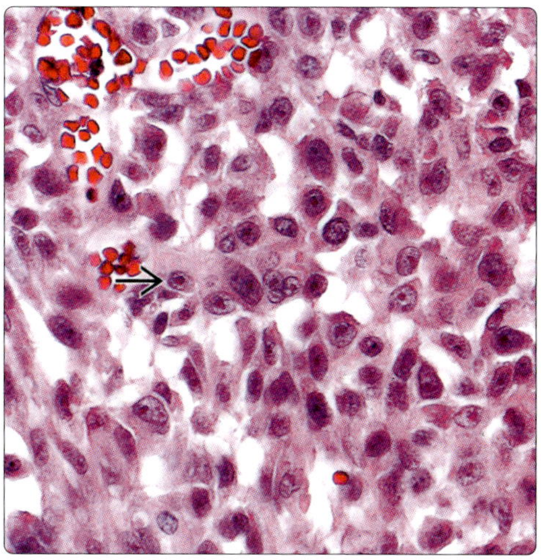

(Left) *Chondroid metaplasia is uncommon in D-TGCT but is more likely in TMJ tumors. It is characterized by geographic areas of pale blue hyaline matrix* →. *Areas of dystrophic calcification can impart a chicken-wire pattern* ↪ *mimicking a chondroblastoma.* **(Right)** *Malignant transformation of TCGT is a rare event that usually follows multiple recurrences. Many cases had prior radiotherapy. Most are high-grade undifferentiated sarcomas, often having sheets of malignant epithelioid cells with prominent nucleoli* →.

Cellular Neurothekeoma

KEY FACTS

TERMINOLOGY

- Rare dermal tumor of uncertain histogenesis composed of epithelioid cells in multiple nests divided by fibrous septa
- Unrelated to dermal nerve sheath myxoma (conventional neurothekeoma)

CLINICAL ISSUES

- Children and young adults (mean age: 25 years)
- Head/neck and upper extremity (mostly on face and shoulder)
- Benign (even if atypical histologic features)

MICROSCOPIC

- Epithelioid to spindled cells with abundant pale eosinophilic cytoplasm arranged in nests divided by dense fibrous septa
- Myxoid change common (30%)
- Multinucleated giant cells (osteoclastic or Touton)
- Nuclear atypia/pleomorphism in 25%
- Mitotic activity common (mean: 3/10 HPF; range: 0-22)
    - Subset have brisk mitotic activity (> 5/10 HPF in 20%; > 10/10 HPF in 5%)
    - Atypical mitotic figures may be seen

ANCILLARY TESTS

- Negative for S100 protein and SOX10
    - Most important IHC; essentially excludes melanocytic
- Often positive for variety of nonspecific markers, including CD63 (NKI/C3), NSE, PGP9.5
    - No specific positive IHC marker

TOP DIFFERENTIAL DIAGNOSES

- Spitz nevus or spitzoid melanoma
- Dermal nerve sheath myxoma (conventional neurothekeoma)
- Plexiform fibrohistiocytic tumor
- Epithelioid fibrous histiocytoma
- Benign cutaneous biphasic (or plexiform) hybrid tumor of perineurioma and cellular neurothekeoma

Cellular Neurothekeoma

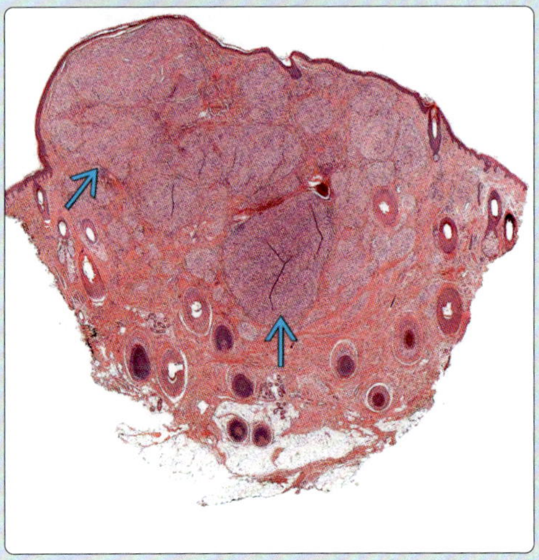

Nests and Aggregates of Tumor Cells

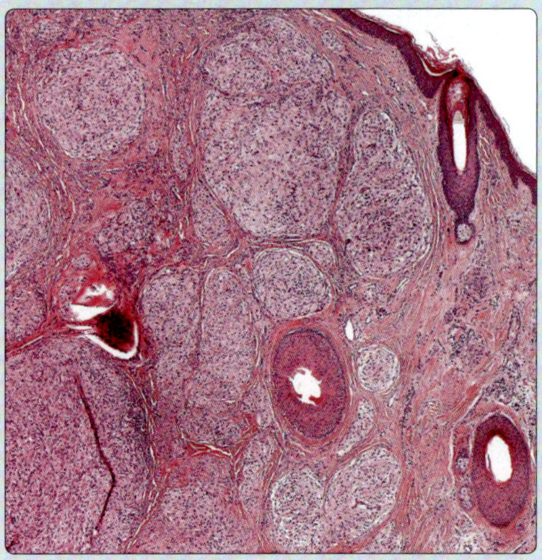

(Left) *Cellular neurothekeoma is a benign tumor of uncertain histogenesis that typically presents as a multilobular tumor ➔ centered in the dermis.* **(Right)** *Cellular neurothekeoma is generally characterized by multiple nests or aggregates of histiocytoid tumor cells divided by intervening fibrous bands.*

Bland Histiocytoid Cells

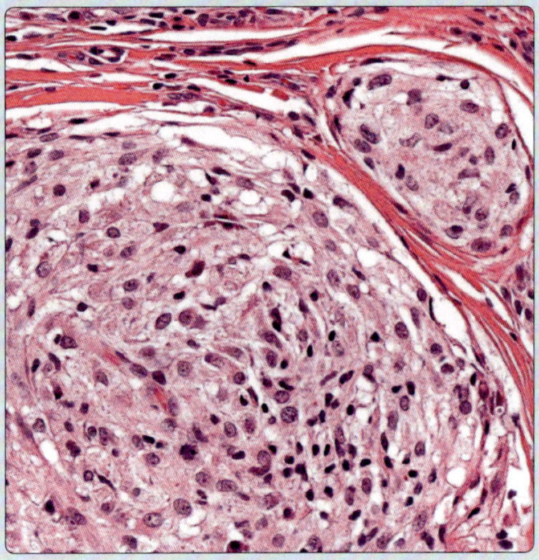

Atypia and Mitotic Activity

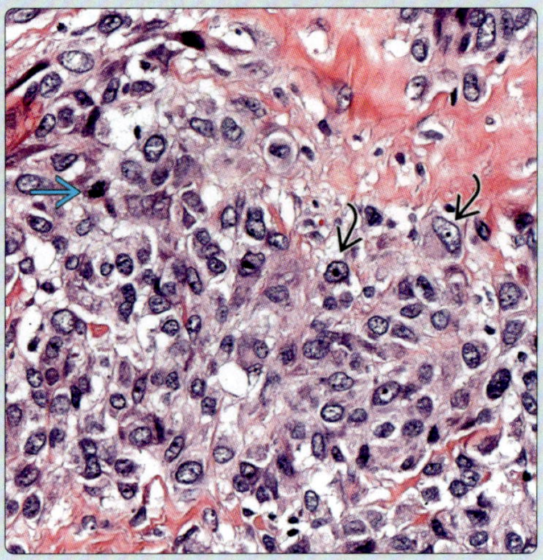

(Left) *Nests are composed of histiocytoid cells with abundant pale cytoplasm and uniform round nuclei.* **(Right)** *Nuclear atypia ➔ or pleomorphism is seen in 25% of cellular neurothekeoma and does not indicate aggressive behavior. Mitotic activity ➔ is common and may be brisk.*

TERMINOLOGY

Definitions

- Rare dermal tumor of uncertain histogenesis composed of epithelioid cells in multiple nests divided by fibrous septa
- Unrelated to dermal nerve sheath myxoma (conventional neurothekeoma)

CLINICAL ISSUES

Site

- Head/neck and upper extremity (mostly on face and shoulder)

Presentation

- Children & young adults (mean: 25 years; most < 40 years)
- Painless solitary skin nodule, often present > 1 year
  - Rarely agminated (cluster of multiple lesions in 1 site)
  - Rarely may occur in oral cavity

Treatment

- Simple but complete excision

Prognosis

- Benign (even if atypical histologic features)
- Small subset recur, especially if incompletely excised

MACROSCOPIC

General Features

- Rounded or dome-shaped skin lesion, usually < 2 cm

MICROSCOPIC

Histologic Features

- Micronodular or lobulated dermal tumor
  - No epidermal involvement
  - Usually has infiltrative borders
  - 50% also involve subcutis
- Epithelioid to spindled cells with abundant pale eosinophilic cytoplasm, arranged in nests divided by dense fibrous septa
- May have plexiform, desmoplastic, or focally sheet-like growth patterns
- Myxoid change common (30%)
  - Spindling more prominent in myxoid areas; may resemble pattern of dermal nerve sheath myxoma (conventional neurothekeoma)
- Multinucleated giant cells (osteoclastic or Touton) in some
- Nuclear atypia/pleomorphism in 25%
  - Atypical multinucleated tumor giant cells may be seen
- Mitotic activity common (mean: 3 mitoses/10 HPF; range: 0-22 mitoses)
  - Subset have brisk mitotic activity (> 5/10 HPF in 20%; > 10/10 HPF in 5%)
  - Atypical mitotic figures may be seen
- Lymphovascular or perineural invasion rarely
- Necrosis rarely

ANCILLARY TESTS

Immunohistochemistry

- Negative for S100 protein and SOX10
  - Most important IHC; essentially excludes melanocytic
- Positive for variety of relatively nonspecific markers
  - CD63 (NKI/C3), NSE, MITF, PGP9.5 (most cases)
  - SMA, p63 (~ 1/2 of cases)
  - Lack of specificity limits utility of these stains
- No specific positive IHC marker
- Also negative: MART-1, HMB-45, desmin, keratin

DIFFERENTIAL DIAGNOSIS

Spitz Nevus or Spitzoid Melanoma

- Small skin nodule, sometimes nonpigmented, on face or extremity of young patients
- Nests of epithelioid to spindled cells with abundant eosinophilic cytoplasm
- Often have intraepidermal component
- Cellular neurothekeoma should always be in differential of **intradermal** atypical spitzoid lesion, especially on face of child or young adult
  - Atypical spitzoid lesions often treated with wider excision ± sentinel lymph node biopsy; sometimes behave aggressively
- S100 protein, SOX10, MART-1, and HMB-45 (+) in Spitzoid lesions; negative in cellular neurothekeoma

Dermal Nerve Sheath Myxoma (Conventional Neurothekeoma)

- Skin nodule of middle-aged adults
- Usually on distal extremities (especially fingers)
- Circumscribed, multilobulated dermal tumor
- Hypocellular myxoid nodules with strands of spindle cells
- Nodules divided by fibrous septa
- S100 protein and SOX10 (+) (100%)

Plexiform Fibrohistiocytic Tumor

- Skin nodule on extremities of children and young adults
- Plexiform pattern of multiple small nodules infiltrating deep dermis and subcutis
- Nodules composed of round histiocytoid cells ± multinucleated giant cells
  - Similar to nested pattern of cellular neurothekeoma
- Usually has fascicles of spindled fibroblasts
- Usually lacks dense collagen septa

Epithelioid Fibrous Histiocytoma

- Often polypoid nodule with epidermal collarette
- Epithelioid histiocytoid cells arranged in sheets (not nests)
- ALK-1(+) in majority

Benign Cutaneous Biphasic (or Plexiform) Hybrid Tumor of Perineurioma and Cellular Neurothekeoma

- Usually perioral
- Biphasic (often plexiform) admixture of cellular neurothekeoma and perineurioma components
- Perineurioma component has whorls of bland spindle cells
- Often EMA(+), claudin-1 (+), GLUT1(+)

SELECTED REFERENCES

1. Fried I et al: SOX-10 and MiTF expression in cellular and 'mixed' neurothekeoma. J Cutan Pathol. 41(8):640-5, 2014
2. Stratton J et al: Cellular neurothekeoma: analysis of 37 cases emphasizing atypical histologic features. Mod Pathol. 27(5):701-10, 2014
3. Hornick JL et al: Cellular neurothekeoma: detailed characterization in a series of 133 cases. Am J Surg Pathol. 31(3):329-40, 2007

Dome-Shaped Nodule

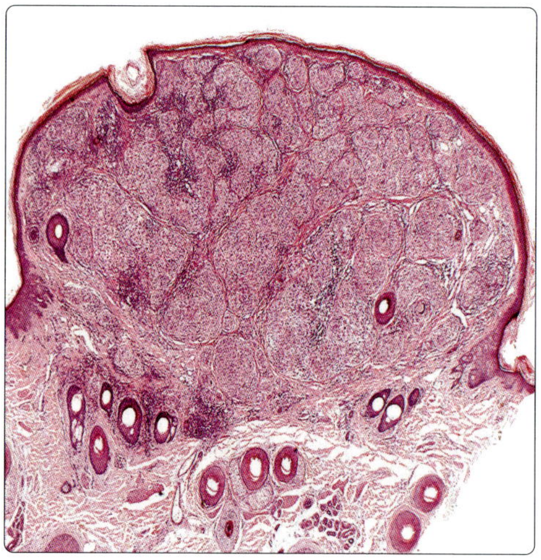

Nested Growth

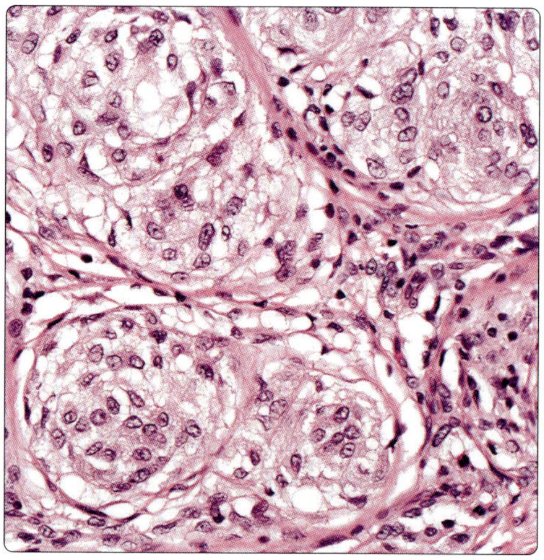

(Left) *Nests of tumor cells fill the dermis, forming a dome-shaped nodule in this low-power H&E of cellular neurothekeoma.* **(Right)** *Nests of histiocytoid cells are separated by thin fibrous septa. The cells have uniform nuclei, a moderate amount of cytoplasm, and indistinct cell margins in this case.*

Myxoid Change

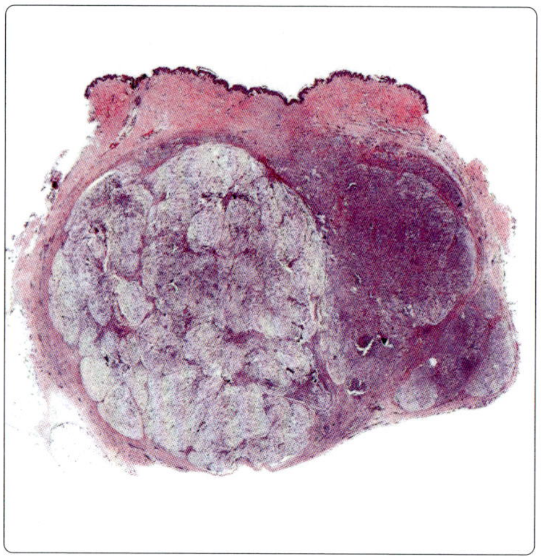

Mimicking Nerve Sheath Myxoma

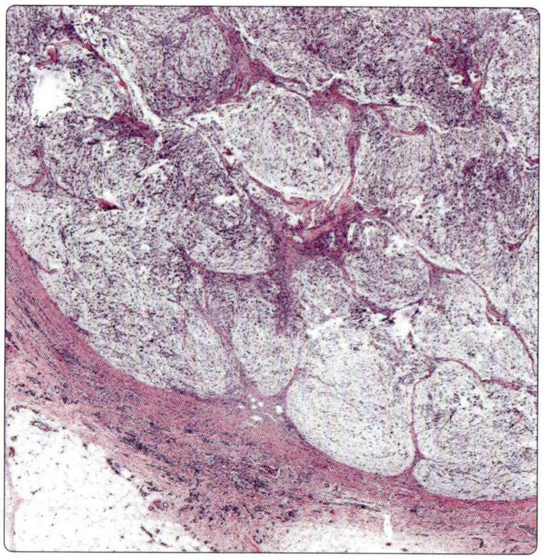

(Left) *Myxoid change is present in 30% of cellular neurothekeoma and may be prominent, as seen here.* **(Right)** *Areas of myxoid change in cellular neurothekeoma may be arranged into myxoid nodules with intervening fibrous septa, an appearance very similar to that of dermal nerve sheath myxoma (conventional neurothekeoma), an unrelated entity.*

Myxoid and Nonmyxoid Zones

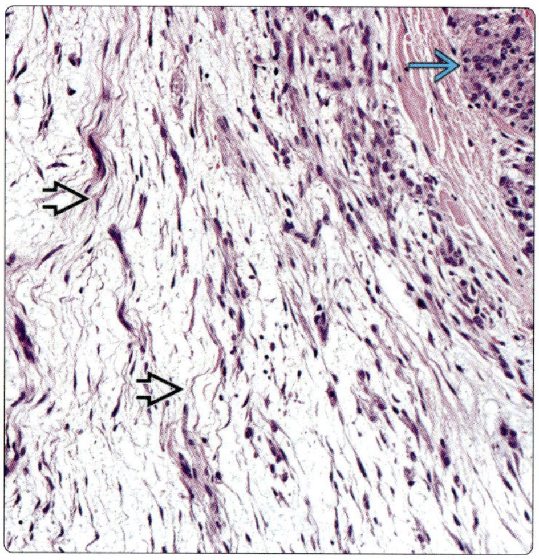

Multinucleated Tumor Giant Cells

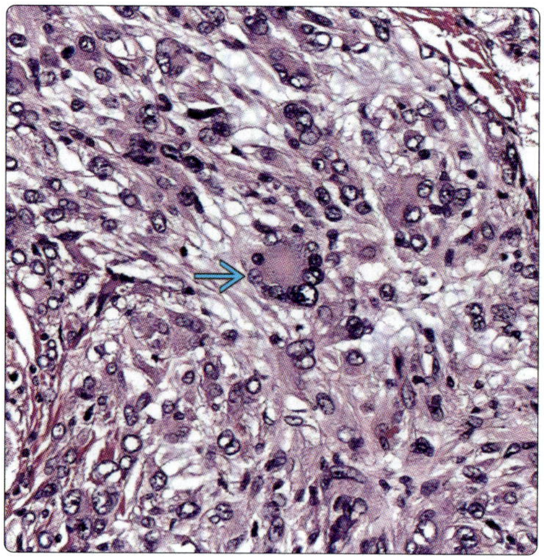

(Left) *Nests of typical nonmyxoid cellular neurothekeoma ➔ transition to myxoid spindled zones resembling nerve sheath myxoma ⇨ in the depicted case.* **(Right)** *Atypical multinucleated tumor giant cells ➔ may be present in cellular neurothekeoma. This is a benign finding not indicative of aggressive behavior. Classic Touton or osteoclastic giant cells may also be seen.*

Mitotic Activity

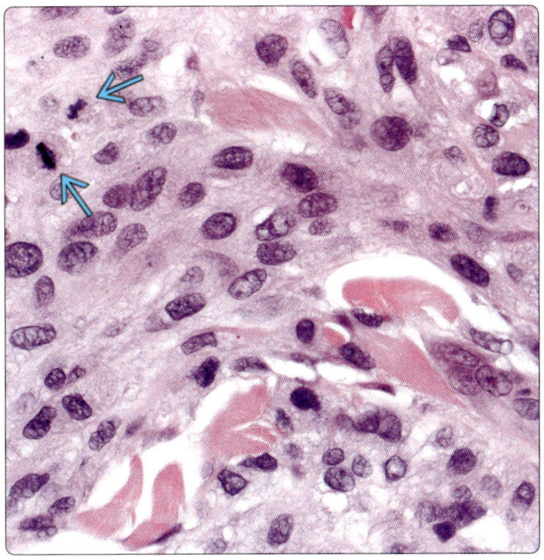

Nests of Atypical Cells

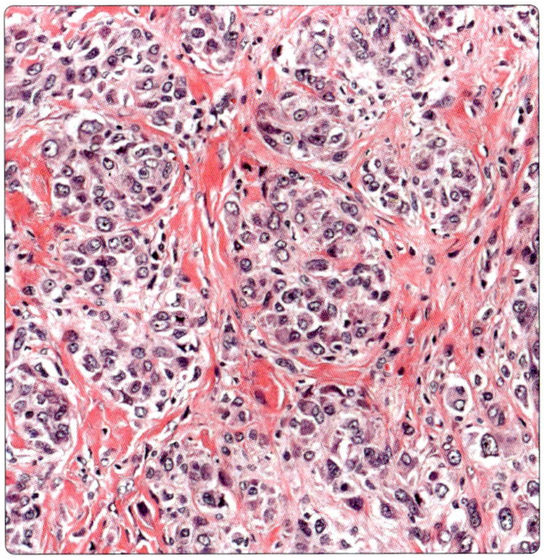

(Left) *Nuclei are oval/round and usually have fine, powdery or pale chromatin. Mitotic activity* → *is common in cellular neurothekeoma and may be brisk (≥ 10 figures/10 HPF).* **(Right)** *This H&E shows a case of cellular neurothekeoma with typical nests of tumor cells but with the additional feature of cellular atypia.*

Pleomorphism

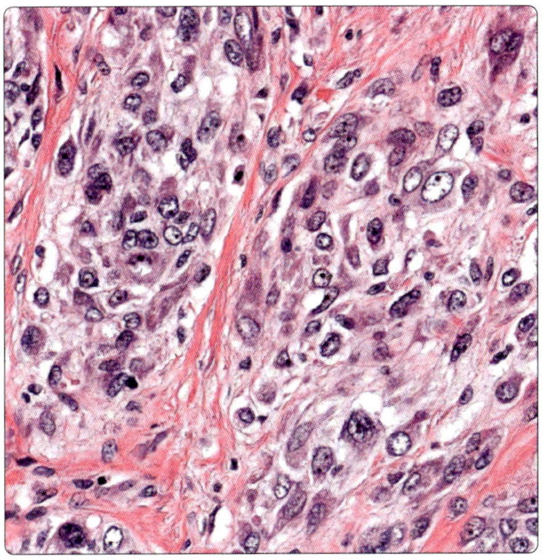

Subcutaneous Involvement

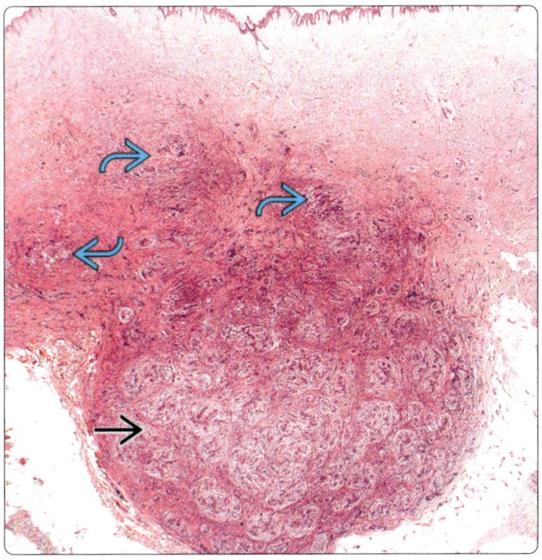

(Left) *Nuclear pleomorphism is a relatively common finding in cellular neurothekeoma; it not does not indicate malignancy or aggressive behavior.* **(Right)** *Subcutaneous involvement* → *is present in 50% of cases of cellular neurothekeoma. Note the focal, small, discrete nests* ↷ *of tumor cells in the overlying dermis.*

Sheet-Like Growth

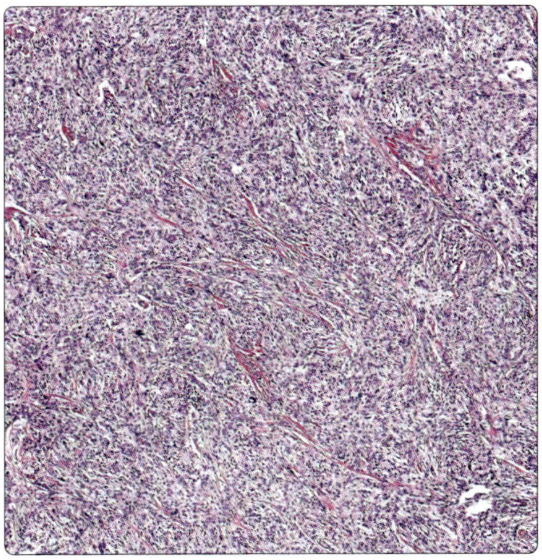

Spindle Cell Areas

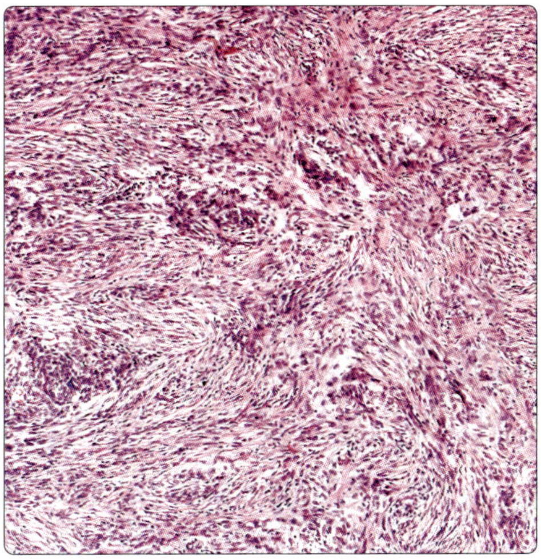

(Left) *Areas of cellular sheet-like growth without nesting may be seen in occasional cases of cellular neurothekeoma, as depicted. More conventional nested or nodular areas are typically seen elsewhere.* **(Right)** *Sheets or fascicles of more spindled tumor cells are occasionally encountered in cellular neurothekeoma.*

Xanthomas

KEY FACTS

TERMINOLOGY

- Reactive, mass-forming collection of lipidized macrophages, usually resulting from altered serum lipid levels
- Several forms
  - Xanthelasma, eruptive, tuberous, tendinous, plane, plexiform

ETIOLOGY/PATHOGENESIS

- Associated with hereditary lipoproteinemias and occasionally secondary lipoproteinemias
- May also occur in normolipemic patients
  - Particularly plexiform xanthoma

CLINICAL ISSUES

- Wide age range (children or adults)
- Usually occur in skin and subcutaneous tissue
- Occasionally arise in deep soft tissues (tendon, synovium, bone)
- Classified based on clinical features and gross appearance
- Treatment: Medical therapy or conservative excision
- Excellent prognosis

MICROSCOPIC

- Specific classification requires clinicopathologic correlation
- Sheets and aggregates of foamy macrophages
- Variable secondary changes, including inflammation, giant cells, fibrosis, and cholesterol cleft formation
- Plexiform xanthoma features multinodular or plexiform growth pattern

TOP DIFFERENTIAL DIAGNOSES

- Localized-type tenosynovial giant cell tumor (giant cell tumor of tendon sheath)
- Solitary (juvenile) xanthogranuloma
- Lipidized-type dermatofibroma (fibrous histiocytoma)
- Verruciform xanthoma
- Plexiform fibrohistiocytic tumor

Xanthelasma

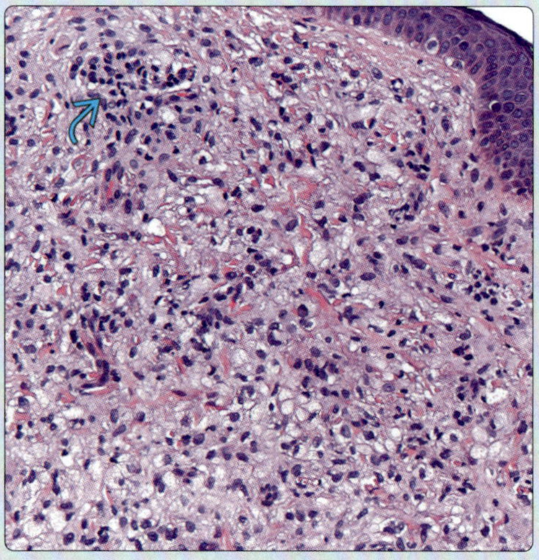

Eruptive Xanthoma

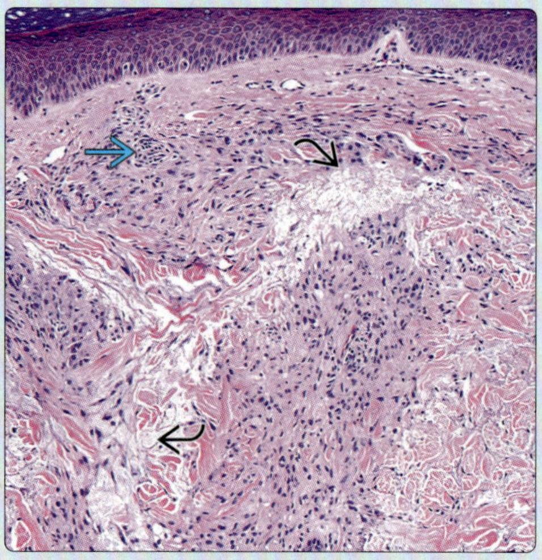

(Left) *Xanthelasmas (and plane xanthomas) consist of a sheet-like infiltrate of foamy macrophages involving the dermis and surrounding adnexal structures. Small areas of chronic inflammation may be present, but fibrosis and cholesterol clefts are not typical.* **(Right)** *Eruptive xanthoma is characterized by sheets of macrophages within the dermis. Extravascular lipid deposits with a blue-gray, amorphous appearance are often seen between dermal collagen bundles. A sparse perivascular inflammatory infiltrate can also be seen.*

Early Eruptive Xanthoma

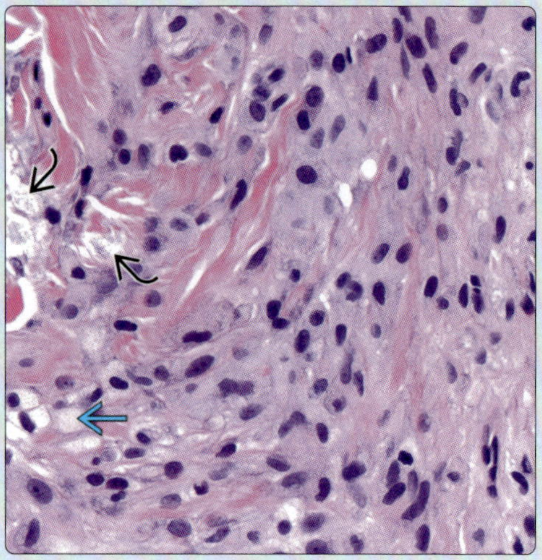

Older Eruptive Xanthoma

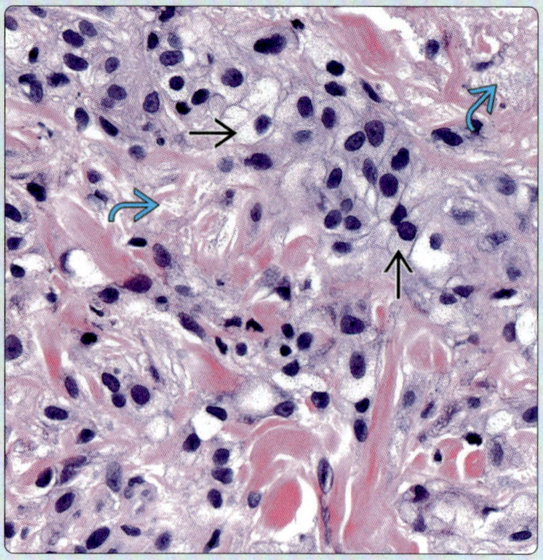

(Left) *In contrast to other forms of xanthoma, the cells in eruptive xanthoma are nonfoamy in early lesions. Note the rare foamy macrophages and extravascular lipid.* **(Right)** *Older eruptive xanthomas accumulate more foamy macrophages and consist of a mixture of foamy and nonfoamy cells. Again, note areas of lace-like, blue-gray extravascular lipid between the dermal collagen bundles.*

TERMINOLOGY

Synonyms

- Plexiform xanthomatous tumor (for plexiform xanthoma)

Definitions

- Reactive, mass-forming collection of lipidized macrophages, usually resulting from altered serum lipid levels
  - Several forms
    - Xanthelasma
    - Eruptive xanthoma
    - Tuberous xanthoma
    - Tendinous xanthoma
    - Planar xanthoma
    - Plexiform xanthoma

ETIOLOGY/PATHOGENESIS

Hereditary or Nonhereditary

- Associated with hereditary lipoproteinemias and occasionally secondary lipoproteinemias (e.g., diabetes, hypothyroidism, primary biliary cirrhosis)
- May also occur in normolipemic patients
  - Particularly plexiform xanthoma

CLINICAL ISSUES

Epidemiology

- Age
  - Wide age range (children or adults)

Presentation

- Usually occur in skin and subcutaneous tissue
- Occasionally arise in deep soft tissues (tendon, synovium, bone)
- Classified based on clinical features
  - **Xanthelasma**
    - Soft, yellow plaques
    - Predilection for eyelids and periorbital skin; often bilateral
  - **Eruptive xanthoma**
    - Sudden onset of small, yellow papules with erythematous halo
    - Predilection for gluteal region, thigh, and shoulders
  - **Tuberous xanthoma**
    - Firm, yellow, subcutaneous nodules and plaques
    - Predilection for elbow, knee, gluteal region, and fingers
  - **Tendinous xanthoma**
    - Soft tissue mass associated with tendons, ligaments, &/or fascia; predilection for hands, feet, and Achilles tendon
    - May impair joint function but often asymptomatic
  - **Planar xanthoma**
    - Variably sized yellow macules; predilection for palmar creases
    - In normolipemic patients, consider underlying reticuloendothelial malignancy
  - **Plexiform xanthoma**
    - Dermal-based cutaneous nodule(s) occurring most often on extremities
      - ▫ Particularly extensor surfaces of elbow and knee regions
    - Usually in males
    - Patients usually normolipemic
  - **Cerebrotendinous xanthomatosis**
    - Rare autosomal recessive disease; sterol 27-hydroxylase gene (*CYP27A1*) mutation
    - Enzyme involved in bile acid synthesis; defect results in accumulation of cholestanol, which is deposited systemically
    - Bilateral Achilles tendon xanthomas and cataracts; CNS symptoms include ataxia, dementia, dysarthria, psychiatric disturbances, and seizures

Treatment

- May regress with medical therapy for hyperlipidemia or underlying cause if secondary
- Conservative excision can be employed for large or symptomatic lesions

Prognosis

- Excellent prognosis
- Surgically treated lesions may recur

MACROSCOPIC

General Features

- Diffuse or circumscribed
  - Plexiform xanthoma may appear grossly multinodular
- Variegated yellow, tan, and white appearance

Size

- Generally few mm to several cm depending on type
- Tendinous xanthomas can be quite large (up to 20 cm)

MICROSCOPIC

Histologic Features

- Specific classification requires clinicopathologic correlation
- Xanthelasma and planar xanthoma
  - Sheets of foamy macrophages
- Eruptive xanthomas
  - Sheets of mostly nonfoamy macrophages with some foamy macrophages
  - Later lesions contain more foamy macrophages
- Tuberous and tendinous xanthoma
  - Nodules of foamy macrophages
  - Chronic inflammation, fibrosis, and cholesterol clefts with giant cells common
- Plexiform xanthoma
  - Multinodular or plexiform growth of nodules of foamy histiocytes separated by fibrous or sclerotic stroma
  - Giant cells
  - Variable chronic inflammation, fibrosis, and cholesterol clefts

ANCILLARY TESTS

Immunohistochemistry

- CD68(+), CD163(+)
- S100 protein (-)

Clinical Forms of Xanthoma

Feature	Xanthelasma	Eruptive	Tuberous	Tendinous	Plane	Plexiform
Lipoprotein association	None or IIa, III	I, III, V, secondary	IIa, III, secondary	IIa, secondary	None, III, secondary	Usually none
Characteristic location	Eyelids	Buttock	Elbow, knee, buttock, finger	Hand, foot, ankle (Achilles)	Palm creases	Elbow, knee, foot/hand
Foamy macrophages	Present	Present (absent in early lesions)	Present	Present	Present	Present
Characteristic histopathology	Foamy macrophages	Foamy and nonfoamy macrophages	Foamy macrophages, cholesterol clefts, giant cells, inflammation, fibrosis	Foamy macrophages, cholesterol clefts, giant cells, inflammation, fibrosis	Foamy macrophages	Plexiform nodules of foamy macrophages; giant cells

Hyperlipoproteinemia (Fredrickson) Classification

Feature	I	IIa	IIb	III	IV	V
Elevated lipoprotein	Chylomicrons	LDL	LDL, VLDL	Chylomicrons, VLDL remnants	VLDL	Chylomicrons, VLDL
Molecular defect	Lipoprotein lipase, apoC-II	LDL receptor, apoB-100	Unknown	ApoE	Unknown	Unknown

DIFFERENTIAL DIAGNOSIS

Localize-Type Tenosynovial Giant Cell Tumor

- Synonym: Giant cell tumor of tendon sheath
- Vast majority arise in digits
- Usually solitary; resembles tendinous xanthoma but contains multinucleated giant cells and hemosiderin
- Contains nonfoamy epithelioid, mononuclear stromal cells
- Osteoclast-like giant cells and hemosiderin common

Solitary (Juvenile) Xanthogranuloma

- Usually young children
- Touton giant cells often present
- Mixed inflammation, including eosinophils and neutrophils

Lipidized-Type Dermatofibroma (Fibrous Histiocytoma)

- Usually lower leg (ankle predominant)
- Demonstrates dermal collagen entrapment

Verruciform Xanthoma

- Most are intraoral or anogenital
- Verrucous epithelium with parakeratin plugs and stromal foam cells

Plexiform Fibrohistiocytic Tumor

- DDx for plexiform xanthoma
- Most common in children and adolescents
- Biphasic appearance
    - Fibromatosis-like fascicles of spindle cells
    - Nodules of epithelioid or histiocytoid cells ± multinucleated giant
- Xanthomatous change rare and usually limited in extent

Plexiform Schwannoma

- DDx for plexiform xanthoma
- Cellular nodules of spindled Schwann cells
- Nuclear palisading common
- Foamy histiocytes may be present but are not usually prominent
- S100(+)

SELECTED REFERENCES

1. Sasamura A et al: A case of late-onset cerebrotendinous xanthomatosis with a novel mutation in the cyp27a1 gene. Intern Med. 57(11):1611-1616, 2018
2. Ghosh SK et al: Tuberous xanthoma as a presenting feature of familial homozygous hypercholesterolemia with aortic regurgitation. J Pediatr. 166(1):198, 2015
3. Blankenship DW et al: Verruciform xanthoma of the upper-extremity in the absence of chronic skin disease or syndrome: a case report and review of the literature. J Cutan Pathol. 40(8):745-52, 2013
4. Shahrabi Farahani S et al: Oral verruciform xanthoma associated with chronic graft-versus-host disease: a report of five cases and a review of the literature. Head Neck Pathol. 5(2):193-8, 2011
5. Reichwaldt I et al: Differential diagnosis of tendon tumors: xanthomas caused by hyperlipidemia in children. J Pediatr Surg. 45(10):e9-12, 2010
6. Oosterveer DM et al: 5-Lipoxygenase activating protein (ALOX5AP) gene variants associate with the presence of xanthomas in familial hypercholesterolemia. Atherosclerosis. 206(1):223-7, 2009
7. Chuang AY et al: Xanthoma of the prostate: a mimicker of high-grade prostate adenocarcinoma. Am J Surg Pathol. 31(8):1225-30, 2007
8. Tsouli SG et al: Pathogenesis, detection and treatment of Achilles tendon xanthomas. Eur J Clin Invest. 35(4):236-44, 2005
9. Moghadasian MH: Cerebrotendinous xanthomatosis: clinical course, genotypes and metabolic backgrounds. Clin Invest Med. 27(1):42-50, 2004
10. Michal M et al: Plexiform xanthomatous tumor: a report of 20 cases in 12 patients. Am J Surg Pathol. 26(10):1302-11, 2002
11. Michal M: Plexiform xanthomatous tumor. A report of three cases. Am J Dermatopathol. 16(5):532-6, 1994
12. Beham A et al: Plexiform xanthoma: an unusual variant. Histopathology. 19(6):565-7, 1991
13. Cruz PD Jr et al: Dermal, subcutaneous, and tendon xanthomas: diagnostic markers for specific lipoprotein disorders. J Am Acad Dermatol. 19(1 Pt 1):95-111, 1988
14. Parker F: Xanthomas and hyperlipidemias. J Am Acad Dermatol. 13(1):1-30, 1985

Tuberous Xanthoma

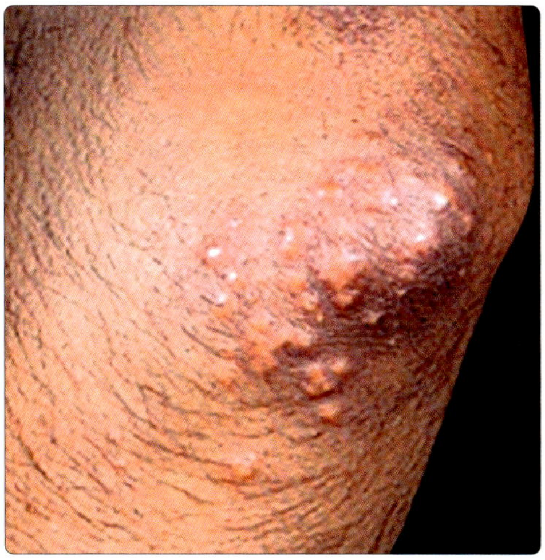

Tuberous Xanthoma

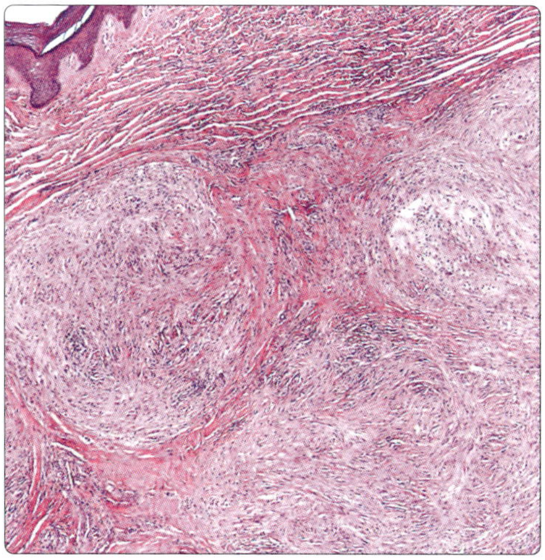

(Left) *Tuberous xanthoma is shown involving the knee. Tuberous xanthomas appear as firm, yellow-red, subcutaneous nodules and occur at pressure areas, such as the buttock and extensor surfaces of the knee and elbow. Smaller nodules often coalesce to form larger nodules or plaques.* **(Right)** *Tuberous xanthomas consists of a nodular infiltrate of foamy macrophages involving the dermis and may be uninodular or multinodular, as in this example.*

Cholesterol Clefts and Giant Cells

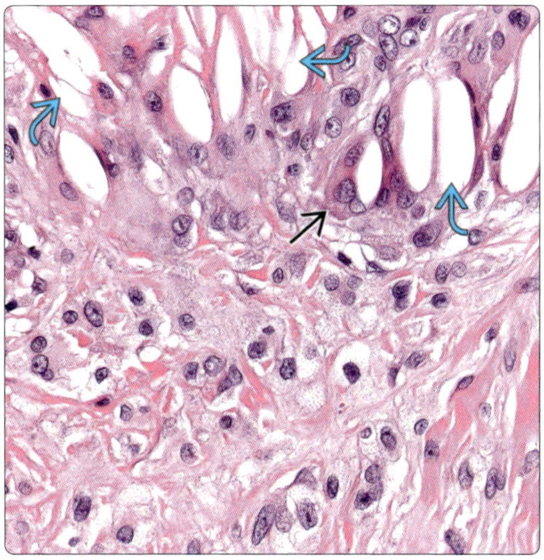

Fibrosis, Necrosis, and Cholesterol Clefts

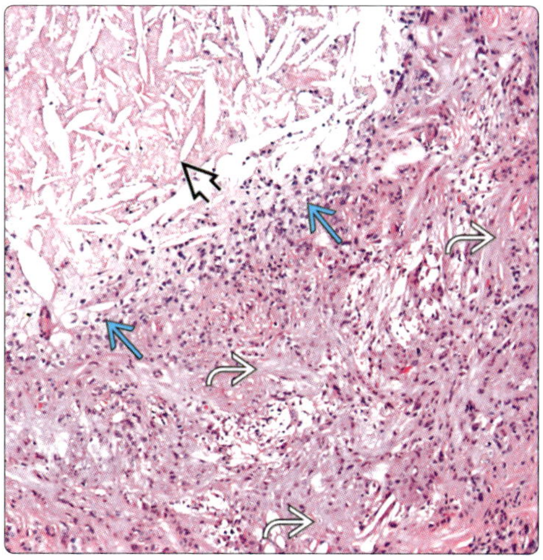

(Left) *Unlike the other forms of xanthoma, tuberous (and tendinous) xanthomas usually have secondary changes, including collections of extracellular cholesterol with cholesterol cleft formation → and associated giant cells →.* **(Right)** *Other secondary changes in tuberous (and tendinous) xanthomas include varying degrees of fibrosis → and foci of necrosis → containing amorphous eosinophilic debris with cholesterol clefts and a surrounding rim of foamy macrophages →.*

Tendinous Xanthoma

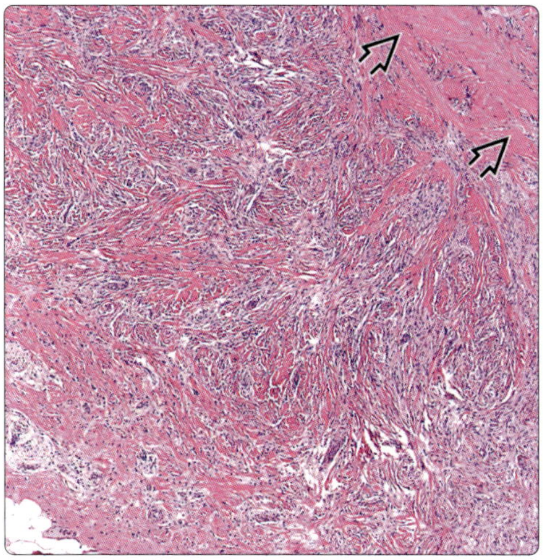

Plexiform Xanthoma

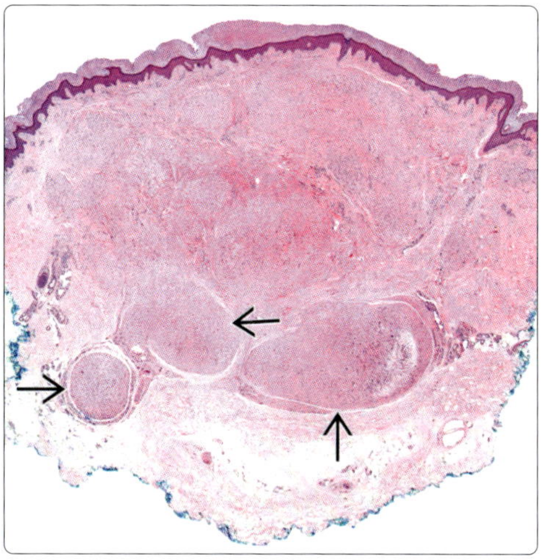

(Left) *Tendinous xanthomas are histologically identical to tuberous xanthomas except that they involve deeper structures, such as tendons → and ligaments.* **(Right)** *A multinodular proliferation with a plexiform architecture filling the dermis is typical of plexiform xanthoma. The deep nodules → tend to be more well developed than the superficial ones.*

Solitary (Juvenile) Xanthogranuloma

KEY FACTS

TERMINOLOGY

- Stable or regressing histiocytic lesion that usually occurs in childhood
  - Form of non-Langerhans histiocytosis

CLINICAL ISSUES

- Majority occur in children < 3 years of age
- Solitary cutaneous lesion in majority of cases
  - Head and neck > trunk > extremities
- Visceral examples almost exclusively in infants and children
- Treatment: Excision
  - Chemotherapy administered to rare patients with systemic disease
- Prognosis usually excellent
  - Most lesions regress or stabilize (including large visceral ones)
- Rare deaths associated with multiorgan disease

MICROSCOPIC

- Mononuclear and spindle cells
- Multinucleated cells ± Touton features
- Inflammatory cell background, often with many eosinophils
- Variable lipid and foamy histiocytes
- Negligible nuclear atypia
- Minimal mitotic activity

ANCILLARY TESTS

- CD68(+), CD163(+)
- CD1a(-), S100(-)

TOP DIFFERENTIAL DIAGNOSES

- Xanthoma
- Fibrous histiocytoma/dermatofibroma
- Langerhans cell histiocytosis
- Rosai-Dorfman disease
- Reticulohistiocytoma

(Left) *This is the typical appearance of a juvenile xanthogranuloma (JXG) at low magnification. The lesion is composed of a nodular, cellular histiocytic proliferation in the dermis with no intervening grenz zone between the tumor and the epidermis.* **(Right)** *This cellular example of JXG shows an inflammatory background composed mostly of mononuclear histiocytic and lymphoid cells.*

Solitary (Juvenile) Xanthogranuloma

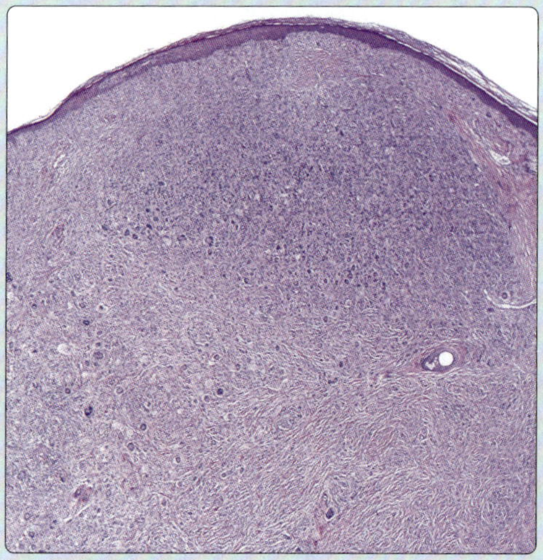

Mononuclear Cells

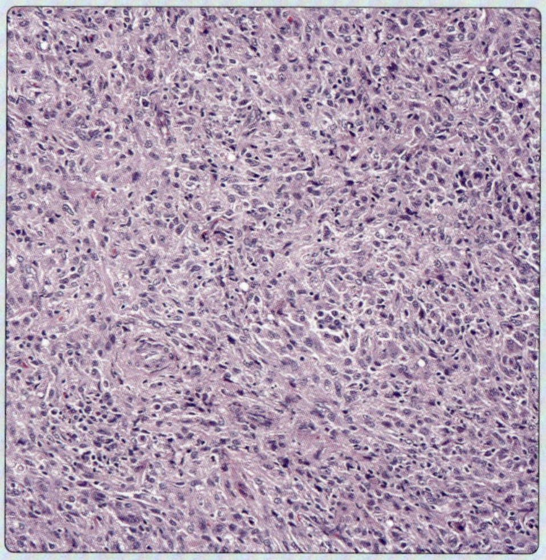

(Left) *Many Touton giant cells with a ring of peripheral nuclei can be seen in this JXG. The background cells are spindled to ovoid with eosinophilic cytoplasm, which shows only minimal lipid in this case.* **(Right)** *High magnification shows eosinophils and foamy histiocytes, which are commonly encountered in JXG.*

Touton Giant Cells

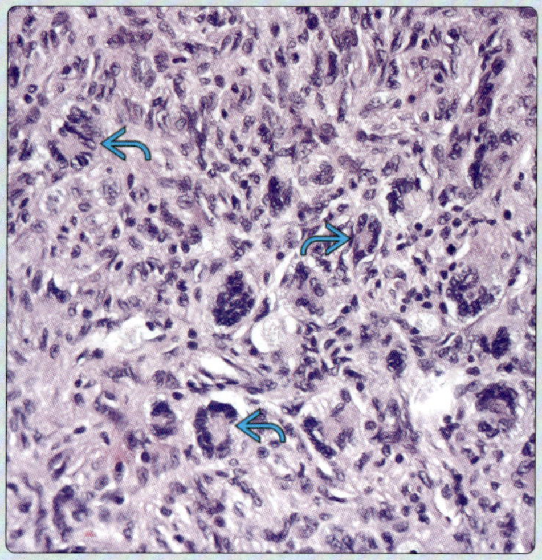

Eosinophils and Foamy Histiocytes

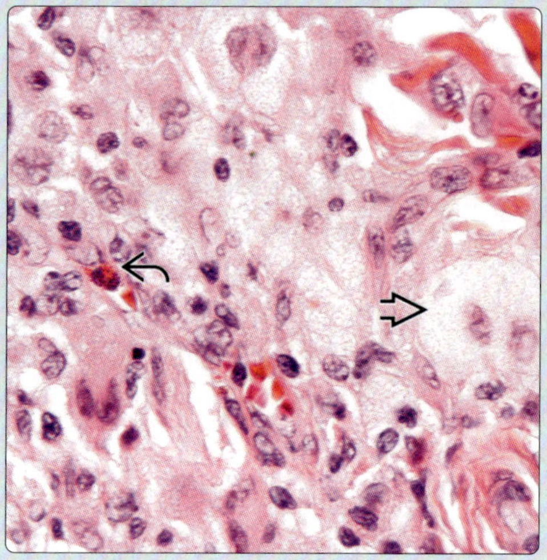

TERMINOLOGY

Abbreviations

- Juvenile xanthogranuloma (JXG)

Definitions

- Stable or regressing histiocytic lesion that usually occurs in childhood
  - Form of non-Langerhans histiocytosis

CLINICAL ISSUES

Epidemiology

- Incidence
  - Rare
- Age
  - Majority under 3 years
    - Visceral examples almost exclusively in infants and children
  - 13-30% in older children and adults
- Sex
  - Slight male predominance

Presentation

- Solitary cutaneous lesion in majority of cases
  - Head and neck > trunk > extremities
- Up to 10% of patients with multiple cutaneous lesions
- Up to 5% of patients with visceral systemic disease

Treatment

- Excision
- Chemotherapy administered to rare patients with systemic disease

Prognosis

- Usually excellent
  - Most lesions regress or stabilize (including large visceral ones)
  - Rare deaths associated with multiorgan disease

MICROSCOPIC

Histologic Features

- Proliferation of numerous mononuclear and multinucleated cells
  - Multinucleated cells may show Touton-type features (ring of peripheral nuclei)
- Spindle cells
  - Variable finely vacuolated cytoplasm
  - Often lightly eosinophilic
- Variable lipid and foamy histiocytes
  - Minimal lipid in early lesions
- Inflammatory cell background
  - Acute and chronic inflammatory cells
    - Eosinophils and lymphocytes are consistently present
    - Neutrophils uncommon
- Negligible nuclear atypia
- Minimal mitotic activity

ANCILLARY TESTS

Immunohistochemistry

- CD68(+), CD163(+)
- CD1a(-), S100(-)

DIFFERENTIAL DIAGNOSIS

Xanthoma

- Proliferation of numerous foamy histiocytes
- No Touton-type giant cells
- Minimal background inflammation
- Can be associated with hyperlipidemia
  - Usually lesions of adults

Fibrous Histiocytoma/Dermatofibroma

- Usually in adults
- Prominent storiform pattern
- Peripheral collagen trapping usually prominent
- Overlying epidermal hyperplasia usually seen
- Intralesional hemorrhage, hemosiderin

Langerhans Cell Histiocytosis

- Usually presents with skeletal disease but also in skin
- Atypical reniform-appearing histiocytic cells
- Background of many eosinophils usually seen
- S100(+), CD1a(+), langerin (+)

Rosai-Dorfman Disease

- a.k.a. sinus histiocytosis with massive lymphadenopathy
- Usually involves lymph nodes but may present in skin and soft tissues
- Large histiocytes with abundant foamy cytoplasm
- Emperipolesis of inflammatory cells (including lymphocytes, plasma cells, and neutrophils) is key diagnostic feature
- Histiocytes are S100(+), CD1a(-)

Reticulohistiocytoma

- Lesions of adults
- Brown-yellow papules at any site
- Nodules of densely eosinophilic or 2-toned histiocytes, some multinucleated
- Nuclear atypia may be present but not clinically significant
- CD68(+), S100(-), CD1a(-)

SELECTED REFERENCES

1. Ladha MA et al: Giant juvenile xanthogranuloma: case report, literature review, and algorithm for classification. J Cutan Med Surg. 1203475418777734, 2018
2. López-Robles J et al: Juvenile xanthogranuloma with angiomatous appearance and a peculiar immunophenotype. Pediatr Dermatol. 35(1):e55-e56, 2018
3. Meyer M et al: Systemic juvenile xanthogranuloma: a case report and brief review. Clin Exp Dermatol. 43(5):642-4, 2018
4. Paxton CN et al: Genetic evaluation of juvenile xanthogranuloma: genomic abnormalities are uncommon in solitary lesions, advanced cases may show more complexity. Mod Pathol. 30(9):1234-40, 2017
5. Song M et al: Structural correlations between dermoscopic and histopathological features of juvenile xanthogranuloma. J Eur Acad Dermatol Venereol. 25(3):259-63, 2011
6. Kaur MR et al: Disseminated clustered juvenile xanthogranuloma: an unusual morphological variant of a common condition. Clin Exp Dermatol. 33(5):575-7, 2008
7. Janssen D et al: Juvenile xanthogranuloma in childhood and adolescence: a clinicopathologic study of 129 patients from the kiel pediatric tumor registry. Am J Surg Pathol. 29(1):21-8, 2005
8. Zelger B et al: Juvenile and adult xanthogranuloma. A histological and immunohistochemical comparison. Am J Surg Pathol. 18(2):126-35, 1994

Reticulohistiocytoma

KEY FACTS

TERMINOLOGY

- Proliferation of histiocytes with abundant dense, glassy-appearing eosinophilic cytoplasm
- Solitary cutaneous reticulohistiocytoma (SCR)

CLINICAL ISSUES

- Usually occurs in adults > 40 years old
- Most commonly in head and neck region, including mucosal sites, but may present at any cutaneous site
- Usually single lesion, but several may be present in some cases
- Often appear red-brown or yellow-brown
- May be preceded by trauma in some cases

MICROSCOPIC

- Dermal-based nodular proliferation of large mononuclear and multinucleated histiocytes
- Cells show characteristic abundant glassy/hyalinized-appearing eosinophilic cytoplasm
- Occasional Touton-type giant cells containing lipid may be present
- Early lesions characterized by more mononuclear cells with lymphocytes
- Cytologic atypia is usually minimal, and mitoses are few and nonatypical

ANCILLARY TESTS

- CD68 (KP1)(+), CD163(+), and lysozyme (+)
- Variable expression of FXIIIA, CD64, and α-1-antitrypsin
- S100(-); rarely focal (+)

TOP DIFFERENTIAL DIAGNOSES

- Multicentric and generalized cutaneous reticulohistiocytosis
- Solitary (juvenile) xanthogranuloma
- Langerhans cell histiocytosis
- Rosai-Dorfman disease

(Left) *At low magnification, reticulohistiocytoma shows a dense, nodular but symmetric and well-circumscribed collection of large histiocytic-appearing cells in the dermis.* **(Right)** *The tumor cells of reticulohistiocytoma show abundant dense, eosinophilic, glassy-appearing cytoplasm and vesicular nuclei ⇒ with prominent nucleoli.*

Reticulohistiocytoma

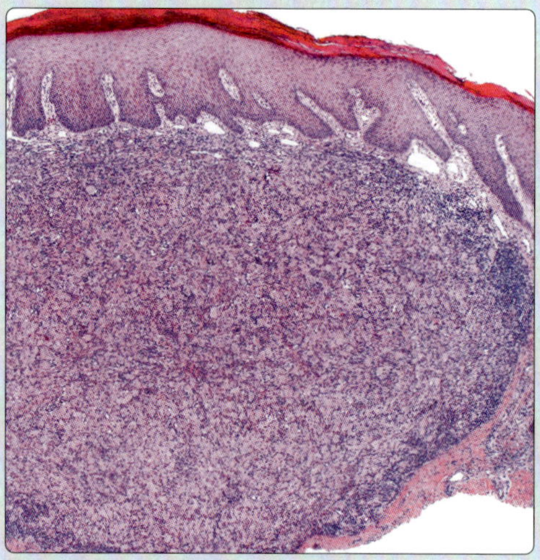

Prominent Nucleoli

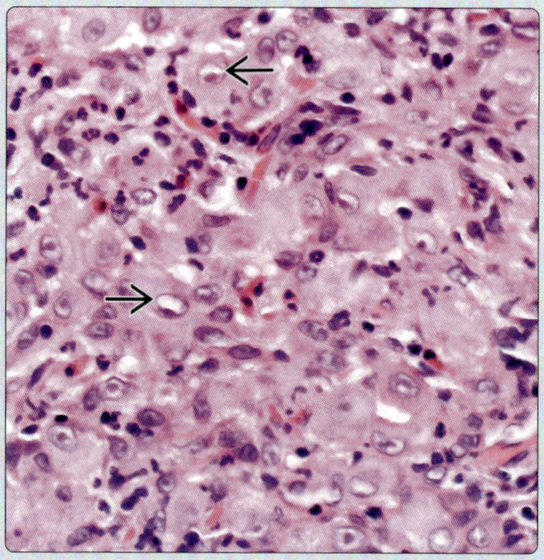

(Left) *Higher power examination shows sheets of eosinophilic cells associated with an inflammatory infiltrate containing lymphocytes, neutrophils ⇒, and eosinophils.* **(Right)** *Another case at high-power examination shows large eosinophilic cells associated with an inflammatory infiltrate with numerous eosinophils ⇒.*

Mixed Inflammatory Infiltrate

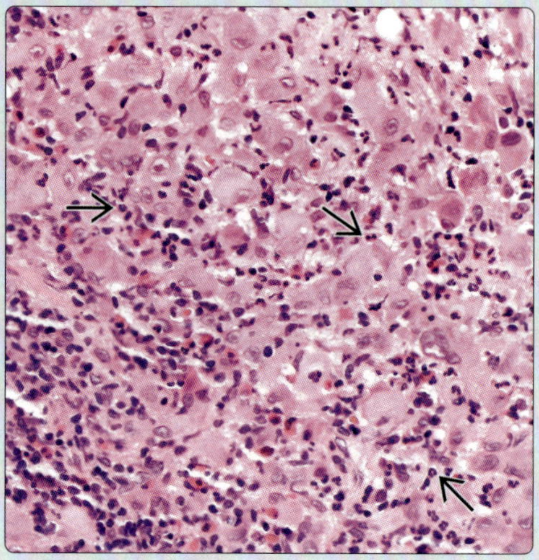

Numerous Eosinophils

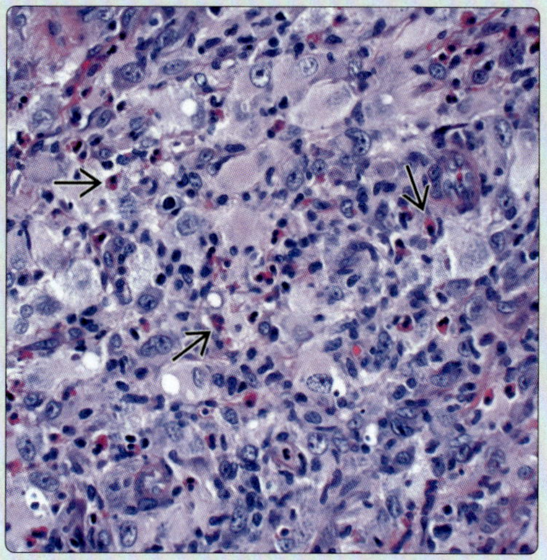

TERMINOLOGY

Synonyms

- Solitary cutaneous reticulohistiocytoma (SCR)
- Reticulohistiocytic granuloma
- Giant cell reticulohistiocytoma

Definitions

- Proliferation of histiocytes with abundant dense, glassy-appearing, eosinophilic to 2-toned cytoplasm

ETIOLOGY/PATHOGENESIS

Environmental Exposure

- May be related to stimuli, such as insect bites, infection, trauma, or ruptured folliculitis or cyst

CLINICAL ISSUES

Epidemiology

- Incidence
  - Rare
- Age
  - Usually occurs in adults > 40 years
    - However, some cases have been reported in adolescents
- Sex
  - M = F

Site

- Usually head and neck region, including mucosal sites
  - However, may present at any cutaneous site

Presentation

- Skin papule or nodule
  - Usually single lesion, but several may be present in some cases
- Firm, rapidly growing lesion
- Usually appear as red-brown or yellow-brown
- May be preceded by trauma in some cases
- Lack of systemic symptoms, including fever, weight loss, or weakness (which may be seen in multicentric reticulohistiocytosis)

Treatment

- Complete conservative excision is curative
  - Usually not required unless lesion is very large or fails to resolve

Prognosis

- Excellent
- Lesions often involute spontaneously
- No definite relationship with more aggressive multicentric reticulohistiocytosis
  - However, multiple skin lesions should suggest possibility of generalized cutaneous reticulohistiocytosis

MACROSCOPIC

General Features

- Dermal-based, nodular, well-circumscribed but unencapsulated lesion

Size

- Lesions typically range in size from 0.5-2.0 cm

MICROSCOPIC

Histologic Features

- Dermal-based nodular proliferation of large mononuclear and multinucleated histiocytes
  - Cells show characteristic abundant glassy/hyalinized-appearing eosinophilic to amphophilic-staining (2-toned) cytoplasm
  - Some cells may show finely granular cytoplasm
  - Occasional Touton-type giant cells (similar to those in juvenile xanthogranuloma) containing lipid may be present but are not prominent
  - Cytologic atypia is usually minimal, and mitoses are few and nonatypical
  - No infiltrative features are present
- Overlying epidermis may show atrophy/thinning
  - Often grenz zone separating infiltrate from epidermis
- Early lesions characterized by background inflammatory infiltrate with many small mononuclear cells and lymphocytes
- Later lesions show greater numbers of large mononuclear and multinucleated cells with background infiltrate, including neutrophils and eosinophils
- Phagocytosis of inflammatory cells and collagen may be present
- Occasional bizarre-appearing cells may be present but do not indicate malignancy
- Rare cases may show deep subcutaneous, and even lymph node, involvement

ANCILLARY TESTS

Histochemistry

- PAS-D digestion and Sudan black
  - Reactivity: Positive
  - Staining pattern: Cytoplasmic; highlights granules

Immunohistochemistry

- CD68(+), CD4(+), CD163(+), and lysozyme (+)
- Variable expression of FXIIIA, CD64, and α-1-antitrypsin
- S100(-); rarely focal (+)
- Cells negative for CD1a, CD3, CD20, CD34, actin, desmin, HMB-45, Melan-A

Electron Microscopy

- Large cells showing abundant granular cytoplasm containing numerous mitochondria, phagolysosomes, dense bodies, and myelin figures
  - Also contain so-called pleomorphic cytoplasmic inclusions
    - Highly complex structures consisting mainly of unit membranes, which may surround vesicles
- Birbeck granules are absent

DIFFERENTIAL DIAGNOSIS

Multicentric and Generalized Cutaneous Reticulohistiocytosis

- These entities show different clinical features

- Multicentric cutaneous reticulohistiocytosis (MCR) presents with multiple lesions involving skin, mucosal sites, joints, and occasionally internal organs
  - MCR may show aggressive course with destructive arthropathy and constitutional symptoms
- Generalized cutaneous reticulohistiocytosis (GCR) is characterized by eruption of multiple small cutaneous lesions
  - Some cases may progress to MCR
- Histologically, there is considerable overlap with solitary reticulohistiocytoma, but some differences have been described
  - Solitary lesions may be better circumscribed and show more multinucleated giants cells
  - Neutrophils and xanthomatized cells have been reported to be more common in solitary reticulohistiocytoma
  - FXIIIA expression may be lower in systemic cases

Juvenile Xanthogranuloma

- Typically occurs in children, but some cases occur in adults (adult-type xanthogranuloma)
- Multiple papules are common, and dozens of lesions have been reported in some cases
- Histologically, typically shows more foamy histiocytes and Touton-type giant cells with peripheral wreath-like arrangement of nuclei
  - Cells lack dense glassy eosinophilic cytoplasm of reticulohistiocytoma
- Cells positive by immunohistochemistry for CD68 and CD163, but negative for S100 and CD1a

Langerhans Cell Histiocytosis

- Langerhans cell histiocytosis includes Letterer-Siwe, Hand-Schüller-Christian, eosinophilic granuloma, and congenital self-healing reticulohistiocytosis variants
- Predominantly occur in children
  - Also 2nd peak in elderly adults (usually eosinophilic granuloma variant)
- Typically characterized by multiple skin lesions and systemic involvement (especially bone)
- Histologic examination shows proliferation of mononuclear cells in dermis and occasionally in epidermis
  - Cells show large folded or reniform vesicular nuclei and abundant eosinophilic cytoplasm
  - Cells lack dense eosinophilic or 2-toned cytoplasm of reticulohistiocytoma
  - Background infiltrate often contains numerous eosinophils and variable numbers of lymphocytes
- CD1a, langerin, and S100 are positive in vast majority of cases (all are negative in reticulohistiocytoma)

Rosai-Dorfman Disease

- Also known as sinus histiocytosis with massive lymphadenopathy (SHML)
- Often shows concomitant lymphadenopathy and constitutional symptoms
- Lesions may be solitary or multiple
- Histologic examination shows proliferation of large, pale-staining histiocytes with emperipolesis of lymphocytes, plasma cells, and erythrocytes
  - Cells lack dense, glassy, 2-toned cytoplasm of reticulohistiocytoma
- S100(+) (negative in reticulohistiocytoma), CD1a(-)

DIAGNOSTIC CHECKLIST

Pathologic Interpretation Pearls

- Nodular proliferation of large mononuclear and multinucleated histiocytes
  - Cells show characteristic abundant glassy/hyalinized-appearing eosinophilic cytoplasm
  - Occasional Touton-type giant cells containing lipid may be present but are not prominent (as in juvenile xanthogranuloma)
- Cells are typically positive for CD68, CD163, and lysozyme
- Cells are negative for S100, CD1a, CD3, CD20, and CD34

SELECTED REFERENCES

1. Shen WC et al: Co-existence of Langerhans cell histiocytosis and reticulohistiocytosis with initial presentation of skull lesions: a case report. J Cutan Pathol. 46(1):62-6, 2019
2. Aasano T et al: The utility of FDG-PET/CT imaging in the evaluation of multicentric reticulohistiocytosis: a case report. Medicine (Baltimore). 97(33):e11449, 2018
3. Delorenze LM et al: Dermoscopy of solitary cutaneous reticulohistiocytoma. G Ital Dermatol Venereol. 153(4):579-80, 2018
4. Gru AA et al: Cutaneous hematolymphoid and histiocytic proliferations in children. Pediatr Dev Pathol. 21(2):208-51, 2018
5. Güleç AT: Solitary reticulohistiocytoma with arborizing vessels: a new mimicker of basal cell carcinoma. J Am Acad Dermatol. 74(1):e5-6, 2016
6. Cohen PR et al: Adult-onset reticulohistiocytoma presenting as a solitary asymptomatic red knee nodule: report and review of clinical presentations and immunohistochemistry staining features of reticulohistiocytosis. Dermatol Online J. 20(3), 2014
7. Kandiah DA: Multicentric reticulohistiocytosis. Mayo Clin Proc. 89(8):e73, 2014
8. Saba R et al: Multicentric reticulohistiocytosis presenting with papulonodular skin lesions and arthritis mutilans. Case Rep Rheumatol. 2013:201563, 2013
9. Caputo R et al: Unusual variants of non-Langerhans cell histiocytoses. J Am Acad Dermatol. 57(6):1031-45, 2007
10. Chen CH et al: Multicentric reticulohistiocytosis presenting with destructive polyarthritis, laryngopharyngeal dysfunction, and a huge reticulohistiocytoma. J Clin Rheumatol. 12(5):252-4, 2006
11. Miettinen M et al: Reticulohistiocytoma (solitary epithelioid histiocytoma): a clinicopathologic and immunohistochemical study of 44 cases. Am J Surg Pathol. 30(4):521-8, 2006
12. Wang KH et al: Cutaneous Rosai-Dorfman disease: clinicopathological profiles, spectrum and evolution of 21 lesions in six patients. Br J Dermatol. 154(2):277-86, 2006
13. Nguyen TT et al: Expression of CD163 (hemoglobin scavenger receptor) in normal tissues, lymphomas, carcinomas, and sarcomas is largely restricted to the monocyte/macrophage lineage. Am J Surg Pathol. 29(5):617-24, 2005
14. Bakri SJ et al: Recurrent solitary reticulohistiocytoma of the eyelid. Ophthal Plast Reconstr Surg. 19(2):162-4, 2003
15. Busam KJ et al: Immunohistochemical distinction of epithelioid histiocytic proliferations from epithelioid melanocytic nevi. Am J Dermatopathol. 22(3):237-41, 2000
16. Burgdorf WH et al: The non-Langerhans' cell histiocytoses in childhood. Cutis. 58(3):201-7, 1996
17. Suwabe H et al: Reticulohistiocytoma involving the skin, subcutaneous tissue and a regional lymph node. Pathol Int. 46(7):531-7, 1996
18. Hunt SJ et al: Solitary reticulohistiocytoma in pregnancy: immunohistochemical and ultrastructural study of a case with unusual immunophenotype. J Cutan Pathol. 22(2):177-81, 1995
19. Zelger B et al: Reticulohistiocytoma and multicentric reticulohistiocytosis. Histopathologic and immunophenotypic distinct entities. Am J Dermatopathol. 16(6):577-84, 1994
20. Caputo R et al: Solitary reticulohistiocytosis (reticulohistiocytoma) of the skin in children: report of two cases. Arch Dermatol. 128(5):698-9, 1992
21. Davies BT et al: The so-called reticulohistiocytoma of the skin; a comparison of two distinct types. Br J Dermatol. 67(6):205-11, 1955

Reticulohistiocytoma

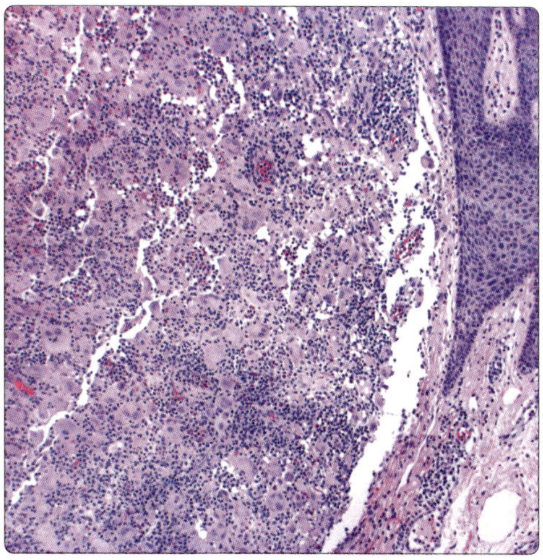

High Magnification

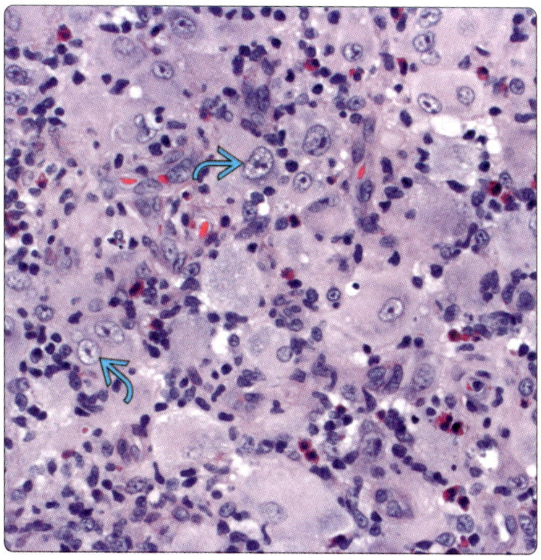

(Left) *The edge of this nodular reticulohistiocytoma shows a well-circumscribed collection of large histiocytic-appearing cells in the dermis, associated with many lymphocytes and eosinophils.* **(Right)** *High magnification of the same tumor shows large histiocytic cells with abundant dense eosinophilic to amphophilic (2-toned) cytoplasm and large, vesicular-appearing nuclei →.*

CD163 Expression

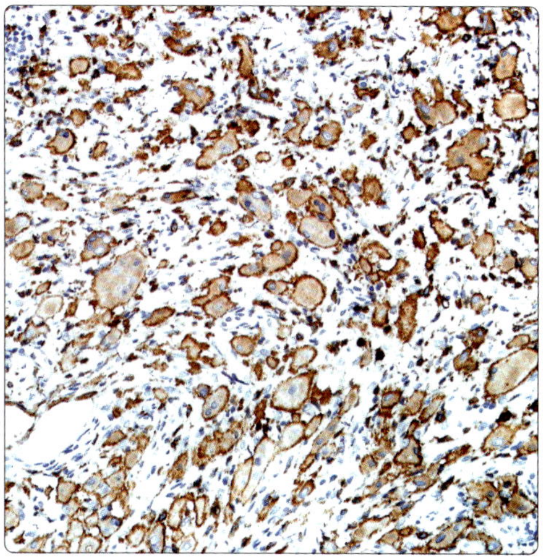

S100 Immunohistochemical Stain

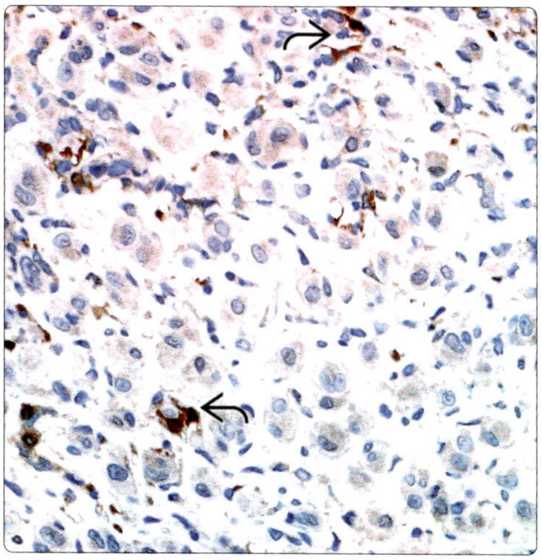

(Left) *CD163 immunohistochemical stain is strongly and diffusely positive in reticulohistiocytoma, highlighting the tumor cell cytoplasm and membranes.* **(Right)** *S100 protein is essentially negative in reticulohistiocytoma with only very weak cytoplasmic, and no nuclear, staining. A few background dendritic cells are strongly positive →.*

Differential Diagnosis: Multicentric Reticulohistiocytosis

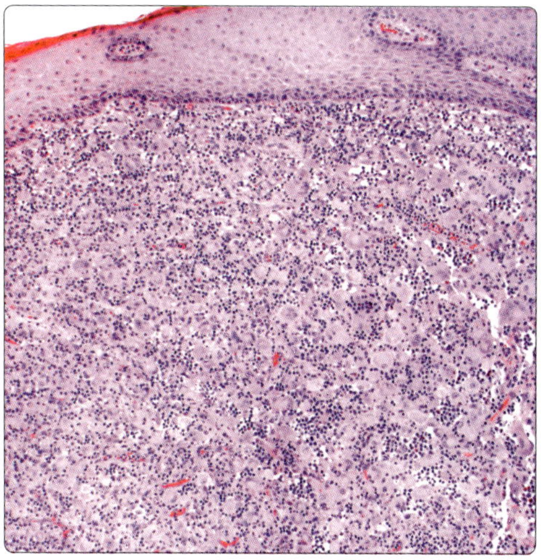

Differential Diagnosis: Multicentric Reticulohistiocytosis

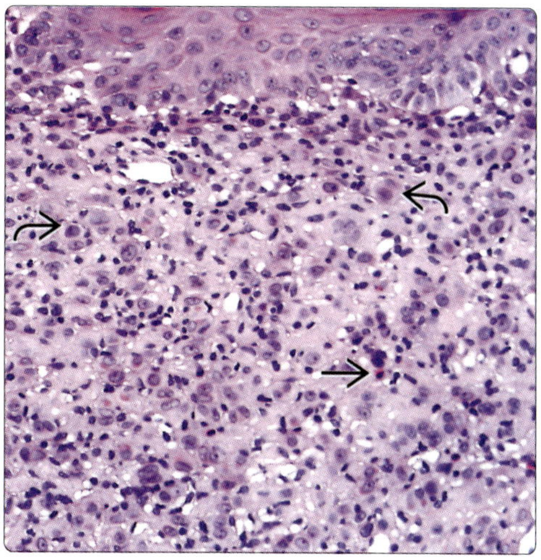

(Left) *Multicentric reticulohistiocytosis (MCR) shows a nodular proliferation of enlarged histiocytic cells in the dermis. The findings are very similar to those in solitary reticulohistiocytoma, and clinical history/description are essential in differentiating between these conditions.* **(Right)** *Higher magnification of MCR shows a proliferation of numerous enlarged, histiocytic-appearing cells → associated with a background of mixed inflammatory infiltrate containing scattered eosinophils →.*

Deep Granuloma Annulare

KEY FACTS

TERMINOLOGY

- Synonyms: Subcutaneous granuloma annulare (GA), pseudorheumatoid nodule

CLINICAL ISSUES

- Children and young adults (mean age: 4 years old)
- 2:1 female predominance
- Painless subcutaneous nodules
- Lower legs (especially tibial), forearms/hands, face, scalp, buttocks
- Some also have cutaneous papules of conventional GA
- No association with rheumatoid arthritis
- Benign
- No consistently effective treatment; variable response to steroids
- Lesions often regress within several years but recurrence seen in 20% or more

MICROSCOPIC

- Multiple nodular subcutaneous granulomas with necrobiosis and blue mucin, surrounded by palisading histiocytes at periphery
- Typical GA in overlying dermis (25%)
- Often with surrounding inflammation and fibrosis

ANCILLARY TESTS

- Alcian blue (pH 2.5) and colloidal iron highlight mucin
- CD68(+), CD163(+)
- Keratin (-), EMA(-)
- Retained nuclear INI1

TOP DIFFERENTIAL DIAGNOSES

- Rheumatoid nodule
- Epithelioid sarcoma
- Infectious granulomas
- Necrobiosis lipoidica diabeticorum

Deep Granuloma Annulare

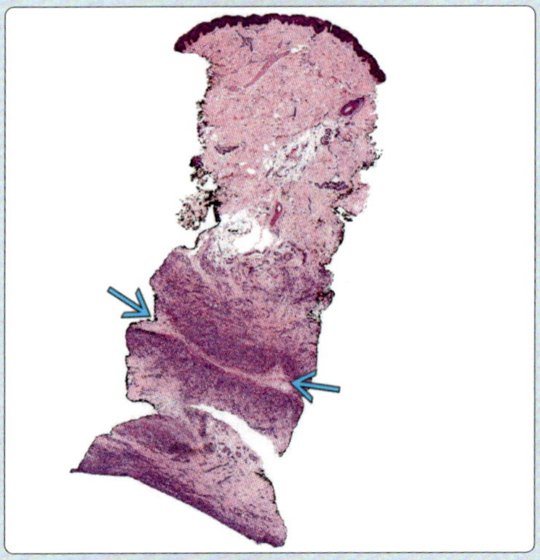

Central Necrobiosis

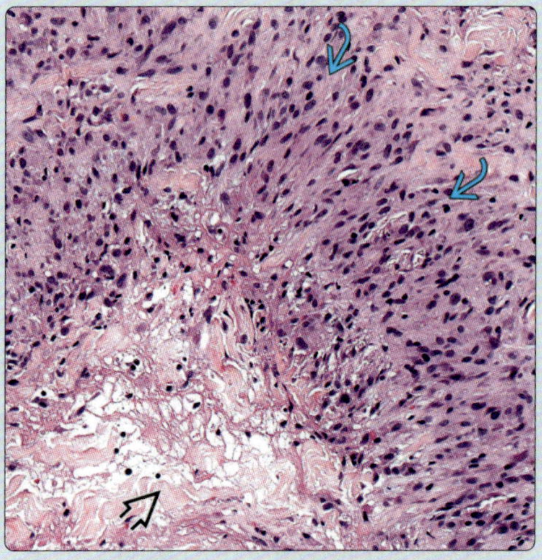

(Left) *Deep granuloma annulare is composed of palisaded granulomas centered in the deep dermis or subcutis. Central zones of necrobiosis are evident even from low magnification.* **(Right)** *Bland, spindled and epithelioid histiocytes are radially arranged (palisading) around a central zone of degenerated collagen bundles (necrobiosis).*

Blue Granulomas

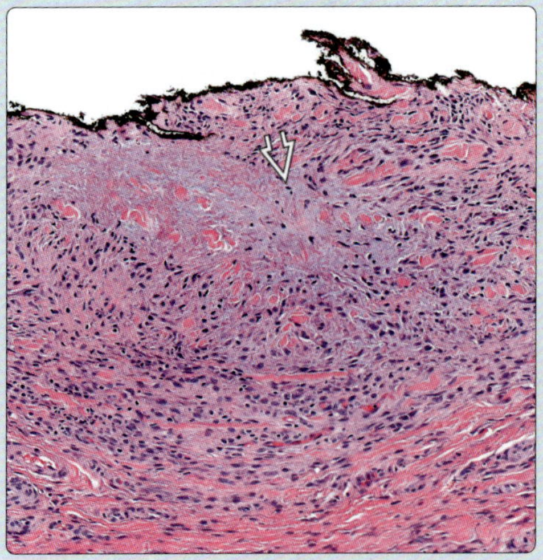

Mimicking Rheumatoid Nodule

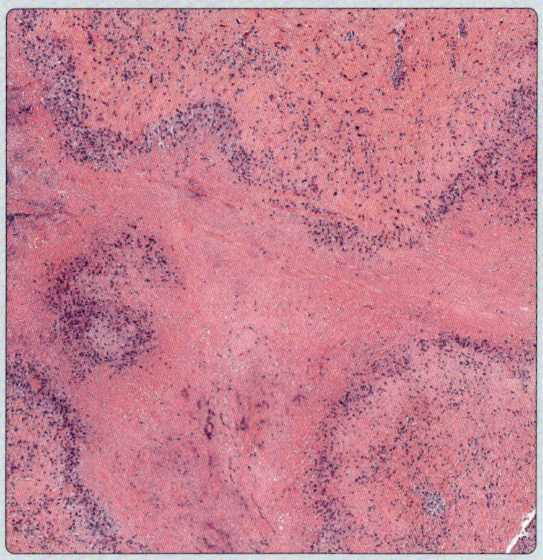

(Left) *Blue acid mucopolysaccharides (mucin) are often deposited within the palisading granulomas. This is a useful feature in distinguishing deep granuloma annulare (blue granulomas) from rheumatoid nodule (red granulomas).* **(Right)** *Some deep granuloma annulare have abundant red fibrin but minimal blue mucin, as depicted, and can look essentially identical to rheumatoid nodule. Clinical history is critical; this case is from a 6-year-old boy without rheumatoid arthritis.*

Deep Granuloma Annulare

TERMINOLOGY

Abbreviations

- Granuloma annulare (GA)

Synonyms

- Subcutaneous GA, pseudorheumatoid nodule, palisading subcutaneous granuloma

Definitions

- Nodules due to deep dermal and subcutaneous necrobiotic granulomas in children

CLINICAL ISSUES

Epidemiology

- Children and young adults (mean age: 4 years old)
- 2:1 female predominance

Site

- Lower legs (especially tibial), forearms/hands, face, scalp, buttocks

Presentation

- Painless subcutaneous nodules
  - Often involve periosteum
  - May be juxtaarticular
- Some also have cutaneous papules of conventional GA
- No association with rheumatoid arthritis

Treatment

- No consistently effective treatment
- Topical or systemic corticosteroids used most often with variable success

Prognosis

- Benign
- Lesions often regress within several years, but recurrence seen in 20% or more

MICROSCOPIC

Histologic Features

- Multiple nodular subcutaneous granulomas
  - Center of granuloma
    - Necrobiosis (basophilic collagen degeneration)
    - "Blue granuloma" due to mucin deposition (acid mucopolysaccharide)
      - Usually abundant but sometimes scant or absent
    - Sometimes red fibrin (like rheumatoid nodule)
    - Sometimes karyorrhectic nuclear debris
  - Periphery of granuloma
    - Rim of palisading spindled or epithelioid histiocytes
    - No atypia, but mitoses may be seen
    - Often with surrounding fibrosis and inflammation (lymphocytes, eosinophils, multinucleated giant cells)
    - Tight sarcoid-like granulomas may be seen
- Typical GA in overlying dermis (25%)
  - Palisading histiocytes around necrobiotic dermal collagen and mucin
  - Interstitial histiocytes between individual dermal collagen fibers

ANCILLARY TESTS

Histochemistry

- Alcian blue (pH 2.5) and colloidal iron highlight mucin
- PAS, GMS, Fite stains negative for organisms

Immunohistochemistry

- CD68(+), CD163(+), and other histiocytic markers
- Keratin (-), EMA(-)
- Retention of nuclear SMARCB1/INI1 expression

DIFFERENTIAL DIAGNOSIS

Rheumatoid Nodule

- Subcutaneous nodules in adults with rheumatoid arthritis
- Usually red granuloma due to abundant fibrin
- Most lack blue mucin seen in GA (most useful feature)
- Some deep GA can look identical; clinical info essential

Epithelioid Sarcoma

- Rare aggressive sarcoma with over 50% mortality
  - Misdiagnosis as deep GA or rheumatoid nodule disastrous pitfall
- Often subcutaneous nodule on distal extremity of young adults
- Tumor nodule with central zonal necrosis mimics necrobiotic granuloma at low power
  - Peripheral rim of epithelioid tumor cells
    - Large atypical nuclei with vesicular chromatin
    - Abundant dense eosinophilic cytoplasm
  - Central zone of coagulative tumor cell necrosis
    - Resembles fibrin but contains necrotic tumor cells
- Keratin (+), EMA(+); loss of nuclear SMARCB1/INI1

Infectious Granulomas

- Fungal or mycobacterial organisms identified by culture or PAS, GMS, or Fite stains
- Clinical features suspicious for infection
- Usually abundant neutrophils
- Usually lack mucin or fibrin deposition

Necrobiosis Lipoidica Diabeticorum

- Atrophic yellowish plaques on lower legs of adults
- Often associated with diabetes
- Dermal-based, rather than subcutaneous, process
- Multiple layers of fibrin, necrobiosis, fibrosis, and inflammation fill dermis
  - Layered cake or parfait appearance
  - Abundant plasma cells usually
- Lacks nodular subcutaneous granulomas

SELECTED REFERENCES

1. Fathi K et al: Subcutaneous granuloma annulare of the penis associated with a urethral anomaly: case report and review of the literature. Pediatr Dermatol. 31(4):e100-3, 2014
2. Lynch JM et al: Collagenolytic (necrobiotic) granulomas: part 1–the "blue" granulomas. J Cutan Pathol. 31(5):353-61, 2004
3. Grogg KL et al: Subcutaneous granuloma annulare in childhood: clinicopathologic features in 34 cases. Pediatrics. 107(3):E42, 2001
4. McDermott MB et al: Deep granuloma annulare (pseudorheumatoid nodule) in children: clinicopathologic study of 35 cases. Pediatr Dev Pathol. 1(4):300-8, 1998
5. Felner EI et al: Subcutaneous granuloma annulare: a review of 47 cases. Pediatrics. 100(6):965-7, 1997

Rheumatoid Nodule

KEY FACTS

TERMINOLOGY

- Nodules due to subcutaneous necrobiotic granulomas in adults with rheumatoid arthritis (RA)

CLINICAL ISSUES

- Asymptomatic smooth, firm, subcutaneous nodules
- Solitary or numerous lesions
- Size: From mm up to 5 cm
- Occur in 20-30% of adults with RA
- Elbow, extensor forearms, hands, feet, scalp, back, buttocks, and many other sites, including lung and heart
- Nodules may indicate severe RA (high titer of rheumatoid factor, severe erosive arthritis, &/or vasculitis)

MICROSCOPIC

- Multiple nodular subcutaneous granulomas
- May extend into overlying dermis and occasionally even perforate epidermis
- Central necrobiosis (collagen degeneration) with abundant red fibrin (red granuloma); usually lack blue mucin
- Surrounded at periphery by palisading spindled and epithelioid histiocytes
- No atypia, but mitoses may be seen
- Often with surrounding inflammation, granulation tissue, fibrosis
- Mixed infiltrate with plasma cells, lymphocytes

ANCILLARY TESTS

- Alcian blue (pH 2.5) and colloidal iron negative for mucin
- PAS, GMS, Fite stains (-) for organisms
- Keratin, EMA (-); retention of nuclear INI1

TOP DIFFERENTIAL DIAGNOSES

- Deep granuloma annulare
- Epithelioid sarcoma
- Infectious granulomas
- Necrobiosis lipoidica diabeticorum

Rheumatoid Nodule

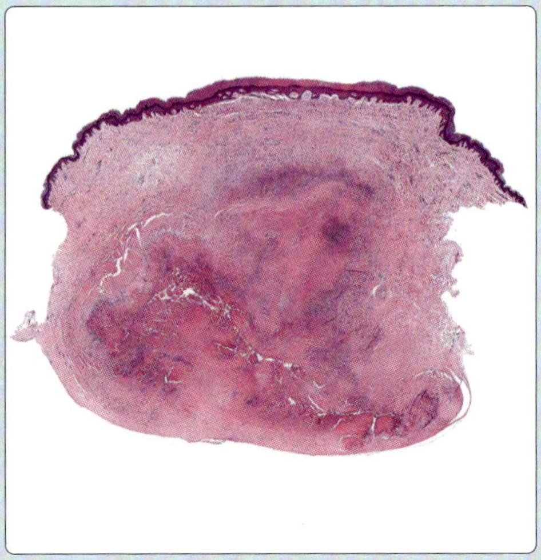

Red Granulomas

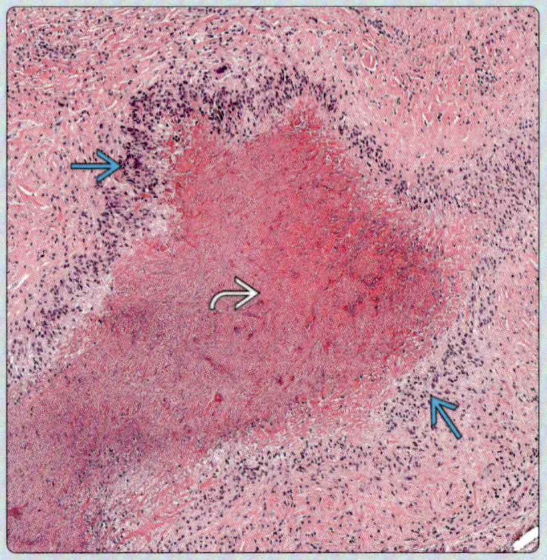

(Left) *Rheumatoid nodules are palisading granulomas centered in the subcutis but often with involvement of the overlying dermis. The distinctive red granuloma appearance is due to abundant central fibrin deposition.* **(Right)** *Histiocytes form a distinct palisading rim around the central zone of necrobiosis and bright red fibrin.*

Lymphoplasmacytic Infiltrate

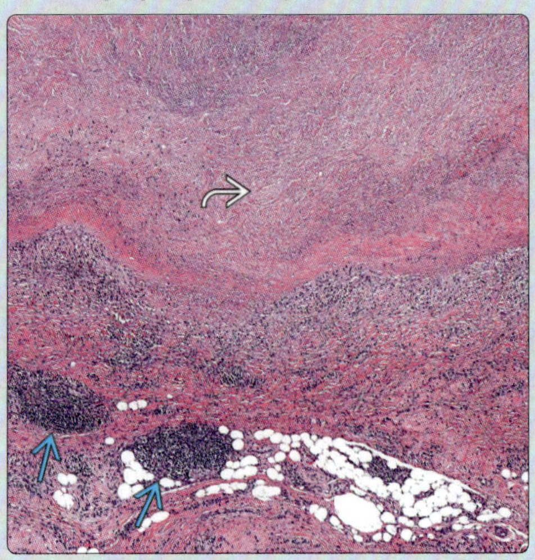

Neutrophils and Nuclear Dust

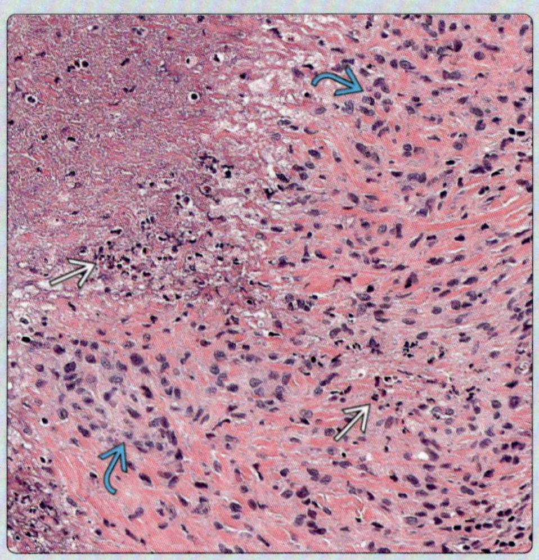

(Left) *Fibrosis and mixed inflammation are commonly seen adjacent to rheumatoid nodules. Lymphocytic aggregates and prominent plasma cells are often present.* **(Right)** *Bland histiocytes with indistinct cytoplasm surround the necrobiotic center of the granuloma. Scattered neutrophils &/or nuclear dust are sometimes seen.*

TERMINOLOGY

Definitions

- Nodules due to subcutaneous necrobiotic granulomas in adults with rheumatoid arthritis (RA)

CLINICAL ISSUES

Site

- Elbow, extensor forearms, hands, feet, scalp, back, buttocks, and many other sites, including lung and heart
  - Often arise near joints, pressure points, sites of trauma
  - Often involve fascia or periosteum

Presentation

- Asymptomatic smooth, firm, subcutaneous nodules
  - Solitary or numerous lesions
  - Size: From millimeters up to 5 cm
  - Occur in 20-30% of adults with RA
  - May occur in other connective tissue or immune diseases (systemic lupus erythematosus, ankylosing spondylitis, scleroderma)

Treatment

- No standard treatment; recommendations vary
- Most nodules asymptomatic and do not require treatment
- Treatment of RA with methotrexate, infliximab, or letrozole may lead to multiple small skin nodules (cutaneous nodulosis)
  - Treatment with etanercept may rarely lead to extensive pulmonary nodules (pulmonary nodulosis)

Prognosis

- Nodules may indicate severe RA (high titer of rheumatoid factor, severe erosive arthritis, &/or vasculitis)

MICROSCOPIC

Histologic Features

- Multiple nodular subcutaneous granulomas
  - May extend into overlying dermis and occasionally even perforate epidermis
- Central necrobiosis (collagen degeneration) with abundant red fibrin (red granuloma); usually lack blue mucin
  - Sometimes karyorrhectic nuclear debris
  - May have clefts or cystic degeneration
- Surrounded at periphery by palisading spindled and epithelioid histiocytes
  - No atypia, but mitoses may be seen
- Often with surrounding inflammation, granulation tissue, fibrosis
  - Mixed infiltrate with plasma cells, lymphocytes
- Leukocytoclastic vasculitis sometimes present

ANCILLARY TESTS

Histochemistry

- Alcian blue (pH 2.5) and colloidal iron stains (-) for mucin (usually)
- PAS, GMS, Fite stains (-) for organisms

Immunohistochemistry

- CD68(+), CD163(+), and other histiocytic markers
- Keratin, EMA (-)
- Retained nuclear SMARCB1/INI1 expression

DIFFERENTIAL DIAGNOSIS

Deep Granuloma Annulare

- Painless subcutaneous nodules in children and young adults
- Blue granulomas featuring abundant mucin (most useful feature)
- Some have red fibrin, look identical to rheumatoid nodule
  - Clinical info essential; no association with RA

Epithelioid Sarcoma

- Rare aggressive sarcoma with over 50% mortality
  - Misdiagnosis as deep granuloma annulare or rheumatoid nodule disastrous pitfall
- Often subcutaneous nodule on distal extremity of young adults
- Tumor nodule with central zonal necrosis mimics necrobiotic granuloma at low power
  - Peripheral rim of epithelioid tumor cells
    - Large, atypical nuclei with vesicular chromatin
    - Abundant, dense eosinophilic cytoplasm
  - Central zone of coagulative tumor cell necrosis
    - Red-like fibrin, but individual necrotic tumor cells seen
- Keratin (+), EMA(+)
- Loss of nuclear SMARCB1/INI1 expression

Infectious Granulomas

- Fungal or mycobacterial organisms identified by culture or by PAS, GMS, or Fite stains
- Clinical features suspicious for infection
- Usually abundant neutrophils
- Usually lack mucin or fibrin deposition

Necrobiosis Lipoidica Diabeticorum

- Atrophic, yellowish plaques on lower legs of adults
- Often associated with diabetes
- Dermal-based rather than subcutaneous process
- Multiple layers of fibrin, necrobiosis, fibrosis, and inflammation fill dermis
  - Layered cake or parfait appearance
  - Abundant plasma cells usually
- Lacks nodular subcutaneous granulomas

SELECTED REFERENCES

1. Prasad NK et al: A new pattern of lipomatosis of nerve: case report. J Neurosurg. 126(3):933-937, 2017
2. Munns JJ et al: Rheumatoid nodules. J Hand Surg Am. 39(4):765-7; quiz 767, 2014
3. Chao J et al: Accelerated cutaneous nodulosis associated with aromatase inhibitor therapy in a patient with rheumatoid arthritis. J Rheumatol. 36(5):1087-8, 2009
4. van Ede A et al: Etanercept-related extensive pulmonary nodulosis in a patient with rheumatoid arthritis. J Rheumatol. 34(7):1590-2, 2007
5. Lynch JM et al: Collagenolytic (necrobiotic) granulomas: part II–the 'red' granulomas. J Cutan Pathol. 31(6):409-18, 2004
6. Mackley CL et al: Accelerated cutaneous nodulosis during infliximab therapy in a patient with rheumatoid arthritis. J Clin Rheumatol. 10(6):336-8, 2004
7. Veys EM et al: Rheumatoid nodules: differential diagnosis and immunohistological findings. Ann Rheum Dis. 52(9):625-6, 1993
8. Smith ML et al: Rheumatoid papules: lesions showing features of vasculitis and palisading granuloma. J Am Acad Dermatol. 20(2 Pt 2):348-52, 1989
9. Patterson JW: Rheumatoid nodule and subcutaneous granuloma annulare. A comparative histologic study. Am J Dermatopathol. 10(1):1-8, 1988

Langerhans Cell Histiocytosis

KEY FACTS

TERMINOLOGY

- Clonal neoplastic proliferation of modified dendritic cells (Langerhans cells)
- Synonyms: Histiocytosis X, eosinophilic granuloma, Hand-Schüller-Christian disease, Letterer-Siwe disease

CLINICAL ISSUES

- Common
- Usually children and young adults
  - 3.5:1.0 male predominance
- Occurs in solitary, multifocal unisystem and disseminated multisystem forms
  - Bony sites most common in solitary and multifocal forms
    - Soft tissue extension common
  - Skin, bone, liver, lung, spleen, and bone marrow in disseminated form
- Treatment: Surgical excision
  - Chemotherapy for disseminated disease
- Excellent prognosis for solitary lesions
  - High mortality for disseminated disease

MICROSCOPIC

- Sheets or nests of uniform, ovoid, or epithelioid cells
  - Irregular nuclei with grooves, folds, or indentations
- Prominent eosinophilic infiltrate
- Osteoclast-like multinucleated giant cells are common

ANCILLARY TESTS

- CD1a(+), S100 protein (+), langerin/CD207 (+)
- CD163(-), CD21(-), CD68 (variable)
- EM: Presence of characteristic Birbeck granules (tennis racket-shaped)
- Molecular: *BRAF* V600E mutations common

TOP DIFFERENTIAL DIAGNOSES

- Langerhans cell sarcoma
- Histiocytic sarcoma
- Extranodal Rosai-Dorfman disease
- Granulomatous inflammation

Langerhans Cell Histiocytosis

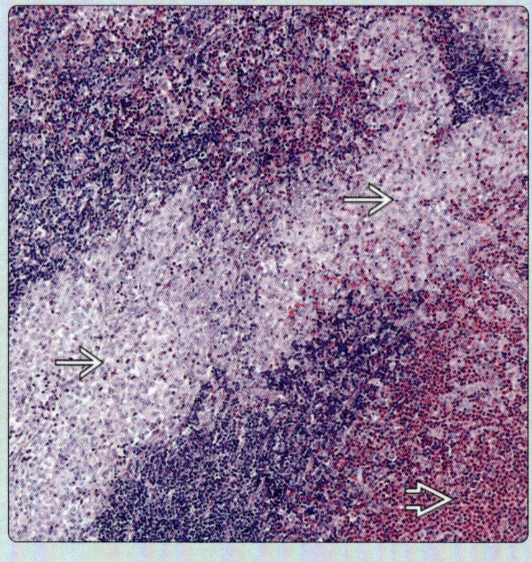

Prominent Eosinophils

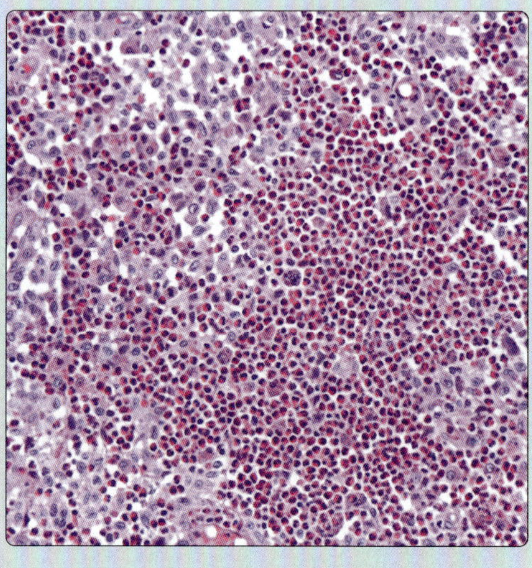

(Left) *Langerhans cell histiocytosis (LCH) is characterized by sheets ➡ and aggregates of palely eosinophilic ovoid Langerhans cells in a background of mixed chronic inflammatory cells, particularly eosinophils ➡.* **(Right)** *Eosinophils are very common in LCH and are often quite prominent. Eosinophilic microabscesses may even be formed, and in occasional cases, Charcot-Leyden crystals may be present.*

Nuclear Grooves and Folds

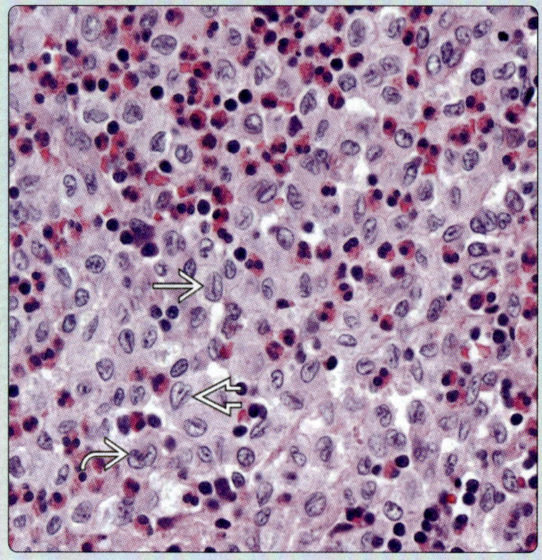

Osteoclast-Like Giant Cells

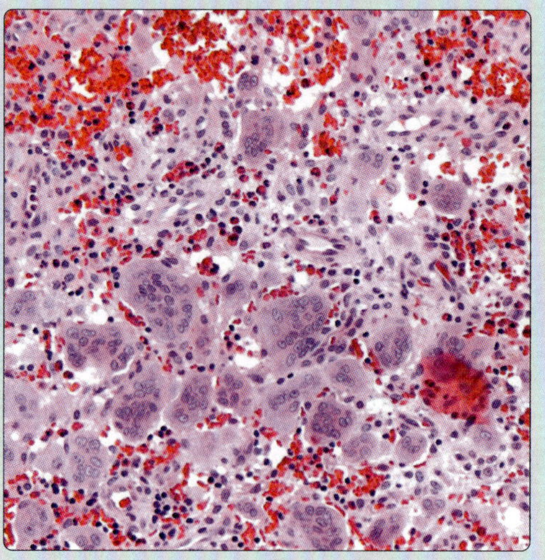

(Left) *Nuclear grooves ➡, folds ➡, or indentations ➡ are characteristic cytologic findings in cases of LCH. Atypia is minimal. Note the numerous eosinophils.* **(Right)** *Osteoclast-like multinucleated giant cells are often seen in LCH and may be sparsely distributed or found in clusters. A background eosinophilic infiltrate can also be seen in this H&E.*

Langerhans Cell Histiocytosis

TERMINOLOGY

Abbreviations

- Langerhans cell histiocytosis (LCH)

Synonyms

- Histiocytosis X
- Eosinophilic granuloma
  - Isolated lesions
- Hand-Schüller-Christian disease
  - Multifocal bony lesions ± proptosis, diabetes insipidus
- Letterer-Siwe disease
  - Disseminated multiorgan involvement

Definitions

- Clonal neoplastic proliferation of modified dendritic cells (Langerhans cells)

CLINICAL ISSUES

Epidemiology

- Incidence
  - Common
- Age
  - Children and young adults
    - Disseminated multisystem disease usually in infants
- Sex
  - 3.5:1.0 male predominance

Site

- Solitary and multifocal forms
  - Bony sites most common (may extend into soft tissue)
    - Skull, mandible, femur, ribs, vertebra, others
  - In solitary form, also lymph nodes, skin
- Disseminated form (multiorgan involvement)
  - Skin, bone, liver, lung, spleen, and bone marrow

Presentation

- Solitary and multifocal forms
  - Usually lytic bone lesion(s) with cortical disruption
- Disseminated form
  - Fever, cytopenia, hepatosplenomegaly, skin lesions

Treatment

- Surgical excision
- Disseminated disease may be treated with chemotherapy

Prognosis

- Excellent for solitary lesions
- High mortality rate in infants with multisystem disease who do not respond to chemotherapy

MACROSCOPIC

Size

- Variable

MICROSCOPIC

Histologic Features

- Sheets or nests of uniform, ovoid, or epithelioid cells
  - Pale eosinophilic cytoplasm
  - Irregular nuclei with grooves, folds, or indentations
  - Vesicular chromatin ± small nucleoli
    - Minimal nuclear atypia
- Prominent eosinophilic infiltrate
  - May form eosinophilic microabscesses
  - Other inflammatory cells may be variably present (lymphocytes, neutrophils, foamy histiocytes, neutrophils)
- Variable mitotic rate; no atypical forms
- Osteoclast-like multinucleated giant cells are common

ANCILLARY TESTS

Immunohistochemistry

- CD1a(+), S100 protein (+), langerin/CD207 (+)
- Cyclin-D1 (+)
- CD163(-), CD21(-), CD68 (variable)

Electron Microscopy

- Presence of characteristic Birbeck granules (tennis racket-shaped)

Molecular Genetics

- *BRAF* V600E mutations common
  - Also, *MAP2K1* mutations reported in BRAF (-) tumors

DIFFERENTIAL DIAGNOSIS

Langerhans Cell Sarcoma

- Extremely rare
  - Most reported cases occur in adults
- Overtly malignant cytology
- Nuclear grooves and eosinophilic infiltrate may be present
- Similar immunophenotype to LCH

Histiocytic Sarcoma

- Diffuse sheets of enlarged epithelioid histiocytes, often with prominent nucleoli
- Marked atypia/pleomorphism present, at least focally
- CD163(+), CD1a(-), langerin (-)

Extranodal Rosai-Dorfman Disease

- Large sheets of polygonal to spindled histiocytes with pale cytoplasm
- Emperipolesis is often present
- Plasma cells common; eosinophils rare
- Osteoclast-like giant cells rare
- S100 protein (+), CD163(+), CD1a(-), langerin (-)

Granulomatous Inflammation

- Well-formed aggregates of syncytial histiocytes
- CD163(+), CD1a(-), S100(-)

SELECTED REFERENCES

1. Xerri L et al: CDKN2A/B Deletion and double-hit mutations of the MAPK pathway underlie the aggressive behavior of Langerhans cell tumors. Am J Surg Pathol. 42(2):150-159, 2018
2. Shanmugam V et al: Cyclin D1 is expressed in neoplastic cells of Langerhans cell histiocytosis but not reactive Langerhans cell proliferations. Am J Surg Pathol. 41(10):1390-1396, 2017
3. Morimoto A et al: Recent advances in Langerhans cell histiocytosis. Pediatr Int. ePub, 2014
4. Roden AC et al: BRAF V600E expression in Langerhans cell histiocytosis: clinical and immunohistochemical study on 25 pulmonary and 54 extrapulmonary cases. Am J Surg Pathol. 38(4):548-51, 2014

Extranodal Rosai-Dorfman Disease

KEY FACTS

TERMINOLOGY

- Nonneoplastic, chronic inflammatory process of uncertain etiology characterized by distinctive histiocytic proliferation that presents with lymphadenopathy &/or extranodal disease

CLINICAL ISSUES

- Wide range (4th-5th decades most common)
- Multiple sites often involved simultaneously
- Skin and subcutaneous tissue of extremities, trunk, head/neck most common sites
  - Also nasal cavity, paranasal sinuses, eye/orbit, bone
- Treatment: Local excision for isolated lesions
- Benign; overall excellent prognosis for extranodal cases

MACROSCOPIC

- May be multiple
- Usually 2-5 cm

MICROSCOPIC

- Clusters, sheets, and syncytia of large histocytes
  - Can be spindled and form storiform architectures
  - May contain intracytoplasmic inflammatory cells (emperipolesis)
  - Minimal to mild cytologic atypia
- Plasma cell aggregates (polyclonal) and reactive lymphocytes common and characteristic
- Variable stromal collagen deposition and fibrosis

ANCILLARY TESTS

- S100 protein (+) in large histiocytes
- CD1a(-)

TOP DIFFERENTIAL DIAGNOSES

- Histiocytic sarcoma
- Langerhans cell histiocytosis
- Miscellaneous histiocytic proliferations
- Undifferentiated pleomorphic sarcoma

Extranodal Rosai-Dorfman Disease

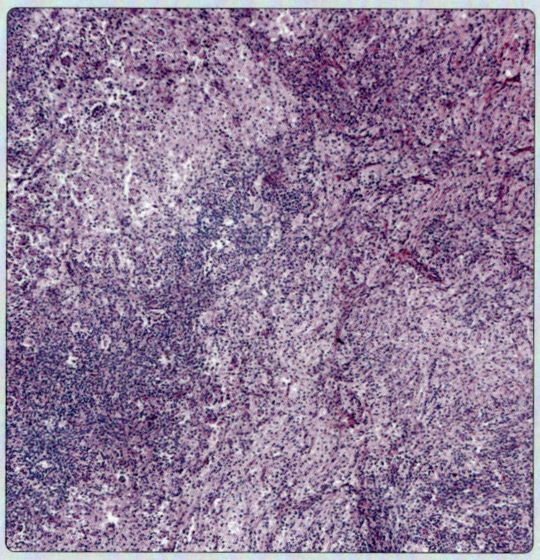

Subcutaneous Adipose Tissue

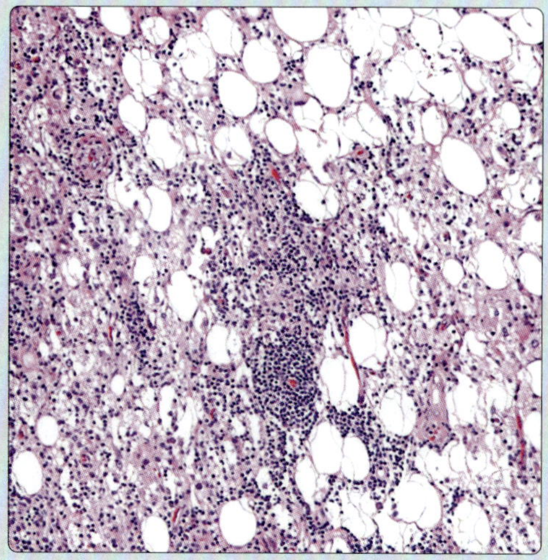

(Left) *Rosai-Dorfman disease (RDD) most commonly presents as nodal disease ± involvement of various extranodal sites. Isolated soft tissue involvement is even rarer. At low magnification, RDD is composed of a mixture of pink to clear histiocytic areas and darker lymphoplasmacytic aggregates.* **(Right)** *Although well marginated grossly, most cases of extranodal RDD show at least focal intratumoral subcutaneous adipose tissue, giving it the appearance of a locally infiltrative process.*

Pale Eosinophilic Histiocytes

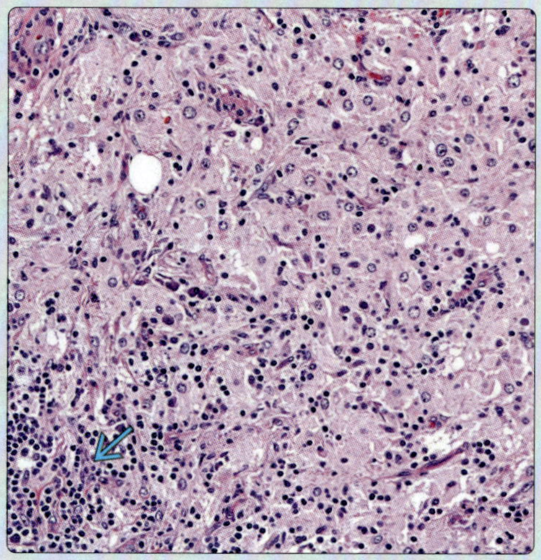

Emperipolesis

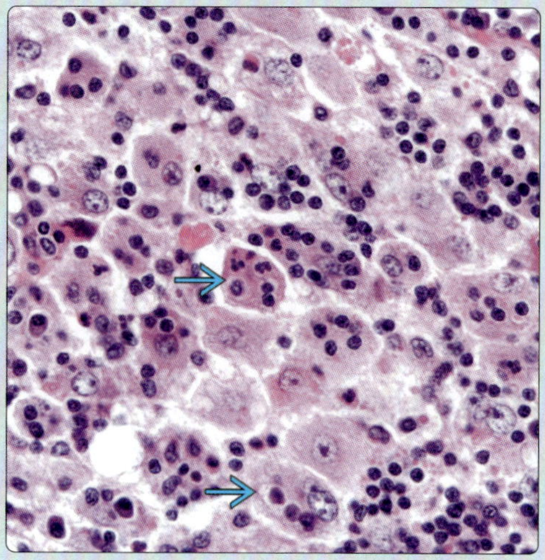

(Left) *The lesional histocytes of RDD are polygonal to spindled and typically demonstrate pale eosinophilic cytoplasm. Cell borders are often inconspicuous. A reactive lymphoid ➡ and plasmacytic infiltrate is commonly present and may be prominent.* **(Right)** *The presence of inflammatory cells (particularly lymphocytes) within the cytoplasm of the histiocytes (emperipolesis ➡) is characteristic of RDD; however, it is seen much less frequently in extranodal tumors.*

TERMINOLOGY

Abbreviations

- Rosai-Dorfman disease (RDD)

Synonyms

- Soft tissue RDD
- Sinus histiocytosis with massive lymphadenopathy (SHML)
  - Not applied to extranodal disease

Definitions

- Nonneoplastic, chronic inflammatory process of uncertain etiology characterized by distinctive histiocytic proliferation that presents with lymphadenopathy &/or extranodal disease

ETIOLOGY/PATHOGENESIS

Under Investigation

- Etiology still uncertain

Infectious Agents

- Various infections associated with cases of RDD/SHML, but none as yet proven to be etiologic infectious agent
  - Simian virus 40 (SV40, polyomavirus) in several extranodal cases
  - Also parvovirus, Epstein-Barr virus, HHV-6 in nodal cases

CLINICAL ISSUES

Epidemiology

- Incidence
  - Rare
  - Most patients with extranodal involvement also have nodal disease
    - Extranodal involvement is seen in ~ 10% of cases
      - Rarely sole manifestation of disease
- Age
  - Wide range (4th-5th decades most common)
    - Patients with extranodal disease are often older than those without
- Sex
  - May be more common in females

Site

- Multiple sites often involved simultaneously
- Extranodal
  - Skin and subcutaneous tissue
    - Extremities, trunk, head/neck most common
  - Also nasal cavity, paranasal sinuses, eye/orbit, bone, salivary gland, central nervous system, many others
- Nodal
  - Cervical lymph nodes involved in 90% of cases

Presentation

- Varies with site of involvement
  - Painful or painless papules, nodules, or masses in skin/soft tissue
  - Painless lymphadenopathy with concomitant nodal disease (most frequent presenting symptom overall)
    - Hepatosplenomegaly uncommon

Treatment

- Conservative surgical excision for isolated lesions

Prognosis

- Benign
- Overall excellent prognosis for pure extranodal RDD
  - No deaths or metastases yet reported
- Isolated skin lesions may spontaneously resolve
- Rare reports of aggressive clinical course in nodal disease, often with widespread dissemination, involvement of kidneys or lower respiratory tract, &/or associated with immunologic abnormalities

MACROSCOPIC

General Features

- Well circumscribed, often multinodular
- Tan-yellow, firm
- May be multiple

Size

- Usually 2-5 cm

MICROSCOPIC

Histologic Features

- Extranodal RDD
  - Admixed subcutaneous fat often present
  - Clusters, sheets, and syncytia of large histocytes
    - Cytoplasm ranges from clear and foamy to variably eosinophilic
    - May contain intracytoplasmic inflammatory cells (emperipolesis)
      - Generally much less conspicuous than in nodal RDD
    - Histiocytes may be spindled and form storiform architectures
    - Minimal to mild cytologic atypia
    - Rare to no mitotic figures
  - Plasma cell aggregates (polyclonal) common and characteristic
  - Reactive B-cell aggregates and T-cell infiltrates common
  - Neutrophils may be seen ± microabscess formation
  - Variable stromal collagen deposition and fibrosis
  - Rare findings: Focal Touton giant cells, focal necrosis, scattered eosinophils
- Nodal RDD (SHML)
  - Expanded sinuses contain histiocytic cells with abundant cytoplasm, sometimes multinucleated
  - Emperipolesis often striking feature

ANCILLARY TESTS

Immunohistochemistry

- S100 protein (+) in large histiocytes
  - Often helps highlight emperipolesis
- CD68(+), CD163(+)
- CD1a(-)
- Plasma cells are polyclonal

Electron Microscopy

- Lacks Birbeck granules

DIFFERENTIAL DIAGNOSIS

Histiocytic Sarcoma

- Marked cytologic atypia
- Conspicuous mitotic activity
- S100 protein (-)
- Aggressive clinical course

Langerhans Cell Histiocytosis

- Clusters and sheets of pale, pink epithelioid cells with nuclear grooves
- Usually associated with significant eosinophilic infiltrate, including abscesses
- CD1a(+), S100 protein (+)

Miscellaneous Histiocytic Proliferations

- Secondary to infection
  - Usually contains well-formed granulomas, at least focally, often with necrosis
  - Lacks emperipolesis
  - Organisms can be detected by culture/special stains
  - S100 protein (-)
- Malakoplakia
  - Usually identified in bladder or GI tract
  - Sheets of small or medium-sized eosinophilic histiocytes, some of which contain targetoid Michaelis-Guttman bodies
  - S100 protein (-)

Myxoinflammatory Fibroblastic Sarcoma

- Often contains prominent stromal inflammatory component
- Typically contains population of large histiocyte-like cells, which may contain inflammatory cells
- Bizarre nuclear atypia, including smudgy heterochromatin and prominent macronucleoli

Undifferentiated Pleomorphic Sarcoma

- Often contains subtle admixed histiocytic population
- Usually significant and bizarre nuclear pleomorphism
- Mitoses, including atypical forms, and coagulative necrosis common
- S100 protein (-)

Sarcoidosis

- Well-formed, confluent, nonnecrotizing granulomas associated with fibrosis
- Pulmonary involvement common
- Lacks emperipolesis
- S100 protein (-)

Follicular Dendritic Cell Sarcoma

- May involve lymph nodes, nodal tissue, or extranodal sites
- Oval to spindle cells with eosinophilic cytoplasm forming syncytial sheets or storiform/whorling arrays
- Tumor cells intimately admixed with small lymphocytes, with prominent perivascular cuffing
- CD21(+), CD25(+), D2-40 (podoplanin) (+)
- May express focal S100 protein

Juvenile Xanthogranuloma

- Most common in pediatric age groups
- Head/neck most common site
- Often cutaneous; rarely subcutaneous or intramuscular
- Histiocytic cells with variable population of Touton giant cells
- Variable stromal eosinophilic infiltrate
- S100 protein (-)

SELECTED REFERENCES

1. Meindl A et al: Extranodal Rosai-Dorfman disease with mucosal involvement of the stomach in a background of autoimmune atrophic Gastritis. Int J Surg Pathol. 26(7):671-675, 2018
2. Heidarian A et al: Extranodal Rosai-Dorfman disease arising in the heart: clinical course and review of literature. Cardiovasc Pathol. 31:1-4, 2017
3. Mantilla JG et al: Extranodal Rosai-Dorfman disease: clinicopathologic series of 10 patients with radiologic correlation and review of the literature. Am J Clin Pathol. 145(2):211-21, 2016
4. Komaragiri M et al: Extranodal Rosai-Dorfman disease: a rare soft tissue neoplasm masquerading as a sarcoma. World J Surg Oncol. 11:63, 2013
5. Liu L et al: Relationship between Rosai-Dorfman disease and IgG4-related disease: study of 32 cases. Am J Clin Pathol. 140(3):395-402, 2013
6. Al-Daraji W et al: Soft tissue Rosai-Dorfman disease: 29 new lesions in 18 patients, with detection of polyomavirus antigen in 3 abdominal cases. Ann Diagn Pathol. 14(5):309-16, 2010
7. Gaitonde S: Multifocal, extranodal sinus histiocytosis with massive lymphadenopathy: an overview. Arch Pathol Lab Med. 131(7):1117-21, 2007
8. Mehraein Y et al: Parvovirus B19 detected in Rosai-Dorfman disease in nodal and extranodal manifestations. J Clin Pathol. 59(12):1320-6, 2006
9. Wang KH et al: Cutaneous Rosai-Dorfman disease: clinicopathological profiles, spectrum and evolution of 21 lesions in six patients. Br J Dermatol. 154(2):277-86, 2006
10. Maric I et al: Histologic features of sinus histiocytosis with massive lymphadenopathy in patients with autoimmune lymphoproliferative syndrome. Am J Surg Pathol. 29(7):903-11, 2005
11. Hindermann W et al: [Extranodal Rosai Dorfman disease (sinus histiocytosis with massive lymphadenopathy). Report of 5 cases.] Pathologe. 25(3):222-8, 2004
12. Rodriguez-Galindo C et al: Extranodal Rosai-Dorfman disease in children. J Pediatr Hematol Oncol. 26(1):19-24, 2004
13. Anders RA et al: Rosai-Dorfman disease presenting in the gastrointestinal tract. Arch Pathol Lab Med. 127(2):E74-5, 2003
14. Sneller MC et al: Autoimmune lymphoproliferative syndrome. Curr Opin Rheumatol. 15(4):417-21, 2003
15. Andriko JA et al: Rosai-Dorfman disease isolated to the central nervous system: a report of 11 cases. Mod Pathol. 14(3):172-8, 2001
16. Lauwers GY et al: The digestive system manifestations of Rosai-Dorfman disease (sinus histiocytosis with massive lymphadenopathy): review of 11 cases. Hum Pathol. 31(3):380-5, 2000
17. Green I et al: Breast involvement by extranodal Rosai-Dorfman disease: report of seven cases. Am J Surg Pathol. 21(6):664-8, 1997
18. Levine PH et al: Detection of human herpesvirus 6 in tissues involved by sinus histiocytosis with massive lymphadenopathy (Rosai-Dorfman disease). J Infect Dis. 166(2):291-5, 1992
19. Montgomery EA et al: Rosai-Dorfman disease of soft tissue. Am J Surg Pathol. 16(2):122-9, 1992
20. Eisen RN et al: Immunophenotypic characterization of sinus histiocytosis with massive lymphadenopathy (Rosai-Dorfman disease). Semin Diagn Pathol. 7(1):74-82, 1990
21. Foucar E et al: Sinus histiocytosis with massive lymphadenopathy (Rosai-Dorfman disease): review of the entity. Semin Diagn Pathol. 7(1):19-73, 1990
22. Foucar E et al: Sinus histiocytosis with massive lymphadenopathy. An analysis of 14 deaths occurring in a patient registry. Cancer. 54(9):1834-40, 1984
23. Walker PD et al: The osseous manifestations of sinus histiocytosis with massive lymphadenopathy. Am J Clin Pathol. 75(2):131-9, 1981
24. Rosai J et al: Sinus histiocytosis with massive lymphadenopathy. A newly recognized benign clinicopathological entity. Arch Pathol. 87(1):63-70, 1969

Occasional Distinct Cell Borders

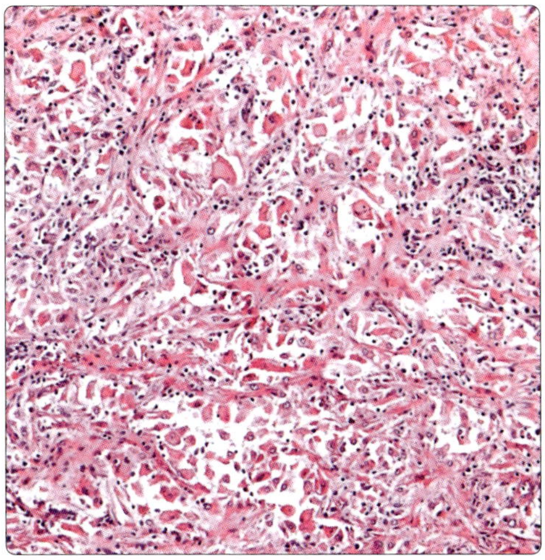

Foamy Cytoplasm

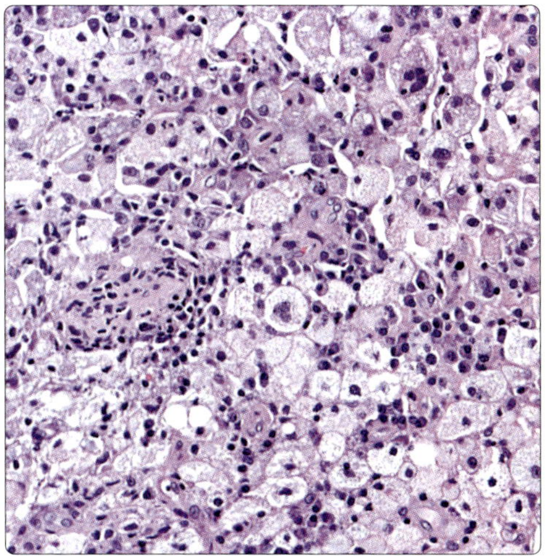

(Left) *In some foci, the lesional histiocytes of extranodal RDD have more prominent eosinophilic cytoplasm and more distinct cell borders, imparting somewhat of a pseudoalveolar appearance.* **(Right)** *Some of the lesional histiocytes of extranodal RDD may show foamy, somewhat clear cytoplasm. This finding is often particularly prominent in RDD of bone.*

Spindled Storiform Growth

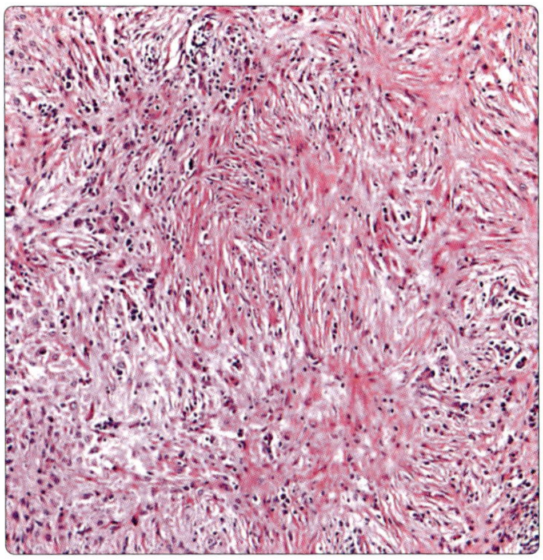

Subtle Histiocytic Morphology

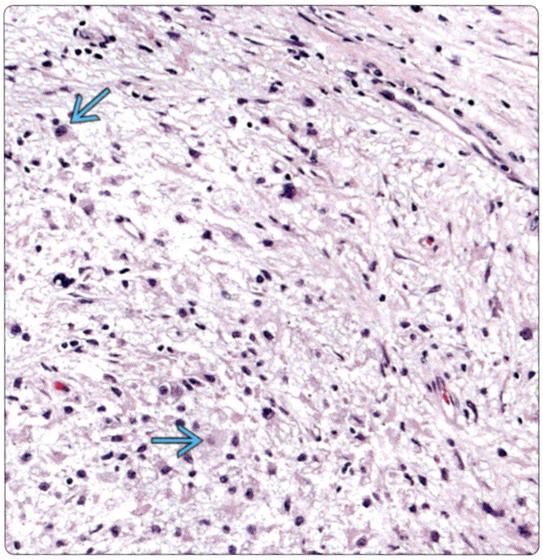

(Left) *Storiform or whorled growth by spindled histiocytes is a common morphologic pattern in extranodal RDD and may lead to confusion with a fibrohistiocytic neoplasm.* **(Right)** *In some cases of extranodal RDD, the histiocytes are small and subtle in foci and may be mistaken for fibroconnective tissue. Note that the pale eosinophilic cytoplasm → is still evident.*

Stromal Collagen

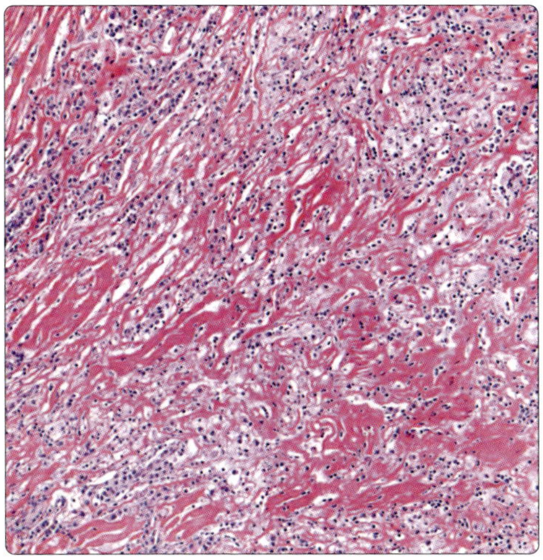

S100 Protein Expression

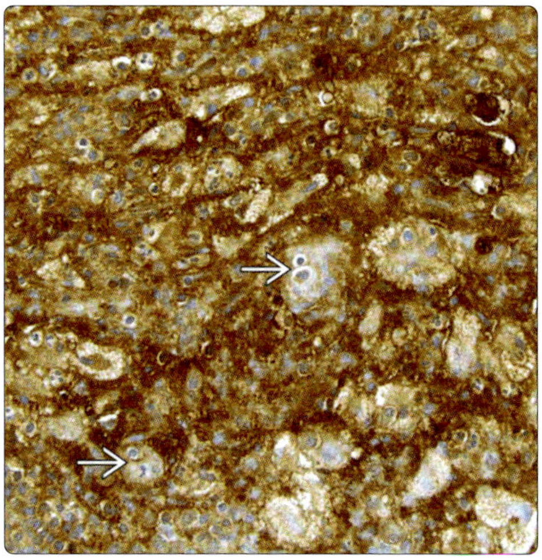

(Left) *Stromal collagen deposition or sclerosis is a common finding in extranodal RDD but is usually not extensive. Sclerotic foci, such as the one shown, may be mistaken for nonspecific chronic inflammation, particularly on small samples.* **(Right)** *S100 protein expression by the lesional histiocytes is characteristic of RDD. Note that intracytoplasmic lymphocytes (emperipolesis →) may be more easily demonstrated using this immunostain.*

Crystal-Storing Histiocytosis

KEY FACTS

TERMINOLOGY

- Nonneoplastic histiocytic proliferation containing crystalline material, usually associated with underlying lymphoproliferative or plasmacytic disorder

ETIOLOGY/PATHOGENESIS

- Lymphoproliferative or plasma cell disorder most common
  - Lymphoplasmacytic lymphoma, MALT lymphoma, extranodal marginal zone lymphoma, others
  - MGUS, myeloma, plasmacytoma
- Rarely associated with chronic inflammatory conditions or clofazimine use
- Crystals most commonly derived from immunoglobulins

CLINICAL ISSUES

- Middle-aged to older adults
- May be localized/solitary or generalized/systemic
- Wide variety of sites, including soft tissue and visceral organs
- May have signs of underlying lymphoproliferative disorder, such as lymphadenopathy or hepatosplenomegaly
- Treatment and prognosis relate to underlying disease

MICROSCOPIC

- Sheets of polygonal, epithelioid, or spindled histiocytes
  - Eosinophilic cytoplasm containing elongated crystals
  - Occasionally, cells are multinucleated
- Associated lymphoproliferative or plasmacytic neoplasm often present

ANCILLARY TESTS

- CD68(+), S100 protein (-), desmin (-), myogenin (-)

TOP DIFFERENTIAL DIAGNOSES

- Rhabdomyoma
- Granular cell histiocytosis
- Granular cell tumor
- Malakoplakia
- Mycobacterial pseudotumor

(Left) *Crystal-storing histiocytosis (CSH) is a nonneoplastic proliferation of spindled or epithelioid, eosinophilic histiocytes that is most commonly associated with a lymphoplasmacytic neoplasm. This case involved the lung, evidenced by entrapped normal structures ➙.* **(Right)** *The lesional histiocytes of CSH demonstrate eosinophilic cytoplasm and contain variably prominent clusters of elongated crystalline material ➙. These crystals are most commonly composed of immunoglobulin.*

Crystal-Storing Histiocytosis

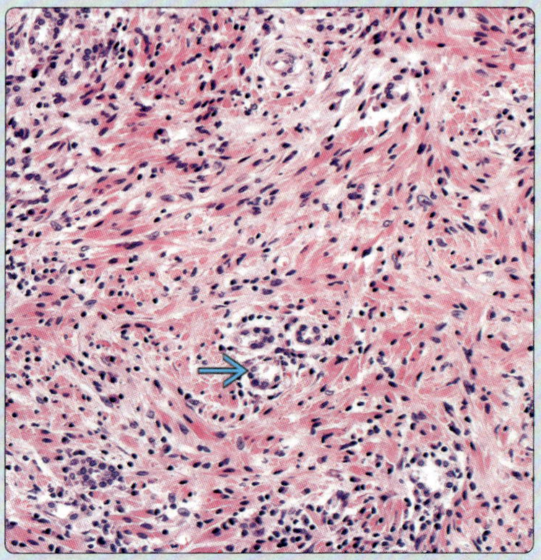

Crystalline Structures

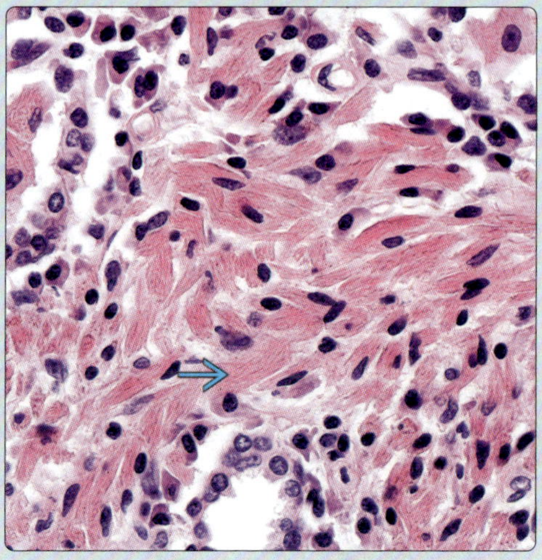

(Left) *The rod-shaped intracytoplasmic crystals ➙ are numerous and easily identified by light microscopy in this case of pulmonary CSH.* **(Right)** *Although spindled histiocytes are a common finding in CSH, in some cases they may predominate and exist within a loosely collagenous stroma with a mild chronic inflammatory infiltrate.*

Polygonal Histiocytes

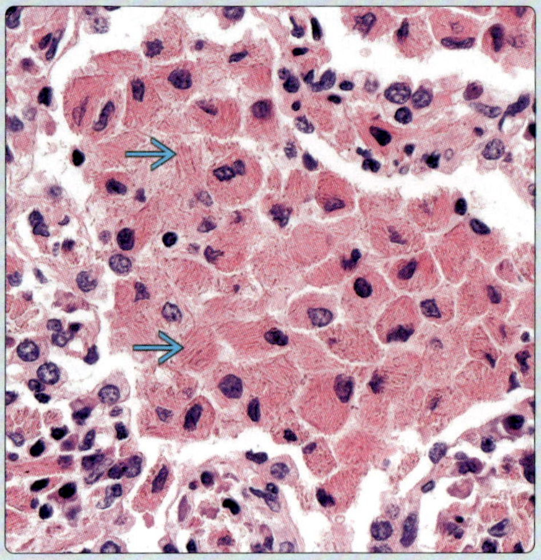

Spindled Histiocytes

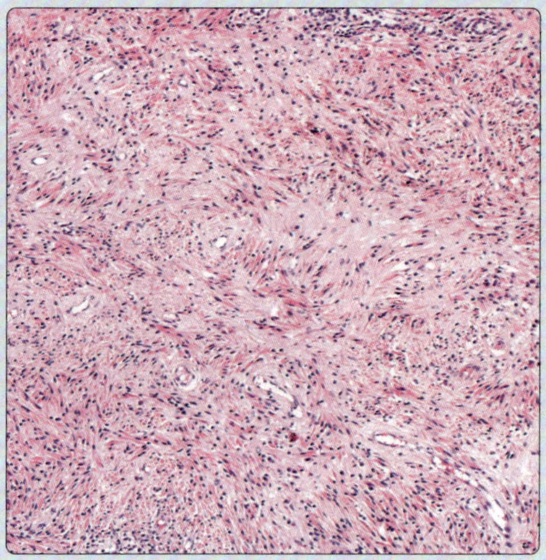

TERMINOLOGY

Abbreviations

- Crystal-storing histiocytosis (CSH)

Definitions

- Nonneoplastic histiocytic proliferation containing crystalline material, usually associated with underlying lymphoproliferative or plasmacytic disorder

ETIOLOGY/PATHOGENESIS

Paraneoplastic Phenomenon

- By far most common etiology overall
- Lymphoproliferative or plasma cell disorder
  - Lymphoplasmacytic lymphoma
  - Chronic lymphocytic leukemia
  - Extranodal marginal zone lymphoma
  - MALT lymphoma
  - Plasma cell dyscrasias
    - Monoclonal gammopathy of undetermined significance (MGUS)
    - Myeloma
    - Plasmacytoma
- Systemic mastocytosis

Inflammatory Disease

- Eosinophilic colitis
- Rheumatoid arthritis, Crohn disease

Iatrogenic

- Treatment of lepromatous leprosy with clofazimine

Pathogenesis

- Crystals are formed from
  - Immunoglobulins (most common)
  - Eosinophil cytoplasmic granules (Charcot-Leyden)
    - Eosinophilic colitis or systemic mastocytosis
  - Clofazimine
- Crystals are phagocytosed by histiocytes
- Histiocytes aggregate to form ill-defined mass
  - Infiltrate adjacent tissues

CLINICAL ISSUES

Epidemiology

- Incidence
  - Very rare
- Age
  - Middle-aged to older adults

Site

- Wide variety of locations, including soft tissue
- Also visceral organs
- May be localized/solitary or generalized/systemic

Presentation

- Painless mass or swelling (in soft tissue)
- May have signs of underlying lymphoproliferative disorder, such as lymphadenopathy or hepatosplenomegaly
  - Rare cases precede development of or are unassociated with lymphoplasmacytic disorder
- Visceral lesions be incidentally detected by imaging

Prognosis

- Relates to underlying disease

MACROSCOPIC

General Features

- Usually ill-defined, tan-yellow mass

Size

- Often small (most < 3 cm)

MICROSCOPIC

Histologic Features

- Sheets of polygonal, epithelioid, or spindled histiocytes
  - Eosinophilic cytoplasm containing variably prominent clusters of elongated crystals
    - Cells may be markedly distended
  - Occasionally cells are multinucleated
- Fibrosis and chronic inflammatory cells may be present
- Associated lymphoproliferative or plasmacytic neoplasm often present
  - May be overshadowed by histiocytic component

ANCILLARY TESTS

Immunohistochemistry

- CD68(+)
- S100 protein (-), desmin (-), myogenin (-), CD1a(-)

DIFFERENTIAL DIAGNOSIS

Rhabdomyoma

- Granular eosinophilic cytoplasm
- Desmin (+), myogenin (+)

Granular Cell Histiocytosis

- Site of previous surgery
- Granular cytoplasm without crystals

Granular Cell Tumor

- Granular cytoplasm without crystals
- Diffuse S100 protein (+)

Malakoplakia

- Epithelioid, eosinophilic histiocytes without intracytoplasmic crystals
- Michaelis-Gutmann bodies characteristic

Mycobacterial Pseudotumor

- Immunocompromised patients
- Abundant acid-fast bacilli

SELECTED REFERENCES

1. Kokuho N et al: Localized pulmonary crystal-storing histiocytosis complicating pulmonary mucosa-associated lymphoid tissue lymphoma presenting with multiple mass lesions. Hum Pathol. 65:180-186, 2017
2. Kanagal-Shamanna R et al: Crystal-storing histiocytosis: a clinicopathological study of 13 cases. Histopathology. 68(4):482-91, 2016
3. Rossi G et al: Localized pleuropulmonary crystal-storing histiocytosis: 5 cases of a rare histiocytic disorder with variable clinicoradiologic features. Am J Surg Pathol. 37(6):906-12, 2013
4. Dogan S et al: Crystal-storing histiocytosis: report of a case, review of the literature (80 cases) and a proposed classification. Head Neck Pathol. 6(1):111-20, 2012

Plexiform Fibrohistiocytic Tumor

KEY FACTS

TERMINOLOGY

- Rarely metastasizing dermal-subcutaneous mesenchymal neoplasm composed of variable mixture of fibroblasts and histiocyte-like cells

CLINICAL ISSUES

- Children and young adults
- Most common in upper extremity
  - Most arise at dermal-subcutaneous interface
- Also lower extremity, trunk, head and neck
- Painless, slow-growing mass or plaque
- Treatment: Wide surgical excision with negative margins
- Local recurrence in up to 40%
- Low metastatic potential (6%)

MACROSCOPIC

- Multinodular, poorly delineated, tan-white
- Usually < 3 cm (range 0.3-8.5 cm)

MICROSCOPIC

- Poorly circumscribed with infiltrative growth pattern
- Morphologically subdivided into 3 types (fibroblastic, histiocytic, mixed)
- Fascicles of spindled fibroblastic cells
- Nodules or aggregates of epithelioid histiocytoid cells
  - Osteoclast-like giant cells common
- Multinodular and plexiform growth
- Low mitotic rate; usually no cellular pleomorphism

ANCILLARY TESTS

- Spindle cells: SMA(+); histiocytes CD68(+) and CD163(+)
- Negative for S100 protein, CD34, desmin, keratin, MITF

TOP DIFFERENTIAL DIAGNOSES

- Cellular neurothekeoma
- Giant cell tumor of soft tissue
- Fibromatosis
- Low-grade myofibroblastic sarcoma

Plexiform Fibrohistiocytic Tumor

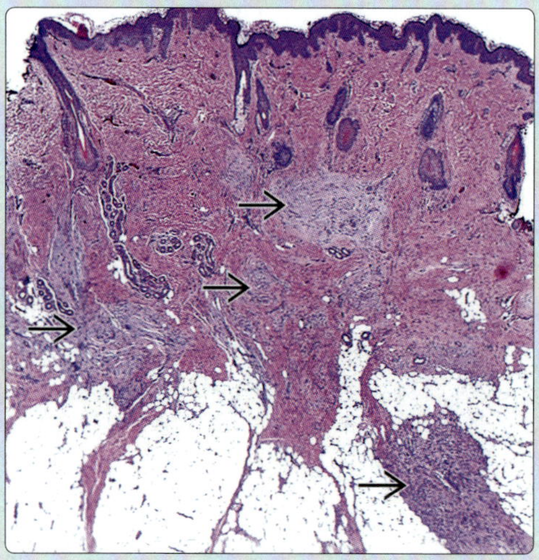

Infiltrative Growth

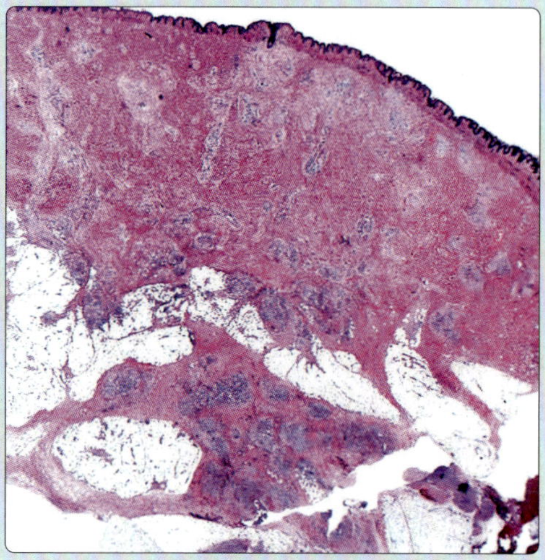

(Left) *Plexiform fibrohistiocytic tumor (PFHT) is an unusual, infiltrative mesenchymal neoplasm ⇨ that typically arises near the dermal-subcutaneous junction, as depicted. Tumors are characterized by fascicles or sheets of spindled fibroblasts &/or nests of histiocytoid cells in a nodular and plexiform growth pattern.* **(Right)** *Most cases of PFHT are infiltrative and characteristically show extensions or projections of tumor into the subcutaneous adipose tissue.*

Mixed-Type Plexiform Fibrohistiocytic Tumor

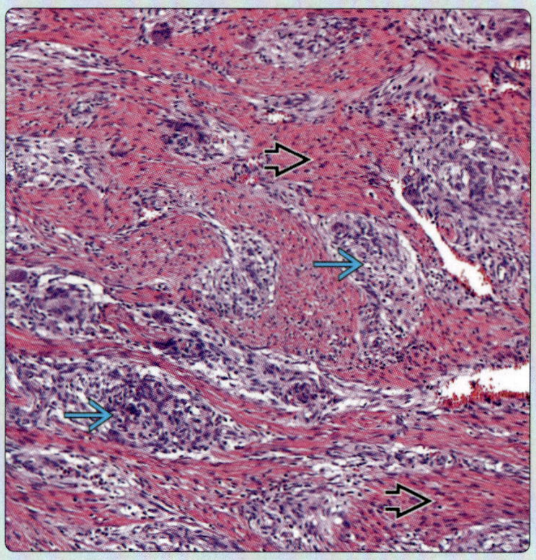

Histiocytoid Nests

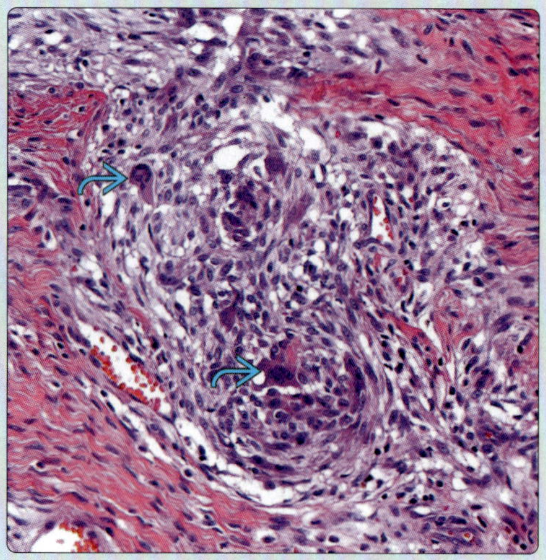

(Left) *The mixed subtype of PFHT shows a complex mixture of nests ⇨ of histiocytoid cells with short fascicles of bland spindled cells ⇨.* **(Right)** *The characteristic nests and aggregates of PFHT, when present, contain plump to epithelioid mononuclear histiocytoid cells. Multinucleated giant cells ⇨ may or may not be present.*

Plexiform Fibrohistiocytic Tumor

TERMINOLOGY

Abbreviations

- Plexiform fibrohistiocytic tumor (PFHT)

Definitions

- Rarely metastasizing dermal-subcutaneous mesenchymal neoplasm composed of variable mixture of fibroblasts and histiocyte-like cells

CLINICAL ISSUES

Epidemiology

- Incidence
  - Rare
- Age
  - Most common in children and young adults
    - Overall wide range: 1-77 years

Site

- Upper extremity (particularly forearm and hand)
- Also lower extremity, trunk, head and neck
- Most arise at dermal-subcutaneous interface
  - May also be purely dermal or subcutaneous
    - Subcutaneous tumors may involve skeletal muscle

Presentation

- Painless, slow-growing mass or plaque

Treatment

- Wide surgical excision or reexcision with negative margins
- Examination of regional lymph nodes may be warranted
- Indefinite clinical follow-up recommended

Prognosis

- Local recurrence in up to 40%
- Low metastatic potential (6%)
  - Regional lymph nodes
  - Systemic metastases very rare (lung)

MACROSCOPIC

General Features

- Multinodular, poorly delineated, tan-white

Size

- Usually < 3 cm (range 0.3-8.5 cm)

MICROSCOPIC

Histologic Features

- Most are located near dermal-subcutaneous interface
- Poorly circumscribed with infiltrative growth pattern
  - Adnexa often spared
- Morphologically subdivided into 3 types
  - Fibroblastic
    - Predominantly spindled fibroblastic cells
    - Plexiform to infiltrative fascicular growth
      - Ray-like extensions into subcutis
    - Chronic inflammatory infiltrate common
  - Histiocytic
    - Epithelioid histiocytoid cells
    - Cannonball-like, multinodular growth
      - Nodules may show hemorrhage
    - Osteoclast-like giant cells common
  - Mixed type
    - Histiocytoid nodules separated by fascicles
- Cellular and nuclear pleomorphism is usually absent
- Stromal can show dense hyalinization or myxoid change
  - Rare metaplastic bone formation
- Usually low mitotic rate (very rare atypical mitoses)
- Necrosis absent
- Rare focal lymphovascular invasion

ANCILLARY TESTS

Immunohistochemistry

- Spindle cells are SMA(+), at least focally
- Histiocytes are CD68(+) and CD163(+)
- Negative for S100 protein, CD34, desmin, keratin
- Negative for MITF (may be focally positive)

DIFFERENTIAL DIAGNOSIS

Cellular Neurothekeoma

- Can show significant morphologic overlap with PFHT
  - Entities may be closely related
- 1/3 of cases arise in head/neck
- MITF(+), usually diffuse

Giant Cell Tumor of Soft Tissue

- Prominent nodularity with abundant osteoclast-like giant cells
- Lacks infiltrative spindle cell component
- Peripheral shell of woven bone in 50%

Fibromatosis

- Lacks nodules of histiocytoid and osteoclast-like giant cells
- Characteristic elongated stromal vasculature
- Nuclear β-catenin (+)

Low-Grade Myofibroblastic Sarcoma

- Most common in head/neck and extremities
- Usually arise in deep subcutaneous tissue or skeletal muscle
- Highly infiltrative, often with checkerboard pattern
- At least focal nuclear enlargement, hyperchromasia

SELECTED REFERENCES

1. Liu CY et al: Myxoid plexiform fibrohistiocytic tumor masquerading as ganglion cyst: a case report and literature review. Case Rep Pathol. 2017:5370894, 2017
2. Fox MD et al: Expression of MiTF may be helpful in differentiating cellular neurothekeoma from plexiform fibrohistiocytic tumor (histiocytoid predominant) in a partial biopsy specimen. Am J Dermatopathol. 34(2):157-60, 2012
3. Luzar B et al: Cutaneous fibrohistiocytic tumours - an update. Histopathology. 56(1):148-65, 2010
4. Jaffer S et al: Neurothekeoma and plexiform fibrohistiocytic tumor: mere histologic resemblance or histogenetic relationship? Am J Surg Pathol. 33(6):905-13, 2009
5. Moosavi C et al: An update on plexiform fibrohistiocytic tumor and addition of 66 new cases from the Armed Forces Institute of Pathology, in honor of Franz M. Enzinger, MD. Ann Diagn Pathol. 11(5):313-9, 2007
6. Remstein ED et al: Plexiform fibrohistiocytic tumor: clinicopathologic analysis of 22 cases. Am J Surg Pathol. 23(6):662-70, 1999
7. Fisher C: Atypical plexiform fibrohistiocytic tumour. Histopathology. 30(3):271-3, 1997
8. Enzinger FM et al: Plexiform fibrohistiocytic tumor presenting in children and young adults. An analysis of 65 cases. Am J Surg Pathol. 12(11):818-26, 1988

(Left) *Osteoclast-like multinucleated giant cells are often seen within histiocytoid nodules in PFHT; however, they are absent in a subset of cases. Note also that the cells at the periphery of the nests may be spindled and appear to encircle the plumper epithelioid cells.* **(Right)** *The histiocytoid nodules of PFHT may lack multinucleated giant cells, as depicted. In the histiocytic subtype, this absence of giant cells may lead to an overall impression of cellular neurothekeoma, an entity that may be related to PFHT.*

Multinucleated Giant Cells

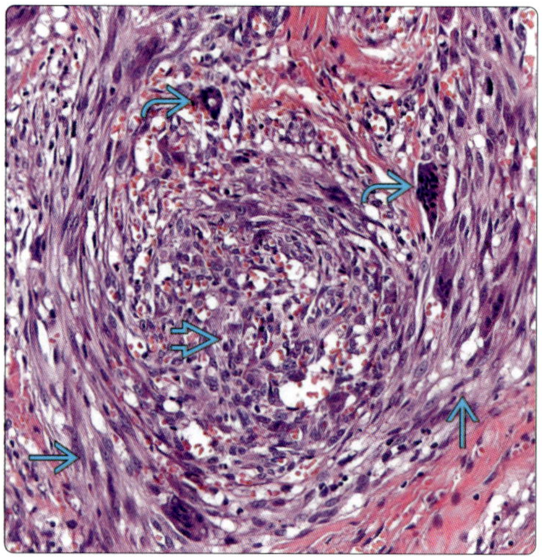

Histiocytoid Nodules

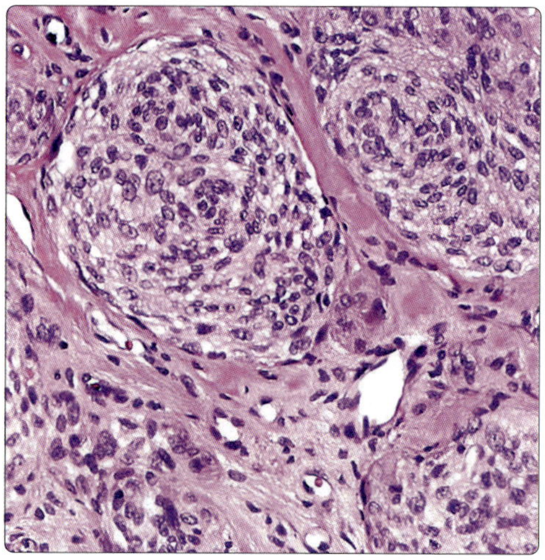

(Left) *Hemorrhage may be seen within PFHT and, when present, is often localized to histiocytoid nodules and nests, particularly if osteoclast-like multinucleated giant cells are present. This appearance can lead to consideration of a soft tissue giant cell tumor.* **(Right)** *The fibroblastic component of PFHT is characterized by fascicles and sheets of spindled cells within a variably collagenous stroma. Histiocytoid nodules ± giant cells are also seen in mixed subtypes.*

Intranodular Hemorrhage

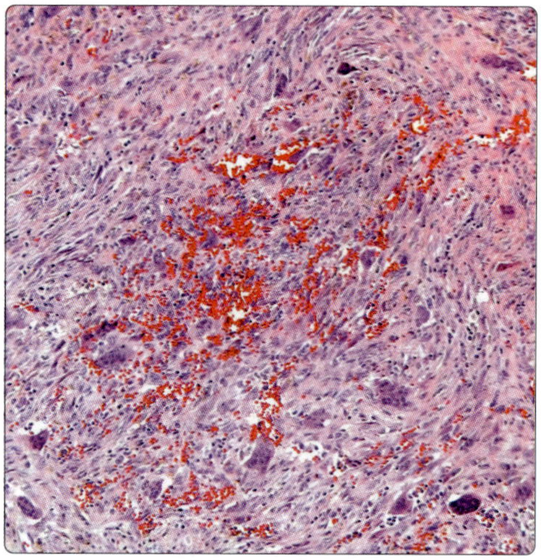

Fibroblastic Component

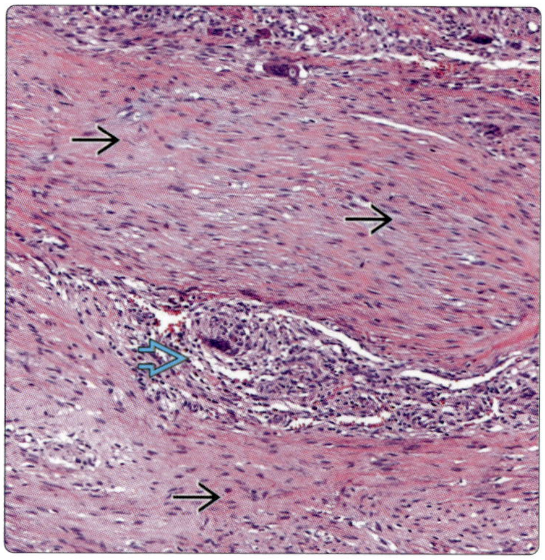

(Left) *The spindled fibroblastic cells of PFHT are generally cytologically banal and are associated with a variable amount of stromal collagen. In some cases, the stroma can be densely hyalinized or even focally myxoid.* **(Right)** *This case of PFHT shows areas of fibroblastic morphology with densely hyalinized stroma.*

Fibroblastic Component

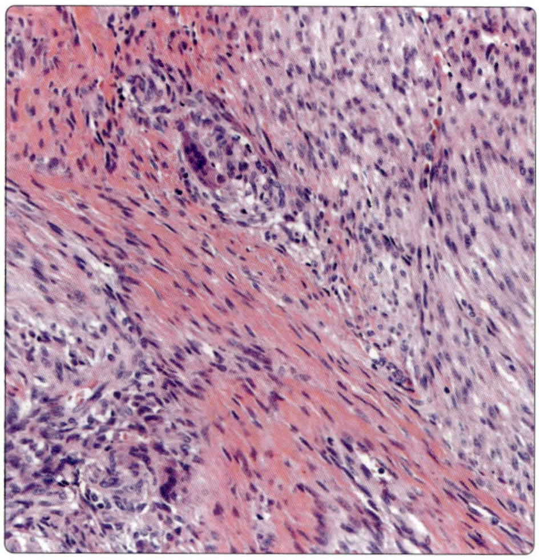

Fibroblastic Component

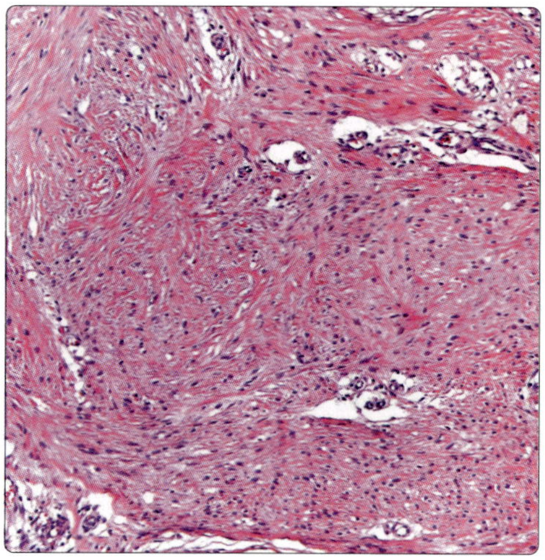

Cytologic Features

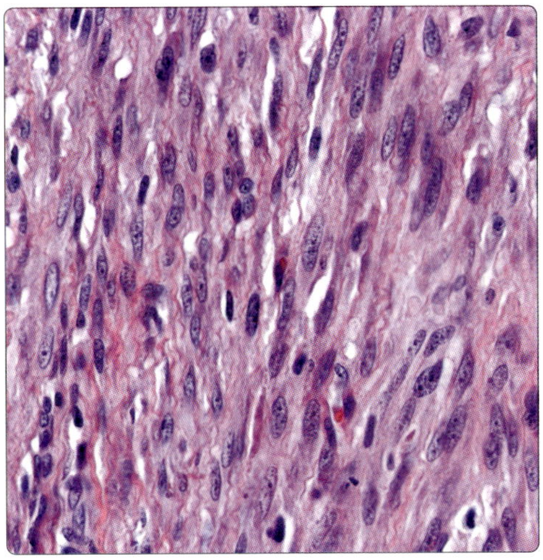

Fibroblastic-Type Plexiform Fibrohistiocytic Tumor

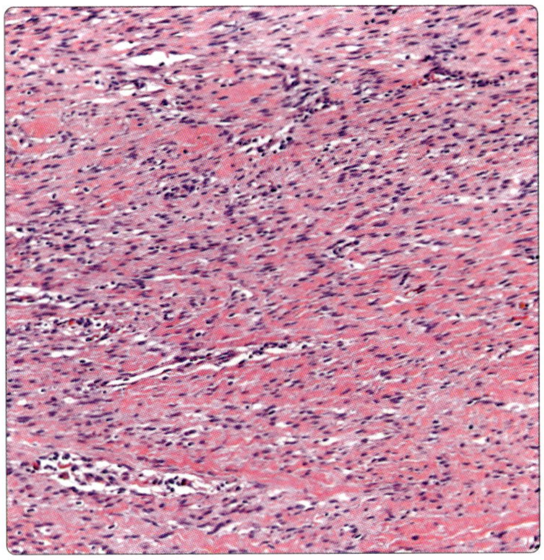

(Left) *The lesional cells of PFHT usually lack significant cytologic atypia, and mitotic activity is often low. Rare tumors, however, can show nuclear pleomorphism &/or rare atypical mitoses.* **(Right)** *The fibroblastic subtype of PFHT is composed predominantly, or entirely, of short fascicles and sheets of bland spindle cells with few to no histiocytic nests. Together with the infiltrative growth pattern, this subtype morphologically resembles fibromatosis.*

Histiocytic-Type Plexiform Fibrohistiocytic Tumor

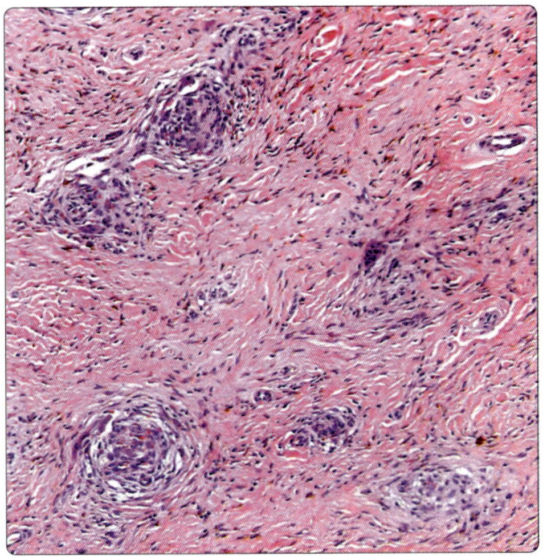

Infiltrative Growth

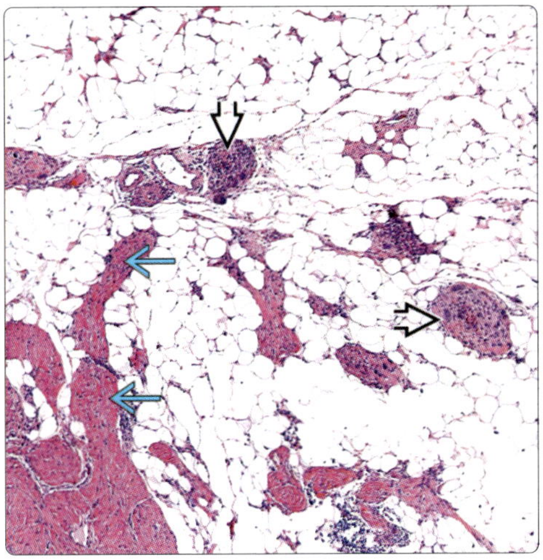

(Left) *The histiocytic subtype of PFHT is composed of infiltrating clusters and nests of plump histiocytoid cells ± giant cells. The surrounding connective tissue may appear reactive and contain inflammatory cells &/or hemosiderin pigment.* **(Right)** *Infiltrative growth is characteristic of PFHT, and the fibroblastic component, if present, often projects out into surrounding tissues as finger-like or ray-like extensions ⇨. Isolated nodules ⇨ of histiocytoid cells and giant cells may also be seen within fat.*

Increased Cellularity

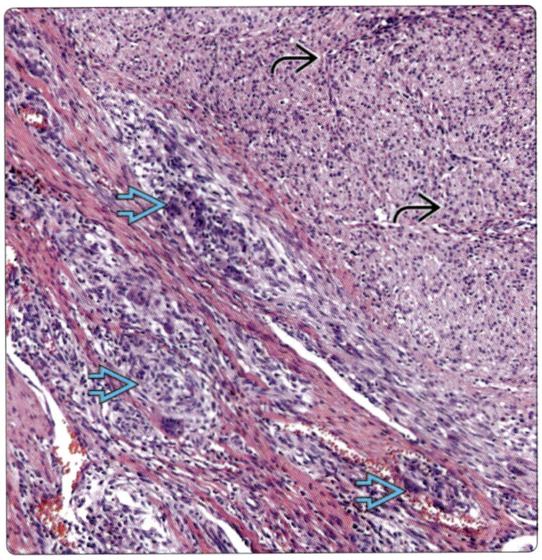

Increased Cellularity

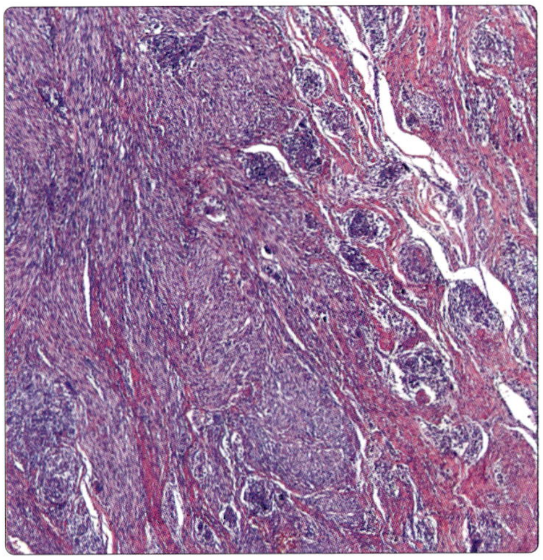

(Left) *Rare cases of PFHT show an increase in cellularity in the spindled fibroblastic component ↷ that may be easily mistaken for frank sarcoma. Note the compressed histiocytic nodules ⇨, some of which contain osteoclast-like giant cells and hemorrhage.* **(Right)** *Image of a cellular example of PFHT shows a mixture of fibroblastic elements (left) and histiocytoid nodules (right).*

Giant Cell Tumor of Soft Tissue

KEY FACTS

TERMINOLOGY

- Benign soft tissue neoplasm composed of mononuclear stromal cells, osteoclastic giant cells, and metaplastic bone
- Microscopically identical to giant cell tumor of bone
- Genetically distinct from giant cell tumor of bone
  - Lacks *H3F3A* mutation

CLINICAL ISSUES

- Average age: ~ 40 years; wide range: 1-86 years
- Superficial (subcutaneous) in 2/3
- Arm, thigh, and calf most common sites
- Local recurrence ~ 10%
- No established reports of metastasis

MACROSCOPIC

- Average size: 3.5 cm
  - Range: 0.7-10.0 cm

MICROSCOPIC

- Multinodular with fibrous septa
- Peripheral rim of metaplastic ossification
  - Can extend into center of tumor
- Hemorrhage and cystic hemorrhage
- Aneurysmal bone cyst-like changes
- Mononuclear stromal cells
  - Oval to spindle-shaped nuclei
  - No significant cytological atypia
- Osteoclastic giant cells
  - Evenly distributed throughout tumor
- Mitotic rate 2-5/10 HPF; rare tumors with > 30/10 HPF
- Xanthoma cells in some

TOP DIFFERENTIAL DIAGNOSES

- Tenosynovial giant cell tumor
- Undifferentiated pleomorphic sarcoma (with giant cells)
- Extraskeletal recurrence of giant cell tumor of bone

Giant Cell Tumor of Soft Tissue

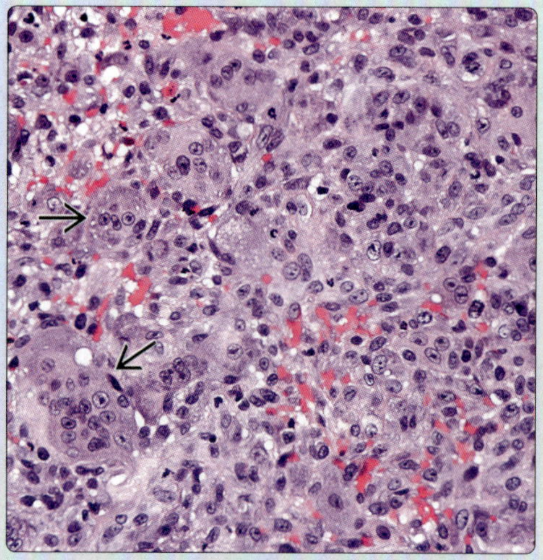

Soft Tissue Mass of Shoulder

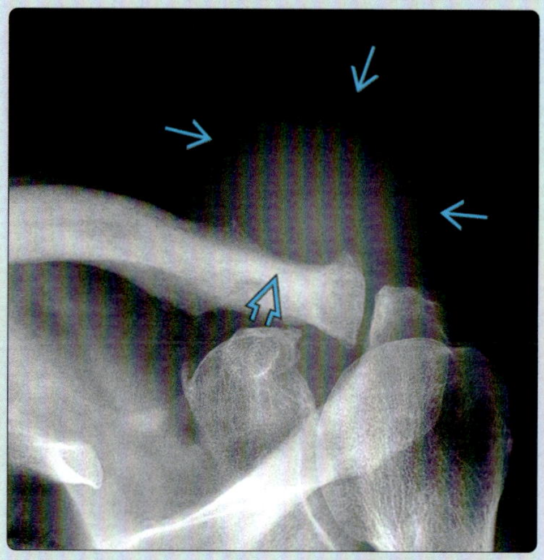

(Left) *Microscopically, giant cell tumor of soft tissue (GCTST) is identical to giant cell tumor of bone composed of mononuclear stromal cells and multinuclear osteoclastic giant cells ➡ that are evenly distributed throughout the tumor.* **(Right)** *Radiographically, GCTST presents as a soft tissue mass ➡. Although most occur in the subcutis, 1/3 involve the deep soft tissue, such as this tumor that saucerizes the clavicle ⇨. GCTST can be associated with Paget disease of bone, as in this 64-year-old man.*

Ossification

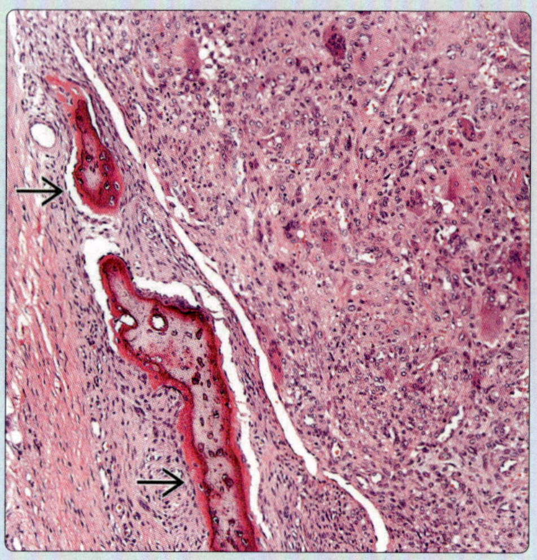

Cytological Features

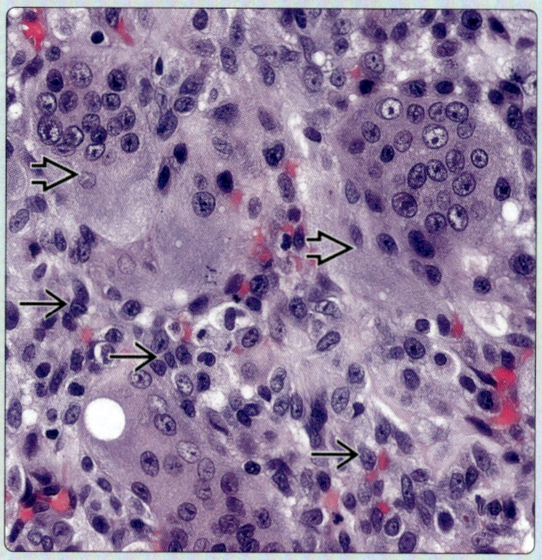

(Left) *Metaplastic ossification is present in ~ 1/2 of GCTST. It typically forms a peripheral rind of woven bone ➡. However, ossification can also be found in the center of the mass.* **(Right)** *GCTST is composed of uniform mononuclear stromal cells with round to oval nuclei and ill-defined cytoplasmic borders ➡. Osteoclastic giant cells ⇨ are abundant and evenly distributed throughout the tumor. Although mitoses are readily identified in most tumors, none are atypical.*

TERMINOLOGY

Abbreviations

- Giant cell tumor of soft tissue (GCTST)

Synonyms

- Soft tissue giant cell tumor of low malignant potential

Definitions

- Benign soft tissue neoplasm composed of mononuclear stromal cells, osteoclastic giant cells, and metaplastic bone
  - Microscopically identical to giant cell tumor of bone
  - Genetically distinct from giant cell tumor of bone
    - Lacks *H3F3A* mutation

CLINICAL ISSUES

Epidemiology

- Incidence
  - Rare; exact incidence unknown
- Age
  - Average: ~ 40 years (wide range: 1-86 years)
- Sex
  - F = M

Site

- Arm, thigh, and calf most common sites
  - Others: Hand, shoulder, foot, buttock, groin, hip, head and neck, abdominal wall, chest wall, flank, back, ischiorectal fossa, presacrum, peripancreas, mediastinum, intracranium, retroperitoneum, breast
- Superficial (subcutaneous) in 2/3, deep (subfascial) in 1/3

Presentation

- Painless mass
- Can be associated with Paget disease of bone

Treatment

- Complete surgical excision

Prognosis

- Very good; benign
- Local recurrence ~ 10%
- No established reports of metastasis

IMAGING

Radiographic Findings

- Soft tissue mass
- Peripheral mineralization in some
- Deep-seated tumors can saucerize underlying bone

MACROSCOPIC

General Features

- Most tumors well circumscribed
- Multinodular
- Red-brown
- Peripheral rim of ossification in 1/2
- Hemorrhagic cystic spaces

Size

- Average: 3.5 cm (range: 0.7-10.0 cm)

MICROSCOPIC

Histologic Features

- Multinodular with fibrous septa
- Peripheral rim of metaplastic ossification
  - Can extend into center of tumor
- Storiform pattern in some
- Hemorrhage and cystic hemorrhage
  - Aneurysmal bone cyst-like changes
  - Hemosiderin deposition
- Variable stromal fibrosis
- Vascular invasion in 1/3

Cytologic Features

- Mononuclear stromal cells
  - Oval to spindle-shaped nuclei
  - Ill-defined cytoplasm and cytoplasmic boundaries
  - No significant cytologic atypia
  - Mitoses readily identified
    - Rate = 2-5/10 HPF; rare tumors with > 30/10 HPF
    - No atypical mitotic figures
- Osteoclastic giant cells
  - Evenly distributed throughout tumor
- Xanthoma cell (foamy macrophages) in some

ANCILLARY TESTS

Immunohistochemistry

- Mononuclear cells p63(+)

DIFFERENTIAL DIAGNOSIS

Tenosynovial Giant Cell Tumor

- Synovial-based or intraarticular tumor
- More heterogeneous population of cells
- Epithelioid cells with eccentric, vesicular nuclei

Undifferentiated Pleomorphic Sarcoma (With Giant Cells)

- High-grade sarcoma with numerous osteoclastic giant cells
- Pleomorphic stromal cells, atypical mitotic figures, necrosis

Extraskeletal Recurrence of Giant Cell Tumor of Bone

- Grossly and microscopically indistinguishable from GCTST

SELECTED REFERENCES

1. Lee JC et al: Giant cell tumor of soft tissue is genetically distinct from its bone counterpart. Mod Pathol. 30(5):728-33, 2017
2. Mishra SS et al: Intracranial giant cell tumor of soft tissue: mimicking a glioma. Neurol India. 61(2):192-3, 2013
3. Lau YS et al: Phenotypic and molecular studies of giant-cell tumors of bone and soft tissue. Hum Pathol. 36(9):945-54, 2005
4. O'Connell JX et al: Giant cell tumors of soft tissue: a clinicopathologic study of 18 benign and malignant tumors. Am J Surg Pathol. 24(3):386-95, 2000
5. Oliveira AM et al: Primary giant cell tumor of soft tissues: a study of 22 cases. Am J Surg Pathol. 24(2):248-56, 2000
6. Galed-Placed I et al: Giant-cell tumor in soft parts in a patient with osseous Paget's disease: diagnosis by fine-needle aspiration. Diagn Cytopathol. 19(5):352-4, 1998

(Left) *In the absence of clinical and radiographic correlation, GCTST is indistinguishable from giant cell tumor of bone, consisting of sheets of mononuclear stromal cells with oval to spindle-shaped nuclei admixed with uniformly distributed osteoclastic giant cells* ⇨. **(Right)** *Most often, GCTST presents as a well-circumscribed mass. This low-power micrograph illustrates sharp demarcation between tumor* ⇨ *and surrounding fibroadipose tissue by a thick fibrous pseudocapsule* ⇨.

Giant Cell Tumor of Soft Tissue

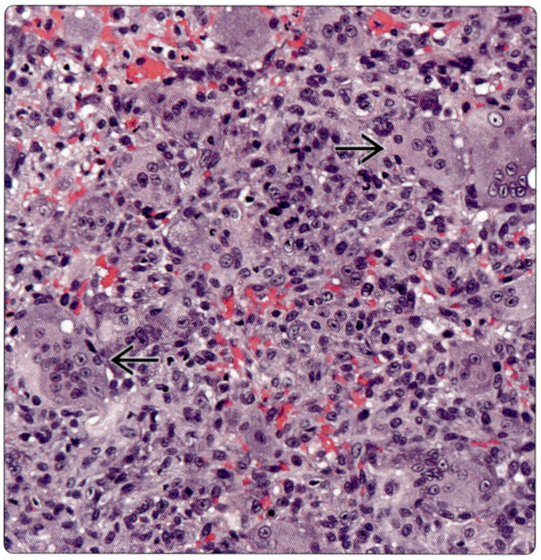

Circumscribed Border

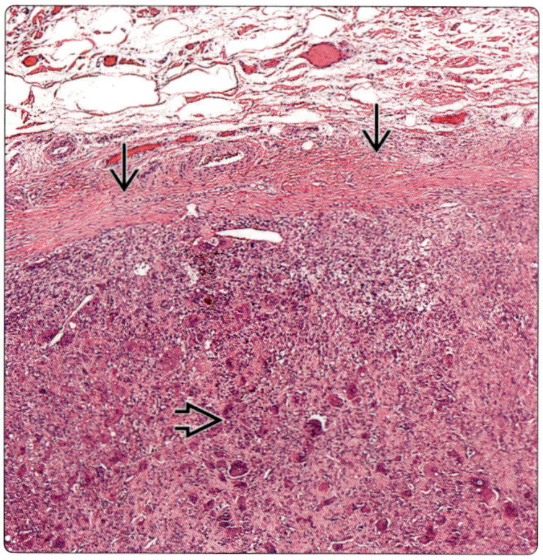

(Left) *Most tumors have a multinodular architecture defined by fibrous septa* ⇨ *that divide it into cellular nodules* ⇨. *Numerous osteoclastic giant cells* ⇨ *are easily identified even at low power.* **(Right)** *Similar to giant cell tumor of bone, the osteoclastic giant cells in GCTST can be very large and harbor very many nuclei, as indicated by this huge giant cell with > 50 nuclei* ⇨.

Nodular Architecture

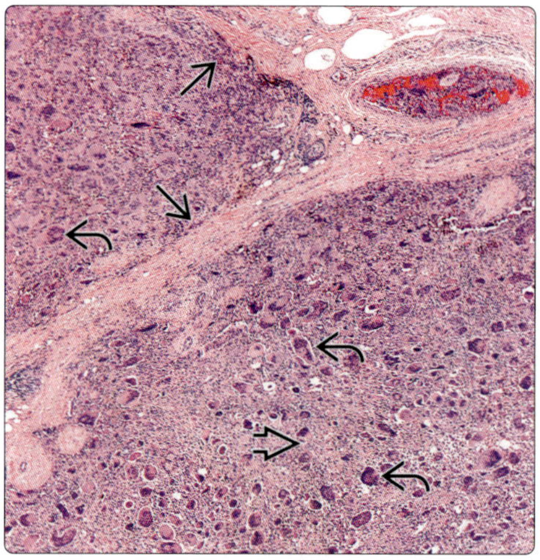

Large Osteoclastic Giant Cells

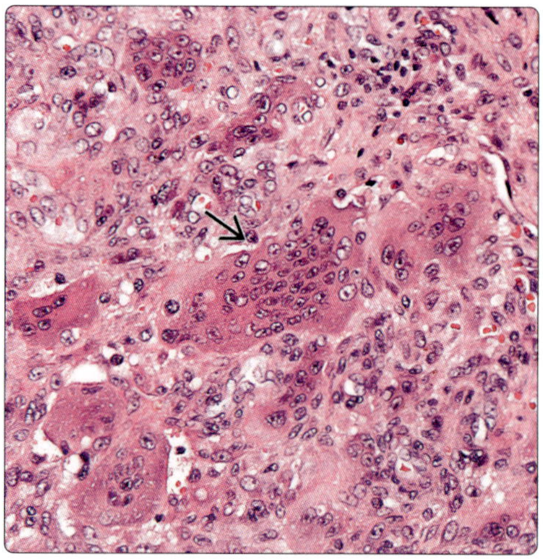

(Left) *Like giant cell tumor of bone, GCTST can have a storiform architecture, as depicted by short curvilinear fascicles of plump spindle cells that intersect to form a pinwheel pattern.* **(Right)** *Stromal hemorrhage is common, often presenting as blood-filled cystic spaces or aneurysmal bone cyst-like change. This micrograph depicts aneurysmal bone cyst-like change in a giant cell tumor characterized by blood pools* ➡ *separated by an edematous fibromyxoid trabecula* ⇨ *containing giant cells* ⇨.

Storiform Pattern

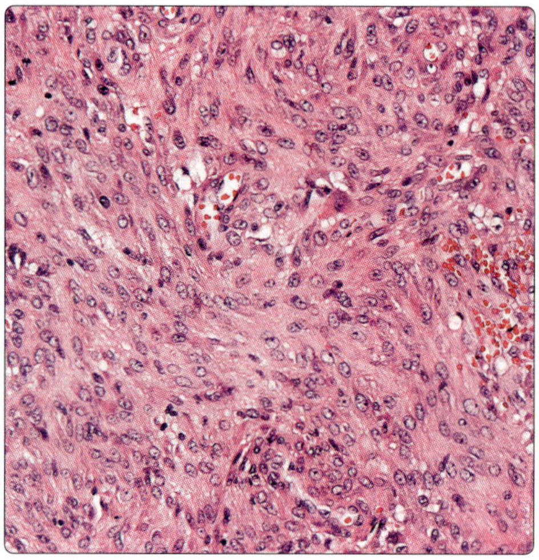

Aneurysmal Bone Cyst-Like Change

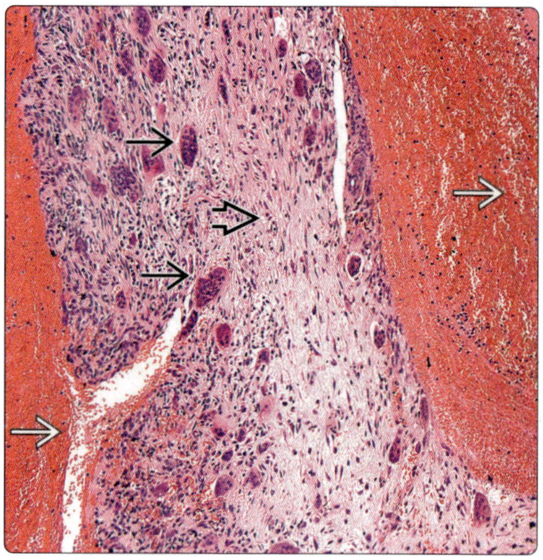

Giant Cell Tumor of Soft Tissue of Finger

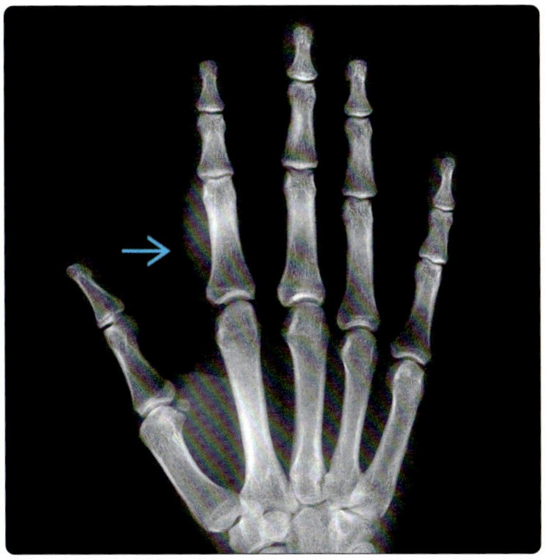

MR

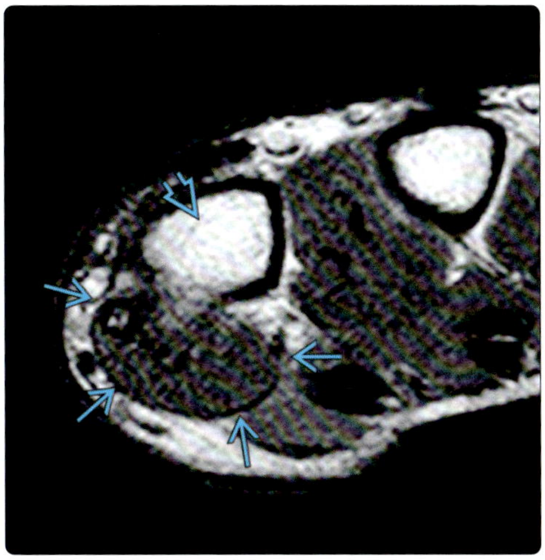

(Left) *Although most common in the arm, thigh, and calf, GCTST has a wide anatomic distribution, including the fingers, as depicted in this radiograph, which shows an extraskeletal soft tissue mass* → *in the index finger of a 21-year-old man. Differential diagnosis would include tenosynovial giant cell tumor.* **(Right)** *This MR from the same patient reveals a well-circumscribed mass adjacent* → *to, but not directly involving, the bony phalanx* ⇨.

Hemosiderin Deposits

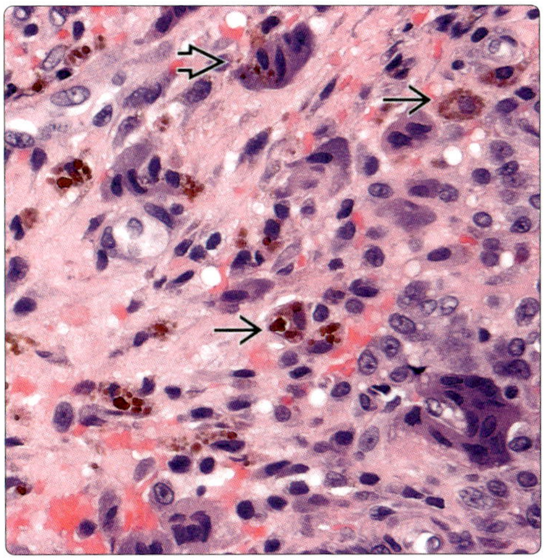

Fibrosis

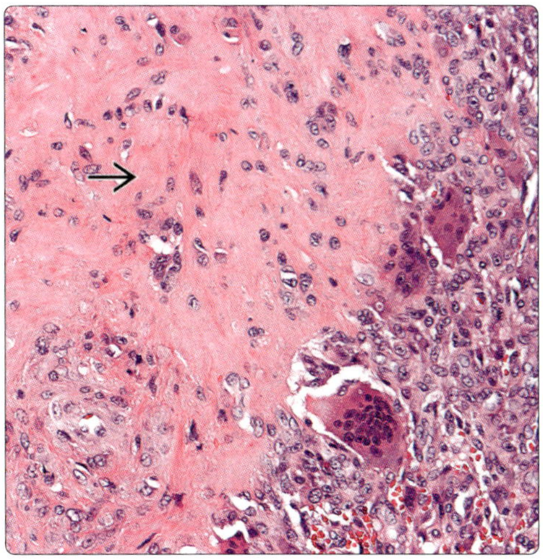

(Left) *Stromal hemorrhage is common in GCTST with subsequent hemosiderin deposition. This micrograph illustrates hemosiderin pigment within macrophages* → *as well as within osteoclastic giant cells* ⇨. **(Right)** *Stromal fibrosis is common in GCTST and is highly variable in its extent. It can sometimes form large sheets of hyalinized collagenous matrix, as depicted* →.

Xanthoma Cells

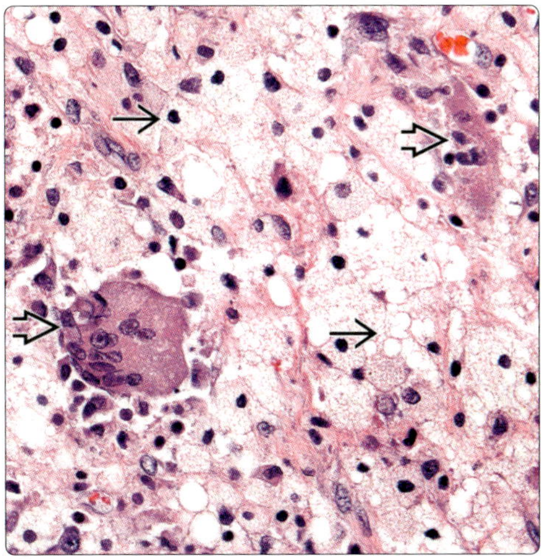

Vascular Invasion

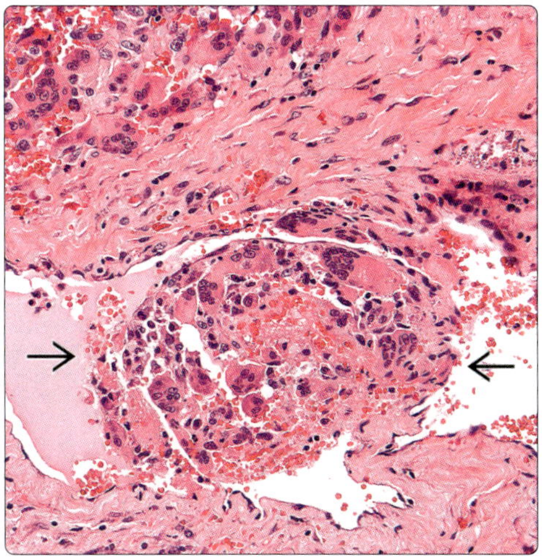

(Left) *Areas containing sheets of xanthoma cells (foamy macrophages) can be seen in GCTST. These cells contain abundant phagocytized lipid material, which imparts a microvacuolar cytoplasm* →. *Here, they are admixed with osteoclastic giant cells* ⇨. **(Right)** *Vascular invasion* → *can be seen in ~ 1/3 of GCTST. As in giant cell tumor of bone, vascular invasion does not have prognostic value nor does it indicate an increased risk of metastasis.*

Histiocytic Sarcoma

KEY FACTS

TERMINOLOGY

- Malignant neoplasm showing morphologic and immunophenotypic evidence of histiocytic differentiation

CLINICAL ISSUES

- Wide age range (median: 50 years)
- Superficial or deep soft tissues of the extremities
- Also skin, gastrointestinal tract, other sites
- Treatment: Complete surgical resection with postoperative chemotherapy or radiotherapy
- Aggressive clinical course with overall poor prognosis
  - Small, localized tumors that are completely removed may have better clinical outcome

MACROSCOPIC

- Most 5-10 cm

MICROSCOPIC

- Infiltrative periphery
- Diffuse sheets of medium to large epithelioid cells with eosinophilic or foamy cytoplasm and irregular, vesicular nuclei with prominent nucleoli
- Mitoses and necrosis common
- Admixed inflammatory infiltrate common and may be abundant

ANCILLARY TESTS

- CD45, CD68, and CD163 (+)
- S100 protein (+), usually focal
- Negative for keratin, CD20, HMB45, CD21, CD30

TOP DIFFERENTIAL DIAGNOSES

- Non-Hodgkin lymphoma
- Metastatic carcinoma/melanoma
- Dedifferentiated liposarcoma
- Extranodal Rosai-Dorfman disease
- Gastrointestinal stromal tumor

Histiocytic Sarcoma

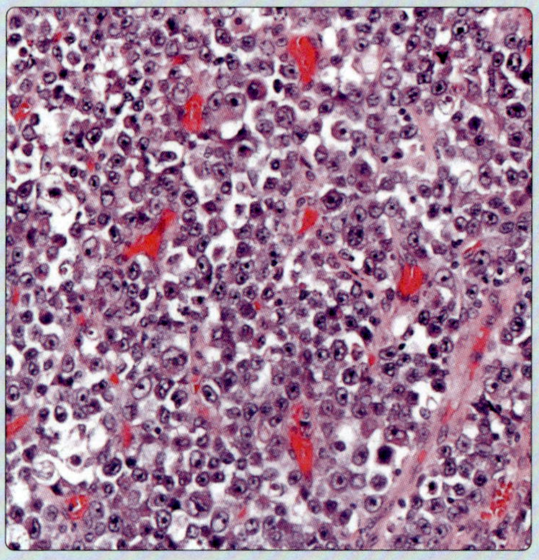

Foamy Cytoplasm

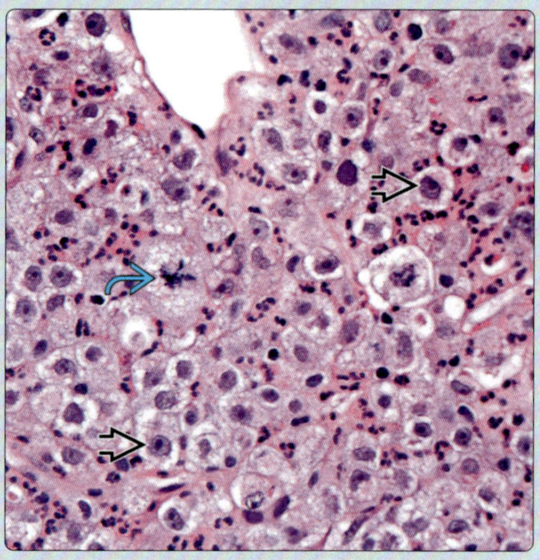

(Left) *Histiocytic sarcoma (HS) is an aggressive malignant neoplasm that is classically composed of sheets of epithelioid histiocytic cells with pale eosinophilic cytoplasm and vesicular nuclei with prominent nucleoli. Mitoses and necrosis are common.* **(Right)** *Some tumor cells in HS show foamy cytoplasm and may be confused for nonneoplastic histiocytes; however, the prominent nucleoli and mitoses support HS. Note also the background neutrophilic inflammatory infiltrate.*

Binucleated and Multinucleated Cells

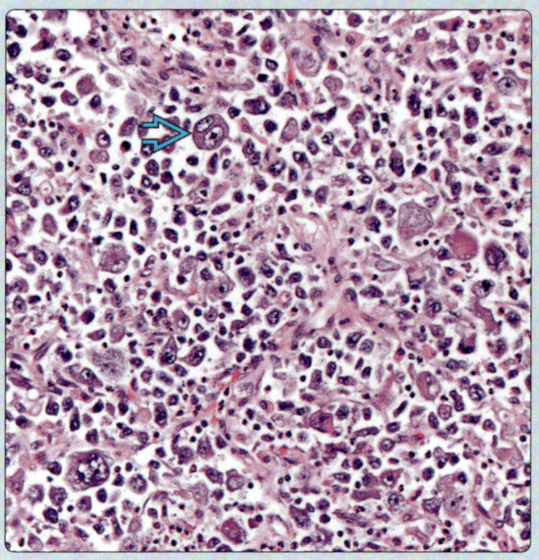

Histiocytic Immunophenotype

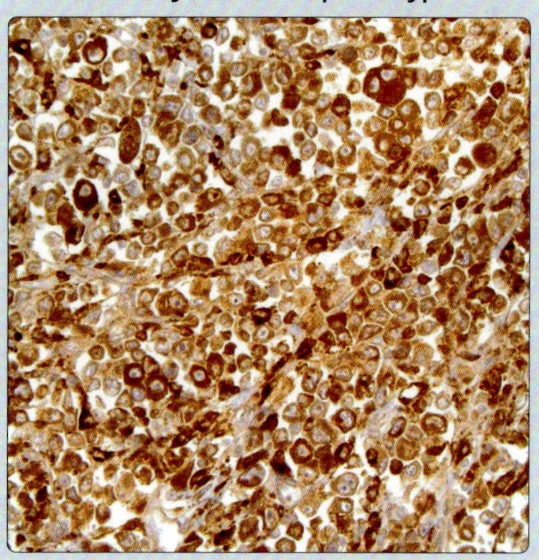

(Left) *Binucleated and multinucleated tumor cells are a relatively common finding in HS. The case depicted in this image also shows cellular and nuclear pleomorphism. Note also the dyscohesive nature of the cells; however, in some cases, the cells are densely packed.* **(Right)** *Histiocytic sarcoma shows immunoexpression of antigens typically seen in mature histiocytes, such as CD68 (shown) and lysozyme. CD163 is also expressed in HS and is a better, more specific marker of histiocytic origin.*

TERMINOLOGY

Abbreviations

- Histiocytic sarcoma (HS)

Definitions

- Malignant neoplasm showing morphologic and immunophenotypic evidence of histiocytic differentiation

CLINICAL ISSUES

Epidemiology

- Incidence
  - Very rare
- Age
  - Wide range (median: 50 years)

Site

- Superficial or deep soft tissues of extremities
  - May arise in skin
- Gastrointestinal tract
- Lymph nodes, spleen, central nervous system, and others

Presentation

- Often solitary, painless mass
- Site-specific symptoms
  - Skin: Rash
  - GI tract: Abdominal pain, obstruction
- May have weight loss and other systemic symptoms
- Prior history of lymphoma (e.g., follicular, mantle cell) may exist

Treatment

- Complete surgical resection with postoperative chemotherapy or radiotherapy

Prognosis

- Overall poor prognosis
- Most show aggressive clinical course
  - Metastases common (usually to lymph nodes, lung, bone)
- Small, localized tumors that are completely removed may have better clinical outcome

MACROSCOPIC

General Features

- Tan-yellow, soft, fleshy cut surface
- Hemorrhage and necrosis common

Size

- Most 5-10 cm

MICROSCOPIC

Histologic Features

- Infiltrative periphery
- Diffuse sheets of medium to large epithelioid cells
  - Abundant pale eosinophilic or foamy cytoplasm
  - Irregular, vesicular nuclei with prominent nucleoli
    - Binucleation and multinucleation are common
    - Mitoses frequent
  - Cellular pleomorphism may be seen
- Necrosis common
- Admixed inflammatory infiltrate common and may be abundant
  - Usually neutrophils or lymphocytes
- Spindled morphology may be present in some cases

ANCILLARY TESTS

Immunohistochemistry

- CD45, CD68, and CD163 (+)
- CD4, CD31, and lysozyme (+)
- S100 protein (+), often focal
- Negative for keratin, CD20, CD1a, CD21, CD30, HMB45, ALK, myeloperoxidase

DIFFERENTIAL DIAGNOSIS

Non-Hodgkin Lymphoma

- Usually diffuse large B-cell lymphoma or anaplastic large cell lymphoma
- Utilization of immunohistochemistry and flow cytometry often necessary for distinction from HS

Metastatic Carcinoma/Melanoma

- Usually easily excluded through use of immunohistochemistry
- History of previous diagnosis may be available

Dedifferentiated Liposarcoma

- Often contain areas of well-differentiated liposarcoma
- May show prominent admixed inflammatory component
- MDM2 amplification by fluorescence in situ hybridization (FISH) analysis
- MDM2 or CDK4 overexpression by immunohistochemistry

Extranodal Rosai-Dorfman Disease

- Histiocytes lack prominent nucleoli and nuclear atypia
- No mitoses or necrosis

Gastrointestinal Stromal Tumor

- Most show spindled morphology; less commonly epithelioid
- Prominent nucleoli not usually a feature
- CD117 and DOG1(+)

SELECTED REFERENCES

1. Magro CM et al: Primary cutaneous histiocytic sarcoma: a report of five cases with primary cutaneous involvement and review of the literature. Ann Diagn Pathol. 32:56-62, 2018
2. Hung YP et al: Histiocytic sarcoma: new insights into FNA cytomorphology and molecular characteristics. Cancer Cytopathol. 125(8):604-614, 2017
3. Takahashi E et al: Histiocytic sarcoma : an updated literature review based on the 2008 WHO classification. J Clin Exp Hematop. 53(1):1-8, 2013
4. Sundersingh S et al: Multifocal histiocytic sarcoma of the gastrointestinal tract. Indian J Pathol Microbiol. 55(2):233-5, 2012
5. Vos JA et al: Histiocytic sarcoma: a study of five cases including the histiocyte marker CD163. Mod Pathol. 18(5):693-704, 2005
6. Hornick JL et al: Extranodal histiocytic sarcoma: clinicopathologic analysis of 14 cases of a rare epithelioid malignancy. Am J Surg Pathol. 28(9):1133-44, 2004
7. Lau SK et al: CD163: a specific marker of macrophages in paraffin-embedded tissue samples. Am J Clin Pathol. 122(5):794-801, 2004
8. Mikami M et al: Monocyte/macrophage-specific marker CD163+ histiocytic sarcoma: case report with clinical, morphologic, immunohistochemical, and molecular genetic studies. Int J Hematol. 80(4):365-9, 2004

Follicular Dendritic Cell Sarcoma

KEY FACTS

TERMINOLOGY

- Neoplastic proliferation of cells showing morphologic and immunophenotypic features of follicular dendritic cells

CLINICAL ISSUES

- Young and middle-aged adults
- Female predominance in inflammatory pseudotumor-like variant
- Majority involve lymph nodes, particularly cervical
- > 1/3 arise in extranodal sites (GI tract, soft tissue, etc.)
- Treatment: Complete surgical excision ± chemotherapy or radiotherapy
- Generally protracted clinical course
  - Up to 50% recur locally
  - Up to 25% metastasize, often late

MICROSCOPIC

- Spindled to ovoid cells in sheets, fascicles, or storiform whorls
  - Indistinct cell borders, eosinophilic cytoplasm
  - Nuclei with finely dispersed, speckled chromatin and nucleolus
- Lymphocytic infiltrate common
- Some cases show significant cytologic atypia and pleomorphism
- Morphologic variant: Inflammatory pseudotumor-like

ANCILLARY TESTS

- CD21(+), CD23(+), CD35(+)
- Clusterin (+), fascin (+), vimentin (+)
- EMA (variable), S100 (variable), CD68 (variable)
- CD45(-), CD34(-), keratin (-), desmin (-), CD1a(-), HMB-45(-)

TOP DIFFERENTIAL DIAGNOSES

- Interdigitating dendritic cell sarcoma
- Metastatic sarcomatoid carcinoma
- Inflammatory myofibroblastic tumor

Follicular Dendritic Cell Sarcoma

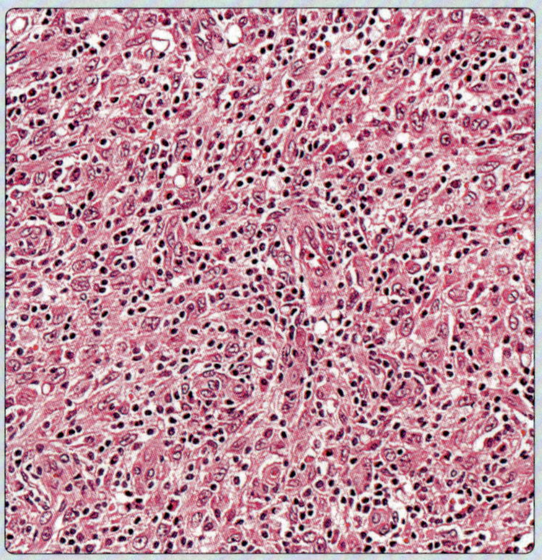

Whorling Architecture

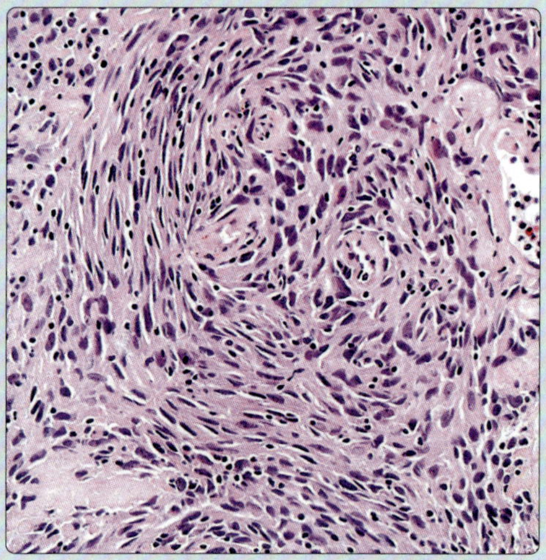

(Left) *Follicular dendritic cell sarcoma (FDCS) may be impossible to distinguish from interdigitating dendritic cell sarcoma histologically and often requires immunohistochemistry. In this slide, sheets of ovoid tumor cells are associated with admixed lymphocytes and capillary blood vessels.* **(Right)** *Architecturally, FDCS typically shows a storiform or whorling growth pattern, at least focally. Other patterns include fascicular, nests, and sheet-like growth.*

Cytologic Features

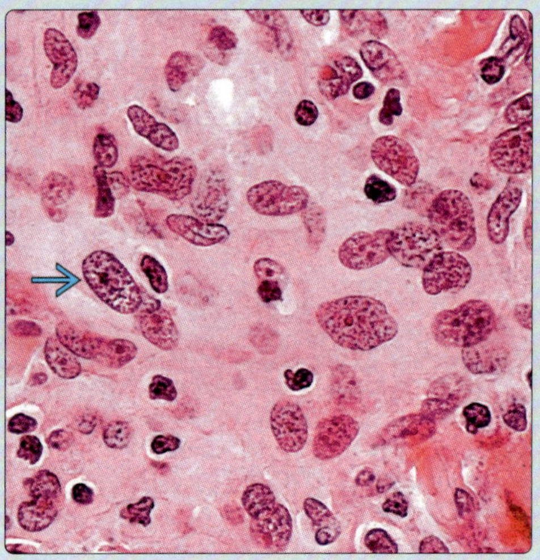

CD23 Expression

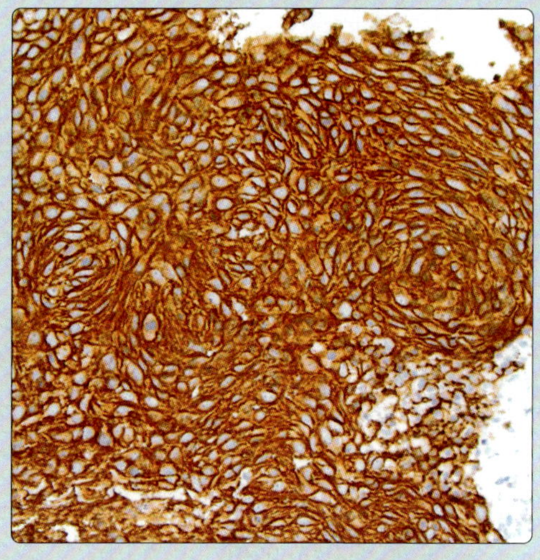

(Left) *The neoplastic dendritic cells of FDCS have distinctive oval nuclei with speckled chromatin, small nucleoli, and prominent nuclear membrane* ➡*. Indistinct cell margins give a syncytial appearance to the tumor.* **(Right)** *The lesional cells of FDCS express markers of follicular dendritic cell origin, including CD21, CD23 (shown), and CD35, although expression of each varies from case to case. Keratins and S100 protein are generally negative.*

Follicular Dendritic Cell Sarcoma

TERMINOLOGY

Abbreviations

- Follicular dendritic cell sarcoma (FDCS)

Synonyms

- Follicular dendritic reticulum cell sarcoma

Definitions

- Neoplastic proliferation of cells showing morphologic and immunophenotypic features of follicular dendritic cells

ETIOLOGY/PATHOGENESIS

Varied Etiologies

- Most cases arise de novo
- 10-15% arise in hyaline-vascular-type Castleman disease
  - Antecedent dendritic cell hyperplasia and dysplasia
- Inflammatory pseudotumor-like variant associated with EBV

CLINICAL ISSUES

Epidemiology

- Age
  - Young and middle-aged adults
- Sex
  - M = F
    - Female predominance in inflammatory pseudotumor-like variant

Site

- Majority involve lymph nodes
  - Cervical node involved most commonly
- Inflammatory pseudotumor-like variant
  - Liver or spleen characteristic
- > 1/3 arise in extranodal sites
  - GI tract, tonsil, mediastinum, skin, soft tissue, others

Presentation

- Slow-growing, painless mass
- Systemic symptoms (e.g., fever) uncommon
  - Exception: Inflammatory pseudotumor-like variant
- Rare patients have paraneoplastic pemphigus or myasthenia gravis

Treatment

- Complete surgical excision ± chemotherapy or radiotherapy

Prognosis

- Generally protracted clinical course
  - Up to 50% recur locally
  - Up to 25% metastasize
    - Often later in disease course
  - Up to 20% of patients die of disease, often after long period of time
- High-grade cytologic features, necrosis, size > 6 cm, or intraabdominal location often indicate greater potential for aggressive behavior

MACROSCOPIC

Size

- Mean: 5 cm

MICROSCOPIC

Histologic Features

- Spindled to ovoid cells in sheets, fascicles, or storiform whorls
  - Indistinct cell borders, eosinophilic cytoplasm
  - Nuclei distinctive
    - Ovoid or elongated
    - Finely dispersed, speckled chromatin with nucleolus
    - Pseudoinclusions common
    - Multinucleated cells often seen
- Lymphocytic infiltrate common
- Mitotic rate usually < 10 per 10 HPF
- Some cases show significant cytologic atypia and pleomorphism
  - More likely to contain atypical mitoses and coagulative necrosis
- Rare features: Myxoid stroma, clear cells, oncocytic cells, epithelioid cells, cystic spaces, osteoclast-like giant cells

Morphologic Variants

- Inflammatory pseudotumor-like variant
  - Spindled to ovoid cells associated with prominent lymphoplasmacytic infiltrate
  - Necrosis and hemorrhage common
  - Fibrinoid vascular changes

ANCILLARY TESTS

Immunohistochemistry

- CD21(+), CD23(+), CD35(+)
- Clusterin (+), fascin (+), vimentin (+)
- EMA (variable), S100 (variable), CD68 (variable)
- EBER(+) in inflammatory pseudotumor-like variant
- CD45(-), CD34(-), keratin (-), desmin (-), CD1a(-), HMB-45(-)

DIFFERENTIAL DIAGNOSIS

Interdigitating Dendritic Cell Sarcoma

- May be histologically indistinguishable from FDCS
- Immunohistochemistry helpful
  - S100(+), CD21(-), CD23(-), CD35(-), clusterin (-)

Metastatic Sarcomatoid Carcinoma

- Clinical history of primary tumor elsewhere
- Keratin (+)

Inflammatory Myofibroblastic Tumor

- Can mimic inflammatory pseudotumor-like FDCS
- SMA (+); ALK-1(+) in up to 50% of cases
- CD21(-) and EBER(-)

SELECTED REFERENCES

1. Wu A et al: Follicular dendritic cell sarcoma. Arch Pathol Lab Med. 140(2):186-90, 2016
2. Pang J et al: Follicular dendritic cell sarcoma of the head and neck: case report, literature review, and pooled analysis of 97 cases. Head Neck. ePub, 2015
3. Choe JY et al: Inflammatory pseudotumor-like follicular dendritic cell sarcoma of the spleen: a report of six cases with increased IgG4-positive plasma cells. Pathol Int. 63(5):245-51, 2013
4. Soriano AO et al: Follicular dendritic cell sarcoma: a report of 14 cases and a review of the literature. Am J Hematol. 82(8):725-8, 2007

Interdigitating Dendritic Cell Sarcoma

KEY FACTS

TERMINOLOGY

- Neoplastic proliferation of cells with immunophenotype similar to normal interdigitating dendritic cells

CLINICAL ISSUES

- Very rare
- Most patients are adults (median: 6th-7th decades)
- Usually arises in single lymph node
  - Less commonly arises in extranodal sites
- Slow-growing, asymptomatic mass
  - Systemic symptoms (e.g., fever) occur in subset
- Treatment: Surgical resection ± radiation for localized disease
- Prognosis is variable and largely unpredictable
  - 40-50% of patients develop disseminated disease

MICROSCOPIC

- Partial or complete replacement of lymph node architecture
  - Paracortical localization of tumor cells is common
- Spindled-to-ovoid, eosinophilic cells forming sheets, fascicles, whorls
  - Vesicular nuclei with small or prominent nucleoli
- Nuclei uniform to pleomorphic
- Mitotic rate usually < 5 per 10 HPF
- Infiltrate of small lymphocytes common

ANCILLARY TESTS

- S100(+), SOX10(+)
- Variable CD45(+), CD163(+), and CD68(+)
- CD21(-), CD23(-), CD35(-), CD1a(-), clusterin (-), EMA(-), keratin (-), melanocytic markers (-)

TOP DIFFERENTIAL DIAGNOSES

- Follicular dendritic cell sarcoma
- Metastatic melanoma
- Histiocytic sarcoma

Interdigitating Dendritic Cell Sarcoma

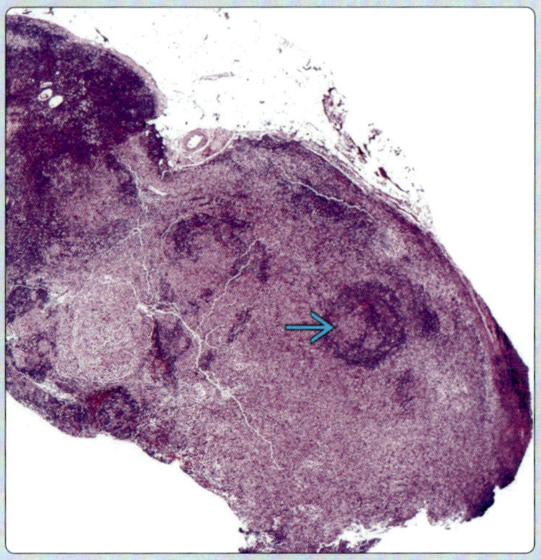

Cytologic Features

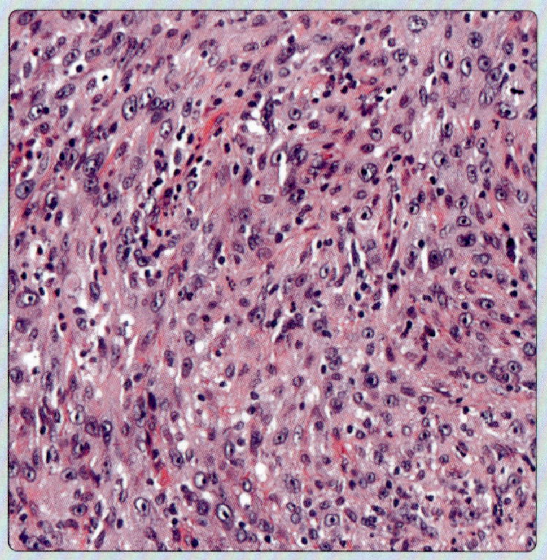

(Left) *Interdigitating dendritic cell sarcoma (IDCS) usually arises in lymph nodes and typically shows a paracortical distribution with sparing of lymphoid follicles ➔.* **(Right)** *Cytologically, the cells of IDCS are spindled to ovoid with eosinophilic cytoplasm and indistinct borders. Nuclei are often vesicular and contain small-to-prominent nucleoli. A chronic inflammatory infiltrate, particularly lymphocytes, is common.*

Cytologic Features

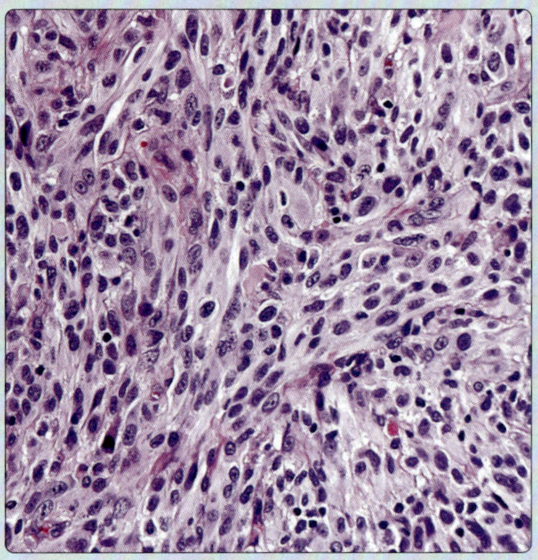

Nuclear Pleomorphism

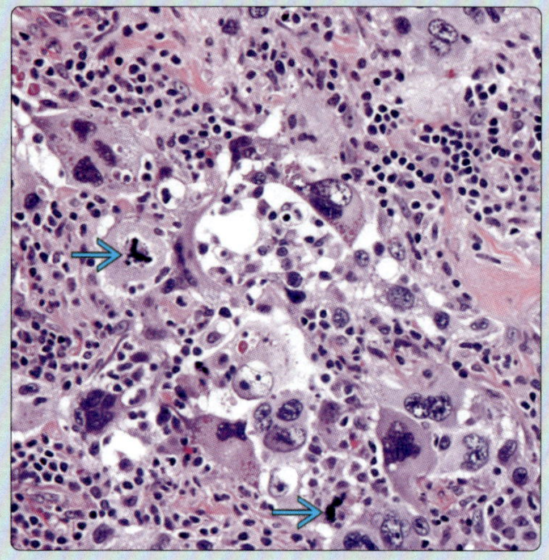

(Left) *This example of IDCS is more cellular but still shows typical cytologic features. Mitoses are usually low. Immunohistochemistry is often very helpful in establishing the diagnosis.* **(Right)** *Some cases of IDCS may show marked nuclear atypia and pleomorphism as well as increased mitoses ➔. These findings have not been confirmed to portend a more adverse prognosis.*

Interdigitating Dendritic Cell Sarcoma

TERMINOLOGY

Abbreviations

- Interdigitating dendritic cell sarcoma (IDCS)

Synonyms

- Interdigitating dendritic cell tumor
- Interdigitating dendritic reticulum cell sarcoma

Definitions

- Neoplastic proliferation of cells with immunophenotype similar to normal interdigitating dendritic cells

CLINICAL ISSUES

Epidemiology

- Incidence
  - Very rare
- Age
  - Most patients are adults; median: 6th-7th decades

Site

- Usually arises in single lymph node
  - Usually cervical, axillary, or inguinal lymph node groups
- Extranodal sites can be involved
  - Skin and soft tissue most common
  - Liver, spleen, other viscera

Presentation

- Slow-growing, asymptomatic mass
- Systemic symptoms (e.g., fever) occur in subset
- Rare hepatosplenomegaly, generalized lymphadenopathy
- May rarely arise in patients with history of low-grade B-cell lymphoma or T-cell lymphoma

Treatment

- Surgical resection ± radiation for localized disease
- No current established chemotherapy regimen due to rarity of disease

Prognosis

- Variable, largely unpredictable clinical course
  - 40-50% of patients develop disseminated disease with poor outcome

MACROSCOPIC

General Features

- Lobulated mass with firm or fleshy cut surface

Size

- Usually < 10 cm

MICROSCOPIC

Histologic Features

- Partial or complete replacement of lymph node architecture
  - Paracortical localization of tumor cells is common
    - Spares lymphoid follicles
  - Sinusoidal pattern of involvement can be prominent
- Spindled-to-ovoid cells forming sheets, fascicles, whorls
  - Vesicular nuclei with small or prominent nucleoli
    - Nuclear membrane indentations may be seen
  - Abundant eosinophilic cytoplasm; indistinct cell borders
  - Occasional epithelioid morphology
- Nuclei may be relatively uniform or occasionally pleomorphic
  - Mitotic rate is variable, but usually < 5 per 10 HPF
  - Occasional multinucleated cells
- Scattered infiltrate of small lymphocytes common
  - Less commonly plasma cells, eosinophils

ANCILLARY TESTS

Immunohistochemistry

- S100(+), SOX10(+), fascin (+)
- Variable CD45(+), CD163(+), and CD68(+)
- CD21(-), CD23(-), CD35(-), CD1a(-), clusterin (-), EMA(-), keratin (-), melanocytic markers (-)

DIFFERENTIAL DIAGNOSIS

Follicular Dendritic Cell Sarcoma

- May be histologically indistinguishable from IDCS
- Whorled or storiform architecture prominent
- Nuclear pseudoinclusions
- Immunohistochemistry helpful
  - CD21(+), CD23(+), CD35(+), clusterin (+), D2-40(+)
  - S100(-), but may be focally (+)

Metastatic Melanoma

- Can closely simulate IDCS both histologically and immunohistochemically
  - Prior history of melanoma may be crucial for diagnosis
- More often cytologically atypical than IDCS
- CD45(-)
- HMB-45, melan-A, and tyrosinase variably positive but may be negative

Histiocytic Sarcoma

- Epithelioid morphology is dominant, often with prominent nucleoli
- Strongly CD163(+), CD68(+)
- S100 (variable)

Langerhans Cell Sarcoma

- Nuclear grooves may be present
- Eosinophilic infiltrate
- S100(+), CD1a(+), langerin (+)

SELECTED REFERENCES

1. Ninkovic S et al: Interdigitating dendritic cell sarcoma: diagnostic pitfalls, treatment challenges and role of transdifferentation in pathogenesis. Pathology. 49(6):643-646, 2017
2. Nguyen CM et al: Primary cutaneous interdigitating dendritic cell sarcoma: a case report and review of the literature. Am J Dermatopathol. 38(8):628-31, 2016
3. Stowman AM et al: Spindle cell melanoma and interdigitating dendritic cell sarcoma: do they represent the same process? Am J Surg Pathol. 40(9):1270-9, 2016
4. Ohtake H et al: Interdigitating dendritic cell sarcoma and follicular dendritic cell sarcoma: histopathological findings for differential diagnosis. J Clin Exp Hematop. 53(3):179-84, 2013
5. Perkins SM et al: Interdigitating and follicular dendritic cell sarcomas: a SEER analysis. Am J Clin Oncol. 36(4):395-8, 2013
6. Orii T et al: Differential immunophenotypic analysis of dendritic cell tumours. J Clin Pathol. 63(6):497-503, 2010
7. Gaertner EM et al: Interdigitating dendritic cell sarcoma. A report of four cases and review of the literature. Am J Clin Pathol. 115(4):589-97, 2001

SECTION 7

Smooth Muscle Tumors

Benign

Smooth Muscle Hamartoma 332
Superficial Leiomyoma 334
Deep Leiomyoma 338

Intermediate

Epstein-Barr Virus-Associated Smooth Muscle Tumor 342

Malignant

Leiomyosarcoma 344

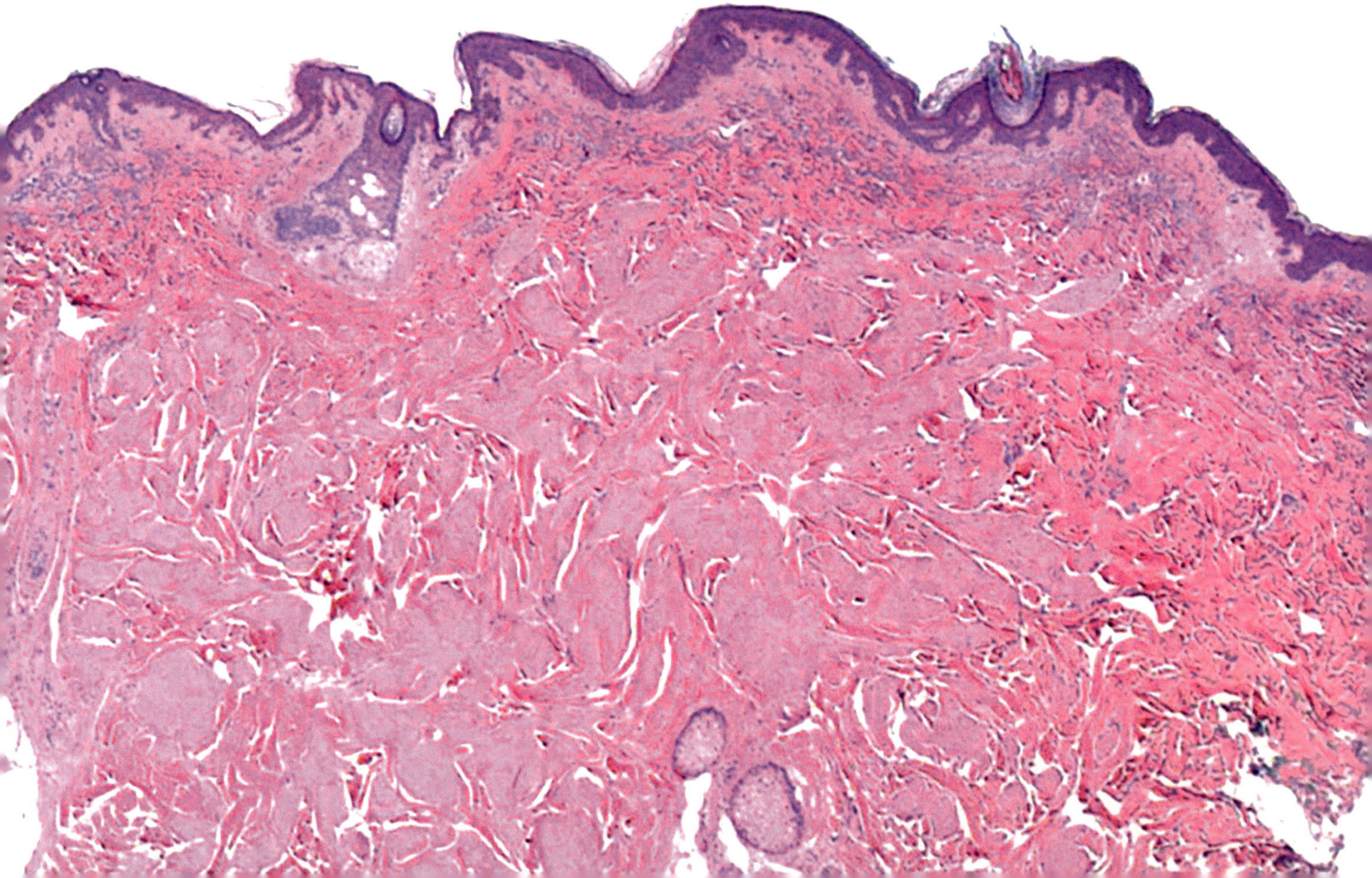

Smooth Muscle Hamartoma

KEY FACTS

TERMINOLOGY

- Synonym: Congenital smooth muscle hamartoma
- Rare, benign smooth muscle proliferation presenting in infants
- Horizontal band-like dermal proliferation of haphazard smooth muscle bundles
- Probably on spectrum with Becker nevus
- Probably unrelated to acquired smooth muscle hamartoma of scrotum (reactive smooth muscle hyperplasia) despite similar histologic features

CLINICAL ISSUES

- Lumbosacral area and proximal extremities
- Macule or slightly indurated plaque
- Often hyperpigmented
- Usually with increased &/or coarse hair (> 80%)
- Pseudo-Darier sign: Rubbing lesion produces temporary induration or piloerection

MICROSCOPIC

- Horizontal band-like proliferation of smooth muscle in dermis
- Haphazardly arranged bundles of benign smooth muscle
- Each bundle has similar appearance to arrector pili
- Lacks pleomorphism, mitoses, necrosis
- Often overlying epidermal hyperplasia with basal hyperpigmentation
- If lentiginous junctional melanocytes also present = Becker nevus

TOP DIFFERENTIAL DIAGNOSES

- Cutaneous leiomyoma (pilar leiomyoma)
- Cutaneous leiomyosarcoma (atypical intradermal smooth muscle neoplasm)
- Acquired smooth muscle "hamartoma" of scrotum
- Combined blue nevus/smooth muscle hamartoma
- Normal skin from special sites (nipple, vulva, or scrotum)

(Left) *Smooth muscle hamartoma is composed of haphazardly arranged smooth muscle bundles that form a horizontal band-like proliferation* ⇒ *in the dermis and superficial subcutis.* **(Right)** *Smooth muscle bundles* ⇒ *are arranged haphazardly in the dermis in smooth muscle hamartoma. This lesion lacks the areas of solid growth more typical of cutaneous (pilar) leiomyoma.*

Horizontal Band-Like Proliferation

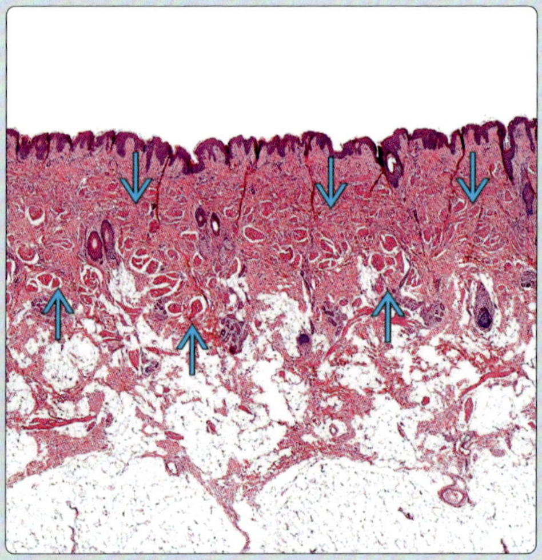

Haphazard Bundles

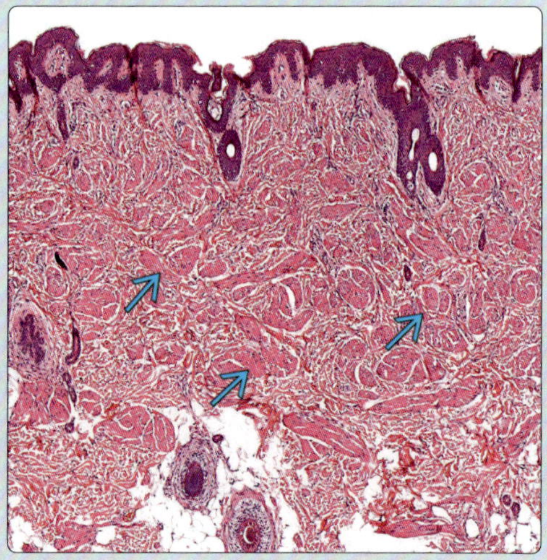

(Left) *The smooth muscle bundles in smooth muscle hamartoma are very similar to normal arrector pili. There may be a thin clefting artifact between the bundles and the surrounding dermal collagen* ⇒. **(Right)** *The spindled nuclei are bland, and mitoses are usually not seen. There is abundant eosinophilic fibrillary cytoplasm typical of normal smooth muscle.*

Resemblance to Arrector Pili Muscles

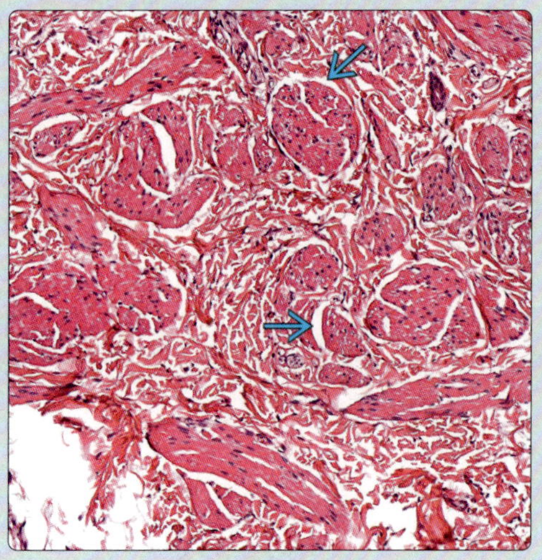

Minimal Atypia and Mitotic Activity

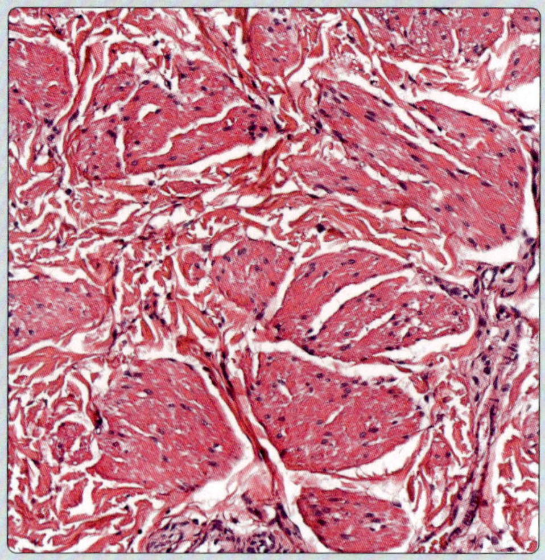

TERMINOLOGY

Synonyms

- Congenital smooth muscle hamartoma

Definitions

- Rare, benign smooth muscle proliferation presenting in infants
- Horizontal band of haphazard smooth muscle bundles in dermis
- Probably at one end of spectrum that includes Becker nevus
- Probably unrelated to acquired smooth muscle hamartoma of scrotum (reactive smooth muscle hyperplasia) despite similar histologic features

CLINICAL ISSUES

Site

- Lumbosacral area and proximal extremities
- Occasionally scrotum (debatable)
  - Some reported scrotal cases are actually reactive smooth muscle hyperplasia rather than true hamartomas

Presentation

- Macule or slightly indurated plaque
  - Present since birth/infancy
  - Often hyperpigmented
  - Usually with increased &/or coarse hair (> 80%)
  - Sometimes with perifollicular papules but lacking prominent hair
  - Rarely linear with perifollicular papules
  - Usually < 10 cm (sometimes much larger)
- Pseudo-Darier sign
  - Rubbing lesion produces temporary induration or piloerection
- Rarely generalized (subset of "Michelin tire baby" cases)
- Rarely multiple
- Rarely familial
- Rarely admixed with port-wine stain (nevus flammeus)

Treatment

- Simple excision

Prognosis

- Excellent (completely benign)

MICROSCOPIC

Histologic Features

- Horizontal band-like proliferation of smooth muscle in dermis and superficial subcutis
- Haphazardly arranged bundles of benign smooth muscle
  - Bundles are similar to arrector pili
  - May be cleft artifact between bundle and surrounding dermis
  - Bland spindled nuclei
  - Abundant stringy eosinophilic cytoplasm
  - Lacks pleomorphism, mitoses, necrosis
- Often overlying epidermal hyperplasia with basal hyperpigmentation
  - If lentiginous junctional melanocytes also present = Becker nevus

ANCILLARY TESTS

Immunohistochemistry

- Desmin, actins, other smooth muscle markers (+)
- Abundant CD34(+) dendritic cells may be seen in dermis

DIFFERENTIAL DIAGNOSIS

Cutaneous Leiomyoma (Pilar Leiomyoma)

- Young adults rather than infants
- Papules/nodules, sometimes multiple, sometimes coalescing into plaques
- More abundant muscle bundles forming solid nodule with irregular borders (not horizontal band)

Cutaneous Leiomyosarcoma (Atypical Intradermal Smooth Muscle Neoplasm)

- Dermal nodule of atypical smooth muscle cells in intersecting fascicles
- Marked nuclear atypia and increased mitoses
- More abundant muscle bundles forming solid nodule with irregular borders (not horizontal band)

Acquired Smooth Muscle "Hamartoma" of Scrotum

- Similar histologic appearance; adults
- Reactive hyperplasia of scrotal smooth muscle (not true hamartoma)
  - Often secondary to chronic lymphedema

Combined Blue Nevus/Smooth Muscle Hamartoma

- Haphazard benign smooth muscle bundles in dermis
- Admixed benign pigmented spindled melanocytes and melanophages (blue nevus)
- Sometimes with nests of benign epithelioid melanocytes (as in common nevi)

Normal Skin From Special Sites

- Abundant smooth muscle bundles normally present in nipple, vulva, and scrotum

SELECTED REFERENCES

1. Jain S et al: Multiple acquired smooth muscle hamartomas with thick-walled blood vessels on scalp. J Cutan Pathol. 45(8):629-32, 2018
2. Fernandez-Flores A et al: Combined cutaneous smooth muscle hamartoma and nevus flammeus. J Cutan Pathol. 41(7):612-6, 2014
3. Tzu J et al: Combined blue nevus-smooth muscle hamartoma: a series of 12 cases. J Cutan Pathol. 40(10):879-83, 2013
4. Holland KE et al: Generalized congenital smooth muscle hamartoma presenting with hypertrichosis, excess skin folds, and follicular dimpling. Pediatr Dermatol. 25(2):236-9, 2008
5. Kharfi M et al: Michelin tire syndrome: a report of two siblings. Pediatr Dermatol. 22(3):245-9, 2005
6. van Kooten EO et al: Acquired smooth-muscle hamartoma of the scrotum: a histological simulator? J Cutan Pathol. 31(5):388-92, 2004
7. Gualandri L et al: Multiple familial smooth muscle hamartomas. Pediatr Dermatol. 18(1):17-20, 2001
8. Jang HS et al: Linear congenital smooth muscle hamartoma with follicular spotted appearance. Br J Dermatol. 142(1):138-42, 2000
9. Koizumi H et al: CD34-positive dendritic cells are an intrinsic part of smooth muscle hamartoma. Br J Dermatol. 140(1):172-4, 1999
10. Gagné EJ et al: Congenital smooth muscle hamartoma of the skin. Pediatr Dermatol. 10(2):142-5, 1993
11. Zvulunov A et al: Congenital smooth muscle hamartoma. Prevalence, clinical findings, and follow-up in 15 patients. Am J Dis Child. 144(7):782-4, 1990
12. Johnson MD et al: Congenital smooth muscle hamartoma. A report of six cases and a review of the literature. Arch Dermatol. 125(6):820-2, 1989

Superficial Leiomyoma

KEY FACTS

TERMINOLOGY

- Benign dermal smooth muscle neoplasm
  - Pilar type (piloleiomyoma) arises from arrector pili
  - Genital type arises from specialized genital smooth muscle

ETIOLOGY/PATHOGENESIS

- Hereditary leiomyomatosis and renal cell cancer syndrome (HLRCC)
  - Multiple leiomyomas of skin and uterus
  - Subsets develop renal cell carcinoma (RCC)
  - Mutations in fumarate hydratase (*FH*) gene (autosomal dominant)

CLINICAL ISSUES

- Pilar leiomyoma: Multiple painful pink/brown papules/nodules, most < 2 cm
- Genital leiomyoma: Solitary painless nodule on scrotum, penis, vulva, or nipple of adults

MICROSCOPIC

- Pilar leiomyoma
  - Ill-defined dermal nodule composed of haphazardly arranged smooth muscle bundles/fascicles
  - Bland, blunt-ended, spindled nuclei
  - Abundant fibrillary eosinophilic cytoplasm
  - Focal atypia and occasional mitoses (up to 1/10 HPF) acceptable
  - Fascicles often dissect between dermal collagen
- Genital leiomyoma
  - Usually more circumscribed, cellular, and histologically heterogeneous (e.g., myxoid change, hyalinization, epithelioid cells) than pilar leiomyoma

TOP DIFFERENTIAL DIAGNOSES

- Superficial leiomyosarcoma
- Congenital smooth muscle hamartoma
- Angioleiomyoma
- Dermatomyofibroma

Cutaneous Leiomyomas and HLRCC

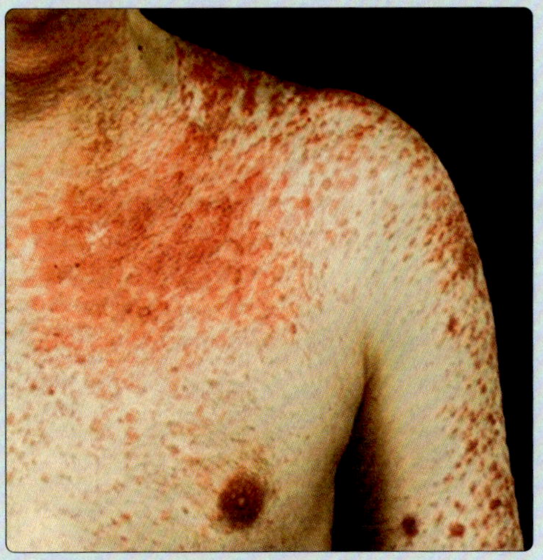

Pilar Leiomyoma

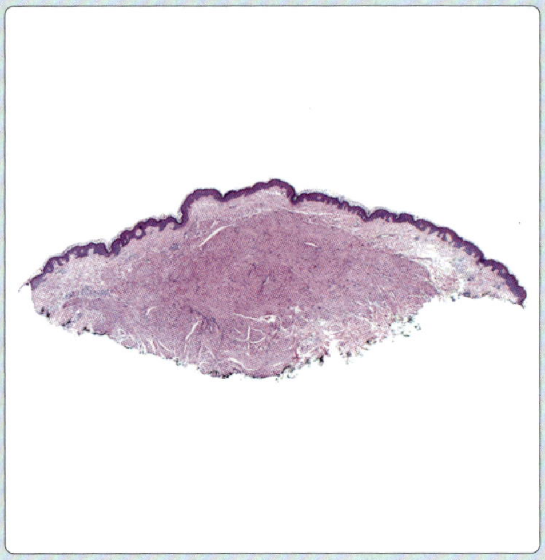

(Left) *Clinical photo shows cutaneous leiomyomas in a patient with hereditary leiomyomatosis and renal cell cancer (HLRCC). Numerous red/brown papules coalescing into plaques are present on the chest, lower neck, shoulder, and upper arm.* ***(Right)*** *The pilar type of superficial leiomyoma is an ill-defined dermal nodule composed of multiple eosinophilic smooth muscle bundles.*

Resemblance to Arrector Pili Muscles

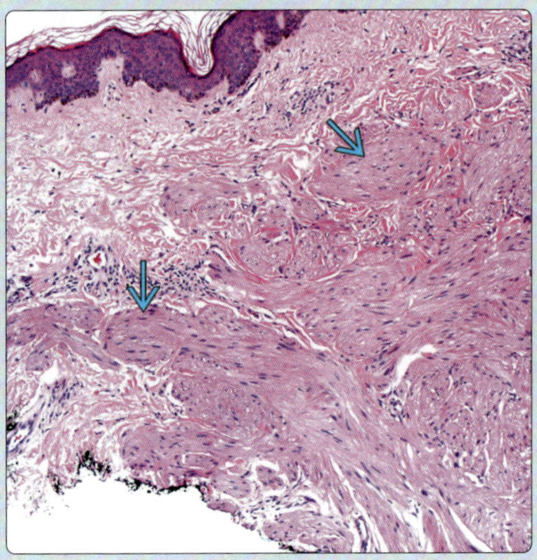

Smooth Muscle Cytology

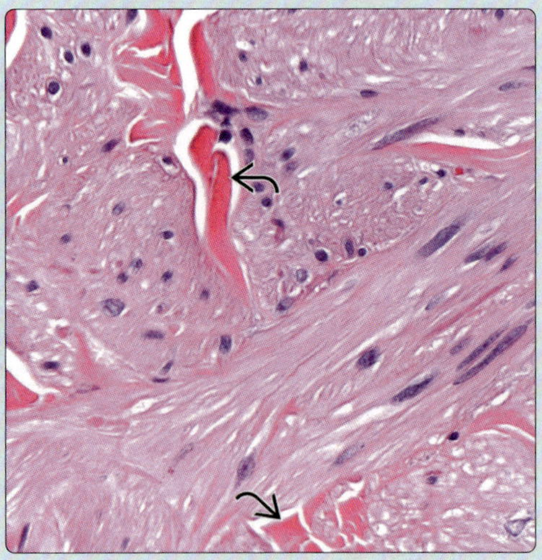

(Left) *The individual eosinophilic smooth muscle bundles* ➡ *of pilar leiomyoma resemble normal arrector pili muscles.* ***(Right)*** *The smooth muscle fascicles/bundles of pilar leiomyoma consist of elongated spindled cells with abundant fibrillary eosinophilic cytoplasm. Nuclei are oval with blunt ends (cigar-shaped) and show little cytologic atypia or mitotic activity. Note the characteristic pattern of fascicles dissecting between dermal collagen bundles* ↷*.*

Superficial Leiomyoma

TERMINOLOGY

Synonyms

- Cutaneous leiomyoma, leiomyoma cutis

Definitions

- Benign dermal smooth muscle neoplasm
  - Pilar type (piloleiomyoma) arises from arrector pili
  - Genital type arises from specialized genital smooth muscle

ETIOLOGY/PATHOGENESIS

Hereditary Leiomyomatosis and Renal Cell Cancer Syndrome (HLRCC)

- Synonyms: Multiple cutaneous and uterine leiomyomatosis syndrome, Reed syndrome
- Multiple leiomyomas of skin and uterus, risk of renal cell carcinoma (RCC)
- Familial autosomal dominant germline loss of function mutations in fumarate hydratase (*FH*) gene
  - Most with multiple cutaneous leiomyomas have *FH* mutation
  - Most women with *FH* mutation have uterine leiomyomas
- Features of uterine leiomyomas in HLRCC
  - Multiple; 1-8 cm; presenting at young age
  - Increased cellularity and nuclear atypia
  - Unique prominent eosinophilic inclusion-like nucleoli surrounded by clear halo
    - Similar distinct nucleoli seen in RCC occurring in HLRCC
    - These nucleoli not present in cutaneous leiomyomas of HLRCC
- Subset of HLRCC patients develop RCC
  - Often more aggressive; usually papillary, tubulopapillary, or collecting duct types
  - Distinct large eosinophilic nucleoli with clear halo

CLINICAL ISSUES

Presentation

- Pilar leiomyoma
  - Most arise in adolescents or young adults
  - Multiple painful pink/brown papules/nodules, most < 2 cm
    - Rare cases are solitary and painless
  - Papules may coalesce into nodules/plaques
  - Extensor surfaces of extremities, trunk, head, and neck
    - Often 2 or more body sites affected
- Genital leiomyoma
  - Solitary painless nodule on scrotum, penis, vulva, or nipple of adults

Treatment

- Depends on number of lesions and symptomatology
- Excision for localized or symptomatic lesions
- Conservative management for extensive lesions
- Imaging of kidneys and uterus if multiple skin lesions
- Cryotherapy and laser ablation: Mixed results

Prognosis

- Benign; does not undergo malignant transformation
- Excised lesions may recur (or new lesions may develop)

MICROSCOPIC

Histologic Features

- Pilar leiomyoma
  - Ill-defined dermal nodule composed of haphazardly arranged smooth muscle bundles/fascicles
  - Bland, blunt-ended, spindled nuclei
  - Abundant fibrillary eosinophilic cytoplasm
  - Focal atypia and occasional mitoses (up to 1 figure per 10 HPF) acceptable
    - Numerous mitoses, diffuse/marked atypia, high cellularity, &/or necrosis: Leiomyosarcoma
  - Fascicles often dissect between dermal collagen
  - Rare cases are circumscribed
- Genital leiomyoma
  - Usually more circumscribed, cellular, and histologically heterogeneous (e.g., myxoid change, hyalinization, epithelioid cells) than pilar leiomyoma
- "Symplastic" pilar and genital leiomyoma (very rare, use caution): Scattered pleomorphism but no mitoses

ANCILLARY TESTS

Immunohistochemistry

- Strong, diffuse desmin (+) (best), SMA(+), MSA(+)
- Leiomyoma in HLRCC often (-) fumarate hydratase by IHC (not 100% sensitive or specific)

DIFFERENTIAL DIAGNOSIS

Superficial Leiomyosarcoma

- Usually solitary; marked atypia, hypercellularity, mitoses

Congenital Smooth Muscle Hamartoma

- Usually solitary lumbosacral plaque in child, often with increased hair and pigmentation
- Horizontal band-like dermal proliferation of haphazard smooth muscle bundles

Angioleiomyoma

- Solitary painful subcutaneous nodule, usually in lower extremity of middle-aged women
- Sharply circumscribed; smooth muscle intimately admixed with thick-walled vessels; usually lacks discrete bundles; dermal involvement rare

Dermatomyofibroma

- Solitary plaque on shoulder/trunk of young adult
- Fascicles of spindled (myo)fibroblasts arranged parallel to epidermis; lacks smooth muscle bundles
- Despite name, often lack desmin and actin staining

SELECTED REFERENCES

1. Jones C et al: Incidence of mature adipocytic component within cutaneous smooth muscle neoplasms. J Cutan Pathol. 43(10):866-71, 2016
2. Llamas-Velasco M et al: Fumarate hydratase immunohistochemical staining may help to identify patients with multiple cutaneous and uterine leiomyomatosis (MCUL) and hereditary leiomyomatosis and renal cell cancer (HLRCC) syndrome. J Cutan Pathol. 41(11):859-65, 2014
3. Matoso A et al: Symplastic leiomyomas of the scrotum: a comparative study to usual leiomyomas and leiomyosarcomas. Am J Surg Pathol. 38(10):1410-7, 2014

(Left) *Superficial leiomyomas (pilar type) are usually under 2 cm and appear as multiple pink or brown papules or nodules. Clinically, they tend to elicit pain and are often distributed in a dermatomal fashion.* (Right) *Low-power H&E shows a superficial (pilar type) leiomyoma involving the majority of the dermis. The lesion is unencapsulated and vaguely circumscribed but does have an irregular border → with displacement of dermal appendages ⇨.*

Multiple Pilar Leiomyomas

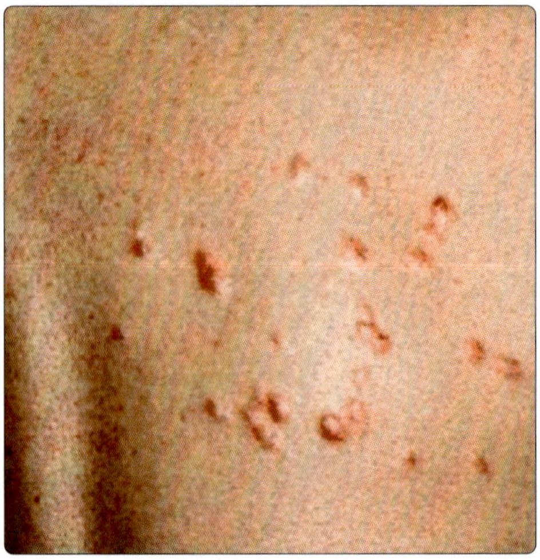

Ill-Defined Dermal Nodule

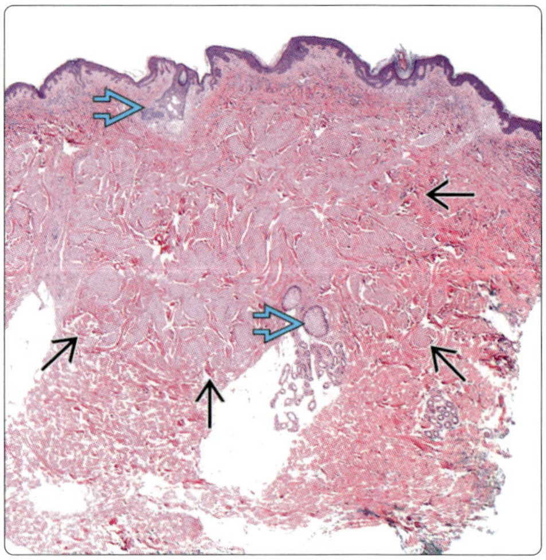

(Left) *At higher power, superficial leiomyomas consist of short fascicles or bundles of smooth muscle → haphazardly arranged within the dermis and tend to dissect between dermal collagen bundles ↷.* (Right) *Many superficial leiomyomas have a grenz zone ⇨ and epidermal hyperplasia with elongated rete pegs adjacent to normal epidermis →.*

Collagen Bundles

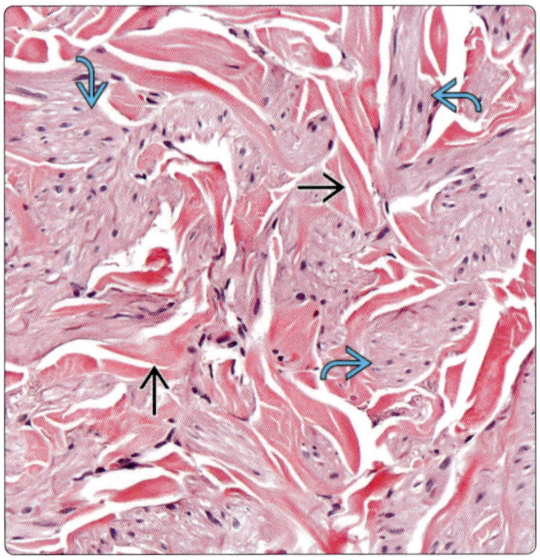

Grenz Zone

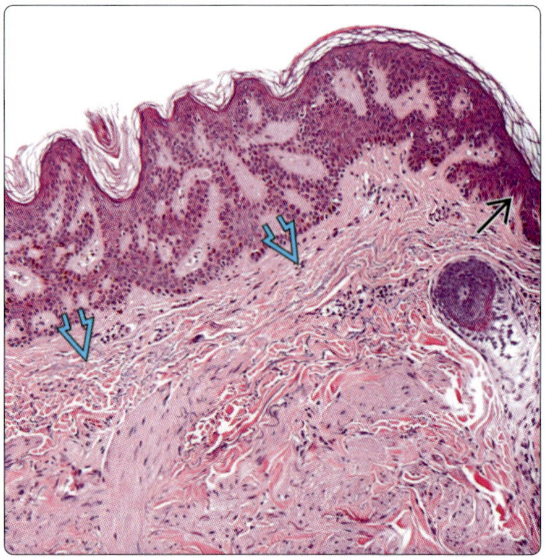

(Left) *Surgical specimens often reveal incipient pilar leiomyomas ↗ adjacent to the primary tumor. The primary tumor in this example does show areas of circumscription ⇨, but other areas have the more typical infiltrative pattern →.* (Right) *Rare examples of superficial leiomyoma are well circumscribed, such as this solitary lesion, which shows only focal areas with an irregular border ↷. Solitary lesions, such as the example shown, often present without pain symptoms.*

Incipient Pilar Leiomyoma

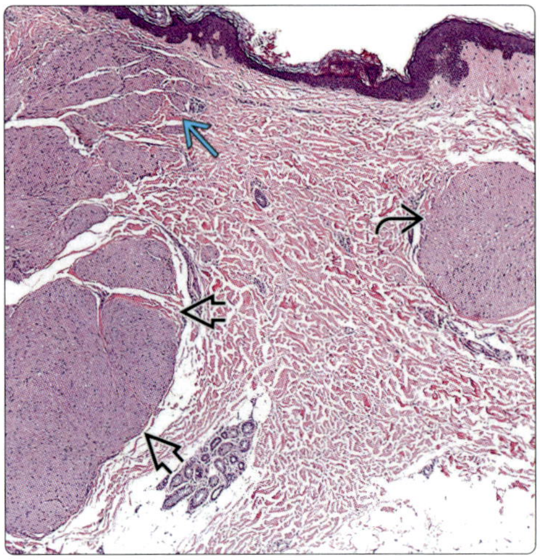

Rare Sharp Circumscription

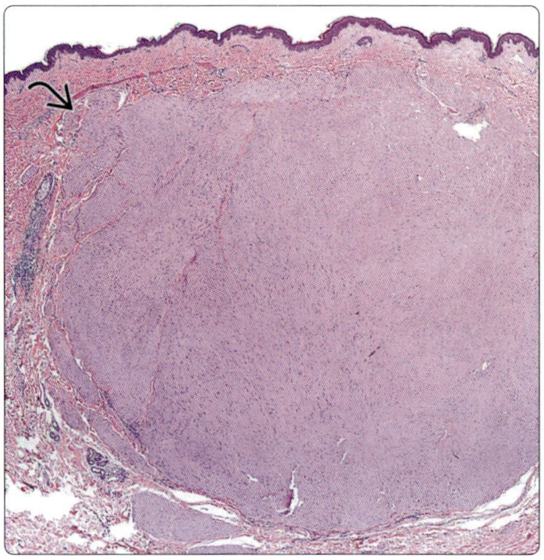

Solitary, Circumscribed Leiomyoma

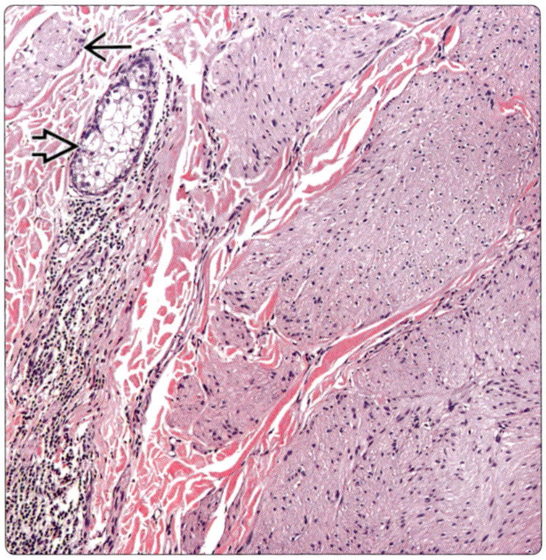

Solitary Leiomyoma

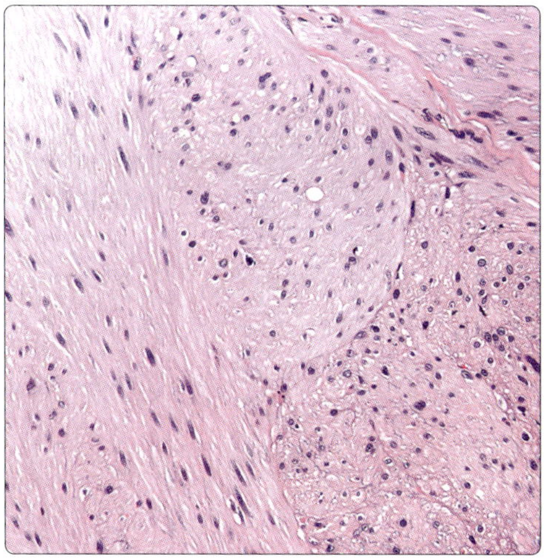

(Left) *Similar to typical superficial leiomyomas, solitary and circumscribed cutaneous leiomyomas can arise from the pilar smooth muscle. This solitary and circumscribed tumor was located adjacent to a sebaceous gland ⇨ and pilar smooth muscle bundle →, indicating likely origin from this pilosebaceous unit.* **(Right)** *Compared to typical pilar leiomyomas, solitary superficial leiomyomas are more often solid and less often characterized by small smooth muscle fascicles intersecting between dermal collagen.*

DDx: Angioleiomyoma

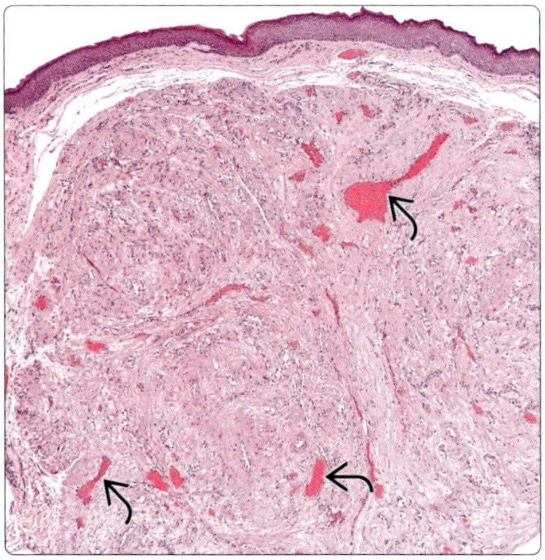

Vessels in Angioleiomyoma

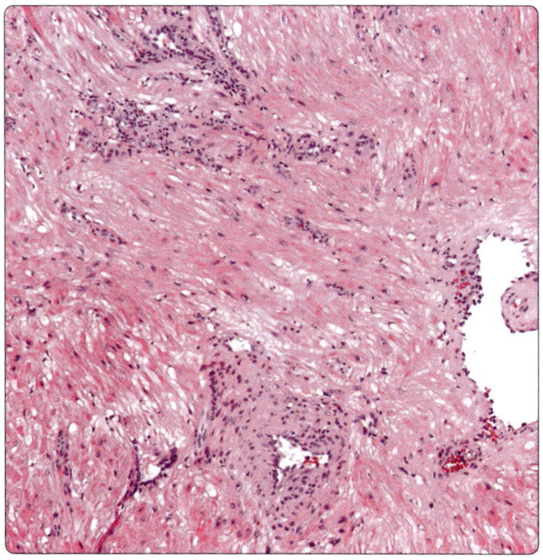

(Left) *In contrast to superficial leiomyoma, angioleiomyoma is usually circumscribed and contains numerous variably sized vascular channels that stand out at low power ↶. In addition, it is usually solitary and located in the lower extremity.* **(Right)** *Sheets of smooth muscle cells with abundant fibrillary eosinophilic cytoplasm intimately associated with thick-walled, often slit-like vascular channels characterize angioleiomyoma at higher power.*

DDx: Superficial Leiomyosarcoma

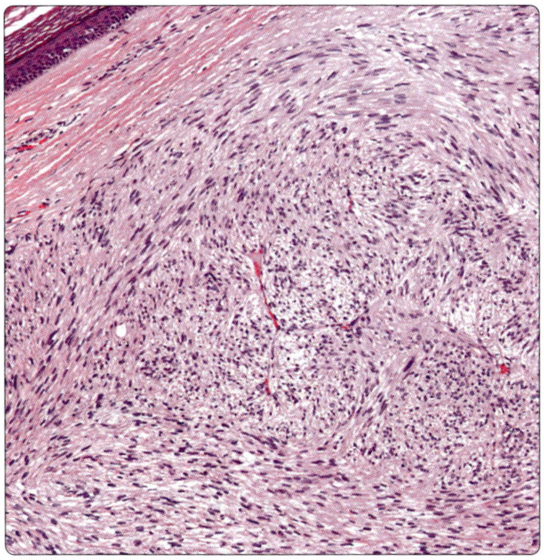

Atypia and Mitoses in Leiomyosarcoma

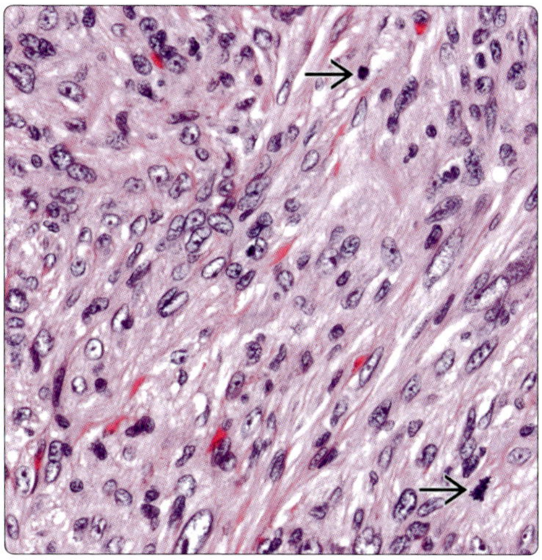

(Left) *Superficial (or cutaneous) leiomyosarcoma also consists of fascicles of cells with abundant fibrillary eosinophilic cytoplasm with blunt-ended, oval nuclei. However, this tumor is more cellular and demonstrates less dissection of dermal collagen. It is also usually larger than superficial leiomyoma.* **(Right)** *At higher power, superficial leiomyosarcoma usually features moderate to marked nuclear atypia with a higher nuclear:cytoplasmic ratio than leiomyoma. Mitotic figures → are also generally more frequent.*

Deep Leiomyoma

KEY FACTS

TERMINOLOGY

- Benign smooth muscle neoplasm arising in deep soft tissue of extremities (somatic), retroperitoneum, or abdominopelvic cavity

CLINICAL ISSUES

- 4th-6th decades of life most common
- Strong female predominance for retroperitoneal/pelvic tumors
- Treatment: Simple surgical excision
- Benign tumor if correctly diagnosed
  - Recurrence rare (more likely in retroperitoneum/pelvis)

MACROSCOPIC

- Well circumscribed with gray/white, firm cut surface
- 3-20 cm (wide size range)

MICROSCOPIC

- Short fascicles or aggregates of uniform spindle cells with abundant eosinophilic cytoplasm and blunt-ended nuclei
- Other findings: Myxoid change, fibrosis, cystic changes, rare epithelioid or clear cell morphology
- No significant nuclear pleomorphism, mitotic activity, or necrosis
  - Low mitotic rates allowed in retroperitoneal/pelvic tumors in women

ANCILLARY TESTS

- Diffuse SMA(+), MSA(+), desmin (+)
- ER, PR, and WT1 often expressed in retroperitoneal and abdominopelvic tumors in women; rare in deep somatic tumors

TOP DIFFERENTIAL DIAGNOSES

- Leiomyosarcoma
- Gastrointestinal stromal tumor
- Cellular schwannoma
- PEComa

(Left) *Deep leiomyoma is a well-circumscribed (but nonencapsulated) benign smooth muscle tumor of deep somatic soft tissue and the retroperitoneum/abdominopelvis. Myxoid stromal changes* ➔ *and fibrosis may be seen in some cases, similar to gynecologic leiomyomas.* **(Right)** *Similar to those that occur in other sites, leiomyoma of deep soft tissue commonly shows variably sized bundles of well-differentiated smooth muscle cells.*

Deep Leiomyoma

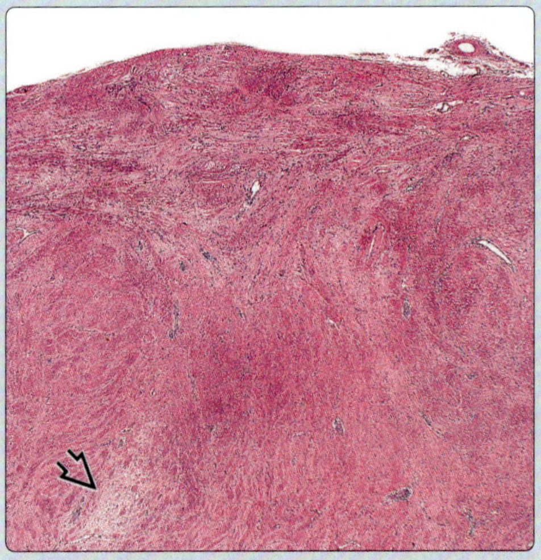

Smooth Muscle Bundles

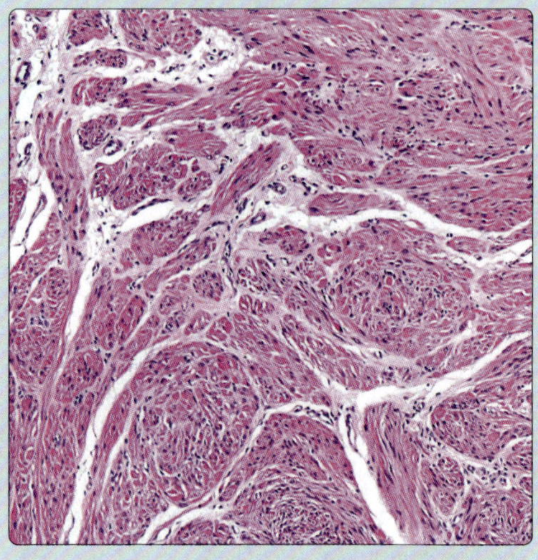

(Left) *Deep leiomyoma shows classic cytologic features of smooth muscle differentiation, including abundant eosinophilic cytoplasm and uniform nuclei with blunt ends (cigar-shaped). Varying degrees of fascicular growth is also typical.* **(Right)** *Most cases of deep leiomyoma show diffuse cytoplasmic immunoreactivity for smooth muscle actin, muscle specific actin, and desmin (shown). A subset of tumors may show focal keratin expression as well.*

Smooth Muscle Cytology

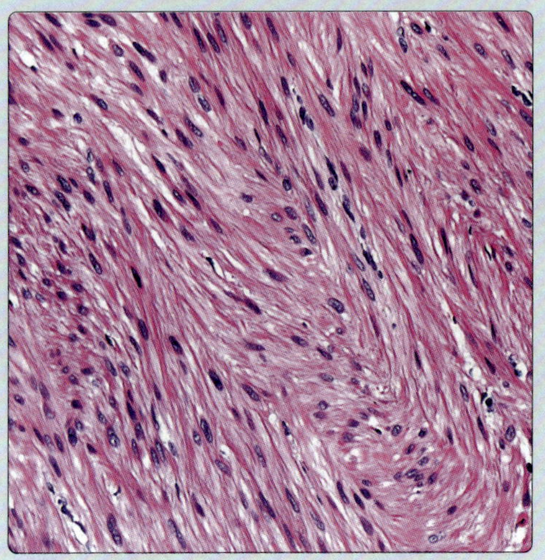

Myogenic Marker Expression

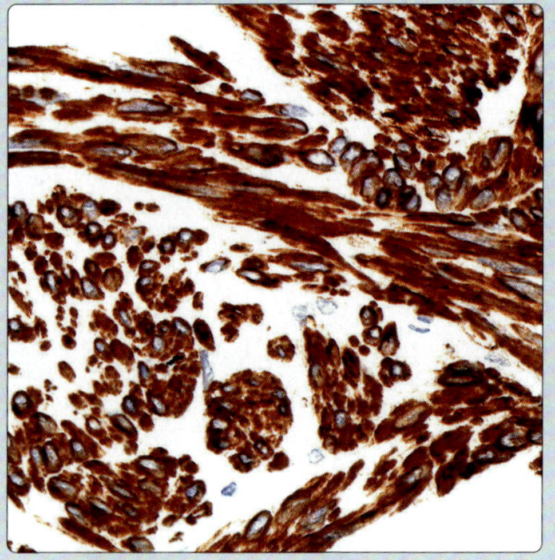

Deep Leiomyoma

TERMINOLOGY

Definitions

- Benign smooth muscle neoplasm arising in deep soft tissue of extremities (somatic), retroperitoneum, or abdominopelvic cavity
  - Gynecologic smooth muscle neoplasms are different and have well-established criteria for predicting behavior

CLINICAL ISSUES

Epidemiology

- Incidence
  - Rare overall
  - More common in retroperitoneum/pelvis than deep soft tissue (somatic)
- Age
  - 4th-6th decades most common
- Sex
  - M = F for deep soft tissue (somatic) tumors
  - Female predominance for retroperitoneal/pelvic tumors

Site

- Most in retroperitoneum or abdominopelvic cavity
- Deep subcutis or intramuscularly in extremities (somatic)

Presentation

- Slow-growing painless mass

Treatment

- Simple surgical excision

Prognosis

- Benign tumor if correctly diagnosed
  - Tumors with certain levels of mitotic activity may recur and are better classified as smooth muscle tumors of uncertain malignant potential (SMTUMP)
- Possibility of metastasis from uterine or abdominopelvic leiomyosarcoma should always be excluded clinically

MACROSCOPIC

General Features

- Well circumscribed with gray/white, firm cut surface
- Calcification not uncommon

Size

- 3-20 cm (wide range)

MICROSCOPIC

Histologic Features

- Short fascicles or aggregates of uniform spindle cells
  - Abundant eosinophilic cytoplasm
  - Blunt-ended nuclei (cigar-shaped)
- No significant nuclear pleomorphism
  - Focal degenerative atypia may be present (symplastic change)
  - More than minimal true nuclear pleomorphism ± mitoses should be classified as leiomyosarcoma
- Mitotic rate should be absent or low, depending on site and sex of patient
  - < 1 per 50 HPF in deep soft tissues of extremities (somatic)
    - Between 1 and 5 per 50 HPF in this location should be classified as SMTUMP
  - < 5 per 50 HPF in retroperitoneum/abdominopelvic cavity in women
    - Between 5 and 10 per 50 HPF in this location should be classified as SMTUMP
  - < 1 per 50 HPF in retroperitoneum/abdominopelvic cavity in men
    - Between 1 and 5 per 50 HPF in this location should be classified as SMTUMP
- Necrosis is absent
- Calcification common in deep somatic tumors
- Other findings: Myxoid change, fibrosis, mature adipose tissue, clear cell change, osteoclast-like giant cells

ANCILLARY TESTS

Immunohistochemistry

- Diffuse SMA(+), MSA(+), desmin (+), h-caldesmon (+)
- Subset express patchy keratin/EMA
- ER, PR, and WT1 often expressed in retroperitoneal/abdominopelvic tumors in women

DIFFERENTIAL DIAGNOSIS

Leiomyosarcoma

- Necrosis &/or nuclear pleomorphism ± mitotic activity
- If no nuclear pleomorphism or necrosis
  - Presence of > 5 mitoses per 50 HPF in deep soft tissue (somatic) tumors
  - > 10 mitoses per 50 HPF in retroperitoneal/abdominopelvic tumors in females
  - > 5 mitoses per 50 HPF in retroperitoneal/abdominopelvic tumors in males

Gastrointestinal Stromal Tumor

- Most cases arise from muscular wall of gastrointestinal tract
- CD117(+), DOG1(+)
- SMA, desmin expression occur but are uncommon

Cellular Schwannoma

- Diffuse S100 protein (+)
- SMA(-) and desmin (-)

PEComa

- Spindled to ovoid and epithelioid cells with clear or finely granular eosinophilic cytoplasm
- SMA(+), HMB-45(+), MART-1(+)
  - May show desmin (+)

SELECTED REFERENCES

1. Panagopoulos I et al: Genetic heterogeneity in leiomyomas of deep soft tissue. Oncotarget. 8(30):48769-48781, 2017
2. Miettinen M: Smooth muscle tumors of soft tissue and non-uterine viscera: biology and prognosis. Mod Pathol. 27 Suppl 1:S17-29, 2014
3. Miettinen M et al: Evaluation of biological potential of smooth muscle tumours. Histopathology. 48(1):97-105, 2006
4. Hornick JL et al: Criteria for malignancy in nonvisceral smooth muscle tumors. Ann Diagn Pathol. 7(1):60-6, 2003
5. Paal E et al: Retroperitoneal leiomyomas: a clinicopathologic and immunohistochemical study of 56 cases with a comparison to retroperitoneal leiomyosarcomas. Am J Surg Pathol. 25(11):1355-63, 2001

(Left) *Calcification ⇨ is generally a common finding in deep leiomyoma and varies from small and psammomatous to large and chunky. Clear cell change may occasionally be associated with the calcification.* **(Right)** *Small concentric or psammomatous calcifications ⇨ may be seen in some cases of deep leiomyoma, particularly in cases with other degenerative features.*

Calcification

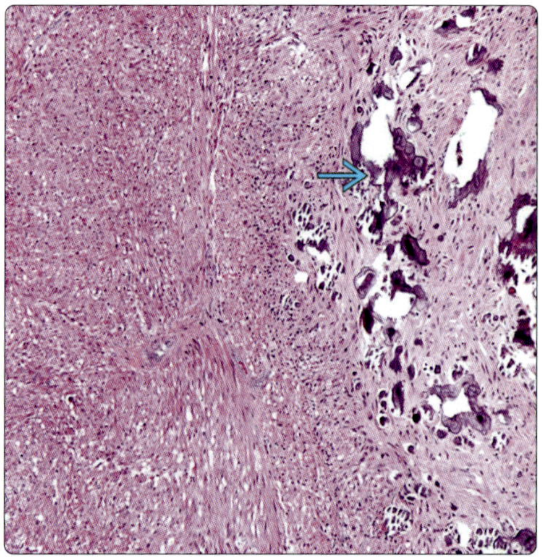

Calcification

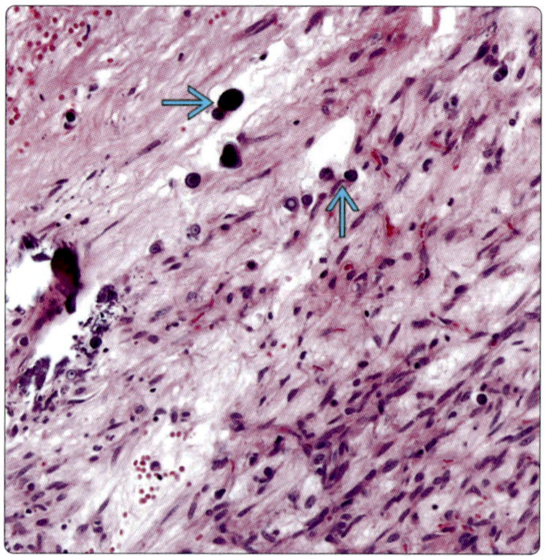

(Left) *Scattered, separated, eosinophilic smooth muscle cells ⇨ are evident at lower magnification in this H&E from a deep leiomyoma with areas of prominent stromal edema.* **(Right)** *Focal myxoid stromal change is common in deep leiomyoma and may occasionally be prominent. Rare cases are entirely myxoid.*

Stromal Edema

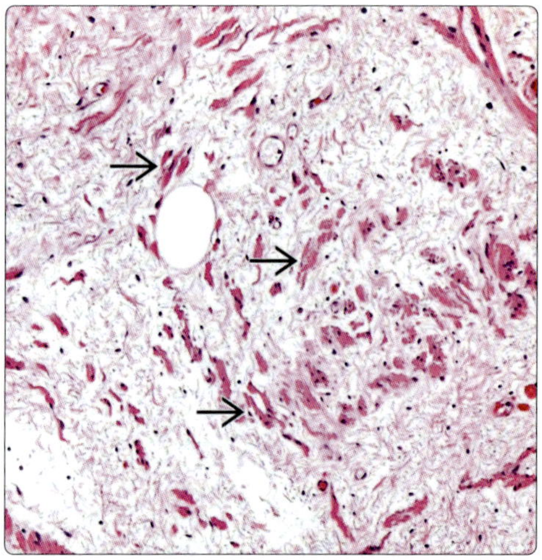

Myxoid Stromal Change

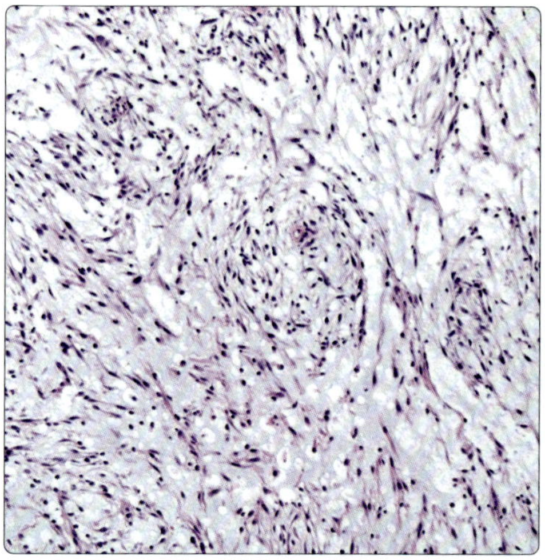

(Left) *Stromal hyalinization and hypocellularity is another common finding in leiomyoma and may be focal or diffuse. This finding is typical of longstanding tumors and may also be associated with stromal calcification.* **(Right)** *Nuclear palisading is an uncommon but well-described finding in deep leiomyoma. It is often a focal finding when present, but rare cases have been described with diffuse palisading.*

Stromal Hyalinization

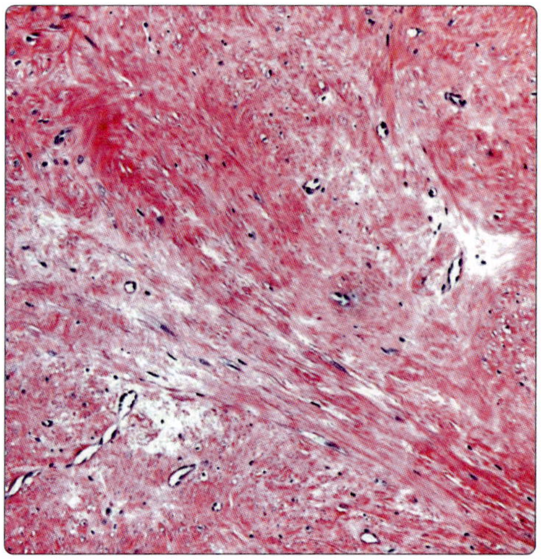

Nuclear Palisading

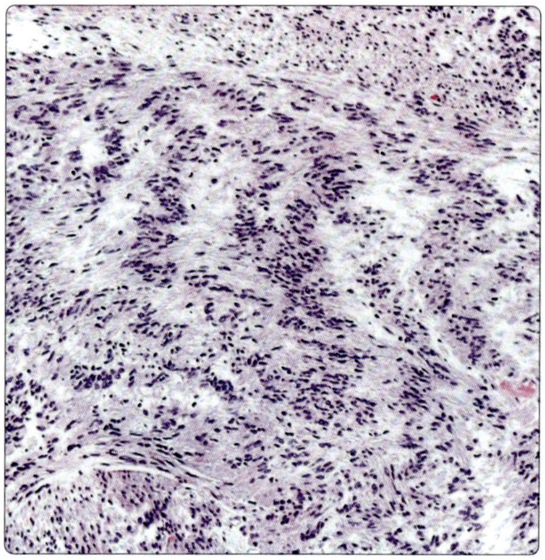

Macrotrabecular Architecture

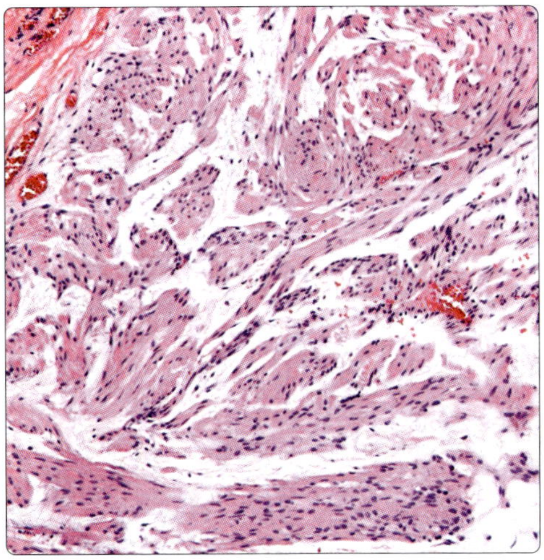

Microtrabecular Architecture

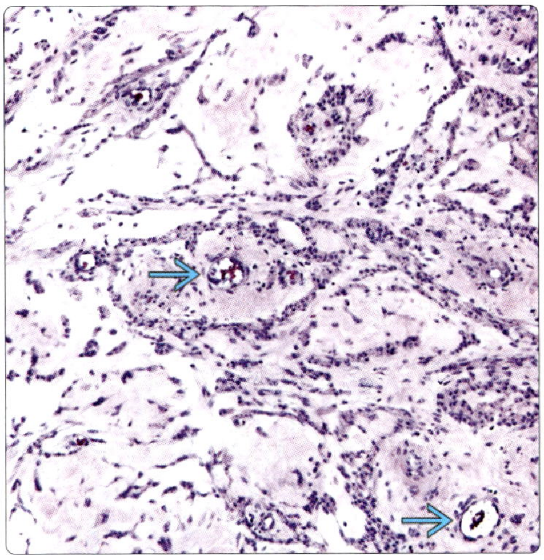

(Left) *Macrotrabecular growth in deep leiomyoma is characterized by thick, elongated bundles of smooth muscle cells within a loose myxoid or edematous stroma.* **(Right)** *Microtrabecular growth in deep leiomyoma is characterized by thin bundles or cords of smooth muscle cells within a loose myxoid or edematous stroma. Organization around blood vessels ➡ is often apparent.*

Microtrabecular Architecture

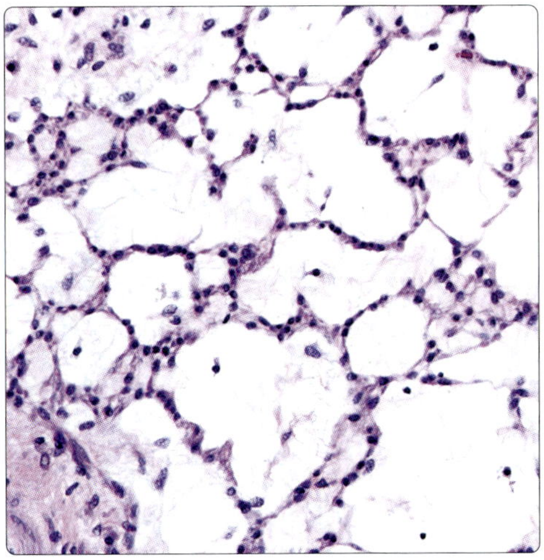

Epithelioid Morphology

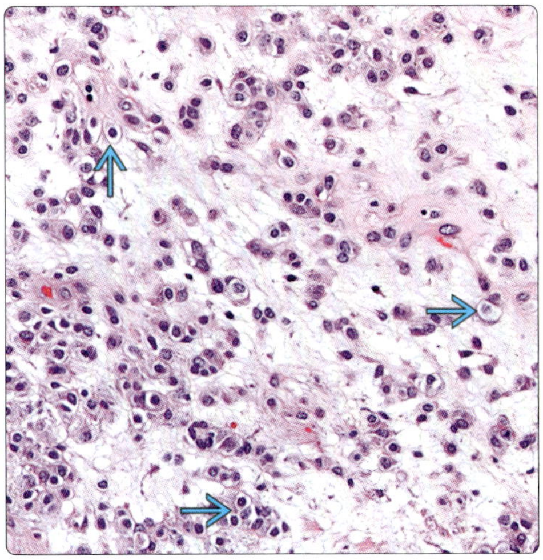

(Left) *Deep leiomyoma with a microtrabecular growth pattern may also show areas with a variably complex reticular appearance.* **(Right)** *Epithelioid cytomorphology is an uncommon finding in deep leiomyoma and is often focal. Clear cell change ➡ may also be seen but is likewise usually focal and, in some cases, associated with calcification.*

Epithelioid Morphology

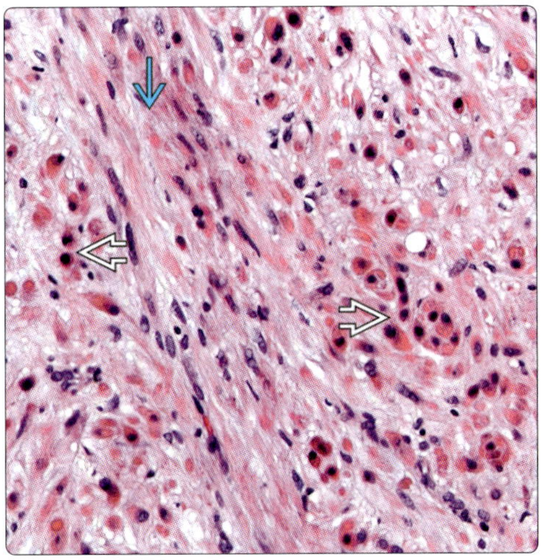

Mature Adipose Tissue

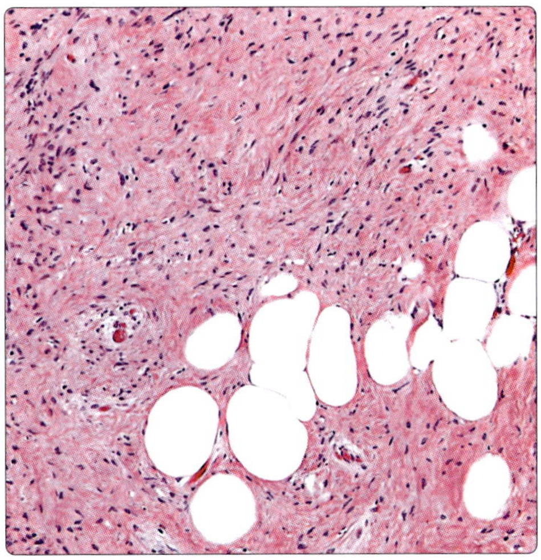

(Left) *H&E of a retroperitoneal deep leiomyoma shows a mixture of conventional spindled smooth muscle cells ➡ and epithelioid smooth muscle cells ➡ with more prominent eosinophilic cytoplasm.* **(Right)** *Mature adipose tissue is occasionally encountered in deep leiomyoma and is often focal. When prominent, classification as an extrauterine lipoleiomyoma or myolipoma may be warranted.*

Epstein-Barr Virus-Associated Smooth Muscle Tumor

KEY FACTS

TERMINOLOGY

- Well-differentiated smooth muscle tumor associated with Epstein-Barr virus, often multifocal, occurring in immunocompromised patients

CLINICAL ISSUES

- Adults and children (median age: 30 years)
- Pain and organ dysfunction
- Late complication of transplantation/immunosuppression
- Arises in visceral organs, skin, and soft tissue
  - HIV related (50%): CNS most common
  - Post transplant (45%): Liver most common
  - Congenital immunodeficiency related (5%): Lung/larynx most common
- Multifocal in > 50% of cases
- Surgical excision is 1st-line therapy
- Reduction of immunosuppressive agents
- Efficacy of chemotherapy, antiviral therapy, radiotherapy unproven
- Most patients survive with persistent disease (80%)
- HIV-related disease and intracranial tumors have worse overall survival
- Prognosis determined by immune condition of patient, not by histology

MACROSCOPIC

- Median: 3-4 cm (range: 0.7-21.0 cm)

MICROSCOPIC

- Well circumscribed
- Fascicles of well-differentiated smooth muscle cells
- Primitive rounded cells in 50%
- Tumor infiltrating T cells
- Mitotic rate = 1-3 mitotic figures per 10 HPF
- Only rare tumors with malignant (sarcoma-like) features

TOP DIFFERENTIAL DIAGNOSES

- Leiomyoma
- Leiomyosarcoma

EBV-Associated Smooth Muscle Tumor

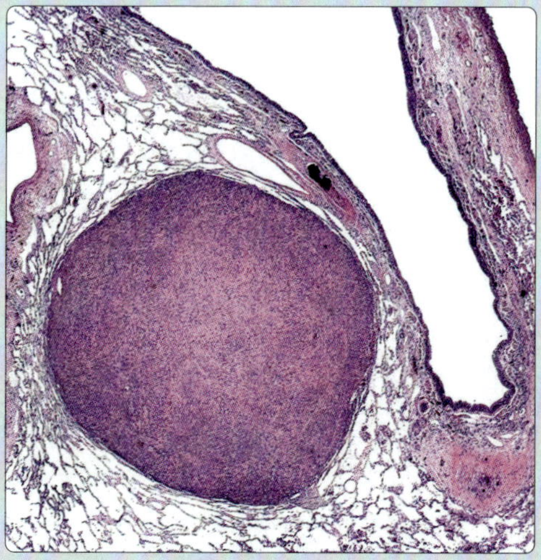

Low-Power Appearance

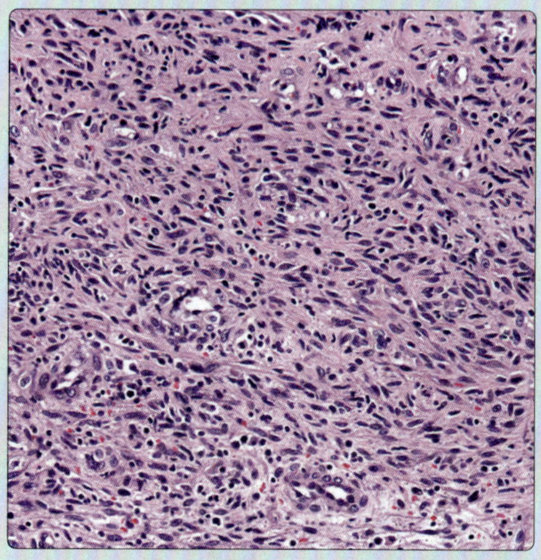

***(Left)** Epstein-Barr virus-associated smooth muscle tumor (EBV-SMT) typically presents as a visceral tumor in an immunocompromised host as exemplified by this lung tumor in a postrenal transplant patient. The tumors are well circumscribed and often multifocal. **(Right)** Most EBV-SMTs are comprised by sheets or fascicles of well-differentiated smooth muscle cells with uniform nuclei, low mitotic activity, and no necrosis. Only rare sarcoma-like tumors occur, which have not been found to have prognostic significance.*

Fascicles of Smooth Muscle Cells

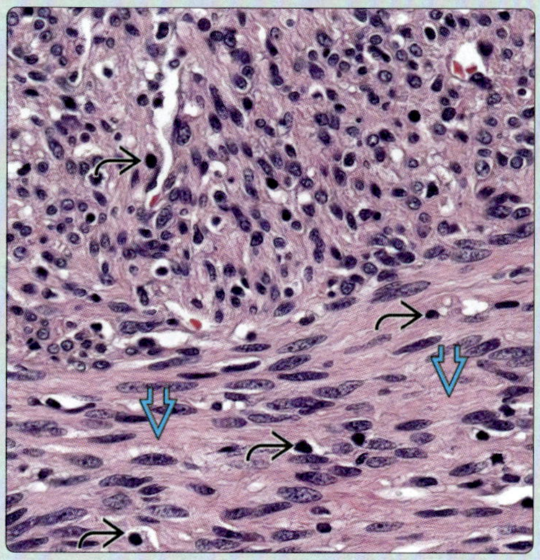

EBER In Situ Hybridization

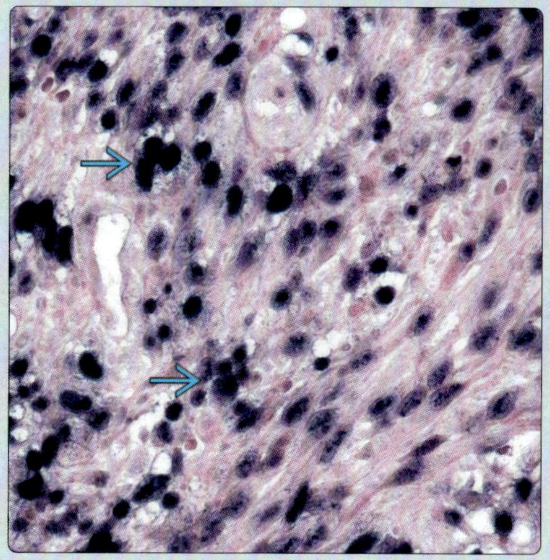

***(Left)** The cells of EBV-SMT are usually arranged in fascicles ⇩ and have low-grade cytologic atypia as illustrated. Tumor-infiltrating T cells ↗ are common. Primitive round cells (not shown) are present in 50% of cases. **(Right)** The diagnosis of EBV-SMT is confirmed by detection of Epstein-Barr-encoded RNA (EBER) by in situ hybridization, as depicted by diffuse, dark blue nuclear stippling ⇨.*

Epstein-Barr Virus-Associated Smooth Muscle Tumor

TERMINOLOGY

Abbreviations

- Epstein-Barr virus-associated smooth muscle tumor (EBV-SMT)

Definitions

- Well-differentiated SMT associated with EBV, often multifocal, occurring in immunocompromised patients

ETIOLOGY/PATHOGENESIS

Infectious Agents

- EBV (EBV-1 and EBV-2)

CLINICAL ISSUES

Epidemiology

- Age
  - Adults and children (median: 30 years; range: 1-66 years)
- Sex
  - F > M (55-67%)

Site

- Visceral organs, skin, soft tissue
- Varies by clinical subtype
  - HIV related (50%)
    - CNS most common, followed by GI, liver, skin, lungs
  - Post transplant (45%)
    - Liver most common, followed by lungs/larynx, GI/spleen, CNS
  - Congenital immunodeficiency related (5%)
    - Lungs/larynx most common, followed by CNS, liver, adrenal, spleen

Presentation

- Pain and organ dysfunction
- Late complication of transplantation/immunosuppression (median: 48 months)
- Multifocal in > 50% of cases
  - Distinct clones
    - Indicates multiple infections, not metastases

Treatment

- Surgical excision is 1st-line therapy
  - Most effective in unifocal disease
- Reduction of immunosuppressive agents
  - Risk of transplant organ rejection
- Antiviral agents recommended for HIV patients
- Efficacy of chemotherapy, antiviral therapy, radiotherapy unproven

Prognosis

- Most patients survive with persistent disease (80%)
  - Most patients who die succumb to infections
  - Only rare patients die of disease
- HIV-related disease and intracranial tumors have worse overall survival
- Prognosis determined by immune condition of patient, not by histology

MACROSCOPIC

General Features

- Circumscribed, solid or cystic

Size

- Median: 3-4 cm (range: 0.7-21.0 cm)

MICROSCOPIC

Histologic Features

- Well circumscribed
- Fascicles of well-differentiated smooth muscle cells
- Primitive rounded cells in 50%
- Small tumor seedlings often found next to main tumor
- Tumor infiltrating T cells
- Mitotic rate = 1-3 mitotic figures per 10 HPF
  - Higher in HIV-related disease
- Only rare tumors with malignant (sarcoma-like) features
  - More common in HIV-related disease

ANCILLARY TESTS

Immunohistochemistry

- Smooth muscle actin (+) in all cases
- Desmin (+) in 50%
- CD21(+) also common

In Situ Hybridization

- EBV-encoded RNA (EBER)

DIFFERENTIAL DIAGNOSIS

Leiomyoma

- Histologically indistinguishable from EBV-SMT in most cases
  - Lacks primitive round cells
- Rare in visceral organs outside uterus
- EBER(-)

Leiomyosarcoma

- Most EBV-SMT are histologically bland
- Rare sarcoma-like tumors, usually in HIV-related disease
- EBER(-)

Angioleiomyoma

- Prominent muscular vascular stroma
- Soft tissues in extremities
- Rare in visceral organs

Myopericytoma

- Smaller cells, prominent pericytomatous vascular stroma
- Soft tissues in extremities
- Rare in visceral organs

SELECTED REFERENCES

1. Hussein K et al: Clinico-pathological characteristics of different types of immunodeficiency-associated smooth muscle tumours. Eur J Cancer. 50(14):2417-24, 2014
2. Issarachaikul R et al: Epstein-Barr virus-associated smooth muscle tumors in AIDS patients: a largest case (series). Intern Med. 53(20):2391-6, 2014
3. Deyrup AT et al: Epstein-Barr virus-associated smooth muscle tumors are distinctive mesenchymal tumors reflecting multiple infection events: a clinicopathologic and molecular analysis of 29 tumors from 19 patients. Am J Surg Pathol. 30(1):75-82, 2006

Leiomyosarcoma

KEY FACTS

TERMINOLOGY

- Malignant neoplasm composed of cells exhibiting true smooth muscle differentiation

CLINICAL ISSUES

- Most common in middle-aged to older adults
- Female predilection in retroperitoneum/pelvis
- Retroperitoneum most common site
  - Also inferior vena cava, extremities, head/neck
- Vena caval tumors may cause Budd-Chiari syndrome
- Treatment: Complete surgical resection
- Overall poor prognosis
  - Local recurrence and metastasis common
  - Retroperitoneal tumors have worst prognosis
- Lung is most common site of metastasis
  - Can also metastasize to skin, lymph nodes, bone, and other soft tissue sites

MICROSCOPIC

- Well-defined, cellular, intersecting fascicles or bundles of spindle cells
- Eosinophilic cytoplasm with elongated, blunt-ended nuclei
  - Nuclear pleomorphism and hyperchromasia common
  - Mitotic rate varies but is often high
- Variants: Myxoid, pleomorphic

ANCILLARY TESTS

- SMA(+), usually diffuse and cytoplasmic
- Variable desmin and caldesmon expression

TOP DIFFERENTIAL DIAGNOSES

- Leiomyoma
- PEComa
- Desmoid fibromatosis
- Malignant peripheral nerve sheath tumor
- Undifferentiated pleomorphic sarcoma

(Left) *Leiomyosarcoma (LMS) of soft tissue is a malignant smooth muscle neoplasm that most commonly arises in the retroperitoneum or is associated with a large vessel (shown), particularly the inferior vena cava. It arises less frequently in the extremities and head/neck region. Uterine LMS has separate defined diagnostic criteria and is not addressed in this text.* **(Right)** *LMS ⇒ is often associated with (and arises from) the muscular wall of larger blood vessels (note the vein → in this image).*

Leiomyosarcoma

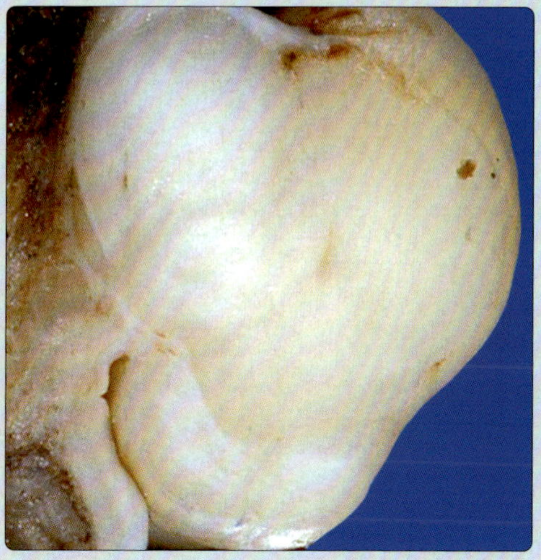

Large Vessel Association

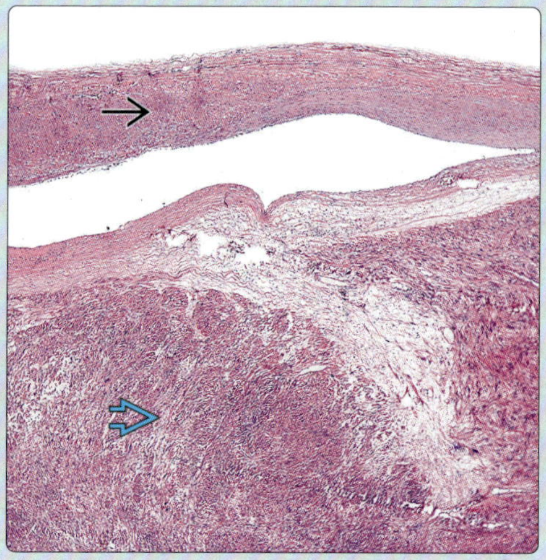

(Left) *The classic morphology of LMS is that of cellular fascicles and bundles of prominently eosinophilic spindle cells. Not infrequently, fascicles appear to be arranged perpendicularly to each other, both longways → and en face ⇒, as depicted.* **(Right)** *As is the case with benign true smooth muscle tumors, tumor cell nuclei in LMS are generally elongated with blunted ends (cigar shaped). Note the characteristic eosinophilic fibrillary cytoplasm.*

Fascicles and Bundles

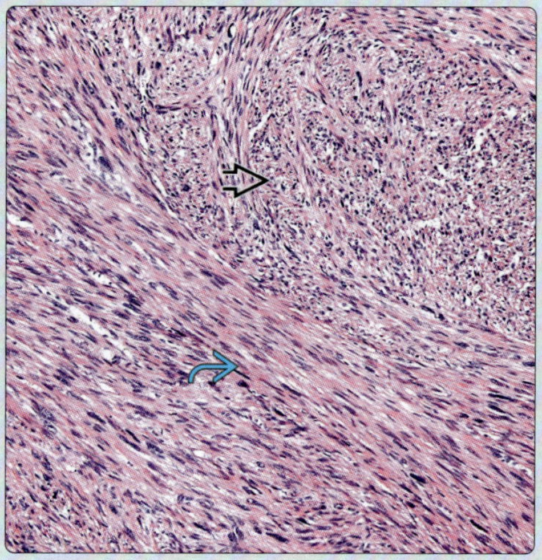

Cytologic Features

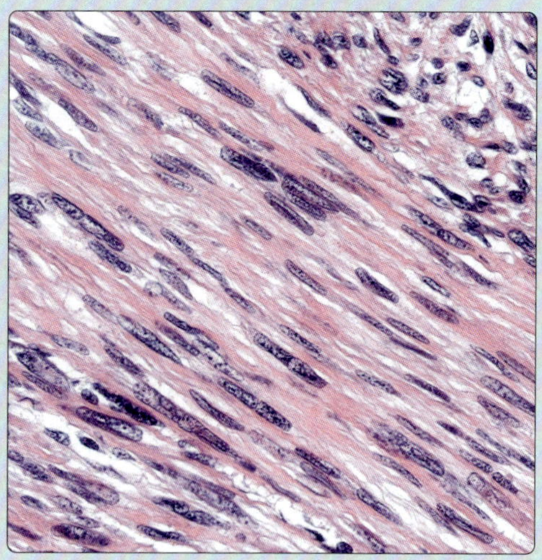

TERMINOLOGY

Abbreviations

- Leiomyosarcoma (LMS)

Definitions

- Malignant neoplasm composed of cells exhibiting true smooth muscle differentiation
- Primary uterine/gynecologic and gastrointestinal LMS not considered in this chapter

CLINICAL ISSUES

Epidemiology

- Age
  - Most common in middle-aged to older adults
    - Rarely arise in children
- Sex
  - No gender preference overall
    - Retroperitoneal and pelvic tumors show clear female predilection

Site

- Retroperitoneum (including pelvis) most common
- Large blood vessels (particularly inferior vena cava)
- Extremities (particularly lower limb) and head/neck region
- Visceral organs

Presentation

- Solitary, often large mass
  - Extremity lesions often smaller compared to other sites
- Retroperitoneal lesions can be associated with abdominal pain
  - Vena cava examples often symptomatic
    - Upper portion: Budd-Chiari syndrome (hepatomegaly, jaundice, ascites)
    - Mid portion: Renal obstruction and dysfunction
    - Lower portion: Lower extremity edema
- In extremities, may arise in subcutaneous fat or muscle
  - Often relatively asymptomatic

Treatment

- Complete surgical resection
- Radiation &/or chemotherapy

Prognosis

- Overall poor prognosis
  - Outcome depends on site and stage
    - Retroperitoneum
      - Very poor prognosis
      - Difficult to resect completely
      - ~ 80% of patients die of disease, typically with metastases
    - Inferior vena cava
      - 5- and 10-year survival: 50% and 30%, respectively
    - Extremities and head/neck
      - Somewhat better prognosis, likely due to increased chance of complete resection
      - Up to 30-50% of tumors metastasize
      - Subcutaneous tumors have been associated with improved survival over deep (subfascial) tumors in some studies
    - Lesions restricted to dermis/cutis can recur but almost never metastasize
      - Some observers have advocated classification as atypical intradermal smooth muscle neoplasm
- Lung is most common site of metastasis
  - Can also spread to skin, bone, lymph nodes, and other soft tissue sites
- Adverse prognostic factors: Larger size, high histologic grade, bone/vascular involvement

MACROSCOPIC

General Features

- Firm to fleshy, tan-gray cut surface
- Hemorrhage &/or necrosis common

Size

- Wide range (often large)
  - Retroperitoneal tumors are frequently > 10 cm
  - Superficial tumors of somatic soft tissue often < 5 cm

MICROSCOPIC

Histologic Features

- Peripheral border may be sharply circumscribed and "pushing" or irregular and infiltrative
- Well-defined, cellular, intersecting fascicles or bundles of spindle cells
  - Usually prominent, brightly eosinophilic cytoplasm
  - Elongated blunt-ended (cigar-shaped) nuclei
    - Nuclear pleomorphism and hyperchromasia common but variable in extent
    - Mitotic rate variable, but often high
      - Atypical forms frequently seen
- Coagulative necrosis common but variable in extent
- Stromal myxoid change or fibrosis/hyalinization
- Many cases are histologically high grade with prominent atypia, mitoses, and necrosis
  - Low-grade tumors have minimal to no atypia, low mitotic indices, and no necrosis
- Large, ectatic staghorn vasculature occasionally present
- Some cases feature prominent inflammatory cell infiltrate
  - May be extensive and obscuring
- Osteoclast-like multinucleated giant cells in some cases
- Focal palisaded architecture rare

Morphologic Variants

- Epithelioid LMS
  - Sheets and nests of small cells with minimal cytoplasm or large eosinophilic cells with macronucleoli
  - Myxoid &/or hyalinized stroma can be seen
- Myxoid LMS
  - Extensively myxoid stroma
  - Tends to be of low histologic grade
  - Areas of conventional LMS usually present at least focally
- Pleomorphic LMS
  - Contains large, sheet-like areas of markedly pleomorphic tumor cells, similar to undifferentiated pleomorphic sarcoma
  - Prominent cytoplasmic eosinophilia
  - Identification of more conventional areas of LMS often necessary for diagnosis

ANCILLARY TESTS

Immunohistochemistry

- SMA(+), usually diffuse and cytoplasmic
- Variable desmin and caldesmon expression
  - Higher grade tumors more likely to be negative for these markers
- Focal keratin (+) or EMA(+) in some tumors
- Generally CD117, ALK1, S100 protein, CD34, HMB-45, MART-1, p63 (-)

DIFFERENTIAL DIAGNOSIS

Leiomyoma

- Well circumscribed
  - Superficial (pilar) leiomyoma is not well circumscribed but is small and superficial
- Variable cellularity, often low
- Generally lack significant nuclear atypia
  - However, rare cases with symplastic (degenerative) atypia
- Degenerative changes (e.g., calcification, fibrosis) common
- Mitoses rare to absent
  - Deep leiomyomas of retroperitoneum/abdominopelvic cavity in females may show up to 5 mitoses per 50 HFP
- Strong diffuse SMA(+), desmin (+), and caldesmon (+)

Malignant Peripheral Nerve Sheath Tumor

- May demonstrate clinical or histologic origin from nerve
- Can arise in association with benign nerve sheath tumor (usually neurofibroma) or within context of NF1
- Alternating regions of varying cellularity
- Increased perivascular tumor cell density
- S100(+) &/or SOX10(+) in 50% of cases (often focal)
- Loss of nuclear H3K27me3
- SMA and desmin (-)
  - Desmin and myogenin expression seen in rhabdomyoblastic elements, if present (malignant Triton tumor)

PEComa

- May show morphologic overlap with LMS
  - Can arise in similar locations (including uterus and bladder)
- Sheets and fascicles of spindled to epithelioid cells with clear to eosinophilic "stringy" cytoplasm
- May show focal association with walls of larger blood vessels
- Characteristic myomelanocytic immunophenotype
  - Variable expression of SMA, desmin, HMB-45, MART-1/Melan-A, MITF
    - Exact expression pattern varies case by case
- Minor subset shows nuclear TFE3(+)

Desmoid Fibromatosis

- Long fascicles of slender spindle cells without atypia
- Prominent collagenous stroma
- Nuclear β-catenin (+) in majority

Gastrointestinal Stromal Tumor

- Significant nuclear pleomorphism uncommon in spindled tumors
- CD117(+), CD34(+), DOG1(+)
- Minor subset expresses SMA
- Desmin (-)
- *KIT* or *PDGFRA* mutations

Inflammatory Myofibroblastic Tumor

- Most common in children and young adults
- Some tumors show prominent fascicular growth
- Admixed chronic inflammatory component common (particularly plasma cells)
- Variable SMA(+) and desmin (+)
- ALK1(+) by IHC
- 2p23 rearrangements involving *ALK* gene

Synovial Sarcoma (Monophasic)

- Cytologically monomorphic (lacks significant nuclear pleomorphism)
- Strong, diffuse nuclear TLE1(+)
- Negative for SMA, desmin, and caldesmon
- t(X;18) with *SS18 (SYT)* gene fusions

Sarcomatoid Squamous Cell Carcinoma

- May be associated with in situ dysplastic component
- May contain foci showing more conventional epithelial architectures (e.g., nests)
- p63(+), p40(+)

Cellular Fibrous Histiocytoma (Dermatofibroma)

- Can show morphologic overlap with superficial LMS
- Primarily dermal based but often shows extension into subcutaneous fat
- May feature overlying epidermal alterations, such as basal cell hyperplasia
- Focal SMA(+), if any; no diffuse expression
- Negative for both desmin and caldesmon

Undifferentiated Pleomorphic Sarcoma

- Can be indistinguishable from pleomorphic LMS
- Lacks areas of conventional LMS
- SMA expression usually limited to focal positivity, at most
- Negative for both desmin and caldesmon

SELECTED REFERENCES

1. Arbajian E et al: Inflammatory leiomyosarcoma is a distinct tumor characterized by near-haploidization, few somatic mutations, and a primitive myogenic gene expression signature. Mod Pathol. 31(1):93-100, 2018
2. Schneider N et al: The adequacy of core biopsy in the assessment of smooth muscle neoplasms of soft tissues: implications for treatment and prognosis. Am J Surg Pathol. 41(7):923-31, 2017
3. Gupta S et al: Renal leiomyoma and leiomyosarcoma: a study of 57 cases. Am J Surg Pathol. 40(11):1557-63, 2016
4. Liau JY et al: Leiomyosarcoma with alternative lengthening of telomeres is associated with aggressive histologic features, loss of ATRX expression, and poor clinical outcome. Am J Surg Pathol. 39(2):236-44, 2015
5. Baltz RG et al: Cutaneous scalp metastases from retroperitoneal leiomyosarcoma: a case report. J Cutan Pathol. 41(8):680-5, 2014
6. Miettinen M: Smooth muscle tumors of soft tissue and non-uterine viscera: biology and prognosis. Mod Pathol. 27 Suppl 1:S17-29, 2014
7. Bathan AJ et al: Diagnosis, prognosis, and management of leiomyosarcoma: recognition of anatomic variants. Curr Opin Oncol. 25(4):384-9, 2013
8. Oda Y et al: Pleomorphic leiomyosarcoma: clinicopathologic and immunohistochemical study with special emphasis on its distinction from ordinary leiomyosarcoma and malignant fibrous histiocytoma. Am J Surg Pathol. 25(8):1030-8, 2001
9. Rubin BP et al: Myxoid leiomyosarcoma of soft tissue, an underrecognized variant. Am J Surg Pathol. 24(7):927-36, 2000

Intersecting Fascicles

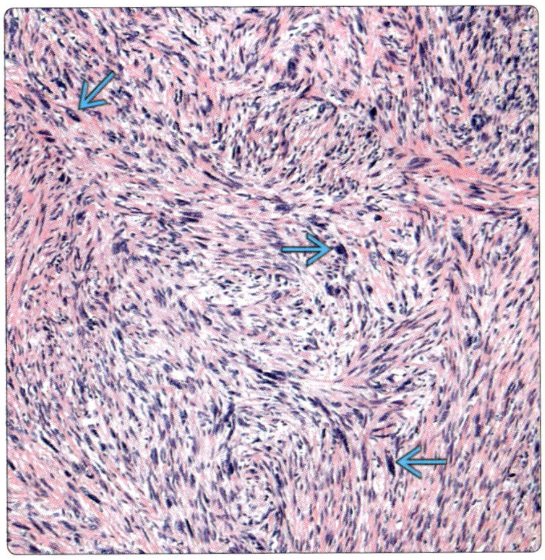

Mitotic Activity

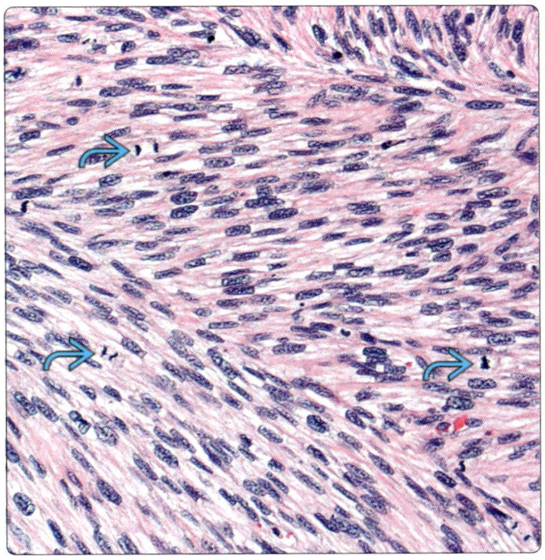

(Left) *Intersecting fascicles and bundles are a common architectural arrangement in LMS, as shown in this image. This morphology is not well developed in all tumors, however. Note the presence of scattered pleomorphic and hyperchromatic nuclei, a frequent, but not invariable, finding in LMS.* **(Right)** *The mitotic rate in LMS varies from tumor to tumor, but figures are generally easy to find in most cases and include both normal and abnormal forms.*

Paranuclear Vacuoles

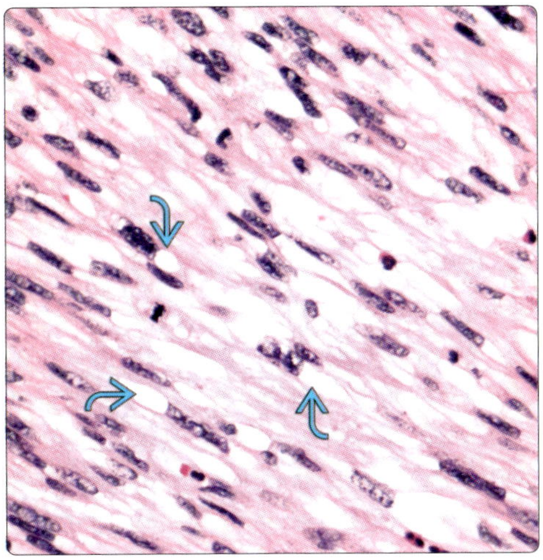

Coagulative Necrosis

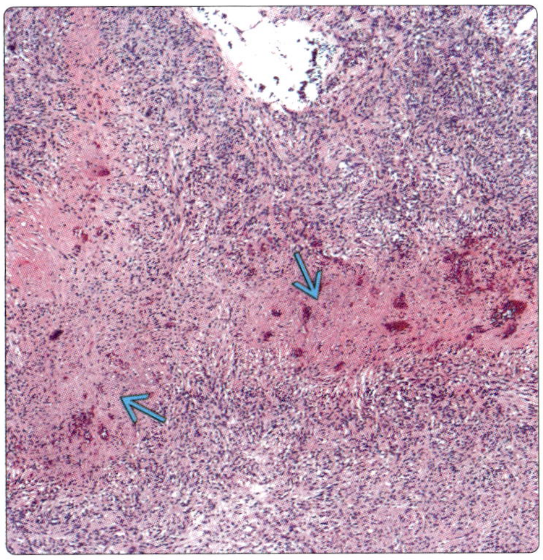

(Left) *Some tumoral smooth muscle cells in LMS feature a perinuclear vacuole that may or may not indent the adjacent nucleus. A similar finding is seen in gastrointestinal stromal tumor.* **(Right)** *Coagulative tumor necrosis is common in LMS and is more frequently seen in tumors that are larger &/or of higher histologic grade. Stromal fibrosis and hyalinization may also be present ± necrosis.*

Circumscribed Border

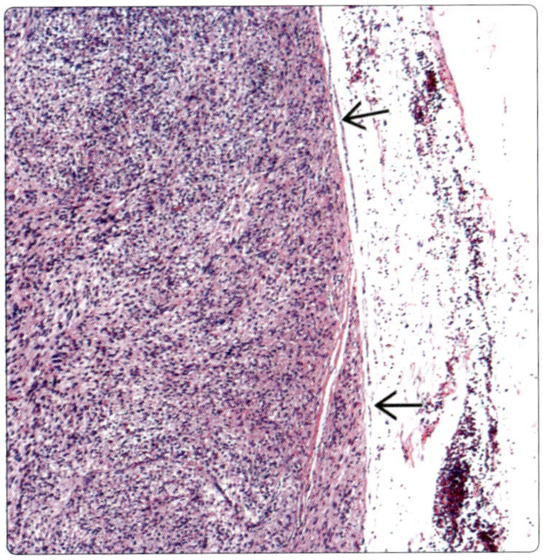

Infiltrative Growth

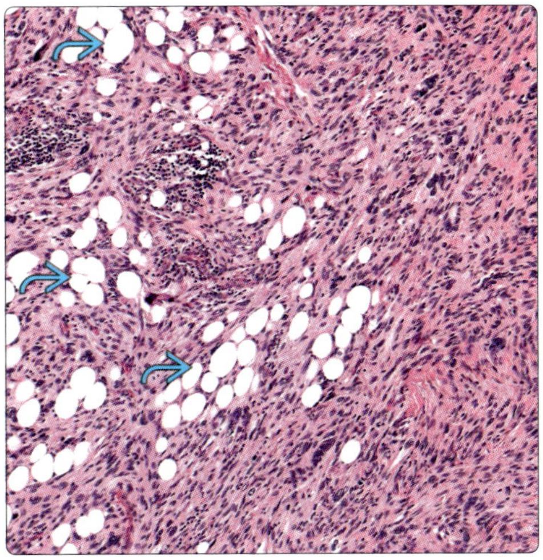

(Left) *Not infrequently, LMS shows a well-circumscribed, expansile, or "pushing" border with the surrounding soft tissue, as depicted. An irregular, infiltrative periphery can be seen in other tumors, however.* **(Right)** *Despite the apparent circumscription seen in many cases of LMS, microscopic evidence of infiltrative growth, including entrapped adipocytes or muscle fibers, is often present.*

(Left) *Based on the dermal confinement and lack of involvement of the subcutaneous adipose tissue, a favorable prognosis would be anticipated for this cutaneous example of LMS. In fact, some observers have suggested diagnosing such superficial lesions as atypical intradermal smooth muscle neoplasm given that they may recur but essentially never metastasize.* **(Right)** *Discrete bundles of collagen ⇨ may be conspicuous in LMS, particularly superficial (dermal/subcutaneous) tumors.*

Cutaneous Leiomyosarcoma

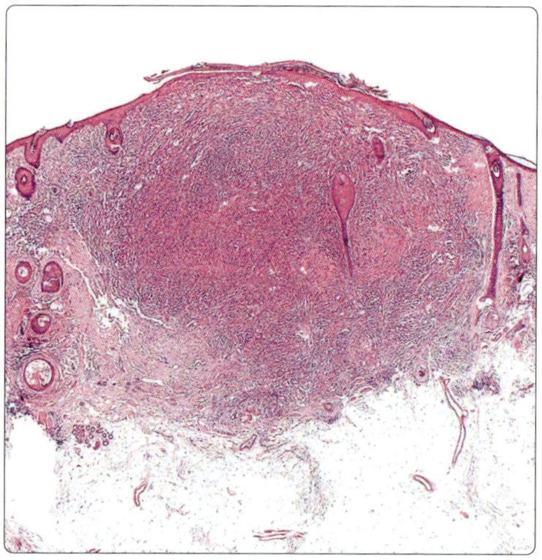

Stromal Collagen

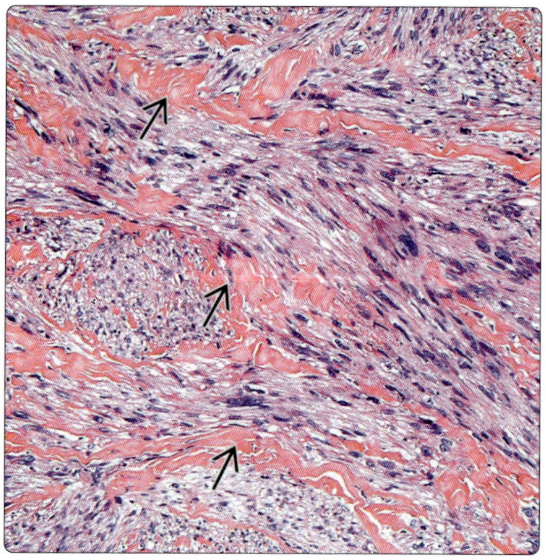

(Left) *Foci of stromal myxoid change or hyalinization may be seen in LMS. Some tumors may even have large, paucicellular, sclerotic zones. At times, the collagen ⇨ may resemble osteoid deposits and raise considerations of extraskeletal osteosarcoma.* **(Right)** *Myxoid stromal change is not uncommon in LMS but is often patchy or focal. Occasional tumors are predominantly myxoid. Of note, cytologic atypia and mitotic activity are often milder/lower in this variant compared to conventional LMS.*

Stromal Changes

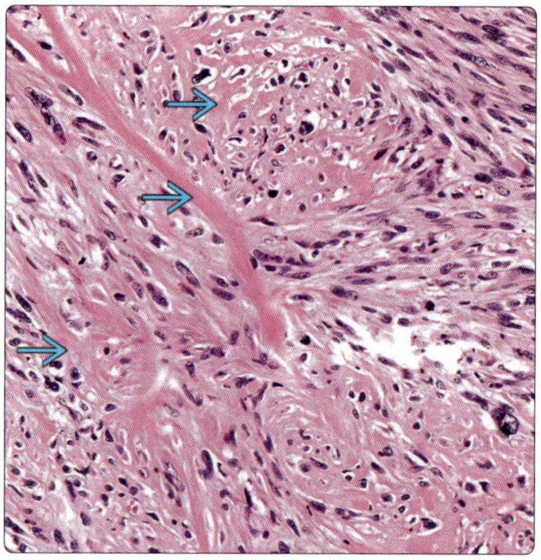

Myxoid Leiomyosarcoma

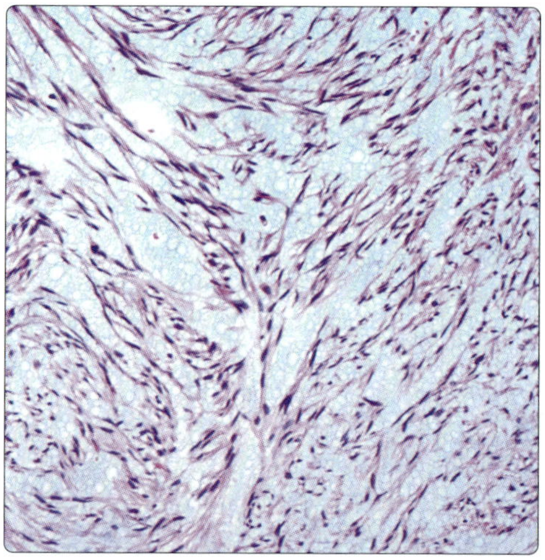

(Left) *A mixed chronic inflammatory infiltrate may be seen in LMS. In rare cases, this infiltrate is prominent (inflammatory LMS) and may obscure other typical diagnosis features of LMS.* **(Right)** *Areas of severe cytologic atypia and pleomorphism, as depicted, may be seen in otherwise typical LMS. In occasional cases, the majority or entirety of the neoplasm is pleomorphic and resembles undifferentiated pleomorphic sarcoma (UPS). Cytoplasmic eosinophilia is often more prominent in pleomorphic LMS than UPS, however.*

Inflammatory Leiomyosarcoma

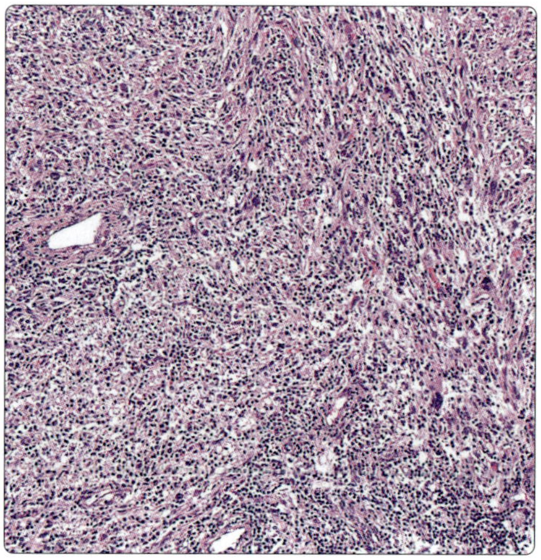

Pleomorphic Leiomyosarcoma

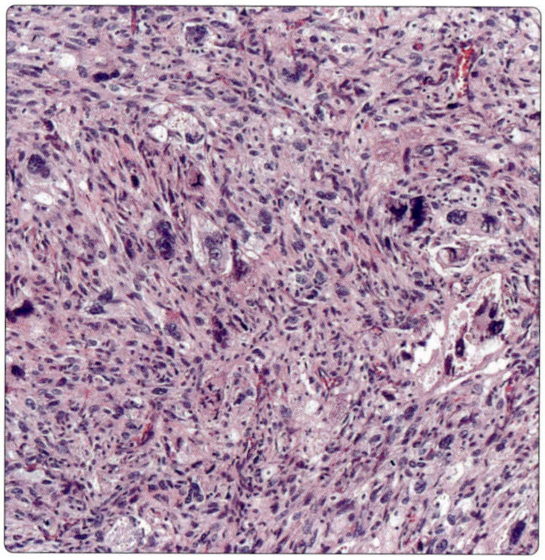

Epithelioid Leiomyosarcoma

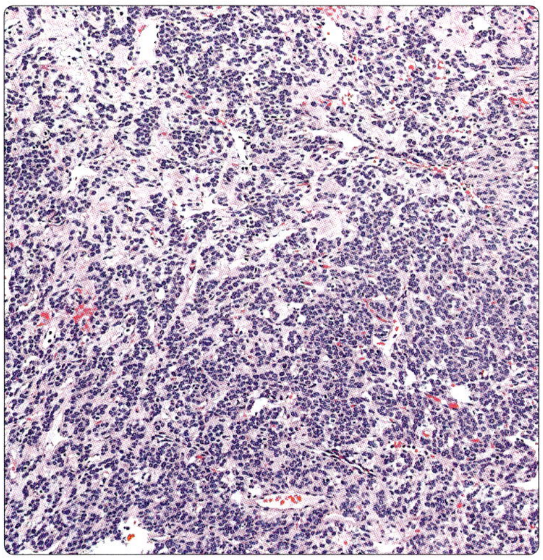

Epithelioid Leiomyosarcoma

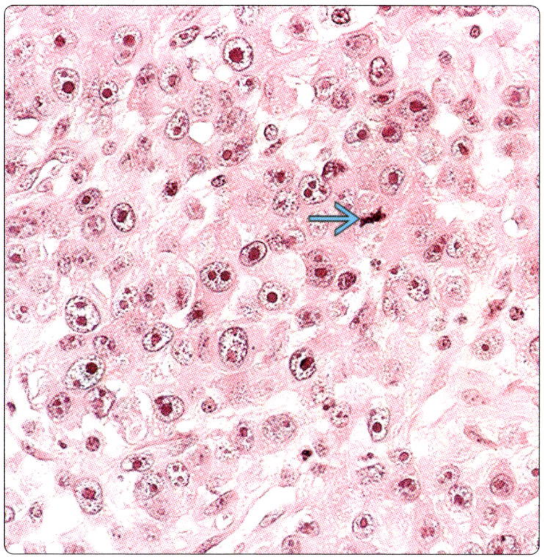

(Left) *Epithelioid change in LMS, if present, is often focal, but it can be prominent in rare tumors. This variant is composed of sheets and cords of either small blue tumor cells (shown) or larger pink cells with prominent nucleoli. Malignant cytologic features and mitotic activity are consistent findings.* **(Right)** *This epithelioid LMS is composed of large rounded cells with abundant eosinophilic cytoplasm and prominent nucleoli. A mitotic figure ⇨ is also present.*

Highly Cellular Leiomyosarcoma

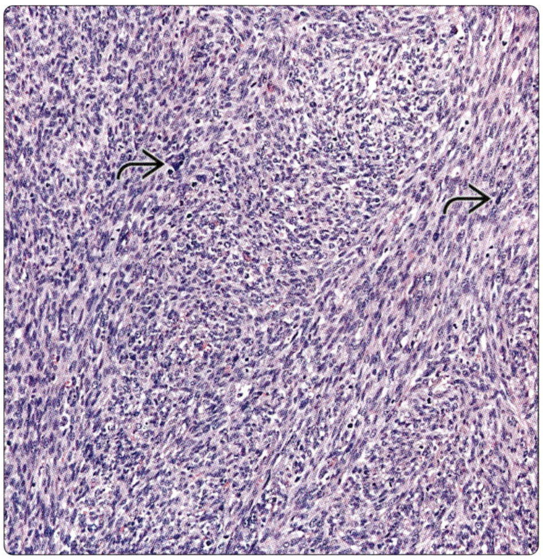

Focal Nuclear Palisading

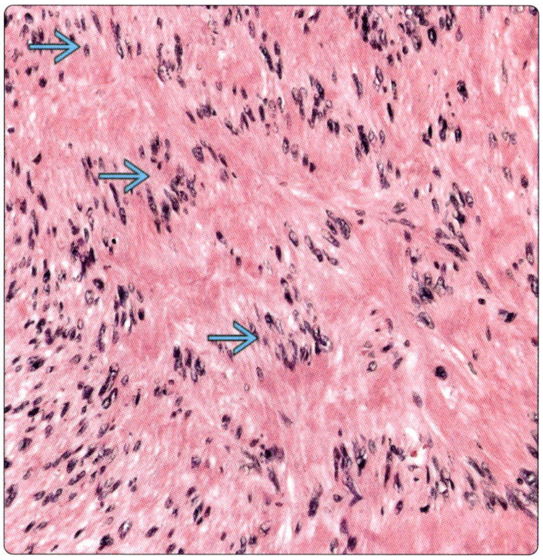

(Left) *Occasional cases of LMS show marked cellularity with comparatively less abundant eosinophilic cytoplasm, as depicted. These cases may be confused for other spindle cell sarcomas, including malignant peripheral nerve sheath tumor or synovial sarcoma, the latter particularly when nuclear pleomorphism ↪ is focal or absent.* **(Right)** *As is the case with leiomyoma, LMS may show foci of palisading nuclei ⇨. This feature is more common (and generally more prominent) in neural tumors.*

SMA Expression

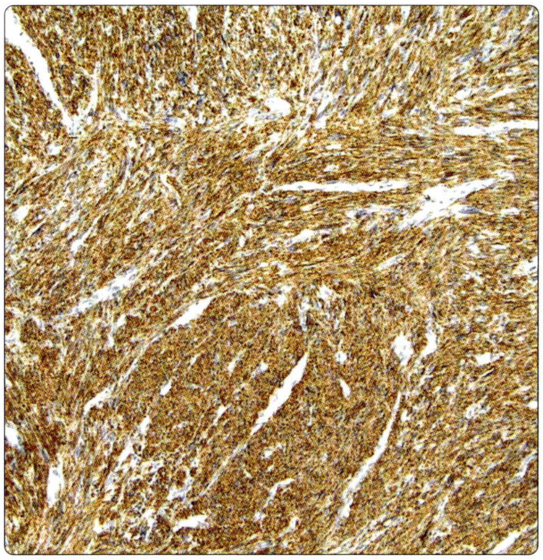

Desmin Expression

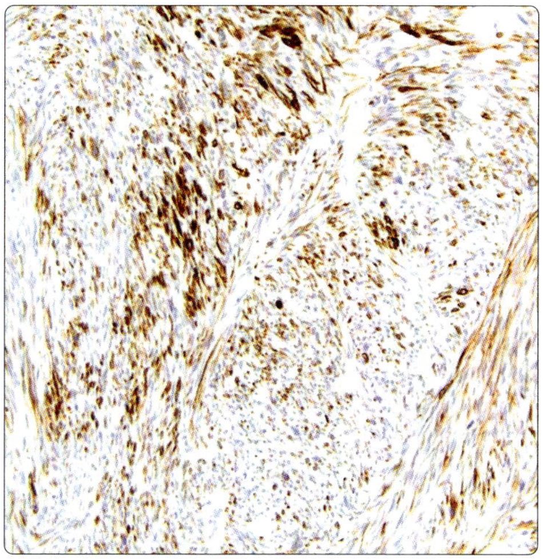

(Left) *Diffuse cytoplasmic expression of smooth muscle actin (SMA) is a characteristic finding in most cases of LMS; however, patchy expression may also be seen. Loss of expression may be seen in markedly pleomorphic areas. Note that the pattern of SMA expression differs from myofibroblastic tumors in which it is often finer and more wispy.* **(Right)** *Desmin expression is usually strong in LMS but is often patchy or focal in extent and may be absent in higher grade tumors.*

SECTION 8

Pericytic (Perivascular) Tumors

Benign

Glomus Tumors (and Variants) 352
Myopericytoma 358
Myofibroma and Myofibromatosis 362
Angioleiomyoma 366

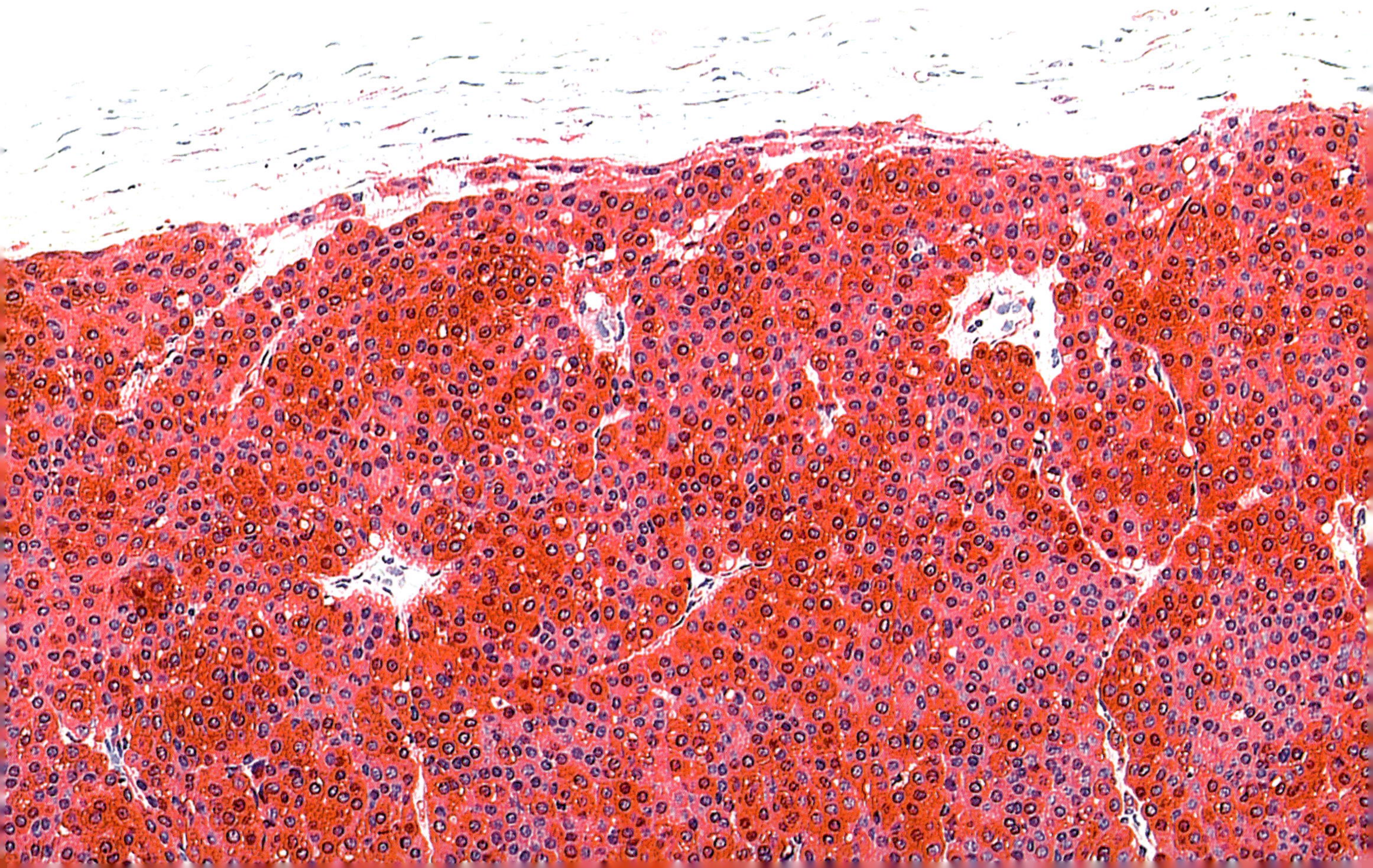

Glomus Tumors (and Variants)

KEY FACTS

TERMINOLOGY

- Perivascular mesenchymal neoplasm composed of cells closely resembling modified smooth muscle cells of normal glomus body
  - Considered to fall on morphologic spectrum with myopericytoma, myofibroma, and angioleiomyoma

CLINICAL ISSUES

- Most common in young adults (20-40 years)
- Female predilection in subungual tumors
- Most common in distal extremities (particularly nail bed)
- Typically small, red-blue nodule, often solitary and painful
- Most arise in skin or subcutis
- Treatment: Complete surgical excision
- Excellent prognosis in conventional glomus tumor (GT)
- Malignant GT is clinically aggressive

MACROSCOPIC

- Most are < 1 cm in size

MICROSCOPIC

- Typically solid nests of round cells closely associated with variably sized blood vessels
  - Characteristic centralized, rounded, uniform nuclei
- Hyalinized to myxoid stroma
- No mitotic activity or necrosis
- Variants: Glomangioma, glomangiomyoma, glomangiomatosis, symplastic GT
- Malignant forms exist but are very rare

ANCILLARY TESTS

- SMA(+), caldesmon (+)
- Desmin, S100 protein, keratin, synaptophysin (-)

TOP DIFFERENTIAL DIAGNOSES

- Myopericytoma
- Benign adnexal tumors
- Dermal melanocytic nevus
- Paraganglioma

Glomus Tumor

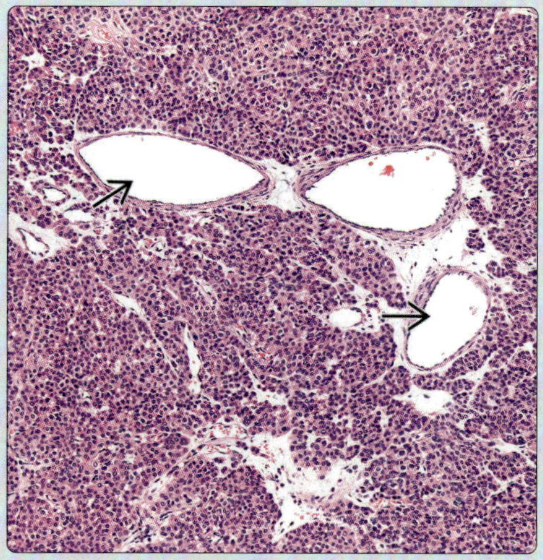

Circumscription

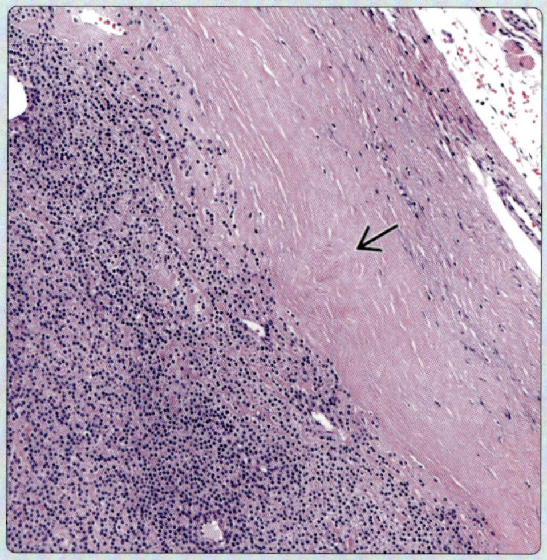

(Left) *Glomus tumor (GT) is a rare, benign tumor that may arise almost anywhere but shows a predilection for the distal extremities, particularly under the nail bed (subungual). It is histologically characterized by sheets and nests of uniform, round to epithelioid cells arranged around a conspicuous vasculature* →. **(Right)** *Most cases of solid GT are well circumscribed and may or may not feature a variably thickened, fibrous pseudocapsule* →.

Monotonous Nuclei

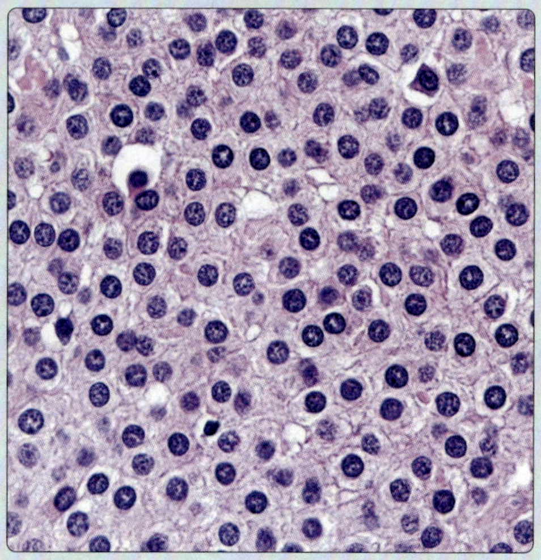

SMA Expression

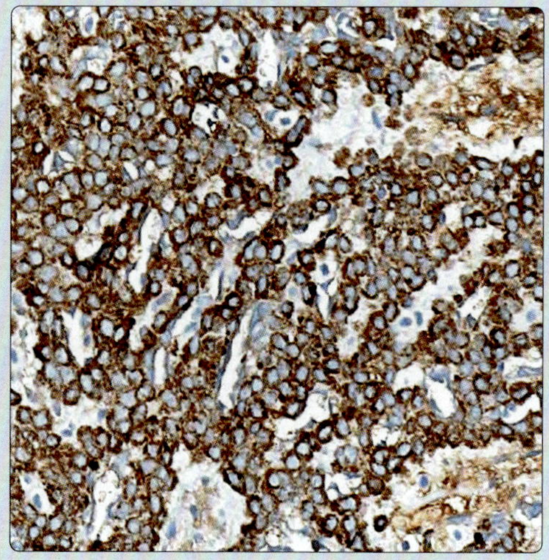

(Left) *The distinctive nuclei in GT are strikingly monomorphic and feature a sharply defined, round, nuclear contour. They are often described as being punched-out. Cytoplasmic borders vary in prominence and may be easy or difficult to visualize, depending upon the individual tumor. Mitotic figures are absent.* **(Right)** *Strong, diffuse cytoplasmic expression of SMA is characteristic of GT. Caldesmon is also typically positive. Desmin is negative.*

TERMINOLOGY

Abbreviations

- Glomus tumor (GT)

Definitions

- Perivascular mesenchymal neoplasm composed of cells closely resembling modified smooth muscle cells of normal glomus body
  - Considered to fall on morphologic spectrum with myopericytoma, myofibroma, and angioleiomyoma
- Several morphologic variants exist, including glomangioma (glomuvenous malformation), glomangiomyoma, glomangiomatosis, and symplastic GT

ETIOLOGY/PATHOGENESIS

Small Subset Are Inherited

- Often feature multiple lesions
- Multiple familial GT
  - Inactivation of *GLMN* gene
- Neurofibromatosis type 1 (NF1)
  - Biallelic inactivation of *NF1* gene

CLINICAL ISSUES

Epidemiology

- Incidence
  - Rare
    - Malignant GT extremely rare
- Age
  - Most common in young adults (20-40 years)
    - Overall wide range
    - Glomangioma variant more common in childhood
- Sex
  - Female predilection in subungual tumors

Site

- Overall wide distribution
- Most common in distal extremities
  - Particularly subungual location
- Rarely in other anatomic locations, including visceral organs (particularly GI tract), bone, mediastinum

Presentation

- Typically small, red-blue nodule, often solitary
  - Multiple in up to 10% of cases
    - Multifocality also seen within setting of NF1
- Most arise in skin or subcutis
  - Rarely in deep soft tissues and viscera
- Usually painful
  - Long history of pain
  - Pain with exposure to cold &/or tactile stimulation

Treatment

- Complete surgical excision
- Clinical follow-up for malignant GT and GT of uncertain malignant potential

Prognosis

- Excellent in conventional GT
  - < 10% recur locally
  - Includes symplastic forms, glomangiomatosis, and other variants
- Malignant GT is clinically aggressive
  - Metastases and death of patients in up to 40% of cases
- Large, visceral GT have potential for aggressive behavior regardless of histology

MACROSCOPIC

General Features

- Red-blue nodular lesions

Size

- Most are < 1 cm
  - Deeper lesions may be larger

MICROSCOPIC

Histologic Features

- Well circumscribed ± fibrous pseudocapsule
  - Small nests of glomus cells associated with small vessels may be identified around periphery of main tumor
- Typically solid nests of cells within highly vascularized stroma
  - Vessels range from small to large and ectatic ("staghorn")
  - Tumor cells arranged around vessels, often as cuffs
  - Diffuse, nodular, sheet-like appearance in highly cellular tumors
- Characteristic small, round, uniform tumor cells with pale, eosinophilic to amphophilic cytoplasm
  - Each cell contains single centralized small, round, uniform nucleus
    - Sometimes described as punched-out
    - Absence of nuclear atypia and significant mitotic activity
  - Occasionally cases feature oncocytic or epithelioid cytomorphology
  - Each cell surrounded by basal lamina
- Hyalinized to myxoid stroma
- No necrosis
- Rare intravascular growth

Morphologic Variants

- Glomangioma (glomuvenous malformation)
  - 20% of cases
  - Less well circumscribed
  - Large, gaping veins surrounded by clusters of glomus cells
    - Resembles vascular spaces of cavernous hemangioma
    - Secondary thrombosis may occur
- Symplastic GT
  - Prominent degenerative atypia in form of marked nuclear hyperchromasia and pleomorphism
    - Lacks mitotic activity and necrosis
    - Lacks other atypical features (e.g., large size, deep location)
  - Otherwise typical features of GT
- Glomangiomyoma
  - Typical GT or glomangioma with additional component of spindled cells resembling smooth muscle
  - Rare

- Glomangiomatosis
  - Diffuse, infiltrative growth pattern resembling angiomatosis
  - Nests of glomus cells around vessels
  - Very rare

Malignant Glomus Tumor (Glomangiosarcoma)

- Preexisting conventional GT may or may not be present
- Criteria for malignancy
  - Tumors showing marked nuclear atypia **and** any degree of mitotic activity **or**
  - Tumor showing atypical mitotic figures
- 2 main morphologies
  - Spindled cells in bundles or fascicles, often resembling leiomyosarcoma or fibrosarcoma
  - Sheets of small round cells with high-grade nuclei
  - Mitoses frequent

Glomus Tumor of Uncertain Malignant Potential

- Reserved for tumors that do not fulfill above criteria for malignancy but that show at least 1 atypical feature other than nuclear pleomorphism
- Also includes deeply situated tumors that are > 2 cm

ANCILLARY TESTS

Immunohistochemistry

- SMA(+), caldesmon (+)
- Variable CD34(+)
- Abundant pericellular type IV collagen (+)
- Desmin, S100 protein, keratin, synaptophysin (-)
- Recent report suggests frequent TLE-1 positivity in benign GT

Molecular Genetics

- NOTCH gene rearrangements (*NOTCH1*, *NOTCH2*, or *NOTCH3*) reported in recent series of benign and malignant GTs
  - 1 case of *NOTCH3-MIR143* fusion reported
- *BRAF* (V600E) and *KRAS* (G12A) mutations reported in some cases of sporadic GT
  - *BRAF* (V600E) may be associated with increased risk of aggressive behavior

DIFFERENTIAL DIAGNOSIS

Myopericytoma

- Exists on morphologic spectrum with GT
- Pure forms lack uniform, round cell component of GT
- Characteristic perivascular, concentric growth of ovoid to spindled tumor cells

Benign Adnexal Tumors

- e.g., nodular hidradenoma, spiradenoma
- Epithelial, ductal/glandular, or sebaceous differentiation should be identifiable
- Keratin (+)
- SMA(-)

Paraganglioma

- Deceptively termed glomus tympanicum in ear and glomus jugulare in neck
- Prominent nested zellballen growth pattern common
- Synaptophysin (+), chromogranin (+)
- S100 protein(+) in sustentacular cells
- SMA (-)

Dermal Melanocytic Nevus

- Nests of melanocytic cells, ± pigmentation
- Intranuclear pseudoinclusions common
- Cells lack close association with blood vessels
- Expression of melanocytic markers (e.g., S100, Melan-A)
- SMA, caldesmon (-)

Angioleiomyoma

- Predominantly composed of bundles of mature, eosinophilic smooth muscle cells
- Lacks prominent uniform round cell component of GT
- SMA(+), desmin (+)
- Often painful

Carcinoid Tumor

- Visceral organs
- Can show close architectural overlap with GT
- Speckled or salt and pepper chromatin pattern
- SMA(-)
- Keratin (+), synaptophysin (+), chromogranin (+)

SELECTED REFERENCES

1. Luzar B et al: Cutaneous malignant glomus tumours: applicability of currently established malignancy criteria for tumours occurring in the skin. Pathology. ePub, 2018
2. Bozdogan N et al: Transducing-like enhancer of split 1: a potential immunohistochemical marker for glomus tumor. Am J Dermatopathol. 39(7):524-527, 2017
3. Karamzadeh Dashti N et al: BRAF V600E mutations occur in a subset of glomus tumors, and are associated with malignant histologic characteristics. Am J Surg Pathol. 41(11):1532-1541, 2017
4. Kumar R et al: Glomangiomatosis of the sciatic nerve: a case report and review of the literature. Skeletal Radiol. 46(6):807-815, 2017
5. Damavandy AA et al: Malignant glomus tumor arising in a long standing precursor lesion. Am J Dermatopathol. 38(5):384-7, 2016
6. Weissferdt A et al: Intrathoracic glomus tumors and glomangiosarcomas: a clinicopathological and immunohistochemical study of 14 cases with emphasis on anatomic distribution. Virchows Arch. 469(5):541-546, 2016
7. Mravic M et al: Clinical and histopathological diagnosis of glomus tumor: an institutional experience of 138 cases. Int J Surg Pathol. 23(3):181-8, 2015
8. Kumar MG et al: Glomus tumors in individuals with neurofibromatosis type 1. J Am Acad Dermatol. 71(1):44-8, 2014
9. Mosquera JM et al: Novel MIR143-NOTCH fusions in benign and malignant glomus tumors. Genes Chromosomes Cancer. 52(11):1075-87, 2013
10. Chakrapani A et al: BRAF and KRAS mutations in sporadic glomus tumors. Am J Dermatopathol. 34(5):533-5, 2012
11. Sheehan JP et al: Gamma Knife surgery for the management of glomus tumors: a multicenter study. J Neurosurg. 117(2):246-54, 2012
12. Semaan MT et al: Current assessment and management of glomus tumors. Curr Opin Otolaryngol Head Neck Surg. 16(5):420-6, 2008
13. Brouillard P et al: Four common glomulin mutations cause two thirds of glomuvenous malformations ("familial glomangiomas"): evidence for a founder effect. J Med Genet. 42(2):e13, 2005
14. Mentzel T et al: CD34-positive glomus tumor: clinicopathologic and immunohistochemical analysis of six cases with myxoid stromal changes. J Cutan Pathol. 29(7):421-5, 2002
15. Folpe AL et al: Atypical and malignant glomus tumors: analysis of 52 cases, with a proposal for the reclassification of glomus tumors. Am J Surg Pathol. 25(1):1-12, 2001
16. Hiruta N et al: Malignant glomus tumor: a case report and review of the literature. Am J Surg Pathol. 21(9):1096-103, 1997
17. Van Geertruyden J et al: Glomus tumours of the hand. A retrospective study of 51 cases. J Hand Surg [Br]. 21(2):257-60, 1996
18. Gould EW et al: Locally infiltrative glomus tumors and glomangiosarcomas. A clinical, ultrastructural, and immunohistochemical study. Cancer. 65(2):310-8, 1990
19. Slater DN et al: Oncocytic glomus tumour: a new variant. Histopathology. 11(5):523-31, 1987

Variable Stromal Hyalinization

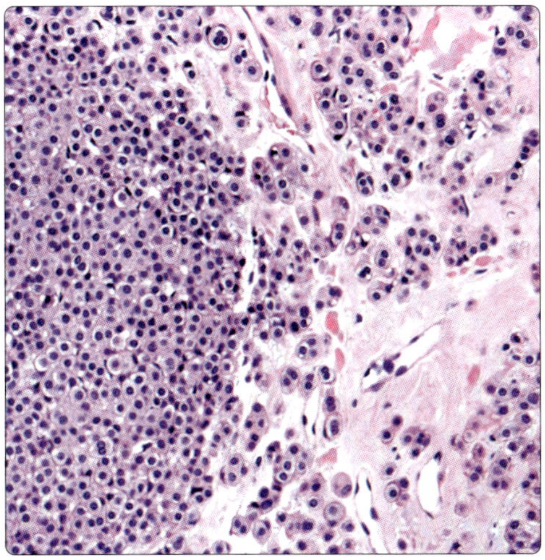

Peritumoral Glomus Proliferations

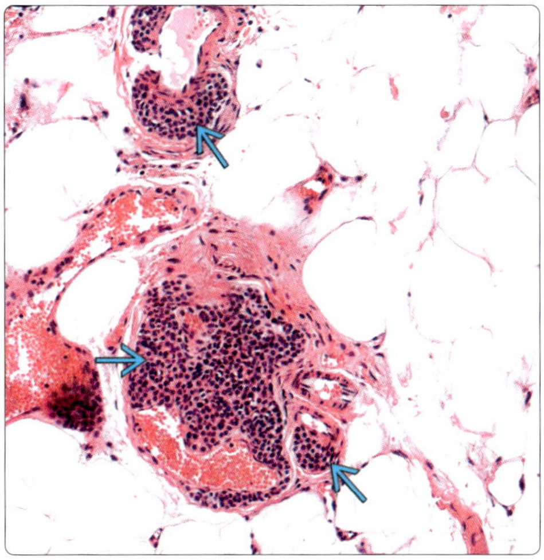

(Left) *The stroma in GT varies from hyalinized to myxoid. Some zones of prominent hyalinization or sclerosis can feature tumor cells arranged singly or in small aggregate or cords (right).* **(Right)** *In some cases of GT, small vessels at the periphery of the tumor may contain a subtle or conspicuous glomus cell proliferation →. This finding can be diagnostically helpful in distinguishing a solid GT from an adnexal tumor.*

Sheet-Like Growth

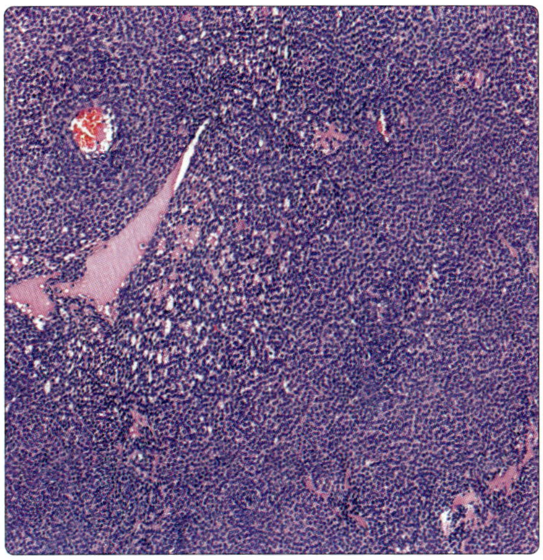

Conspicuous Vasculature

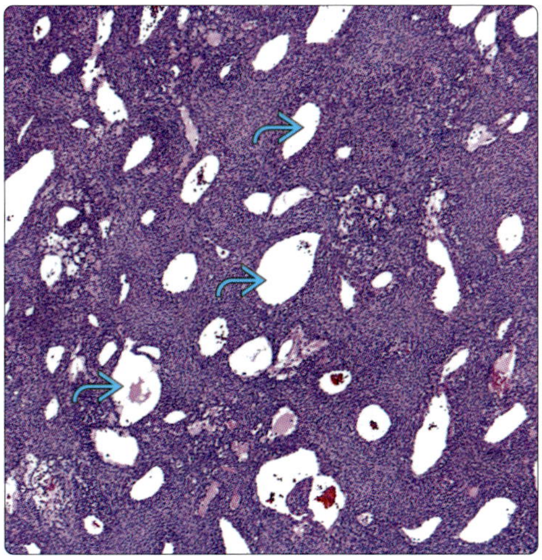

(Left) *Some GTs may feature a strikingly solid growth pattern with a less prominent vasculature, as depicted here. These tumors can closely mimic a cutaneous adnexal neoplasm.* **(Right)** *The stromal vasculature ↷ can be very prominent in some cases of GT and may also adopt irregular or staghorn shapes. This morphology can lead to consideration of a cellular solitary fibrous tumor.*

Pericellular Type IV Collagen

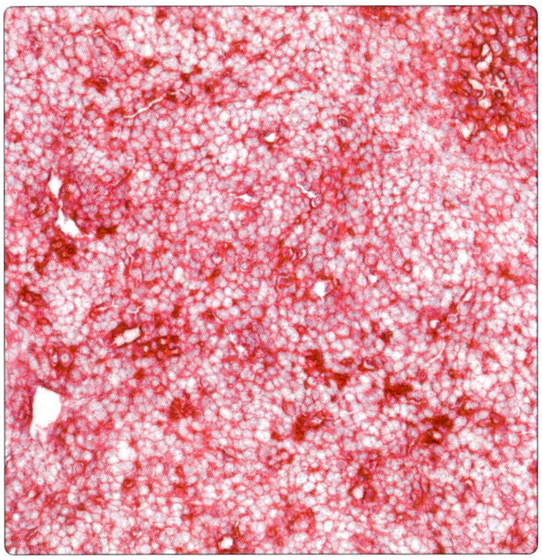

Oncocytic Change

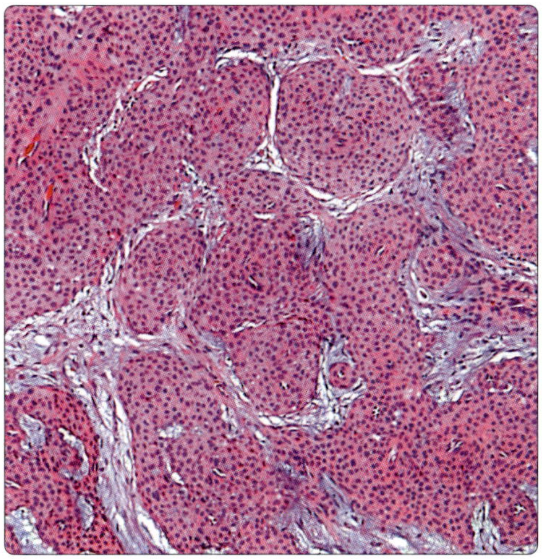

(Left) *Although not widely utilized in general practice, a collagen IV (or laminin) immunostain can nicely highlight the pericellular basement membrane material characteristic of GT.* **(Right)** *Oncocytic change is an occasional finding in GT and is characterized by tumor cells with abundant granular cytoplasm, as depicted here. This particular tumor also features a myxoid stroma.*

(Left) *Glomangioma is a variant of GT that features larger, dilated vascular spaces lined by the characteristic tumor cells. Compared to conventional GT, glomangioma is often less well circumscribed and is more common in children and in familial cases.* **(Right)** *The large, dilated spaces of glomangioma are always lined by arrays of neoplastic glomus cells; however, this lining can vary widely in thickness from field to field.*

Glomangioma

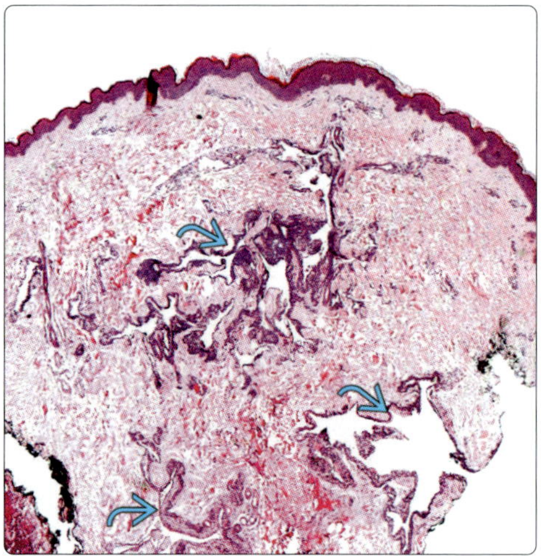

Prominent Dilated Vessels

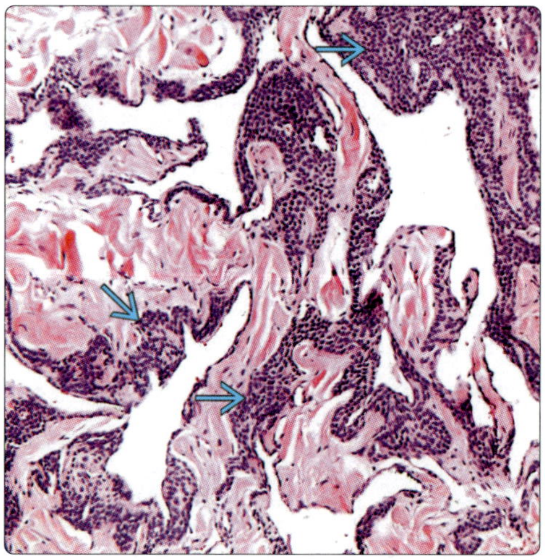

(Left) *As shown in this H&E, vascular spaces in glomangioma may be markedly expanded and closely resemble those of cavernous hemangioma. However, the glomus cell lining is distinctive. Also note that large thrombi or phleboliths may be present in some cases.* **(Right)** *Rare cases of GT (or any of its other variants) may contain scattered pleomorphic nuclei, suggesting malignancy. Mitoses and other atypical features are absent, however. These changes are likely degenerative in nature.*

Cavernous Vascular Pattern

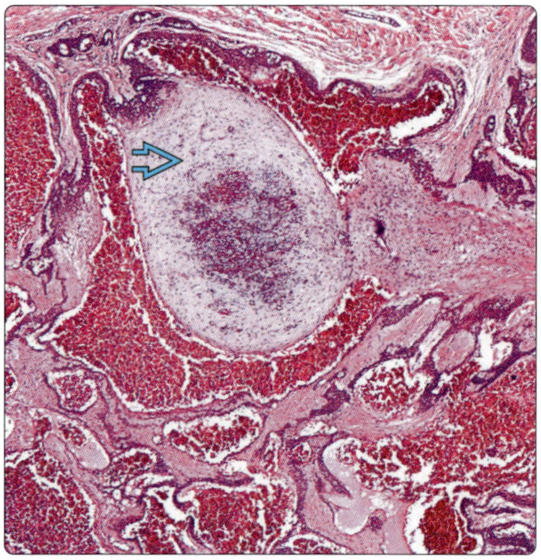

Symplastic Glomangioma

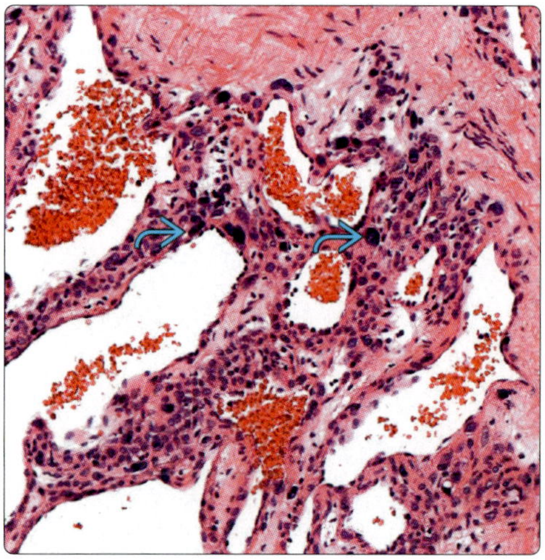

(Left) *Glomangiomyoma is a variant of GT that features a smooth muscle component in addition to areas of otherwise conventional-appearing GT or glomangioma. Note the small areas of rounded glomus cells.* **(Right)** *Glomangiomatosis is a rare, benign, diffuse variant of GT that resembles the pattern seen in angiomatosis; however, small vessels in glomangiomatosis feature glomus cell proliferations.*

Glomangiomyoma

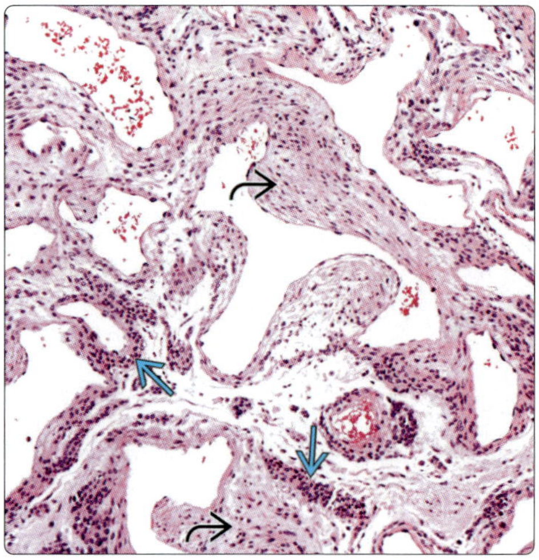

Glomangiomatosis

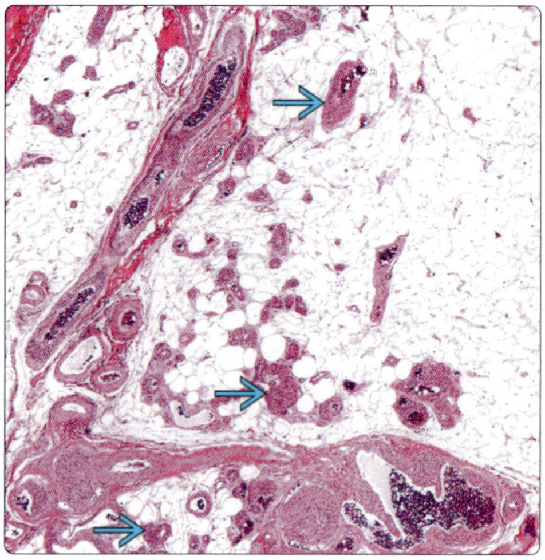

Interface Between Benign and Malignant Glomus Tumor

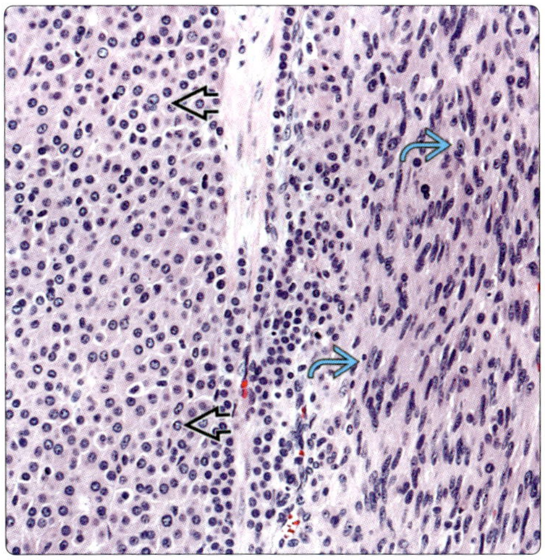

Malignant Spindle Cell Morphology

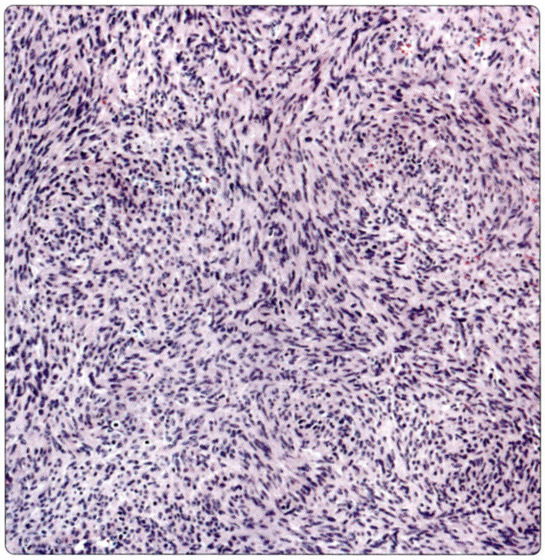

(Left) *Malignant GT ↷ is rare. A preexisting component of conventional benign-appearing GT ⇨ may or may not be present. In the latter situation, inununohlstochemistry is often needed to support the diagnosis.* **(Right)** *The spindled morphology of malignant GT often resembles other spindle cell sarcomas, such as leiomyosarcoma or fibrosarcoma. Short fascicles and whorls are common. Mitoses are usually numerous.*

Malignant Round Cell Morphology

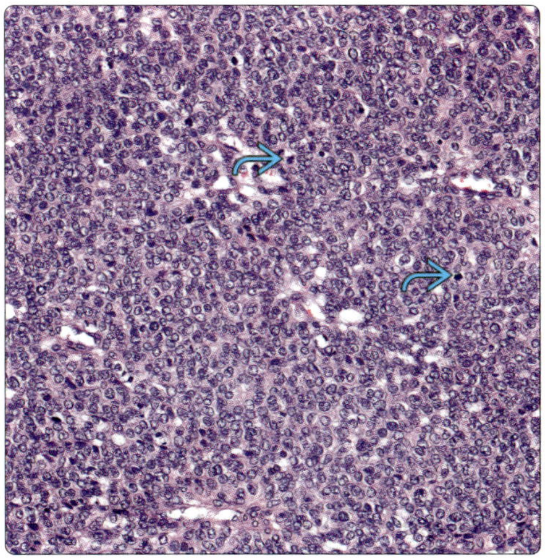

Nuclear Atypia and Mitoses

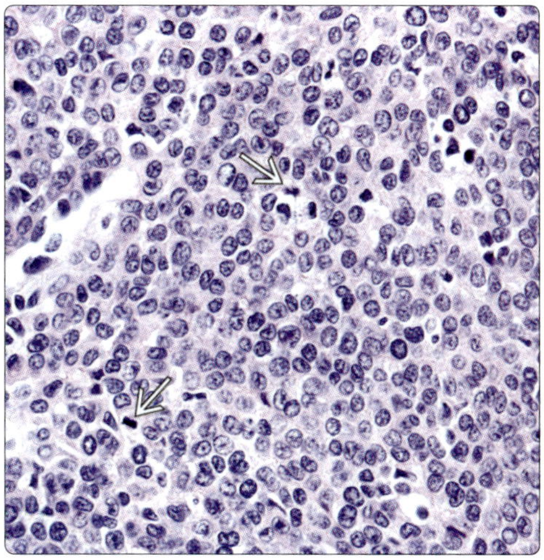

(Left) *The round cell morphology of malignant GT mimics somewhat conventional GT in architecture; however, the nuclei often show a high degree of atypia, and mitoses ↷ are easily identified.* **(Right)** *Malignant GT with a round cell pattern shows increased nuclear atypia, including prominent nucleoli in some cases. Note the mitoses ➡.*

Nuclear Pleomorphism

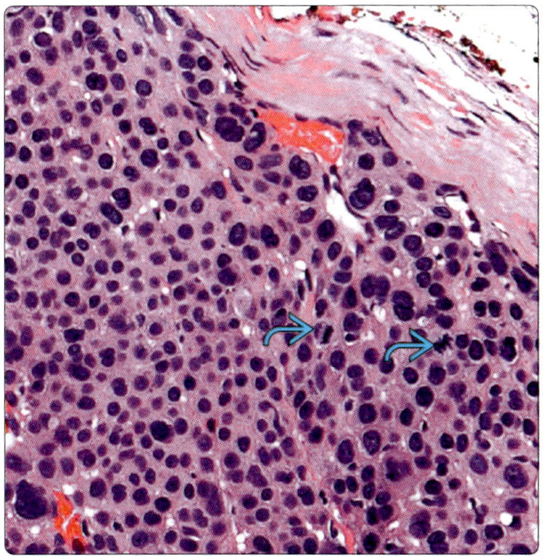

Multinodularity and Vascular Invasion

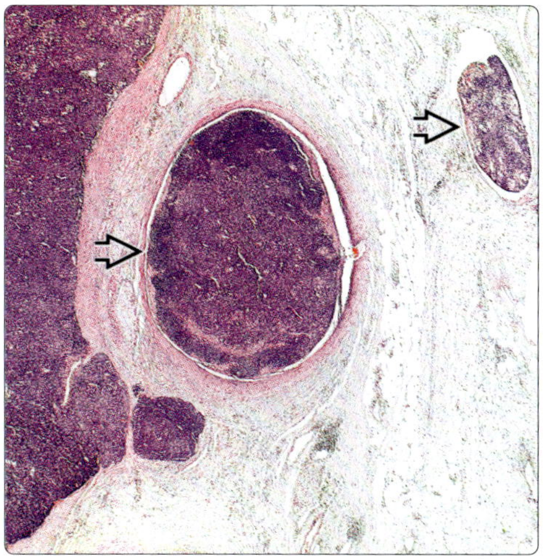

(Left) *Some cases of malignant GT feature marked nuclear pleomorphism &/or hyperchromasia. Distinction from symplastic GT is possible through identification of other atypical features, including multiple mitoses ↷.* **(Right)** *Malignant GT can show a more prominent multinodular growth pattern compared to conventional GT. Vascular invasion ⇨ may also be seen.*

Myopericytoma

KEY FACTS

TERMINOLOGY

- Benign perivascular myoid neoplasm with prominent vascularity
  - Forms morphologic spectrum with angioleiomyoma, myofibroma, and glomus tumor

CLINICAL ISSUES

- Wide age range (most common in middle-aged adults)
- Most common in dermal or subcutaneous tissue of distal extremities
- Usually solitary and slow growing; rarely multiple
- Treatment: Simple surgical excision
- Excellent prognosis: Local recurrence rare
  - Very rare malignant forms are clinically aggressive

MACROSCOPIC

- Usually < 2 cm

MICROSCOPIC

- Characteristic multilayered concentric growth of myoid tumor cells around thin-walled blood vessels
- Mitoses are rare
- Some hybrid cases have focal features of glomus tumor, angioleiomyoma, or myofibroma

ANCILLARY TESTS

- SMA(+), h-caldesmon (+)
- Negative for desmin, CD31, CD34, S100 protein, keratin
- *PDGFRB* alterations identified in both myopericytoma, myopericytomatosis, and myofibroma

TOP DIFFERENTIAL DIAGNOSES

- Myofibroma
- Angioleiomyoma
- Solitary fibrous tumor
- Glomus tumor

Myopericytoma

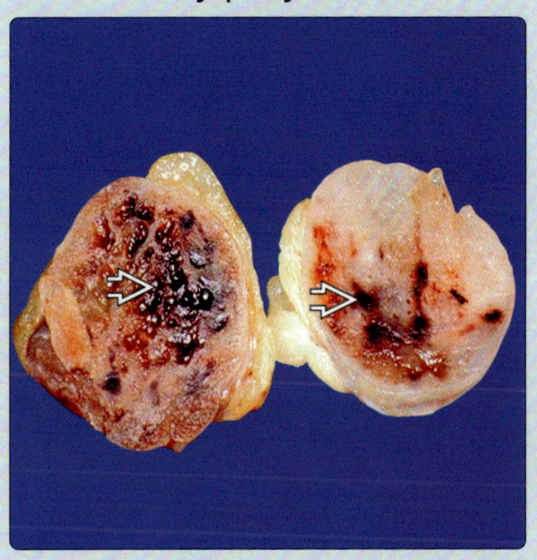

Well Circumscribed

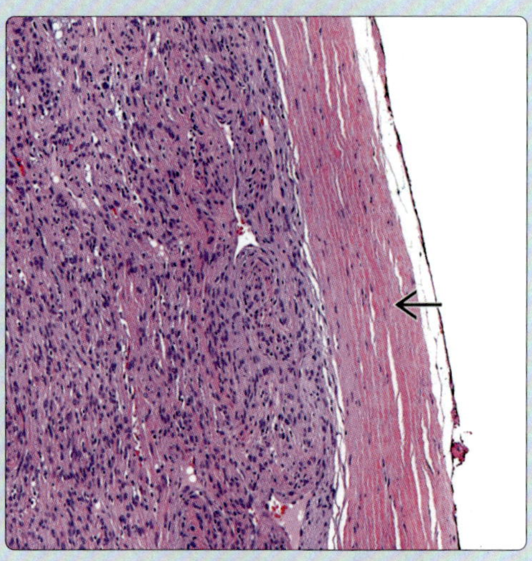

(Left) *Grossly, myopericytoma is characterized by a nodular, well-circumscribed neoplasm with numerous vessels ➡ and a tan-white cut surface.* **(Right)** *Myopericytoma is a benign perivascular neoplasm that is generally small, well circumscribed, and unencapsulated; however, some tumors may show a compressed pseudocapsule ➡.*

Concentric Perivascular Growth

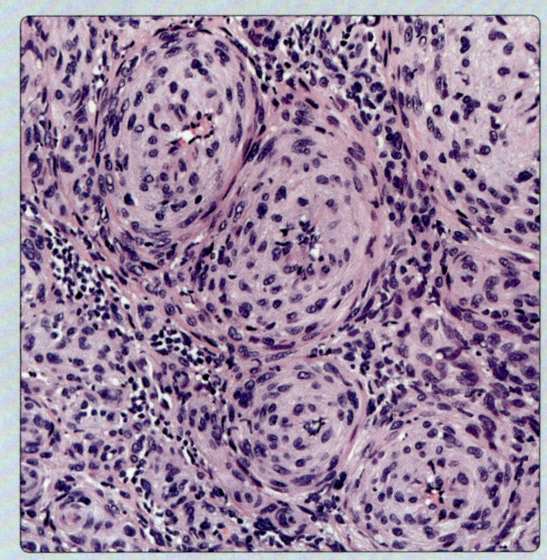

Smooth Muscle Actin Expression

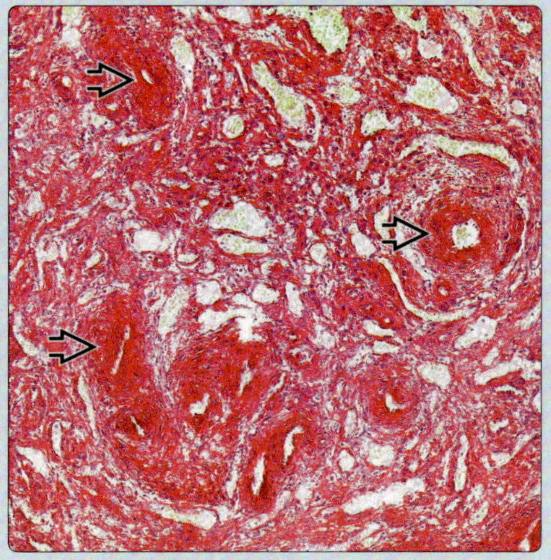

(Left) *A characteristic feature of myopericytoma is multilayered, concentric perivascular growth by the lesional cells, as depicted. The prominence of this finding varies from case to case, but is often easy to spot. Note that the nuclei are relatively uniform, and mitoses are rare.* **(Right)** *Homogeneous expression of SMA (red chromogen shown) is characteristic of myopericytoma (and related pericytic neoplasms) and highlights the striking perivascular growth ➡ of neoplastic cells.*

TERMINOLOGY

Definitions

- Benign perivascular myoid neoplasm with prominent vascularity
  - Forms morphologic spectrum with angioleiomyoma, myofibroma, and glomus tumor
- Myopericytomatosis
  - Diffuse involvement of dermis and subcutaneous tissue by microscopic myopericytomatous nodules

CLINICAL ISSUES

Epidemiology

- Age
  - Wide age range (most common in middle-aged adults)
- Sex
  - Male predominance

Site

- Most common in dermal or subcutaneous tissue
  - Rarely in deep soft tissues
- Distal extremities are most frequently involved
  - Less commonly proximal extremities, neck, trunk

Presentation

- Usually solitary, slow-growing mass
  - Rarely multiple

Treatment

- Simple surgical excision

Prognosis

- Benign
- Local recurrence rare
  - Additional, new tumors may arise in same region
- Very rare malignant myopericytomas are often clinically aggressive

MACROSCOPIC

General Features

- Well-circumscribed, nodular/lobular mass
- Tan-white firm cut surface with evidence of vascularity

Size

- Usually < 2 cm
  - Deeply situated lesions can be larger

MICROSCOPIC

Histologic Features

- Generally well circumscribed, unencapsulated
- Uniform, plump spindled and ovoid cells
  - Eosinophilic cytoplasm and elongated, bland nuclei
  - Mitoses are rare
- Characteristic multilayered concentric growth of myoid tumor cells around thin-walled blood vessels
  - Vessels often numerous and variable in size
  - Some vessels are large, dilated, and irregular ("staghorn")
    - Extensive hemangiopericytoma-like vasculature may be seen in some cases
  - Nearby blood vessels peripheral to tumor may show similar concentric growth of myoid cells
- Cellularity varies widely
- Degenerative changes in longstanding tumors
  - Scattered atypical nuclei, myxoid stroma, hyalinization, hemorrhage, infarction, metaplastic bone formation
- Some hybrid cases have focal features of glomus tumor, angioleiomyoma, or myofibroma
- May show intramural or intravascular growth
- Myopericytomatosis
  - Diffuse involvement of dermis and subcutaneous tissue by microscopic myopericytomatous nodules
- Very rare malignant forms
  - Prominent nuclear atypia and numerous mitoses
  - Evidence of perivascular growth usually present

ANCILLARY TESTS

Immunohistochemistry

- SMA(+), h-caldesmon (+)
- Negative for desmin, CD31, CD34, S100, keratin, STAT6

In Situ Hybridization

- *PDGFRB* alterations identified in both myopericytoma, myopericytomatosis, and myofibroma
  - Includes mutations and low-level amplification

DIFFERENTIAL DIAGNOSIS

Myofibroma

- Can show morphologic overlap with myopericytoma
- More common in pediatric age group than myopericytoma
- Shows conspicuous areas of myoid nodule formation

Angioleiomyoma

- Can show morphologic overlap with myopericytoma
- Predominance of plump, eosinophilic spindle cells in bundles and fascicles
  - Cytologic features of smooth muscle
- Desmin (+), SMA(+)

Glomus Tumor

- Usually sheets of rounded, strikingly monomorphic cells arranged around ectatic vasculature

Solitary Fibrous Tumor

- No concentric, multilayered, perivascular growth
- Diffuse CD34(+), STAT6(+); negative for SMA and desmin

SELECTED REFERENCES

1. Hung YP et al: Myopericytomatosis: clinicopathologic analysis of 11 cases with molecular identification of recurrent PDGFRB alterations in myopericytomatosis and myopericytoma. Am J Surg Pathol. 41(8):1034-44, 2017
2. Dray MS et al: Myopericytoma: a unifying term for a spectrum of tumours that show overlapping features with myofibroma. A review of 14 cases. J Clin Pathol. 59(1):67-73, 2006
3. Mentzel T et al: Myopericytoma of skin and soft tissues: clinicopathologic and immunohistochemical study of 54 cases. Am J Surg Pathol. 30(1):104-13, 2006
4. McMenamin ME et al: Malignant myopericytoma: expanding the spectrum of tumours with myopericytic differentiation. Histopathology. 41(5):450-60, 2002

Perivascular Myxoid Change

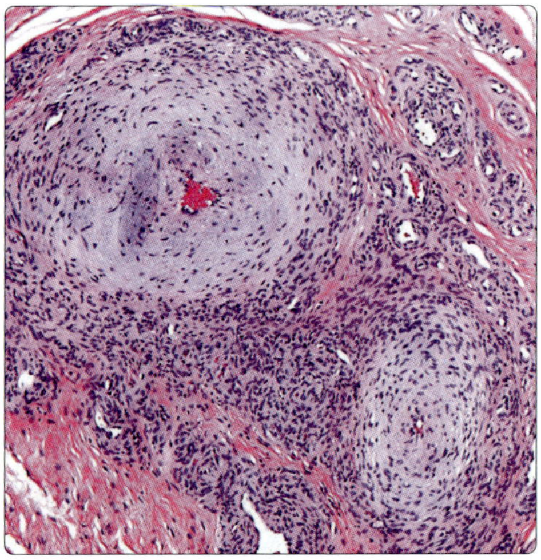

Solid Growth

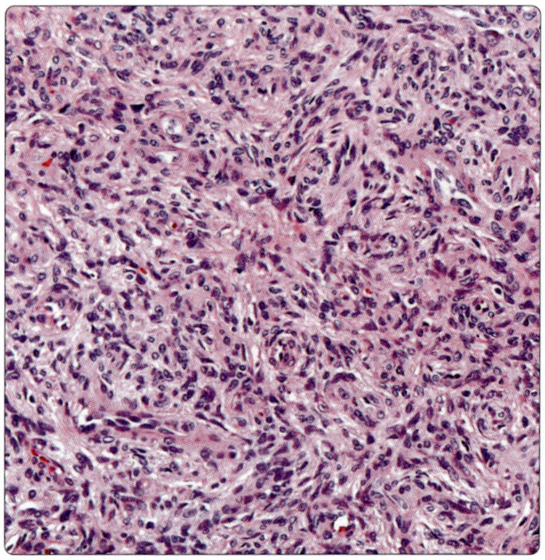

(Left) *In some cases of myopericytoma, the immediate region around the blood vessels is myxoid and less cellular than the surrounding areas. Note that a concentric, perivascular growth is readily identified.* **(Right)** *In other areas of myopericytoma, concentric vascular growth is not as overtly conspicuous, and tumor cells appear to form haphazard sheets of variable cellularity.*

Ectatic Vascular Channels

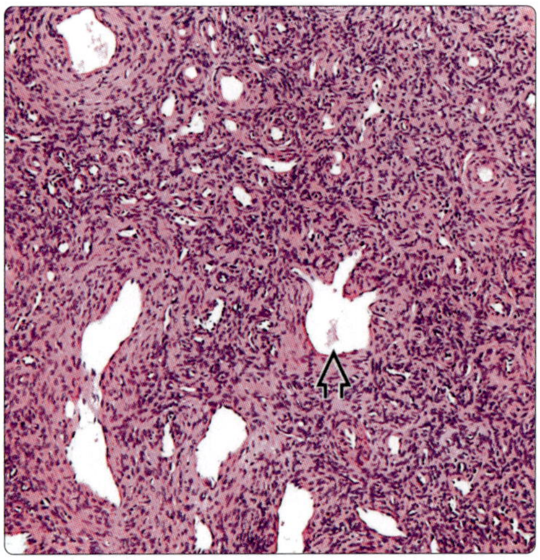

Hemangiopericytoma-Like Growth

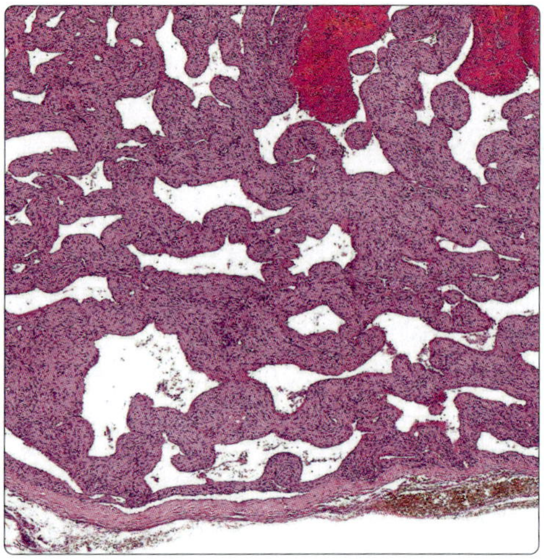

(Left) *Ectatic, "staghorn" vascular channels ➲ are a common finding in myopericytoma and may be prominent. This appearance can suggest solitary fibrous tumor (SFT); however, the concentric, perivascular tumor cell arrangement of myopericytoma is not a typical feature of SFT.* **(Right)** *A prominent, visually striking hemangiopericytoma-like vascular pattern may be seen in some cases of myopericytoma, as depicted. The lesional cells express SMA and are negative for CD34.*

Angioleiomyoma-Like Areas

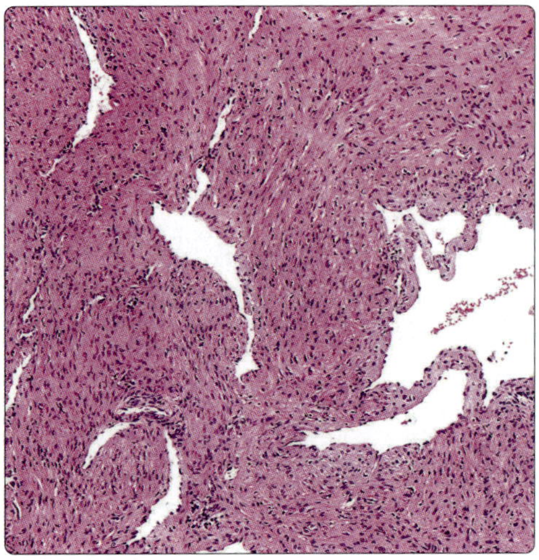

Focal Myoid Bundles

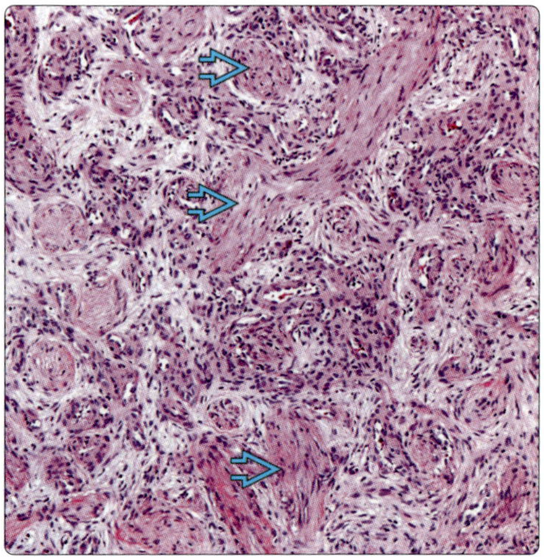

(Left) *Some cases of myopericytoma contain areas that are cytomorphologically similar to the smooth muscle cells of angioleiomyoma, which is considered to be another perivascular neoplasm related to myopericytoma.* **(Right)** *Myopericytoma may contain myoid nodules ➲ similar to what is seen in myofibroma. There is significant histologic overlap between these 2 entities; however, classification as myofibroma is more appropriate in the setting of a significant myoid component.*

Degenerative Changes

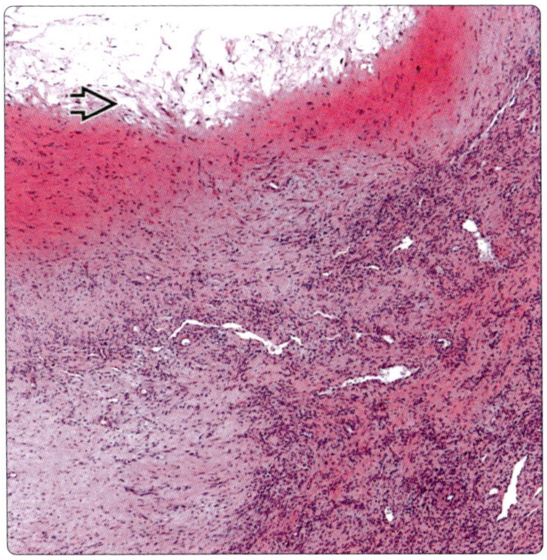

Degenerative Changes

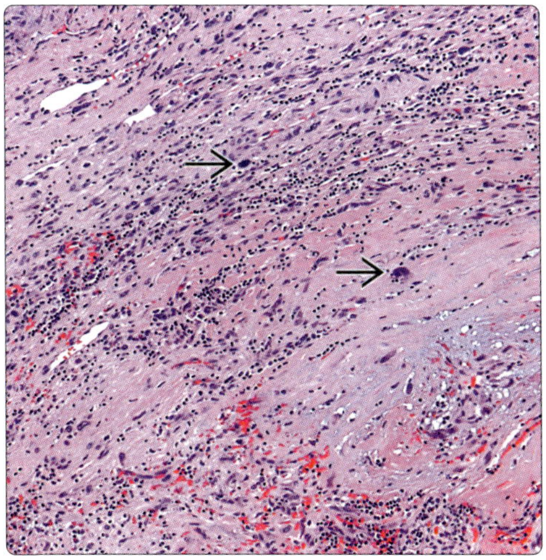

(Left) *Degenerative changes are not uncommon in myopericytoma and include hemorrhage, cystic change ⇨, fibrosis, and stromal hyalinization. These changes may be so extensive that the underlying diagnosis is obscured.* **(Right)** *Other degenerative changes that occur in myopericytoma include stromal myxoid change, chronic inflammation, and scattered hyperchromatic nuclei with "smudgy" chromatin →.*

Intravascular Growth

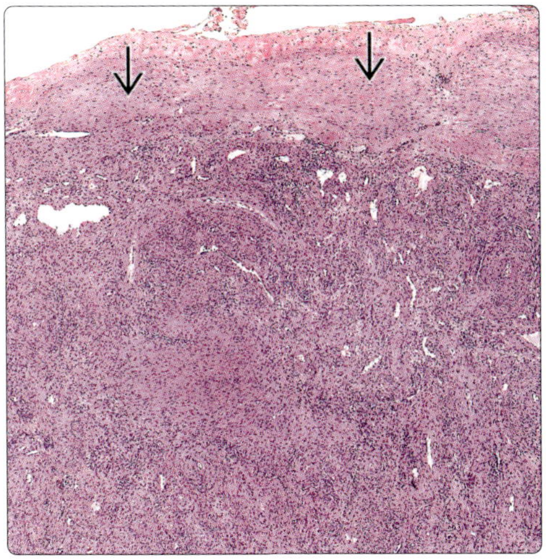

Peritumoral Vessels

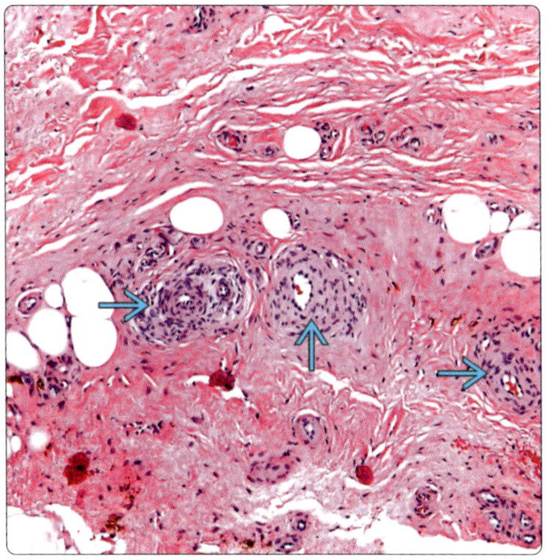

(Left) *Intravascular and intramural growth is an occasional finding in myopericytoma. Note the muscular wall → of the involved blood vessel at the periphery.* **(Right)** *An interesting finding noted in some cases of myopericytoma is the presence of a subtle, concentric proliferation of pericytic cells around the blood vessels → located peripherally in the vicinity of the main tumor.*

Malignant Myopericytoma

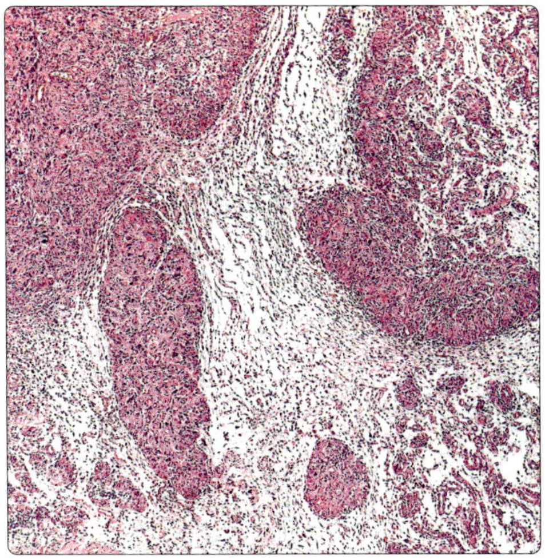

Malignant Myopericytoma

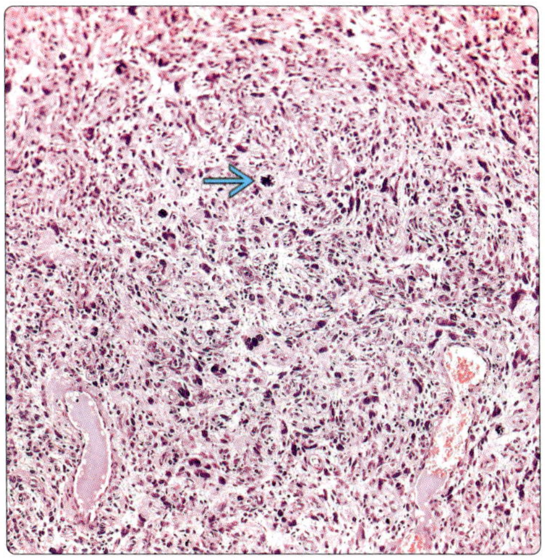

(Left) *Malignant forms of myopericytoma are extremely rare and are usually characterized by significant nuclear atypia, pleomorphism, and mitotic activity. Of note, a perivascular arrangement of the tumor cells is usually maintained, at least focally.* **(Right)** *This case of a malignant myopericytoma showed extensive nuclear pleomorphism and numerous mitoses, including atypical forms →.*

Myofibroma and Myofibromatosis

KEY FACTS

TERMINOLOGY

- Benign pericytic neoplasm classically composed of lobules of myoid cells separated by cellular, vascularized zones
  - Solitary form (myofibroma); multicentric form (myofibromatosis)

CLINICAL ISSUES

- Wide age range (most common in infants and children)
- Solitary form most common in dermis and subcutis of head and neck, trunk, and extremities
- Multicentric form occurs in dermis, subcutis, muscle, bones, and visceral organs
- Treatment: Simple conservative excision
  - Both nonvisceral solitary and multicentric forms often spontaneously regress
- All forms are benign
  - Excellent prognosis without visceral organ involvement
  - Extensive visceral organ involvement may be fatal

MICROSCOPIC

- Most lesions are small and well marginated
- Classic biphasic pattern
  - Myoid nodules separated by cellular zones of ovoid cells with hemangiopericytoma-like *NTRK3* (biphasic pattern)
    - Variable amounts of each component (vascular zones more prominent in children and less so in adults)
- Hypercellular variant often shows long fascicles and resembles fibrosarcoma

ANCILLARY TESTS

- SMA(+); desmin and S100 protein (-)

TOP DIFFERENTIAL DIAGNOSES

- Leiomyoma
- Fibromatosis
- Nodular fasciitis
- Infantile fibrosarcoma

Myofibroma

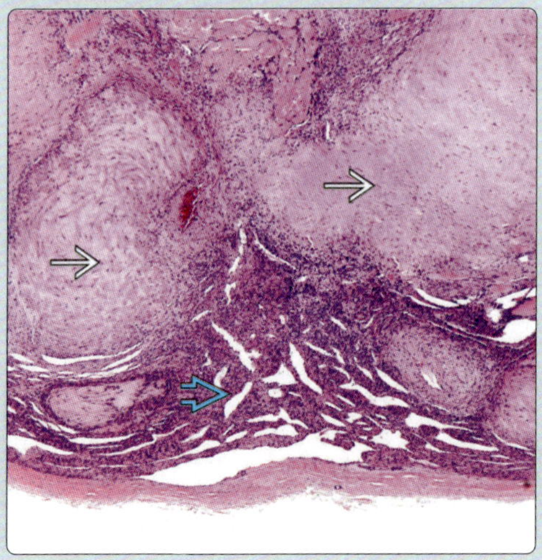

Myoid Nodules

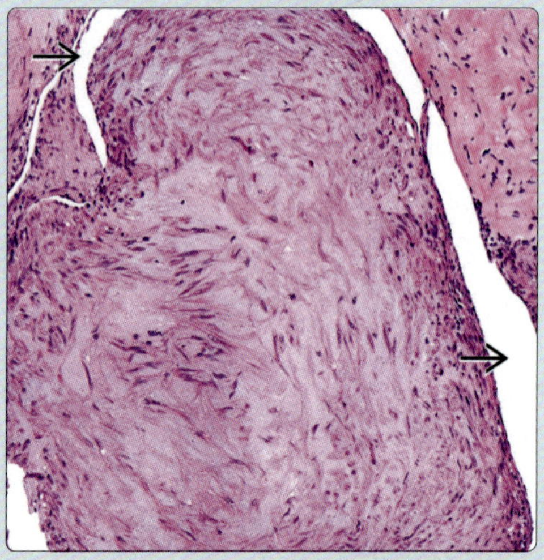

(Left) *The classic case of myofibroma shows a biphasic morphology consisting of vague nodules* ➡ *of myoid cells admixed with more cellular zones demonstrating a pericytomatous (hemangiopericytoma-like) vasculature* ⇨. **(Right)** *The myoid cells are thin to plump, elongated spindle cells with eosinophilic cytoplasm, often within myxoid matrix. These cells may be loosely arranged or may form short fascicles or whorls. Note that the myoid nodules may project or extend into thin-walled vascular channels* ➡.

Cytologic Features

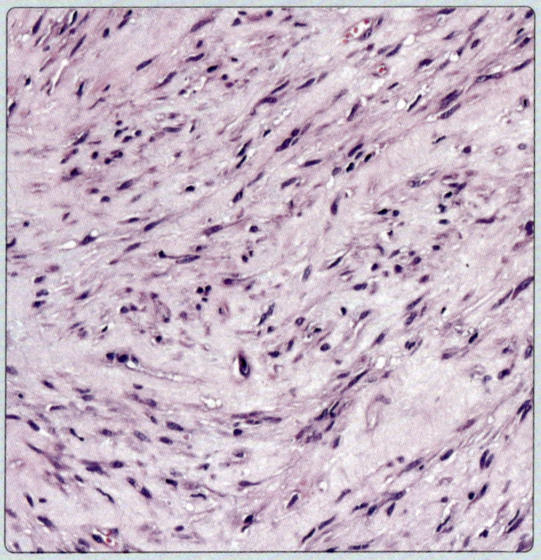

Cellular Vascular Zones

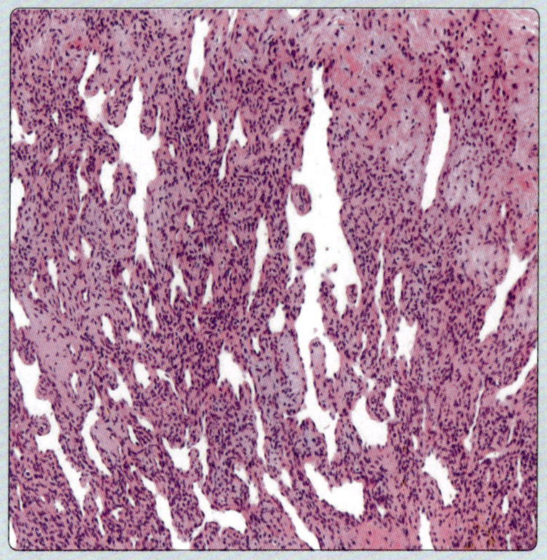

(Left) *Cytologically, the cells of myofibroma are bland and relatively uniform. Significant nuclear pleomorphism is not a feature of this tumor. The mitotic index is generally low and without atypical figures.* **(Right)** *The centralized or internodular vascular zones are composed of smaller, ovoid tumor cells between irregularly shaped, small to large vessels, many of which have a staghorn appearance. The overall appearance is often described as hemangiopericytoma-like.*

TERMINOLOGY

Synonyms

- Infantile myofibroma/myofibromatosis

Definitions

- Benign, biphasic neoplasm classically composed of lobules of myoid cells separated by cellular, vascularized zones
  - Solitary form (myofibroma)
  - Multicentric form (myofibromatosis)
- Currently considered to be pericytic neoplasm related to myopericytoma

CLINICAL ISSUES

Epidemiology

- Incidence
  - Solitary form more common than multicentric form
- Age
  - Wide range (most common in infants and children)
- Sex
  - 2:1 male predominance

Site

- Solitary
  - Dermis and subcutaneous tissue
  - Most common in head and neck region
  - Also lower and upper extremities and trunk
  - Occasional intraosseous examples
- Multicentric form
  - Dermis, subcutaneous tissue, muscle, bones
  - Also visceral sites (gastrointestinal tract, lung, heart, others)

Presentation

- Small, painless growth
  - Superficial nodules may appear purple, clinically simulating hemangioma
  - Larger tumors may ulcerate overlying epidermis

Treatment

- Both nonvisceral solitary and multicentric forms often spontaneously regress
- Simple conservative excision

Prognosis

- All forms are benign
- Excellent prognosis in solitary and multicentric forms without visceral organ involvement
  - Solitary form recurrence rate ~ 10%
- Extensive visceral organ involvement may be fatal in infants and young children

MACROSCOPIC

Size

- Usually small (1-5 cm)

MICROSCOPIC

Histologic Features

- Most lesions are well marginated
  - Can be locally infiltrative and with intravascular growth
- Classic biphasic pattern
  - Myoid nodules separated by cellular zones of ovoid cells with pericytomatous (hemangiopericytoma-like) vascular pattern
  - Variable amounts of each component (vascular zones more prominent in children and less so in adults)
- Myoid nodules
  - More common at periphery of tumor
  - Bland spindle cells with pale eosinophilic cytoplasm and elongated nuclei arranged in short fascicles or whorls
  - Myxoid change or hyalinization
  - Absence of nuclear pleomorphism
- Cellular hemangiopericytoma-like vascular zones
  - Round to ovoid cells without nuclear pleomorphism
  - Prominent small, irregular vascular spaces
  - May contain area of coagulative necrosis or hemorrhage
- Hypercellular variant
  - Overall higher cellularity with long fascicle formation
  - Hemangiopericytoma-like vascular component often minimal or absent
- Mitotic rate is generally low

ANCILLARY TESTS

Immunohistochemistry

- Smooth muscle actin (+)
- Desmin, caldesmon, CD34, S100 protein, keratins, STAT6 (-)

Genetic Testing

- *PDGFRB* gene alterations

DIFFERENTIAL DIAGNOSIS

Leiomyoma

- Perpendicularly oriented fascicles of pink spindled cells
- Lacks hemangiopericytoma-like zones

Fibromatosis

- Highly infiltrative growth pattern
- Prominent stromal collagen
- Nuclear β-catenin expression in 70%

Nodular Fasciitis

- Rare in infants
- Often very myxoid; lacks hemangiopericytoma-like areas

Infantile Fibrosarcoma

- Often large mass in extremity of newborns/infants
- t(12;15)(p13;q25) with *ETV6-NTRK3* fusion

SELECTED REFERENCES

1. Agaimy A et al: Recurrent somatic PDGFRB mutations in sporadic infantile/solitary adult myofibromas but not in angioleiomyomas and myopericytomas. Am J Surg Pathol. 41(2):195-203, 2017
2. Arts FA et al: PDGFRB gain-of-function mutations in sporadic infantile myofibromatosis. Hum Mol Genet. 26(10):1801-1810, 2017
3. Linos K et al: Myofibromas with atypical features: expanding the morphologic spectrum of a benign entity. Am J Surg Pathol. 38(12):1649-54, 2014
4. Oudijk L et al: Solitary, multifocal and generalized myofibromas: clinicopathological and immunohistochemical features of 114 cases. Histopathology. 60(6B):E1-11, 2012
5. Granter SR et al: Myofibromatosis in adults, glomangiopericytoma, and myopericytoma: a spectrum of tumors showing perivascular myoid differentiation. Am J Surg Pathol. 22(5):513-25, 1998

(Left) *In the vascular zones of myofibroma, the tumor cells are smaller and more primitive-appearing, and the overall cellularity is higher than the myoid areas. In occasional tumors, where the vessels are not as prominent, this cellularity may be alarming and lead to consideration of a sarcoma.* **(Right)** *In some areas, the appearance of plump eosinophilic cells forming bundles and short fascicles closely resembles smooth muscle tissue, particularly if the fascicles are cut in cross section.*

Cellular Vascular Zones

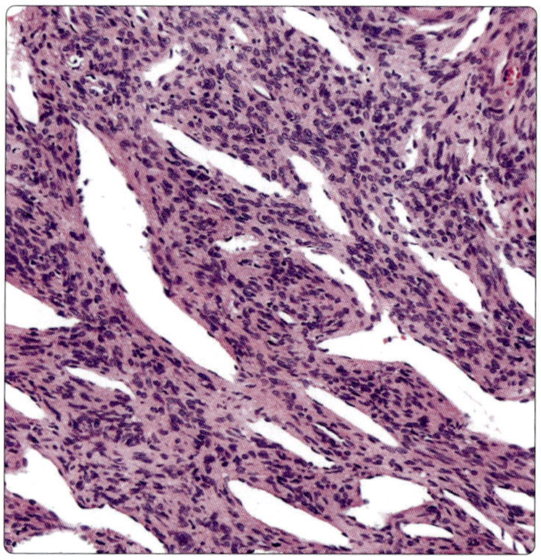

Myoid Morphology

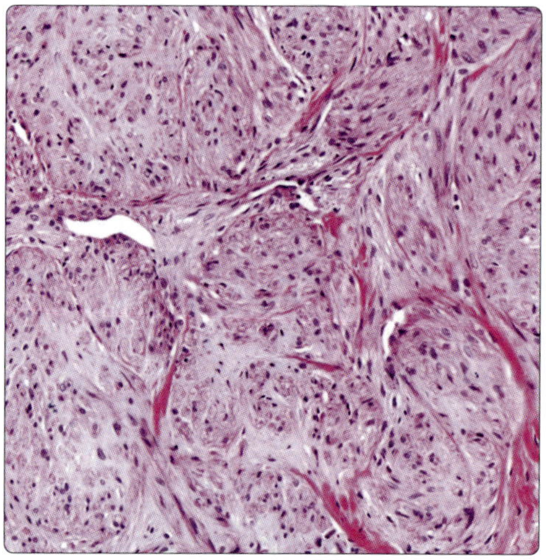

(Left) *In some cases, the myoid zones are paucicellular and contain a chronic inflammatory infiltrate, resembling a reactive myofibroblastic process. Identification of a low-power nodular growth pattern or presence of a pericytomatous vascular component is helpful.* **(Right)** *Stromal collagen and hyalinization are seen in some cases of myofibroma and may be present in either zone.*

Myoid Zones

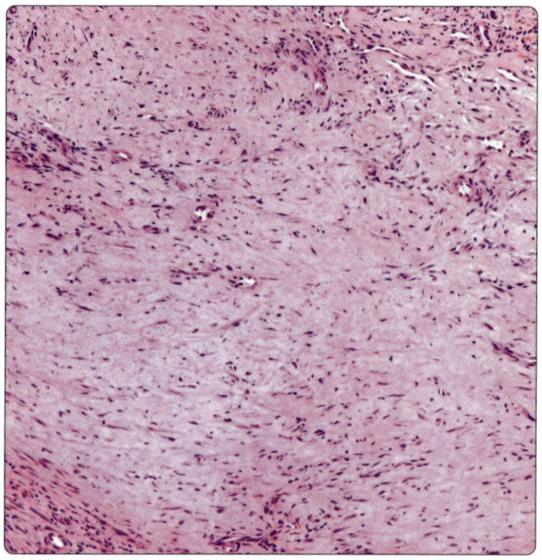

Stromal Hyalinization

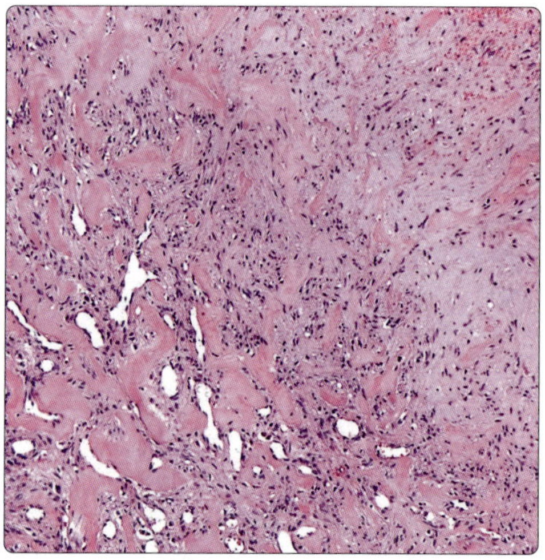

(Left) *Myoid zones may show extensive stromal hyalinization. When these areas are larger, it may be difficult to recognize the lesion as a myofibroma, particularly if a more cellular pericytomatous component is inconspicuous or absent.* **(Right)** *The lesional cells of myofibroma commonly express smooth muscle actin and are almost always negative for desmin, in contrast to benign smooth muscle tumors.*

Stromal Hyalinization

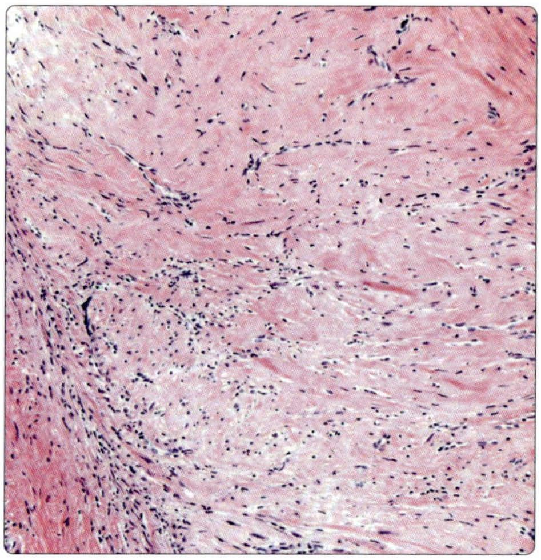

Smooth Muscle Actin

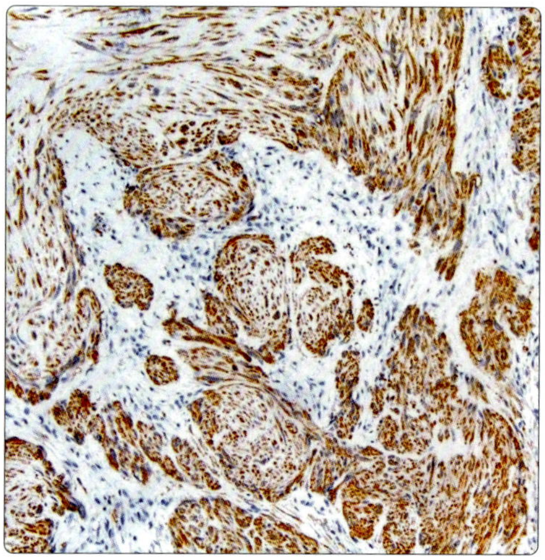

Multinucleated Giant Cells

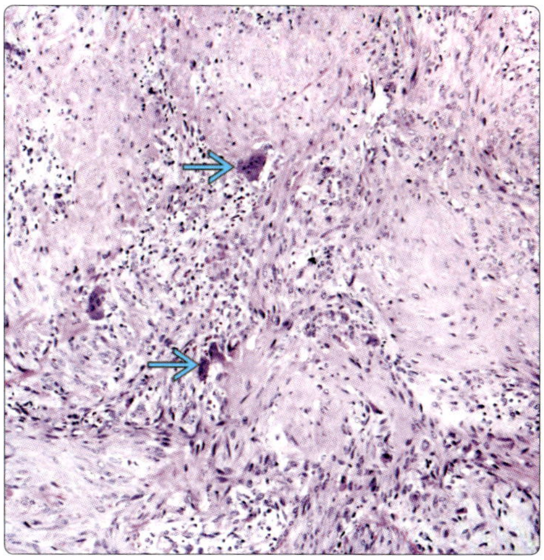

Necrosis

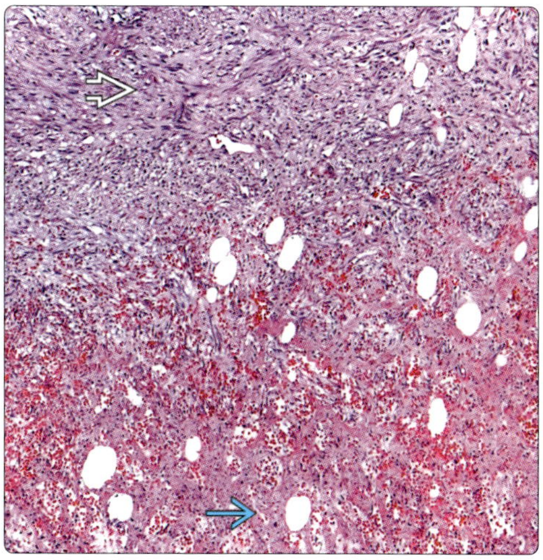

(Left) *Multinucleated giant cells ➡ are rarely seen in myofibroma but are more likely to be seen in intraosseous cases. When present in soft tissue lesions, a diagnosis of nodular fasciitis may be considered.* **(Right)** *Coagulative necrosis ➡ may be seen in some cases of myofibroma and is usually localized to the cellular vascular component, particularly when prominent and centrally located. Hemorrhage and calcification may also be seen. Note the peripheral myoid area ⇨.*

Prominent Vascularity

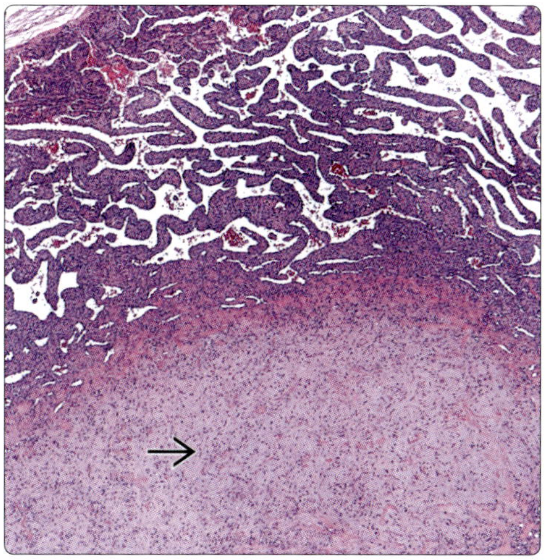

Vascular Intimal Involvement

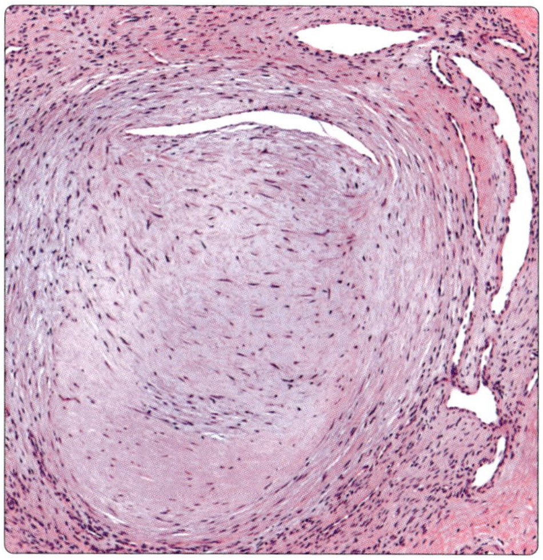

(Left) *Myofibroma is currently thought to be related to other pericytic tumors, such as myopericytoma, glomus tumor, and angioleiomyoma, and may show overlapping features with 1 or more of these entities. Tumors with a conspicuous myoid component → are probably best classified as myofibroma.* **(Right)** *Intimal involvement of peripheral blood vessels is not uncommon in myofibroma and appears to have no significant prognostic importance. This finding is also commonly seen in myopericytoma.*

Increased Cellularity

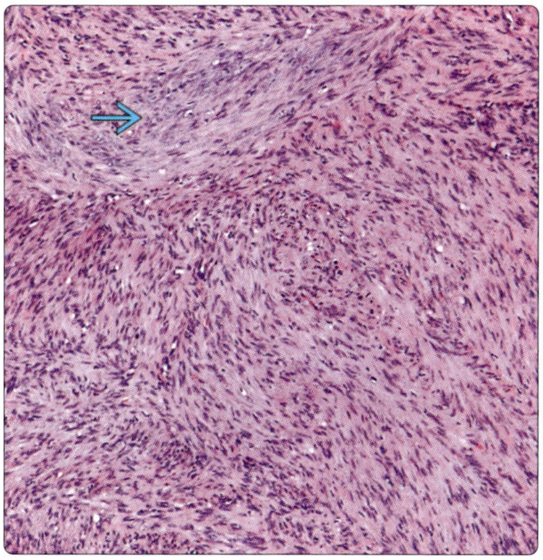

Hypercellularity

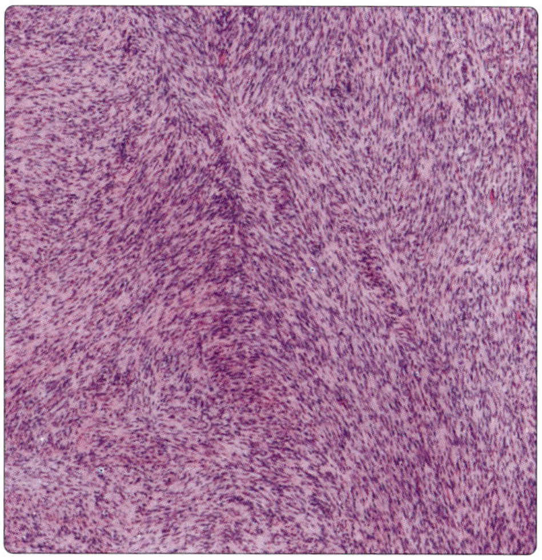

(Left) *Rare cases of myofibroma show a relatively significant increase in cellularity and may mimic a sarcoma. Most of these cases, however, show myoid nodule ➡ formation, at least focally. Despite the cellularity, significant nuclear atypia is not seen.* **(Right)** *Prominent fascicular growth may be seen in hypercellular regions of myofibroma. In these cases, a variety of spindle cell sarcomas, such as infantile fibrosarcoma and spindle cell rhabdomyosarcoma, must be diligently excluded first.*

Angioleiomyoma

KEY FACTS

TERMINOLOGY

- Benign, well-circumscribed neoplasm composed of mature smooth muscle cells arranged around prominent blood vessels
- Synonyms: Vascular leiomyoma, angiomyoma

CLINICAL ISSUES

- Wide range (40-70 years most common)
- Upper and lower extremities (most common in lower leg)
- Usually small, solitary, subcutaneous nodule
  - More than 50% are painful
- Treatment: Simple, conservative excision
- Excellent prognosis; very rarely recurs

MACROSCOPIC

- Usually < 2 cm

MICROSCOPIC

- Sharp circumscription
- 3 types described: Solid (most common), venous, and cavernous
- Well-differentiated smooth muscle component
- Prominent component of medium- to large-sized blood vessels with dilated or compressed lumina
  - Smooth muscle cells can show concentric, perivascular accentuation in some cases
- No significant nuclear atypia or mitotic activity
- Mature adipose tissue, stromal hyalinization, myxoid changes, or calcification may be present

ANCILLARY TESTS

- Strong, diffuse SMA(+) and h-caldesmon (+)
- Desmin (+) but varies in extent

TOP DIFFERENTIAL DIAGNOSES

- Myopericytoma
- Hemangioma
- PEComa

Angioleiomyoma

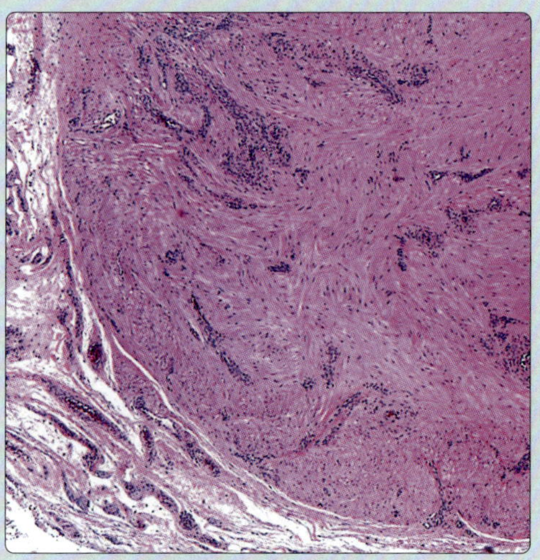

Perivascular Growth

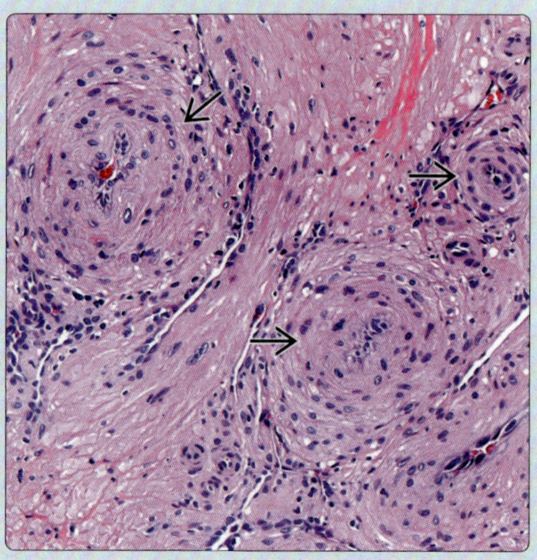

(Left) *Angioleiomyoma is a small, sharply circumscribed smooth muscle neoplasm containing a prominent component of stromal blood vessels. These vessels vary in size and may be compressed (solid variant, shown) or markedly dilated/ectatic (venous and cavernous variants).* **(Right)** *Perivascular arrangement* → *of the lesional smooth muscle cells is a common finding in angioleiomyoma and creates morphologic overlap with myopericytoma. This finding, however, may be focal or absent in some cases.*

Mature Smooth Muscle Cells

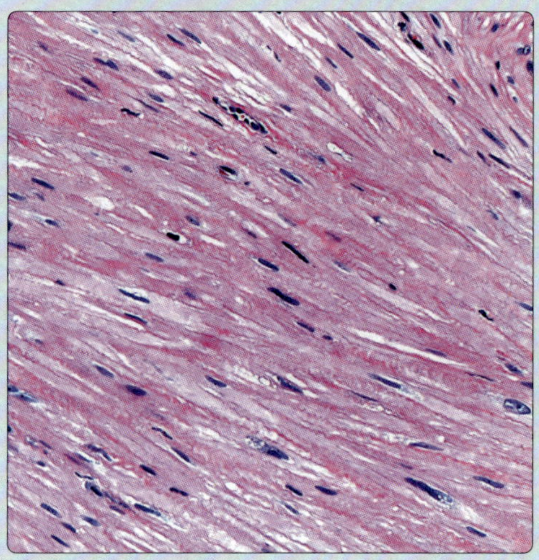

Cavernous Morphology

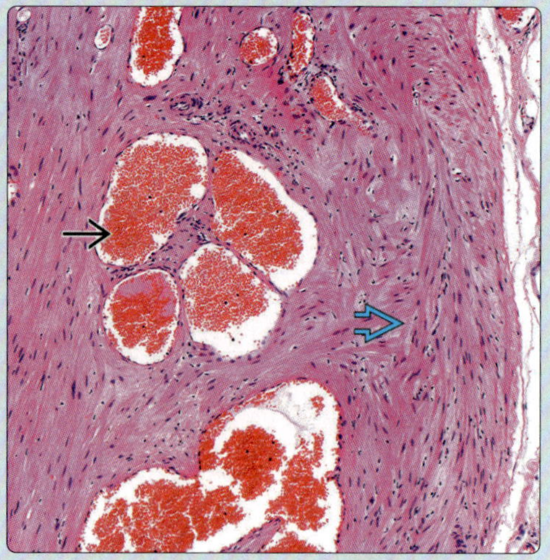

(Left) *The well-differentiated smooth muscle cells of angioleiomyoma show classic cytologic features, including prominent eosinophilic cytoplasm and elongated, blunt, cigar-shaped nuclei. They are also typically arranged in bundles and fascicles, as seen in other smooth muscle neoplasms.* **(Right)** *The cavernous type of angioleiomyoma has thin-walled, dilated vascular channels* → *arranged in small clusters within a stroma composed of smooth muscle fibers* ⇨ *that form branching fascicles.*

Angioleiomyoma

TERMINOLOGY

Synonyms

- Vascular leiomyoma
- Angiomyoma

Definitions

- Benign, well-circumscribed neoplasm composed of mature smooth muscle cells arranged around prominent blood vessels
  - Now classified as tumor of pericytic (perivascular) origin (2013 WHO Classification)
  - Considered to exist on morphologic spectrum with myopericytoma

CLINICAL ISSUES

Epidemiology

- Age
  - Wide range (40-70 years most common)
- Sex
  - Male predominance in upper extremity
  - Female predominance in lower extremity

Site

- Upper and lower extremities (most common in lower leg)
- Head and neck (particularly oral cavity, lip, palate)
- Rare on trunk

Presentation

- Usually small, solitary, subcutaneous nodule
- Often slow growing
- More than 50% are painful
  - May be exacerbated by pregnancy, menses, or change in temperature

Treatment

- Simple, conservative excision

Prognosis

- Excellent
- Recurrences very rare

MACROSCOPIC

General Features

- Small, well circumscribed
- White, rubbery cut surface
  - Calcified examples may be gritty

Size

- Usually < 2 cm

MICROSCOPIC

Histologic Features

- Sharp circumscription
- 3 morphologic forms described
  - Solid type (most common)
    - Bundles and fascicles of spindled, well-differentiated smooth muscle cells
    - Intervening compressed, slit-like vessels
  - Venous type
    - Mature smooth muscle arranged around dilated, thick-walled vascular channels
      - Smooth muscle cells often show concentric, perivascular accentuation
  - Cavernous type (least common)
    - Resembles cavernous hemangioma
    - Intervascular septa contain smooth muscle cells
- Occasional cases show some morphologic overlap with myopericytoma
- No significant nuclear atypia or mitotic activity
  - Focal (likely degenerative) atypia may be present in older lesions
- Mature adipose tissue, stromal hyalinization, or myxoid changes may be present
- Calcification is more common in older lesions
- Small nerve twigs are occasionally identifiable within or at periphery of lesion

ANCILLARY TESTS

Immunohistochemistry

- Strong, diffuse SMA(+) and h-caldesmon (+)
- Desmin (+) but varies in extent
- Negative for HMB-45

DIFFERENTIAL DIAGNOSIS

Myopericytoma

- May show morphologic overlap with angioleiomyoma
- Prominent perivascular growth
- Lesional cells lack mature smooth muscle cytomorphology
- SMA(+), desmin (-)

Hemangioma

- Vascular (capillary or cavernous) channels are numerous
- Lacks prominent intervascular smooth muscle cell proliferation

PEComa (a.k.a. Perivascular Epithelioid Cell Tumor)

- Tumor cell cytoplasm varies from eosinophilic to clear
- Variably sclerotic stroma
- May contain fat (angiomyolipoma)
- Most coexpress SMA and melanocytic markers (HMB-45, MART-1, etc.)

SELECTED REFERENCES

1. Rawal SY et al: Angioleiomyoma (vascular leiomyoma) of the oral cavity. Head Neck Pathol. 12(1):123-126, 2018
2. Marco VS et al: Acral angioleiomyoma with tumoral calcinosis: a complication of the insertional Achilles tendinopathy. J Cutan Pathol. ePub, 2017
3. Agaimy A et al: Angioleiomyoma of the sinonasal tract: analysis of 16 cases and review of the literature. Head Neck Pathol. 9(4):463-73, 2015
4. Liu Y et al: Angioleiomyomas in the head and neck: a retrospective clinical and immunohistochemical analysis. Oncol Lett. 8(1):241-247, 2014
5. Houdek MT et al: Angioleiomyoma of the upper extremity. J Hand Surg Am. 38(8):1579-83, 2013
6. Matsuyama A et al: Angioleiomyoma: a clinicopathologic and immunohistochemical reappraisal with special reference to the correlation with myopericytoma. Hum Pathol. 38(4):645-51, 2007
7. Fox SB et al: Angioleiomyomas: an immunohistological study. Histopathology. 16(5):495-6, 1990
8. Hachisuga T et al: Angioleiomyoma. A clinicopathologic reappraisal of 562 cases. Cancer. 54(1):126-30, 1984

SECTION 9

Tumors of Skeletal Muscle

Benign

Focal Myositis 370
Adult Rhabdomyoma 372
Fetal Rhabdomyoma 374
Genital Rhabdomyoma 376
Cardiac Rhabdomyoma 378

Malignant

Embryonal Rhabdomyosarcoma 380
Alveolar Rhabdomyosarcoma 386
Spindle Cell Rhabdomyosarcoma 392
Sclerosing Rhabdomyosarcoma 396
Pleomorphic Rhabdomyosarcoma 400
Epithelioid Rhabdomyosarcoma 404

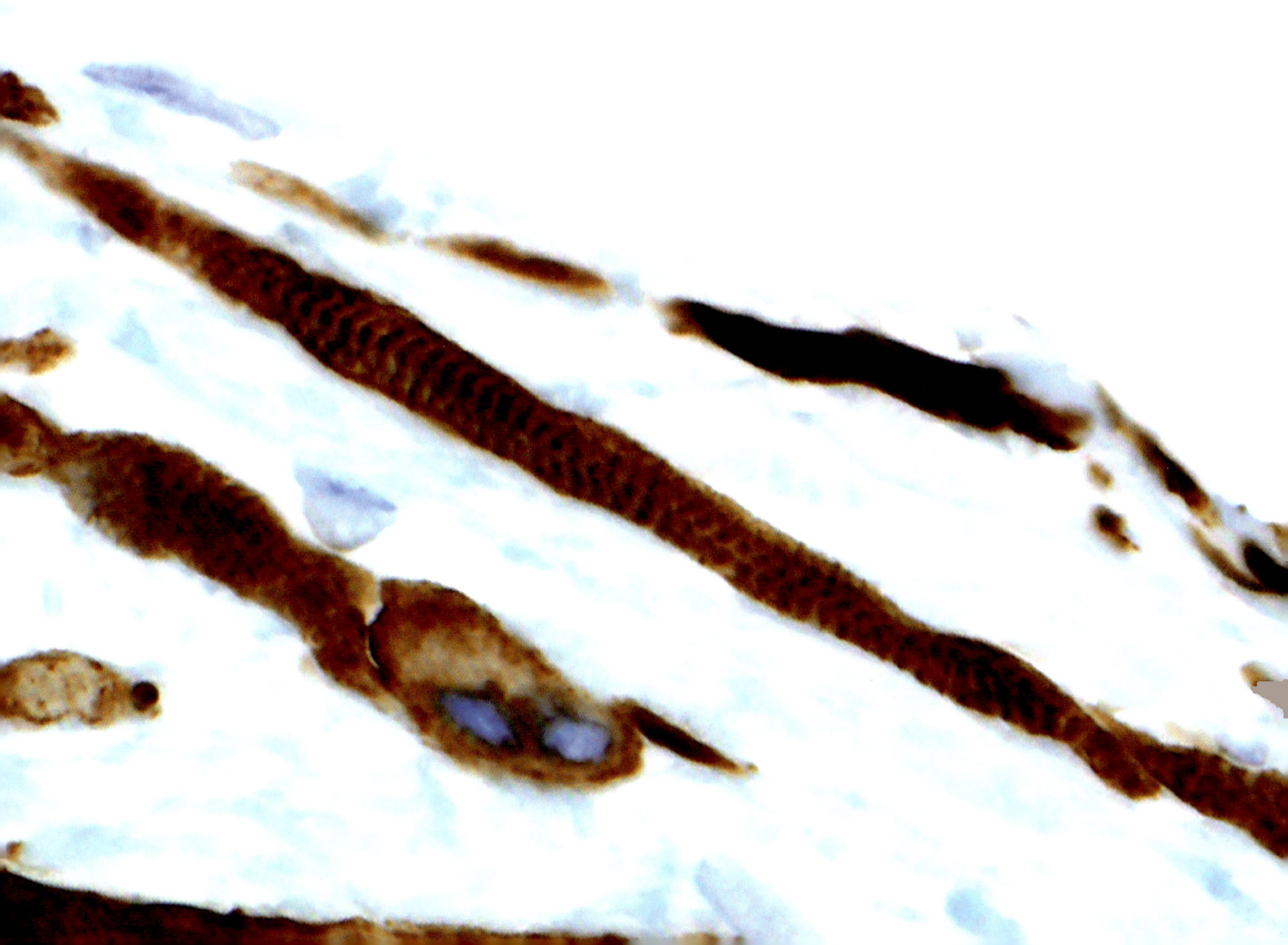

Focal Myositis

KEY FACTS

TERMINOLOGY

- Benign self-limiting, intramuscular inflammatory pseudotumor

CLINICAL ISSUES

- Wide range (median: 36 years)
- Single muscle involvement is typical
- Limbs most common site, especially lower extremities
- Rapidly appearing and growing mass
  - Generally asymptomatic
  - Weakness is rare, and joint involvement is not present
- Treatment usually not required
  - Many cases spontaneously regress
- Excellent prognosis

MACROSCOPIC

- Between 1-20 cm in size (median: 3 cm)

MICROSCOPIC

- Skeletal muscle with marked variation in size of individual myocytes
- Dense fibrosis common (endomysial more prominent than perimysial)
- Chronic inflammatory infiltrate, particularly lymphocytes
- Regenerative myocytes with basophilic cytoplasm and large vesicular nuclei with nucleoli
- Focal denervation changes
- Variable fatty replacement of muscle
- No atypia, calcification, or ossification

TOP DIFFERENTIAL DIAGNOSES

- True inflammatory myopathies
- Proliferative myositis
- Lymphoma
- Myositis ossificans
- Inflammatory myofibroblastic tumor

Focal Myositis

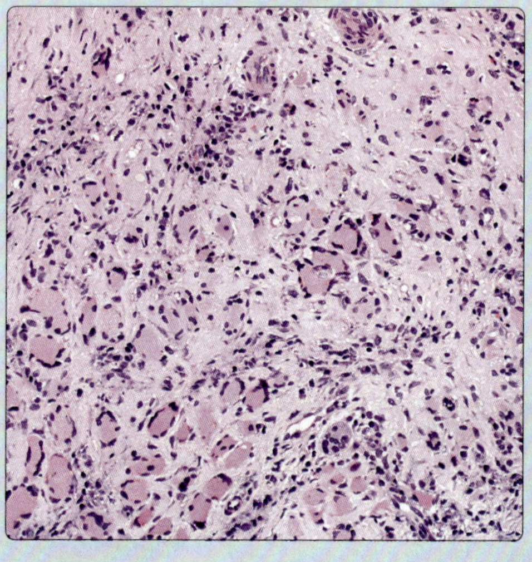

Focal Myositis

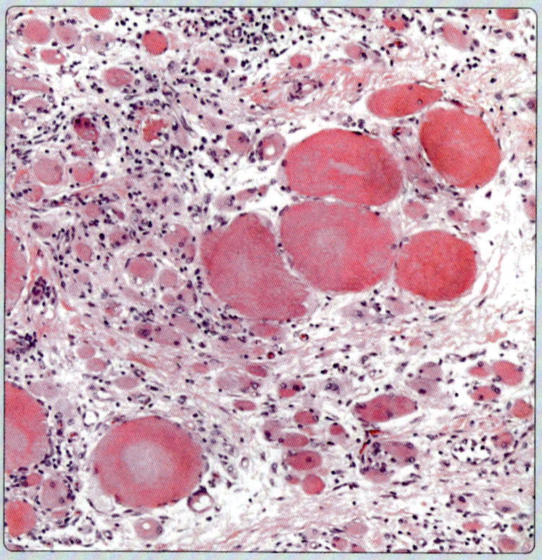

(Left) *Focal myositis is a benign, nonneoplastic inflammatory pseudotumor that classically arises as a rapidly growing, solitary mass affecting 1 muscle. Histologically, it is characterized in most cases by skeletal muscle with variable inflammation, fibrosis, and myopathic/neurogenic changes.* **(Right)** *Variation in size of myocytes is a common finding in focal myositis, and it is not unusual to see hypertrophic fibers immediately adjacent to small- or normal-sized ones.*

Inflammatory Component

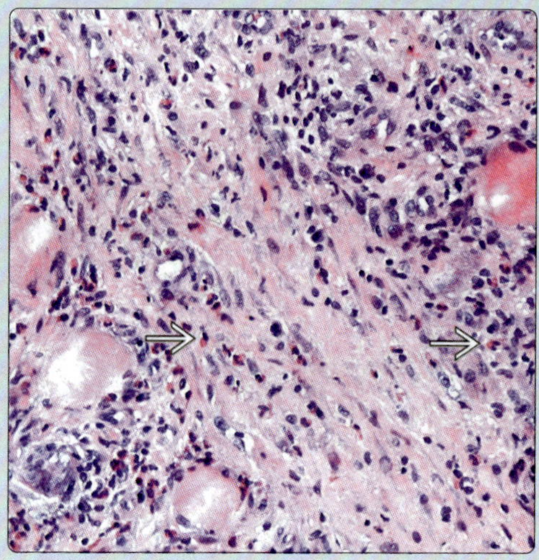

Endomysial Fibrosis

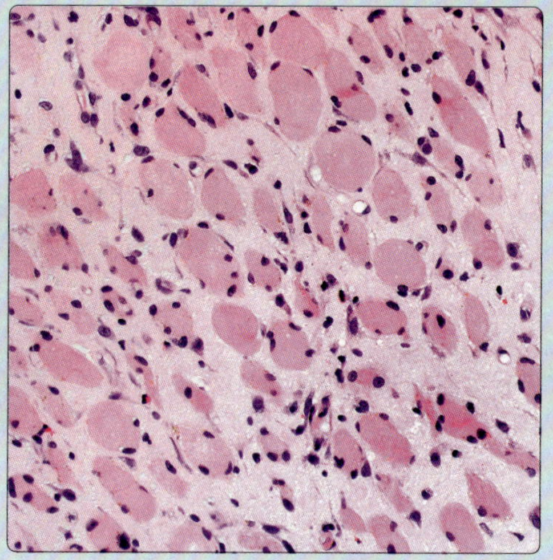

(Left) *Chronic inflammatory cells are seen in the vast majority of cases of focal myositis, with lymphocytes generally dominating the distribution. Plasma cells, histiocytes, and eosinophils ➡ may also be seen.* **(Right)** *Fibrosis is a common finding in focal myositis and tends to predominate in the endomysium, separating individual myofibers.*

Focal Myositis

TERMINOLOGY

Definitions

- Benign self-limiting, intramuscular inflammatory pseudotumor

ETIOLOGY/PATHOGENESIS

Idiopathic

- Exact cause(s) uncertain
- Some cases may be related to previous trauma
- Infectious etiologies and relationship to transient autoimmune disease have been suggested

CLINICAL ISSUES

Epidemiology

- Incidence
  - Uncommon
- Age
  - Wide range (median: 36 years)

Site

- Single muscle involvement
- Limbs most common, especially lower extremities
  - Particularly gastrocnemius and vastus lateralis
- Also head/neck, trunk, other

Presentation

- Rapidly appearing and growing mass
- Generally asymptomatic
  - Most are painless
- Weakness is rare, and joint involvement is not present

Treatment

- None required
  - Surgery is generally not indicated

Prognosis

- Excellent
- Most cases regress over time
  - Rare cases recur

MACROSCOPIC

General Features

- Ovoid, unencapsulated, firm mass
- No involvement of tendons, fascia, or subcutaneous fat

Size

- Between 1-20 cm (median: 3 cm)

MICROSCOPIC

Histologic Features

- Skeletal muscle with marked variation in size of individual myocytes
- Fibrosis common (endomysial more prominent than perimysial)
  - Dense fibrosis in older lesions
- Regenerative myocytes with basophilic cytoplasm and large vesicular nuclei with nucleoli
- Patchy necrosis of single myofibers may be seen
- Chronic inflammatory infiltrate common
  - Mainly lymphocytes
  - Plasma cells, histiocytes, and eosinophils are less common
- Focal denervation changes
  - Axonal swelling, demyelination, endoneurial fibrosis
- Variable fatty replacement of muscle
- No atypia, calcification, or ossification

DIFFERENTIAL DIAGNOSIS

True Inflammatory Myopathies

- Polymyositis, dermatomyositis, inclusion body myositis
- Typical presentation: Progressive weakness on both sides of body
  - Proximal muscles often affected 1st
- Only rare reported cases of solitary mass-like involvement
- Histologic overlap with focal myositis is common

Proliferative Myositis

- Checkerboard pattern, less muscle fiber damage
- Ganglion cell-like myofibroblasts characteristic
  - Not feature of focal myositis

Lymphoma

- Sheet-like growth of atypical lymphocytes
- B- or T-cell clonality present

Myositis Ossificans

- Shows central fasciitis-like morphology and evidence of woven bone formation with maturation
- No intratumoral damaged muscle fibers

Inflammatory Myofibroblastic Tumor

- Spindled myofibroblasts with prominent stromal inflammatory infiltrate, particularly plasma cells
- Lacks myopathic and neurogenic changes
- ALK(+) in 50% of cases

Rhabdomyoma

- Involvement of extremities rare
- Sheets of large polygonal eosinophilic cells with nucleoli
- Fibrosis and chronic inflammation are not typical features

SELECTED REFERENCES

1. Gallay L et al: Focal myositis: new insights on diagnosis and pathology. Neurology. ePub, 2018
2. Auerbach A et al: Focal myositis: a clinicopathologic study of 115 cases of an intramuscular mass-like reactive process. Am J Surg Pathol. 33(7):1016-24, 2009
3. Georgalas C et al: Inflammatory focal myositis of the sternomastoid muscle: is there an absolute indication for biopsy? A case report and review of the literature. Eur Arch Otorhinolaryngol. 263(2):149-51, 2006
4. Smith AG et al: Clinical and pathologic features of focal myositis. Muscle Nerve. 23(10):1569-75, 2000
5. Moskovic E et al: Benign mimics of soft tissue sarcomas. Clin Radiol. 46(4):248-52, 1992
6. Moskovic E et al: Focal myositis, a benign inflammatory pseudotumour: CT appearances. Br J Radiol. 64(762):489-93, 1991
7. Vercelli-Retta J et al: Focal myositis and its differential diagnosis. A case report and review of the literature. Ann Pathol. 8(1):54-6, 1988
8. Heffner RR Jr et al: Denervating changes in focal myositis, a benign inflammatory pseudotumor. Arch Pathol Lab Med. 104(5):261-4, 1980
9. Heffner RR Jr et al: Focal myositis. Cancer. 40(1):301-6, 1977

Adult Rhabdomyoma

KEY FACTS

TERMINOLOGY

- Extracardiac lobular neoplasm composed of polygonal, differentiated skeletal muscle cells

CLINICAL ISSUES

- Usually adults (mean age: 50 years)
- Predilection for men (4:1)
- Predominantly head and neck region
- Solitary, painless, slow-growing mass
- Treatment: Surgical excision
- Benign but local recurrence in up to 40%

MACROSCOPIC

- Well-circumscribed, lobulated red/brown/gray mass
- 1-10 cm (median: 3 cm)

MICROSCOPIC

- Sheets and large nests of large, polygonal tumor cells with granular eosinophilic or vacuolated cytoplasm
    - Scattered "spider cells" may be seen
- Cytoplasmic cross striations &/or rod-like crystalline structures may be identified
- Mitotic figures and necrosis are not seen

ANCILLARY TESTS

- Strongly PAS(+) but diastase resistant
- Positive for diffuse desmin, myogenin, and MYOD1
- Negative for keratin, CD68, CD163, TFE3, synaptophysin, and chromogranin

TOP DIFFERENTIAL DIAGNOSES

- Cardiac rhabdomyoma
- Granular cell tumor
- Alveolar soft part sarcoma
- Hibernoma
- Crystal-storing histiocytosis
- Paraganglioma

Adult Rhabdomyoma

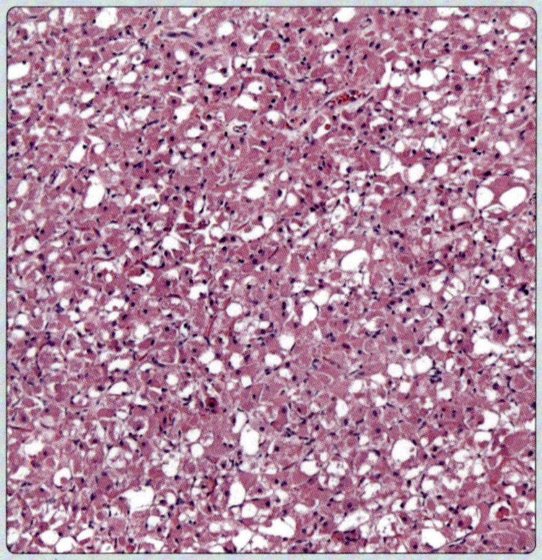

Fine Capillary Network

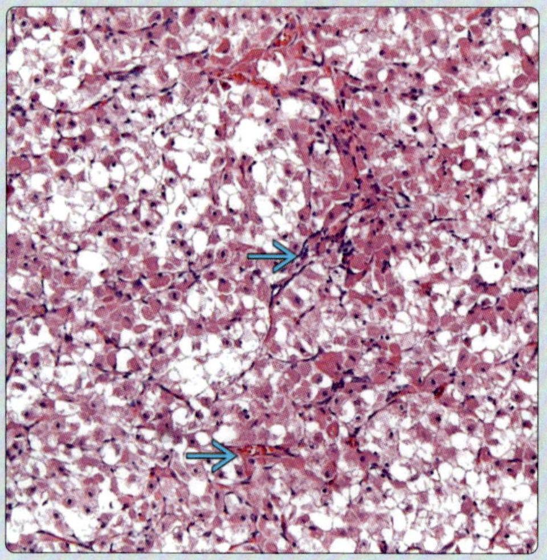

(Left) *Adult rhabdomyoma is a benign tumor of differentiated skeletal muscle cells that typically occurs in the head and neck region of adults. It is composed of sheets and lobules of eosinophilic and clear, vacuolated cells.* **(Right)** *Adult rhabdomyoma also contains a fine capillary network →, which may impart an overall nested appearance reminiscent of alveolar soft part sarcoma or a high-grade clear cell renal cell carcinoma.*

Eosinophilic Polygonal Cells

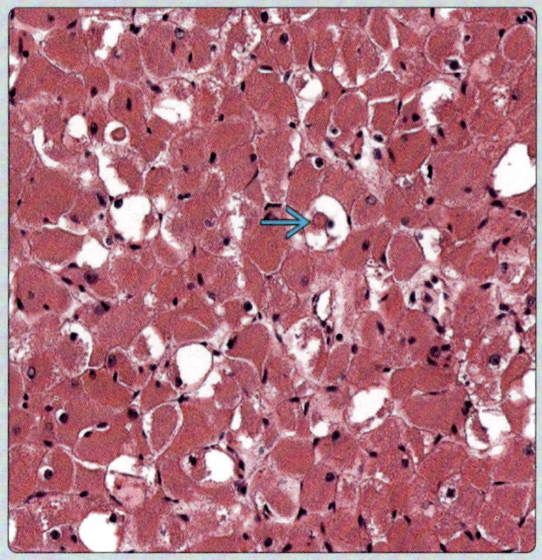

Cross Striations and Inclusions

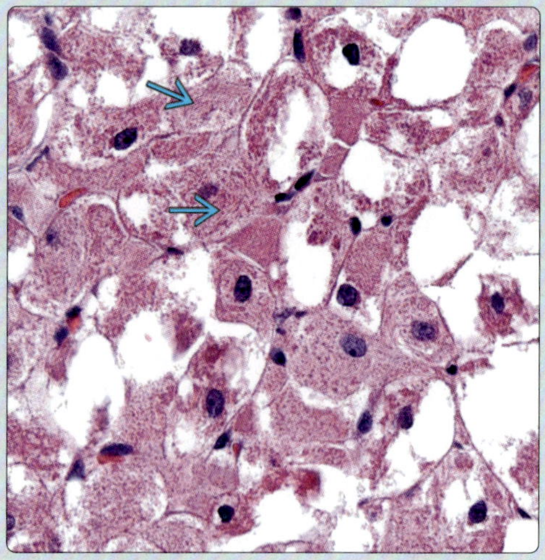

(Left) *In most cases of adult rhabdomyoma, the predominant tumor cell is large and polygonal and contains prominent eosinophilic cytoplasm. Tumor cells may also contain cytoplasmic vacuolizations and appear completely clear or demonstrate a retracted "spider cell" morphology →.* **(Right)** *Cytoplasmic cross striations → or rod-like inclusions may be seen in scattered tumor cells in adult rhabdomyoma. Tumor cells also commonly show prominent nucleoli.*

TERMINOLOGY

Definitions

- Extracardiac lobular neoplasm composed of polygonal, differentiated skeletal muscle cells

CLINICAL ISSUES

Epidemiology

- Incidence
  - Rare but most common type of extracardiac rhabdomyoma
- Age
  - Usually adults (mean age: 50 years)
    - Rare cases reported in children
- Sex
  - Predilection for men (4:1)

Site

- Predominantly head and neck region
  - Particularly in region of pharynx, larynx, base of tongue, and floor of mouth
- Rare cases reported all over body

Presentation

- Solitary, painless, slow-growing mass
  - Minority of cases (20%) are multifocal, usually in neck
- Hoarseness or symptoms related to airway obstruction may be present

Treatment

- Surgical excision

Prognosis

- Benign
- Local recurrence in up to 40%
  - May recur multiple times or many years after initial excision
- Spontaneous regression has not been reported

MACROSCOPIC

General Features

- Well-circumscribed, lobulated mass
  - May be pedunculated
- Red/brown/gray coloration

Size

- 1-10 cm (median: 3 cm)

MICROSCOPIC

Histologic Features

- Sheets and large nests of large, polygonal tumor cells
  - Most cells have finely granular eosinophilic cytoplasm
  - Subset of cells have cytoplasmic vacuolizations and appear optically clear
    - Cells with retracted cytoplasm ("spider cells") may be seen
- 1 or 2 central or peripherally located nuclei, often with prominent nucleoli
- Cytoplasmic cross striations &/or rod-like inclusions may be identified
- Mitotic figures and necrosis are not seen
- Fine stromal capillary vascular network

ANCILLARY TESTS

Histochemistry

- Strong PAS staining that is diastase sensitive (due to prominent intracytoplasmic glycogen)

Immunohistochemistry

- Positive for diffuse desmin, myogenin, and MYOD1
- S100 protein and SMA may be focally (+) but not diffuse
- Negative for keratin, CD68, CD163, pax-8, TFE3, synaptophysin, and chromogranin

DIFFERENTIAL DIAGNOSIS

Cardiac Rhabdomyoma

- Usually occurs in association with tuberous sclerosis
- Most tumor cells are vacuolated, and spider cells are common

Granular Cell Tumor

- Lacks cytoplasmic vacuolizations
- Diffuse PAS(+) but diastase resistant (phagolysosomes)
- Diffuse S100 protein (+)

Alveolar Soft Part Sarcoma

- Large tumors, usually with prominent nested architecture
- Nuclear TFE3(+), desmin (-), myogenin (-)
- Presence of t(X;17) unbalanced translocation

Hibernoma

- Eosinophilic cells containing numerous tiny intracytoplasmic lipid vacuoles
- Often show obvious component of adipocytic differentiation
- Desmin (-), myogenin (-)

Crystal-Storing Histiocytosis

- Lesional cells are histiocytes, not myocytes
- Accompanying lymphoplasmacytic infiltrate is typically clonal/neoplastic
- CD68(+), CD163(+), desmin (-), myogenin (-)

Paraganglioma

- Prominent nested or organoid growth
- Synaptophysin (+), desmin (-), myogenin (-)

SELECTED REFERENCES

1. Dermawan JK et al: Cytologic findings of an adult rhabdomyoma in the parapharyngeal space: a report of a case and review of the literature. Diagn Cytopathol. 46(5):419-24, 2018
2. Altissimi G et al: Adult-type rhabdomyoma of the larynx: clinicopathologic study of an uncommon tumor in a rare location. Case Rep Otolaryngol. 2017:7186768, 2017
3. Zhang GZ et al: Intraoral multifocal and multinodular adult rhabdomyoma: report of a case. J Oral Maxillofac Surg. 70(10):2480-5, 2012
4. Hansen T et al: Rhabdomyoma of the head and neck: morphology and differential diagnosis. Virchows Arch. 447(5):849-54, 2005
5. Willis J et al: Extracardiac rhabdomyomas. Semin Diagn Pathol. 11(1):15-25, 1994
6. Kapadia SB et al: Adult rhabdomyoma of the head and neck: a clinicopathologic and immunophenotypic study. Hum Pathol. 24(6):608-17, 1993

Fetal Rhabdomyoma

KEY FACTS

TERMINOLOGY

- Benign rhabdomyoblastic tumor demonstrating immature skeletal muscle differentiation

ETIOLOGY/PATHOGENESIS

- Subset arise in association with nevoid basal cell carcinoma syndrome (Gorlin syndrome)

CLINICAL ISSUES

- Very rare
- Usually in children < 3 years of age
  - Male predilection
- Head and neck region most common
- Treatment: Complete surgical excision
- Excellent prognosis

MACROSCOPIC

- Well circumscribed
- Median size: 3 cm (range: 1.0-12.5 cm)

MICROSCOPIC

- Well circumscribed; infiltrative growth always absent
- Classic (myxoid) type
  - Loose bundles of eosinophilic spindled fetal myotubules
  - Prominent myxoid stroma
- Intermediate (juvenile) type
  - Greater cellularity and mitotic activity than classic type
  - Greater degree of rhabdomyoblastic differentiation
- Both types lack nuclear atypia, atypical mitoses, and necrosis

ANCILLARY TESTS

- Desmin (+), myogenin (+)

TOP DIFFERENTIAL DIAGNOSES

- Embryonal rhabdomyosarcoma
- Spindle cell rhabdomyosarcoma
- Genital rhabdomyoma

Fetal Rhabdomyoma

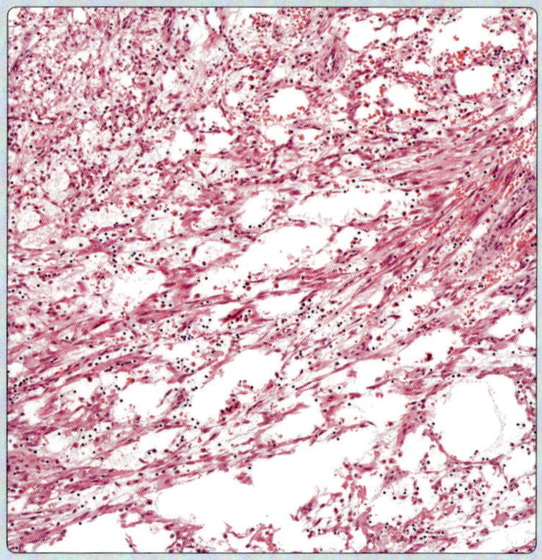

Absence of Nuclear Pleomorphism

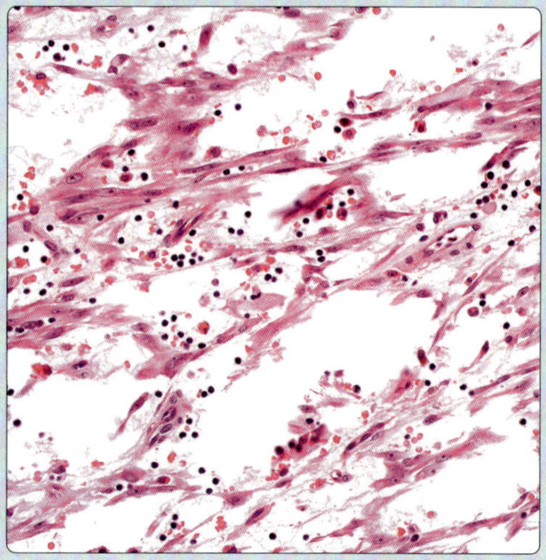

(Left) *Fetal rhabdomyoma is a well-circumscribed tumor with a predilection for arising in the head and neck region of infants and young children. It is characterized by loose bundles and fascicles of spindled eosinophilic cells within a prominent myxoid stroma.* **(Right)** *Similar to other forms of rhabdomyoma, fetal rhabdomyoma lacks significant nuclear atypia, atypical mitoses, and necrosis. These pertinent negative findings help in the distinction from rhabdomyosarcoma.*

Fetal Rhabdomyoma (Intermediate Type)

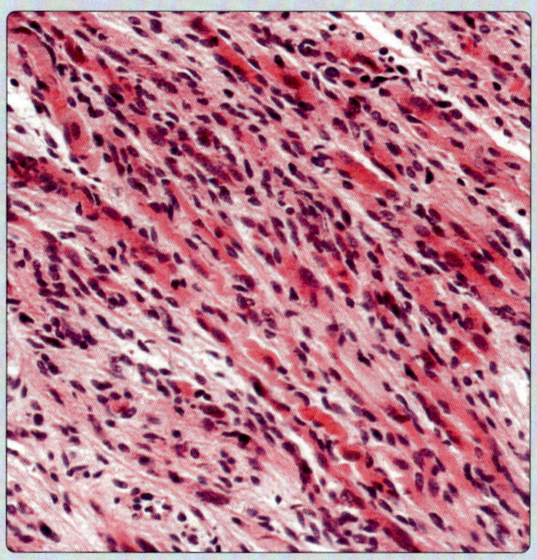

Cross Striations

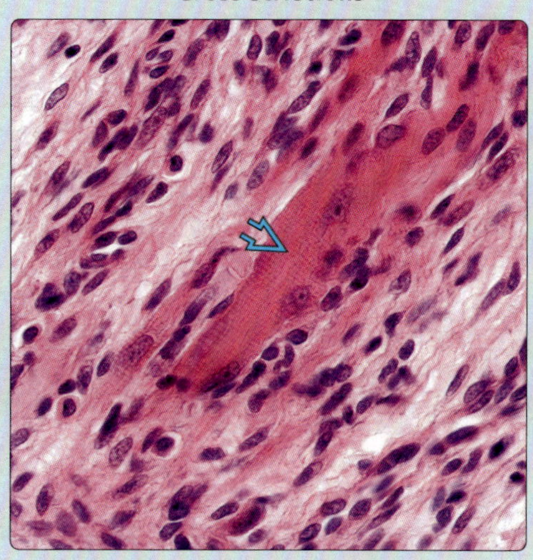

(Left) *The intermediate (or juvenile) type of fetal rhabdomyoma is more uniformly cellular than the classic type and can show increased mitotic activity. Cellular differentiation also resembles late-stage embryonic skeletal muscle. Nuclei still lack pleomorphism and there are no atypical mitoses or necrosis.* **(Right)** *Cytoplasmic cross-striations ⇨, characteristic of skeletal muscle differentiation, are apparent in some of the tumor cells in fetal rhabdomyoma.*

Fetal Rhabdomyoma

TERMINOLOGY

Definitions

- Benign rhabdomyoblastic tumor demonstrating immature skeletal muscle differentiation

ETIOLOGY/PATHOGENESIS

Genetics

- Subset arise in association with nevoid basal cell carcinoma syndrome (Gorlin syndrome)
  - *PTCH1* mutations

CLINICAL ISSUES

Epidemiology

- Incidence
  - Very rare
- Age
  - Usually in children < 3 years
    - 1/2 arise within 1st year, including congenitally
    - Overall wide range; rare in adults
- Sex
  - Male predilection

Site

- Head and neck region most common
  - Particularly postauricular area
  - Oral cavity, oropharynx, nasal cavity
- Occasionally elsewhere

Presentation

- Vast majority arise in subcutaneous tissue
- Solitary, slow-growing mass
  - Multifocal/multicentric tumors in Gorlin syndrome
- Oropharyngeal lesions may create obstructive breathing difficulties

Treatment

- Complete surgical excision

Prognosis

- Excellent prognosis
- Generally does not recur
- No metastatic potential

MACROSCOPIC

General Features

- Well circumscribed
- Sessile or polypoid in mucosal sites

Size

- Median: 3 cm (range: 1.0-12.5 cm)

MICROSCOPIC

Histologic Features

- Well circumscribed; infiltrative growth always absent
- 2 main forms
  - Classic (myxoid) type
    - Loose bundles of eosinophilic spindled fetal myotubules
    - Prominent myxoid stroma
    - Elongated rhabdomyoblasts (strap cells) with cross striations
    - No significant nuclear atypia
    - Mitotic rate usually low
  - Intermediate (juvenile) type
    - Greater cellularity and mitotic activity than classic type
    - Myxoid stroma less prominent
    - Greater degree of rhabdomyoblastic differentiation
    - May contain cells with smooth muscle differentiation
    - No significant nuclear atypia
    - Lacks atypical mitoses and necrosis

ANCILLARY TESTS

Immunohistochemistry

- Desmin (+), myogenin (+)
- May also express SMA and S100 protein
- Negative for keratin, CD68, and CD163

DIFFERENTIAL DIAGNOSIS

Embryonal Rhabdomyosarcoma

- Nuclear atypia
- Infiltrative growth; lacks circumscription
- Atypical mitoses &/or necrosis
- Cellular cambium layer in botryoid-type tumors

Spindle Cell Rhabdomyosarcoma

- Often displays cellular, prominently fascicular growth
- Nuclear atypia
- Head and neck common site in adults

Genital Rhabdomyoma

- Stroma is loose and fibrous rather than prominently myxoid
- Can show morphologic overlap with classic fetal rhabdomyoma
- Arises in genital sites rather than head and neck
- Strong female predilection

SELECTED REFERENCES

1. Thompson LD: Ear fetal rhabdomyoma. Ear Nose Throat J. 96(9):358, 2017
2. Zheng L et al: Paratesticular fetal-type rhabdomyoma in a 12-year-old boy: a case report and literature review. Urology. 82(5):1150-2, 2013
3. Fletcher DM et al: WHO Classification of Tumours of Soft Tissue and Bone. Lyon: IARC, 2013
4. Yang S et al: Mediastinal fetal rhabdomyoma in nevoid basal cell carcinoma syndrome: a case report and review of the literature. Virchows Arch. 459(2):235-8, 2011
5. Walsh SN et al: Cutaneous fetal rhabdomyoma: a case report and historical review of the literature. Am J Surg Pathol. 32(3):485-91, 2008
6. Hansen T et al: Rhabdomyoma of the head and neck: morphology and differential diagnosis. Virchows Arch. 447(5):849-54, 2005
7. Watson J et al: Nevoid basal cell carcinoma syndrome and fetal rhabdomyoma: a case study. Ear Nose Throat J. 83(10):716-8, 2004
8. Crotty PL et al: Juvenile rhabdomyoma. An intermediate form of skeletal muscle tumor in children. Arch Pathol Lab Med. 117(1):43-7, 1993
9. Kapadia SB et al: Fetal rhabdomyoma of the head and neck: a clinicopathologic and immunophenotypic study of 24 cases. Hum Pathol. 24(7):754-65, 1993
10. DiSanto S et al: Fetal rhabdomyoma and nevoid basal cell carcinoma syndrome. Pediatr Pathol. 12(3):441-7, 1992

Genital Rhabdomyoma

KEY FACTS

TERMINOLOGY
- Benign neoplasm of rhabdomyoblastic origin arising in genital tract
- Synonym: Vaginal rhabdomyoma

CLINICAL ISSUES
- Rare
- Usually adults
  - Occasionally children or adolescents
- Strong female predilection
- Females: Vagina (most common), vulva, cervix
- Males: Paratesticular region, including spermatic cord and tunica vaginalis
- Treatment: Conservative surgical excision
- Excellent prognosis
  - Generally does not recur
  - Does not metastasize

MACROSCOPIC
- Usually small (< 3 cm)

MICROSCOPIC
- Hypocellular proliferation of differentiated rhabdomyoblasts within loose fibrous stroma
  - Spindled (strap cells) or polygonal rhabdomyoblasts
- No cytologic atypia, mitoses, or necrosis
- Morphologic variant: Sclerosing rhabdomyoma

ANCILLARY TESTS
- Desmin (+), myogenin (+)
- S100 protein (-), keratin (-)

TOP DIFFERENTIAL DIAGNOSES
- Embryonal rhabdomyosarcoma
- Fetal rhabdomyoma
- Fibroepithelial stromal polyp
- Spindle cell rhabdomyosarcoma

Genital Rhabdomyoma

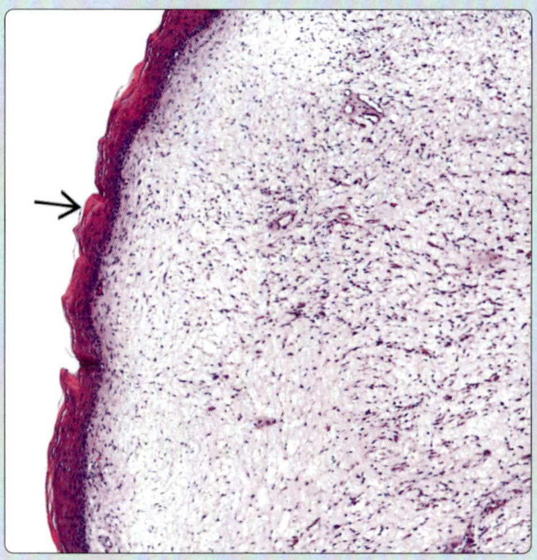

Hypocellular Proliferation

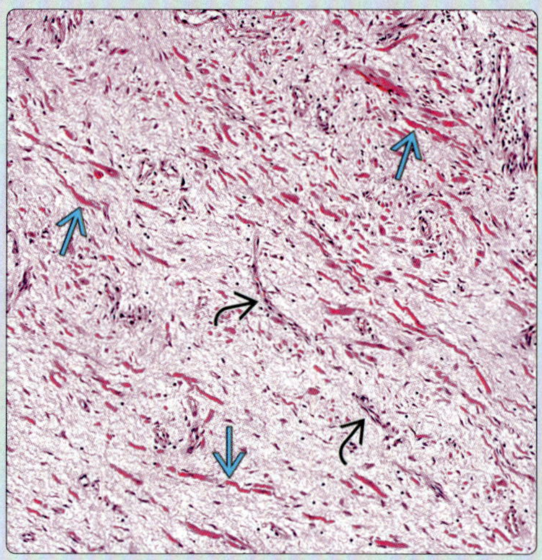

(Left) *Genital rhabdomyoma is the rarest form of rhabdomyoma. It usually arises in adult women (particularly in the vagina) but can also be seen in men and in children. In women, lesions are generally polypoid, as depicted, with overlying squamous epithelium. Note the absence of a cambium layer.* **(Right)** *Genital rhabdomyoma features a hypocellular proliferation of mature rhabdomyoblastic elements within a loose fibrous stroma. Small vessels are often conspicuous.*

Differentiated Rhabdomyoblasts

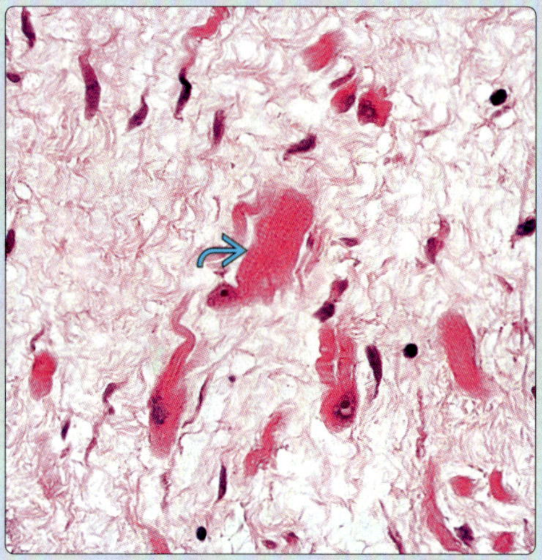

DDx: Botryoid-Type ERMS

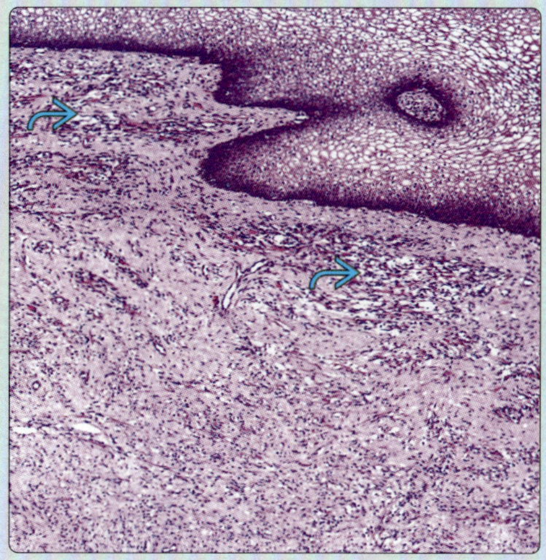

(Left) *Rhabdomyoblastic elements are well differentiated in genital rhabdomyoma and show an elongated or polygonal morphology. Cytoplasmic cross striations are common. Mitotic figures are absent.* **(Right)** *Botryoid-type ERMS may mimic genital rhabdomyoma, particularly following treatment with chemotherapy. Note however, that botryoid-type ERMS is generally more cellular and often shows a cellular, subepithelial cambium layer.*

TERMINOLOGY

Synonyms

- Vaginal rhabdomyoma

Definitions

- Benign neoplasm of rhabdomyoblastic origin arising in genital tract

CLINICAL ISSUES

Epidemiology

- Incidence
  - Rare
- Age
  - Usually adults
    - Occasionally children or adolescents
- Sex
  - Strong female predilection

Site

- Females
  - Vagina (most common)
  - Vulva
  - Cervix
- Males
  - Paratesticular region, including spermatic cord and tunica vaginalis

Presentation

- Slow growing
- Painless

Treatment

- Conservative surgical excision

Prognosis

- Excellent prognosis
- Generally does not recur
- No metastatic potential

MACROSCOPIC

General Features

- Firm, well-circumscribed, lobulated mass
- Often polypoid in females
  - Covered by mucosa

Size

- Usually small (< 3 cm)

MICROSCOPIC

Histologic Features

- Hypocellular proliferation of differentiated rhabdomyoblasts within loose fibrous stroma
  - Spindled (strap cells) or polygonal rhabdomyoblasts
- In females, lesion shows overlying squamous epithelium
- Small stromal vessels often prominent
- No cytologic atypia
- No mitoses
- No necrosis

Morphologic Variants

- Sclerosing rhabdomyoma
  - Arises in paratesticular region of young men
  - Features mature rhabdomyoblastic elements within abundant dense collagenous stroma
  - No atypia, mitoses, or necrosis

ANCILLARY TESTS

Immunohistochemistry

- Desmin (+), myogenin (+)
- S100 protein (-), keratin (-)

DIFFERENTIAL DIAGNOSIS

Embryonal Rhabdomyosarcoma

- Often forms larger lesions
- Wide range of cellularity
  - Postchemotherapy embryonal rhabdomyosarcoma (ERMS) can mimic genital rhabdomyoma
    - Hypocellular and with mature rhabdomyoblastic elements
- Cytologic atypia, mitoses, &/or necrosis
- Botryoid-type ERMS usually features cellular subepithelial layer (cambium layer)

Fetal Rhabdomyoma

- Myxoid rather than fibrous stroma
- Predilection for head and neck region
- Some cases can show morphologic overlap with genital rhabdomyoma

Fibroepithelial Stromal Polyp

- Similar clinical presentation to genital rhabdomyoma
- Lacks rhabdomyoblasts

Teratoma

- Epithelial elements common
- May contain skeletal muscle or rhabdomyoblastic elements
- In males, often intratesticular rather than paratesticular

Spindle Cell Rhabdomyosarcoma

- Paratesticular region is common site
- Generally far more cellular than genital rhabdomyoma
  - Fascicular growth common
- Atypia and mitoses common

SELECTED REFERENCES

1. Schoolmeester JK et al: Genital rhabdomyoma of the lower female genital tract: a study of 12 cases with molecular cytogenetic findings. Int J Gynecol Pathol. 37(4): 349-55, 2018
2. Jo VY et al: Paratesticular rhabdomyoma: a morphologically distinct sclerosing variant. Am J Surg Pathol. 37(11):1737-42, 2013
3. Lu DY et al: Genital rhabdomyoma of the urethra in an infant girl. Hum Pathol. 43(4):597-600, 2012
4. Cooper CL et al: Paratesticular rhabdomyoma. Pathology. 39(3):367-9, 2007
5. Wehner MS et al: Epididymal rhabdomyoma: report of a case, including histologic and immunohistochemical findings. Arch Pathol Lab Med. 124(10):1518-9, 2000
6. Tanda F et al: Rhabdomyoma of the tunica vaginalis of the testis: a histologic, immunohistochemical, and ultrastructural study. Mod Pathol. 10(6):608-11, 1997
7. Iversen UM: Two cases of benign vaginal rhabdomyoma. Case reports. APMIS. 104(7-8):575-8, 1996
8. Suarez Vilela D et al: Vaginal rhabdomyoma and adenosis. Histopathology. 16(4):393-4, 1990

Cardiac Rhabdomyoma

KEY FACTS

TERMINOLOGY

- Benign cardiac neoplasm composed of fetal cardiac myoblasts

ETIOLOGY/PATHOGENESIS

- Most arise within setting of tuberous sclerosis complex

CLINICAL ISSUES

- Most common primary pediatric cardiac tumor
- Occurs primarily in infants and young children
- Right and left ventricular walls are most common sites
  - Multifocality is common
- May be asymptomatic or cause arrhythmia, ventricular outflow obstruction, tachycardia, Wolff-Parkinson-White syndrome, sudden death
- Treatment: Usually nonsurgical and conservative
  - Many cases regress spontaneously over time

MACROSCOPIC

- Relatively well demarcated
- Usually 0.1-3.0 cm

MICROSCOPIC

- Sheets of large polygonal cells with large, clear vacuoles
- Some cells have eosinophilic cytoplasm that is retracted away from cell membrane ("spider cells")

ANCILLARY TESTS

- Immunophenotype: Desmin (+), myogenin (+), MYOD1(+)
- Mutations in *TSC2* (tuberin) on chromosome 16 and *TSC1* (hamartin) on chromosome 9

TOP DIFFERENTIAL DIAGNOSES

- Adult-type rhabdomyoma
- Cardiac fibroma

Cardiac Rhabdomyoma

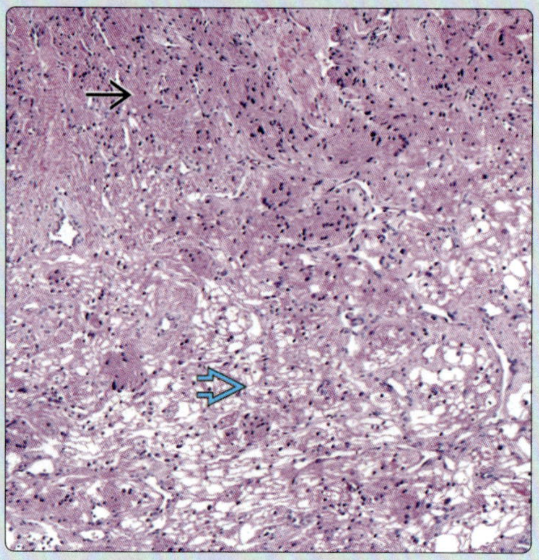

Prominent Clear Cell Morphology

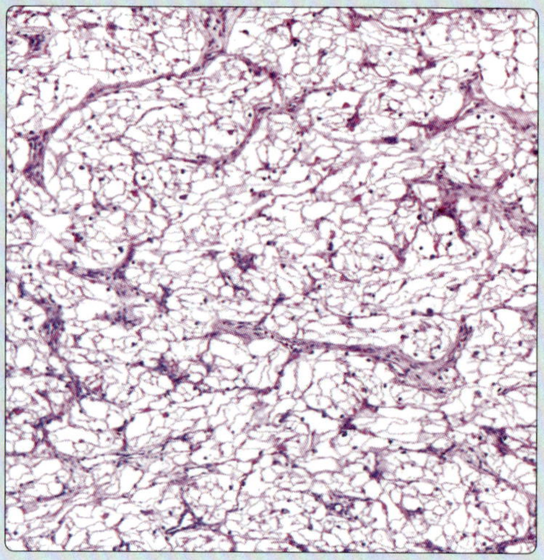

(Left) *Cardiac rhabdomyoma is the most common primary pediatric neoplasm of the heart and is associated with the tuberous sclerosis syndrome in most cases. Histologically, it can be readily distinguished from normal cardiac muscle ➔ by the prominent cytoplasmic vacuolization/clearing ➩.* **(Right)** *Cardiac rhabdomyoma is composed predominantly of large polygonal cells containing prominent cytoplasmic vacuolizations, imparting a clear cell morphology.*

Vacuolated Tumor Cells

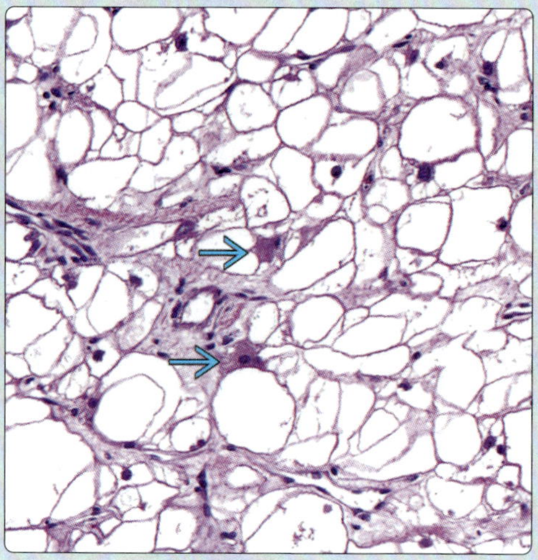

"Spider Cells"

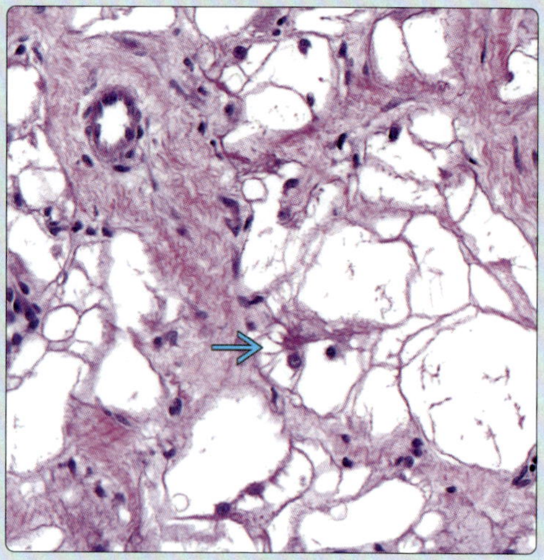

(Left) *Although most of the tumor cells in cardiac rhabdomyoma are heavily vacuolated clear cells, some cells are less vacuolated and show eosinophilic cytoplasm ➔.* **(Right)** *The combination of eosinophilic cytoplasm and intracytoplasmic vacuolizations often gives the appearance of centralized cells with radially oriented cytoplasmic extensions ➔. These cells are aptly described as "spider cells."*

Cardiac Rhabdomyoma

TERMINOLOGY

Definitions

- Benign cardiac neoplasm composed of fetal cardiac myoblasts

ETIOLOGY/PATHOGENESIS

Genetics

- Most arise within setting of tuberous sclerosis (TS)
  - More than 1/2 of patients with TS have 1 or more cardiac rhabdomyoma
- May also arise in association with congenital abnormalities, such as ventricular or valvular malformations

CLINICAL ISSUES

Epidemiology

- Incidence
  - Most common primary pediatric cardiac tumor
- Age
  - Infants and young children
    - Most common in 1st year of life
- Sex
  - Slight male predilection

Site

- Right and left ventricular walls most common
  - Rarely intraventricular septum or atrial walls
- Multifocality is common

Presentation

- May cause arrhythmia, ventricular outflow obstruction, tachycardia, Wolff-Parkinson-White syndrome, or sudden death
- May be asymptomatic

Treatment

- Usually conservative
  - Medical therapy for arrhythmias
  - Surgical excision is often utilized in tumors causing outflow obstruction or those that are refractive to medical therapy
  - Everolimus (mTOR inhibitor) may have role in facilitating regression

Prognosis

- Benign
- Many cases regress spontaneously over time

IMAGING

General Features

- Often multiple intramural lesions
- May be detected antenatally on ultrasound

MACROSCOPIC

General Features

- Relatively well demarcated
- Pale pink-tan cut surface

Size

- Usually 0.1-3.0 cm

MICROSCOPIC

Histologic Features

- Sheets of large polygonal cells with large, clear vacuoles
  - Vacuoles result from glycogen accumulation
- Some cells have eosinophilic cytoplasm that is retracted away from cell membrane
  - Described as "spider cells"
- Cytoplasmic cross striations rare
- Small nuclei with irregular contours; may show nucleoli
- Mitoses rare
- Necrosis absent

ANCILLARY TESTS

Immunohistochemistry

- Desmin (+), myogenin (+), MYOD1(+)
- HMB-45(+) reported in some cases

Genetic Testing

- Mutations in *TSC2* (tuberin) on chromosome 16
- Mutations in *TSC1* (hamartin) on chromosome 9

DIFFERENTIAL DIAGNOSIS

Adult-Type Rhabdomyoma

- Extracardiac in nearly all cases
  - Very rare intracardiac cases reported
- Cellular sheets of polygonal eosinophilic cells
- "Spider cells" not usually prominent

Cardiac Fibroma

- Composed of loose fascicles of spindled fibroblastic cells
- SMA(+), desmin (-), myogenin (-)

SELECTED REFERENCES

1. Bejiqi R et al: Prenatally diagnosis and outcome of fetuses with cardiac rhabdomyoma - single centre experience. Open Access Maced J Med Sci. 5(2):193-6, 2017
2. Chang JS et al: Regression of neonatal cardiac rhabdomyoma in two months through low-dose everolimus therapy: a report of three cases. Pediatr Cardiol. 38(7):1478-84, 2017
3. Sciacca P et al: Rhabdomyomas and tuberous sclerosis complex: our experience in 33 cases. BMC Cardiovasc Disord. 14:66, 2014
4. Chaurasia AK et al: Cardiac rhabdomyoma in familial tuberous sclerosis. J Cardiovasc Thorac Res. 5(2):71-2, 2013
5. Kutluk T et al: Cardiac rhabdomyomas in childhood: six cases from a single institution. Turk J Pediatr. 55(1):69-73, 2013
6. Benyounes N et al: Cardiac rhabdomyomas in tuberous sclerosis patients: a case report and review of the literature. Arch Cardiovasc Dis. 105(8-9):442-5, 2012
7. Demir HA et al: Everolimus: a challenging drug in the treatment of multifocal inoperable cardiac rhabdomyoma. Pediatrics. 130(1):e243-7, 2012
8. Madueme P et al: Tuberous sclerosis and cardiac rhabdomyomas: a case report and review of the literature. Congenit Heart Dis. 6(2):183-7, 2011
9. Tiberio D et al: Regression of a cardiac rhabdomyoma in a patient receiving everolimus. Pediatrics. 127(5):e1335-7, 2011
10. Burke A, Virmani R. Pediatric heart tumors. Cardiovasc Pathol. 2008 Jul-Aug;17(4):193-8.
11. Burke AP et al: Cardiac rhabdomyoma: a clinicopathologic study. Mod Pathol. 4(1):70-4, 1991

Embryonal Rhabdomyosarcoma

KEY FACTS

TERMINOLOGY

- Malignant primitive mesenchymal neoplasm that shows variable differentiation toward embryonic skeletal muscle
  - May originate in epithelial-lined viscera (botryoid type)

CLINICAL ISSUES

- Embryonal rhabdomyosarcoma (ERMS) is most common subtype (60-70%)
- Most occur in 1st decade of life
- Most arise in head/neck region or genitourinary system
- Suddenly enlarging mass
  - Botryoid-type ERMS arises as polypoid growth in mucosal sites (e.g., vagina, bladder)
- Treatment: Multimodality therapy
- Main prognostic parameters are histologic type, disease stage, age, and site
  - ERMS has significantly better prognosis than alveolar rhabdomyosarcoma (ARMS)

MICROSCOPIC

- Patternless sheets of spindled, stellate, and ovoid cells
  - Widely variable cellularity
- Myxoid stromal matrix is common
- Rhabdomyoblastic differentiation often conspicuous but variable
- Variants: Botryoid, anaplastic

ANCILLARY TESTS

- Diffuse desmin (+)
- Nuclear myogenin (+) and MYOD1(+)
- Molecular: Absence of *FOXO1* translocations

TOP DIFFERENTIAL DIAGNOSES

- Rhabdomyoma
- ARMS
- Malignant peripheral nerve sheath tumor with rhabdomyoblastic differentiation
- Neuroblastoma

Embryonal Rhabdomyosarcoma

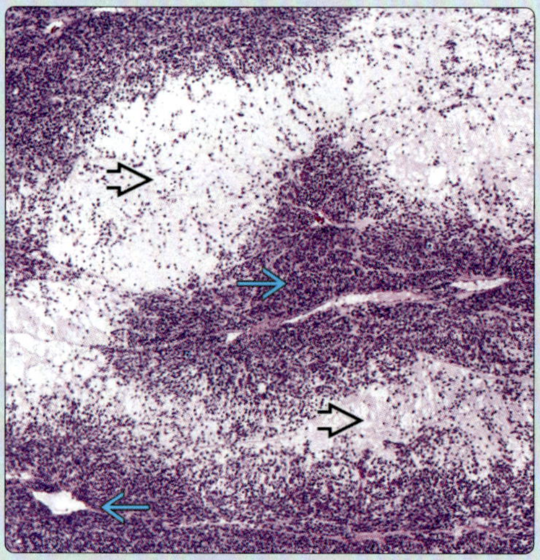

Variable Cellularity

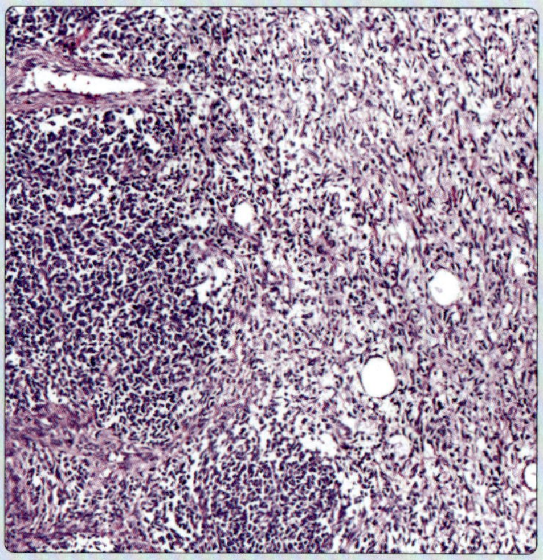

(Left) *Embryonal rhabdomyosarcoma (ERMS) often shows a somewhat marbled appearance due to regional variations in cellularity; however, some cases are more or less evenly hypo- or hypercellular. Of note, perivascular regions* → *are often more cellular than the adjacent looser myxoid zones* ⇨*.* **(Right)** *This higher power image shows a loose, more myxoid zone transitioning into a denser, less myxoid area. The cells vary from spindled or stellate to ovoid.*

Rhabdomyoblastic Differentiation

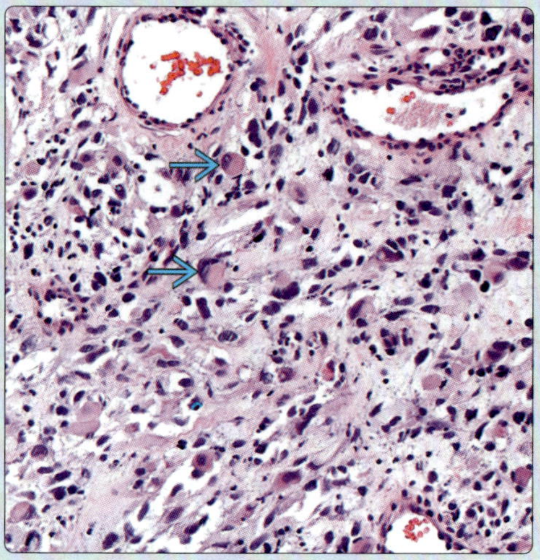

Myogenin Expression

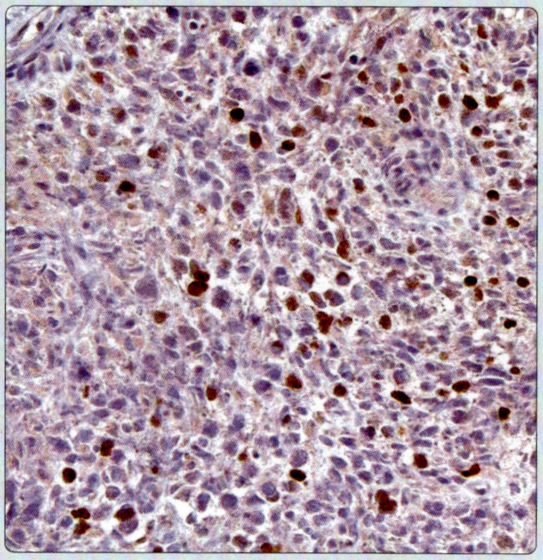

(Left) *Rhabdomyoblastic differentiation is usually evident in most cases of ERMS and is heralded by development of dense eosinophilic cytoplasm in tumor cells. Some cells show a rounded epithelioid morphology with an eccentric nucleus* →*.* **(Right)** *Myogenin expression is usually seen in ERMS; however, in contrast to alveolar rhabdomyosarcoma (ARMS), it is often sparse, focal, or patchy. Only nuclear expression should be counted, as cytoplasmic expression is nonspecific.*

TERMINOLOGY

Abbreviations

- Embryonal rhabdomyosarcoma (ERMS)

Definitions

- Malignant primitive mesenchymal neoplasm that shows variable differentiation toward embryonic skeletal muscle
  - May originate in epithelial-lined viscera (botryoid type)
- Spindle cell rhabdomyosarcoma is now provisionally listed as rhabdomyosarcomas (RMS) subtype, separate and distinct from ERMS (2013 WHO Classification)

CLINICAL ISSUES

Epidemiology

- Incidence
  - RMS are most frequent soft tissue sarcomas in children and young adults
    - ERMS is most common subtype (60-70%)
- Age
  - Most occur in 1st decade of life
    - Majority in children < 5 years
      - Occasional cases congenital
  - Less common in adolescence
    - Rare in adults

Site

- Most arise in head/neck region or genitourinary system
  - Periorbital soft tissues, sinonasal tract, oral cavity, auditory canal
  - Bladder, prostate, paratesticular soft tissue
- Less frequent sites
  - Biliary tract, retroperitoneum, abdomen/pelvis
- Rare involvement of trunk and extremities

Presentation

- Suddenly enlarging mass
  - Local symptoms pertaining to site of origin
  - Botryoid-type ERMS arises as polypoid growth in mucosal sites (e.g., vagina, bladder)
- May be associated with variety of genetic syndromes
  - Neurofibromatosis type 1, Noonan syndrome, Costello syndrome
  - Also Beckwith-Wiedemann syndrome, Li-Fraumeni syndrome, Gorlin syndrome, others
  - Pleuropulmonary blastoma syndrome associated with ERMS of uterine cervix

Treatment

- Multimodality therapy with chemotherapy in conjunction with surgery &/or radiotherapy

Prognosis

- Main prognostic parameters are histologic type, disease stage, age, and site
  - ERMS has significantly better prognosis than alveolar rhabdomyosarcoma (ARMS)
    - Likely related to absence of *FOXO1* fusions
  - Botryoid-type ERMS associated with better prognosis
  - Anaplasia in ERMS associated with worse outcome
  - Intergroup Rhabdomyosarcoma Study Group (IRSG) surgicopathologic grouping is predictive of outcome
  - Children generally show better outcome than infants, adolescents, and adults
  - Favorable sites are orbital, paratesticular, and bile duct
    - Parameningeal and extremities unfavorable

MACROSCOPIC

General Features

- Poorly demarcated, friable mass
- Tan-white, fleshy or rubbery cut surface
- Hemorrhage or necrosis may be present
- Botryoid-type RMS
  - Exophytic, polypoid, grape like
  - Often gelatinous cut surface

MICROSCOPIC

Histologic Features

- Patternless sheets of spindled, stellate, and ovoid cells
  - Hyperchromatic nuclei
  - Cytoplasm ranges from scant and amphophilic to more prominent and eosinophilic
- Myxoid stromal matrix is common
- Widely variable cellularity
  - Often show alternating hyper- and hypocellular zones (marbled pattern)
    - Cellularity is often higher around stromal blood vessels
  - Hypercellular dense zones may resemble ARMS
- Rhabdomyoblastic differentiation often conspicuous, but variable
  - Rounded or spindled cells with eccentric nuclei and prominent eosinophilic cytoplasm
  - May show cytoplasmic cross striations &/or multinucleation
  - Includes strap cells, tadpole cells, and spider cells
- Mitoses common
- Variable coagulative necrosis
- Multinucleated wreath cells absent
- Some composite (mixed-type) tumors show features of both ERMS and ARMS
  - Previously classified automatically as ARMS
  - Current recommendation: Greater than 50% alveolar elements needed to designate as ARMS
  - Determination of fusion status through molecular analysis recommended in mixed-type cases
- Occasional tumors have histologic features of both ERMS and spindle cell RMS
- Postchemotherapy changes
  - Residual cells often appear less primitive and more differentiated
  - Prominent fibrosis, myxoid change, necrosis

Morphologic Variants

- Botryoid type
  - Arises at mucosal sites underneath epithelial surface lining
  - Presence of cambium layer characteristic
    - Tightly packed cellular layer of tumor cells closely abutting epithelial surface

- Otherwise loose myxoid stroma and variable cellularity
- Anaplastic
  - Singly scattered, clusters, or sheets of markedly atypical cells
    - Enlarged, hyperchromatic, pleomorphic nuclei
    - Atypical mitotic figures common
  - Areas of more typical ERMS present

ANCILLARY TESTS

Immunohistochemistry

- Diffuse desmin (+)
  - Can highlight cytoplasmic cross striations
- Nuclear myogenin (+) and MYOD1(+)
  - Cytoplasmic staining is nonspecific and should be disregarded
  - Expression often focal or patchy (unlike ARMS)
- Variable SMA(+)
- May show focal aberrant keratin (+)

Molecular Genetics

- Absence of *PAX3-FOXO1* and *PAX7-FOXO1* fusions
- Complex karyotypes
  - Often gains of chromosomes 2, 8, 12, and 13
- Loss of heterozygosity at 11p15.5 considered hallmark of ERMS

DIFFERENTIAL DIAGNOSIS

Rhabdomyoma

- Head and neck predilection, especially fetal type
- Fetal-type rhabdomyoma
  - No significant nuclear atypia, necrosis, or infiltrative margins
  - Mitoses may be conspicuous but are not atypical
- Adult-type rhabdomyoma
  - Middle-aged adults, often men
  - Sheets of large polygonal, eosinophilic cells
- Genital-type rhabdomyoma
  - Mostly middle-aged women; genital region
  - Bland strap cells in loose fibrous stroma; no mitoses

Alveolar Rhabdomyosarcoma

- Nests of tumor cells divided by fibrous septa (pseudoalveolar pattern)
  - Solid areas may be nearly indistinguishable from dense foci of ERMS
- Most common in extremities and trunk in adolescents and young adults
- Diffuse nuclear myogenin (+)
- Characteristic translocations between *FOXO1* and *PAX3* or *PAX7*

Spindle Cell Rhabdomyosarcoma

- Most common in paratesticular region of children or head/neck region of adults
- Predominantly fascicles of spindled cells; rhabdomyoblasts often sparse

Malignant Peripheral Nerve Sheath Tumor With Rhabdomyoblastic Differentiation

- a.k.a. malignant triton tumor
- Occur mostly in adults
- Can be associated with neurofibromatosis type 1
- Predominantly shows histologic features of malignant peripheral nerve sheath tumor (MPNST)
  - Contains foci of rhabdomyoblastic cells with prominent eosinophilic cytoplasm
    - Desmin (+), myogenin (+) in rhabdomyoblastic cells only

Pleomorphic Rhabdomyosarcoma

- Almost exclusively in adults
- Most common in extremities
- Diffuse, overtly malignant, pleomorphic, high-grade cytomorphology

Neuroblastoma

- Intraabdominal sympathetic chain, adrenal gland
- Variable amount of neurofibrillary matrix
- NB84(+), desmin (-), myogenin (-)

Pleuropulmonary Blastoma

- Occurs in peripheral lung, pleura, chest wall
- Small primitive blastemal cells with focal differentiation toward other mesenchymal lineages, including skeletal muscle

Infantile Fibrosarcoma

- Usually occurs in extremities in first 2 years of life
- Intersecting fascicles of primitive ovoid and spindled tumor cells
- Desmin (-), myogenin (-)
- Characteristic t(12;15) with *NTRK3-ETV6* fusion

Ectomesenchymoma

- Usually in infants; very rare
- ERMS admixed with neuronal or neural component
  - e.g., ganglion cells, ganglioneuroma, neuroblastoma, MPNST

SELECTED REFERENCES

1. Rekhi B et al: Clinicopathologic features of 300 rhabdomyosarcomas with emphasis upon differential expression of skeletal muscle specific markers in the various subtypes: single institutional experience. Ann Diagn Pathol. 36:50-60, 2018
2. McInturff M et al: Embryonal rhabdomyosarcoma of the oral cavity. Head Neck Pathol. 11(3):385-8, 2017
3. Rudzinski ER et al: The World Health Organization Classification of Skeletal Muscle Tumors in Pediatric Rhabdomyosarcoma: a report from the Children's Oncology Group. Arch Pathol Lab Med. 139(10):1281-7, 2015
4. Rudzinski ER et al: Myogenin, AP2β, NOS-1, and HMGA2 are surrogate markers of fusion status in rhabdomyosarcoma: a report from the soft tissue sarcoma committee of the children's oncology group. Am J Surg Pathol. 38(5):654-9, 2014
5. Li RF et al: Embryonal rhabdomyosarcoma (botryoid type) of the uterine corpus and cervix in adult women: report of a case series and review of the literature. Am J Surg Pathol. 37(3):344-55, 2013
6. Rudzinski ER et al: Dense pattern of embryonal rhabdomyosarcoma, a lesion easily confused with alveolar rhabdomyosarcoma: a report from the Soft Tissue Sarcoma Committee of the Children's Oncology Group. Am J Clin Pathol. 140(1):82-90, 2013
7. Raney RB et al: Results of the Intergroup Rhabdomyosarcoma Study Group D9602 protocol, using vincristine and dactinomycin with or without cyclophosphamide and radiation therapy, for newly diagnosed patients with low-risk embryonal rhabdomyosarcoma: a report from the Soft Tissue Sarcoma Committee of the Children's Oncology Group. J Clin Oncol. 29(10):1312-8, 2011
8. Davicioni E et al: Molecular classification of rhabdomyosarcoma–genotypic and phenotypic determinants of diagnosis: a report from the Children's Oncology Group. Am J Pathol. 174(2):550-64, 2009

Prominent Myxoid Stroma

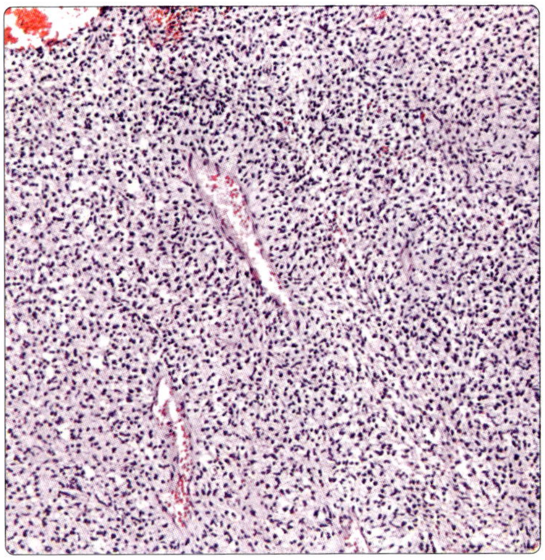

Bland Cytomorphology

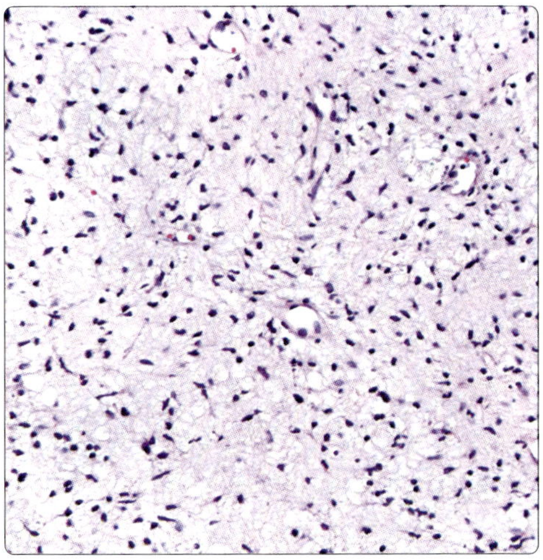

(Left) *Myxoid stroma is a characteristic feature of ERMS and is especially prominent in less cellular cases.* **(Right)** *In addition to the prominent myxoid matrix, some cases of ERMS may show paradoxically bland cytologic features, potentially leading to confusion with a myxoma or myxoid neurofibroma.*

Perivascular Accentuation

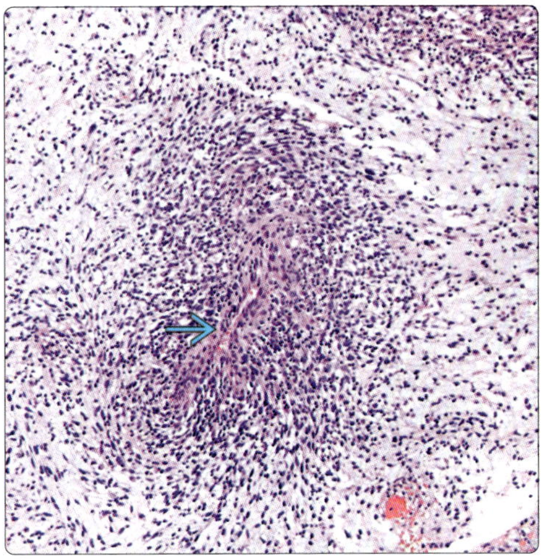

Focal Fascicular Morphology

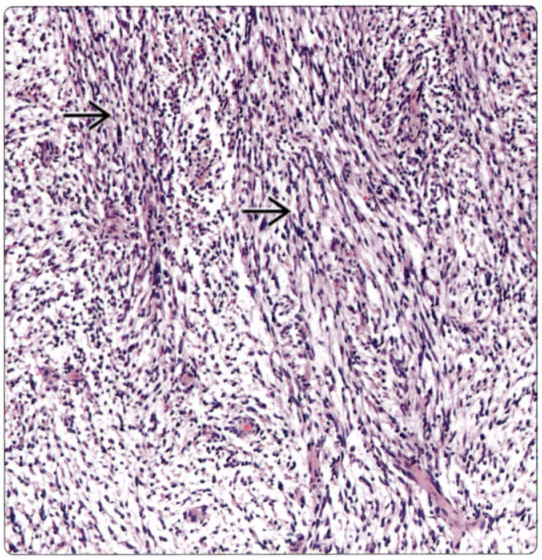

(Left) *Tumor cell condensation around a stromal blood vessel* ➙ *is a feature of some cases of ERMS and contrasts nicely with the less cellular adjacent areas.* **(Right)** *Typical examples of ERMS may show focal areas of increased cellularity with loose fascicular growth* ➙*. Tumors with extensive fascicular growth are best considered spindle cell rhabdomyosarcomas.*

Increased Cellularity

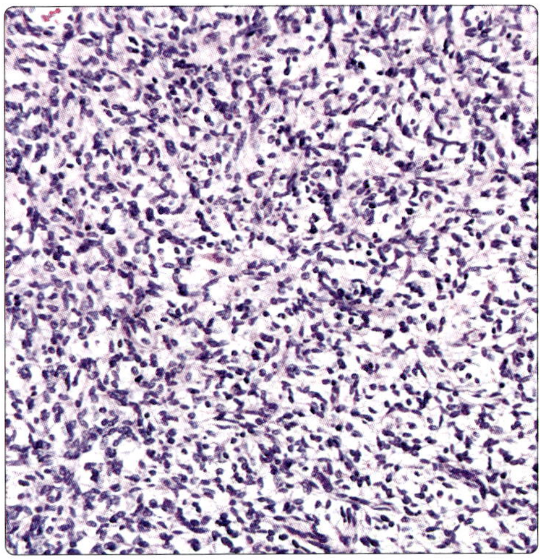

Hypercellularity

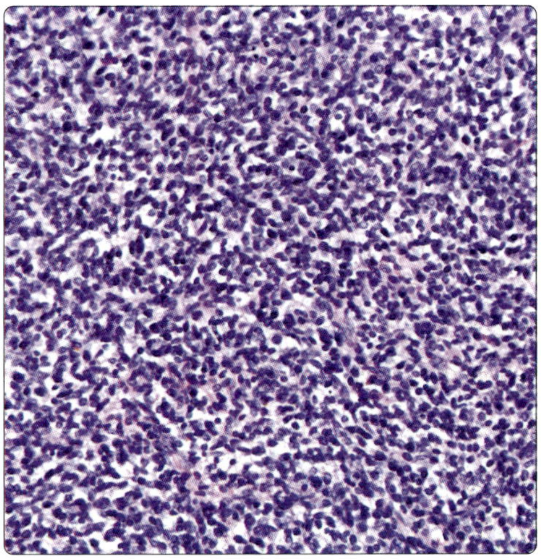

(Left) *Cellularity varies widely in ERMS from patient to patient and even within the same patient. This image shows increased cellularity within a still prominent myxoid matrix.* **(Right)** *This image shows a hypercellular focus in ERMS with extensive nuclear overlapping. Note the lack of nuclear pleomorphism despite the marked cellularity.*

(Left) *The tumor cells may show a more ovoid cytomorphology with rounded nuclei in some cases of ERMS. This morphology may simulate solid growth in ARMS if myxoid stroma is limited.* **(Right)** *Rhabdomyoblastic cells are generally easier to identify in ERMS compared to other forms of rhabdomyosarcoma. In addition to larger epithelioid cells ⇨, some cells are more elongated and myofiber-shaped and may be referred to as strap cells → or tadpole cells. Cross striations may also be evident.*

Ovoid Cellular Morphology

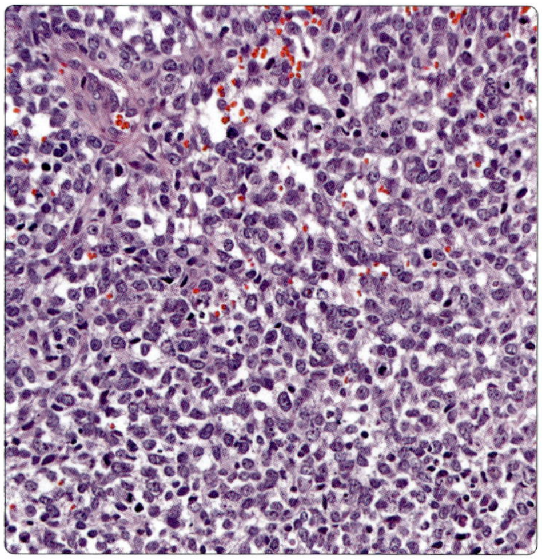

Rhabdomyoblasts

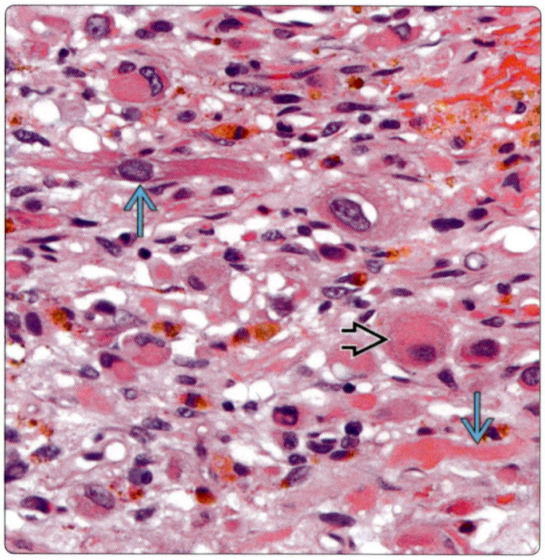

(Left) *Occasional rhabdomyoblastic cells in ERMS show centralized cytoplasmic retraction and have been referred to as spider cells.* **(Right)** *Focal pseudoalveolar growth may be present in otherwise conventional ERMS and currently no longer warrants immediate classification as ARMS. However, if suspicions are high, molecular studies to evaluate for FOXO1 fusions are warranted.*

Rhabdomyoblasts

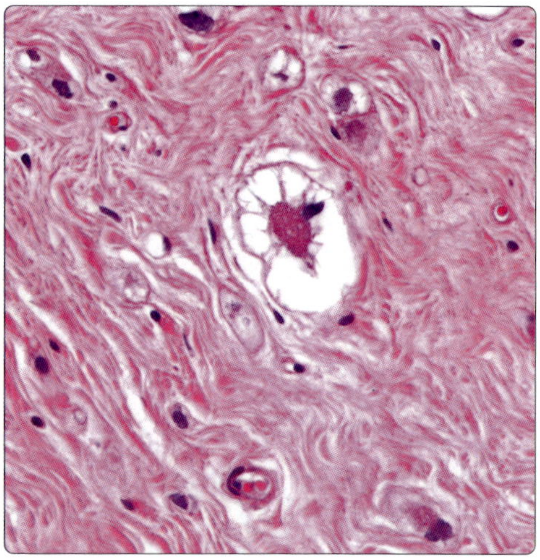

Focal Pseudoalveolar Growth

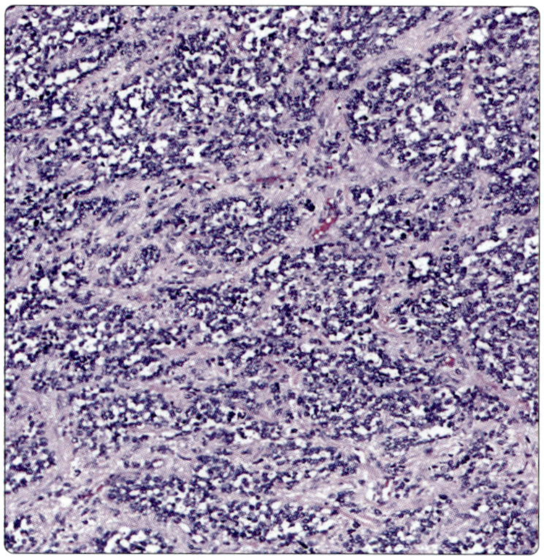

(Left) *Coagulative necrosis is a common finding in ERMS and usually manifests as small pockets of dead or dying cells; however, extensive zones of necrosis with perivascular sparing may also be seen.* **(Right)** *This unusual case of otherwise conventional ERMS showed foci of intratumoral cystic change with hemorrhage, somewhat reminiscent of the pattern seen in aneurysmal bone cyst.*

Necrosis

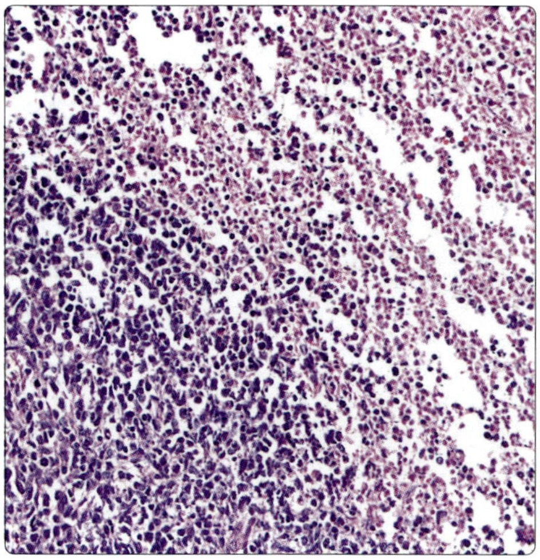

Focal Cystic Change

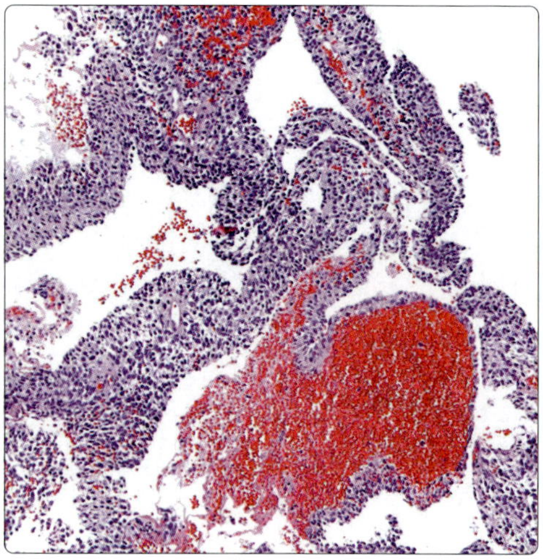

Anaplasia

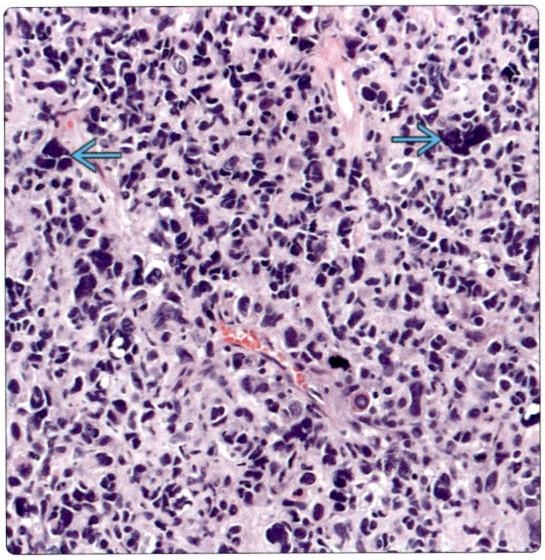

Botryoid-Type Embryonal Rhabdomyosarcoma

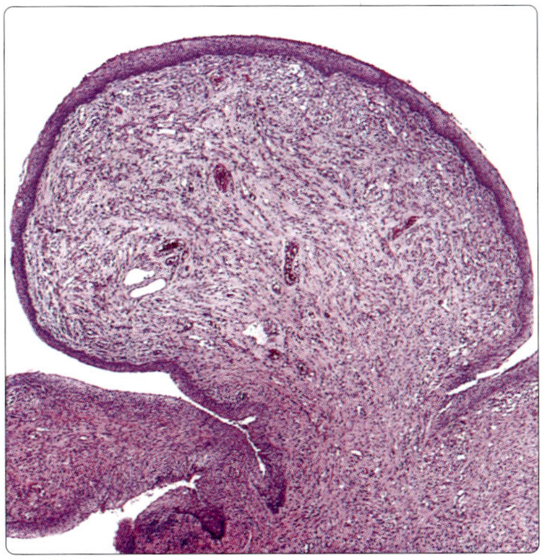

(Left) *The presence of scattered enlarged tumor cells with hyperchromatic and pleomorphic nuclei are seen in some cases of ERMS and is termed anaplasia* ⇒. *Some variants show diffuse anaplasia and contain atypical mitotic figures. In either case, the presence of anaplasia portends a worsened prognosis.* **(Right)** *Botryoid-type ERMS presents as an exophytic, polypoid growth from underneath a mucosal surface and, in some cases, resembles a bunch of grapes macroscopically.*

Cambium Layer

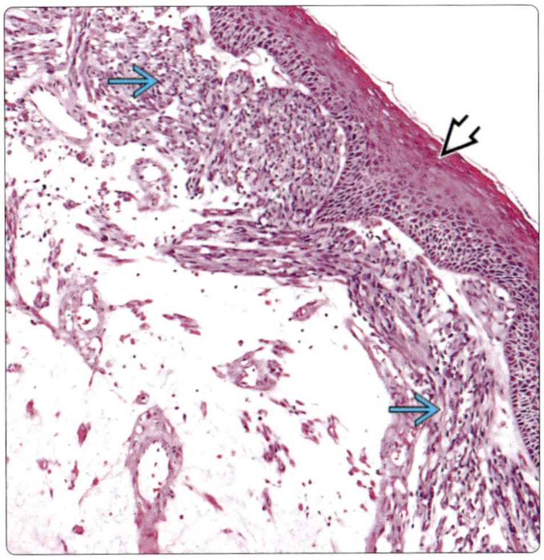

Reactive Appearance

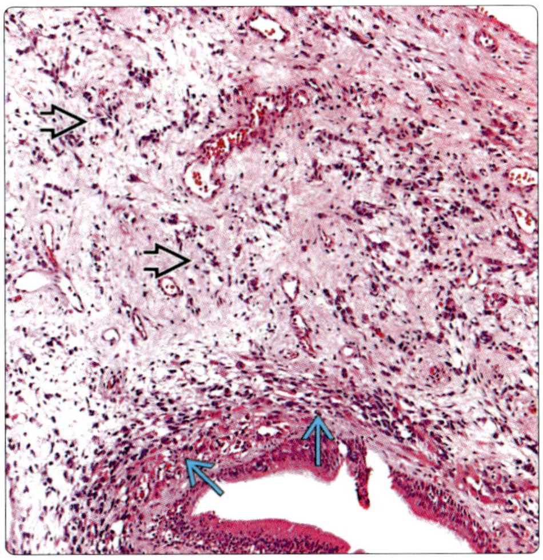

(Left) *A characteristic finding in botryoid-type ERMS is the presence of a superficial zone* ⇒ *of increased cellular density underneath the epithelial surface* ⇒. *This zone is termed the cambium layer.* **(Right)** *In some cases of botryoid-type ERMS, the neoplastic cells* ⇒ *deep to the surface are small and relatively innocuous appearing and may be mistaken for inflammatory cells or reactive tissue. Hypocellularity further complicates the issue. However, note the cambium layer* ⇒.

Posttherapy Changes

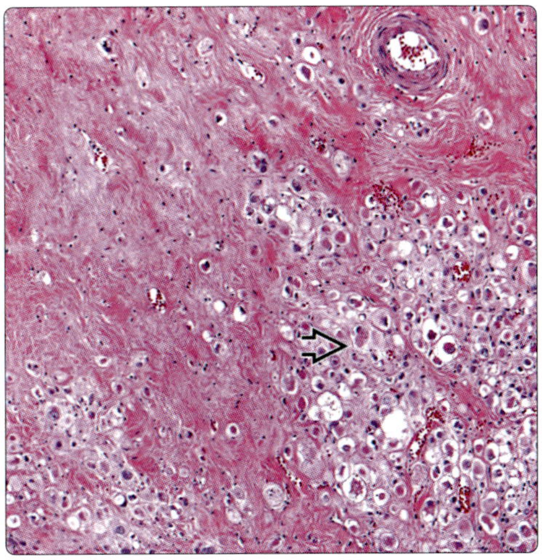

Posttherapy Maturation

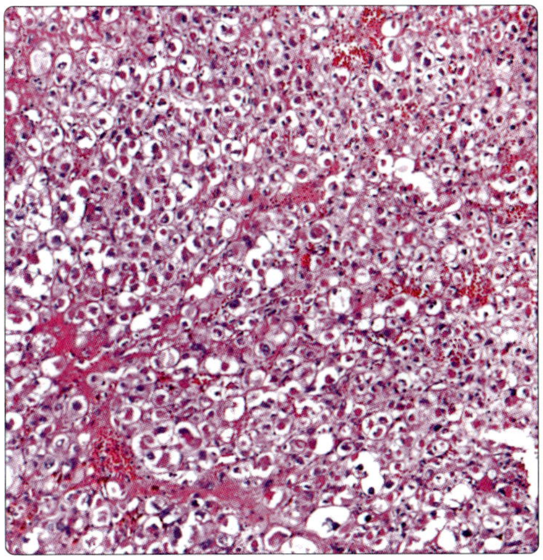

(Left) *Following chemotherapy, ERMS often shows prominent stromal fibrosis with areas of myxoid change. Of note, islands of more mature/differentiated rhabdomyoblasts* ⇒ *are not uncommon.* **(Right)** *Occasional cases of ERMS may show a highly differentiated appearance following chemotherapy and may closely resemble an adult-type rhabdomyoma.*

Alveolar Rhabdomyosarcoma

KEY FACTS

TERMINOLOGY

- Cellular, malignant neoplasm composed of primitive round cells with evidence of skeletal muscle differentiation

CLINICAL ISSUES

- Most common between 10-25 years of age
- Most frequent in deep soft tissues of extremities
- Often high stage at presentation
- Treatment: Multimodality approach
- Fully malignant, high-grade sarcoma
  - Overall, worse prognosis than embryonal rhabdomyosarcoma (ERMS)
  - Recent evidence suggests that prognosis may be related to fusion status

MICROSCOPIC

- Generally, highly cellular
- Nests and sheets of primitive rounded cells separated by variably prominent fibrous septa
  - Nests show central loss of cellular cohesion
- Rhabdomyoblasts may be seen
- Distinctive multinucleate tumor giant cells ("wreath cells") in some cases
- Some tumors show both alveolar and embryonal features
- Morphologic variant: Solid type

ANCILLARY TESTS

- Usually diffuse desmin (+), myogenin (+), MyoD1(+)
- May show focal expression of keratin, CD99, neuroendocrine markers
- Molecular: 2 characteristic recurrent chromosomal translocations (80% of cases)
  - t(2;13)(*PAX3-FOXO1*) or t(1;13)(*PAX7-FOXO1*)

TOP DIFFERENTIAL DIAGNOSES

- ERMS
- Sclerosing rhabdomyosarcoma (RMS)
- Various small round blue cell tumors

Alveolar Rhabdomyosarcoma

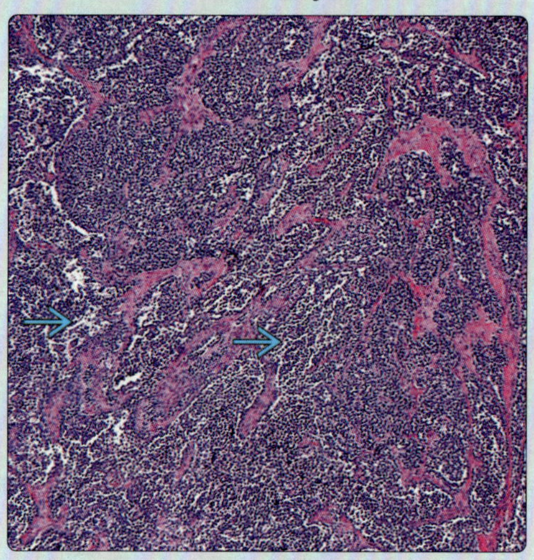

Pseudoalveolar Pattern

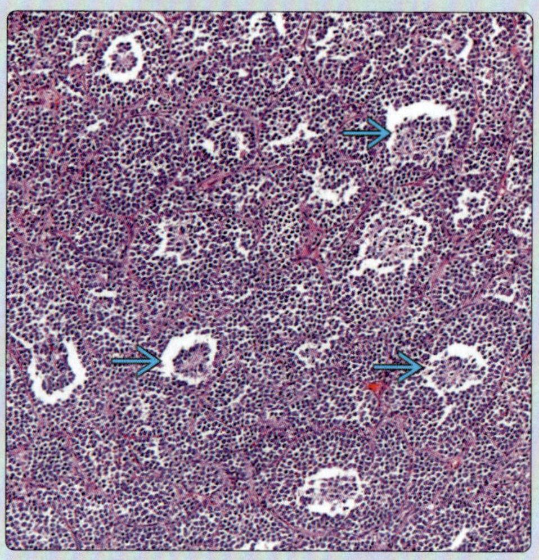

(Left) *Alveolar rhabdomyosarcoma (ARMS) is a high-grade, malignant neoplasm composed of nests and sheets of primitive rounded cells within a fibrovascular stroma. At least focal cellular dyscohesion ➔ is usually evident at low magnification.* **(Right)** *In ARMS, a pseudoalveolar pattern ➔ is imparted by the central loss of cellular cohesion and viability within the tumor nests.*

Pseudoalveolar Pattern

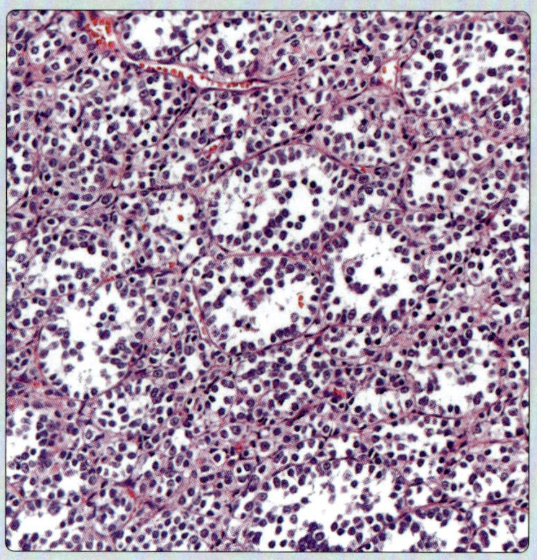

Cytologic Features

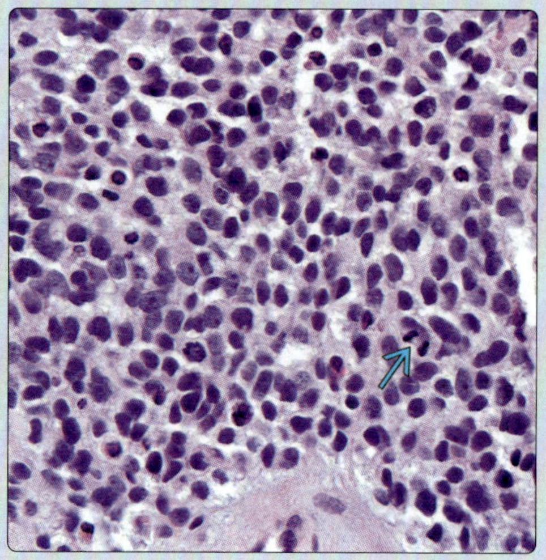

(Left) *Despite the loss of cellular cohesion in the center of the nests, the peripheral cells often remain attached to the fibrous septa, an appearance somewhat resembling alveoli. This pattern is similar to what is seen in alveolar soft-part sarcoma.* **(Right)** *The lesional cells of ARMS are medium-sized with relatively monomorphic nuclei and usually little eosinophilic cytoplasm. Small, centralized nucleoli may or may not be present. Mitoses ➔ are common.*

TERMINOLOGY

Abbreviations

- Alveolar rhabdomyosarcoma (ARMS)

Definitions

- Cellular, malignant neoplasm composed of primitive, monomorphic round cells with evidence of skeletal muscle differentiation

CLINICAL ISSUES

Epidemiology

- Incidence
  - 2nd most common type of rhabdomyosarcoma (RMS) [after embryonal rhabdomyosarcoma (ERMS)]
- Age
  - Predominantly adolescents and young adults (most common 10-25 years)
    - Less common than ERMS in children
    - Rare in adults > 45 years
    - Very rare cases are congenital
- Sex
  - M = F
- Ethnicity
  - No ethnic or geographical predilections

Site

- Most common in deep soft tissues of extremities
- Also head and neck, trunk, paraspinal, perineal, retroperitoneum

Presentation

- Usually rapidly enlarging mass
  - Local symptoms pertaining to site of origin
    - Proptosis or cranial nerve deficits (head and neck)
    - Paresthesia or paresis (paraspinal areas of trunk)
    - Constipation (perineal region)
  - Can present with widespread dissemination
    - Lymphadenopathy or marrow infiltration
    - Rarely may present without obvious primary
- Often high stage at presentation

Treatment

- Multimodality approach
  - Surgery, chemotherapy, &/or radiotherapy
    - RMS is sensitive to both chemotherapy and radiation therapy

Prognosis

- Fully malignant, high-grade sarcoma
  - Overall, worse prognosis than ERMS
  - Intergroup Rhabdomyosarcoma Study (IRS) stage grouping is predictive of outcome
- Recent evidence suggests that prognosis may be related to fusion status
  - ARMS with *PAX3-FOXO1* or *PAX7-FOXO1* fusion shows worse outcome than ERMS and fusion; negative ARMS
    - *PAX3-FOXO1*-fusion ARMS may have worse outcome than *PAX7-FOXO1*-fusion ARMS
  - Fusion-negative ARMS shows similar outcome to ERMS

MACROSCOPIC

General Features

- Tan-gray-white with fleshy cut surface
- Hemorrhage &/or necrosis may be present

MICROSCOPIC

Histologic Features

- Generally highly cellular
- Nests and sheets of primitive rounded cells separated by variably prominent fibrous septa
  - Lesional cells are relatively monomorphic and medium sized with minimal cytoplasm
    - Hyperchromatic nuclei ± small nucleoli
    - Mitotic figures often abundant
  - Sheets and nests characteristically show central loss of cellular cohesion
    - Forms alveolar-like (pseudoalveolar) spaces
    - Central cells often poorly preserved and necrotic
      - Many appear freely floating
    - Layer of cells cling to fibrous septa
  - Fibrous septa vary in thickness
    - Fibrous stroma may appear abundant in some cases
- Rhabdomyoblasts may be seen (less frequent than ERMS)
  - Usually round or oval
    - Elongated, strap cells less common
- Distinctive multinucleate tumor giant cells in some cases
  - Peripheral or wreath-like arrangement of nuclei
- Variable tumor necrosis
- Rare findings
  - Clear cell change
  - Scattered pleomorphic cells (anaplasia)
- Some composite tumors show features of both ARMS and ERMS (mixed type)
  - Previously classified automatically as ARMS
  - Current recommendation: > 50% alveolar elements needed to designate as ARMS
    - Determination of fusion status through molecular analysis recommended in mixed-type cases

Morphologic Variants

- Solid-type ARMS
  - Similar in appearance to conventional ARMS but lacks pseudoalveolar pattern
  - Fibrous stroma/septa may or may not be conspicuous
  - Cytomorphology similar to conventional type

ANCILLARY TESTS

Immunohistochemistry

- Desmin (+) and MSA(+), usually diffuse
- Myogenin (+), MyoD1(+)
  - Only nuclear expression counts
  - Characteristically diffuse (in contrast to ERMS)
- May show focal/patchy keratin (+), particularly in sinonasal ARMS
- Variable expression of neuroendocrine markers (CD56, synaptophysin)
- Patchy, variable CD99(+)

Molecular Genetics

- 2 characteristic recurrent chromosomal translocations (80% of cases)
  - t(2;13)(q35;q14)
    - *PAX3* on chromosome 2 and *FOXO1* on chromosome 13
    - Most common translocation
  - t(1;13)(p36;q14)
    - *PAX7* on chromosome 1 and *FOXO1* on chromosome 13
- ~ 20% of cases of ARMS are fusion (-) by routine RT-PCR
  - Fusion (-) ARMS is genetically heterogeneous
    - May have alternate fusions with other genes (*NCOA1, INO80D*)
    - Some may be truly fusion (-)
- Histologic appearances of ARMS do not predict presence or type of gene fusion
  - However, solid growth or mixed embryonal/alveolar patterns show higher incidence of fusion negativity

DIFFERENTIAL DIAGNOSIS

Embryonal Rhabdomyosarcoma

- More common in urogenital or head and neck sites
- Overall, affects younger age group than in ARMS
- More morphologically heterogeneous
- Spindle morphology and myxoid stroma common
- Rhabdomyoblastic differentiation usually more pronounced
- Desmin and myogenin expression less diffuse than in ARMS
- Absence of *FOXO1* translocations

Sclerosing Rhabdomyosarcoma

- Abundant hyalinizing matrix
- Absence of *FOXO1* translocations
- Pronounced MyoD1(+); weaker expression of myogenin
- Desmin (+), often perinuclear dot like

Alveolar Soft Part Sarcoma

- Shows similar pseudoalveolar growth
- Large, rounded oncocytic cells rather than small blue cells
- Nuclear TFE3(+); nuclear myogenin (-)
- PAS(+), diastase-resistant cytoplasmic crystals
- Presence of t(X;17) translocation
- Absence of *FOXO1* translocations

Lymphoma/Leukemia

- Often systemic involvement by disease ± lymphadenopathy
- Architecture dispersed and sheet like rather than nested
- Expression of hematolymphoid markers
- Desmin (-), myogenin (-)
- Absence of *FOXO1* translocations

Ewing Sarcoma

- Can show morphologic overlap with ARMS
- Many cases CD99(+) with strong, membranous expression
- Desmin (-), myogenin (-), MyoD1(-)
- Usually CD56(-)
- Characteristic translocations involving *EWSR1*

Desmoplastic Small Round Cell Tumor

- Intraabdominal location common
- Prominent stromal fibroplasia
- Keratin (+), desmin (+), myogenin (-), MyoD1(-)
- Characteristic *EWSR1-WT1* gene fusion

Neuroblastoma

- Younger age group affected
- Often in characteristic locations
  - Adrenal gland
  - Intraabdominal sympathetic chain
- Variable amount of neurofibrillary matrix
- Homer Wright rosettes in some cases
- NB84(+), desmin (-), myogenin (-)
- Absence of *FOXO1* translocations

Extrarenal Rhabdoid Tumor

- Affects infants and very young children
- Larger cells with eccentric nuclei and hyaline cytoplasmic inclusions
  - Some tumors are composed of smaller cells with scant cytoplasm
- Keratin (+), desmin (-), myogenin (-)
- Loss of nuclear INI1 expression
- Absence of *FOXO1* translocations

SELECTED REFERENCES

1. Rekhi B et al: Clinicopathologic features of 300 rhabdomyosarcomas with emphasis upon differential expression of skeletal muscle specific markers in the various subtypes: a single institutional experience. Ann Diagn Pathol. 36:50-60, 2018
2. Thompson LDR et al: Sinonasal tract alveolar rhabdomyosarcoma in adults: a clinicopathologic and immunophenotypic study of fifty-two cases with emphasis on epithelial immunoreactivity. Head Neck Pathol. 12(2):181-92, 2018
3. Chen E et al: Head and neck rhabdomyosarcoma: clinical and pathologic characterization of seven cases. Head Neck Pathol. 11(3):321-6, 2017
4. Charville GW et al: PAX7 expression in rhabdomyosarcoma, related soft tissue tumors, and small round blue cell neoplasms. Am J Surg Pathol. 40(10):1305-15, 2016
5. Shern JF et al: Comprehensive genomic analysis of rhabdomyosarcoma reveals a landscape of alterations affecting a common genetic axis in fusion-positive and fusion-negative tumors. Cancer Discov. 4(2):216-31, 2014
6. Parham DM et al: Classification of rhabdomyosarcoma and its molecular basis. Adv Anat Pathol. 20(6):387-97, 2013
7. Skapek SX et al: PAX-FOXO1 fusion status drives unfavorable outcome for children with rhabdomyosarcoma: a children's oncology group report. Pediatr Blood Cancer. 60(9):1411-7, 2013
8. Liu J et al: FOXO1-FGFR1 fusion and amplification in a solid variant of alveolar rhabdomyosarcoma. Mod Pathol. 24(10):1327-35, 2011
9. Williamson D et al: Fusion gene-negative alveolar rhabdomyosarcoma is clinically and molecularly indistinguishable from embryonal rhabdomyosarcoma. J Clin Oncol. 28(13):2151-8, 2010
10. Downs-Kelly E et al: The utility of FOXO1 fluorescence in situ hybridization (FISH) in formalin-fixed paraffin-embedded specimens in the diagnosis of alveolar rhabdomyosarcoma. Diagn Mol Pathol. 18(3):138-43, 2009
11. Sullivan LM et al: PAX immunoreactivity identifies alveolar rhabdomyosarcoma. Am J Surg Pathol. 33(5):775-80, 2009
12. Yasuda T et al: Alveolar rhabdomyosarcoma of the head and neck region in older adults: genetic characterization and a review of the literature. Hum Pathol. 40(3):341-8, 2009
13. Bahrami A et al: Aberrant expression of epithelial and neuroendocrine markers in alveolar rhabdomyosarcoma: a potentially serious diagnostic pitfall. Mod Pathol. 21(7):795-806, 2008
14. Parham DM et al: Correlation between histology and PAX/FKHR fusion status in alveolar rhabdomyosarcoma: a report from the Children's Oncology Group. Am J Surg Pathol. 31(6):895-901, 2007
15. Sorensen PH et al: PAX3-FKHR and PAX7-FKHR gene fusions are prognostic indicators in alveolar rhabdomyosarcoma: a report from the children's oncology group. J Clin Oncol. 20(11):2672-9, 2002
16. Dias P et al: Strong immunostaining for myogenin in rhabdomyosarcoma is significantly associated with tumors of the alveolar subclass. Am J Pathol. 156(2):399-408, 2000

Rhabdomyoblasts

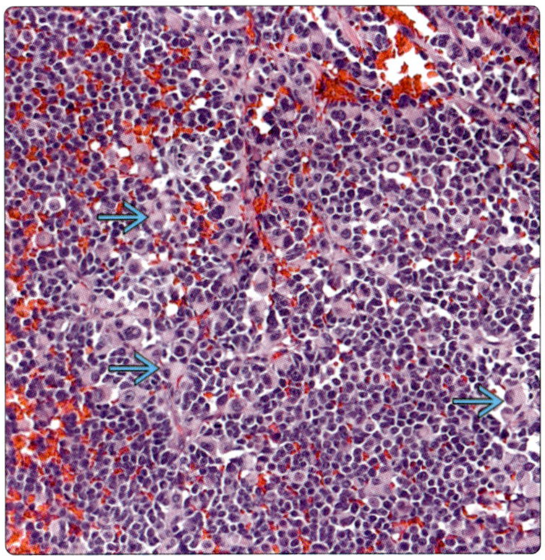

Rhabdomyoblasts

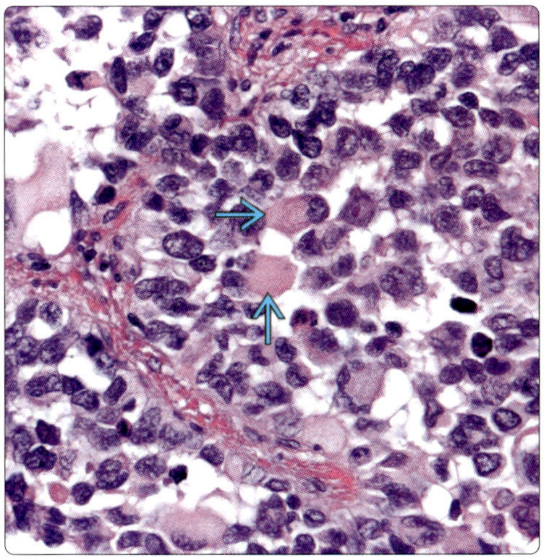

(Left) *Rhabdomyoblasts → in ARMS vary widely in number from case to case and may be identified singly or in clusters. When present, they are usually round or polygonal rather than spindled or elongated.* **(Right)** *Ovoid or rounded rhabdomyoblasts → typically show eccentric nuclei and prominent cytoplasmic eosinophilia. Spindled strap cells and cytoplasmic cross-striations are uncommon in ARMS.*

Multinucleated Tumor Giant Cells

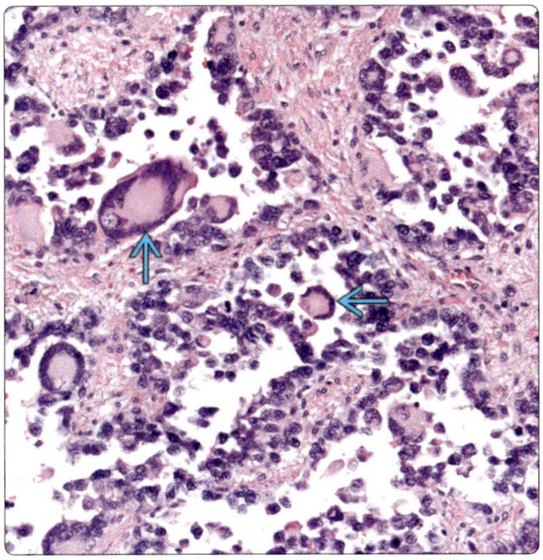

Clear Cell Change

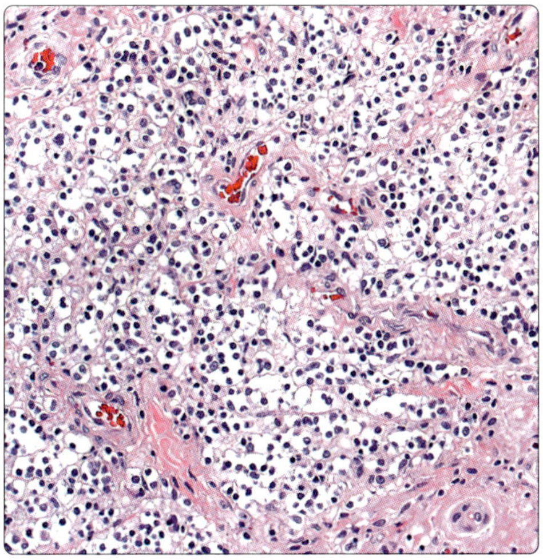

(Left) *A distinctive finding in some cases of ARMS is the presence of multinucleated tumor giant cells →. These cells classically show a peripheral or wreath-like arrangement of nuclei and abundant eosinophilic cytoplasm.* **(Right)** *Clear cell change is an uncommon but well-documented finding in ARMS. It is usually focal but may be extensive. This morphology may lead to confusion with Ewing sarcoma, and immunohistochemistry is often helpful.*

Thick Fibrous Septa

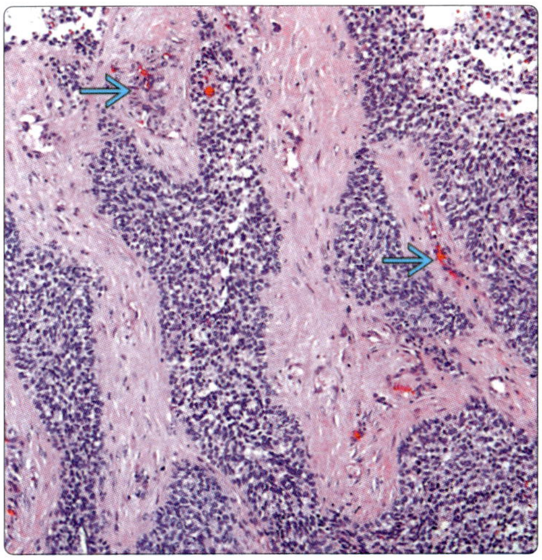

Thick Fibrous Septa

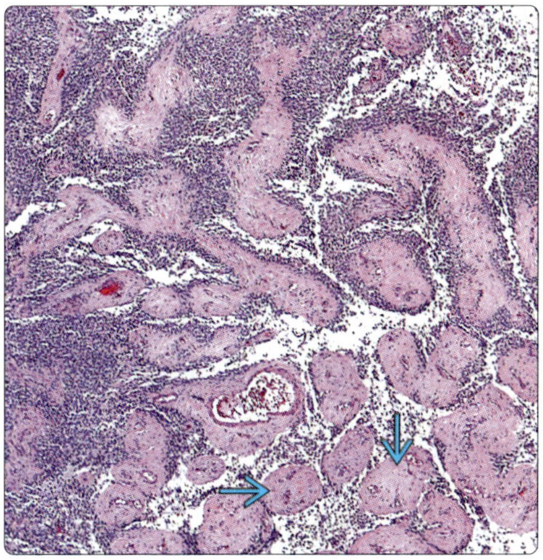

(Left) *The fibrous septa of ARMS vary in thickness and may be quite striking in some cases. Variably dilated vascular channels → are commonly present within the septa.* **(Right)** *The combination of thickened or sclerotic fibrous septa and loss of cellular cohesion may impart a pseudopapillary appearance in ARMS. The illusion of discrete fibrovascular nodules → may be seen in some foci.*

Ramifying Fibrous Septa

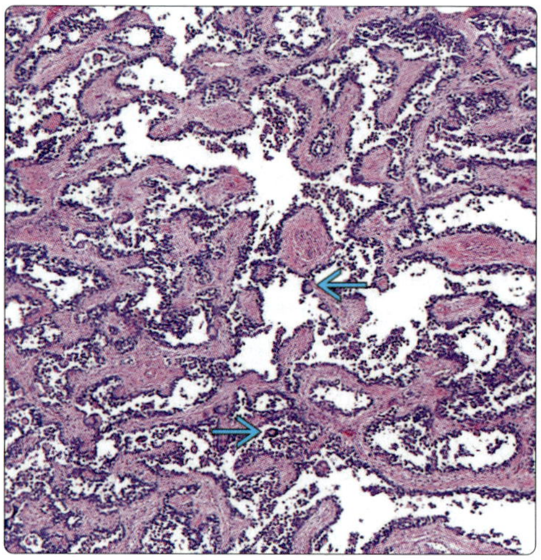

Diffuse Dyscohesion

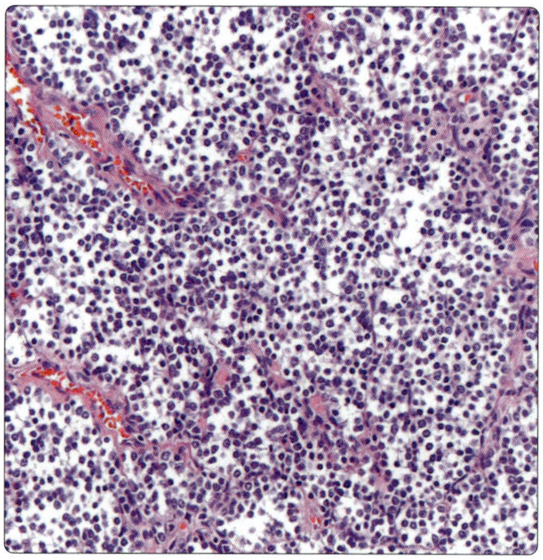

(Left) *This case of ARMS shows extensive cellular drop out and at low magnification appears as ramifying and interconnecting fibrous cords or trabeculae. Note that a thin layer of tumor cells remain attached to the septa. Scattered "wreath cells"* ➔ *can also be seen.* **(Right)** *This ARMS shows diffuse cellular dyscohesion with thin fibrovascular septa, reminiscent of a germ cell neoplasm.*

Hemorrhage

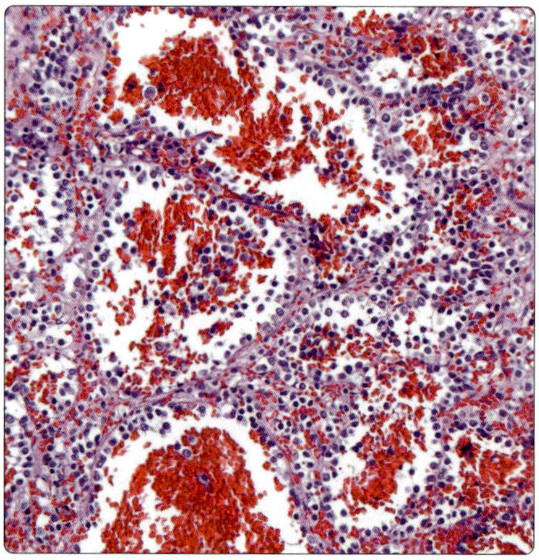

Unusual Corded Growth

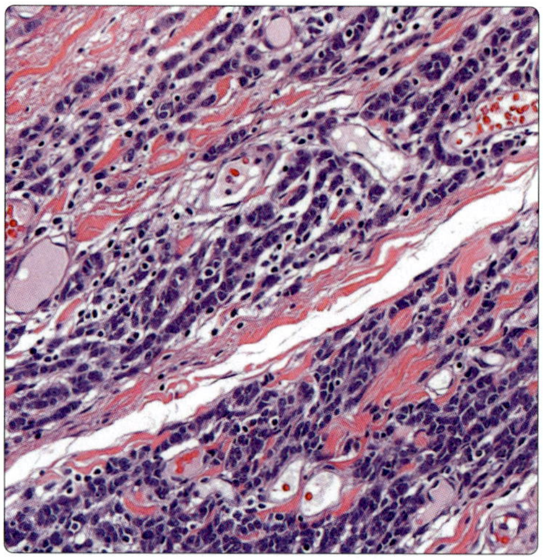

(Left) *Foci of intratumoral hemorrhage may be seen in ARMS and may appear mostly within nests of tumor cells, mimicking vascular channels or vascularized carcinomas such as renal cell carcinoma.* **(Right)** *This case of otherwise conventional ARMS contained rare, peripherally located foci demonstrating tumor cells with a corded growth pattern. This finding is not well described in ARMS but mimics carcinoma.*

Solid Variant

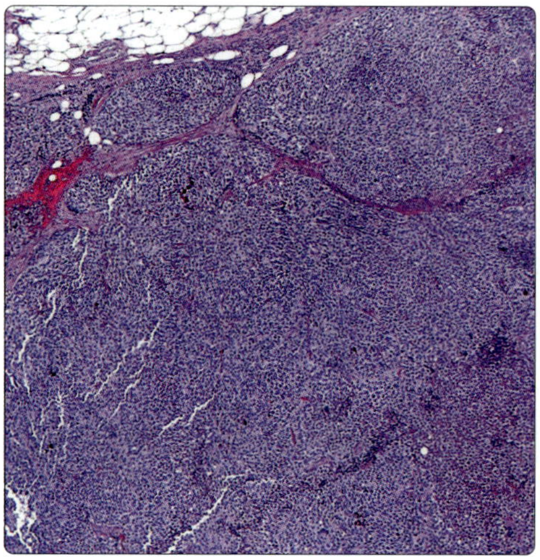

Solid Variant

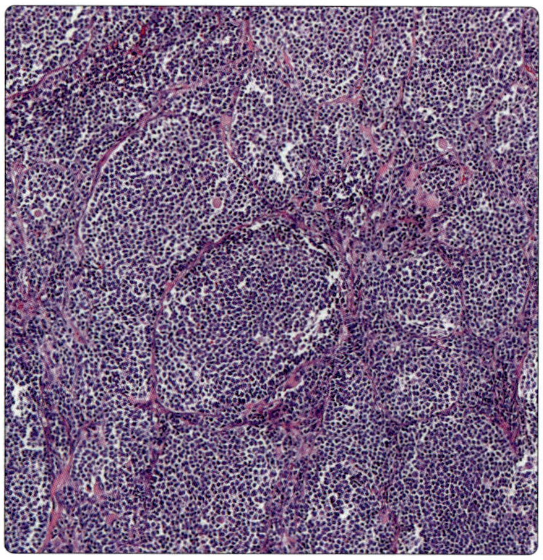

(Left) *The solid variant of ARMS shows large nodules and diffuse sheets of lesional cells within minimal to no fibrous septation and an absence of pseudoalveolar growth. To qualify for this designation, this solid growth should reflect the majority of the tumor. This variant appears to show a higher incidence of fusion negativity than conventional ARMS.* **(Right)** *Solid ARMS may show areas of nested growth with thin fibrous septa; however, a pseudoalveolar pattern is absent.*

Myoinvasion

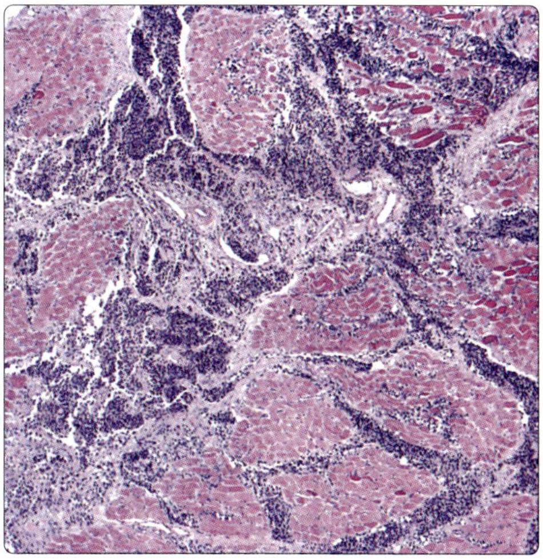

Procedure Artifact

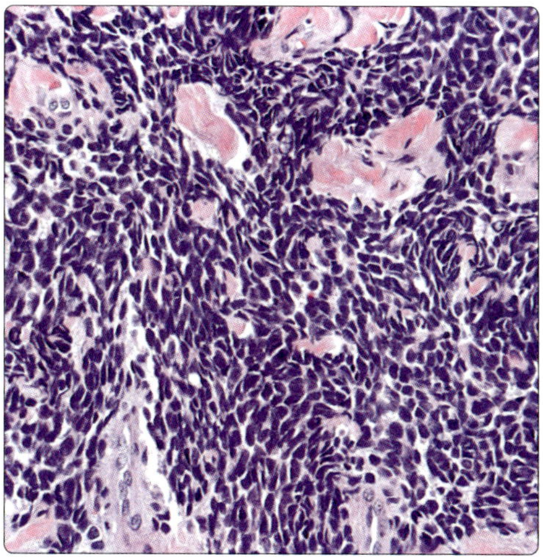

(Left) *ARMS most commonly arises in deep soft tissues of the extremities. In some cases, infiltration of skeletal muscle is prominent and resembles the myoinvasive pattern of lymphoma.* **(Right)** *Cauterized or crushed tumor samples of ARMS may be impossible to distinguish histologically from a variety of other small round blue cell tumors, such as small cell carcinoma, lymphoma, Ewing sarcoma, desmoplastic small round cell tumor, and others.*

Mixed Morphology

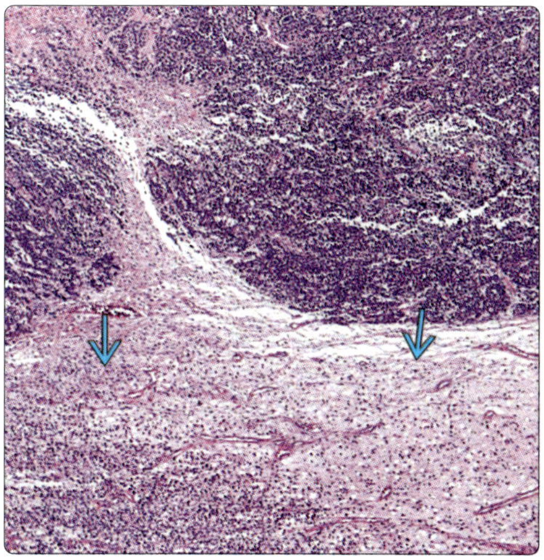

Cutaneous Involvement

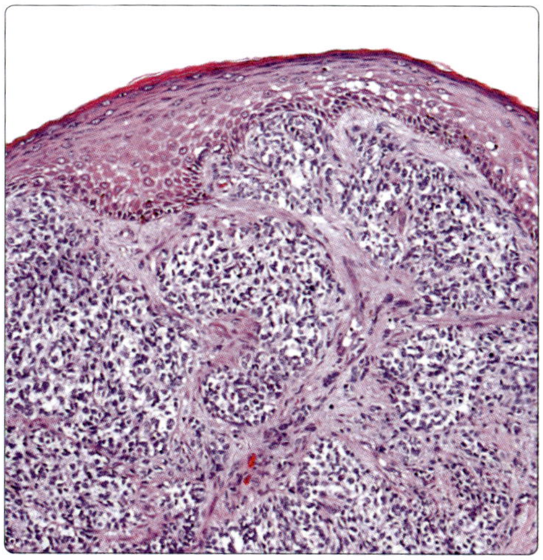

(Left) *Some cases of ARMS contain areas → morphologically compatible with embryonal rhabdomyosarcoma (ERMS). These composite or mixed-type tumors are more likely to be fusion negative than pure ARMS and may, therefore, be more closely related to ERMS than ARMS.* **(Right)** *ARMS may grow and extend to involve the skin and can be mistaken for a variety of other lesions including nevi and malignant melanoma. Immunohistochemistry is often discriminatory in a small biopsy.*

Desmin

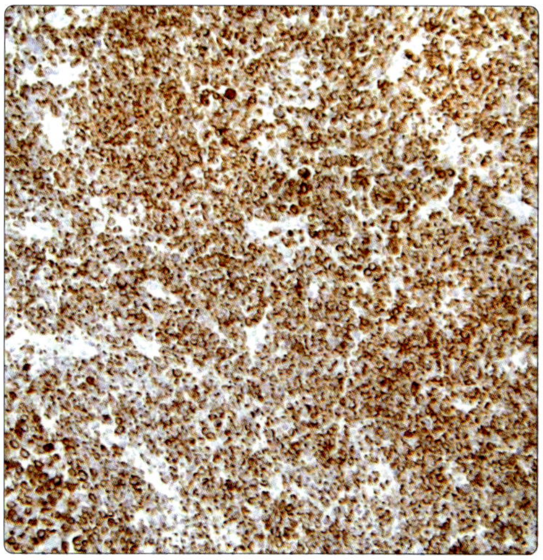

Myogenin

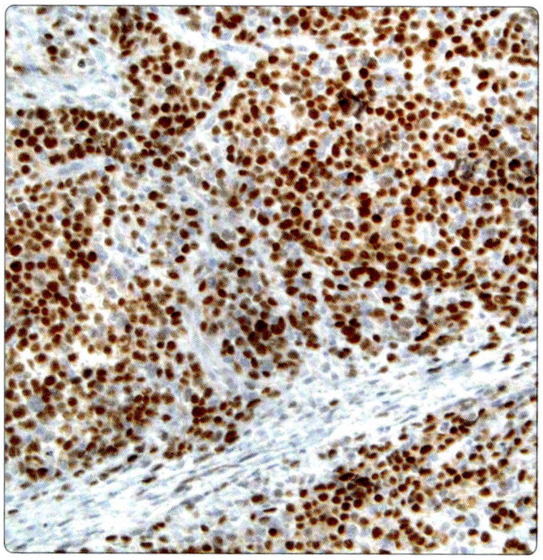

(Left) *Diffuse cytoplasmic expression of desmin is characteristic of ARMS.* **(Right)** *Nuclear expression of myogenin (shown) or MyoD1 is a consistent finding in ARMS. Of note, the expression is often diffuse and prominent in ARMS, whereas it is often patchy or focal in ERMS. Importantly, only nuclear expression counts for these markers, as cytoplasmic staining is nonspecific and should be ignored.*

Spindle Cell Rhabdomyosarcoma

KEY FACTS

TERMINOLOGY

- Subtype of rhabdomyosarcoma (RMS) affecting both children and adults that features prominent fascicular spindle cell morphology
  - Currently considered to be very closely related to sclerosing RMS and not embryonal RMS (2013 WHO classification)

CLINICAL ISSUES

- Affects both children and adults
  - Strong male predilection
- Most common sites
  - Paratesticular region in children
  - Head and neck region in adults
- Differences in behavior and outcome depending upon age group
  - Overall good prognosis in children (< 10 years)
  - Clinically aggressive in adults

MICROSCOPIC

- Cellular proliferation of relatively uniform spindle cells
  - Mitotic figures common
- Fascicular growth is usually prominent
- Variable number of rhabdomyoblasts
- Prominent collagenous stroma in some tumors

ANCILLARY TESTS

- Desmin (+), myogenin (+), MYOD1(+)
- SMA(+) and MSA(+) common
- Molecular: Recurrent *MYOD1* mutations
  - *VGLL2* and *NCOA2* rearrangements in infancy

TOP DIFFERENTIAL DIAGNOSES

- Synovial sarcoma (monophasic)
- Malignant peripheral nerve sheath tumor
- Low-grade myofibroblastic sarcoma
- Infantile fibrosarcoma
- Leiomyosarcoma

Spindle Cell Rhabdomyosarcoma

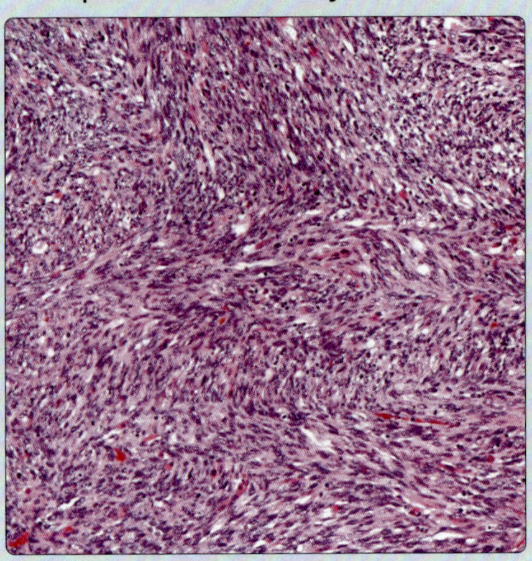

Rhabdomyoblasts

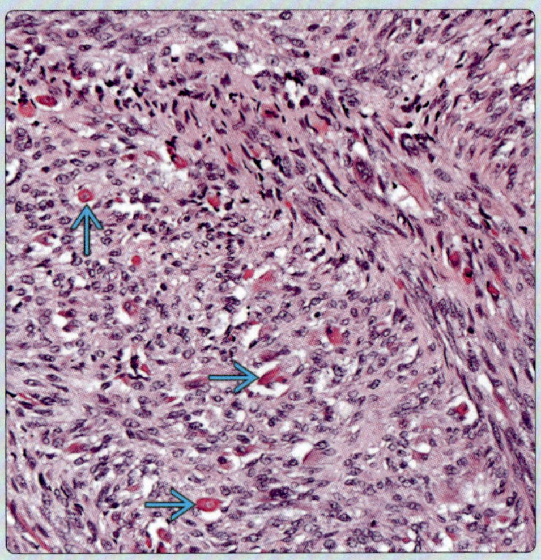

(Left) *Spindle cell rhabdomyosarcoma (SCRMS) is a distinctive subtype of RMS that affects both children and adults. It appears to be both morphologically and genetically related to sclerosing RMS. As shown on this H&E, most cases of SCRMS feature prominent fascicular growth with moderate to high cellularity.* **(Right)** *Rhabdomyoblasts → are often seen in SCRMS but vary in number and distribution from case to case. Both polygonal and spindled (strap cell) forms may be seen.*

Herringbone Architecture

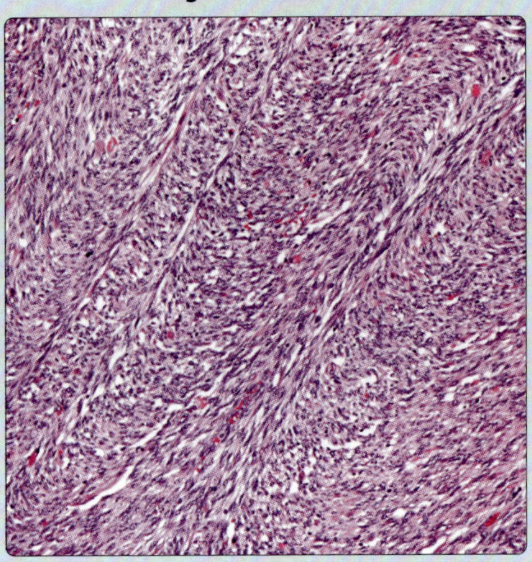

Myogenin Expression

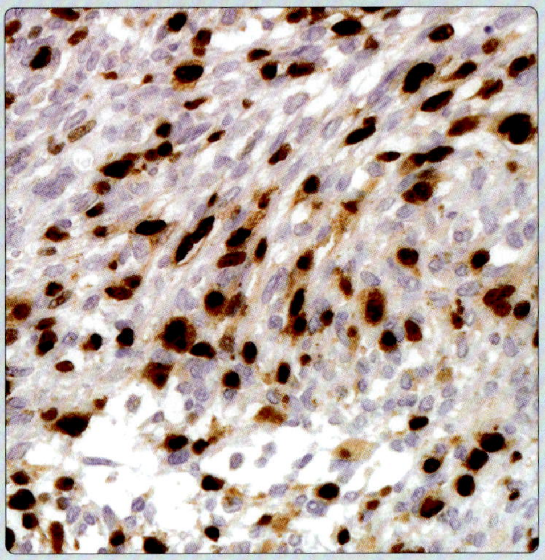

(Left) *A herringbone architectural pattern can be encountered in SCRMS, as depicted, and may lead to morphologic overlap with a variety of other mesenchymal spindle cell neoplasms.* **(Right)** *Strong myogenin expression is typical of SCRMS; however, in general, expression of this antigen is patchy or focal rather than diffuse and widespread. Cytoplasmic staining is nonspecific and should be disregarded.*

Spindle Cell Rhabdomyosarcoma

TERMINOLOGY

Abbreviations

- Spindle cell rhabdomyosarcoma (SCRMS)

Definitions

- Subtype of rhabdomyosarcoma (RMS) affecting both children and adults that features prominent fascicular spindle cell morphology
  - Currently considered to be very closely related to sclerosing RMS and not embryonal RMS (2013 WHO classification)

CLINICAL ISSUES

Epidemiology

- Age
  - Affects both children and adults
    - Children (< 10 years)
    - Adults (median: 30 years)
- Sex
  - Strong male predilection

Site

- Children
  - Most frequently arise in paratesticular region
- Adults
  - Head and neck region (> 50% of cases)
  - Occasionally other sites, including extremities, retroperitoneum, trunk

Presentation

- Usually deeply situated, often painless mass
  - Local symptoms pertaining to site of origin

Prognosis

- Significant differences in behavior and outcome depending upon age group
  - Overall good prognosis in children (< 10 years)
    - Usually low stage at presentation
    - > 95% survival at 5 years
  - Clinically aggressive in adults
    - Recurrence and metastasis in up to 50%
  - Metastases to lymph nodes, lungs, other sites

MACROSCOPIC

General Features

- Generally well circumscribed
- Firm, tan-white, fibrous cut surface
- Hemorrhage &/or necrosis infrequent

Size

- Wide range (mean: 6 cm)
  - Tumors > 30 cm reported

MICROSCOPIC

Histologic Features

- Cellular proliferation of relatively uniform spindle cells
  - Ovoid, elongated, or wavy and vesicular or hyperchromatic nuclei ± nucleoli
    - Frank pleomorphism absent
  - Scant, pale, eosinophilic or amphophilic cytoplasm
    - Cross striations may be seen
  - Mitotic figures common
- Fascicular growth is usually prominent
  - Can show herringbone pattern
  - Storiform growth in some tumors
- Variable number of rhabdomyoblasts
  - Spindled (strap cell) or polygonal
  - Brightly eosinophilic cytoplasm and hyperchromatic nucleus
  - May be sparse in adult tumors
- Less cellular tumors may show more prominent collagenous stroma
  - Collagen may be densely hyalinized
    - Areas may be indistinguishable from sclerosing RMS
- Necrosis may be present but is uncommon

ANCILLARY TESTS

Immunohistochemistry

- Desmin (+)
  - Characteristically strong, diffuse cytoplasmic expression
- Myogenin (+) and MYOD1(+)
  - Nuclear expression
  - Variable in extent (may be focal)
- SMA(+) and MSA(+) common
- Generally S100 protein, keratin, caldesmon, CD34, TLE1, β-catenin (-)

Molecular Genetics

- Lacks genetic features of embryonal and alveolar RMS
- Recurrent *MYOD1* mutations reported in SCRMS as well as sclerosing RMS
  - Supports relationship between these 2 entities
- *VGLL2* and *NCOA2* gene rearrangements reported in cases of infantile/congenital SCRMS

DIFFERENTIAL DIAGNOSIS

Synovial Sarcoma (Monophasic)

- Cellular fascicular of monomorphic spindled cells
- Stromal calcifications common
- Rhabdomyoblasts absent
- Keratin (+), EMA(+), typically patchy/focal
- Diffuse nuclear TLE1(+)
- Desmin, myogenin, MYOD1 (-)
- t(X;18) with fusions involving *SS18* (SYT)

Malignant Peripheral Nerve Sheath Tumor

- May arise from large nerves, preexisting benign nerve sheath tumors, or within setting of neurofibromatosis type 1
- Buckled, wavy, or bullet-shaped nuclei
- Increased perivascular cellularity common
- Necrosis common (can show perivascular preservation)
- S100 protein (+) in 60% of cases, classically focal
- May contain rhabdomyoblasts (a.k.a. malignant triton tumor)
  - Expression of desmin, myogenin, MYOD1 restricted to rhabdomyoblasts

Low-Grade Myofibroblastic Sarcoma

- Common in head and neck region of adults
- Prominent infiltrative growth
- Stromal collagen often abundant
- Rhabdomyoblasts absent
- Variable SMA(+), desmin (+)
- Myogenin (-), MYOD1(-)

Infantile Fibrosarcoma

- Can show morphologic overlap with SCRMS
- Rhabdomyoblasts absent
- Desmin, myogenin, MYOD1 (-)
- t(12;15) with *ETV6-NTRK3* fusion

Embryonal Rhabdomyosarcoma

- Most common in head/neck and genitourinary tract
- Cambium layer in epithelial-lined mucosal sites
- Myxoid stroma common
- Lacks prominent fascicular architecture
- Similar expression of myogenic markers to SCRMS

Fetal Rhabdomyoma

- Predilection for head and neck
- Bland spindled cells without atypia
- Mitoses usually absent; no necrosis

Desmoid Fibromatosis

- Low to moderate cellularity with prominent stromal collagen
- Nuclear atypia absent
- Distinctive thin-walled blood vessels, often with mild perivascular edema
- Rhabdomyoblasts absent
- Nuclear β-catenin (+) in 70%
- Desmin, myogenin, MYOD1 (-)

Leiomyosarcoma

- Characteristic smooth muscle cytology
  - Prominent cytoplasmic eosinophilia
  - Elongated nuclei with blunted ends (cigar-shaped)
- Strong diffuse SMA(+) and caldesmon (+) in most cases
- Variable desmin (+)
- Myogenin (-), MYOD1(-)

Myofibroma

- Cellular variant can show prominent fascicular growth
- Rhabdomyoblasts absent
- SMA(+)
- Desmin, myogenin, MYOD1 (-)

Fibrosarcomatous Dermatofibrosarcoma Protuberans

- Prominent fascicular growth in fibrosarcomatous areas
- Lower grade areas of conventional storiform dermatofibrosarcoma protuberans often present
- Rhabdomyoblasts absent
- Variable CD34(+)
- Desmin, myogenin, MYOD1 (-)
- t(17;22) with *COL1A1-PDGFRB* fusion

Inflammatory Myofibroblastic Tumor

- Myxoid stroma common
- Prominent chronic inflammatory cell infiltrate
- Rhabdomyoblasts absent
- *ALK* gene rearrangements in ~ 50% of cases
  - ALK(+) by immunohistochemistry
- Myogenin (-), MYOD1(-)

Adult-Type Fibrosarcoma

- Diagnosis of exclusion
- Prominent fascicular growth and herringbone pattern
- Rhabdomyoblasts absent
- Desmin, myogenin, MYOD1 (-)

Sarcomatoid Carcinoma

- Overlying epithelium may show dysplastic or in situ changes
- History of carcinoma may be present
- Keratin (+), EMA(+)
- Desmin, myogenin, MYOD1 (-)

Spindle Cell Melanoma

- Junctional component may be present in epidermis
- Diffuse S100 protein (+)
- Variable expression of melanocytic markers
- Desmin, myogenin, MYOD1 (-)

Cellular Schwannoma

- Most common in retroperitoneum, posterior mediastinum, pelvis
- Admixed lymphocytes and sheets of foamy histiocytes may be seen
- Lacks rhabdomyoblasts
- Strong, diffuse S100 protein (+)
- Desmin, myogenin, MYOD1 (-)

SELECTED REFERENCES

1. Smith MH et al: Rhabdomyosarcoma, spindle cell/sclerosing variant: a clinical and histopathological examination of this rare variant with three new cases from the oral cavity. Head Neck Pathol. 11(4):494-500, 2017
2. Alaggio R et al: A molecular study of pediatric spindle and sclerosing rhabdomyosarcoma: identification of novel and recurrent VGLL2-related fusions in infantile cases. Am J Surg Pathol. 40(2):224-35, 2016
3. Rekhi B et al: MYOD1 (L122R) mutations are associated with spindle cell and sclerosing rhabdomyosarcomas with aggressive clinical outcomes. Mod Pathol. 29(12):1532-1540, 2016
4. Agaram NP et al: Recurrent MYOD1 mutations in pediatric and adult sclerosing and spindle cell rhabdomyosarcomas: evidence for a common pathogenesis. Genes Chromosomes Cancer. 53(9):779-87, 2014
5. Rekhi B et al: Histopathological, immunohistochemical and molecular cytogenetic analysis of 21 spindle cell/sclerosing rhabdomyosarcomas. APMIS. 122(11):1144-52, 2014
6. Szuhai K et al: Transactivating mutation of the MYOD1 gene is a frequent event in adult spindle cell rhabdomyosarcoma. J Pathol. 232(3):300-7, 2014
7. Yasui N et al: Clinicopathologic analysis of spindle cell/sclerosing rhabdomyosarcoma. Pediatr Blood Cancer. 62(6):1011-6, 2014
8. Carroll SJ et al: Spindle cell rhabdomyosarcoma: a brief diagnostic review and differential diagnosis. Arch Pathol Lab Med. 137(8):1155-8, 2013
9. Mosquera JM et al: Recurrent NCOA2 gene rearrangements in congenital/infantile spindle cell rhabdomyosarcoma. Genes Chromosomes Cancer. 52(6):538-50, 2013
10. Stock N et al: Adult-type rhabdomyosarcoma: analysis of 57 cases with clinicopathologic description, identification of 3 morphologic patterns and prognosis. Am J Surg Pathol. 33(12):1850-9, 2009
11. Mentzel T et al: Spindle cell rhabdomyosarcoma in adults: clinicopathological and immunohistochemical analysis of seven new cases. Virchows Arch. 449(5):554-60, 2006
12. Parham DM et al: Rhabdomyosarcomas in adults and children: an update. Arch Pathol Lab Med. 130(10):1454-65, 2006
13. Nascimento AF et al: Spindle cell rhabdomyosarcoma in adults. Am J Surg Pathol. 29(8):1106-13, 2005

Cytologic Features

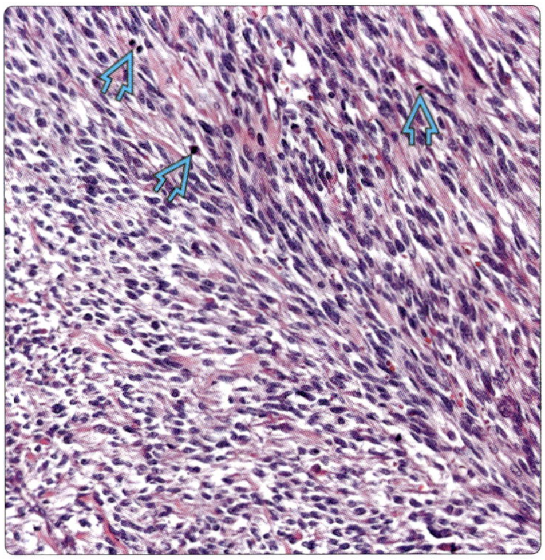

Desmin Expression

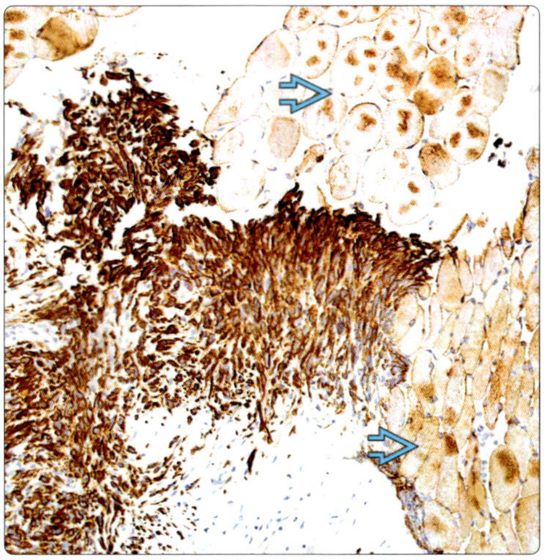

(Left) *Tumor cells in SCRMS are generally relatively uniform and may show ovoid, elongated, or wavy forms; however, nuclear atypia varies widely from case to case. Mitotic figures ➡ are often easily identified.* **(Right)** *Strong, diffuse cytoplasmic expression of desmin is characteristic of SCRMS. Weaker staining is seen within the fascicles of normal skeletal muscle ➡ in this stain.*

Infiltrative Borders

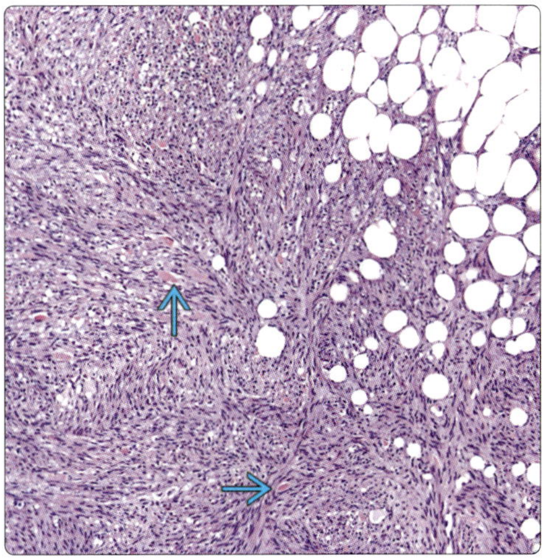

Variable Cellularity

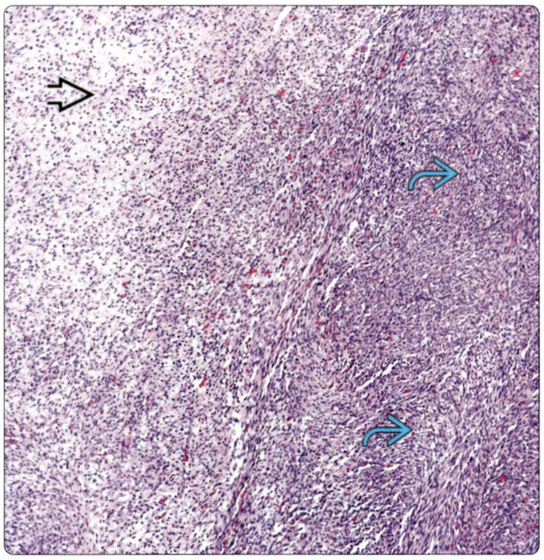

(Left) *SCRMS often shows an infiltrative peripheral border, as evidenced on this H&E by entrapped subcutaneous adipose tissue. Note the scattered rhabdomyoblasts ➡. H&E also shows a mixture of fascicular and storiform growth patterns.* **(Right)** *Many cases of SCRMS are highly cellular ➡; however, areas of lower cellularity ➡ and increased stromal collagen are not uncommon.*

Stromal Collagen

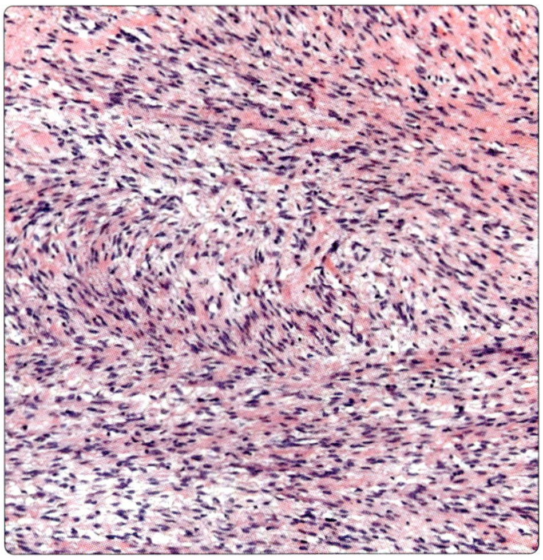

Densely Hyalinized Foci

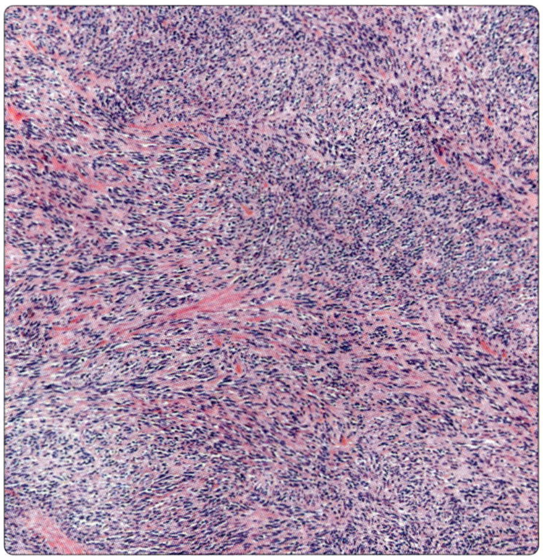

(Left) *H&E shows an area of SCRMS with a lower degree of cellularity and more prominent stromal collagen than is usually seen. A fascicular growth pattern is still present, but no obvious rhabdomyoblasts are seen in this field.* **(Right)** *Some cases of SCRMS contain minor foci showing densely hyalinized stromal collagen and a pseudovascular morphology, identical to what is seen in the related entity, sclerosing RMS.*

Sclerosing Rhabdomyosarcoma

KEY FACTS

TERMINOLOGY

- Synonym: Sclerosing pseudovascular rhabdomyosarcoma (RMS)
- Distinctive subtype of RMS featuring prominent hyalinized stroma and primitive-appearing tumor cells arranged predominantly in cords and nests
  - Currently considered to be very closely related to spindle cell RMS, not embryonal RMS (2013 WHO classification)

CLINICAL ISSUES

- Wide age range (median: 30 years)
- Most common in extremities
- Treatment: Wide surgical excision with negative margins
- Overall poor prognosis, particularly in adults
  - Recurrence and metastasis in up to 50%

MICROSCOPIC

- Primitive round, ovoid, or spindled tumor cells arranged predominantly in cords or nests
- Characteristic prominent hyaline collagenous stroma
  - Often imparts pseudovascular appearance
- Rhabdomyoblasts are generally uncommon
- Areas of fascicular growth may be seen
  - Indistinguishable from spindle cell RMS

ANCILLARY TESTS

- MYOD1(+), typically diffuse
- Variable desmin (+), myogenin (+)
  - Both/either may be very focally expressed
- Molecular: Recurrent *MYOD1* mutations
- Lacks genetic features of embryonal and alveolar RMS

TOP DIFFERENTIAL DIAGNOSES

- Alveolar RMS
- Sclerosing epithelioid fibrosarcoma
- Metastatic carcinoma
- Angiosarcoma

(Left) *Sclerosing rhabdomyosarcoma (SRMS) is an aggressive sarcoma that may affect both children and adults. It is morphologically and genetically related to spindle cell rhabdomyosarcoma (RMS). At low power, the hyalinized/sclerotic collagenous stroma is one of the more characteristic features of this tumor.* **(Right)** *Densely hyalinized or sclerotic stroma classically leads to cellular dyscohesion* → *in SRMS, which in turn can resemble infiltrating vascular channels of angiosarcoma.*

Sclerosing Rhabdomyosarcoma

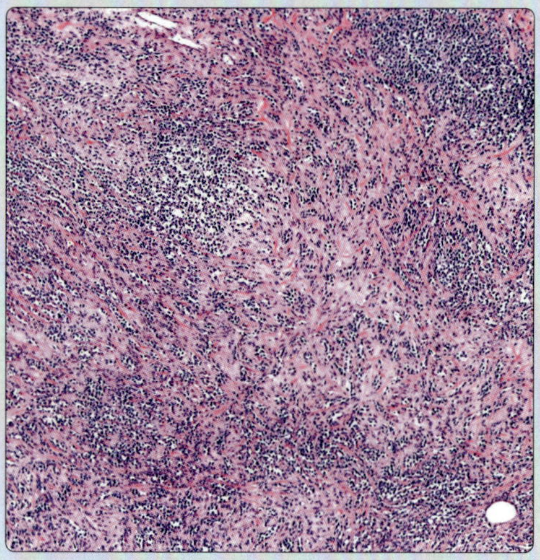

Pseudovascular Appearance

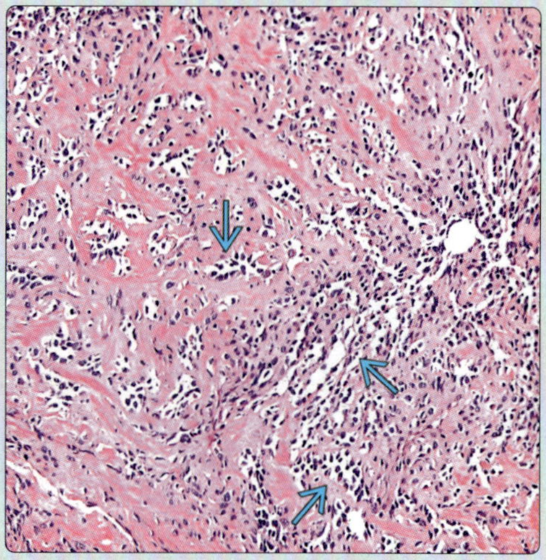

(Left) *Tumor cells in SRMS are usually arranged in small nests and cords within the hyalinized collagenous stroma. Some smaller nests may show central dyscohesion, imparting a microalveolar appearance* →. **(Right)** *MYOD1 expression (shown) is characteristically strong and diffuse in SRMS. In contrast, expression of myogenin is much more variable and can be very focal. Of note, only nuclear expression of MYOD1 (and myogenin) should be considered positive.*

Cords and Nests

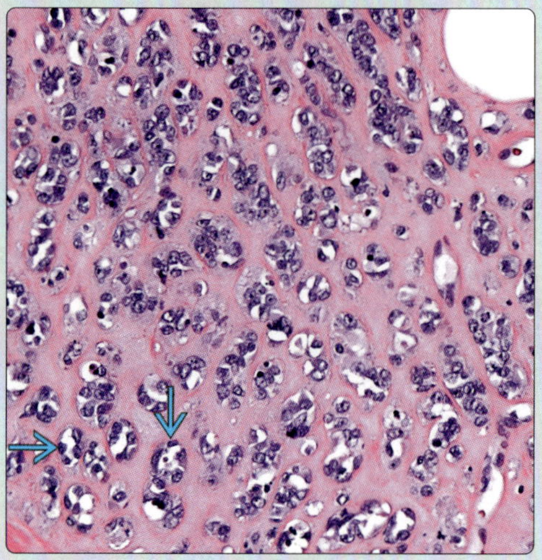

Myogenic Immunophenotype

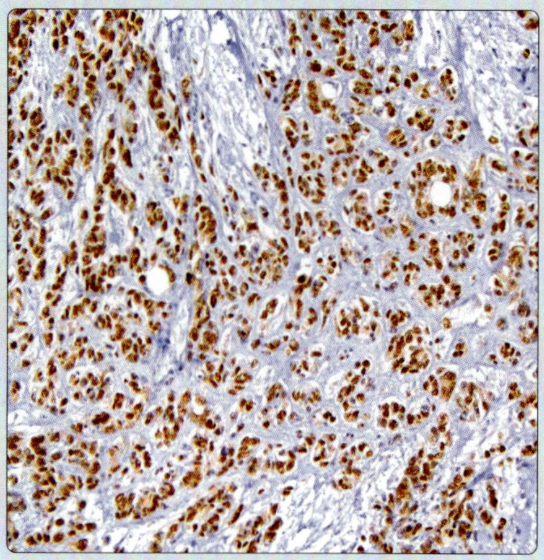

TERMINOLOGY

Abbreviations

- Sclerosing rhabdomyosarcoma (SRMS)

Synonyms

- Sclerosing pseudovascular rhabdomyosarcoma (RMS)

Definitions

- Distinctive subtype of RMS featuring prominent hyalinized stroma and primitive-appearing tumor cells arranged predominantly in cords and nests
  - Currently considered to be very closely related to spindle cell RMS and not embryonal RMS (2013 WHO classification)

CLINICAL ISSUES

Epidemiology

- Age
  - Wide range (median: 30 years)
- Sex
  - Strong male predilection

Site

- Most common in extremities
- Also head/neck region

Presentation

- Painless, often deep-seated mass

Treatment

- Wide surgical excision with negative margins, if possible
  - May require amputation
- Chemotherapy &/or radiotherapy

Prognosis

- Overall poor prognosis, particularly in adults
  - Recurrence and metastasis in up to 50%
- Worse prognosis reported in presence of *MYOD1* mutation

MACROSCOPIC

General Features

- White to tan, firm to fleshy, hemorrhagic areas

Size

- Wide range (median: 6 cm)

MICROSCOPIC

Histologic Features

- Infiltrative borders
- Primitive round, ovoid, or spindled tumor cells arranged predominantly in cords or nests
  - Scant eosinophilic or clear cytoplasm
  - Mitoses frequent
- Characteristic prominent hyaline collagenous stroma
  - Can mimic osteoid
  - Often imparts pseudovascular appearance
- Solid, cellular areas present in some tumors
- Rhabdomyoblasts are generally uncommon
- Areas of fascicular growth may be seen
  - Indistinguishable from spindle cell RMS

ANCILLARY TESTS

Immunohistochemistry

- Variable desmin (+), myogenin (+)
  - Expression of either/both may be very focal
  - Desmin may show perinuclear, dot-like expression
- MYOD1(+), typically diffuse
- SMA(+) in subset of cases
- Keratin, S100 protein, SATB2, CD31, CD34 (-)

Molecular Genetics

- Lacks genetic features of embryonal and alveolar RMS
- Recurrent *MYOD1* mutations reported in SRMS as well as spindle cell RMS
  - Supports relationship between these 2 entities
- Also *PIK3CA* mutations

DIFFERENTIAL DIAGNOSIS

Alveolar Rhabdomyosarcoma

- Generally lacks densely hyalinized stroma of SRMS
- Wreath-like multinucleated giant cells
- Lacks spindle cell component
- Myogenin (+) characteristically diffuse
- t(2;13) or t(1;13) rearrangement with *FOXO1* fusion

Sclerosing Epithelioid Fibrosarcoma

- Bland tumor cell nuclei
- MUC4(+)
- Desmin, myogenin, MYOD1 (-)
- *EWSR1* and *CREB3L2* rearrangements

Angiosarcoma

- More complex branching architecture
- CD31, CD34, ERG (+)
- Desmin, myogenin, MYOD1 (-)

Metastatic Carcinoma

- Keratin (+)
- Desmin, myogenin, MYOD1 (-)

Extraskeletal Osteosarcoma

- Often features sheets of large pleomorphic cells
- SATB2(+)
- Desmin, myogenin, MYOD1 (-)

SELECTED REFERENCES

1. Smith MH et al: Rhabdomyosarcoma, spindle cell/sclerosing variant: a clinical and histopathological examination of this rare variant with three new cases from the oral cavity. Head Neck Pathol. 11(4):494-500, 2017
2. Rekhi B et al: MYOD1 (L122R) mutations are associated with spindle cell and sclerosing rhabdomyosarcomas with aggressive clinical outcomes. Mod Pathol. 29(12):1532-1540, 2016
3. Rekhi B et al: Histopathological, immunohistochemical and molecular cytogenetic analysis of 21 spindle cell/sclerosing rhabdomyosarcomas. APMIS. 122(11):1144-52, 2014
4. Robinson JC et al: Sclerosing rhabdomyosarcoma: report of a case arising in the head and neck of an adult and review of the literature. Head Neck Pathol. 7(2):193-202, 2013
5. Wang J et al: Sclerosing rhabdomyosarcoma: a clinicopathologic and immunohistochemical study of five cases. Am J Clin Pathol. 129(3):410-5, 2008
6. Chiles MC et al: Sclerosing rhabdomyosarcomas in children and adolescents: a clinicopathologic review of 13 cases from the Intergroup Rhabdomyosarcoma Study Group and Children's Oncology Group. Pediatr Dev Pathol. 8(1):141, 2005

(Left) *Tumors cells in SRMS are cytologically variable and may feature nuclear atypia that ranges from mild to marked. Mitotic figures* ⇒*, however, are generally abundant.* **(Right)** *Rhabdomyoblasts are often sparse and difficult to find in SRMS; however, in rare cases, they are more readily identified. As is often the case in other forms of RMS, these cells have abundant, deeply eosinophilic cytoplasm and are polygonal* → *or fusiform-shaped* ↗*.*

Cytologic Features

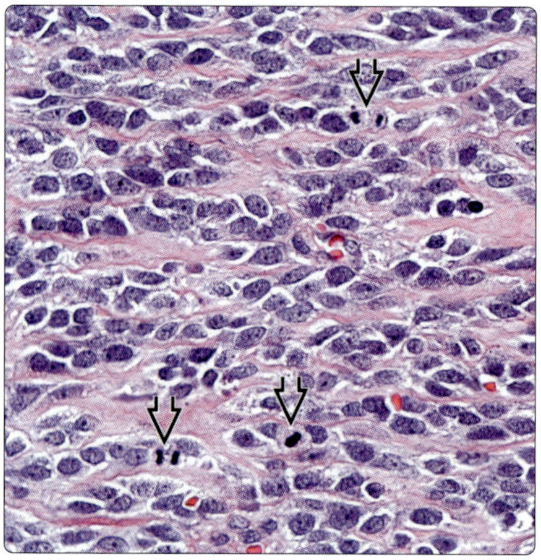

Rhabdomyoblasts

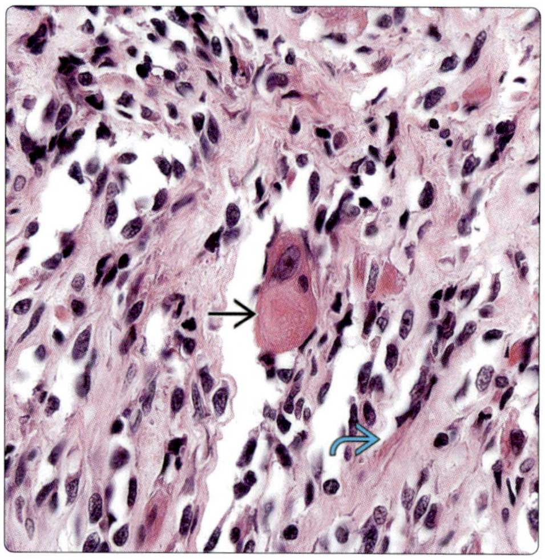

(Left) *Corded or trabecular growth is common in SRMS and may be quite prominent in some cases, as depicted. Note the densely hyalinized stroma between the cords.* **(Right)** *H&E shows a case of SRMS in which the cords of tumor cells are more compressed, subsequently creating a more cellular overall appearance. Note, however, that the characteristic hyalinized stroma can still be appreciated, even at low magnification.*

Prominent Corded Morphology

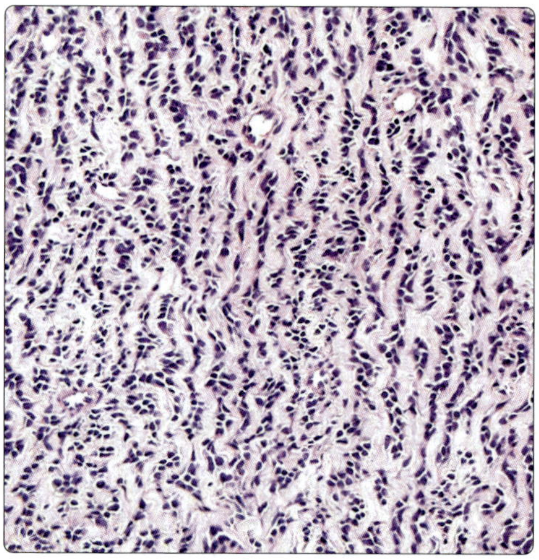

Cellular Corded Morphology

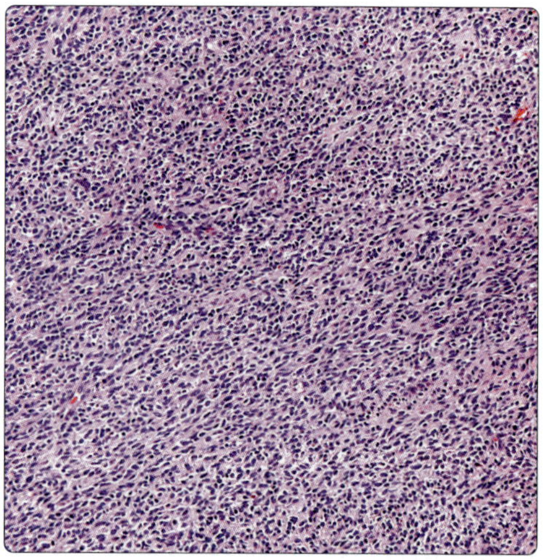

(Left) *A microalveolar pattern is a common finding in SRMS and may cause confusion with alveolar RMS. It is characterized by clusters and nests of loosely cohesive tumor cells* → *with central spaces, reminiscent of small pulmonary alveoli. These spaces are smaller than what is typically seen in alveolar RMS, and wreath-like multinucleated cells are absent.* **(Right)** *Areas of more densely cellular and sheet-like growth may be seen in SRMS; however, these areas are generally not extensive.*

Microalveolar Pattern

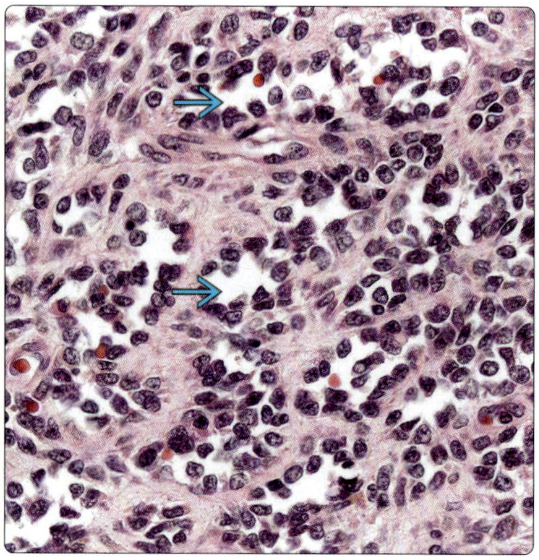

Cellular, Solid Foci

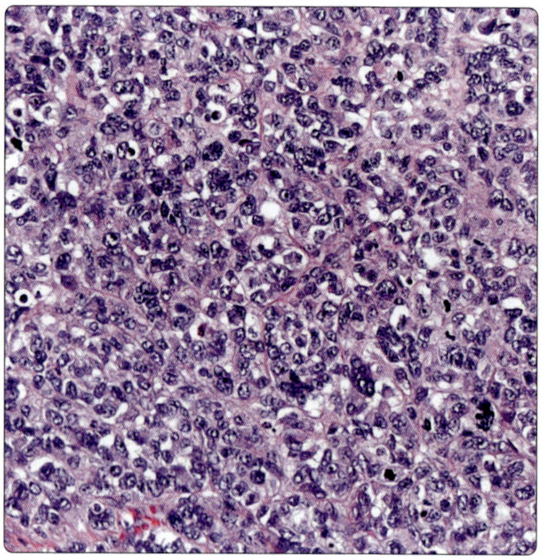

Clear Cell Change

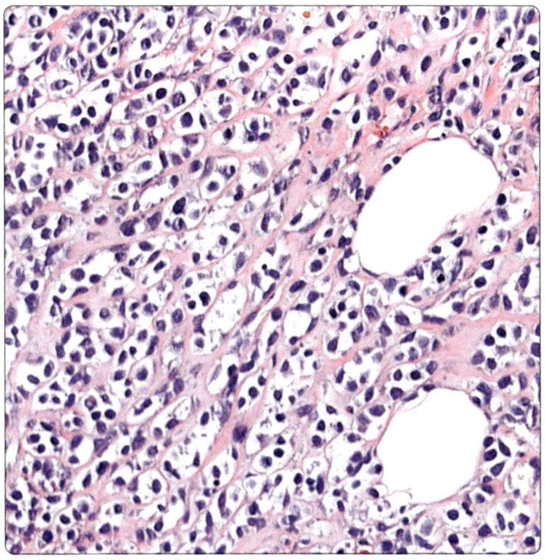

Infiltrative Growth

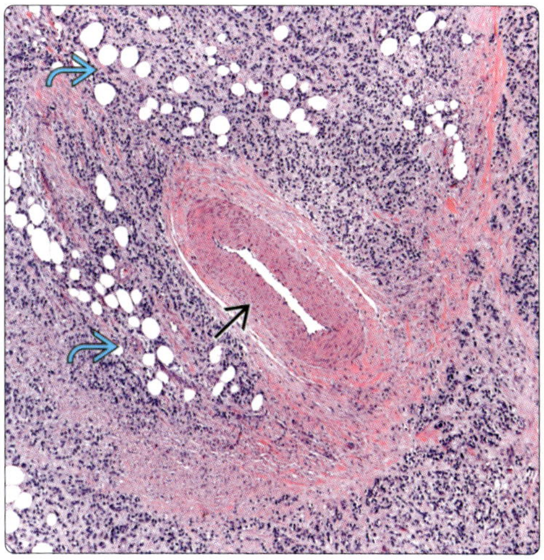

(Left) *Tumor cells with clear cytoplasm can be seen in SRMS. In conjunction with the sclerotic stroma, this appearance may easily lead to confusion with sclerosing epithelioid fibrosarcoma. Immunohistochemistry may be needed to make the distinction.* **(Right)** *Most cases of SRMS show an infiltrative pattern of growth, and tumors can contain areas of entrapped adipose tissue ↪, nerves, muscle, or large vessels →. Involvement of the latter may complicate or preclude local resection.*

Diffusely Hyalinized Zones

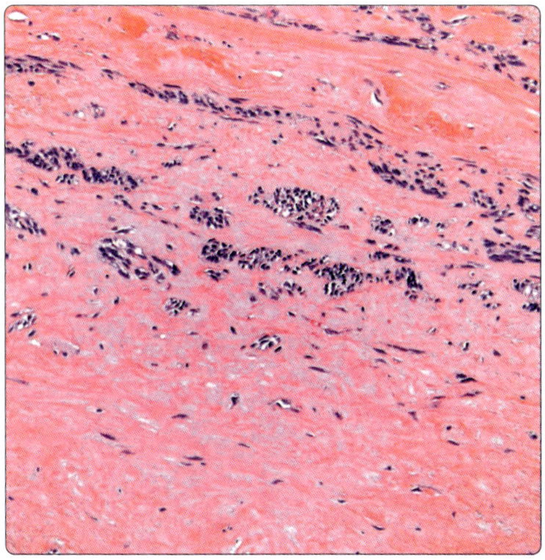

Spindle Cell Morphology

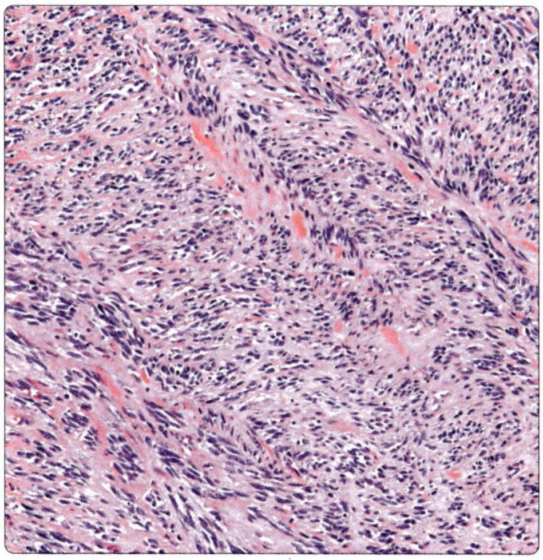

(Left) *Paucicellular hyalinized zones may be present in SRMS but are usually not a dominant feature.* **(Right)** *Spindled tumor cells (± fascicular growth) are not uncommon in SRMS and serve to establish a morphologic link with the related entity spindle cell RMS. Note the densely hyalinized stroma.*

Fascicular Growth

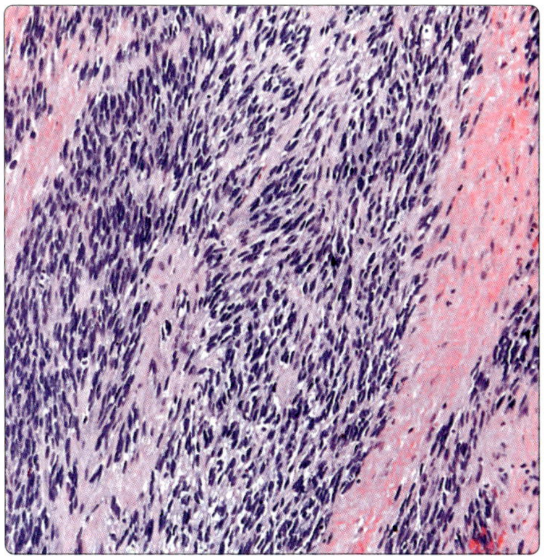

Desmin Expression

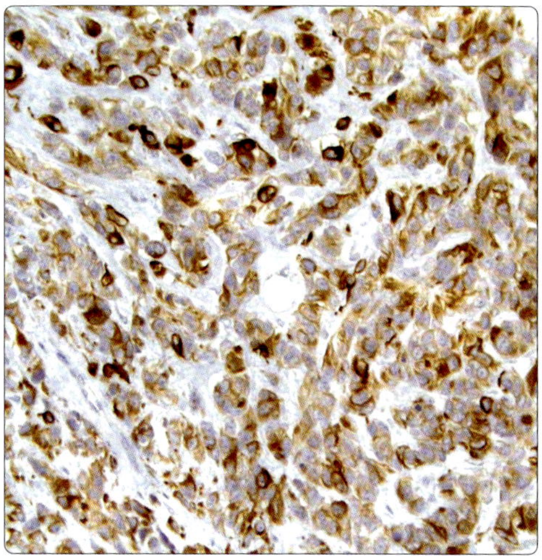

(Left) *Prominent fascicular growth by spindled tumor cells, as depicted, is seen in some cases of SRMS. These areas may be morphologically indistinguishable from spindle cell RMS, which is related to SRMS.* **(Right)** *Desmin expression is highly variable in SRMS and can range from focal to extensive. Notably, in some cases, it may show a perinuclear, dot-like pattern of expression.*

Pleomorphic Rhabdomyosarcoma

KEY FACTS

TERMINOLOGY

- High-grade sarcoma of adulthood composed of varying numbers of pleomorphic rhabdomyoblasts

CLINICAL ISSUES

- Almost exclusively in adults > 45 years
- Deep soft tissue of lower extremity, particularly thigh
- Aggressive disease with frequent early metastasis

MICROSCOPIC

- Variable numbers of pleomorphic rhabdomyoblasts: Large polygonal cells with pleomorphic nuclei and abundant, deeply eosinophilic cytoplasm
- Frequent mitoses with atypical mitotic forms
- Geographic tumor necrosis often present
- 3 main histologic patterns
  - Classic
    - Diffuse sheets of pleomorphic rhabdomyoblasts
  - Round cell
    - Clusters of pleomorphic rhabdomyoblasts
    - Background of medium-sized round cells with slight pleomorphism
  - Spindle cell
    - Pleomorphic spindle cells predominate
    - Storiform or fascicular growth pattern
    - Only scattered pleomorphic rhabdomyoblasts

ANCILLARY TESTS

- Strong desmin (+)
- Strong nuclear myogenin (+) and MYOD1(+)
- No consistent molecular abnormality

TOP DIFFERENTIAL DIAGNOSES

- Other pleomorphic sarcomas
- Alveolar or embryonal rhabdomyosarcoma
- Epithelioid rhabdomyosarcoma
- Undifferentiated or metastatic carcinoma
- Melanoma

Pleomorphic Rhabdomyosarcoma

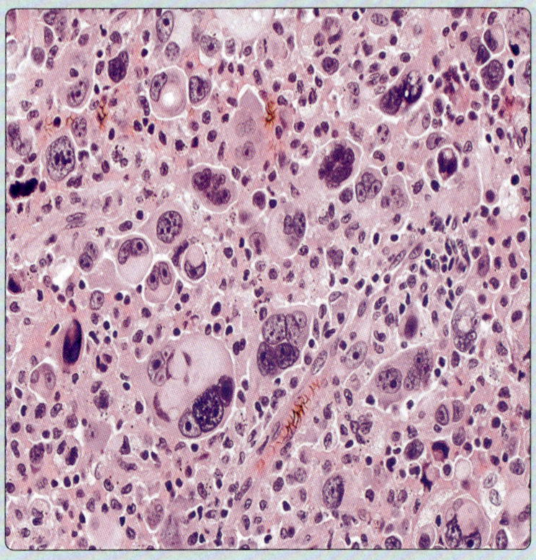

Pleomorphic Rhabdomyoblasts

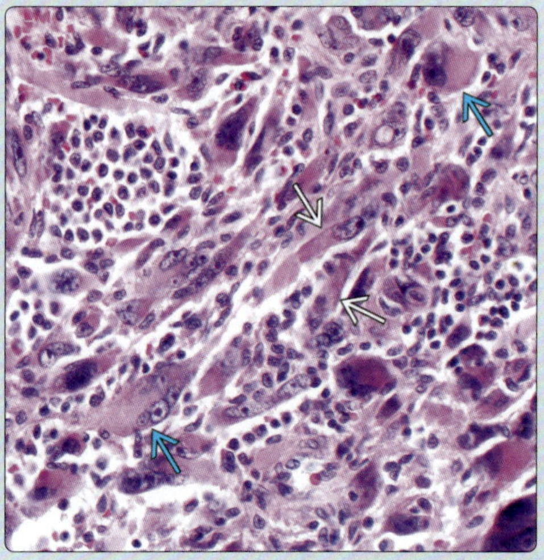

(Left) *Pleomorphic rhabdomyosarcoma (RMS) is a high-grade, adult-type sarcoma composed of a variable number of pleomorphic rhabdomyoblasts. Pleomorphic rhabdomyoblasts are large polygonal cells with markedly atypical nuclei and abundant, deeply eosinophilic cytoplasm. These cells are the hallmark of pleomorphic RMS.* **(Right)** *Pleomorphic rhabdomyoblasts may display a variety of appearances, including large, multinucleated polygonal cells and elongated, strap-like cells.*

Pleomorphic Rhabdomyoblasts

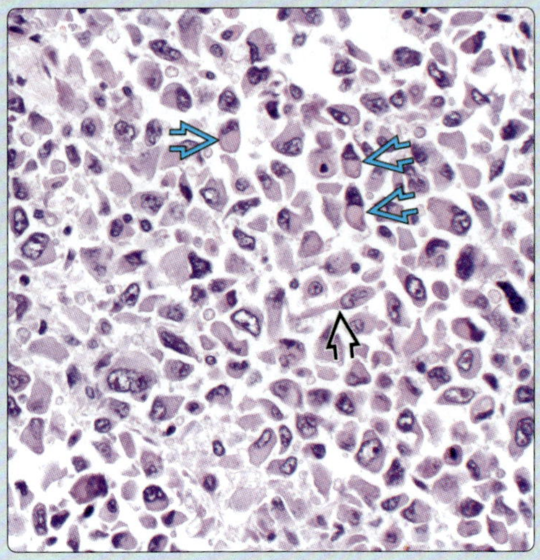

Pleomorphic Rhabdomyoblasts

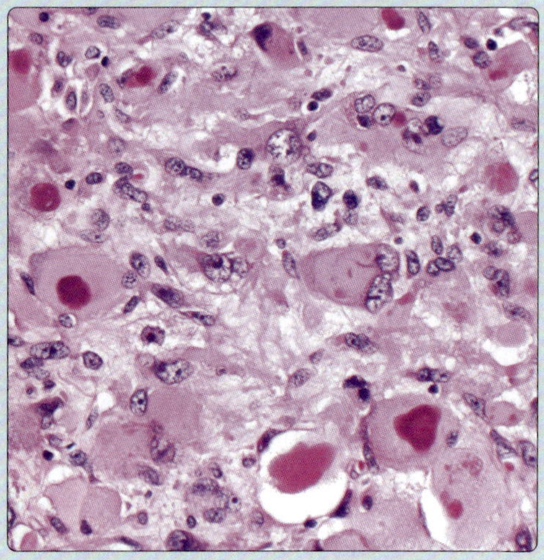

(Left) *Pleomorphic rhabdomyoblasts exhibit a diverse array of shapes and sizes. Some are tadpole- or racquet-shaped. Rhabdoid cells with an eccentric nucleus and a dense eosinophilic globule in the paranuclear cytoplasm are uncommon in pleomorphic RMS but may be seen.* **(Right)** *These pleomorphic rhabdomyoblasts display unusual dense, eosinophilic inclusions within their abundant cytoplasm.*

Pleomorphic Rhabdomyosarcoma

TERMINOLOGY

Definitions

- High-grade sarcoma of adulthood composed of varying numbers of pleomorphic rhabdomyoblasts

CLINICAL ISSUES

Epidemiology

- Age
  - Almost exclusively in adults > 45 years
    - Median: 6th-7th decades
  - Vanishingly rare in childhood
- Sex
  - M > F

Site

- Deep soft tissue of lower extremity, particularly thigh
- Less common sites
  - Retroperitoneum
  - Abdominal wall or chest wall
  - Spermatic cord and testes
  - Upper extremity
  - Visceral organs
  - Skin

Presentation

- Rapidly growing mass

Prognosis

- Aggressive disease with frequent early metastasis
- Mortality approaches 70% in some series

MACROSCOPIC

General Features

- Usually large (> 10-cm), circumscribed mass in deep skeletal muscle
- Fleshy cut surface often with extensive necrosis

MICROSCOPIC

Histologic Features

- Variable numbers of pleomorphic rhabdomyoblasts: Large polygonal cells with pleomorphic nuclei and abundant, deeply eosinophilic cytoplasm
  - Rhabdomyoblasts may be tadpole- or racquet-shaped as in embryonal rhabdomyosarcoma (RMS) but are usually larger and more irregular
    - Cross striations are rare
- 3 main histologic patterns
  - Classic
    - Diffuse sheets of pleomorphic rhabdomyoblasts
  - Round cell
    - Clusters of pleomorphic rhabdomyoblasts
    - Background of medium-sized round cells with slight pleomorphism
  - Spindle cell
    - Pleomorphic spindle cells predominate; arranged in storiform or fascicular (less common) pattern
    - Only scattered pleomorphic rhabdomyoblasts
- Frequent mitoses with atypical mitotic forms
- Geographic tumor necrosis often present
- Only rarely display "rhabdoid" features (eccentric nucleus, dense paranuclear eosinophilic globule)

ANCILLARY TESTS

Immunohistochemistry

- Strong desmin (+) but may be focal
- Strong nuclear myogenin (+) and MYOD1(+)
  - Often more focal than in pediatric (embryonal and alveolar) RMS
- Other myogenic markers (e.g., actins) variably expressed
- May express keratin focally

DIFFERENTIAL DIAGNOSIS

Other Pleomorphic Sarcomas

- Pleomorphic leiomyosarcoma
  - Lower grade areas with intersecting fascicles
  - Myogenin (-) and MYOD1(-)
- Pleomorphic liposarcoma
  - Must have pleomorphic lipoblasts
- Undifferentiated pleomorphic sarcoma
  - Desmin (-), myogenin (-), and MYOD1(-)

Alveolar or Embryonal Rhabdomyosarcoma

- Children and adolescents
- May have pleomorphic foci resembling pleomorphic RMS
  - Diffuse, marked pleomorphism absent
- Areas of classic alveolar or embryonal RMS usually present
- Characteristic translocation in alveolar RMS

Epithelioid Rhabdomyosarcoma

- Affects children and adults
- Large, monomorphic cells; lacks prominent nuclear and cytologic pleomorphism
- Obvious evidence of rhabdomyoblastic differentiation (e.g., rhabdomyoblasts, strap cells) usually absent

Anaplastic Large Cell Lymphoma

- Expresses CD30, ALK1, some T-cell markers

Undifferentiated or Metastatic Carcinoma

- Clinical scenario/history favoring carcinoma over sarcoma
- Often at least focally (+) for cytokeratin, EMA, or p63/p40

Melanoma

- S100 and SOX10 (+)
- Often HMB-45 and MART-1 (+), but some are (-)

SELECTED REFERENCES

1. Nishijima Y et al: Pleomorphic rhabdomyosarcoma arising in the anterior mediastinum: a case report with cytological features of imprint and liquid-based cytology specimens. Diagn Cytopathol. 45(4):333-8, 2017
2. Marburger TB et al: Primary cutaneous rhabdomyosarcoma: a clinicopathologic review of 11 cases. J Cutan Pathol. 39(11):987-95, 2012
3. Li G et al: Cytogenetic and real-time quantitative reverse-transcriptase polymerase chain reaction analyses in pleomorphic rhabdomyosarcoma. Cancer Genet Cytogenet. 192(1):1-9, 2009
4. Furlong MA et al: Pleomorphic rhabdomyosarcoma in adults: a clinicopathologic study of 38 cases with emphasis on morphologic variants and recent skeletal muscle-specific markers. Mod Pathol. 14(6):595-603, 2001
5. Furlong MA et al: Pleomorphic rhabdomyosarcoma in children: four cases in the pediatric age group. Ann Diagn Pathol. 5(4):199-206, 2001

(Left) *Pleomorphic RMS is often relatively circumscribed with a smooth, pushing border and dense fibrous pseudocapsule separating the tumor from adjacent skeletal muscle. Focal inflammation is also present.* **(Right)** *Geographic zones of tumor necrosis are usually present in pleomorphic RMS.*

Circumscribed With Pseudocapsule

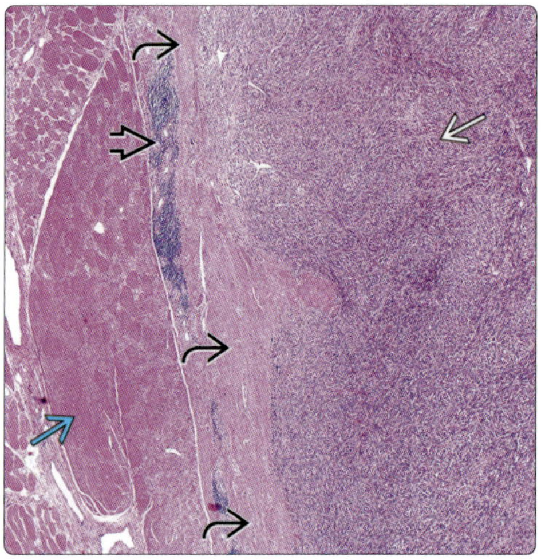

Geographic Necrosis

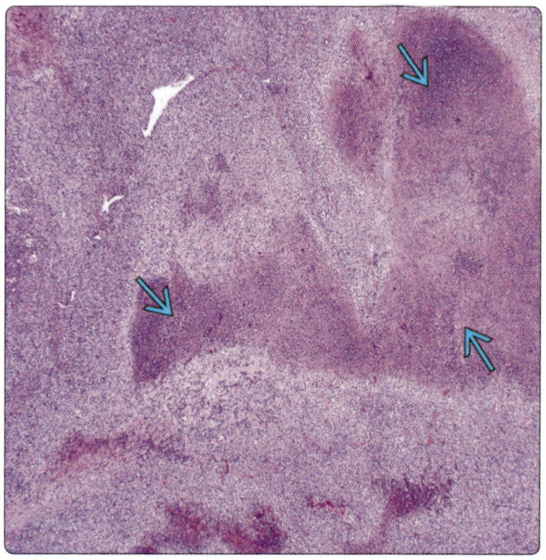

(Left) *Pleomorphic rhabdomyoblasts are arranged in diffuse sheets in the classic pattern of pleomorphic RMS. The degree of atypia can be severe in some cases and easily suggest a diagnosis of undifferentiated pleomorphic sarcoma at first.* **(Right)** *There is marked nuclear atypia with pleomorphism and prominent nucleoli in pleomorphic RMS. Mitotic figures are usually abundant.*

Classic Pattern

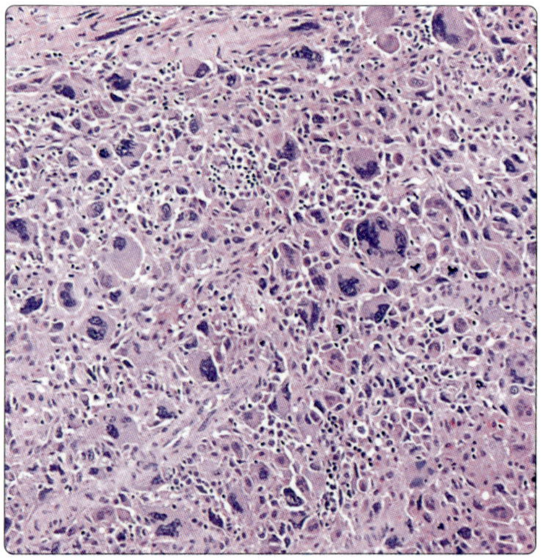

Pleomorphism and Mitoses

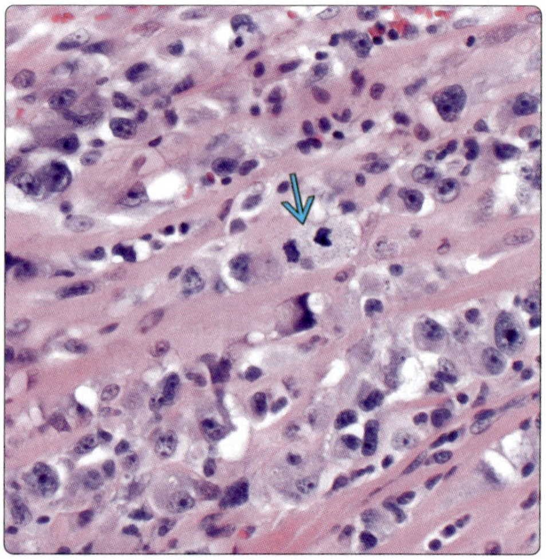

(Left) *Large pleomorphic rhabdomyoblasts are distributed in a background of smaller oval/round cells in the round cell pattern of pleomorphic RMS.* **(Right)** *Large pleomorphic rhabdomyoblasts are distributed in a background of smaller round cells in the round cell pattern of pleomorphic RMS. The smaller cells have oval/round, slightly pleomorphic nuclei and scant amounts of deeply eosinophilic cytoplasm.*

Round Cell Pattern

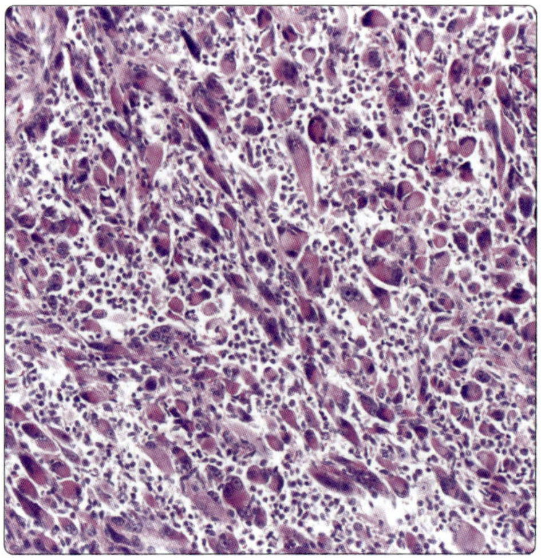

Round Cell Pattern

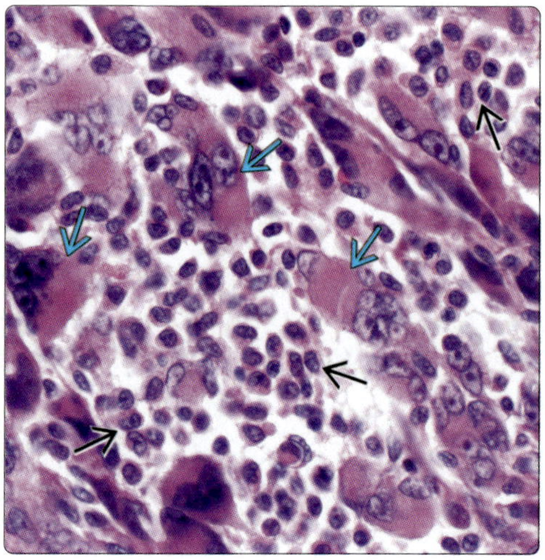

Spindle Cell Pattern

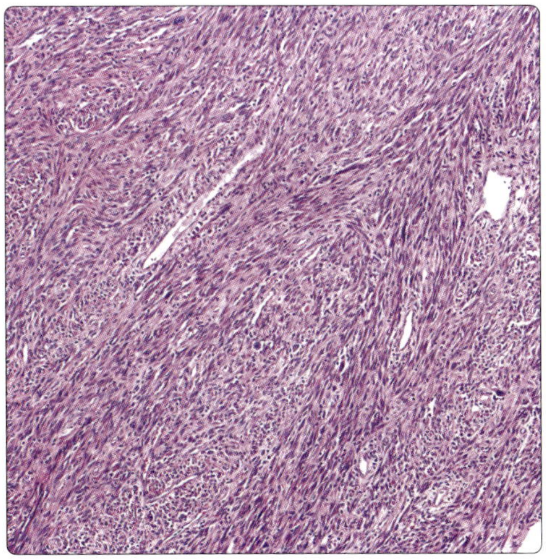

Spindle Cell Pattern

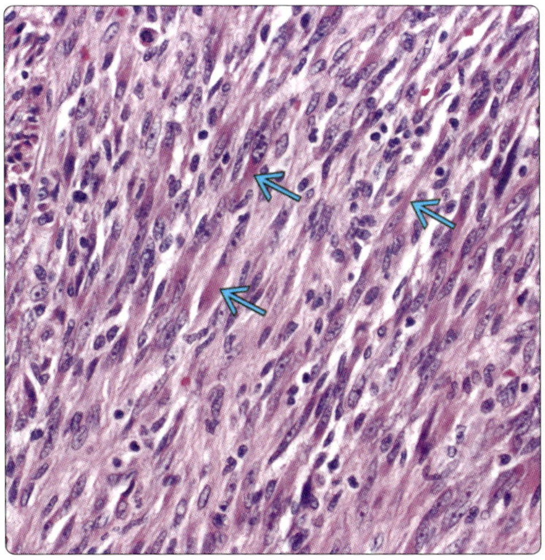

(Left) *Atypical spindle cells predominate over pleomorphic rhabdomyoblasts in the spindle cell pattern of pleomorphic RMS. The spindle cells may be arranged in long, intersecting fascicles, as shown here.* **(Right)** *Some of the spindle cells are elongated pleomorphic rhabdomyoblasts with abundant, deeply eosinophilic cytoplasm* ➡.

Storiform Areas

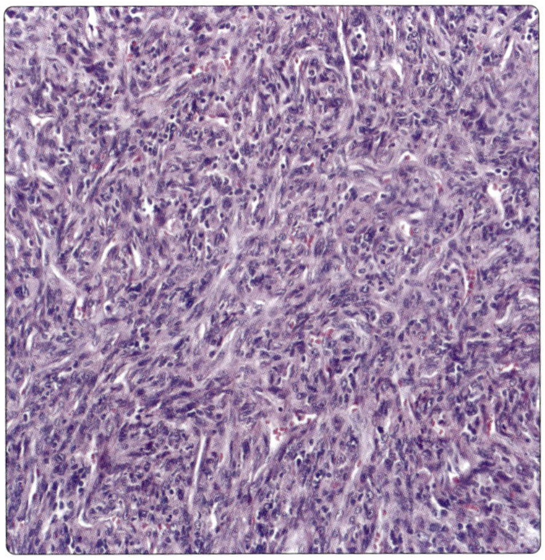

Multinucleated Rhabdomyoblasts

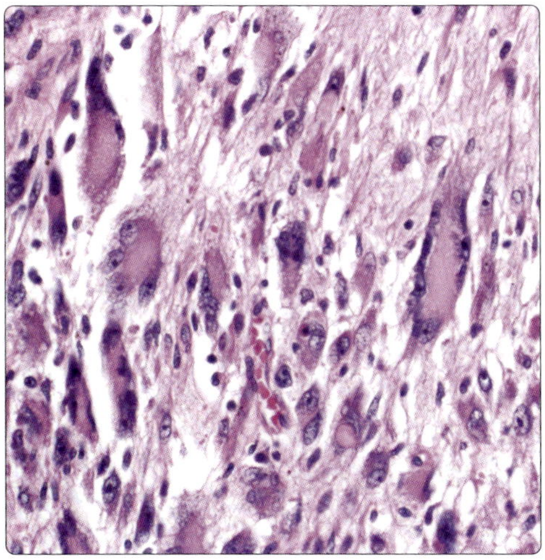

(Left) *Atypical spindle cells predominate over pleomorphic rhabdomyoblasts in the spindle cell pattern of pleomorphic RMS. The spindle cells may be arranged in a storiform pattern, as shown here.* **(Right)** *Multinucleated pleomorphic rhabdomyoblasts may be seen in pleomorphic RMS.*

Desmin Expression

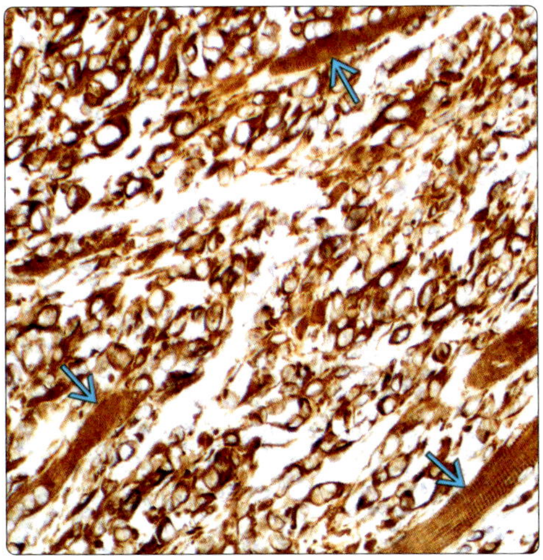

Myogenin Expression

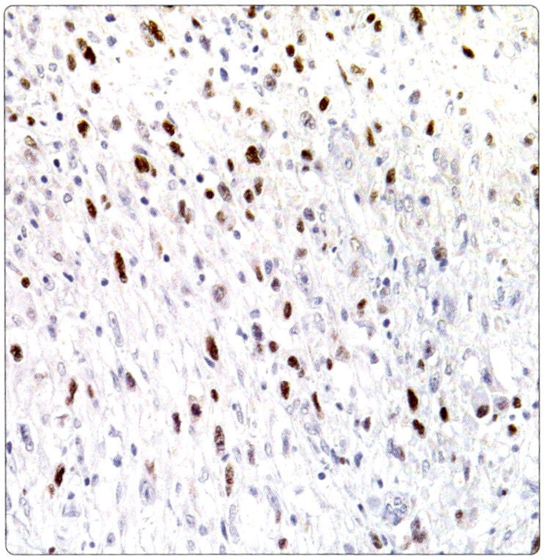

(Left) *The tumor cells of pleomorphic RMS display diffuse, strong cytoplasmic expression of desmin. The intervening normal skeletal muscle fibers are also positive* ➡. **(Right)** *Strong nuclear expression of myogenin is usually seen, but it may be more focal than in the pediatric forms of RMS.*

Epithelioid Rhabdomyosarcoma

KEY FACTS

TERMINOLOGY

- Distinctive rhabdomyosarcoma (RMS) variant characterized by uniform epithelioid cytomorphology

CLINICAL ISSUES

- Very rare
- Wide age reported (6-78 years)
  - Often in older or elderly adults
- Male predilection
- Deep soft tissues of the extremities, head/neck, trunk
  - Occasionally, superficial or cutaneous sites
- Treatment: Combination of surgery and chemotherapy &/or radiation
- Favorable prognosis and outcome in children
- Aggressive clinical course in adults
  - Recurrence and metastases common
  - Very poor 5-year survival rate

MICROSCOPIC

- Relatively uniform epithelioid cells with abundant eosinophilic cytoplasm
  - Large, vesicular nuclei often with prominent nucleoli
  - Intracytoplasmic rhabdoid inclusions may be seen
- Diffuse, sheet-like growth pattern
- Mitotic figures abundant, including atypical forms
- Necrosis common

ANCILLARY TESTS

- Desmin (+), myogenin (+), MYOD1(+)
- Retention of nuclear INI1 expression

TOP DIFFERENTIAL DIAGNOSES

- Carcinoma or melanoma
- Myoepithelial carcinoma (malignant myoepithelioma)
- Epithelioid sarcoma
- Pleomorphic RMS
- Epithelioid angiosarcoma

Epithelioid Rhabdomyosarcoma

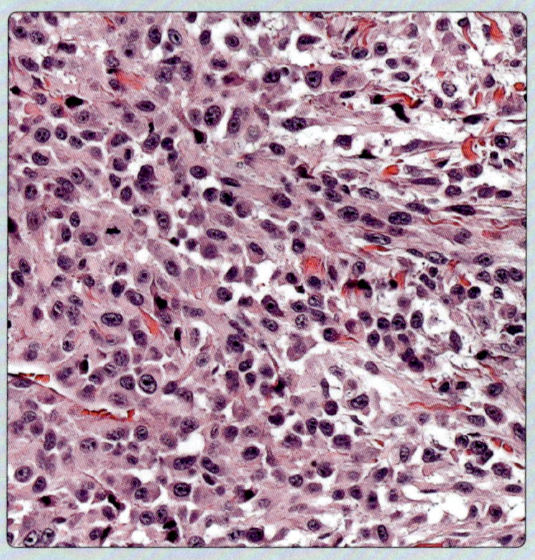

Rhabdoid Morphology

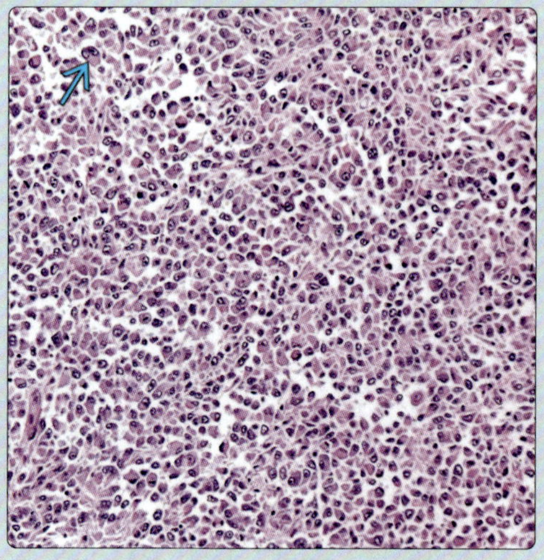

(Left) *Epithelioid rhabdomyosarcoma (RMS) is a distinctive subtype that features sheets of epithelioid tumor cells with abundant eosinophilic cytoplasm and often prominent nucleoli. Cells and nuclei are relatively uniform.* **(Right)** *Rhabdoid cytomorphology may be seen in epithelioid RMS, as depicted; however, overt features of rhabdomyoblastic differentiation (e.g., strap cells) are generally absent. Note that occasional multinucleated tumor cells* ➙ *can also be seen.*

Prominent Nucleoli

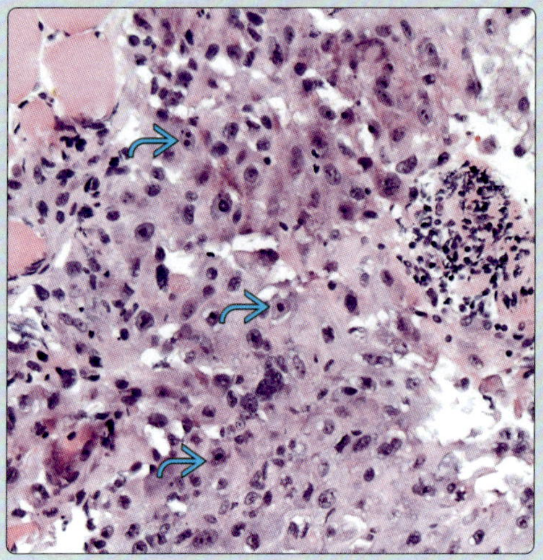

Myogenic Marker Expression

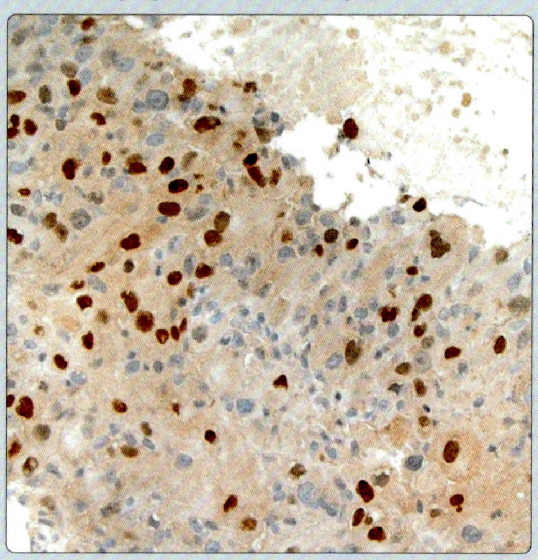

(Left) *Nuclei are relatively uniform in size in epithelioid RMS and often show 1 or more prominent nucleoli* ➙*. Immunohistochemistry is essentially required to prove myogenic differentiation and exclude carcinoma and melanoma.* **(Right)** *Similar to other forms of RMS, epithelioid RMS expresses desmin, myogenin (shown), and MYOD1. In general, myogenin positivity is less diffuse than in alveolar RMS but much more prominent than in pleomorphic RMS.*

TERMINOLOGY

Definitions

- Distinctive rhabdomyosarcoma (RMS) variant characterized by relatively uniform epithelioid cytomorphology

CLINICAL ISSUES

Epidemiology

- Incidence
  - Very rare
- Age
  - Wide age reported (6-78 years)
    - Often in older or elderly adults
- Sex
  - Male predilection

Site

- Deep soft tissues of extremities, head/neck, trunk
  - Less common in superficial tissues (subcutis or dermis)

Presentation

- Painful mass, usually of short clinical duration
- Metastases may be present at time of presentation

Treatment

- Limited data
- Most reported cases treated by combination of surgery and chemotherapy &/or radiation
- Reported childhood cases respond well to established chemotherapy regimens for high-risk RMS

Prognosis

- Favorable prognosis and outcome in children
- Aggressive clinical course in adults
  - Recurrence and metastases common
    - Lymph nodes and lung
  - Very poor 5-year survival rate

MACROSCOPIC

General Features

- Poorly circumscribed, nodular mass
- Fleshy cut surface
- Necrosis common

Size

- Range: 3-15 cm

MICROSCOPIC

Histologic Features

- Infiltrative appearance
- Diffuse, sheet-like growth pattern
- Relatively uniformly sized epithelioid cells with abundant eosinophilic cytoplasm
  - Intracytoplasmic "glassy" rhabdoid inclusions can be seen
- Large, vesicular nuclei often with prominent nucleoli
  - Minimal to mild cytologic pleomorphism only
  - Rare multinucleated tumor cells
- Overt features of rhabdomyoblastic differentiation (e.g., strap cells) absent
- Usually numerous mitotic figures, including atypical forms
- Necrosis frequent

ANCILLARY TESTS

Immunohistochemistry

- Desmin (+), usually strong and diffuse
- Nuclear myogenin (+) and MYOD1(+)
  - Extent of expression varies
- Rare focal keratin (+)
- Retention of nuclear INI1 expression
- Negative for S100 protein, CD31, CD34, HMB-45, Melan-A

Molecular Genetics

- Lacks characteristic genetic features of other types of RMS

DIFFERENTIAL DIAGNOSIS

Poorly Differentiated Carcinoma

- Diffuse keratin (+)
- Negative for desmin, myogenin, MYOD1

Melanoma

- Can show significant morphologic overlap with epithelioid RMS
- Expression of S100 protein and melanocytic markers
- Negative for desmin, myogenin, MYOD1

Myoepithelial Carcinoma (Malignant Myoepithelioma)

- Can show significant morphologic overlap with epithelioid RMS
- Variable expression of keratin, S100 protein, calponin, SMA, desmin, others
- Negative for myogenin, MYOD1

Epithelioid Sarcoma

- Diffuse keratin (+)
- CD34(+) in 50% of cases
- Loss of nuclear INI1 expression
- Negative for desmin, myogenin, MYOD1

Pleomorphic Rhabdomyosarcoma

- Characterized by pronounced nuclear and cytologic pleomorphism
- May contain areas showing epithelioid cytomorphology

Extrarenal Rhabdoid Tumor

- Affects infants and children
- Loss of nuclear INI1 expression
- Keratin (+); negative for myogenic markers

SELECTED REFERENCES

1. Jokoji R et al: Epithelioid rhabdomyosarcoma; a case report with immunohistochemical and molecular study. Diagn Pathol. 10:124, 2015
2. Feasel PC et al: Primary cutaneous epithelioid rhabdomyosarcoma: a rare, recently described entity with review of the literature. J Cutan Pathol. 41(7):588-91, 2014
3. Zin A et al: Epithelioid rhabdomyosarcoma: a clinicopathologic and molecular study. Am J Surg Pathol. 38(2):273-8, 2014
4. Marburger TB et al: Primary cutaneous rhabdomyosarcoma: a clinicopathologic review of 11 cases. J Cutan Pathol. 39(11):987-95, 2012
5. Bowe SN et al: Primary intranodal epithelioid rhabdomyosarcoma. Am J Clin Pathol. 136(4):587-92, 2011
6. Jo VY et al: Epithelioid rhabdomyosarcoma: clinicopathologic analysis of 16 cases of a morphologically distinct variant of rhabdomyosarcoma. Am J Surg Pathol. 35(10):1523-30, 2011

SECTION 10

Vascular Tumors (Including Lymphatics)

Benign

Papillary Endothelial Hyperplasia 408
Bacillary Angiomatosis 410
Congenital Hemangioma 412
Infantile Hemangioma 416
Lobular Capillary Hemangioma 420
Epithelioid Hemangioma 422
Spindle Cell Hemangioma 426
Intramuscular Hemangioma 430
Hobnail Hemangioma 434
Acquired Tufted Angioma 436
Microvenular Hemangioma 438
Sinusoidal Hemangioma 440
Glomeruloid Hemangioma 442
Angiomatosis 444
Lymphangioma 446
Massive Localized Lymphedema 450
Atypical Vascular Lesion 452

Intermediate (Locally Aggressive)

Kaposiform Hemangioendothelioma 454

Intermediate (Rarely Metastasizing)

Papillary Intralymphatic Angioendothelioma 456
Retiform Hemangioendothelioma 458
Composite Hemangioendothelioma 460
Pseudomyogenic Hemangioendothelioma 462

Malignant

Epithelioid Hemangioendothelioma 466
Angiosarcoma 470
Kaposi Sarcoma 476

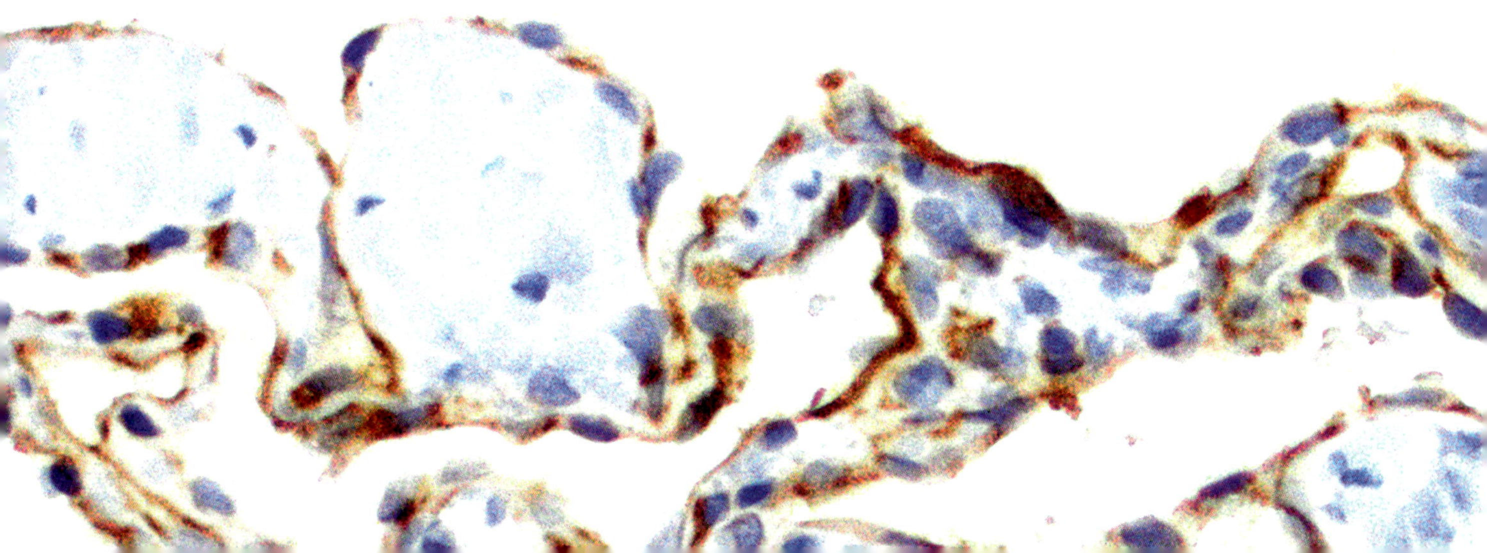

Papillary Endothelial Hyperplasia

KEY FACTS

TERMINOLOGY

- Synonym: Masson tumor
- Benign, reactive intravascular papillary endothelial proliferation

ETIOLOGY/PATHOGENESIS

- Manifestation of organizing intravascular thrombus
- Papillary endothelial hyperplasia-like changes may be present in preexisting hemangiomas or vascular malformations

CLINICAL ISSUES

- Wide site distribution; located in deep dermis or subcutaneous tissue
  - Common sites includes head and neck, fingers, trunk
- Clinically presents as painless mass
- Excision is curative
- Excellent prognosis

MACROSCOPIC

- Small, cystic lesions with red-purple discoloration
  - Usually < 2 cm
- Often surrounded by pseudocapsule

MICROSCOPIC

- Circumscribed lesion with pseudocapsule
- Fibrin thrombi often present
- Papillary structures lined by endothelial cells
- Significant nuclear pleomorphism is absent
- Endothelial cells in single layer
- Vessel rupture may lead to extension of papillary endothelial proliferation into adjacent soft tissue

TOP DIFFERENTIAL DIAGNOSES

- Angiosarcoma
- Hemangiomas
- Arteriovenous malformation
- Hematoma

Papillary Endothelial Hyperplasia

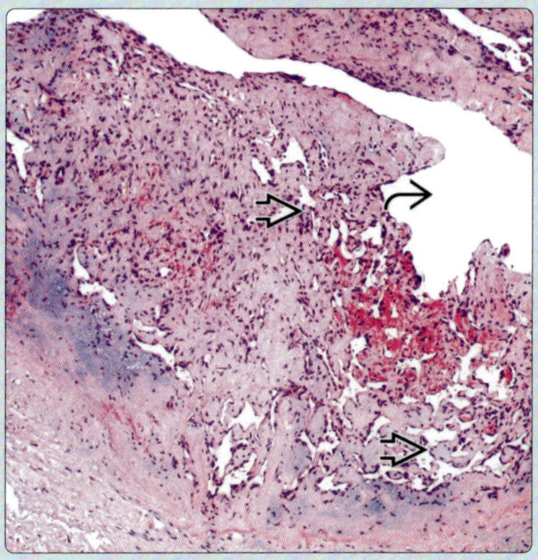

Fibrin Thrombi and Fibrous Papillary Cores

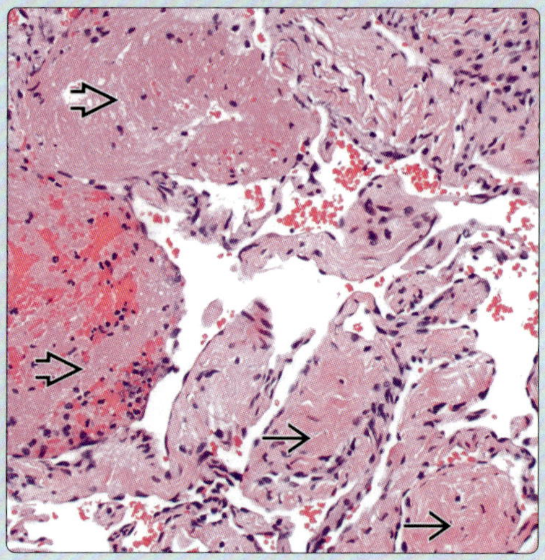

(Left) *Papillary endothelial hyperplasia (PEH) is a well-circumscribed, reactive lesion in which papillary fronds ⇨ lined by a single layer of endothelial cells proliferate within a vascular lumen ↪.* **(Right)** *Fibrin thrombi ⇨ are apparent in early stages and with time are replaced by papillary fronds with a fibrous core → characteristic of PEH.*

Prominent Papillary Fronds

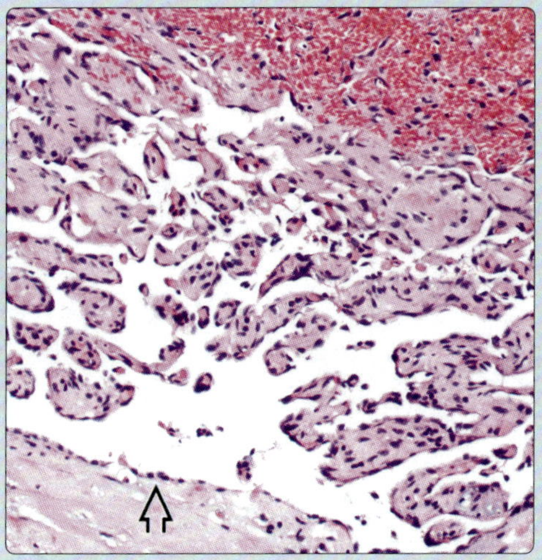

Intravascular Localization

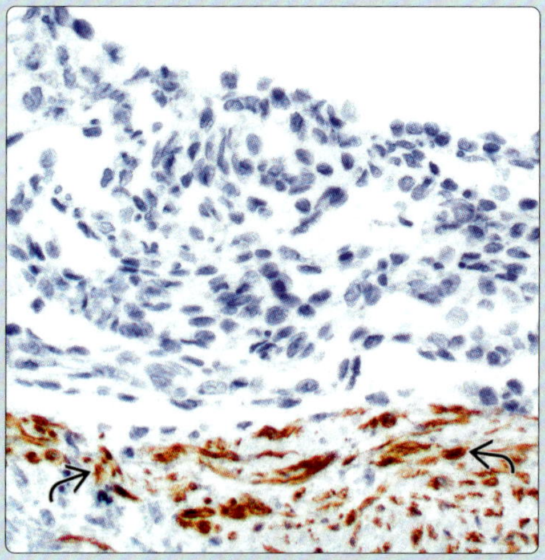

(Left) *PEH with prominent papillary fronds can be mistaken for the anastomosing and dissecting vascular spaces of low-grade angiosarcoma. However, note the endothelial lining ⇨ of the blood vessel lumen.* **(Right)** *Desmin immunohistochemical stain highlights remnants of smooth muscle in the blood vessel wall ↪, confirming the intravascular location of PEH.*

Papillary Endothelial Hyperplasia

TERMINOLOGY

Abbreviations

- Papillary endothelial hyperplasia (PEH)

Synonyms

- Masson tumor
- Intravascular angiomatosis

Definitions

- Benign intravascular papillary endothelial proliferation

ETIOLOGY/PATHOGENESIS

Reactive Vascular Proliferation

- Manifestation of organizing intravascular thrombus
- PEH-like changes may be present in preexisting hemangiomas or vascular malformations

CLINICAL ISSUES

Site

- Wide distribution
- Common sites include
  - Head and neck, fingers, trunk

Presentation

- Painless mass
- Located in deep dermis or subcutaneous tissue

Treatment

- Excision is curative

Prognosis

- Excellent
- Cases with underlying hemangioma or vascular malformation may recur

MACROSCOPIC

General Features

- Cystic mass with red-purple discoloration
- Often surrounded by pseudocapsule

Size

- Mostly small in size (< 2 cm)

MICROSCOPIC

Histologic Features

- Circumscribed lesion with pseudocapsule
  - Residual smooth muscle or elastic lamina of preexisting vessel may be apparent
- Fibrin thrombi often seen
- Papillary structures lined by endothelial cells
  - Endothelial cells in single layer
    - May appear plump or hobnail in appearance
    - Significant nuclear pleomorphism is absent
  - Papillae form anastomosing network
- Papillary cores may consist of fibrin or fibrous connective tissue
- Vessel rupture may lead to extension of papillary endothelial proliferation into adjacent soft tissue
- Rare examples of extravascular variant in soft tissue have been reported
  - Represent reactive endothelial proliferation in organizing hematoma

Cytologic Features

- Enlarged endothelial cells but lack significant cytologic atypia or pleomorphism

DIFFERENTIAL DIAGNOSIS

Angiosarcoma

- Angiosarcoma is infiltrative process that involves surrounding tissue, unlike PEH, which is intraluminal
- Even PEH cases with soft tissue extension have bulk of lesion confined to vascular lumen
- PEH lacks nuclear atypia, tumor cell necrosis, and mitotic activity present in angiosarcoma

Hemangiomas

- PEH-like changes may occur in hemangiomas complicated by thrombosis

Arteriovenous Malformations

- PEH-like changes may occur in arteriovenous malformations
- Important to recognize, since these may recur

Hematoma

- Soft tissue hematomas may have foci of PEH
- May be mistaken for angiosarcoma

DIAGNOSTIC CHECKLIST

Clinically Relevant Pathologic Features

- Intravascular process

Pathologic Interpretation Pearls

- Intravascular papillary proliferation lined by endothelial cells without significant nuclear atypia

SELECTED REFERENCES

1. Díaz-Flores L et al: Sinusoidal hemangioma and intravascular papillary endothelial hyperplasia: interrelated processes that share a histogenetic piecemeal angiogenic mechanism. Acta Histochem. 120(3):255-62, 2018
2. Vicensoto Moreira Milhan N et al: A mixed form of intravascular papillary endothelial hyperplasia in an uncommon location: case and literature review. Dermatol Online J. 24(2), 2018
3. Gupta A et al: Intravascular papillary endothelial hyperplasia presenting as a cystic mass in the scalp with underlying bone involvement: A Rare Entity. Int J Appl Basic Med Res. 7(4):269-71, 2017
4. Liné A et al: Papillary endothelial hyperplasia (Masson's tumor) in children. Ann Chir Plast Esthet. 62(3):232-7, 2017
5. Shah HC et al: Intravascular papillary endothelial hyperplasia (Masson's tumor) of the scalp with intracranial extension. J Pediatr Neurosci. 9(3):260-2, 2014
6. Handa U et al: Cytologic diagnosis of intravascular papillary endothelial hyperplasia: a report of two cases and review of cytologic literature. Acta Cytol. 56(2):199-203, 2012
7. Inoue H et al: Intravascular papillary endothelial hyperplasia of the oral cavity. J Oral Sci. 53(4):475-80, 2011
8. Branton PA et al: Papillary endothelial hyperplasia of the breast: the great impostor for angiosarcoma: a clinicopathologic review of 17 cases. Int J Surg Pathol. 11(2):83-7, 2003
9. Hashimoto H et al: Intravascular papillary endothelial hyperplasia. A clinicopathologic study of 91 cases. Am J Dermatopathol. 5(6):539-46, 1983
10. Kuo T et al: Masson's "vegetant intravascular hemangioendothelioma:" a lesion often mistaken for angiosarcoma: study of seventeen cases located in the skin and soft tissues. Cancer. 38(3):1227-36, 1976

Bacillary Angiomatosis

KEY FACTS

TERMINOLOGY

- Bacillary angiomatosis (BA)
- Reactive vascular proliferation associated with *Bartonella* bacterial infection

ETIOLOGY/PATHOGENESIS

- Most patients are immunocompromised, especially HIV/AIDS
- Also associated with organ transplantation, systemic steroids, and leukemia

CLINICAL ISSUES

- May involve any cutaneous site; uncommonly involves mucosal sites, deep soft tissues
  - Internal organ involvement rare but may affect liver (peliosis hepatis)

MICROSCOPIC

- Nodular to dome-shaped/polypoid dermal-based vascular proliferation
- May have overlying epidermal ulceration and collarette (similar to pyogenic granuloma)
- Vessels are arranged in loose lobular configuration
- Deeper parts of lesion may show greater cellularity and crowding of vessels
- Background stroma shows fibrosis, edema, and mixed inflammatory infiltrate

TOP DIFFERENTIAL DIAGNOSES

- Pyogenic granuloma
  - Polypoid dermal-based lesion composed of lobular collection of capillary-type vessels
  - Overlying ulceration and peripheral epidermal collarette are typically present, similar to BA
- Kaposi sarcoma
  - Plaque-like or nodular dermal collection of slit-like vessels lined by atypical spindle cells
  - Inflammatory infiltrate is typically composed of lymphocytes and plasma cells, not neutrophils

Bacillary Angiomatosis

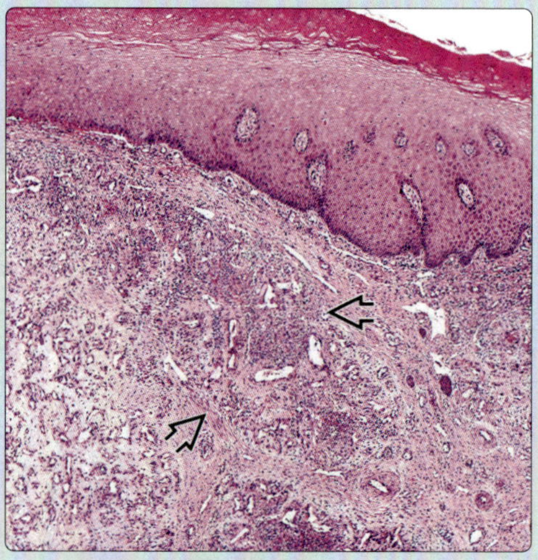

Blood Vessels and Inflammation

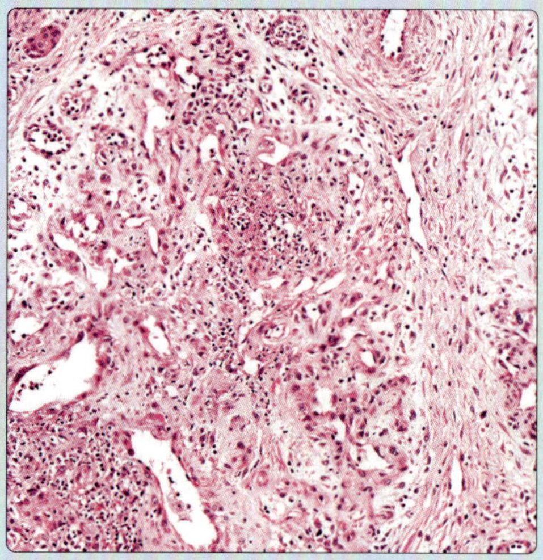

(Left) *Low-power examination of bacillary angiomatosis (BA) demonstrates a superficial dermal proliferation of blood vessels in a lobular configuration* ⇨ *associated with edema and inflammation.* **(Right)** *Intermediate magnification of BA shows a proliferation of small blood vessels arranged in a vaguely lobular configuration with prominent stromal edema, mild fibrosis, and mixed inflammatory infiltrate.*

Acute Inflammation

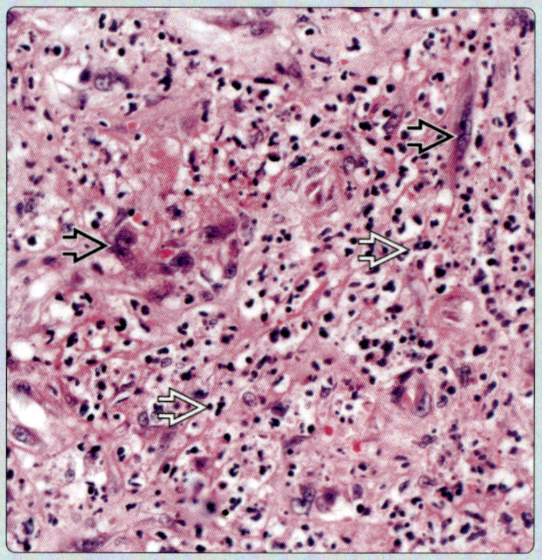

Warthin-Starry Stain

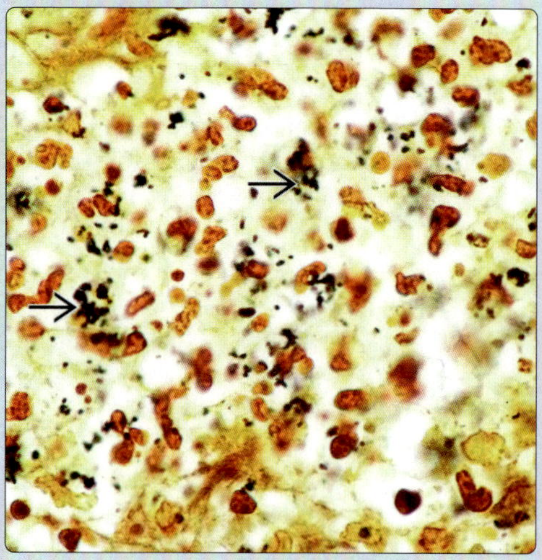

(Left) *High magnification of bacillary angiomatosis demonstrates a proliferation of small blood vessels with swollen endothelial cells* ⇨ *surrounded by edema and acute inflammation with leukocytoclasia* ➡. **(Right)** *Warthin-Starry stain demonstrates positive staining of numerous clusters* ⇨ *and single bacterial organisms.*

Bacillary Angiomatosis

TERMINOLOGY

Abbreviations

- Bacillary angiomatosis (BA)

Synonyms

- Epithelioid angiomatosis

Definitions

- Reactive vascular proliferation associated with *Bartonella* bacterial infection

ETIOLOGY/PATHOGENESIS

Infectious Agents

- Caused by infection with *Bartonella* (gram-negative coccobacilli) species, usually *B. henselae* or *B. quintana*
  - Most patients have history of cat exposure (and may have preceding scratch or bite)
- Most patients are immunocompromised, especially due to HIV/AIDS
  - Also has been associated with organ transplantation, systemic steroids, and leukemia

CLINICAL ISSUES

Epidemiology

- Age
  - May occur in both adults and children

Site

- Can involve any cutaneous site; uncommonly may involve mucosal sites and deep soft tissues
  - Internal organ involvement rare but may affect liver (peliosis hepatis), spleen, lungs

Presentation

- Skin nodules or, less likely, plaques
  - Typically present with multiple lesions, often pyogenic granuloma-like

Treatment

- Drugs
  - Antibiotics typically lead to resolution of lesions

Prognosis

- Typically good, but depends on patient's immune status and sites involved

MACROSCOPIC

General Features

- Reddish-brown, dermal-based nodular, hemorrhagic lesion

MICROSCOPIC

Histologic Features

- Typically nodular to dome-shaped/polypoid dermal-based vascular proliferation
  - May have overlying epidermal ulceration and collarette (similar to pyogenic granuloma)
- Vessels are arranged in loose lobular configuration
  - Endothelial cells show mild enlargement and oval to epithelioid shape
  - Deeper parts of lesion may show greater cellularity and crowding of vessels
  - No significant cytologic atypia or atypical mitotic activity
- Background stroma shows fibrosis, edema, and mixed inflammatory infiltrate
  - Infiltrate is rich in neutrophils with leukocytoclasia, macrophages, lymphocytes, and may show focal collections of basophilic granular material (clumps of bacteria)
    - Neutrophils are more plentiful in deeper lesions

ANCILLARY TESTS

Histochemistry

- Warthin-Starry
  - Reactivity: Positive
  - Staining pattern: Granular (coccobacillary organisms)
- Gomori methenamine silver
  - Reactivity: Positive
  - Staining pattern: Granular (coccobacillary organisms)

PCR

- PCR for *Bartonella* species may be ordered if organisms are not identified on histochemical stains

DIFFERENTIAL DIAGNOSIS

Pyogenic Granuloma

- Polypoid dermal-based lesion composed of lobular collections of capillary-type vessels
- Overlying ulceration and peripheral epidermal collarette are typically present, similar to BA
- No organisms identified on H&E or special stains

Kaposi Sarcoma

- Plaque-like or nodular collection of slit-like vessels lined by atypical spindle cells
- Inflammatory infiltrate is typically composed mostly of lymphocytes and plasma cells, not neutrophils
- No bacterial organisms identified
- HHV8(+) is diagnostic

DIAGNOSTIC CHECKLIST

Pathologic Interpretation Pearls

- Proliferation of vessels associated with neutrophils and clumps of bacterial organisms

SELECTED REFERENCES

1. Nikam BP et al: Bacillary angiomatosis in an immunocompetent individual. Indian Dermatol Online J. 9(3):205-6, 2018
2. Eyer-Silva WA et al: An unusual case of bacillary angiomatosis in the oral cavity of an AIDS patient who had no concomitant tegumentary lesions - case report and review. Rev Inst Med Trop Sao Paulo. 59:e59, 2017
3. Diniz LM et al: Bacillary angiomatosis with bone invasion. An Bras Dermatol. 91(6):811-4, 2016
4. Moulin C et al: Cutaneous bacillary angiomatosis in renal transplant recipients: report of three new cases and literature review. Transpl Infect Dis. 14(4):403-9, 2012
5. Amsbaugh S et al: Bacillary angiomatosis associated with pseudoepitheliomatous hyperplasia. Am J Dermatopathol. 28(1):32-5, 2006
6. LeBoit PE et al: Bacillary angiomatosis. The histopathology and differential diagnosis of a pseudoneoplastic infection in patients with human immunodeficiency virus disease. Am J Surg Pathol. 13(11):909-20, 1989

Congenital Hemangioma

KEY FACTS

TERMINOLOGY

- 2 major clinicopathologic subtypes
  - Rapidly involuting congenital hemangioma (RICH)
  - Noninvoluting congenital hemangioma (NICH)

CLINICAL ISSUES

- Antenatal or congenital presentation of exophytic or plaque-like soft tissue mass at birth
  - Fully developed at birth without accelerated postnatal growth
- Most common sites of involvement: Head, neck, and extremities in close proximity to joints
- RICH: Spontaneous, rapid involution complete by 8-14 months of age
- NICH: Postnatal growth proportionate with child
  - Does not regress and persists indefinitely
- Excellent prognosis for uncomplicated lesions

MICROSCOPIC

- Well-defined lobules of capillaries with central draining vessels and separated by fibrous tissue
- RICH
  - Focal hemosiderin and extramedullary hematopoiesis
  - Involutional changes: Increased interstitial fibrosis, cysts, and microthrombi
- NICH
  - Focal hobnailed endothelial cells
  - Interlobular stroma with prominent dysplastic vessels

ANCILLARY TESTS

- GLUT1(-)

TOP DIFFERENTIAL DIAGNOSES

- Infantile hemangioma
- Vascular malformation
- Tufted angioma
- Kaposiform hemangioendothelioma

Congenital Hemangioma

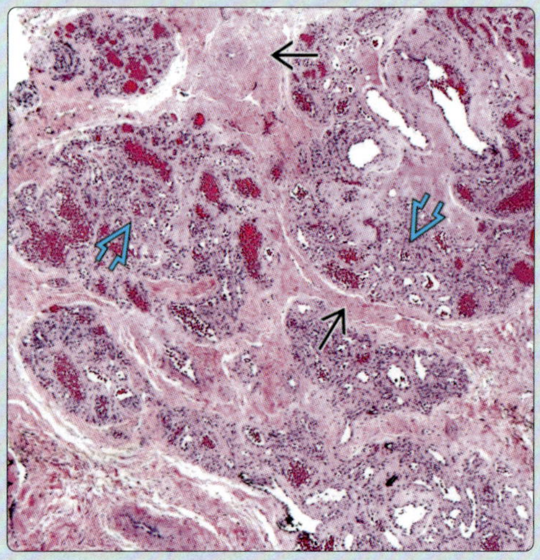

Central Draining Vessel

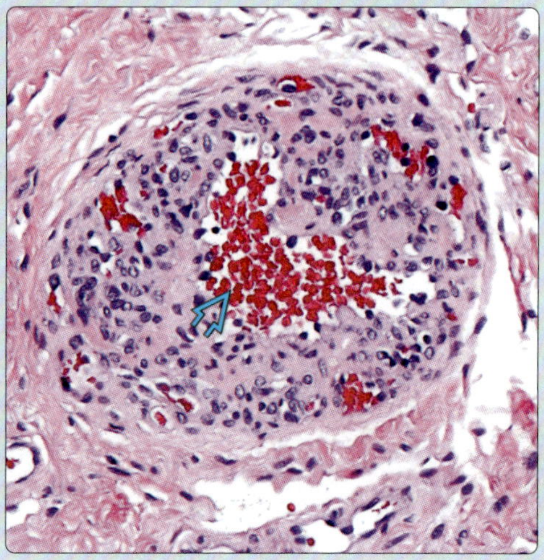

(Left) *Congenital hemangiomas are characterized by a dermal &/or subcutaneous proliferation of capillaries growing in lobules, which are separated by dense fibrous tissue.* **(Right)** *Within both subtypes of congenital hemangioma [rapidly involuting congenital hemangioma (RICH) and noninvoluting congenital hemangioma (NICH)], the cellular lobules contain prominent centrally placed draining vessels. The endothelial cells and pericytes are moderately plump with bland cytologic features.*

Interlobular Stromal Vessels

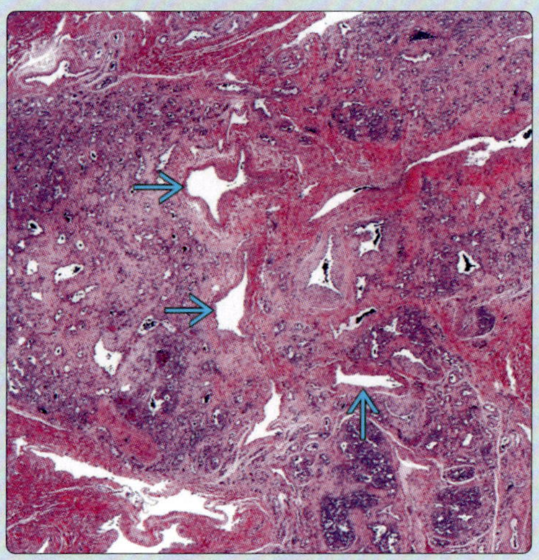

GLUT1 Negative

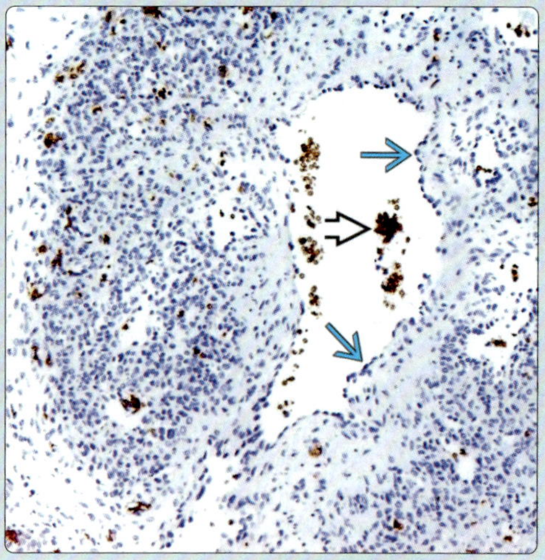

(Left) *The lobules within NICH are typically larger than those seen in RICH. In addition, the interlobular stroma contains an increased number of large, irregular vessels.* **(Right)** *In contrast to infantile hemangiomas, the endothelial cells in RICH and NICH are negative for GLUT1. This immunophenotypic difference is a useful marker for differentiating between the 2 entities, which have overlapping morphologic features. Of note, erythrocytes are positive for GLUT1, allowing them to serve as an internal control.*

TERMINOLOGY

Synonyms

- Congenital nonprogressive hemangioma
- Rapidly involuting congenital hemangioma (RICH)
- Noninvoluting congenital hemangioma (NICH)

Definitions

- Benign congenital vascular neoplasm that is fully developed at birth and does not display accelerated postnatal growth

ETIOLOGY/PATHOGENESIS

Developmental Anomaly

- Lesions arise and proliferate in utero
- Relationship to infantile hemangioma is heavily debated and controversial
  - Presence of reported cases of congenital hemangioma and infantile hemangioma arising in same patient may suggest lesions are part of clinical spectrum
  - Differential protein and mRNA expression in congenital vs. infantile hemangiomas may suggest these are distinct entities
    - Congenital hemangiomas demonstrate higher levels of expression of FLT-1 (VEGFR-R1) and lower levels of IGF-2 than infantile hemangiomas

Genetics

- Associated with somatic activating mutations in *GNAQ* and *GNA11*

CLINICAL ISSUES

Epidemiology

- **Incidence**
  - Affects 0.3% of infants
  - RICH is more common than NICH
- **Demographics**
  - Newborns (presentation at birth)
  - No gender predilection

Site

- Most common sites of involvement are head, neck, and extremities in close proximity to joints
- RICH may demonstrate hepatic involvement ± skin lesions

Presentation

- 2 major clinicopathologic subtypes: RICH and NICH
- Antenatal or congenital presentation at birth
  - May be detected as early as 12 weeks of gestation by prenatal ultrasonography
- Usually solitary lesions
- Solitary, exophytic, or bossed plaque-like soft tissue mass
  - Violaceous overlying skin with telangiectasia and peripheral draining veins
- Natural course varies by subtype
- Rare reports of RICH occurring in setting of PHACE syndrome
  - PHACE syndrome: Posterior fossa abnormalities, hemangiomas, arterial lesions, cardiac and eye abnormalities, sternal clefting or supraumbilical raphe
- Potential complications
  - Ulceration relatively frequent in large lesions during involution
  - Transient thrombocytopenia and coagulopathy in large RICH prior to regression
    - Self-limited and minor, in contrast to Kasabach-Merritt phenomenon (most commonly associated kaposiform hemangioendothelioma)
    - Usually resolves by 2 weeks of age without treatment
  - High-output cardiac failure secondary to arteriovenous shunting in large RICH prior to regression

Natural History

- Both subtypes have reached or passed their proliferative peak at birth
  - Proliferative phase occurs in utero
- RICH
  - Stable size at birth with subsequent spontaneous and rapid involution early in postnatal period
  - Involution begins within few days to weeks after birth
  - Majority of lesions completely involute by 8-14 months of age
  - Rare reports of rapid involution in utero with complete regression prior to birth
  - Following involution, skin is anetodermic with dermal or subcutaneous atrophy in area of lesion
- NICH
  - Stable size at birth with static course
    - Rare reported cases of growth and expansion during adolescence
  - Demonstrates postnatal growth proportionate with somatic growth of child
  - Does not spontaneously regress and persists indefinitely throughout adulthood
- Minor subset of RICH lesions demonstrate initial rapid but incomplete involution resulting in persistent residual vascular plaque that is indistinguishable from NICH
  - Raises possibility that NICH represents RICH in arrested growth phase

Treatment

- RICH
  - Observation as 1st-line treatment
  - Surgical excision reserved for cases complicated by persistent/repeated ulceration, severe hemorrhage, or congestive heart failure secondary to arteriovenous shunting
  - Cosmetic repair of residual skin changes after involution
- NICH
  - Pulsed dye laser therapy
  - Surgical excision ± preoperative embolization for large or symptomatic lesions

Prognosis

- RICH
  - Excellent for uncomplicated lesions
  - Vast majority of lesions completely regress without treatment
  - High mortality rate associated with rare complication of high-output heart failure
- NICH
  - Favorable with no risk of recurrence following excision
  - Persists indefinitely without surgical intervention

MACROSCOPIC

General Features

- Red to violaceous nodule or plaque
- Telangiectasia of overlying skin (more prominent in NICH)
- Peripheral white or bluish pallor producing halo effect (more characteristic of RICH)
- May have central ulceration, fissure, or depression (more characteristic of RICH)
- Typically solitary

Size

- Average diameter: 5-6 cm at birth

MICROSCOPIC

Histologic Features

- Early RICH and NICH lesions (prior to involution) demonstrate similar morphologic features
  - Usually best distinguished using clinical features
- RICH
  - Well-defined, variably sized lobules of capillaries within dermis and subcutaneous tissue
  - Prominent, thin-walled centrilobular, draining vessels
  - Dense, interlobular fibrous tissue
  - Focal hemosiderin and extramedullary hematopoiesis commonly seen
  - Mitoses may be present
    - No atypical figures
  - No significant cytologic atypia
  - Involutional changes initially occur in center of lesion
    - Decreased numbers of lobules with progressive interstitial fibrosis, cystic spaces, and vascular thrombi
    - No fibrofatty residuum after involution (in contrast to infantile hemangioma)
- NICH
  - Well-defined, large lobules of capillaries within dermis and subcutaneous tissue
  - Centrilobular draining vessels appear larger, stellate, and more ectatic than in RICH
  - Focal hobnailed appearance of endothelial cells with small, hyperchromatic nuclei bulging into lumen
  - Round, eosinophilic globules may be present in cytoplasm of endothelial cells
  - Interlobular fibrovascular stroma with arteries, large dysplastic veins, and lymphatic-like structures
    - Prominence of large interlobular vessels may be misleading and confused for vascular malformation
  - Rare mitoses
  - No significant cytologic atypia

ANCILLARY TESTS

Histochemistry

- Elastin stain highlights deficient or excessive elastic tissue in walls of interlobular dysplastic vessels

Immunohistochemistry

- Endothelial cells express CD31, CD34, factor VIII-related antigen, and WT-1
- Typically GLUT1(-), but rare focal reactivity has been reported in RICH

DIFFERENTIAL DIAGNOSIS

Infantile Hemangioma

- Majority are not present at birth (presents within few weeks after birth)
- Demonstrates accelerated postnatal growth
  - Growth rate of lesion exceeds that of child
- GLUT1(+)

Vascular Malformation

- Congenital lesions that grow proportionately with child and persist without regression
- Not hypercellular and nonproliferative endothelial cells
- WT1(-)

Tufted Angioma

- Slow, indolent growth over months to years followed by stabilization &/or regression
- Randomly dispersed compact nodules of capillaries in cannonball configuration

Kaposiform Hemangioendothelioma

- Infiltrating spindled endothelial cells forming slit-like vascular spaces and glomeruloid-like nests
- Associated with Kasabach-Merritt phenomenon
- Periphery of lobules D2-40(+)
  - Lobular component of congenital hemangiomas typically D2-40(-)
    - Interlobular or perilesional lymphatic channels may be immunoreactive

SELECTED REFERENCES

1. Lewis D et al: Rapidly involuting congenital haemangioma of the liver. BMJ Case Rep. 2018
2. Ayturk UM et al: Somatic activating mutations in GNAQ and GNA11 are associated with congenital hemangioma. Am J Hum Genet. 98(6):1271, 2016
3. Nasseri E et al: Partially involuting congenital hemangiomas: a report of 8 cases and review of the literature. J Am Acad Dermatol. 70(1):75-9, 2014
4. Patrick LM et al: Rapid involuting congenital hemangioma in the setting of PHACE association. Pediatrics. 133(6):e1777-80, 2014
5. Bruder E et al: Vascular and perivascular lesions of skin and soft tissues in children and adolescents. Pediatr Dev Pathol. 15(1 Suppl):26-61, 2012
6. Kanada KN et al: A prospective study of cutaneous findings in newborns in the United States: correlation with race, ethnicity, and gestational status using updated classification and nomenclature. J Pediatr. 161(2):240-5, 2012
7. Roebuck D et al: Rapidly involuting congenital haemangioma (RICH) of the liver. Pediatr Radiol. 42(3):308-14, 2012
8. Fadell MF 2nd et al: Prenatal diagnosis and postnatal follow-up of rapidly involuting congenital hemangioma (RICH). Pediatr Radiol. 41(8):1057-60, 2011
9. Niimi R et al: Epithelioid hemangioendothelioma after radiotherapy for congenital hemangioma: a case report. Med Oncol. 27(1):130-3, 2010
10. Ozcan UA: Rapidly involuting congenital hemangioma: a case of complete prenatal involution. J Clin Ultrasound. 38(2):85-8, 2010
11. Moukaddam H et al: MRI characteristics and classification of peripheral vascular malformations and tumors. Skeletal Radiol. 38(6):535-47, 2009
12. Picard A et al: IGF-2 and FLT-1/VEGF-R1 mRNA levels reveal distinctions and similarities between congenital and common infantile hemangioma. Pediatr Res. 63(3):263-7, 2008

Dense Interlobular Fibrosis

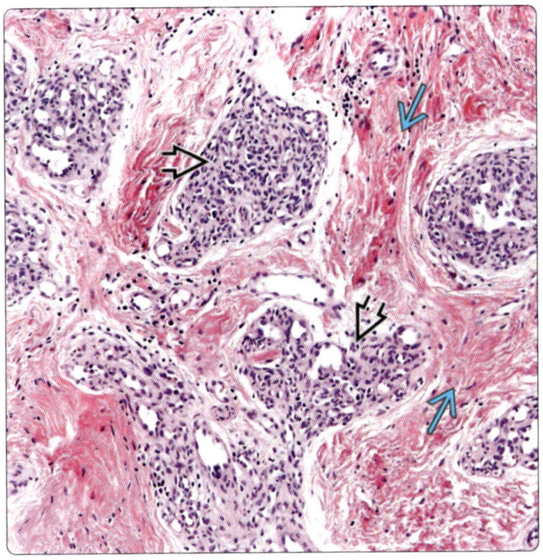

Vascular Microthrombi

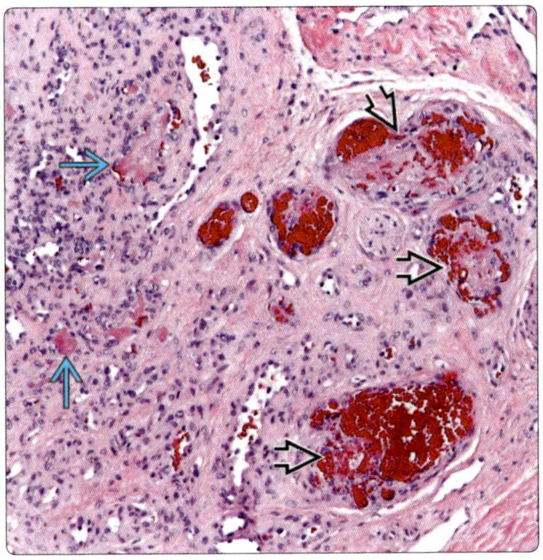

(Left) *RICH is composed of well-defined, variably sized lobules of capillaries ⇨ that are separated by dense fibrous tissue →. The interlobular vascular component is oftentimes less prominent than that seen in NICH.* **(Right)** *Although they can be seen in both subtypes of congenital hemangioma, the lobular vessels within RICH more frequently contain organizing fibrin thrombi → with evidence of recanalization ⇨.*

Eosinophilic Globules

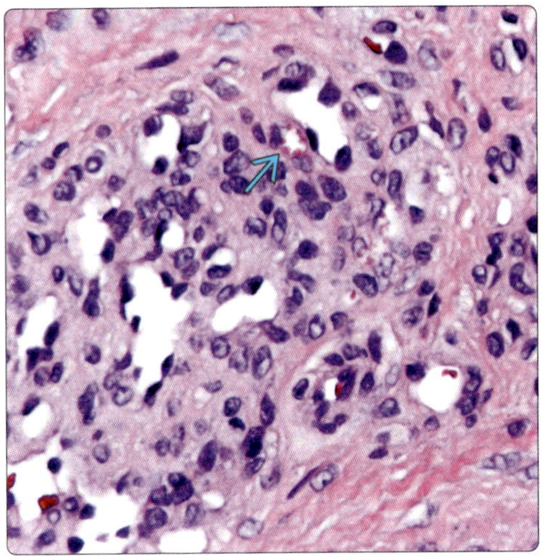

Hobnailed Endothelium

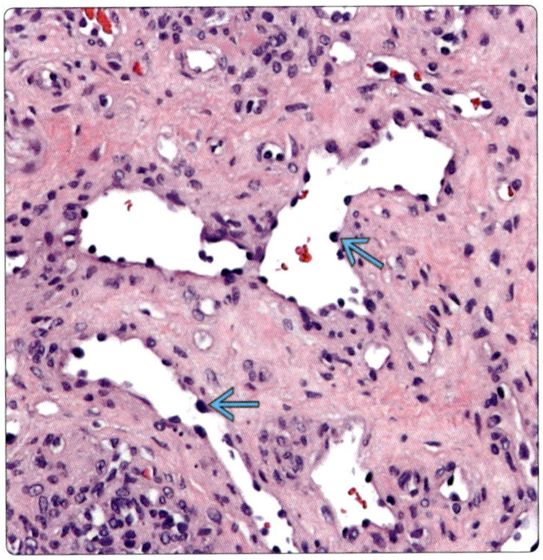

(Left) *Lobular endothelial cells of NICH may contain foci of intracytoplasmic eosinophilic globules, which tend to cluster →.* **(Right)** *The lobular endothelial cells within NICH are often small, hyperchromatic, and bulge into the vascular lumen, imparting a hobnailed appearance →.*

Prominent Interlobular Vessels

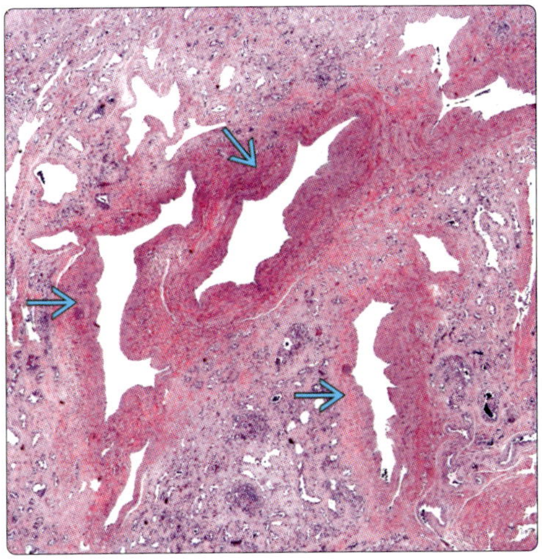

Dysplastic Vessels

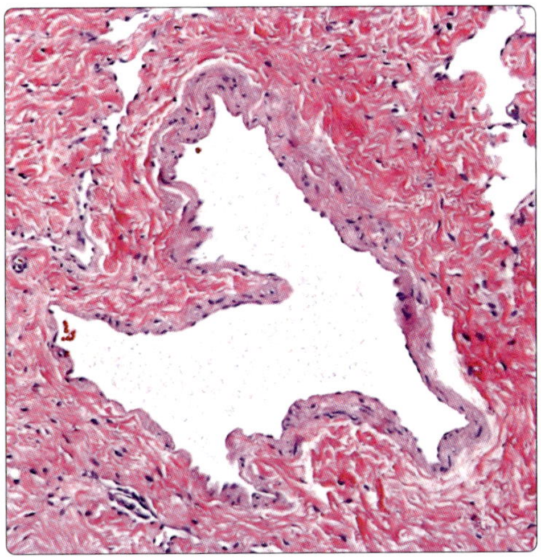

(Left) *The interlobular stroma of NICH frequently contains abundant large and irregularly shaped venous, arterial, and lymphatic-like structures →. These vessels can be a dominant feature and may lead to misdiagnosis as a vascular malformation.* **(Right)** *Many of the interlobular vessels in NICH are distorted in shape and composition. This stellate-shaped, venous-like structure has poorly developed media with variable areas of thickness and deficient smooth muscle and elastic tissue.*

Infantile Hemangioma

KEY FACTS

TERMINOLOGY

- Juvenile hemangioma
- Hemangioma of infancy

CLINICAL ISSUES

- Most common vascular tumor of infancy (usually present within 1st few weeks of life)
- Most common sites of involvement: Skin and soft tissue of face, head, and neck
- Multifocal disease associated with visceral involvement
- Syndromic associations: PHACE and LUMBAR syndrome
- Characteristic proliferative and involutional growth phases
  - Proliferative phase: Occurs in 1st several months with rapid enlargement
  - Involutional phase: Proceeding 1-12 years of life
- Excellent prognosis with complete spontaneous regression occurring in 80-90% of cases

MICROSCOPIC

- Proliferative phase
  - Tightly packed lobules of capillaries lined by plump endothelial cells and pericytes
  - Early lesions densely cellular and mitotically active
- Involutional phase
  - Dilated capillaries with flattened endothelial cells
  - Progressive fibrosis and fatty replacement

ANCILLARY TESTS

- Endothelial cells (+) for GLUT1, Lewis-Y antigen, and IGF-2
  - GLUT1 is most reliable and specific marker

TOP DIFFERENTIAL DIAGNOSES

- Congenital hemangioma
- Lobular capillary hemangioma (pyogenic granuloma)
- Tufted angioma
- Kaposiform hemangioendothelioma
- Vascular malformation

Infantile Hemangioma

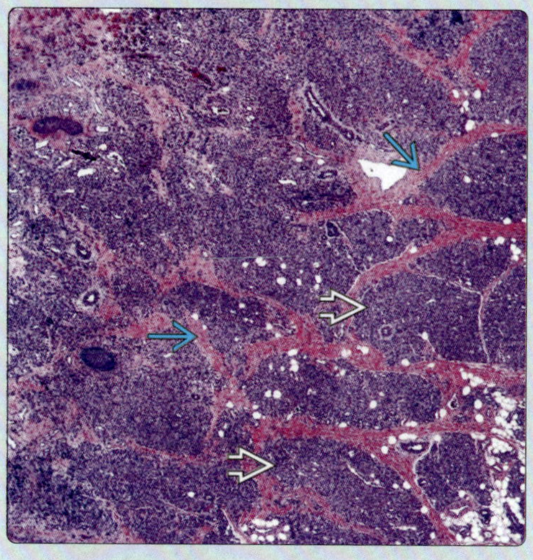

Proliferative Phase: Dense Cellularity

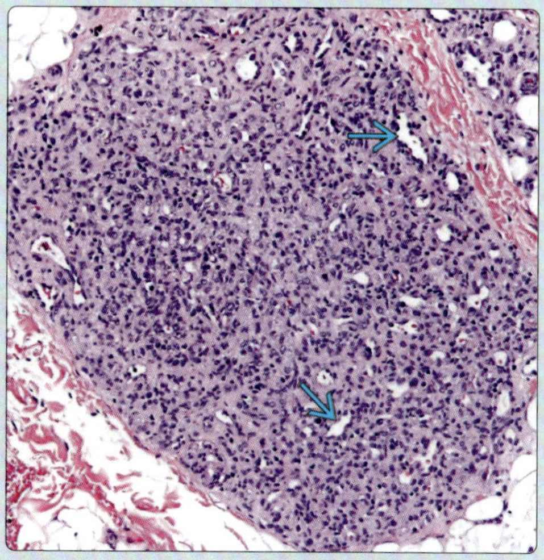

(Left) *Infantile hemangioma is characterized by a dermal &/or subcutaneous proliferation of tightly packed capillaries growing in lobules ➡, which are separated by thin, fibrous bands ⇨.* **(Right)** *The proliferative phase demonstrates increased cellularity with dense, solid-appearing areas containing inconspicuous vascular lumina ⇨. These solid-appearing areas are composed of plump endothelial cells and pericytes.*

Involution Phase: Dilated Vessels

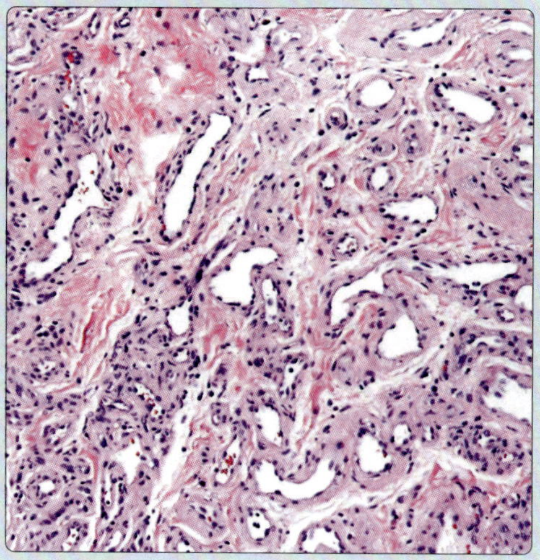

GLUT1 Positive

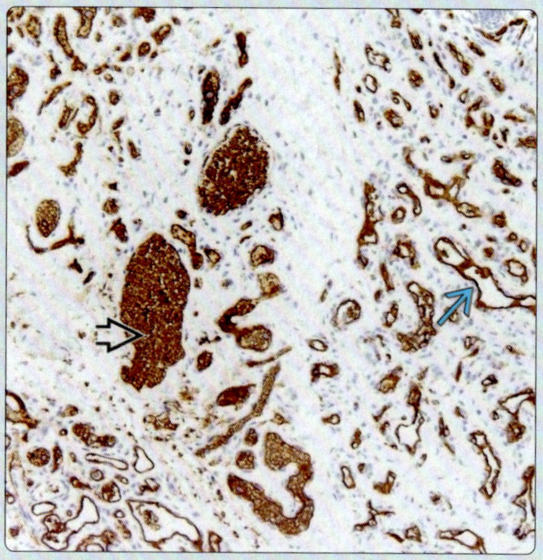

(Left) *During the involution phase of infantile hemangioma, the capillaries become more dilated, and the endothelial cells are flattened.* **(Right)** *Infantile hemangiomas are immunoreactive with GLUT1, which stains the cytoplasm of the endothelial cells in all phases of development ⇨. As such, it is the most reliable and specific marker for this entity. Erythrocytes are also immunoreactive for GLUT1 and serve as an internal control ➡.*

TERMINOLOGY

Synonyms

- Juvenile hemangioma
- Hemangioma of infancy

Definitions

- Benign vascular neoplasm of infancy with characteristic proliferative and involutional phases

ETIOLOGY/PATHOGENESIS

Developmental Anomaly/Environmental Exposure

- Postulated to result from hypoxia-induced stimulation of endothelial progenitor cells and angiogenic peptides or clonal expansion of placental emboli
  - VEGF, β-adrenergic, and NOTCH signaling pathways have been implicated
- Risk factors include prematurity, low birth weight, and product of multiple gestations

Genetics/Inheritance

- Most cases are sporadic
- Rare reports of autosomal-dominant pattern of inheritance with linkage to 5q31-33 (region containing *FLT4* and *FGFR4*)

CLINICAL ISSUES

Epidemiology

- Incidence
  - Affects 4-5% of infants
  - Most common vascular tumor of infancy
- **Demographics**
  - Neonates and infants (present at birth or within 1st few weeks of life)
  - Female predominance (M:F = 3-5:1)
  - Caucasians more commonly affected

Site

- Skin and soft tissue of face, head, and neck are most common sites of involvement (60%)
- Other sites: Trunk, extremities, and viscera (central nervous system, liver, lungs, eyes, and kidneys)
- Typically solitary lesion (85%) but can be variable in distribution
  - Localized, segmental, or multifocal
  - Multifocal disease defined as > 5 lesions
    - Associated with visceral involvement

Presentation

- Superficial lesions present at birth and are telangiectatic in appearance early on
  - Appear as bright red plaques or nodules when fully formed
- Deep lesions appear later (at 2-3 months of age) as subcutaneous bluish swellings
- Segmental lesions may be associated with congenital anomalies
  - PHACE syndrome presents in 20-31% of those with large segmental facial lesions
    - Posterior fossa abnormalities, hemangiomas, arterial lesions, cardiac and eye abnormalities, sternal clefting, or supraumbilical raphe
  - LUMBAR syndrome presents in 10% of those with perineal or reticular hemangiomas
    - Lower body hemangiomas, urogenital anomalies, myelopathy, bony abnormalities, anorectal malformations or arterial anomalies, and renal anomalies

Natural History

- Characteristic proliferative and involutional growth phases
- Proliferative growth phase occurs in 1st several months, during which lesion rapidly enlarges in noncommensurate manner
  - Proliferation after 1st year of life is uncommon
  - Deep lesions tend to have longer proliferative phase than superficial ones
- Spontaneous involution occurs over proceeding 1-12 years
- Clinical variant: Infantile hemangioma with minimal or arrested growth (IH-MAG)
  - Minor subset that fails to proliferate beyond precursor telangiectatic stage
  - Usually located on lower body (associated with LUMBAR syndrome)

Treatment

- Close observation of small lesions
- Pharmacotherapy: Systemic or topical corticosteroids, β-blockers, imiquimod, or interferon-α
- Pulsed dye laser therapy
- Surgical excision usually reserved for involuted lesions with residual skin abnormalities

Prognosis

- Excellent
- Complete regression in 80-90% without medical or surgical intervention
- Rare case report of malignant transformation to angiosarcoma

MACROSCOPIC

General Features

- Superficial lesions: Bright red, lobulated nodules or plaques
- Deep lesions: Bluish color with telangiectasia of overlying skin

Size

- Variable in size (ranging from pinpoint lesions to > 20 cm)

MICROSCOPIC

Histologic Features

- Variable histologic appearance based on growth phase
- Proliferative phase
  - Tightly packed syncytial aggregates of small capillaries lined by plump endothelial cells and pericytes
  - Lobules of capillaries separated by thin bands of fibrous tissue
  - Replacement or displacement of normal dermal structures
  - Early lesions are densely cellular with inconspicuous vascular lumina and solid-appearing areas
  - Abundant typical mitotic figures may be present during early proliferative phase

- No atypical mitotic figures or significant cytologic atypia
- Involutional phase
  - Dilated capillaries with flattened endothelial cells
  - Progressive interstitial fibrosis and increasing amounts of adipose tissue
  - More pronounced lobular architecture
  - Increased number of mast cells and apoptotic bodies
  - Thickening and hyalinization of vessel walls
- End stage
  - Fibrofatty replacement with sparse vessels
  - Residual larger feeder vessels and draining veins
- IH-MAG variant
  - Proliferative component comprises < 25% of total surface area of lesion **and**
  - Patient is > 2 years of age

ANCILLARY TESTS

Immunohistochemistry

- Endothelial cells express GLUT1, IGF-2, CD31, CD34, factor VIII-related antigen, Lewis-Y antigen, and WT1
  - GLUT1 is most reliable and specific marker
    - Positive in all growth phases
    - Negative in most other vascular tumors
- Pericytes are SMA(+)
- Loss of immunoreactivity for CD31, CD34, and factor VIII-related antigen in fully involuted lesions

DIFFERENTIAL DIAGNOSIS

Congenital Hemangioma

- In utero growth with fully developed lesions present at birth
- Rapidly involuting type regresses faster than infantile hemangiomas
- Noninvoluting type does not regress and grows commensurately with child
- Hemosiderin and extramedullary hematopoiesis commonly present
- GLUT1(-)

Lobular Capillary Hemangioma (Pyogenic Granuloma)

- Usually older children and adolescents (mean age: 6 years in pediatric population)
- Polypoid or sessile mass ± ulceration
- Lobule(s) of capillaries surrounded by epidermal/mucosal collarette
- GLUT1(-)

Tufted Angioma

- Slow, indolent growth over months to years followed by stabilization &/or regression
- Randomly dispersed compact nodules of capillaries in cannonball configuration
- GLUT1(-)

Kaposiform Hemangioendothelioma

- Infiltrating spindled endothelial cells forming slit-like vascular spaces and glomeruloid-like nests
- Associated with Kasabach-Merritt phenomenon
- GLUT1(-)
- Periphery of lobules D2-40(+)
  - Lobular component of infantile hemangiomas typically D2-40(-)
    - Perilesional lymphatic channels may be immunoreactive

Vascular Malformation

- Congenital lesions that grow proportionately with child and persist without regression
- Not hypercellular and nonproliferative endothelial cells
- GLUT1(-)

SELECTED REFERENCES

1. Adams DM et al: Infantile hemangiomas in the head and neck region. Otolaryngol Clin North Am. 51(1):77-87, 2018
2. Valdivielso-Ramos M et al: Infantile hemangioma with minimal or arrested growth as the skin manifestation of PHACE syndrome. Pediatr Dermatol. 35(5):622-627, 2018
3. Yin RR et al: Expression and correlation of MMP-9, VEGF, and p16 in infantile hemangioma. Eur Rev Med Pharmacol Sci. 22(15):4806-4811, 2018
4. Darrow DH et al: Diagnosis and management of infantile hemangioma: executive summary. Pediatrics. 136(4):786-91, 2015
5. Bellaud G et al: PHACE syndrome, a series of six patients: clinical and morphological manifestations, propranolol efficacy, and safety. Int J Dermatol. 54(1):102-7, 2014
6. Jeng MR et al: Malignant transformation of infantile hemangioma to angiosarcoma: response to chemotherapy with bevacizumab. Pediatr Blood Cancer. 61(11):2115-7, 2014
7. Kwon SH et al: Effect of early long-pulse pulsed dye laser treatment in infantile hemangiomas. Dermatol Surg. 40(4):405-11, 2014
8. Sethuraman G et al: Management of infantile hemangiomas: current trends. J Cutan Aesthet Surg. 7(2):75-85, 2014
9. Chen TS et al: Infantile hemangiomas: an update on pathogenesis and therapy. Pediatrics. 131(1):99-108, 2013
10. Greenberger S et al: Pathogenesis of infantile haemangioma. Br J Dermatol. 169(1):12-9, 2013
11. Lee KC et al: Update on infantile hemangiomas. Semin Perinatol. 37(1):49-58, 2013
12. Malik MA et al: Effect of propranolol vs prednisolone vs propranolol with prednisolone in the management of infantile hemangioma: a randomized controlled study. J Pediatr Surg. 48(12):2453-9, 2013
13. Reddy KK et al: Retrospective study of the treatment of infantile hemangiomas using a combination of propranolol and pulsed dye laser. Dermatol Surg. 39(6):923-33, 2013
14. Bischoff J: Progenitor cells in infantile hemangioma. J Craniofac Surg. 20 Suppl 1:695-7, 2009
15. Calicchio ML et al: Identification of signaling systems in proliferating and involuting phase infantile hemangiomas by genome-wide transcriptional profiling. Am J Pathol. 174(5):1638-49, 2009
16. Kilcline C et al: Infantile hemangiomas: how common are they? A systematic review of the medical literature. Pediatr Dermatol. 25(2):168-73, 2008
17. Haggstrom AN et al: Prospective study of infantile hemangiomas: clinical characteristics predicting complications and treatment. Pediatrics. 118(3):882-7, 2006
18. Nguyen VA et al: Infantile hemangioma is a proliferation of LYVE-1-negative blood endothelial cells without lymphatic competence. Mod Pathol. 19(2):291-8, 2006
19. North PE et al: infancy and childhood: beyond capillary hemangioma. Cardiovasc Pathol. 2006 Nov-Dec;15(6):303-17. 15(6):303-17,
20. Dadras SS et al: Infantile hemangiomas are arrested in an early developmental vascular differentiation state. Mod Pathol. 17(9):1068-79, 2004
21. Pagliai KA et al: Pyogenic granuloma in children. Pediatr Dermatol. 21(1):10-3, 2004
22. Walter JW et al: Somatic mutation of vascular endothelial growth factor receptors in juvenile hemangioma. Genes Chromosomes Cancer. 33(3):295-303, 2002
23. North PE et al: immunohistochemical marker for juvenile hemangiomas. Hum Pathol. 2000 Jan;31(1):11-22. 31(1):11-22,

Bland Endothelium

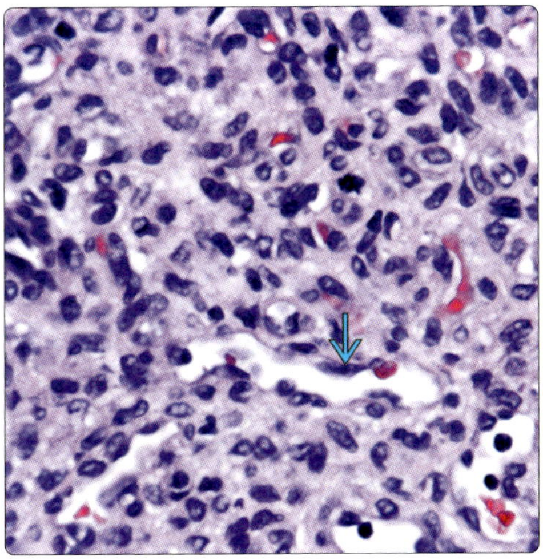

Mitotic Activity

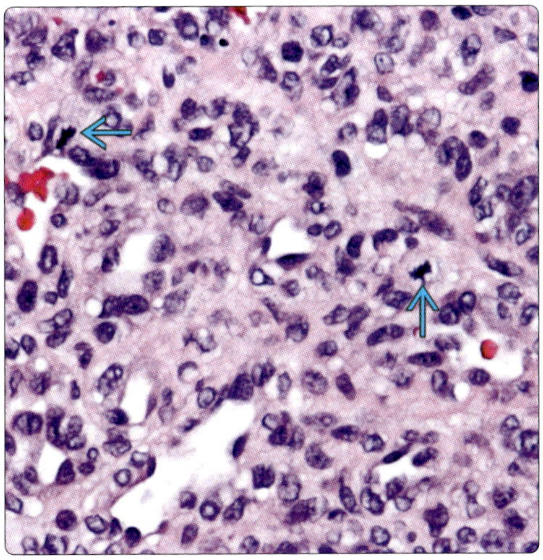

(Left) *During the proliferative phase, the endothelial cells and pericytes are plump with bland cytologic features ⇒.* **(Right)** *Early proliferative lesions may be mitotically active with multiple mitotic figures observed per HPF ⇒. However, no atypical mitoses, significant nuclear pleomorphism, or frank atypia are present.*

Mixed Phases

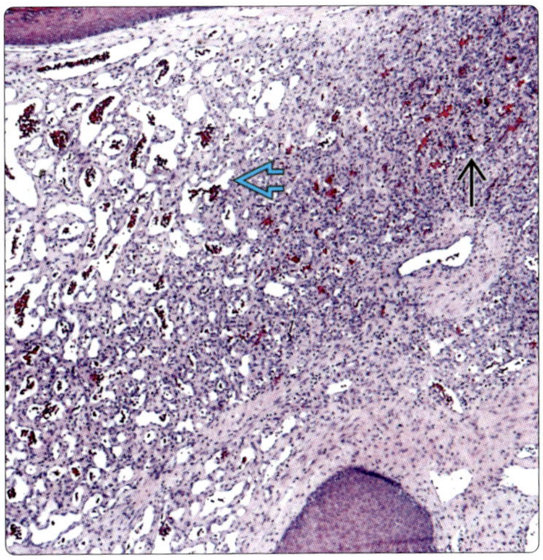

Interstitial Fibrosis

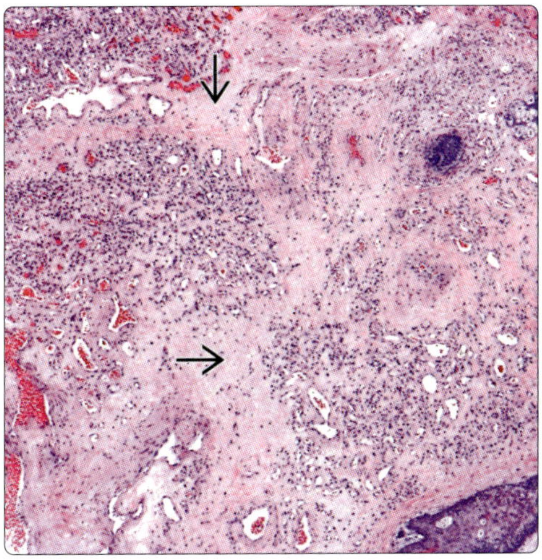

(Left) *The periphery of infantile hemangiomas involute first with eventual involution of the remainder of the lesion. As such, within the same specimen, features of both the proliferative ⇒ and involution phases ⇒ may be evident.* **(Right)** *During involution, the overall cellularity of the lesion decreases secondary to progressively increasing interstitial fibrosis ⇒.*

Thick, Hyalinized Vessels

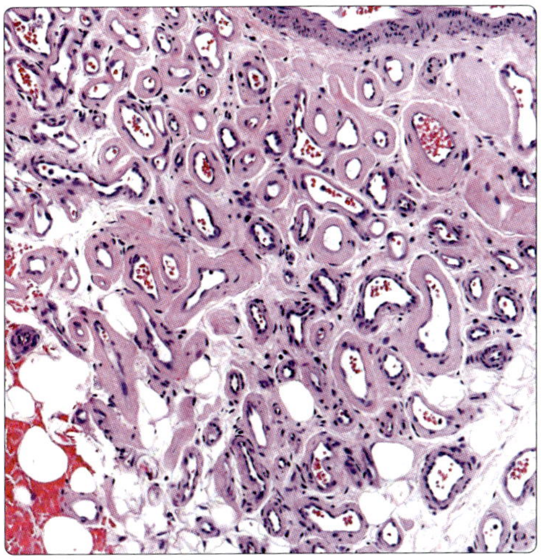

Fibrofatty Replacement

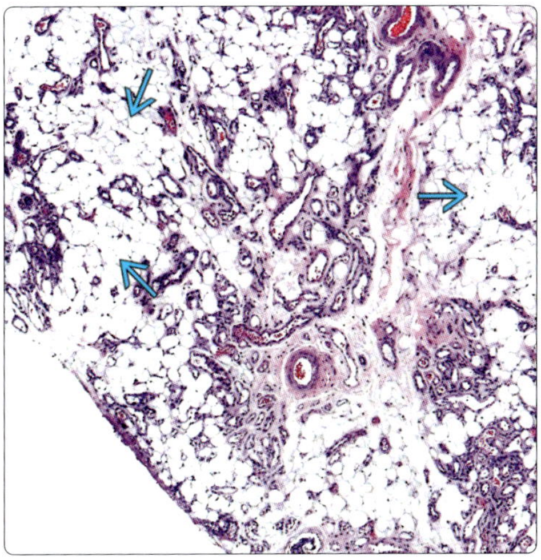

(Left) *Late in the involution phase, the remaining vessels often develop thickened basement membranes with subsequent hyalinization of the vessel walls.* **(Right)** *Toward the end stage of involution, the vascular component of infantile hemangiomas are progressively replaced by fibrous and fatty tissue ⇒. A few small lobules of capillaries may persist.*

Lobular Capillary Hemangioma

KEY FACTS

TERMINOLOGY

- Clinically distinctive benign vascular lesion characterized by vague lobules of capillary channels arranged around larger "feeder" vessels
- Synonym: Pyogenic granuloma

CLINICAL ISSUES

- Wide age range (common in children and young adults)
- Occurs in superficial skin and mucosal sites
  - Head and neck most common (particularly lip, gingiva, nasal cavity)
- Small (< 2.5 cm), red-purple, rapidly growing exophytic nodule
  - Overlying mucosal surface often atrophic or ulcerated
  - May occur during pregnancy (granuloma gravidarum)
- Treatment: Simple excision
- Benign
  - Local recurrence is rare

MICROSCOPIC

- Well circumscribed or demarcated
- Overlying squamous mucosa is often ulcerated with acute and chronic inflammation
- Vague lobules of capillary channels organized around larger "feeder" vessels
- Edematous to fibromyxoid stroma
- Mitotic rate may be brisk
- Intravascular variant exists

ANCILLARY TESTS

- CD31(+), CD34(+), ERG(+) in endothelial cells
- SMA(+) pericytic cell population
- GLUT1 and D2-40 (-)

TOP DIFFERENTIAL DIAGNOSES

- Bacillary angiomatosis
- Angiofibroma of soft tissue
- Angiosarcoma

Lobular Capillary Hemangioma

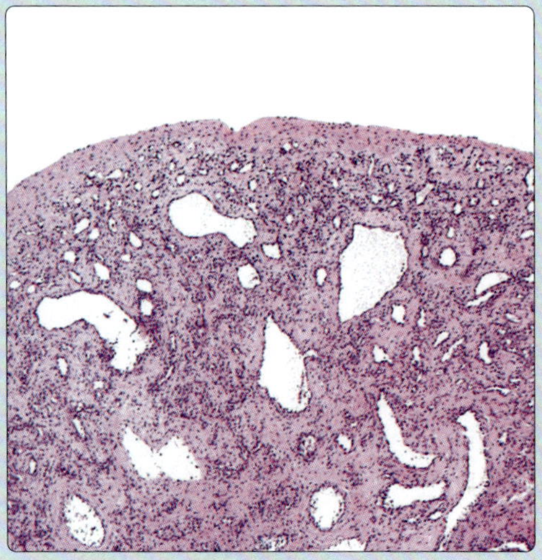

Central Ectatic Vessels

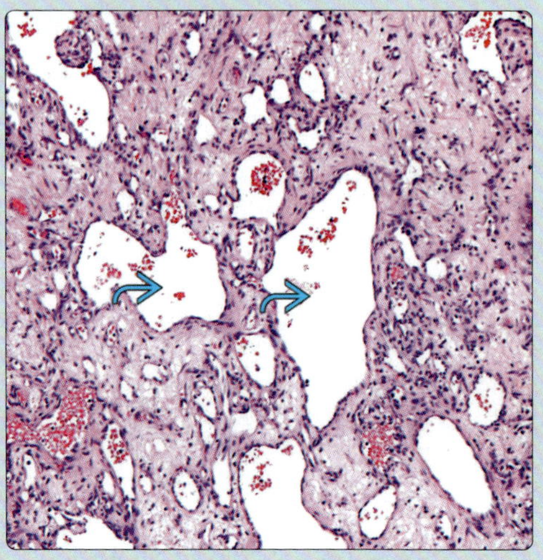

(Left) *Lobular capillary hemangioma, also commonly referred to as pyogenic granuloma, is a common benign vascular lesion that has a predilection for the head and neck region of children and young adults. Tumors are well circumscribed or demarcated and often show surface mucosal atrophy or ulceration.* **(Right)** *A characteristic finding in lobular capillary hemangioma is the presence of capillary channels arranged around larger, dilated "feeder" vessels ➡.*

Bland Endothelial Cell Lining

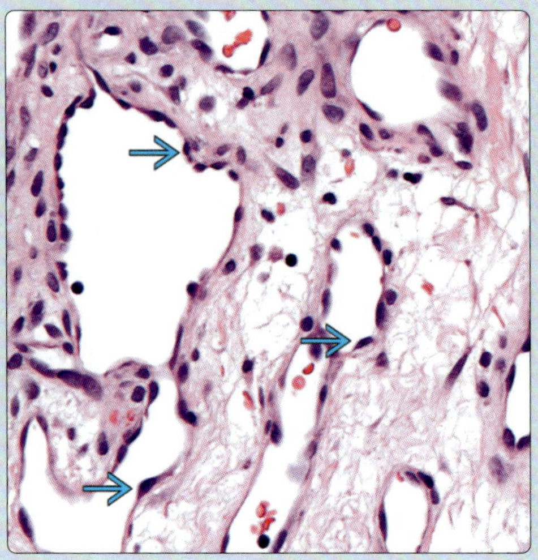

Compressed Capillary Lumina

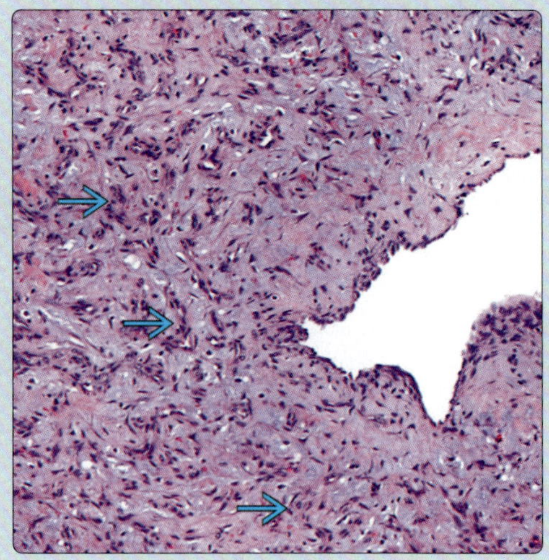

(Left) *The capillary channels are lined by small, benign endothelial cells ➡ that may show, at most, mild nuclear atypia. Mitotic activity can be brisk, particularly in cases associated with ulceration.* **(Right)** *Vascular lumina may not be readily apparent in some cases of lobular capillary hemangioma due to compression of the capillary channels ➡. This change varies in extent and may be diffuse in larger cases.*

TERMINOLOGY

Synonyms

- Pyogenic granuloma (PG)

Definitions

- Clinically distinctive benign vascular lesion characterized by vague lobules of capillary channels arranged around larger "feeder" vessels

CLINICAL ISSUES

Epidemiology

- Incidence
  - Common
- Age
  - Wide range (common in children and young adults)
- Sex
  - Slight male predominance

Site

- Superficial skin and mucosal sites
  - Rarely subcutaneous or intravascular
- Head and neck most common (particularly lip, gingiva, nasal cavity)
- Also upper extremity (mainly subcutaneous and intravascular variants) and other sites

Presentation

- Small, red-purple, rapidly growing exophytic nodule
  - Overlying mucosal surface often atrophic or ulcerated
- Most are solitary; rarely multifocal
- Minority of cases associated with trauma
- May occur during pregnancy (granuloma gravidarum)

Treatment

- Simple excision

Prognosis

- Benign
  - Do not generally spontaneously regress
    - Exception is granuloma gravidarum, which often regresses following parturition
- Local recurrence is rare

MACROSCOPIC

General Features

- Soft red lesion, often with friable overlying mucosa

Size

- Usually < 2.5 cm
  - Nasal cavity lesions may be larger

MICROSCOPIC

Histologic Features

- Well circumscribed or demarcated
- Overlying squamous mucosa is often ulcerated with acute and chronic inflammation
  - May show peripheral epidermal collarette
- Vague lobules of capillary channels organized around larger "feeder" vessels
  - Endothelial cells usually bland but may show mild nuclear atypia
  - Capillaries may be compressed and lack visible lumina
- Edematous to fibromyxoid stroma
- Mitotic rate may be brisk
- Intravascular variant
  - Usually occurs within small veins
  - Histologically similar to conventional types

ANCILLARY TESTS

Immunohistochemistry

- CD31(+), CD34(+), ERG(+), WT1(+) in endothelial cells
- SMA(+) pericytic cell population
- GLUT1 and D2-40 (-)

DIFFERENTIAL DIAGNOSIS

Bacillary Angiomatosis

- May appear histologically similar to lobular capillary hemangioma but with more solid growth pattern
- Plump endothelial cells with focally clear cytoplasm
- Characteristically contains stromal neutrophilic microabscesses and foci of amorphous eosinophilic extracellular material (contains bacillary organisms)

Angiofibroma of Soft Tissue

- Most occur in extremities (rare in head and neck)
- Usually larger lesions than PG
- t(5;8) (p15;q13) with *AHRR* and *NCOA2* genes

Angiosarcoma

- Usually poorly circumscribed with infiltrative growth
- Malignant cytologic features

Cavernous Hemangioma

- Usually large and can occur in wide variety of locations, including viscera
- Contain large, dilated, thin-walled vessels separated by thin bands of fibroconnective tissue
- Thrombosis and calcification are common

SELECTED REFERENCES

1. Johnson EF et al: Vascular tumors in infants: case report and review of clinical, histopathologic, and immunohistochemical characteristics of infantile hemangioma, pyogenic granuloma, noninvoluting congenital hemangioma, tufted angioma, and kaposiform hemangioendothelioma. Am J Dermatopathol. 40(4):231-239, 2018
2. Wollina U et al: Pyogenic granuloma - a common benign vascular tumor with variable clinical presentation: new findings and treatment options. Open Access Maced J Med Sci. 5(4):423-426, 2017
3. Handra-Luca A et al: CD99 expression in nasal lobular capillary haemangioma. Histopathology. 65(4):583-5, 2014
4. Puxeddu R et al: Lobular capillary hemangioma of the nasal cavity: a retrospective study on 40 patients. Am J Rhinol. 20(4):480-4, 2006
5. Truss L et al: Deletion (21)(q21.2q22.12) as a sole clonal cytogenetic abnormality in a lobular capillary hemangioma of the nasal cavity. Cancer Genet Cytogenet. 170(1):69-70, 2006
6. Epivatianos A et al: Pyogenic granuloma of the oral cavity: comparative study of its clinicopathological and immunohistochemical features. Pathol Int. 55(7):391-7, 2005
7. Toida M et al: Lobular capillary hemangioma of the oral mucosa: clinicopathological study of 43 cases with a special reference to immunohistochemical characterization of the vascular elements. Pathol Int. 53(1):1-7, 2003
8. Patrice SJ et al: Pyogenic granuloma (lobular capillary hemangioma): a clinicopathologic study of 178 cases. Pediatr Dermatol. 8(4):267-76, 1991

Epithelioid Hemangioma

KEY FACTS

TERMINOLOGY

- Synonym: Angiolymphoid hyperplasia with eosinophilia
- Definition: Benign, likely neoplastic vascular proliferation featuring epithelioid endothelial cells and usually associated with stromal eosinophils

CLINICAL ISSUES

- Wide age range (most common: 20-50 years)
- Head and neck most common region (particularly around ear)
  - Also distal extremities (digits)
- Usually solitary subcutaneous or dermal nodule
  - May be multifocal
- Treatment: Complete surgical excision
- Benign; local recurrence in up to 30%

MACROSCOPIC

- Usually small size (0.5-2.0 cm)

MICROSCOPIC

- Lobular proliferation of capillaries, often surrounding central vessel
  - Capillaries lined by plump, epithelioid endothelial cells
    - May appear to project into lumen of dilated channels (hobnail or tombstone appearance)
- Usually abundant stromal chronic inflammation, particularly eosinophils
- No necrosis; mitotic figures uncommon

ANCILLARY TESTS

- CD31(+), CD34(+), nuclear ERG(+) in endothelial cells
- *FOS* or *FOSB* gene rearrangements in subset

TOP DIFFERENTIAL DIAGNOSES

- Kimura disease
- Epithelioid hemangioendothelioma
- Epithelioid angiosarcoma

Epithelioid Hemangioma

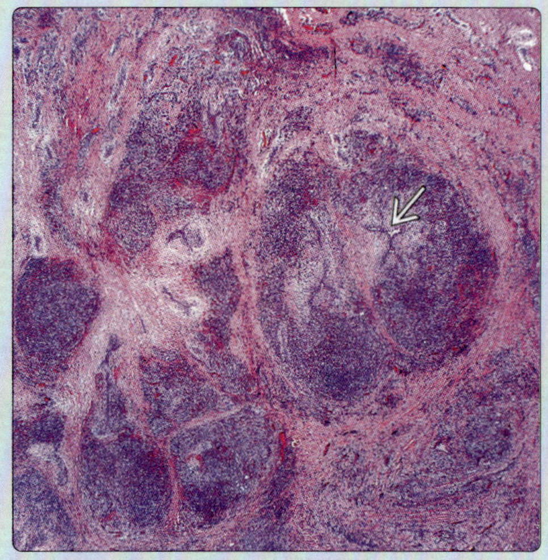

Typical Features

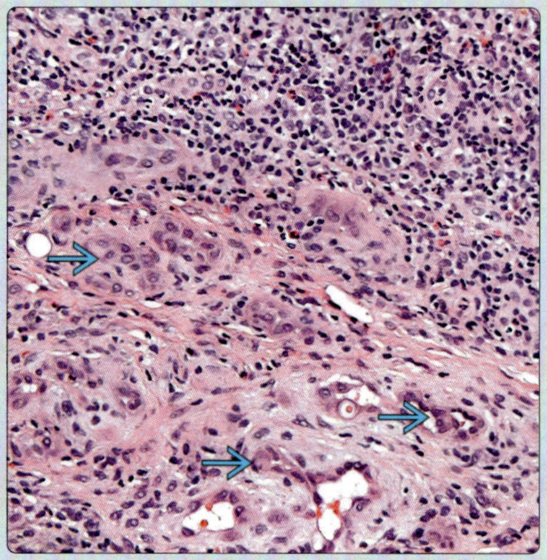

(Left) *Epithelioid hemangioma (EH) is a benign vascular tumor that occurs most commonly in the head and neck region. At low power, it typically shows a vaguely lobular growth pattern and may be associated with a small artery or vein* ➡. **(Right)** *The lesional endothelial cells* ➡ *of EH are usually plump and epithelioid and have eosinophilic or amphophilic cytoplasm. An associated brisk chronic inflammatory infiltrate is typical.*

Epithelioid Cytomorphology

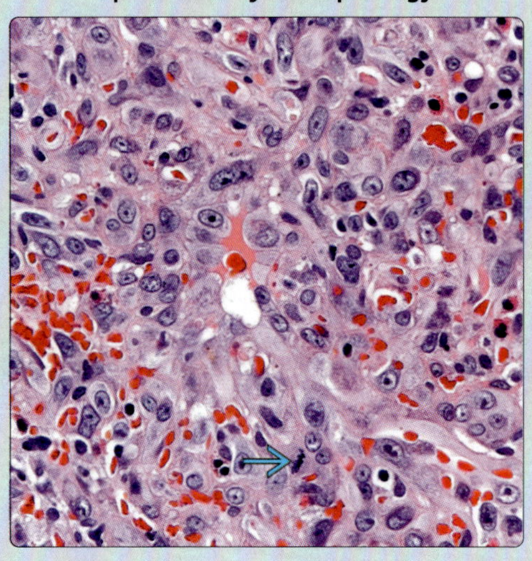

Eosinophils

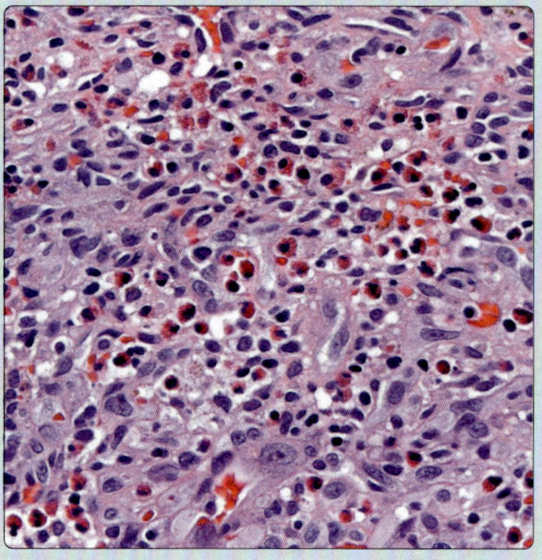

(Left) *The lesional cells of EH are plump and ovoid/epithelioid and show a single nucleus with a central nucleolus. Mitotic figures* ➡ *are usually sparse and inconspicuous. Erythrocytes are common given the vascular origin of the tumor.* **(Right)** *A brisk eosinophilic infiltrate is characteristic of EH; however, the eosinophils may be sparse in some cases (particularly dermal lesions). Mast cells and plasma cells may also be identified.*

Epithelioid Hemangioma

TERMINOLOGY

Abbreviations

- Epithelioid hemangioma (EH)

Synonyms

- Angiolymphoid hyperplasia with eosinophilia
- Histiocytoid hemangioma

Definitions

- Benign, likely neoplastic vascular proliferation featuring epithelioid endothelial cells and usually associated with stromal eosinophils

CLINICAL ISSUES

Epidemiology

- Age
  - Wide range (most common: 20-50 years)
- Sex
  - Slight female predominance

Site

- Head and neck most common region
  - Particularly around ear
- Also distal extremities (digits)
- Other sites include bone, penis, oral cavity, lymph node

Presentation

- Usually solitary subcutaneous or dermal nodule
  - May be multiple within same region
  - Rare lesions arise in deep soft tissue
- Slow growing; may be ulcerated

Treatment

- Complete surgical excision
  - Reexcision of local recurrences

Prognosis

- Benign
  - Local recurrence in up to 30%
  - No distant metastasis reported

MACROSCOPIC

Size

- Usually small (0.5-2.0 cm)

MICROSCOPIC

Histologic Features

- Most are nodular and well demarcated
- Lobular proliferation of capillaries, often surrounding central vessel
  - Capillaries lined by plump, epithelioid endothelial cells
    - Abundant eosinophilic or amphophilic cytoplasm
      - Can show vacuolization, ± erythrocytes
    - May appear to project into lumen of dilated channels (hobnail or tombstone appearance)
    - Single large nucleus with fine chromatin and central nucleolus
      - Nuclear pleomorphism usually absent
      - Mitotic figures uncommon
    - Epithelioid endothelial cells not always prominent
      - Lesional vascular channels may be lined by more typical flattened endothelial cells
  - Increased cellularity/density may be seen centrally in some cases
    - Rare spindled cellular morphology
  - Necrosis very rare
- Usually abundant stromal chronic inflammation (may obscure vascular channels)
  - Brisk eosinophilic infiltrate characteristic of most lesions
  - Mostly lymphocytes but also mast cells, plasma cells
    - Lymphoid tissue may form reactive germinal centers, particularly at periphery of lesion
- Rare tumors arise intravascularly
- Atypical features can be seen in *FOSB*-rearranged cases
  - Solid growth, increased cellularity, focal necrosis, decreased inflammation, nuclear pleomorphism
- Dermal lesions
  - Less well defined at low magnification
  - Endothelial cells may be less plump
  - Centralized vessels usually not present
  - Inflammatory infiltrate may be sparse

ANCILLARY TESTS

Immunohistochemistry

- CD31(+), CD34(+), nuclear ERG(+) in endothelial cells
- May show focal keratin (+)

Molecular Genetics

- *FOS* gene rearrangements reported in up to 30% of cases
- Also, *FOSB*, *FOSL1*, and *FOSL2* rearrangements

DIFFERENTIAL DIAGNOSIS

Kimura Disease

- Endemic in Asian population
- Associated with lymphadenopathy, peripheral eosinophilia, elevated serum IgE
- Prominent eosinophils; lacks epithelioid endothelial cells

Epithelioid Hemangioendothelioma

- Usually larger tumors
- Cords of tumor cells in myxohyaline matrix
- Well-formed, dilated capillary channels and chronic inflammatory component are not features

Epithelioid Angiosarcoma

- Frank nuclear atypia, prominent macronucleoli, and conspicuous mitotic activity
- Lacks characteristic inflammatory component of EH
- More conventional, complex interanastomosing or dissecting growth pattern may be present

SELECTED REFERENCES

1. Ortins-Pina A et al: FOSB immunoreactivity in endothelia of epithelioid hemangioma (angiolymphoid hyperplasia with eosinophilia). J Cutan Pathol. 45(6):395-402, 2018
2. Huang SC et al: Frequent FOS gene rearrangements in epithelioid hemangioma: a molecular study of 58 cases with morphologic reappraisal. Am J Surg Pathol. 39(10):1313-21, 2015
3. Antonescu CR et al: ZFP36-FOSB fusion defines a subset of epithelioid hemangioma with atypical features. Genes Chromosomes Cancer. 53(11):951-9, 2014

(Left) *Dilated vascular channels in EH may be lined by cuboidal or epithelioid endothelial cells, imparting a hobnail or tombstone appearance. This finding is a helpful clue to the diagnosis, but it is not present in every case.* **(Right)** *Cytoplasmic vacuolization ⇾ is a common finding in EH and may be focally prominent. The additional presence of erythrocytes ⇨ indicates early vasoformation.*

Hobnail Nuclei

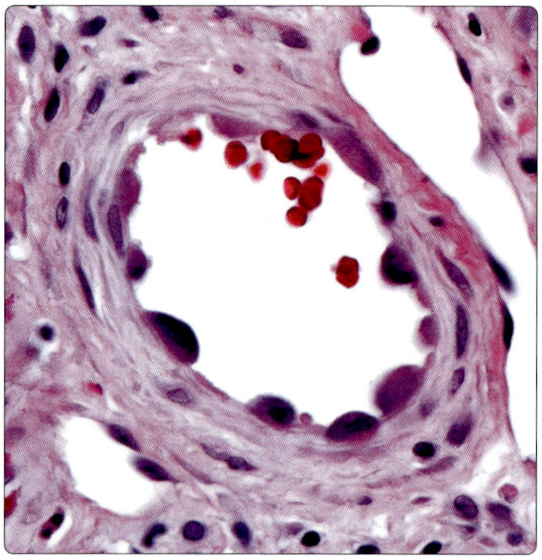

Cytoplasmic Vacuolization

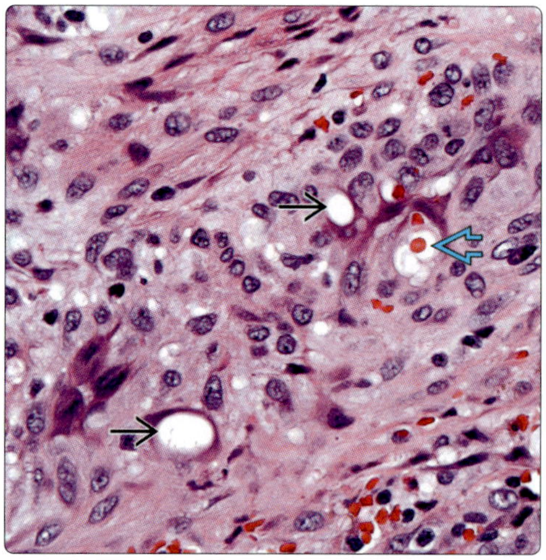

(Left) *Although the vessels appear immature in EH, they are well formed, and all cases show an intact layer of myopericytic/smooth muscle cells. In some cases, the endothelial cells are more flattened than epithelioid.* **(Right)** *Some cases of EH contain cellular foci that appear as relatively solid aggregates of epithelioid cells. These foci, when present, are more likely to be seen centrally within the lesion.*

Myopericytic Layer Present

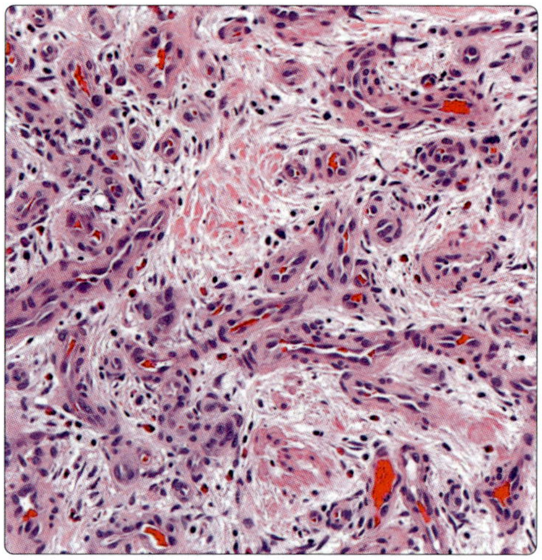

Cellular Foci

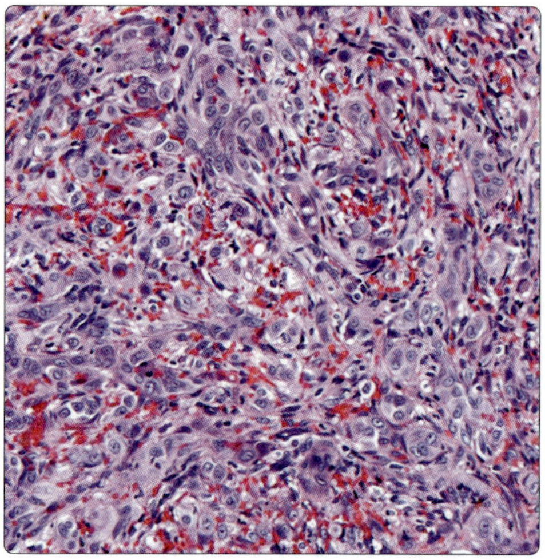

(Left) *A spindled tumor cell morphology ⇨ is a rare finding in EH and is usually focal when present. This morphology is much more common in EH of bone.* **(Right)** *Lobules of lesional tissue may be associated with an artery or vein in EH. These vessels may appear damaged or show evidence of rupture.*

Rare Spindled Foci

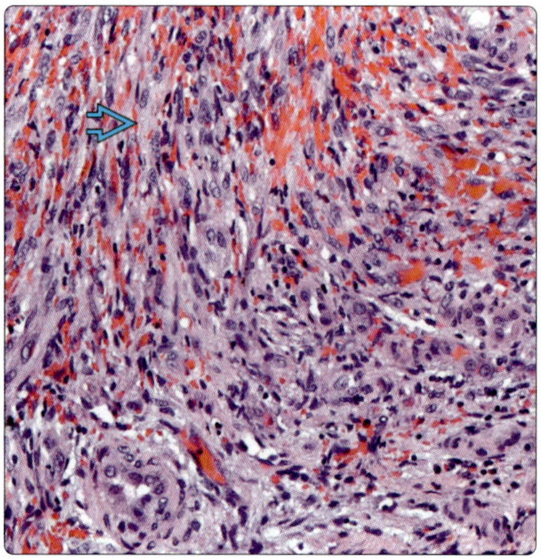

Large Vessel Involvement

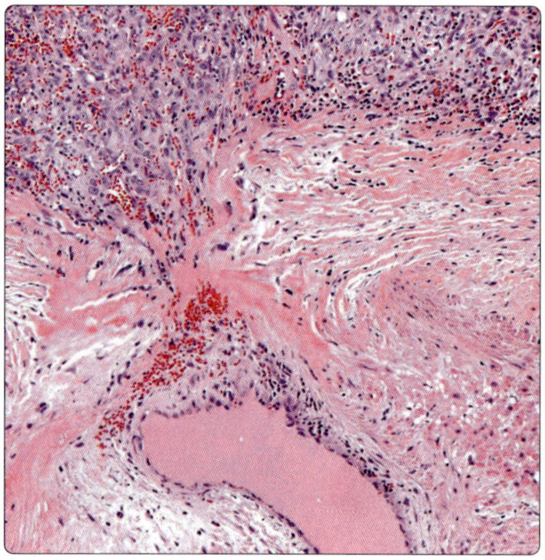

Vessel Involvement

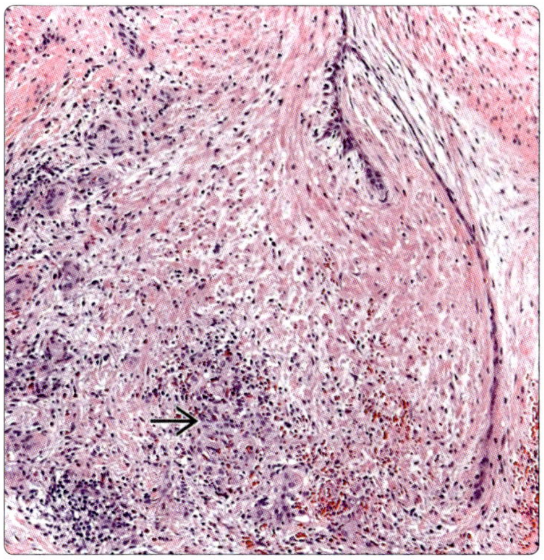

Dilated Vascular Lumina

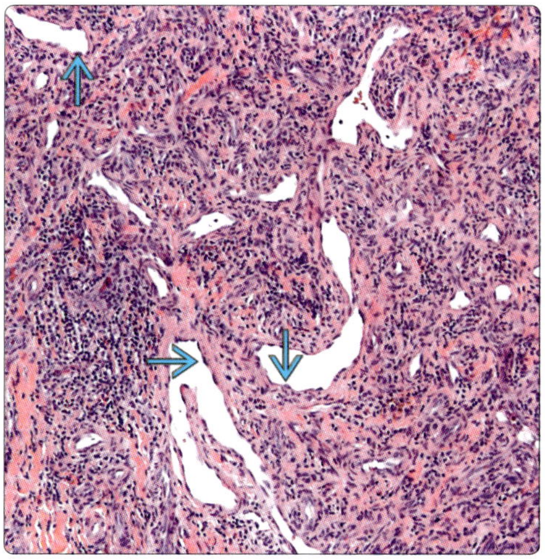

(Left) *The epithelioid endothelial-lined vascular channels* ⊡ *may also be seen within the muscular wall of the involved vessel and may even communicate with the lumen in some cases.* **(Right)** *This H&E shows an EH with prominent dilated and irregular vascular channels, reminiscent of the "staghorn" vessels of a solitary fibrous tumor. Hobnailed nuclei* ⊡ *are somewhat apparent at this magnification.*

Vascular Lumina

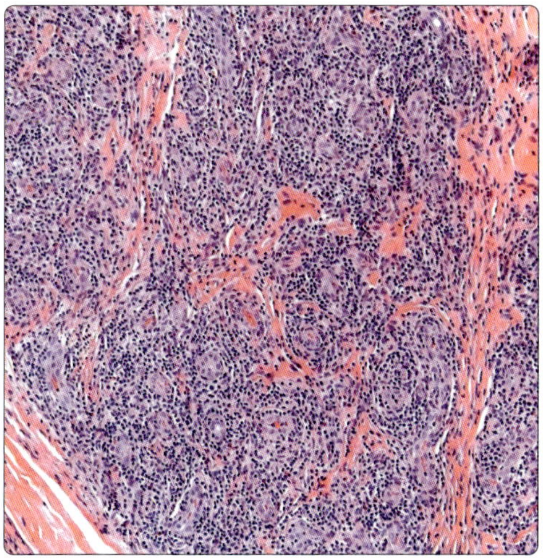

Chronic Inflammatory Infiltrate

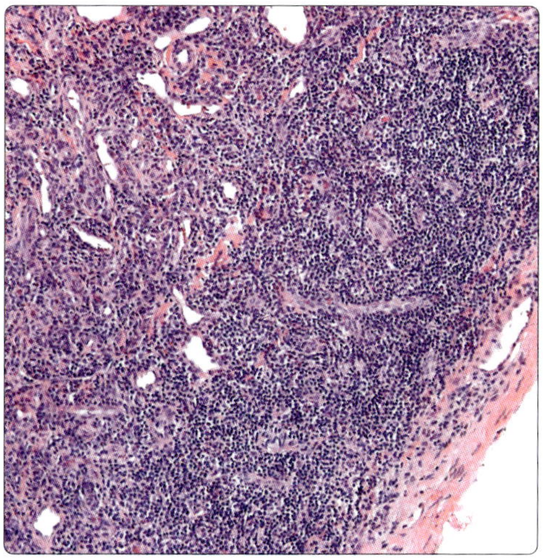

(Left) *Well-defined vascular lumina are not always identified in EH, as shown in this H&E, and vascular origin may be difficult to discern in these cases.* **(Right)** *A chronic inflammatory infiltrate is common in EH and may be quite prominent, particularly at the periphery of the lesion. Most of the cells are lymphocytes, but eosinophils are also usually prominent.*

Eosinophils

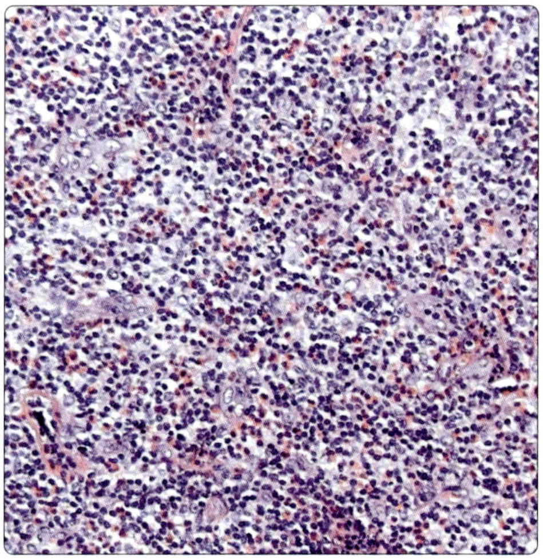

Reactive Germinal Centers

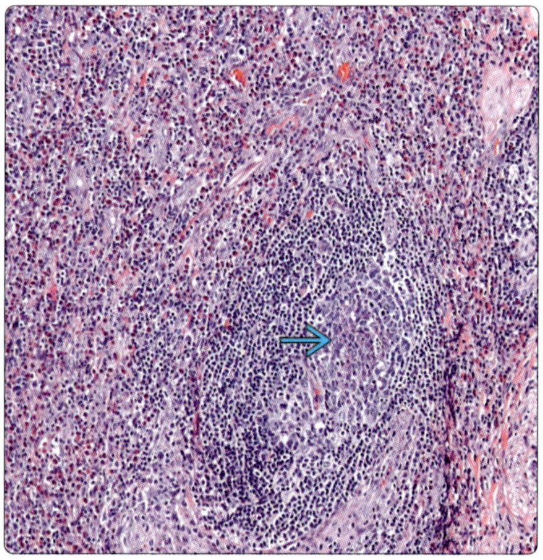

(Left) *The inflammatory stromal infiltrate may appear diffuse in some foci of EH and obscure the characteristic epithelioid endothelial cells. Note the admixed brisk infiltrate of eosinophils, a finding that should always raise the possibility of EH.* **(Right)** *The lymphoid tissue in EH may show a formation of reactive germinal centers* ⊡. *This feature may be very prominent and is often seen at the periphery of the lesion.*

Spindle Cell Hemangioma

KEY FACTS

TERMINOLOGY

- Benign vascular tumor featuring both cavernous and cellular, predominantly spindled zones
- Synonym: Spindle cell hemangioendothelioma (obsolete)

CLINICAL ISSUES

- Young adults
- Distal extremities, often acral
- Subcutaneous mass
- Often multifocal
- May be associated with Maffucci syndrome (multiple enchondromas + spindle cell hemangioma)

MICROSCOPIC

- 2 zones
  - Large, dilated cavernous spaces
  - Solid areas of bland spindled and epithelioid endothelial cells with slit-like vascular spaces
- Clear endothelial vacuoles common, often grouped resembling clusters of small adipocytes
- Often arises from vessel; may be intravascular
- Minimal atypia or mitotic activity
- Large calcified thrombi (phleboliths) may be present

ANCILLARY TESTS

- Expression of vascular markers (CD31, CD34, ERG)
- Often have *IDH1* (or *IDH2*) mutation

TOP DIFFERENTIAL DIAGNOSES

- Kaposi sarcoma (tumor stage)
- Kaposiform hemangioendothelioma
- Epithelioid hemangioendothelioma
- Organizing thrombus/intravascular papillary endothelial hyperplasia
- Cavernous hemangioma (venous malformation)

Spindle Cell Hemangioma

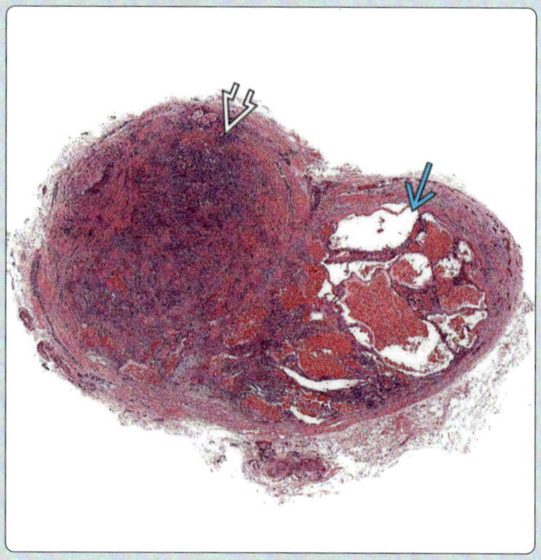

Cavernous and Cellular Zones

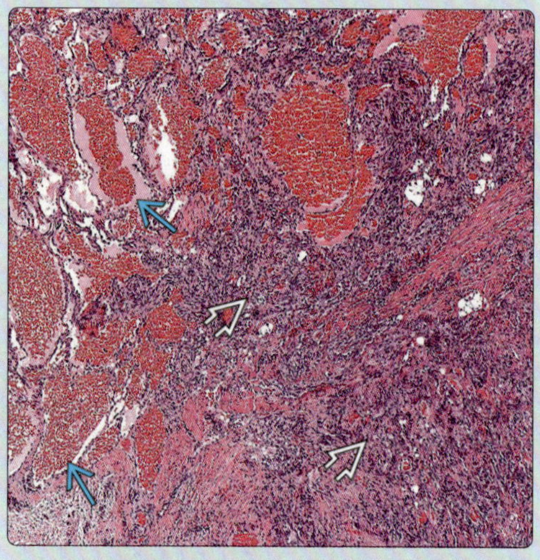

(Left) *Spindle cell hemangioma (SCH) is classically characterized by cavernous vascular spaces adjacent to more cellular zones of spindle and epithelioid endothelial cells.* **(Right)** *The cavernous vascular channels of SCH are essentially identical to those of cavernous hemangioma. The cellular zones are composed of sheets of plump, spindled, and epithelioid endothelial cells that may bear some resemblance to Kaposi sarcoma.*

Vacuolated Endothelial Cells

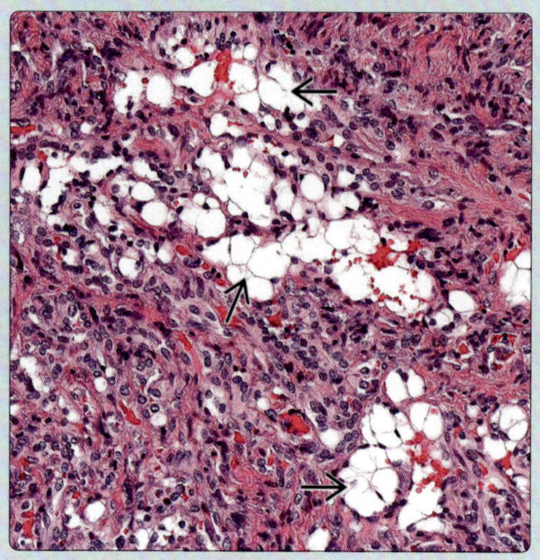

Kaposi-Like Cellular Zones

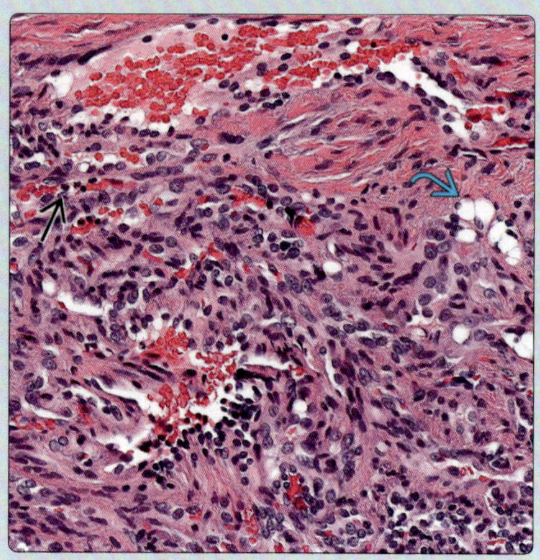

(Left) *Some of the endothelial cells display clear cytoplasmic vacuoles and are often clustered together within the cellular zones creating a striking resemblance to entrapped groups of miniaturized adipocytes. This is a characteristic feature of SCH.* **(Right)** *Cellular zones of plump spindled and epithelioid endothelial cells lack atypia or significant mitotic activity in SCH. Compressed vascular channels may resemble the slit-like vascular spaces of Kaposi sarcoma. Note the vacuolated endothelial cells.*

Spindle Cell Hemangioma

TERMINOLOGY

Abbreviations

- Spindle cell hemangioma (SCH)

Synonyms

- Spindle cell hemangioendothelioma (obsolete term)

Definitions

- Benign vascular tumor featuring both cavernous and cellular, predominantly spindled zones

CLINICAL ISSUES

Epidemiology

- Age
  - Young adults

Site

- Distal extremities, often acral

Presentation

- Subcutaneous mass
- Often multifocal
- May be associated with Maffucci syndrome (multiple enchondromas + SCH), Klippel-Trenaunay syndrome, varicosities, and congenital lymphedema

Treatment

- Simple surgical excision

Prognosis

- Regional "recurrence" most likely multifocal disease and not true recurrence
- No metastatic potential

MICROSCOPIC

Histologic Features

- 2 distinct zones characteristic
  - Large, dilated cavernous spaces
    - Large thrombi, often calcified (phleboliths), may be present
  - Solid, cellular areas of bland, spindled, and epithelioid endothelial cells with slit-like vascular spaces
    - Clear endothelial vacuoles common, often grouped resembling clusters of small adipocytes
- Often arises from vessel; may be intravascular
- Minimal atypia or mitotic activity

ANCILLARY TESTS

Immunohistochemistry

- CD34(+), CD31(+), ERG(+)
- HHV-8(-)

Genetic Testing

- *IDH1* (or *IDH2*) mutation common in both sporadic and Maffucci-associated SCH
  - These mutations are absent in other vascular lesions

DIFFERENTIAL DIAGNOSIS

Kaposi Sarcoma (Tumor Stage)

- Usually dermal based rather than subcutaneous
- Usually in either HIV(+) patients or in elderly
- Cavernous vascular channels are uncommon
- Greater cytologic atypia and more mitoses than SCH
- More prominent slit/sieve-like vascular channels with abundant erythrocyte extravasation
- Plasma cells almost always present
- HHV-8 (LANA1) (+) by immunohistochemistry

Kaposiform Hemangioendothelioma

- Almost exclusively in children
- Glomeruloid nodules of spindled endothelial cells
- Usually lacks cavernous areas
- Associated with Kasabach-Merritt phenomenon

Epithelioid Hemangioendothelioma

- Cords of epithelioid endothelial cells; usually lacks well-formed vascular channels
- Endothelial vacuoles contain erythrocyte fragments ("blister" cells)
- Characteristic myxohyaline stroma
- Lacks cavernous spaces

Organizing Thrombus/Intravascular Papillary Endothelial Hyperplasia

- Spindled areas have myxoid background and merge with fibrin
- Spindled areas are within cavernous vascular spaces rather than adjacent
- Papillary architecture of endothelial cells overlying fibrin cores
- Lacks clusters of adipocyte-like vacuoles

Cavernous Hemangioma (Venous Malformation)

- Lacks cellular spindled and epithelioid zone

DIAGNOSTIC CHECKLIST

Pathologic Interpretation Pearls

- 2 zones
  - Cavernous spaces
  - Cellular spindled and epithelioid cells
- Clustered vacuoles resemble miniature fat cells; very characteristic

SELECTED REFERENCES

1. Ten Broek RW et al: Mutational analysis using Sanger and next generation sequencing in sporadic spindle cell hemangiomas: a study of 19 cases. Genes Chromosomes Cancer. 56(12):855-60, 2017
2. Kurek KC et al: R132C IDH1 mutations are found in spindle cell hemangiomas and not in other vascular tumors or malformations. Am J Pathol. 182(5):1494-500, 2013
3. Perkins P et al: Spindle cell hemangioendothelioma. An analysis of 78 cases with reassessment of its pathogenesis and biologic behavior. Am J Surg Pathol. 20(10):1196-204, 1996
4. Fanburg JC et al: Multiple enchondromas associated with spindle-cell hemangioendotheliomas. An overlooked variant of Maffucci's syndrome. Am J Surg Pathol. 19(9):1029-38, 1995
5. Fletcher CD et al: Spindle cell haemangioendothelioma: a clinicopathological and immunohistochemical study indicative of a non-neoplastic lesion. Histopathology. 18(4):291-301, 1991
6. Weiss SW et al: Spindle cell hemangioendothelioma. A low-grade angiosarcoma resembling a cavernous hemangioma and Kaposi's sarcoma. Am J Surg Pathol. 10(8):521-30, 1986

(Left) *SCH may present as a dermal or subcutaneous mass, usually on the distal extremities. More superficial lesions like this example may have a violaceous appearance. (Courtesy C. Montgomery, MD.)* **(Right)** *The cavernous vascular channels of SCH are lined by bland endothelium. They are essentially identical to those seen in cavernous hemangioma.*

Violaceous Dermal Papule

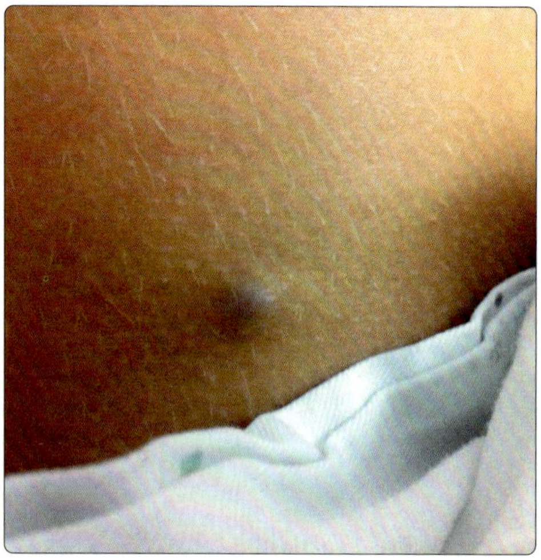

Cavernous Spaces

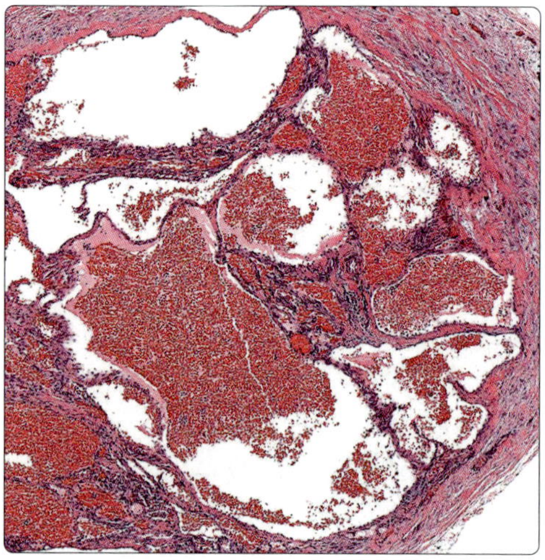

(Left) *Large fibrin thrombi with secondary calcification (phleboliths) are commonly present within the cavernous spaces ➡ of SCH.* **(Right)** *SCH often arises from a thick-walled muscular vessel ⇨. Intravascular tumor growth ↷ may be seen; this is not an indication of malignancy or aggressive behavior.*

Calcified Thrombi (Phleboliths)

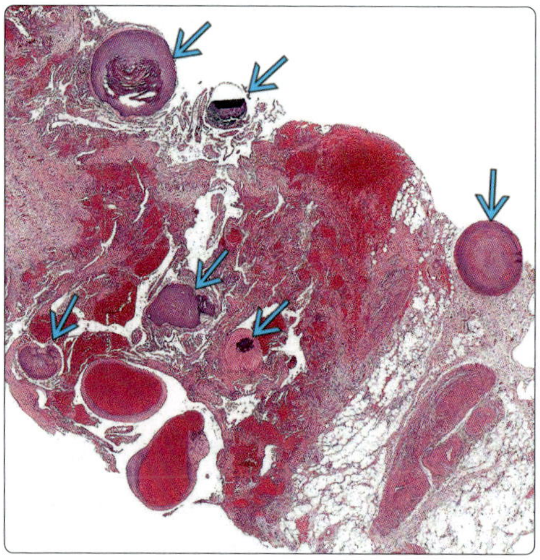

Origin From Thick-Walled Vessel

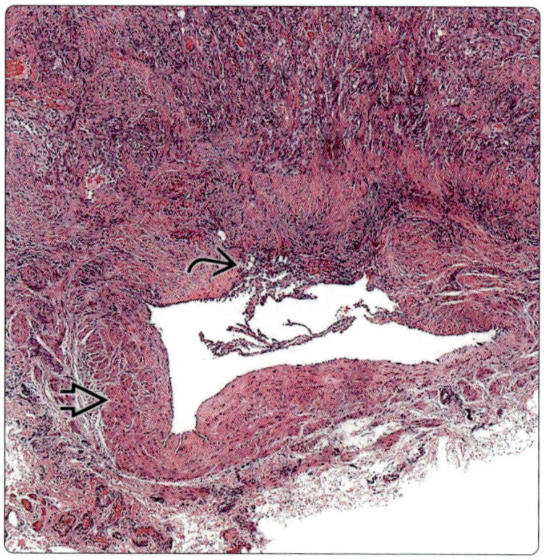

(Left) *In the cellular areas of SCH, the spindled and epithelioid endothelial cells often display clear cytoplasmic vacuoles →. These should not be confused with the vacuolated "blister" cells of epithelioid hemangioendothelioma, which are usually smaller and can contain erythrocyte fragments.* **(Right)** *Vacuolated endothelial cells can occasionally be quite numerous and prominent in SCH, as depicted in this H&E.*

Clear Cytoplasmic Vacuoles

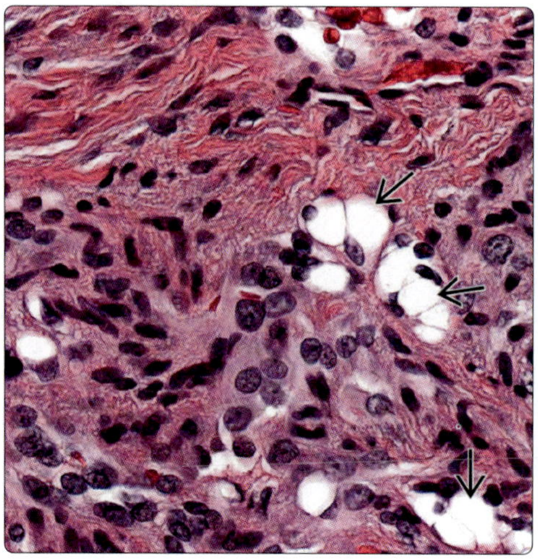

Vacuolated Endothelial Cells

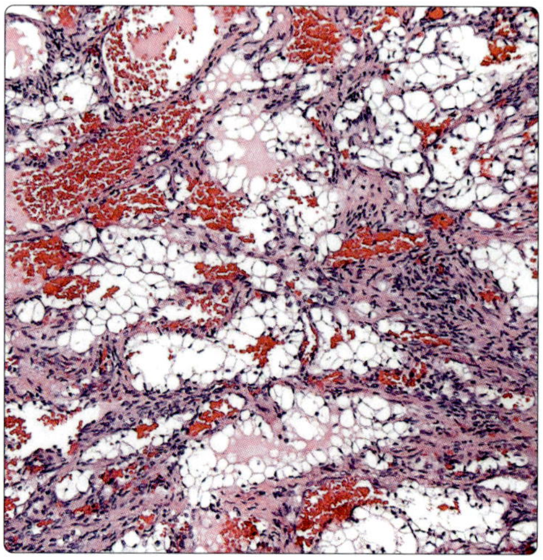

Kaposi-Like Areas

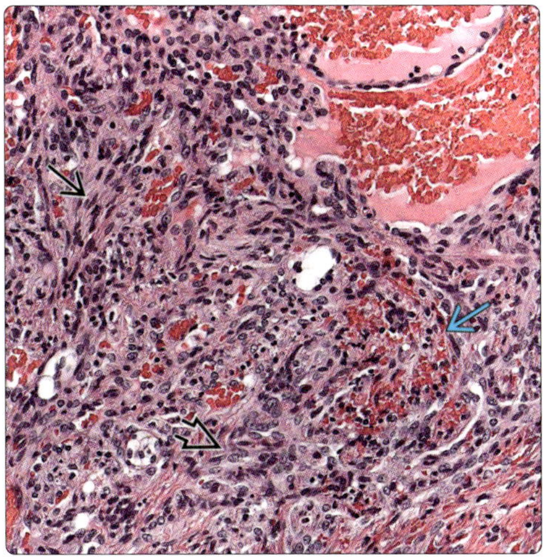

Kaposi-Like Areas

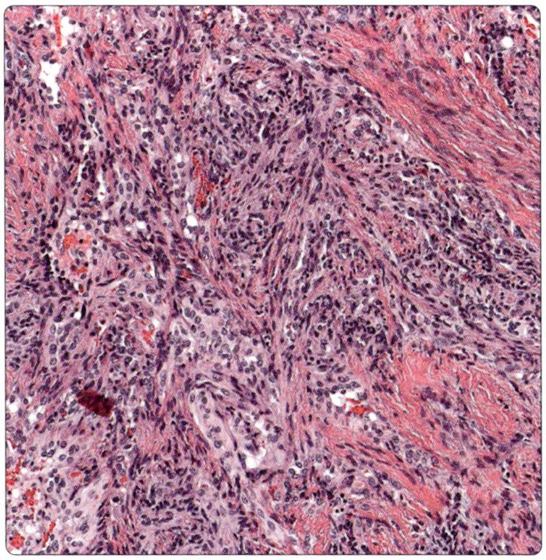

(Left) *The cellular zones of SCH are composed of both spindled → and epithelioid ⇨ endothelial cells. Blood-filled compressed vascular channels are seen →, but unlike Kaposi sarcoma, extravasation of erythrocytes is usually minimal.* **(Right)** *Even in the absence of detectable vasoformation, relatively solid areas like this can resemble the infiltrative spindled morphology of Kaposi sarcoma.*

Maffucci Syndrome

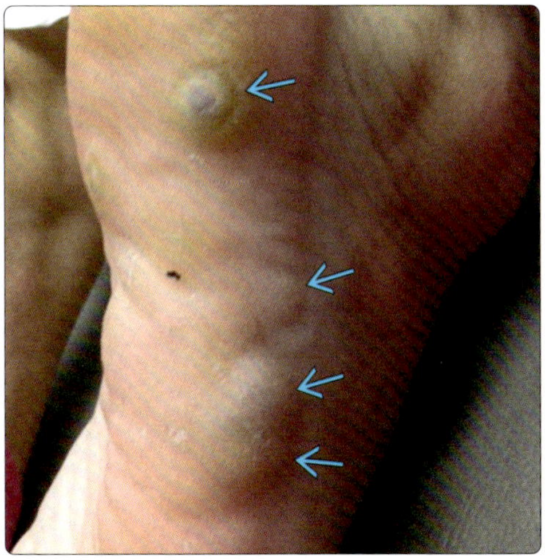

Maffucci Syndrome

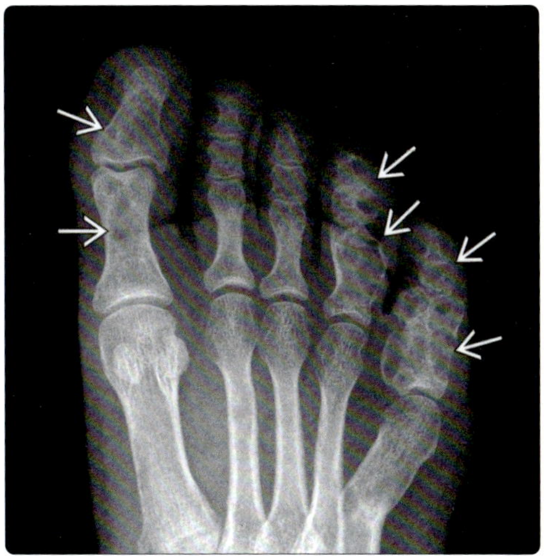

(Left) *This patient with Maffucci syndrome has multiple SCHs of the right foot →. Radiographic studies also revealed multiple enchondromas in the foot, leg, and pelvis. (Courtesy C. Montgomery, MD.)* **(Right)** *Plain radiograph of the foot in a patient with Maffucci syndrome shows multiple expansile lytic bone lesions consistent with enchondromas in the phalanges →.*

Maffucci Syndrome

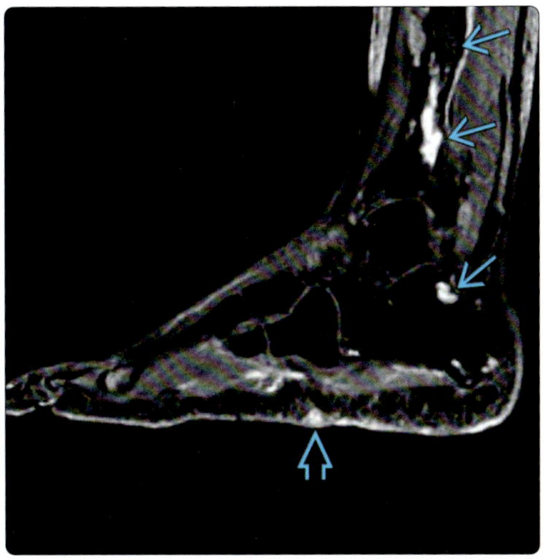

MR of Maffucci Syndrome

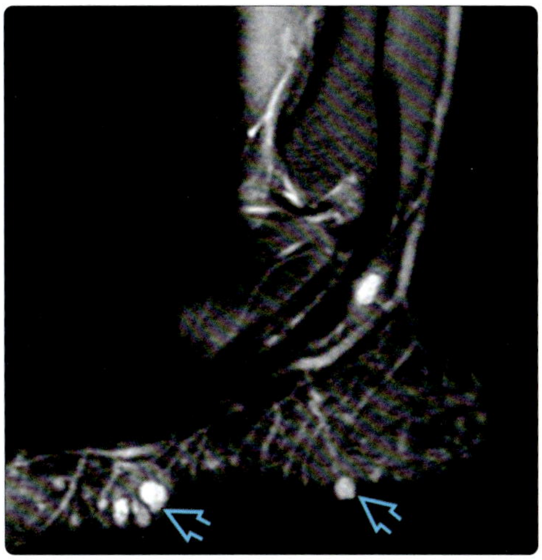

(Left) *MR of a patient with Maffucci syndrome displays hyperintense bone lesions consistent with enchondromas → in the calcaneus and distal tibia. The hyperintense plantar subcutaneous nodule is an SCH ⇨.* **(Right)** *STIR MR of a patient with Maffucci syndrome suppresses the subcutaneous fat signal, allowing for better visualization of multiple subcutaneous SCHs of the lateral plantar foot ⇨.*

Intramuscular Hemangioma

KEY FACTS

TERMINOLOGY

- Benign vascular proliferation located within skeletal muscle with varying amounts of mature adipose tissue
- Synonyms: Infiltrating (intramuscular) angiolipoma, intramuscular angioma

ETIOLOGY/PATHOGENESIS

- Likely represents vascular malformation

CLINICAL ISSUES

- 85% diagnosed prior to 30 years of age
- Most commonly arises in skeletal muscle of thigh
  - Other common sites: Head and neck, upper extremities, trunk
- Deep-seated, slow-growing mass
  - Frequently associated with pain
- Treatment: Complete surgical excision
- Significant recurrence rate (30-50%)

MACROSCOPIC

- Ill-defined mass within skeletal muscle
- Wide size range: 1-29 cm; mean size: 6.5 cm

MICROSCOPIC

- Vary greatly in histologic appearance
- Typically consist of mixture of thick-walled veins; arteries; capillaries; and ectatic, thin-walled vascular spaces
  - Historically classified into capillary, cavernous, and mixed types
- Associated with varying amounts of mature adipose tissue
- Vascular and adipose elements infiltrate among skeletal muscle fibers

TOP DIFFERENTIAL DIAGNOSES

- Angiosarcoma
- Angiomatosis
- Angiolipoma

Intramuscular Hemangioma

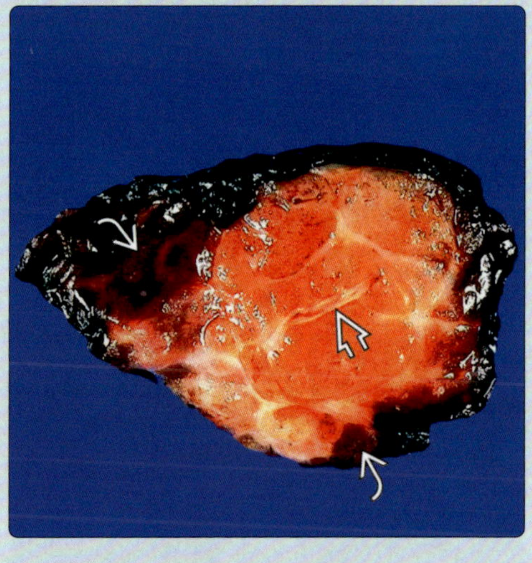

Intramuscular Hemangioma

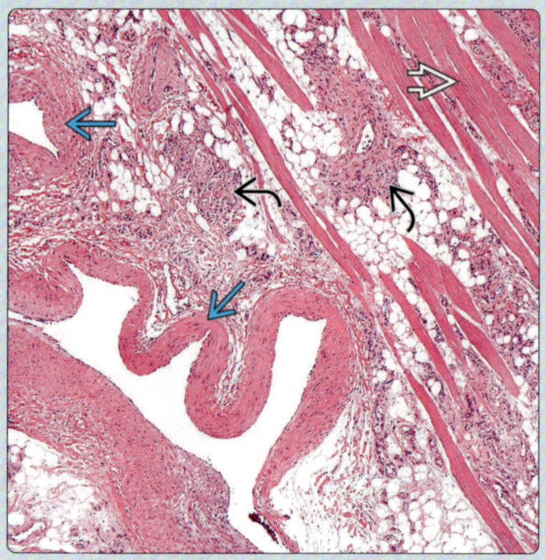

(Left) *Gross photograph of intramuscular hemangioma (IMH) demonstrates a solid, tan mass involving skeletal muscle. The lesion has an irregular border with the muscle, and there are grossly evident, large vascular structures.* **(Right)** *The typical case of IMH shows a complex mixture of blood vessels, including large, ectatic vessels and capillaries and adipose tissue that appears to infiltrate skeletal muscle.*

Skeletal Muscle Infiltration

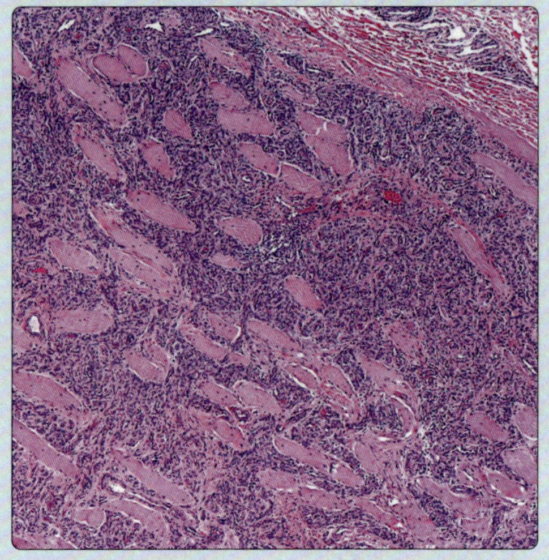

Mature Adipose Tissue

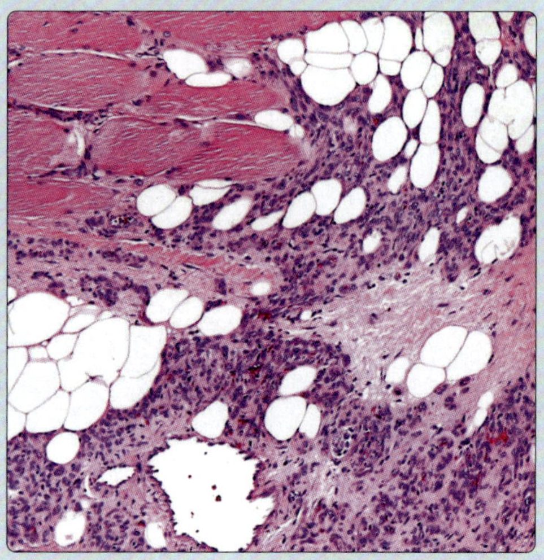

(Left) *Infiltration of skeletal muscle is a common feature of IMH with capillary-sized vessels arranged in between skeletal muscle fibers. Note the overall checkerboard appearance, a common occurrence.* **(Right)** *Mature adipose tissue is a common feature of IMH and may be abundant in some cases. The presence of fat accounts for the previous designation as an infiltrating or intramuscular angiolipoma.*

Intramuscular Hemangioma

TERMINOLOGY

Abbreviations

- Intramuscular hemangioma (IMH)

Synonyms

- Intramuscular angioma
- Infiltrating/intramuscular angiolipoma

Definitions

- Benign vascular proliferation located within skeletal muscle with varying amounts of mature adipose tissue

ETIOLOGY/PATHOGENESIS

Developmental Anomaly

- Likely represents vascular malformation
- No relation to trauma

CLINICAL ISSUES

Epidemiology

- Incidence
  - Uncommon
- Age
  - Most occur in young adults, but all ages affected
    - 85% diagnosed prior to 30 years

Site

- Most frequent in skeletal muscle of lower extremities
  - Thigh is most common site
- Other common sites: Head and neck, upper extremities, trunk
- Can also arise in cardiac muscle

Presentation

- Deep-seated, slow-growing mass
- Frequently associated with pain
  - Pain often occurs during exercise

Treatment

- Complete surgical excision

Prognosis

- Benign; no risk of malignant transformation
- Significant recurrence rate (30-50%)
  - Often secondary to incomplete excision
  - Histologic parameters (e.g., vessel type) not predictive of recurrence risk

IMAGING

Radiographic Findings

- Intramuscular soft tissue mass
  - Fatty areas will appear low density on CT
- Frequently show foci of calcification
  - Phleboliths or metaplastic ossification

MACROSCOPIC

General Features

- Ill-defined mass within skeletal muscle
- Color varies depending on cellularity, vessel type, and amount of adipose tissue

Size

- Wide range: 1-29 cm; mean: 6.5 cm

MICROSCOPIC

Histologic Features

- Vary greatly in histologic appearance
  - Typically consist of mixture of thick-walled veins; arteries; capillaries; and ectatic, thin-walled vascular spaces
    - Tumors may also have lymphatic component
  - Associated with varying amounts of mature adipose tissue
  - Vascular and adipose elements infiltrate among skeletal muscle fibers
    - Pattern of infiltration may appear checkerboard-like
    - Muscle atrophy and degenerative sarcolemmal changes may be seen
- Historically classified into capillary, cavernous, and mixed types (latter most common)
  - Capillary type
    - More frequent in head and neck sites
    - Composed of numerous small (capillary-sized) vessels
    - Lumen formation typically apparent
    - Solid growth akin to juvenile hemangiomas may be seen
    - Endothelial cells are plump and cytologically bland with rare mitoses
  - Cavernous type
    - More common in trunk locations
    - Endothelial cells are attenuated and cytologically bland
- Presurgical embolization may result in secondary changes and presence of embolization material

DIFFERENTIAL DIAGNOSIS

Angiosarcoma

- Very uncommon in deep-seated locations
- Complex anastomosing vascular channels
- Multilayered endothelial cells, often with pleomorphic and hyperchromatic nuclei

Angiomatosis

- Histologically identical to IMH in many cases, so distinction is clinical
- Usually congenital
- Involves large region of body and multiple tissues (e.g., skin, muscle, and bone)

Angiolipoma

- Small and well circumscribed; often multiple
- Arises in subcutaneous tissue
- Capillary channels contain fibrin thrombi

SELECTED REFERENCES

1. Patnaik S et al: Intramuscular arteriovenous hemangioma of thigh: a case report and review of literature. J Orthop Case Rep. 6(5):20-23, 2016
2. Yilmaz S et al: Intramuscular capillary-type hemangioma: radiologic-pathologic correlation. Pediatr Radiol. 44(5):558-65, 2014
3. Beham A et al: Intramuscular angioma: a clinicopathological analysis of 74 cases. Histopathology. 18(1):53-9, 1991
4. Cohen AJ et al: Intramuscular hemangioma. JAMA. 249(19):2680-2, 1983

(Left) *Hematoxylin and eosin of IMH demonstrates scattered large blood vessels mixed in with dense zones of small capillary channels, all proliferating around and in between mature skeletal muscle fibers.* **(Right)** *Capillary- and mixed-types IMH may show large zones of dense capillary channels, which at low magnification can raise concerns for a sarcoma. The impression of infiltrated adipose tissue and skeletal muscle may amplify this concern if the pathologist is not aware of this entity.*

Intramuscular Hemangioma

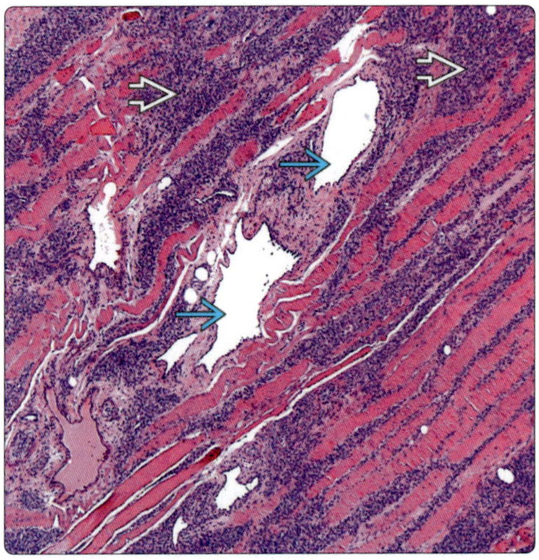

Dense Growth

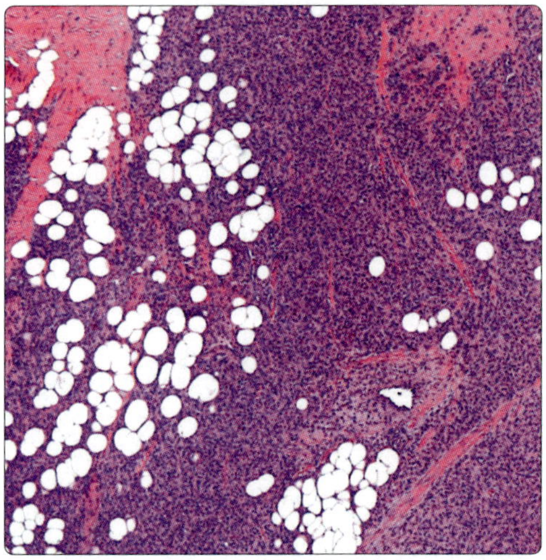

(Left) *The endothelial cells in all types of IMH are cytologically bland and lack nuclear pleomorphism and malignant atypia. In some cases, capillary lumina are inconspicuous, as in this hematoxylin and eosin.* **(Right)** *Some cases of IMH contain abundant mature adipose tissue and a comparatively small vascular component, potentially leading to consideration of an intramuscular lipoma or an angiolipoma.*

Benign Cytologic Features

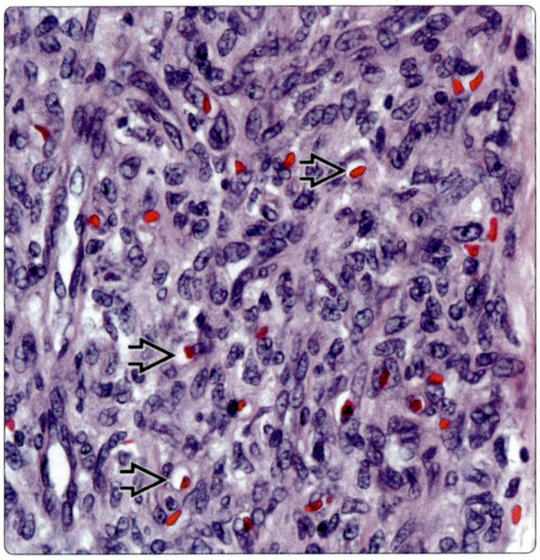

Abundant Mature Adipose Tissue

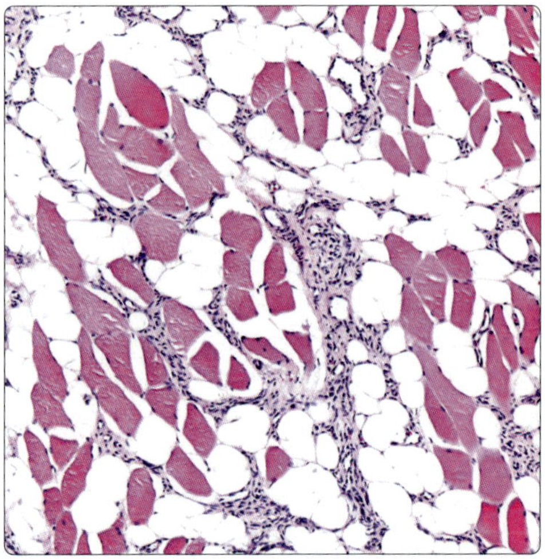

(Left) *Small, entrapped myocytes with degenerative/reactive sarcolemmal changes may be seen in some cases of IMH.* **(Right)** *High-power examination shows the features of a degenerative/reactive myocyte in IMH, including dense eosinophilic cytoplasm and multiple, small hyperchromatic nuclei in clusters ("grapes") and peripheral ring-like arrangements. This finding can also be seen in other intramuscular tumors.*

Degenerative Skeletal Muscle Fibers

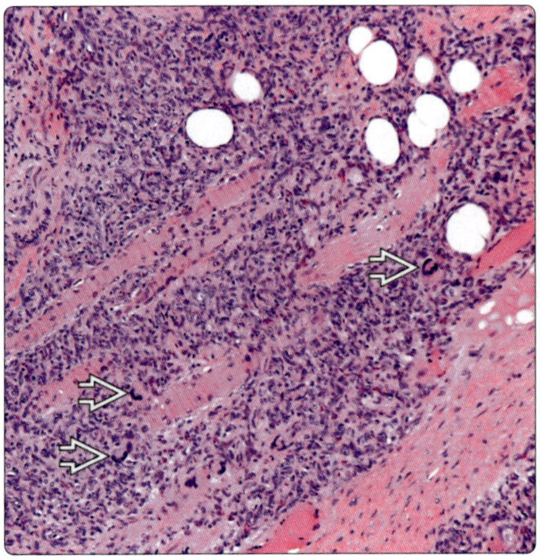

Degenerative Skeletal Muscle Fibers

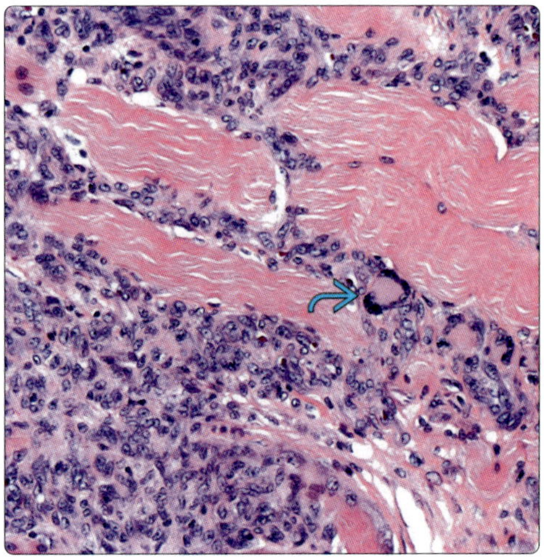

Cavernous Intramuscular Hemangioma

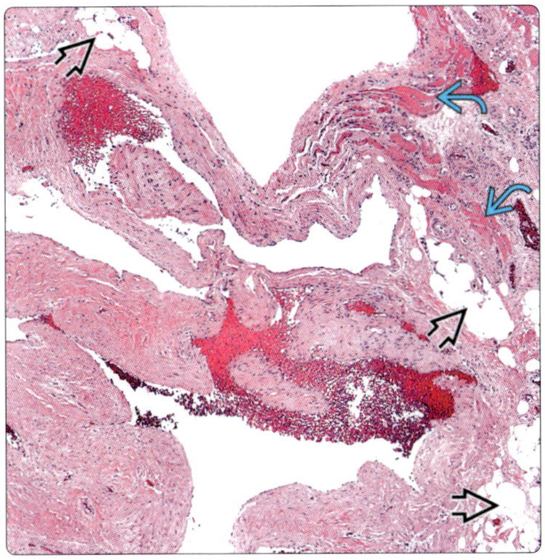

Cavernous Intramuscular Hemangioma

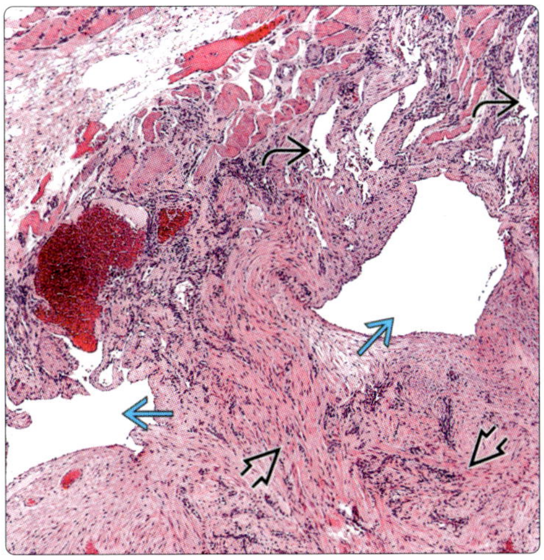

(Left) *Cavernous IMH is characterized by ectatic, thin-walled vascular spaces with associated adipose tissue and infiltrating within degenerating skeletal muscle.* **(Right)** *Cavernous IMHs are frequently associated with an irregular proliferation of smooth muscle bundles and smaller, slit-like vascular channels at the periphery of the larger, ectatic vessels.*

Lobulated Growth

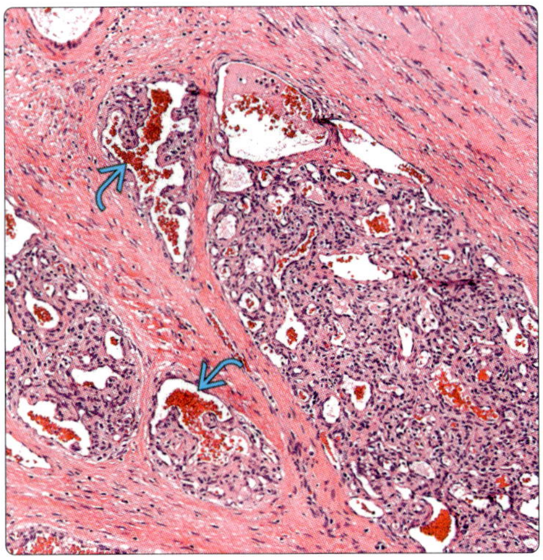

Secondary Changes

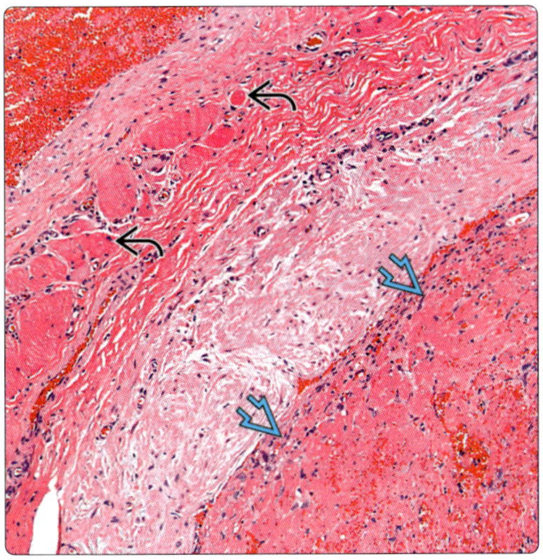

(Left) *Some IMHs have a lobulated appearance, imparting a resemblance to lobular capillary hemangioma. The lobules in this example are composed of numerous small capillaries with larger, feeder-type vascular channels.* **(Right)** *Secondary changes are common in IMH. Note the compressed and atrophic skeletal muscle bundles in this cavernous IMH. Cavernous examples frequently develop thrombi that may calcify and become phleboliths.*

Embolization Material

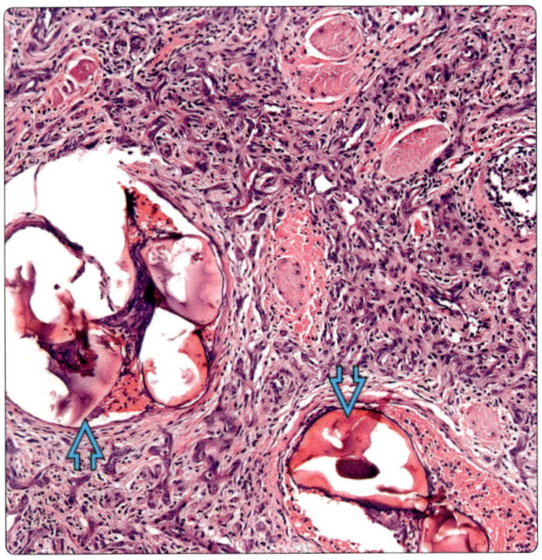

Imaging Characteristics

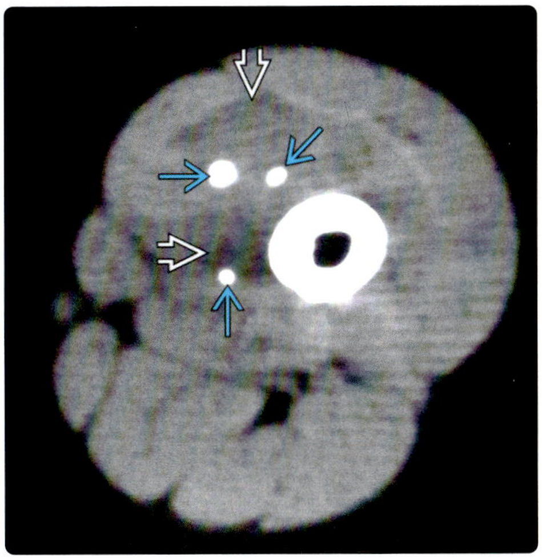

(Left) *Many cases of suspected IMH are embolized prior to resection and show embolization material and thrombus formation in vessels with secondary inflammation &/or necrosis.* **(Right)** *Axial CT through the midthigh shows phleboliths within an IMH. The low-density areas represent fat within the lesion.*

Hobnail Hemangioma

KEY FACTS

TERMINOLOGY

- Synonym: Targetoid hemosiderotic hemangioma
- Definition: Benign vascular proliferation, typically wedge-shaped, showing intravascular papillae and hobnail endothelial cells

ETIOLOGY/PATHOGENESIS

- Postulated to represent traumatized lymphangioma or hemangioma

CLINICAL ISSUES

- Typically presents on lower extremities; may also occur on upper extremities, rarely in oral cavity
- Young to middle-aged adults
- More common in male patients
- Often pigmented due to hemosiderin deposition
- May show halo (targetoid appearance) in minority of cases
- Excellent prognosis

MICROSCOPIC

- Vascular proliferation with wedge-shaped appearance
- Superficial vessels are dilated and thin walled
- Deeper vessels are progressively smaller
- Vessels are lined by small, bland-appearing endothelial cells with hobnail appearance
- Focal papillary projections with fibrous cores may be present
- Hemorrhage and hemosiderin deposition are typically prominent
- Inflammation is usually minimal

TOP DIFFERENTIAL DIAGNOSES

- Progressive lymphangioma
- Kaposi sarcoma
- Microvenular hemangioma
- Retiform hemangioendothelioma

(Left) *Low magnification of a hobnail hemangioma shows superficial dilated vascular spaces ⇨ in the papillary dermis with deeper small blood vessels and stromal hemosiderin deposits →.* **(Right)** *Higher magnification of the superficial portion of the tumor shows small endothelial cells protruding into the dilated vascular spaces ⇨.*

Hobnail Hemangioma

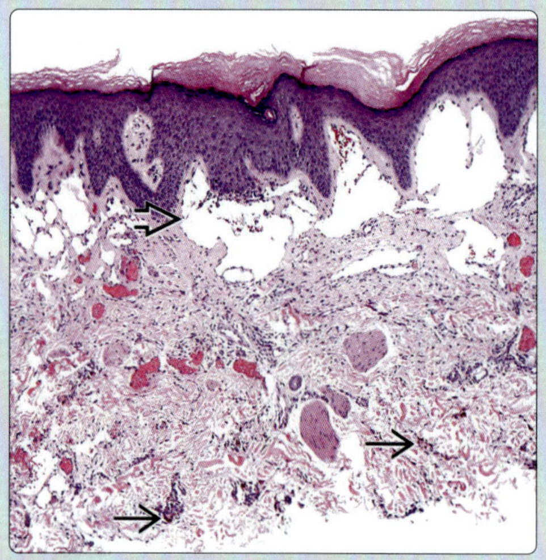

Dilated Vascular Spaces

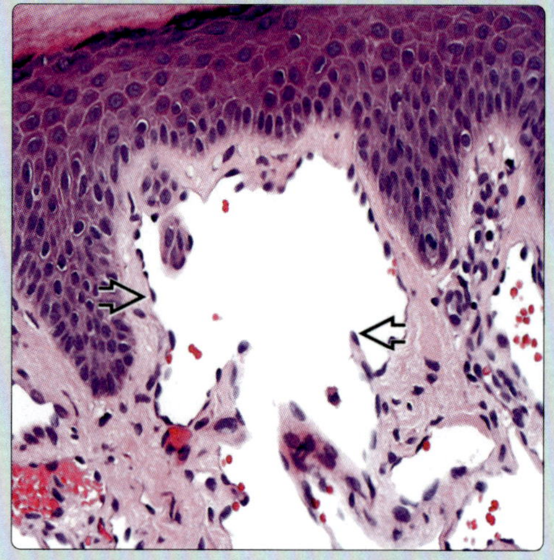

(Left) *High-power examination demonstrates superficial dilated vessels lined by small endothelial cells protruding into the lumina → and showing nuclear hyperchromasia.* **(Right)** *Histologic examination of the deeper aspect of the lesion shows smaller blood vessels ⇨ and prominent hemosiderin deposition in the stroma →.*

Hobnail Endothelial Cells

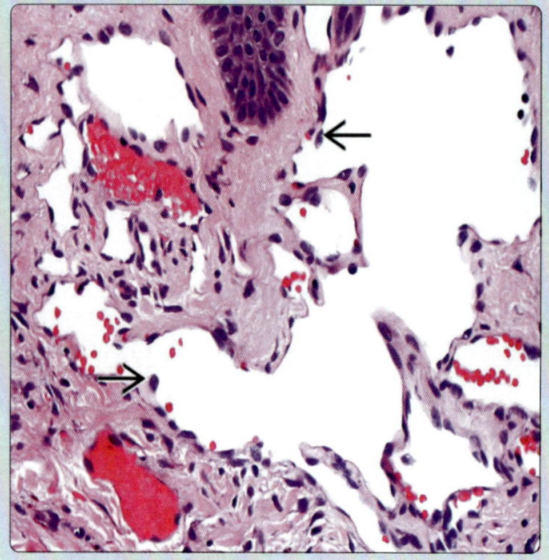

Hemosiderin Deposition

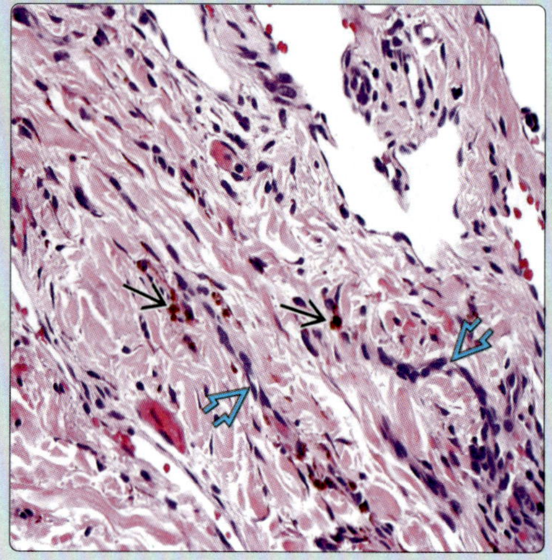

TERMINOLOGY

Abbreviations

- Hobnail hemangioma (HH)

Synonyms

- Targetoid hemosiderotic hemangioma (clinical term)

Definitions

- Benign vascular proliferation, typically wedge-shaped, showing intravascular papillae and hobnailed endothelial cells

ETIOLOGY/PATHOGENESIS

Unknown

- Trauma has been implicated in some cases
    - Postulated to represent traumatized lymphangioma or hemangioma

CLINICAL ISSUES

Epidemiology

- Age
    - Young to middle-aged adults
- Sex
    - M > F

Site

- Typically presents on lower extremities; also may occur on upper extremities, rarely in oral cavity

Presentation

- Skin papule or nodule
    - Often pigmented due to hemosiderin deposition
    - May show halo (targetoid appearance) but only in minority of cases

Treatment

- Complete, conservative excision

Prognosis

- Excellent with no tendency for local recurrence

MACROSCOPIC

General Features

- Dermal-based, reddish-brown lesion with hemorrhage

Size

- Small, usually < 2 cm

MICROSCOPIC

Histologic Features

- Vascular proliferation with wedge-shaped appearance
- Superficial vessels are dilated and thin walled
    - Some vessels may resemble lymphatics
    - Focal papillary projections with fibrous cores may be present
    - Vessels are lined by small, uniform, bland-appearing endothelial cells with hobnail appearance (nuclei project into lumina)
    - Mitoses usually not present
- Deeper vessels are progressively smaller and show narrow lumina
- Hemorrhage and hemosiderin deposition are typically prominent
- Inflammation is usually minimal

DIFFERENTIAL DIAGNOSIS

Progressive Lymphangioma

- Thin-walled, dilated, superficial vascular spaces with narrower deeper vessels
- Lacks hobnail endothelial cell morphology and hemosiderin deposition of HH

Kaposi Sarcoma

- Shows proliferation of slit-like spaces lined by atypical spindle cells
- Typically lacks superficial, dilated vascular spaces and hobnail cells
- HHV8(+) by immunohistochemistry

Microvenular Hemangioma

- Proliferation of small, round to slit-like, thin-walled vessels involving reticular dermis
- Lacks superficial, dilated vascular spaces, hobnail cells, and hemosiderin deposition

Retiform Hemangioendothelioma

- Dermal and subcutaneous tumor characterized by proliferation of arborizing vessels lined by hobnail endothelial cells
- Typically prominent lymphoid infiltrate, which is lacking in HH
- HH is usually more superficial, and deeper vessels are smaller and compact

DIAGNOSTIC CHECKLIST

Pathologic Interpretation Pearls

- Wedge-shaped vascular proliferation
- Dilated, superficial vessels, deeper small/collapsed vessels
- Intravascular papillae and hobnail endothelial cells
- Prominent hemosiderin deposition

SELECTED REFERENCES

1. Biondo G et al: A pigmented papule acting like a playful ghost: dermoscopy of three targetoid hemosiderotic hemangiomas. G Ital Dermatol Venereol. 153(5):685-91, 2018
2. Porriño-Bustamante ML et al: Hobnail hemangioma with an unusual clinical presentation. J Cutan Med Surg. 21(2):164-6, 2017
3. Joyce JC et al: Superficial hemosiderotic lymphovascular malformation (hobnail hemangioma): a report of six cases. Pediatr Dermatol. 31(3):281-5, 2014
4. Kim DS et al: Multiple hobnail hemangiomas. Int J Dermatol. 53(4):e240-2, 2014
5. Hejnold M et al: Hobnail hemangioma: a immunohistochemical study and literature review. Pol J Pathol. 63(3):189-92, 2012
6. Trindade F et al: Hobnail hemangioma reclassified as superficial lymphatic malformation: a study of 52 cases. J Am Acad Dermatol. 66(1):112-5, 2012
7. Fernandez-Flores A et al: Clinical changes in "true" hobnail hemangioma during menstruation. Bratisl Lek Listy. 109(3):141-3, 2008
8. Franke FE et al: Hobnail hemangiomas (targetoid hemosiderotic hemangiomas) are true lymphangiomas. J Cutan Pathol. 31(5):362-7, 2004
9. Pabuccuoğlu U et al: Hobnail haemangioma occurring on the nasal dorsum. Br J Dermatol. 146(1):162-4, 2002
10. Santonja C et al: Hobnail hemangioma. Dermatology. 191(2):154-6, 1995

Acquired Tufted Angioma

KEY FACTS

TERMINOLOGY

- Acquired tufted angioma (ATA)
- Synonym: Angioblastoma (of Nakagawa)
- Definition: Multiple cannonball-like, cellular collections of small vessels in dermis

ETIOLOGY/PATHOGENESIS

- Most cases sporadic; rare familial cases described
- Some cases associated with pregnancy or liver transplantation

CLINICAL ISSUES

- Rare tumors
- Mostly occur in children and young adults
- Neck, shoulders, and upper trunk most common sites
- Slowly growing erythematous macules and plaques
- May be associated with Kasabach-Merritt syndrome (consumptive coagulopathy)

MICROSCOPIC

- Scattered, lobular collections of small, capillary-type vessels throughout dermis; may involve subcutis
- Cleft-like lumina often present around capillary tufts; may impart glomerular appearance
- Cells are oval to spindle-shaped
- Mitoses may be present but cells lack significant cytologic atypia or pleomorphism
- Hemosiderin deposition may be seen
- Inflammation typically not present

TOP DIFFERENTIAL DIAGNOSES

- Lobular capillary hemangioma
- Glomeruloid hemangioma
- Infantile (juvenile) hemangioma
- Kaposiform hemangioendothelioma
- Kaposi sarcoma

Acquired Tufted Angioma

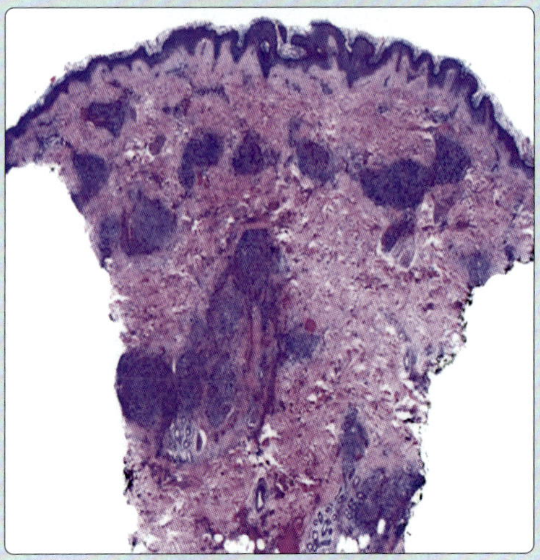

Lobules and Nests of Vessels

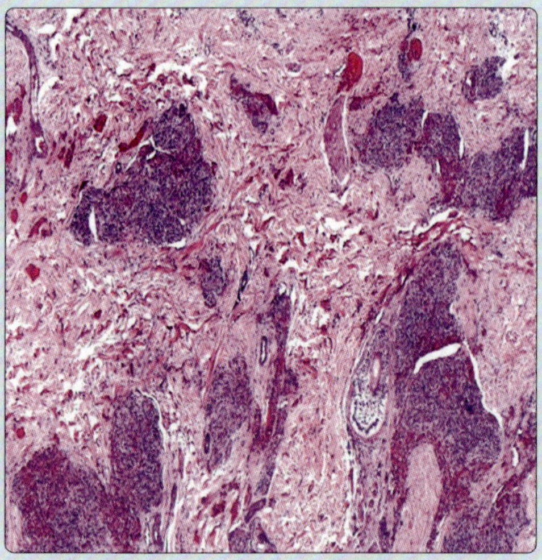

(Left) *Acquired tufted angioma (ATA) is a benign vascular proliferation that usually arises in the dermis. At low magnification, ATA shows a diffuse, lobular, dermal proliferation of blood vessels.* **(Right)** *Intermediate-magnification view of ATA shows a diffuse, dermal proliferation of small, lobular or nested clusters of blood vessels. A cannonball-like appearance, as depicted, is typical.*

Collapsed, Slit-Like Lumina

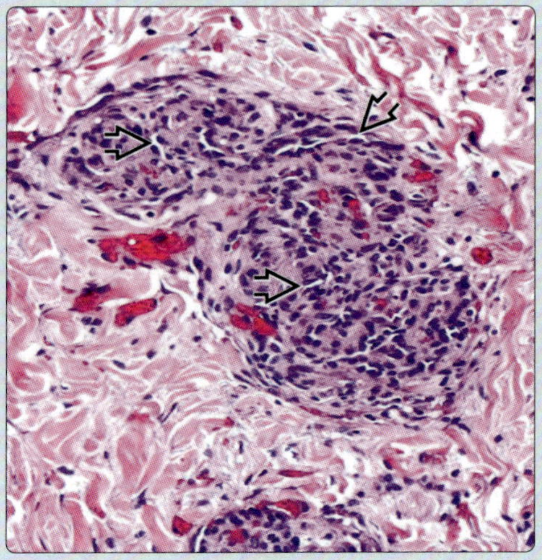

Bland Cytologic Features

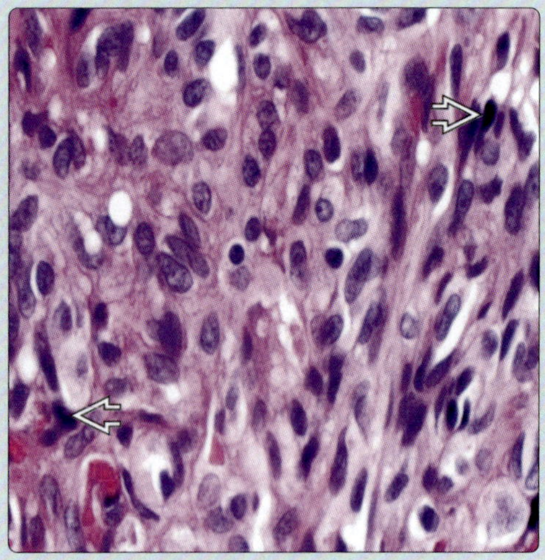

(Left) *Higher magnification shows a lobular cluster of blood vessels lined by small, oval to spindle-shaped cells. Lumina are collapsed and slit-like ⇨.* **(Right)** *High-power view shows bland cytologic features of the tufted angioma endothelial cells. Some of the cells show mild nuclear hyperchromasia ➡, but no significant cytologic atypia is identified.*

Acquired Tufted Angioma

TERMINOLOGY

Abbreviations

- Acquired tufted angioma (ATA)

Synonyms

- Tufted angioma, angioblastoma (of Nakagawa)

Definitions

- Multiple scattered, cannonball-like, cellular collections of small vessels in dermis

ETIOLOGY/PATHOGENESIS

Unknown

- Most cases sporadic; rare familial cases described
- Some cases associated with pregnancy or liver transplantation

CLINICAL ISSUES

Epidemiology

- Incidence
  - Rare tumors
- Age
  - Children and young adults

Site

- Neck, shoulders, and upper trunk most common

Presentation

- Slow growing; erythematous macules and plaques

Prognosis

- Excellent; completely benign behavior
- May be associated with Kasabach-Merritt syndrome (consumptive coagulopathy)

MACROSCOPIC

General Features

- Reddish brown, nonencapsulated, dermal lesion

Size

- Typically small papules but may be large plaque

MICROSCOPIC

Histologic Features

- Multiple scattered, lobular collections of small, capillary-type vessels throughout dermis
  - Typical cannonball-like appearance at low magnification
  - Collections are larger in middle and lower dermis
  - Cleft-like lumina often present around capillary tufts; may impart glomerular appearance
  - Capillaries may be so closely packed that lumina may be inconspicuous
  - Cells are oval to spindle-shaped
  - May show nuclear hyperchromasia but lack significant cytologic atypia or pleomorphism
  - A few mitoses may be present
- Hemosiderin deposition may be seen
- Inflammation typically not present
- Subcutaneous tissue usually not involved

DIFFERENTIAL DIAGNOSIS

Lobular Capillary Hemangioma

- Shows exophytic appearance and epidermal collarette, often ulcerated and acutely inflamed
- Proliferation of small, capillary-type blood vessels typically arranged in a few larger, nodular collections rather than multiple smaller, dispersed collections seen in ATA

Glomeruloid Hemangioma

- Usually associated with Castleman disease or POEMS syndrome (**p**olyneuropathy, **o**rganomegaly, **e**ndocrinopathy, **M**-protein, **s**kin changes)
- Smaller, capillary-like collections inside vascular spaces with clefts around them
- PAS(+) cytoplasmic globules (immunoglobulin aggregates)

Infantile (Juvenile) Hemangioma

- Cellular, dermal nodules composed of lobular collections of oval endothelial cells
- Vascular lumina often small and slit-like, become larger, later stage lesions
- GLUT1(+)

Kaposiform Hemangioendothelioma

- May exist on clinical and morphologic spectrum with ATA
  - Similar or identical histologic features to ATA; very similar demographics & clinical features between both entities
    - However, kaposiform hemangioendothelioma often larger than ATA and may be deeply located

Kaposi Sarcoma

- Proliferation of interlacing bundles of spindle cells forming slit-like, vascular spaces
- Cytoplasmic hyalinized globules, plasma cells, and hemosiderin deposits typically present
- HHV8(+) by immunohistochemistry

DIAGNOSTIC CHECKLIST

Pathologic Interpretation Pearls

- Multiple scattered, cannonball-like, lobular collections of small-capillary-type vessels throughout dermis

SELECTED REFERENCES

1. Marušić Z et al: Histopathology of spindle cell vascular tumors. Surg Pathol Clin. 10(2):345-66, 2017
2. Croteau SE et al: The clinical spectrum of kaposiform hemangioendothelioma and tufted angioma. Semin Cutan Med Surg. 35(3):147-52, 2016
3. Pesapane F et al: A case of acquired tufted angioma in adulthood. An Bras Dermatol. 90(3 Suppl 1):16-8, 2015
4. Omori M et al: Acquired tufted angioma in pregnancy showing expression of estrogen and progesterone receptors. Eur J Dermatol. 23(6):898-9, 2013
5. Arai E et al: Usefulness of D2-40 immunohistochemistry for differentiation between kaposiform hemangioendothelioma and tufted angioma. J Cutan Pathol. 33(7):492-7, 2006
6. Igarashi M et al: The relationship between angioblastoma (Nakagawa) and tufted angioma: report of four cases with angioblastoma and a literature-based comparison of the two conditions. J Dermatol. 27(8):537-42, 2000
7. Kleinegger CL et al: Acquired tufted angioma: a unique vascular lesion not previously reported in the oral mucosa. Br J Dermatol. 142(4):794-9, 2000

Microvenular Hemangioma

KEY FACTS

TERMINOLOGY

- Synonym: Microcapillary angioma
- Definition: Slow-growing, benign vascular proliferation composed of small, collapsed vessels

ETIOLOGY/PATHOGENESIS

- Some cases reportedly related to pregnancy or contraceptives

CLINICAL ISSUES

- Young to middle-aged adults
- Typically occurs on upper extremities, especially forearms
- Slow-growing papule or nodule
  - Often present only several weeks to months at presentation
- Simple excision is curative but not necessary
- Benign; excellent prognosis

MICROSCOPIC

- Poorly circumscribed dermal proliferation of small blood vessels that diffusely involve reticular dermis
  - Branching vessels typically present
  - Most vessels show narrow or collapsed lumina
- Endothelial cells may be slightly enlarged but lack significant cytologic atypia
- Tufted groups of vessels may be seen in deep dermis
- Background of mild dermal sclerosis
- Inflammation and hemosiderin deposition typically lacking

TOP DIFFERENTIAL DIAGNOSES

- Kaposi sarcoma
- Stasis changes/stasis dermatitis
- Hobnail hemangioma (targetoid hemosiderotic hemangioma)
- Early scar

Microvenular Hemangioma

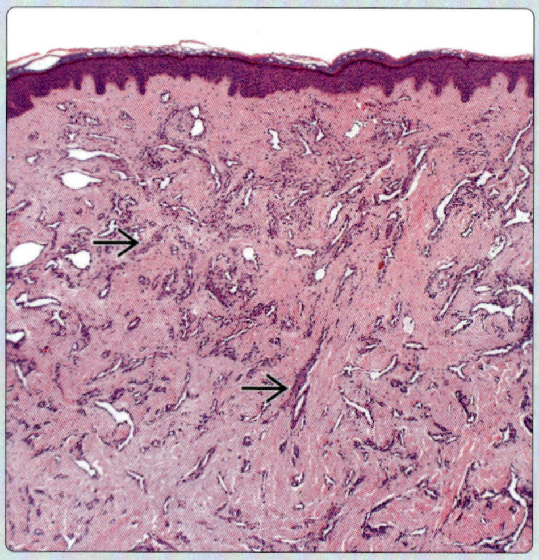

Branching and Narrow Lumina

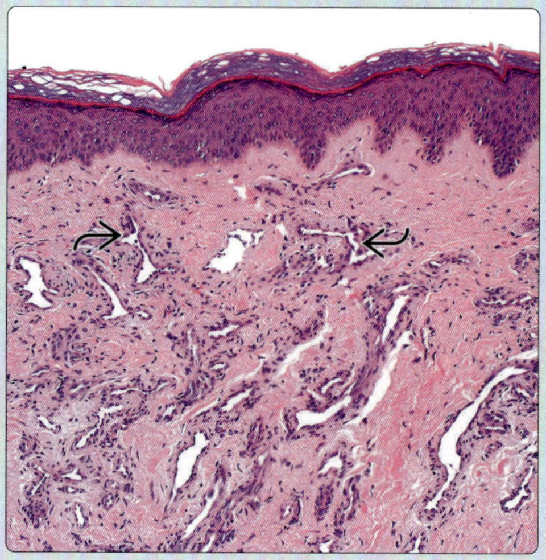

(Left) *Scanning magnification shows a diffuse dermal proliferation of small, elongated blood vessels with narrow to collapsed lumina and a background of dermal sclerosis.* **(Right)** *Higher magnification shows increased numbers of small blood vessels in the superficial dermis with irregular branching and narrow lumina.*

Sclerotic Stroma

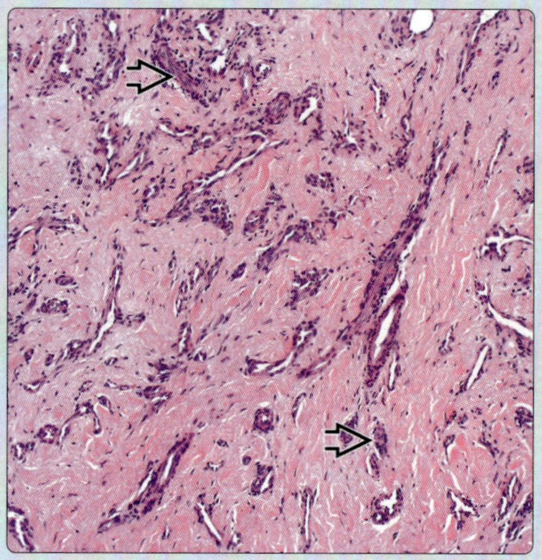

Bland Cytologic Features

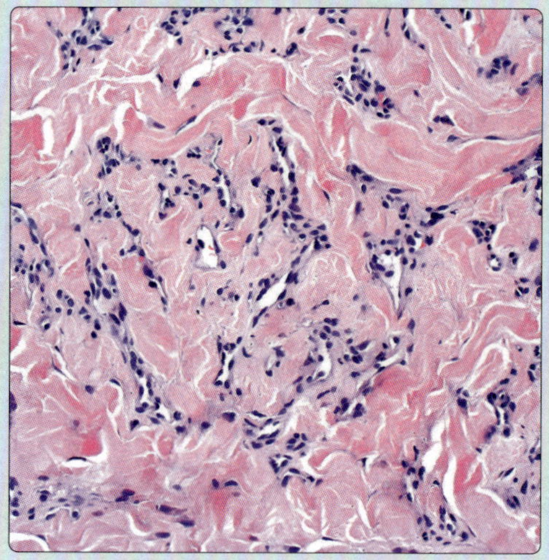

(Left) *Higher magnification of microvenular hemangioma shows a proliferation of small blood vessels with thin walls and small to collapsed lumina associated with a sclerotic stroma.* **(Right)** *High-power examination of microvenular hemangioma shows bland cytologic features of the endothelial cells with small, hyperchromatic-staining nuclei. No evidence of mitotic activity or necrosis are identified.*

Microvenular Hemangioma

TERMINOLOGY

Abbreviations

- Microvenular hemangioma (MVH)

Synonyms

- Microcapillary angioma

Definitions

- Slow-growing, benign vascular proliferation composed of small, collapsed vessels

ETIOLOGY/PATHOGENESIS

Unknown

- In most cases

Hormonal Influence

- Some cases reportedly related to pregnancy or contraceptives

CLINICAL ISSUES

Epidemiology

- Age
  - Young to middle-aged adults
- Sex
  - Occurs in both male and female patients about equally

Site

- Typically occurs on upper extremities, especially forearms

Presentation

- Slow-growing papule or nodule

Natural History

- Often present for only several weeks to months at presentation

Treatment

- Simple excision is curative but not necessary, as these are benign lesions

Prognosis

- Excellent

MACROSCOPIC

Size

- Small, typically < 1 cm

MICROSCOPIC

Histologic Features

- Poorly circumscribed dermal proliferation of small blood vessels that diffusely involve reticular dermis
  - Branching vessels typically present
  - Most vessels show narrow or collapsed lumina
    - Several erythrocytes may be present with lumina
  - Endothelial cells may be slightly enlarged, but they show bland nuclei without significant atypia or pleomorphism
  - Some cases may show large epithelioid cells resembling those seen in epithelioid (histiocytoid) hemangiomas
- Tufted groups of vessels may be seen in deep dermis
- Background of mild dermal sclerosis
- Inflammation and hemosiderin deposition typically lacking

ANCILLARY TESTS

Immunohistochemistry

- HHV8 and D2-40 (podoplanin) (-)

DIFFERENTIAL DIAGNOSIS

Kaposi Sarcoma

- Usually shows infiltrative, thin-walled vessels
- Irregular anastomosing spaces lined by atypical spindle cells
- Plasma cells and hyaline globules are seen (lacking in MVH)
- HHV-8(+) by immunohistochemistry

Targetoid Hemosiderotic Hemangioma (Hobnail Hemangioma)

- While deeper small vessels are similar to those in MVH, superficial vessels are larger and dilated
- Hobnailed endothelial cells project into vascular lumina
- Hemosiderin deposition is typically very prominent

Stasis Changes/Stasis Dermatitis

- Superficial proliferation of clustered small, thick-walled blood vessels
- Usually shows hemosiderin deposition throughout dermis (lacking in MVH)
- Often shows more inflammation and overlying spongiosis (stasis dermatitis)
- Clinical presentation distinctive: Lower extremities of elderly adults

Early Scar

- Angiogenesis in early scars may mimic MVH
- Typically greater fibrosis, inflammation, extravasated red blood cells, and hemosiderin deposition in scars

DIAGNOSTIC CHECKLIST

Pathologic Interpretation Pearls

- Benign vascular proliferation composed of small, collapsed vessels
- Branching vessels typically present
- Endothelial cells may be enlarged but lack cytologic atypia
- Background of mild dermal sclerosis

SELECTED REFERENCES

1. Giacaman A et al: Microvenular hemangioma: morphological study of 3 cases. Actas Dermosifiliogr. 109(4):381-4, 2018
2. Juan YC et al: A microvenular hemangioma with a rare expression of progesterone receptor immunocreativity and a review of the literature. J Cutan Pathol. 45(11):847-50, 2018
3. Mansur AT et al: An unusual lesion on the nose: microvenular hemangioma. Dermatol Pract Concept. 8(1):7-11, 2018
4. Napekoski KM et al: Microvenular hemangioma: a clinicopathologic review of 13 cases. J Cutan Pathol. 41(11):816-22, 2014
5. Linos K et al: Microvenular hemangioma presenting with numerous bilateral macules, patches, and plaques: a case report and review of the literature. Am J Dermatopathol. 35(1):98-101, 2013
6. Chang SE et al: Microvenular hemangioma in a boy with acute myelogenous leukemia. Pediatr Dermatol. 20(3):266-7, 2003
7. Kim YC et al: Microvenular hemangioma. Dermatology. 206(2):161-4, 2003
8. Rikihisa W et al: Microvenular haemangioma in a patient with Wiskott-Aldrich syndrome. Br J Dermatol. 141(4):752-4, 1999
9. Hunt SJ et al: Acquired benign and "borderline" vascular lesions. Dermatol Clin. 10(1):97-115, 1992
10. Hunt SJ et al: Microvenular hemangioma. J Cutan Pathol. 18(4):235-40, 1991

Sinusoidal Hemangioma

KEY FACTS

TERMINOLOGY

- Acquired vascular lesion in adults with features similar to venous malformation (cavernous hemangioma)

ETIOLOGY/PATHOGENESIS

- May represent reactive vascular proliferation rather than true neoplastic process

CLINICAL ISSUES

- Typically occurs in adult female patients
- Painless bluish or red nodule
- Often occurs on extremities, trunk, or breast
- Complete excision is curative but not necessary given benign nature of lesions
- Excellent prognosis, no malignant potential

MACROSCOPIC

- Typically < 2 cm

MICROSCOPIC

- Well-circumscribed vascular proliferation
- Vessels are thin-walled and closely packed with little intervening stroma
- Lining cells are small endothelial cells with nuclear hyperchromasia
- Pseudopapillary pattern may be seen (due to tangential sectioning)
- Some cases may show smooth muscle in vessel walls
- Thrombosis may occur and be associated with Masson tumor/change

TOP DIFFERENTIAL DIAGNOSES

- Venous malformation (cavernous hemangioma)
- Cherry angioma
- Arteriovenous hemangioma (malformation)
- Glomeruloid hemangioma

(Left) *Histologic section shows the superficial portion of a cutaneous sinusoidal hemangioma with large, dilated vascular spaces.* **(Right)** *High-magnification examination of sinusoidal hemangioma demonstrates the cytologic features of the endothelial cells, which show small, uniform nuclei with hyperchromasia ➙ and inconspicuous nucleoli.*

Sinusoidal Hemangioma

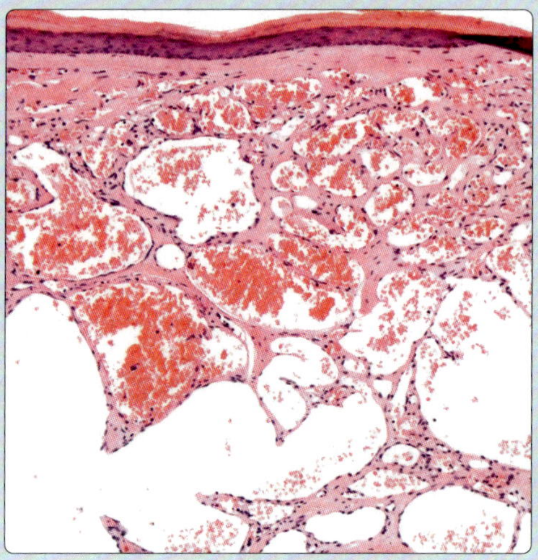

Cytologic Features

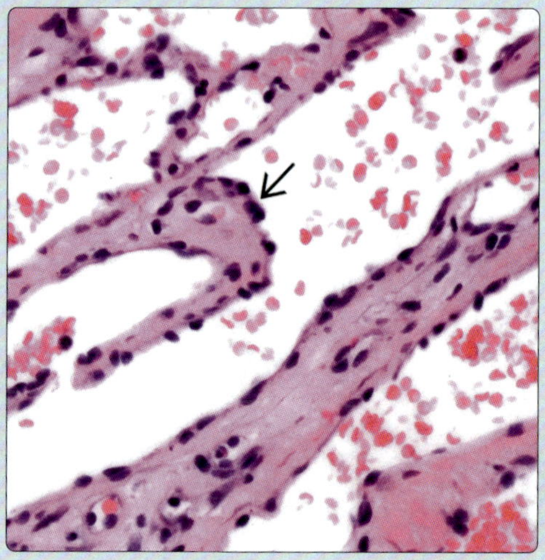

(Left) *High magnification shows sinusoidal vascular spaces with thrombosis ➙, a finding often seen in sinusoidal hemangioma.* **(Right)** *Another example of a sinusoidal hemangioma shows hemorrhage, thrombosis ➙, and intravascular papillary endothelial hyperplasia (a.k.a. Masson tumor or change).*

Thrombosis

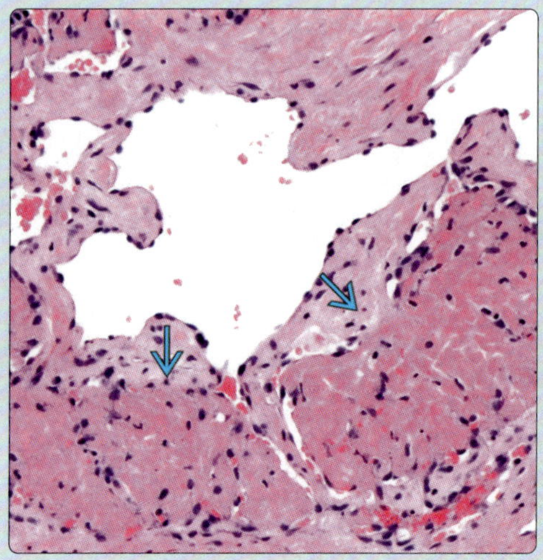

Masson Change

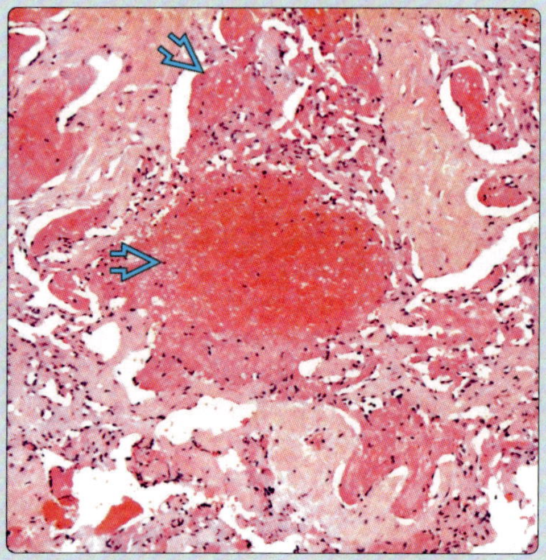

Sinusoidal Hemangioma

TERMINOLOGY

Abbreviations

- Sinusoidal hemangioma (SH)

Synonyms

- Cavernous hemangioma (variant of)

Definitions

- Acquired vascular lesion in adults; features similar to cavernous hemangioma/venous malformation

ETIOLOGY/PATHOGENESIS

Unknown

- May represent reactive vascular proliferation rather than true neoplastic process

CLINICAL ISSUES

Epidemiology

- Incidence
  - Rare
- Age
  - Typically occurs in adults
- Sex
  - More common in female patients

Site

- Often occurs on extremities, trunk, or breast

Presentation

- Subcutaneous or dermal mass
  - Solitary, painless, bluish (deep) or red (superficial) nodule
    - Freely movable

Treatment

- Complete excision is curative but not necessary given benign nature of lesions

Prognosis

- Excellent, no malignant potential

MACROSCOPIC

Size

- Typically < 2 cm

MICROSCOPIC

Histologic Features

- Proliferation of numerous thin-walled, anastomosing vessels
  - Well-circumscribed proliferation of vessels in sinusoidal pattern
  - Vessels are thin walled and closely packed with little intervening stroma
    - Occasional cases may show smooth muscle in vessel walls
    - Pseudopapillary pattern may be seen (due to tangential sectioning)
    - Thrombosis may occur and be associated with intravascular papillary endothelial hyperplasia (Masson tumor)
  - Lining cells are small endothelial cells with nuclear hyperchromasia
  - Mitotic figures typically not seen
  - Calcifications may rarely be present

Cytologic Features

- Nuclei are hyperchromatic but show regular borders and uniform chromatin

DIFFERENTIAL DIAGNOSIS

Venous Malformation (Cavernous Hemangioma)

- Typically occurs in children
- Often larger and more poorly circumscribed than SH
- No ramified pattern and less tightly packed vessels

Cherry Angioma

- Very common small papular lesions occurring in adults
- Superficial papillary dermal lesions, as opposed to SH (which is typically deep dermal or subcutaneous)

Arteriovenous Hemangioma (Malformation)

- Typically occurs on lips, perioral skin, or nose of young adults
- Proliferation of large, thick-walled blood vessels with smooth muscle in their walls, which mostly represent veins
- Feeder vessel (ascending muscular artery) may be present in some cases

Glomeruloid Hemangioma

- Associated with Castleman syndrome and **p**olyneuropathy, **o**rganomegaly, **e**ndocrinopathy, **m**onoclonal paraproteinemia, and **s**kin lesions (POEMS) syndrome
- Typically presents as multiple eruptive lesions on trunk and limbs
- Dilated vascular spaces filled by grape-like clusters of capillaries, reminiscent of renal glomeruli

DIAGNOSTIC CHECKLIST

Pathologic Interpretation Pearls

- Closely packed lobular proliferation of vessels in deep dermis or subcutis

SELECTED REFERENCES

1. Díaz-Flores L et al: Sinusoidal hemangioma and intravascular papillary endothelial hyperplasia: interrelated processes that share a histogenetic piecemeal angiogenic mechanism. Acta Histochem. 120(3):255-62, 2018
2. Salemis NS: Sinusoidal hemangioma of the breast: diagnostic evaluation management and literature review. Gland Surg. 6(1):105-9, 2017
3. Konda P et al: Intramuscular sinusoidal haemangioma with secondary Masson's phenomenon. BMJ Case Rep. 2016, 2016
4. Halawar SS et al: Intramuscular sinusoidal hemangioma with Masson's lesion. J Oral Maxillofac Pathol. 17(2):315-7, 2013
5. Ban M et al: Giant sinusoidal hemangioma revealing diffuse ancient change: hyalinization and organized thrombi. Int J Dermatol. 49(5):589-90, 2010
6. Nakamura M et al: Calcifying sinusoidal haemangioma on the back. Br J Dermatol. 141(2):377-8, 1999
7. Ruck P et al: Diffuse sinusoidal hemangiomatosis of the spleen. A case report with enzyme-histochemical, immunohistochemical, and electron-microscopic findings. Pathol Res Pract. 190(7):708-14; discussion 715-7, 1994
8. Calonje E et al: New entities in cutaneous soft tissue tumours. Pathologica. 85(1095):1-15, 1993
9. Calonje E et al: Sinusoidal hemangioma. A distinctive benign vascular neoplasm within the group of cavernous hemangiomas. Am J Surg Pathol. 15(12):1130-5, 1991

Glomeruloid Hemangioma

KEY FACTS

TERMINOLOGY

- Benign proliferation of small vessels mimicking renal glomeruli
- Synonym: Glomeruloid angioma

ETIOLOGY/PATHOGENESIS

- Association with **p**olyneuropathy, **o**rganomegaly, **e**ndocrinopathy, **M**-protein, **s**kin changes (POEMS) or multicentric Castleman syndrome in most cases
- Rare cases not associated with POEMS syndrome

CLINICAL ISSUES

- More common in Asian (especially Japanese) patients
- More common in female patients
- Typically presents as multiple red to purple eruptive papules (POEMS syndrome)
  - Single lesions may occur in patients without POEMS
- Excellent prognosis, no malignant potential

MICROSCOPIC

- Vessels show distinctive grape-like clusters mimicking renal glomeruli
- Endothelial cells are mildly enlarged, and many show cytoplasmic eosinophilic globules
  - Cytoplasmic globules represent secondary lysosomes containing immunoglobulins
- Few mitoses; no necrosis or infiltrative features

ANCILLARY TESTS

- PAS(+) cytoplasmic globules

TOP DIFFERENTIAL DIAGNOSES

- Acquired tufted hemangioma
- Lobular capillary hemangioma (pyogenic granuloma)
- Hobnail hemangioma (targetoid hemosiderotic hemangioma)
- Kaposi sarcoma

Glomeruloid Hemangioma

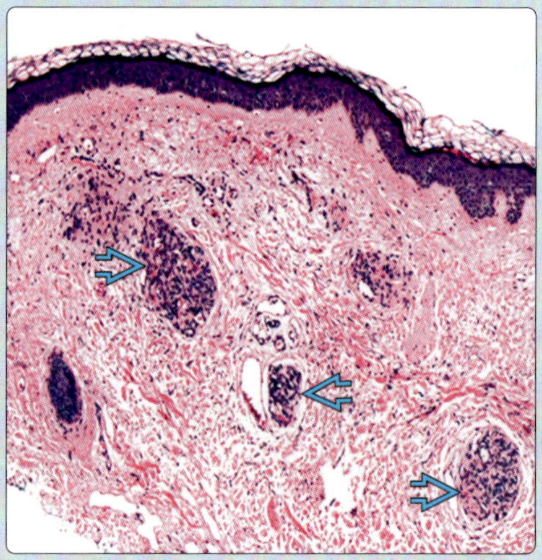

Glomeruloid Vascular Structures

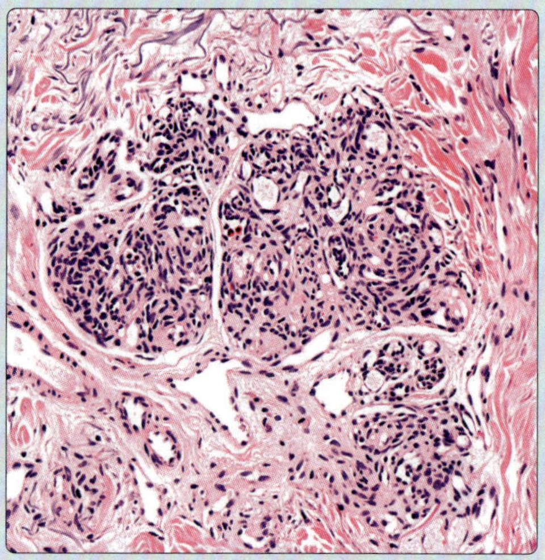

(Left) *Low-power H&E of glomeruloid hemangioma shows a superficial dermal proliferation of small clusters of vessels ⇨ with a glomeruloid pattern.* **(Right)** *The characteristic vasculature of glomeruloid hemangioma features a grape-like pattern of clustered, small vessels mimicking renal glomeruli, as depicted here.*

Glomeruloid Vascular Structures

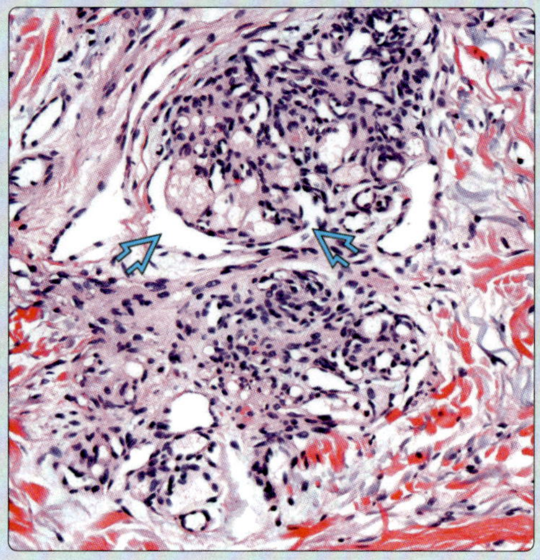

Cytologic Features and Eosinophilic Globules

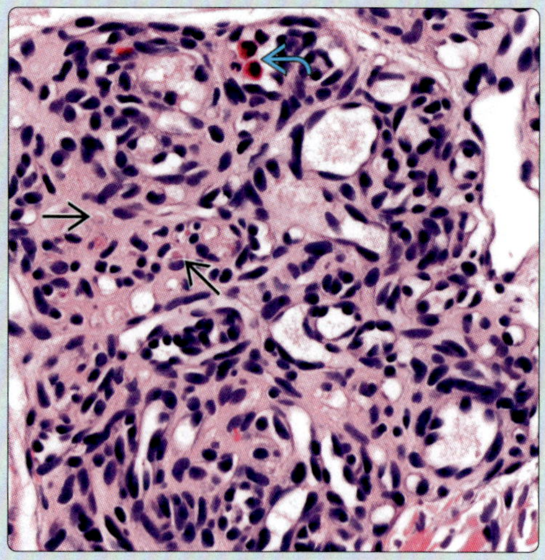

(Left) *High-power H&E of glomeruloid hemangioma shows small, grape-like clusters of vessels projecting into vascular lumina (with peripheral crescentic spaces ⇨).* **(Right)** *The vessels in glomeruloid hemangioma contain endothelial cells with oval- to spindle-shaped nuclei. Cytoplasmic eosinophilic globules (containing immunoglobulins) are present focally →. A few intraluminal eosinophils are also seen ⇨ in this image.*

TERMINOLOGY

Abbreviations

- Glomeruloid hemangioma (GH)

Synonyms

- Glomeruloid angioma

Definitions

- Benign proliferation of small vessels mimicking renal glomeruli

ETIOLOGY/PATHOGENESIS

Paraneoplastic Syndromes

- Association with **p**olyneuropathy, **o**rganomegaly, **e**ndocrinopathy, **M**-protein, **s**kin changes (POEMS syndrome) or multicentric Castleman disease in almost all cases

Unknown

- Rare cases not associated with POEMS syndrome

CLINICAL ISSUES

Epidemiology

- Incidence
  - Rare
- Sex
  - More common in female patients
- Ethnicity
  - More common in Asian (especially Japanese) patients

Site

- Trunk and extremities

Presentation

- Multiple red to purple eruptive papules (POEMS syndrome)
  - Most patients also have diffuse skin hyperpigmentation
- Single lesions reported in patients without POEMS

Treatment

- Surgical excision is curative, but not necessary in most cases
- Treatment of underlying plasma cell disorder may lead to regression of lesions

Prognosis

- Excellent; no malignant potential

MACROSCOPIC

General Features

- Dermal-based, well-circumscribed, unencapsulated lesions

Size

- Small; typically only a few millimeters

MICROSCOPIC

Histologic Features

- Dermal-based proliferation of vascular spaces containing small capillary-type vessels
- Vessels show distinctive grape-like clusters projecting into lumina, mimicking renal glomeruli
- Endothelial cells are mildly enlarged, and many show cytoplasmic eosinophilic globules
  - Cytoplasmic globules represent secondary lysosomes containing immunoglobulins
- Endothelial cells may show nuclear hyperchromasia but do not show significant cytologic atypia
- Few mitoses, no necrosis or infiltrative features

ANCILLARY TESTS

Histochemistry

- PAS(+) cytoplasmic globules

DIFFERENTIAL DIAGNOSIS

Acquired Tufted Hemangioma (Angioblastoma)

- Slowly spreading macules and plaques in young children and adults
- Multiple dermal and subcutaneous vascular lobules composed of spindled and polygonal-shaped cells
- Some cases may show overlapping features with GH

Lobular Capillary Hemangioma (Pyogenic Granuloma)

- Often shows polypoid configuration with epidermal collarette
- Lobular proliferation typically associated with ulceration, edema, and acute inflammation

Targetoid Hemosiderotic Hemangioma (Hobnail Hemangioma)

- Superficial dilated vessels and smaller, narrow, deeper vessels lined by plump (hobnailed) cells
- Extravasated red blood cells and prominent stromal hemosiderin deposition

Kaposi Sarcoma

- Clinical history distinctive
  - HIV positive with multiple lesions, or lower extremity lesion in elderly Mediterranean male
- Cords or fascicles of spindled cells with slit-like lumina associated with hemosiderin deposition and plasma cells
- HHV8(+)
  - Not reported in GH

DIAGNOSTIC CHECKLIST

Pathologic Interpretation Pearls

- Dermal proliferation of vessels showing distinctive glomeruloid morphology

SELECTED REFERENCES

1. Shinozaki-Ushiku A et al: Glomeruloid hemangioma associated with TAFRO syndrome. Hum Pathol. ePub, 2018
2. Gali VL et al: Cutaneous glomeruloid hemangioma: a report on two cases and a review of literature. S D Med. 70(6):250-1, 2017
3. Lee JY et al: Glomeruloid hemangioma as a marker for the early diagnosis of POEMS syndrome. Ann Dermatol. 29(2):249-51, 2017
4. Jacobson-Dunlop E et al: Glomeruloid hemangiomas in the absence of POEMS syndrome. J Cutan Pathol. 39(4):402-3, 2012
5. Rongioletti F et al: Glomeruloid hemangioma. A cutaneous marker of POEMS syndrome. Am J Dermatopathol. 16(2):175-8, 1994
6. Chan JK et al: Glomeruloid hemangioma. A distinctive cutaneous lesion of multicentric Castleman's disease associated with POEMS syndrome. Am J Surg Pathol. 14(11):1036-46, 1990

Angiomatosis

KEY FACTS

TERMINOLOGY

- Definition: Diffuse, benign, vascular lesion of soft tissue affecting large segments of body or multiple tissue planes in contiguous fashion

ETIOLOGY/PATHOGENESIS

- Likely represents congenital vascular malformation

CLINICAL ISSUES

- Most present in early childhood
- Lower extremities (> 50%)
- Treatment: Conservative but complete excision
- Benign lesion with frequent recurrences and persistent disease

MACROSCOPIC

- Predominant fatty appearance
- Wide size range (3-26 cm)

MICROSCOPIC

- 2 common patterns
    - Haphazard arrangement of venous-, cavernous-, and capillary-sized vessels
    - Infiltrating nodules of capillary vessels
- May involve multiple tissue planes (vertical involvement)
    - Dermis, subcutis, muscle, and bone
    - May also involve only single tissue type
- Lacks distinct lobular pattern
- Osseous involvement can occur

ANCILLARY TESTS

- GLUT1(-)

TOP DIFFERENTIAL DIAGNOSES

- Glomangiomatosis
- Infantile hemangioma
- Intramuscular hemangioma

(Left) *This example of angiomatosis shows a diffuse vascular proliferation involving the papillary and reticular dermis → and extending down into the subcutaneous adipose tissue →. In some cases, involvement of muscle and bone may also be seen.* **(Right)** *A large cavernous vessel with an irregular wall → is surrounded by numerous small to medium-sized capillaries →.*

Angiomatosis

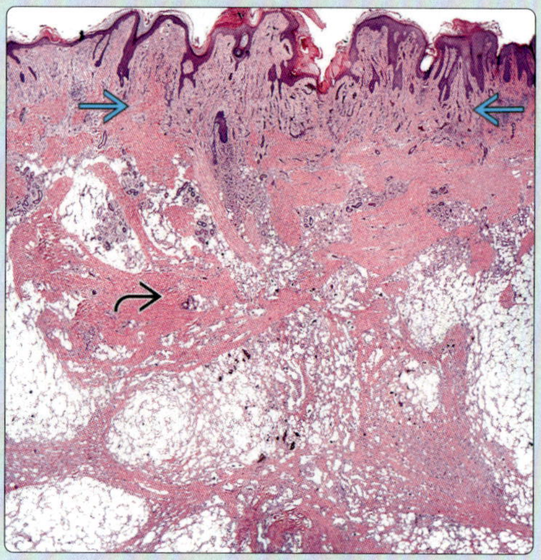

Capillary Vascular Pattern

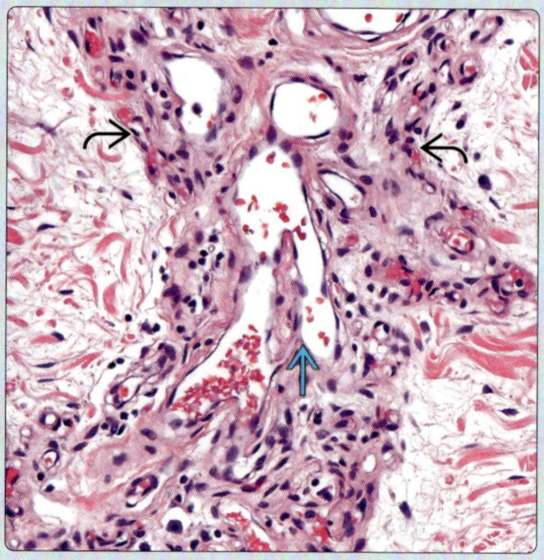

(Left) *Numerous small and dilated capillaries → are shown infiltrating the fibrous connective tissue and extending down into the adjacent adipose tissue.* **(Right)** *Scattered vessels of varying size and wall thickness are seen within the fibrous connective tissue and lobules of mature adipose tissue, consisting of muscular venous- →, cavernous- →, and capillary-type vessels →.*

Infiltrating Capillary Hemangioma Pattern

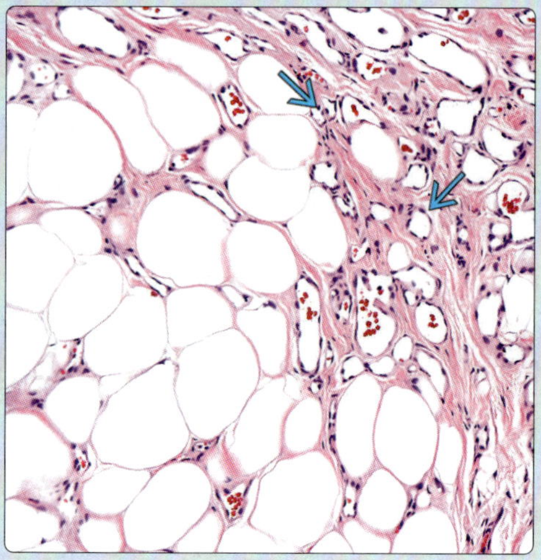

Various Vessel Types

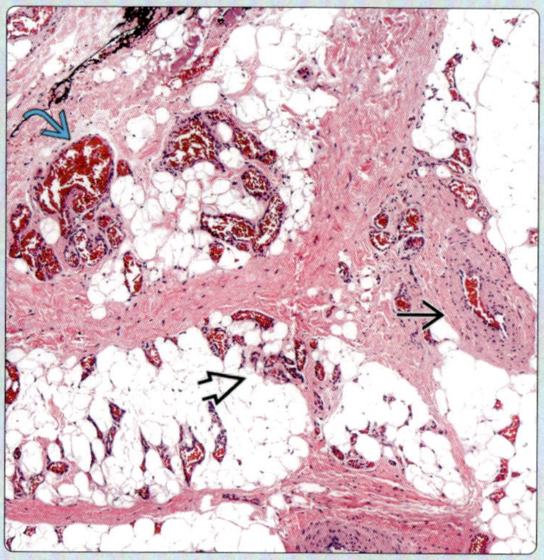

TERMINOLOGY

Synonyms

- Diffuse hemangioma, vascular malformation, infiltrating angiolipoma

Definitions

- Diffuse, benign, vascular lesion of soft tissue affecting large segments of body or multiple tissue planes in contiguous fashion

ETIOLOGY/PATHOGENESIS

Developmental Anomaly

- Benign congenital/developmental vascular malformation
  - Thought to arise in early intrauterine life during limb bud formation
  - Disease associations: Von Hippel Lindau, Klippel-Trénaunay-Weber, and Sturge-Weber syndromes

CLINICAL ISSUES

Epidemiology

- Age
  - Most present in early childhood
  - 2/3 develop by 2nd decade of life
- Sex
  - Females affected slightly more than males

Site

- Lower extremities (> 50%)
- Chest wall, abdomen, and upper extremities

Presentation

- Diffuse and persistent swelling; worsened by strenuous exercise
- Pain and discoloration

Treatment

- Conservative but complete excision

Prognosis

- Benign lesion with frequent recurrences and persistent disease
  - Majority will develop recurrences (60-90%)
  - Multiple recurrences (40%)
- Prognosis depends on size and location
  - Death may occur due to complications of renal or brain involvement
  - Blindness
- Metastases or malignant transformation not reported

IMAGING

CT Findings

- Ill-defined, nonhomogeneous mass
- Serpiginous densities within low-density areas corresponding to tortuous vessels

MACROSCOPIC

General Features

- Ill-defined mass

Size

- 3-26 cm

Gross Features

- Variable coloration
- Most have predominantly fatty appearance

MICROSCOPIC

Microscopic Features

- 2 common patterns
  - Haphazard arrangement of venous-, cavernous-, and capillary-sized vessels
    - Most common and most characteristic pattern
    - Irregular and thick to attenuated walls with herniations and intimal redundancies
    - Clusters of capillary vessels within or adjacent to vein walls
    - Large amounts of mature adipose tissue
  - Infiltrating nodules of capillary vessels
    - Nodules infiltrate into soft tissue
    - Large amounts of mature adipose tissue
    - Previously referred to as infiltrating angiolipoma
- May involve multiple tissue planes (vertical involvement)
  - Dermis, subcutis, muscle, and bone
- May involve only single tissue type
  - Multiple muscles
- Lacks distinct lobular pattern

ANCILLARY TESTS

Immunohistochemistry

- CD31(+), CD34(+), GLUT1(-)

DIFFERENTIAL DIAGNOSIS

Glomangiomatosis

- Diffusely infiltrating
- Well-formed vessels of varying size surrounded by clusters of glomus cells
- Often accompanied by mature adipose tissue

Infantile Hemangioma

- Distinct lobular pattern
- Lacks extensive involvement
- GLUT1(+)

Intramuscular Hemangioma

- Homogeneous cellular groups of capillary-sized vessels
- Usually lacks mixture of vessel sizes
- May require clinical correlation to make distinction

SELECTED REFERENCES

1. Khan S et al: Angiomatosis: a rare vascular proliferation of head and neck region. J Cutan Aesthet Surg. 8(2):108-10, 2015
2. Rao VK et al: Angiomatosis of soft tissue. An analysis of the histologic features and clinical outcome in 51 cases. Am J Surg Pathol. 16(8):764-71, 1992
3. Howat AJ et al: Angiomatosis: a vascular malformation of infancy and childhood. Report of 17 cases. Pathology. 19(4):377-82, 1987
4. Koblenzer PJ et al: Angiomatosis (hamartomatous hem-lymphangiomatosis). Report of a case with diffuse involvement. Pediatrics. 28:65-76, 1961

Lymphangioma

KEY FACTS

TERMINOLOGY

- Benign proliferation of lymphatic vessels; may be superficial, deep, or diffusely involve organ systems
  - Includes lymphangioma circumscriptum (LAC) (superficial lymphangioma), lymphangiomatosis (systemic angiomatosis), cystic lymphangioma, and deep lymphangioma

ETIOLOGY/PATHOGENESIS

- Most cases considered developmental malformations/hamartomas, **not** true neoplasms
- Associated with trisomies and other genetic syndromes, including Turner (cystic hygroma), Noonan, and Maffucci

CLINICAL ISSUES

- More common in children (6% of benign childhood tumors); present at birth or within first 2 years of life
- Typically presents as large, slow-growing, painless mass (deep lymphangioma) or as multiple small, grouped, superficial vesicular lesions (LAC)
- Excellent prognosis in most cases
- Recurrence rate is high if removal incomplete

MICROSCOPIC

- Variably sized anastomosing vascular spaces lined by small, bland-appearing endothelial cells
  - Endothelial cells are small with uniform, bland-appearing, oval to flattened, hyperchromatic nuclei
- Often contain abundant proteinaceous debris, scattered lymphocytes, and erythrocytes
- Walls show stromal fibrosis (older lesions) and may contain smooth muscle

TOP DIFFERENTIAL DIAGNOSES

- Hemangioma
- Progressive lymphangioma
- Secondary lymphangiectasia
- Atypical vascular proliferation
- Lymphangioma-like Kaposi sarcoma

Lymphangioma

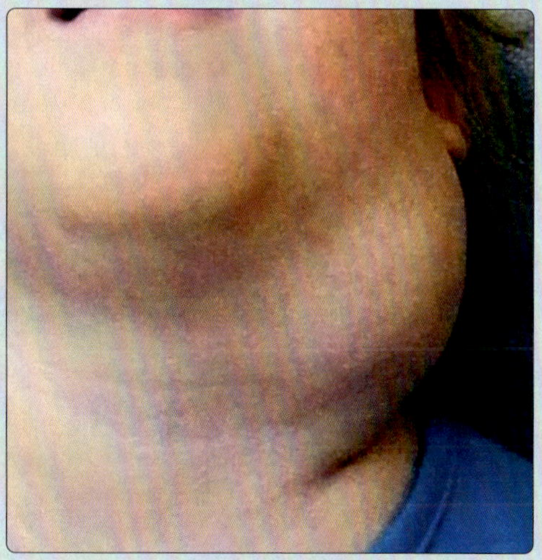

Gross Photograph of Lymphangioma

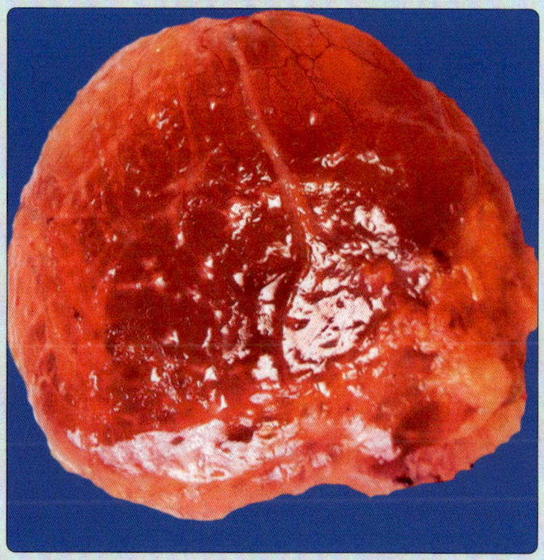

(Left) *Clinical photograph shows a large, deep cystic lymphangioma on the lateral neck of a child. In this location, this lesion is also known as cystic hygroma.* **(Right)** *Macroscopic view of a lymphangioma shows a reddish/brown translucent cystic mass. Small vessels are noted within the lining, and the cyst was filled with clear, watery fluid.*

Lymphangioma at Low Magnification

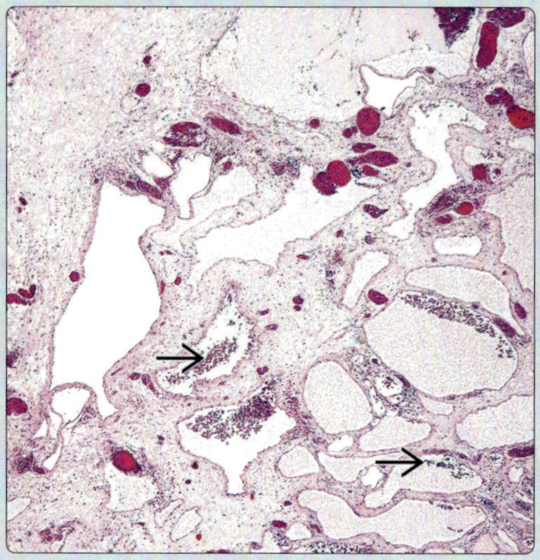

Bland Endothelial Cell Lining

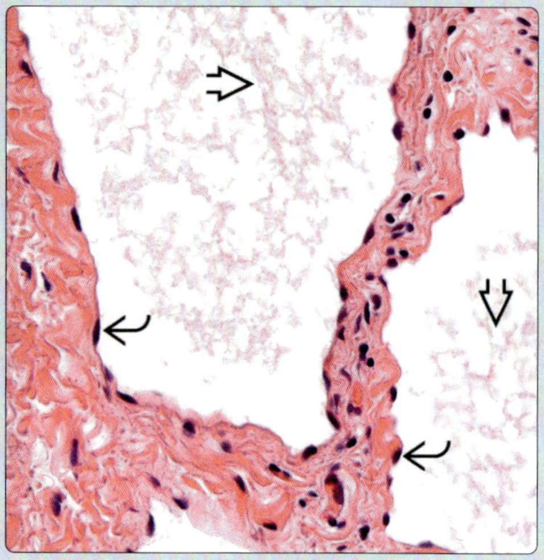

(Left) *Histologic examination of lymphangioma shows multiple dilated, cystic, endothelial-lined channels. There are small collections of lymphocytes → within the lumina along with proteinaceous lymphatic fluid and erythrocytes.* **(Right)** *The spaces of lymphangioma are lined by a thin layer of cytologically bland endothelial cells ↩. Note the granular, eosinophilic proteinaceous material (lymph ⇨) within the lumina.*

Lymphangioma

TERMINOLOGY

Synonyms

- Lymphatic malformation
- Lymphangioma circumscriptum (superficial cutaneous lymphangioma) (LAC)
- Cystic lymphangioma (cystic hygroma)
- Deep lymphangioma (cavernous lymphangioma)
- Lymphangiomatosis (generalized lymphangioma, systemic angiomatosis) (LAS)

Definitions

- Benign proliferation of lymphatic vessels; may be
  - Superficial (LAC)
  - Deep (cavernous lymphangioma)
  - Diffusely involving most organ systems (LAS)

ETIOLOGY/PATHOGENESIS

Developmental Anomaly

- Most cases of lymphangioma considered developmental or congenital malformations/hamartomas, **not** true neoplasms
  - Maldevelopment of embryonic lymphangiogenesis most likely etiology
    - Leads to sequestered lymphatics that fail to communicate with normal lymphovascular system
  - LAS considered congenital in most cases

Genetics

- Associated with genetic syndromes, including Turner syndrome (cystic hygroma), Noonan syndrome, Maffucci syndrome, trisomies 13, 18, 21
- Mutations in *FLT4 (VEGFR-3)*, *PROX1*, *FOXC2*, and *SOX18* genes implicated

Acquired

- Rare acquired cases occur in adults

CLINICAL ISSUES

Epidemiology

- Incidence
  - More common in children: Estimated 6% of benign childhood tumors
- Age
  - Often present at birth or within first 2 years of life (~ 90% of cases)
  - LAS usually presents within first 2 decades of life
- Sex
  - Intraabdominal lymphangiomas have slight male predominance
  - LAS has no sex predilection

Site

- Head and neck most common site for cystic lymphangiomas
  - Usually posterior triangle but can occur in anterior triangle
  - Also occur in axillae, abdomen, and internal organs
- Cavernous type more frequent in oral cavity, upper trunk, limbs, and abdominal sites
  - Intraabdominal lymphangiomas occur in mesentery, omentum, and retroperitoneum
- LAC: Axillary folds, neck, and trunk are most common sites
- LAS: Can affect any organ system but often involves bones, soft tissues, and skin

Presentation

- Cystic mass lesion; may be superficial or deep
  - Typically presents as large, slow-growing, painless mass (deep lymphangioma) or as multiple small, grouped, superficial vesicular lesions (LAC)
  - LAS presents with numerous cystic lesions, both superficial and deep
- Soft and fluctuant swellings on palpation
- Intraabdominal cases may present with abdominal distension, mass on palpation
  - May also develop abdominal obstruction, volvulus, and infarction
- Generalized LAS: Depends on affected site
  - Bone: Pathologic fractures
  - Lungs: Dyspnea, wheezing due to chylothorax, chylous ascites
  - Spleen: Splenomegaly, left upper quadrant pain

Treatment

- Surgical resection may be indicated in large, deep lesions, especially if symptomatic
  - LAS not amenable to surgical excision
- Intralesional injection of sclerosing agents, including bleomycin and OK-432

Prognosis

- Excellent in most cases, although LAS may be fatal if involving mediastinum or internal organs, especially lungs
- Recurrence rate high with incomplete removal
- No malignant transformation reported

IMAGING

Ultrasonographic Findings

- Unilocular or multilocular anechoic mass
- Can be used in utero to detect cystic lymphangioma (associated with hydrops fetalis, Turner syndrome, and high death rate)

CT Findings

- Nonenhancing cystic lesions with homogeneous attenuation
- Visceral and osseous lesions often show contrast enhancement
- May displace surrounding organs

MACROSCOPIC

General Features

- Multiple cystic spaces with clear to whitish fluid

MICROSCOPIC

Histologic Features

- Variably sized anastomosing vascular spaces lined by endothelial cells

- Endothelial cells are small with uniform, bland-appearing, oval to flattened, hyperchromatic nuclei
- Dilated lumina
  - Often contain abundant eosinophilic proteinaceous debris, scattered lymphocytes, and erythrocytes
- Walls show stromal fibrosis (older lesions) and occasional myxoid change
  - Often contain lymphoid infiltrates
    - May show occasional reactive germinal centers
  - Mast cells are common
  - Hemosiderin deposition in stroma may be seen
- Large vessels may contain smooth muscle in their walls
- Cavernous lymphangioma has infiltrative margins and often extends into surrounding tissues

ANCILLARY TESTS

Immunohistochemistry

- Endothelial lining cells show variable positivity with vascular markers CD31, CD34, and FVIIIRAg
- Newer lymphatic markers, including D2-40 (podoplanin), VEGFR-3, and LYVE-1, typically (+)

DIFFERENTIAL DIAGNOSIS

Hemangiomas

- Most cases show smaller vascular spaces with more red blood cells, less proteinaceous material, and fewer lymphocytes
- Often well-circumscribed, noninfiltrative borders

Progressive Lymphangioma

- Form of cutaneous lymphangioma with distinct clinical findings
  - Typically presents on lower extremities of adults as slow-growing patches or plaques
- Histologic findings very similar to other forms of lymphangioma
  - Superficially dilated spaces that become progressively smaller with deep extension

Secondary Lymphangiectasia

- May be due to local factors, such as obstruction (e.g., due to tumor), scarring, or previous radiation therapy
- Identical histologic findings; can only be distinguished by clinical history or other findings (if present)

Atypical Vascular Proliferation

- Radiation induced; most frequent in breast
- Clinically, presents as multiple small vesicles in radiation field
- Irregularly dilated vascular spaces lined by atypical endothelial cells

Lymphangioma-Like Kaposi Sarcoma

- Usually shows at least focal areas of more typical Kaposi sarcoma
  - Infiltrative, slit-like spaces lined by hyperchromatic, spindle-shaped cells
  - Stromal hemosiderin deposition and inflammatory infiltrate containing plasma cells
- HHV8(+) is diagnostic

Angiosarcoma

- Highly atypical vascular proliferation showing irregular, anastomosing vascular spaces
- Poorly circumscribed, infiltrative neoplasm
- Endothelial cells typically show epithelioid or spindle cell features, prominent nuclear enlargement, and atypia with enlarged nucleoli
  - Endothelial multilayering often present
  - Mitotic figures easily identified

DIAGNOSTIC CHECKLIST

Clinically Relevant Pathologic Features

- Margins
  - High recurrence rate with positive margins

Pathologic Interpretation Pearls

- Proliferation of superficial &/or deep dilated vascular spaces lined by bland, oval or flattened endothelial cells

SELECTED REFERENCES

1. Akhavan S et al: Congenital lymphangioma circumscriptum of vulva presenting as multiple giant mass lesions: a case report and literature review. J Obstet Gynaecol Res. 44(5):978-982, 2018
2. Taylor D et al: A supernumerary nipple-like clinical presentation of lymphangioma circumscriptum. Case Rep Dermatol Med. 2018:6925105, 2018
3. Patoulias D et al: Cystic lymphangioma of the chest wall in a 5-year-old male patient: a rare and atypical localization-a case report and comprehensive review of the literature. Case Rep Pediatr. 2017:2083204, 2017
4. Salman A et al: Acquired progressive lymphangioma: case report with partial response to imiquimod 5% cream. Pediatr Dermatol. 34(6):e302-e304, 2017
5. Massa AF et al: Cutaneous Lymphangioma circumscriptum - dermoscopic features. An Bras Dermatol. 90(2):262-4, 2015
6. Oiso N et al: Cutaneous lymphangioma circumscriptum with marked blood presence: histopathologic evaluation of the endothelial cells. Eur J Dermatol. 24(1):127-8, 2014
7. Flucke U et al: Radiation-induced vascular lesions of the skin: an overview. Adv Anat Pathol. 20(6):407-15, 2013
8. Wang L et al: Benign lymphangioendothelioma: a clinical, histopathologic and immunohistochemical analysis of four cases. J Cutan Pathol. 40(11):945-9, 2013
9. Blei F: Lymphangiomatosis: clinical overview. Lymphat Res Biol. 9(4):185-90, 2011
10. Gupta SS et al: Cystic lymphangioma of the breast in an 8-year-old boy: report of a case with a review of the literature. Surg Today. 41(9):1314-8, 2011
11. Ji RC et al: Multiple expressions of lymphatic markers and morphological evolution of newly formed lymphatics in lymphangioma and lymph node lymphangiogenesis. Microvasc Res. 80(2): 195-201, 2010
12. Chen EY et al: Similar histologic features and immunohistochemical staining in microcystic and macrocystic lymphatic malformations. Lymphat Res Biol. 7(2):75-80, 2009
13. Gedikbasi A et al: Multidisciplinary approach in cystic hygroma: prenatal diagnosis, outcome, and postnatal follow up. Pediatr Int. 51(5):670-7, 2009
14. Patel GA et al: Cutaneous lymphangioma circumscriptum: frog spawn on the skin. Int J Dermatol. 48(12):1290-5, 2009
15. Patel GA et al: Zosteriform lymphangioma circumscriptum. Acta Dermatovenerol Alp Panonica Adriat. 18(4):179-82, 2009
16. Richmond B et al: Adult presentation of giant retroperitoneal cystic lymphangioma: case report. Int J Surg. 7(6):559-60, 2009
17. Edwards JR et al: Lymphatics and bone. Hum Pathol. 39(1):49-55, 2008
18. François M et al: Sox18 induces development of the lymphatic vasculature in mice. Nature. 456(7222):643-7, 2008
19. Santo S et al: Prenatal ultrasonographic diagnosis of abdominal cystic lymphangioma: a case report. J Matern Fetal Neonatal Med. 21(8):565-6, 2008
20. Norgall S et al: Elevated expression of VEGFR-3 in lymphatic endothelial cells from lymphangiomas. BMC Cancer. 7:105, 2007
21. Wilting J et al: The transcription factor Prox1 is a marker for lymphatic endothelial cells in normal and diseased human tissues. FASEB J. 16(10):1271-3, 2002

Dilated Lymphatic Spaces

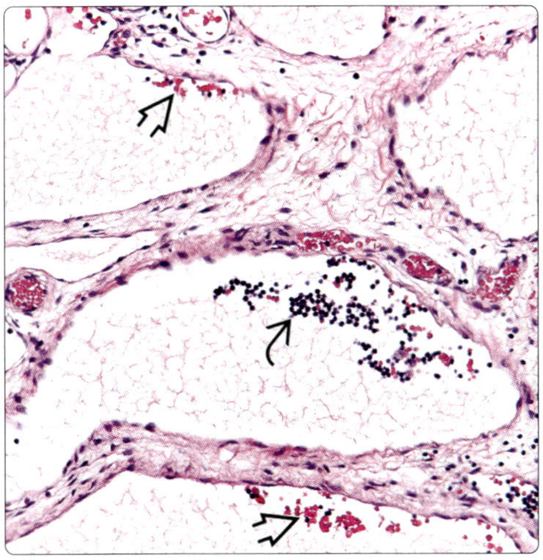

Lymphoid Aggregates in Lymphangioma

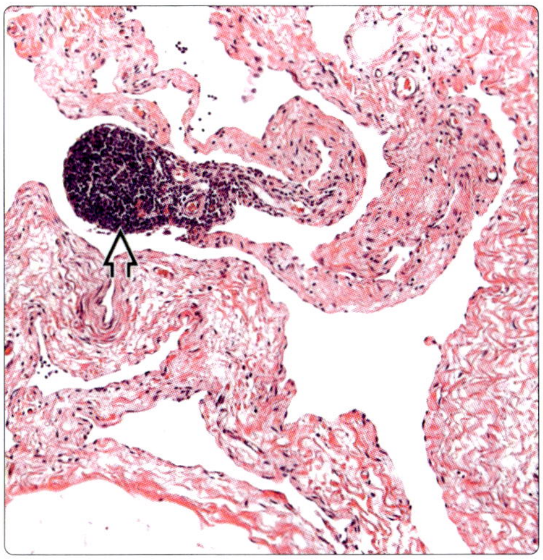

(Left) *Deep lymphangioma shows large vascular channels filled with proteinaceous material, a few lymphocytes* ↗*, and scattered erythrocytes* ⇨*.* **(Right)** *Lymphocytes* ⇨ *may be seen not only within the dilated spaces of lymphangioma but also within the septa, as depicted in this H&E. In some cases, reactive germinal centers may also be present.*

Intraabdominal Lymphangioma

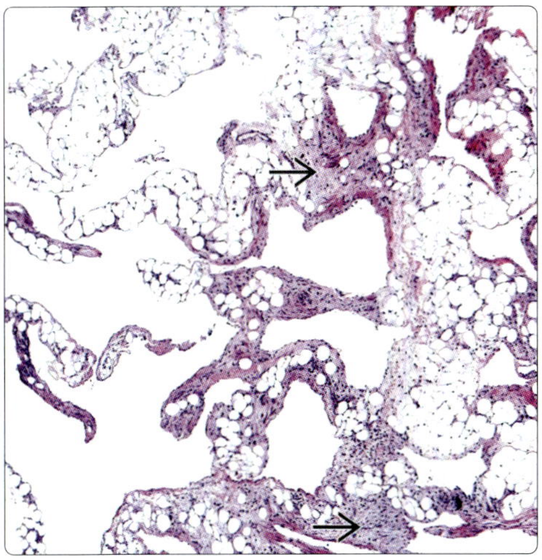

Superficial Lymphangioma

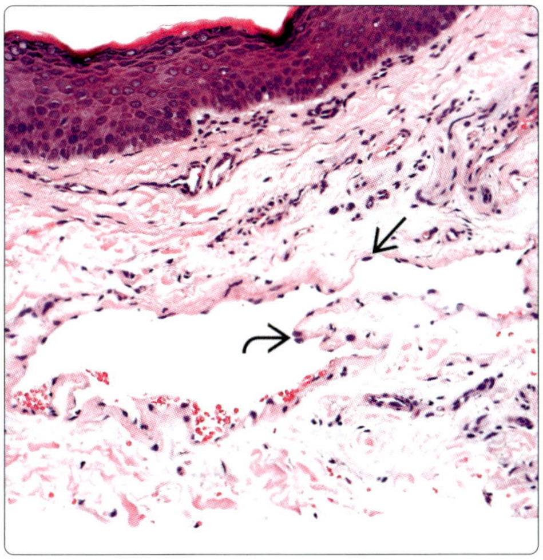

(Left) *Lymphangiomas that arise within the abdominal cavity often contain mature adipose tissue within the septa. Note the numerous cystically dilated lymphatic spaces. Stromal myxoid change* → *can also be appreciated in this H&E.* **(Right)** *Examination of a superficial lymphangioma shows the dilated vascular spaces lined by small, bland endothelial cells with uniform, hyperchromatic-staining, oval* ↗ *to flattened* → *nuclei.*

Superficial Lymphangioma With Papillary Projections

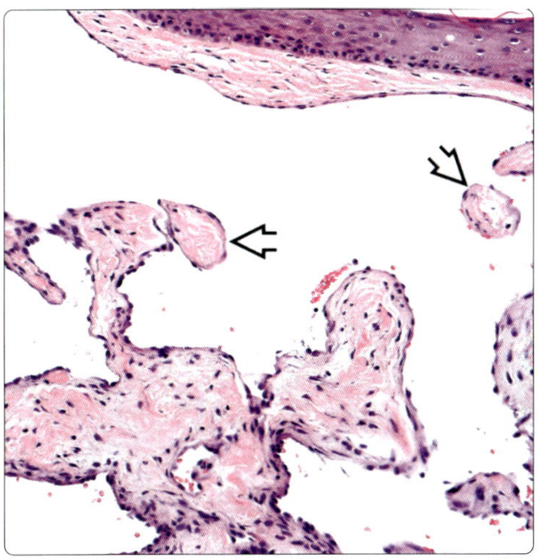

Superficial Lymphangioma With Red Cells

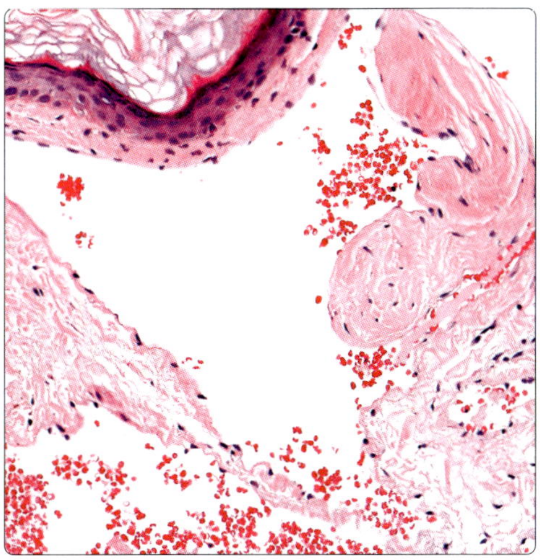

(Left) *Superficial lymphangioma shows widely dilated spaces in the superficial dermis. The lumina show several papillary projections* ⇨ *with slightly fibrinous cores lined by small, hyperchromatic endothelial cells.* **(Right)** *H&E of superficial lymphangioma shows a large, irregularly dilated space lined by thin endothelial cells containing scattered red blood cells in the superficial dermis.*

Massive Localized Lymphedema

KEY FACTS

TERMINOLOGY

- Pseudoneoplastic process related to localized lymphatic obstruction

CLINICAL ISSUES

- Seen in morbidly obese patients (> 300 lb)
- Medial thigh is most common site
  - Also lower abdominal wall, scrotum, proximal arm
- Usually middle aged (range: 30-60 years)
- More common in women
- Benign
- Recurrences are common

MACROSCOPIC

- Typically large specimens (> 20 cm)
- Overlying skin has thickened, indurated peau d'orange appearance
- Cut surface shows pronounced connective tissue septa in subcutaneous fat
- May weep serous fluid

MICROSCOPIC

- Overlying skin is often thickened
- Fibrous thickening of dermis with dilated lymphatics surrounded by lymphocytic infiltrate
- Expanded subcutaneous septa between lobules of mature adipose tissue
  - Prominent septal edema
  - Preserved lobular architecture of subcutaneous fat
- Reactive capillary vascular proliferation often seen at interface of subcutaneous septa and lobules

TOP DIFFERENTIAL DIAGNOSES

- Atypical lipomatous tumor/well-differentiated liposarcoma
- Myxoid liposarcoma
- Myxofibrosarcoma (low grade)

Massive Localized Lymphedema

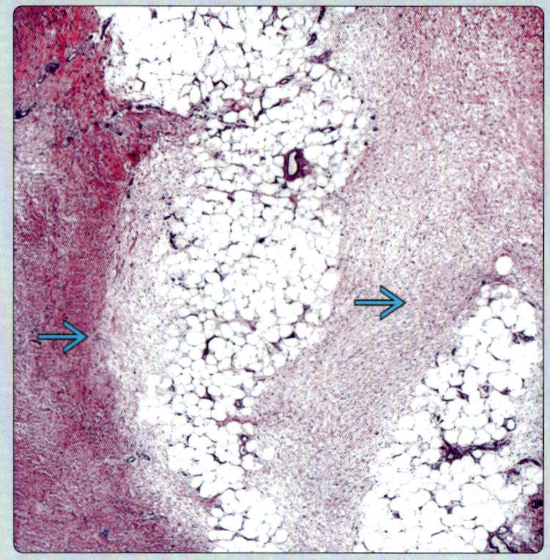

Neovascularization

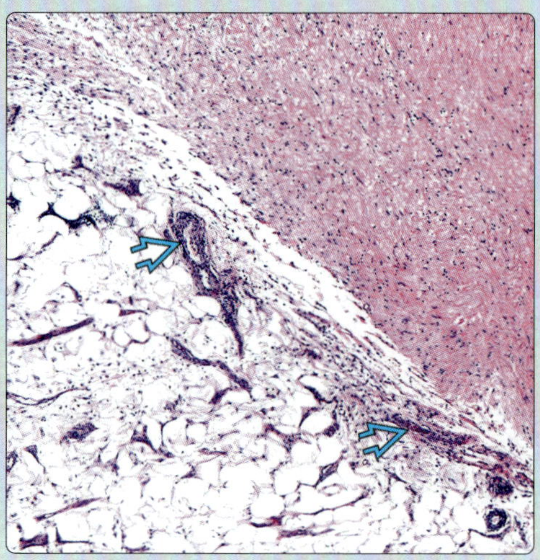

(Left) *Massive localized lymphedema (MLL) is a large soft tissue pseudotumor that occurs secondary to obstruction of lymphatic drainage in morbidly obese patients. At low magnification, MLL is characterized by lobules of adipose tissue separated by expanded, edematous interlobular connective tissue septa* ➡. **(Right)** *In many cases of MLL, the fat lobules characteristically show a proliferation of reactive capillary vessels* ⇨ *near the interface with the interlobular septa.*

Bland, Reactive Fibroblasts

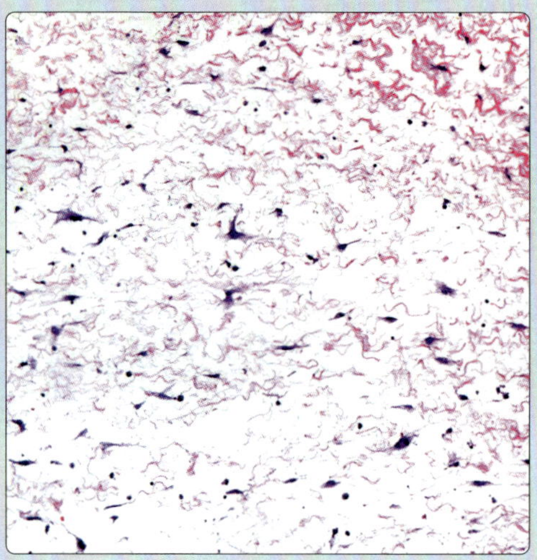

Lymphoid Aggregates

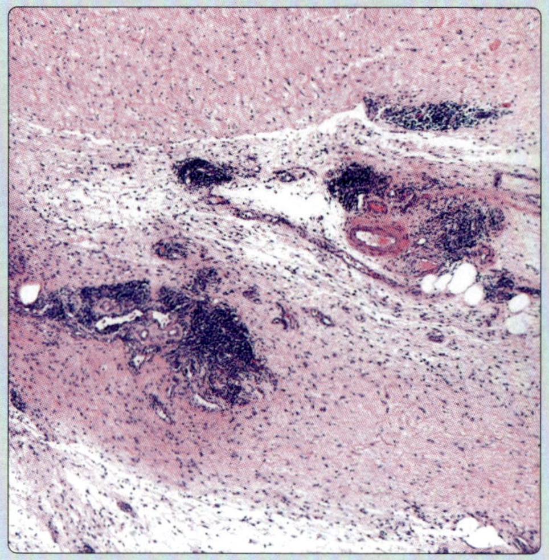

(Left) *The septal fibroblasts in MLL are spindled to stellate and generally appear mildly atypical but reactive. Occasional cells may be enlarged and multinucleated and may even resemble the "floret cells" seen in well-differentiated liposarcoma. In general, however, there are no atypical cells or lipoblasts within the adipose tissue lobules in MLL.* **(Right)** *Lymphoid aggregates, particularly around lymphatic channels and blood vessels, are common in MLL.*

Massive Localized Lymphedema

TERMINOLOGY

Synonyms

- Lymphatic pseudotumor
- Pseudosarcoma

Definitions

- Pseudoneoplastic process related to localized lymphatic obstruction

ETIOLOGY/PATHOGENESIS

Mechanical

- Lymphatic obstruction by enlarged folds of fat

Other

- May also be seen secondary to lymphatic damage during surgery or trauma
- Hypothyroidism may play role in some patients

CLINICAL ISSUES

Epidemiology

- Age
  - Usually middle aged (range: 30-60 years)
- Sex
  - More common in women

Site

- Medial thigh is most common
  - May be bilateral
- Also lower abdominal wall, scrotum, proximal arm

Presentation

- Morbidly obese patients (> 300 lb)
- Large, painless mass
- May be multiple

Prognosis

- Benign
  - Recurrence or persistence common

IMAGING

CT Findings

- Soft tissue streaking due to expanded subcutaneous septa
- Cysts
- No discrete mass

MACROSCOPIC

General Features

- Overlying skin has thickened, indurated peau d'orange appearance
- Cut surface shows pronounced connective tissue septa in subcutaneous fat
- Edematous adipose tissue may weep serous fluid
- May show small cysts of varying sizes containing serous fluid

Size

- Typically large specimens (> 20 cm)

MICROSCOPIC

Histologic Features

- Overlying skin is often thickened
- Fibrous thickening of dermis with dilated lymphatic surrounded by lymphocytic infiltrate
- Expanded subcutaneous septa between lobules of mature adipose tissue
  - Prominent septal edema
  - Increased mildly atypical fibroblasts
    - May be multinucleated and with "floret cell" morphology
  - Preserved lobular architecture of subcutaneous fat
    - Fat lacks lipoblasts and hyperchromatic atypical cells
    - Pseudocyst formation in adipose tissue may be seen
- Mild perivascular lymphocytic infiltrate
- Reactive capillary vascular proliferation often seen at interface of subcutaneous septa and lobules
- Other findings may include calcification, metaplastic bone

DIFFERENTIAL DIAGNOSIS

Atypical Lipomatous Tumor/Well-Differentiated Liposarcoma

- Lacks characteristic skin changes of lymphedema
- Thickened fibrous bands with atypical hyperchromatic "smudge" cells
- Usually marked variation in size of adipocytes
- Lipoblasts may be identified
- *MDM2* amplification

Myxofibrosarcoma (Low Grade)

- Hyperchromatic spindled cells
- Variable nuclear pleomorphism and mitotic activity
- Well-developed, arcing, "curvilinear" vasculature
- Prominent myxoid stroma

Myxoid Liposarcoma

- Hyperchromatic, small, monomorphic, spindled and ovoid cells
- Uni- and multivacuolated lipoblasts are common
- Delicate plexiform (chicken-wire) capillary vasculature
- Abundant myxoid stroma with variable microcyst formation
- t(12;16) translocation with *FUS-DDIT3* fusion

SELECTED REFERENCES

1. Kurt H et al: Massive localized lymphedema: a clinicopathologic study of 46 patients with an enrichment for multiplicity. Mod Pathol. 29(1):75-82, 2016
2. Porrino J et al: Massive localized lymphedema of the thigh mimicking liposarcoma. Radiol Case Rep. 11(4):391-397, 2016
3. Chopra K et al: Massive localized lymphedema revisited: a quickly rising complication of the obesity epidemic. Ann Plast Surg. 74(1):126-32, 2013
4. Lee S et al: Massive localized lymphedema of the male external genitalia: a clinicopathologic study of 6 cases. Hum Pathol. 44(2):277-81, 2013
5. Bogusz AM et al: Massive localized lymphedema with unusual presentations: report of 2 cases and review of the literature. Int J Surg Pathol. 19(2):212-6, 2011
6. Bogusz AM et al: Massive localized lymphedema with unusual presentations: report of two cases and review of the literature. Int J Surg Pathol. 19(2):212-6, 2008
7. Wu D et al: Massive localized lymphedema: additional locations and association with hypothyroidism. Hum Pathol. 31(9):1162-8, 2000

Atypical Vascular Lesion

KEY FACTS

TERMINOLOGY

- Synonym: Atypical vascular proliferation
- Benign cutaneous vascular lesion presenting as small papule or patch in radiated skin, comprised of thin-walled lymphatic vessels, usually limited to dermis

ETIOLOGY/PATHOGENESIS

- Median latency 3 years post radiotherapy

CLINICAL ISSUES

- Wide age range; median in late 50s
- Skin of breast or chest wall most common following radiotherapy for breast cancer
- Small, flesh-colored papule or erythematous patch
- Solitary or multiple
- Most lesions pursue benign course
- New lesions frequently appear
- Only rare reports of transformation to angiosarcoma
- Complete excision of all lesions recommended

MICROSCOPIC

- Dermal based, small, symmetrical, often wedge shaped
- Usually confined to superficial dermis
- Thin-walled lymphatic capillary vessels
- Dilated or jagged, anastomosing vascular structures
- Dissects preexisting dermal collagen
- Rarely extends into subcutis
- Lacks endothelial multilayering and significant atypia
- Mitoses rarely present
- No amplification of *MYC*

TOP DIFFERENTIAL DIAGNOSES

- Well-differentiated angiosarcoma
- Hobnail hemangioma
- Lymphangioma circumscriptum
- Progressive lymphangioma (benign lymphangioendothelioma)

Atypical Vascular Lesion

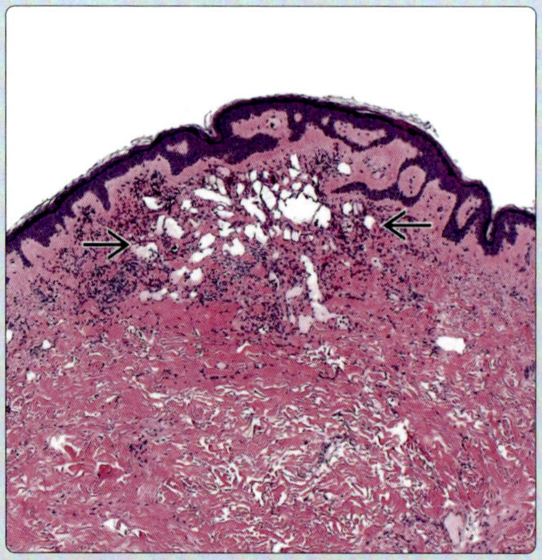

Clinical Appearance

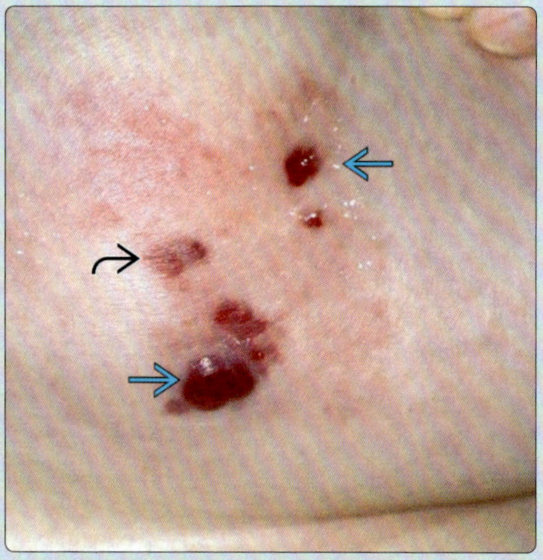

(Left) *An atypical vascular lesion (AVL) typically appears as a symmetrical, wedge-shaped lesion → in the superficial dermis. It is composed of variably dilated and narrow lymphatic channels devoid of red blood cells. AVL is usually confined to the dermis; however, rare lesions can infiltrate the underlying subcutis.* **(Right)** *An AVL typically presents as small papules → and patches → in radiated skin at a median time of 3 years post radiotherapy. Breast or chest wall are most common sites. The lesions can be solitary or multiple.*

Dissecting Growth Pattern

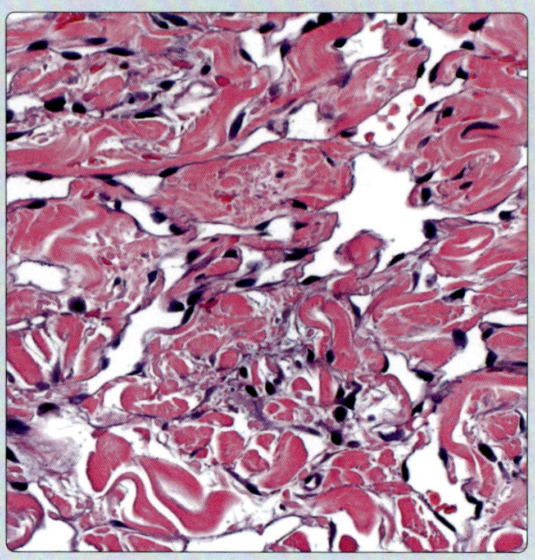

Cytologic Features

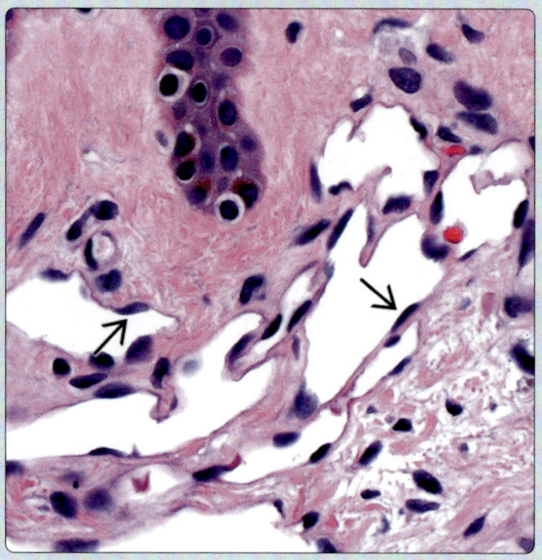

(Left) *AVLs often have a dissecting growth pattern consisting of jagged, anastomosing channels that infiltrate dermal collagen; a pattern that mimics well-differentiated angiosarcoma. Unlike angiosarcoma, however, there is no significant nuclear atypia, no multilayering of cells, and rarely any mitotic activity.* **(Right)** *The lymphatic channels of AVL, although irregular in contour, are lined by a single layer of endothelial cells → that lack significant nuclear atypia.*

Atypical Vascular Lesion

TERMINOLOGY

Abbreviations

- Atypical vascular lesion (AVL)

Synonyms

- Atypical vascular proliferation

Definitions

- Benign cutaneous vascular lesion presenting as small papule(s) or patch(es) in radiated skin, composed of thin-walled lymphatic vessels, usually limited to dermis

ETIOLOGY/PATHOGENESIS

Environmental Exposure

- Radiation (40-60 Gy)
- Median latency: 3 years post radiotherapy

CLINICAL ISSUES

Epidemiology

- Incidence
  - Exact incidence unknown
- Age
  - Wide age range; median in late 50s
  - Usually 1 decade earlier than radiation-associated cutaneous angiosarcoma

Site

- Skin of breast or chest wall most common site, following radiotherapy for breast cancer
- Less frequent in radiation fields associated with gynecological and other malignancies

Presentation

- Small, flesh-colored papule or erythematous patch
- Solitary or multiple

Treatment

- Complete excision of all lesions recommended

Prognosis

- Most lesions pursue benign course
- New lesions frequently appear
- Only rare reports of transformation to angiosarcoma
  - Usually following multiple recurrences

MICROSCOPIC

Histologic Features

- Dermal based, small, symmetrical, often wedge shaped
- Usually confined to superficial dermis
  - Rarely extends into subcutis
- Thin-walled lymphatic capillary vessels
- Dilated or jagged, anastomosing vascular structures
- Dissects preexisting dermal collagen
- Single layer of slightly enlarged endothelial cells
- Lacks endothelial multilayering and significant cytologic atypia
- Mitoses rarely present

DIFFERENTIAL DIAGNOSIS

Well-Differentiated Angiosarcoma

- Clinically presents as large, erythematous plaque (median: 7 cm)
- Anastomosing and infiltrating vascular structures
- Endothelial multilayering and nuclear atypia
- Mitotic figures often present
- Evidence of *MYC* amplification by FISH or immunohistochemistry

Hobnail Hemangioma

- Solitary papule or nodule
- Biphasic pattern (dilated superficial vessels; narrow deep vessels)
- Hobnail endothelial cells
- Stromal fibrosis, hemosiderin deposits

Lymphangioma Circumscriptum

- Clinically, groups of small vesicles containing clear fluid
- Small and superficially located lesion
- Large, ectatic lymphatic channels
- Represents developmental malformation (infants, adults)
- Similar lesion seen in radiated skin

Progressive Lymphangioma (Benign Lymphangioendothelioma)

- Presents clinically as large, slowly increasing, pink to red-brown plaque
- Infiltrating, dissecting lymphatic channels
- Lymphatics orientated horizontally in dermis
- Similar lesion seen in radiated skin

DIAGNOSTIC CHECKLIST

Clinically Relevant Pathologic Features

- Symptom time frame
- Gross appearance

SELECTED REFERENCES

1. Fernandez AP et al: FISH for MYC amplification and anti-MYC immunohistochemistry: useful diagnostic tools in the assessment of secondary angiosarcoma and atypical vascular proliferations. J Cutan Pathol. 39(2):234-42, 2012
2. Manner J et al: MYC high level gene amplification is a distinctive feature of angiosarcomas after irradiation or chronic lymphedema. Am J Pathol. 176(1):34-9, 2010
3. Lucas DR: Angiosarcoma, radiation-associated angiosarcoma, and atypical vascular lesion. Arch Pathol Lab Med. 133(11):1804-9, 2009
4. Patton KT et al: Atypical vascular lesions after surgery and radiation of the breast: a clinicopathologic study of 32 cases analyzing histologic heterogeneity and association with angiosarcoma. Am J Surg Pathol. 32(6):943-50, 2008
5. Gengler C et al: Vascular proliferations of the skin after radiation therapy for breast cancer: clinicopathologic analysis of a series in favor of a benign process: a study from the French Sarcoma Group. Cancer. 109(8):1584-98, 2007
6. Brenn T et al: Radiation-associated cutaneous atypical vascular lesions and angiosarcoma: clinicopathologic analysis of 42 cases. Am J Surg Pathol. 29(8):983-96, 2005
7. Requena L et al: Benign vascular proliferations in irradiated skin. Am J Surg Pathol. 26(3):328-37, 2002
8. Fineberg S et al: Cutaneous angiosarcoma and atypical vascular lesions of the skin and breast after radiation therapy for breast carcinoma. Am J Clin Pathol. 102(6):757-63, 1994

Kaposiform Hemangioendothelioma

KEY FACTS

CLINICAL ISSUES

- Usually occurs in infants and children
    - 50% in 1st year of life
    - Less common in teenagers
- Cutaneous lesions present as violaceous plaques
- Deep tumors often multinodular
- Associated with Kasabach-Merritt syndrome (especially retroperitoneal tumors)
    - Consumptive coagulopathy
    - Thrombocytopenia
- Treated with surgical excision
    - Adjuvant therapy in some cases
- Mortality ~ 10%
    - Due to local effects of tumor or Kasabach-Merritt syndrome
- Rare regional lymph node metastasis
- No distant metastasis

MICROSCOPIC

- Lobular architecture
- Spindle cell areas resemble Kaposi sarcoma
- Capillary hemangioma-like areas
- Glomeruloid structures
- Associated with peripheral lymphatic channels (or lymphangioma) in some cases
- Minimal atypia

ANCILLARY TESTS

- CD31(+), CD34(+), ERG(+), PROX1(+), D2-40 (podoplanin) (+)
- GLUT1(-) and HHV8(-)

TOP DIFFERENTIAL DIAGNOSES

- Infantile hemangioma
- Kaposi sarcoma
- Acquired tufted angioma
- Spindle cell hemangioma

(Left) *Kaposiform hemangioendothelioma (KHE) is a rare vascular tumor that usually presents during early childhood. Deep-seated tumors, such as this one, present as nodular masses and are more prone to develop Kasabach-Merritt syndrome than superficial tumors (especially retroperitoneal tumors).* **(Right)** *Solid spindle cell areas account for the major component of most examples of KHE. These areas resemble Kaposi sarcoma consisting of long fascicles of closely spaced spindle cells, yet lack atypia.*

Kaposiform Hemangioendothelioma

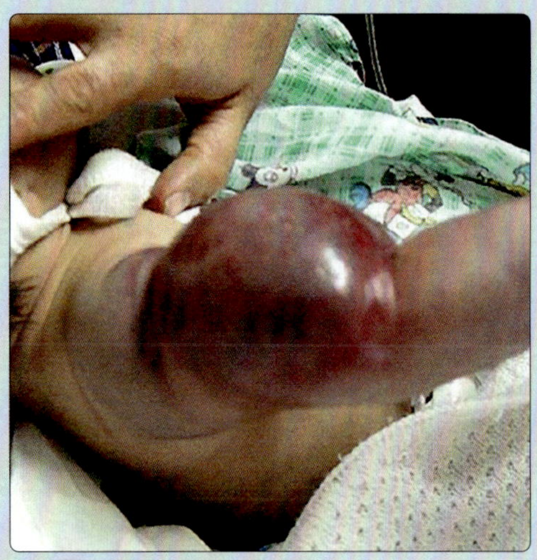

Spindle Cell Kaposiform Areas

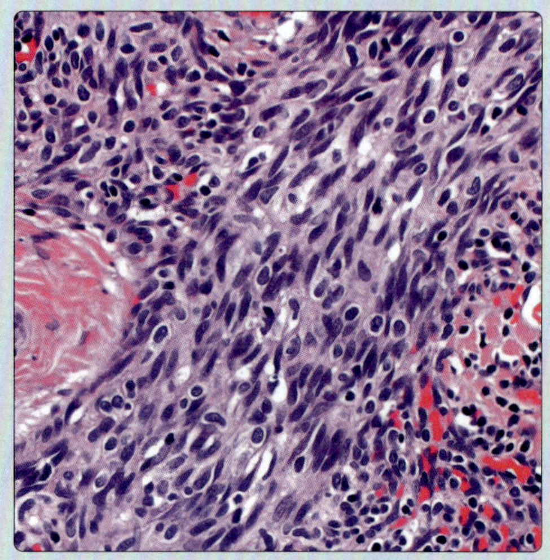

(Left) *H&E depicts an interface between spindle cell → and hemangioma-like areas → in KHE. The tumor shows an overall lobular architecture, as indicated by the fibrous septum → traversing the lesion.* **(Right)** *Glomeruloid structures are a very characteristic attribute of KHE. They are composed of tangles of endothelial cells and pericytes arranged in lobulated, whorling structures that resemble renal glomeruli. Entrapped thrombi may or may not be evident.*

Capillary Hemangioma-Like Areas

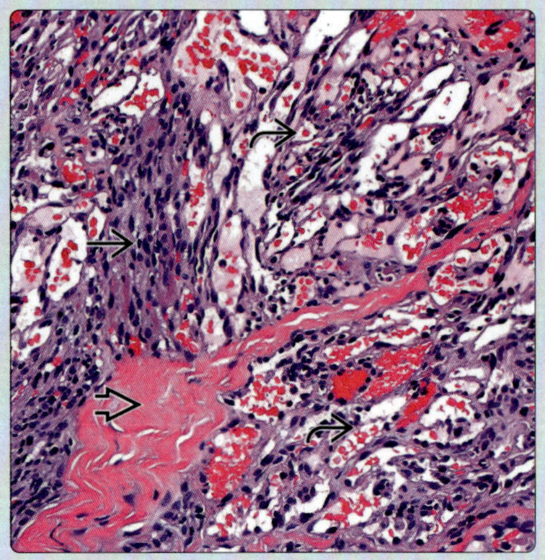

Glomeruloid Structure

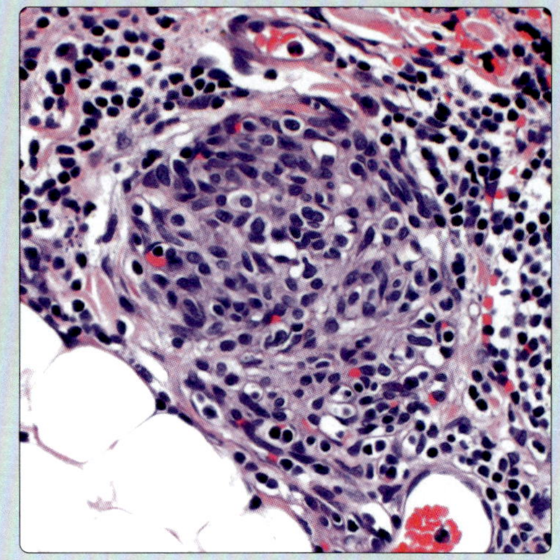

Kaposiform Hemangioendothelioma

TERMINOLOGY

Abbreviations

- Kaposiform hemangioendothelioma (KHE)

Definitions

- Vascular neoplasm associated with development of Kasabach-Merritt syndrome and demonstrates features reminiscent of both Kaposi sarcoma and capillary hemangioma

CLINICAL ISSUES

Epidemiology

- Age
  - Majority present in childhood to teen years
    - 50% in 1st year of life

Site

- Most common in extremities
  - Also retroperitoneum

Presentation

- Painful or painless mass
  - Presents as superficial or deep mass
  - Cutaneous lesions present as violaceous plaques
  - Deep tumors often multinodular and desmoplastic
  - Associated with Kasabach-Merritt syndrome (especially retroperitoneal tumors)
    - Consumptive coagulopathy and thrombocytopenia
    - Majority of cases of Kasabach-Merritt syndrome associated with KHE

Treatment

- Wide surgical excision, best option when feasible
- Medical therapy (sirolimus, steroids, cytotoxic agents, α-interferon) in some cases

Prognosis

- Rare regional lymph node metastasis
- No distant metastasis
- Mortality ~ 10%, related to local effects of tumor or Kasabach-Merritt syndrome

MICROSCOPIC

Histologic Features

- Lobular architecture
- Spindle cell areas resemble Kaposi sarcoma
- Capillary hemangioma-like areas
- Glomeruloid structures characteristic
- Associated with peripheral lymphatic channels (or lymphangioma) in some cases
- Mitoses but minimal atypia

ANCILLARY TESTS

Immunohistochemistry

- CD31(+), CD34(+), ERG(+)
- Also PROX1(+) and D2-40 (podoplanin) (+) (especially in peripheral lymphatic component)
- GLUT1(-) and HHV8(-)

DIFFERENTIAL DIAGNOSIS

Infantile Hemangioma

- Early postnatal period
- Lobular capillary architecture
- Lacks spindle cell areas
- GLUT1(+)
- Regresses spontaneously

Kaposi Sarcoma

- Older or immunocompromised patients
- Very rare in children, except in Africa
- Nodular phase composed of solid spindle cell areas
- Lacks capillary hemangioma-like areas
- HHV8(+)

Acquired Tufted Angioma

- Similar demographics as KHE
- Small, cutaneous lesion
- Histologically almost indistinguishable from KHE
  - Nodular proliferation of closely packed capillaries in dermis (cannonball pattern)
- Kasabach-Merritt syndrome in some cases

Spindle Cell Hemangioma

- Occurs in adults in distal extremities
- Often partially intravascular
- Ectatic vessels and spindle cell areas
- Vacuolated endothelial cells ("blister" cells)
- May have areas of thrombosis or phleboliths

DIAGNOSTIC CHECKLIST

Clinically Relevant Pathologic Features

- Age distribution
  - Vast majority occur in children
- Symptom complex
  - Kasabach-Merritt syndrome

Pathologic Interpretation Pearls

- Vascular tumor in child, composed predominantly of spindled endothelial cells: Consider KHE

SELECTED REFERENCES

1. Schmid I et al: Kaposiform hemangioendothelioma in children: a benign vascular tumor with multiple treatment options. World J Pediatr. 14(4):322-9, 2018
2. Miettinen M et al: ERG transcription factor as an immunohistochemical marker for vascular endothelial tumors and prostatic carcinoma. Am J Surg Pathol. 35(3):432-41, 2011
3. Cheuk W et al: Immunostaining for human herpesvirus 8 latent nuclear antigen-1 helps distinguish Kaposi sarcoma from its mimickers. Am J Clin Pathol. 121(3):335-42, 2004
4. Lyons LL et al: Kaposiform hemangioendothelioma: a study of 33 cases emphasizing its pathologic, immunophenotypic, and biologic uniqueness from juvenile hemangioma. Am J Surg Pathol. 28(5):559-68, 2004
5. Brasanac D et al: Retroperitoneal kaposiform hemangioendothelioma with tufted angioma-like features in an infant with Kasabach-Merritt syndrome. Pathol Int. 53(9):627-31, 2003
6. Mentzel T et al: Kaposiform hemangioendothelioma in adults. Clinicopathologic and immunohistochemical analysis of three cases. Am J Clin Pathol. 108(4):450-5, 1997
7. Zukerberg LR et al: Kaposiform hemangioendothelioma of infancy and childhood. An aggressive neoplasm associated with Kasabach-Merritt syndrome and lymphangiomatosis. Am J Surg Pathol. 17(4):321-8, 1993

Papillary Intralymphatic Angioendothelioma

KEY FACTS

TERMINOLOGY

- Also known as Dabska tumor
- Low-grade malignant vascular tumor composed of hobnailed endothelial cells

ETIOLOGY/PATHOGENESIS

- May be associated with vascular or lymphatic tumor/malformation

CLINICAL ISSUES

- Typically occur in children (minority in adults)
- Distal extremities most common, but may occur in other sites
- High rate of local recurrence, rare metastasis
- Complete surgical excision recommended to prevent metastasis (rare) or recurrence

MACROSCOPIC

- Dermal-based infiltrative tumor with extension into subcutis

MICROSCOPIC

- Dermal proliferation of vessels with papillary projections lined by enlarged, cuboidal endothelial cells
- Endothelial cells show prominent hobnail features with plump, rounded profiles protruding into lumina
  - Hobnail cells show high N:C ratio but lack significant atypia or mitotic activity
- Typically associated with surrounding lymphoid infiltrate and sclerotic collagen
- Vessels often extend into subcutaneous tissues

ANCILLARY TESTS

- CD31 and CD34 (+)

TOP DIFFERENTIAL DIAGNOSES

- Retiform hemangioendothelioma
- Composite hemangioendothelioma
- Kaposi sarcoma
- Angiosarcoma

Papillary Intralymphatic Angioendothelioma

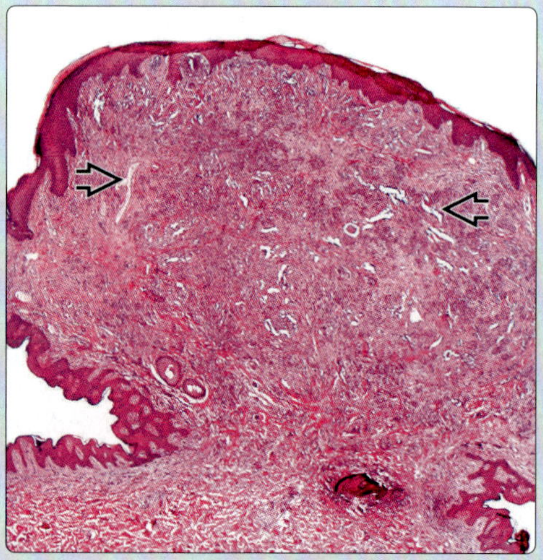

Dilated Vascular Spaces

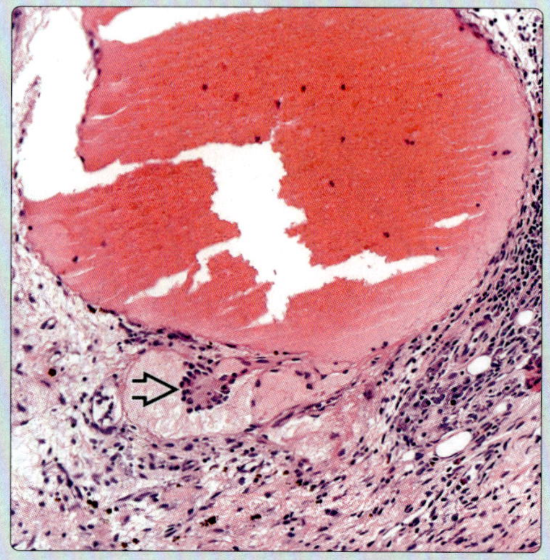

(Left) *Scanning magnification view of a papillary intralymphatic angioendothelioma (PILA) (Dabska tumor) shows a polypoid lesion in the skin with irregular dilated vascular spaces ➡.* **(Right)** *This shows a dilated vascular space filled with red blood cells overlying a smaller space with a prominent papillary intralymphatic projection lined by hobnailed cells ➡.*

Intraluminal Papillary Structures

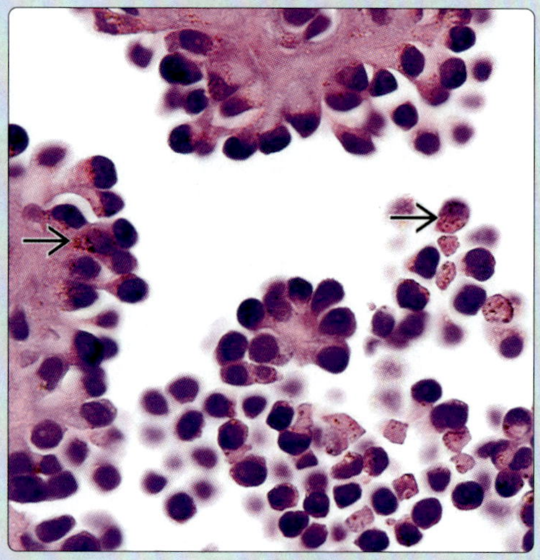

Hobnail Cells

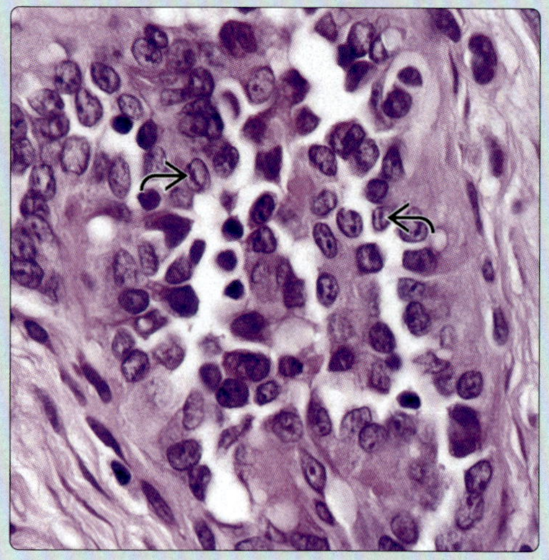

(Left) *Prominent intralymphatic projections of papillary structures with hyaline cores are lined by plump hyperchromatic-staining cells, some of which contain cytoplasmic hemosiderin pigment ➡.* **(Right)** *Another example at high-power examination shows papillae lined by mildly enlarged hobnailed cells projecting into the vascular lumina. The cells show vesicular chromatin, small nucleoli, and occasional grooves ➡.*

TERMINOLOGY

Abbreviations

- Papillary intralymphatic angioendothelioma (PILA)

Synonyms

- Dabska tumor
- Endovascular papillary angioendothelioma

Definitions

- Low-grade malignant vascular tumor composed of hobnailed endothelial cells

ETIOLOGY/PATHOGENESIS

Unknown

- May be associated with vascular or lymphatic tumor/malformation

CLINICAL ISSUES

Epidemiology

- Incidence
  - Rare tumors
- Age
  - Typically occur in children (minority in adults)
- Sex
  - Slight female predominance

Site

- Distal extremities most common but may occur in other sites

Presentation

- Plaque-like lesion of dermis + subcutis
  - May show overlying violaceous skin discoloration

Treatment

- Complete surgical excision recommended

Prognosis

- High rate of local recurrence, rare metastasis (to lymph nodes)

MACROSCOPIC

General Features

- Dermal-based infiltrative tumor with extension into subcutis

Size

- Can be quite large (average: 7 cm)

MICROSCOPIC

Histologic Features

- Dermal proliferation of vessels lined by enlarged, cuboidal endothelial cells
  - Intravascular papillary projections with hyaline cores
  - Endothelial cells show prominent hobnail features with plump, rounded profiles protruding into lumina
    - Hobnail cells show high N:C ratio; nuclei may show grooves
  - Cytoplasmic vacuolation may be seen
  - Mitotic figures absent or rare
- Typically associated with surrounding lymphoid infiltrate and sclerotic collagen
- Vessels often extend into subcutaneous tissues
- Associated lymphatic or vascular tumor or malformation in some cases

ANCILLARY TESTS

Immunohistochemistry

- CD31, CD34, and FVIIIRAg (+)
- Most cases also show expression of lymphatic markers D2-40 and VEGFR-3

DIFFERENTIAL DIAGNOSIS

Retiform Hemangioendothelioma

- Most cases occur in adults, but some present in children
- Proliferation of vessels forming distinct elongated rete-like structures lined by hobnail cells
- Some cases of retiform hemangioendothelioma (RHE) show significant overlap with PILA, with prominent papillary structures

Composite Hemangioendothelioma

- By definition, composed of at least 2 distinct types of hemangioendothelioma
  - Predominant histologic components usually are epithelioid hemangioendothelioma and RHE

Kaposi Sarcoma

- Much more common, associated with HIV infection and AIDS in most cases
- Proliferation of small, slit-like vascular spaces lined by spindle cells, lacking papillary pattern of PILA
- HHV8(+)

Angiosarcoma

- Typically occurs in older adults or post mastectomy
- Proliferation of atypical spindled or epithelioid endothelial cells forming anastomosing vascular spaces and showing infiltrative features

DIAGNOSTIC CHECKLIST

Pathologic Interpretation Pearls

- Dermal proliferation of vessels with papillary projections lined by enlarged, cuboidal endothelial cells

SELECTED REFERENCES

1. Gambarotti M et al: Intraosseous papillary intralymphatic angioendothelioma (PILA): one new case and review of the literature. Clin Sarcoma Res. 8:1, 2018
2. Kugler A et al: Papillary intralymphatic angioendothelioma (PILA), also referred to as Dabska tumour, in an 83-year-old woman. J Eur Acad Dermatol Venereol. 30(10):e59-e61, 2016
3. Neves RI et al: Endovascular papillary angioendothelioma (Dabska tumor): underrecognized malignant tumor in childhood. J Pediatr Surg. 46(1):e25-8, 2011
4. Emanuel PO et al: Dabska tumor arising in lymphangioma circumscriptum. J Cutan Pathol. 35(1):65-9, 2008
5. Fukunaga M: Expression of D2-40 in lymphatic endothelium of normal tissues and in vascular tumours. Histopathology. 46(4):396-402, 2005
6. Fanburg-Smith JC et al: Papillary intralymphatic angioendothelioma (PILA): a report of twelve cases of a distinctive vascular tumor with phenotypic features of lymphatic vessels. Am J Surg Pathol. 23(9):1004-10, 1999
7. Dabska M: Malignant endovascular papillary angioendothelioma of the skin in childhood. Clinicopathologic study of 6 cases. Cancer. 24(3):503-10, 1969

Retiform Hemangioendothelioma

KEY FACTS

TERMINOLOGY

- Synonym: Hobnail hemangioendothelioma
- Low-grade malignant vascular tumor composed of elongated vessels resembling rete testis

CLINICAL ISSUES

- Typically presents in middle-aged adults but may occur in children
- More common in females
- Treatment: Wide local excision
- Local recurrences common if not completely excised
- Very rare metastases reported (regional lymph nodes)

MACROSCOPIC

- Typically poorly circumscribed dermal &/or subcutaneous tumor

MICROSCOPIC

- Distinctive, elongated, arborizing blood vessels resembling rete testis
- Often show papillary-like intraluminal projections, some of which may have hyaline core
- Vascular spaces are lined by endothelial cells with characteristic hobnail morphology
  - Hobnail cells with oval nuclei with mild hyperchromasia
- Very prominent lymphocytic infiltrate in most cases
- Some cases show significant overlap with papillary intralymphatic angioendothelioma (Dabska tumor)

ANCILLARY TESTS

- Vascular markers: CD31(+), CD34(+), and FVIIIRAg(+)
- Usually D2-40(-) and VEGFR-3(-)

TOP DIFFERENTIAL DIAGNOSES

- Papillary intralymphatic angioendothelioma (Dabska tumor)
- Composite hemangioendothelioma
- Kaposi sarcoma
- Angiosarcoma

(Left) *This cutaneous retiform hemangioendothelioma (RHE) shows superficial dermal involvement by elongated, irregularly branching vascular spaces. Focal papillary structures are present.* **(Right)** *RHE features a proliferation of elongated vessels lined by hyperchromatic-staining hobnailed endothelial cells. The surrounding stroma shows fibrosis and scattered lymphocytes.*

Retiform Hemangioendothelioma

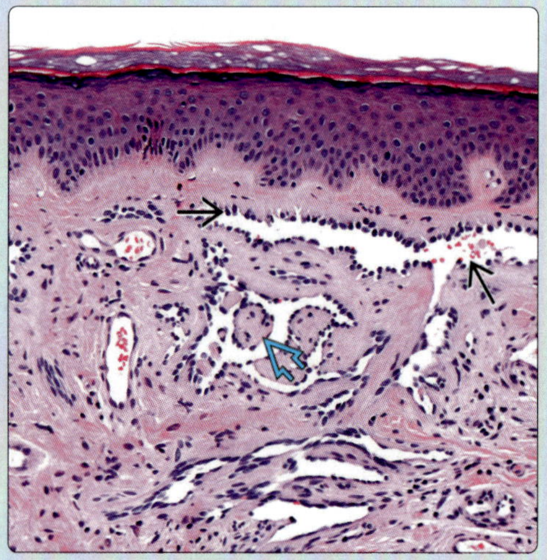

Hobnailed Endothelial Cells

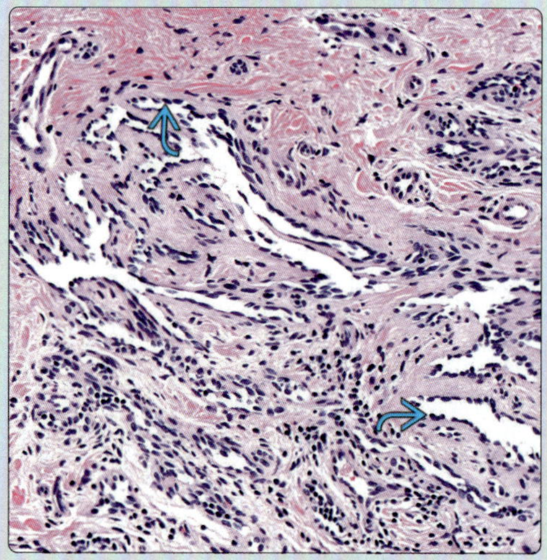

(Left) *High-magnification view of RHE shows hyperchromatic endothelial cells with hobnail features, nuclear crowding, and focally enlarged nucleoli.* **(Right)** *H&E of the deep aspect of a RHE shows elongated vascular spaces surrounded by prominent lymphoid aggregates. Note the hobnailed endothelial cells.*

Cytologic Features

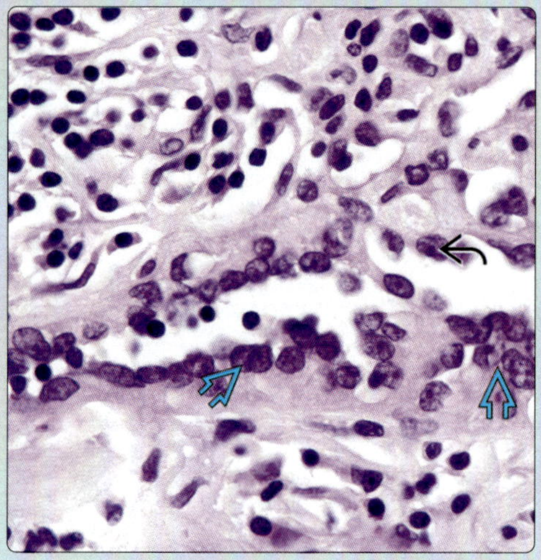

Stromal Lymphocytic Infiltrate

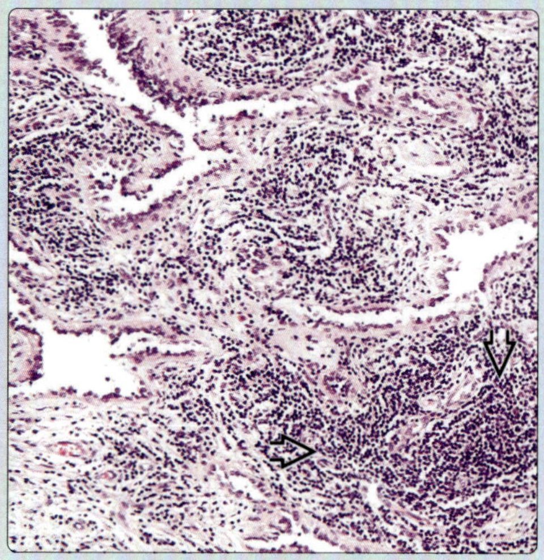

Retiform Hemangioendothelioma

TERMINOLOGY

Abbreviations

- Retiform hemangioendothelioma (RHE)

Synonyms

- Hobnail hemangioendothelioma

Definitions

- Low-grade malignant vascular tumor composed of elongated vessels resembling rete testis

ETIOLOGY/PATHOGENESIS

Unknown

- Rare cases associated with lymphedema or preceding radiation
- 1 case reported to be positive for HHV8

CLINICAL ISSUES

Epidemiology

- Incidence
  - Rare
- Age
  - Typically middle-aged adults but may occur in children
- Sex
  - More common in females

Site

- Trunk or extremities

Presentation

- Large, nodular to plaque-like lesion

Treatment

- Wide local excision is necessary to prevent recurrence

Prognosis

- Locally aggressive, often with multiple recurrences if not completely excised
- Very rare metastases reported (regional lymph nodes)
- No deaths from disease reported

MACROSCOPIC

General Features

- Typically poorly circumscribed dermal &/or subcutaneous tumor

Size

- May be large tumors (up to 12 cm)

MICROSCOPIC

Histologic Features

- Dermal-based infiltrative proliferation of distinctive, elongated, arborizing blood vessels resembling rete testis
- Vascular spaces are lined by endothelial cells with characteristic hobnail morphology
  - Endothelial cells show hyperchromasia, but typically do not show prominent cytologic atypia
  - Hobnail cells with oval nuclei with mild hyperchromasia
  - Mitotic figures may be present but are usually rare
- Very prominent lymphocytic infiltrate reported in most cases
- May show invasion of subcutaneous tissues
- Some cases show significant overlap with Dabska tumor (both have hobnailed cells) with prominent papillary structures and hyaline cores

ANCILLARY TESTS

Immunohistochemistry

- Vascular markers: CD31(+), CD34(+), and FVIIIRAg(+)
- Usually D2-40(-) and VEGFR-3(-)

DIFFERENTIAL DIAGNOSIS

Papillary Intralymphatic Angioendothelioma (Dabska Tumor)

- More common in children, but cases in young adults also reported
- Papillary structures more common
- Typically do not show prominent rete-like, elongated vessels of RHE
- Some cases show significant overlap with RHE (both have hobnailed cells)

Composite Hemangioendothelioma

- By definition, composed of at least 2 distinct hemangioendothelioma types
  - Predominant histologic components usually are epithelioid hemangioendothelioma and RHE

Kaposi Sarcoma

- Much more common, associated with HIV/AIDS or other forms of immunosuppression
- Proliferation of small, slit-like vascular spaces lined by spindle cells lacking rete-like pattern of RHE
- HHV8(+) (only 1 case of RHE reported to be positive)

Angiosarcoma

- Typically occurs in older adults or post mastectomy and irradiation
- Proliferation of atypical spindled or epithelioid endothelial cells, often forming anastomosing vascular spaces and showing infiltrative features

DIAGNOSTIC CHECKLIST

Pathologic Interpretation Pearls

- Proliferation of distinctive elongated blood vessels (lined by hobnail cells) resembling rete testis

SELECTED REFERENCES

1. Kiyohara T et al: Retiform hemangioendothelioma presenting as a pedunculated nodule on the site of an inguinal pyoderma chronica. J Dermatol. ePub, 2018
2. Arriola AG et al: Atypical retiform hemangioendothelioma arising in a patient with Milroy disease: a case report and review of the literature. J Cutan Pathol. 44(1):98-103, 2017
3. Mota A et al: Clinical, dermoscopic and histopathologic findings of retiform hemangioendothelioma. Dermatol Pract Concept. 3(4):11-4, 2013
4. Keiler SA et al: Retiform hemangioendothelioma treated with Mohs micrographic surgery. J Am Acad Dermatol. 65(1):233-5, 2011
5. Parsons A et al: Retiform hemangioendotheliomas usually do not express D2-40 and VEGFR-3. Am J Dermatopathol. 30(1):31-3, 2008

Composite Hemangioendothelioma

KEY FACTS

TERMINOLOGY

- Endothelial neoplasm of low malignant potential composed of admixture of histologically benign, intermediate, and malignant components

ETIOLOGY/PATHOGENESIS

- Can arise from preexisting or congenital vascular malformation

CLINICAL ISSUES

- Very rare
- Acral extremities most common
- Enlarging nodular erythematous or violaceous mass
- Treatment: Wide local excision
- Local recurrence (up to 50%)
- Metastases (15%)
- No reports of death from disease to date

MACROSCOPIC

- Red to purple, nodular or multinodular mass
- Infiltrative border
- Average: 5 cm; range: 1-30 cm

MICROSCOPIC

- Complex admixture of variety of vasoformative patterns
- Retiform hemangioendothelioma (HE) pattern
    - Most common and usually dominant
- Epithelioid HE pattern
    - 2nd most common pattern
- Well-differentiated angiosarcoma pattern
- Spindle cell hemangioma pattern

TOP DIFFERENTIAL DIAGNOSES

- Retiform HE
- Epithelioid HE
- Well-differentiated angiosarcoma
- Spindle cell hemangioma

Composite Hemangioendothelioma

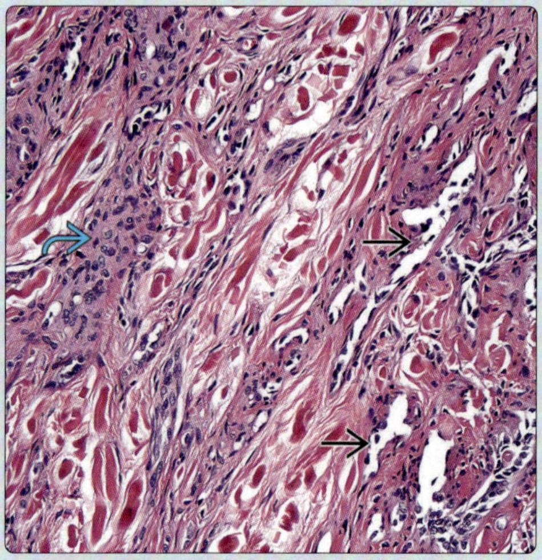

Retiform Hemangioendothelioma Component

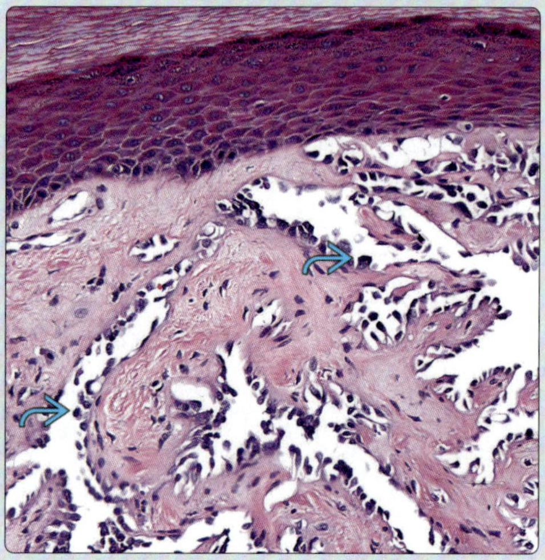

(Left) *Composite hemangioendothelioma (HE) usually presents as a dermal/subcutaneous tumor on an acral extremity. It has complex histology with admixtures of various elements, most often retiform and epithelioid HE.* **(Right)** *Retiform HE is the most common component of composite HE, composed of elongated, thin-walled channels lined by endothelial cells that protrude into the lumen, forming a hobnail pattern.*

Epithelioid Hemangioendothelioma Component

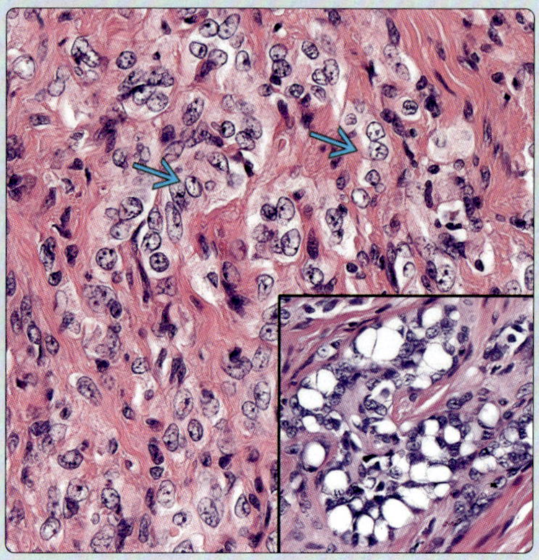

Angiosarcoma-Like Areas

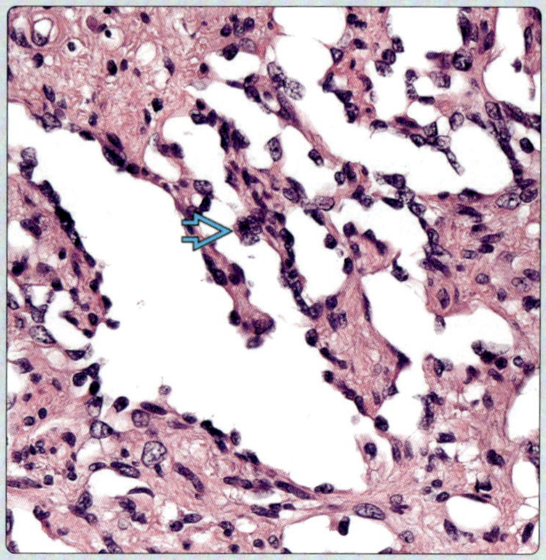

(Left) *An epithelioid HE component is present in most composite HEs and consists of cords of cells with abundant eosinophilic cytoplasm within hyalinized or myxoid matrix. Cells with intracytoplasmic vacuoles mimic lipoblasts (inset).* **(Right)** *Angiosarcoma-like areas are present in some tumors and are characterized by irregular anastomosing channels lined by atypical endothelial cells. This pattern is not associated with a worse prognosis.*

Composite Hemangioendothelioma

TERMINOLOGY

Abbreviations

- Hemangioendothelioma (HE)

Definitions

- Endothelial neoplasm of low malignant potential composed of admixture of histologically benign, intermediate, and malignant components

ETIOLOGY/PATHOGENESIS

Developmental Anomaly

- Can arise from preexisting or congenital vascular malformation

CLINICAL ISSUES

Epidemiology

- Incidence
  - Very rare

Site

- Dermis and subcutis
  - Acral extremities most common
    - Foot/ankle region (50%)
    - Hand/forearm (25%)
- Oral mucosa (12%)
- Other reported sites: Thigh, hip, upper arm, back, inguinal lymph nodes, mediastinum, scalp, kidney, manubrium, neck, nose, spleen, hypopharynx, periaortic tissue, vertebra, pulmonary vein, liver

Presentation

- Enlarging nodular or multinodular erythematous or violaceous mass
  - Satellite nodules, ulceration, bleeding, edema

Natural History

- High local recurrence rate (up to 50%)
  - Often many years after primary excision
- Metastases (15%)
  - Usually to regional lymph nodes

Treatment

- Wide local excision

Prognosis

- No reports of death from disease to date

MACROSCOPIC

General Features

- Red to purple, nodular or multinodular mass with infiltrative border

Size

- Average: 5 cm; range: 1-30 cm

MICROSCOPIC

Histologic Features

- Complex admixture of variety of vasoformative patterns
- Retiform HE pattern
  - Most common and usually dominant
  - Long, branching, thin-walled vessels
  - Single layer of bland endothelial cells that protrude intraluminally (hobnail pattern)
  - Intraluminal papillary structures in some
- Epithelioid HE pattern
  - 2nd most common
  - Cords, strands, or sheets of epithelioid endothelial cells
    - Abundant eosinophilic cytoplasm
    - Intracytoplasmic vacuoles
    - Hyalin or myxoid stroma
- Well-differentiated angiosarcoma pattern
  - Anastomosing spaces lined by atypical cells, often multilayered
  - Dissecting growth pattern
  - Minor component when present
- Spindle cell hemangioma pattern
  - Sheets and fascicles of spindle-shaped endothelial cells
  - Slit-like vascular spaces
  - Cavernous spaces, often with organizing thrombi and phleboliths
- Composite HE with neuroendocrine marker expression
  - Variant tumor with synaptophysin staining and focal nested pattern
  - Usually negative for chromogranin (< 10%) and CD56 (< 50%)
  - Often deep seated
  - More aggressive than convention variant

DIFFERENTIAL DIAGNOSIS

Retiform Hemangioendothelioma

- Skin and soft tissue of acral extremities
- Pure pattern, lacks other vascular components

Epithelioid Hemangioendothelioma

- Various skin, soft tissue, osseous, and visceral sites
- Pure pattern, lacks other vascular components

Well-Differentiated Angiosarcoma

- Most often cutaneous tumor on scalp/face of elderly patient
- Dissecting channels lined by atypical, multilayered endothelial cells

Spindle Cell Hemangioma

- Skin and soft tissue of acral extremities
- Spindle cell, cavernous and epithelioid patterns
- Thrombi and phleboliths

Kaposi Sarcoma

- Fascicles of atypical spindle cells
- Slit-like, blood-filled spaces
- HHV8(+)

SELECTED REFERENCES

1. Perry KD et al: Composite hemangioendothelioma with neuroendocrine marker expression: an aggressive variant. Mod Pathol. 30(11):1589-1602, 2017
2. Requena L et al: Cutaneous composite hemangioendothelioma with satellitosis and lymph node metastases. J Cutan Pathol. 35(2):225-30, 2008
3. Nayler SJ et al: Composite hemangioendothelioma: a complex, low-grade vascular lesion mimicking angiosarcoma. Am J Surg Pathol. 24(3):352-61, 2000

Pseudomyogenic Hemangioendothelioma

KEY FACTS

TERMINOLOGY

- Synonym: Epithelioid sarcoma-like hemangioendothelioma
- Distinctive vascular neoplasm of borderline malignant potential that shows morphologic features reminiscent of myoid neoplasm or epithelioid sarcoma

CLINICAL ISSUES

- Most common in young adults (mean: 30 years)
- Male predilection
- Most arise in extremities (particularly lower limb)
- Multicentric in over 50% of patients
  - May present in superficial &/or deep soft tissue
- Treatment: Complete surgical excision
- Generally indolent clinical course
  - Local recurrence common
  - True metastasis very rare

MACROSCOPIC

- Usually < 3 cm

MICROSCOPIC

- Ill-defined nodules, sheets, and fascicles
- Plump spindled and epithelioid cells with abundant eosinophilic cytoplasm
- Usually scant mitoses
- Brisk neutrophilic infiltrate common
- Well-developed vasoformation absent

ANCILLARY TESTS

- Cytokeratin AE1/AE3(+), ERG(+), FLI-1(+)
- CD31(+) in 50% of cases
- Retained nuclear INI1
- t(7;19)(q22;q13) with *SERPINE1-FOSB* fusion

TOP DIFFERENTIAL DIAGNOSES

- Epithelioid sarcoma
- Sarcomatoid squamous cell carcinoma
- Epithelioid hemangioendothelioma
- Cellular fibrous histiocytoma (fibrous histiocytoma)

Pseudomyogenic Hemangioendothelioma

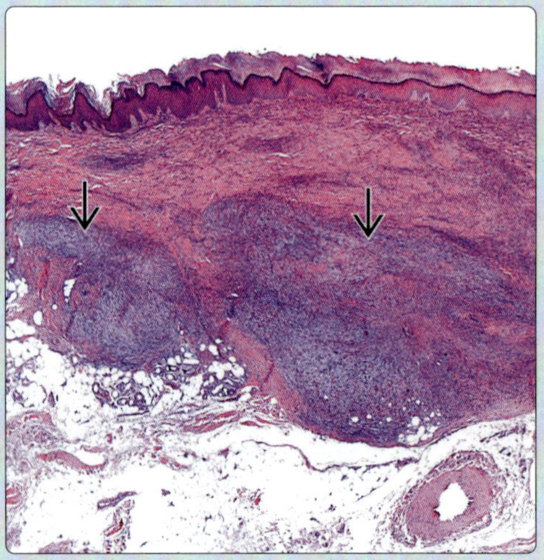

Sheets, Nodules, and Fascicles

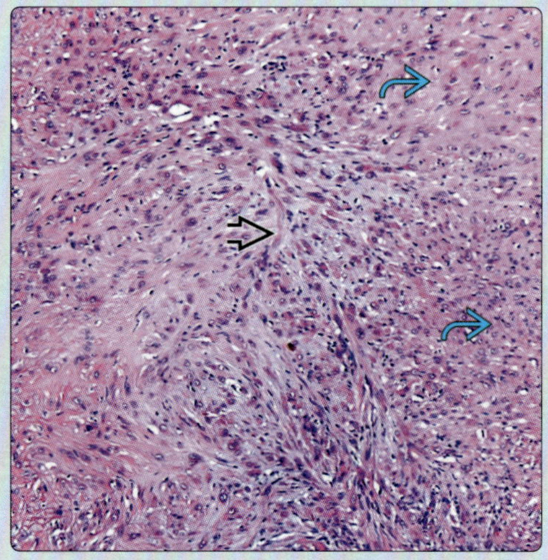

(Left) *Pseudomyogenic hemangioendothelioma (PMH), a.k.a. epithelioid sarcoma-like hemangioendothelioma, is a distinctive vascular neoplasm that, in > 1/2 of cases, shows multicentric/multifocal nodular growth that often involves multiple tissue planes, including dermis, subcutis, muscle, and even bone.* **(Right)** *PMH typically grows in sheets, ill-defined nodules, &/or fascicles. Some areas contain tumor cells that are tightly packed, while others show loose dyscohesion.*

Pseudomyogenic Cells and Neutrophils

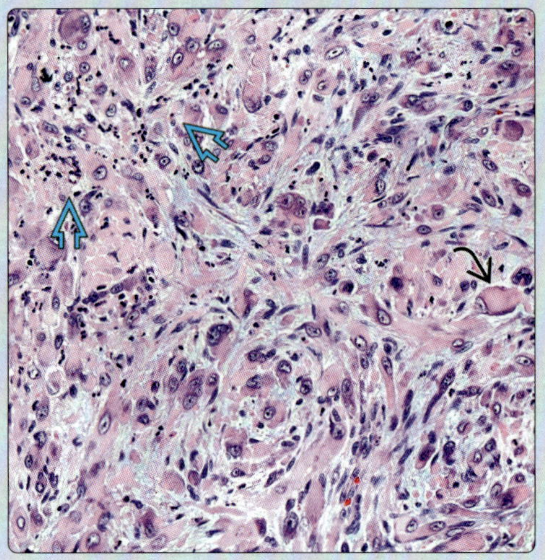

Cytokeratin AE1/AE3 Expression

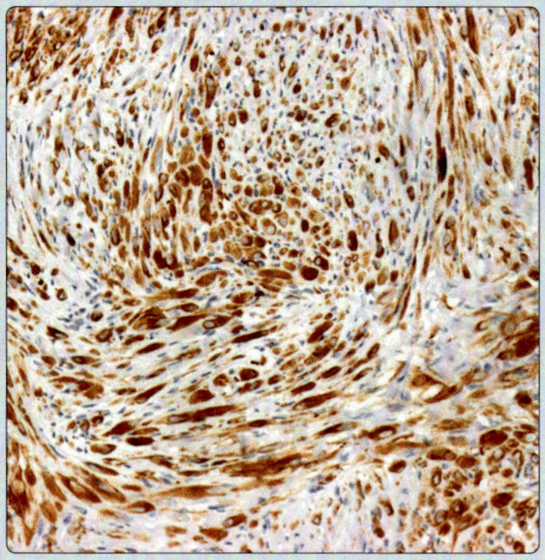

(Left) *Tumor cells in PMH are generally plump and spindled and feature abundant, brightly eosinophilic cytoplasm, reminiscent of myoid cells. Some larger cells can resemble rhabdomyoblasts. A brisk neutrophilic infiltrate is seen in ~ 50% of cases and is a helpful diagnostic feature.* **(Right)** *Strong cytokeratin AE1/AE3 expression is characteristic of PMH and can lead to obvious confusion with epithelioid sarcoma. The latter, however, is positive for CD34 (50% of cases), negative for CD31, and shows loss of INI1.*

TERMINOLOGY

Abbreviations

- Pseudomyogenic hemangioendothelioma (PMH)

Synonyms

- Epithelioid sarcoma-like hemangioendothelioma

Definitions

- Distinctive vascular neoplasm of borderline malignant potential that shows morphologic features reminiscent of myoid neoplasm or epithelioid sarcoma

CLINICAL ISSUES

Epidemiology

- Age
  - Most common in young adults (mean: 30 years)
    - Infrequent > 40 years
- Sex
  - Male predilection

Site

- Most common in lower extremity
- Also upper extremity, trunk, head/neck

Presentation

- Painful or painless nodule(s)
- Multicentric in > 50% of patients
- May present in superficial or deep soft tissue
  - Not uncommon for multiple tissue planes to be involved
    - Skin, subcutis, muscle, &/or bone
  - Cutaneous lesions may be ulcerated

Treatment

- Complete surgical excision

Prognosis

- Generally indolent clinical course
- Local recurrence common
  - Often multiple; can occur over long time period
- True metastasis very rare
  - Reported sites include lung, bone, lymph node, scalp
  - Multicentricity may be mistaken for locoregional metastases

MACROSCOPIC

General Features

- Poorly demarcated
- Tan-white to gray cut surface

Size

- Usually < 3 cm

MICROSCOPIC

Histologic Features

- Infiltrative borders
- Ill-defined nodules, sheets, and fascicles
- Plump spindled and epithelioid cells with abundant eosinophilic cytoplasm
  - Round, vesicular nuclei with variable nucleoli
    - Usually mild to moderate atypia; rarely marked
  - Intracytoplasmic lumen formation rare and usually focal
  - Some cells may resemble rhabdomyoblasts
  - Usually scant mitoses
- Fibrous or desmoplastic stroma; rarely myxoid
- Brisk neutrophilic infiltrate common
- Well-developed vasoformation absent
- Intralesional hemorrhage uncommon
- Some tumors contain foci of necrosis or vascular invasion

ANCILLARY TESTS

Immunohistochemistry

- Cytokeratin AE1/AE3(+), ERG(+), FLI-1(+)
  - Often negative for other keratins
- CD31(+) in 50% of cases
- FOSB(+)
- Retained nuclear INI1
- Focal SMA(+) in up to 30%
- CD34, EMA, S100 protein, desmin, myogenin, CAMTA1 (-)

Molecular Genetics

- Characteristic recurring t(7;19)(q22;q13)
  - Results in *SERPINE1-FOSB* fusion

DIFFERENTIAL DIAGNOSIS

Epithelioid Sarcoma

- Nodular growth predominates, often with necrosis
- Multicentric disease uncommon
- Loss of nuclear INI1
- Keratin (+), EMA(+); CD34(+) in 50% of tumors
- CD31 and FLI-1 (-)

Sarcomatoid Squamous Cell Carcinoma

- Overlying in situ component may be present
- Usually more pronounced cytologic atypia
- p63(+); CD31(-)

Epithelioid Hemangioendothelioma

- Cords and small aggregates of small epithelioid cells
  - Intracytoplasmic lumina common
- Characteristic myxohyaline stroma
- CD31(+), CD34(+), ERG(+), FLI-1(+)
- CAMTA1(+) by immunohistochemistry
- Characteristic t(1;3) with *WWTR1-CAMTA1* fusion

Cellular Fibrous Histiocytoma (Fibrous Histiocytoma)

- Lacks plump, myoid-appearing tumor cells and brisk neutrophilic infiltrate
- Negative for keratin

SELECTED REFERENCES

1. Raftopoulos E et al: Pseudomyogenic hemangioendothelioma: case report and review of the literature. Am J Dermatopathol. 40(8):597-601, 2018
2. Hung YP et al: FOSB is a useful diagnostic marker for pseudomyogenic hemangioendothelioma. Am J Surg Pathol. 41(5):596-606, 2017
3. Walther C et al: A novel SERPINE1-FOSB fusion gene results in transcriptional up-regulation of FOSB in pseudomyogenic haemangioendothelioma. J Pathol. 232(5):534-40, 2014
4. Hornick JL et al: Pseudomyogenic hemangioendothelioma: a distinctive, often multicentric tumor with indolent behavior. Am J Surg Pathol. 35(2):190-201, 2011
5. Billings SD et al: Epithelioid sarcoma-like hemangioendothelioma. Am J Surg Pathol. 27(1):48-57, 2003

(Left) *Sheets of plump eosinophilic spindled cells may naturally bring to mind a myogenic tumor, such as rhabdomyosarcoma or leiomyosarcoma. PMH, however, is negative for desmin and myogenin and does not show diffuse SMA positivity.* **(Right)** *Tumor cell nuclei are mostly round to ovoid, but elongated forms can be seen as well. They contain vesicular chromatin with variably prominent nucleoli. Atypia is generally mild, but occasional cases can show focal marked atypia or nuclear pleomorphism.*

Myoid Appearance

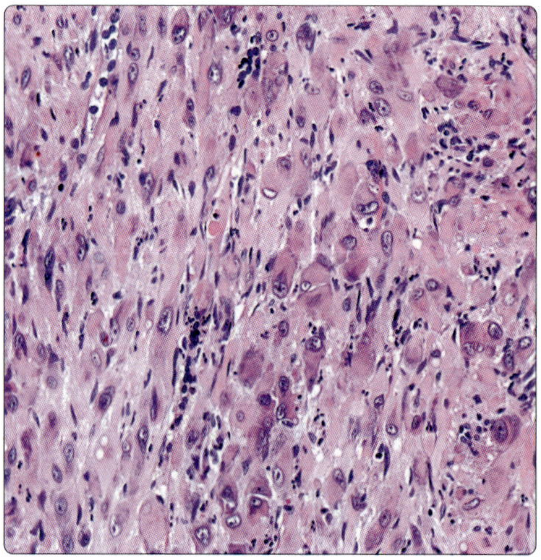

Cytologic Features

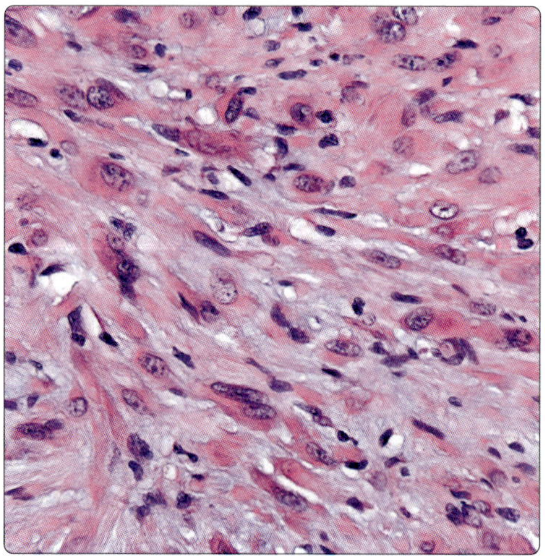

(Left) *In addition to tightly packed, cellular areas, foci of apparent cellular dyscohesion are common in PMH. The stroma varies from fibrous to myxoid and can appear desmoplastic, as depicted.* **(Right)** *Myxoid stroma may be seen in PMH but is usually focal. Note the prominent eosinophilic cytoplasm of the tumor cells in this H&E.*

Loosely Cellular Areas

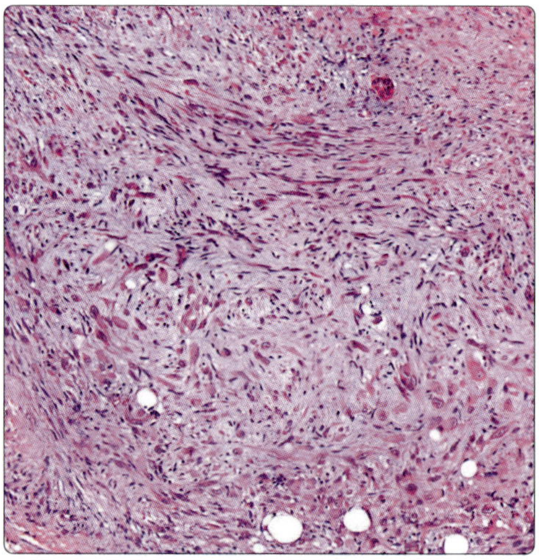

Myxoid Stroma

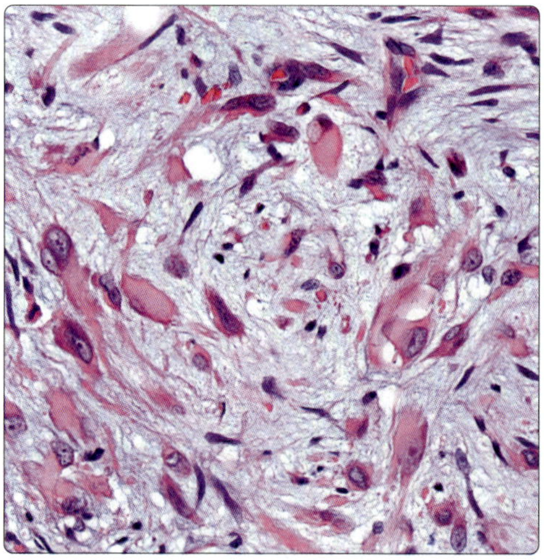

(Left) *A loose fascicular architecture is common in PMH and can result in the tumor being misinterpreted as a spindled epithelioid sarcoma (fibroma-like variant). Fascicles may be better developed in some tumors but rarely to the degree that a fibroblastic sarcoma is considered. Vague storiform growth may also be seen.* **(Right)** *Tumor cells in this fascicular area of PMH are more slender than plump, but more typical cells* ➔ *can still be identified upon close inspection. Note the subtle scattered neutrophils* ↗.

Fascicular Growth

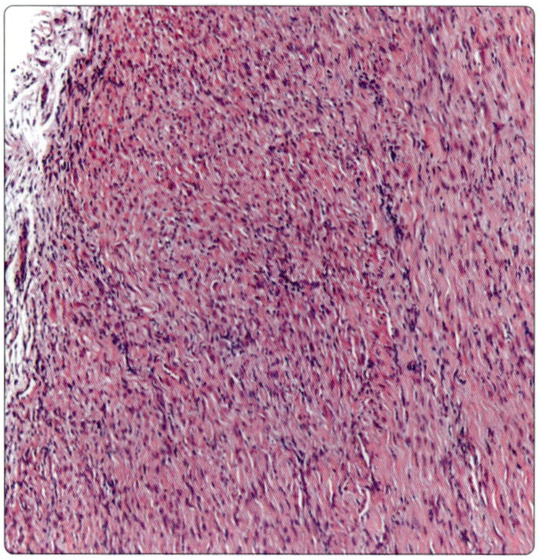

Thinner Spindled Cells

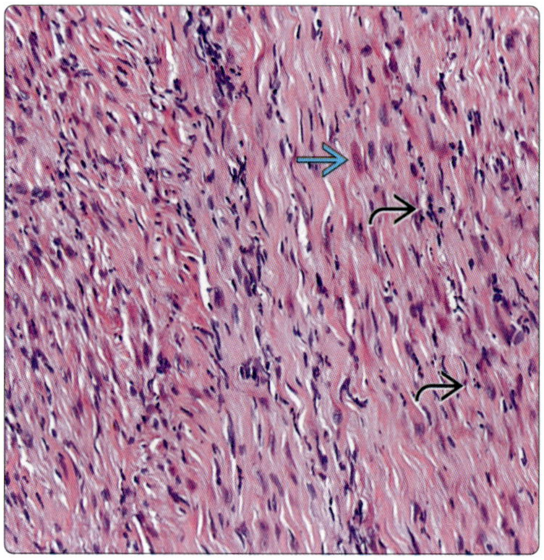

Deceptively Bland Areas

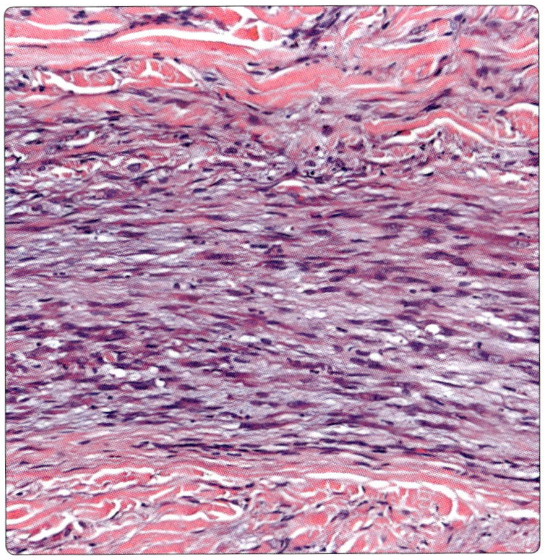

Bony Involvement

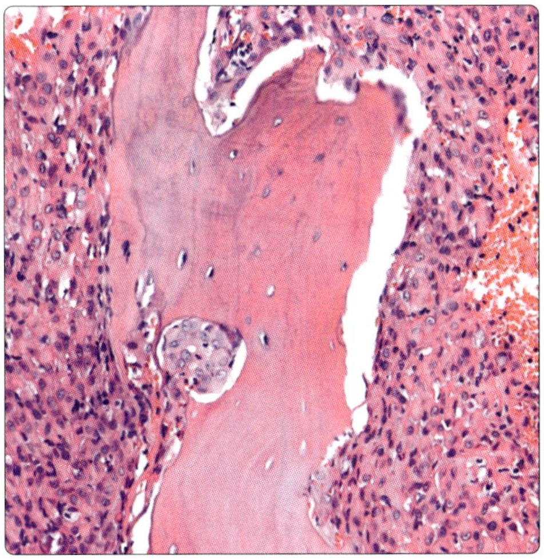

(Left) *Several foci containing slender, spindled tumor cells, as depicted, were found adjacent to the main tumor nodule in this case of PMH. At low power, these areas may be misconstrued as reactive fibroblastic proliferations and not taken into consideration when evaluating the margin status.* **(Right)** *PMH can involve superficial and deep soft tissues, including bone, as depicted. This patient had separate discontiguous tumor nodules in the skin, subcutis, muscle, and bone of the foot and ankle.*

Epithelioid Cytomorphology

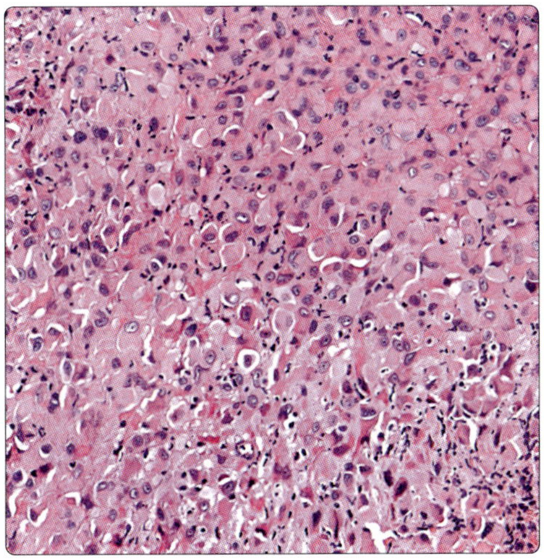

Infiltrative Growth

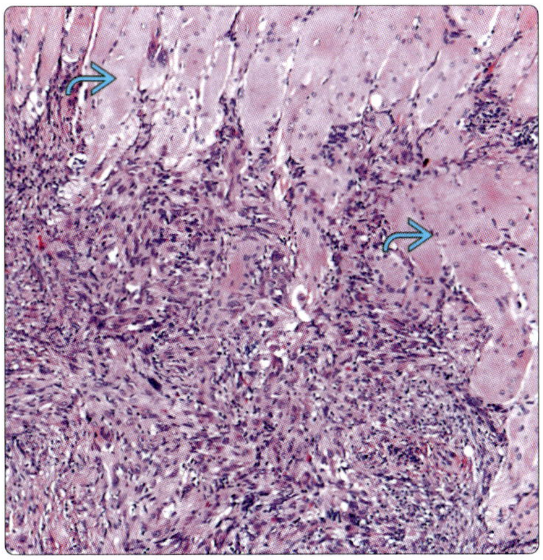

(Left) *A distinct epithelioid cytomorphology is usually present in PMH but is often focal. In conjunction with cytokeratin AE1/AE3 expression, squamous cell carcinoma and epithelioid sarcoma are potential serious misdiagnoses.* **(Right)** *Tumor nodules in PMH are generally poorly defined and often show infiltrative borders microscopically. This H&E shows an intramuscular mass featuring an irregular border with surrounding mature skeletal muscle* ↪.

Frozen Section Tissue

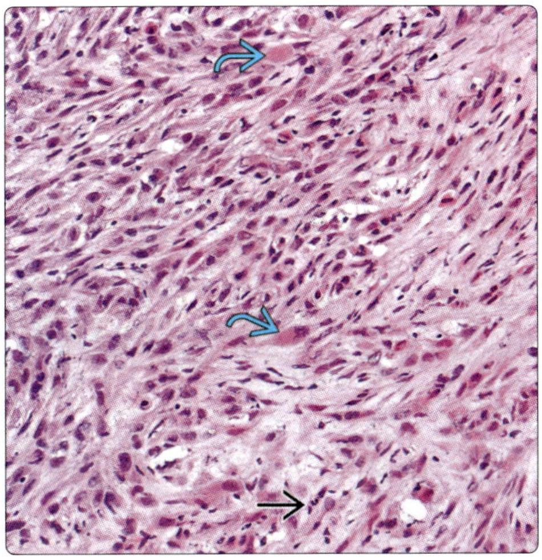

CD31 Expression

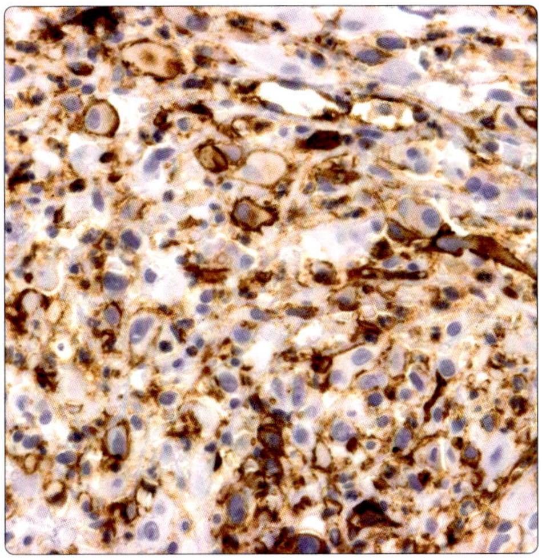

(Left) *Characteristic features of PMH can often be identified even on frozen section. Note the plump tumor cells, scattered rhabdomyoblast-like cells* ↪, *and scattered neutrophils* →. **(Right)** *CD31 positivity is seen in 50% of cases of PMH and shows a true endothelial pattern of expression (strong, linear membranous staining) in contrast to weak, granular staining in histiocytes. ERG and FLI-1 are also positive in PMH; however, CD34 is negative.*

Epithelioid Hemangioendothelioma

KEY FACTS

TERMINOLOGY

- Malignant angiocentric vascular neoplasm composed of epithelioid endothelial cells within characteristic myxohyaline stromal matrix

CLINICAL ISSUES

- Most common: 30-50 years
- Wide distribution in soft tissue
- Also visceral organs (particularly liver and lung)
- Solitary, often painful mass
  - Multicentricity at presentation likely represents locoregional metastases
- Treatment: Wide surgical excision with negative margins
- Indolent clinical course in majority of cases
- Metastases in 20-30%
- Overall mortality rate of 10-20%
  - High-risk tumors are > 3 cm with > 3 mitoses/50 HPF
    - Associated with significant decrease in survival

MICROSCOPIC

- Infiltrative growth with absence of defined lobularity
- Epithelioid eosinophilic cells arranged in cords, nests
  - Intracytoplasmic vacuoles common ("blister cells")
- Well-formed vascular channels typically absent
- Characteristic myxoid to hyaline stromal matrix
- Involvement of larger vessels common

ANCILLARY TESTS

- CD31, CD34, ERG, FLI-1, CAMTA1 (+)
- Nuclear TFE3(+) observed in distinctive genetic subset
- Keratin (+) in up to 35% of cases, often focal
- Molecular: t(1;3)(p36;q25) with *WWTR1-CAMTA1*
  - Distinctive subset contains *YAP1-TFE3* fusion

TOP DIFFERENTIAL DIAGNOSES

- Epithelioid hemangioma
- Epithelioid angiosarcoma
- Composite hemangioendothelioma

(Left) *Epithelioid hemangioendothelioma (EHE) is a distinctive malignant vascular neoplasm characterized by predominant cords of epithelioid tumor cells within a characteristic myoid to hyaline matrix.* **(Right)** *Another characteristic finding in EHE is the presence of intracytoplasmic vacuoles ⇗. Despite their resemblance to fat cells, these spaces actually represent immature vascular lumina and may at times contain erythrocytes →.*

Epithelioid Hemangioendothelioma

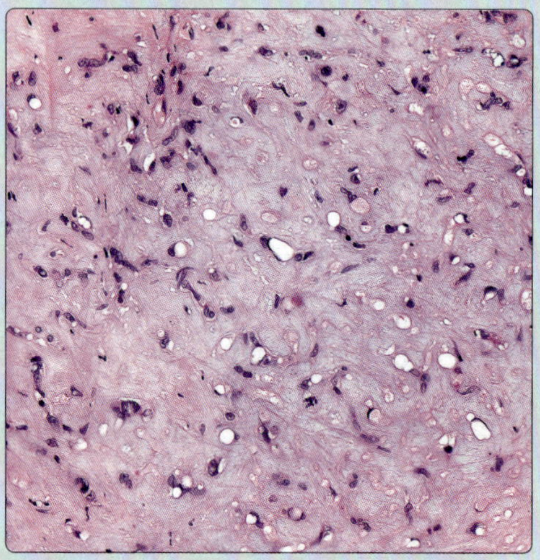

Intracytoplasmic Vacuoles

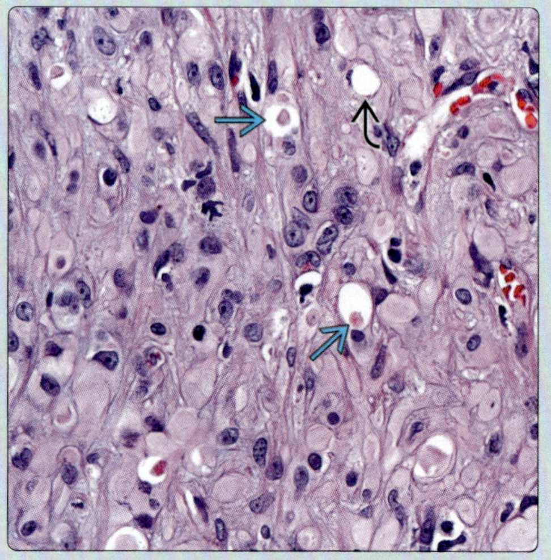

(Left) *EHE is an angiocentric neoplasm, and evidence of origin from a larger vessel may be evident histologically. Note the residual smooth muscle wall → in this hematoxylin and eosin. Tumor cells often extend outward from the involved vessel into the surrounding tissues.* **(Right)** *EHE shows expression of endothelial markers, including CD31 (shown), CD34, ERG, and FLI-1. Nuclear CAMTA1(+) is also present in tumors with CAMTA1 gene fusion. Focal keratin positivity is seen in up to 1/3 of cases.*

Vessel Involvement

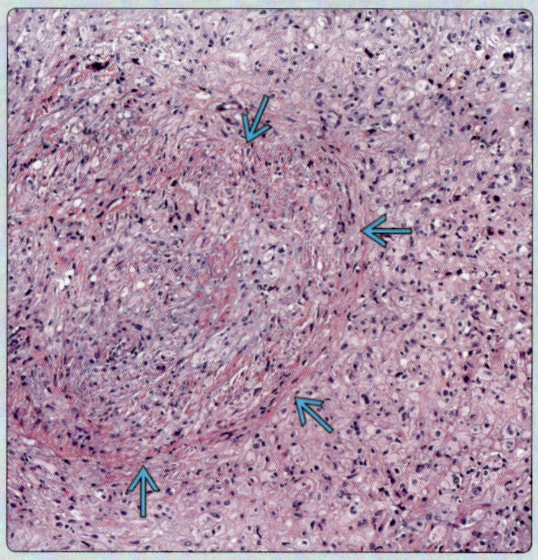

Endothelial Marker Expression

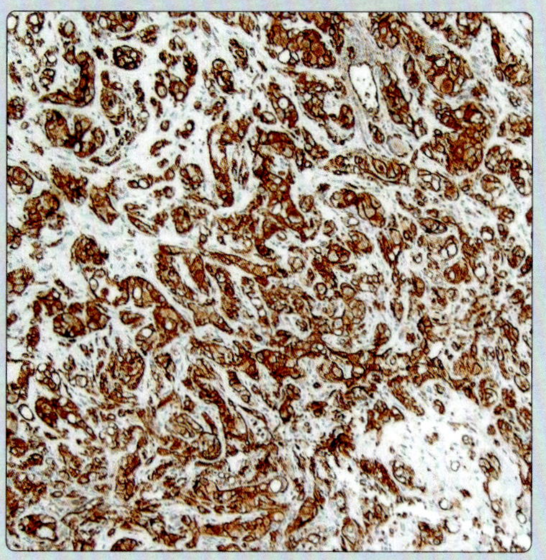

Epithelioid Hemangioendothelioma

TERMINOLOGY

Abbreviations

- Epithelioid hemangioendothelioma (EHE)

Synonyms

- Intravascular bronchioloalveolar tumor (lung)

Definitions

- Malignant angiocentric vascular neoplasm composed of epithelioid endothelial cells within characteristic myxohyaline stromal matrix

CLINICAL ISSUES

Epidemiology

- Incidence
  - Rare
- Age
  - Wide range affected
    - Most common: 30-50 years
    - Rare in childhood
- Sex
  - Slight female predominance

Site

- Wide distribution in soft tissue
  - Extremities, head/neck region, others
- Visceral organs (particularly liver and lung)

Presentation

- Solitary, often painful mass
  - Superficial or deep
  - Rarely cutaneous
- Apparent multicentricity at time of presentation (up to 50% of cases)
  - Recent molecular data supports conclusion of locoregional metastases over multiple primary lesions
- Occlusion of vessels
  - 30-50% of cases arise in or are associated with preexisting vessel
  - May cause more profound vasoocclusive symptoms, including edema

Treatment

- Wide surgical excision with negative margins
- No proven role for adjuvant chemo-/radiotherapy

Prognosis

- Indolent clinical course in majority of cases
  - Local recurrence in 10-15%
- Metastases in 20-30%
  - Usually liver, bone, lungs
  - Occasionally regional lymph nodes
- Overall mortality rate of 10-20%
- Proposed risk assessment
  - High-risk EHE features size > 3 cm and > 3 mitoses per 50 HPF
    - Significant decrease in survival in these cases

MACROSCOPIC

General Features

- Well-circumscribed nodular lesion
- Firm, tan-gray cut surface
- Intravascular tumors may simulate organizing thrombi

Size

- Wide range
  - Mean: 2.5 cm in one large series

MICROSCOPIC

Histologic Features

- Infiltrative growth with absence of defined lobularity
- Epithelioid cells arranged in cords, singly, and in small aggregates or nests
  - Pale to densely eosinophilic cytoplasm
    - Intracytoplasmic vacuoles representing primitive vascular lumina (blister cells)
      - May contain erythrocytes
  - Small, vesicular nuclei ± small nucleoli
    - Occasional tumors show marked nuclear pleomorphism and hyperchromasia
  - Mitotic rate usually low (< 3 figures per 50 HPF)
  - Occasional spindled cytomorphology
- Well-formed vascular channels typically absent
- Characteristic myxoid to hyaline stromal matrix
  - Contains sulfated acid mucopolysaccharides
- Involvement of larger vessels common
  - Obliteration of lumina
  - Outward growth of tumor cells into surrounding tissue
- Metaplastic calcification &/or ossification in some cases
- Necrosis infrequent
- Site-specific unique features (visceral EHE)
  - Lung
    - Characteristic alveolar-filling pattern
    - Central necrosis common
  - Liver
    - Distinct tumor nodules common
    - Entrapped hepatocytes and bile ducts common

Morphologic/Genetic Variant

- EHE with *YAP1-TFE3* fusion
  - Tumor cells often feature more abundant eosinophilic cytoplasm
  - Vasoformation more developed

ANCILLARY TESTS

Immunohistochemistry

- CD31, CD34, ERG, FLI-1 (+)
- CAMTA1(+) in tumors with *CAMTA1* fusion
  - Nuclear TFE3(+) observed in *YAP1-TFE3* fusion subset
- Keratin (+) in up to 35% of cases, often focal
- FOSB, S100 protein, SMA, desmin, CD117, EMA, HMB-45 (-)

Molecular Genetics

- Characteristic t(1;3)(p36;q25) in most cases (90%)
  - Results in *WWTR1-CAMTA1* fusion
- Distinctive subset (5%) contains *YAP1-TFE3* fusion

DIFFERENTIAL DIAGNOSIS

Epithelioid Hemangioma

- Lobular architecture
- Well-formed vascular channels present; plump endothelial cells
- Complete rim of SMA(+) pericytes
- Characteristic mixed chronic inflammatory infiltrate, particularly eosinophils
- FOSB(+) by immunohistochemistry
- Lacks genetic signatures of EHE

Epithelioid Angiosarcoma

- Background of conventional angiosarcoma often present
- Large epithelioid tumor cells in nests or lining irregular vascular spaces
- Mitoses common, include atypical forms
- Frequent tumor necrosis

Composite Hemangioendothelioma

- Rare tumor
- Most occur on distal extremities, particularly hands and feet
- Contains components of at least 2 vascular neoplasms
  - Often retiform hemangioendothelioma and EHE
  - Also, well-differentiated angiosarcoma, spindle cell hemangioma, others

Pseudomyogenic Hemangioendothelioma

- Sheets and fascicles of predominantly plump spindled cells
- Neutrophilic infiltrate common
- Keratin (+) usually diffuse; CD34(-)
- FOSB(+) by immunohistochemistry

Myoepithelioma of Soft Tissue

- Epithelial differentiation evidence in subset (mixed tumor)
- Lacks angiocentric growth
- Usually diffuse keratin (+)
- S100 protein (+) in most cases
- Variable expression of SMA, GFAP, several other markers
- CD31, CD34, ERG (-)

Epithelioid Sarcoma

- Most common in distal extremities of younger patients
- May show granuloma-like growth pattern with centralized necrosis
- Diffuse expression of keratins and EMA
- CD31 (-)
- Loss of nuclear INI1 expression

Extraskeletal Myxoid Chondrosarcoma

- Prominent lobular growth with fibrous septa
- Fibrous pseudocapsule common
- Small, rounded to spindled tumor cells with uniform nuclei
- Prominent myxoid, hypovascular stroma
- Keratin, CD31, CD34, ERG (-)
- Fusions involving *NR4A3* (most commonly to *EWSR1*)

Metastatic Carcinoma

- Clinical history of primary tumor
- Usually higher degree of atypia
- Strong, diffuse keratin (+)
- CD31 and CD34 (-)

Chondroid Lipoma

- Lobular, often encapsulated
- Conspicuous lipogenic component (mature adipocytes, lipoblasts)
- CD31, CD34, keratins (-)

SELECTED REFERENCES

1. Studer LL et al: Hepatic epithelioid hemangioendothelioma. Arch Pathol Lab Med. 142(2):263-267, 2018
2. Thway K et al: Multicentric visceral epithelioid hemangioendothelioma, with extremity dermal deposits, unusual late recurrence on the nasal bridge, and TFE3 gene rearrangement. Hum Pathol. 72:153-159, 2018
3. Sugita S et al: Diagnostic utility of FOSB immunohistochemistry in pseudomyogenic hemangioendothelioma and its histological mimics. Diagn Pathol. 11(1):75, 2016
4. Anderson T et al: Thoracic epithelioid malignant vascular tumors: a clinicopathologic study of 52 cases with emphasis on pathologic grading and molecular studies of WWTR1-CAMTA1 fusions. Am J Surg Pathol. 39(1):132-9, 2015
5. Doyle LA et al: Nuclear expression of CAMTA1 distinguishes epithelioid hemangioendothelioma from histologic mimics. Am J Surg Pathol. 40(1):94-102, 2015
6. Patel NR et al: Molecular characterization of epithelioid haemangioendotheliomas identifies novel WWTR1-CAMTA1 fusion variants. Histopathology. 67(5):699-708, 2015
7. Puls F et al: YAP1-TFE3 epithelioid hemangioendothelioma: a case without vasoformation and a new transcript variant. Virchows Arch. 466(4):473-8, 2015
8. Shibuya R et al: CAMTA1 is a useful immunohistochemical marker for diagnosing epithelioid hemangioendothelioma. Histopathology. 67(6):827-35, 2015
9. Flucke U et al: Epithelioid Hemangioendothelioma: clinicopathologic, immunhistochemical, and molecular genetic analysis of 39 cases. Diagn Pathol. 9:131, 2014
10. Antonescu CR et al: Novel YAP1-TFE3 fusion defines a distinct subset of epithelioid hemangioendothelioma. Genes Chromosomes Cancer. 52(8):775-84, 2013
11. Chevreau C et al: Sorafenib in patients with progressive epithelioid hemangioendothelioma: a phase 2 study by the French Sarcoma Group (GSF/GETO). Cancer. 119(14):2639-44, 2013
12. Mistry AM et al: Diagnostic and therapeutic challenges in hepatic epithelioid hemangioendothelioma. J Gastrointest Cancer. 43(4):521-5, 2012
13. Wang LR et al: Clinical experience with primary hepatic epithelioid hemangioendothelioma: retrospective study of 33 patients. World J Surg. 36(11):2677-83, 2012
14. Murali R et al: Cytologic features of epithelioid hemangioendothelioma. Am J Clin Pathol. 136(5):739-46, 2011
15. Woelfel C et al: Molecular cytogenetic characterization of epithelioid hemangioendothelioma. Cancer Genet. 204(12):671-6, 2011
16. Gill R et al: Utility of immunohistochemistry for endothelial markers in distinguishing epithelioid hemangioendothelioma from carcinoma metastatic to bone. Arch Pathol Lab Med. 133(6):967-72, 2009
17. Clarke LE et al: Cutaneous epithelioid hemangioendothelioma. J Cutan Pathol. 35(2):236-40, 2008
18. Deyrup AT et al: Epithelioid hemangioendothelioma of soft tissue: a proposal for risk stratification based on 49 cases. Am J Surg Pathol. 32(6):924-7, 2008
19. Celikel C et al: Epithelioid hemangioendothelioma with multiple organ involvement. APMIS. 115(7):881-8, 2007
20. Bagan P et al: Prognostic factors and surgical indications of pulmonary epithelioid hemangioendothelioma: a review of the literature. Ann Thorac Surg. 82(6):2010-3, 2006
21. Tsarouha H et al: Chromosome analysis and molecular cytogenetic investigations of an epithelioid hemangioendothelioma. Cancer Genet Cytogenet. 169(2):164-8, 2006
22. Mendlick MR et al: Translocation t(1;3)(p36.3;q25) is a nonrandom aberration in epithelioid hemangioendothelioma. Am J Surg Pathol. 25(5):684-7, 2001
23. Quante M et al: Epithelioid hemangioendothelioma presenting in the skin: a clinicopathologic study of eight cases. Am J Dermatopathol. 20(6):541-6, 1998
24. Mentzel T et al: Epithelioid hemangioendothelioma of skin and soft tissues: clinicopathologic and immunohistochemical study of 30 cases. Am J Surg Pathol. 21(4):363-74, 1997
25. Weiss SW et al: Epithelioid hemangioendothelioma: a vascular tumor often mistaken for a carcinoma. Cancer. 50(5):970-81, 1982

Nested Growth

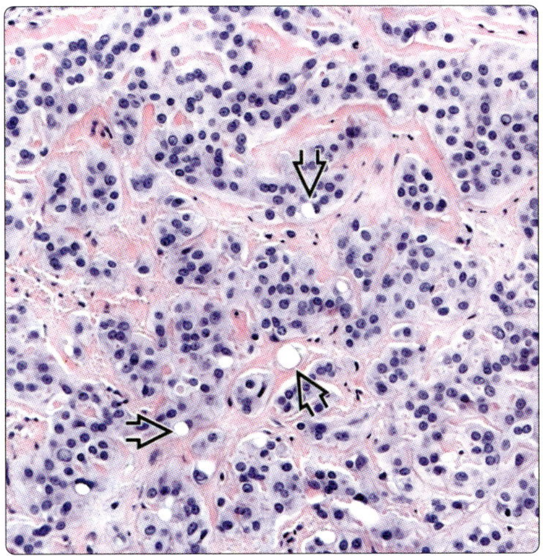

Increased Cellularity

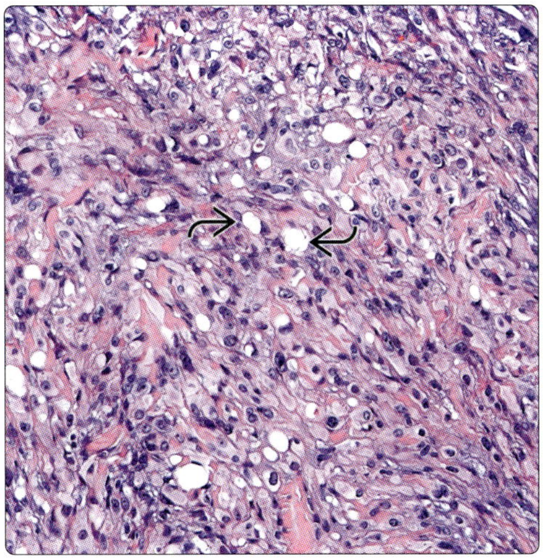

(Left) *In addition to growth in cords and chains, tumor cells in EHE may also be arranged in small aggregates and nests, as depicted. Note the intracytoplasmic vacuoles* ⇨*. Also note that the stroma is more hyaline than myxoid in this hematoxylin and eosin.* **(Right)** *Some cases of EHE feature areas of increased cellularity, as depicted. Note also that some tumor cells can appear to contain multiple intracytoplasmic vacuoles* ➔*, mimicking true lipoblastic cells.*

Spindled Cytomorphology

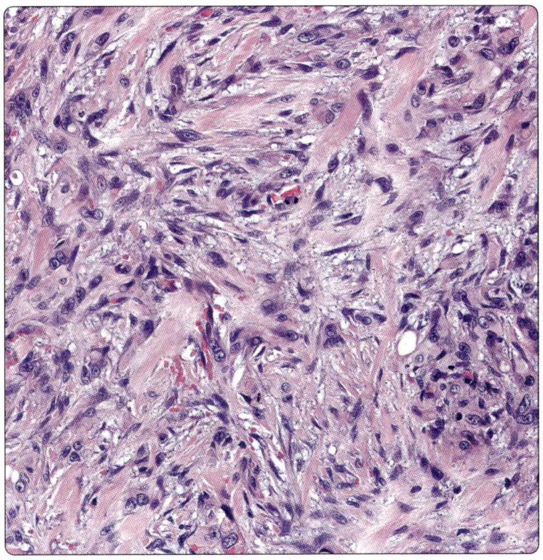

Metaplastic Bone Formation

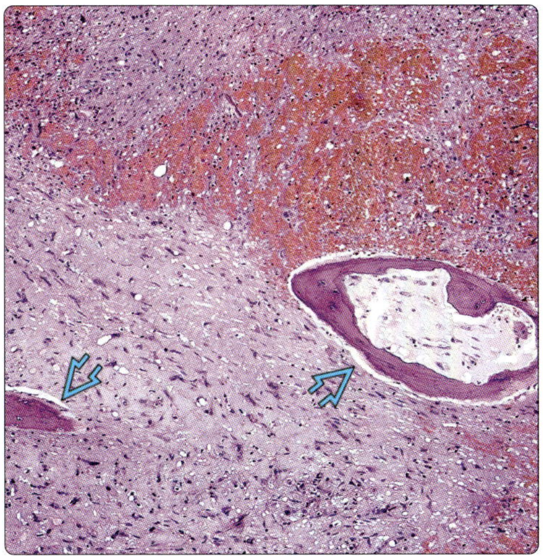

(Left) *Spindling of tumor cells is seen in a minor proportion of cases of EHE. Areas of more conventional epithelioid morphology are usually also present. Increased nuclear atypia may also be seen but does not correlate well with more aggressive behavior. In contrast, increased size and mitotic activity do appear to correlate with reduced survival.* **(Right)** *Foci of metaplastic ossification* ⇨ *may be seen in up to 10% of EHE.*

Hepatic Epithelioid Hemangioendothelioma

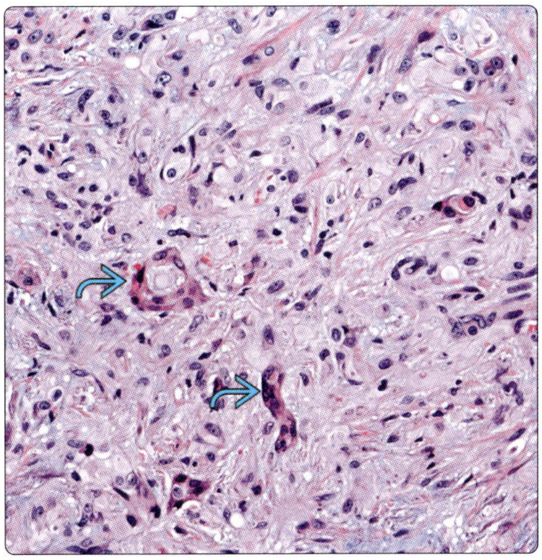

Pulmonary Epithelioid Hemangioendothelioma

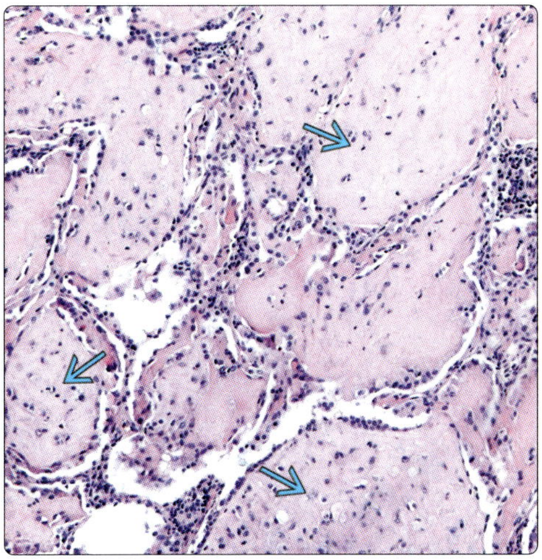

(Left) *Hepatic EHE shows a similar morphology to soft tissue EHE; however, entrapped hepatocytes and reactive bile ducts* ➔ *are often present. Growth as multiple distinct nodules is also more common in this site.* **(Right)** *Pulmonary EHE shows a characteristic alveolar-filling pattern by tumor nodules* ➔*. Central necrosis within tumor nodules is also relatively common.*

Angiosarcoma

KEY FACTS

TERMINOLOGY

- Malignant neoplasm showing morphologic &/or immunophenotypic evidence of vascular/endothelial differentiation

ETIOLOGY/PATHOGENESIS

- Subsets associated with prior radiotherapy, chronic lymphedema, exposure to certain chemicals, certain syndromes

CLINICAL ISSUES

- Wide age range overall (more common in adults)
- Various clinical features depending upon subset
  - Cutaneous scalp/face in elderly, cutaneous breast with history of radiotherapy or chronic lymphedema, parenchymal breast in young women
  - Deep soft tissue forms most common in lower extremity
- Treatment: Aggressive surgical resection with widely negative margins
- Overall poor prognosis (overall survival rate: 30%)
  - Epithelioid angiosarcoma is often more aggressive

MICROSCOPIC

- Infiltrative tumors with dissecting growth through fat and collagen characteristic
- Histologic appearance depends upon degree of vasoformation
- Lesional endothelial cells show variable nuclear atypia; often multilayering
- Morphologic variant: Epithelioid angiosarcoma

ANCILLARY TESTS

- CD31(+), CD34(+), ERG(+), FLI-1(+)
- Keratin (+) in significant subset of epithelioid angiosarcoma

TOP DIFFERENTIAL DIAGNOSES

- Hemangioma
- Atypical vascular lesion
- Kaposi sarcoma

Angiosarcoma

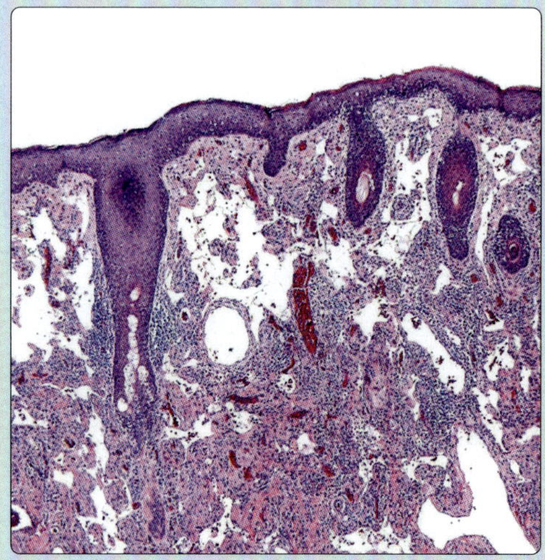

Angiosarcoma

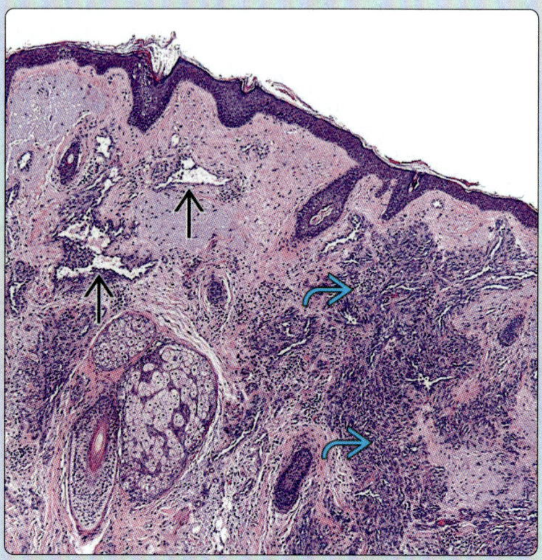

(Left) *Angiosarcoma is an aggressive vascular malignancy that occurs most commonly in adults, especially in cutaneous sites (particularly the scalp and face), but can also involve the breast, deep soft tissues, bone, and visceral organs.* **(Right)** *Depending upon the degree of vasoformation in a given case, some areas of angiosarcoma may appear more clearly vascular (with luminal spaces ➡), and others may appear less well differentiated ➡.*

Infiltrating, Dissecting Growth

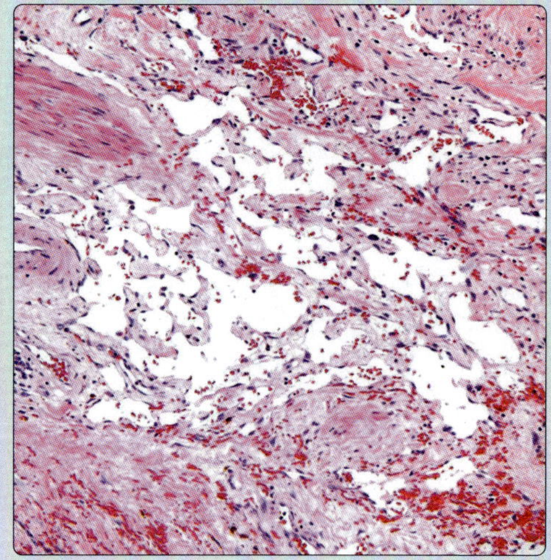

Atypical Endothelial Cells

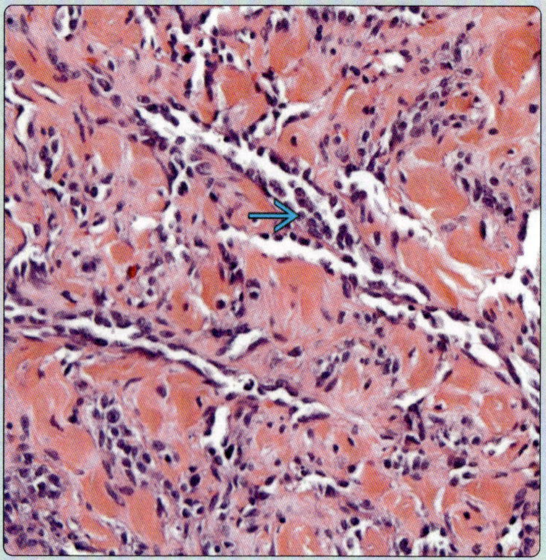

(Left) *Infiltrative and dissecting growth through collagenous connective tissue and adipose tissue by irregularly shaped and anastomosing vascular channels is a characteristic feature of angiosarcoma. The depth and extent of infiltration can be striking.* **(Right)** *The lesional endothelial cells in many cases of angiosarcoma show at least mild nuclear enlargement and hyperchromasia. Multilayering ➡ &/or tufting of nuclei is also a common feature.*

TERMINOLOGY

Synonyms

- Hemangiosarcoma
- Malignant hemangioendothelioma

Definitions

- Malignant neoplasm showing morphologic &/or immunophenotypic evidence of vascular/endothelial differentiation
- Many clinicopathologic subsets (cutaneous, deep soft tissue, radiation or lymphedema associated, breast parenchymal, others)

ETIOLOGY/PATHOGENESIS

Developmental Anomaly

- Develops rarely in association with genetic syndromes
  - Klippel-Trenaunay, Maffucci, neurofibromatosis
  - Often deep soft tissue angiosarcoma

Environmental Exposure

- Associated with exposure to radiation or certain chemicals (e.g., polyvinyl chloride)
- Can arise within setting of chronic lymphedema
- Rarely develops adjacent to foreign material or synthetic vascular grafts

Tumor Associations

- May rarely arise in benign nerve sheath tumors, malignant nerve sheath tumors, germ cell tumors, others

CLINICAL ISSUES

Epidemiology

- Incidence
  - Rare (< 1-2% of all sarcomas)
    - Cutaneous angiosarcoma is most common form
- Age
  - Wide age range overall
    - Cutaneous: 60-80 years most common
    - Breast parenchymal: 30-40 years most common
  - Rare in childhood
- Sex
  - Male predominance in nonbreast cutaneous and deep soft tissue
  - Female predominance in breast (cutaneous and parenchymal)

Site

- Most common site overall is scalp and face (cutaneous type)
  - Superficial cutaneous tumors may also arise elsewhere, including breast and lower extremity
- Deep soft tissue tumors are most common in deep muscles of lower extremity
  - Also retroperitoneum, abdominal cavity, mesentery
- Also arises in breast parenchyma, spleen, liver, heart, bone, other viscera

Presentation

- Cutaneous
  - Dark red or purple nodules, plaques, or bruise-like areas
  - May be multifocal
- Breast
  - May be cutaneous or parenchymal
    - Cutaneous
      - Macroscopically similar to other cutaneous forms
      - Often history of irradiation to breast or chest wall area (short latency, usually < 7 years)
      - Occurrence in setting of postsurgical lymphedema (Stewart-Treves syndrome)
    - Parenchymal
      - Solitary or multiple breast masses
      - May show purple discoloration of overlying skin
- Deep soft tissue
  - Slow-growing, often large, painful mass
  - Hematologic abnormalities (e.g., coagulopathy) in up to 1/3 of cases
  - May also arise within field of previous irradiation

Treatment

- Aggressive surgical resection with widely negative margins
- Chemotherapy

Prognosis

- Overall poor prognosis (overall survival rate: 30%)
  - Local recurrences and distant metastases common
    - Cutaneous disease is often more extensive than clinically/macroscopically apparent
    - Metastases to lung, brain, bone, soft tissue sites, others
  - High mortality rate
- In general, prognosis unrelated to histologic grade
  - Possible exception: Breast parenchymal tumors
- Adverse prognostic factors for deep soft tissue cases: Older age, larger size, high proliferation rate, retroperitoneal origin
- Tumors with prominent epithelioid morphology are often more clinically aggressive than conventional forms

MACROSCOPIC

General Features

- Poorly demarcated or nodular
- Red to brown hemorrhagic cut surface

Size

- Highly variable but often large

MICROSCOPIC

Histologic Features

- Often highly infiltrative and not well demarcated
  - Poorly differentiated areas are often more nodular and better demarcated
- Apparent multifocality within same tissue section is common
- Morphologic appearance depends heavily upon degree of vasoformation
  - Formation of irregular, anastomosing vascular channels in well-differentiated areas
    - Vessels characteristically appear to dissect through collagen, fat, and other soft tissues
      - May entrap fragments of collagen and form intraluminal papillary structures

- Endothelial cell lining may show multilayering or intraluminal tufting
  - Nuclear atypia varies, but hyperchromasia, enlargement, and irregularity are often present
  - Mitotic activity variable, often conspicuous
  - Intracytoplasmic lumina may be present focally
- Back-to-back vascular channels may appear sieve-like
- Solid growth in more poorly differentiated areas
  - Cells may be spindled, epithelioid, or pleomorphic
- Intraluminal erythrocytes and hemorrhage common
- Stromal lymphoid infiltrate may be present
- Pericytes usually absent
- Rare findings: Solid spindle, granular, clear cell, or foamy cell morphology; prominent inflammation

Morphologic Variants

- Epithelioid angiosarcoma
  - More frequent in deep soft tissues
  - Predominantly large epithelioid cells in nests and sheets
    - Abundant eosinophilic cytoplasm
    - Large vesicular nuclei with prominent macronucleoli
  - Irregular vascular spaces lined by protuberant epithelioid cells may also be seen
  - Mitoses often numerous; necrosis common

ANCILLARY TESTS

Immunohistochemistry

- Endothelial differentiation
  - CD31(+), CD34(+), ERG(+), FLI-1(+)
    - Multistain panel recommended, as sensitivity varies
  - Variable D2-40 (podoplanin)
- Keratin (+) in significant subset of epithelioid angiosarcoma
- SMA, desmin, HHV8, CAMTA1 (-)
- Retention of nuclear INI1 expression

Molecular Genetics

- High-level *MYC* (8q24) amplification in radiation-/lymphedema-associated (secondary) tumors
- *FLT4* (VEGFR3) (5q35) amplification in 25% of secondary tumors

DIFFERENTIAL DIAGNOSIS

Hemangioma

- Well-defined lobular architecture
  - No peripheral infiltrative or dissecting growth
- Well-formed vascular channels with bland endothelial cells
  - No endothelial multilayering and tufting

Atypical Vascular Lesion

- Small, solitary, or multiple lesion(s) in previously irradiated skin
  - Small size (median 0.5 cm) of atypical vascular lesion is helpful feature
- Histologically resemble lymphangioma
- Usually no multilayering or significant nuclear atypia

Kaposi Sarcoma

- Predominantly spindled cellular morphology
- Vasoformation generally less developed than in angiosarcoma
- Characteristically HHV8(+)

Retiform Hemangioendothelioma

- Most common in extremities of younger patients
- Slit-like spaces lined by hobnail tumor cells
- Absence of nuclear pleomorphism and multilayering

Atypical Fibroxanthoma

- Small lesion; lacks vasoformation
- CD31, CD34, ERG (-)
  - CD31 stains histiocytes

Papillary Endothelial Hyperplasia

- Generally small lesions
- Bulk of lesion confined to lumen of vessel
- Lacks nuclear atypia, mitoses, and necrosis

Giant Cell Fibroblastoma

- Most common in children
- Cleft-like pseudovascular spaces lined by mononuclear and multinucleated giant cells
- CD34(+) but CD31 and ERG (-)
- Related to dermatofibrosarcoma protuberans

Epithelioid Hemangioendothelioma

- Included in differential diagnosis of epithelioid angiosarcoma
- Lacks well-developed vasoformation
- Characteristic chondromyxoid stroma
- Recurrent t(1;3) involving *CAMTA1* and *WWTR1*

Metastatic Carcinoma or Melanoma

- Can resemble epithelioid angiosarcoma
- Lacks vasoformation
- Diffuse keratin (+) in carcinoma
- Diffuse S100 protein (+) in melanoma

Epithelioid Sarcoma (Proximal Type)

- Can resemble epithelioid angiosarcoma
- Diffuse keratin (+); CD34(+) in 50% of cases
- May express ERG but CD31(-)
- Loss of nuclear INI1 expression

SELECTED REFERENCES

1. Requena C et al: Immunohistochemical and fluorescence in situ hybridization analysis of MYC in a series of 17 cutaneous angiosarcomas: A Single-center study. Am J Dermatopathol. 40(5):349-354, 2018
2. Gervais MK et al: Clinical outcomes in breast angiosarcoma patients: a rare tumor with unique challenges. J Surg Oncol. 116(8):1056-1061, 2017
3. Shustef E et al: Cutaneous angiosarcoma: a current update. J Clin Pathol. 70(11):917-925, 2017
4. Patel SH et al: Angiosarcoma of the scalp and face: the Mayo Clinic experience. JAMA Otolaryngol Head Neck Surg. 141(4):335-40, 2015
5. Suchak R et al: Primary cutaneous epithelioid angiosarcoma: a clinicopathologic study of 13 cases of a rare neoplasm occurring outside the setting of conventional angiosarcomas and with predilection for the limbs. Am J Surg Pathol. 35(1):60-9, 2011
6. Lucas DR: Angiosarcoma, radiation-associated angiosarcoma, and atypical vascular lesion. Arch Pathol Lab Med. 133(11):1804-9, 2009
7. Nascimento AF et al: Primary angiosarcoma of the breast: clinicopathologic analysis of 49 cases, suggesting that grade is not prognostic. Am J Surg Pathol. 32(12):1896-904, 2008
8. Fayette J et al: Angiosarcomas, a heterogeneous group of sarcomas with specific behavior depending on primary site: a retrospective study of 161 cases. Ann Oncol. 18(12):2030-6, 2007
9. Meis-Kindblom JM et al: Angiosarcoma of soft tissue: a study of 80 cases. Am J Surg Pathol. 22(6):683-97, 1998

Subtle Nuclear Atypia

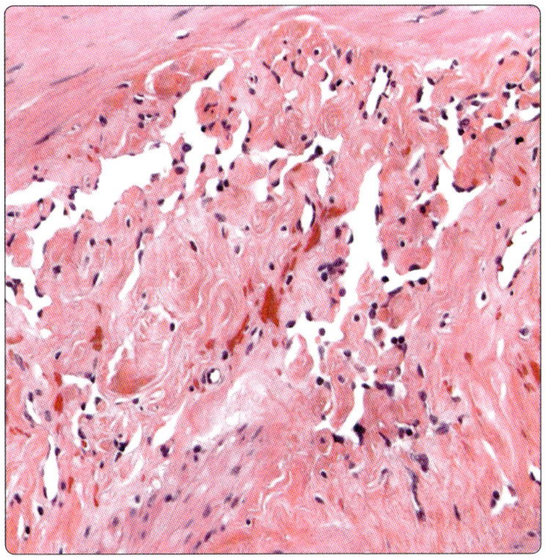

Papillary-Like Structures

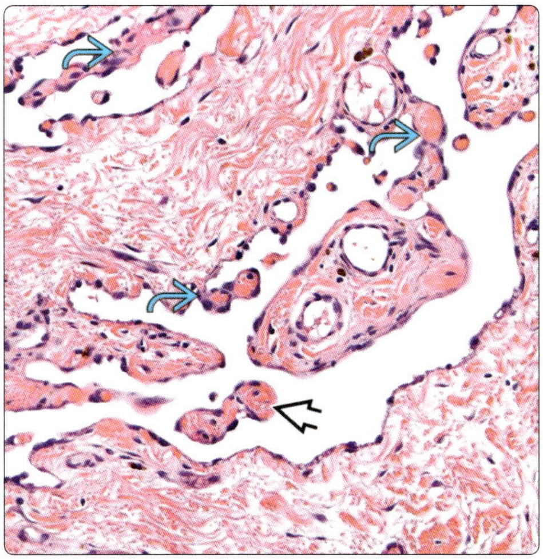

(Left) *In highly differentiated areas of angiosarcoma, the lesional endothelial cells may show very little atypia; however, the irregular and dissecting growth can help establish the diagnosis.* **(Right)** *A common finding in angiosarcoma is variably sized, papillary-like structures composed of collagen lined by lesional endothelial cells. These structures can also appear to float freely within the open vascular spaces.*

Papillary-Like Structures

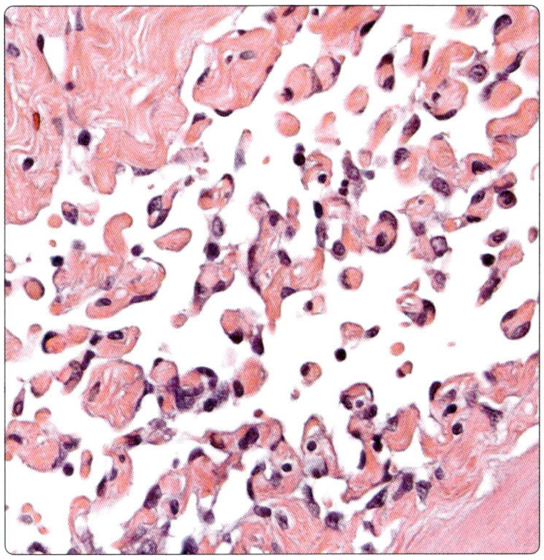

Infiltration of Adipose Tissue

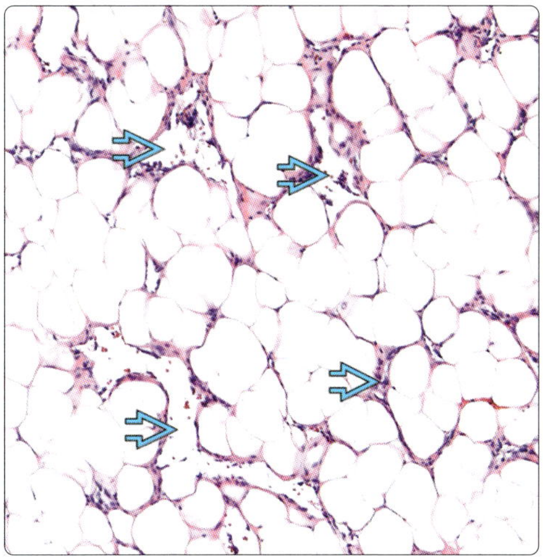

(Left) *In some areas, the papillary-like structures may be abundant and resemble papillary endothelial hyperplasia.* **(Right)** *Angiosarcoma can infiltrate normal subcutaneous adipose tissue and may show extensive or subtle involvement. Note the irregular, infiltrating vascular channels.*

Infiltration of Adipose Tissue

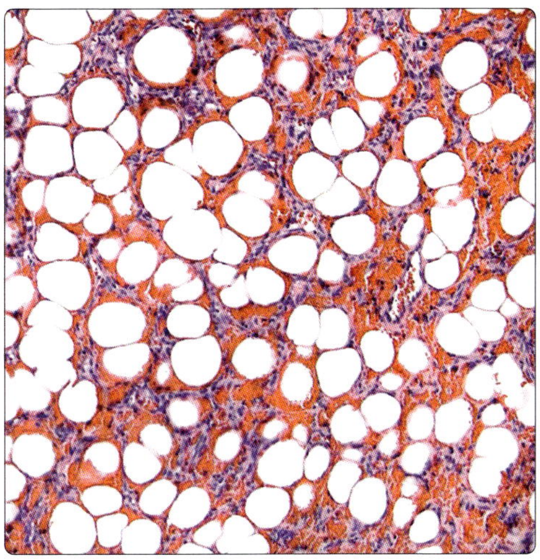

Subtle Cutaneous Involvement

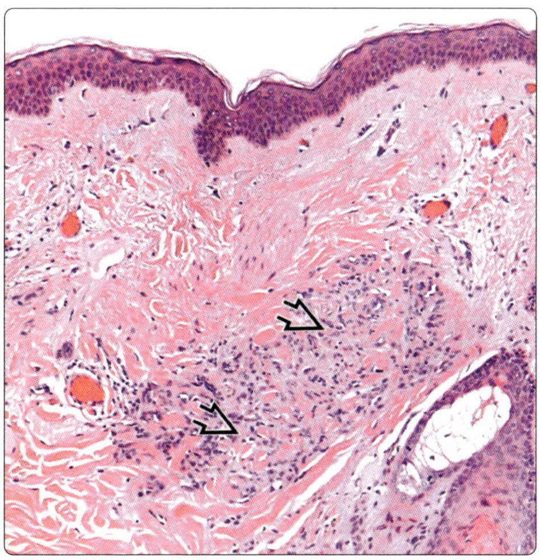

(Left) *H&E of angiosarcoma shows a highly fat-infiltrative tumor with extensive hemorrhage, somewhat obscuring the malignant tumor cells.* **(Right)** *Conspicuous vascular lumina are not present in all areas of angiosarcoma, and identification of subtle tumor foci can be challenging. This appearance can be problematic when evaluating margins by frozen section at the time of surgery.*

(Left) *In some cases of angiosarcoma, the lesional endothelial cells show a much greater degree of nuclear enlargement and hyperchromasia.* **(Right)** *In occasional cases, there is marked nuclear pleomorphism in angiosarcoma. This may lead to consideration of other malignant entities in solid areas in a small biopsy.*

Prominent Nuclear Atypia

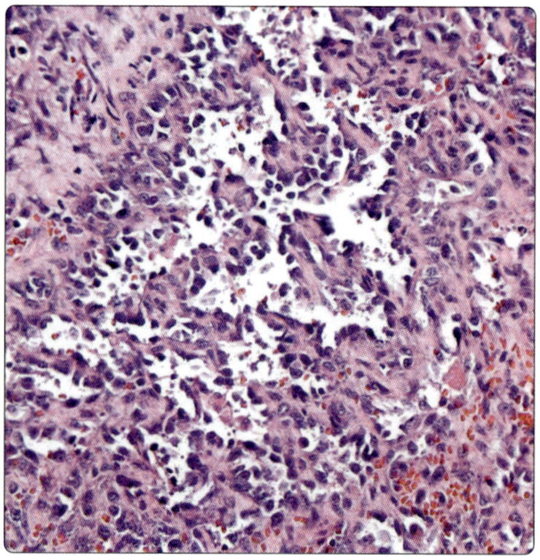

Marked Nuclear Pleomorphism

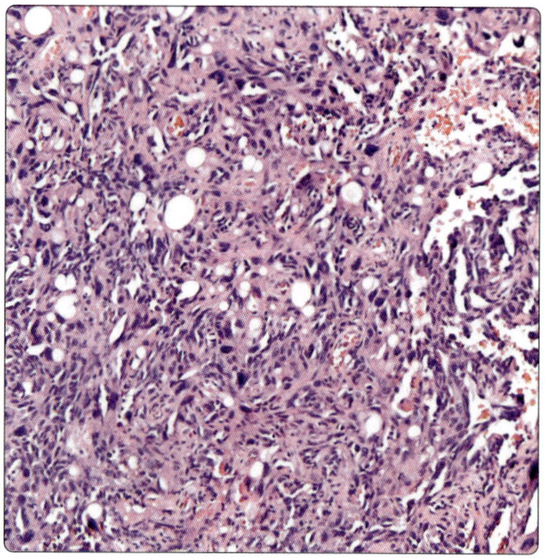

(Left) *A variable degree of vasoformation is a common occurrence in angiosarcoma. Note the more well-differentiated, vasoformative areas (right) and less-differentiated, more solid areas (left).* **(Right)** *Poorly differentiated areas of angiosarcoma often show a greater degree of solid growth; however, vasoformation ➡ is still evident, at least focally.*

Variable Vasoformation

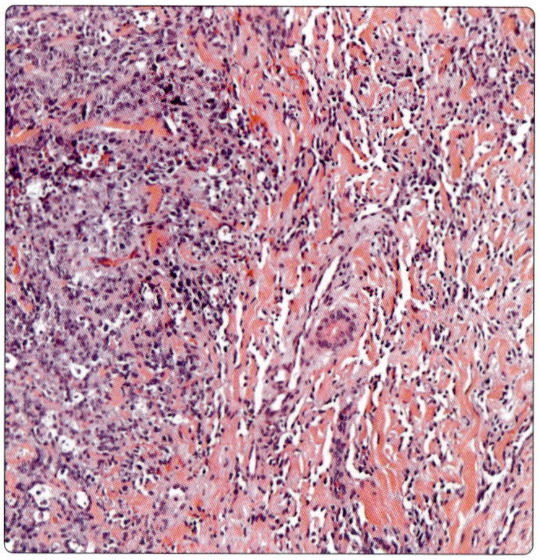

Solid Growth

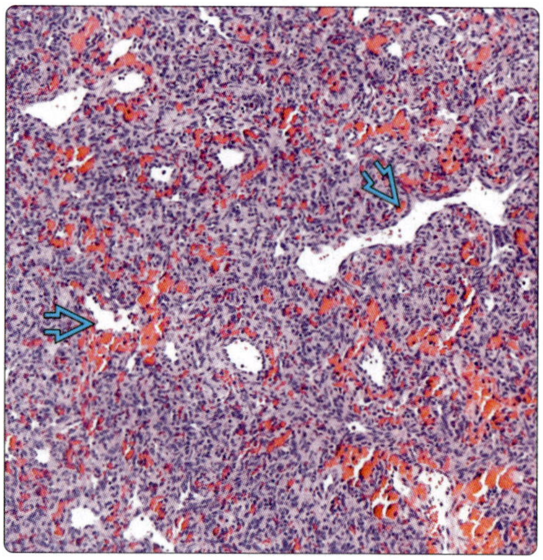

(Left) *A sieve-like or lattice-like growth pattern may be seen in some areas of angiosarcoma. These back-to-back channels may also contain abundant erythrocytes.* **(Right)** *Hemorrhage is not uncommon in angiosarcoma and may be prominent in some cases. It can occasionally be so extensive that the neoplastic cells are obscured and underrecognized.*

Sieve-Like Pattern

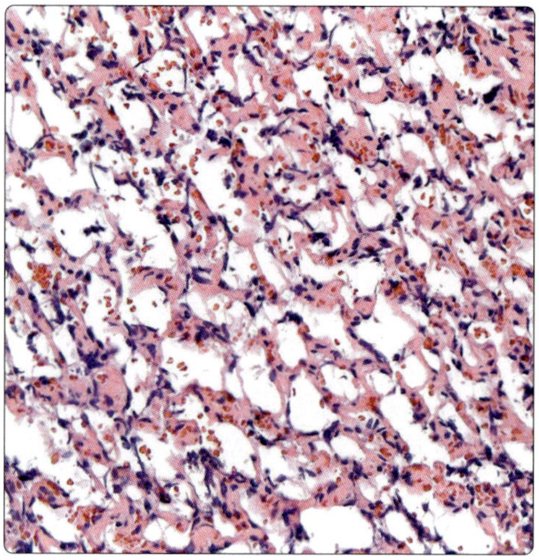

Hemorrhage

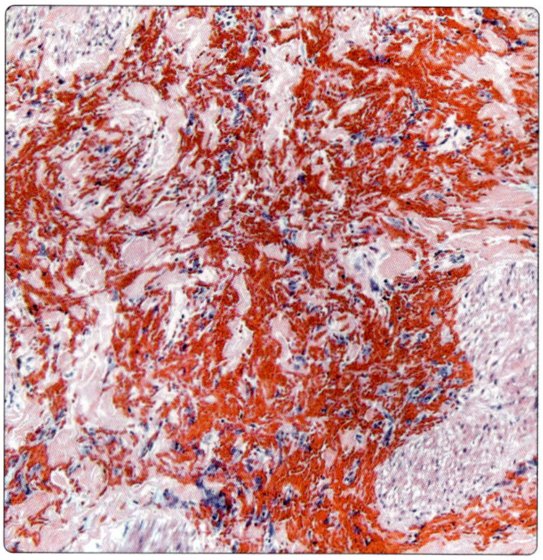

Spindled Morphology

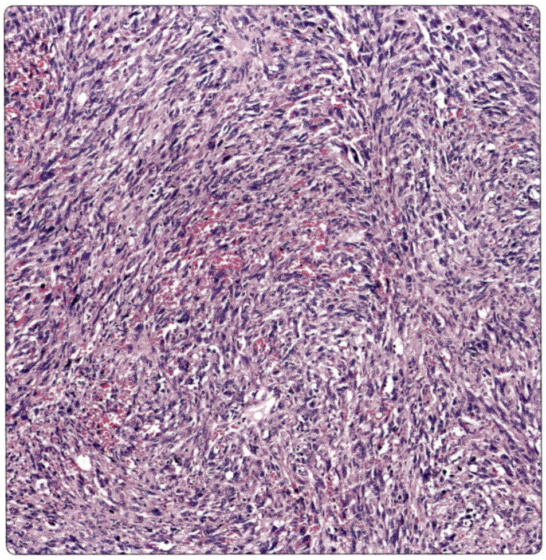

Prominent Inflammation

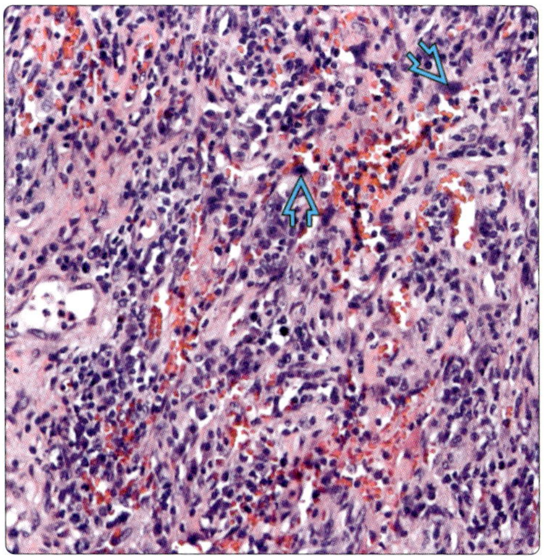

(Left) *A spindled morphology may be seen in poorly differentiated areas of angiosarcoma. It can also be the dominant pattern in rare tumors.* **(Right)** *Stromal chronic inflammatory cells, particularly lymphocytes and plasma cells, may be seen in angiosarcoma, particularly in cutaneous forms. When extensive, it may obscure the underlying neoplasm. Note the hyperchromatic endothelial cell nuclei* ⇨.

Epithelioid Angiosarcoma

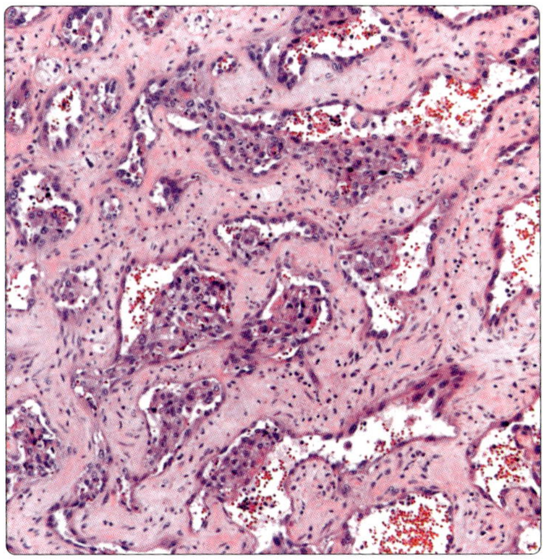

Prominent Epithelioid Morphology

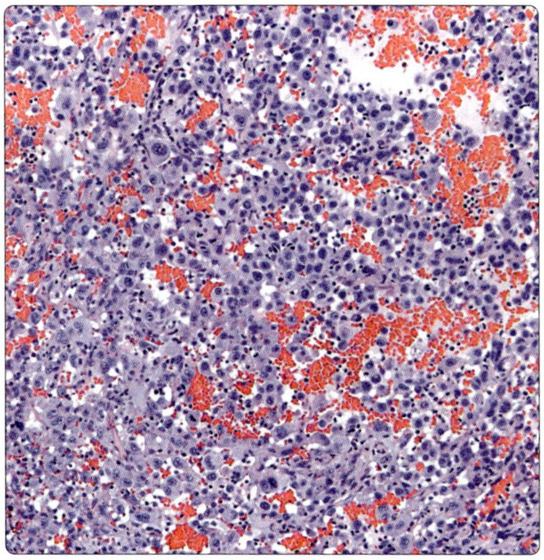

(Left) *The lesional endothelial cells of angiosarcoma may show an epithelioid morphology in some cases; rarely, is it a predominant feature of the tumor. In the latter scenario, the term epithelioid angiosarcoma is often utilized.* **(Right)** *Epithelioid angiosarcoma may mimic a variety of epithelioid neoplasms, including, carcinoma, melanoma, and epithelioid sarcoma. Immunohistochemistry is often necessary.*

Macronucleoli

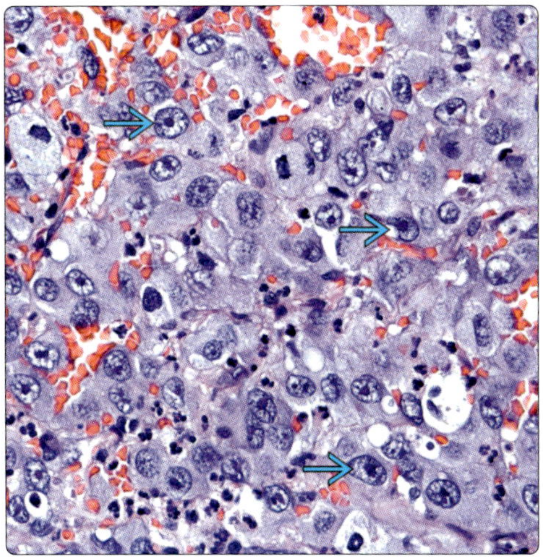

Epithelioid Angiosarcoma

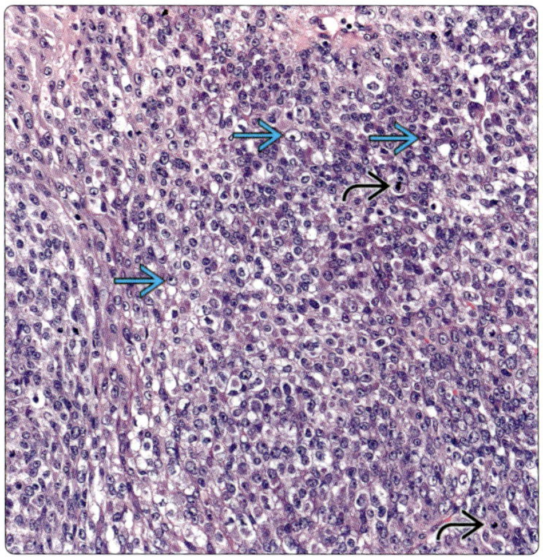

(Left) *A characteristic finding in epithelioid angiosarcoma is the presence of enlarged vesicular nuclei with prominent macronucleoli* →. **(Right)** *In some cases of epithelioid angiosarcoma, the malignant cells form diffuse sheets. Prominent nucleoli* → *and mitotic figures* ↪ *are evident even at this magnification.*

Kaposi Sarcoma

KEY FACTS

TERMINOLOGY

- Vascular neoplasm (usually low grade) caused by HHV8

CLINICAL ISSUES

- Sites: Skin (majority), mucosa, lymph nodes, organs
- Clinical variants
  - Classic: Lower legs/feet of elderly (M > F); indolent
  - African/endemic: Children/adults in equatorial Africa
  - Iatrogenic: Immunosuppressed patients of any age
  - AIDS associated: Aggressive (often disseminated)
- Many modalities for symptom control but no cure

MICROSCOPIC

- Patch stage
  - Infiltrative interconnected vascular channels dissect dermal collagen; scattered plasma cells (useful clue)
- Plaque stage
  - Spindle cell proliferation infiltrating dermis and invading/destroying eccrine glands
- Tumor stage
  - Nodules with intersecting fascicles of spindle cells
  - Blood-filled, slit-/sieve-like spaces between spindle cells

ANCILLARY TESTS

- Positive HHV8 (LANA1) in essentially 100%

TOP DIFFERENTIAL DIAGNOSES

- Angiosarcoma
- Severe vascular stasis (acroangiodermatitis)
- Hobnail (targetoid hemosiderotic) hemangioma
- Microvenular hemangioma
- Spindle cell hemangioma
- Kaposiform hemangioendothelioma
- Acquired tufted angioma
- Progressive lymphangioma
- Cellular fibrous histiocytoma
- Leiomyosarcoma (cutaneous)

(Left) *Classic Kaposi sarcoma is shown presenting as diffuse erythematous and hyperpigmented plaques and nodules on the lower extremities of this elderly male patient. (Courtesy J. McMichael, MD.)* **(Right)** *Earlier lesions of Kaposi sarcoma display increased numbers of irregular vascular channels infiltrating the dermis. Hemorrhage is evident even at low power* ➡*.*

Classic Kaposi Sarcoma

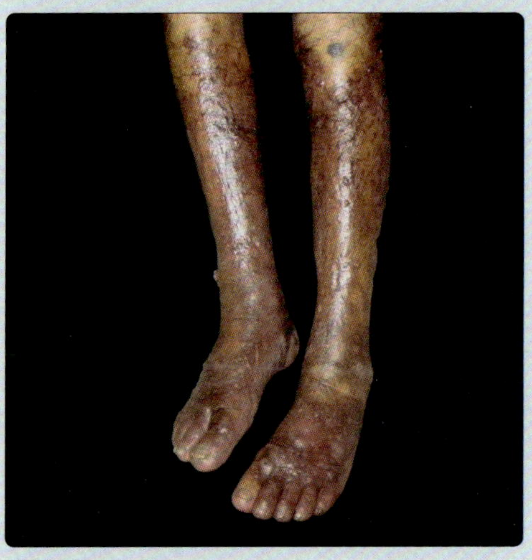

Infiltrating Vascular Channels

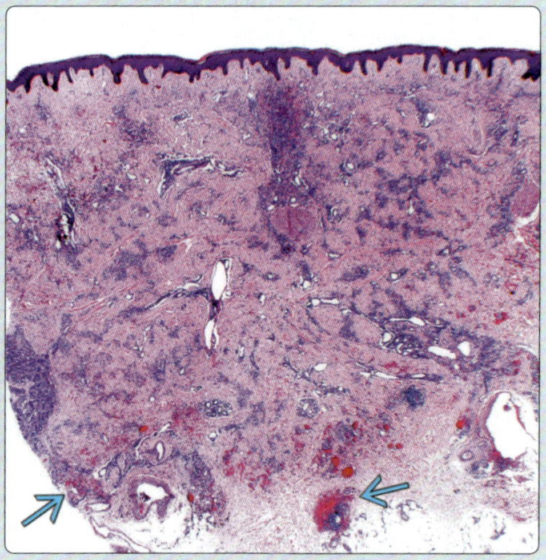

(Left) *In addition to vascular channels, infiltrative spindle cells with hemorrhage are present in the plaque stage of Kaposi sarcoma. These have a tendency to infiltrate and destroy the eccrine sweat coils.* **(Right)** *In later stage lesions of Kaposi sarcoma, spindled endothelial cells form fascicles with intervening slit- and sieve-like vascular spaces containing numerous erythrocytes.*

Infiltrative Growth

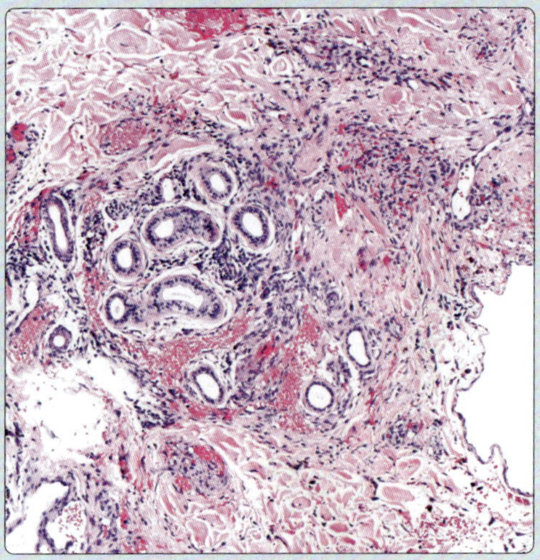

Slit- and Sieve-Like Spaces

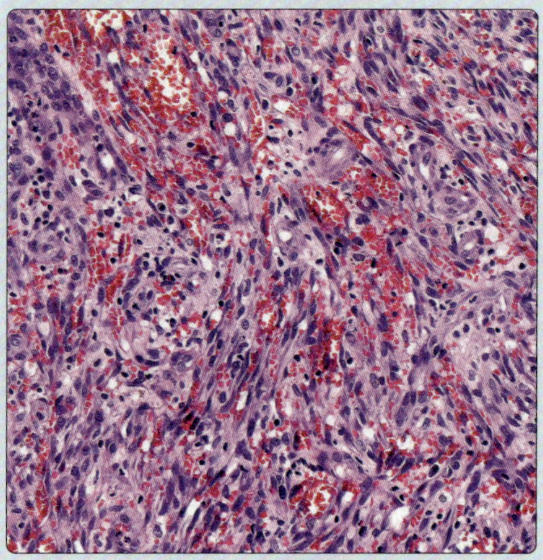

TERMINOLOGY

Abbreviations

- Kaposi sarcoma (KS)

Definitions

- Locally aggressive vascular proliferation (usually low grade) caused by human herpes virus 8 (HHV8)

ETIOLOGY/PATHOGENESIS

Infectious Agents

- All forms of KS are caused by HHV8
  - HHV8 detectable in 100% of KS
  - HHV8 present in tumor cells and peripheral blood

CLINICAL ISSUES

Presentation

- Most cases involve skin
  - Also can involve mucosa, lymph nodes, visceral organs
- Multiple lesions may arise in different sites simultaneously
  - Multifocality does not necessarily represent metastatic spread in a classic sense
- 3 stages
  - Patch stage: Red or violaceous macules coalescing into patches
  - Plaque stage: Thickened red/blue/purple/brown plaques
  - Tumor stage: Larger nodules arise from plaques; may ulcerate and simulate pyogenic granuloma clinically
- Stages are same regardless of clinical variant of KS; stages may coexist with one another

Natural History

- Clinical variants of KS
  - Classic
    - Elderly men (90%), usually nodules/plaques on feet and lower legs
    - Most prevalent regions: Mediterranean, East European, and central equatorial Africa
      - Rare in USA
    - Often associated with underlying malignancy, usually hematologic
    - Indolent behavior: Slow growth over years
      - Lymph node or organ involvement uncommon
  - African (endemic)
    - Young children and middle-aged adults in equatorial Africa
    - May be associated with podoconiosis (endemic lymphedema from barefoot soil exposure)
    - **Not** associated with HIV
    - Multiple skin nodules/tumors of lower legs progressing over many years
    - Aggressive, often fatal, disease if lymph node involvement (lymphadenopathic form)
  - Iatrogenic
    - Occurs in immunosuppressed patients of any age
    - Skin and mucosal involvement common; may be disseminated with organ involvement
    - Variable behavior
  - AIDS associated
    - Occurs in patients coinfected by HIV-1 and HHV8
      - Specific predilection for homosexual men and IV drug users with HIV
      - In Africa, has equal M:F incidence among HIV-positive patients
    - Usually patch stage at presentation with subsequent progression
    - Predilection for skin of face, genitals, lower extremities
    - Frequently disseminated with involvement of mucosa, lymph nodes, organs
    - Most aggressive type of KS

Treatment

- No cure for KS
- Wide variety of treatment options for symptom reduction, prevention of disease progression, &/or cosmesis
  - Surgical excision (only for individual more symptomatic lesions, not for complete excision of all lesions)
  - External beam radiation
  - Cryo-, laser, or photodynamic therapy
  - Topical or intralesional drugs
  - Systemic chemotherapy only in more severe scenarios
- In AIDS-associated KS, lesions may regress or flare with antiretroviral therapy
- In Iatrogenic KS, lesions may regress (sometimes entirely) once immunosuppression removed

Prognosis

- Depends on epidemiological/clinical type of KS
- Strongly related to stage of disease
- Strongly related to coexisting infectious diseases

MICROSCOPIC

Histologic Features

- Differ by stage of disease but not by clinical/epidemiological type
- Distinction of stages not required by pathologist but are useful for recognition of varying histologic patterns in KS
- Patch stage
  - Increased "jagged" interconnected vascular channels in reticular dermis
    - Dissecting/wrapping collagen bundles
    - Growing around adnexa
    - Growing around normal vessels ("promontory" sign is characteristic but uncommon finding)
    - Lined by uniform endothelial cells with minimal atypia
  - Scattered plasma cells (very useful clue) and lymphocytes
  - Extravasated erythrocytes and hemosiderin deposits
- Plaque stage
  - More extensive vascular proliferation
  - Increased inflammatory infiltrate with plasma cells
  - Spindle cell proliferation infiltrating dermis and invading/destroying eccrine glands
- Tumor stage
  - Nodules of spindle cells arranged in intersecting fascicles
  - Blood-filled slit- and sieve-like spaces between spindle cells
    - When blood-filled spaces absent, may be difficult to recognize as vascular tumor

- Mitoses often prominent, but nuclear atypia only mild-moderate usually
  - If severe atypia, consider spindled angiosarcoma
  - In AIDS, KS may have more atypical areas similar to angiosarcoma
- Intracytoplasmic hyaline globules in spindle cells
  - Some suggest these are degenerated erythrocytes
- Inflammatory infiltrate with plasma cells usually present

- Other unique histologic variants
  - Lymphangioma-like: Bulla-like clinical appearance, dilated lymphatic-like channels similar to lymphangioma
  - Hemangioma-like: Larger dilated blood-filled spaces similar to hemangioma
  - Poorly differentiated: Pleomorphism and numerous mitoses (more common in Africa)

ANCILLARY TESTS

Immunohistochemistry

- Positive for endothelial and lymphatic markers
  - CD31, CD34, ERG, D2-40 (podoplanin), PROX1, FLI1
- Nuclear HHV8 (LANA1) positive in essentially 100% (punctate, speckled, or granular pattern of nuclear staining is classic)
  - Essentially all other vascular proliferations are HHV8 negative

DIFFERENTIAL DIAGNOSIS

Angiosarcoma

- Different clinical scenario
- Anastomosing infiltrating vascular channels lined by markedly atypical endothelium with multilayering
  - Negative for HHV8

Severe Vascular Stasis (Acroangiodermatitis)

- Very similar clinical and histologic appearance to KS
  - Violaceous plaques on lower extremities
  - Increased vascular channels and spindle cells in dermis
  - Extravasated RBCs and hemosiderin
- Dermal spindle cells are fibroblasts (not spindled endothelial cells like KS)
  - Negative for vascular markers: CD31, ERG, etc.
- Negative for HHV8 (in vessels and spindle cells)

Hobnail (Targetoid Hemosiderotic) Hemangioma

- Solitary vascular lesion of skin
- Dilated lymphatic-like channels with bland hobnail endothelium in superficial dermis
- Compressed vessels trickle into underlying dermis
  - Apparently "infiltrative" thin vessels can mimic KS
- Negative for HHV8

Microvenular Hemangioma

- Solitary vascular lesion of skin
- Compressed vascular channels trickle between dermal collagen (similar to hobnail hemangioma)
  - Apparently "infiltrative" thin vessels can mimic KS
- Negative for HHV8

Spindle Cell Hemangioma

- Subcutaneous (or dermal) nodule(s), usually in leg
- Biphasic pattern
  - Cavernous zone: Similar to cavernous hemangioma
  - Cellular zone: Spindled endothelium and compressed vascular spaces can resemble KS
    - No mitoses, hemorrhage, plasma cells
    - Epithelioid endothelium with vacuoles resembling miniature adipocytes (not seen in KS)
- Negative for HHV8

Kaposiform Hemangioendothelioma

- Infants and young children (vast majority)
  - Very rare in skin of adults
- Whorled nodules of spindled endothelium with slit-like vascular channels
  - No mitoses, hemorrhage, plasma cells
  - Whorled nodular pattern not seen in KS
- Negative for HHV8

Acquired Tufted Angioma

- Solitary skin lesion in adults
- Histologically identical to kaposiform hemangioendothelioma
- Negative for HHV8

Progressive Lymphangioma (Benign Lymphangioendothelioma)

- Slowly growing, solitary, patch or plaque
- Infiltrative channels with bland lymphatic endothelium
- No spindle cells, hemorrhage, plasma cells
- Negative for HHV8

Cellular Fibrous Histiocytoma (Cellular Dermatofibroma)

- Dermatofibroma with intersecting hypercellular fascicles
  - Similar fascicles in paucivascular tumor stage KS
- Epidermal hyperplasia, peripheral collagen trapping, and other features of dermatofibroma present
- Lacks infiltrative vascular channels
- Negative for HHV8 and vascular markers

Leiomyosarcoma (Superficial/Cutaneous)

- Intersecting fascicles of atypical smooth muscle cells
  - Similar fascicles in paucivascular tumor stage KS
- SMA and desmin positive
- Negative for HHV8 and vascular markers

SELECTED REFERENCES

1. Vangipuram R et al: Epidemiology of Kaposi sarcoma: review and description of the nonepidemic variant. Int J Dermatol. ePub, 2018
2. Schnebelen AM et al: Benign lymphangioendothelioma presenting as a giant flank mass. J Cutan Pathol. 42(3):217-21, 2015
3. Chadburn A et al: Molecular and immunohistochemical detection of Kaposi sarcoma herpesvirus/human herpesvirus-8. Methods Mol Biol. 999:245-56, 2013
4. Dittmer DP et al: Kaposi sarcoma associated herpesvirus pathogenesis (KSHV)–an update. Curr Opin Virol. 3(3):238-44, 2013
5. Radu O et al: Kaposi sarcoma. Arch Pathol Lab Med. 137(2):289-94, 2013
6. Miettinen M et al: Prox1 transcription factor as a marker for vascular tumors-evaluation of 314 vascular endothelial and 1086 nonvascular tumors. Am J Surg Pathol. 36(3):351-9, 2012
7. Rosado FG et al: Utility of immunohistochemical staining with FLI1, D2-40, CD31, and CD34 in the diagnosis of acquired immunodeficiency syndrome-related and non-acquired immunodeficiency syndrome-related Kaposi sarcoma. Arch Pathol Lab Med. 136(3):301-4, 2012
8. Grayson W et al: Histological variants of cutaneous Kaposi sarcoma. Diagn Pathol. 3:31, 2008

Nodules of Classic Kaposi Sarcoma

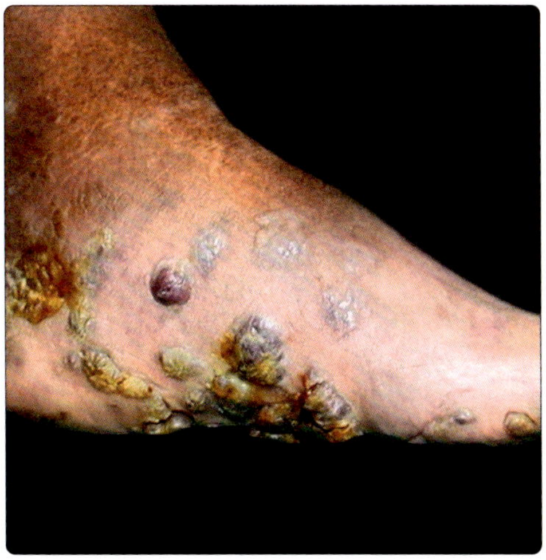

AIDS-Associated Kaposi Sarcoma

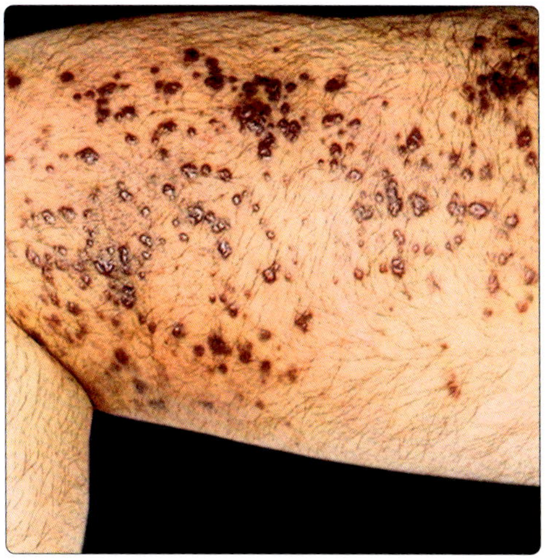

(Left) *Classic Kaposi sarcoma arising in an elderly man who presented with multiple violaceous and hyperkeratotic nodules on the foot.* **(Right)** *Photograph shows an HIV-positive patient exhibiting multiple erythematous to violaceous patches and coalescing papules on the thigh.*

Early Kaposi Sarcoma

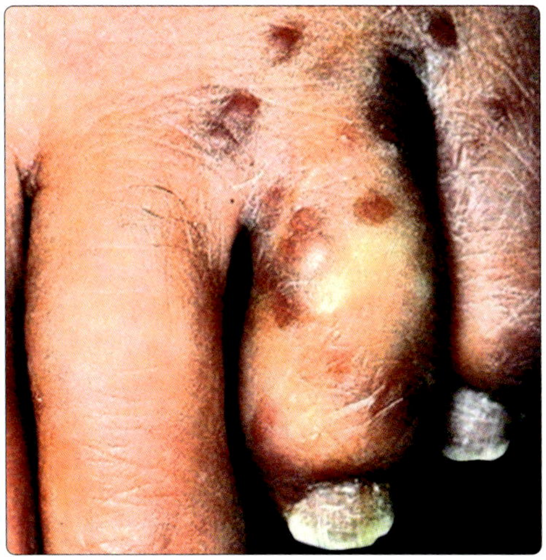

Patch Stage Kaposi Sarcoma

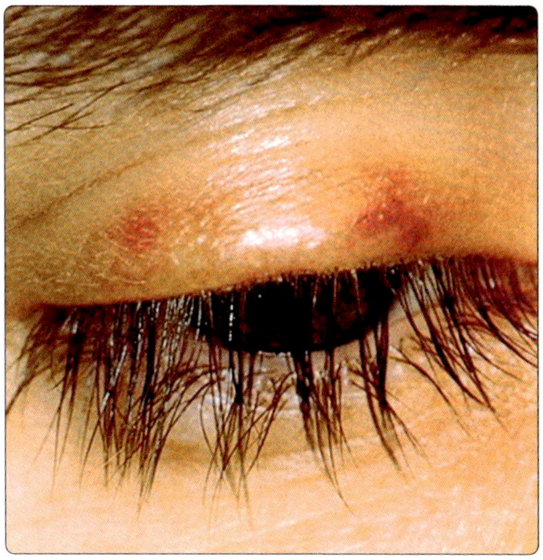

(Left) *Early forms of Kaposi sarcoma may be subtle and difficult to diagnose clinically. This elderly patient developed multiple erythematous macules and slightly elevated papules on the toe.* **(Right)** *Patients with AIDS-associated Kaposi sarcoma may present with lesions at unusual anatomic sites, as did this young patient who developed small erythematous patches on his upper eyelid.*

Classic Kaposi Sarcoma

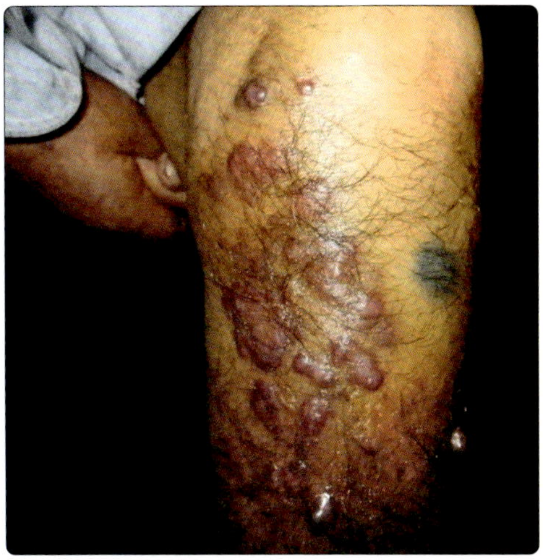

Patch Stage Kaposi Sarcoma

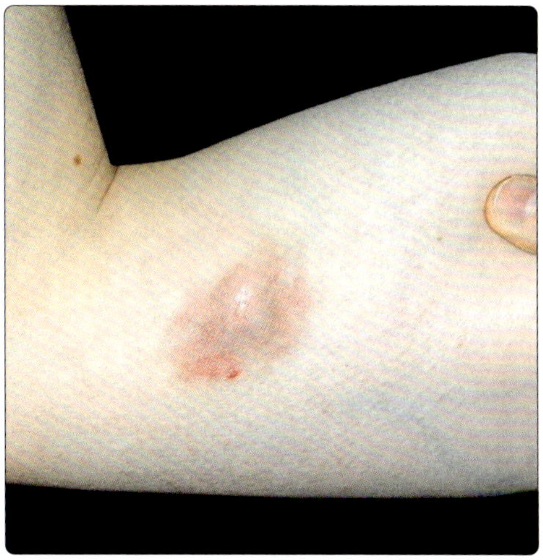

(Left) *Photograph shows multiple erythematous nodules and plaques of classic Kaposi sarcoma in an elderly male patient. (Courtesy J. McMichael, MD.)* **(Right)** *A 30-year-old male patient with HIV presented with an irregularly shaped erythematous to violaceous patch on the upper arm. The lesion proved to be Kaposi sarcoma.*

Increased Numbers of Vessels

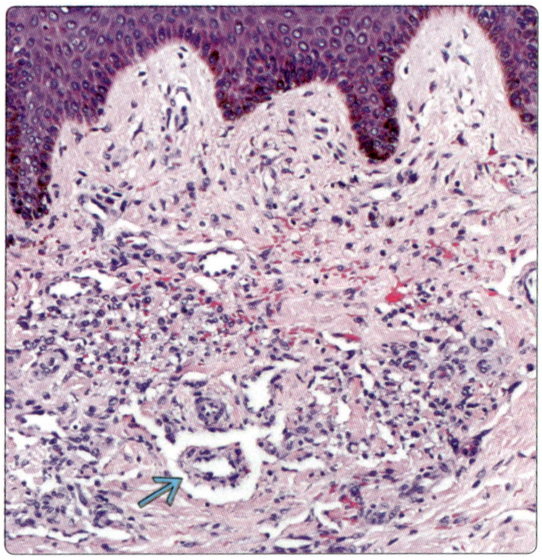

Inflammation

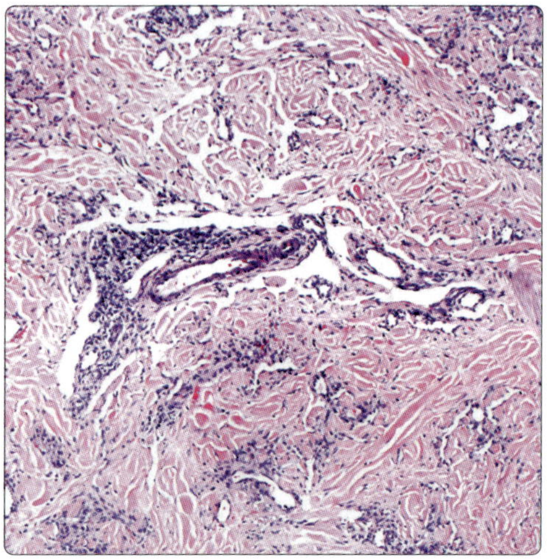

(Left) *Earlier lesions of Kaposi sarcoma display increased numbers of irregular vascular channels and spindle cells infiltrating the dermis. Hemorrhage is present. Some preexisting dermal vessels protrude into the lumen of dilated Kaposi sarcoma vascular channels (promontory sign)* →. **(Right)** *Increased numbers of irregular vascular channels infiltrate the dermis. Mixed inflammation is also present.*

Promontory Sign

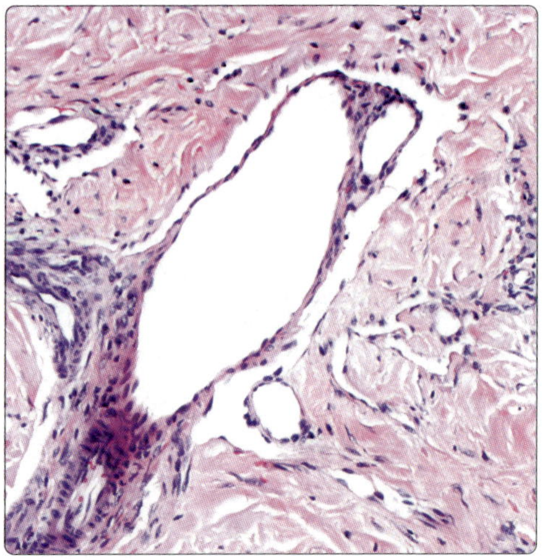

Infiltrative Spindle Cells

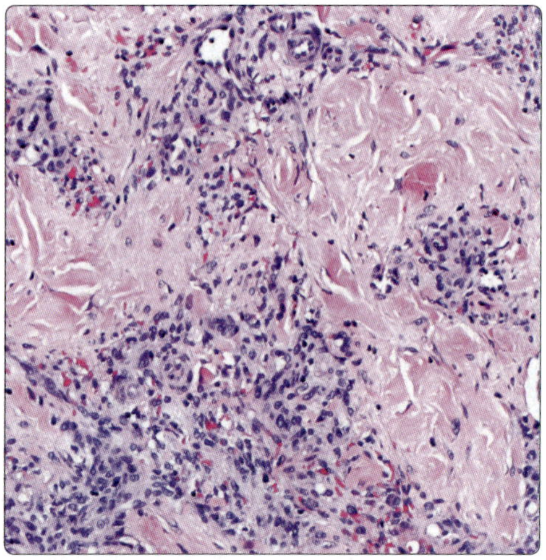

(Left) *Vessels protrude into the lumen of larger vascular channels (promontory sign) giving a vessel within a vessel appearance. This finding is characteristic of Kaposi sarcoma, although it is relatively uncommon.* **(Right)** *Bland spindle cells with associated hemorrhage infiltrate the dermis in plaque-stage Kaposi sarcoma. Most of these are endothelial cells, not fibroblasts, and will thus be highlighted on IHC by CD31, ERG, CD34, and other vascular markers.*

Infiltration of Eccrine Coils

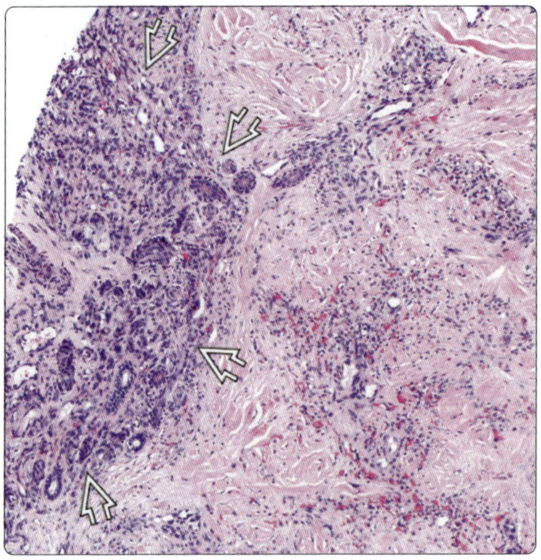

Disruption of Eccrine Coils

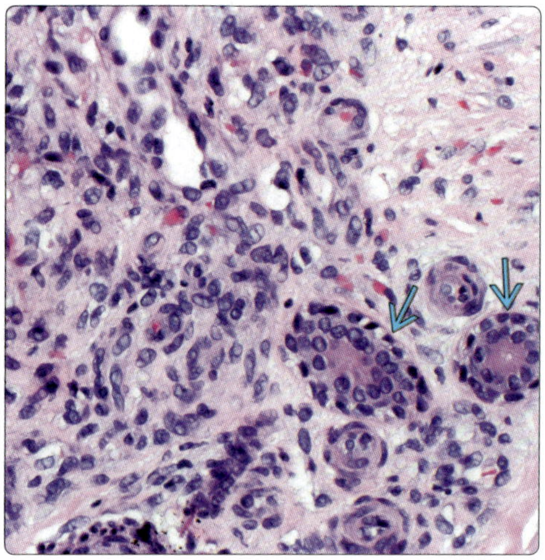

(Left) *Spindled endothelial cells often infiltrate and disrupt the eccrine coils* ➡*, a very characteristic finding in Kaposi sarcoma.* **(Right)** *Bland spindled endothelial cells infiltrate and disrupt the eccrine coils in Kaposi sarcoma, intervening between individual eccrine ducts* →*. Scattered extravasated erythrocytes are present.*

Kaposi Sarcoma

Early Kaposi Sarcoma

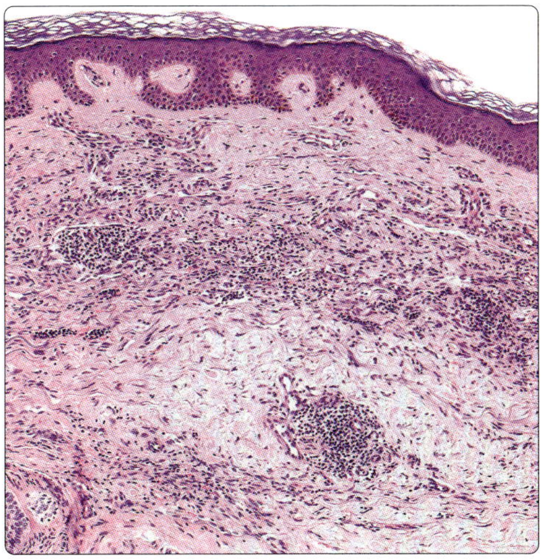

Spindle Cells and Inflammation

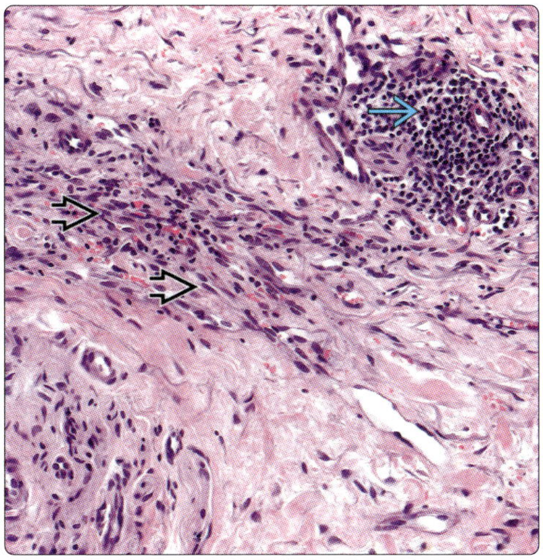

(Left) *Early Kaposi sarcoma displays infiltrating, irregular, thin-walled vascular channels; scattered spindle cells; and brisk inflammation.* **(Right)** *Spindled endothelial cells infiltrate the dermis. Extravasated erythrocytes are present, and there are aggregates of lymphocytes and plasma cells.*

Mitoses

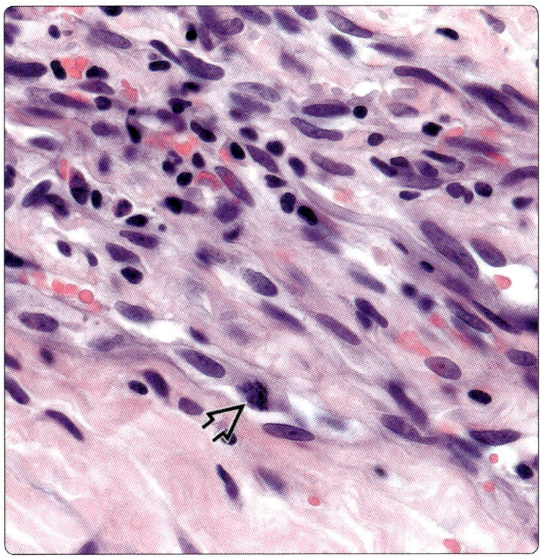

Plasma Cells

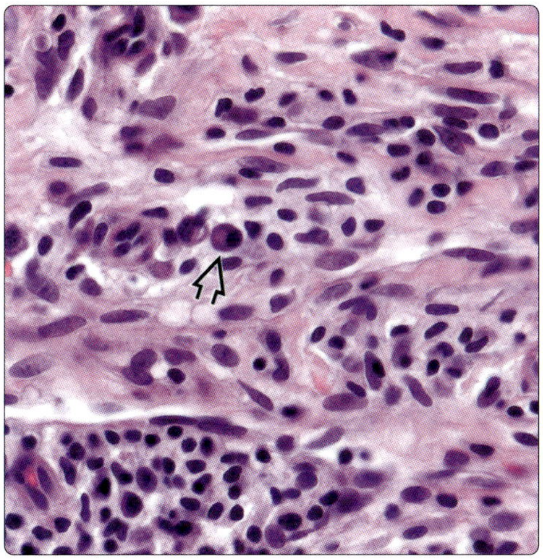

(Left) *At high-power magnification, narrow vascular spaces and cytologically bland spindled cells are seen. Note the presence of inflammatory cells and scattered mitoses.* **(Right)** *The inflammatory infiltrate in Kaposi sarcoma usually contains plasma cells.*

Dilated Cavernous Channels

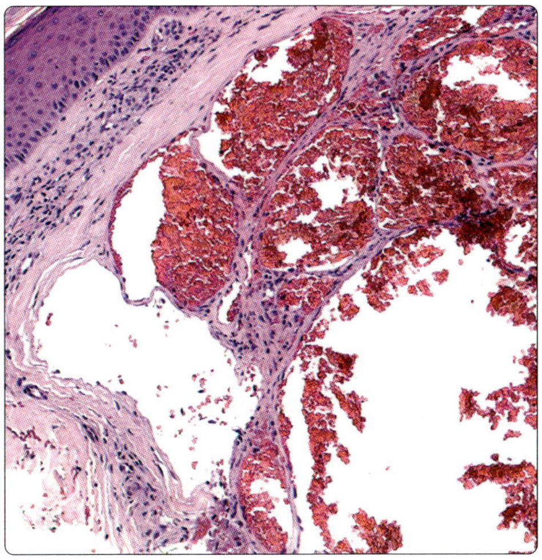

Dissection of Dermal Collagen

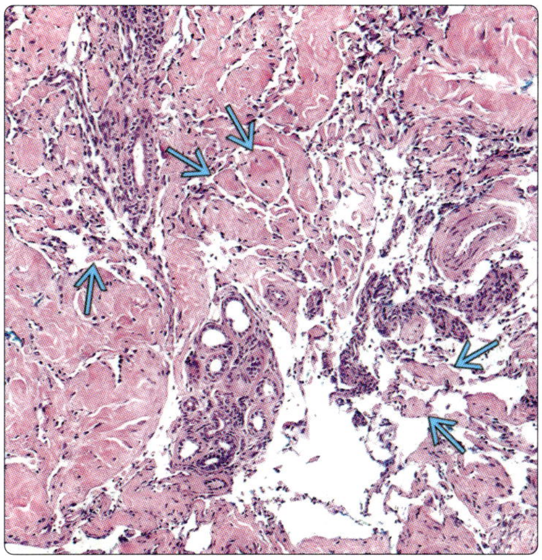

(Left) *Larger, dilated, blood-filled vessels may be present in some cases of Kaposi sarcoma, as depicted. These unique cases have been described as hemangioma-like variants of Kaposi sarcoma.* **(Right)** *Infiltrative, dilated vascular channels dissect between dermal collagen in this H&E. This growth may be so extensive that individual collagen bundles appear to be suspended within empty spaces. Angiosarcoma can also produce this pattern.*

(Left) *Low-power view of tumor-stage Kaposi sarcoma shows an ulcerated, exophytic, pedunculated, and hypercellular dermal nodule with hemorrhage.* **(Right)** *Tumor-stage Kaposi sarcoma displays cellular fascicles of relatively uniform spindle cells with intervening slit- or sieve-like spaces filled with erythrocytes.*

Tumor-Stage Kaposi Sarcoma

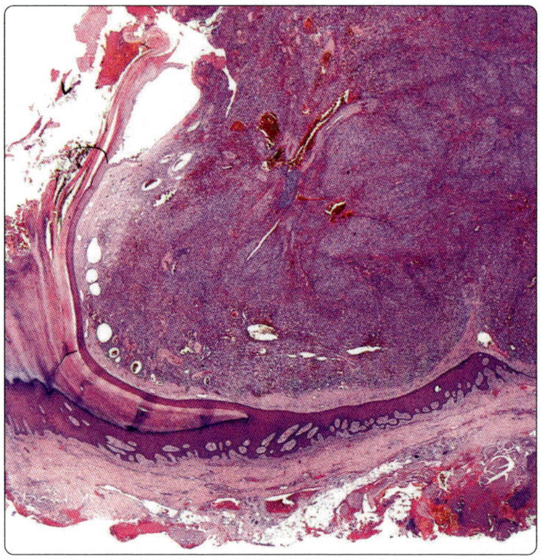

Cellular Fascicles of Spindle Cells

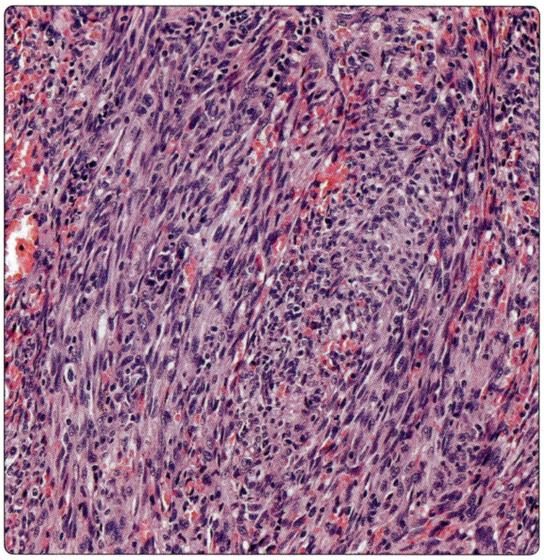

(Left) *Short fascicles of spindle cells intersect one another in tumor-stage Kaposi sarcoma. Abundant erythrocytes are present between tumor cells.* **(Right)** *Kaposi sarcoma displays tumor cells with relatively uniform, spindled nuclei that typically have minimal nuclear atypia. Mitoses are usually seen ➡. Small, sieve-like spaces containing erythrocytes are seen between the spindled cells →.*

Intersecting Fascicles

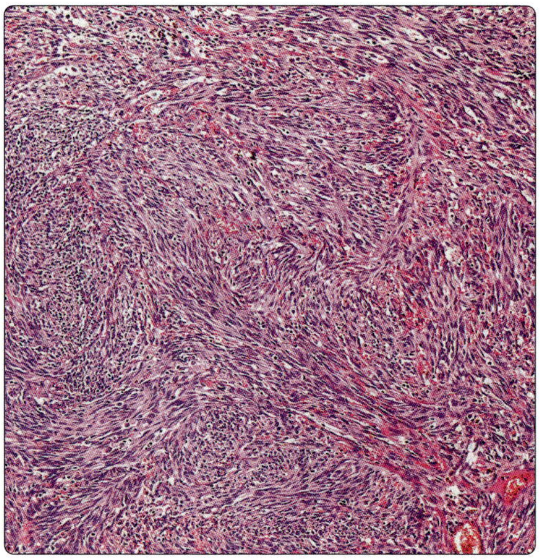

Mitoses but Minimal Nuclear Atypia

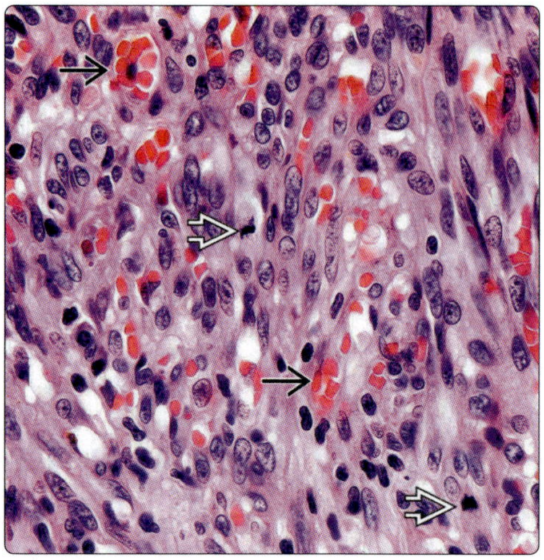

(Left) *Abundant erythrocyte extravasation is seen. Hemosiderin is often present →. Mitoses are readily identified ➡.* **(Right)** *Tumor-stage Kaposi sarcoma sometimes has minimal or completely absent erythrocyte-filled spaces or hemorrhage. These cases may be easily confused with other fascicular-patterned, nonvascular spindle cell tumors.*

Hemorrhage and Hemosiderin

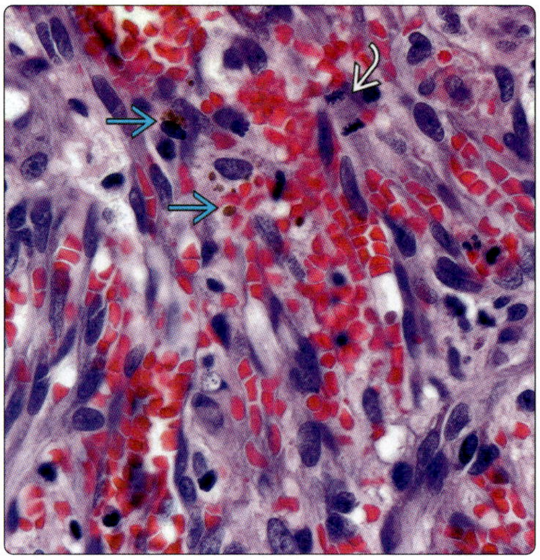

Minimal Hemorrhage

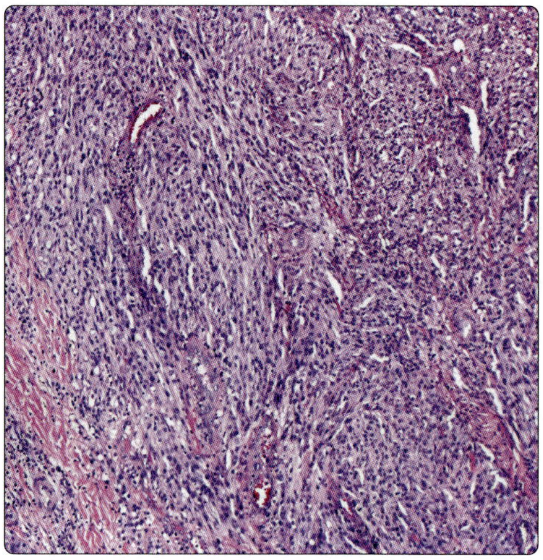

Fascicles Without Erythrocytes

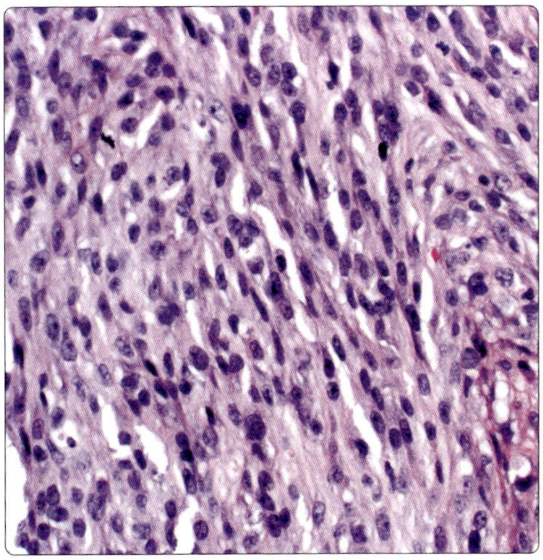

Plasma Cells Characteristic

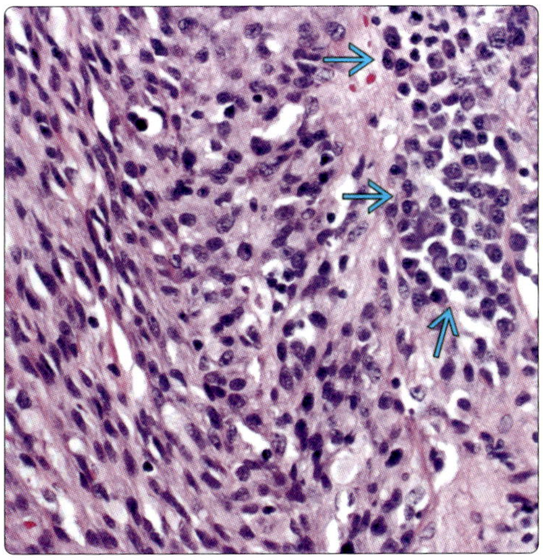

(Left) *This tumor-stage Kaposi sarcoma is composed of cellular fascicles of uniform spindle cells but is essentially devoid of erythrocytes. Recognizing the endothelial nature of these cells is very challenging in areas like this.* **(Right)** *In tumor-stage Kaposi sarcoma lacking erythrocytes, the presence of plasma cells* → *is a very important clue to the diagnosis.*

Nuclear HHV8 Expression

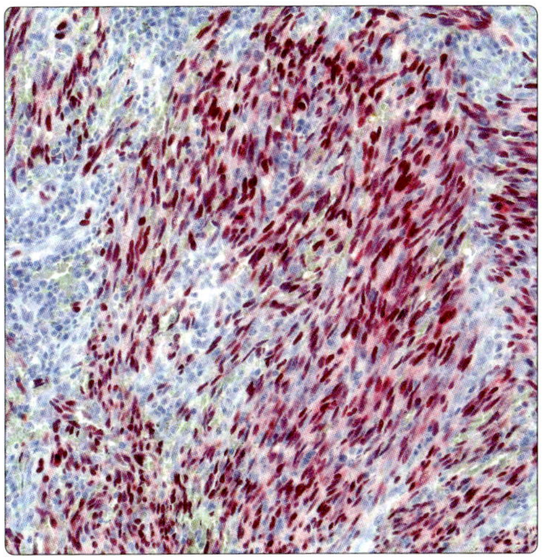

HHV8: Granular Nuclear Staining

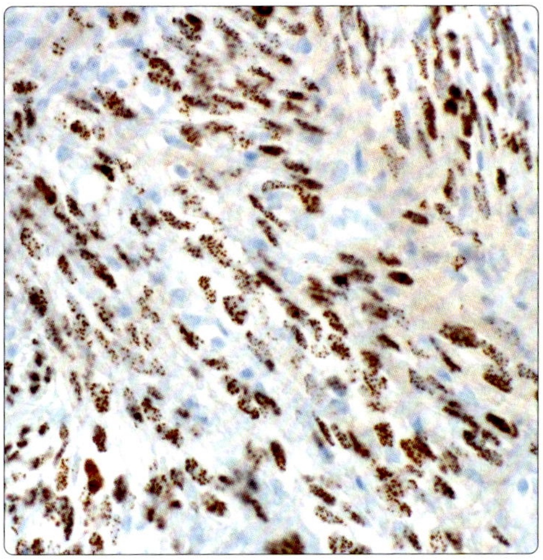

(Left) *Nuclear HHV8 expression is present in essentially 100% of Kaposi sarcoma but is absent in all other vascular proliferations.* **(Right)** *HHV8 immunostain often displays a punctate granular stippled/speckled nuclear staining pattern.*

CD34 Expression

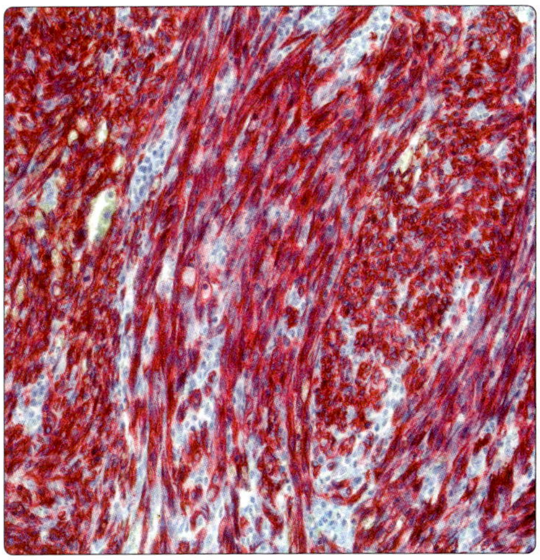

Podoplanin (D2-40) Expression

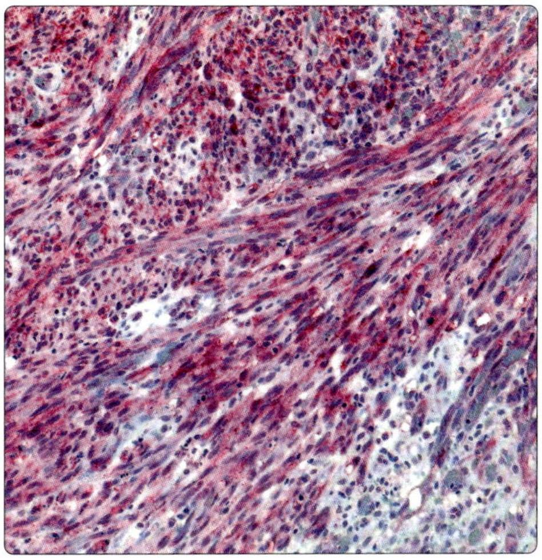

(Left) *Fascicles of spindle cells are diffusely positive for CD34 in this case of tumor-stage Kaposi sarcoma. CD31 is also typically expressed.* **(Right)** *Most cases of Kaposi sarcoma have a lymphatic endothelial phenotype resulting in podoplanin expression detected on D2-40 immunostaining.*

SECTION 11

Chondroosseous Tumors

Benign

Soft Tissue Chondroma 486
Synovial Chondromatosis 492

Malignant

Extraskeletal Osteosarcoma 496
Extraskeletal Mesenchymal Chondrosarcoma 500

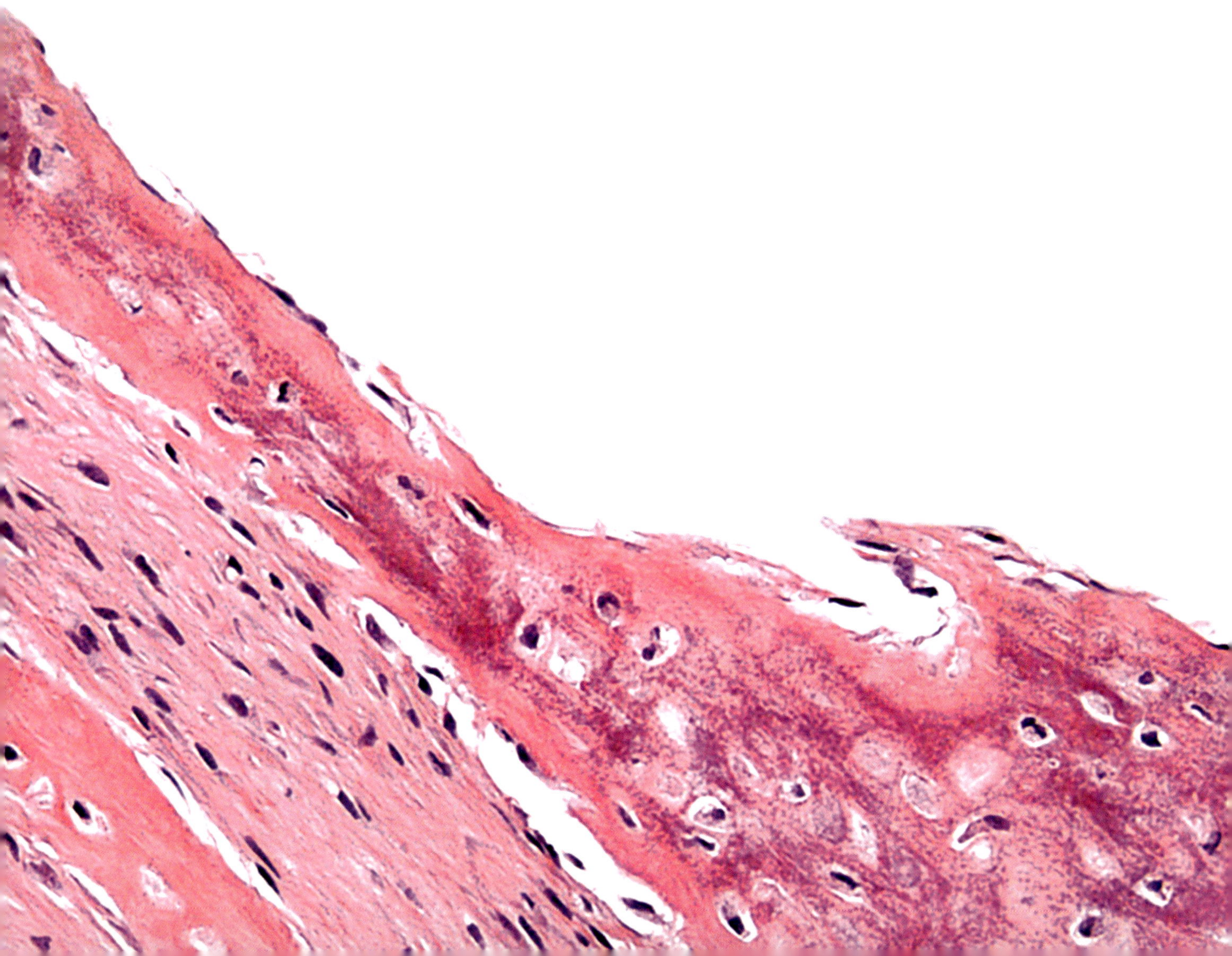

Soft Tissue Chondroma

KEY FACTS

TERMINOLOGY

- Benign hyaline cartilage neoplasm of soft tissue with predilection for hands and feet

CLINICAL ISSUES

- Low recurrence rate (15-20%)
- Recurrences controlled by reexcision

IMAGING

- Small, well demarcated
- Mineralized soft tissue mass
- Acral extremity

MACROSCOPIC

- Median size: 1.6 cm
- Range: 0.3-6.5 cm

MICROSCOPIC

- Well circumscribed and lobulated
- Mostly composed of mature hyaline cartilage
- Variable amounts of calcification
- Ossification common
- Granulomatous inflammation in 15% of cases
- Rare tumors with extensive xanthogranulomatous inflammation
- Myxoid matrix common (myxochondroma)
- Rare tumors with extensive stromal fibrosis (fibrochondroma)
- Morphologic variant: Chondroblastoma-like chondroma

TOP DIFFERENTIAL DIAGNOSES

- Synovial chondromatosis
- Tophaceous pseudogout
- Tumoral calcinosis
- Extraskeletal myxoid chondrosarcoma
- Calcifying aponeurotic fibroma
- Myxochondroid metaplasia of plantar foot
- Cutaneous mixed tumor with chondroid metaplasia
- Tenosynovial giant cell tumor

Soft Tissue Chondroma

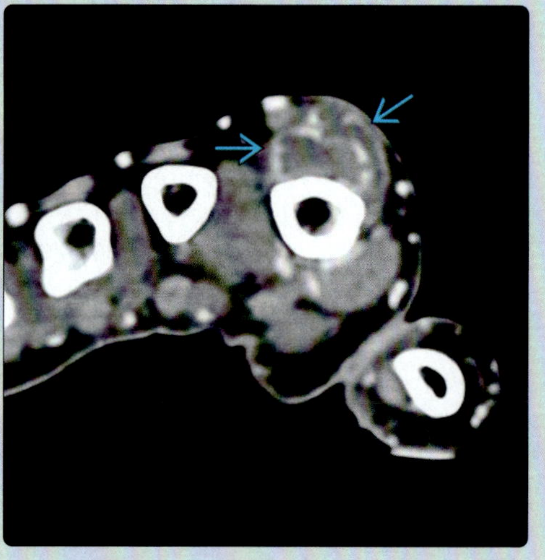

Lobular Architecture

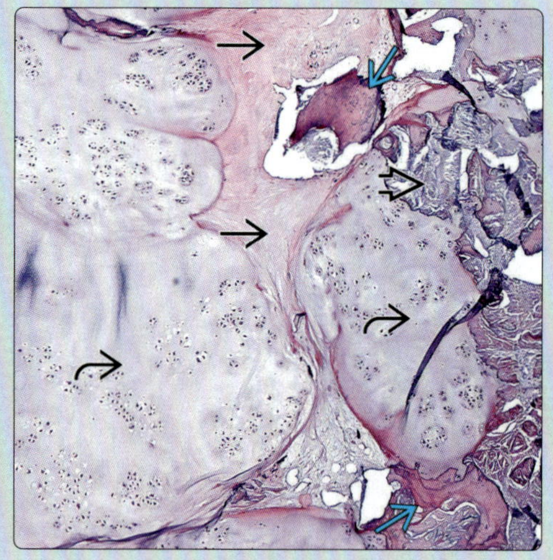

(Left) *Soft tissue chondroma typically occurs in the digits of the hands and feet. It presents as a painless, well-demarcated, mineralized mass, as demonstrated in this CT of a dorsal index finger lesion. Note the peripheral distribution of mineralization* →. **(Right)** *Soft tissue chondroma typically has a lobular architecture with islands of hyaline cartilage* ↷ *separated by fibrous bands* →. *Matrix calcification* ⇒ *and ossification* → *are common.*

Cytologic Features

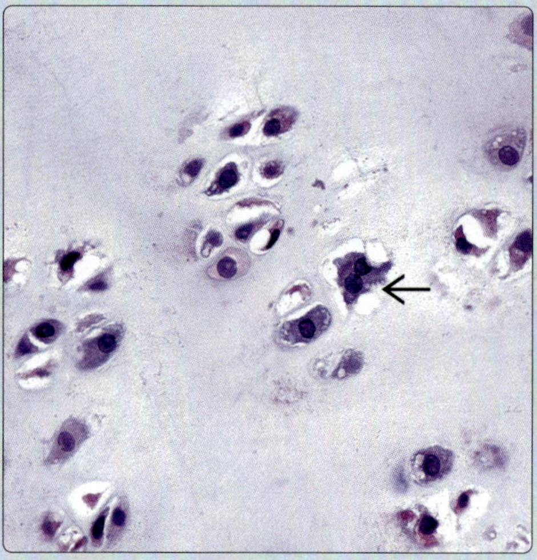

Calcified Hyaline Cartilage

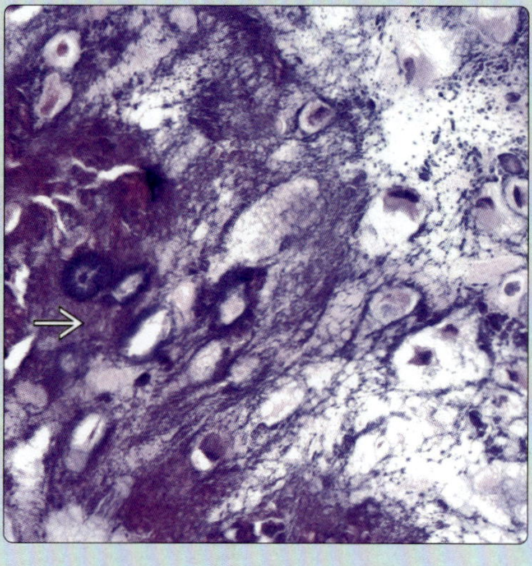

(Left) *High-power micrograph illustrates the typical cytologic features of soft tissue chondroma. The chondrocytes are often arranged in clusters, situated in lacunar spaces within pale blue hyaline matrix, and have uniform, round nuclei and abundant eosinophilic cytoplasm. Rare binucleated cells can be seen* →. *Mitoses are rare.* **(Right)** *Areas of very dense calcification are common, illustrated by heavy basophilic stippling* ➡ *of the cartilage matrix.*

TERMINOLOGY

Synonyms

- Extraskeletal chondroma
- Chondroma of soft parts
- Fibrochondroma
- Osteochondroma
- Myxochondroma
- Chondroblastoma-like chondroma

Definitions

- Benign hyaline cartilage neoplasm of soft tissue with predilection for hands and feet

ETIOLOGY/PATHOGENESIS

Neoplasm

- Rearrangement of 12q13-15
- Trisomy 5
- Aberrations of chromosome 11
- *HMGA2* abnormalities

CLINICAL ISSUES

Epidemiology

- Incidence
  - Uncommon
    - Exact incidence unknown
- Age
  - Median: 4th decade
    - Range: Infancy to 9th decade
- Sex
  - M = F

Presentation

- Painless mass
- Most common in hands and feet (60-95%)
  - Especially in fingers
- Rare sites
  - Proximal extremities, trunk, head and neck, oral cavity, ear, upper aerodigestive tract, dura/extradural, skin, fallopian tube, bladder, scrotum, orbit, eyelid

Treatment

- Simple surgical excision

Prognosis

- Low recurrence rate (15-20%)
  - Recurrences controlled by reexcision
- No reports of malignant degeneration

IMAGING

General Features

- Best diagnostic clue
  - Small, well demarcated
  - Mineralized soft tissue mass
  - Acral extremity
- Location
  - Hands and feet
  - Often in vicinity of joint or tendon
  - No intraarticular or subperiosteal localization by definition
- Morphology
  - Most are calcified or ossified
  - Sometimes erode and deform underlying bone

MACROSCOPIC

General Features

- Well demarcated and bosselated
- Spherical or oval
- Rubbery or hard
- Sometimes soft, friable, gelatinous, or cystic

Size

- Median: 1.6 cm
  - Range: 0.3-6.5 cm

MICROSCOPIC

Histologic Features

- Well circumscribed and lobulated
- Mostly composed of mature hyaline cartilage
- Chondrocytes located in lacunae
  - Arranged diffusely or in small clusters
  - Some have enlarged nuclei and moderate pleomorphism
  - Very low mitotic rate
- Variable amounts of calcification
  - Granular stippled calcification that surrounds chondrocytes in lace-like pattern
  - Some with extensive calcification
    - Deep basophilia of cartilage
- Ossification common
- Granulomatous inflammation in 15% of cases
  - Epithelioid macrophages and osteoclastic giant cells
  - Most pronounced in heavily calcified tumors
- Myxoid areas and cystic degeneration in some
- Rare tumors with extensive xanthogranulomatous inflammation
  - Mimics fibrous histiocytoma or tenosynovial giant cell tumor
- Rare tumors with extensive stromal fibrosis (fibrochondroma)

Morphologic Variant

- Chondroblastoma-like chondroma
  - Abundant myxoid matrix
  - Immature chondrocytes
    - Resemble cells of chondroblastoma of bone
      - Polygonal or elongated cells
      - Abundant eosinophilic or vacuolated cytoplasm
      - Eccentrically located, grooved or reniform nuclei

ANCILLARY TESTS

Immunohistochemistry

- S100 and ERG (+)
- Keratin and SMA (-)

DIFFERENTIAL DIAGNOSIS

Synovial Chondromatosis

- Larger tumors
- Most often in synovium of large joints, especially knee

- Also found in tenosynovium of acral extremities
- More discrete lobular architecture and chondrocyte clusters
- Intrarticular loose bodies

Tophaceous Pseudogout

- Wide distribution, including acral extremities
  - Predilection for temporomandibular joint
- Heavily calcified lesions with metaplastic cartilage formation
- Rhomboid-shaped calcium pyrophosphate dihydrate (CPPD) crystals
  - Positive birefringence under polarized light

Tumoral Calcinosis

- Predilection for large joints
- Calcium hydroxyapatite crystals (psammomatous)
- Histiocytic giant cells with intracytoplasmic calcifications
- Familial and nonfamilial cases

Extraskeletal Myxoid Chondrosarcoma

- Large, lobulated soft tissue mass
- Abundant myxoid matrix
- Thick fibrous septa
- Interconnecting cords of neoplastic cells
- Lacks true cartilage
- Necrosis

Calcifying Aponeurotic Fibroma

- Hands and feet
  - Especially palms of children
- Geographic areas of calcification surrounded by chondroid cells
- Fibromatous areas

Myxochondroid Metaplasia of Plantar Foot

- All reports from plantar foot, including toes
- Fibromyxoid background
- Areas with distinct stromal basophilia and chondroid appearance
- Cystic change common
- Reactive, nonneoplastic

Cutaneous Mixed Tumor With Chondroid Metaplasia

- Massive chondroid metaplasia
- Epithelial glandular structures

Tenosynovial Giant Cell Tumor

- Similar location, most common in fingers
- Calcified soft tissue chondromas can have extensive granulomatous inflammation
- Osteoclastic giant cells
- Xanthoma cells

DIAGNOSTIC CHECKLIST

Clinically Relevant Pathologic Features

- Predilection for acral extremities

Pathologic Interpretation Pearls

- Features that can lead to misdiagnosis
  - Chondrocyte atypia
  - Increased cellularity
  - Extensive calcification and ossification
  - Granulomatous or xanthogranulomatous reaction
  - Fibrous and myxoid areas
  - Chondroblastoma-like features

SELECTED REFERENCES

1. Sugiura Y et al: Convexity dural chondroma: a case report with pathological and molecular analysis. Clin Neuropathol. 34(1):13-8, 2015
2. Pace J et al: Extradural chondroma presenting as lumbar mass with compressive neuropathy. J Craniovertebr Junction Spine. 5(3):131-3, 2014
3. Shon W et al: ERG expression in chondrogenic bone and soft tissue tumours. J Clin Pathol. 68(2):125-9, 2014
4. Vescovi P et al: Soft tissue chondroma of the oral cavity: an extremely rare tumour localized on the hard palate. Case Rep Med. 2014:414861, 2014
5. Choi Y et al: A case of auricular chondroma. Korean J Audiol. 17(3):156-8, 2013
6. Choi Y et al: Extraskeletal chondroma of the scalp: an atypical location. Indian J Dermatol Venereol Leprol. 79(3):435-6, 2013
7. Raparia K et al: Chondroblastoma-like chondroma of soft tissue: report of the first case in the base of skull. Ann Diagn Pathol. 17(3):298-301, 2013
8. Shon W et al: Myxochondroid metaplasia of the plantar foot: a distinctive pseudoneoplastic lesion resembling nuchal fibrocartilaginous pseudotumor and the equine digital cushion. Mod Pathol. 26(12):1561-7, 2013
9. Smith EJ et al: Case presentation of soft tissue parapharyngeal chondroma in a pediatric patient. Am J Otolaryngol. 34(6):720-3, 2013
10. Thompson J et al: Cutaneous mixed tumor with extensive chondroid metaplasia: a potential mimic of cutaneous chondroma. Dermatol Online J. 18(3):9, 2012
11. Kim HS et al: A true chondroma cutis. J Eur Acad Dermatol Venereol. 23(5):612-3, 2009
12. Khedhaier A et al: Soft tissues chondromas of the hand: a report of five cases. Acta Orthop Belg. 73(4):458-61, 2007
13. Hondar Wu HT et al: Imaging and pathological correlation of soft-tissue chondroma: a serial five-case study and literature review. Clin Imaging. 30(1):32-6, 2006
14. Dahlén A et al: Fusion, disruption, and expression of HMGA2 in bone and soft tissue chondromas. Mod Pathol. 16(11):1132-40, 2003
15. Fetsch JF et al: Tenosynovial (extraarticular) chondromatosis: an analysis of 37 cases of an underrecognized clinicopathologic entity with a strong predilection for the hands and feet and a high local recurrence rate. Am J Surg Pathol. 27(9):1260-8, 2003
16. Tallini G et al: Correlation between clinicopathological features and karyotype in 100 cartilaginous and chordoid tumours. A report from the Chromosomes and Morphology (CHAMP) Collaborative Study Group. J Pathol. 196(2):194-203, 2002
17. Cates JM et al: Chondroblastoma-like chondroma of soft tissue: an underrecognized variant and its differential diagnosis. Am J Surg Pathol. 25(5):661-6, 2001
18. Ishida T et al: Tophaceous pseudogout (tumoral calcium pyrophosphate dihydrate crystal deposition disease). Hum Pathol. 26(6):587-93, 1995
19. Pollock L et al: Childhood soft tissue chondroma: a case report. Pediatr Pathol Lab Med. 15(3):437-41, 1995
20. Bridge JA et al: Biologic and clinical significance of cytogenetic and molecular cytogenetic abnormalities in benign and malignant cartilaginous lesions. Cancer Genet Cytogenet. 69(2):79-90, 1993
21. Humphreys S et al: Soft tissue chondroma–a study of 15 tumours. Histopathology. 10(2):147-59, 1986
22. Chung EB et al: Chondroma of soft parts. Cancer. 41(4):1414-24, 1978
23. Dahlin DC et al: Cartilaginous tumors of the soft tissues of the hands and feet. Mayo Clin Proc. 49(10):721-6, 1974

Soft Tissue Chondroma

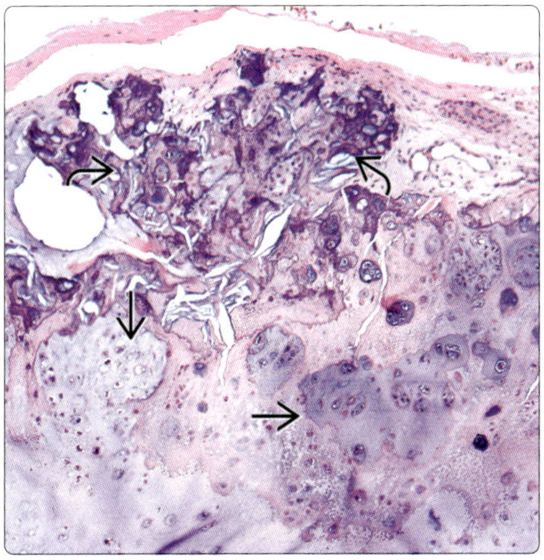

Calcification

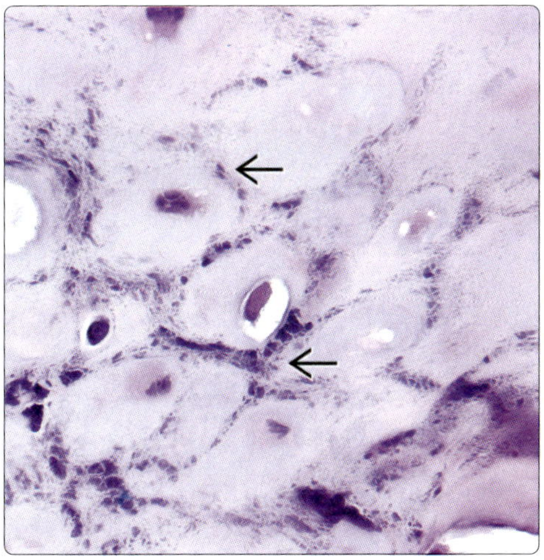

(Left) *Soft tissue chondroma is typically a well-circumscribed tumor composed of hyaline cartilage lobules →, areas of calcification →, and sharp demarcation from adjacent soft tissue (top).* **(Right)** *Calcification is very common in soft tissue chondroma. It appears as granular basophilic stippling of the matrix, which often surrounds individual chondrocytes to form a reticular pattern →.*

Dense Calcification

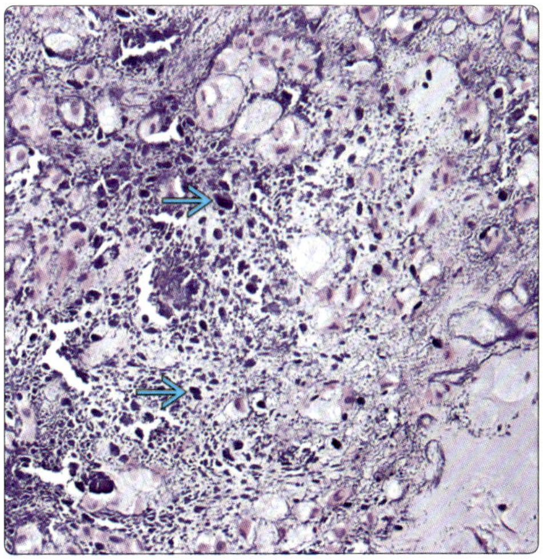

Granulomatous Inflammation and Giant Cells

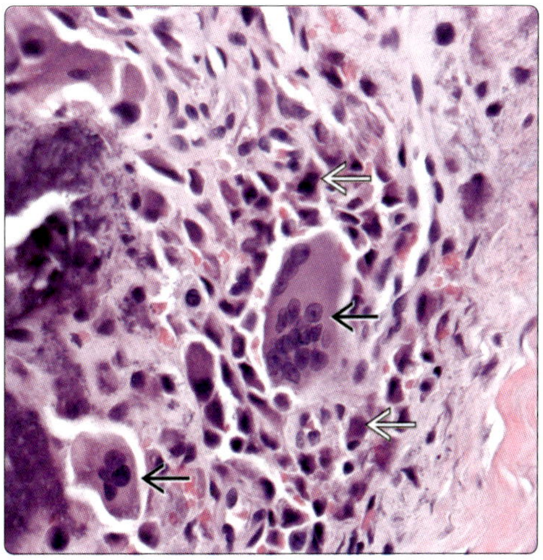

(Left) *This medium-power micrograph depicts very dense mineralization of the cartilage matrix, consisting of coarse, basophilic particles of calcium →.* **(Right)** *Granulomatous inflammation is often present in heavily calcified tumors. This micrograph illustrates epithelioid macrophages → and osteoclastic giant cells → in a calcified tumor. When extensive, it mimics tenosynovial giant cell tumor.*

Xanthogranulomatous Inflammation

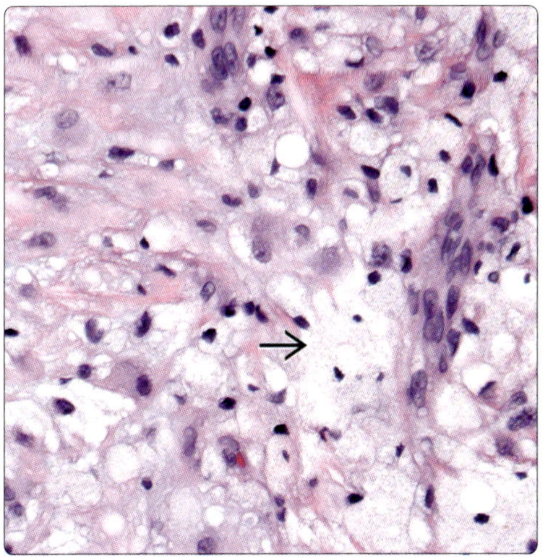

Ossification

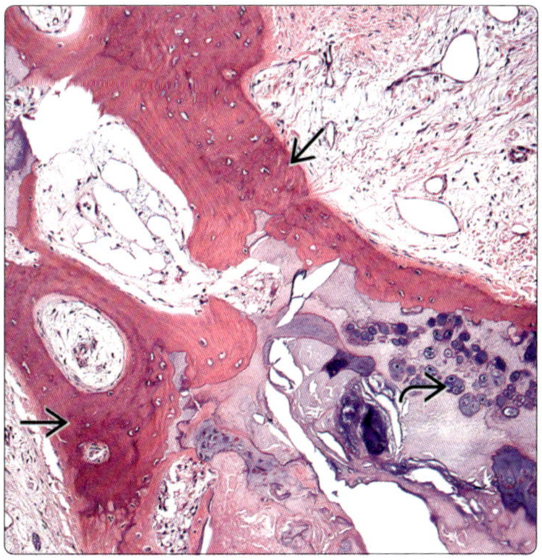

(Left) *Xanthogranulomatous inflammation can be present in soft tissue chondroma, consisting of sheets or clusters of foamy histiocytes →. When extensive, such a tumor can be mistaken for fibrous histiocytoma or tenosynovial giant cell tumor.* **(Right)** *Ossification → is common in soft tissue chondroma and can sometimes be extensive, as illustrated here. It can be located either at the center or periphery of the tumor and is formed via endochondral ossification of calcified cartilage matrix →.*

(Left) *CT depicts a mineralized soft tissue chondroma → involving the plantar soft tissue adjacent to the 4th metatarsal. Soft tissue chondroma has a predilection for the hands and feet, often near a joint or tendon.* **(Right)** *This low-power micrograph illustrates well-defined, lobular architecture in a soft tissue chondroma, consisting of cartilaginous lobules → separated by fibrous bands ↪. Note the deeply basophilic calcium deposits within the center of the lobules →.*

Soft Tissue Chondroma of Foot

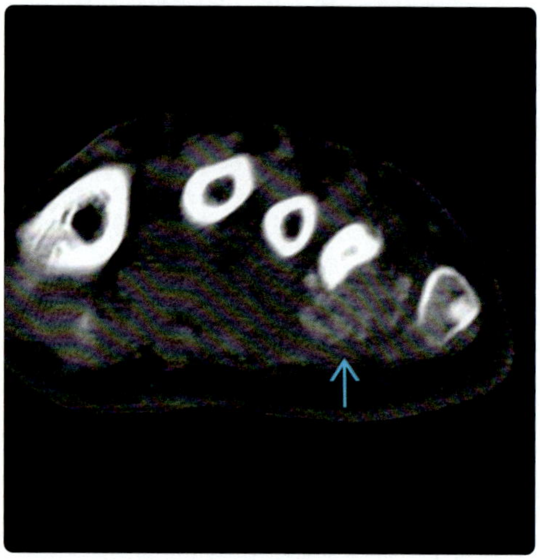

Lobular Architecture and Calcification

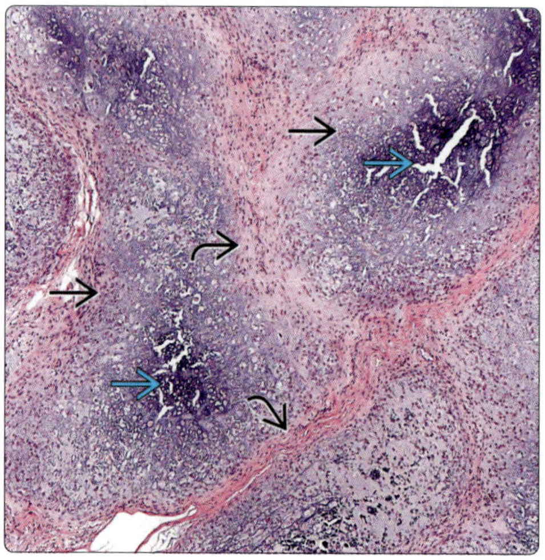

(Left) *This high-power micrograph of a densely calcified tumor depicts finely granular → and coarse ↪ calcium deposits. The hyaline matrix is degenerated, and the chondrocytes → are no longer contained within lacunae.* **(Right)** *Some tumors have extensive myxoid matrix where chondrocytes assume elongated and stellate configurations, sometimes interconnecting with each other to form a network, mimicking extraskeletal myxoid chondrosarcoma. Such tumors have been called myxochondromas.*

Calcified Cartilage Matrix

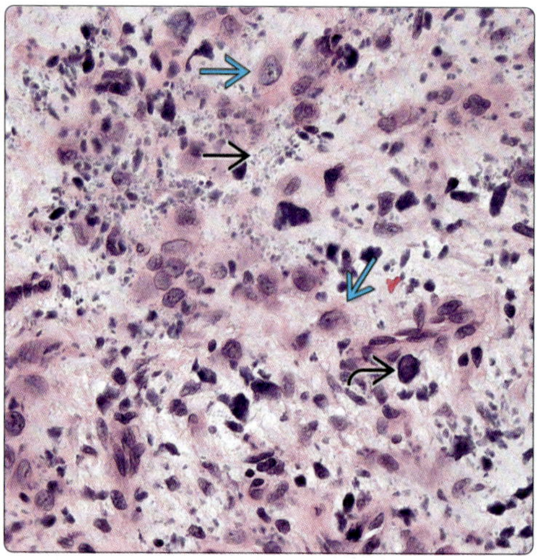

Myxoid Matrix

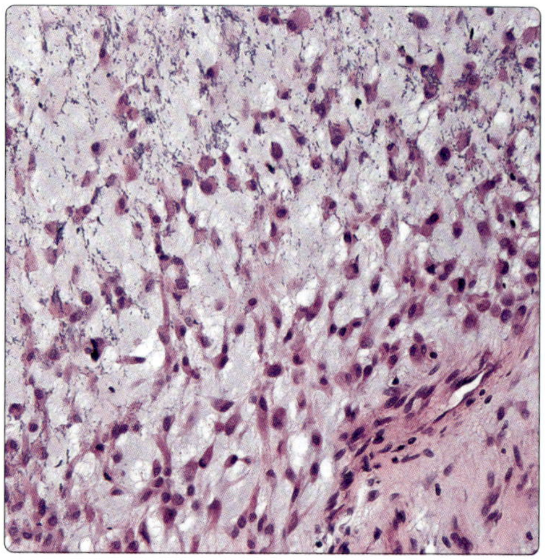

(Left) *In myxoid areas, the chondrocytes lose their lacunae and assume stellate shapes → and rounded cells that resemble chondroblasts with abundant eosinophilic cytoplasm and eccentric grooved or reniform nuclei ↪.* **(Right)** *Soft tissue chondroma can have extensive fibrosis exemplified by numerous collagen bundles traversing this tumor →. Tumors with extensive fibrosis are sometimes referred to as fibrochondromas.*

Stellate and Chondroblastoma-Like Cells

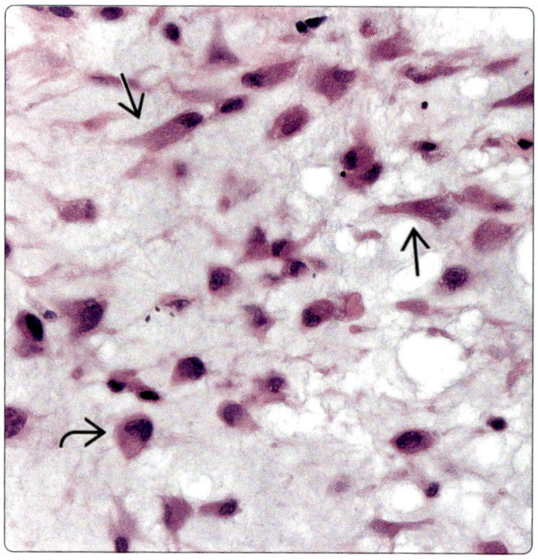

Fibrocollagenous Matrix

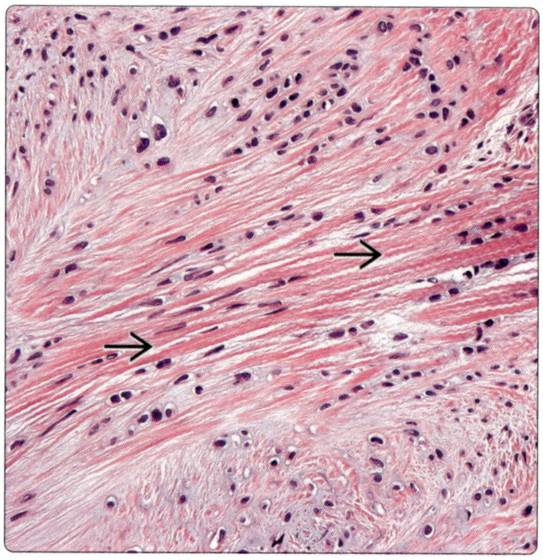

Circumscription and Lobular Architecture

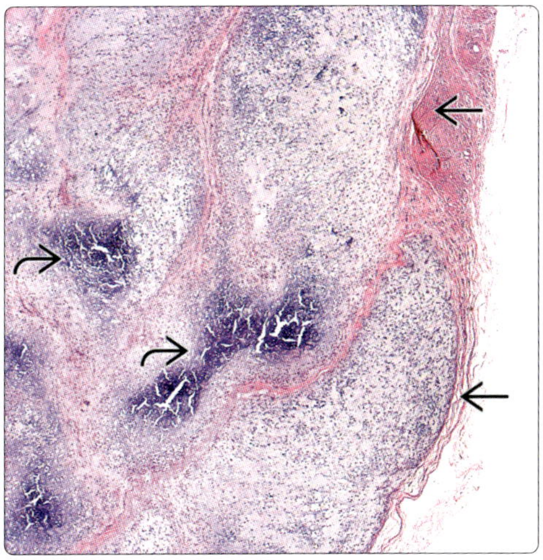

Calcification and Increased Cellularity

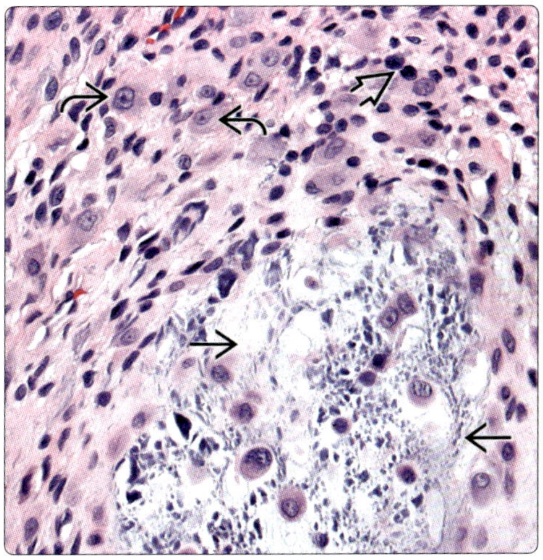

(Left) *Soft tissue chondroma is well circumscribed and well demarcated from adjacent soft tissues* →*. It typically has a multilobular architecture, as shown, and zones of calcification* ↷*.* **(Right)** *This micrograph illustrates a zone of calcified matrix* → *surrounded by an area of increased cellularity. The cellular area is composed by a mixture of chondrocytes devoid of lacunae* ⇗ *and mononuclear inflammatory cells* ↷ *and resembles tenosynovial giant cell tumor.*

Increased Cellularity

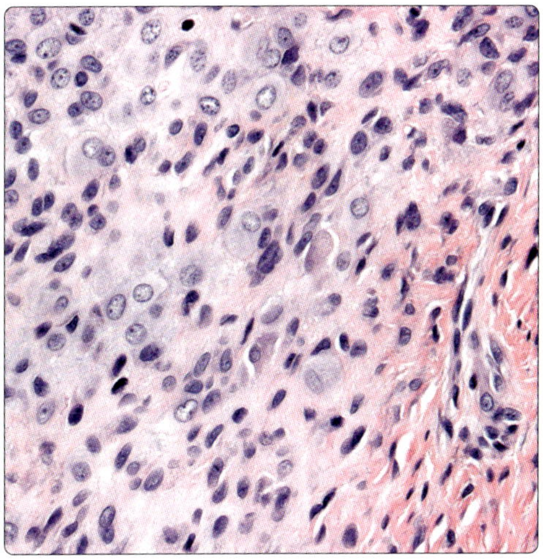

Cellular Atypia

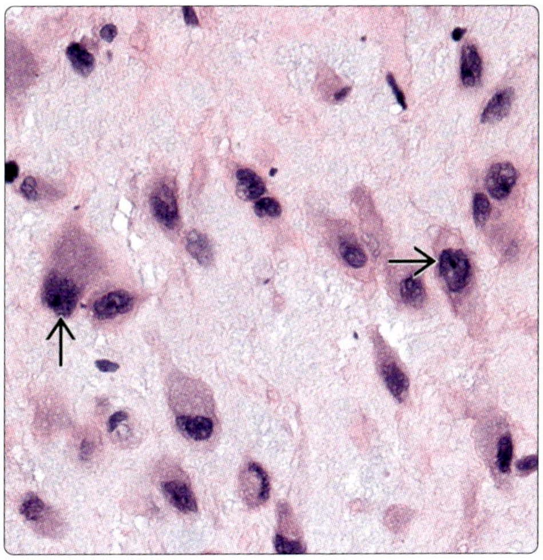

(Left) *Areas of increased cellularity can be present in soft tissue chondroma, as exemplified, and does not portend a more aggressive behavior.* **(Right)** *Degenerative cytologic atypia is not uncommon in soft tissue chondroma. This high-power micrograph illustrates chondrocytes with nuclear enlargement* → *and pleomorphism, which, out of context, would be suspicious for chondrosarcoma.*

Chondroblastoma-Like Features

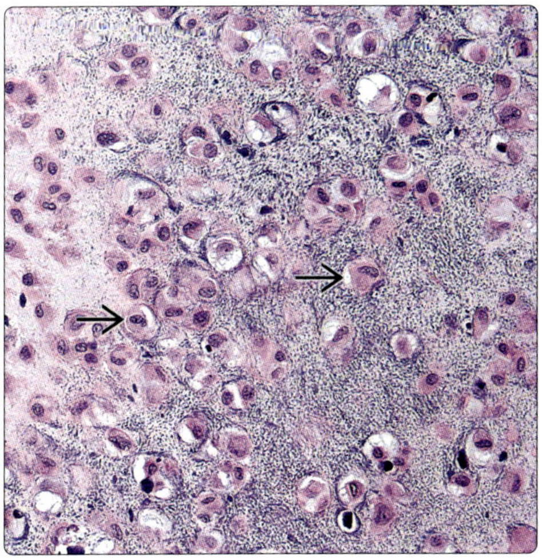

Cystic Degeneration

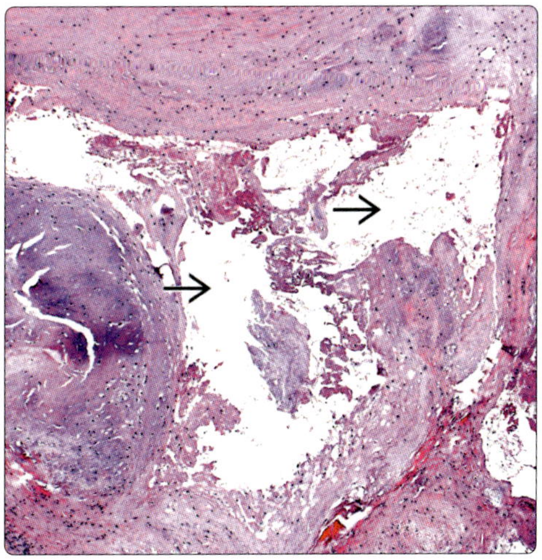

(Left) *This heavily calcified soft tissue chondroma contains cells with abundant eosinophilic cytoplasm and eccentric nuclei with reniform and grooved shapes* →*, resembling the cells of a chondroblastoma.* **(Right)** *Cystic degeneration can occur in some tumors consisting of liquefaction of the hyaline cartilage matrix, as seen in this foot lesion* →*.*

Synovial Chondromatosis

KEY FACTS

TERMINOLOGY

- Benign, multinodular proliferation of hyaline cartilage within articular synovium, tendon sheath, or bursa
- Usually diffuse and associated with loose bodies

CLINICAL ISSUES

- Site
  - Knee, hip, and elbow most common
  - Temporomandibular joint
  - Tenosynovium of acral extremities
- Benign with propensity for local recurrence
- Very rare chondrosarcomatous transformation

IMAGING

- Diffuse, punctate and ring-like calcifications
- Intense T2 signal on MR

MACROSCOPIC

- Multiple small, cartilaginous nodules (0.1-1.0 cm) that coalesce into larger conglomerates
- Diffuse lesions stud synovial membrane

MICROSCOPIC

- Multiple discrete nodules of hyaline cartilage
- Chondrocytes arranged in small clusters
- Cytologic atypia and increased cellularity in some
- Matrix usually hyaline but may be myxoid or heavily calcified
- Can undergo endochondral ossification
- Temporomandibular joint tumors often calcified and have cytological atypia

TOP DIFFERENTIAL DIAGNOSES

- Osteocartilaginous loose bodies
- Soft tissue chondroma
- Synovial chondrosarcoma

(Left) *Synovial chondromatosis has a well-defined, multinodular architecture, characterized by discrete nodules of hyaline cartilage within subsynovial tissue. The chondrocytes are arranged in small clusters →.* **(Right)** *The knee is the most common site of synovial chondromatosis. Radiographically, it appears as periarticular punctate calcifications →. Other common sites are the hip, elbow, shoulder, and temporomandibular joint (TMJ).*

Synovial Chondromatosis

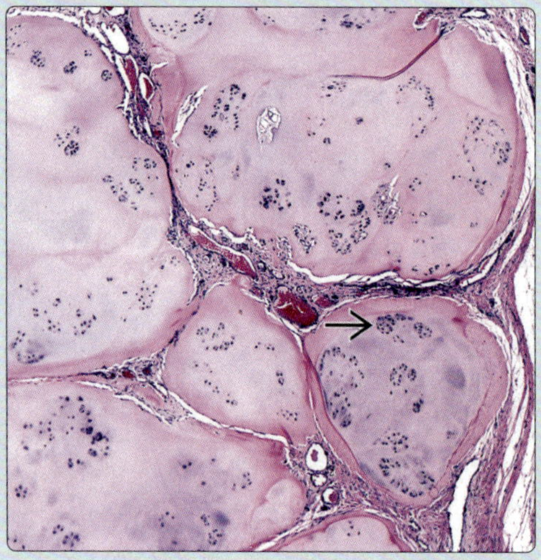

Radiology

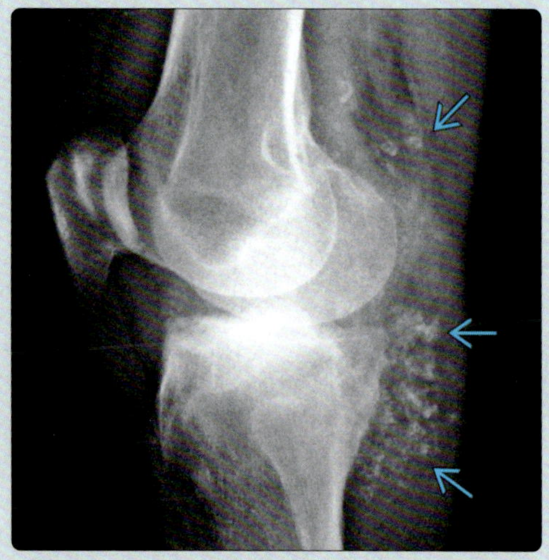

(Left) *Proliferating cells are benign-appearing chondrocytes with uniform, small nuclei situated within lacunar spaces. Note the clustered arrangement of the cells and occasional lacunae containing 2 cells →.* **(Right)** *Grossly, synovial chondromatosis has a very distinctive multinodular pattern characterized by small, opalescent, cartilaginous nodules, which coalesce into larger conglomerates.*

High-Power Features

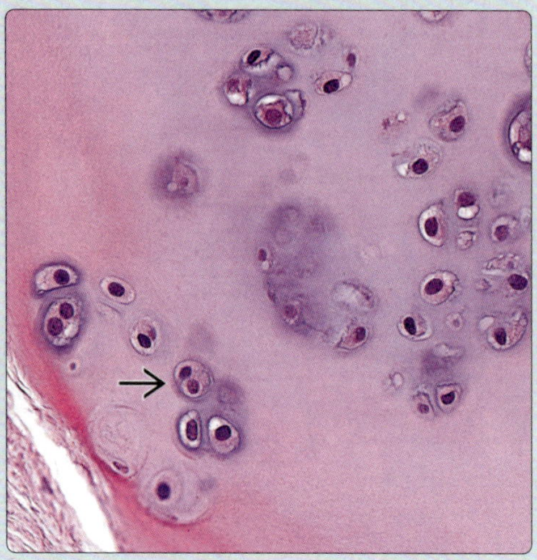

Gross Appearance

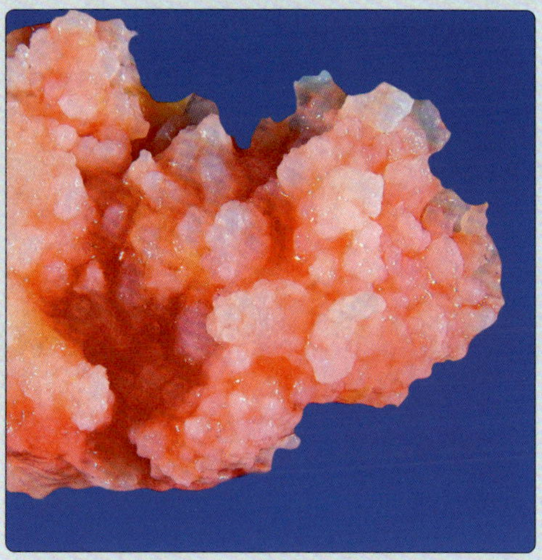

TERMINOLOGY

Synonyms

- Primary synovial chondromatosis, synovial osteochondromatosis, synovial chondroma, synovial chondrometaplasia

Definitions

- Benign, multinodular proliferation of hyaline cartilage within articular synovium, tendon sheath, or bursa
  - Usually diffuse and associated with loose bodies, with propensity for local recurrence

CLINICAL ISSUES

Epidemiology

- Incidence
  - Rare but exact incidence unknown
- Age
  - Peak age: 5th decade but wide variation (1st-7th decades)
- Sex
  - M:F = 2:1
- Etiology
  - Unknown, possibly neoplastic
    - Clonal chromosomal changes, chromosome 6, 1, 5 abnormalities reported
  - *IDH1* and *IDH2* mutations absent

Site

- Virtually any joint may be involved
  - Knee is most common site
  - Hip, elbow, and shoulder common
  - Temporomandibular joint
- Soft tissue around joints
  - Tenosynovium of acral extremities
  - Bursae
- Can be multifocal

Presentation

- Painful or painless mass
- Impaired range of motion

Treatment

- Synovectomy and removal of loose bodies

Prognosis

- Benign; 15-20% local recurrence rate
- Chondrosarcomatous transformation very rare

IMAGING

Radiographic Findings

- Multifocal, punctate and ring-like calcifications involving joint, tendon sheath, or bursa
  - Early lesions lack calcification
  - Older lesions may become heavily mineralized with ossified bodies
  - Can erode adjacent bone

MR Findings

- Lobulated mass with intense T2 signal

MACROSCOPIC

General Features

- Multiple small, cartilaginous nodules (0.1-1.0 cm) that coalesce into larger conglomerates
  - Diffuse lesions stud synovial membrane
  - Detached loose bodies

MICROSCOPIC

Histologic Features

- Multiple nodules of hyaline cartilage
- Nodules underlie flattened synovium
- Chondrocytes arranged in small clusters
  - Binucleation common
  - Cytologic atypia and increased cellularity in some lesions
- Hyaline cartilage matrix
  - Can be focally myxoid
  - Calcification common
    - Some lesions heavily calcified
  - Nodules may undergo endochondral ossification

DIFFERENTIAL DIAGNOSIS

Osteocartilaginous Loose Bodies

- Concentric laminations of variably calcified/ossified cartilage
- Associated with degenerative joint disease, trauma, osteochondritis dissecans

Soft Tissue Chondroma

- Lacks well-defined, multinodular architecture
- Predilection for hands and feet

Juxtaarticular Chondroma

- Most common in subpatellar knee
- Often heavily ossified

Synovial Chondrosarcoma

- Very rare
- May arise within synovial chondromatosis or de novo
- Loss of clustered growth, prominent myxoid matrix, necrosis, peripheral spindling

DIAGNOSTIC CHECKLIST

Clinically Relevant Pathologic Features

- Tissue distribution

Pathologic Interpretation Pearls

- Multinodularity
- Clustered chondrocytes

SELECTED REFERENCES

1. Shah SB et al: Synovial chondromatosis of temporomandibular joint: journey through 25 decades and a case report. J Oral Maxillofac Surg. 69(11):2795-814, 2011
2. Fetsch JF et al: Tenosynovial (extraarticular) chondromatosis: an analysis of 37 cases of an underrecognized clinicopathologic entity with a strong predilection for the hands and feet and a high local recurrence rate. Am J Surg Pathol. 27(9):1260-8, 2003
3. Sciot R et al: Synovial chondromatosis: clonal chromosome changes provide further evidence for a neoplastic disorder. Virchows Arch. 433(2):189-91, 1998

(Left) *Low-power micrograph depicts the characteristic well-defined, multinodular architecture of synovial chondromatosis consisting of hyaline cartilage nodules that contain clusters of chondrocytes* →. **(Right)** *Low-power micrograph depicts discrete nodules of synovial chondromatosis within subsynovial tissue. Note the overlying synovial membrane* ↷ *and nodules of cartilage with sharp borders, separated by fibrovascular tissue* →.

Multinodular Architecture

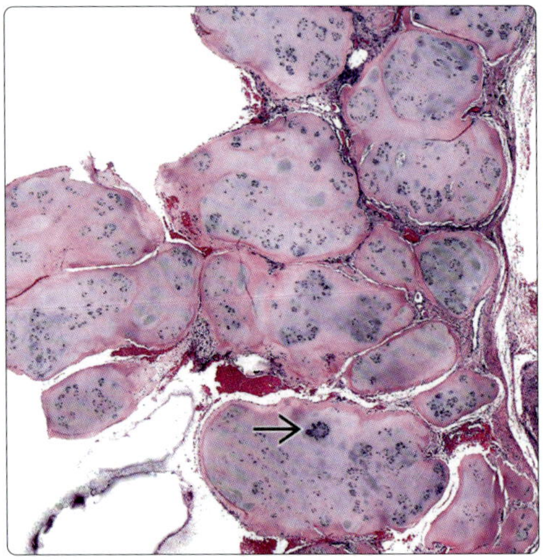

Subsynovial Location

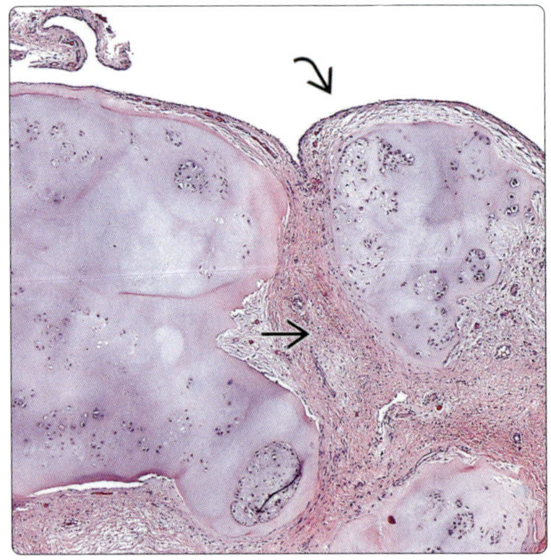

(Left) *In most cases of synovial chondromatosis, the matrix consists of pale blue or pink hyaline cartilage, and the chondrocytes are arranged in small clusters, as shown.* **(Right)** *Intraarticular loose bodies frequently occur in synovial chondromatosis. Unlike the osteocartilaginous loose bodies associated with degenerative joint disease, they lack concentric laminations and maintain the clustered arrangement of chondrocytes.*

Hyaline Cartilage Matrix and Cell Clusters

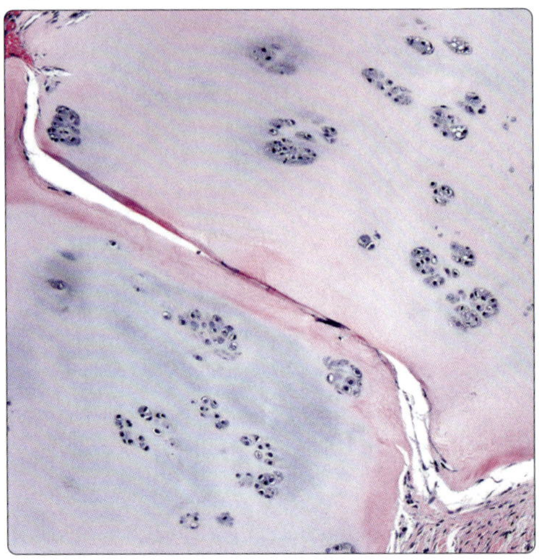

Intraarticular Loose Bodies

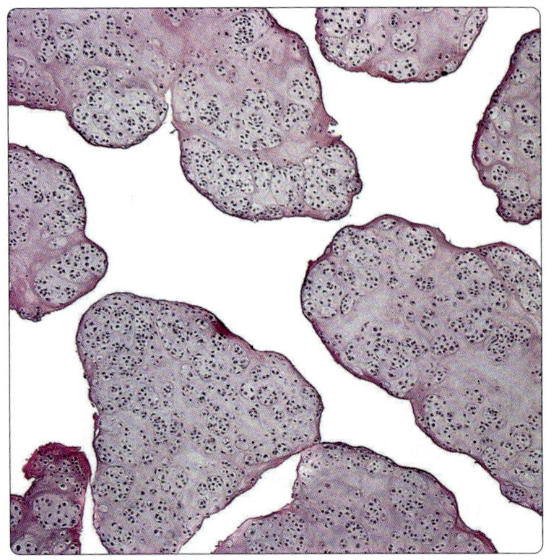

(Left) *Calcification is common in synovial chondromatosis* →*, as depicted. This pattern correlates with the punctate calcifications seen on radiographs.* **(Right)** *Calcified nodules may be transformed into ring-like, ossified structures via endochondral ossification. Note the remnants of calcified cartilage* → *peripheral to the bone* ↷*. Such ossified nodules correspond to the ring-like structures seen on radiographs.*

Calcification

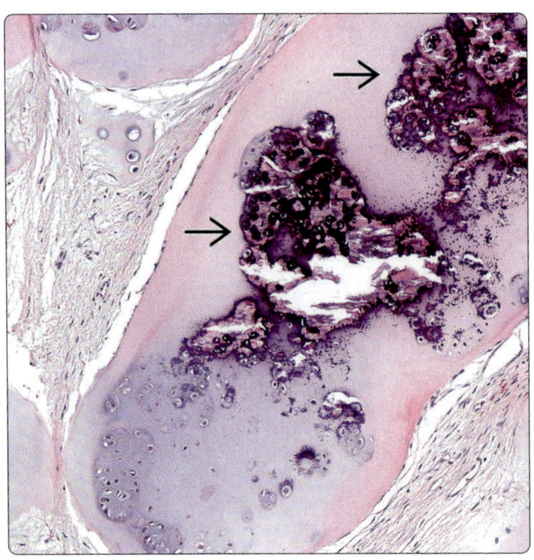

Endochondral Ossification

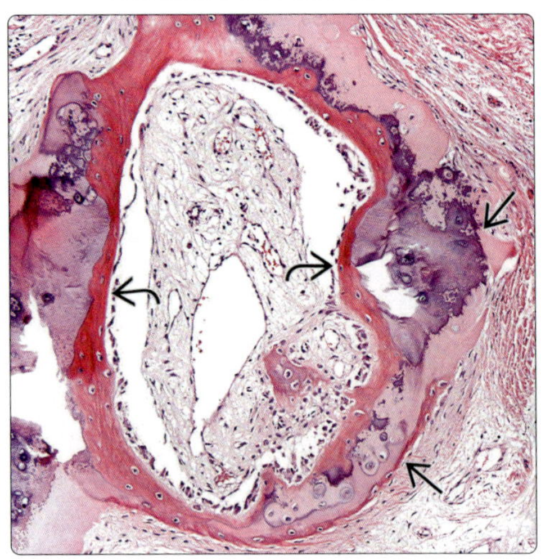

Cytological Atypia

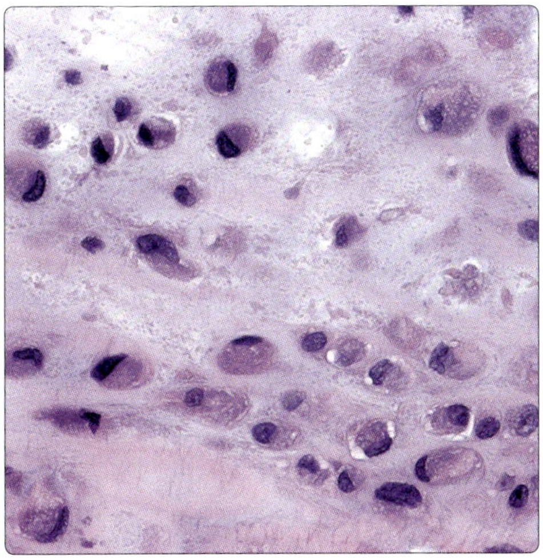

Synovial Chondromatosis of Hip

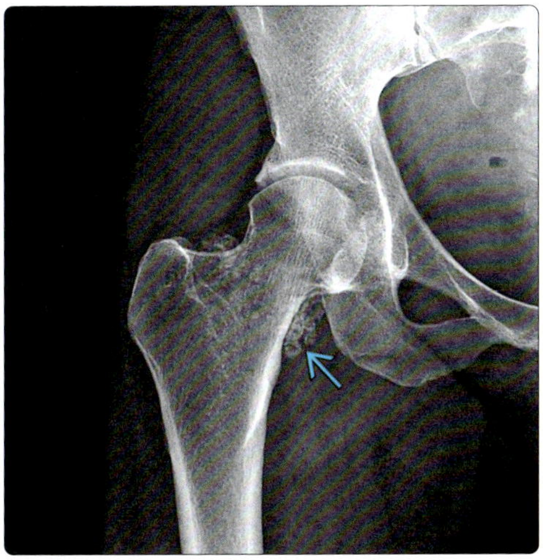

(Left) *Degenerative cytological atypia may be seen in synovial chondromatosis. This high-power micrograph depicts large chondrocytes with eccentric cytoplasm and pleomorphic nuclei with smudged chromatin.* **(Right)** *Synovial chondromatosis typically presents as a calcified mass in a large, weight-bearing joint, such as the hip. It usually presents as multiple diffuse punctate or ring-like calcifications →.*

Gross Appearance

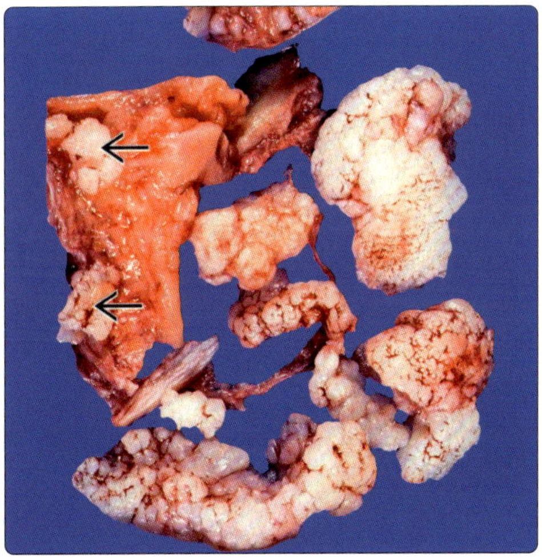

Nodules Separated by Fibrous Stroma

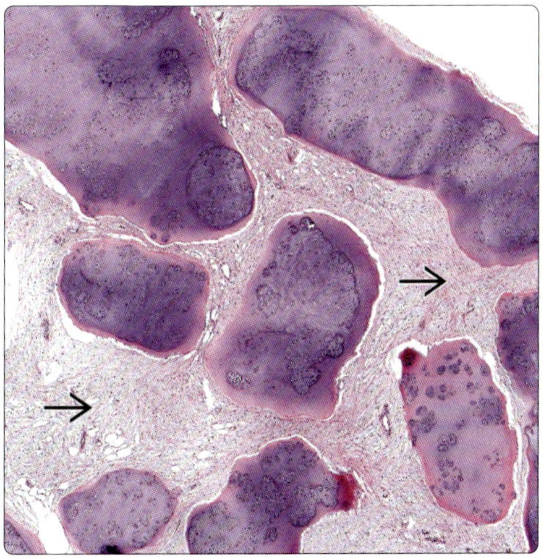

(Left) *Gross photograph depicts tissue removed at knee synovectomy. Note the characteristic multinodular appearance as well as how it studs the synovial membrane →. Detached loose bodies typically accompany such specimens.* **(Right)** *In some cases, the cartilaginous nodules are separated by abundant fibrous stroma →, as depicted in this low-power micrograph. Note the sharp demarcation between the nodules and stroma.*

Temporomandibular Joint Tumor

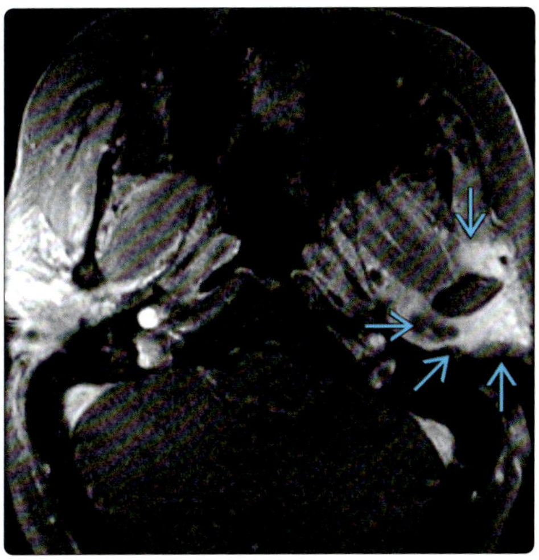

Synovial Chondromatosis of Temporomandibular Joint

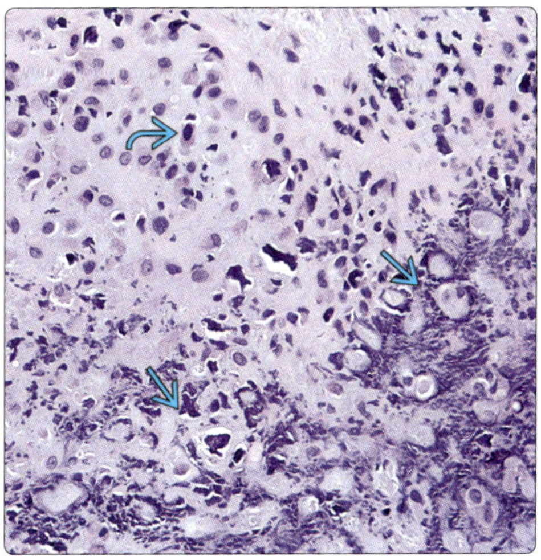

(Left) *T2-weighted MR depicts bright signaling in a case of synovial chondromatosis → of the TMJ. In this location, synovial chondromatosis presents with pain, swelling, and deviation. It frequently recurs and rarely can invade intracranially.* **(Right)** *Synovial chondromatosis of the TMJ is often heavily calcified → and has increased cellularity and degenerative cytologic atypia ↗, as is seen in this H&E.*

Extraskeletal Osteosarcoma

KEY FACTS

TERMINOLOGY

- Soft tissue sarcoma in which neoplastic cells produce osteoid or bone

ETIOLOGY/PATHOGENESIS

- Radiation associated (10%)

CLINICAL ISSUES

- 1-2% of soft tissue sarcomas
- Affects adults almost exclusively
- Mostly deep seated (70-90%)
- Thigh most common site (30-50%)
- Upper extremity, including shoulder girdle (20%)
- Retroperitoneum (10%)
- Poor prognosis: 5-year survival (30%)
  - Local recurrence (35-50%)
  - Metastasis (60%)
  - Age < 40 years and smaller tumor size associated with better prognosis

IMAGING

- Calcification in 50%
  - Spotty to massive

MACROSCOPIC

- Average size: 8 cm; range: 1-50 cm

MICROSCOPIC

- Wide histologic variation; mixed patterns common
  - Osteoblastic, chondroblastic, fibroblastic
  - Giant cell rich, small cell
  - Well differentiated

TOP DIFFERENTIAL DIAGNOSES

- Undifferentiated pleomorphic sarcoma
- Dedifferentiated liposarcoma
- Sarcomatoid carcinoma
- Myositis ossificans

(Left) *Extraskeletal osteosarcoma (ESOS) is a rare soft tissue tumor found almost exclusively in adult patients. It is histologically identical to skeletal osteosarcoma, consisting of irregular, lace-like osteoid matrix ➡ and high-grade malignant cells with brisk mitotic activity ➡.* **(Right)** *ESOS typically presents as a massive soft tissue tumor, most commonly in the thigh, as shown in this CT scan. Calcifications ➡ are common and highly variable in extent.*

Extraskeletal Osteosarcoma

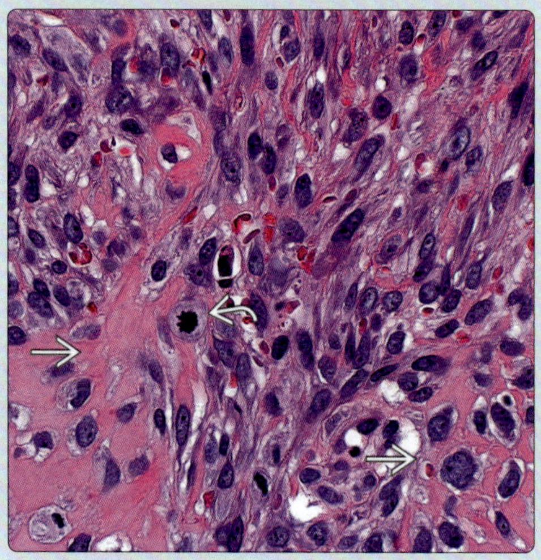

Radiographic Appearance

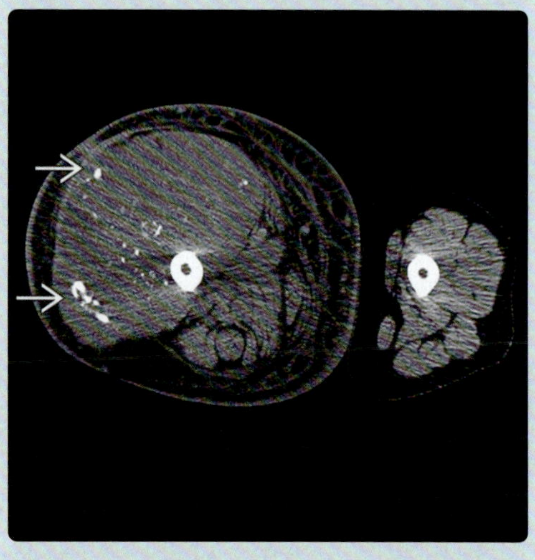

(Left) *Most ESOS are high-grade sarcomas and are characterized by direct production of malignant osteoid and bone by the neoplastic cells. Note the lace-like pattern of mineralization ➡.* **(Right)** *Fibroblastic ESOS resembles undifferentiated pleomorphic or spindle cell sarcoma. Identification of osteoid ➡ is required for diagnosis. However, it can be sparse and hard to distinguish from hyalinized fibrous matrix. Osteoclastic giant cells ➡ are often present.*

Malignant Bone Formation

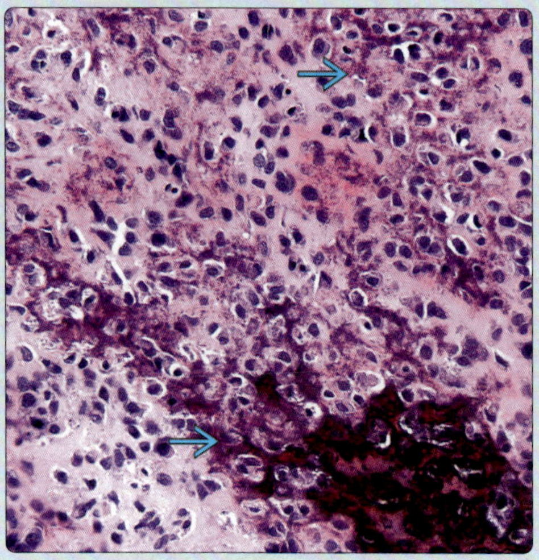

Fibroblastic Osteosarcoma

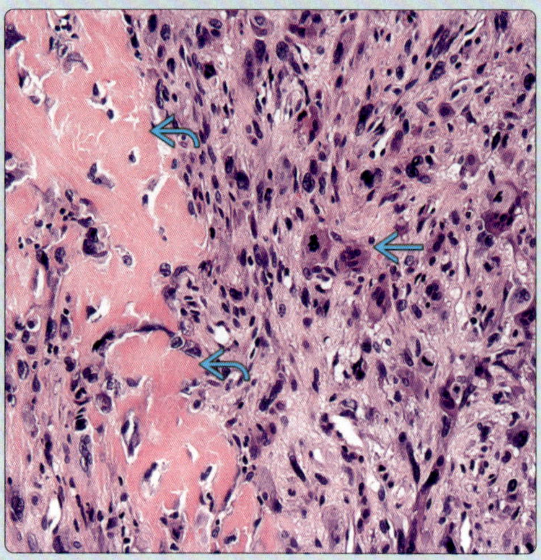

TERMINOLOGY

Abbreviations

- Extraskeletal osteosarcoma (ESOS)

Synonyms

- Soft tissue osteosarcoma
- Extraosseous osteogenic sarcoma

Definitions

- Soft tissue sarcoma in which neoplastic cells produce osteoid or bone
  - Can produce cartilage in addition to osseous matrix
  - No other lines of differentiation

ETIOLOGY/PATHOGENESIS

Environmental Exposure

- Radiation associated (10%)
- Trauma history in some
- Rare tumors arise in myositis ossificans

CLINICAL ISSUES

Epidemiology

- Incidence
  - 1-2% of soft tissue sarcomas
  - 2-4% of osteosarcomas
- Age
  - Affects adults almost exclusively
    - Average: 50 years; range: 20-80 years
- Sex
  - M:F = 2:1

Site

- Mostly deep seated (70-90%)
- Lower extremity (50-70%)
  - Thigh most common site (30-50%)
  - Pelvic girdle, buttocks, leg
- Upper extremity (20%)
  - Shoulder girdle and upper arm common
- Retroperitoneum (10%)
- Rare sites: Hand, foot, larynx, tongue, spermatic cord, penis, pleura, lung, heart, breast, colon, CNS, liver, pancreas, skin

Presentation

- Painless mass
- Progressive enlargement

Treatment

- Wide local excision, resection, or amputation
- Radiation therapy may be used for local control or palliation
- Efficacy of chemotherapy not proven

Prognosis

- Poor; 5-year survival: 30%
- Local recurrence: 35-50%
- Metastasis: 60%
  - Occurs within 2-3 years
  - Lungs most common site
  - Also bone, soft tissue, lymph nodes, liver, brain
- Favorable prognostic factors: Size < 5 cm, age < 40 years, chondroblastic histology, low MIB-1

IMAGING

General Features

- Large mass
- Calcifications in 50%
- May secondarily involve periosteum or bone

MACROSCOPIC

General Features

- Circumscribed or infiltrative
- Firm, fleshy, gritty, or hard
  - Ossification
    - Diffuse, focal, or undetectable
    - Tends to be located in center of tumor
- Cystic hemorrhagic spaces &/or geographic necrosis
- Satellite nodules

Size

- Average: 8 cm; range: 1-50 cm

MICROSCOPIC

Histologic Features

- Identical to skeletal osteosarcoma
- Vast majority are high grade
- Striking variation in amount of osteoid
- Wide histologic variation, mixed patterns common
  - Osteoblastic
    - Polygonal cells with eccentric nuclei
    - Abundant malignant osteoid or bone
    - Fine, lace-like osteoid
    - Wide osseous trabeculae
  - Fibroblastic
    - Resembles undifferentiated pleomorphic sarcoma or fibrosarcoma
    - Osteoid can be sparse
  - Chondroblastic
    - Pleomorphic chondrocytes within lobules of hyaline cartilage
    - Peripheral lobular hypercellularity
    - Often mixed with osteoblastic areas
  - Giant cell rich
    - Pleomorphic sarcoma with numerous osteoclastic giant cells
    - Osteoclasts may obscure underlying malignant histology
    - Osteoid can be sparse
  - Telangiectatic
    - Very rare in pure form
    - Telangiectatic or cystic hemorrhagic areas common in conventional ESOS
  - Well differentiated
    - Very rare
    - Cytologically bland, fibrogenic spindle cells
    - Wide seams of osteoid and woven bone
    - Resembles parosteal or low-grade central osteosarcoma
  - Small cell
    - Very rare
    - Resembles Ewing sarcoma

ANCILLARY TESTS

Immunohistochemistry

- Osteocalcin and SATB2 are sensitive and specific markers for general osteoblastic differentiation
  - Not specific for osteosarcoma
- Variable, nonspecific expression of SMA, CD99, EMA, desmin

Cytogenetics

- Complex karyotype

DIFFERENTIAL DIAGNOSIS

Undifferentiated Pleomorphic Sarcoma

- Can show significant morphologic overlap with ESOS
- Stromal hyalinization can mimic osteoid
- Can have osteoclast-like giant cells
- Distinction from fibroblastic ESOS sometimes arbitrary

Dedifferentiated Liposarcoma

- Heterologous osteosarcomatous differentiation sometimes present
  - Usually in retroperitoneal tumors
- Identification of well-differentiated liposarcomatous component rules out ESOS
- *MDM2* and *CDK4* amplification detectable by immunohistochemistry or fluoroscopic in situ hybridization (FISH)

Extraskeletal Mesenchymal Chondrosarcoma

- Small round blue or spindle cell tumor
- Neoplastic cells produce cartilage that can ossify
- Pericytic vascular pattern

Extraskeletal Ewing Sarcoma

- Small round blue cell tumor
- Fibrinous matrix can mimic osteoid
- CD99(+) characteristically diffuse and membranous
- Cytogenetic [t(11;22), t(7;22), t(21;22), t(2;22)] and molecular (EWS-FLI-1, EWS-ERG) confirmation

Giant Cell Tumor of Soft Tissue

- Numerous osteoclastic giant cells and mononuclear stromal cells
- Can produce bone, usually at periphery of tumor
- Lacks high-grade cytologic atypia and atypical mitoses
- Lacks lace-like osteoid

Myositis Ossificans

- Nonneoplastic, usually post trauma
- Benign, reactive myofibroblasts and osteoblasts
  - Can have brisk mitotic activity
  - Lacks malignant cytologic atypia
- Temporal and peripheral bony maturation
  - Increased bone formation and maturation with time
  - More mature bone forms at periphery of tumor

Fibroosseous Pseudotumor of Digits

- Affects digits
- Benign, reactive fibroblasts and osteoblasts
- Often lack peripheral zonal maturation

Synovial Sarcoma

- Uniform spindle cells
- May have stromal fibrosis with heterotopic ossification
- TLE1, CD99, cytokeratin, and EMA (+) in most
- Cytogenetic t(X;18) and molecular (SSX-SYT) confirmation

Malignant Peripheral Nerve Sheath Tumor

- Hyperchromatic spindle cells in fascicles
- May have heterologous osseous, chondroid, or osteosarcomatous elements
- Usually S100(+) (50-60%)
- Frequent history of neurofibromatosis type 1 (50%)

Osteogenic Melanoma

- Rare melanoma with heterologous osteosarcomatous element
- S100(+)
- Often HMB-45(+) or Melan-A(+)

Ossifying Fibromyxoid Tumor

- Ovoid mesenchymal cells arranged in cords and clusters
- Fibromyxoid stroma
- Usually encased by peripheral shell of bone
- Usually bland but can show cytologic atypia

Sarcomatoid Carcinoma

- Uterus, kidney, lung, others
- Cytokeratin in most
  - However, some osteosarcomas express cytokeratin

DIAGNOSTIC CHECKLIST

Clinically Relevant Pathologic Features

- Tissue distribution

Pathologic Interpretation Pearls

- Microscopically identical to skeletal osteosarcoma

SELECTED REFERENCES

1. Longhi A et al: Extraskeletal osteosarcoma: a European Musculoskeletal Oncology Society study on 266 patients. Eur J Cancer. 74:9-16, 2017
2. Choi LE et al: Analysis of outcomes in extraskeletal osteosarcoma: a review of fifty-three cases. J Bone Joint Surg Am. 96(1):e2, 2014
3. von Baer A et al: Immunohistochemical and FISH analysis of MDM2 and CDK4 in a dedifferentiated extraskeletal osteosarcoma arising in the vastus lateralis muscle: differential diagnosis and diagnostic algorithm. Pathol Res Pract. 210(10):698-703, 2014
4. Conner JR et al: SATB2 is a novel marker of osteoblastic differentiation in bone and soft tissue tumours. Histopathology. 63(1):36-49, 2013
5. Kyriazoglou AI et al: 12q amplification defines a subtype of extraskeletal osteosarcoma with good prognosis that is the soft tissue homologue of parosteal osteosarcoma. Cancer Genet. 205(6):332-6, 2012
6. Yang JY et al: Small cell extraskeletal osteosarcoma. Orthopedics. 32(3):217, 2009
7. Konishi E et al: Extraskeletal osteosarcoma arising in myositis ossificans. Skeletal Radiol. 30(1):39-43, 2001
8. Fanburg-Smith JC et al: Osteocalcin and osteonectin immunoreactivity in extraskeletal osteosarcoma: a study of 28 cases. Hum Pathol. 30(1):32-8, 1999
9. Lucas DR et al: Osteogenic melanoma. A rare variant of malignant melanoma. Am J Surg Pathol. 17(4):400-9, 1993
10. Chung EB et al: Extraskeletal osteosarcoma. Cancer. 60(5):1132-42, 1987
11. Allan CJ et al: Osteogenic sarcoma of the somatic soft tissues. Clinicopathologic study of 26 cases and review of literature. Cancer. 27(5):1121-33, 1971

Extraskeletal Osteosarcoma

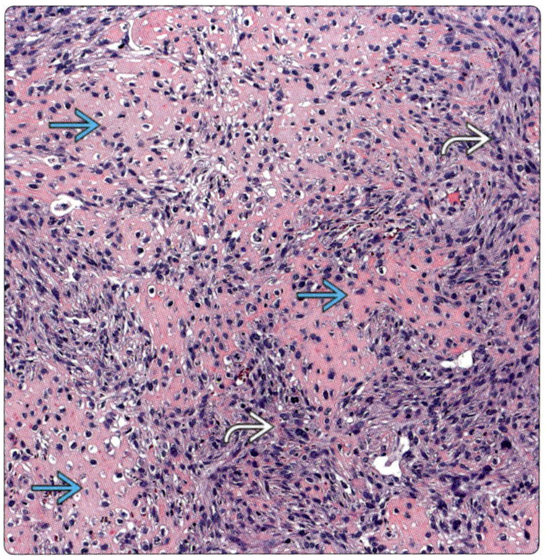

Osteoblastic Osteosarcoma

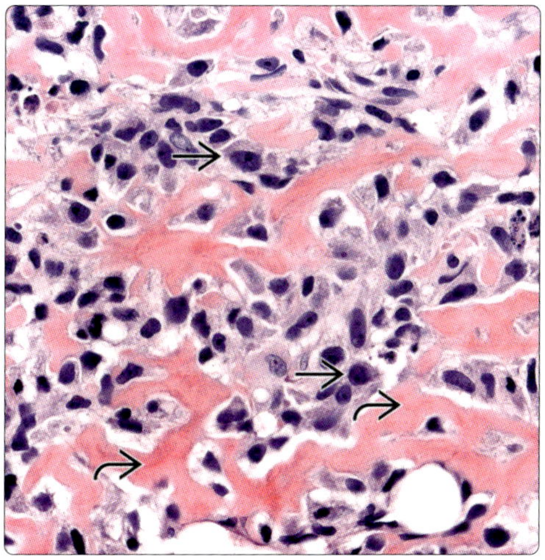

(Left) *This low-power micrograph shows a flank mass in a 42-year-old man. It depicts classic features of osteosarcoma comprised by solid sheets and lace-like configurations of osteoid and large, pleomorphic spindle cells arranged in fascicles and storiform arrays.* **(Right)** *Osteoblastic osteosarcoma is characterized by polygonal osteoblastic cells with eccentric nuclei that produce osteoid or woven bone, often with an irregular, lace-like pattern as shown.*

Chondroblastic Osteosarcoma

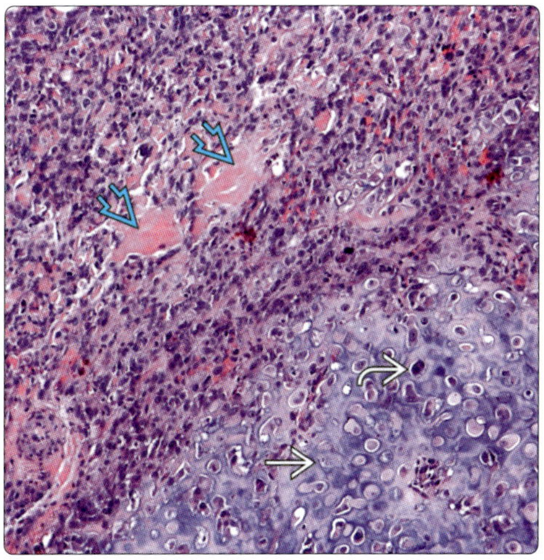

Hemorrhagic Cystic Spaces

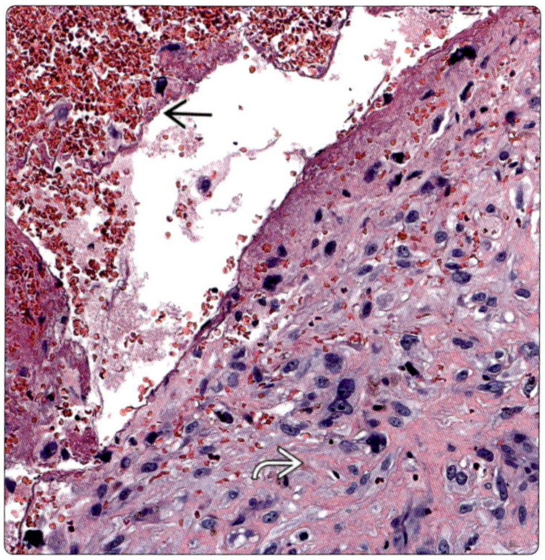

(Left) *Chondroblastic osteosarcoma has pleomorphic chondrocytes in lacunar spaces embedded within a pale blue chondroid matrix. This pattern is often admixed with others, such as osteoblastic or fibroblastic patterns.* **(Right)** *Large, blood-filled cystic spaces are often found in ESOS. This micrograph depicts a space filled with red blood cells adjacent to tumor. Note the lace-like osteoid matrix.*

Giant Cell-Rich Osteosarcoma

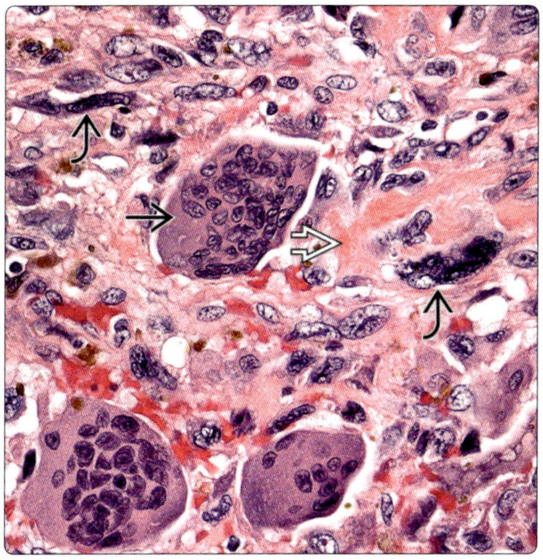

Well-Differentiated Osteosarcoma

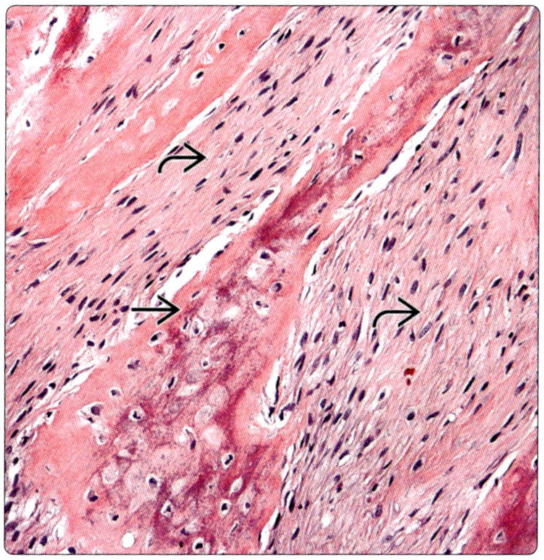

(Left) *Giant cell-rich osteosarcoma contains numerous benign osteoclastic giant cells. In such tumors, one needs to search carefully for atypical cells, atypical mitotic figures (not shown), and osteoid to establish the diagnosis.* **(Right)** *Only a handful of well-differentiated ESOS have been reported. These tumors are microscopically identical to parosteal or low-grade central osteosarcomas, composed of cytologically bland, fibrogenic spindle cells in between a broad trabeculae of woven bone.*

Extraskeletal Mesenchymal Chondrosarcoma

KEY FACTS

TERMINOLOGY

- Bimorphic soft tissue sarcoma characterized by undifferentiated small round or spindle cells, islands of well-differentiated hyaline cartilage, and recurrent *HEY1-NCOA2* fusion

CLINICAL ISSUES

- Rare: < 1% of soft tissue sarcomas
- Age: Mostly 2nd and 3rd decades
- Wide range of soft tissue and visceral locations
- Common locations
  - Head and neck region
  - Cranial and spinal dura
- Clinical course can be protracted

IMAGING

- Calcifications in most

MICROSCOPIC

- Bimorphic pattern
- Small round or spindle cells
- Hyperchromatic coarse chromatin
- Thin-walled, branching (pericytomatous) vascular pattern
- Hyaline cartilage islands
- Calcifications and endochondral ossification
- CD99(+) and SOX9(+)

TOP DIFFERENTIAL DIAGNOSES

- Ewing sarcoma
- Synovial sarcoma
- Solitary fibrous tumor (cellular/malignant)
- Osteosarcoma
- Malignant peripheral nerve sheath tumor with heterologous cartilage
- Atypical teratoid rhabdoid tumor
- Sclerosing rhabdomyosarcoma

Extraskeletal Mesenchymal Chondrosarcoma

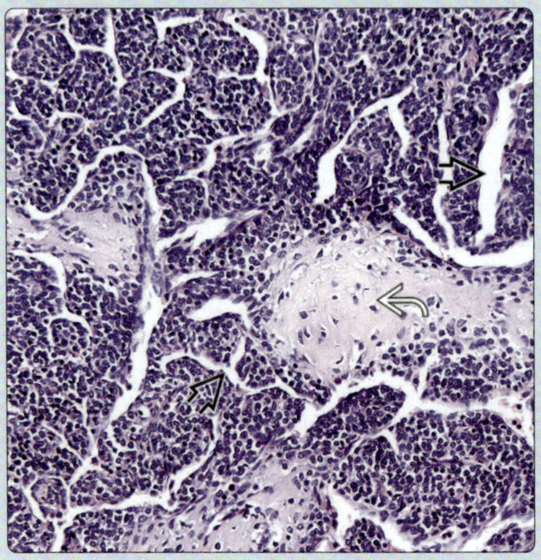

Radiographic Appearance

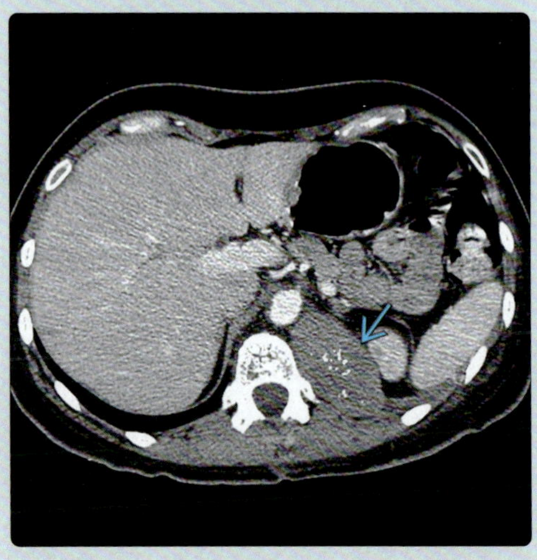

(Left) *Extraskeletal mesenchymal chondrosarcoma (EMC) has a bimorphic histology consisting of small round cell areas and islands of hyaline cartilage ➡. Most tumors have a prominent pericytomatous vascular pattern ⇨.* **(Right)** *EMC typically presents as a circumscribed, calcified mass. Although most common in cranial and spinal meninges, it occurs at widely variable sites. In this case, CT shows a tumor ⇨ in the retrocrural area with stippled calcification.*

Cytologic Features

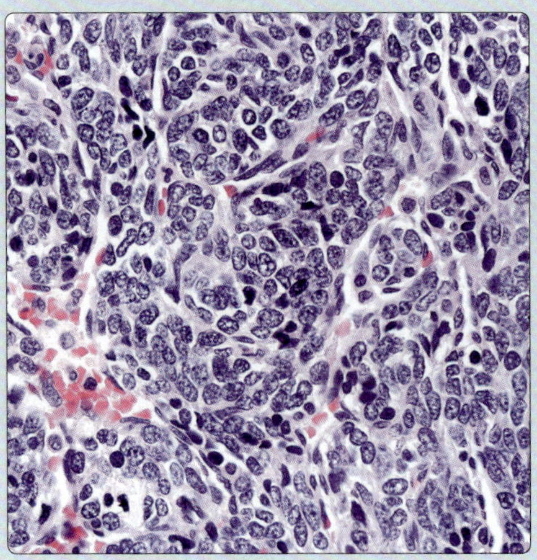

CD99

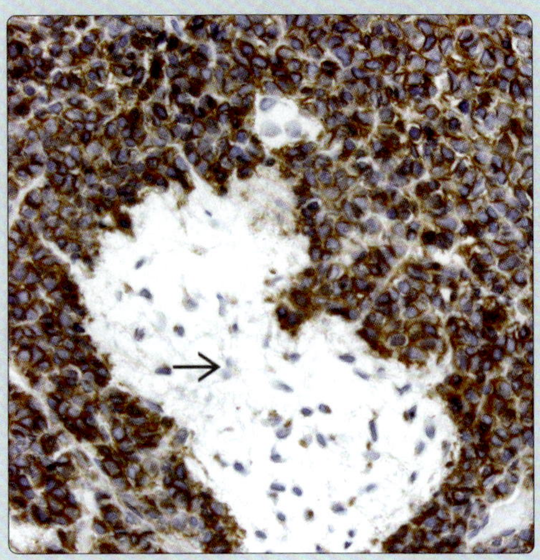

(Left) *Most EMCs are composed of closely spaced small cells with rather distinctive cytologic features consisting of round or oval nuclei with dense, coarse chromatin and scant, indistinct cytoplasm.* **(Right)** *Diffuse, strong CD99 immunoreactivity characterizes EMC. In this example, anti-CD99 shows a cytoplasmic membrane staining pattern, which can lead to a misdiagnosis of Ewing sarcoma. Note that the cells within the cartilage island are negative →.*

Extraskeletal Mesenchymal Chondrosarcoma

TERMINOLOGY

Abbreviations

- Extraskeletal mesenchymal chondrosarcoma (EMC)

Definitions

- Bimorphic soft tissue (or bone) sarcoma characterized by undifferentiated small round or spindle cells, islands of well-differentiated hyaline cartilage, and *HEY1-NCOA2* fusion
  - Microscopically identical to primary skeletal mesenchymal chondrosarcoma

CLINICAL ISSUES

Epidemiology

- Incidence
  - Rare: < 1% of soft tissue sarcomas
  - Only 1/3 of EMCs present as primary soft tissue tumors
    - Most are primary bone tumors
- Age
  - Wide range: 0-70 years
    - Mostly 2nd and 3rd decades
    - Average: 30 years
    - Rare congenital cases
- Sex
  - Women and men equally affected

Site

- Head and neck region
  - Cranial dura
    - Most common extraskeletal site
  - Orbit
- Lower extremities
- Reported in wide array of soft tissue and visceral locations

Presentation

- Painful or painless mass in extremity tumors
- Headache and neurologic symptoms in meningeal tumors
- Proptosis and visual changes in orbital tumors

Natural History

- Fully malignant and aggressive
- Frequent metastases
  - Lungs most common
  - Can have late metastases
    - Up to 20 years following initial presentation
- Behavior regarded as unpredictable

Treatment

- Complete surgical resection when possible
- Role of chemotherapy poorly defined
- Radiation may benefit local control

Prognosis

- Overall poor outcome
  - 50% 5-year survival
  - 25% 10-year survival
- Clinical course can be protracted

IMAGING

Radiographic Findings

- Well-defined soft tissue mass
- Dural-based intracranial/intraspinal tumor
- Calcifications in most
  - Stipples, rings and arcs, streaks

MACROSCOPIC

General Features

- Multilobulated and well circumscribed
- Periphery soft and fleshy
- Center often with gritty texture or cartilaginous foci
- Necrosis and hemorrhage in some

Size

- Variable: 2-37 cm

MICROSCOPIC

Histologic Features

- Bimorphic pattern
  - Small round or spindle cells
    - Clusters or fascicles
    - Uniform round, oval, or spindle-shaped nuclei
      - Hyperchromatic coarse chromatin
      - Scant cytoplasm (may be clear in some cells)
      - Variable mitotic rate
    - Thin-walled branching (pericytomatous) vascular pattern
    - Necrosis or hemorrhage in some
  - Hyaline cartilage
    - Variable-sized islands
    - Large sheets in some
    - Small hyperchromatic cells in lacunar spaces
    - Often low-grade or bland cytologic features
    - Calcifications and endochondral ossification common
      - Bone formation sometimes extensive
    - Sharp demarcation or gradual transition between cellular areas and cartilage

ANCILLARY TESTS

Immunohistochemistry

- CD99(+), SOX9(+), desmin (+) in 50%, EMA(+) in 35%
- S100 protein and ERG expressed in cartilage only
- Osteocalcin expressed in areas of ossification only
- β-catenin may be expressed at interface of cartilage and tumor cells
- Retention of nuclear SNF5 (INI1)
- Negative for FLI-1, STAT6, CD45, SMA, GFAP, keratin, myogenin (very rare focal positivity), MYOD1 (very rare focal positivity)

Molecular Genetics

- Recurrent *HEY1-NCOA2* fusion detectable by RT-PCR (or FISH)
  - *IRF2BP2-CDX1* fusion reported

DIFFERENTIAL DIAGNOSIS

Ewing Sarcoma

- Uniform small round cells
- Softer, less coarse chromatin
- Lacks cartilage
- Lacks pericytomatous vascular pattern
- Glycogen-rich clear cell cytoplasm in most
- CD99(+), FLI-1(+), ERG(+)
- SOX9(+/-)
- *EWSR1* break-apart by FISH
- *EWS-FLI1* or *EWS-ERG* fusion by RT-PCR

Synovial Sarcoma

- Spindle or small round cells
- Softer, less coarse chromatin
- Pericytomatous vascular pattern
- Hyalinized and calcified stroma
- Metaplastic ossification in some
- Lacks hyaline cartilage
- Keratin (+), EMA(+), CD99(+), TLE1(+), SOX9(+)
- *SYT* break-apart by FISH
- *SSX-SYT* fusion by RT-PCR

Solitary Fibrous Tumor (Cellular/Malignant)

- Spindle cells in haphazard or storiform arrays
- Wire-like collagen bundles
- Pericytomatous vascular pattern
- Occurs in meninges, as does EMC
- Lacks hyaline cartilage
- CD99(+)
- CD34(+/-)
- CD10(+)
- STAT6(+)

Osteosarcoma

- Can have small cell or chondroblastic features
- Rare as primary soft tissue tumor
- SOX9(-)
- Osteocalcin (+)

Malignant Peripheral Nerve Sheath Tumor

- Rare cases featuring heterologous cartilage
- Fascicular spindle cell pattern most common
- Can have small round cell pattern
- Can have pericytomatous vascular pattern
- S100 protein (+) in 50% of tumors, usually focal

Atypical Teratoid Rhabdoid Tumor

- Intracranial location
- Small round cells
- More abundant eosinophilic cytoplasm
- Lacks cartilage
- Keratin (+)
- Loss of nuclear SNF5 (INI1)

Sclerosing Rhabdomyosarcoma

- Small round or spindle cells
- Hyalinized matrix can mimic cartilage; well-formed cartilage absent
- Rhabdomyoblasts often sparse
- Desmin (-), MYOD1(+), myogenin (+/-)
  - EMC desmin (+) in 50% of cases
  - Very rare EMCs reported as focally positive for MYOD1 or myogenin

Extraskeletal Myxoid Chondrosarcoma

- Abundant myxoid matrix
- Epithelioid or spindle cells arranged in cords
- Well-formed hyaline cartilage rarely present
- SOX9(-)

SELECTED REFERENCES

1. Arora K et al: Extraskeletal mesenchymal chondrosarcoma. Arch Pathol Lab Med. 142(11):1421-4, 2018
2. Frezza AM et al: Mesenchymal chondrosarcoma: prognostic factors and outcome in 113 patients. A European Musculoskeletal Oncology Society study. Eur J Cancer. 51(3):374-81, 2015
3. Andersson C et al: Primary spinal intradural mesenchymal chondrosarcoma with detection of fusion gene HEY1-NCOA2: a paediatric case report and review of the literature. Oncol Lett. 8(4):1608-12, 2014
4. Cheah AL et al: STAT6 rabbit monoclonal antibody is a robust diagnostic tool for the distinction of solitary fibrous tumour from its mimics. Pathology. 46(5):389-95, 2014
5. Kawaguchi S et al: Radiation therapy is associated with fewer recurrences in mesenchymal chondrosarcoma. Clin Orthop Relat Res. 472(3):856-64, 2014
6. Moriya K et al: Mesenchymal chondrosarcoma diagnosed on FISH for HEY1-NCOA2 fusion gene. Pediatr Int. 56(5):e55-7, 2014
7. Panagopoulos I et al: Chromosome aberrations and HEY1-NCOA2 fusion gene in a mesenchymal chondrosarcoma. Oncol Rep. 32(1):40-4, 2014
8. Fritchie KJ et al: Are meningeal hemangiopericytoma and mesenchymal chondrosarcoma the same?: a study of HEY1-NCOA2 fusion. Am J Clin Pathol. 140(5):670-4, 2013
9. Nakayama R et al: Detection of HEY1-NCOA2 fusion by fluorescence in-situ hybridization in formalin-fixed paraffin-embedded tissues as a possible diagnostic tool for mesenchymal chondrosarcoma. Pathol Int. 62(12):823-6, 2012
10. Shakked RJ et al: Mesenchymal chondrosarcoma: clinicopathologic study of 20 cases. Arch Pathol Lab Med. 136(1):61-75, 2012
11. Wang L et al: Identification of a novel, recurrent HEY1-NCOA2 fusion in mesenchymal chondrosarcoma based on a genome-wide screen of exon-level expression data. Genes Chromosomes Cancer. 51(2):127-39, 2012
12. Cajaiba MM et al: Sox9 expression is not limited to chondroid neoplasms: variable occurrence in other soft tissue and bone tumors with frequent expression by synovial sarcomas. Int J Surg Pathol. 18(5):319-23, 2010
13. Fanburg-Smith JC et al: Immunoprofile of mesenchymal chondrosarcoma: aberrant desmin and EMA expression, retention of INI1, and negative estrogen receptor in 22 female-predominant central nervous system and musculoskeletal cases. Ann Diagn Pathol. 14(1):8-14, 2010
14. Fanburg-Smith JC et al: Reappraisal of mesenchymal chondrosarcoma: novel morphologic observations of the hyaline cartilage and endochondral ossification and beta-catenin, Sox9, and osteocalcin immunostaining of 22 cases. Hum Pathol. 41(5):653-62, 2010
15. Dantonello TM et al: Mesenchymal chondrosarcoma of soft tissues and bone in children, adolescents, and young adults: experiences of the CWS and COSS study groups. Cancer. 112(11):2424-31, 2008
16. Gengler C et al: Desmin and myogenin reactivity in mesenchymal chondrosarcoma: a potential diagnostic pitfall. Histopathology. 48(2):201-3, 2006
17. Wehrli BM et al: Sox9, a master regulator of chondrogenesis, distinguishes mesenchymal chondrosarcoma from other small blue round cell tumors. Hum Pathol. 34(3):263-9, 2003
18. Granter SR et al: CD99 reactivity in mesenchymal chondrosarcoma. Hum Pathol. 27(12):1273-6, 1996
19. Nakashima Y et al: Mesenchymal chondrosarcoma of bone and soft tissue. A review of 111 cases. Cancer. 57(12):2444-53, 1986
20. Bertoni F et al: Mesenchymal chondrosarcoma of bone and soft tissues. Cancer. 52(3):533-41, 1983
21. Huvos AG et al: Mesenchymal chondrosarcoma. A clinicopathologic analysis of 35 patients with emphasis on treatment. Cancer. 51(7):1230-7, 1983

Pericytomatous Vascular Pattern

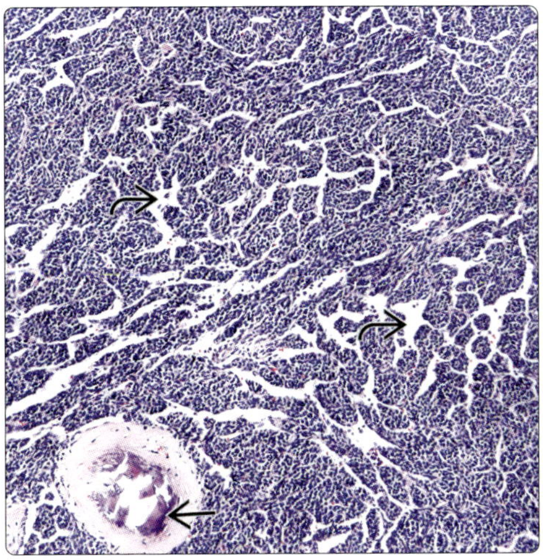

Large Area of Hyaline Cartilage

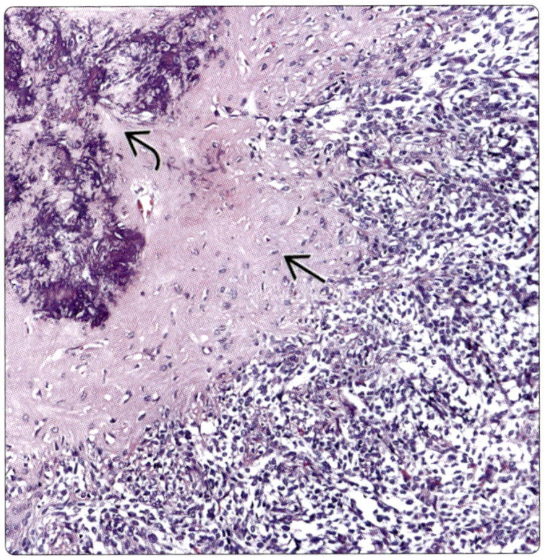

(Left) *The amount of cartilage → is variable in EMC. In most tumors, cellular areas predominate as depicted. Note the prominent pericytomatous vascular pattern ↷ and central calcification of the cartilage.* **(Right)** *In some EMCs, hyaline cartilage forms the predominant element, as depicted →. The cartilage is often pink instead of light blue and can be heavily mineralized ↶.*

Ossification

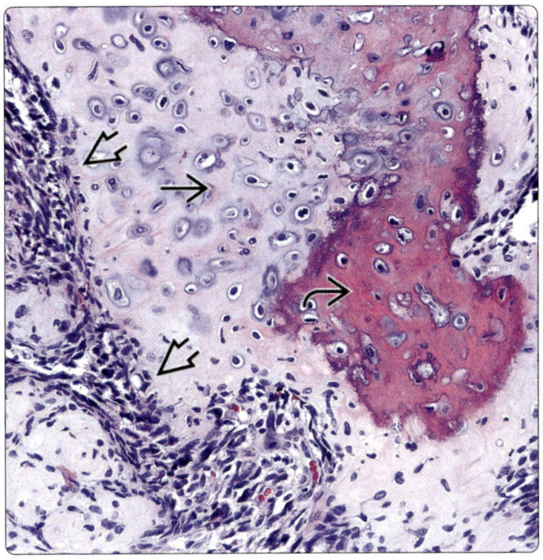

Round Cells Admixed With Chondroid Matrix

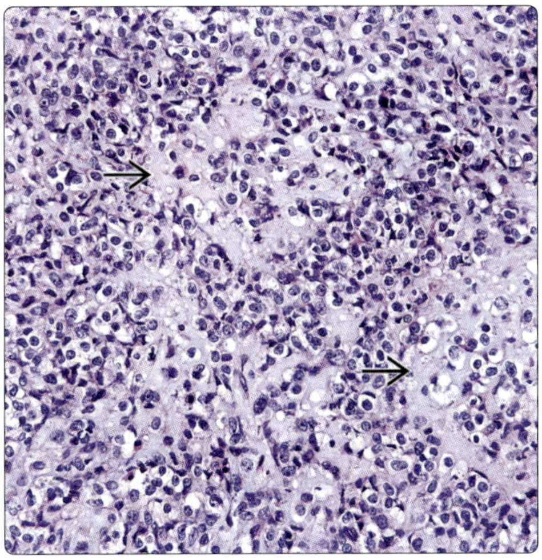

(Left) *Endochondral ossification is often seen in EMC. This micrograph depicts an island of neoplastic hyaline cartilage → transitioning into woven bone ↷. Such tumors can sometimes be misdiagnosed as osteosarcoma. Note the sharp interface between cellular area and cartilage ⇨.* **(Right)** *In some tumors, the malignant cells are intimately admixed with chondroid matrix →, which appears pale blue in the tumor.*

Islands of Hyaline Cartilage

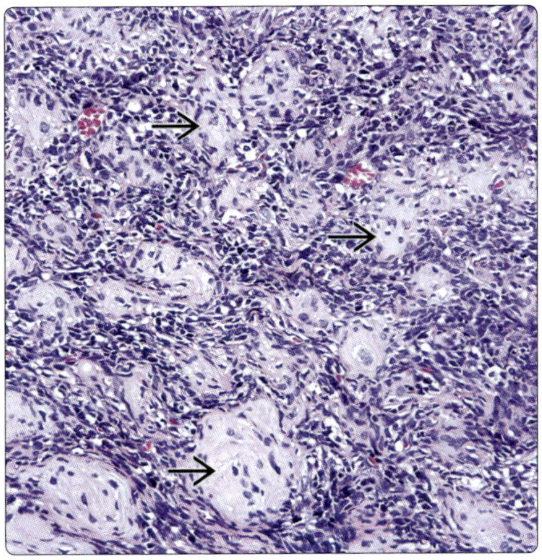

Spindle Cells

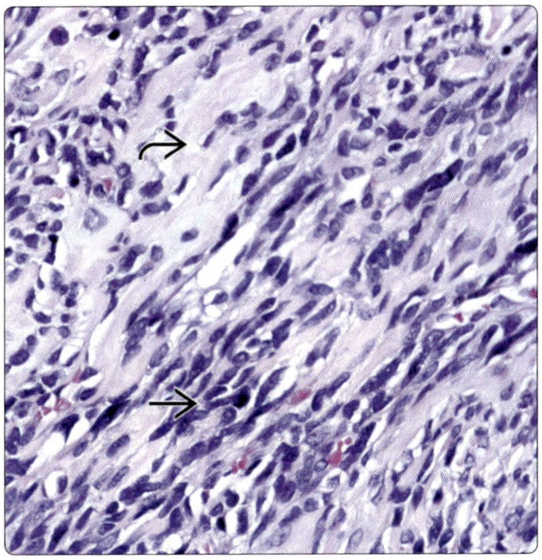

(Left) *Multiple small islands of hyaline cartilage → blend with small round cells in this EMC, creating a multinodular pattern.* **(Right)** *In some tumors, the cells are spindle-shaped and arranged in fascicles →. However, spindle cell areas generally account for only a portion of a given tumor. Fibrotic stroma is also occasionally seen as illustrated ↷.*

SECTION 12

Peripheral Nerve Sheath Tumors

Benign

Solitary Circumscribed Neuroma 506
Schwannoma 508
Neurofibroma 522
Perineurioma 530
Hybrid Nerve Sheath Tumor 536
Granular Cell Tumor 540
Dermal Nerve Sheath Myxoma 546
Ganglioneuroma 550
Neuromuscular Choristoma 554

Intermediate

Melanotic Schwannoma 556

Malignant

Malignant Peripheral Nerve Sheath Tumor 558
Epithelioid Malignant Peripheral Nerve Sheath Tumor 566
Ectomesenchymoma 570

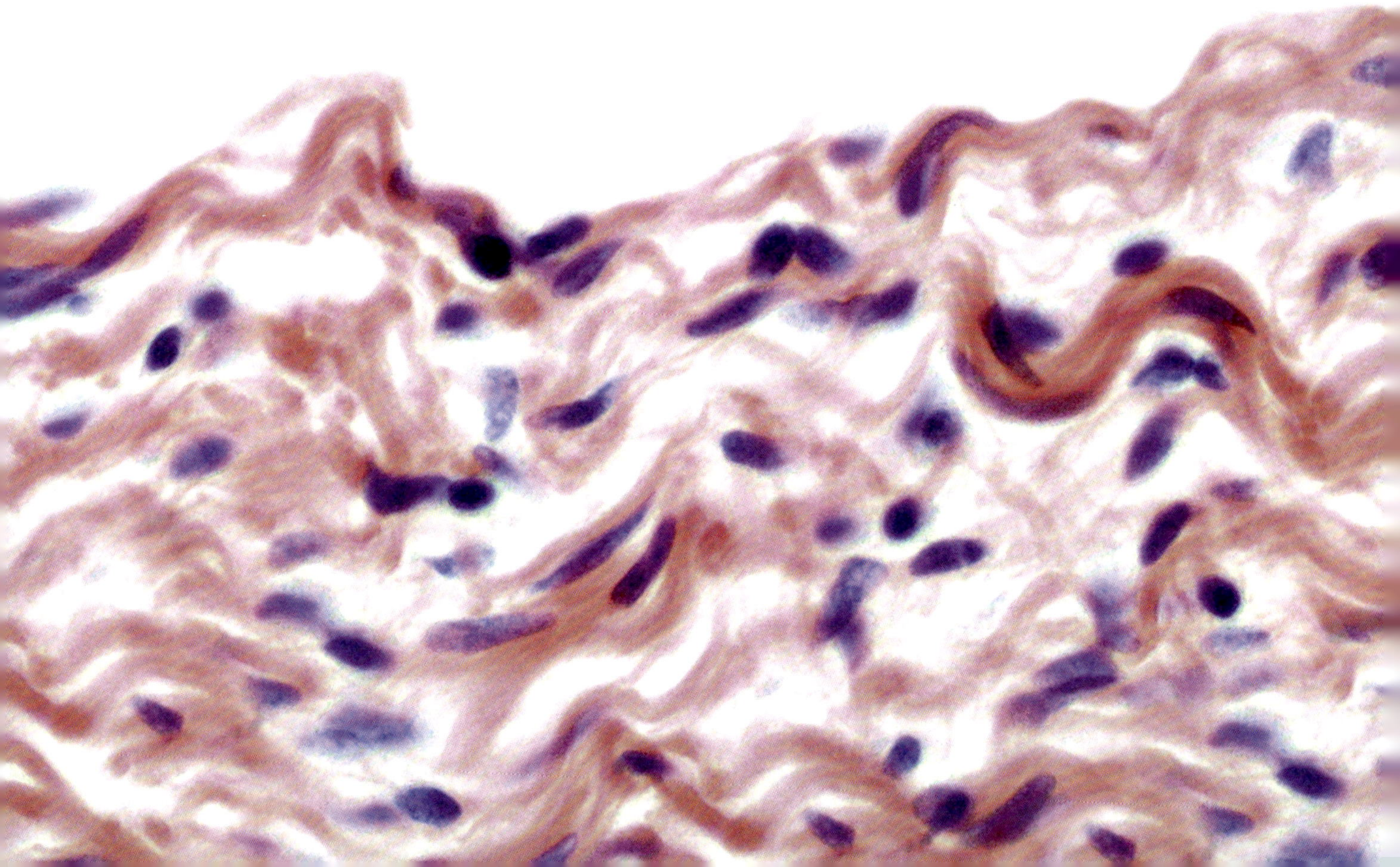

Solitary Circumscribed Neuroma

KEY FACTS

TERMINOLOGY

- Synonym: Palisaded encapsulated neuroma
- Benign dermal/subcutaneous intraneural proliferation of Schwann cells and axons

CLINICAL ISSUES

- Common
- Middle-aged to elderly adults
- Most common sites: Face, especially cheeks, nasolabial folds, and nose
- Less common sites: Oral mucosae, acral skin, eyelid, penis
- Completely benign
- No association with NF1 or MEN 2B

MICROSCOPIC

- Sharply circumscribed dermal nodule with thin capsule
  - May be plexiform or multinodular
- Composed of Schwann cells arranged into short fascicles/bundles with intervening clefting artifact
- Relatively uniform cellularity
- Cells may form vague palisades
  - Usually not as dramatic as seen in Verocay bodies
- Usually only minimal focal myxoid change
- Often connected to nerve
- Likely intraneural proliferation that distends and expands nerve

ANCILLARY TESTS

- S100 protein and SOX10 (+) Schwann cells
- Neurofilament (+) axons throughout lesion
- EMA, claudin-1, GLUT-1 (+) perineurial cells in capsule

TOP DIFFERENTIAL DIAGNOSES

- Schwannoma
- Mucosal neuroma
- Traumatic neuroma
- Plexiform neurofibroma

(Left) *Solitary circumscribed neuroma (SCN) usually presents as a sharply demarcated dermal nodule composed of bundles or fascicles of spindled Schwann cells.* **(Right)** *Bland spindled Schwann cells are arranged in fascicles/bundles, which are divided from one another by very characteristic artifactual clefts →. The spindle cells may form palisades →, although these are usually less well developed in SCN than those of a schwannoma.*

Solitary Circumscribed Dermal Nodule

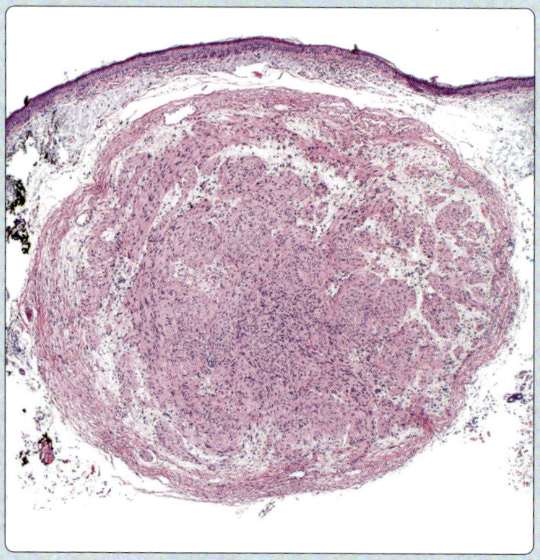

Characteristic Clefting Artifact

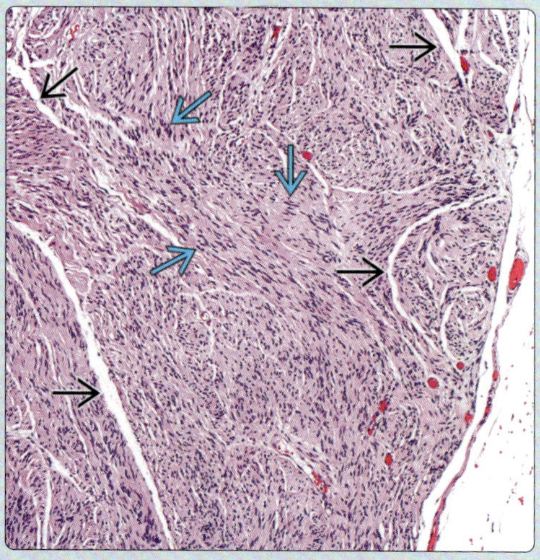

(Left) *Bland spindled Schwann cells may form vague palisades → in SCN. A thin peripheral layer ("capsule") of perineurium often surrounds the lesion →.* **(Right)** *The plexiform pattern of SCN is composed of multiple circumscribed nodules, each of which has the typical features of conventional SCN. Clefting artifact is visible here even from low power →.*

Palisading and Peripheral "Capsule"

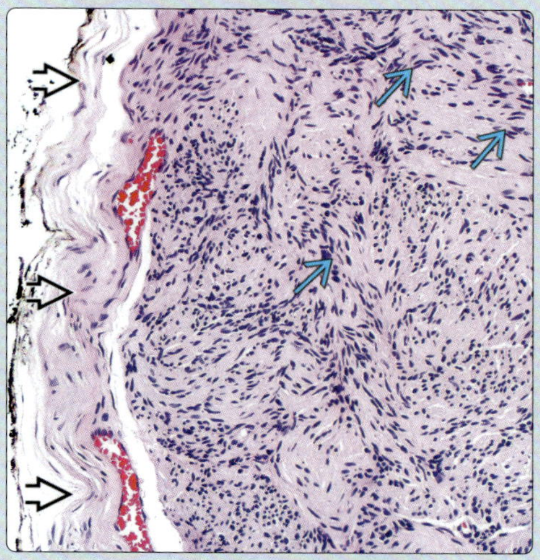

Plexiform Growth Pattern

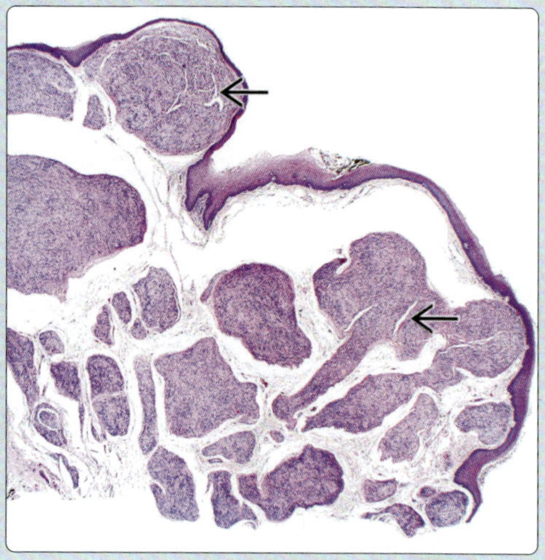

TERMINOLOGY

Abbreviations

- Solitary circumscribed neuroma (SCN)

Synonyms

- Palisaded encapsulated neuroma

Definitions

- Benign dermal/subcutaneous intraneural proliferation of Schwann cells and axons

CLINICAL ISSUES

Epidemiology

- Incidence
  - Common
- Middle-aged to elderly adults

Site

- Face most common site, especially
  - Cheeks
  - Nasolabial folds
  - Nose
- Less common sites
  - Oral mucosa
  - Acral skin
  - Eyelid
  - Penis

Presentation

- Skin-colored papule (may mimic basal cell carcinoma clinically)
- Usually asymptomatic

Treatment

- Simple excision usually curative

Prognosis

- Completely benign
- No association with NF1 or MEN 2B
- Rare plexiform SCN on acral skin may be associated with Cowden syndrome (*PTEN* mutation)

MICROSCOPIC

Histologic Features

- Sharply circumscribed dermal nodule
  - May be plexiform or multinodular
  - May extend into subcutis
  - Thin, peripheral capsule of perineurium
    - Mass often only partially surrounded by perineurium
- Composed of Schwann cells arranged into short fascicles/bundles
  - Intervening clefting artifact between bundles is very characteristic
  - Relatively uniform cellularity
  - Cells have buckled nuclei and scant cytoplasm
  - Majority of cells are bland but may be hyperchromatic
    - As with other Schwann cell proliferations, focal degenerative nuclear pleomorphism may be seen
  - Mitotic activity is very low
  - Cells may form vague palisades
    - Not usually striking palisading like Verocay bodies of schwannoma
  - Usually only minimal focal myxoid change
- Often connected to nerve
  - Likely represents intraneural proliferation that distends and expands nerve

ANCILLARY TESTS

Immunohistochemistry

- S100 protein and SOX10 (+) in Schwann cells
- Neurofilament protein (+) axons throughout lesion
- Perineurial cells in capsule (+) for EMA, claudin-1, GLUT1
- GFAP, SMA, keratin (-)

DIFFERENTIAL DIAGNOSIS

Schwannoma

- Alternating hyper- and hypocellular areas
- Hyalinized or myxoid stromal change
- Hyalinized vessel walls
- More prominent palisading (Verocay bodies)
- Lacks bundles with intervening clefting artifact
- May have some axons
  - Axons usually limited to area beneath capsule

Mucosal Neuroma

- Neural proliferations of oral cavity and gastrointestinal tract
- Thickened tortuous nerve bundles scattered throughout submucosa
- Poorly circumscribed
- May be associated with MEN 2B
- Rare hybrid lesions show overlap between SCN and mucosal neuroma; unclear if these are related to MEN 2B

Traumatic Neuroma

- Neural proliferations in dermis near site of injury or amputation
- Thickened nerve bundles intertwined with one another
- Often poorly circumscribed

Plexiform Neurofibroma

- Can mimic multinodular pattern of SCN
- Less cellular and less organized than SCN
- More myxoid background, scattered disorganized spindle cells
- Virtually diagnostic of NF1
  - Very important to not confuse plexiform neurofibroma with SCN or vice versa

SELECTED REFERENCES

1. Harris E et al: Acral plexiform palisaded encapsulated neuromas as the initial cutaneous manifestation of Cowden syndrome. Pediatr Dermatol. 34(4):e219-20, 2017
2. Jokinen CH et al: Expanding the clinicopathologic spectrum of palisaded encapsulated neuroma. J Cutan Pathol. 37(1):43-8, 2010
3. Koutlas IG et al: Palisaded encapsulated ("solitary circumscribed") neuroma of the oral cavity: a review of 55 cases. Head Neck Pathol. 4(1):15-26, 2010
4. Megahed M: Palisaded encapsulated neuroma (solitary circumscribed neuroma). A clinicopathologic and immunohistochemical study. Am J Dermatopathol. 16(2):120-5, 1994
5. Argenyi ZB: Immunohistochemical characterization of palisaded, encapsulated neuroma. J Cutan Pathol. 17(6):329-35, 1990
6. Fletcher CD: Solitary circumscribed neuroma of the skin (so-called palisaded, encapsulated neuroma). Am J Surg Pathol. 13(7):574-80, 1989

Schwannoma

KEY FACTS

TERMINOLOGY

- Encapsulated, benign peripheral nerve sheath tumor composed predominantly of Schwann cells

CLINICAL ISSUES

- Any age
  - Most common: 20-50 years
- Most occur in superficial soft tissues of head/neck and upper or lower extremities
  - Also retroperitoneum, posterior mediastinum, and viscera [gastrointestinal (GI) tract, kidney, etc.]
- Surgical excision is generally curative and recurrences are rare

MICROSCOPIC

- Well-circumscribed, nodular mass with fibrous capsule
- Hallmark: Variable amounts of hypercellular Antoni A and hypocellular Antoni B areas
- Morphologic variants: Ancient, cellular, plexiform, epithelioid, pseudoglandular, neuroblastoma-like, microcystic/reticular
- Schwannomas in neurofibromatosis type 2 (NF2) and schwannomatosis
  - Similar morphologically to sporadic tumors

ANCILLARY TESTS

- Diffuse, strong S100(+) and SOX10(+) is characteristic of all schwannoma variants
- Type IV collagen is present around individual cells and small groups of cells
- Cytokeratin AE1/AE3 and GFAP expression common in tumors of retroperitoneum, posterior mediastinum, and GI tract

TOP DIFFERENTIAL DIAGNOSES

- Neurofibroma
- Malignant peripheral nerve sheath tumor
- Pleomorphic hyalinizing angiectatic tumor

Schwannoma

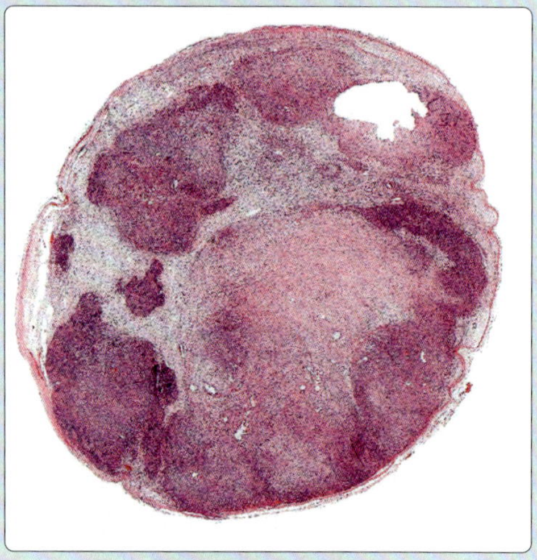

Encapsulation Common

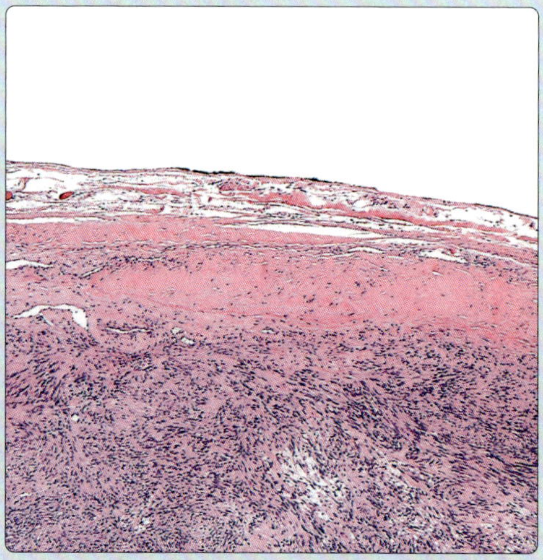

(Left) *Schwannoma is a well-circumscribed, encapsulated peripheral nerve sheath tumor that, in its conventional form, shows a variable admixture of zones of high and low cellularity, imparting a somewhat marbled appearance at low magnification.* **(Right)** *Most schwannomas are surrounded by a thick or thin fibrous capsule that contains epineurium and residual nerve fibers.*

Classic Alternating Cellularity

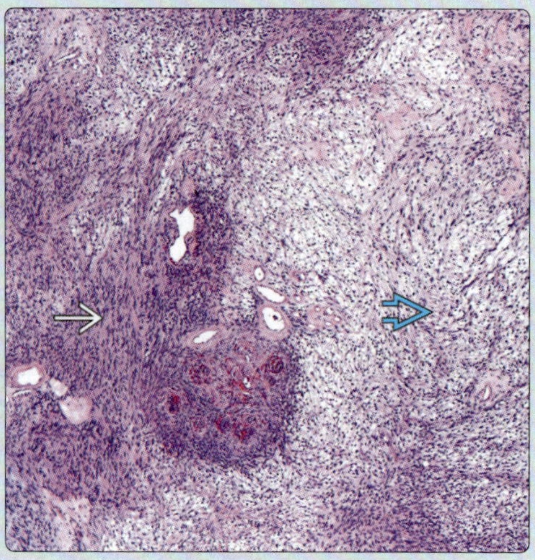

Antoni A and Antoni B Zones

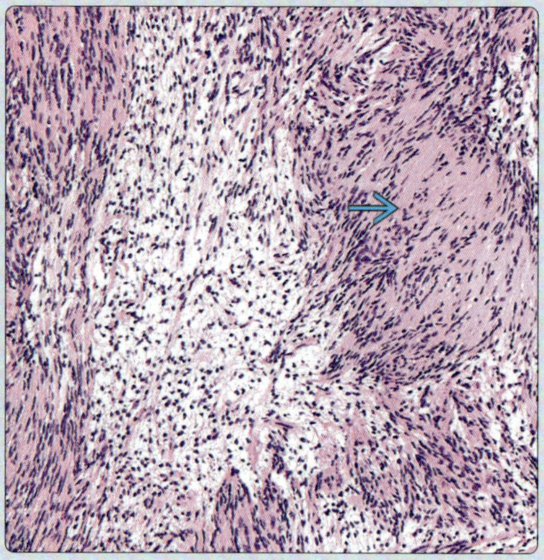

(Left) *The classic marbled appearance of schwannoma is created by interfaces between the cellular Antoni A zones ➡ and the loose edematous or myxoid Antoni B zones ⇨. This interface may be discretely abrupt or a gradual transition.* **(Right)** *Antoni A zones ➡ are more cellular and organized than Antoni B zones. Most schwannomas show a complex admixture of these 2 types of zones, but occasional cases are composed predominantly of either Antoni A or B.*

TERMINOLOGY

Synonyms

- Neurilemmoma

Definitions

- Encapsulated, benign peripheral nerve sheath tumor composed predominantly of Schwann cells

ETIOLOGY/PATHOGENESIS

Molecular Aberrations

- Somatic *NF2* gene mutations present in most tumors
- Bilateral vestibular schwannomas occur in setting of germline *NF2* gene mutations

Associated Syndromes

- Neurofibromatosis type 2 (NF2)
  - Inactivating germline mutations of *NF2* gene on chromosome 22
  - Autosomal dominant condition
    - Incidence around 1:30,000-40,000
  - Bilateral vestibular schwannomas are characteristic and diagnostic
    - Schwannomas involving other cranial nerves may be present
  - CNS tumors, such as meningioma, ependymoma, and gliomas, are also part of disease spectrum
  - Schwannomas in NF2 resemble their sporadic counterparts
    - Of note, plexiform schwannomas are **not** diagnostic of NF2
- Schwannomatosis
  - Rare sporadic or familial (autosomal dominant) condition characterized by formation of multiple peripheral schwannomas
    - Familial cases that follow autosomal dominant inheritance with reduced penetrance occur but are less common
    - Schwannomatosis locus identified on chromosome 22 proximal to *NF2* gene
    - Not associated with germline mutations in *NF1* or *NF2* genes
    - Some cases of inherited and sporadic schwannomatosis may be associated with germline *SMARCB1* mutations
  - By definition, patients do not have bilateral vestibular schwannomas and lack other criteria for NF2
  - Morphology similar to sporadic schwannomas

CLINICAL ISSUES

Epidemiology

- Incidence
  - 90% are sporadic
  - 10% are syndromic
    - ~ 3% with NF2
    - 2% with schwannomatosis
    - 5% with multiple meningiomas
    - Very rarely in association with NF1
- Age
  - All ages
    - Common between 20-50 years
- Sex
  - Affects male and female patients equally

Site

- Most occur in superficial soft tissues of head/neck and upper or lower extremities
  - Deep-seated soft tissue tumors much less common
- Retroperitoneum and mediastinum (often large)
- May also be seen in gastrointestinal (GI) tract and parenchymal organs (kidney, pancreas, etc.)
- May involve cranial nerve VIII in setting of NF2 (vestibular/acoustic neuroma)

Presentation

- Slow-growing, painless mass
  - Large tumors may be painful
- Cystic tumors may show fluctuation in size
- Examples that occur in neck often confused clinically for lymph nodes

Treatment

- Surgical excision, often nerve sparing

Prognosis

- Benign
- Excision is generally curative, and recurrences are rare (usually deep-seated tumors)

MACROSCOPIC

General Features

- Surrounded by true capsule consisting of epineurium
- Eccentric growth off of large nerve, or less likely, as nodular or fusiform mass seemingly unassociated with nerve
  - Dumbbell-shaped tumors occur in vertebral canal, usually in posterior mediastinum
- Variable size (often < 5 cm)
- Cut surface is gray-tan-white to yellow
- Large tumors may show cystic change, hemorrhage, or calcification on cut section

MICROSCOPIC

Histologic Features

- Well-circumscribed, nodular mass with fibrous capsule
- Hallmark: Variable amounts of admixed cellular Antoni A and hypocellular Antoni B areas
  - Antoni A
    - Spindle cells in short or interconnecting fascicles, loosely or tightly formed
    - Generally indistinct cytoplasmic borders
    - Nuclear palisading or whorling is common
      - Verocay bodies: Compact rows of palisaded nuclei separated by fibrillary processes
    - May contain lymphocytic infiltrate
  - Antoni B
    - Less orderly than Antoni A
    - Spindle or ovoid cells with indistinct cytoplasmic borders
    - Loose edematous or myxoid matrix with cystic change and inflammatory cells, particularly lymphocytes and histiocytes

- Presence of scattered collagen bundles may impart resemblance to neurofibroma
  - Large vessels with thick hyalinized walls and luminal thrombi ± hemosiderin deposition
- Nuclei are either thin and elongated with buckled or carrot-like shape or plump and ovoid
  - Intranuclear inclusions may be seen
- Mitotic rate is generally low to absent with no atypical forms
  - Cellular schwannomas may show more conspicuous mitotic activity
- Longstanding lesions often show degenerative changes
  - Nuclear atypia (ancient change) but without increase in mitotic activity
  - Cystic change may be focal or widespread with abundant hemorrhage
  - Stromal hyalinization or marked hypocellularity
  - Calcification ± metaplastic bone formation
  - Infarct-type necrosis may be present
    - True coagulative necrosis is rarely seen in cellular schwannoma (usually focal)
- Malignant transformation in schwannomas extremely rare
  - Usually epithelioid malignant peripheral nerve sheath tumor (MPNST), also epithelioid angiosarcoma

Morphologic Variants

- **Ancient schwannoma**
  - Demonstrates marked nuclear atypia of degenerative type (often "smudgy")
  - Lacks mitotic activity
  - Cystic change, hemorrhage, calcification, and hyalinization present
  - Usually seen in tumors of long duration (particularly deep-seated cases)
- **Cellular schwannoma**
  - By definition, composed almost exclusively of hypercellular Antoni A areas, which lack Verocay bodies
  - Encapsulated tumors; some may be multinodular or plexiform in architecture
    - Many show subcapsular &/or intratumoral lymphoid aggregates
  - Short to long sweeping fascicles of spindle-shaped cells
    - Cells may appear round/ovoid in fascicles that are cut in cross section
  - Mitotic activity is low (< 4/10 HPF)
  - Small foci of necrosis may be present
  - More common in mediastinum, retroperitoneum, and GI tract
- **Plexiform schwannoma**
  - Encapsulated tumors with striking multinodular or plexiform architecture
  - Often more cellular than ordinary schwannoma
    - Highly cellular examples reported in infants and children (cellular plexiform schwannoma)
  - Usually occur in skin or superficial soft tissues
  - Most common in head and neck region; infrequent in deeper locations
  - Association with NF syndromes is weak (unlike plexiform neurofibroma)
- **Epithelioid schwannoma**
  - Epithelioid or polygonal Schwann cells with sharp cell borders and variable amount of eosinophilic cytoplasm
  - Arranged in clusters, cords, or as single cells in variably myxoid or collagenous stroma
  - Foci of conventional schwannoma may be present
  - Small, bland nuclei
    - Degenerative nuclear atypia may be seen
  - Lacks mitotic activity
- **Pseudoglandular schwannoma**
  - Contains cystic spaces that are lined by small round tumor cells, resembling epithelial surfaces
    - Cells may show "apical" cytoplasm
      - May mimic glandular or ductal epithelium
  - Often contains areas of conventional schwannoma
- **Neuroblastoma-like schwannoma**
  - Contains rosette-like structures composed of round to ovoid Schwann cells around acellular collagen cores
    - Collagen cores may lack peripheral cells
    - Structures may be centered around small vessels
  - Mimics rosettes seen in neuroblastoma
- **Microcystic/reticular schwannoma**
  - Anastomosing strands of eosinophilic spindle cells in myxoid, fibrillary, or collagenous matrix
  - Predilection for visceral locations, particularly GI tract
  - Foci of conventional schwannoma or other schwannoma variants may be present

ANCILLARY TESTS

Immunohistochemistry

- Diffuse, strong S100 protein (+) is characteristic
  - Applies to all morphologic variants
  - SOX10 shows similar diffuse expression in nuclei
- Type IV collagen is present around individual cells and small groups of cells
- Loss of nuclear INI1 in up to 1/2 of epithelioid schwannomas
- Nuclear H3K27me3 expression generally intact
- Neurofilament protein expression is often limited to entrapped axons at periphery of tumor but may be also seen within tumor in some cases
- Cytokeratin AE1/AE3 and GFAP expression common in tumors of retroperitoneum, posterior mediastinum, and GI tract
  - In peripheral sites, GFAP expression is rare, and CK AE1/AE3 has not been reported
  - CK AE1/AE3 expression due to cross reactivity with GFAP
- CD34, EMA, claudin-1, GLUT1 (-)
  - Mixed expression of S100 protein with 1 or more of these markers may indicate hybrid peripheral nerve sheath tumor
  - EMA expression often seen in capsule of schwannoma

DIFFERENTIAL DIAGNOSIS

Neurofibroma

- Unencapsulated and lacks Antoni A areas
  - Antoni B areas of schwannoma can look very similar to neurofibroma
- Composed of mixture of Schwann cells, fibroblasts, and perineurial cells

- S100 protein is diffusely positive but less striking overall compared to schwannoma (due to lower cellularity)
- CD34 is commonly positive in admixed population of fibroblasts

Malignant Peripheral Nerve Sheath Tumor

- Often larger and more deep seated than schwannoma
- Cytology varies from monomorphic to highly pleomorphic, and mitotic activity is generally high and conspicuous
- Tumor necrosis common
- S100 protein expression is characteristically negative or at most focal
  - Lower grade MPNST may show more extensive S100 positivity
  - Very rare cases of high-grade MPNST are diffusely S100(+)
- Loss of nuclear H3K27me3 expression by IHC in majority of cases
- Most likely to be confused with cellular, plexiform, and ancient schwannoma variants
  - Cellular examples of plexiform schwannoma may be mistaken for MPNST arising in plexiform neurofibroma
- Epithelioid MPNST is larger and more cellular than epithelioid schwannoma and contains larger nuclei with prominent macronucleoli

Malignant/Metastatic Melanoma

- Always consider in dermal tumors and in patients with history of melanoma
- Lack admixed Antoni A and Antoni B zones
- Primary melanoma often contains cutaneous junctional component
- Spindle cell melanoma may be relatively bland but often shows at least focal nuclear atypia and mitotic activity
- Epithelioid melanoma cells are often cytologically malignant with prominent, eosinophilic, cherry red nucleoli
- Strong expression of S100 protein and SOX10; often diffuse
- Variable expression of melanocytic markers (HMB-45, MART1/melan-A, MITF, tyrosinase)
  - Focal expression is significant in HMB-45 and MART1/melan-A and can be easily missed
  - Desmoplastic melanomas are characteristically HMB-45 and MART-1 (-)

Pleomorphic Hyalinizing Angiectatic Tumor

- Can show markedly similar appearance to ancient schwannoma
- S100 protein (-); CD34(+) (~ 50% of cases)
- Predilection for foot, ankle, and leg
- Significant risk of local recurrence with simple excision

Leiomyoma

- Generally very pink microscopic appearance
- Lack admixed Antoni A and Antoni B zones
- Composed of fascicles of plump, eosinophilic spindle cells with cigar-shaped nuclei
  - May show epithelioid morphology
- SMA, caldesmon, and desmin expression
- S100 protein (-)

SELECTED REFERENCES

1. Jo VY et al: SMARCB1/INI1 loss in epithelioid schwannoma: a clinicopathologic and immunohistochemical study of 65 cases. Am J Surg Pathol. 41(8):1013-22, 2017
2. Hart J et al: Epithelioid schwannomas: an analysis of 58 cases including atypical variants. Am J Surg Pathol. 40(5):704-13, 2016
3. Luzar B et al: Cutaneous microcystic/reticular schwannoma: a poorly recognized entity. J Cutan Pathol. 43(2):93-100, 2015
4. Pekmezci M et al: Morphologic and immunohistochemical features of malignant peripheral nerve sheath tumors and cellular schwannomas. Mod Pathol. 28(2):187-200, 2014
5. Zong S et al: Treatment results in the differential surgery of intradural extramedullary schwannoma of 110 cases. PLoS One. 8(5):e63867, 2013
6. Carter JM et al: Epithelioid malignant peripheral nerve sheath tumor arising in a schwannoma, in a patient with "neuroblastoma-like" schwannomatosis and a novel germline SMARCB1 mutation. Am J Surg Pathol. 36(1):154-60, 2012
7. Harder A et al: Hybrid neurofibroma/schwannoma is overrepresented among schwannomatosis and neurofibromatosis patients. Am J Surg Pathol. 36(5):702-9, 2012
8. Rezanko T et al: Epithelioid schwannoma of soft tissue: unusual morphological variant causing a diagnostic dilemma. Ann Diagn Pathol. 16(6):521-6, 2012
9. Voltaggio L et al: Gastric schwannoma: a clinicopathologic study of 51 cases and critical review of the literature. Hum Pathol. 43(5):650-9, 2012
10. Chetty R: Reticular and microcystic schwannoma: a distinctive tumor of the gastrointestinal tract. Ann Diagn Pathol. 15(3):198-201, 2011
11. Gaudi S et al: Intravascular schwannoma. Am J Dermatopathol. 33(8):850-4, 2011
12. Agaimy A et al: Peripheral nerve sheath tumors of the gastrointestinal tract: a multicenter study of 58 patients including NF1-associated gastric schwannoma and unusual morphologic variants. Virchows Arch. 456(4):411-22, 2010
13. Küsters-Vandevelde HV et al: Improved discrimination of melanotic schwannoma from melanocytic lesions by combined morphological and GNAQ mutational analysis. Acta Neuropathol. 120(6):755-64, 2010
14. Santos PP et al: Clinicopathologic analysis of 7 cases of oral schwannoma and review of the literature. Ann Diagn Pathol. 14(4):235-9, 2010
15. Trufant JW et al: Melanotic schwannoma arising in association with nevus of Ota: 2 cases suggesting a shared mechanism. Am J Dermatopathol. 31(8):808-13, 2009
16. Liegl B et al: Microcystic/reticular schwannoma: a distinct variant with predilection for visceral locations. Am J Surg Pathol. 32(7):1080-7, 2008
17. Fanburg-Smith JC et al: Keratin expression in schwannoma; a study of 115 retroperitoneal and 22 peripheral schwannomas. Mod Pathol. 19(1):115-21, 2006
18. MacCollin M et al: Diagnostic criteria for schwannomatosis. Neurology. 64(11):1838-45, 2005
19. Woodruff JM et al: Congenital and childhood plexiform (multinodular) cellular schwannoma: a troublesome mimic of malignant peripheral nerve sheath tumor. Am J Surg Pathol. 27(10):1321-9, 2003
20. McMenamin ME et al: Expanding the spectrum of malignant change in schwannomas: epithelioid malignant change, epithelioid malignant peripheral nerve sheath tumor, and epithelioid angiosarcoma: a study of 17 cases. Am J Surg Pathol. 25(1):13-25, 2001
21. Antinheimo J et al: Population-based analysis of sporadic and type 2 neurofibromatosis-associated meningiomas and schwannomas. Neurology. 54(1):71-6, 2000
22. Kindblom LG et al: Benign epithelioid schwannoma. Am J Surg Pathol. 22(6):762-70, 1998
23. Chan JK et al: Pseudoglandular schwannoma. Histopathology. 29(5):481-3, 1996
24. Goldblum JR et al: Neuroblastoma-like neurilemoma. Am J Surg Pathol. 18(3):266-73, 1994
25. Brooks JJ et al: Benign glandular schwannoma. Arch Pathol Lab Med. 116(2):192-5, 1992
26. Carney JA: Psammomatous melanotic schwannoma. A distinctive, heritable tumor with special associations, including cardiac myxoma and the Cushing syndrome. Am J Surg Pathol. 14(3):206-22, 1990
27. Fletcher CD et al: Cellular schwannoma: a distinct pseudosarcomatous entity. Histopathology. 11(1):21-35, 1987
28. Fletcher CD et al: Benign plexiform (multinodular) schwannoma: a rare tumour unassociated with neurofibromatosis. Histopathology. 10(9):971-80, 1986

(Left) *Antoni A zones of schwannoma are cellular and relatively organized. Not all Antoni A zones exhibit nuclear palisading, Verocay body formation, or whorling.* **(Right)** *The spindle cells in Antoni A zones of schwannoma typically show indistinct cytoplasmic borders and elongated, buckled, wavy, or twisted nuclei. The matrix is fine, fibrillary, and eosinophilic.*

Antoni A Zones

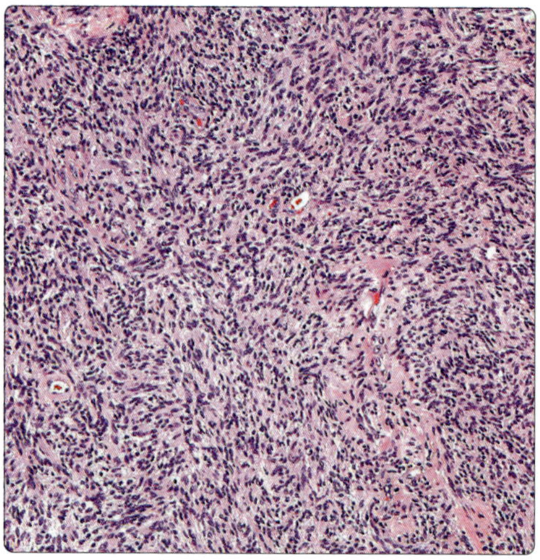

Antoni A Cytologic Features

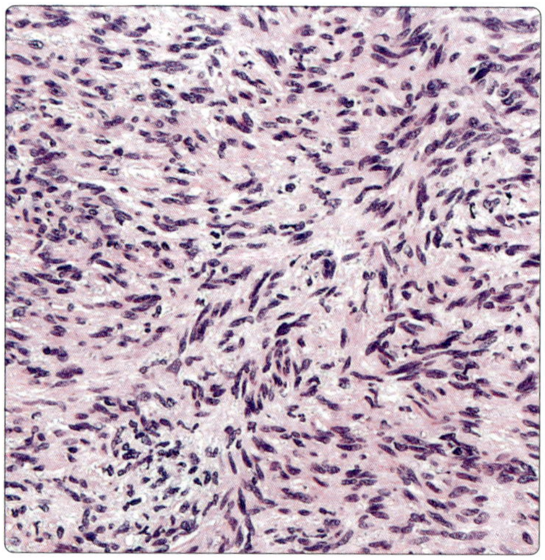

(Left) *A characteristic finding in some Antoni A zones of schwannoma is the presence of focal to prominent nuclear palisading* ➜*. This finding is not pathognomonic, however, as other unrelated tumors can show similar morphology.* **(Right)** *In schwannoma, the term Verocay body is used to describe the finding of eosinophilic fibrillary cell processes* ➜ *between 2 rows of palisading Schwann cell nuclei.*

Nuclear Palisading in Antoni A

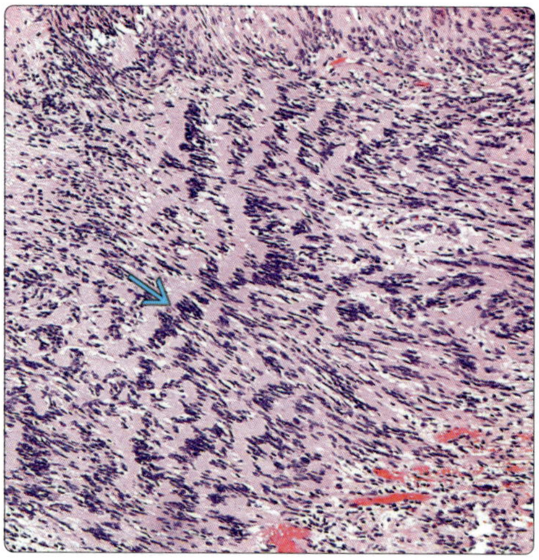

Morphology of Verocay Bodies

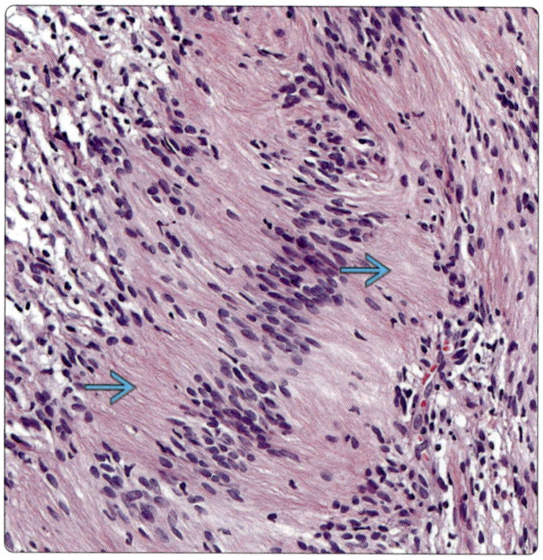

(Left) *In addition to nuclear palisading, a whorling architecture may be identified within Antoni A zones of schwannoma.* **(Right)** *Cytologically, most Schwann cell nuclei are bland, elongated, and often tapered at one or both ends. Nucleoli are inconspicuous. Clear nuclear pseudoinclusions (not pictured) are also seen in some cases. Mitotic figures* ➜ *are rarely identified in schwannoma and, if present, are never atypical.*

Whorling Architecture in Some Cases

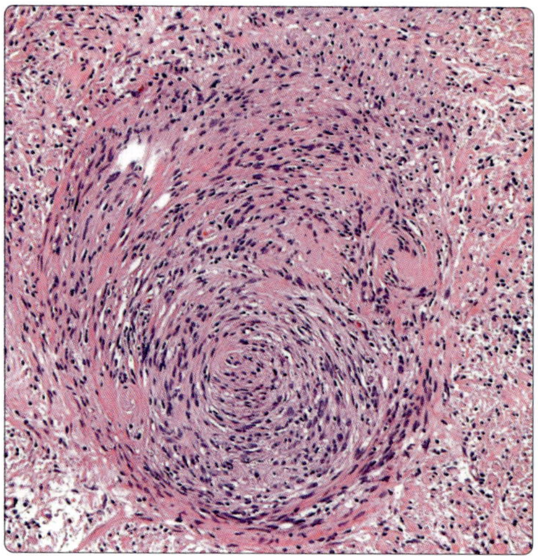

Schwann Cell Nuclear Features

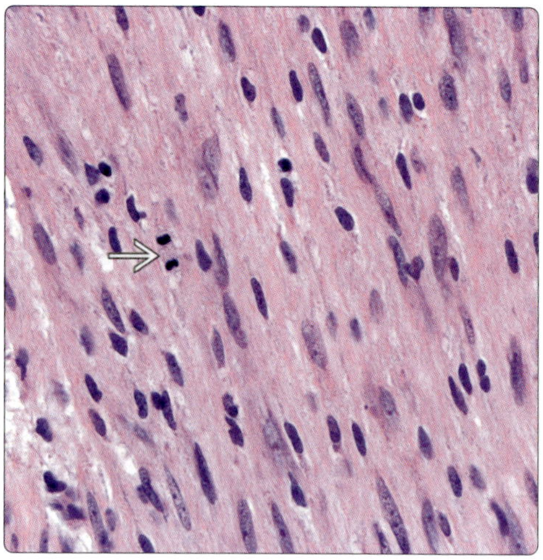

Stromal Inflammation Common

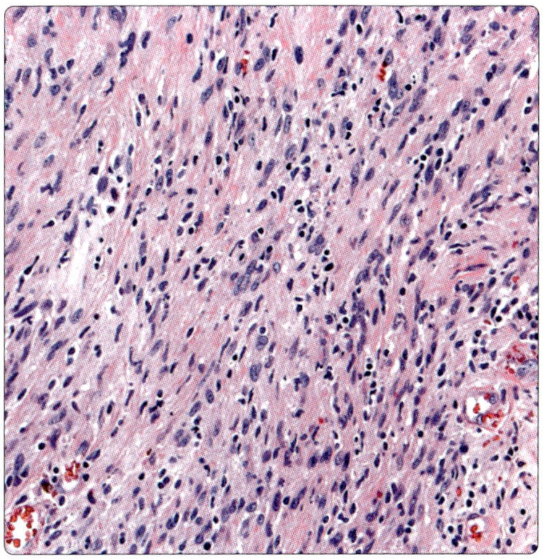

Variable Stromal Collagen

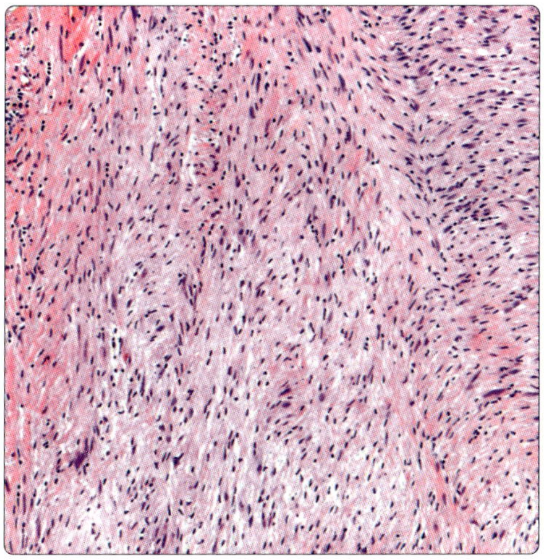

(Left) *A chronic inflammatory infiltrate is not uncommon in schwannoma and usually consists of predominantly reactive lymphocytes. This finding varies in prominence and may be seen in both Antoni A and Antoni B zones.* **(Right)** *Some areas in a schwannoma may show a typical loose fascicular growth of Antoni A but with increased stromal collagen. This finding is a feature of some cellular schwannomas.*

Antoni B Zones

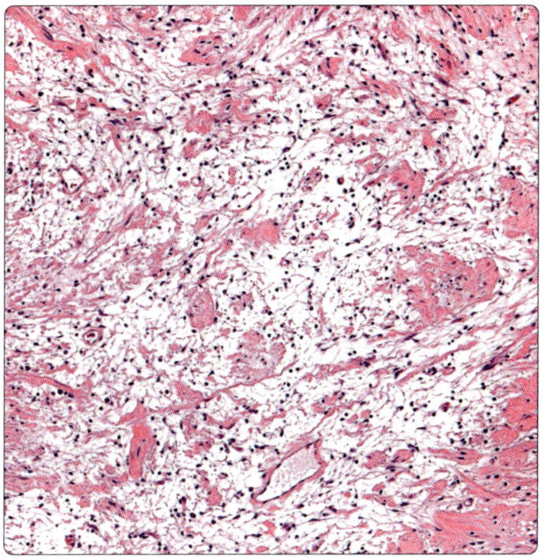

Antoni B Collagen Distribution

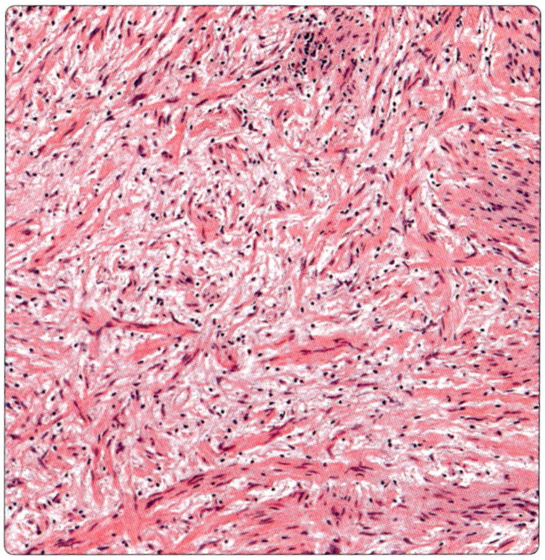

(Left) *Antoni B zones in schwannoma are distinctly less cellular than Antoni A zones and demonstrate a loose edematous or myxoid matrix with scattered collagen fibers.* **(Right)** *In some areas of schwannoma, the distribution of collagen fibers in Antoni B zones may closely resemble that of a neurofibroma, particularly the plexiform type; however, the characteristic multinodular growth pattern of the latter is generally absent.*

Hypocellularity or Myxoid Change in Antoni B

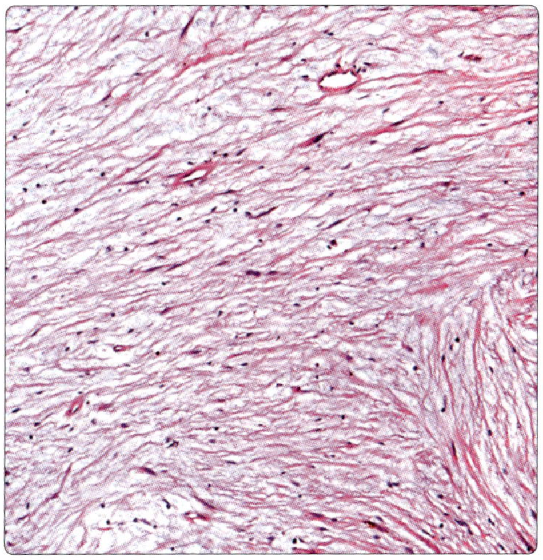

Strong and Diffuse S100 Protein Expression

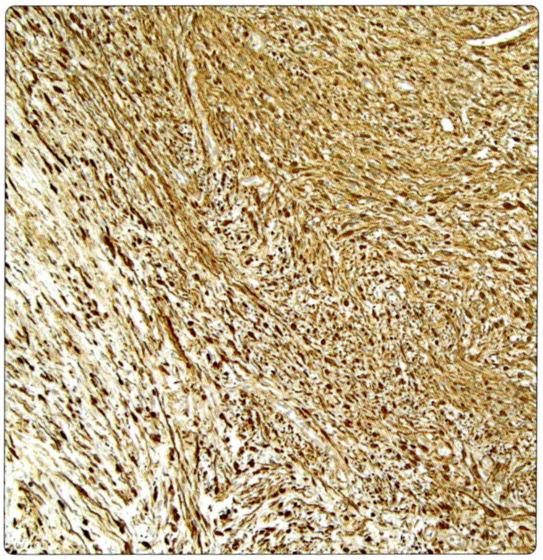

(Left) *Antoni B zones in schwannoma may be significantly myxoid and hypocellular and easily confused with a variety of other low-grade myxoid neoplasms, such as myxoma or neurofibroma.* **(Right)** *S100 protein expression is essentially always strong and diffuse in schwannoma and characteristic of all variants. The staining pattern is typically both nuclear and cytoplasmic.*

(Left) *An often conspicuous and characteristic finding in schwannoma is the presence of single or clusters of irregular vascular channels with hyalinized walls. These vessels predominate in Antoni B zones but may occasionally be identified in cellular Antoni A zones.* **(Right)** *A variety of benign vascular changes may be identified in the vessels of schwannoma, including papillary endothelial hyperplasia and thrombosis.*

Hyalinized Vessels Characteristic

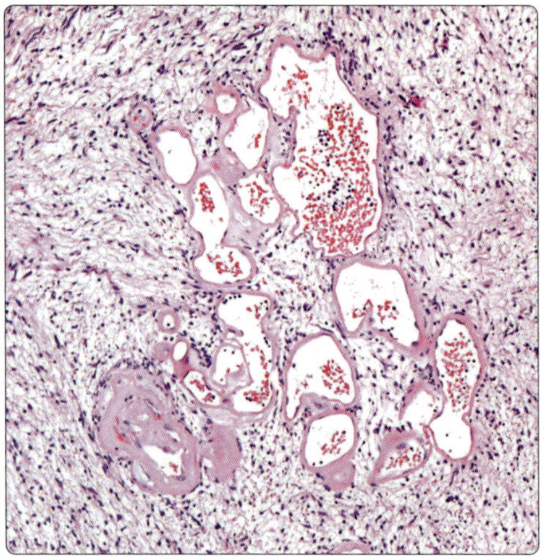

Hyperplastic Vascular Changes in Some Tumors

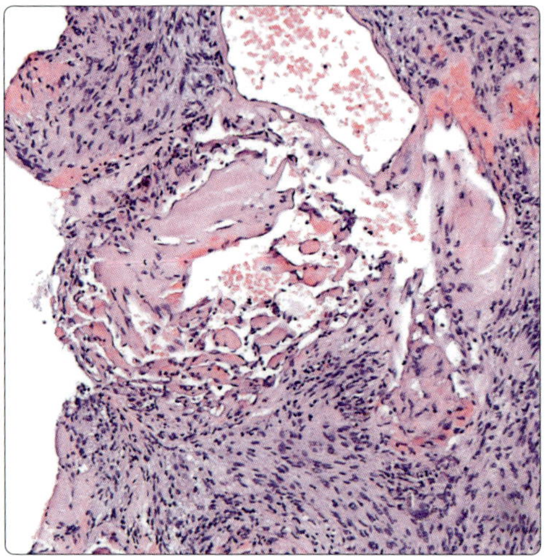

(Left) *Occasional vessels in schwannoma may show fibrinoid change in the wall ± thrombosis. This finding is most commonly seen in ancient schwannoma. Similar vascular changes can be seen in other tumors, particularly pleomorphic hyalinizing angiectatic tumor.* **(Right)** *Some examples of schwannoma show an interesting morphologic arrangement of relatively eosinophilic Antoni A zones and highly myxoid Antoni B. The overall marbled pattern is characteristic of most cases of conventional schwannoma.*

Occasional Vessels With Fibrinoid Changes

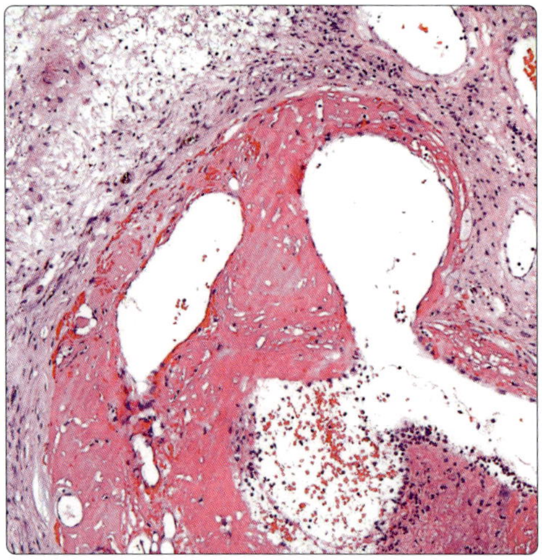

Myxoid Areas in Schwannoma

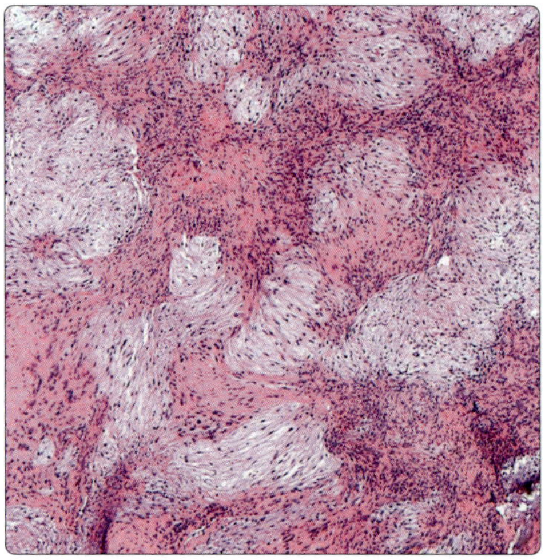

(Left) *This particular case of schwannoma shows large areas of myxoid matrix, resembling other low-grade myxoid neoplasms. S100 protein positivity was helpful in supporting the diagnosis of schwannoma.* **(Right)** *Antoni B zones in schwannoma may be markedly hyalinized and hypocellular, particularly longstanding tumors or those with abundant other degenerative features.*

Rare, Prominent Myxoid Stroma

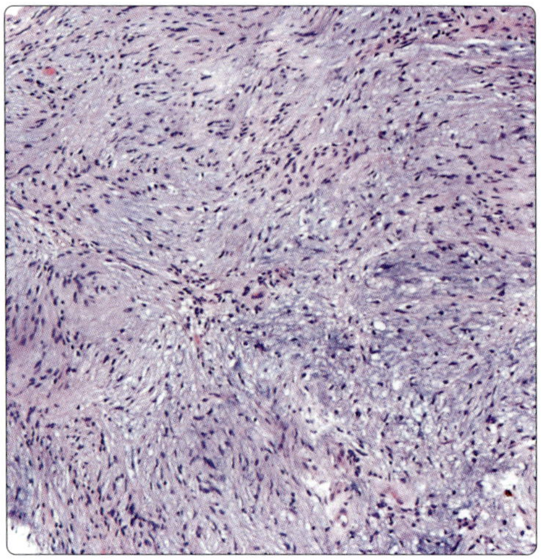

Stromal Hyalinization in Antoni B

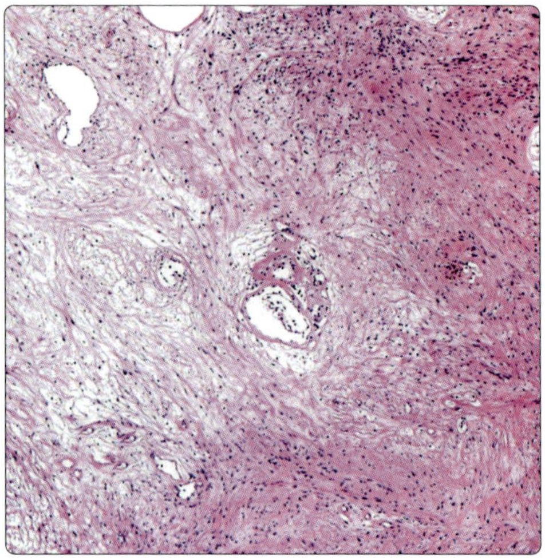

Diffuse Stromal Sclerosis in Older Tumors

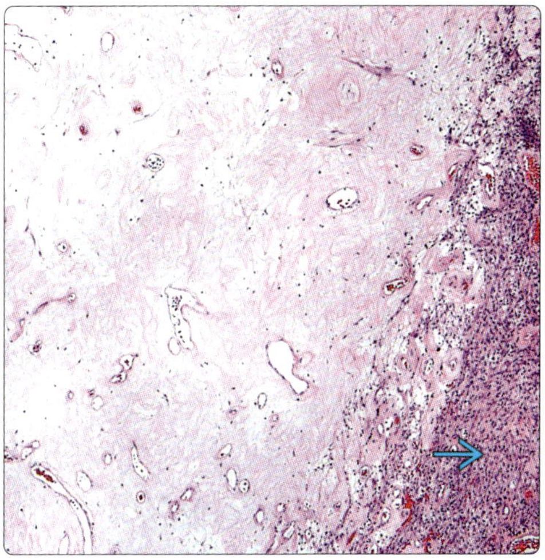

Calcification in Degenerative Schwannoma

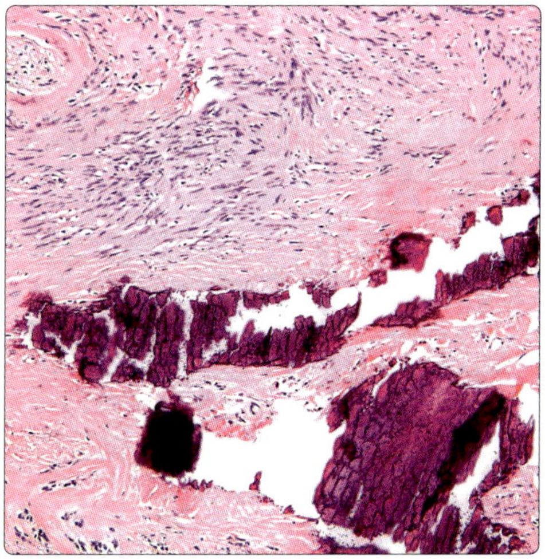

(Left) *Diffuse stromal hyalinization or sclerosis may be seen in degenerative schwannoma, and areas of conventional morphology* ➡ *may be focal or absent altogether.* **(Right)** *Calcification is not uncommon in schwannoma and is often associated with other degenerative changes, including vascular hyalinization, stromal sclerosis, cystic change, and hemosiderin deposition.*

Metaplastic Bone Formation Uncommon

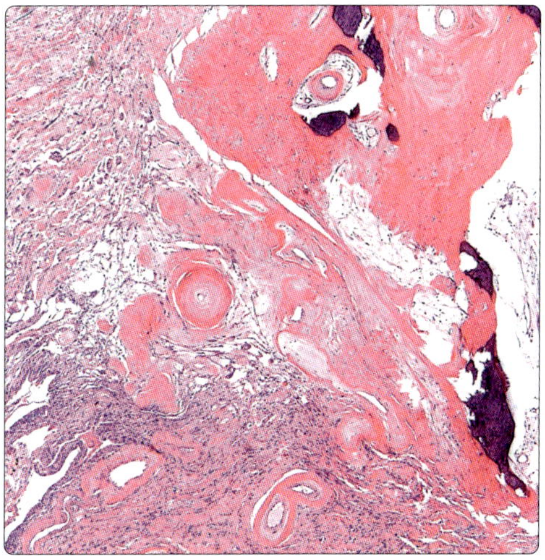

Foamy Histiocytes

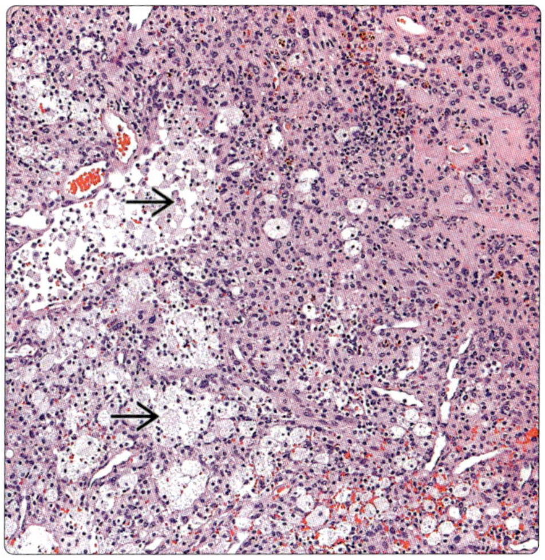

(Left) *Metaplastic bone formation is an uncommon event in schwannoma but is more likely to be seen in longstanding cases.* **(Right)** *Foamy histiocytes* ➡ *may be identified in some cases of schwannoma, particularly cellular variants. They can also be seen as a component of Antoni B zones.*

Cystic Change in Degenerative Schwannoma

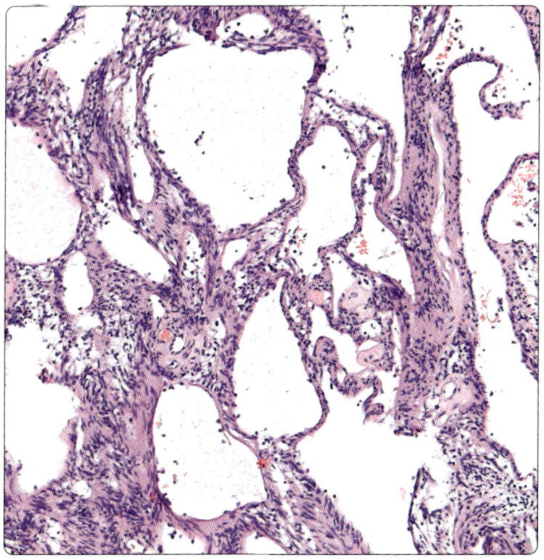

Rare Prominent Cystic Change

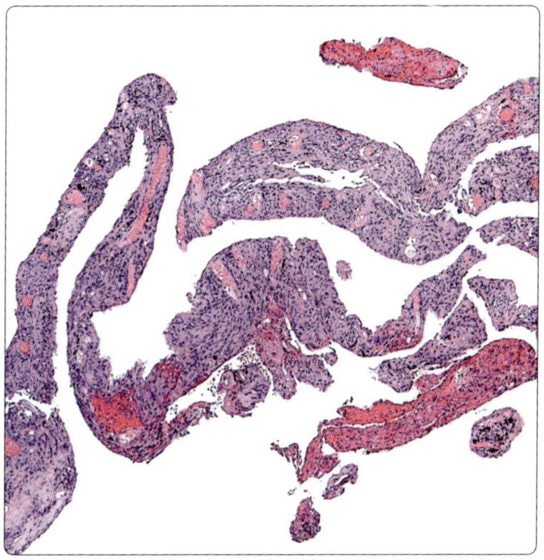

(Left) *Cystic change is not uncommon in schwannoma but is more frequently encountered in ancient/degenerative tumors. Clinically larger schwannomas are more likely to have central cystic hemorrhage.* **(Right)** *Rare cases of schwannoma are predominantly or exclusively cystic and may be challenging to diagnose. This type of schwannoma is usually very hemorrhagic intraoperatively, clinically suggesting a vascular neoplasm.*

(Left) *Hemosiderin deposition ⇨ is common in schwannoma, particularly cases with intratumoral hemorrhage. Rare cases show abundant hemosiderin and blood, simulating a hematoma or vascular neoplasm.* (Right) *Microcystic stromal changes may be seen in some cases of schwannoma. The microcysts vary in size and are often more prominent around large cystic spaces. Note the hyalinized vessels ⇨.*

Hemosiderin Deposition Common

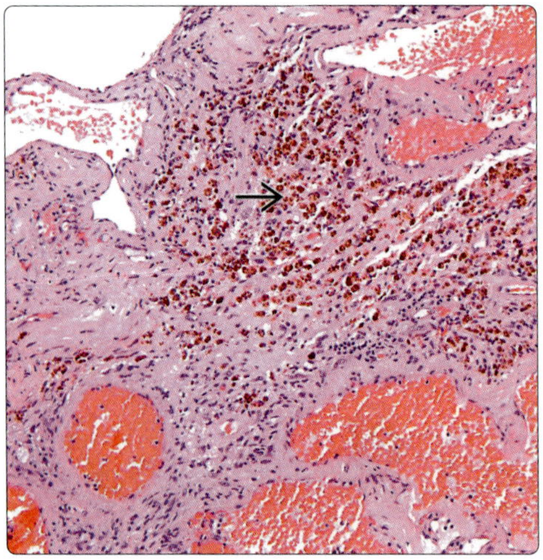

Degenerative Microcystic Stromal Change

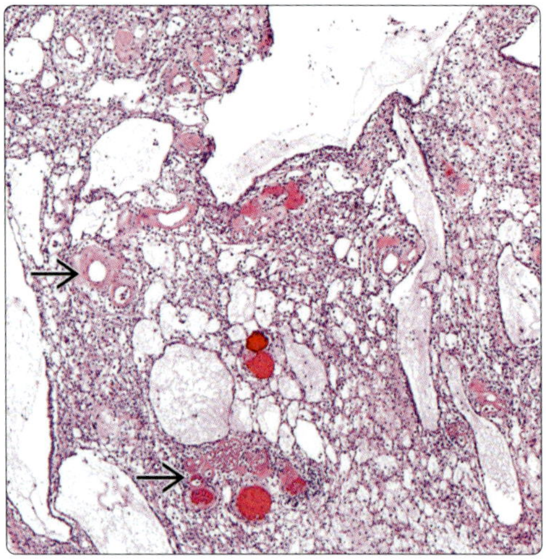

(Left) *Microcystic stromal change in degenerative schwannomas may be associated with a brisk chronic inflammatory infiltrate as well as hyalinized vessels and histiocytes.* (Right) *A common finding in many schwannomas is the presence of scattered enlarged cells with hyperchromatic, "smudgy" nuclei ➡, termed ancient change. Another common finding in these cases is lipofuscin pigment ⇨.*

Microcystic Stromal Change Associated With Inflammation

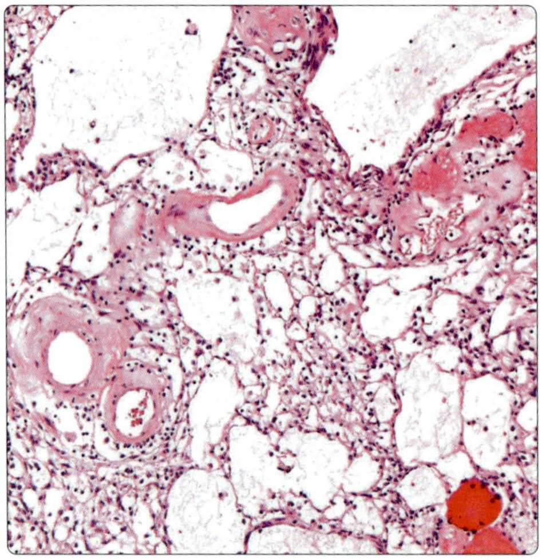

"Smudgy" Degenerative Nuclear Changes

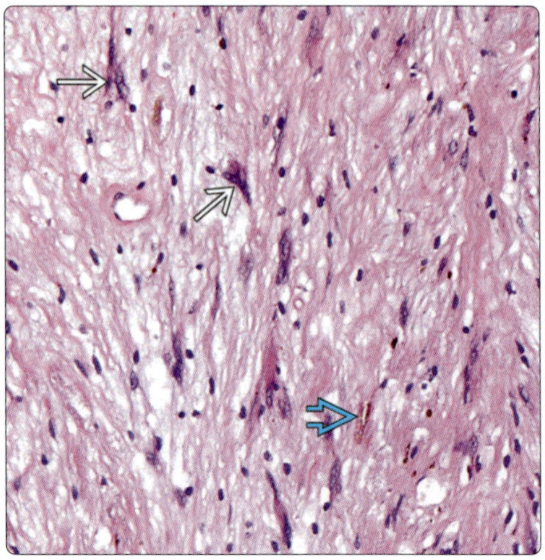

(Left) *Ancient change in a schwannoma may be very prominent in some cases, mostly in Antoni B areas but even in Antoni A zones. This finding may lead one to suspect malignancy; however, mitoses are discrepantly rare, and there is no tumor necrosis.* (Right) *At high magnification, the degenerative nuclei are often hyperchromatic and irregular with "smudgy" contours and may show nuclear vacuolization. Mitoses are inconspicuous or absent.*

Ancient Schwannoma Variant

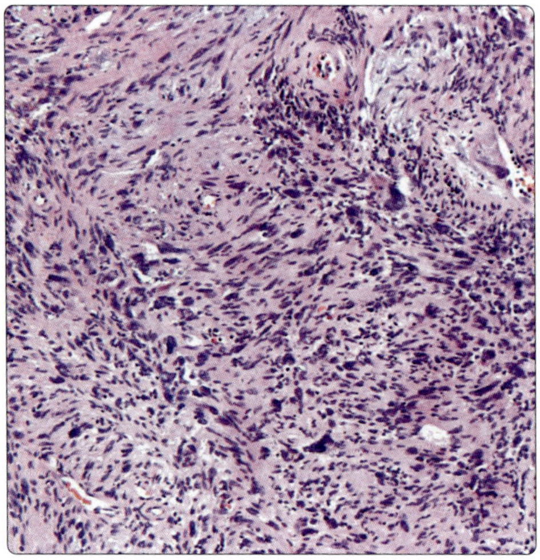

Atypical, "Smudgy" Nuclei in Schwannoma

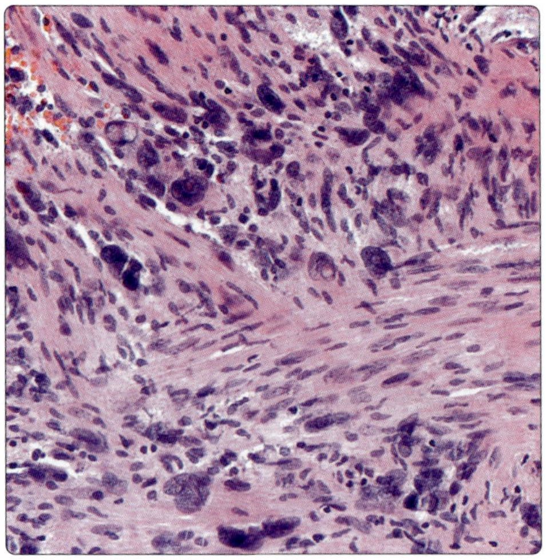

Cellular Schwannoma Variant

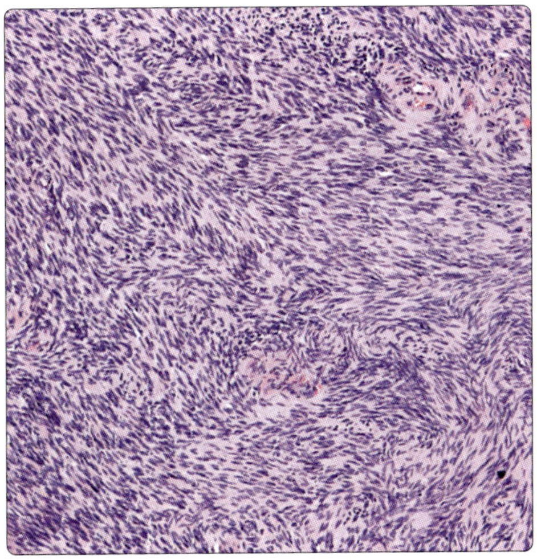

Short Fascicles and Whorls

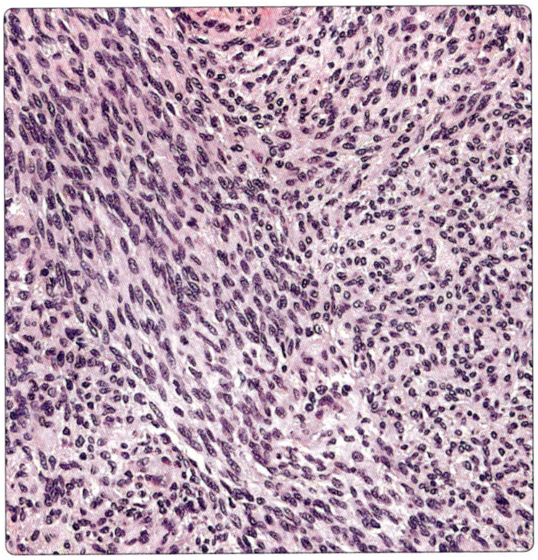

(Left) *The cellular variant of schwannoma is defined as being composed exclusively or predominantly of Antoni A zones. Focal Antoni B zones may be identified but usually do not comprise > 10% of the tumor.* **(Right)** *Cellular schwannoma often shows the formation of short fascicular or vague whorling architectures. Mitoses are more likely to be identified in this variant; however, they are generally not numerous.*

Cellular Whorls

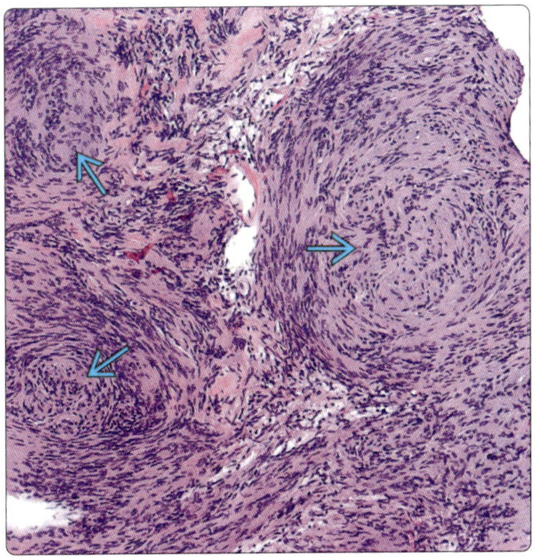

Stromal Collagen in Cellular Schwannoma

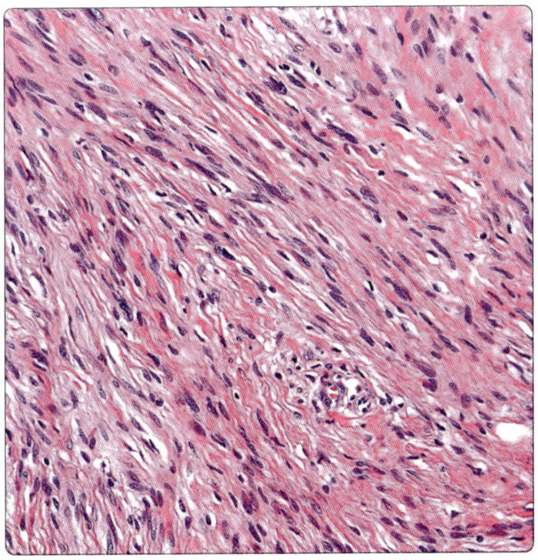

(Left) *A notable finding in some cases of cellular schwannoma is the formation of cellular whorls ⇨ by the tumor cells. This finding may also be seen in malignant peripheral nerve sheath tumor; however, it is uncommon.* **(Right)** *Some examples of cellular schwannoma show increased stromal collagen and are overall more eosinophilic in appearance. Gastrointestinal schwannomas in particular routinely show this morphology.*

Rare Nuclear Palisading in Cellular Tumors

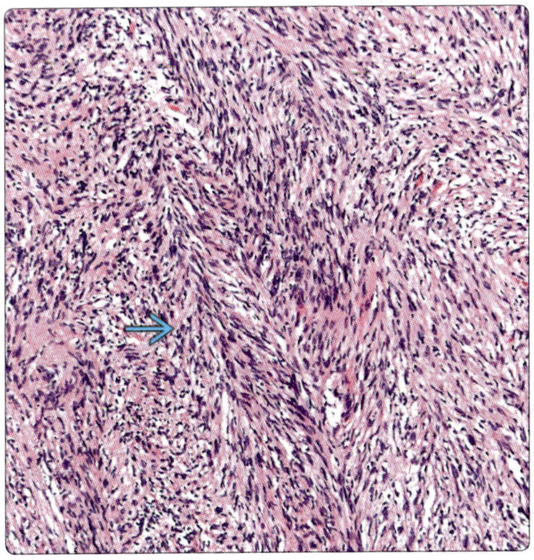

Microtrabecular Pattern in Cellular Schwannoma

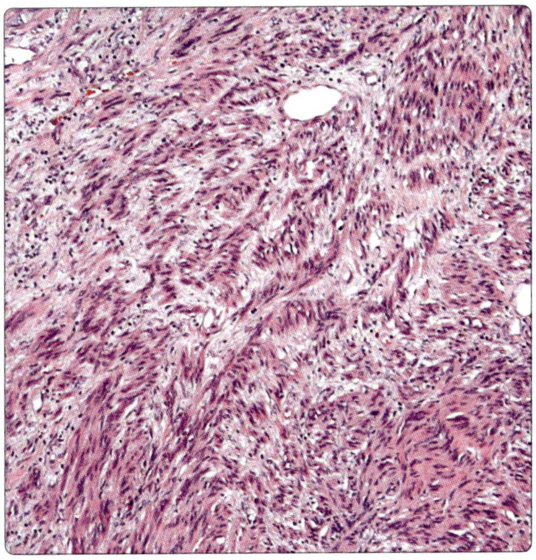

(Left) *In contrast to Antoni A zones in conventional schwannoma, those of cellular schwannoma often lack distinct nuclear palisading and Verocay body formation. Rare herringbone fascicular architecture ⇨ may be identified focally in some cases.* **(Right)** *A microtrabecular architecture is another interesting and recurrent pattern that can be seen in cellular schwannoma. It is characterized by discrete, small clusters or rows of spindled Schwann cells.*

(Left) *Collections or aggregates of foamy histiocytes are a common finding in cellular schwannoma and can be diagnostically helpful in identifying this particular variant.* **(Right)** *Lymphoid aggregates are a very common and characteristic feature of most cellular schwannomas. These aggregates are often subcapsular, pericapsular, or intratumoral and may show reactive germinal center formation.*

Collections of Foamy Histiocytes

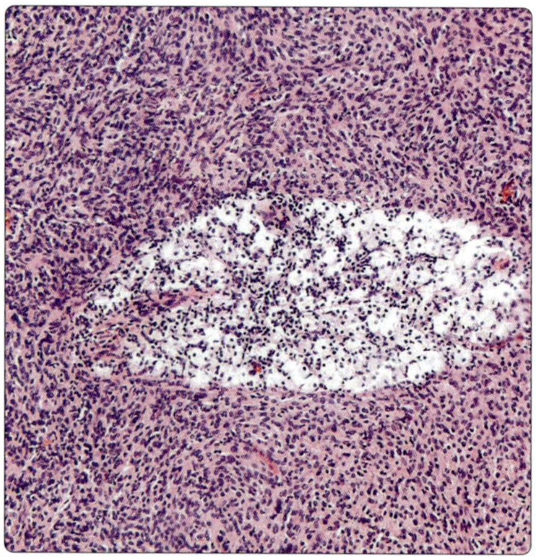

Lymphoid Aggregates Common

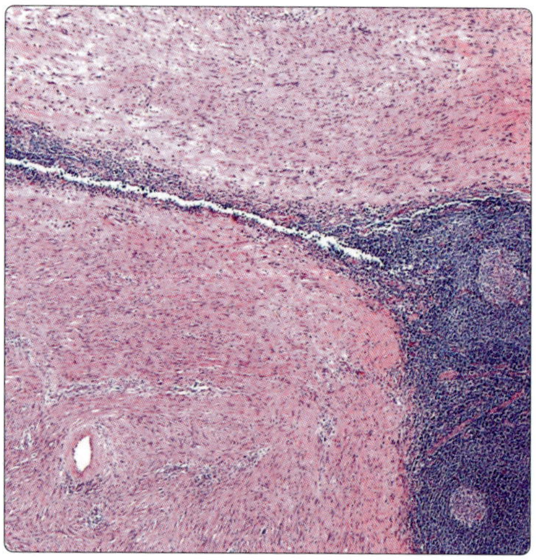

(Left) *The plexiform variant of schwannoma has a distinct multinodular or serpentine growth pattern. It shows a predilection for the skin and is rarely at deep sites. Unlike plexiform neurofibroma, plexiform schwannoma is not diagnostic of neurofibromatosis type 1.* **(Right)** *Plexiform schwannoma generally contains minimal Antoni B and therefore has an overall cellular appearance. Typical features of Antoni A, including nuclear palisading* ➙*, may be seen.*

Plexiform Schwannoma Variant

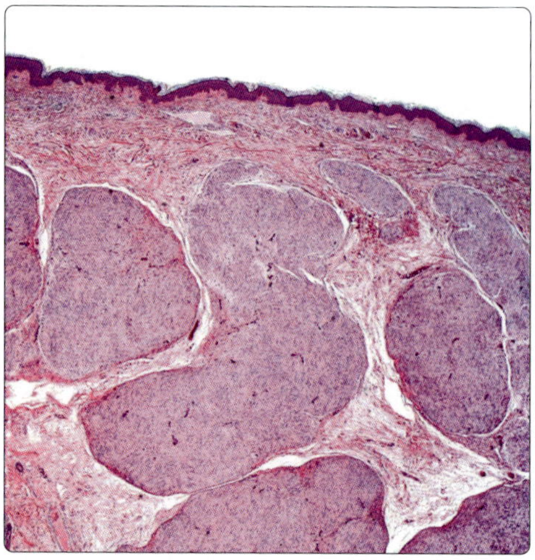

Plexiform Schwannoma With Palisading

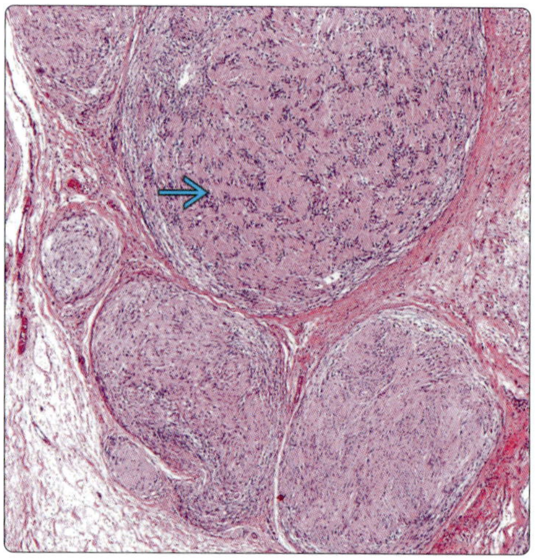

(Left) *Some examples of plexiform schwannoma may show diffuse cellularity without nuclear palisading. In the context of a plexiform growth pattern, this appearance may lead to misdiagnosis of malignant peripheral nerve sheath tumor in a plexiform neurofibroma; however, mitotic activity is low, and there is no tumor necrosis.* **(Right)** *Epithelioid cellular change in a schwannoma is seen focally in many cases. Rarely, this morphology may be diffuse and warrant classification as an epithelioid schwannoma.*

Plexiform Schwannoma Without Palisading

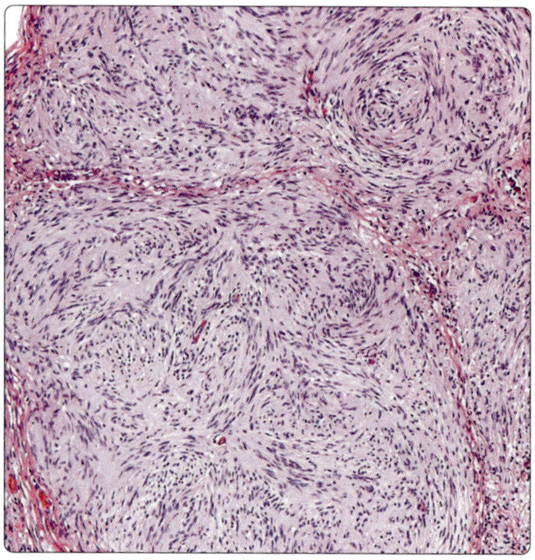

Epithelioid Schwannoma Variant

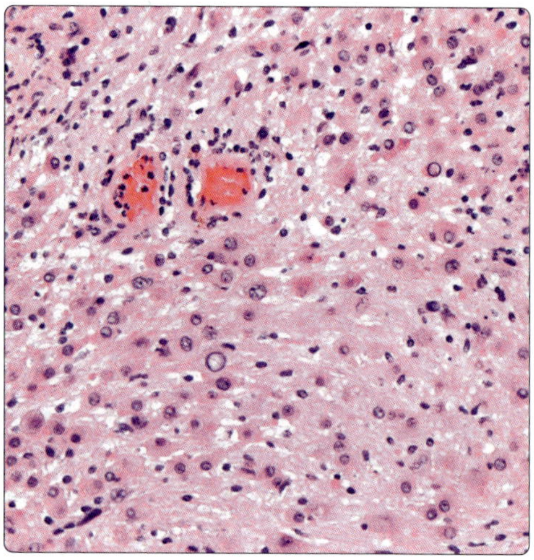

Epithelioid Schwannoma With Clusters of Small Cells

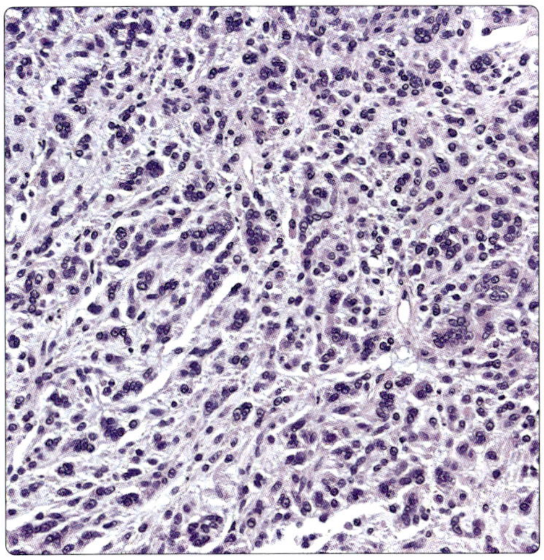

Bland Nuclei in Epithelioid Tumors

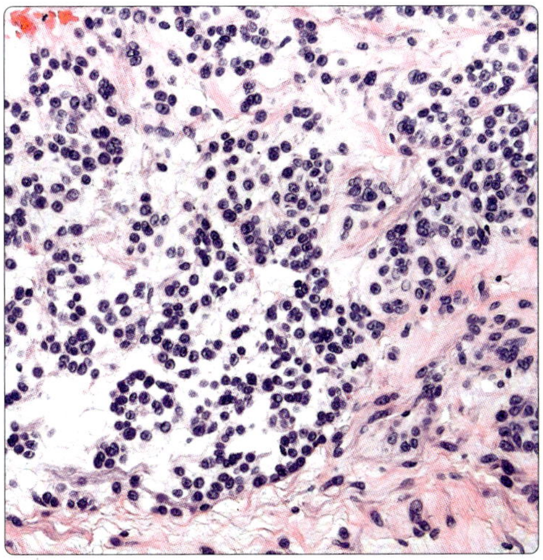

(Left) *Epithelioid schwannoma may show clusters of small, bland tumor cells in small clusters or linear arrays within a myxoid matrix. Mitotic figures are rare or absent.* **(Right)** *Cytologically, the cells of epithelioid schwannoma are generally small and show bland nuclei. Features of epithelioid malignant peripheral nerve sheath tumor, including enlarged nuclei with prominent macronucleoli and conspicuous mitoses, are not seen.*

Mixed Epithelioid and Spindled Cells

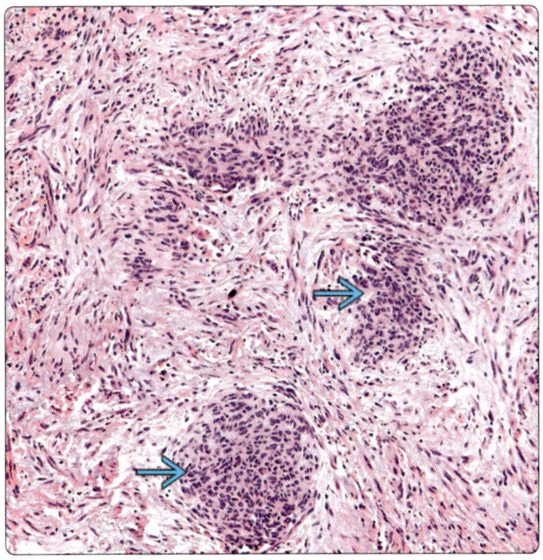

Pseudoglandular Spaces in Schwannoma

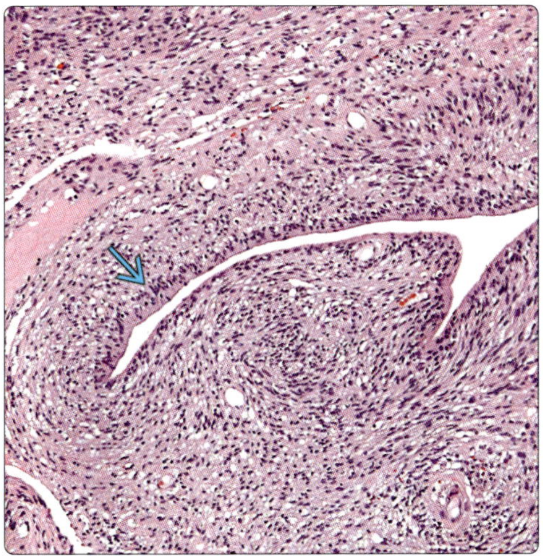

(Left) *Foci of epithelioid Schwann cells* → *may be seen in the background of an otherwise typical spindle cell schwannoma.* **(Right)** *Schwannomas with cystic change may show a lining* → *that is very reminiscent of glandular epithelium. This lining is clearly schwannian, as evidenced by strong S100 protein expression and negative keratin staining. Also, there is an absence of intracytoplasmic mucin.*

Schwann Cell Lining Resembles Gland Formation

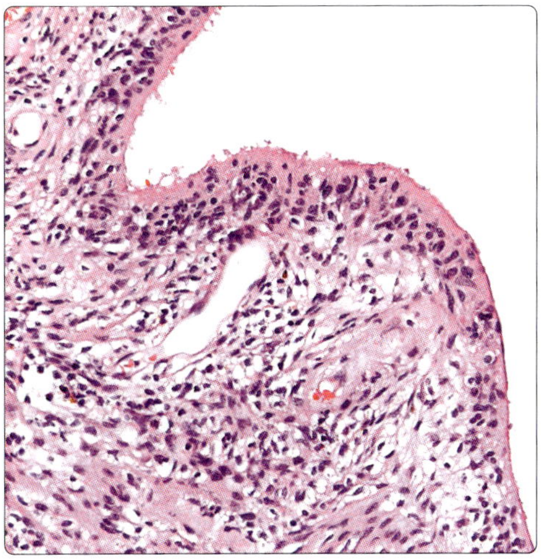

Pseudoglandular Schwannoma Variant

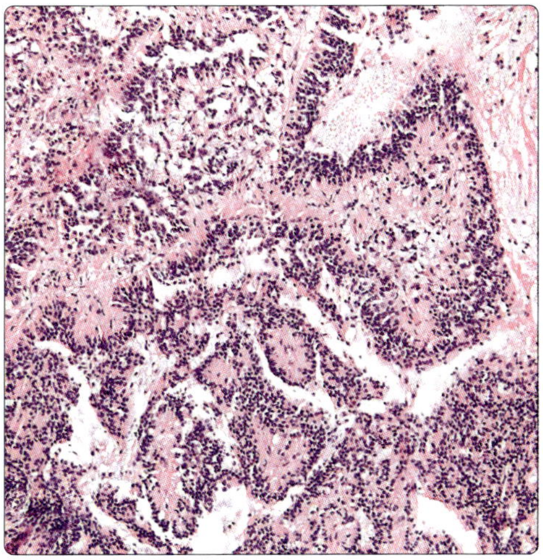

(Left) *The basal polarity of the Schwann cell nuclei lining the cystic spaces helps impart a pseudoglandular appearance.* **(Right)** *In some rare cases of schwannoma, the pseudoglandular change is extensive or predominant, warranting classification as a pseudoglandular schwannoma. Other areas of more typical schwannoma are often present.*

(Left) *Variably sized, hyalinized, rosette-like structures lined by peripheral Schwann cell nuclei are a rare finding in schwannoma and may be numerous.* **(Right)** *The neuroblastoma-like rosettes seen in rare cases of schwannoma are formed by rounded Schwann cells radially oriented around a collagen core. The nuclei of these cells are cytologically banal.*

Neuroblastoma-Like Schwannoma Variant

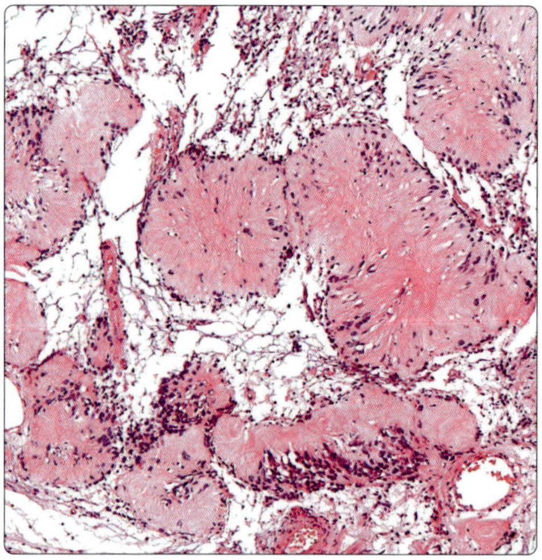

Radial Cellular Arrangement in Rosettes

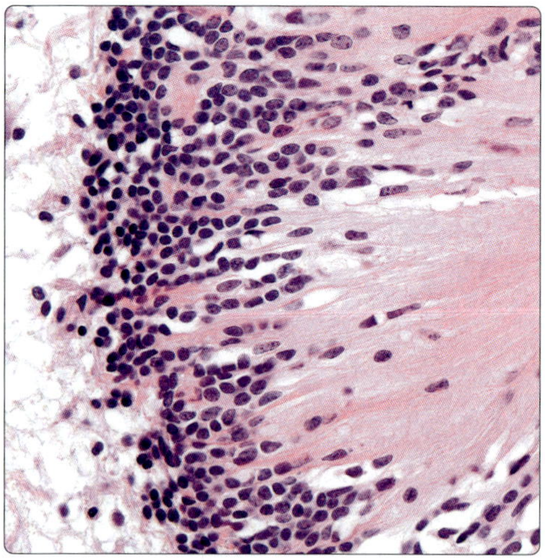

(Left) *In some cases of neuroblastoma-like schwannoma, the rosette structures are formed around what appear to be tiny vascular channels* ⇒. **(Right)** *The radially oriented cells of neuroblastoma-like schwannoma may rarely be spindled rather than epithelioid, warranting consideration of low-grade fibromyxoid sarcoma (hyalinizing spindle cell tumor with giant rosette morphology).*

Focal Perivascular Arrangement

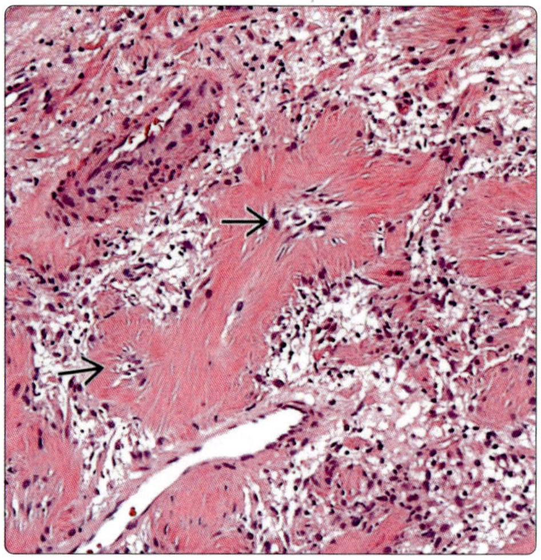

Rosettes With Spindled Cells in Schwannoma

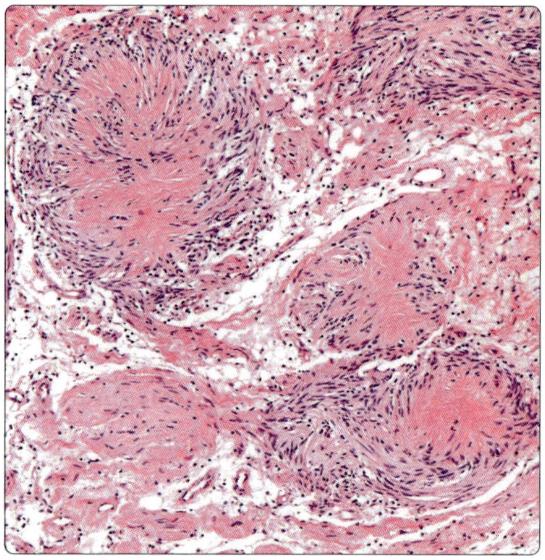

(Left) *Rare cases of schwannoma show a striking reticular growth pattern in a myxoid to hyalinized stroma. This morphology may be predominant or associated with areas of more conventional schwannoma morphology.* **(Right)** *The cytoplasmic eosinophilia is more conspicuous in this example of microcystic/reticular schwannoma.*

Microcystic/Reticular Schwannoma Variant

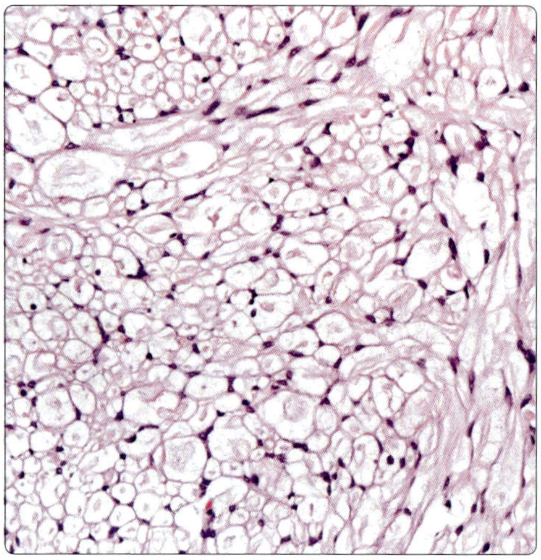

Cytoplasmic Eosinophilia in Reticular Schwannoma

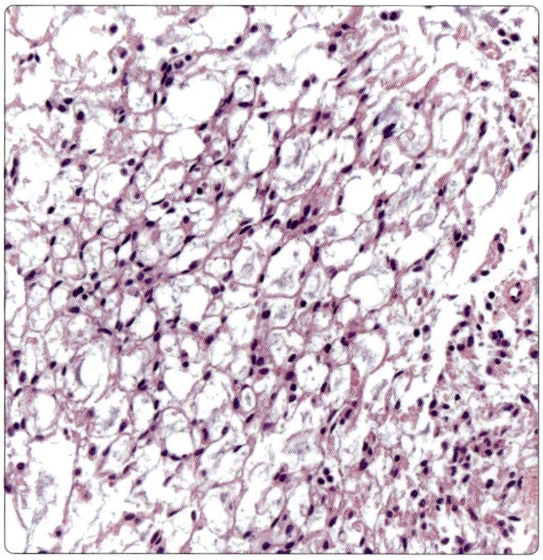

Microcyst Formation

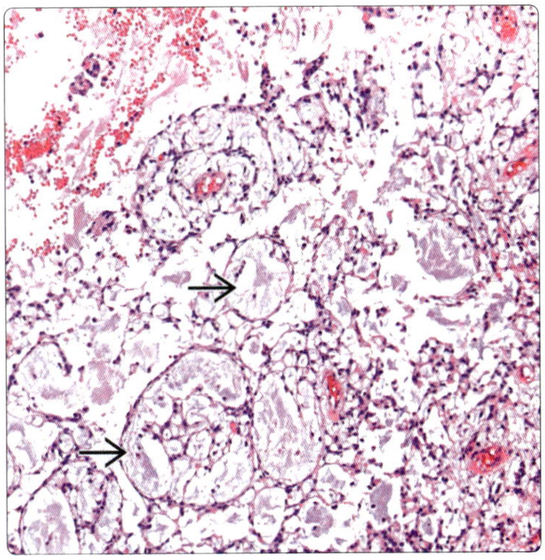

Focal Microcystic/Reticular Change in Otherwise Typical Schwannoma

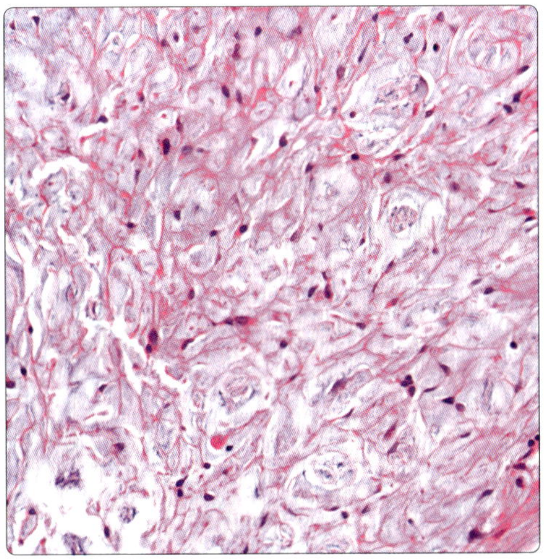

(Left) *Microcyst formation* ⇒ *may also be identified in association with the reticular morphology in some schwannomas. Similar to other forms of schwannoma, this morphologic variant strongly and diffusely expresses S100 protein.* **(Right)** *This case of schwannoma showed small focal areas demonstrating reticulated growth within a myxoid stroma intermixed with areas of more conventional schwannoma.*

Rare Presence of Eosinophilic Granular Bodies

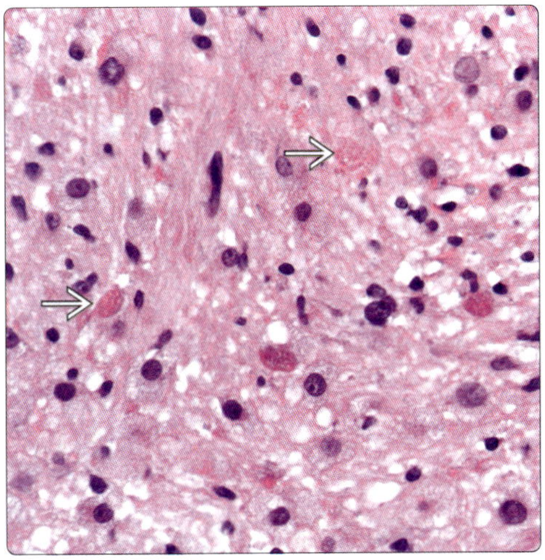

Direct Association With Nerve

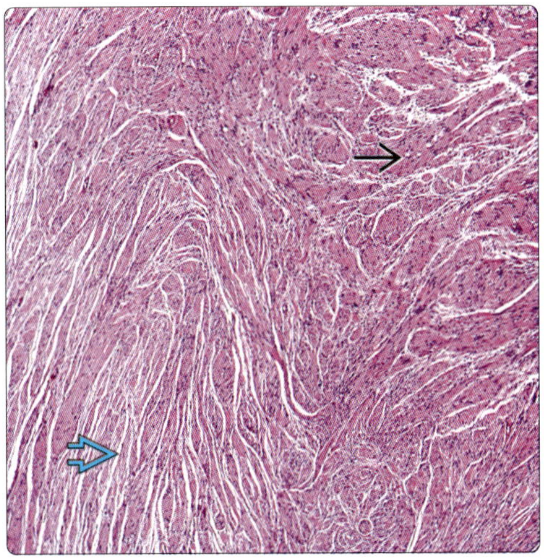

(Left) *Eosinophilic, granular body-like structures* ➡ *are a rare finding in schwannoma but appear to be more prevalent in schwannomas of the vestibulocochlear nerve (acoustic schwannoma) along with Rosenthal fibers.* **(Right)** *Occasionally, a small or incipient schwannoma may be detected intraoperatively as a small nodule growing on an otherwise unremarkable nerve. This H&E shows the tumor* ⇒ *arising in a background of peripheral nerve* ⇒.

Adjacent Ganglion in Schwannoma Mimicking Ganglioneuroma

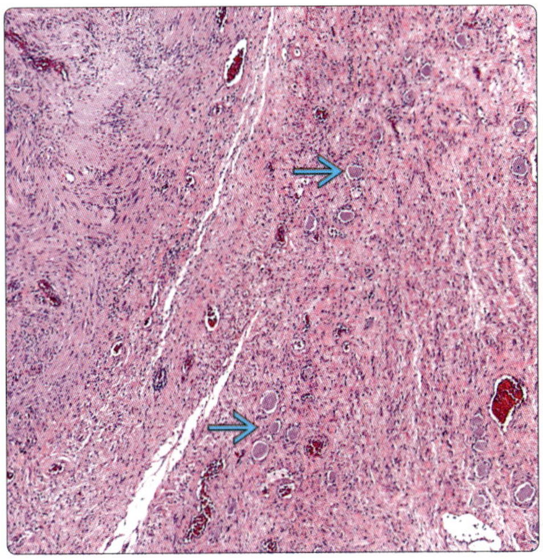

Very Rare Malignant Change in Schwannoma

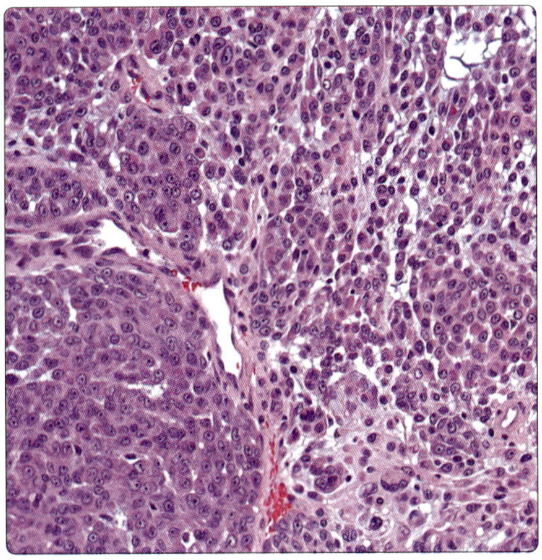

(Left) *Schwannomas that arise in the immediate vicinity of a ganglion will often show scattered collections of benign ganglion cells* ⇒ *in or adjacent to the peripheral capsule. This pattern differs from a true ganglioneuroma, in which ganglion cells are widely scattered throughout the tumor.* **(Right)** *Malignant change in schwannoma is an extremely rare event. Most well-documented cases of this transformation are in the form of an epithelioid malignant peripheral nerve sheath tumor (pictured) or epithelioid angiosarcoma.*

Neurofibroma

KEY FACTS

TERMINOLOGY

- Benign peripheral nerve sheath tumor composed of Schwann cells, fibroblasts, perineurial-like cells, and residual nerve axons within extracellular matrix

CLINICAL ISSUES

- Most common peripheral nerve sheath tumor
  - 3 main types: Localized (cutaneous or intraneural), diffuse, and plexiform
    - Plexiform type is essentially pathognomonic for neurofibromatosis type 1 (NF1)
- Wide age range
  - Diffuse and plexiform types most common in young
- Most (90%) neurofibromas are sporadic
- Benign; very rare local recurrence
- Malignant transformation usually occurs in setting of NF1 (up to 10% of patients)

MICROSCOPIC

- Loosely arranged spindle cells in haphazard arrangement
  - Small, hyperchromatic, wavy or buckled nuclei
  - Variable myxoid to collagenous matrix
- Diffuse type: Ill-defined, dermal and subcutaneous proliferation that entraps adnexa
  - Pseudomeissnerian bodies are characteristic
- Plexiform: Multinodular/serpentine growth pattern
- Malignant transformation: Combination of increased cellularity, nuclear atypia, mitotic activity, &/or necrosis

ANCILLARY TESTS

- Mixture of S100(+), CD34(+), and EMA(+) cells

TOP DIFFERENTIAL DIAGNOSES

- Malignant peripheral nerve sheath tumor
- Dermatofibrosarcoma protuberans
- Schwannoma
- Perineurioma

(Left) *Grossly, neurofibroma often appears as an ovoid or fusiform mass and usually shows a pale, wavy to gelatinous cut surface. The gross degenerative changes often seen in schwannomas are seldom present in neurofibroma. Note the transected nerve fibers ➡ at both ends of the mass.* **(Right)** *Localized cutaneous neurofibroma forms a well-circumscribed, but unencapsulated, dermal proliferation. This lesion may also occur in the nerve (intraneural localized neurofibroma).*

Neurofibroma

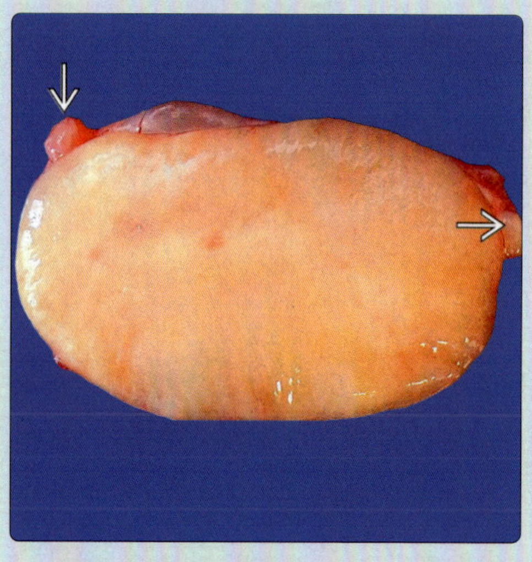

Localized Neurofibroma

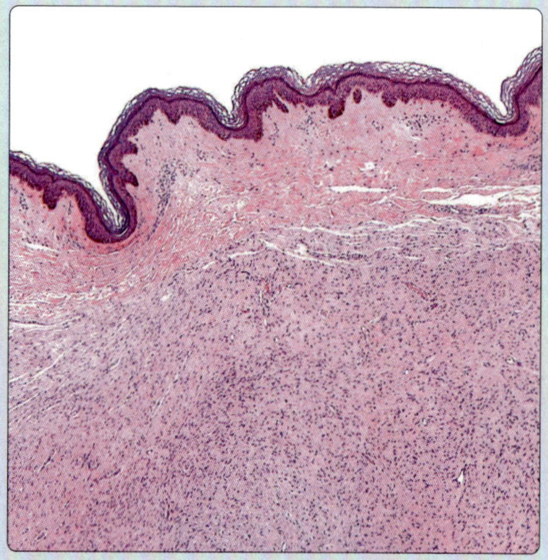

(Left) *All forms of neurofibroma are cytologically similar and are characterized by small, elongated spindled cells in a variably collagenous background stroma. Rare tumors show epithelioid features (not shown).* **(Right)** *Consistent S100 protein expression is seen in all forms of neurofibroma; however, it is usually less impressive than that seen in schwannoma due to the lower overall cellularity and mixture of cell types in the former (e.g., fibroblasts, perineurial-like cells).*

Small Elongated Spindle Cells

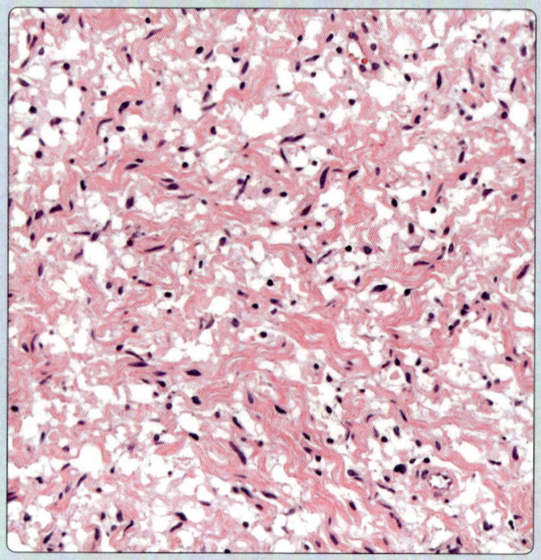

S100 Expression in Schwann Cells

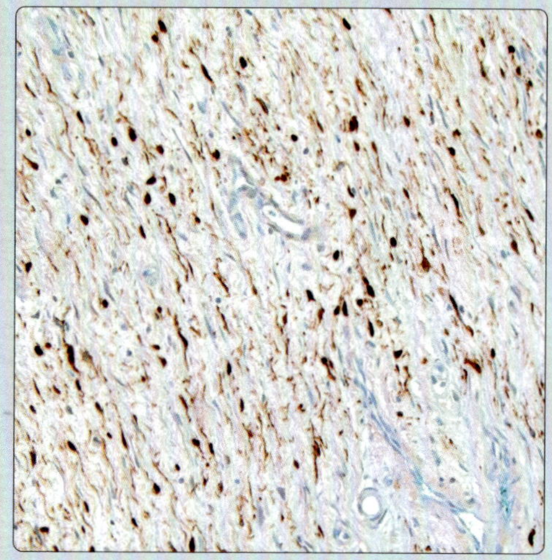

TERMINOLOGY

Definitions

- Benign peripheral nerve sheath tumor composed of Schwann cells, fibroblasts, perineurial-like cells, and residual nerve axons within extracellular matrix
  - 4 major types: Localized cutaneous, localized intraneural, diffuse, and plexiform
    - Plexiform neurofibroma is essentially pathognomonic of neurofibromatosis type 1 (NF1)

ETIOLOGY/PATHOGENESIS

Histogenesis

- Sporadic in ~ 90% of cases; others are syndromic in association with NF1
  - NF1 results from germline mutation in *NF1* gene on chromosome 17q11.2
    - *NF1* gene encodes for neurofibromin protein, which is GTPase-activating protein
  - Sporadic tumors arise from somatic mutations in *NF1*

CLINICAL ISSUES

Epidemiology

- Incidence
  - Most common peripheral nerve sheath tumor
    - Localized type most common among neurofibromas
- Age
  - Wide range (most common in young to middle-aged adults)
    - Plexiform and diffuse variants occur more often in younger age groups, including children
- Sex
  - M = F

Site

- Localized
  - Usually skin of trunk, head/neck, extremities
  - Less common in deeply situated nerves, nerve plexi, major nerve trunks, viscera
- Diffuse
  - Skin &/or subcutaneous tissue of head/neck
- Plexiform
  - Superficial or deep soft tissues, large nerve trunks
  - Head/neck, trunk, extremities

Presentation

- Most (90%) neurofibromas are sporadic and unassociated with NF1
- Usually slow-growing masses overall
  - Rapid growth in preexisting neurofibroma is worrisome for malignant transformation
- Localized
  - Usually small, sporadic, solitary mass
    - Deep lesions may be large
  - Rarely associated with NF1
    - Numerous localized neurofibromas; however, usually indicate NF1
  - Intraneural tumors present as fusiform swellings
    - Often cause sensory or motor disturbances related to affected nerve
- Diffuse type
  - Poorly defined, plaque-like growth, often large
  - 10% of cases associated with NF1
- Plexiform
  - Considered pathognomonic for NF1
    - Occurs in up to 40% of NF1 patients
  - Irregular, nodular mass with bag of worms appearance
  - Entire extremity may be involved (elephantiasis neuromatosa)
- Rare, massive soft tissue neurofibromas may result in large, pendulous folds of neurofibromatous tissue (localized gigantism)

Treatment

- Complete surgical excision

Prognosis

- Benign
  - All forms (including atypical/bizarre neurofibroma)
- Local recurrence very rare
- Malignant transformation
  - Usually occurs in setting of NF1 (rare in sporadic tumors)
    - Seen in 5-10% of NF1 patients
  - Plexiform and localized intraneural types are most frequent precursors to malignant peripheral nerve sheath tumor (MPNST)
    - Essentially no risk for localized cutaneous type
    - Very low risk for diffuse type

MACROSCOPIC

General Features

- Most are well circumscribed or well demarcated
  - Diffuse type is ill defined, plaque-like, cutaneous growth
- Unencapsulated
- Gray-tan firm/fibrous to gelatinous cut surface
- Generally lack degenerative changes (hemorrhage, cystic change)

Size

- Wide range
  - Localized cutaneous types usually small (< 2 cm)
  - Diffuse type often large
  - Rare tumors may be massive

MICROSCOPIC

Histologic Features

- Localized type (cutaneous or intraneural)
  - Well circumscribed, unencapsulated; grenz zone in skin
    - Intraneural tumors may have peripheral rim of perineurium or thickened epineurium
  - Usually low or moderate cellularity
  - Loosely arranged spindle cells in haphazard arrangement
    - Poorly defined cytoplasmic borders/processes
    - Small, hyperchromatic, wavy or buckled nuclei
    - Scattered nuclei may show degenerative changes (pleomorphic, hyperchromatic, "smudgy" nuclei)
      - Described as atypical (or bizarre) neurofibroma
  - Variable myxoid to collagenous matrix
    - Coarse collagen bundles often described as having shredded-carrot appearance

- Mast cells are common
- Rarely contain small nerve twigs
- Many rare variants described: Cellular, epithelioid, lipomatous, granular cell, dendritic cell, others

- Diffuse type
  - Ill-defined, expansive dermal and subcutaneous proliferation
    - Proliferates around cutaneous adnexal structures, entrapping them
      - Entrapped nerve twigs are often hypertrophic or edematous
    - Extends into subcutaneous tissue along connective tissue septa and infiltrates fat
  - Loosely arranged spindle cells in haphazard arrangement
    - Small, hyperchromatic, wavy or buckled nuclei
    - Some cases have epithelioid cytomorphology, at least focally
  - Evenly distributed, fibrillar collagenous stroma
    - May be myxoid
  - Pseudomeissnerian bodies are characteristic
    - Individual or aggregates of whorled eosinophilic fibrillary clusters
    - Vary in number and distribution
  - Rare cases show scattered dendritic cells containing melanin pigment
- Plexiform
  - Defined by growth pattern
    - Multiple, irregularly arranged structures resembling hypertrophic nerve fascicles
      - Imparts mixed multinodular and serpentine appearance
      - Usually markedly myxoid or edematous with abundant collagen bundles
  - May also show areas indistinguishable from diffuse-type neurofibroma
  - May show scattered nuclear atypia (degenerative) without increased mitoses or necrosis
- Hybrid neurofibroma/schwannoma
  - Schwannoma-like nodules within otherwise typical neurofibroma
  - Identified in some patients with NF1, per recent reports
- Malignant transformation (MPNST)
  - Many cases are clear cut and high grade with increased cellularity, generalized nuclear pleomorphism and hyperchromasia, high mitotic activity, &/or necrosis
  - Low-grade MPNST can be challenging to diagnose
    - Cases of neurofibroma with nuclear atypia alone are not MPNST
    - One study (Miettinen 2017) has proposed term "atypical neurofibromatous neoplasm of uncertain biologic potential" (ANNUBP)
      - Defined as neurofibroma with 2 of following 4 features: Nuclear atypia, loss of neurofibroma architecture, high cellularity, mitotic activity > 1/50 HPF but < 3/10 HPF
      - Tumors with features of ANNUBP but with 3-9 mitoses per 10 HPF and no necrosis considered low-grade MPNST
      - ANNUBP associated with local recurrence but not metastasis

ANCILLARY TESTS

Immunohistochemistry

- S100(+) and SOX10(+) in ~ 50% of total cells (Schwann cells)
- CD34(+) admixed spindled fibroblasts
- EMA(+) admixed perineurial cells
- Neurofilament protein highlights intratumoral axons
- Ki-67, p53, and p16 markers are of limited utility

DIFFERENTIAL DIAGNOSIS

Malignant Peripheral Nerve Sheath Tumor

- Usually large, deep tumors
- Variable combination of high cellularity with nuclear atypia, mitotic figures, &/or necrosis
- Perivascular tumor cell accentuation
- May contain peripheral component of preexisting neurofibroma
- Diffuse loss of h3k27me3 by IHC

Dermatofibrosarcoma Protuberans

- Cellular, highly infiltrative tumor with honeycomb infiltration of subcutaneous fat
- Usually prominent storiform architecture
- Diffuse CD34(+), S100(-)
- *PDGFB* rearrangements

Schwannoma

- Biphasic, encapsulated tumor with Antoni A and Antoni B areas
- Verocay body formation, perivascular hyalinization
- Diffuse, uniform S100(+) and SOX10(+)
- Cellular plexiform schwannoma may be mistaken for MPNST arising in plexiform neurofibroma

Desmoplastic Melanoma

- Junctional component may be present
- HMB-45(+), MART-1(+)
- p53(+) by IHC

Perineurioma

- Usually prominent storiform, whorling, or lamellar architecture
- EMA(+), claudin-1 (+), GLUT1(+)
  - Expression is often more diffuse than in neurofibroma (focal, patchy)
- S100(-), CD34(+/-)

SELECTED REFERENCES

1. Elsensohn A et al: Distinguishing neurofibroma from desmoplastic melanoma: the value of p53. Am J Surg Pathol. 42(3):372-5, 2018
2. Miettinen MM et al: Histopathologic evaluation of atypical neurofibromatous tumors and their transformation into malignant peripheral nerve sheath tumor in neurofibromatosis 1 patients - a consensus overview. Hum Pathol. 67:1-10, 2017
3. Jokinen CH et al: Atypical neurofibroma of the skin and subcutaneous tissue: clinicopathologic analysis of 11 cases. J Cutan Pathol. 37(1):35-42, 2010
4. Magro G et al: Multinucleated floret-like giant cells in sporadic and NF1-associated neurofibromas: a clinicopathologic study of 94 cases. Virchows Arch. 456(1):71-6, 2010
5. Spurlock G et al: Molecular evolution of a neurofibroma to malignant peripheral nerve sheath tumor (MPNST) in an NF1 patient: correlation between histopathological, clinical and molecular findings. J Cancer Res Clin Oncol. 136(12):1869-80, 2010

Classic Neural Cytologic Features

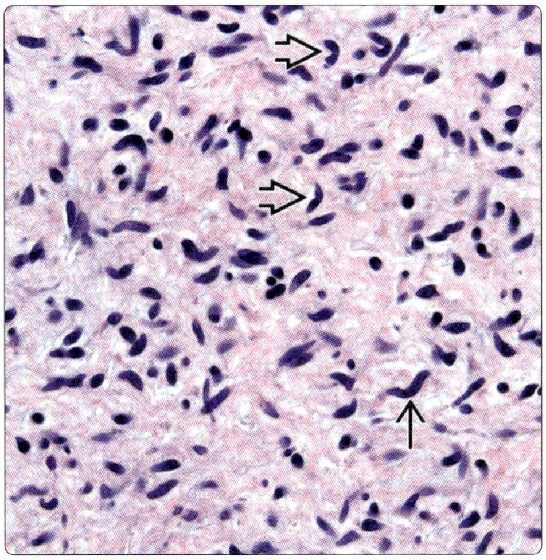

Mast Cells

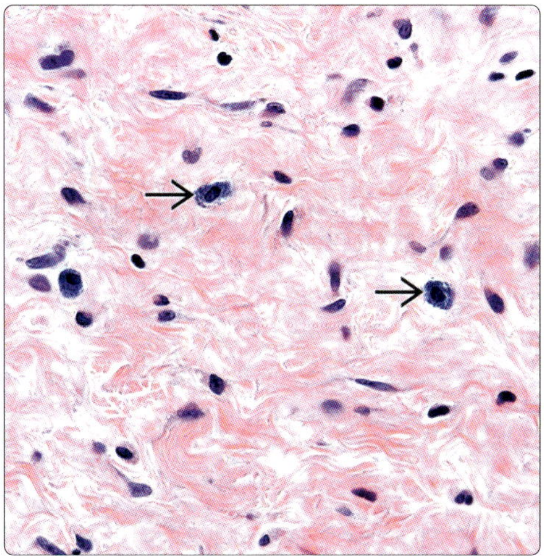

(Left) *The lesional Schwann cell nuclei of neurofibroma are generally elongated with pointed or tapered ends and often appear wavy →or buckled (comma-shaped ⇒). Mitotic activity is essentially nonexistent.* **(Right)** *Mast cells → are commonly identified in neurofibromas, particularly localized and diffuse forms. They may be sparse or relatively abundant.*

Low to Moderate Cellularity

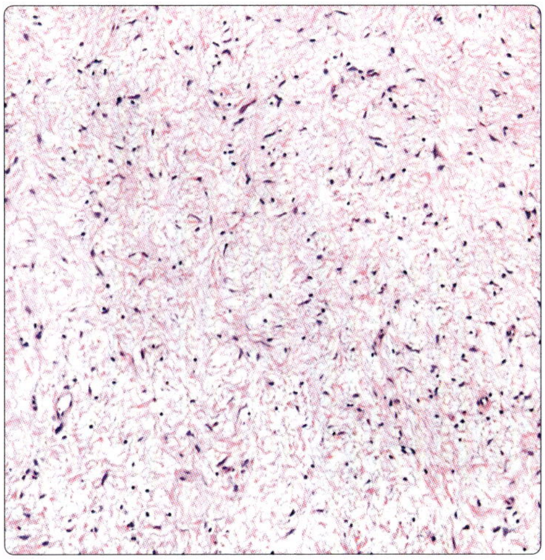

Myxoid Stromal Change

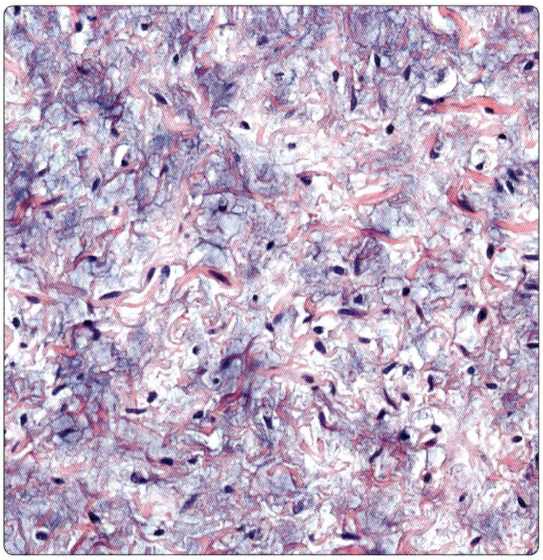

(Left) *Neurofibroma is generally a low to moderately cellular neoplasm. Some cases are heavily edematous (shown). Even at low power, the characteristic wavy nuclei are apparent.* **(Right)** *Myxoid stromal change is not uncommon in neurofibroma. Note the numerous separated pink collagen fibers, which somewhat resemble shredded carrots. Examples in which myxoid change is extensive may show morphologic overlap with myxoma or spindle cell lipoma.*

Rare, Multinucleated, Floret-Like Giant Cells

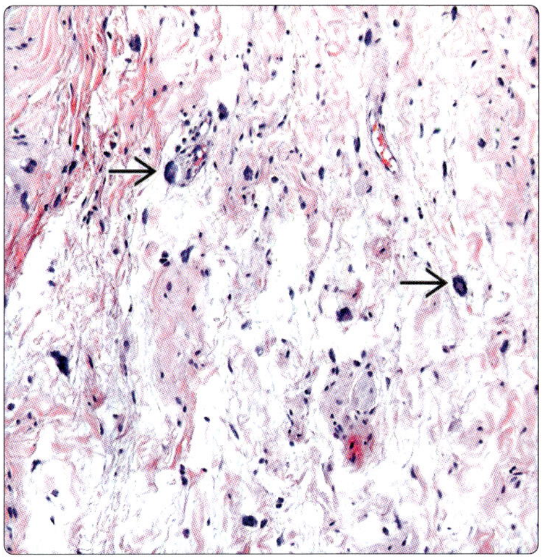

Rare Tumor With Increased Cellularity

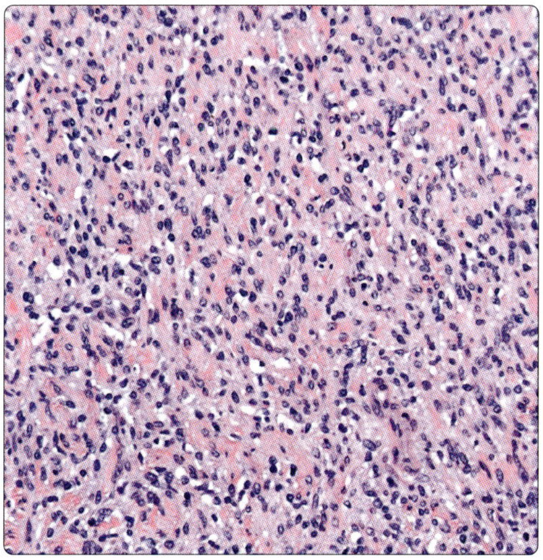

(Left) *Multinucleated, floret-like giant cells →, similar to those seen in pleomorphic lipoma, are occasionally encountered in neurofibroma. They are seen in both sporadic tumors and those associated with neurofibromatosis type 1 (NF1) and are typically CD34(+) and S100(-).* **(Right)** *Rare cases of neurofibroma show increased cellularity. Importantly, mitotic activity and high-grade cytologic atypia are absent.*

(Left) *Diffuse-type neurofibroma usually presents as an ill-defined, cutaneous plaque in the head and neck. It is characteristically highly infiltrative and grows around normal anatomic structures.* **(Right)** *Intralesional adipose tissue may rarely be identified within localized cutaneous neurofibroma; however, it is far more common in diffuse-type neurofibroma (due to peripheral infiltration of subcutaneous fat).*

Diffuse-Type Neurofibroma

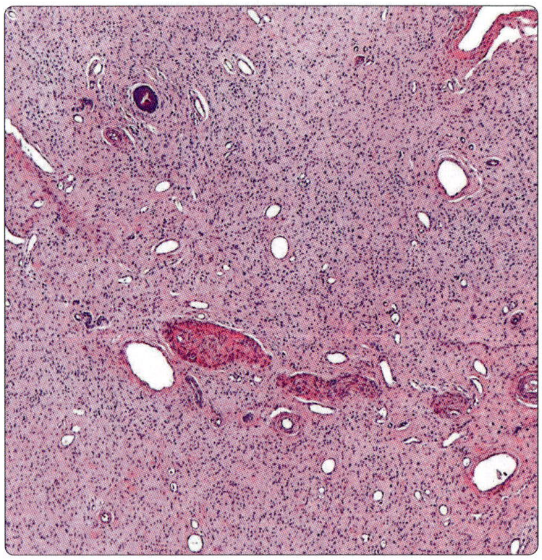

Intralesional Adipose Tissue

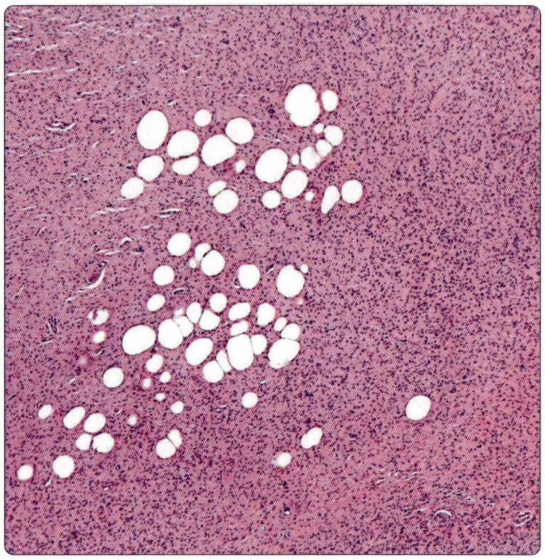

(Left) *The lesional tissue of diffuse-type neurofibroma characteristically grows around and entraps cutaneous adnexa, such as hair follicles and eccrine structures (shown). Note that there is no destruction of these normal structures.* **(Right)** *Infiltration of peripheral soft tissues, including fat and skeletal muscle, is commonly seen in diffuse-type neurofibroma.*

Entrapment of Cutaneous Adnexa

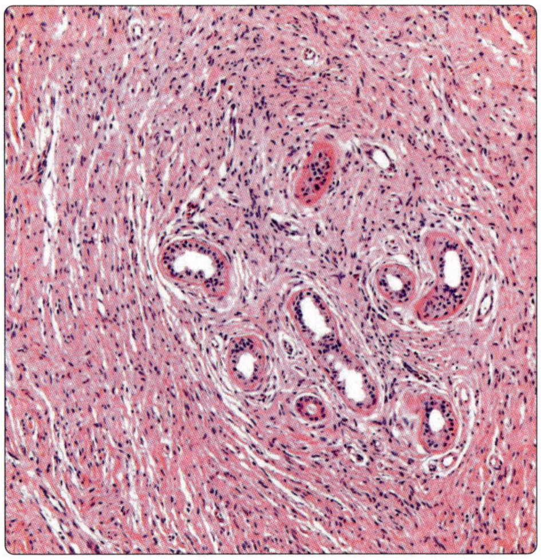

Infiltration of Fat and Muscle

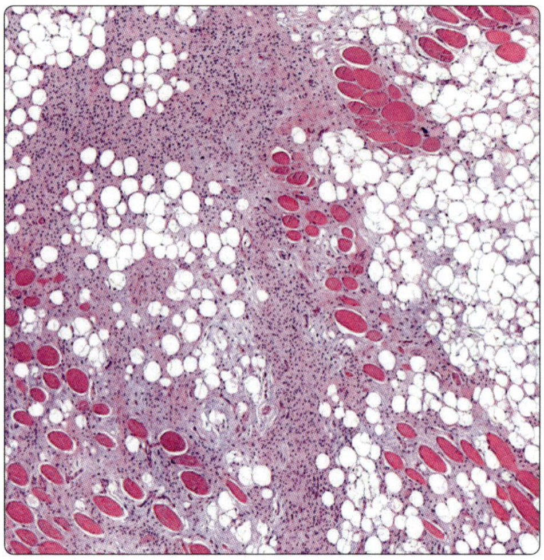

(Left) *Some cases of diffuse-type neurofibroma grow as thin rays* → *of lesional tissue within abundant fat, resembling fibrous septa. This morphology can mimic lipofibromatosis or fibrolipoma.* **(Right)** *The nuclei of Schwann cells in diffuse-type neurofibroma are identical to those of other forms. Note the admixed non-schwannian nuclei, which are larger* → *and paler.*

Infiltration of Fat

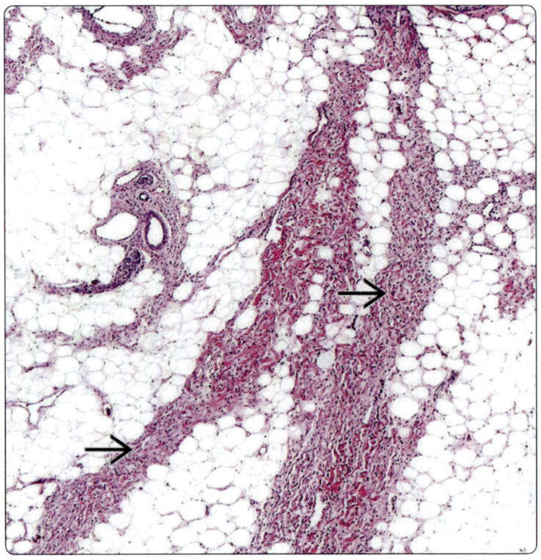

Diffuse-Type Neurofibroma Cytology

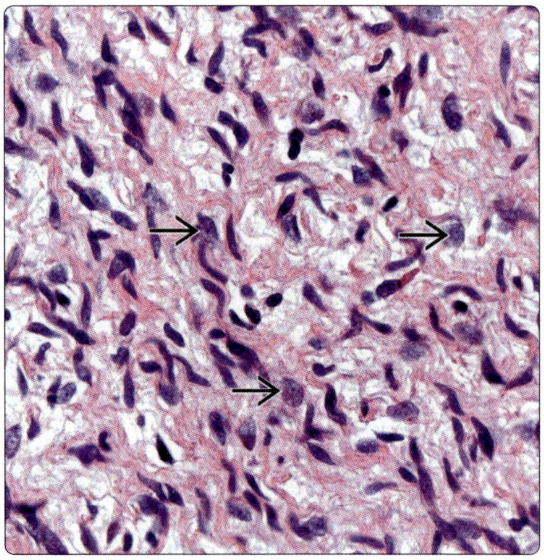

Rounded Nuclei

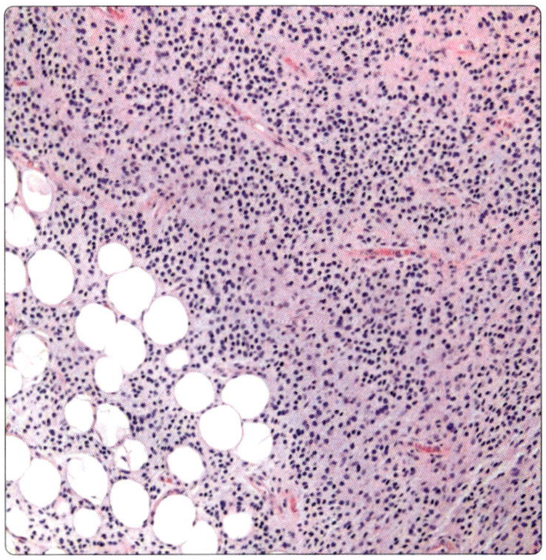

Very Rare Nuclear Palisading

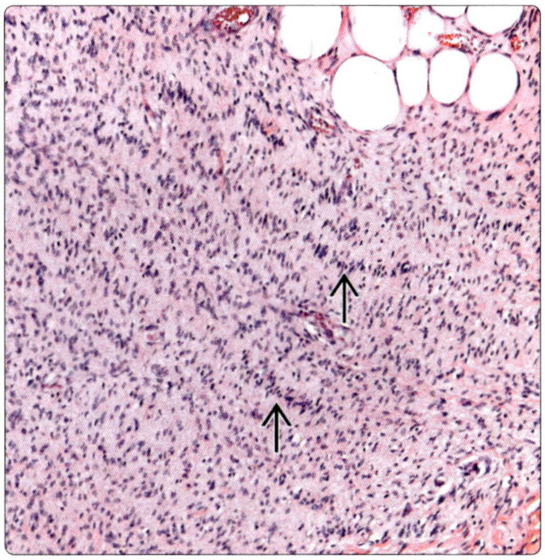

(Left) *Lesional Schwann cells with a rounded nuclear profile may be seen in some cases of diffuse-type neurofibroma. This appearance is more common in this subtype than in the others.* **(Right)** *Nuclear palisading is very uncommon in neurofibroma. This unusual case of otherwise typical diffuse-type neurofibroma had focal areas of increased cellularity with vague palisading ⇨.*

Wagner-Meissner Bodies

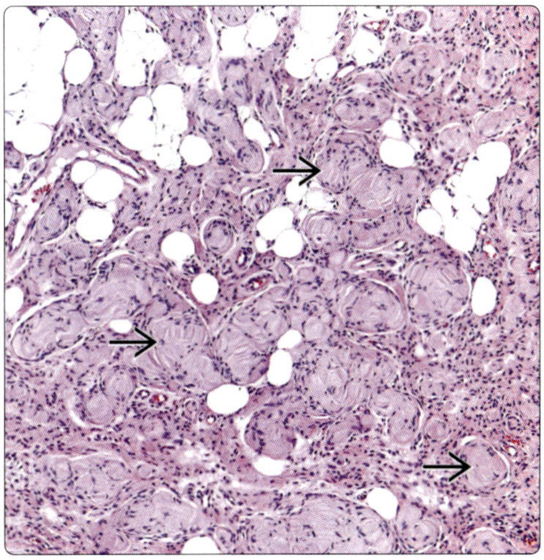

Morphology of Wagner-Meissner Bodies

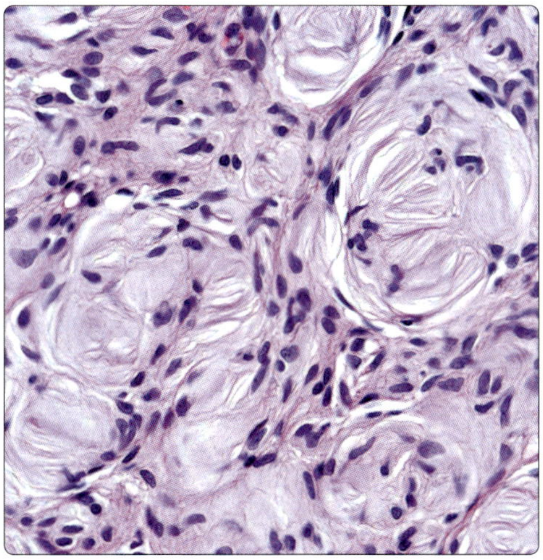

(Left) *Wagner-Meissner (pseudomeissnerian) bodies ⇨ are very characteristic of diffuse-type neurofibroma and may arrange in small aggregates, linear arrays, or larger sheets.* **(Right)** *Wagner-Meissner (pseudomeissnerian) bodies are composed of spherical, layered clusters of thin and elongated spindled cells with long delicate cytoplasmic processes. They resemble Meissner corpuscles.*

Scattered Wagner-Meissner Bodies

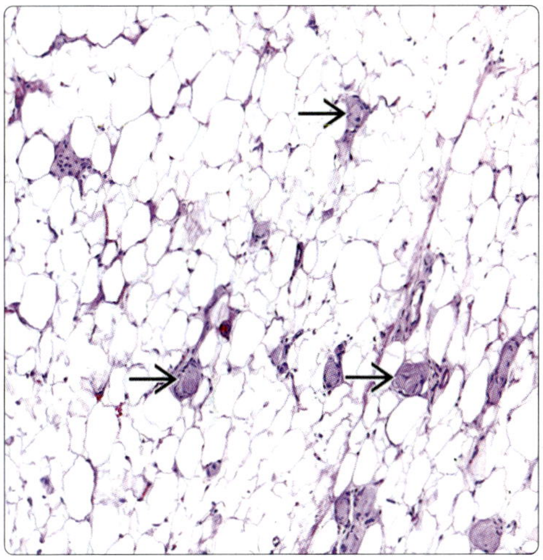

Pigmented Neurofibroma

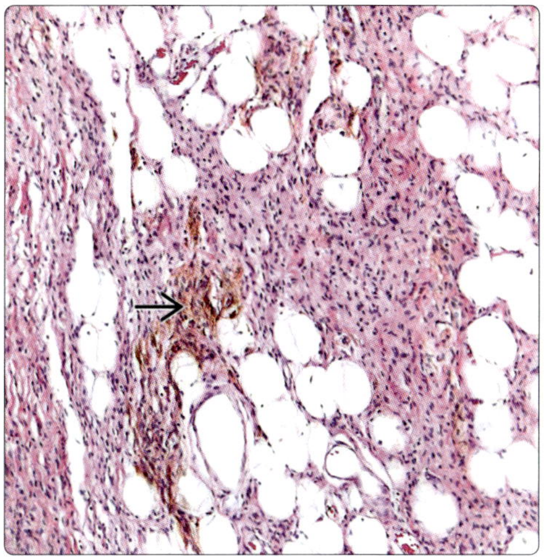

(Left) *Diffuse-type neurofibroma may contain large zones of predominantly mature adipose tissue with scattered small Wagner-Meissner bodies ⇨. This finding may be the only clue to the diagnosis in a small biopsy.* **(Right)** *Rare cases of diffuse-type neurofibroma contain collections of pigmented Schwann cells ⇨ with intracytoplasmic melanin. Most of these tumors occur in the setting of NF1, and some may also show a plexiform morphology.*

(Left) *Plexiform neurofibroma is identified by a characteristic irregular, multinodular, and serpentine growth pattern of expanded nerves. This variant usually first arises in childhood and is virtually diagnostic of NF1.* **(Right)** *Many of the expanded nerves in plexiform neurofibroma contain a centralized core* ➡ *of residual nerve within otherwise typical neurofibromatous tissue.*

Plexiform Neurofibroma

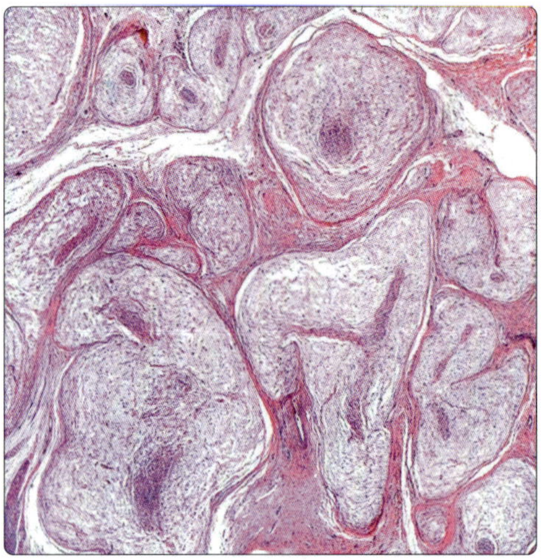

Expanded Nerves

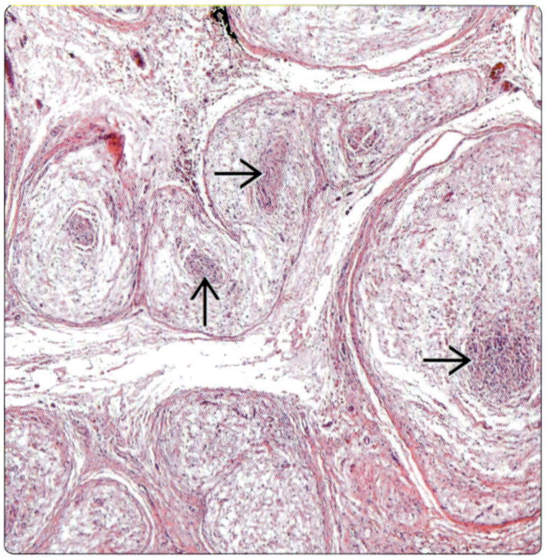

(Left) *Myxoid change is common in plexiform neurofibroma, and collagen fibers are typically splayed apart throughout each expanded nerve, reminiscent of shredded carrots. This morphology is similar to other forms of neurofibroma.* **(Right)** *Collagen fibers may be thicker in some foci of plexiform neurofibroma. Note the small core* ➡ *of centralized residual nerve.*

Myxoid Change

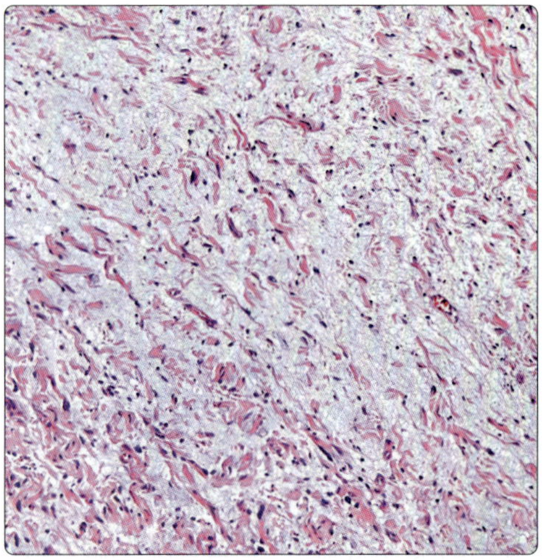

Collagen Fibers

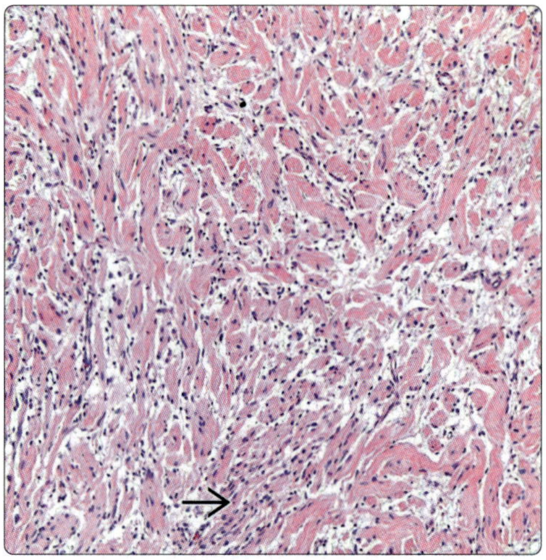

(Left) *This example of plexiform neurofibroma shows foci with extensive bundled collagen between clusters of lesional spindled cells.* **(Right)** *Many cases of plexiform neurofibroma show extension* ➡ *of lesional tissue out of the expanded nerves* ⇨ *in plexiform areas and into the surrounding tissue. The morphology of this extraneural tissue is indistinguishable from diffuse-type neurofibroma.*

Prominent Collagen

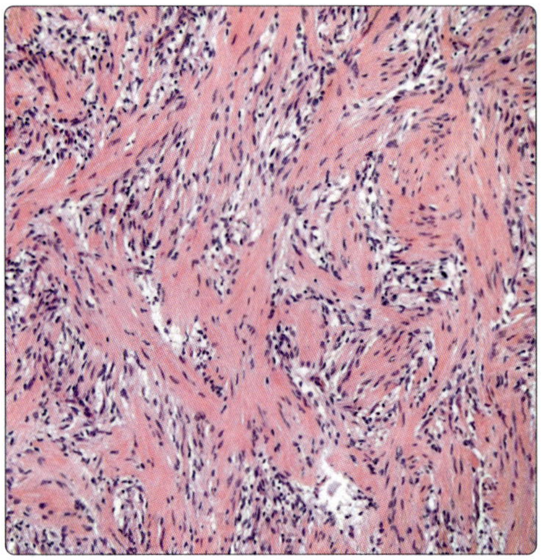

Combined Diffuse and Plexiform Morphologies

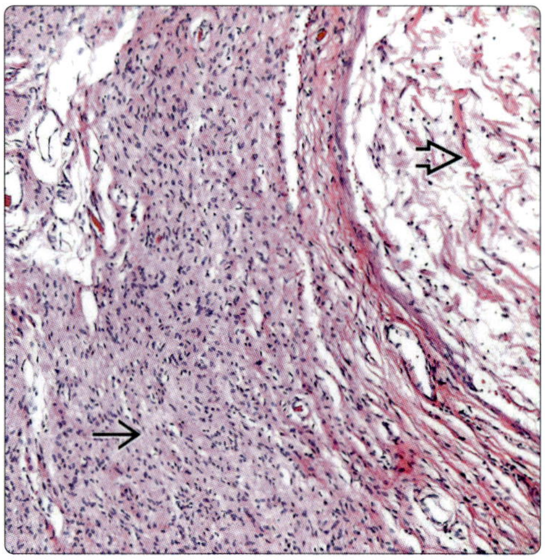

Degenerative Nuclear Atypia

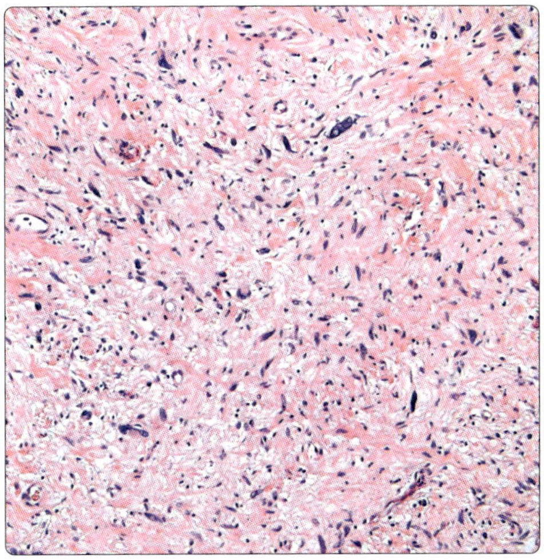

Degenerative Changes Include Foamy Histiocytes

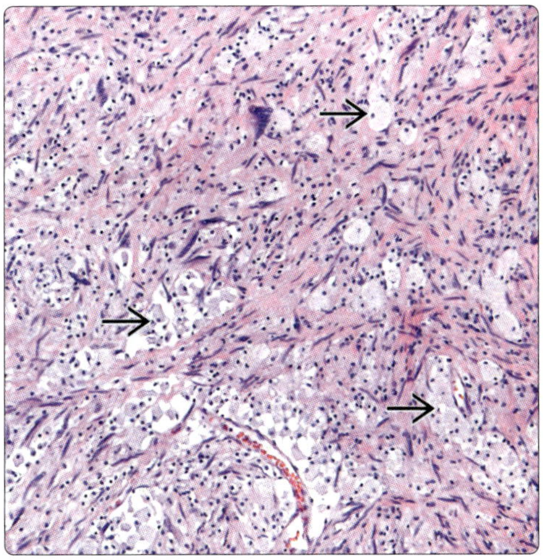

(Left) *Degenerative nuclear atypia, identical to the ancient change seen in schwannoma, may be seen in localized or plexiform neurofibroma. The nuclei generally show "smudgy" chromatin and commonly contain pseudoinclusions. When this change is prominent, these tumors may be referred to as atypical (or bizarre) neurofibroma.* **(Right)** *Collections of foamy histiocytes → may also be seen in degenerative (atypical/bizarre) neurofibromas.*

Central Cellularity in Atypical Neurofibroma

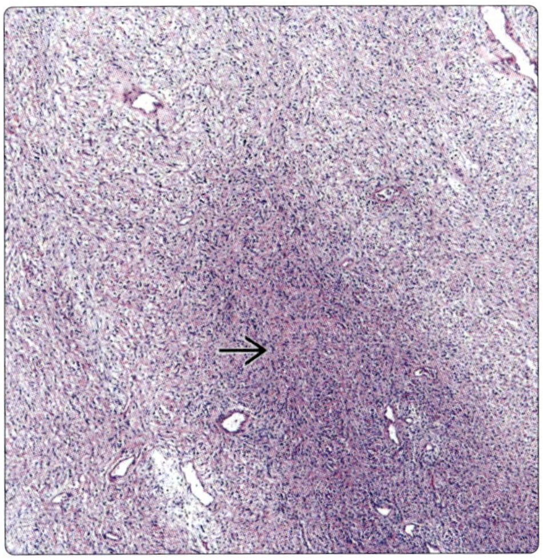

Increased Cellularity in Atypical Neurofibroma

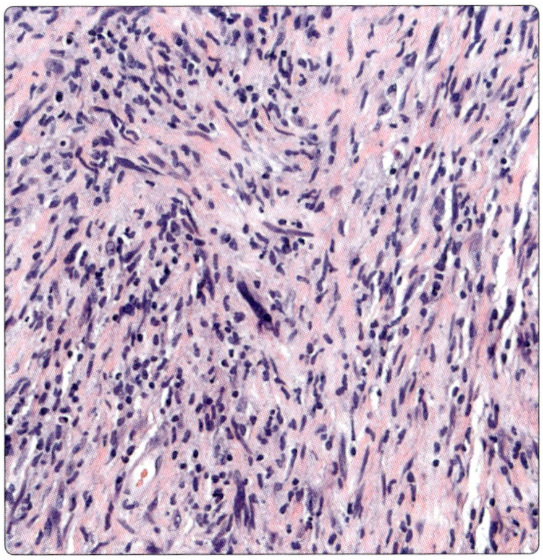

(Left) *Large examples of localized soft tissue neurofibroma may show centralized increases in cellularity →. These areas should be evaluated at higher power for other features that might indicate possible malignant transformation.* **(Right)** *Increased cellularity in atypical (bizarre) neurofibroma does not necessarily imply malignant transformation. However, marked cellularity with generalized nuclear atypia and more than rare mitoses suggests transformation into an MPNST.*

Malignant Transformation in Neurofibroma

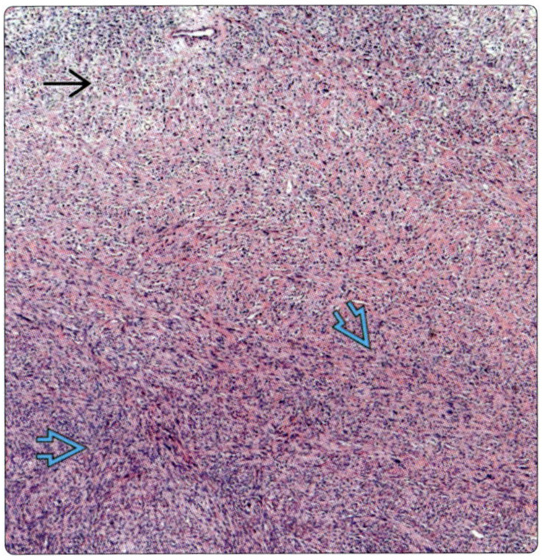

MPNST Arising in Neurofibroma

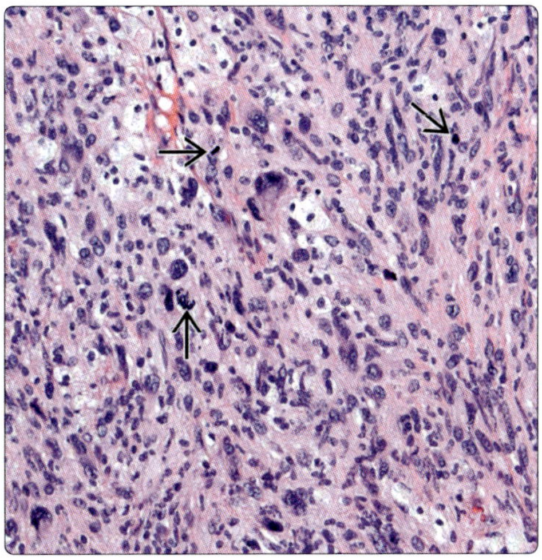

(Left) *This image shows transformation of a localized soft tissue neurofibroma → into an MPNST ⇨. Note the marked increase in cellularity from benign to malignant zones.* **(Right)** *This image shows the MPNST portion of a neurofibroma with malignant transformation, as evidenced by the significant nuclear atypia and several mitotic figures → in 1 field. Necrosis may or may not be present (not shown).*

Perineurioma

KEY FACTS

TERMINOLOGY

- Benign mesenchymal neoplasm composed exclusively of perineural cells

CLINICAL ISSUES

- Wide age range (usually adults)
- Sclerosing perineurioma shows marked male predilection
- Usually occurs in superficial soft tissues of extremities or trunk
  - Sclerosing perineurioma very common in hands/fingers
- Solitary, slow-growing, usually painless mass
- No clear association with neurofibromatosis syndromes
- Treatment: Complete, but conservative surgical excision
- Benign; excellent prognosis

MACROSCOPIC

- Well circumscribed, nodular
- Wide size range (mean: 4 cm)

MICROSCOPIC

- Well circumscribed and unencapsulated
- Bland, elongated spindle cells in various growth patterns (storiform, whorling, lamellar, fascicular)
  - Nuclei range from thin and wavy to round and pale
- Collagenous to myxoid stroma
- Variants: Intraneural, sclerosing, reticular, plexiform

ANCILLARY TESTS

- EMA(+), claudin-1 (+), GLUT-1(+)
- Variable CD34(+)
- Negative for S100 protein, keratin, SMA, desmin, MUC4

TOP DIFFERENTIAL DIAGNOSES

- Hybrid nerve sheath tumor
- Dermatofibrosarcoma protuberans
- Schwannoma
- Neurofibroma
- Low-grade fibromyxoid sarcoma

(Left) *Perineurioma is a rare, well-circumscribed peripheral nerve sheath tumor of perineurial origin. It often contains abundant stromal blood vessels ➙ easily identified at low magnification. Rare cases show microscopically infiltrative margins.* **(Right)** *A storiform architecture is commonly identified in soft tissue perineurioma along with lamellar and fascicular patterns. Although certainly not pathognomonic, this morphologic pattern should always engender consideration of perineurioma.*

Perineurioma

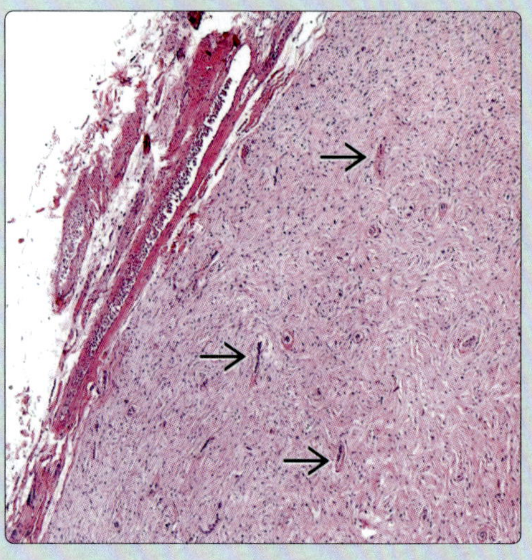

Storiform Whorling Growth

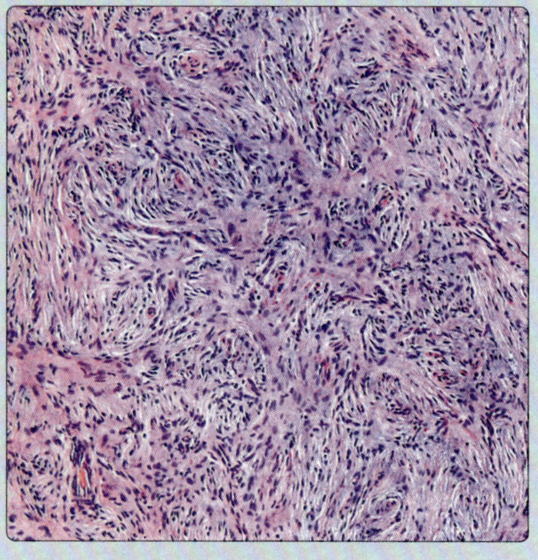

(Left) *Architectural whorls, particularly around small blood vessels ⇨, is highly characteristic of perineurioma and should always lead to consideration of the diagnosis.* **(Right)** *The lesional cells of perineurioma are cytologically banal and vary from slender and elongated ↪ to rounded and pale ⇨. An admixed mild lymphocytic infiltrate may be present in some cases, and occasionally mast cells are seen.*

Whorls

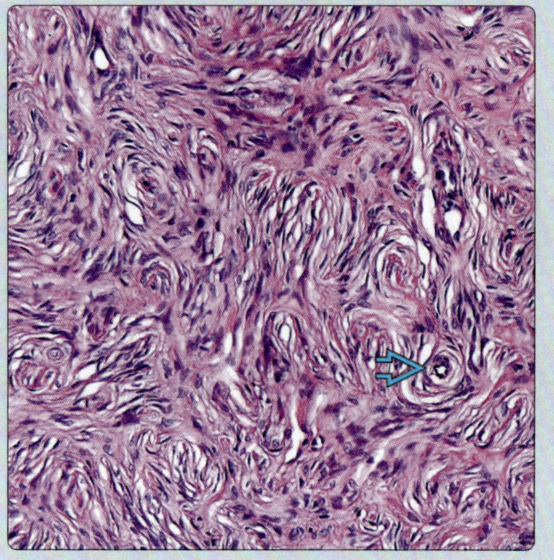

Bland Cytologic Features

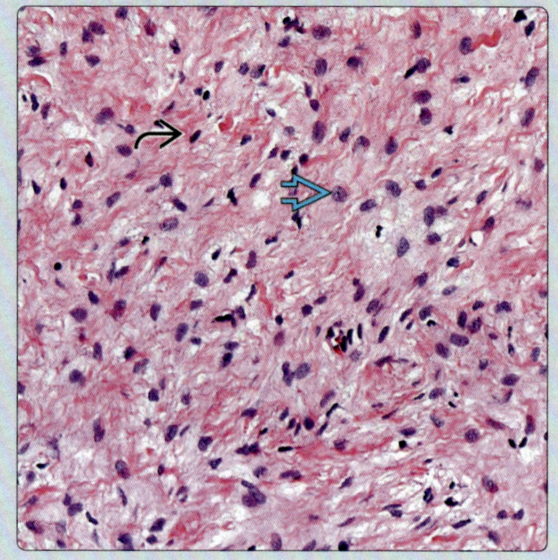

TERMINOLOGY

Synonyms

- Extraneural soft tissue perineurioma
- Storiform perineural fibroma
- Localized hypertrophic neuropathy of limbs (intraneural perineurioma)

Definitions

- Benign mesenchymal neoplasm composed exclusively of perineural cells

CLINICAL ISSUES

Epidemiology

- Age
  - Wide range (usually adults)
    - Intraneural and sclerosing perineuriomas occur in younger age group
    - Rare in children
- Sex
  - Sclerosing perineurioma shows marked male predilection
    - M = F for most other types

Site

- Usually superficial soft tissues of extremities or trunk
  - Up to 30% arise in deep soft tissues or visceral locations
  - Occasional dermal origin
- Sclerosing perineurioma very common in hands/fingers

Presentation

- Solitary, slow-growing, usually painless mass
- No clear association with neurofibromatosis syndromes
- Intraneural perineurioma often presents with symptoms related to neurologic defects
  - Fusiform segmental enlargement of affected nerve

Treatment

- Complete but conservative surgical excision
- Excision with nerve grafting may be attempted in intraneural perineurioma

Prognosis

- Benign (including variants)
- Local recurrence is very rare
- Predictive histologic features
  - Mildly atypical features (scattered pleomorphic cells, infiltrative growth) do not appear to affect excellent prognosis
  - Overtly malignant cytologic features and high mitotic rate diffusely present in large perineurioma indicates increased risk of aggressive behavior and malignant potential

MACROSCOPIC

General Features

- Well circumscribed, nodular
- Tan-white fibrous to gelatinous cut surface

Size

- Wide size range (mean: 4 cm)

MICROSCOPIC

Histologic Features

- Well circumscribed and unencapsulated
  - Rare tumors have infiltrative growth
- Bland, elongated spindle cells in various growth patterns (storiform, whorling, lamellar, fascicular)
  - Nuclei range from thin and wavy to round and pale
  - Nuclear pseudoinclusions common
  - Scattered cells with nuclear atypia may occasionally be present (likely degenerative)
  - Mitotic figures usually rare
- Overall cellularity varies widely
- Collagenous to myxoid stroma
- Unusual findings: Intratumoral mature adipose tissue, metaplastic bone/cartilage, granular cell change, pseudolipoblastic morphology
- Very rare cases show overtly malignant cytologic atypia, numerous mitotic figures, &/or necrosis
  - May be referred to as malignant perineurioma or perineurial malignant peripheral nerve sheath tumor

Morphologic Variants

- Intraneural perineurioma
  - Hypercellular, expanded nerve tissue with bland perineurial cells forming concentric layers around preexisting nerve axons ("onion-bulb" structures)
    - Identified in histologic cross sections of lesion
- Sclerosing perineurioma
  - Plump spindled &/or epithelioid tumor cells in corded, trabecular, or whorled patterns
  - Diffusely hyalinized stroma containing thin-walled blood vessels
- Reticular perineurioma
  - Anastomosing cords of thin, fusiform spindle cells in lace-like pattern
    - Pseudocystic spaces may be present
  - Usually prominent myxedematous stroma
- Plexiform perineurioma
  - Multinodular, serpentine growth pattern
  - Standard histologic features of perineurioma

ANCILLARY TESTS

Immunohistochemistry

- EMA(+), claudin-1 (+), GLUT1(+)
  - EMA expression may be weak &/or focal, requiring careful examination
  - Use of 2 or 3 markers recommended for screening
- Variable CD34(+)
- Negative for S100 protein, keratin, SMA, desmin, MUC4
  - SMA may be (+) in sclerosing variants

Molecular Genetics

- Abnormalities involving chromosome 22q most frequent finding
  - 17q deletions less common
- Rearrangements &/or deletions of 10q in sclerosing perineurioma
- Frequent *TRAF7* mutations in intraneural perineurioma

DIFFERENTIAL DIAGNOSIS

Hybrid Nerve Sheath Tumor

- Most commonly perineurioma-schwannoma hybrid
  - Overall cytoarchitectural features of perineurioma
    - Immunohistochemistry usually required for diagnosis
- S100 protein (+) in Schwann cells
- EMA(+), claudin-1 (+) in perineurial cells

Neurofibroma

- Usually less cellular than perineurioma
- S100 protein (+)
- May show scattered EMA(+) intratumoral perineurial cells

Schwannoma

- Most are encapsulated
- Antoni A and B regions
- Diffuse S100 protein (+)
- EMA(-), claudin-1 (-)
  - May be (+) in peripheral capsule

Ectopic Meningioma

- Occurs predominantly in head and neck sites
- Often shows significant morphologic overlap with soft tissue perineurioma
- EMA(+), progesterone receptor (+)
- Usually claudin-1 (-), GLUT-1(-)

Dermatofibrosarcoma Protuberans

- Diffuse infiltration of dermis and subcutis ("honeycomb" infiltration)
- Storiform growth pattern often present, at least focally
- Diffuse CD34(+)
- EMA(-), claudin-1 (-)
- Characteristic t(17;22) translocation involving *COL1A1* and *PDGFB*

Solitary Fibrous Tumor

- Absence of storiform, whorling growth
- Characteristic hemangiopericytoma-like ectatic vasculature
- Diffuse CD34(+), nuclear STAT6(+)
- EMA(-), claudin-1 (-)

Low-Grade Fibromyxoid Sarcoma

- Usually large, deeply located tumors
- Can show histologic overlap with perineurioma
- Cells lack long cytoplasmic processes
- Arcades of small blood vessels may be seen in myxoid areas
- MUC4(+)
- EMA (variable), claudin-1 (variable)
  - Neither are useful for distinguishing from perineurioma
- *FUS* gene fusions

Desmoid Fibromatosis

- Ill-defined, infiltrative neoplasms
- Long fascicles of bland spindled tumor cells; lacks whorling growth
- Nuclear β-catenin (+) in most cases
- EMA(-), claudin-1 (-)

Juxtaarticular Myxoma

- Absence of storiform, whorling growth
- Often shows highly mucoid foci, at least focally
- EMA(-); claudin-1 (-)

Myoepithelioma

- Nests and clusters of epithelioid (less commonly spindled) cells in myxoid to collagenous stroma
- Keratin (+), S100 protein (+) in majority of cases
- *EWSR1* gene translocations in some cases

Extraskeletal Myxoid Chondrosarcoma

- Large, deeply located tumors
- May resemble reticular perineurioma
- EMA(-)
- Translocations involving 9q22.3 [*NR4A3 (TEC)*]

SELECTED REFERENCES

1. Carter JM et al: Recurrent genomic alterations in soft tissue perineuriomas. Am J Surg Pathol. 42(12):1708-14, 2018
2. Klein CJ et al: Genomic analysis reveals frequent TRAF7 mutations in intraneural perineuriomas. Ann Neurol. 81(2):316-21, 2017
3. Torres-Mora J et al: Pseudolipoblastic perineurioma: an unusual morphological variant of perineurioma that may simulate liposarcoma. Hum Pathol. 57:22-7, 2016
4. Agaimy A et al: Comparative study of soft tissue perineurioma and meningioma using a five-marker immunohistochemical panel. Histopathology. 65(1):60-70, 2014
5. Fox MD et al: Extra-acral cutaneous/soft tissue sclerosing perineurioma: an under-recognized entity in the differential of CD34-positive cutaneous neoplasms. J Cutan Pathol. 37(10):1053-6, 2010
6. Hornick JL et al: Hybrid schwannoma/perineurioma: clinicopathologic analysis of 42 distinctive benign nerve sheath tumors. Am J Surg Pathol. 33(10):1554-61, 2009
7. Macarenco AC et al: Cutaneous lipomatous sclerosing perineurioma. Am J Dermatopathol. 30(3):291-4, 2008
8. Macarenco RS et al: Perineurioma: a distinctive and underrecognized peripheral nerve sheath neoplasm. Arch Pathol Lab Med. 131(4):625-36, 2007
9. Hornick JL et al: Soft tissue perineurioma: clinicopathologic analysis of 81 cases including those with atypical histologic features. Am J Surg Pathol. 29(7):845-58, 2005
10. Mentzel T et al: Reticular and plexiform perineurioma: clinicopathological and immunohistochemical analysis of two cases and review of perineurial neoplasms of skin and soft tissues. Virchows Arch. 447(4):677-82, 2005
11. Michal M et al: A benign neoplasm with histopathological features of both schwannoma and retiform perineurioma (benign schwannoma-perineurioma): a report of six cases of a distinctive soft tissue tumor with a predilection for the fingers. Virchows Arch. 445(4):347-53, 2004
12. Yamaguchi U et al: Sclerosing perineurioma: a clinicopathological study of five cases and diagnostic utility of immunohistochemical staining for GLUT1. Virchows Arch. 443(2):159-63, 2003
13. Folpe AL et al: Expression of claudin-1, a recently described tight junction-associated protein, distinguishes soft tissue perineurioma from potential mimics. Am J Surg Pathol. 26(12):1620-6, 2002
14. Graadt van Roggen JF et al: Reticular perineurioma: a distinctive variant of soft tissue perineurioma. Am J Surg Pathol. 25(4):485-93, 2001
15. Fetsch JF et al: Sclerosing perineurioma: a clinicopathologic study of 19 cases of a distinctive soft tissue lesion with a predilection for the fingers and palms of young adults. Am J Surg Pathol. 21(12):1433-42, 1997
16. Giannini C et al: Soft-tissue perineurioma. Evidence for an abnormality of chromosome 22, criteria for diagnosis, and review of the literature. Am J Surg Pathol. 21(2):164-73, 1997

Artifactual Cracking

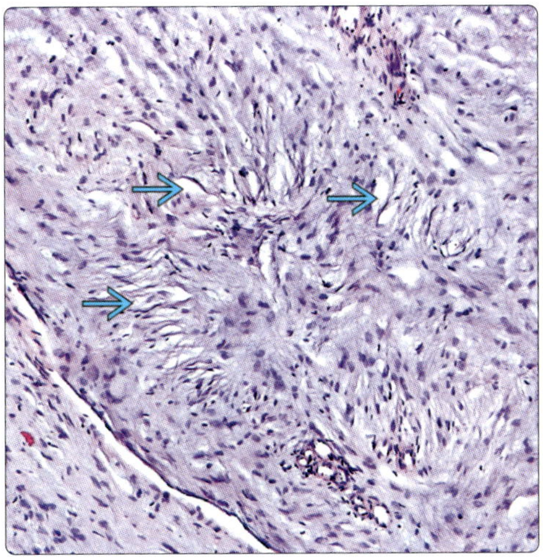

Mixed Elongated and Epithelioid Nuclei

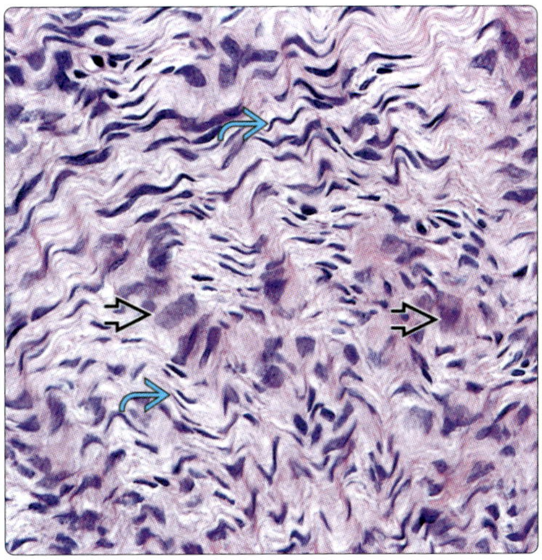

(Left) *Artifactual cracking, or microclefting* → *, of the stroma is not uncommon in perineurioma and may be arranged in a storiform architecture. This finding can be particularly prominent in cases with abundant stromal collagen.* **(Right)** *A useful histologic finding for raising the possibility of perineurioma is the presence of thin, wavy nuclei* ↪ *closely admixed with rounder, pale nuclei* ⇨*.*

Scattered Pleomorphic Nuclei

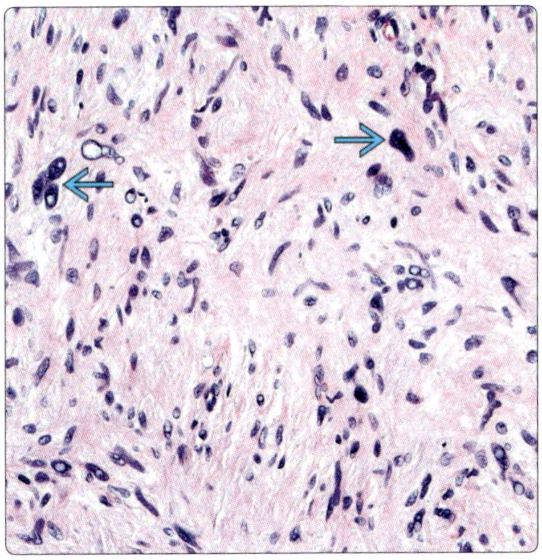

EMA Expression

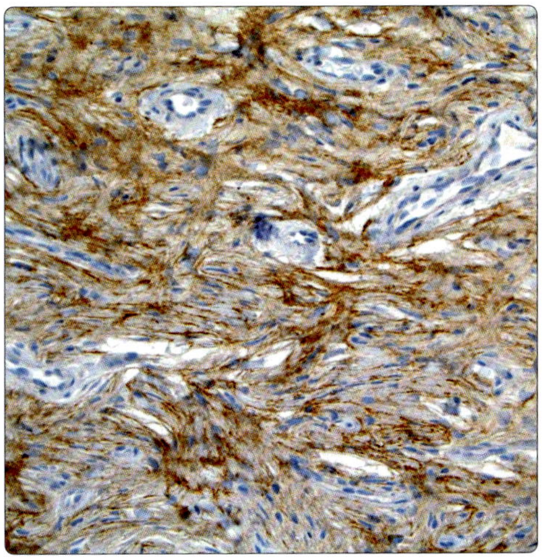

(Left) *Although the vast majority of cases of perineurioma are cytologically banal, rare cases may show scattered pleomorphic nuclei* → *, often with pseudoinclusions. This change is likely degenerative and similar to ancient change seen in schwannoma. Importantly, mitotic figures are rare to absent.* **(Right)** *Epithelial membrane antigen (EMA) expression is present (at least focally) in most cases of perineurioma. However, expression can be weak &/or focal, necessitating careful evaluation.*

Cellular Perineurioma

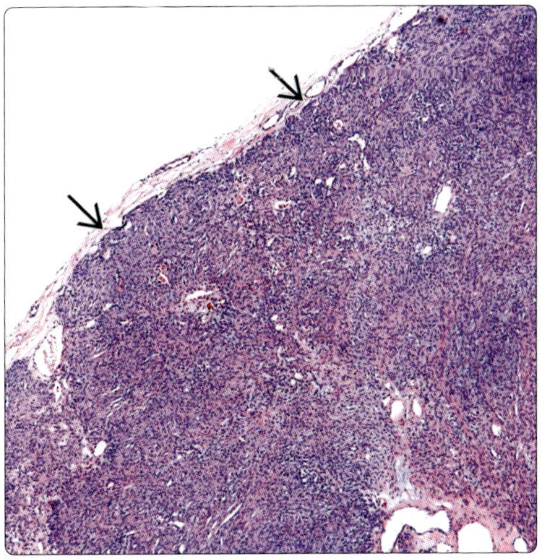

Cellular Perineurioma

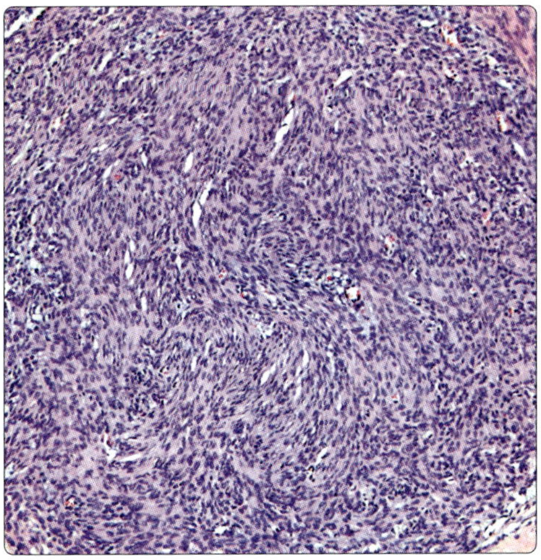

(Left) *Some areas, or cases, of soft tissue perineurioma are quite cellular and may raise differential diagnosis concerns of other neoplasms, including malignancies. Note the sharp circumscription* → *that is characteristic of most examples.* **(Right)** *Storiform, lamellar, and fascicular growth patterns may all be seen in cellular areas of perineurioma. Despite the cellularity, the lesional nuclei of perineurioma are cytologically bland, and mitotic figures are generally rare to absent.*

Nuclear Pseudoinclusions

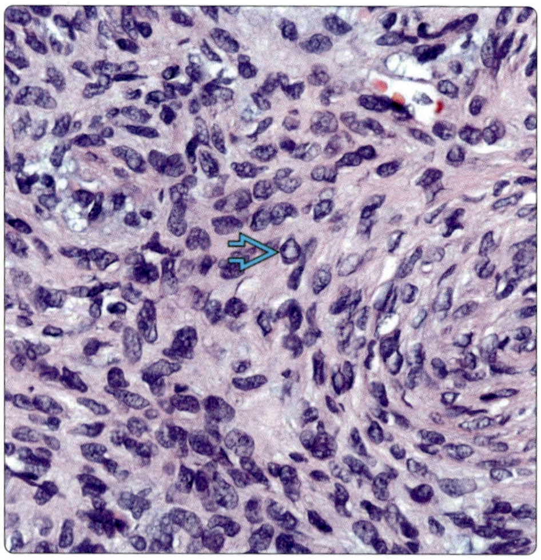

Vague Fascicular Growth

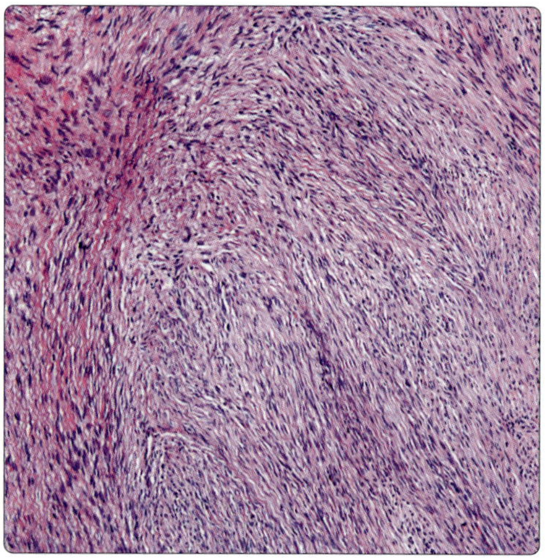

(Left) *Bland nuclear cytology is typical of most cases of perineurioma. Pale to clear nuclear pseudoinclusions ⇨ are also commonly identified.* **(Right)** *This image shows a focal, loose fascicular growth pattern in a soft tissue perineurioma. This pattern may raise considerations of malignant peripheral nerve sheath tumor, synovial sarcoma, or even desmoid fibromatosis.*

Wavy Morphology

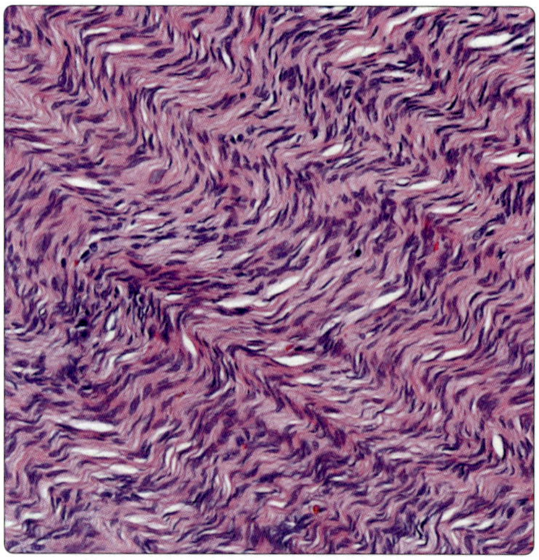

Cellular Whorls

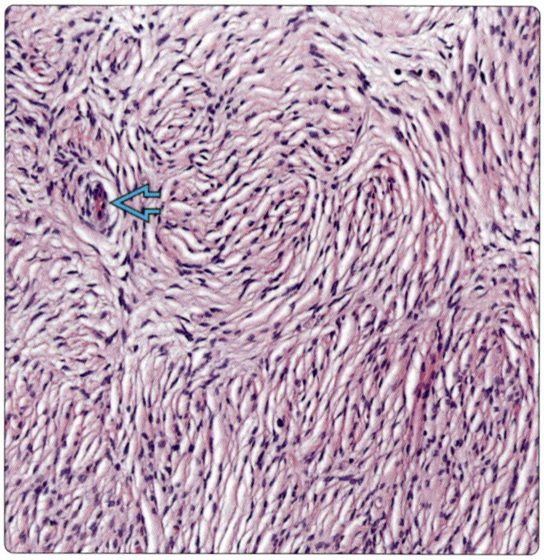

(Left) *Cytologic layering with prominent wavy nuclei is a feature of some cases of perineurioma. This pattern is not unique, however, and can be seen in other neural (and nonneural) tumors.* **(Right)** *Cellular whorls are common features of perineurioma and may be quite diffuse and prominent in some cases. Whorls often arise around small stromal vascular channels ⇨.*

Meningothelial-Like Clusters

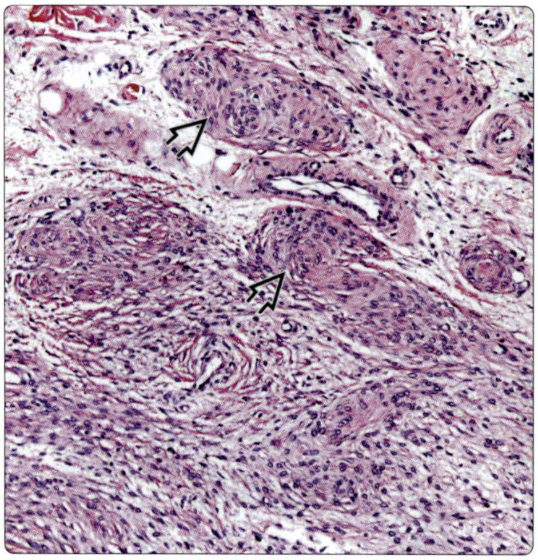

Myxoid Change

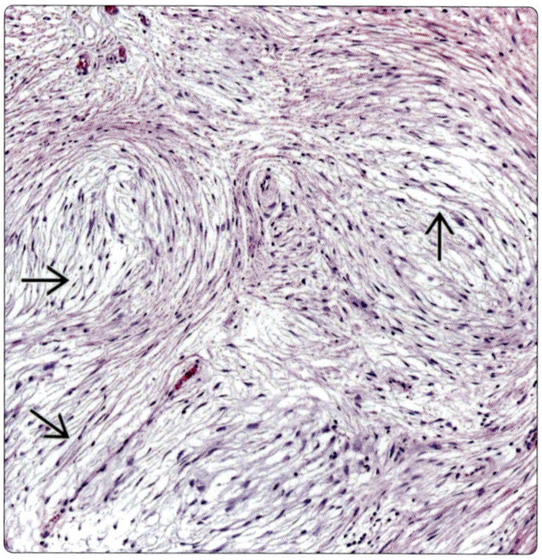

(Left) *Cellular, tightly whorled clusters ⇨ of spindled cells may occasionally be seen in soft tissue perineurioma, somewhat reminiscent of meningioma. Ectopic meningioma tends to occur in locations different from perineurioma, however.* **(Right)** *Myxoid stromal change is not uncommon in perineurioma, but diffusely myxoid tumors are rare. The elongated, fine, cytoplasmic processes of the lesional perineurial cells are nicely evident → in this case.*

Reticular Perineurioma

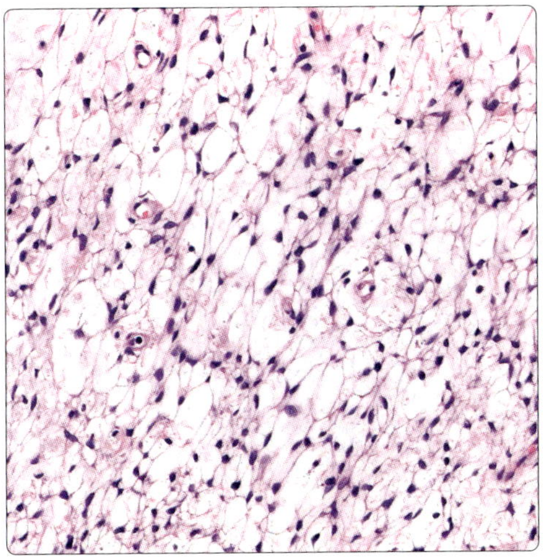

Sclerosing Perineurioma

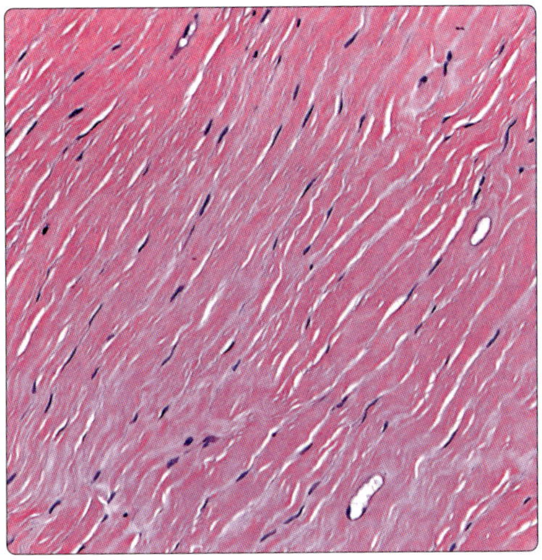

(Left) *Reticular perineurioma is a rare variant of soft tissue perineurioma that is characterized by prominent myxoid stromal changes and lace-like or net-like growth pattern. The neoplastic cells contain very thin and elongated cell processes.* **(Right)** *The sclerosing variant of perineurioma is most common in acral locations and is characterized by an even distribution of abundant stromal collagen. The lesional cells vary from spindled to epithelioid.*

Sclerosing Perineurioma

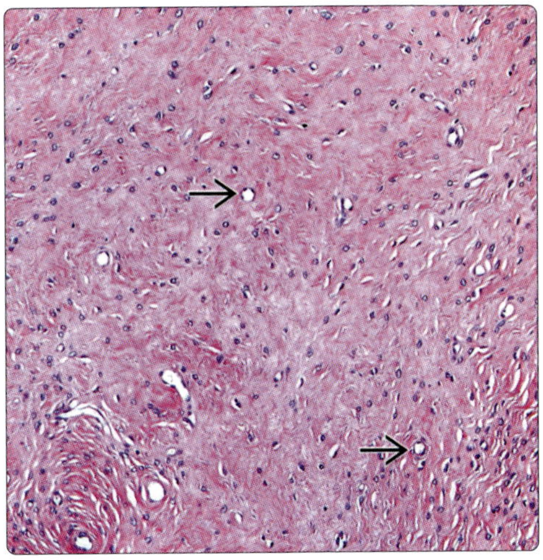

Sclerosing Perineurioma

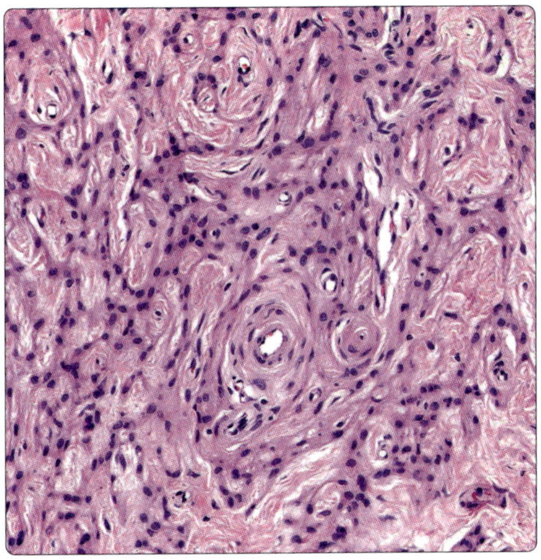

(Left) *This example of sclerosing perineurioma shows scattered lesional cells with round, pale nuclei. Small stromal capillary channels are usually conspicuous in this variant.* **(Right)** *This example of sclerosing perineurioma is composed of rather plump, epithelioid tumor cells set in collagenous, sclerosing stroma. Note the perivascular arrangement of the neoplastic cells.*

Rare Plexiform Perineurioma

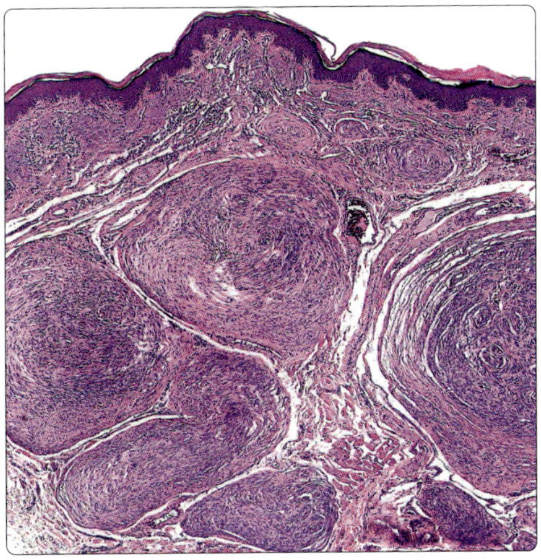

Intraneural Perineurioma

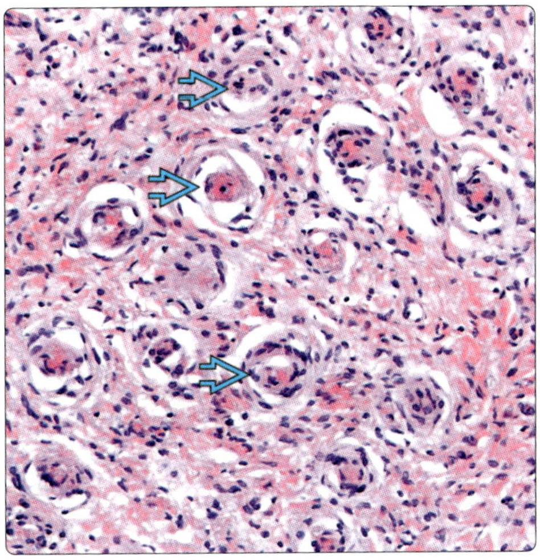

(Left) *Rare cases of plexiform perineurioma have been reported. This case arose on the lower lip of a 60-year-old woman and shows the unique multinodular and serpentine growth pattern.* **(Right)** *The rare intraneural perineurioma usually presents as a fusiform growth within a nerve and is characterized histologically by whorls of perineurial cells around preexisting nerve fibers/axons ("onion bulbs"). These features can only be seen on cross section.*

Hybrid Nerve Sheath Tumor

KEY FACTS

TERMINOLOGY

- Benign composite neoplasm demonstrating morphologic &/or immunohistochemical features of > 1 type of nerve sheath tumor

CLINICAL ISSUES

- Rare, but incidence may be underestimated
- Wide age range
- Wide distribution but most common in extremities
- Most arise in superficial soft tissue, but some are deeply located or visceral
- Slow-growing, often painless mass
- Treatment: Simple surgical excision
- Benign; local recurrence very rare

MACROSCOPIC

- Most < 5 cm in size

MICROSCOPIC

- Usually well circumscribed and unencapsulated
- Morphology depends upon composition
    - Schwannoma, perineurioma, neurofibroma, very rarely others
    - Components may be intimately intermixed or distinct
- Mitoses rare to absent

ANCILLARY TESTS

- S100(+) in Schwann cells
- EMA(+), claudin-1 (+) in perineurial cells

TOP DIFFERENTIAL DIAGNOSES

- Malignant peripheral nerve sheath tumor (low grade)
- Perineurioma
- Schwannoma
- Neurofibroma

(Left) *Hybrid nerve sheath tumors are well circumscribed, unencapsulated, benign neoplasms characterized by mixed features of various nerve sheath tumors. Their incidence is likely underestimated given their morphologic overlap with pure nerve sheath tumors.* **(Right)** *Hybrid perineurioma/schwannoma appears to be the most common hybrid nerve sheath tumor. It often resembles perineurioma architecturally yet contains an admixed Schwann cell component ➔.*

Hybrid Nerve Sheath Tumor

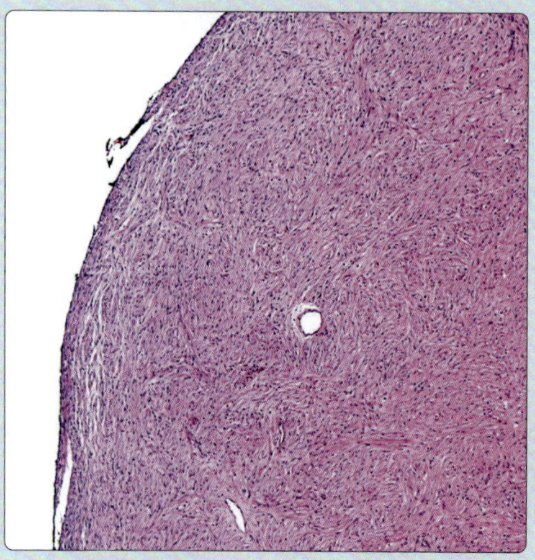

Hybrid Nerve Sheath Tumor

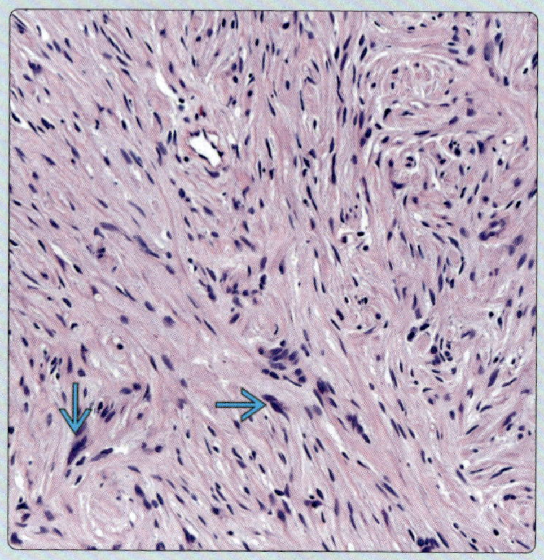

(Left) *S100 protein expression is common in hybrid tumors due to the presence of Schwann cells, as in this example of hybrid perineurioma/schwannoma. Expression is often greater than that of perineurial markers; however, in some cases it is less abundant.* **(Right)** *Claudin-1 (shown) and EMA expression is seen in this case of hybrid perineurioma/schwannoma. Note the Schwann cells in the background that are not staining.*

S100 Protein Expression

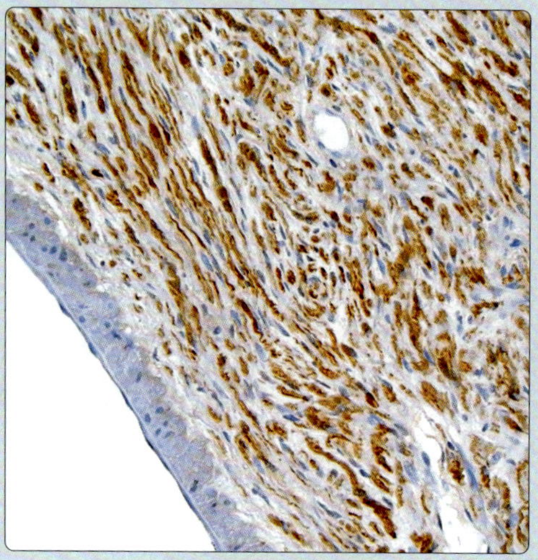

Expression of Perineurial Markers

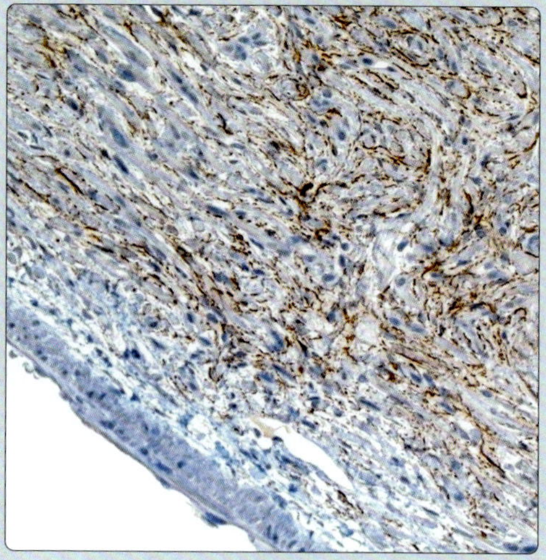

TERMINOLOGY

Definitions

- Benign composite neoplasm demonstrating morphologic &/or immunohistochemical features of > 1 type of nerve sheath tumor
  - Most often schwannoma and perineurioma

CLINICAL ISSUES

Epidemiology

- Incidence
  - Rare
    - However, incidence likely underestimated
- Age
  - Wide range
- Sex
  - No apparent predilection

Site

- Wide distribution but most common in extremities
- Most arise in superficial soft tissue, but some are deeply located or visceral

Presentation

- Slow-growing, often painless mass
- May have clinical features of syndromes, such as neurofibromatosis or schwannomatosis
  - Reports of some cases of hybrid neurofibroma/schwannoma associated with these syndromes

Treatment

- Simple surgical excision

Prognosis

- Benign
- Local recurrence rare

MACROSCOPIC

General Features

- Firm, rubbery mass with tan/white/yellow cut surface

Size

- Most < 5 cm

MICROSCOPIC

Histologic Features

- Usually well circumscribed and unencapsulated
- Morphology depends upon composition
  - Schwannoma/perineurioma (most common)
    - Overall storiform, lamellar, or whorled growth pattern
    - Intimate admixture of spindled Schwann cells with plump nuclei and slender, more inconspicuous perineurial cells with bipolar processes
      - Some cases are composed of discrete areas of one type of nerve sheath tumor within zones of another
    - Variable collagenous or myxoid stroma
    - Degenerative nuclear atypia ("ancient change") &/or multinucleation may be seen
  - Schwannoma/neurofibroma
    - Nodules or zones of typical Antoni A schwannoma within larger zones of neurofibroma
    - May appear plexiform
  - Neurofibroma/perineurioma, granular cell tumor/perineurioma, and perineurioma/cellular neurothekeoma also described
- Mitoses rare to absent
- No coagulative necrosis

ANCILLARY TESTS

Immunohistochemistry

- S100(+) in Schwann cells
- EMA(+), claudin-1 (+), GLUT-1(+) in perineurial cells
- CD34(+) in perineurial cells and fibroblasts (neurofibroma)

DIFFERENTIAL DIAGNOSIS

Malignant Peripheral Nerve Sheath Tumor (Low Grade)

- Areas of increased cellularity with mitotic activity common
- Nuclear atypia that is not degenerative
- Usually EMA(-), claudin-1 (-)

Perineurioma

- Can appear very similar to hybrid perineurioma/schwannoma
- Purely composed of perineurial cells
- EMA(+), claudin-1 (+), CD34 (variable), S100 protein (-)

Schwannoma

- Most are encapsulated
- Most show classic Antoni A and B zonation
  - Also Verocay bodies
- Diffuse S100 protein (+), EMA(-), claudin (-), CD34(-)

Neurofibroma

- Mixture of Schwann cells, fibroblasts, perineurial cells, and variable axons
  - Perineurial component usually minor
- S100 protein (+) but less so than typical schwannoma

SELECTED REFERENCES

1. Ud Din N et al: Hybrid peripheral nerve sheath tumors: report of five cases and detailed review of literature. BMC Cancer. 17(1):349, 2017
2. Kacerovska D et al: Hybrid epithelioid schwannoma/perineurioma. Am J Dermatopathol. 38(7):e90-2, 2016
3. Linos K et al: Benign cutaneous biphasic hybrid tumor of perineurioma and cellular neurothekeoma: a case report expanding the clinical and histopathologic features of a recently described entity. Am J Dermatopathol. 37(4):319-22, 2015
4. Fletcher C et al: WHO Classification of Tumours of Soft Tissue and Bone. Lyon: IARC Press, 2013
5. Kacerovska D et al: Hybrid peripheral nerve sheath tumors, including a malignant variant in type 1 neurofibromatosis. Am J Dermatopathol. 35(6):641-9, 2013
6. Harder A et al: Hybrid neurofibroma/schwannoma is overrepresented among schwannomatosis and neurofibromatosis patients. Am J Surg Pathol. 36(5):702-9, 2012
7. Pusiol T et al: Routine use of immunohisto-chemistry may increase the frequency of hybrid peripheral nerve sheath tumors. Am J Dermatopathol. 33(6):634-6, 2011
8. Hornick JL et al: Hybrid schwannoma/perineurioma: clinicopathologic analysis of 42 distinctive benign nerve sheath tumors. Am J Surg Pathol. 33(10):1554-61, 2009
9. Kazakov DV et al: Hybrid peripheral nerve sheath tumors: schwannoma-perineurioma and neurofibroma-perineurioma. A report of three cases in extradigital locations. Ann Diagn Pathol. 9(1):16-23, 2005

(Left) *The stroma in hybrid nerve sheath tumors varies from collagenous to myxoid. Hybrid schwannoma/perineurioma often contains areas of prominent collagenization ➲, as shown.* **(Right)** *This hybrid nerve sheath tumor showed conspicuous collagen fibers, such as those often seen in neurofibroma. Immunohistochemically, however, EMA and claudin-1 stained the majority of the cells, and a subpopulation expressed S100 protein.*

Stromal Collagen

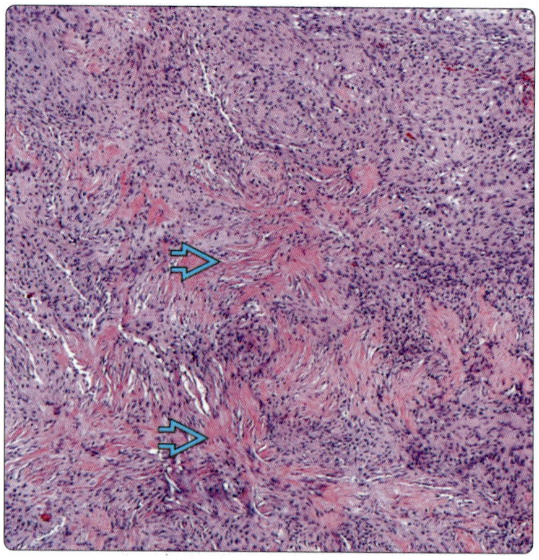

Collagen Fibers

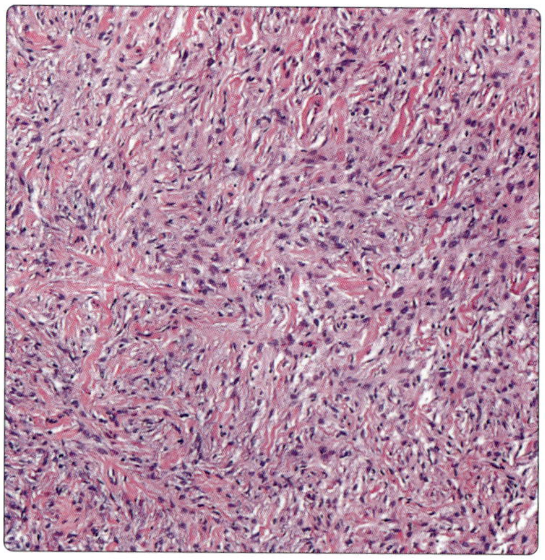

(Left) *Prominent collagen fibers are displayed in this focus of hybrid nerve sheath tumor. Note the appearance of "cracking" due to the presence of slender perineurial cells between the fibers. Immunostains for EMA &/or claudin-1 can highlight these cells.* **(Right)** *Some cases of hybrid nerve sheath tumor are extensively myxoid and may histologically and clinically mimic a myxoma. Stromal collagen ➲, however, is more frequent in hybrid tumors.*

Neurofibroma-Like Appearance

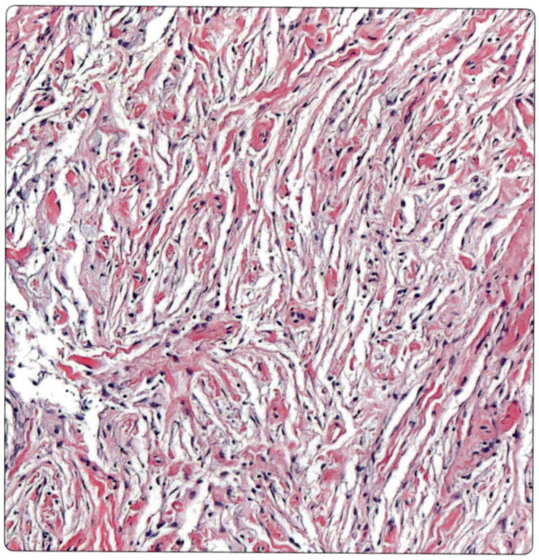

Myxocollagenous Stroma

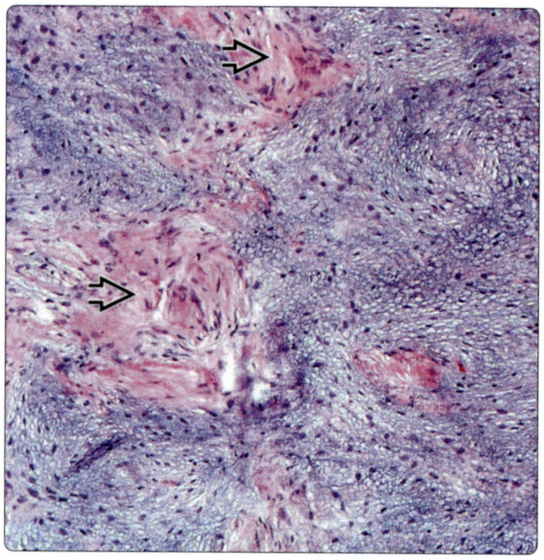

(Left) *This example of a hybrid nerve sheath tumor demonstrates diffuse myxoid stromal change. There is minimal to no cytologic atypia, and there are no mitotic figures or necrosis.* **(Right)** *Areas of hybrid nerve sheath tumor may resemble myxoid neurofibroma, particularly when discrete collagen fibers are present, as depicted in this image.*

Diffuse Myxoid Stroma

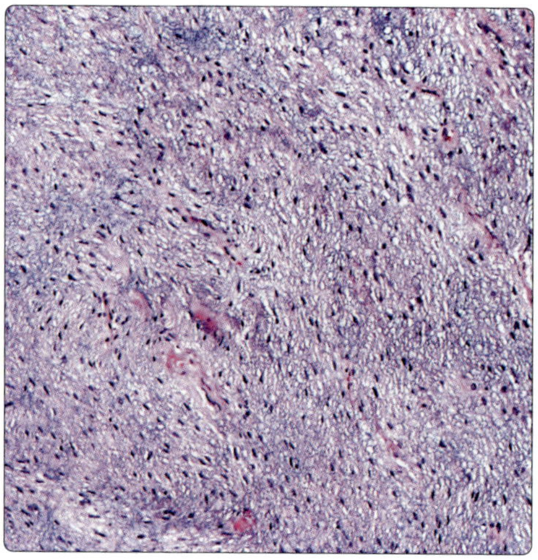

Neurofibroma-Like Areas

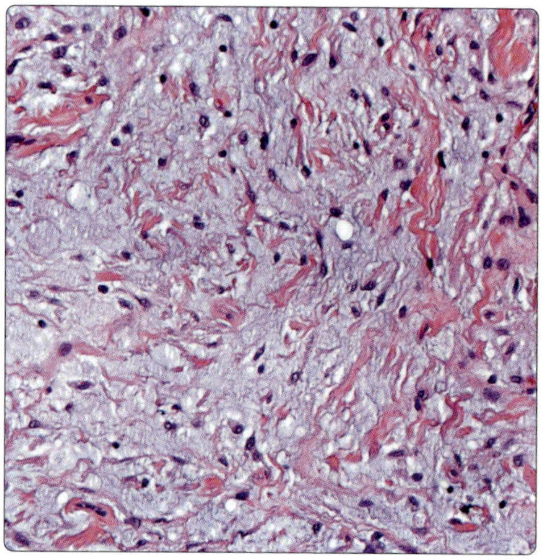

Corded S100 Expression Pattern

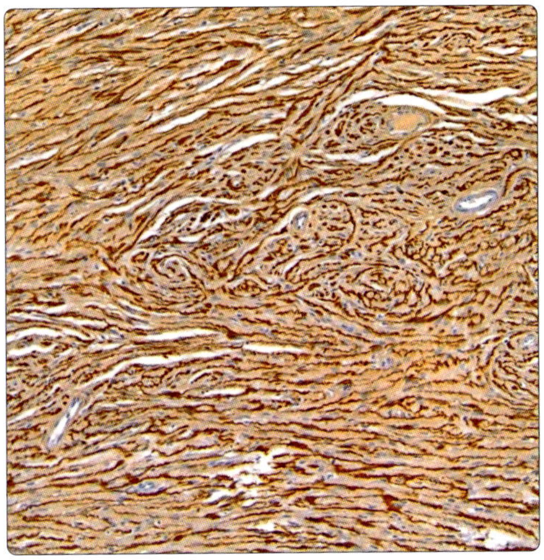

Minor S100 Protein Expression

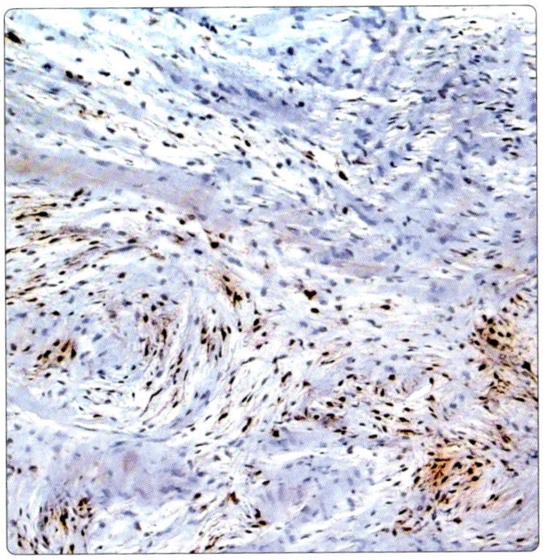

(Left) *A cord-like pattern of S100 protein expression may be seen in hybrid perineurioma/schwannoma due to alternating rows and thin layers of Schwann cells and perineurial cells. A dual chromogen S100/EMA cocktail (not shown) can nicely demonstrate the 2 distinct populations of cells.* **(Right)** *Although it often appears to stain the majority of the cells in hybrid nerve sheath tumor, S100 protein may only be expressed in the minority of cells, as was seen in this case.*

Rare Nodular/Plexiform Growth

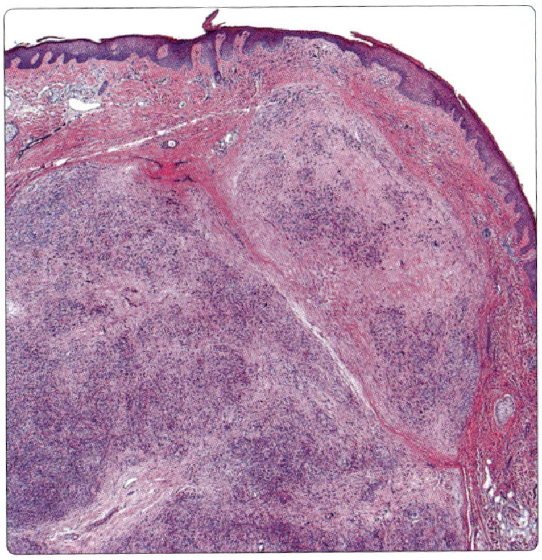

Degenerative Atypia

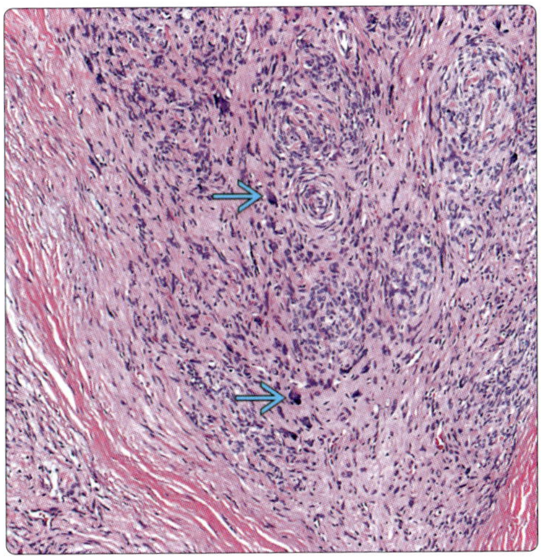

(Left) *This case of superficial hybrid nerve sheath tumor grew in a conspicuous multinodular/plexiform pattern. Other findings included focal multinucleated tumor cells and metaplastic bone (not shown).* **(Right)** *Degenerative nuclear atypia ("ancient change") and multinucleated tumor cells ➔ may be seen in some cases of hybrid nerve sheath tumor, similar to pure nerve sheath tumors. Mitoses are very rare to absent.*

Cellularity

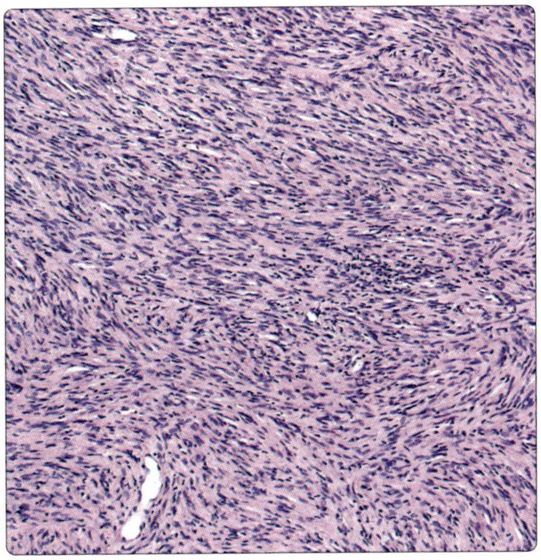

Hybrid Schwannoma/Neurofibroma

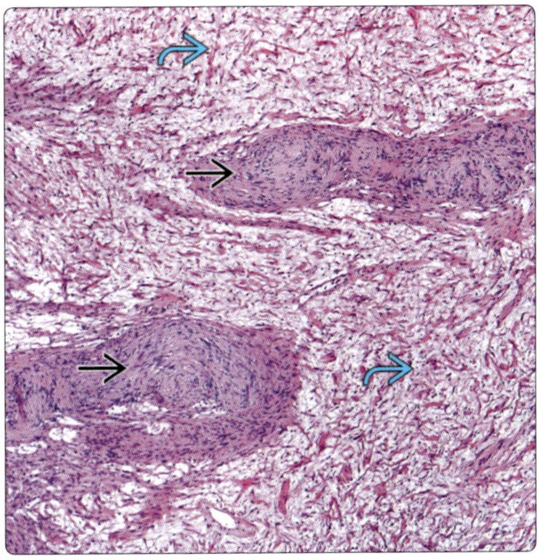

(Left) *Schwannian areas in hybrid nerve sheath tumor may show increased cellularity, similar to cellular schwannomas. A minor component of perineurial cells is often present too, though they are difficult to see without immunostains.* **(Right)** *This tumor had features of schwannoma ➔ and neurofibroma ➔ with a nodular architecture reminiscent of a plexiform growth pattern. Of note, some of these particular tumors may be associated with neurofibromatosis or schwannomatosis.*

Granular Cell Tumor

KEY FACTS

TERMINOLOGY

- Benign tumor of putative schwannian origin composed of cells with abundant granular cytoplasm

CLINICAL ISSUES

- Wide age range (peak: 40-60 years)
  - Female predilection
  - More prevalent in African Americans
- Wide anatomic distribution, usually arises in skin and subcutaneous tissue
  - Head and neck region common (particularly tongue and oral cavity)
- Usually solitary, slowly growing, painless nodule, plaque, or mass
  - Multicentricity in 10% of cases
- Treatment: Complete surgical excision
- Overall excellent prognosis for benign lesions
- Malignant granular cell tumor (GrCT) (rare) metastasizes in up to 50% of cases

MACROSCOPIC

- Usually small (mean: 1-2 cm)

MICROSCOPIC

- Nonencapsulated, usually with irregular borders
- Overlying pseudoepitheliomatous hyperplasia in 30%
- Sheets, nests, and cords of plump, polygonal cells with abundant eosinophilic granular cytoplasm
- Typically prominent collagenous stroma
- Malignant GrCT shows ≥ 3 atypical features (pleomorphism, prominent nucleoli, increased mitoses, etc.)

ANCILLARY TESTS

- PAS(+), diastase-resistant cytoplasmic granules
- Strong, diffuse S100 protein (+), SOX10(+)

TOP DIFFERENTIAL DIAGNOSES

- Congenital granular cell epulis
- Nonneural GrCT

(Left) *Granular cell tumor (GrCT) is a benign tumor of putative Schwann cell origin that occurs at a variety of anatomic sites but shows a predilection for the head and neck region, particularly the tongue and oral cavity. Most cases are dermal or subcutaneous, and some may extend directly up under the overlying epidermis.* **(Right)** *This tumor is composed of sheets, nests, and cords of plump, polygonal cells with abundant eosinophilic granular cytoplasm within a collagenous stroma.*

Granular Cell Tumor

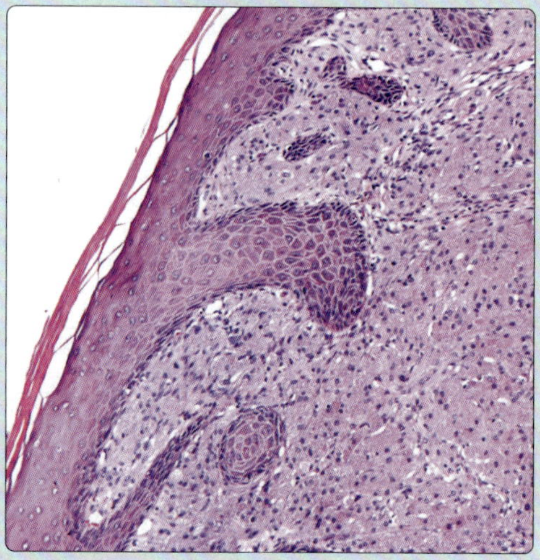

Granular Cell Tumor

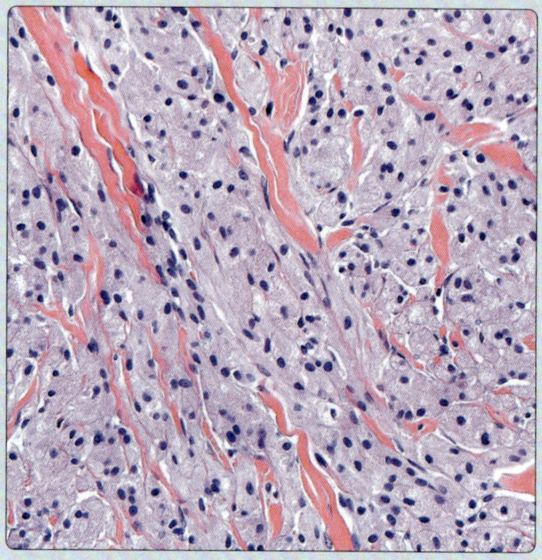

(Left) *Cytologically, the cells of GrCT show prominent granular cytoplasm, which represents numerous lysosomal structures. Nuclei are generally small and may be dark with dense chromatin or vesicular with a small nucleolus. Occasional scattered larger nuclei and nucleoli may be seen in otherwise benign GrCT.* **(Right)** *Strong, diffuse S100 protein expression is characteristic of GrCT and can help to distinguish it from most entities in its differential diagnosis.*

Cytologic Features

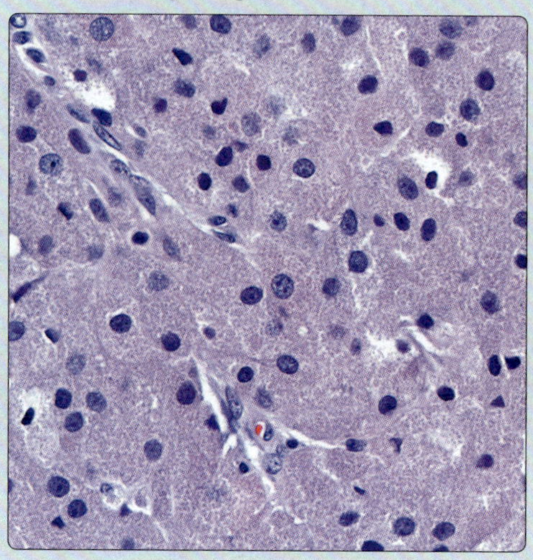

S100 Protein Expression

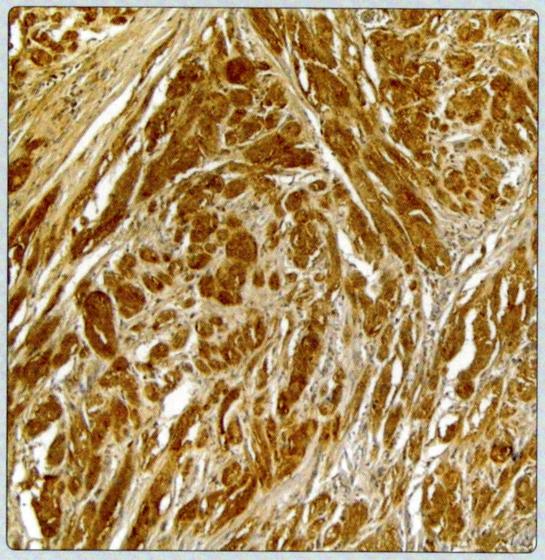

TERMINOLOGY

Abbreviations

- Granular cell tumor (GrCT)

Synonyms

- Granular cell myoblastoma
- Abrikossoff tumor
- Granular cell schwannoma

Definitions

- Benign tumor of putative schwannian origin composed of cells with abundant granular cytoplasm

CLINICAL ISSUES

Epidemiology

- Incidence
  - Benign GrCT not uncommon
    - Malignant GrCT rare
- Age
  - Any (peak: 40-60 years)
- Sex
  - Male predilection
    - Malignant GrCT more frequent in females
- Ethnicity
  - More prevalent in African Americans

Site

- Wide distribution, usually arises in skin and subcutaneous tissue
  - Rarely in deep soft tissue sites
- Head and neck region common
  - Particularly tongue and oral cavity
- Also breast, bronchus, larynx, neurohypophysis, other viscera
- Rarely in nerve, lymph node

Presentation

- Usually solitary, slowly growing, painless nodule, plaque, or mass
  - Multicentric in ~ 10% of cases
    - May appear synchronously or metachronously
    - May rarely arise in association with Noonan syndrome or LEOPARD syndrome
- Oral cavity/tongue lesions may show concurrent candidiasis

Treatment

- Complete surgical excision

Prognosis

- Overall excellent prognosis for benign lesions
  - Local recurrence < 10% of cases
- Multicentric tumors usually benign
- Malignant GrCT
  - Up to 30% recur
  - Up to 50% metastasize
  - Adverse prognostic factors
    - Local recurrence, metastasis
    - Tumor size (> 5 cm), older patient age (> 50 years)

MACROSCOPIC

General Features

- Cutaneous lesions may show hyperplastic/verrucous appearance
- Cut surface firm, pale yellow, or cream colored

Size

- Usually small (mean: 1-2 cm)
  - Deep lesions often larger (5-6 cm)

MICROSCOPIC

Histologic Features

- Nonencapsulated, usually with irregular borders
  - May appear to infiltrate adjacent tissues (dermal collagen, adipose tissue, skeletal muscle)
    - Tumor cells often appear to entrap small nerves
  - Can extend directly up to surface epithelium
    - May incite overlying pseudoepitheliomatous hyperplasia (30% of cases)
      - Can mimic invasive squamous cell carcinoma in superficial biopsies
  - Rare plexiform growth pattern in dermis
- Sheets, nests, and cords of plump, polygonal cells
  - Abundant granular, eosinophilic cytoplasm
    - Enlarged, denser granules with halos (phagolysosomes) frequent
    - Cell membrane often indistinct; appears syncytial
  - Central small nuclei with variable dense to vesicular nuclei
    - Small, subtle nucleoli may be present
    - Mitoses absent
- Typically prominent collagenous stroma
  - May be fibrotic or desmoplastic in longstanding lesions
- Intratumoral lymphoid aggregates in some cases
- Necrosis absent
- Atypical features
  - Pleomorphism, prominent nucleoli, high nuclear:cytoplasmic ratio, spindling of cells
    - Should be prominent in tumor, not focal
  - Mitoses > 2 per 10 HPF
  - Necrosis
- Malignant GrCT shows ≥ 3 atypical features
  - Tumors with 1 or 2 prominent atypical features may be regarded as atypical GrCT

ANCILLARY TESTS

Histochemistry

- PAS(+), diastase-resistant cytoplasmic granules
  - Diffuse, chunky staining

Immunohistochemistry

- Strong, diffuse S100 protein (+) and nuclear SOX10(+)
- Calretinin (+), CD68(+), inhibin (+), nestin (+), MITF (+)
- Nuclear TFE3(+) in majority of cases
- Type IV collagen (+) around nests of cells
- SMA(-), desmin (-), myogenin (-), ALK(-), GFAP(-), HMB-45(-), neurofilament (-)

DIFFERENTIAL DIAGNOSIS

Congenital Granular Cell Epulis

- Can be histologically indistinguishable from GrCT
- Arises in gingiva of newborns (congenital)
- S100 protein and SOX10 (-)

Nonneural Granular Cell Tumor (Primitive Polypoid Granular Cell Tumor)

- Cutaneous lesion, often polypoid with epidermal collarette
- Sheet-like growth of spindled to epithelioid cells with abundant granular, eosinophilic cytoplasm
- Variable nuclear atypia and mitotic activity
- ALK (+); S100 protein and SOX10 (-)

Hibernoma

- Sheets and lobules of multivacuolated brown fat cells
  - Often contains areas of white fat cells
- Most common in subcutis (not cutaneous)
- Cells lack intracytoplasmic phagolysosomes

Malignant Melanoma

- Junctional component usually present
- Melanin pigment in some cases
- Granular cell change rare
- HMB-45(+), MART-1(+) in most cases

Granular Cell Dermatofibroma (Fibrous Histiocytoma)

- Other typical features of dermatofibroma
- Lacks prominent overlying pseudoepitheliomatous hyperplasia
- S100 protein (-)

Reactive Granular Cell Change

- Collections of granular histiocytes
- Occurs at sites of trauma or prior surgical procedures
- Lack diffuse S100 protein expression

Leiomyoma

- Rare granular cell change
- Areas of conventional smooth muscle cytology
- SMA(+) and desmin (+)
- S100 protein (-)

Alveolar Soft Part Sarcoma

- Deep, usually large mass
- Compartmentalized growth; pseudoalveolar pattern common
- Rare granular cell change
- Majority of cases show PAS(+), diastase resistant intracytoplasmic rod-like crystals
- S100 protein, SOX10, and nestin (-)
- Nuclear TFE3(+), like GrCT

Adult-Type Rhabdomyoma

- Sheets of polygonal cells with homogeneous, eosinophilic cytoplasm
- Desmin (+), myogenin (+)
- S100 protein (-)

SELECTED REFERENCES

1. Cohen JN et al: Cutaneous non-neural granular cell tumors harbor recurrent ALK gene fusions. Am J Surg Pathol. 42(9):1133-42, 2018
2. Mirza FN et al: Epidemiology of malignant cutaneous granular cell tumors: a US population-based cohort analysis using the Surveillance, Epidemiology, and End Results (SEER) database. J Am Acad Dermatol. 78(3):490-7.e1, 2018
3. Tsukamoto S et al: Malignant granular cell tumor of the median nerve: a case report with a literature review of 157 cases. Skeletal Radiol. 48(2): 307-16, 2018
4. Fernandez-Flores A et al: Cutaneous dermal non-neural granular cell tumor is a granular cell dermal root sheath fibroma. J Cutan Pathol. 44(6):582-7, 2017
5. Stemm M et al: Typical and atypical granular cell tumors of soft tissue: a clinicopathologic study of 50 patients. Am J Clin Pathol. 148(2):161-6, 2017
6. Battistella M et al: Vascular invasion and other invasive features in granular cell tumours of the skin: a multicentre study of 119 cases. J Clin Pathol. 67(1):19-25, 2014
7. Chamberlain BK et al: Alveolar soft part sarcoma and granular cell tumor: an immunohistochemical comparison study. Hum Pathol. 45(5):1039-44, 2014
8. Gomes CC et al: Evidence for loss of heterozygosity (LOH) at chromosomes 9p and 17p in oral granular cell tumors: a pilot study. Oral Surg Oral Med Oral Pathol Oral Radiol. 115(2):249-53, 2013
9. Izquierdo F et al: Perineurial cells in granular cell tumors and neoplasms with perineural invasion: an immunohistochemical study. Am J Dermatopathol. 34(8):800-9, 2012
10. Covington MF et al: Pituicytoma, spindle cell oncocytoma, and granular cell tumor: clarification and meta-analysis of the world literature since 1893. AJNR Am J Neuroradiol. 32(11):2067-72, 2011
11. Nasser H et al: Malignant granular cell tumor: a look into the diagnostic criteria. Pathol Res Pract. 207(3):164-8, 2011
12. Papalas JA et al: Recurrence risk and margin status in granular cell tumors of the breast: a clinicopathologic study of 13 patients. Arch Pathol Lab Med. 135(7):890-5, 2011
13. Rejas RA et al: The neural histogenetic origin of the oral granular cell tumor: an immunohistochemical evidence. Med Oral Patol Oral Cir Bucal. 16(1):e6-10, 2011
14. Shintaku M: Immunohistochemical localization of autophagosomal membrane-associated protein LC3 in granular cell tumor and schwannoma. Virchows Arch. 459(3):315-9, 2011
15. Papalas JA et al: Isolated and synchronous vulvar granular cell tumors: a clinicopathologic study of 17 cases in 13 patients. Int J Gynecol Pathol. 29(2):173-80, 2010
16. Aldabagh B et al: Plexiform pattern in cutaneous granular cell tumors. J Cutan Pathol. 36(11):1174-6, 2009
17. Rose B et al: Granular cell tumours: a rare entity in the musculoskeletal system. Sarcoma. 2009:765927, 2009
18. Vered M et al: Granular cell tumor of the oral cavity: updated immunohistochemical profile. J Oral Pathol Med. 38(1):150-9, 2009
19. Bhattacharyya I et al: Granular cell leiomyoma of the oral cavity. Oral Surg Oral Med Oral Pathol Oral Radiol Endod. 102(3):353-9, 2006
20. Zarovnaya E et al: Distinguishing pseudoepitheliomatous hyperplasia from squamous cell carcinoma in mucosal biopsy specimens from the head and neck. Arch Pathol Lab Med. 129(8):1032-6, 2005
21. Chrysomali E et al: Immunohistochemical evaluation of cell proliferation antigen Ki-67 and apoptosis-related proteins Bcl-2 and caspase-3 in oral granular cell tumor. Oral Surg Oral Med Oral Pathol Oral Radiol Endod. 96(5):566-72, 2003
22. Becelli R et al: Abrikossoff's tumor. J Craniofac Surg. 12(1):78-81, 2001
23. Philipp K et al: Eagle syndrome produced by a granular cell tumor. Arch Otolaryngol Head Neck Surg. 127(12):1499-501, 2001
24. van der Meij EH et al: Granular cells in oral lichen planus. Oral Dis. 7(2):116-8, 2001
25. Fanburg-Smith JC et al: Malignant granular cell tumor of soft tissue: diagnostic criteria and clinicopathologic correlation. Am J Surg Pathol. 22(7):779-94, 1998
26. Junquera LM et al: Granular-cell tumours: an immunohistochemical study. Br J Oral Maxillofac Surg. 35(3):180-4, 1997
27. Collins BM et al: Multiple granular cell tumors of the oral cavity: report of a case and review of the literature. J Oral Maxillofac Surg. 53(6):707-11, 1995
28. Gordon AB et al: Granular cell tumour of the breast. Eur J Surg Oncol. 11(3):269-73, 1985

Large Intracytoplasmic Granules

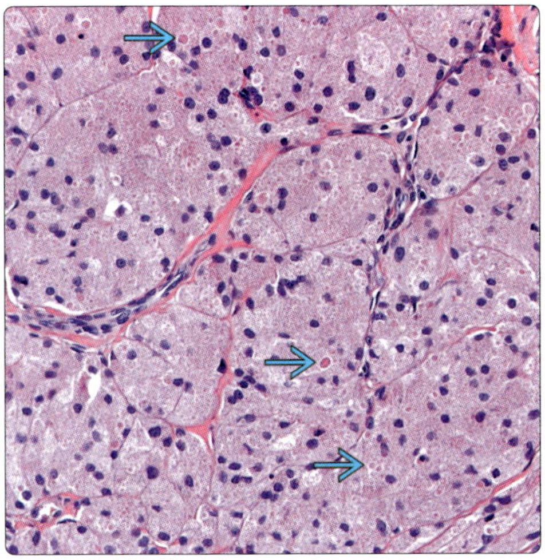

Large Intracytoplasmic Granules

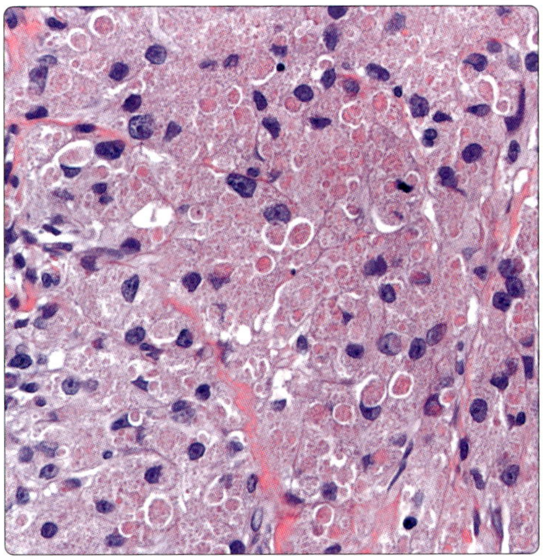

(Left) *A frequent finding in GrCT is the presence of distinctive large granular structures* ➡ *(large lysosomal aggregates) that appear more densely eosinophilic and often show a surrounding clear halo.* **(Right)** *Large intracytoplasmic granular structures are common in GrCT but vary widely in number from case to case. In some tumors, they are abundant.*

Prominent Eosinophilia

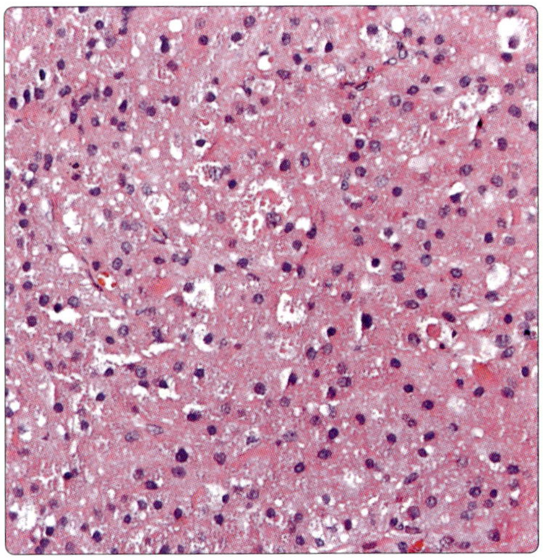

Pale Granular Cells

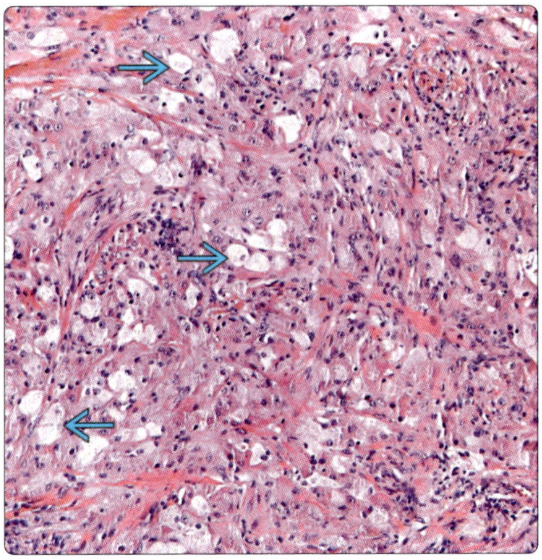

(Left) *Some cases of GrCT show markedly granular and intensely eosinophilic cytoplasm. Note the lack of clear cytoplasmic borders, imparting a syncytial appearance. This lesion arose within the breast parenchyma of a middle-aged woman.* **(Right)** *Occasional cases of GrCT contain scattered tumor cells* ➡ *with pale cytoplasm.*

Entrapped Nerve Fibers

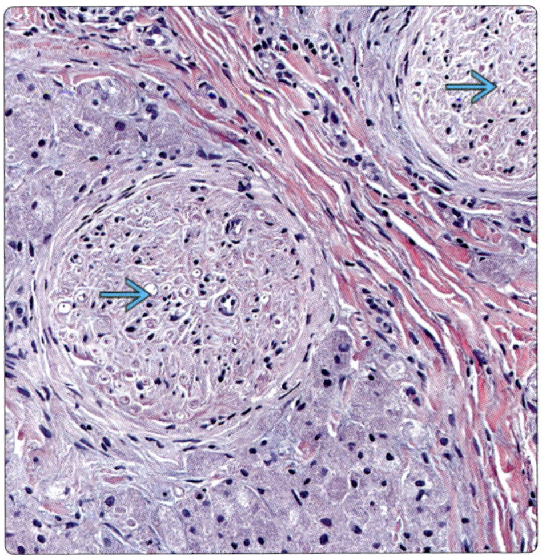

Entrapped Nerve Fibers

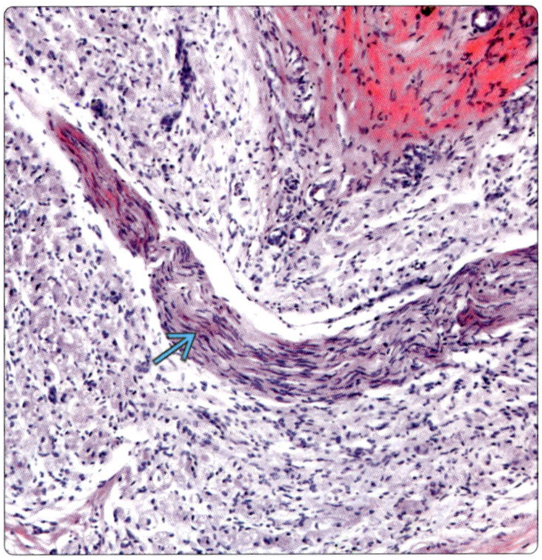

(Left) *In keeping with the likely schwannian origin of this lesion, entrapped nerve fibers* ➡ *are commonly identified in GrCT, both within the tumor and around the periphery. However, to the unwary, this finding may suggest perineural invasion by a malignant process.* **(Right)** *This image of GrCT shows almost complete entrapment of a nerve fiber* ➡ *by lesional tumor cells.*

(Left) *In ~ 1/3 of cases of cutaneous GrCT, the overlying squamous epithelium shows marked hyperplasia and may very closely simulate the appearance of an invasive well-differentiated squamous cell carcinoma. Detection of the GrCT component is critical on a superficial biopsy.* **(Right)** *Note the irregular, small nests of keratinizing squamous epithelial cells* → *that, out of the context of GrCT, would be highly suspicious for invasive carcinoma.*

Pseudoepitheliomatous Hyperplasia

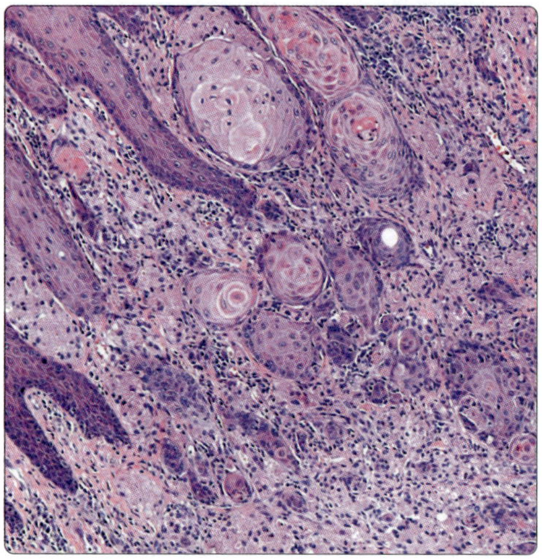

Pseudoepitheliomatous Hyperplasia

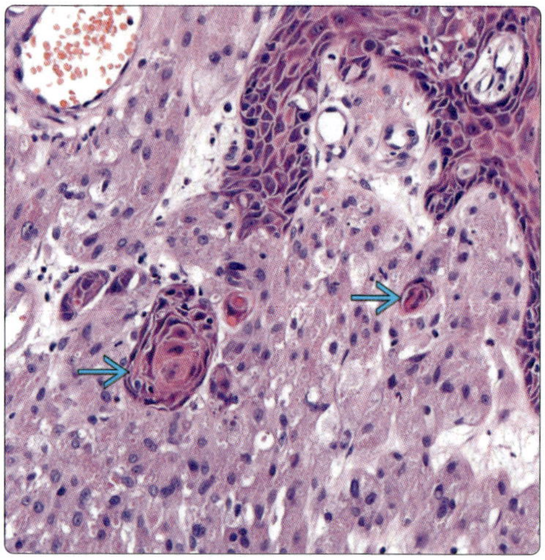

(Left) *Occasional cases of GrCT may show surface ulceration and inflammation and may obscure the actual diagnosis. Note the subtle eosinophilic granular cells* → *underlying the ulceration.* **(Right)** *Some cases of dermal GrCT can show a multinodular growth pattern with satellite nodules. Rarely, an apparent plexiform pattern is seen (shown).*

Surface Ulceration

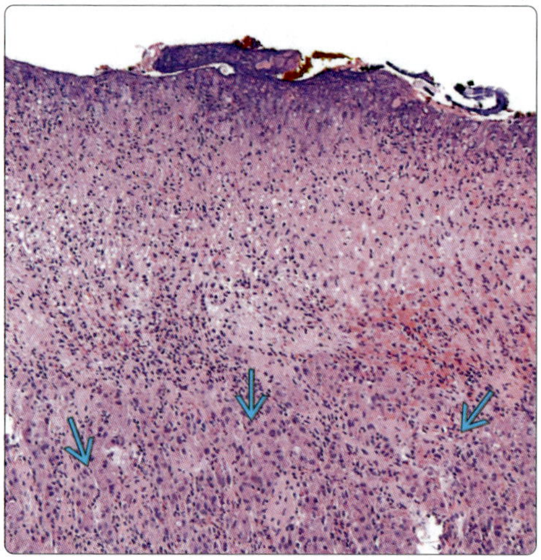

Rare Plexiform Growth

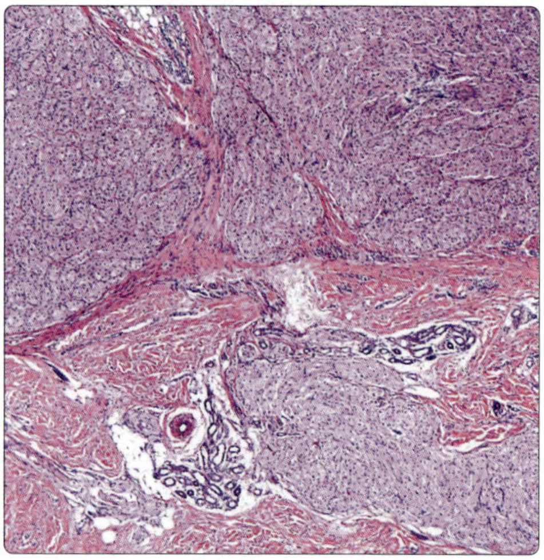

(Left) *Most cases of GrCT are characterized by an ill-defined proliferation of tumor cells that appear to infiltrate adjacent tissues, including dermal collagen, adipose tissue, and skeletal muscle (shown). This finding should not be equated with malignancy.* **(Right)** *Scattered intratumoral lymphoid aggregates may be seen in occasional cases of GrCT, similar to what is seen in some examples of schwannoma.*

Infiltrative Appearance

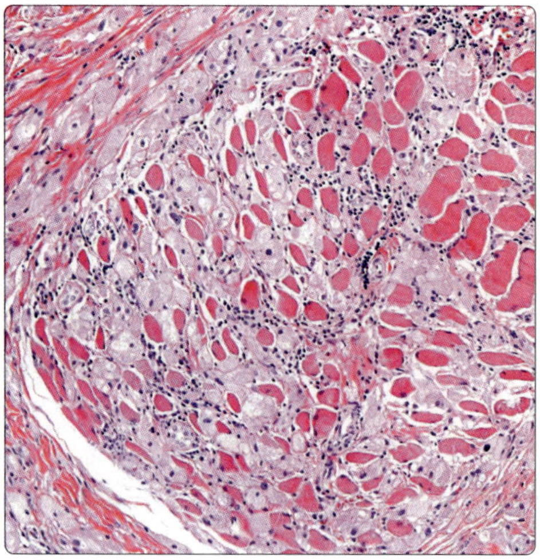

Intratumoral Lymphoid Aggregates

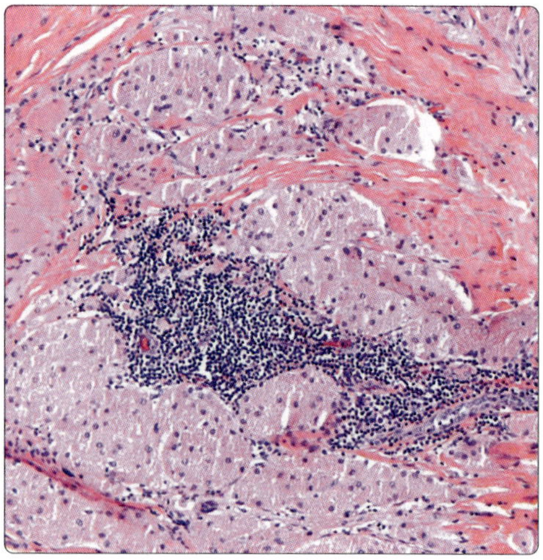

Longstanding Lesions

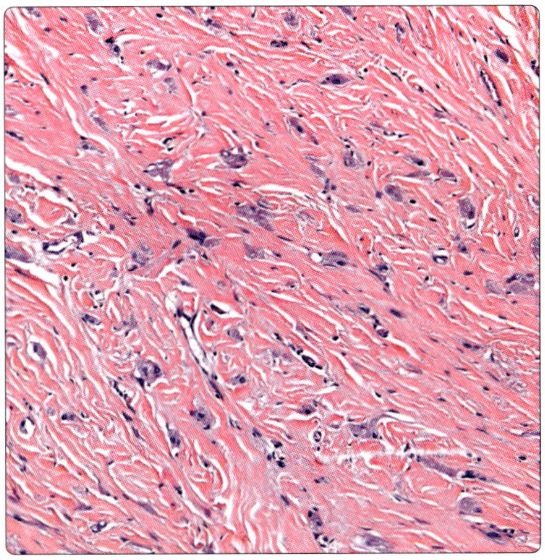

Longstanding Lesions

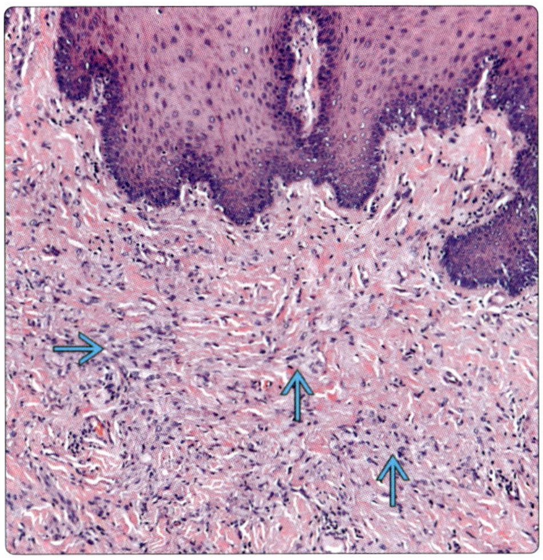

(Left) *The stroma in GrCT is characterized in most cases by prominent, dense collagen. In older lesions, this stroma may appear even more collagenous, fibrotic, or even desmoplastic, and lesional cells may be identified singly &/or in scattered small aggregates or cords.* **(Right)** *Longstanding cases of GrCT may show subtle diagnostic findings that are easily overlooked. This image shows a subtle tumor cell infiltrate → without the classic overlying marked epidermal changes.*

Degenerative Atypia

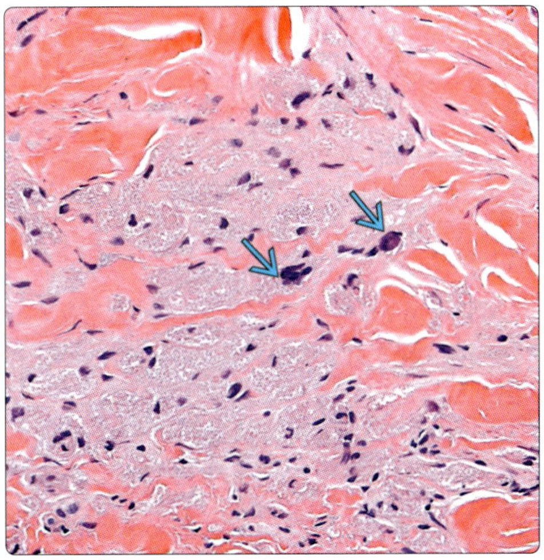

Focal Cellular Spindling

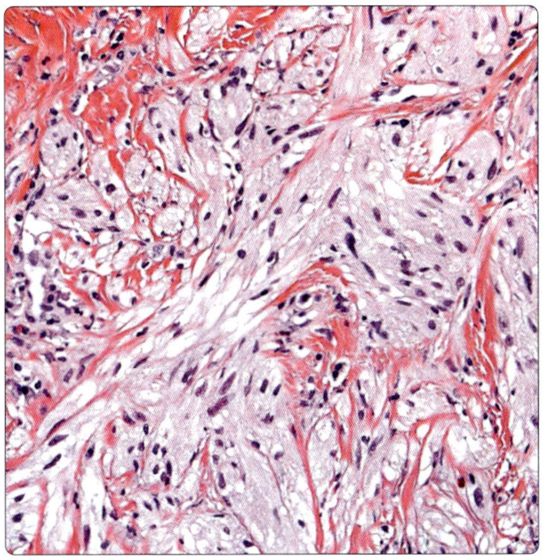

(Left) *Degenerative nuclear atypia → may be seen in occasional cases of GrCT and is rarely prominent. This finding is similar to what is seen in other nerve sheath tumors.* **(Right)** *Although most cases of GrCT are composed of polygonal tumor cells, occasional tumors show focal cellular spindling. This finding, when focal and in isolation, is of no prognostic significance. Of note, spindling is not uncommon in GI tract GrCT.*

Malignant Granular Cell Tumor

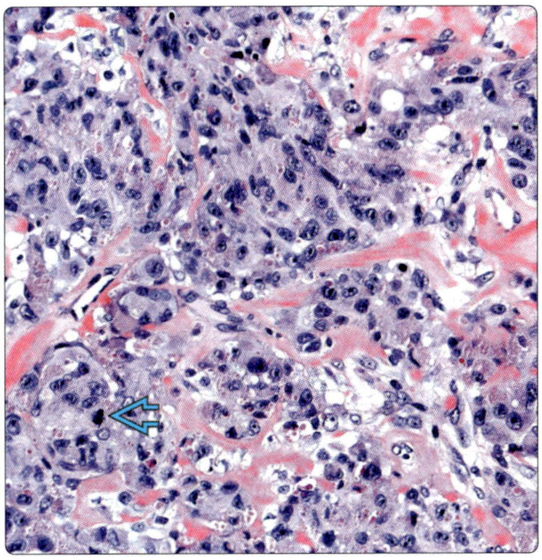

Malignant Granular Cell Tumor

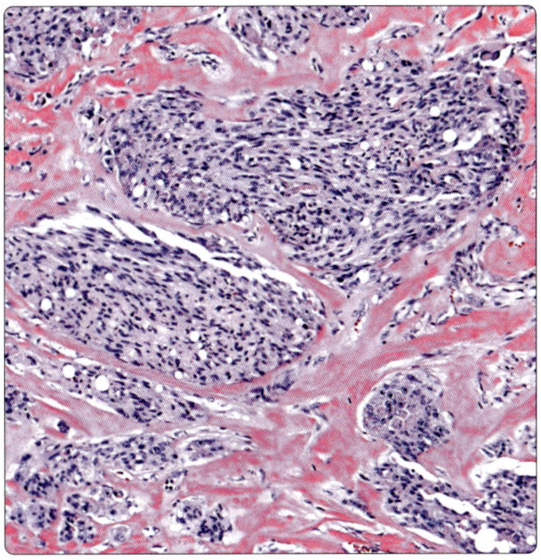

(Left) *Malignant examples of GrCT are extremely rare and usually show diffuse atypical features, such as large vesicular nuclei with prominent nucleoli, high nuclear:cytoplasmic ratio, pleomorphism, and increased mitoses → (> 2 figures per 10 HPF). Necrosis, both single-cell and geographic types, is also common.* **(Right)** *Areas of prominent spindling, increased cellularity, and an overall sarcomatoid appearance are common features of malignant GrCT.*

Dermal Nerve Sheath Myxoma

KEY FACTS

TERMINOLOGY

- Benign, cutaneous nerve sheath tumor with Schwann cell differentiation, abundant myxoid matrix, and well-defined lobular architecture

CLINICAL ISSUES

- Fingers and hand most common sites
  - Pretibial skin also common
  - Uncommon on face
- Benign, but up to 50% recur
- Rare intraoral, orbital, intradural, and paraspinal cases

MICROSCOPIC

- Multiple lobules with abundant myxoid matrix
- Well-defined, lobular architecture and dense fibrous septa
- Usually limited to dermis and subcutis
- Spindle-shaped and epithelioid cells
- Interconnecting cords, networks, syncytial nests, ring-like structures
- Stellate and vacuolated cells common
- No atypia, very low mitotic rate

ANCILLARY TESTS

- Diffuse S100(+)
- GFAP(+) in most
- SMA, desmin, CD68, HMB-45, synaptophysin, chromogranin-A, CD31 (-)

TOP DIFFERENTIAL DIAGNOSES

- Neurothekeoma
- Superficial angiomyxoma
- Digital mucoid cyst
- Myxoid neurofibroma
- Superficial acral fibromyxoma
- Myxoid dermatofibrosarcoma protuberans
- Myxofibrosarcoma (low grade)

(Left) *Dermal nerve sheath myxoma has a very distinctive architecture, consisting of well-defined myxoid lobules. It is typically centered within the dermis and can involve the underlying subcutis as well.* **(Right)** *Dermal nerve sheath myxoma typically presents as a firm papule that varies from 0.5-4.5 cm in size. It usually occurs in adults. Common locations are the fingers, hand, and pretibial skin.*

Dermal Nerve Sheath Myxoma

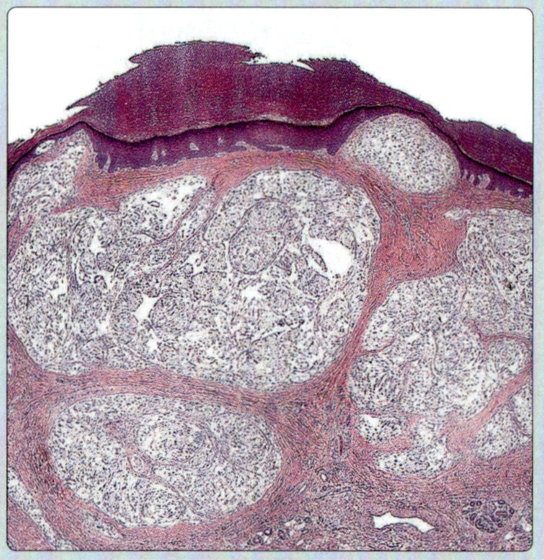

Dermal Papule

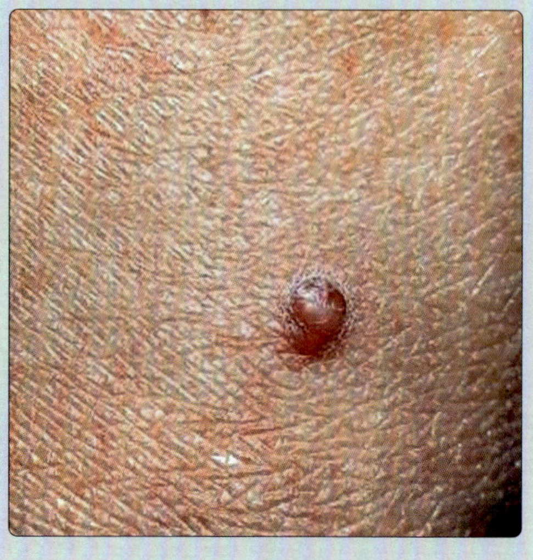

(Left) *The cells in dermal nerve sheath myxoma have schwannian differentiation. They have uniform, spindle-shaped or oval nuclei, evenly distributed chromatin, and long, fibrillary cytoplasmic processes ➔ forming bipolar and stellate configurations.* **(Right)** *Dermal nerve sheath myxomas are strongly S100(+), consonant with Schwann cell differentiation. This immunohistochemically stained section depicts diffuse and intense nuclear ➔ and cytoplasmic ➔ reactivity.*

Schwann Cells

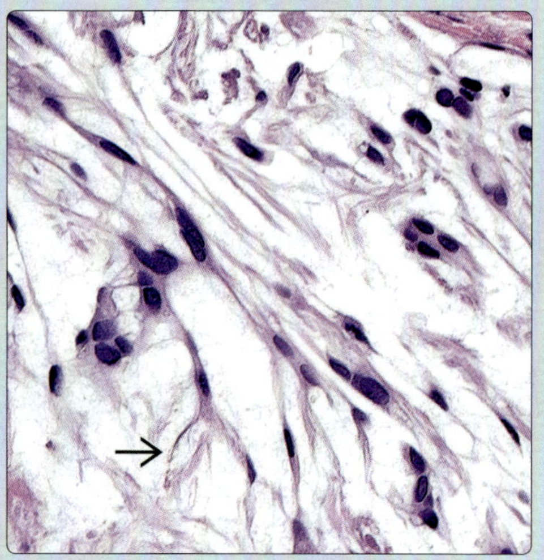

S100 Expression

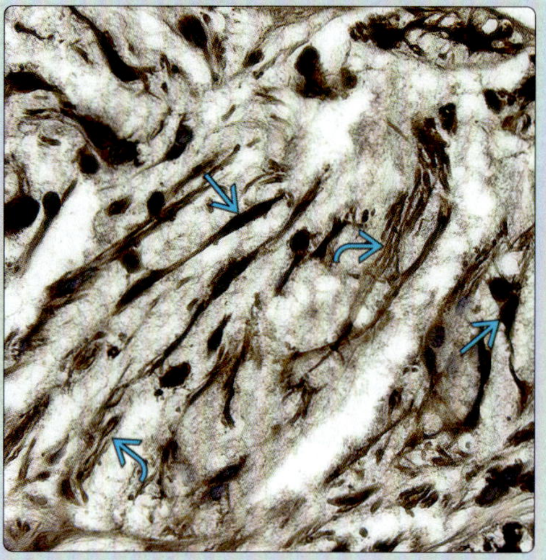

TERMINOLOGY

Definitions

- Benign cutaneous nerve sheath tumor with Schwann cell differentiation, abundant myxoid matrix, and well-defined lobular architecture

CLINICAL ISSUES

Epidemiology

- Incidence
  - Rare; fewer than 100 reports
- Age
  - Mostly adults; median: 34 years

Site

- Extremities
  - Fingers and hand most common
  - Pretibial skin common
- Rare intraoral, orbital, intradural, and paraspinal cases
- Uncommon on face

Presentation

- Slowly growing, painless mass

Prognosis

- Benign and nonaggressive but often excised with positive margins
  - Up to 50% recur

MACROSCOPIC

Size

- 0.5-4.5 cm

MICROSCOPIC

Histologic Features

- Multiple myxoid lobules
  - Well-defined borders separated by dense fibrous septa
- Usually limited to dermis and subcutis
- Paucicellular proliferation of bland spindle cells
  - Interconnecting cords, networks, syncytial nests, ring-like structures, Verocay-like bodies

Cytologic Features

- Spindle-shaped and epithelioid Schwann cells
- Stellate and vacuolated cells
- No atypia, very low mitotic rate

ANCILLARY TESTS

Immunohistochemistry

- S100 diffusely (+) in 100% of tumors
- GFAP(+) in most
- SMA, desmin, CD68, HMB-45, synaptophysin, chromogranin-A, CD31 (-)

DIFFERENTIAL DIAGNOSIS

Neurothekeoma

- Multinodular but less myxoid matrix and less-defined border
- Whorling pattern common
- Spindle and large, plump epithelioid cells; ill-defined cytoplasm
- Lacks cords, syncytial aggregates, vacuolated cells
- S100(-)
- Predilection for face

Superficial Angiomyxoma

- Poorly circumscribed, extends into adjacent tissue
- Fibroblastic cells, often bi- or multinucleated
- Prominent vascularity; small, thin-walled, curvilinear, congested vessels
- Sparse dispersed inflammation, often neutrophils
- S100(-)

Cutaneous Myxoma in Carney Complex

- Indistinguishable from superficial angiomyxoma
- Predilection for ear, eyelid, nipple
- Spotty pigmentation, endocrine overactivity, psammomatous melanotic schwannoma

Digital Mucoid Cyst

- Extruded myxoid material, possibly from underlying joint
- Limited to fingers over dorsal aspect of distal interphalangeal joints

Myxoid Neurofibroma

- Small spindle cells with buckled, wavy nuclei and ill-defined cytoplasm
- Lacks lobular architecture; may be plexiform or diffuse
- Collagen bundles within myxoid stroma

Superficial Acral Fibromyxoma

- Variable fibrous and myxoid areas
- Lacks well-defined lobules
- CD34(+), S100(-)
- Acral extremities, often periungual

Myxoid Dermatofibrosarcoma Protuberans

- Storiform or fascicular, lacks lobular architecture
- Infiltrates subcutis, classic honeycomb pattern
- Plexiform vascular pattern
- CD34(+), S100(-)

Myxofibrosarcoma (Low Grade)

- Variable lobular architecture
- Infiltrative growth into dermis and subcutis
- Pleomorphism and mitotic figures in most cases
- S100(-)

SELECTED REFERENCES

1. Sheth S et al: Differential gene expression profiles of neurothekeomas and nerve sheath myxomas by microarray analysis. Mod Pathol. 24(3):343-54, 2011
2. Nishioka M et al: Nerve sheath myxoma (neurothekeoma) arising in the oral cavity: histological and immunohistochemical features of 3 cases. Oral Surg Oral Med Oral Pathol Oral Radiol Endod. 107(5):e28-33, 2009
3. Fetsch JF et al: Nerve sheath myxoma: a clinicopathologic and immunohistochemical analysis of 57 morphologically distinctive, S-100 protein- and GFAP-positive, myxoid peripheral nerve sheath tumors with a predilection for the extremities and a high local recurrence rate. Am J Surg Pathol. 29(12):1615-24, 2005
4. Carney JA et al: Cutaneous myxomas. A major component of the complex of myxomas, spotty pigmentation, and endocrine overactivity. Arch Dermatol. 122(7):790-8, 1986

Dermal Nerve Sheath Myxoma

(Left) *This scanning-power micrograph of a dermal nerve sheath myxoma illustrates its well-defined, lobular architecture composed of rounded lobules containing copious, pale blue myxoid matrix.* **(Right)** *The lobular architecture in dermal nerve sheath myxoma is defined by thick fibrous septa* ⇨*, which separate the myxoid lobules* ↪*.*

Lobular Architecture

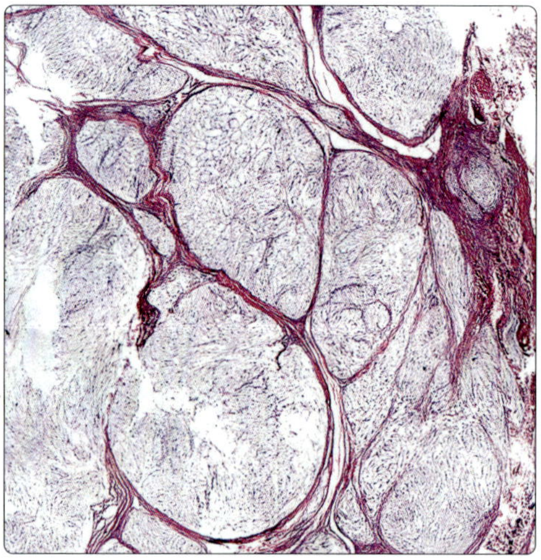

Fibrous Septa

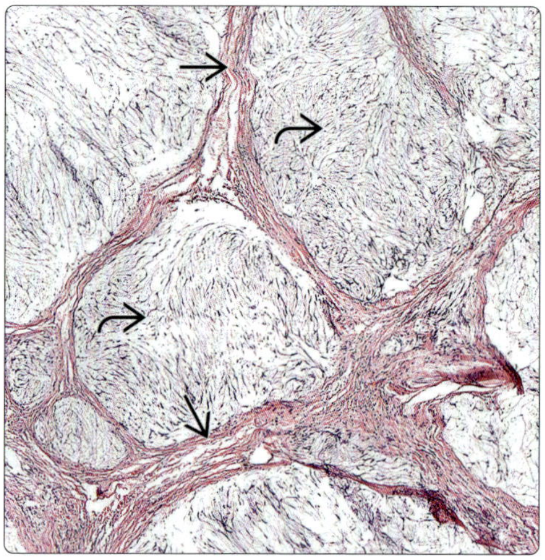

(Left) *This medium-power view of a dermal nerve sheath myxoma depicts a thick fibrous septum composed of dense, mature collagen* ⇨ *in between myxoid lobules.* **(Right)** *Verocay-like bodies consist of parallel arrays of spindle cells* ⇨ *surrounding a fine fibrillary matrix* ↪*. Although rarely seen in dermal nerve sheath myxomas, they provide additional evidence of schwannian differentiation.*

Thick Fibrous Septum

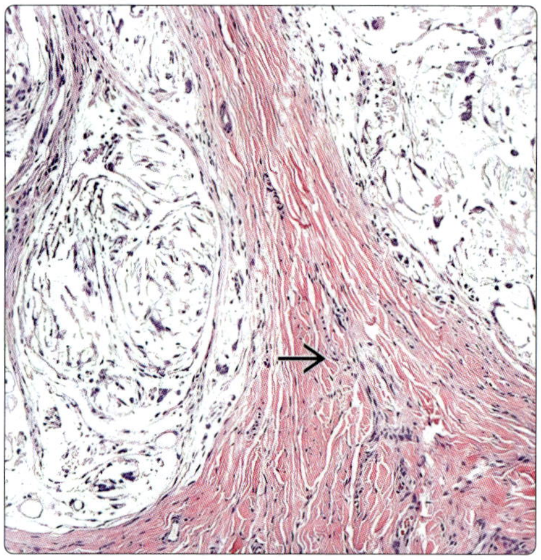

Verocay-Like Body

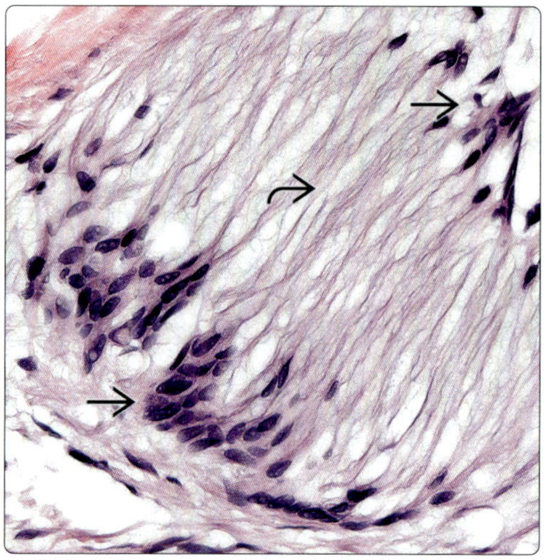

(Left) *The neoplastic cells of nerve sheath myxoma consist of spindle and epithelioid cells with uniform, bland, oval, and elongated nuclei and abundant eosinophilic cytoplasm. They are frequently arranged in syncytial nests and often have intracytoplasmic vacuoles* ⇨*, as depicted.* **(Right)** *The spindle cells may interconnect via elongated cytoplasmic processes to form ring-like structures* ⇨*.*

Syncytial Nests and Vacuoles

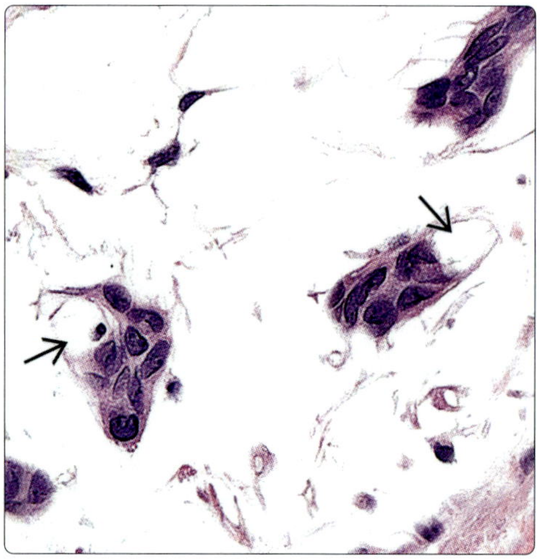

Ring-Like Structures

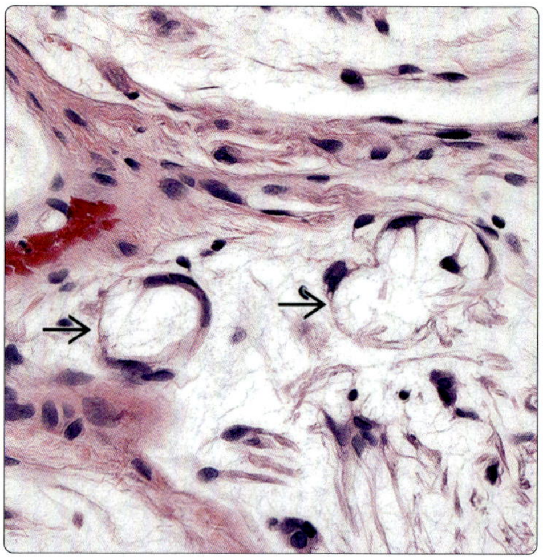

Dermal Nerve Sheath Myxoma

Papule

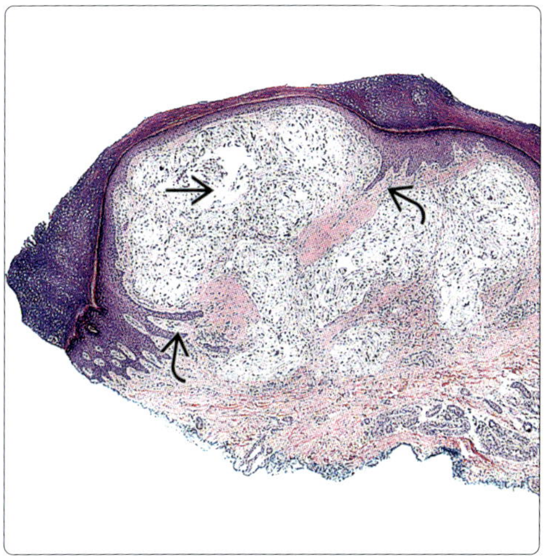

Cohesive Structures

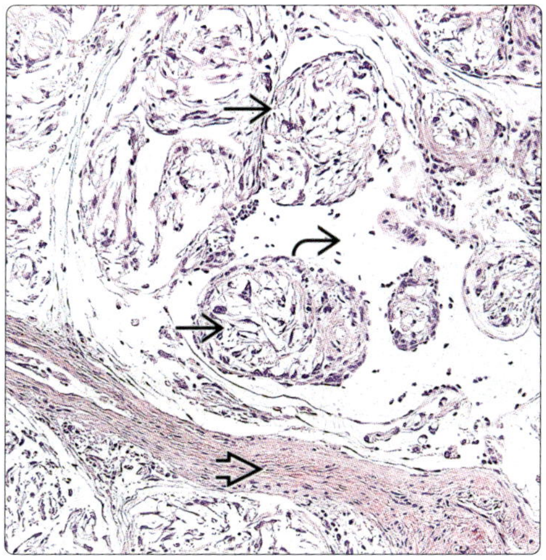

(Left) *This scanning-power micrograph depicts a dermal nerve sheath myxoma with a raised, exophytic pattern due to an expansile myxoid lobule* ➡ *in the superficial dermis. Clinically, it presented as a papule. Note the peripheral epidermal collarette* ↷. **(Right)** *Dermal nerve sheath myxomas often form cohesive structures* ➡ *floating within a myxoid matrix* ↷. *Note the thick fibrous septum at the bottom, which divides the adjacent lobules* ⇨.

Reticulated Pattern

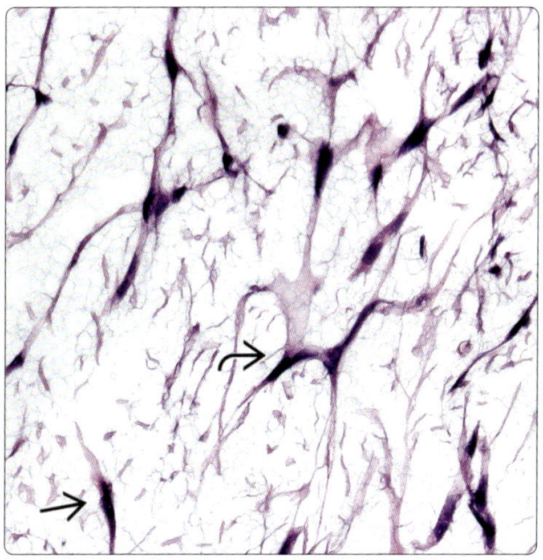

Multilobular and Plexiform Architecture

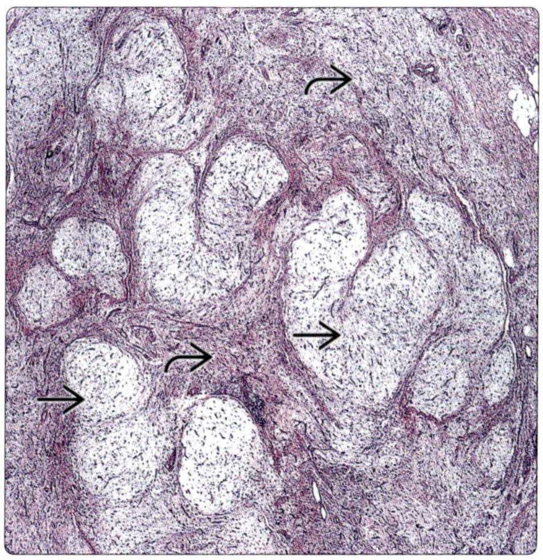

(Left) *This micrograph shows bipolar* ➡ *and stellate* ↷ *spindle cells in a dermal nerve sheath myxoma with abundant eosinophilic cytoplasm and long, interconnecting cell processes, forming a reticulated or network pattern.* **(Right)** *This low-power micrograph highlights a multilobular and plexiform pattern in a dermal nerve sheath myxoma, consisting of sharply demarcated, serpiginous myxoid lobules* ➡ *situated within dense fibroconnective tissue* ↷.

S100 Expression

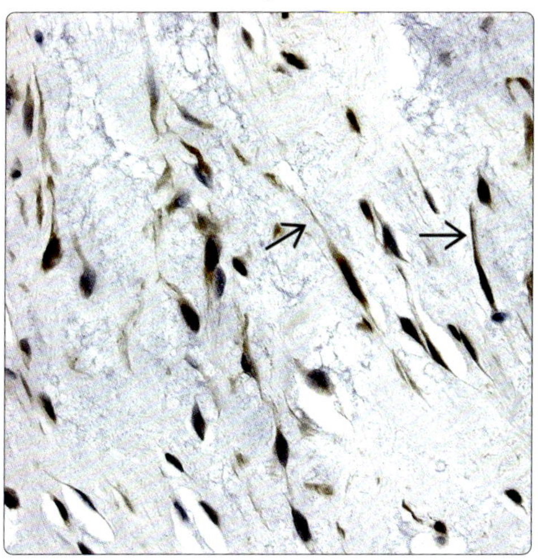

CD34(+) Fibroblasts

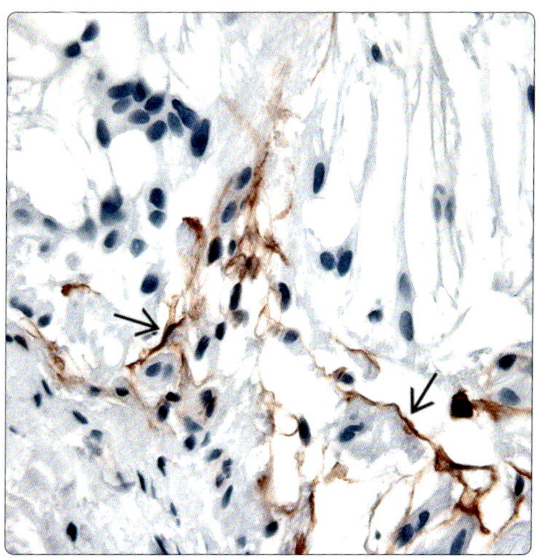

(Left) *S100 immunostain in a dermal nerve sheath myxoma shows diffuse nuclear and cytoplasmic staining, which highlights its long, delicate cytoplasmic processes* ➡. **(Right)** *Immunohistochemical stain for CD34 highlights the long, slender cell processes* ➡ *of intraneurial fibroblasts, which are frequently detected in dermal nerve sheath myxoma. In addition, EMA(+) perineurial cells (not depicted) are also detected in most tumors.*

Ganglioneuroma

KEY FACTS

TERMINOLOGY

- Benign, well-differentiated neoplasm of neural crest origin containing ganglion cells and arising from sympathetic or peripheral nerves

CLINICAL ISSUES

- Most common: 10-30 years of age
- Posterior mediastinum and retroperitoneum most common
  - Less common in adrenal gland
- Usually solitary, painless mass
- Treatment: Complete, conservative excision
- Benign; rare local recurrence
  - Very rare described cases with malignant transformation

MACROSCOPIC

- Wide size range (mean: 8 cm)

MICROSCOPIC

- Uniform spindled Schwann cells in collagenous stroma
  - Fascicles or patternless arrays
  - Elongated or wavy nuclei
- Intermixed ganglion cells of variable size and number
  - Occur in clusters, nests, and singly
- Primitive neuroblasts absent
- May show myxoid stromal change, cystic change, fibrosis, lymphoid aggregates, or calcification

ANCILLARY TESTS

- S100 protein (+) in Schwann cell component
- Synaptophysin (+) in ganglion cells

TOP DIFFERENTIAL DIAGNOSES

- Neurofibroma
- Cellular schwannoma
- Leiomyoma
- Ganglioneuroblastoma

(Left) *Ganglioneuroma is a well-circumscribed, benign neoplasm that occurs most commonly in the posterior mediastinum and retroperitoneum. In the latter location, the tumor ➔ may be extraadrenal (shown) or intraadrenal (much less common). It may or may not have a thin fibrous capsule.* **(Right)** *Ganglioneuroma is composed of ganglion cells ➔ within a mature schwannian stroma.*

Ganglioneuroma

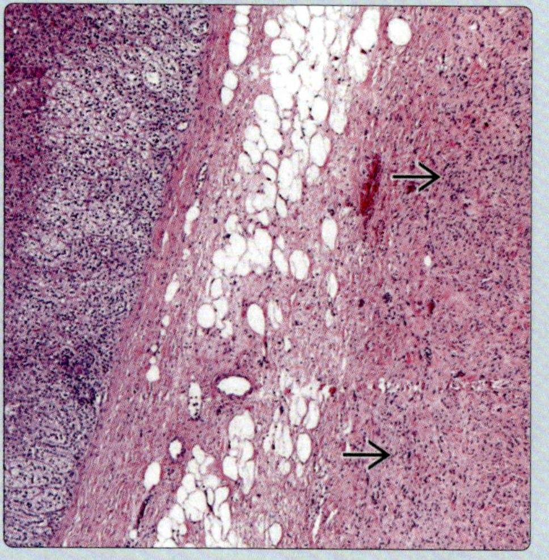

2 Components

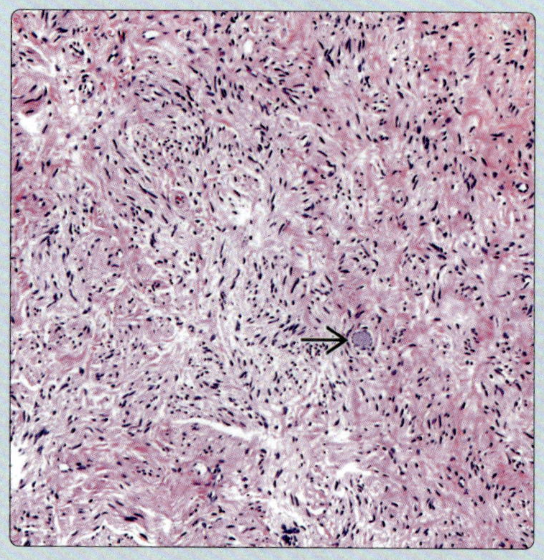

(Left) *The stroma of ganglioneuroma is composed of mature Schwann cells with typical neural cytologic features (elongated nuclei with tapered or pointed ends) within a collagenous and variably edematous background. The overall morphology may closely simulate neurofibroma.* **(Right)** *The number of ganglion cells seen in ganglioneuroma varies from case to case and ranges from sparse or rare to numerous, as is seen in this H&E.*

Schwannian Stroma

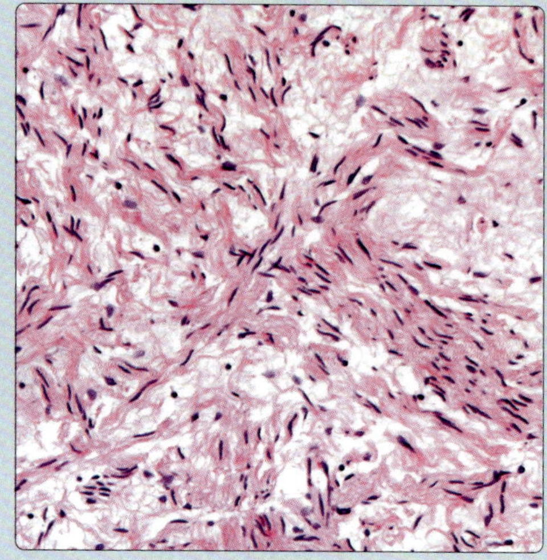

Ganglion Cells

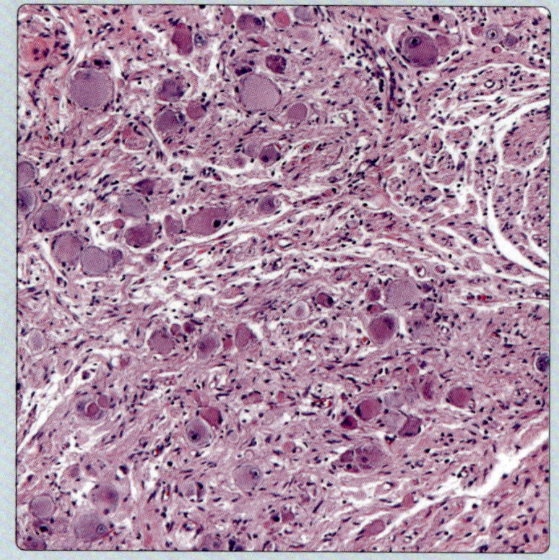

TERMINOLOGY

Abbreviations

- Ganglioneuroma (GN)

Definitions

- Benign, well-differentiated neoplasm of neural crest origin containing ganglion cells and arising from sympathetic or peripheral nerves

ETIOLOGY/PATHOGENESIS

Associated Conditions

- Most develop de novo
- Some develop from maturation of neuroblastoma
- Solitary polypoid GN in gastrointestinal tract may be associated with Cowden syndrome, juvenile polyposis, or tuberous sclerosis
  - Multiple polypoid GN in gastrointestinal tract may be associated with neurofibromatosis type 1 and multiple endocrine neoplasia (MEN) type 2B

CLINICAL ISSUES

Epidemiology

- Age
  - Most common: 10-30 years

Site

- Posterior mediastinum and retroperitoneum most common
  - Less common in adrenal gland
  - Very rarely in skin, parapharynx, and paratestis
- May occur as small polyps in gastrointestinal tract

Presentation

- Usually solitary, painless mass
  - Rarely multifocal
- Rare urinary catecholamine secretion in larger tumors
  - Symptoms: Diarrhea, sweating

Treatment

- Complete, conservative excision

Prognosis

- Benign
  - Rare "metastatic" GN foci described in lymph nodes
    - Presumably represent metastatic neuroblastoma that matured
- Local recurrence is rare
- Very rare described cases with malignant transformation
  - Resembles malignant peripheral nerve sheath tumor (MPNST)

MACROSCOPIC

General Features

- Well-defined, smooth, encapsulated mass
- Gray-white or yellow cut surface
- May have calcification
- Hemorrhage and necrosis absent

Size

- Wide range (mean: 8 cm)

MICROSCOPIC

Histologic Features

- Generally well circumscribed with thin fibrous capsule
  - Rare limited infiltration of surrounding tissue
- Uniform spindled Schwann cells in collagenous stroma
  - Fascicles or patternless arrays
  - Elongated or wavy nuclei
  - May be indistinguishable from neurofibroma
- Intermixed ganglion cells of variable size and number
  - Round, vesicular, sometimes multiple nuclei
    - May show mild to moderate atypia
  - Abundant eosinophilic or amphophilic cytoplasm
  - Occur in clusters, nests, and singly
    - May contain fine granular cytoplasmic pigment
  - Maturation varies
    - Primitive neuroblasts absent
- May show myxoid stromal change, cystic change, fibrosis, lymphoid aggregates, or calcification
- Rare intralesional mature adipose tissue
- Rare composite tumors
  - GN with pheochromocytoma/paraganglioma
- Very rare malignant degeneration to MPNST

ANCILLARY TESTS

Immunohistochemistry

- S100 protein (+) in Schwann cell component
- Neurofilament protein (+) axons
- Synaptophysin (+) in ganglion cells

DIFFERENTIAL DIAGNOSIS

Neurofibroma

- Some areas may be virtually indistinguishable from GN
- Generally lacks discrete bundles of Schwann cells
- Ganglion cells absent
- Most occur in somatic sites

Cellular Schwannoma

- May be seen in retroperitoneum or posterior mediastinum
- Ganglion cells absent
- Strong, diffuse S100 protein (+)

Leiomyoma

- No ganglion cells
- Smooth muscle actin (+), desmin (+)
- S100 protein (-)

Ganglioneuroblastoma

- Contains islands of immature neuroblasts
- Generally seen in younger age group than GN

SELECTED REFERENCES

1. Silveira CRS et al: Magnetic resonance neurography in the diagnosis of a retroperitoneal ganglioneuroma: Case report and literature review. Radiol Case Rep. 13(2):380-385, 2018
2. Gupta S et al: Composite pheochromocytoma/paraganglioma-ganglioneuroma: a clinicopathologic study of eight cases with analysis of succinate dehydrogenase. Endocr Pathol. 28(3):269-275, 2017
3. Hu J et al: Retroperitoneal composite pheochromocytoma-ganglioneuroma : a case report and review of literature. Diagn Pathol. 8:63, 2013

(Left) *Multinucleation* ⇨ *is a common finding in ganglioneuroma, and some cells may show as many as 3 distinct nuclei. Mild to moderate nuclear atypia may be seen.* **(Right)** *Some of the ganglion cells in ganglioneuroma may show accumulation of brown, granular intracytoplasmic pigment* ⇨ *that resembles lipofuscin or neuromelanin.*

Multinucleation

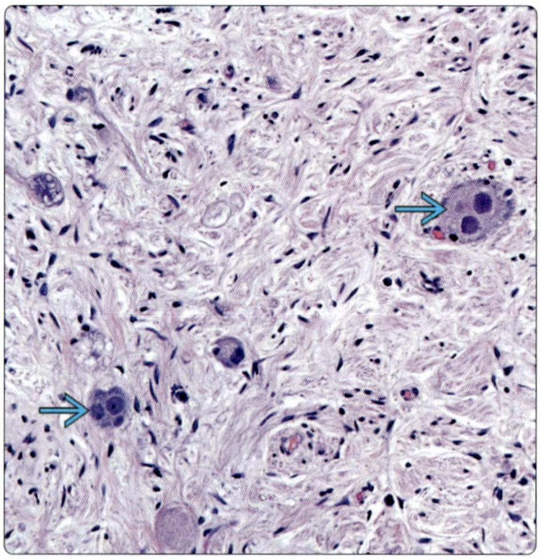

Intracytoplasmic Pigment

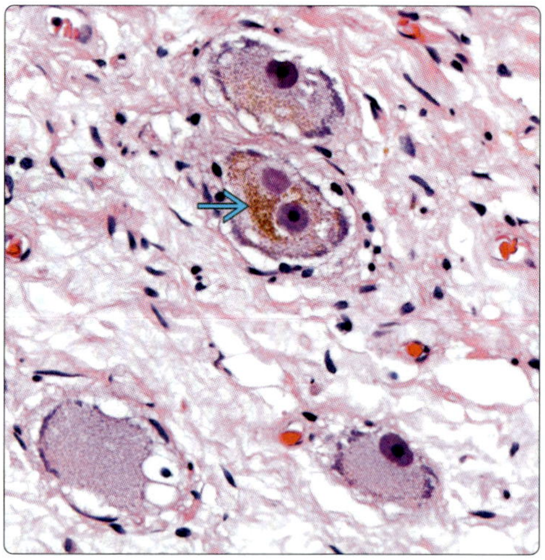

(Left) *Ganglion cells vary widely in size from tumor to tumor, and the cytoplasm ranges from pale to deeply eosinophilic. Most importantly, no immature neuroblastic cells are present.* **(Right)** *Although ganglion cells may be identified singly in many cases of ganglioneuroma, clusters or large nests of ganglion cells are also common.*

Size Variation

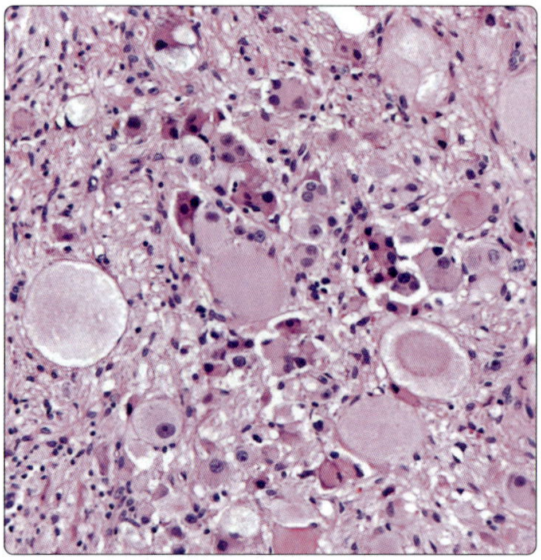

Large Clusters or Nests

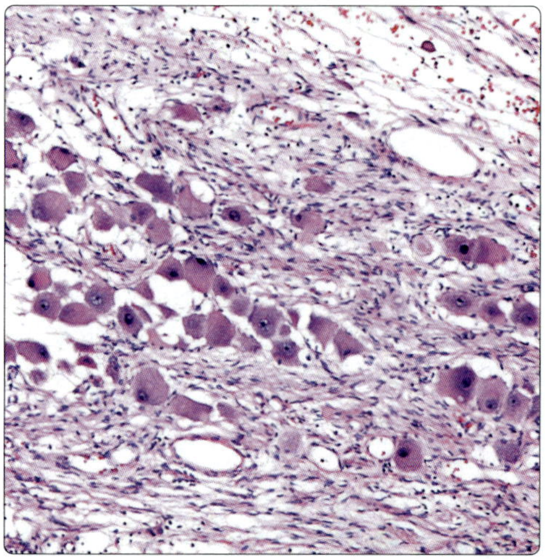

(Left) *The lesional cells of ganglioneuroma may be more compact and bundled in areas, resembling irregular nerve fibers.* **(Right)** *H&E of ganglioneuroma shows fascicular bundles of lesional cells cut in cross section, appearing reminiscent of normal nerve.*

Fascicle Formation

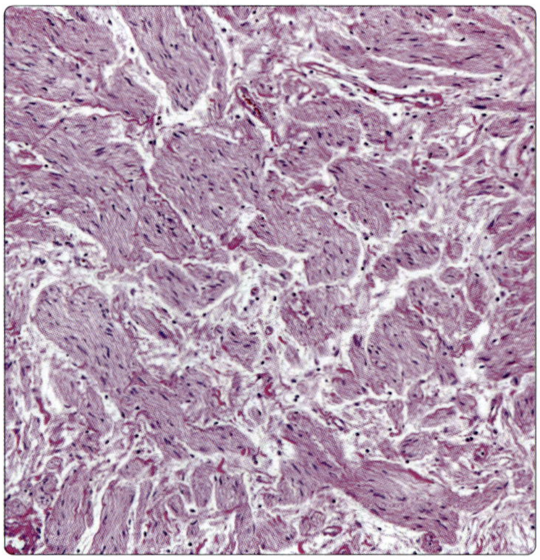

Fascicle Formation (Cross Section)

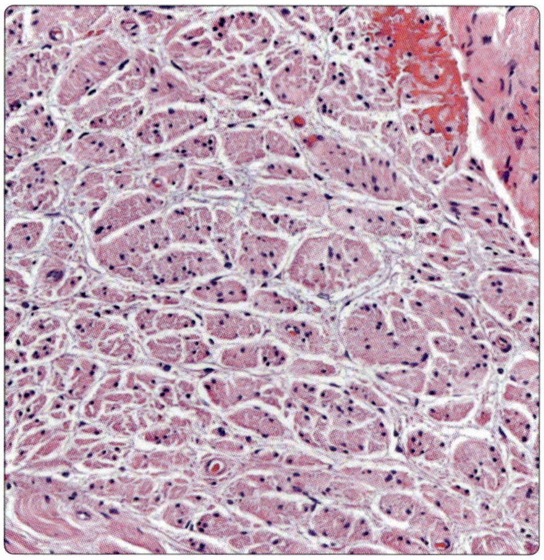

Cellular Fascicles

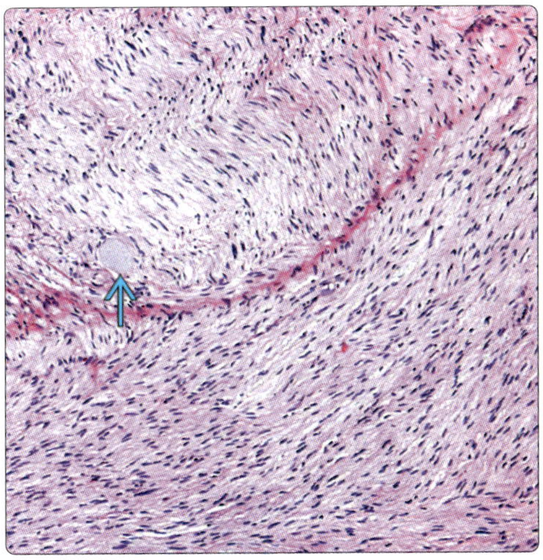

Myxoid Stroma

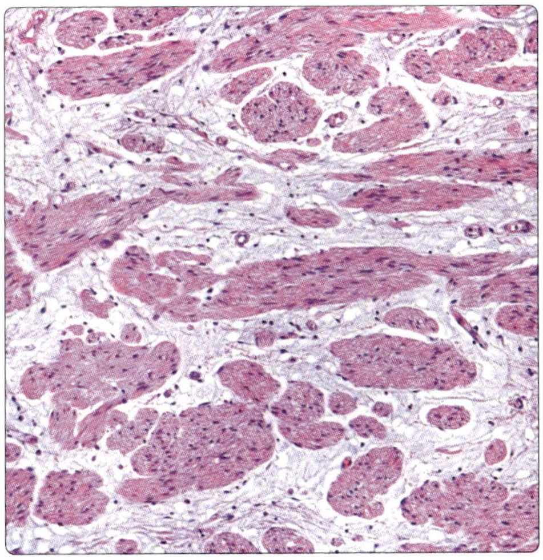

(Left) *Some cases of ganglioneuroma contain more cellular, fascicular foci. This morphology may mimic cellular schwannoma; however, note the presence of a ganglion cell ➡. Also, the nuclei are cytologically bland, and there is no mitotic activity.* **(Right)** *Rare examples of ganglioneuroma demonstrate bundles of lesional Schwann cells separated within a myxoid stroma.*

Myxoid Stromal Change

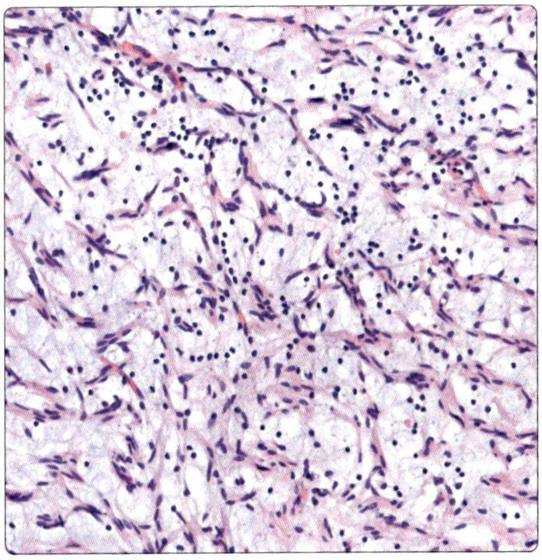

Mild Degenerative Atypia

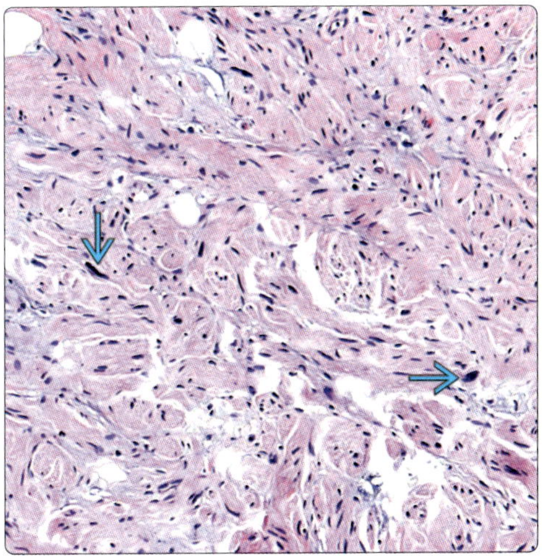

(Left) *H&E shows a myxoid focus of ganglioneuroma in which the lesional cells are individually separated from one another rather than in bundles. A lymphocytic infiltrate is also seen.* **(Right)** *Similar to other benign neural tumors, such as schwannoma and neurofibroma, ganglioneuroma may contain rare, isolated cells with slightly enlarged and hyperchromatic nuclei ➡. This finding is likely degenerative.*

Intralesional Adipose Tissue

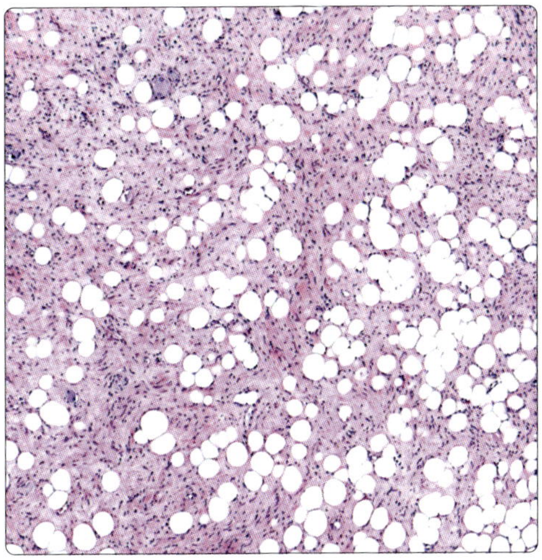

Calcification

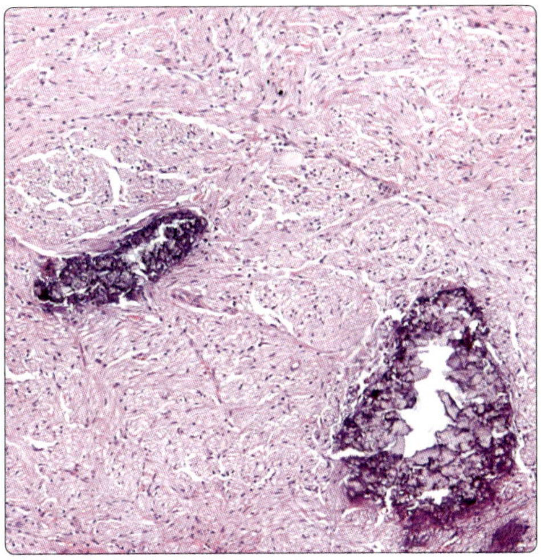

(Left) *A component of mature adipose tissue may be identified within the substance of ganglioneuroma, but it is rare. Fat is more likely to be present near the periphery where the tumor interfaces with surrounding soft tissue.* **(Right)** *Calcification may be seen in ganglioneuroma. It can also be seen in ganglioneuroblastoma, and therefore a thorough search for neuroblastic elements is warranted in these cases.*

Neuromuscular Choristoma

KEY FACTS

TERMINOLOGY

- Benign endoneurial tumor composed of mature skeletal muscle fibers intermixed with peripheral nerve cells often associated with desmoid-type fibromatosis (DTF)
- Synonyms: Benign triton tumor, neuromuscular hamartoma

CLINICAL ISSUES

- Arises in early childhood in most cases
  - Mean age: 10 years (range: Birth to 68 years)
- Affects major peripheral nerves
  - Brachial plexus and sciatic nerve most frequent
- Symptoms related to mass effect, sensory/motor deficits, or musculoskeletal deformity
- Local recurrence in 33%
  - Most recurrent cases associated with DTF

IMAGING

- T1 and T2 signal intensities similar to muscle and nerve
- Low signal in areas of fibrosis/fibromatosis

MACROSCOPIC

- Fusiform expansion of affected nerve with multifascicular involvement

MICROSCOPIC

- Enlarged nerve fascicles containing abundant skeletal muscle fibers
  - Rarely contains smooth muscle fibers
- Surrounded by dense, hypocellular fibrous tissue
- Areas of DTF (18-32% of cases)

ANCILLARY TESTS

- Nuclear β-catenin (+)
- Exon 3 *CTNNB1* mutations

TOP DIFFERENTIAL DIAGNOSES

- Primary DTF
- Lipomatosis of nerve (fibrolipomatous hamartoma)

Neuromuscular Choristoma

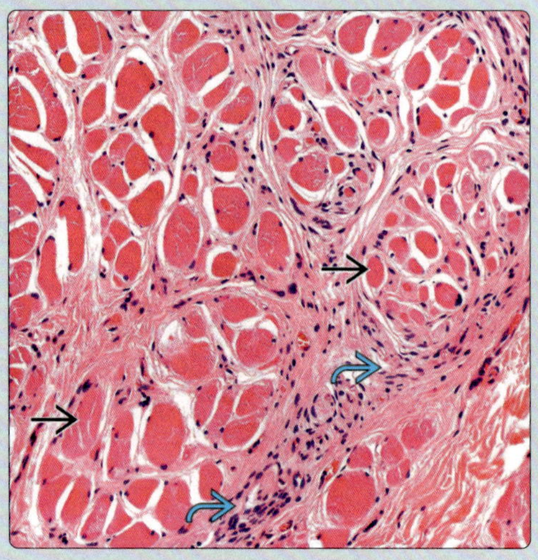

Multifascicular Pattern

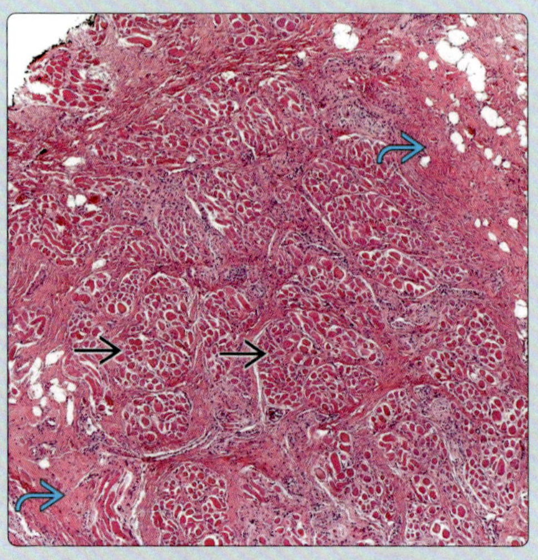

(Left) *Neuromuscular choristoma (NMC) is composed of mature skeletal muscle fibers → admixed with peripheral nerve cells ↷ and has a multifascicular pattern in cross section, as shown. (Courtesy J. Carter, MD, PhD.)* **(Right)** *On cross section of the affected nerve, NMC displays a lobular pattern consisting of fascicles of skeletal muscle fibers → within a peripheral nerve with areas of fibrosis ↷. (Courtesy J. Carter, MD, PhD.)*

Fibrous Area

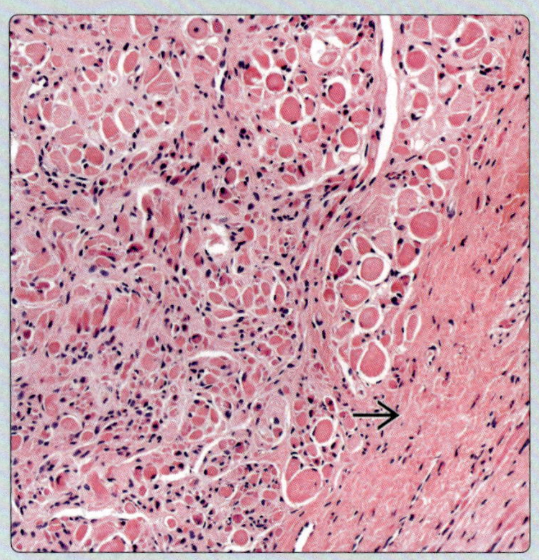

Desmoid-Type Fibromatosis

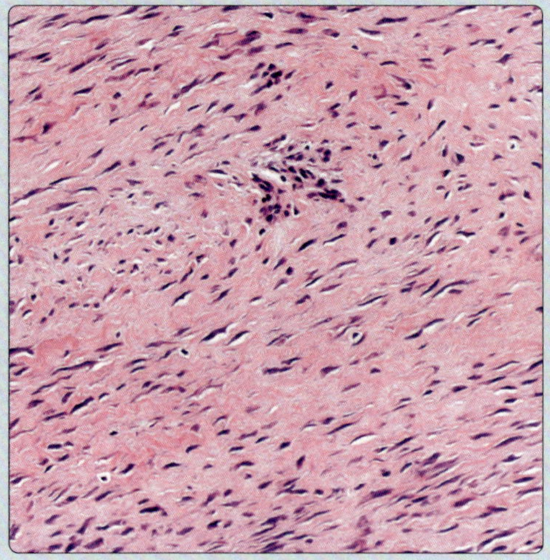

(Left) *In addition to fascicles of skeletal muscle and nerve sheath cells, hypocellular fibrous areas → are common in NMC. (Courtesy J. Carter, MD, PhD.)* **(Right)** *Desmoid-type fibromatosis is often associated with NMC. It may appear de novo or at recurrence and often behaves in an aggressive manner. It is indistinguishable from primary desmoid-type fibromatosis, consisting of fascicles of bland myofibroblasts and fibrous stroma. (Courtesy J. Carter, MD, PhD.)*

TERMINOLOGY

Abbreviations

- Neuromuscular choristoma (NMC)

Synonyms

- Benign triton tumor
- Neuromuscular hamartoma

Definitions

- Benign endoneurial tumor composed of mature skeletal muscle fibers intermixed with peripheral nerve cells often associated with desmoid-type fibromatosis (DTF)

ETIOLOGY/PATHOGENESIS

Developmental Anomaly

- Etiology poorly understood
    - Developmental malformation, most likely

CLINICAL ISSUES

Epidemiology

- Incidence
    - Very rare, only 30 reported cases
- Age
    - Early childhood in most cases
        - Usually before 2 years (mean 10 years)
        - Rare cases in adults
        - Range: Birth to 68 years

Site

- Major peripheral nerves
    - Brachial plexus and sciatic nerve most frequent
    - Head and neck, lumbar plexus, spinal nerves, subcutis

Presentation

- Symptoms related to mass effect or sensory/motor deficits
- Progressive neuropathy or plexopathy
- Secondary musculoskeletal deformity
    - Cavus deformity of foot in sciatic nerve tumors

Treatment

- Complete surgical excision

Prognosis

- Local recurrence in 33%
    - Most recurrent cases are associated with DTF
    - 80% develop DTF in cases with long-term clinical follow-up
    - Development of DTF may be iatrogenically precipitated by biopsy

IMAGING

MR Findings

- T1 and T2 signal intensities similar to muscle and nerve
- Low signal in areas of fibrosis/fibromatosis

MACROSCOPIC

General Features

- Fusiform expansion of affected nerve with multifascicular involvement
- Usually solitary, but may be multifocal

MICROSCOPIC

Histologic Features

- Enlarged nerve fascicles containing abundant skeletal muscle fibers
    - Rarely contain smooth muscle fibers
    - Surrounded by dense, hypocellular fibrous tissue
- Areas of DTF
    - 18-32% of cases
    - Usually in vicinity of NMC
    - May appear in recurrent NMC
    - May be iatrogenically induced by biopsy

ANCILLARY TESTS

Immunohistochemistry

- Both NMC and associated DTF have nuclear β-catenin staining

Genetic Testing

- Most NMC &/or associated DTF have exon 3 *CTNNB1* mutations

DIFFERENTIAL DIAGNOSIS

Primary Desmoid Fibromatosis

- Lacks entrapped NMC

Lipomatosis of Nerve (Fibrolipomatous Hamartoma)

- Usually perineural, not intraneural
- Contains adipose tissue, whereas NMC does not

DIAGNOSTIC CHECKLIST

Clinically Relevant Pathologic Features

- Fusiform enlargement of major nerve
- Early childhood

Pathologic Interpretation Pearls

- Skeletal muscle fibers within nerve fascicle
- Often associated with DTF

SELECTED REFERENCES

1. Stone JJ et al: Recurrent desmoid-type fibromatosis associated with underlying neuromuscular choristoma. J Neurosurg. 1-9, 2018
2. Carter JM et al: CTNNB1 mutations and estrogen receptor expression in neuromuscular choristoma and its associated fibromatosis. Am J Surg Pathol. 40(10):1368-74, 2016
3. Hébert-Blouin MN et al: Fibromatosis: a potential sequela of neuromuscular choristoma. J Neurosurg. 116(2):399-408, 2012
4. Daley TD et al: Benign triton tumor of the tongue. Oral Surg Oral Med Oral Pathol Oral Radiol Endod. 105(6):763-6, 2008
5. Tiffee JC et al: Neuromuscular hamartomas of the head and neck. Arch Otolaryngol Head Neck Surg. 124(2):212-6, 1998
6. Bassett GS et al: Cavus deformity of the foot secondary to a neuromuscular choristoma (hamartoma) of the sciatic nerve. A case report. J Bone Joint Surg Am. 79(9):1398-401, 1997
7. Awasthi D et al: Neuromuscular hamartoma (benign "triton" tumor) of the brachial plexus. Case report. J Neurosurg. 75(5):795-7, 1991
8. O'Connell JX et al: Multiple cutaneous neuromuscular choristomas. Report of a case and a review of the literature. Am J Surg Pathol. 14(1):93-6, 1990
9. Chen KT: Neuromuscular hamartoma. J Surg Oncol. 26(3):158-60, 1984
10. Bonneau R et al: Neuromuscular choristoma. A clinicopathologic study of two cases. Am J Surg Pathol. 7(6):521-8, 1983

Melanotic Schwannoma

KEY FACTS

TERMINOLOGY

- Synonym: Psammomatous melanotic schwannoma
- Unusual Schwann cell neoplasm containing variable melanin pigment and showing potential for malignant behavior

ETIOLOGY/PATHOGENESIS

- Subset of cases associated with Carney complex

CLINICAL ISSUES

- Most common: 20-45 years of age
- Posterior spinal nerve roots (most common)
  - Subset arise in gastrointestinal tract
- Treatment: Complete surgical excision with negative margins
- Local recurrence in 1/3 of cases
- Metastasis in 15-42% of reported cases
- Overall 15% mortality rate
- No correlation between morphology and clinical behavior

MACROSCOPIC

- Variable tan-gray to black cut surface
- Usually < 5 cm

MICROSCOPIC

- Lobular growth but often peripherally infiltrative
- Sheets and fascicles of spindled to epithelioid cells
- Mitoses rare to absent
- Variably prominent melanin pigment
- Psammoma bodies (50% of cases)

ANCILLARY TESTS

- S100 protein (+), SOX10(+), HMB-45(+), MART-1(+)
- Keratin (-), EMA(-), GFAP(-)

TOP DIFFERENTIAL DIAGNOSES

- Metastatic melanoma
- Schwannoma (conventional or gastrointestinal)
- Clear cell sarcoma

Melanotic Schwannoma

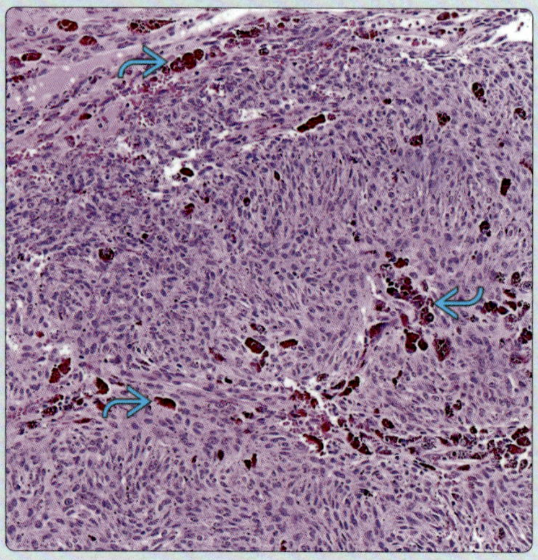

Sheets and Fascicles

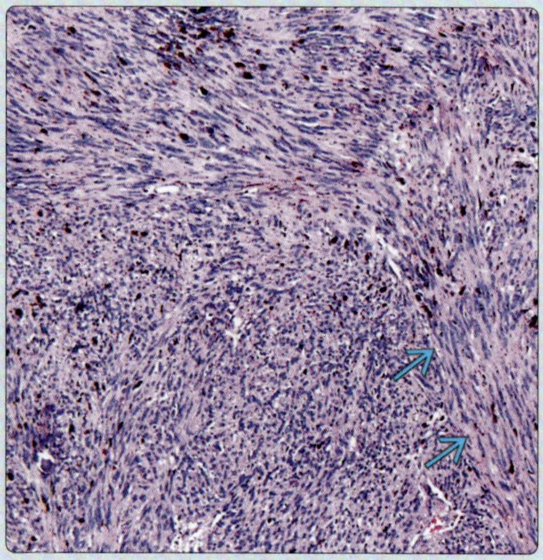

(Left) *Melanotic schwannoma is an unusual neoplasm that shows combined schwannian and melanocytic features and shows a predilection for the posterior spinal nerve roots. Tumor cells are spindled to epithelioid and associated with a highly variable amount of melanin pigment →. Mitoses are rare.* **(Right)** *Tumor cells are arranged in sheets and fascicles and often show mild atypia. Nuclear palisading → may be seen in occasional cases but is usually much less prominent as compared to conventional schwannoma.*

Psammoma Bodies

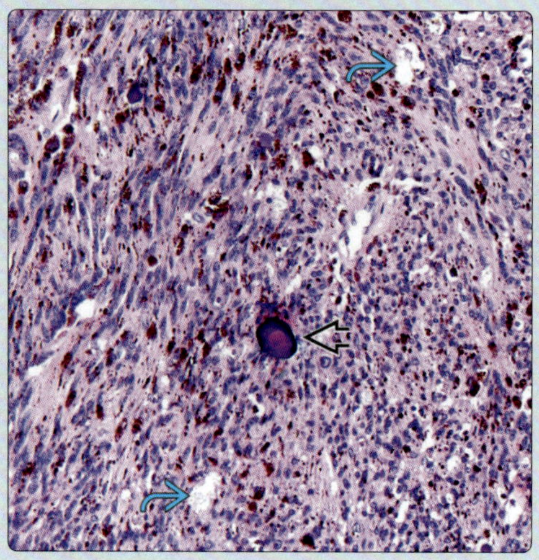

Heavy Melanin Pigment

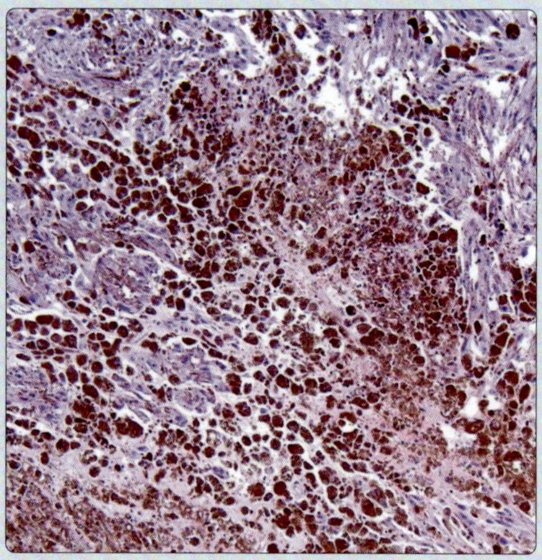

(Left) *Spherical, lamellated calcifications (psammoma bodies) → are seen in up to 50% of cases of melanotic schwannoma and range from sparse to abundant. Cells with cytoplasmic vacuolization → may also be seen in some cases and can mimic adipose tissue when prominent.* **(Right)** *The amount and distribution of melanin pigment is highly variable in melanotic schwannoma. This case showed areas of extensive pigmentation that obscured underlying cytologic features.*

TERMINOLOGY

Synonyms

- Psammomatous melanotic schwannoma
- Malignant melanotic schwannian tumor (proposed)

Definitions

- Unusual Schwann cell neoplasm containing variable melanin pigment and showing potential for malignant behavior

ETIOLOGY/PATHOGENESIS

Common Association With Carney Complex

- Up to 50% of cases (much lower in some series)
- Familial; autosomal dominant
- Other manifestations include myxomas (cutaneous, cardiac), cutaneous hyperpigmentation, and endocrine tumors/abnormalities

CLINICAL ISSUES

Epidemiology

- Incidence
  - Rare
- Age
  - Most common: 20-45 years
- Sex
  - Slight female predominance

Site

- Posterior spinal nerve roots and paraspinal ganglia
  - Particularly cervical and thoracic
- Subset arise in gastrointestinal tract
- Very rarely bone or other sites

Presentation

- May be associated with pain or sensory defects
- Usually solitary
  - May be multicentric in Carney complex

Treatment

- Complete surgical excision with negative margins
- Indefinite, long-term clinical follow-up recommended

Prognosis

- Local recurrence in 1/3 of cases
- Metastasis in 15-42% of reported cases
  - May occur late in clinical course
  - Sites include lung, brain, liver
- Overall 15% mortality rate
- No established correlation between morphology and clinical behavior

MACROSCOPIC

General Features

- Well circumscribed, round to fusiform
- May or may not be encapsulated
- Variable tan-gray to black cut surface

Size

- Usually < 5 cm

MICROSCOPIC

Histologic Features

- Lobular growth but often peripherally infiltrative
- Sheets and fascicles of spindled to epithelioid cells with ample pale eosinophilic cytoplasm
  - Mildly atypical, vesicular nuclei with small nucleoli
    - Nuclear pseudoinclusions or grooves in some cells
  - Occasional cases show nuclear enlargement, multinucleation, or prominent nucleoli
  - Mitoses rare to absent
- Psammoma bodies (50% of cases)
  - Spherical, concentrically laminar calcifications
  - Can range from sparse to numerous
- Variably prominent melanin pigment
  - May be sparse to focal or abundant and obscuring
- Nuclear palisading, scattered hyalinized vessels rare
- Necrosis in minority of cases
- Degenerative changes include stromal fibrosis, myxoid changes, symplastic nuclear atypia, cytoplasmic vacuolizations
- Malignant behavior difficult to predict histologically
  - However, mitotic rate > 2 mitoses/10 HPF may be associated with increased risk

ANCILLARY TESTS

Immunohistochemistry

- Strong, diffuse S100 protein (+), SOX10(+)
  - Rare cases are entirely negative
- HMB-45(+), MART-1(+), tyrosinase (+)
- Pericellular collagen type IV (+) and laminin (+)
- Keratin (-), EMA(-), GFAP(-)

DIFFERENTIAL DIAGNOSIS

Metastatic Melanoma

- Often marked nuclear atypia with abundant mitoses
- Current or prior clinical history
- Lacks psammoma bodies

Schwannoma (Conventional or Gastrointestinal)

- Lacks psammoma bodies and prominent melanin pigment
- No expression of melanocytic markers

Clear Cell Sarcoma

- Most common in distal extremities of young adults
- Lacks psammoma bodies and heavy melanin pigment
- Osteoclast-like multinucleated giant cells common
- *EWSR1* translocations

SELECTED REFERENCES

1. Alexiev BA et al: Pathology of melanotic schwannoma. Arch Pathol Lab Med. ePub, 2018
2. Torres-Mora J et al: Malignant melanotic schwannian tumor: a clinicopathologic, immunohistochemical, and gene expression profiling study of 40 cases, with a proposal for the reclassification of "melanotic schwannoma". Am J Surg Pathol. 38(1):94-105, 2014
3. Chetty R et al: Psammomatous melanotic schwannoma presenting as colonic polyps. Virchows Arch. 451(3):717-20, 2007
4. Carney JA: Psammomatous melanotic schwannoma. A distinctive, heritable tumor with special associations, including cardiac myxoma and the Cushing syndrome. Am J Surg Pathol. 14(3):206-22, 1990

Malignant Peripheral Nerve Sheath Tumor

KEY FACTS

TERMINOLOGY

- Malignant neoplasm showing evidence of nerve sheath (mostly schwannian) cellular differentiation
  - May arise from peripheral nerve or preexisting benign nerve sheath tumor or within context of NF1
- Term malignant triton tumor may be used for MPNST with rhabdomyoblastic differentiation

ETIOLOGY/PATHOGENESIS

- 50% of cases associated with NF1

CLINICAL ISSUES

- Wide age range (most common: 20-50 years)
- Extremities (often proximal), trunk, and head/neck
  - Most (70%) arise in major nerve trunks
- Treatment: Complete surgical resection
- Overall poor prognosis
  - Local recurrence in up to 40%
  - Metastasis: 30-60%

MICROSCOPIC

- Most tumors are histologically high grade
- Fascicles and broad whorls of relatively uniform, spindled cells of variable cellularity
  - Alternating zones of cellularity ("marbled") and perivascular tumor cell accentuation common
  - Hyperchromatic, elongated to pleomorphic nuclei
- Mitoses often numerous and necrosis is common
- May show origin from benign nerve sheath tumor
- Heterologous differentiation in 10-15% of cases

ANCILLARY TESTS

- Focal S100 protein (+) &/or SOX10(+) in up to 50%
- Loss of nuclear H3K27me3 expression by IHC

TOP DIFFERENTIAL DIAGNOSES

- Synovial sarcoma
- Cellular schwannoma
- Atypical neurofibroma

Malignant Peripheral Nerve Sheath Tumor

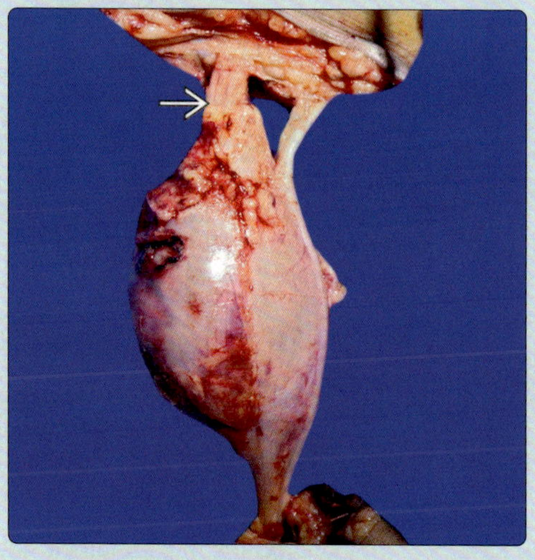

Gross Photograph

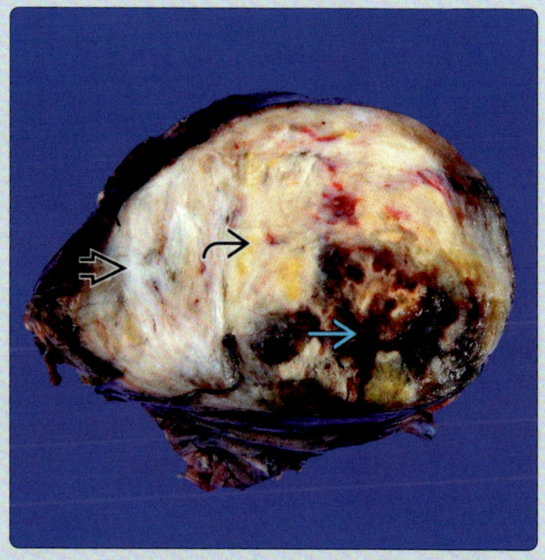

(Left) *Malignant peripheral nerve sheath tumor (MPNST) is a neurogenic neoplasm that may occur sporadically or within the setting of neurofibromatosis type 1. This intraoperative photograph of MPNST shows a large fusiform tumor mass arising from and incorporating the femoral nerve.* **(Right)** *MPNSTs tend to form bulky, circumscribed, and pseudoencapsulated masses often with a variegated cut surface, including firm, white-tan areas of viable tumor, yellow necrotic areas, and cystic hemorrhagic foci.*

Marbled or Tapestry-Like Pattern

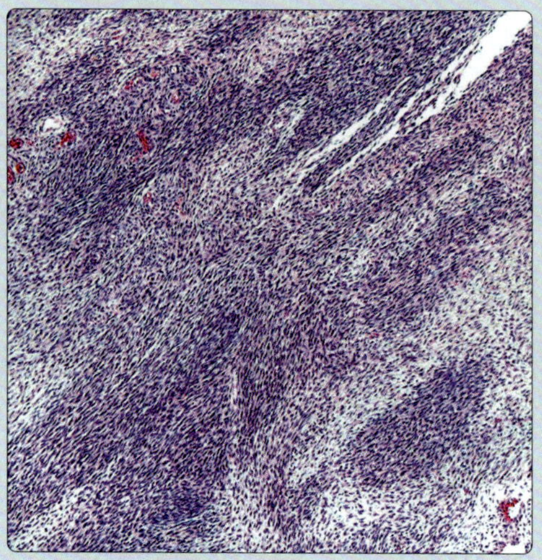

Nuclear Atypia Common

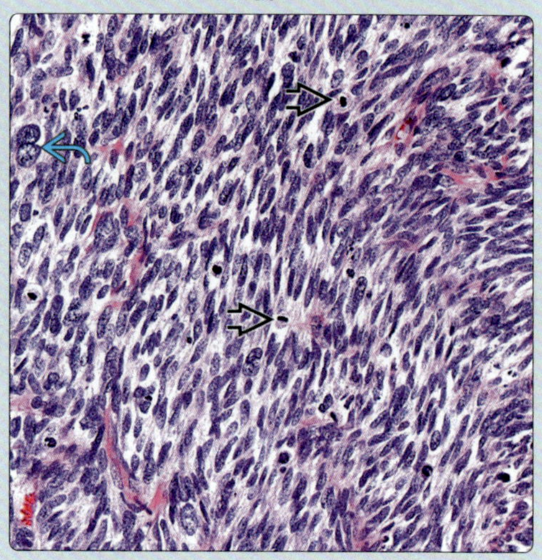

(Left) *Although the morphologic spectrum is relatively broad, the classic low-power appearance of MPNST shows alternating zones of varying cellularity that imparts a marbled or tapestry-like pattern, as depicted.* **(Right)** *Most MPNSTs are high-grade neoplasms, and nuclear atypia and pleomorphism are common. This is in contrast to synovial sarcoma, which shows nuclear monomorphism. Mitotic figures are often easily identified in MPNST as well.*

TERMINOLOGY

Abbreviations

- Malignant peripheral nerve sheath tumor (MPNST)

Synonyms

- Neurofibrosarcoma, malignant schwannoma, neurogenic sarcoma

Definitions

- Malignant neoplasm showing evidence of nerve sheath (mostly schwannian) cellular differentiation
  - Common settings: Origin from peripheral nerve, or preexisting benign nerve sheath tumor, or in patient with neurofibromatosis type 1 (NF1)
    - May also arise outside of these classic settings
- Term malignant triton tumor may be used for MPNST with rhabdomyoblastic differentiation

ETIOLOGY/PATHOGENESIS

Genetic Predisposition

- 50% of cases associated with NF1
  - Lifetime risk: 5-10%
- 40% of cases are sporadic

Molecular Pathogenesis

- NF1 caused by germline mutation of *NF1* tumor suppressor gene (17q11.2)
  - Somatic loss of 2nd *NF1* allele required for tumorigenesis
- Malignant transformation in both NF1-associated and sporadic MPNST often involves *CDKN2A* and *TP53* and their downstream pathways

Environmental Exposure

- 10% of cases associated with history of radiation

CLINICAL ISSUES

Epidemiology

- Incidence
  - Uncommon (5% of soft tissue sarcomas)
- Age
  - Wide range (most common: 20-50 years)
    - Younger average age in NF1 patients
- Sex
  - Male predominance in NF1-associated tumors

Site

- Extremities (often proximal), trunk, and head/neck
  - Most are deep seated
- Most (70%) arise in major nerve trunks
  - Sciatic nerve most common
  - Also brachial plexus, sacral plexus, paraspinal nerves

Presentation

- Enlarging painless or painful mass
  - Rapid enlargement of preexisting nerve sheath tumor in NF1 patient suggests malignant transformation
- Neurogenic symptoms (e.g., weakness, tingling) in some patients

Treatment

- Complete surgical resection
- Postoperative radiotherapy
- Generally poor response to chemotherapy
  - Recent studies suggest efficacy of rapamycin (mTOR inhibitor) ± AKT inhibitors

Prognosis

- Overall poor prognosis
  - Local recurrence in up to 40%
  - Metastasis: 30-60%
    - Lungs, bone, pleura most common
  - 5-year survival rate: 26-60%
    - NF1-associated tumors associated with worse survival than sporadic tumors
- Adverse prognostic factors: Centralized/truncal location, larger size (> 5 cm), high-grade histology, local recurrence
- Malignant triton tumors usually show very aggressive clinical course

MACROSCOPIC

General Features

- Often large, fusiform mass
  - Origin from nerve or benign nerve sheath tumor may be evident
    - Particularly plexiform neurofibroma in NF1
- Tan-white-gray, firm, gelatinous to fleshy cut surface
- Necrosis and hemorrhage common

Size

- Most > 5 cm

MICROSCOPIC

Histologic Features

- Fascicles and broad whorls of relatively uniform, spindled cells
  - Pale eosinophilic cytoplasm with ill-defined cytoplasmic borders
  - Hyperchromatic, elongated nuclei with dispersed coarse chromatin
    - Wavy, tapered, or "buckled" contours in some cells
    - Nuclear pleomorphism not uncommon
      - May rarely be marked and extensive
    - Focal epithelioid cytomorphology may be present
    - Rare primitive, small-cell morphology
- Cellularity characteristically varies
  - Alternating cellular fascicles and hypocellular areas (tapestry or marbled pattern)
    - Cellular areas may show herringbone, palisading, or neuroid whorling patterns
  - Increased cellular density and prominence around some stromal vessels
    - Cells may appear to herniate into vascular lumen
- Vascularized, variable myxoid to collagenous stroma
  - Hemangiopericytoma-like vascular pattern in some
  - Distinct clusters of small vessels may be seen
- Mitoses often numerous
- Coagulative necrosis is common
  - May be geographic with perivascular sparing (peritheliomatous pattern)
- Most are histologically high grade
  - 10-15% are low grade (few mitoses, no necrosis)

- Origin from peripheral nerve may be evident
  - Tumor may track along nerve bundles
- Origin from preexisting benign nerve sheath tumor in some cases
  - Neurofibroma most common
    - Plexiform (in NF1) and solitary soft tissue types; rarely others
    - Transitional areas of increased cellularity and atypia may be seen
  - Rarely schwannoma, ganglioneuroma, ganglioneuroblastoma, or pheochromocytoma
- Heterologous mesenchymal differentiation in 10-15% of cases
  - Rhabdomyoblastic (malignant triton tumor)
  - Osteosarcomatous, chondrosarcomatous
  - Rarely angiosarcomatous, liposarcomatous
- Epithelial elements (e.g., glands) very rare
  - Usually seen within context of NF1

ANCILLARY TESTS

Immunohistochemistry

- S100 protein (+) &/or SOX10 (+) in up to 50%, characteristically focal
  - Diffuse expression very rare (except in low-grade MPNST)
- Loss of nuclear H3K27me3 expression is supportive
  - Usually diffuse loss; rarely heterogeneous
  - Greater sensitivity in sporadic and radiation-induced MPNST than in NF1-related tumors
- Variable CD34(+), GFAP(+)
- Keratin, SMA, desmin, HMB45, MART-1 (-)
  - Heterologous rhabdomyoblasts elements are desmin (+), myogenin (+)

Genetic Testing

- Complex structural and numeric chromosomal abnormalities
  - No consistent differences between NF1-associated and sporadic tumors
- No *MDM2* amplification

DIFFERENTIAL DIAGNOSIS

Synovial Sarcoma (Monophasic)

- Characteristic uniform, cytologic and architectural features
- Presence of stromal "wiry collagen" and calcifications
- Cytokeratin (+) and EMA(+) but usually focal or patchy
- Focal S100(+) in 30% of cases
- Diffuse nuclear TLE1(+)
- Characteristic t(X;18) involving *SS18* (SYT)

Cellular Schwannoma

- Lacks malignant cytological atypia
- Patchy subcapsular lymphoid aggregates &/or foamy macrophages
- Necrosis uncommon but may be present focally
- Strong, diffuse S100(+) and SOX10(+)
- Retention of nuclear H3K27me3 by IHC

Atypical Neurofibroma

- Usually retains cytoarchitectural features of neurofibroma
- Scattered, enlarged nuclei with degenerative, "smudgy" chromatin
- Lacks fascicular growth and marked cellularity
- Mitoses rare to absent

Malignant Melanoma

- May have previous clinical history
- Pure spindled morphology uncommon
- Diffusely S100 protein (+)
- Expression of HMB-45 and other melanocytic markers

Dedifferentiated Liposarcoma

- Heterogeneous morphologic appearance
- Lacks perivascular accentuation of tumor cells
- Identification of well-differentiated liposarcoma component very helpful
- *MDM2* amplification (best supportive test)
- General retention of nuclear H3K27me3 by IHC (lost in rare cases)

Leiomyosarcoma

- Smooth muscle cytomorphology
- SMA(+), variable desmin (+)
- S100 protein (-)

Spindle Cell Rhabdomyosarcoma

- Usually does not arise in association with large nerve or within context of NF1
- Desmin (+), myogenin (+) tumor cells are more evenly distributed

SELECTED REFERENCES

1. Makise N et al: Clarifying the distinction between malignant peripheral nerve sheath tumor and dedifferentiated liposarcoma: a critical reappraisal of the diagnostic utility of MDM2 and H3K27me3 status. Am J Surg Pathol. 42(5):656-64, 2018
2. Le Guellec S et al: Malignant peripheral nerve sheath tumor is a challenging diagnosis: a systematic pathology review, immunohistochemistry, and molecular analysis in 160 patients from the French Sarcoma Group database. Am J Surg Pathol. 40(7):896-908, 2016
3. Prieto-Granada CN et al: Loss of H3K27me3 expression is a highly sensitive marker for sporadic and radiation-induced MPNST. Am J Surg Pathol. 40(4):479-89, 2016
4. Schaefer IM et al: Loss of H3K27 trimethylation distinguishes malignant peripheral nerve sheath tumors from histologic mimics. Mod Pathol. 29(1):4-13, 2016
5. Pekmezci M et al: Morphologic and immunohistochemical features of malignant peripheral nerve sheath tumors and cellular schwannomas. Mod Pathol. 28(2):187-200, 2014
6. Endo M et al: Conventional spindle cell-type malignant peripheral nerve sheath tumor arising in a sporadic schwannoma. Hum Pathol. 44(12):2845-8, 2013
7. Kolberg M et al: Survival meta-analyses for >1800 malignant peripheral nerve sheath tumor patients with and without neurofibromatosis type 1. Neuro Oncol. 15(2):135-47, 2013
8. Wakely PE Jr et al: The cytopathology of malignant peripheral nerve sheath tumor: a report of 55 fine-needle aspiration cases. Cancer Cytopathol. 120(5):334-41, 2012
9. Kroep JR et al: First-line chemotherapy for malignant peripheral nerve sheath tumor (MPNST) versus other histological soft tissue sarcoma subtypes and as a prognostic factor for MPNST: an EORTC soft tissue and bone sarcoma group study. Ann Oncol. 22(1):207-14, 2011
10. Mills AM et al: Endocervical fibroblastic malignant peripheral nerve sheath tumor (neurofibrosarcoma): report of a novel entity possibly related to endocervical CD34 fibrocytes. Am J Surg Pathol. 35(3):404-12, 2011
11. Moretti VM et al: Early outcomes for malignant peripheral nerve sheath tumor treated with chemotherapy. Am J Clin Oncol. 34(4):417-21, 2011
12. Gottfried ON et al: Neurofibromatosis type 1 and tumorigenesis: molecular mechanisms and therapeutic implications. Neurosurg Focus. 28(1):E8, 2010

Cytologic Features

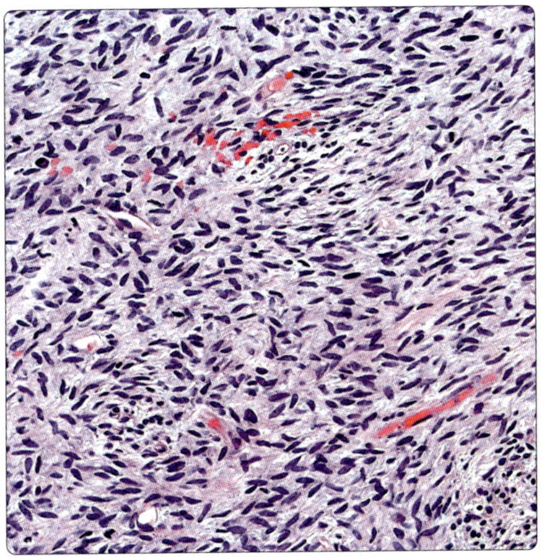

Cytologically Low-Grade Areas

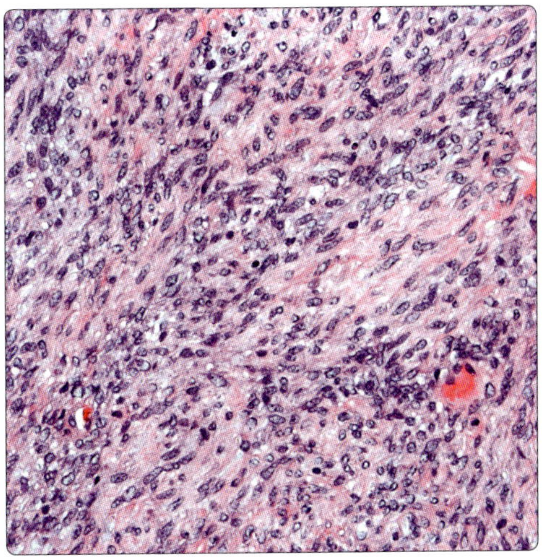

(Left) *General nuclear features of neural tumors, including elongated, tapered/pointed, wavy, or buckled nuclei are often seen at least focally in MPNST. The characteristic cytology may be difficult to appreciate in higher grade areas.* **(Right)** *It is not uncommon for an otherwise high-grade MPNST to contain areas that are cytologically lower grade, as depicted. In a minority of cases, low-grade morphology makes up most or all of the tumor (low-grade or well-differentiated MPNST).*

Perivascular Accentuation

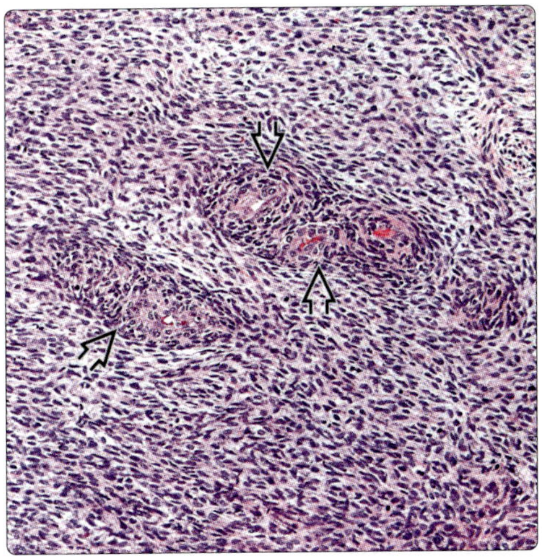

Perivascular Accentuation

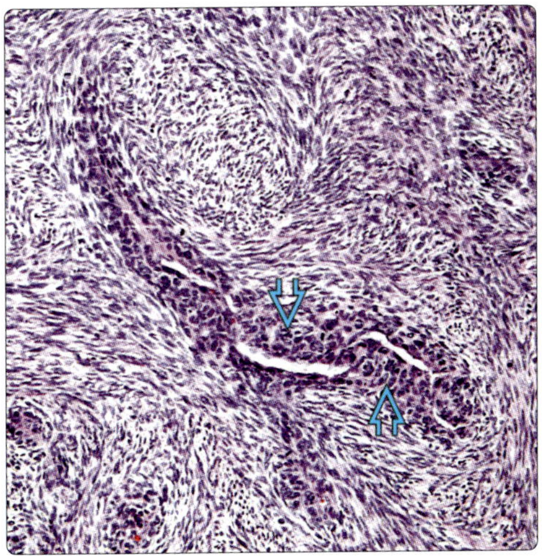

(Left) *A characteristic and helpful diagnostic feature of MPNST is the tendency of tumor cells to become larger and more rounded around the stromal blood vessels ➡. This pattern often makes the vessels stand out at low power and may even superficially resemble epithelial islands/nests.* **(Right)** *In some cases of MPNST, the larger tumor cells around the vessels appear to push ➡ or "herniate" into the lumen.*

Myxoid Stroma

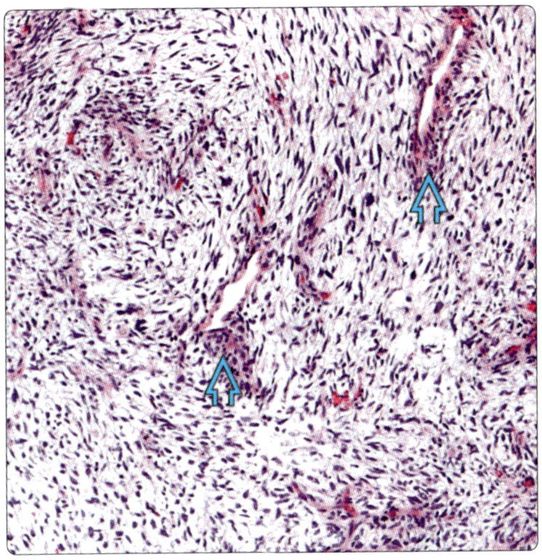

Collagenous Stroma

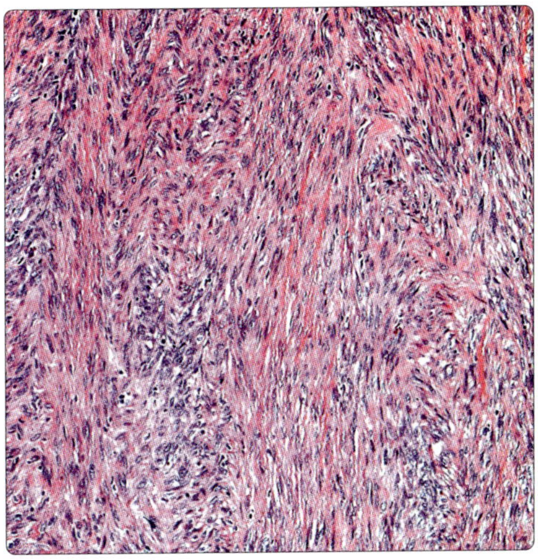

(Left) *This H&E shows a myxoid area of MPNST featuring nuclear pleomorphism, neural cytologic features, and stromal vessels with mild perivascular tumor cell accentuation ➡.* **(Right)** *Some areas of MPNST may contain more stromal collagen and appear more fibroblastic, as depicted, which may lead to consideration of a fibroblastic sarcoma or synovial sarcoma.*

(Left) *Coagulative tumor necrosis ⇨ is common in MPNST.* **(Right)** *Necrosis may be extensive and geographic in MPNST. In these situations, a common finding is the preservation of tumor cells only around vessels ⇨ (peritheliomatous pattern) with necrosis of the intervening cells. Although in no way pathognomonic, this pattern should always raise the possibility of MPNST.*

Coagulative Necrosis

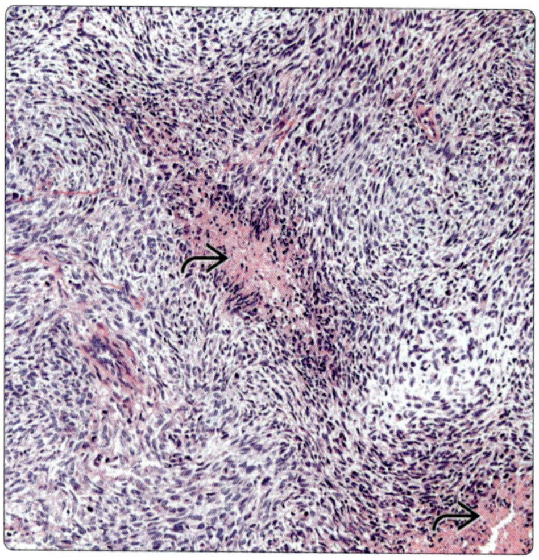

Geographic Necrosis

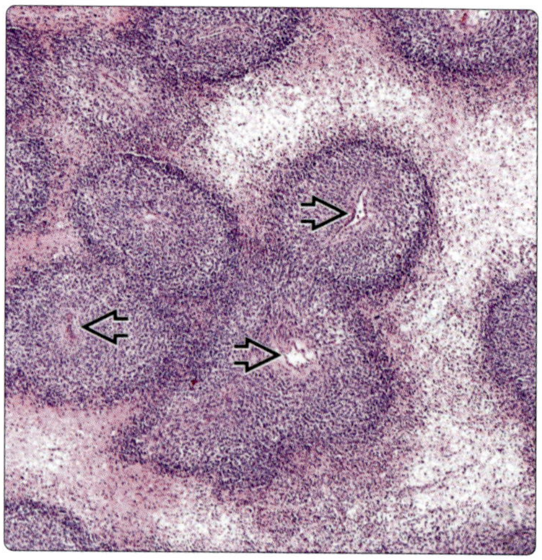

(Left) *A fascicular pattern of growth is common in MPNST. In occasional cases, a herringbone architecture may be identified, as shown. Note the prominent nuclear pleomorphism ⇨, which is not a feature of synovial sarcoma or adult-type fibrosarcoma.* **(Right)** *Fascicular growth may also be seen in areas with more collagenous stroma or myxoid stroma. Note the absence of nuclear pleomorphism in this H&E, which is not uncommon in MPNST.*

Fascicular Growth

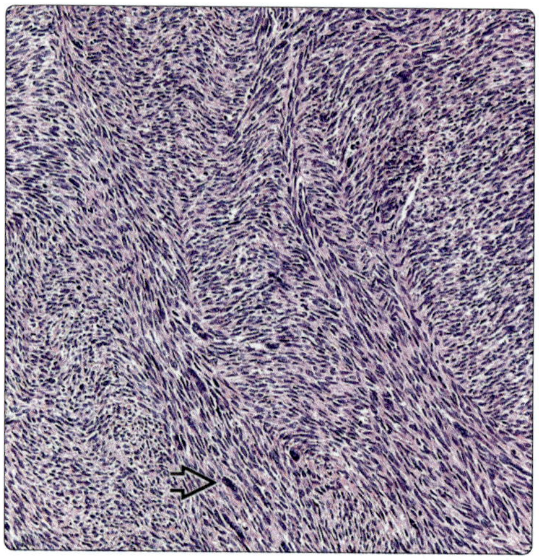

Fascicular Growth

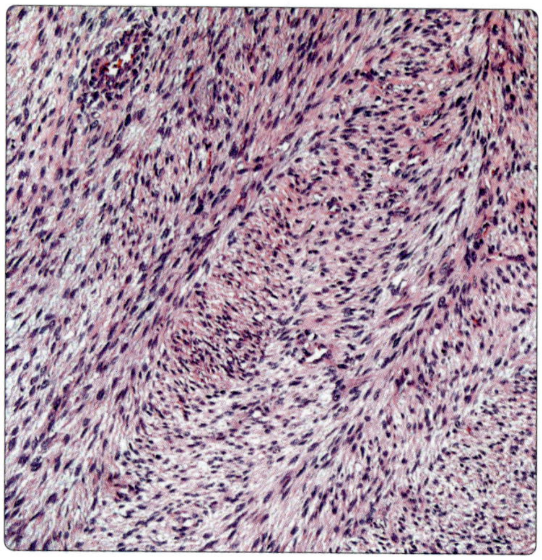

(Left) *Rare cases of MPNST show marked nuclear anaplasia and may mimic other pleomorphic sarcomas. Demonstration of origin from a nerve or benign nerve sheath tumor (mainly neurofibroma) is very helpful.* **(Right)** *A loose, whorling morphology similar to perineurioma may be seen in MPNST and is evidence of perineurial differentiation. IHC (EMA, Claudin-1) can be used to highlight this differentiation, though it is of no clinical significance.*

Marked Anaplasia

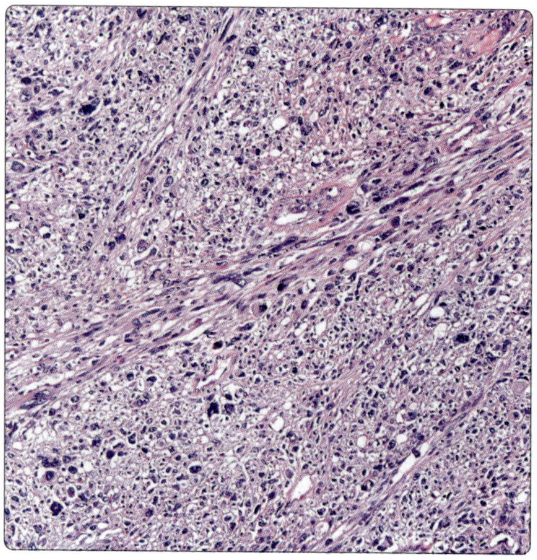

Perineurial Morphology

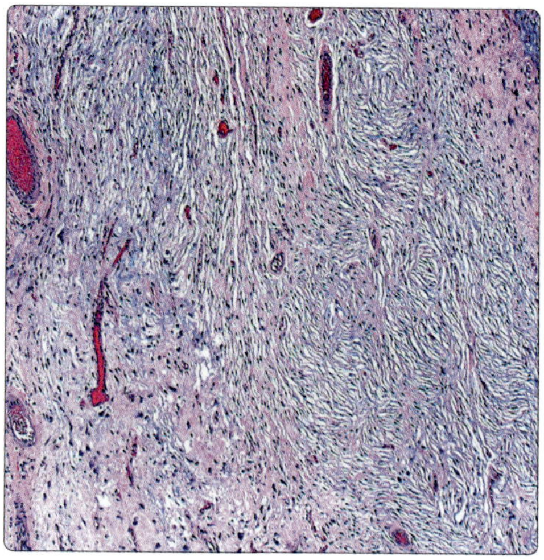

S100 Protein Expression

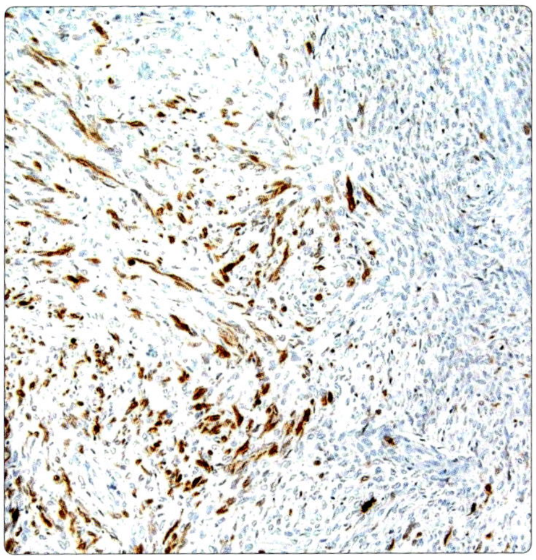

Origin From Nerve

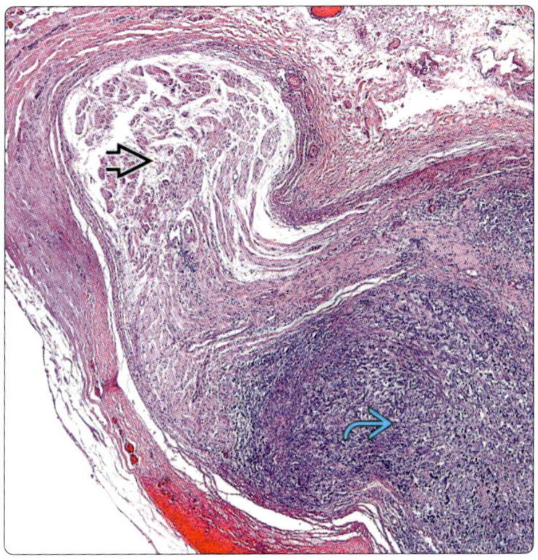

(Left) *S100 protein &/or SOX10 expression is only seen in ~ 50% of cases of MPNST and is characteristically focal or patchy. Diffuse expression of either marker is generally very rare and should raise the possibility of melanoma or cellular schwannoma.* **(Right)** *Origin from a nerve ➩ may be evident grossly &/or histologically in MPNST ➩; however, in some cases, imaging or intraoperative reports can provide this information. In yet other cases, nerve origin cannot be clearly demonstrated.*

Origin From Nerve

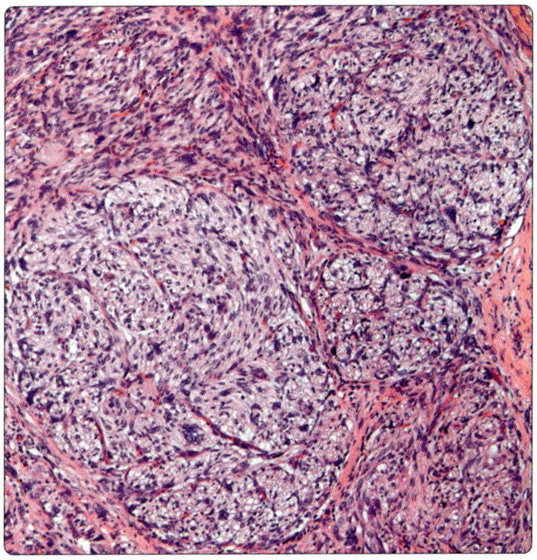

Origin From Neurofibroma

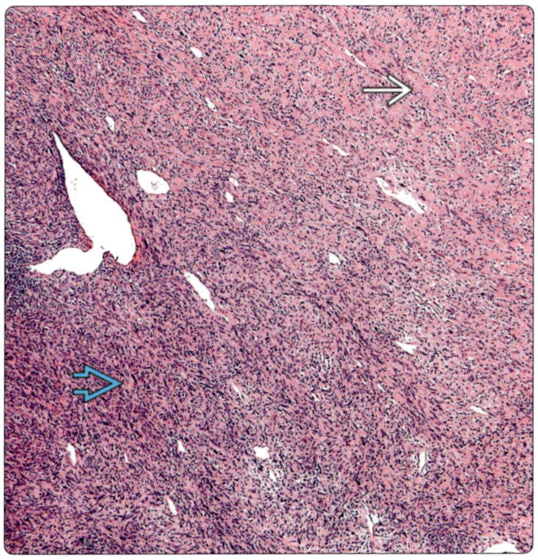

(Left) *This H&E shows cross sections of large nerve fibers being expanded and replaced by MPNST. Note the cellularity and marked pleomorphism.* **(Right)** *Certain forms of neurofibroma (particularly plexiform and large soft tissue ➔ types) are well known to carry a risk for malignant transformation into MPNST. This change ➩ is often heralded by a combination of increased cellularity, nuclear atypia, mitoses, &/or necrosis.*

Origin From Neurofibroma

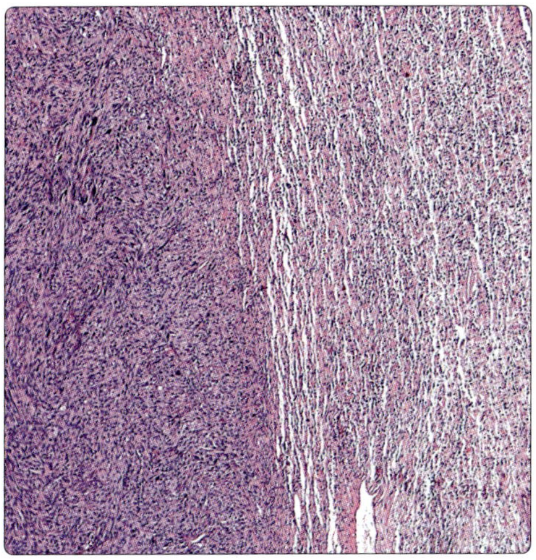

Origin From Neurofibroma

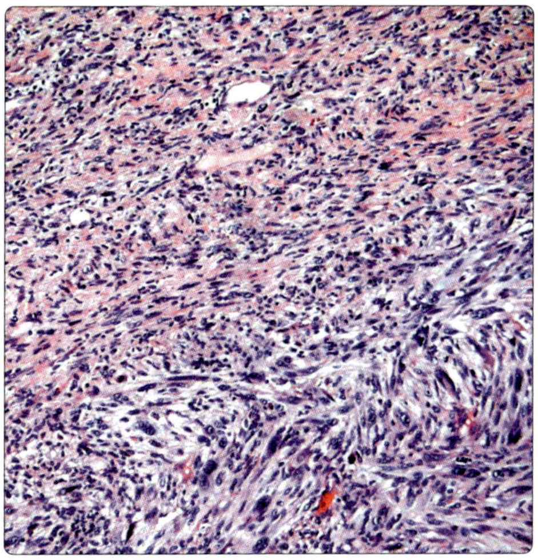

(Left) *This case of MPNST arising in a neurofibroma shows a more abrupt transition between the benign (right) and malignant (left) components.* **(Right)** *At high magnification, the increased cellularity, atypia, and mitoses indicate transformation from neurofibroma (top) into MPNST (bottom).*

(Left) *Up to 15% of cases of MPNST contain evidence of heterologous mesenchymal differentiation. The formation of bone and cartilage can be seen in this example.* **(Right)** *An MPNST with heterologous rhabdomyoblastic elements is also referred to as a malignant triton tumor. This distinction from conventional MPNST is important, as malignant triton tumors are generally more aggressive.*

Heterologous Mesenchymal Elements

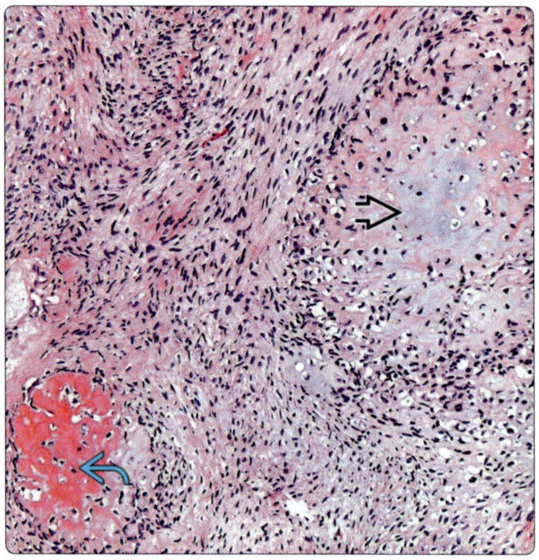

Malignant Triton Tumor

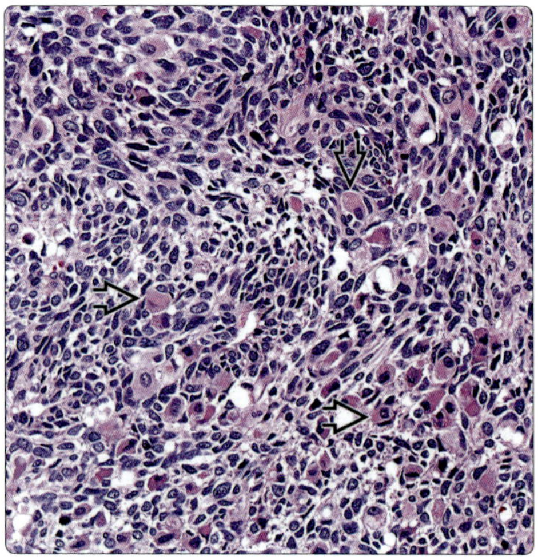

(Left) *Rare cases of MPNST may contain areas of angiosarcoma, as demonstrated in this H&E by irregular vascular channels lined by pleomorphic, hyperchromatic cells. IHC may be utilized to confirm the endothelial origin of the cells [CD31(+) &/or CD34(+)].* **(Right)** *Rarely, MPNST can contain heterologous glandular elements. The glands may or may not show evidence of mucin production and can sometimes show focal neuroendocrine differentiation.*

Heterologous Angiosarcoma

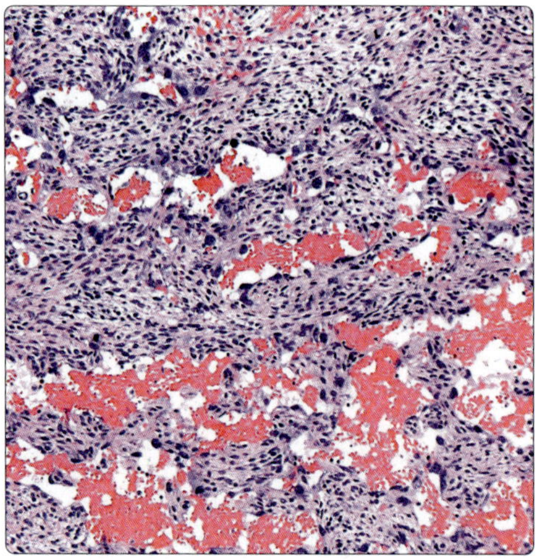

Rare Glandular Elements

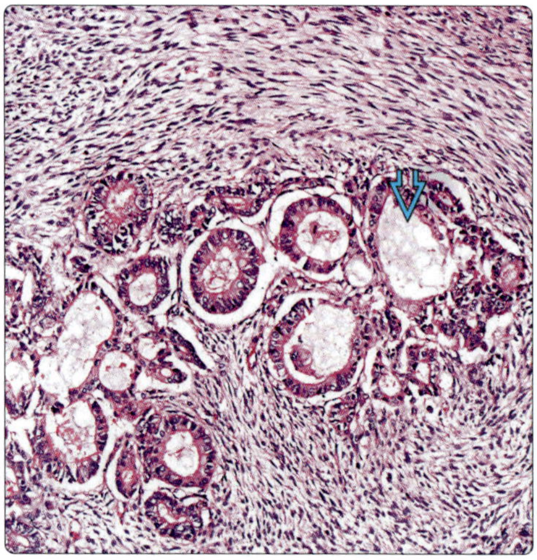

(Left) *The stromal vasculature is generally conspicuous in MPNST and is often highlighted by the characteristic perivascular tumor cell accentuation. Some vessels, however, lack this change, and others may appear more dilated or even staghorn.* **(Right)** *Rare cases of MPNST show a more developed hemangiopericytoma-like vasculature, as depicted, reminiscent of a solitary fibrous tumor.*

Prominent Vasculature

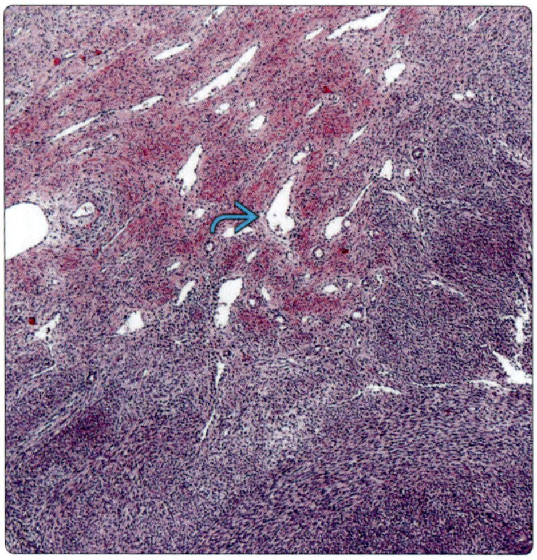

Hemangiopericytoma-Like Vessels

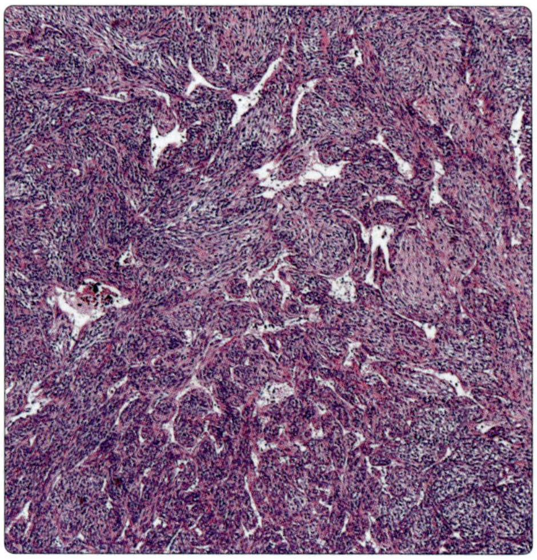

Small Cell Morphology

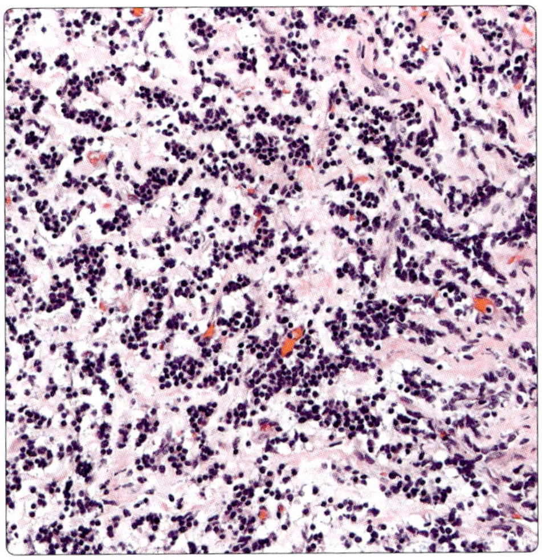

Small Cell Morphology

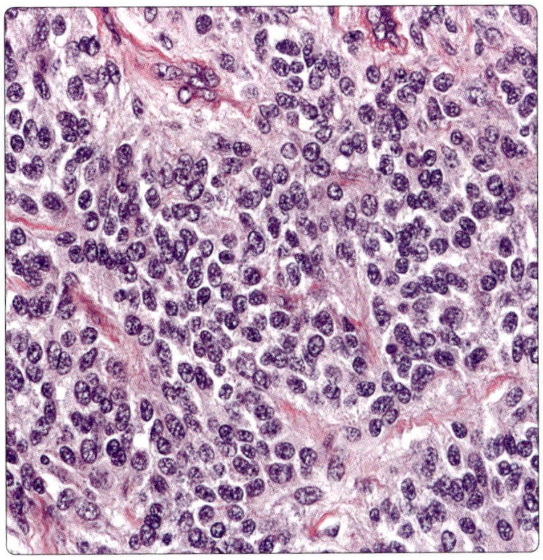

(Left) *Small cell change is an uncommon morphology in MPNST but when present can lead to consideration of a variety of other small round blue cell tumors, particularly on limited biopsy.* **(Right)** *MPNST can have prominent small round blue cell areas, mimicking Ewing sarcoma or poorly differentiated synovial sarcoma. Appropriate use of IHC and molecular analysis can resolve these differential diagnoses in most instances.*

Rare Nuclear Palisading

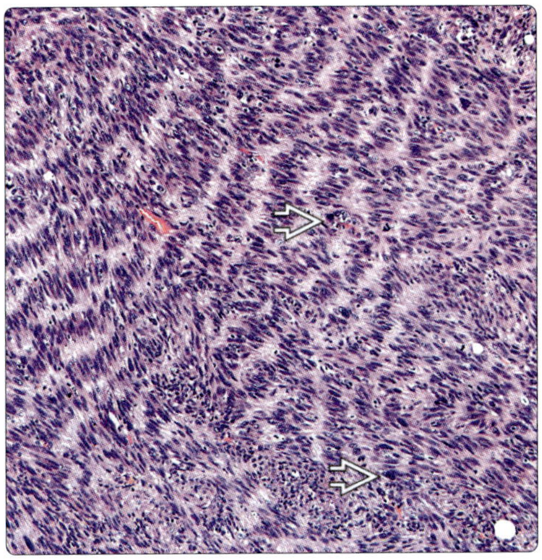

Rare Findings

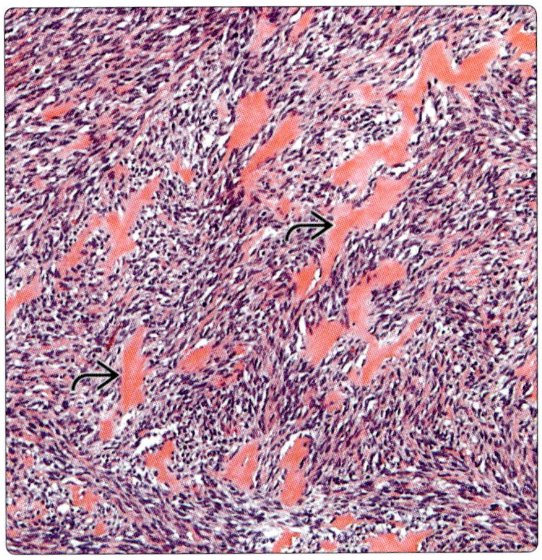

(Left) *Despite the neural origin of MPNST, nuclear palisading is an uncommon finding. Of note, this pattern can also be seen in other entities on the differential of MPNST, including synovial sarcoma and GI stromal tumor. Note the presence of nuclear pleomorphism* ⇨. **(Right)** *Discrete, thickened collagen bundles* ↪ *may rarely be seen in MPNST.*

Rare Findings

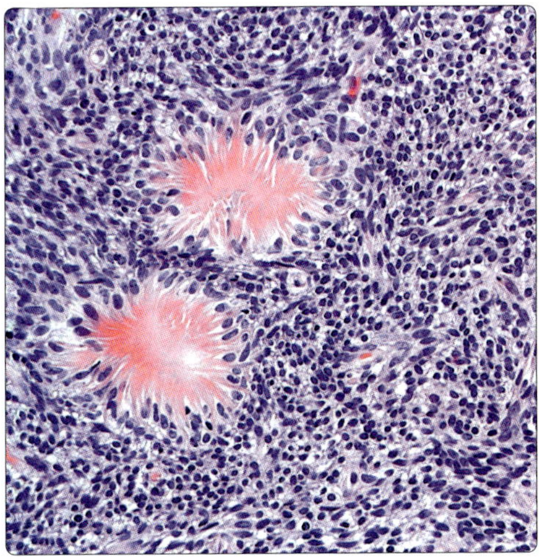

Rare Findings

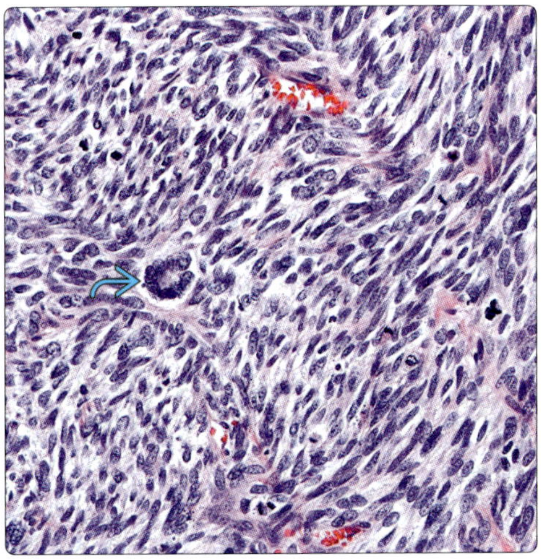

(Left) *Small, rosette-like structures may rarely be seen in MPNST, as depicted. Similar structures may be seen in the neuroblastoma-like variant of schwannoma; however, the latter lacks the other cytologic and architectural features of MPNST.* **(Right)** *Multinucleated giant cells* ↪ *are a very rare finding in MPNST.*

Epithelioid Malignant Peripheral Nerve Sheath Tumor

KEY FACTS

TERMINOLOGY

- Distinctive subtype of malignant peripheral nerve sheath tumor (MPNST) composed predominantly of epithelioid tumor cells and characterized in most cases by strong, diffuse S100 protein expression

ETIOLOGY/PATHOGENESIS

- No association with neurofibromatosis type 1

CLINICAL ISSUES

- Rare subtype of MPNST
- Affects mainly adults (median: 44 years)
- Usually involves extremities or trunk
  - Subcutaneous tissue > deep soft tissue
- Treatment: Complete surgical resection with negative margins
- Prognosis: Potential for aggressive clinical behavior
  - Local recurrence and distant metastasis in subset

MICROSCOPIC

- Lobular or multinodular growth common
- Sheets, nests, and cords of large epithelioid cells
- Large, irregular nucleus with vesicular chromatin and prominent nucleolus
- Variable collagenous to myxoid stroma

ANCILLARY TESTS

- Strong, diffuse S100 protein (+)
- Loss of nuclear INI1 in 50-60% of cases
- HMB-45, MART-1, SMA, desmin, CD31, CD34 (-)
- Intact nuclear expression of H3K27me3

TOP DIFFERENTIAL DIAGNOSES

- Epithelioid schwannoma
- Malignant melanoma
- Clear cell sarcoma
- Malignant myoepithelioma

(Left) *Epithelioid malignant peripheral nerve sheath tumor (EMPNST) is a distinctive subtype of malignant peripheral nerve sheath tumor (MPNST) that shows no clear association with neurofibromatosis type 1. Multinodular growth, as seen in this H&E, is a common feature of these tumors.* **(Right)** *The usual appearance of EMPNST is that of sheets, nests, and cords of large cells with eosinophilic to amphophilic cytoplasm within a myxoid to collagenous matrix.*

Epithelioid Malignant Peripheral Nerve Sheath Tumor

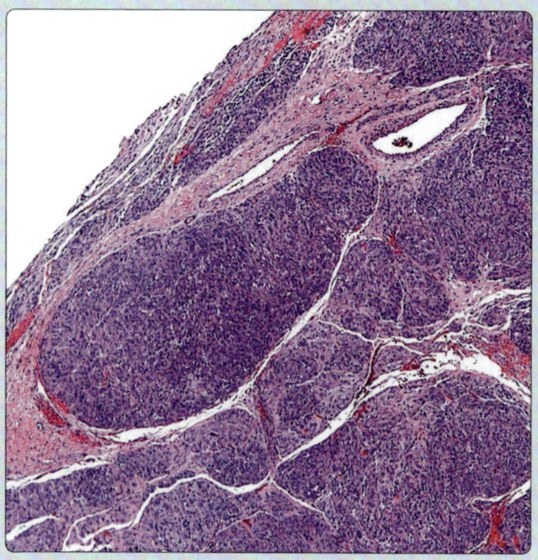

Typical Features

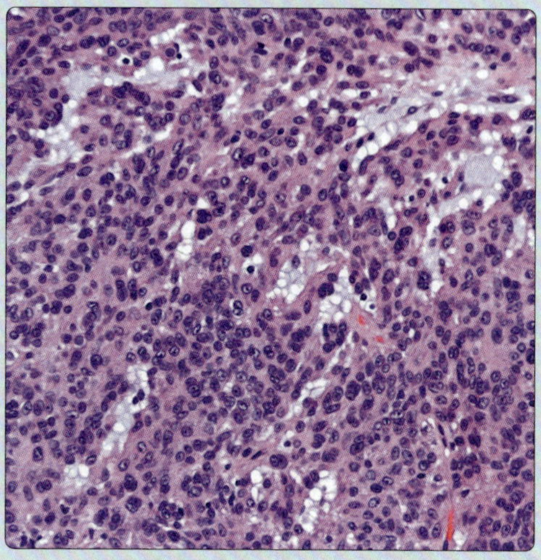

(Left) *The lesional cells of EMPNST characteristically contain a large, vesicular nucleus with a prominent nucleolus. Mitotic figures ➡ are usually easily identified and may be atypical/abnormal.* **(Right)** *In contrast to a conventional MPNST, the epithelioid subtype typically shows strong and diffuse expression of S100 protein, as shown. Due to this feature, epithelioid schwannoma and malignant melanoma must always be considered and excluded.*

Prominent Nucleoli

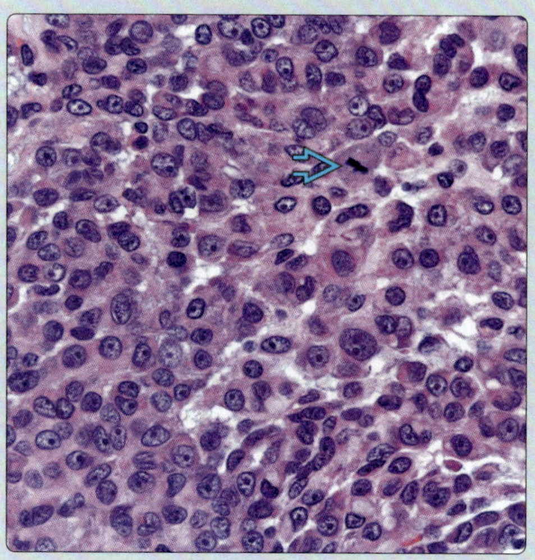

S100 Protein Expression

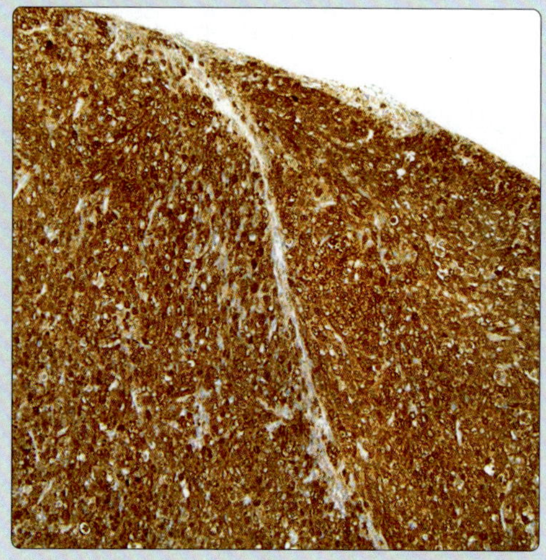

Epithelioid Malignant Peripheral Nerve Sheath Tumor

TERMINOLOGY

Abbreviations

- Epithelioid malignant peripheral nerve sheath tumor (EMPNST)

Synonyms

- Malignant epithelioid schwannoma

Definitions

- Distinctive subtype of malignant peripheral nerve sheath tumor (MPNST) composed predominantly of epithelioid tumor cells and characterized in most cases by strong, diffuse S100 protein expression

ETIOLOGY/PATHOGENESIS

Genetics

- No association with neurofibromatosis type 1

CLINICAL ISSUES

Epidemiology

- Incidence
  - Rare subtype of MPNST
    - ~ 5% of cases
- Age
  - Usually adults (median: 44 years)

Site

- Subcutaneous tissue more common than deep soft tissue
  - May infrequently arise in dermis
- Usually involves extremities (particularly lower)
  - Nearly 1/2 of cases arise in association with large nerve
- Also trunk; occasionally other sites

Presentation

- Slowly growing, painful or painless mass

Treatment

- Complete surgical resection with negative margins
- Postoperative tumor bed radiation may be utilized

Prognosis

- Potential for aggressive clinical behavior
  - Low to moderate risk of local recurrence
  - Distant metastases to lung, pleura, other sites in 10-50%
- Superficial tumors may exhibit better overall prognosis with lower risk of adverse outcome
  - However, recent study suggests that superficial and deep tumors show same potential for aggressive behavior

MACROSCOPIC

General Features

- Multinodular, well demarcated
- Firm, fleshy, tan-gray cut surface

Size

- Median: 3 cm (range: 0.4-20.0 cm)

MICROSCOPIC

Histologic Features

- Lobular or multinodular growth common
  - Superficial tumors may appear encapsulated
- Sheets, nests, and cords of large epithelioid cells
  - Abundant eosinophilic to amphophilic cytoplasm
    - May show rhabdoid cytomorphology
    - Rare clear cell change
  - Large, irregular nucleus with vesicular chromatin and prominent nucleolus
    - Mitoses common
- Minor areas showing spindled morphology may be present
- Variable collagenous to myxoid stroma
- Coagulative necrosis may be present
- May arise in background of benign peripheral nerve sheath tumor, particularly schwannoma
- Rare tumors demonstrate overall low histologic grade

ANCILLARY TESTS

Immunohistochemistry

- Strong, diffuse S100 protein (+) in majority
- Loss of nuclear INI1 in 50-60% of cases
- HMB-45, MART-1, SMA, desmin, CD31, CD34 (-)
- Intact nuclear expression of H3K27me3

DIFFERENTIAL DIAGNOSIS

Epithelioid Schwannoma

- Usually clinically small lesions
- Small nuclei lacking diffuse atypia, macronucleoli, atypical mitoses, and necrosis

Malignant Melanoma

- Clinical history or junctional component may be present
- Often significant nuclear pleomorphism/atypia
- S100 protein (+), HMB-45(+), MART-1(+)

Clear Cell Sarcoma

- S100 protein (+), HMB-45(+), MART-1(+)
- Characteristic t(12;22) with *EWSR1* rearrangement

Malignant Myoepithelioma

- Often keratin (+) &/or EMA(+) as well as S100 protein (+)
  - May also express SMA, GFAP, calponin, desmin, others
- May show formation of epithelial (ductal) structures
- *EWSR1* translocation in 50% of cases

Other Epithelioid Malignancies

- e.g., lymphoma, epithelioid sarcoma, angiosarcoma, extrarenal rhabdoid tumor, rhabdomyosarcoma
- Each can be distinguished by immunohistochemistry

SELECTED REFERENCES

1. Asano N et al: Immunohistochemistry for trimethylated H3K27 in the diagnosis of malignant peripheral nerve sheath tumours. Histopathology. 70(3):385-93, 2017
2. Jo VY et al: Epithelioid malignant peripheral nerve sheath tumor: clinicopathologic analysis of 63 cases. Am J Surg Pathol. 39(5):673-82, 2015
3. Carter JM et al: Epithelioid malignant peripheral nerve sheath tumor arising in a schwannoma, in a patient with "neuroblastoma-like" schwannomatosis and a novel germline SMARCB1 mutation. Am J Surg Pathol. 36(1):154-60, 2012

(Left) *Lobular or nodular architecture is common in EMPNST. In some cases, the tumor cell nodules are separated by thick fibrous septa, as seen in this H&E.* **(Right)** *Solid growth may be seen in EMPNST, either focally or in most of the tumor. Together with the cytologic features, this morphology can raise suspicions for melanoma. Immunohistochemical evaluation with melanocytic markers is often very helpful.*

Lobulated Appearance

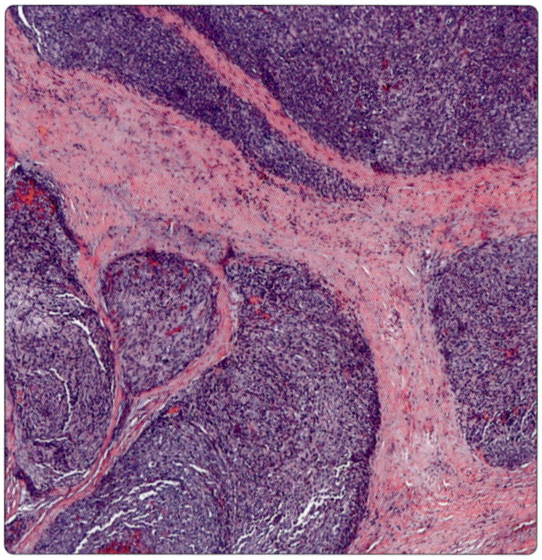

Solid Sheets

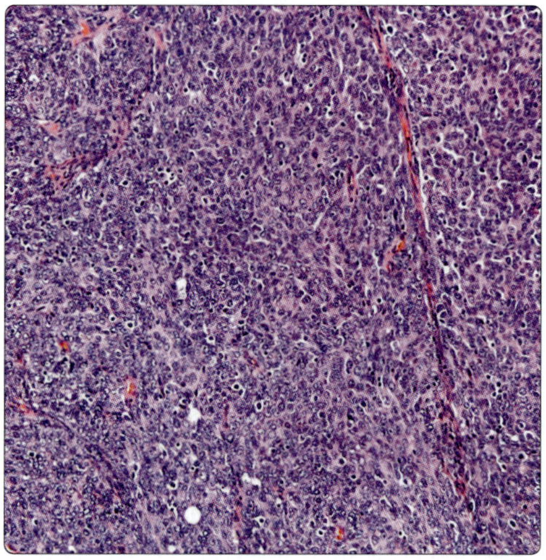

(Left) *Coagulative necrosis may be seen in EMPNST; however, in general, it is not as common as in other high-grade sarcomas. Necrosis may be focal* ⇒*, as depicted, or rarely geographic.* **(Right)** *Myxoid matrix is a relatively common finding in EMPNST and varies widely in amount and distribution. Extensively myxoid examples can closely resemble soft tissue myoepithelioma or myoepithelial carcinoma.*

Necrosis

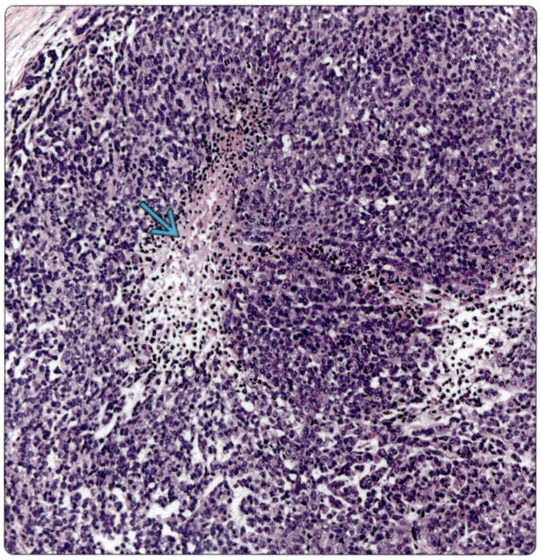

Prominent Myxoid Matrix

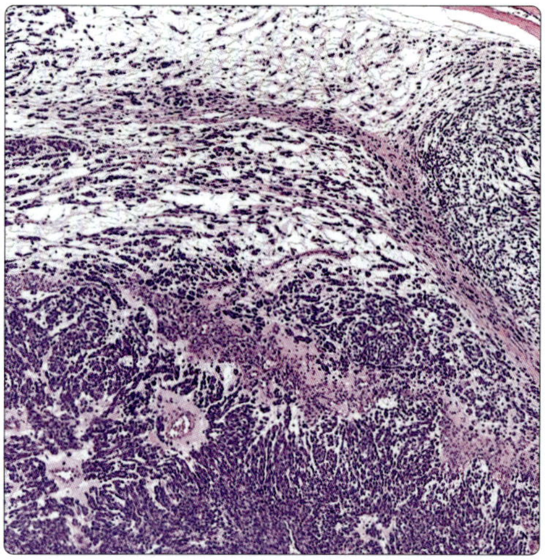

(Left) *Some areas in EMPNST may be less cellular and show small clusters or individual cells within a myxoid or collagenous matrix. Note the prominent nucleoli.* **(Right)** *This case of EMPNST had areas containing nests of tumor cells showing more abundant eosinophilic cytoplasm, all within a loose myxoid matrix.*

Hypocellular Areas

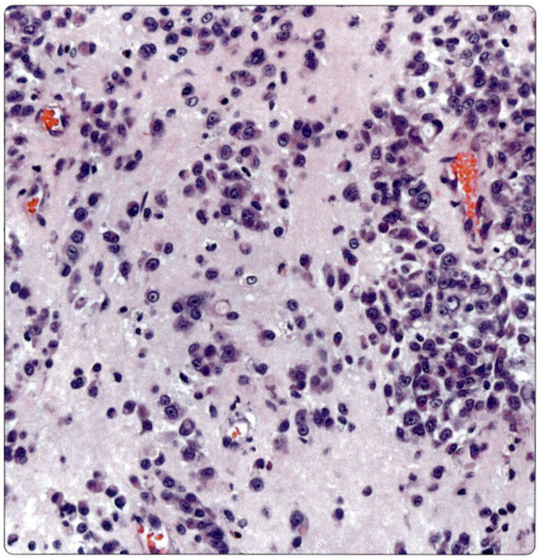

Abundant Cytoplasm

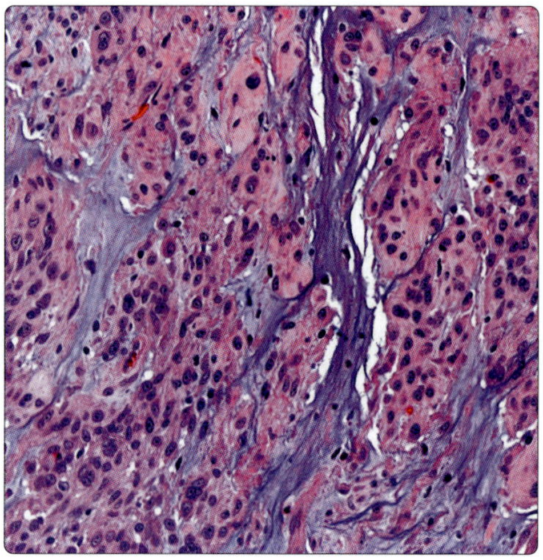

Spindled Morphology

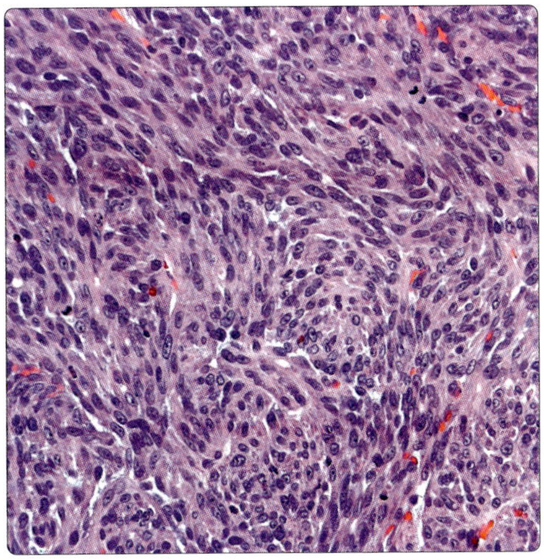

Spindled and Epithelioid Morphology

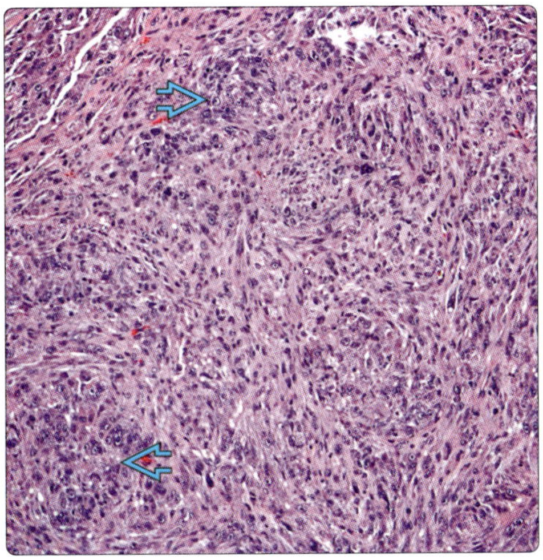

(Left) *The presence of spindling in otherwise cytologically typical tumor cells is not uncommon in EMPNST and can resemble conventional spindle cell MPNST.* **(Right)** *This EMPNST contained minor areas of spindled tumor cells with scattered nests and clusters of epithelioid cells* ⇨. *The majority of the tumor, however, showed a prominent epithelioid morphology.*

Clear Cell Change

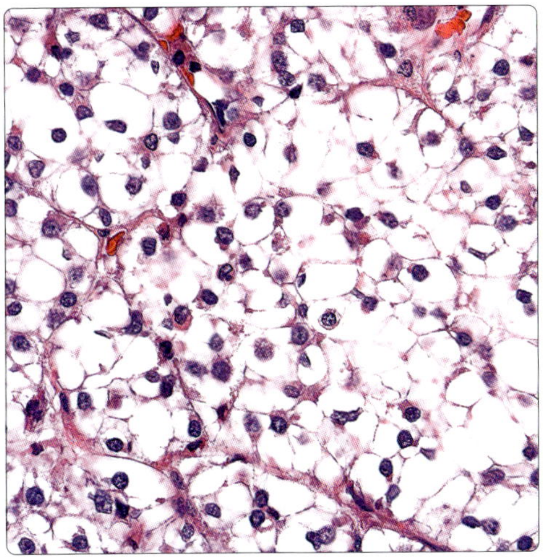

Rhabdoid Cells

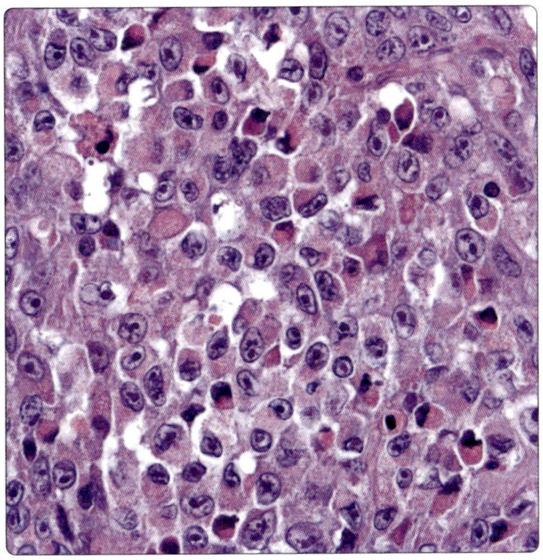

(Left) *Prominent clear cell change may be seen in some cases of EMPNST and may lead to confusion with clear cell sarcoma.* **(Right)** *Rhabdoid cells can be seen in EMPNST and should raise consideration of other tumors that may show a rhabdoid cytomorphology, including melanoma. Of note, ~ 50-60% of cases of EMPNST show loss of nuclear INI1.*

Rare Nuclear Pleomorphism

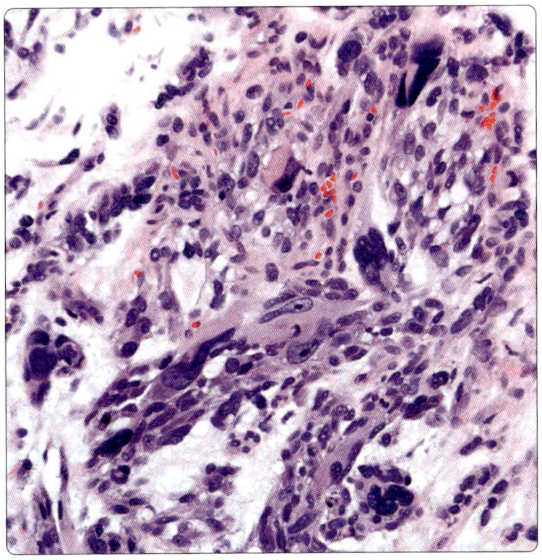

Loss of Nuclear INI1

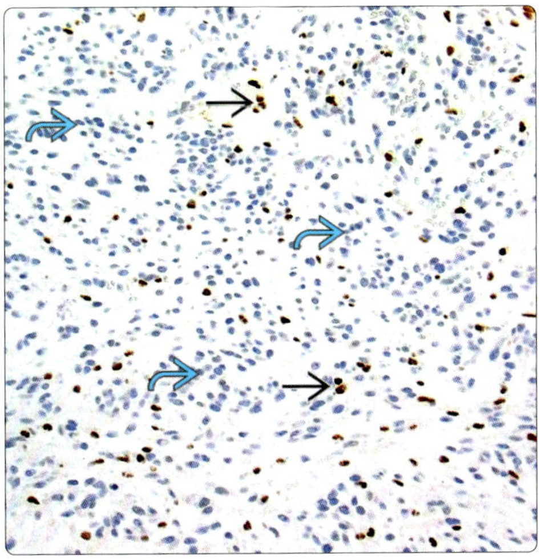

(Left) *Significant nuclear pleomorphism is generally uncommon in EMPNST; however, rare cases may contain cells with bizarre nuclei, as depicted.* **(Right)** *Nuclear loss* ➩ *of INI1 can be seen in 40-60% of cases of EMPNST. Scattered inflammatory cells* → *are often positive for the marker and should be ignored.*

Ectomesenchymoma

KEY FACTS

TERMINOLOGY

- Synonym: Malignant ectomesenchymoma
- Tumor composed of rhabdomyosarcoma (RMS) and neural or neuronal elements

ETIOLOGY/PATHOGENESIS

- Possible origin from pluripotent embryologic migratory neural crest cells

CLINICAL ISSUES

- Usually childhood (< 4 years)
- Head and neck, paratesticular region, abdomen, pelvis
- Treatment: Generally approached like RMS
  - International Rhabdomyosarcoma Group (IRSG) protocol
- Usually aggressive clinical course

MACROSCOPIC

- Median: 5 cm

MICROSCOPIC

- Combination of RMS with variable neural component
  - Components often intermingled
- RMS component often embryonal type
- Variable neural/neuronal component
  - Ganglioneuroma, neuroblastoma, malignant peripheral nerve sheath tumor (MPNST), PNET

ANCILLARY TESTS

- Desmin (+) and myogenin (+) in RMS component
- S100 protein (+) in Schwann cell component
- NB84(+), synaptophysin (+), CD56(+) in neuroblastic component

TOP DIFFERENTIAL DIAGNOSES

- Embryonal RMS
- Malignant triton tumor
- Neuroblastoma
- Ganglioneuroma

Ectomesenchymoma

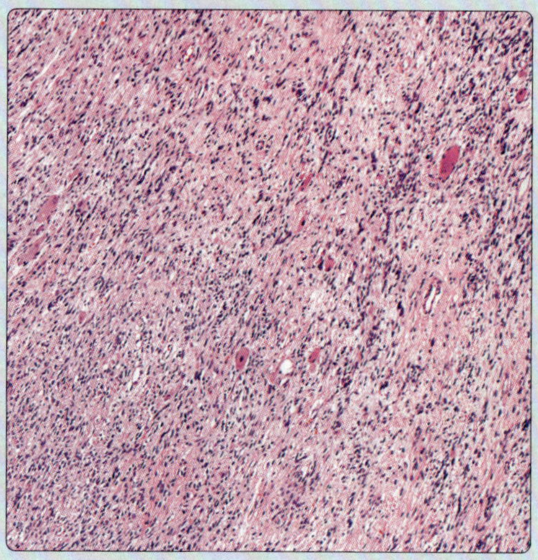

Ectomesenchymoma

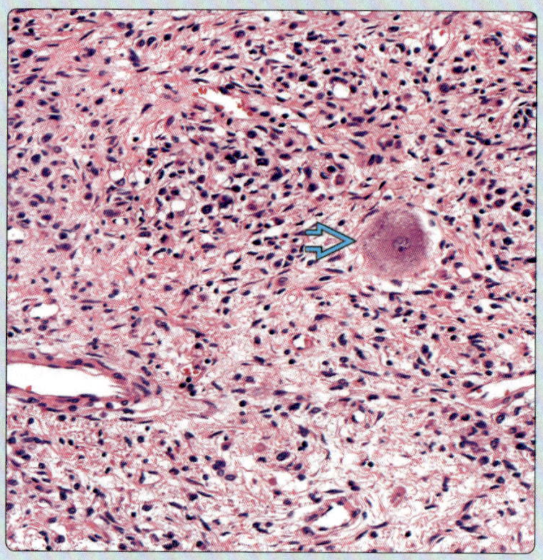

(Left) *Ectomesenchymoma is a very rare and often clinically aggressive tumor that typically features a combination of rhabdomyosarcoma (RMS), usually embryonal type, and neural or neuronal elements (such as ganglion cells or neuroblastic cells).* **(Right)** *This H&E shows a single ganglion cell ➩ amidst rounded cells with small hyperchromatic nuclei dispersed in a fibrillary background. Typically, the elements of ectomesenchymoma are randomly intermingled.*

Rhabdomyoblastic Elements

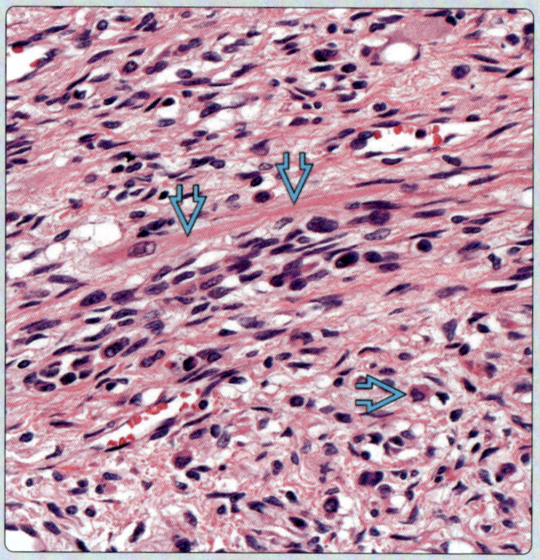

Schwann Cell Component

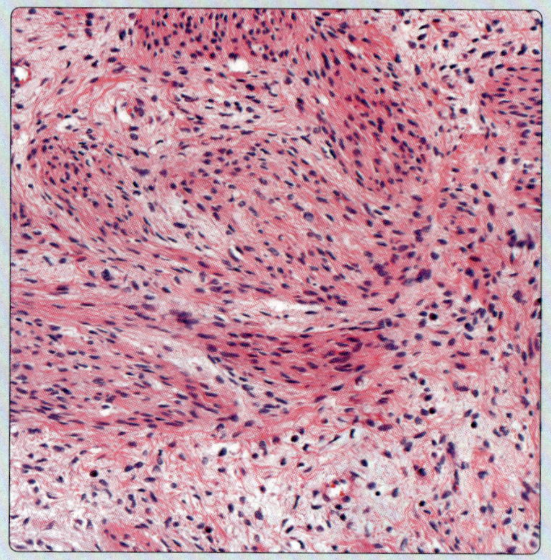

(Left) *The RMS component of ectomesenchymoma is most often embryonal type, but spindle cell and alveolar RMS may also be seen. Rhabdomyoblastic elements ➩ are often readily identifiable.* **(Right)** *Ectomesenchymoma may contain areas showing fascicles of differentiated Schwann cells, as depicted, similar to ganglioneuroma or even cellular schwannoma. S100 protein expression is seen in these areas.*

TERMINOLOGY

Synonyms

- Malignant ectomesenchymoma
- Gangliorhabdomyosarcoma

Definitions

- Tumor composed of rhabdomyosarcoma (RMS) and neural or neuronal elements

ETIOLOGY/PATHOGENESIS

Uncertain Etiology

- Possible origin from pluripotent embryologic migratory neural crest cells
- Possible RMS variant
  - Ganglion cells reported in rare cases of both metastatic and treated RMS
  - Gene expression profiling suggests genetic link to RMS

CLINICAL ISSUES

Epidemiology

- Incidence
  - Extremely rare
- Age
  - Usually childhood (< 4 years)

Site

- Head and neck
  - Nasal cavity, orbit
- Paratesticular region
- Abdomen, pelvis
- CNS

Presentation

- Often, rapidly growing mass
- Superficial or deep soft tissues

Treatment

- Generally approached like RMS
  - Treated per International Rhabdomyosarcoma Group (IRSG) protocols

Prognosis

- Usually aggressive clinical course
- Favorable prognostic factors
  - Tumor size < 10 cm, superficial location, low stage at presentation
  - Absence of alveolar RMS component

MACROSCOPIC

General Features

- Lobular
- Well circumscribed or infiltrative
- Hemorrhage and necrosis

Size

- Median: 5 cm

MICROSCOPIC

Histologic Features

- Combination of RMS with variable neural component
  - Components often intermingled
  - RMS
    - Sheets, nests, or cords of small round cells
      - Can resemble embryonal, alveolar, or spindle cell RMS
    - Spindled or rounded rhabdomyoblasts with eosinophilic cytoplasm
  - Variable neural/neuronal component
    - Ganglioneuroma
      - Ganglion cells in variable numbers
      - Differentiated Schwann cells in fascicles or whorls
    - Neuroblastoma
      - Clusters or nodules of small primitive cells
    - Primitive neuroectodermal tumor
    - Malignant peripheral nerve sheath tumor

ANCILLARY TESTS

Immunohistochemistry

- Desmin (+) and myogenin (+) in RMS component
- S100 protein (+) in Schwann cell component
- NB84(+), synaptophysin (+), CD56(+) in neuroblastic component
- Retained H3K27me3 expression

Genetic Testing

- *HRAS* mutations common

DIFFERENTIAL DIAGNOSIS

Embryonal Rhabdomyosarcoma

- Can be impossible to distinguish from ectomesenchymoma on limited biopsy
  - Embryonal RMS is far more common, however
- Absence of neural/neuroectodermal component

Malignant Triton Tumor

- MPNST with heterologous rhabdomyoblastic elements
  - Rhabdomyoblastic component often discrete rather than diffusely intermingled
- Lacks ganglion cells and other neural/neuroectodermal component

Neuroblastoma

- Arises along sympathetic chain
- Lacks rhabdomyosarcomatous component

Ganglioneuroma

- Mixture of Schwann cells and mature ganglion cells
- Lacks component of RMS or neuroblastoma

SELECTED REFERENCES

1. Griffin BB et al: Malignant ectomesenchymoma: series analysis of a histologically and genetically heterogeneous tumor. Int J Surg Pathol. 1066896917734915, 2017
2. Huang SC et al: Frequent HRAS mutations in malignant ectomesenchymoma: overlapping genetic abnormalities with embryonal rhabdomyosarcoma. Am J Surg Pathol. 40(7):876-85, 2016

SECTION 13

Genital Stromal Tumors

Fibroepithelial Stromal Polyp	574
Angiomyofibroblastoma	576
Cellular Angiofibroma	580
Deep (Aggressive) Angiomyxoma	584

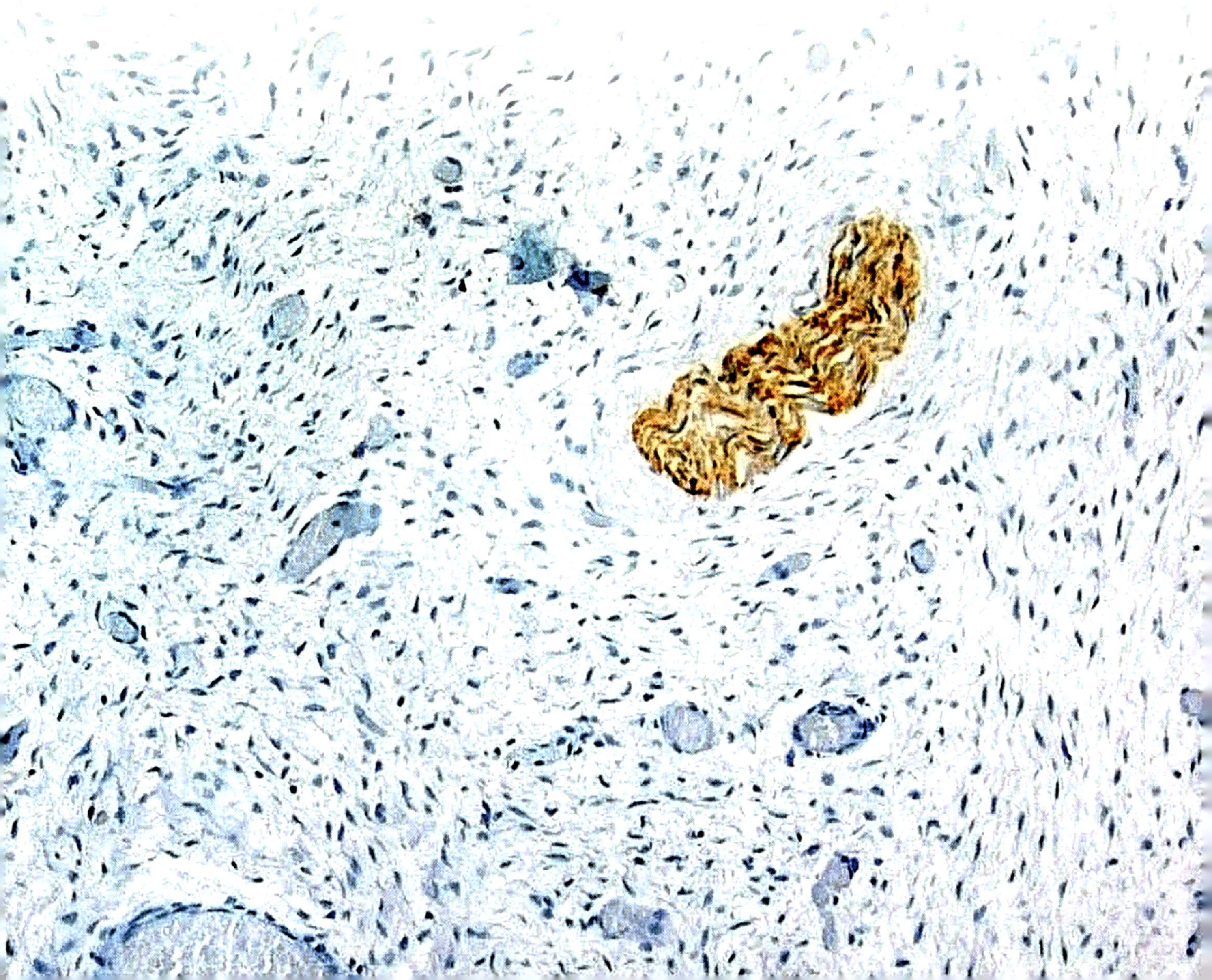

Fibroepithelial Stromal Polyp

KEY FACTS

TERMINOLOGY

- Benign polypoid fibroblastic proliferation, usually involving vagina in women of reproductive age

CLINICAL ISSUES

- Occurs in women, usually in vagina or vulva
- Wide age range (particularly reproductive years)
- 1/2 of patients are asymptomatic
- Significant association with pregnancy
- Treatment: Simple excision
- Benign; rare recurrences

MACROSCOPIC

- Often polypoid
- Usually 1-3 cm

MICROSCOPIC

- No grenz zone between lesion and overlying squamous mucosa
- Spindle to stellate cells
    - Multinucleation and nuclear enlargement common
- Fibrous, edematous, or myxoid stroma
- Can be alarmingly cellular with nuclear pleomorphism and mitotic figures
    - Most often seen in pregnancy

ANCILLARY TESTS

- Immunophenotype
    - Desmin (+), ER(+), PR(+)
    - Variable CD34(+) and SMA(+)
    - Myogenin (-), MYOD1(-)

TOP DIFFERENTIAL DIAGNOSES

- Aggressive angiomyxoma
- Angiomyofibroblastoma
- Cellular angiofibroma
- Botryoid rhabdomyosarcoma
- Genital rhabdomyoma

(Left) *Fibroepithelial stromal polyp (FSP) most often presents as a small, polypoid mass on the vagina or vulva. Most cases are hypocellular and contain a myxoid or edematous stroma. The overlying epidermis is usually unremarkable or reactive.* **(Right)** *A helpful feature for identifying FSP is the absence of a grenz zone (normal subepithelial tissue) between the lesion and overlying squamous mucosa. This is in direct contrast to other benign genital stromal tumors.*

Fibroepithelial Stromal Polyp

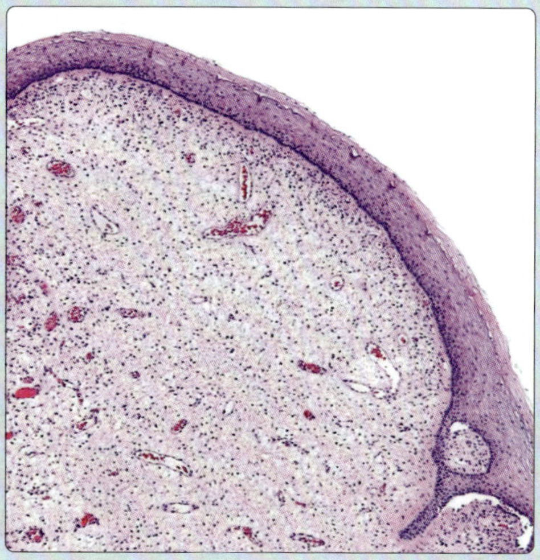

Grenz Zone Absent

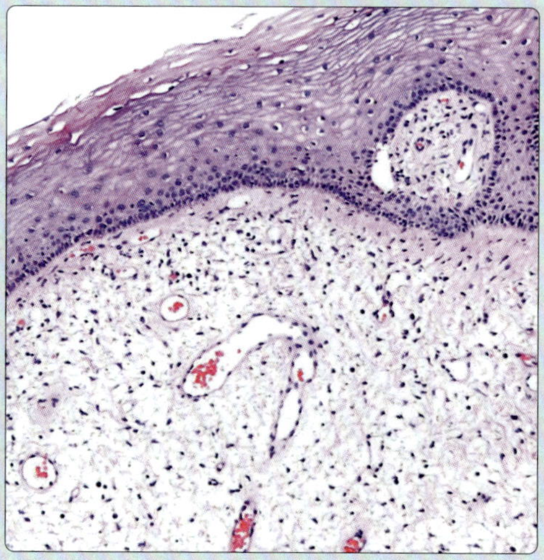

(Left) *The cells of FSP have eosinophilic cytoplasm and are usually spindled with bipolar processes. Stellate and multinucleated forms → are common and are often seen close to the overlying mucosa.* **(Right)** *Occasional cases of FSP (particularly those that occur during pregnancy) show marked cellularity and nuclear pleomorphism. Mitotic figures, including atypical forms, may also be seen. This variant has been described as cellular pseudosarcomatous fibroepithelial stromal polyp. Note the absence of a grenz zone →.*

Nuclear Morphology

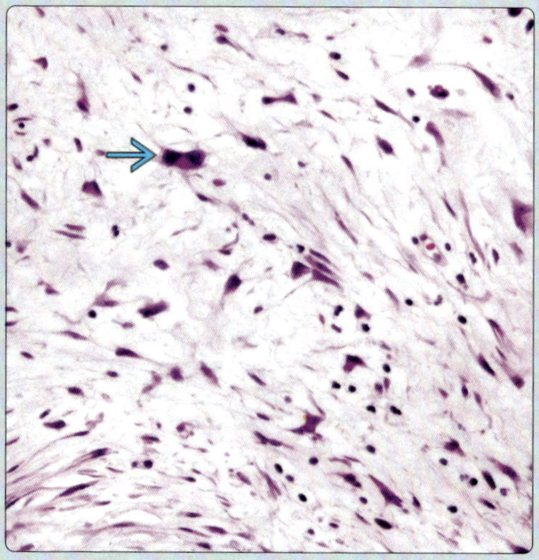

Pseudosarcomatous Change

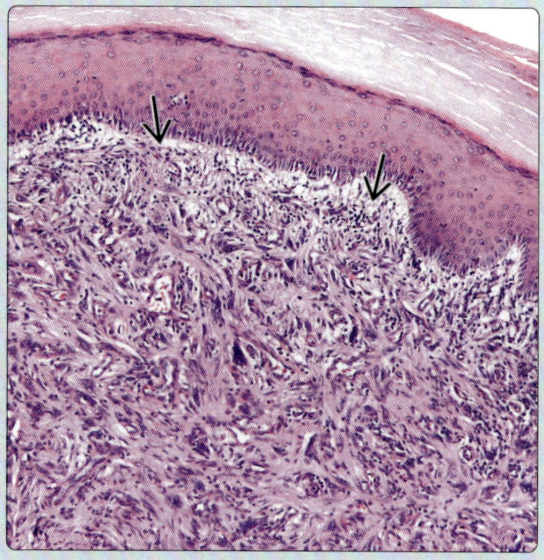

TERMINOLOGY

Abbreviations

- Fibroepithelial stromal polyp (FSP)

Synonyms

- Mesodermal stromal polyp
- Cellular pseudosarcomatous fibroepithelial stromal polyp; pseudosarcoma botryoides

Definitions

- Benign polypoid fibroblastic proliferation, usually involving vagina in women of reproductive age

CLINICAL ISSUES

Epidemiology

- Incidence
  - Relatively common
- Age
  - Wide range (particularly reproductive years)
- Sex
  - Women

Site

- Usually vagina or vulva
  - Rarely cervix

Presentation

- 1/2 of patients are asymptomatic
- May present with vaginal bleeding or local pain
- Association with pregnancy
  - Likely hormone related
  - Polyps may be multiple

Treatment

- Simple excision

Prognosis

- Benign
- Recurrence is rare
  - May be associated with subsequent pregnancies or presence of atypical features
- Regression reported in some infants

MACROSCOPIC

General Features

- Often polypoid
- Smooth or villiform surface

Size

- Usually 1-3 cm

MICROSCOPIC

Histologic Features

- Overlying squamous mucosa is often unremarkable or reactive
  - No grenz zone between lesion and overlying mucosa
- Spindle to stellate cells
  - Tapering cytoplasmic processes
  - Multinucleation and nuclear enlargement common
    - May have wreath-like appearance
- Fibrous, edematous, or myxoid stroma
- Thick- or thin-walled vessels more prominent in center of lesion
- Larger lesions can undergo torsion
  - Imparts striking edema/myxoid change
- Can be alarmingly cellular with nuclear pleomorphism and mitotic figures
  - Most often seen in pregnancy

ANCILLARY TESTS

Immunohistochemistry

- Desmin (+), ER(+), PR(+)
- Variable CD34(+) and SMA(+)
- Myogenin (-), MYOD1(-)

DIFFERENTIAL DIAGNOSIS

Aggressive Angiomyxoma

- Poorly circumscribed, large, deep masses
- Medium- and large-caliber vessels common throughout lesion
- Multinucleated cells uncommon
- Similar immunophenotype to FSP

Angiomyofibroblastoma

- Well-circumscribed mass rather than polyp
- Grenz zone in superficial lesions
- Plump epithelioid to spindled cells proliferating around vessels
- Similar immunophenotype to FSP

Cellular Angiofibroma

- Occurs in both men and women
- Well-circumscribed mass rather than polyp
- Grenz zone in superficial lesions
- Uniformly cellular spindle cells in myxocollagenous stroma
- Medium-sized vessels with hyalinized vessels common
- CD34(+), ER/PR(+); usually desmin (-); loss of Rb protein

Botryoid-Type Embryonal Rhabdomyosarcoma

- Young patients, polypoid masses
- Cellular subepithelial layer ("cambium layer")
- Cytologically malignant cells
- Desmin (+), myogenin (+), MYOD1(+)

Genital Rhabdomyoma

- Similar clinical presentation to FSP
- Contains variable number of rhabdomyoblasts

SELECTED REFERENCES

1. Madueke-Laveaux OS et al: Giant fibroepithelial stromal polyp of the vulva: largest case reported. Ann Surg Innov Res. 7:8, 2013
2. Song JS et al: Cellular pseudosarcomatous fibroepithelial stromal polyp of the vagina during pregnancy: a lesion that is overdiagnosed as a malignant tumor. Korean J Pathol. 46(5):494-8, 2012
3. Wani Y et al: A vulvar fibroepithelial stromal polyp appearing in infancy. Am J Dermatopathol. 31(5):465-7, 2009
4. Nucci MR et al: Vulvovaginal soft tissue tumours: update and review. Histopathology. 36(2):97-108, 2000
5. Nucci MR et al: Cellular pseudosarcomatous fibroepithelial stromal polyps of the lower female genital tract: an underrecognized lesion often misdiagnosed as sarcoma. Am J Surg Pathol. 24(2):231-40, 2000

Angiomyofibroblastoma

KEY FACTS

TERMINOLOGY

- Benign genital stromal tumor composed of fibroblasts oriented around prominent capillary vasculature

CLINICAL ISSUES

- Occurs in women between 35-60 years (median: 46)
- Vulva and vagina most common sites
- Slow-growing, painless mass
- Treatment: Simple local excision
- Benign

MACROSCOPIC

- Superficial, well-circumscribed, solid mass

MICROSCOPIC

- Nonencapsulated
- Alternating zones of cellularity
- Prominent vascular component
- Plump epithelioid, ovoid, or plasmacytoid tumor cells with eosinophilic cytoplasm
  - Cells characteristically cluster around thin-walled capillaries
- In postmenopausal patients, cells are more spindled and overall cellularity is low
- Mature adipose tissue component in minority of cases
- Some cases show morphologic overlap with cellular angiofibroma

ANCILLARY TESTS

- Desmin (+), ER(+), PR(+)
- Usually CD34(-) and SMA(-)

TOP DIFFERENTIAL DIAGNOSES

- Deep (aggressive) angiomyxoma
- Cellular angiofibroma
- Fibroepithelial stromal polyp

(Left) *Angiomyofibroblastoma is a distinctive, benign neoplasm of the lower female genital tract. At low magnification, the classic morphologic pattern is that of irregular zones of cellularity within a myxoid or fibrous stroma.* **(Right)** *Some areas of angiomyofibroblastoma are less myxoid and more fibrous, as seen here. Note the sharp circumscription →, a feature seen in most examples.*

Angiomyofibroblastoma

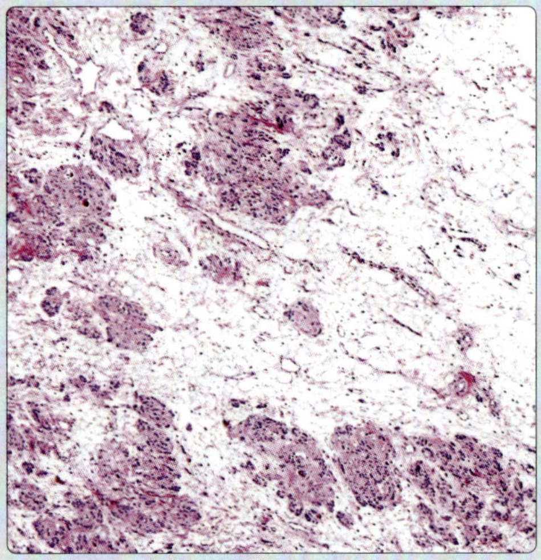

Circumscription

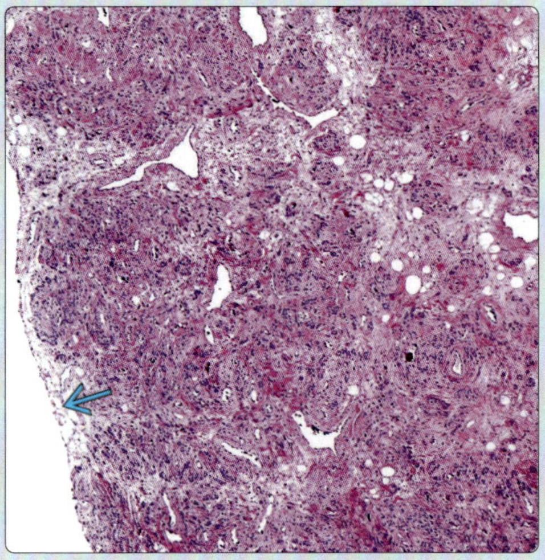

(Left) *The neoplastic cells of angiomyofibroblastoma are characteristically clustered around small thin-walled capillary channels →, which can often be recognized by the presence of intraluminal erythrocytes. The intervening myxoid stroma is hypocellular.* **(Right)** *In classic cases of angiomyofibroblastoma, the tumor cells are epithelioid, ovoid, or plasmacytoid and form small nests or clusters around capillary channels. This perivascular orientation is characteristic of this tumor.*

Alternating Zones of Cellularity

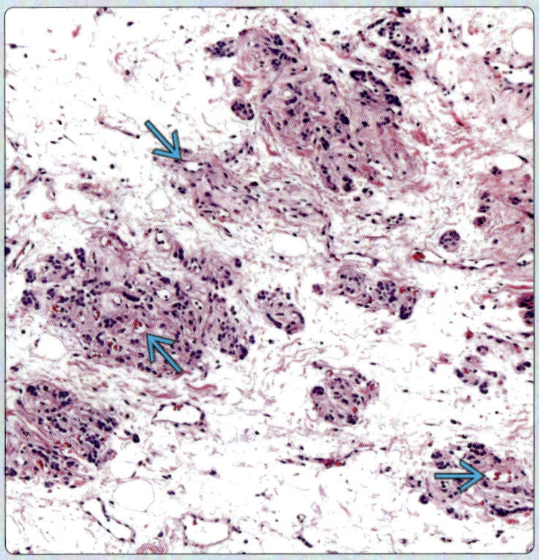

Perivascular Organization

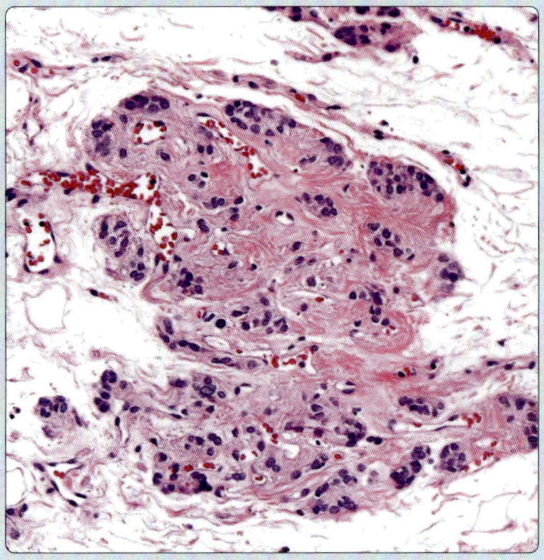

TERMINOLOGY

Abbreviations

- Angiomyofibroblastoma (AMFB)

Definitions

- Benign genital stromal tumor composed of fibroblasts oriented around prominent capillary vasculature

CLINICAL ISSUES

Epidemiology

- Age
  - Generally 35-60 years (median: 46)
- Sex
  - Affects women almost exclusively

Site

- Vulva (most common) and vagina
- Rarely perineum or inguinal region

Presentation

- Slow-growing, painless mass
  - Often mistaken clinically for Bartholin cyst

Treatment

- Simple local excision

Prognosis

- Benign
- Very rare recurrences reported

MACROSCOPIC

General Features

- Well-circumscribed solid mass
- Tan-white coloration
- Rubbery or mucoid cut surface

Size

- Usually < 5 cm

MICROSCOPIC

Histologic Features

- Nonencapsulated
- Alternating zones of cellularity
  - Hypocellular zones often myxoid or edematous
- Prominent vascular component
  - Numerous thin-walled capillaries
- Plump epithelioid, ovoid, or plasmacytoid tumor cells with eosinophilic cytoplasm
  - Singly, in cords, or small nests
  - Cells characteristically cluster around thin-walled capillaries
  - Cells may show multinucleation
- Mast cells common
- In postmenopausal patients
  - Often less cellular
  - Cells are more spindled than epithelioid
  - Increased stromal collagen
- Mature adipose tissue component in minority of cases
- Some cases of AMFB show morphologic overlap with cellular angiofibroma
- Very rare reports describing malignant transformation

ANCILLARY TESTS

Immunohistochemistry

- Desmin (+)
- Often ER(+) and PR(+)
- Usually CD34(-) and SMA(-)
- Negative for keratin and S100 protein
- Retained nuclear Rb1 expression

DIFFERENTIAL DIAGNOSIS

Deep (Aggressive) Angiomyxoma

- Often large and deeply located
- Infiltrative margins
- Uniform cellularity (lacks perivascular orientation of AMFB)
- Contains medium- to large-sized vessels
  - Overall less vascular than AMFB
- Lacks epithelioid cells
- Aberrations involving 12q13-15 (*HMGA2*)

Cellular Angiofibroma

- Some cases may show considerable overlap with AMFB
  - May appropriately classify as "benign genital stromal tumor"
- More uniformly cellular
  - May show formation of short fascicles
- Contains medium-sized vessels, often with hyalinization
  - Overall less vascular than AMFB
- Lacks epithelioid cells with perivascular orientation
- Often CD34(+); most cases desmin negative
- Loss of *RB1* (13q14)

Fibroepithelial Stromal Polyp

- Young to middle-aged women
- Typically very superficial and polypoid
  - Overlying squamous epithelium
  - No grenz zone
- Stellate and multinucleate cells are characteristic
  - Often located beneath epithelial surface at epithelial-stromal interface
- Some cases are associated with pregnancy
  - May contain bizarre nuclear atypia and mitoses (pseudosarcomatous stromal polyp)
- Desmin (+), ER(+), PR(+)

SELECTED REFERENCES

1. Schoolmeester JK et al: Genital soft tissue tumors. J Cutan Pathol. 42(7):441-51, 2015
2. Magro G et al: Vulvovaginal angiomyofibroblastomas: morphologic, immunohistochemical, and fluorescence in situ hybridization analysis for deletion of 13q14 region. Hum Pathol. 45(8):1647-55, 2014
3. Kairi-Vassilatou E et al: Angiomyofibroblastoma of the vulva: a clinicopathological and immunohistochemical analysis of a rare benign mesenchymal tumor. Eur J Gynaecol Oncol. 32(3):353-5, 2011
4. Laskin WB et al: Angiomyofibroblastoma of the female genital tract: analysis of 17 cases including a lipomatous variant. Hum Pathol. 28(9):1046-55, 1997
5. Fletcher CD et al: Angiomyofibroblastoma of the vulva. A benign neoplasm distinct from aggressive angiomyxoma. Am J Surg Pathol. 16(4):373-82, 1992

(Left) *The tumor cell nuclei of angiomyofibroblastoma are cytologically bland and may show small, inconspicuous nucleoli. Multinucleated forms are not uncommon. Mitoses are rare.* **(Right)** *In addition to small clusters and nests, the tumor cells in angiomyofibroblastoma may show a linear, corded growth pattern. This pattern may mimic the growth of lobular carcinoma of the breast or a Sertoli cell tumor.*

Epithelioid Cytomorphology

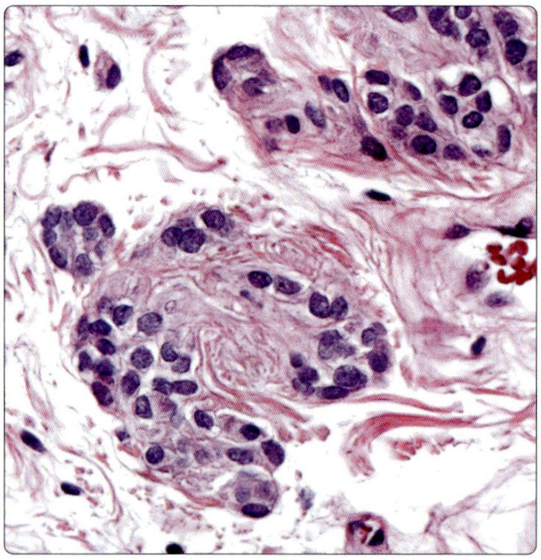

Cording Growth

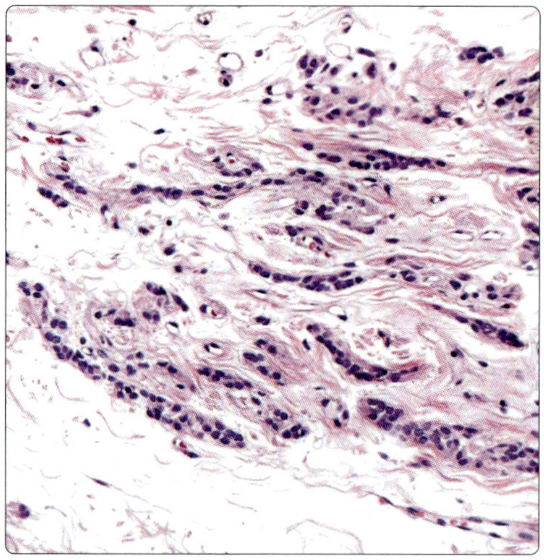

(Left) *A component of mature adipose tissue is seen in a minority (~ 10%) of cases of angiomyofibroblastoma. These tumors have been referred to as "lipomatous angiomyofibroblastoma" when the fat is prominent.* **(Right)** *Although the vast majority of vessels in angiomyofibroblastoma are thin-walled capillaries, larger thicker-walled vessels are occasionally seen.*

Mature Adipose Tissue

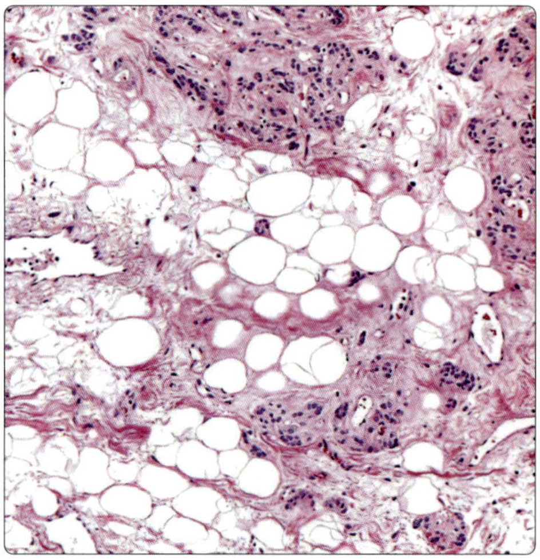

Vasculature

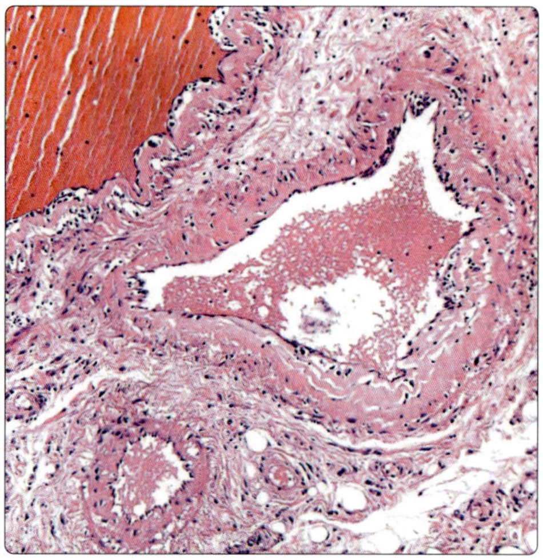

(Left) *In rare cases of angiomyofibroblastoma, larger dilated vessels forming an ectatic "staghorn" pattern may be apparent. This finding is generally nonspecific, but it may raise the consideration of a solitary fibrous tumor.* **(Right)** *A mild chronic inflammatory infiltrate may be seen in angiomyofibroblastoma and tends to be accentuated around the vessels. Mast cells are also a common finding.*

Vasculature

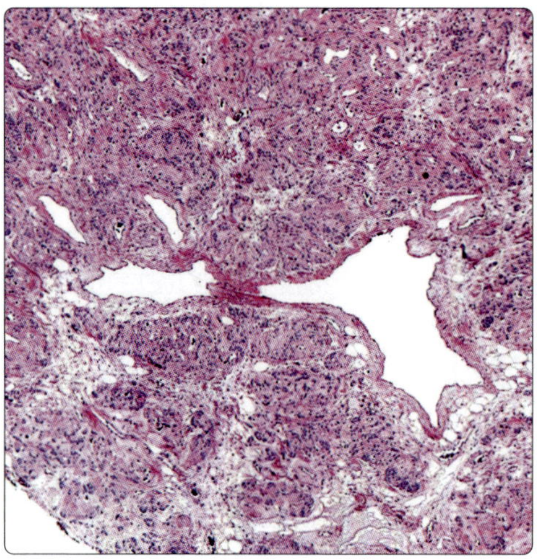

Chronic Inflammatory Infiltrate

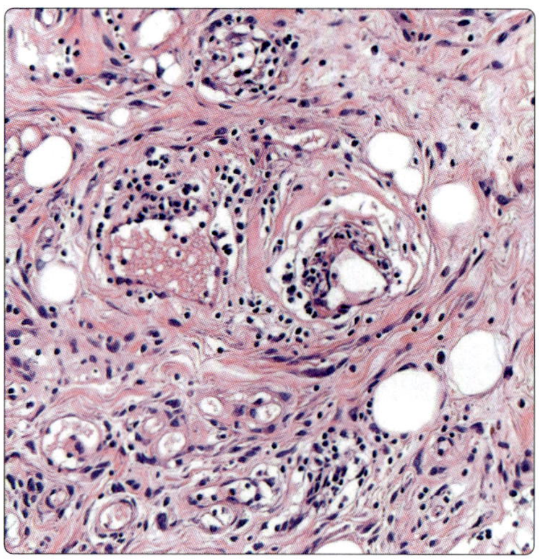

Postmenopausal Angiomyofibroblastoma

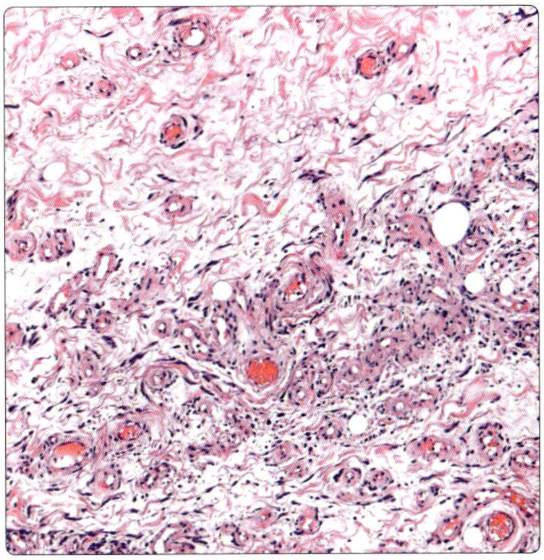

Stromal Collagen

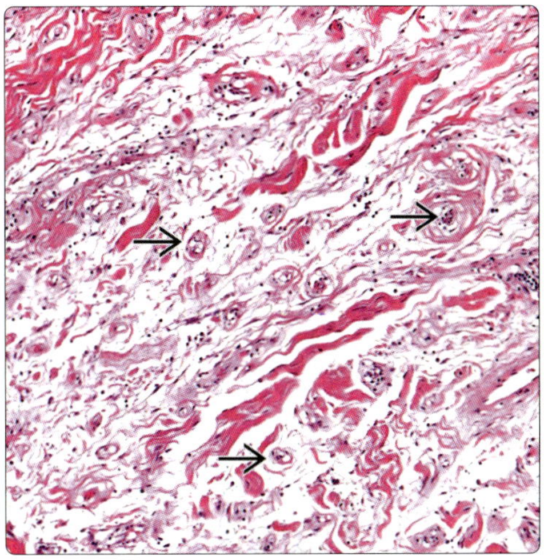

(Left) *In postmenopausal patients, angiomyofibroblastoma often shows a drop in cellularity as well as a tendency for the tumor cells to be more spindled and less epithelioid. Note, however, that the perivascular orientation is still maintained.* **(Right)** *Some examples of postmenopausal angiomyofibroblastoma are markedly hypocellular and may show prominent collagen or hyalinization. Note the numerous thin-walled capillary channels* ➙*.*

Subtle Perivascular Arrangement

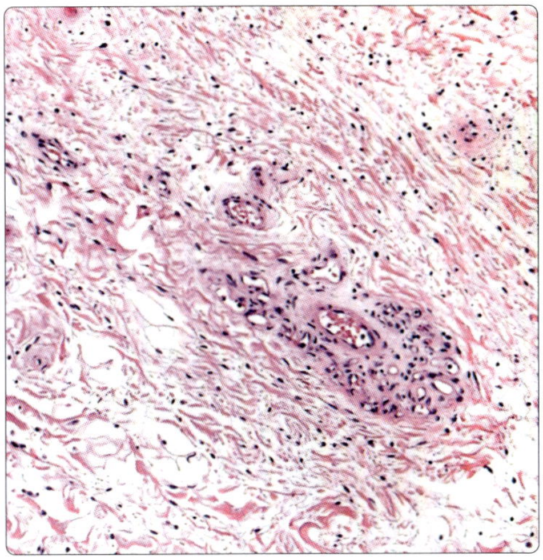

Desmin Expression

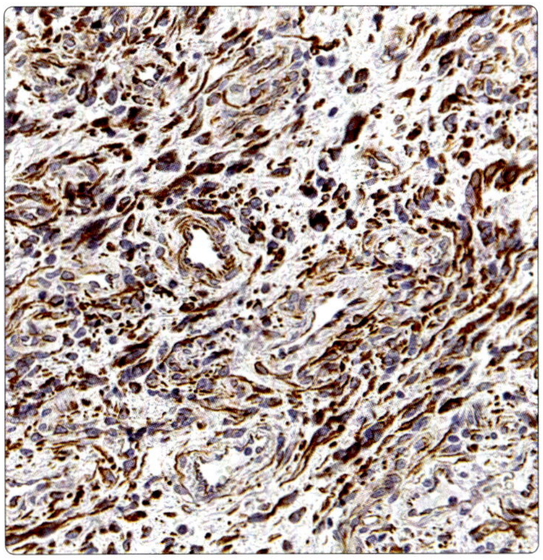

(Left) *This image of angiomyofibroblastoma in a postmenopausal patient demonstrates a marked drop in overall cellularity but also shows how the tumor cells (more spindled rather than epithelioid) congregate around the capillary channels.* **(Right)** *The tumor cells of angiomyofibroblastoma usually show diffuse expression of desmin. Estrogen receptor and progesterone receptor stains are often positive as well. CD34 is usually negative.*

Cellular Angiofibroma

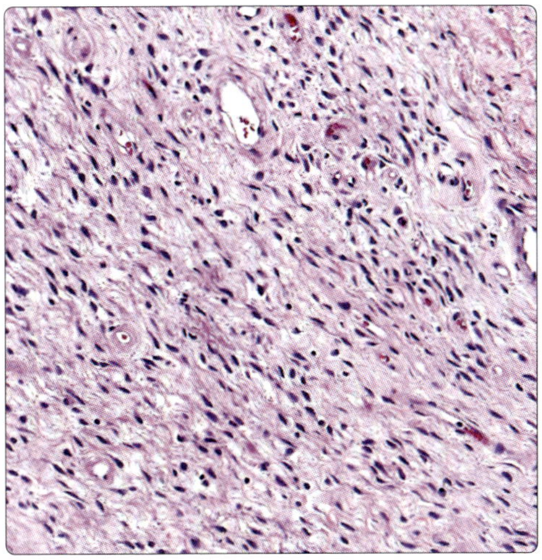

Deep (Aggressive) Angiomyxoma

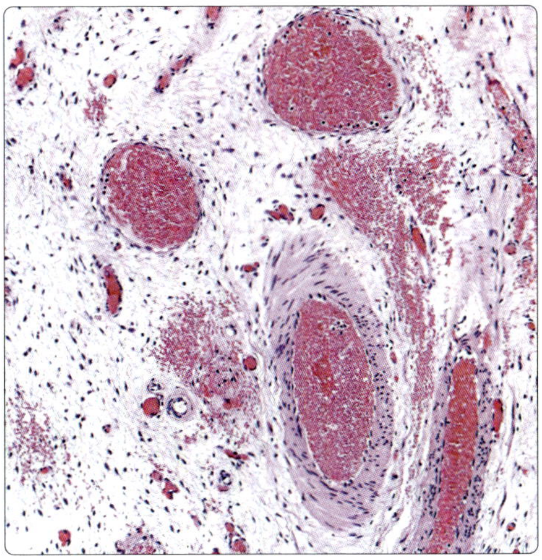

(Left) *In contrast to angiomyofibroblastoma, cellular angiofibroma is more uniformly cellular. The vessels are often of a larger caliber and usually show at least focal hyalinization. CD34 is also typically expressed.* **(Right)** *Deep angiomyxoma differs from angiomyofibroblastoma in that it is often larger, more deeply located, and demonstrates a prominent component of medium- to large-size thick-walled vessels. The uniform hypocellularity and myxoedematous stroma are also characteristic.*

Cellular Angiofibroma

KEY FACTS

TERMINOLOGY

- Synonym: Angiomyofibroblastoma-like tumor of male genital tract
- Benign, often moderately cellular genital stromal neoplasm composed of spindled cells and often containing small- to medium-sized vessels with hyalinized walls

CLINICAL ISSUES

- Middle-aged to older adults (median: 52 years)
- Occurs in both sexes
- Usually subcutaneous tissue of vulva/vagina (women) and inguinoscrotal region (men)
  - Can also arise in anogenital region and pelvic soft tissues in both sexes
- Benign; recurrences rare

MICROSCOPIC

- Well-marginated and evenly cellular bland spindle cell neoplasm
- Prominent component of small- to medium-sized blood vessels, often with hyalinized walls
- May contain component of mature adipose tissue
- Rare examples with atypical or sarcomatous features

ANCILLARY TESTS

- Diffuse CD34(+) in majority of cases
- Loss of nuclear Rb protein expression
- STAT6(-)
- Usually desmin, smooth muscle actin, and S100 protein (-)
- Molecular: Loss of 13q14 region (*RB1*)

TOP DIFFERENTIAL DIAGNOSES

- Aggressive angiomyxoma
- Angiomyofibroblastoma
- Mammary-type myofibroblastoma
- Spindle cell lipoma
- Solitary fibrous tumor

Cellular Angiofibroma

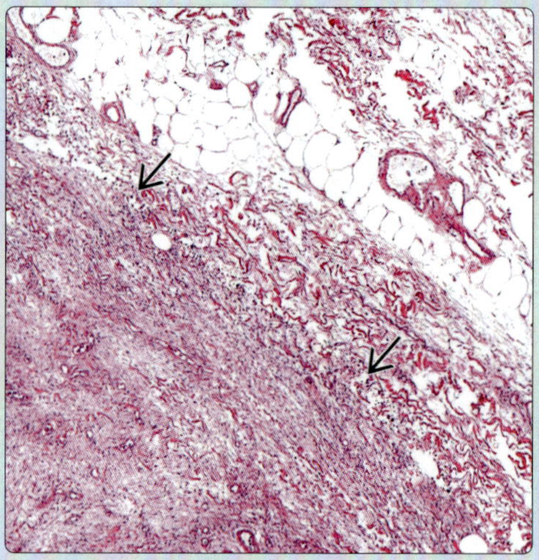

Conspicuous Vasculature

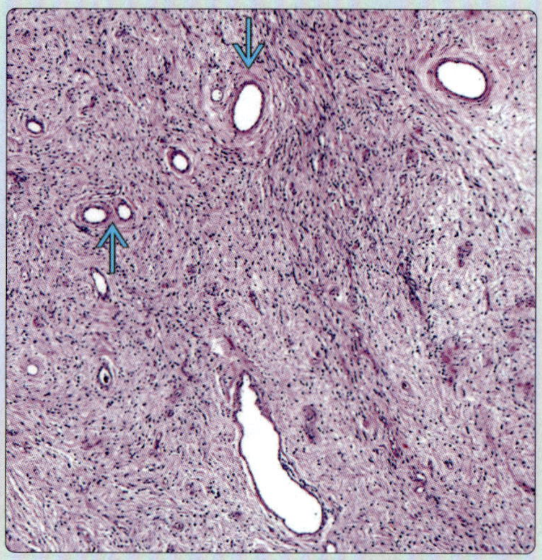

(Left) *Cellular angiofibroma is a well-circumscribed → benign neoplasm of genital stromal fibroblasts. Unlike angiomyofibroblastoma and aggressive angiomyxoma, cellular angiofibroma is well described in men.* **(Right)** *Medium- to large-sized blood vessels are often conspicuous in cellular angiofibroma, and many show some degree of perivascular hyalinization →. Cellularity can vary widely from field to field; however, cells are usually evenly distributed regardless of the overall cellularity.*

Hyalinized Vessels

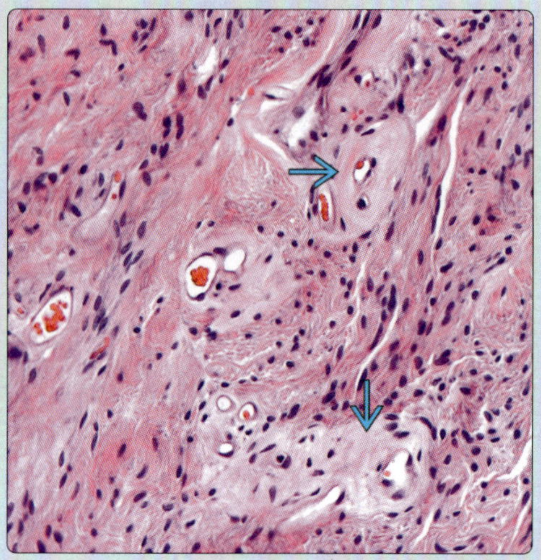

Even Cellular Distribution

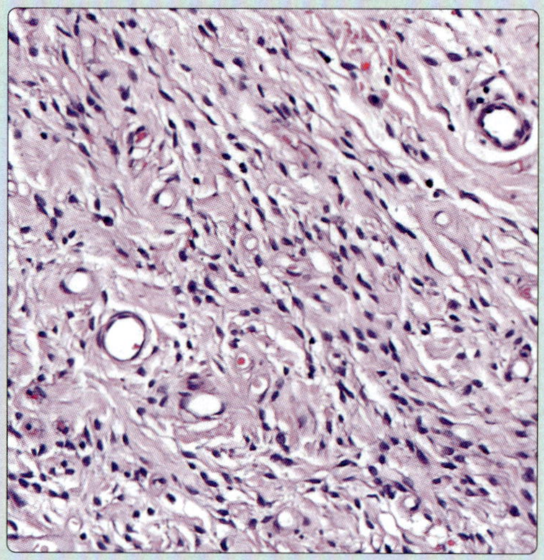

(Left) *Perivascular hyalinization → or fibrosis is seen at least focally in most cases of cellular angiofibroma and may affect both small and larger vessels. In some cases, the extent of change can be striking.* **(Right)** *The cellularity of cellular angiofibroma is generally more evenly distributed than is seen in angiomyofibroblastoma, in which cells tend to cluster around capillary vascular channels.*

TERMINOLOGY

Synonyms

- Angiomyofibroblastoma-like tumor of male genital tract

Definitions

- Benign, often moderately cellular genital stromal neoplasm composed of spindled cells and often containing small vessels with hyalinized walls

CLINICAL ISSUES

Epidemiology

- Age
  - Middle-aged to older adults (median: 52 years)
- Sex
  - Occurs in both sexes

Site

- Women: Usually vulva or vagina
- Men: Scrotal or inguinal region
- Can also arise in anogenital region and pelvic soft tissues in both sexes
- Rare cases reported in retroperitoneum

Presentation

- Well-circumscribed, painless mass
- May simulate Bartholin cyst in women or hernia in men

Prognosis

- Benign
  - Rare examples with sarcomatous features have also exhibited benign behavior
- Recurrences rare

MACROSCOPIC

General Features

- Well circumscribed ("shelled out") and lobulated
- Dermal or subcutaneous
- Firm to rubbery, gray-white cut surface

Size

- Median: 2-3 cm in females
- Median: 6-7 cm in males

MICROSCOPIC

Histologic Features

- Well marginated and variably but evenly cellular
- Uniform spindle cells, often with bipolar processes
  - May be arranged randomly, in loose whorls, in palisades, or in short fascicles
- Fibrous to myxoid stroma with wispy collagen
- Prominent component of small- to medium-sized blood vessels
  - Hyalinized vessels common and characteristic
- Mitotic activity generally low
- Stromal lymphocytes are common
- May contain component of mature adipose tissue
- Rare examples with atypical or sarcomatous features
  - Scattered cells with marked nuclear atypia or foci resembling various pleomorphic sarcomas or well-differentiated liposarcoma

ANCILLARY TESTS

Immunohistochemistry

- Diffuse CD34(+) in majority of cases, rare desmin (+)
- ER(+), PR(+) in most cases in women (less common in men)
- Loss of nuclear Rb protein expression
- Usually smooth muscle actin and S100 protein (-)

Molecular Genetics

- Monoallelic or biallelic loss of 13q14 region (*RB1*)
  - Identical aberration to that seen in spindle cell lipoma and mammary-type myofibroblastoma

DIFFERENTIAL DIAGNOSIS

Deep (Aggressive) Angiomyxoma

- Large, deeply located tumors
- Infiltrative, paucicellular tumor with spindled to stellate cells
- Prominent medium- to large-sized stromal blood vessels
- Desmin (+), CD34 variable

Angiomyofibroblastoma

- Tumor cells are more epithelioid than spindled and cluster around prominent capillary vascular channels
- Alternating zones of cellularity and hypocellularity
- Desmin (+), variable CD34(+)

Mammary-Type Myofibroblastoma

- Can show morphologic and immunohistochemical overlap with cellular angiofibroma
  - However, mammary-type myofibroblastoma is often desmin (+)

Spindle Cell Lipoma

- Can show morphologic and immunohistochemical overlap with cellular angiofibroma
- Commonly arise in region of neck, shoulder, and upper back

Solitary Fibrous Tumor

- Usually prominent component of ectatic "staghorn" blood vessels
- Diffuse CD34(+), STAT6(+), retained Rb protein expression

SELECTED REFERENCES

1. Mandato VD et al: Cellular angiofibroma in women: a review of the literature. Diagn Pathol. 10:114, 2015
2. Chen BJ et al: Loss of retinoblastoma protein expression in spindle cell/pleomorphic lipomas and cytogenetically related tumors: an immunohistochemical study with diagnostic implications. Am J Surg Pathol. 36(8):1119-28, 2012
3. Flucke U et al: Cellular angiofibroma: analysis of 25 cases emphasizing its relationship to spindle cell lipoma and mammary-type myofibroblastoma. Mod Pathol. 24(1):82-9, 2011
4. Chen E et al: Cellular angiofibroma with atypia or sarcomatous transformation: clinicopathologic analysis of 13 cases. Am J Surg Pathol. 34(5):707-14, 2010
5. Iwasa Y et al: Cellular angiofibroma: clinicopathologic and immunohistochemical analysis of 51 cases. Am J Surg Pathol. 28(11):1426-35, 2004
6. Laskin WB et al: Angiomyofibroblastoma-like tumor of the male genital tract: analysis of 11 cases with comparison to female angiomyofibroblastoma and spindle cell lipoma. Am J Surg Pathol. 22(1):6-16, 1998

Bland Spindle Cells

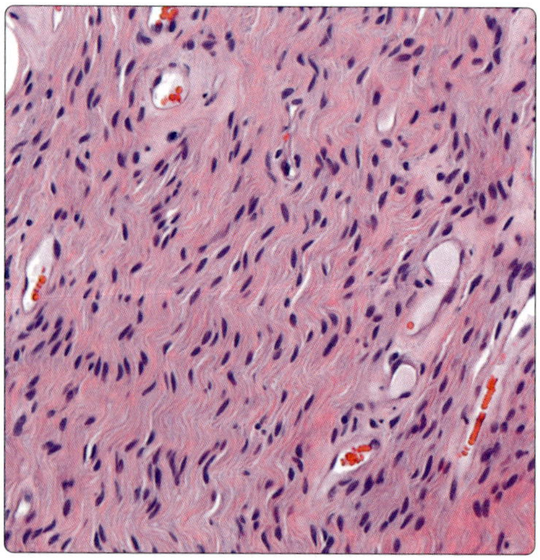

Cytologic Features

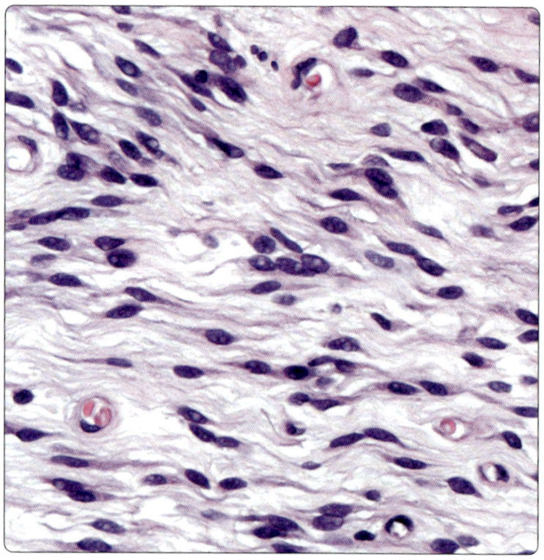

(Left) *The lesional cells of cellular angiofibroma are generally spindled with bipolar processes and may show a wavy, undulating morphology. The background stroma is often filled with fine collagen fibers.* **(Right)** *The spindle cells of cellular angiofibroma are generally devoid of significant nuclear atypia. Nonspecific findings, such as small, pale intranuclear pseudoinclusions or nuclear grooving, may be seen.*

Moderate Cellularity

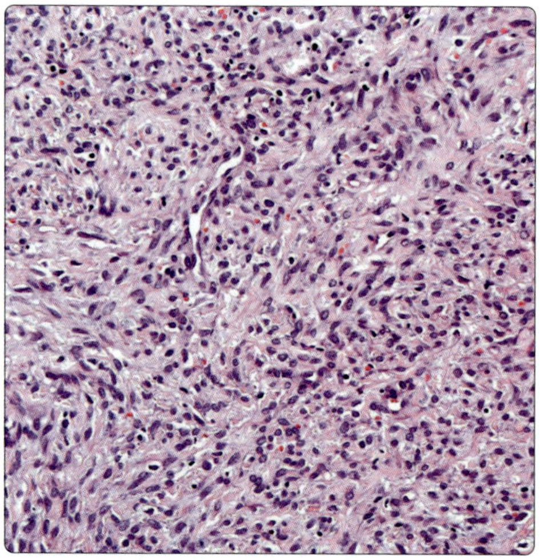

Various Architectural Patterns

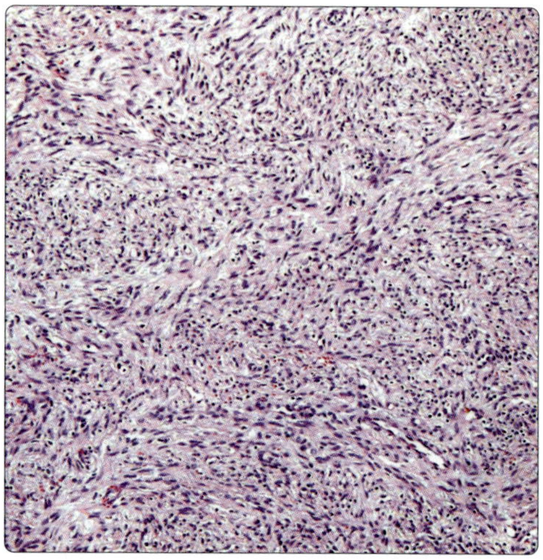

(Left) *Cellular angiofibroma often shows zones of moderate cellularity, which can vary from focal to extensive. In these areas, there is no significant nuclear atypia, and mitotic figures are generally inconspicuous.* **(Right)** *Cellular areas of cellular angiofibroma may show a variety of architectural patterns, including short fascicles, loose whorling/storiform growth, or haphazard arrays.*

Stromal Inflammation

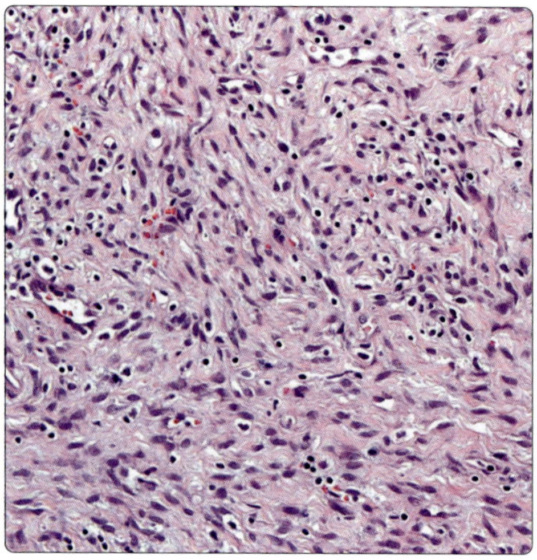

Mast Cells

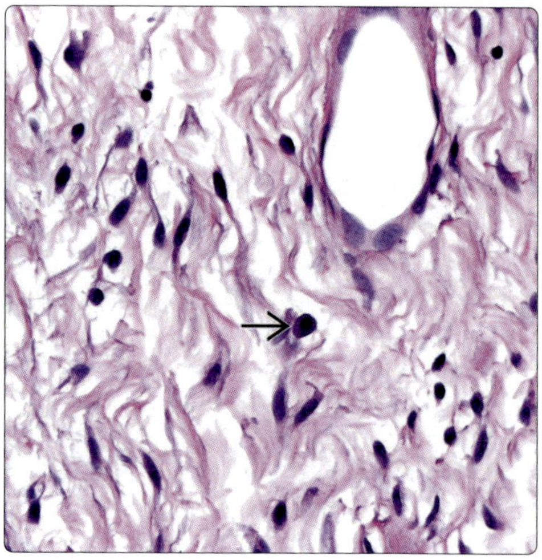

(Left) *A subtle to brisk chronic inflammatory infiltrate is a common finding in cellular angiofibroma and is composed of mostly lymphocytes. Mast cells are also frequently identified.* **(Right)** *As seen in other genital stromal neoplasms, scattered mast cells ⇒ are commonly identified in most cases of cellular angiofibroma. In rare cases, they may be numerous.*

Myxoedematous Stromal Change

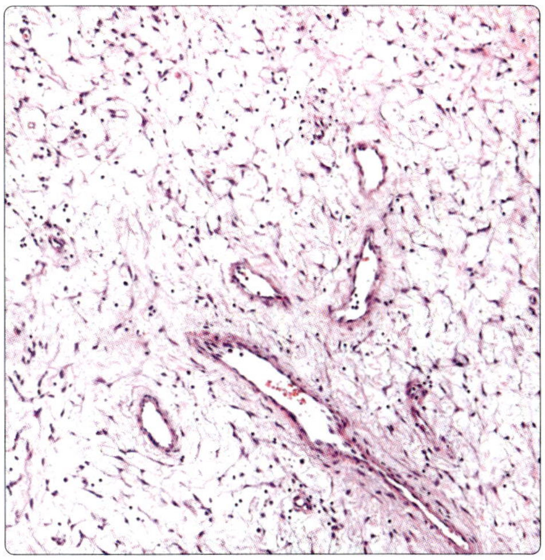

Mature Adipose Tissue

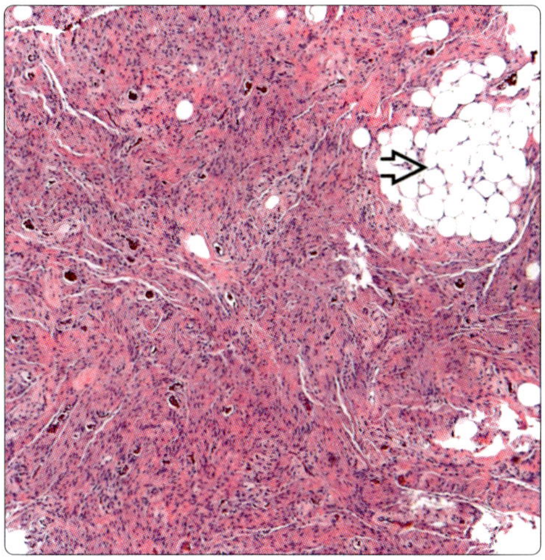

(Left) *Stromal edema or myxoid changes are seen in some cases of cellular angiofibroma and vary in extent. Other typical features, including hyalinized vessels and a chronic inflammatory infiltrate, are often present.* **(Right)** *Mature adipose tissue* ⇨ *may be identified as a component of cellular angiofibroma in a minority of cases (~ 10%) and is usually found near the periphery of the tumor.*

Spindle Cell Lipoma-Like Morphology

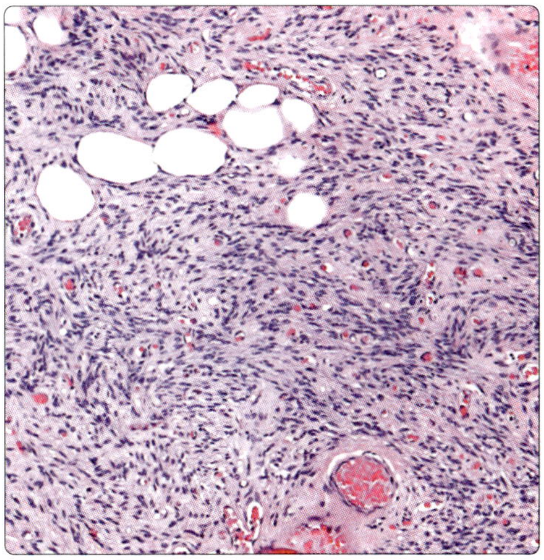

Sarcomatous Features

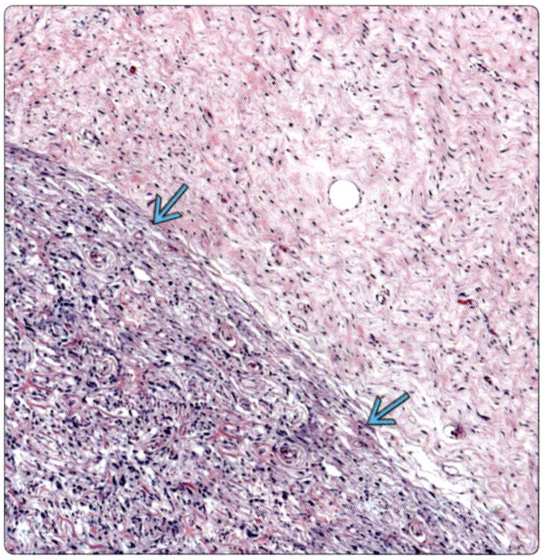

(Left) *Occasional cases of cellular angiofibroma may show cellular regions containing mature adipose tissue, a morphology reminiscent of a spindle cell lipoma. Interestingly, recent evidence suggests that these tumors are histogenetically related.* **(Right)** *Rare cases of otherwise conventional cellular angiofibroma show solitary or multiple nodules of increased cellularity and nuclear atypia, suggestive of pleomorphic sarcoma* ➡*. In fact, in one study, several foci resembled well-differentiated or pleomorphic liposarcoma.*

DDx: Angiomyofibroblastoma

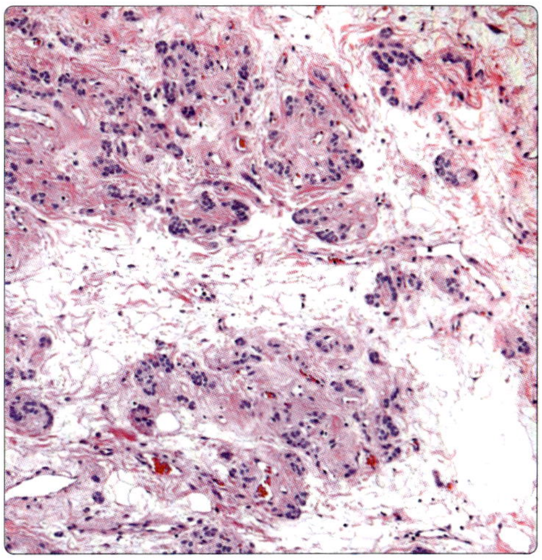

DDx: Deep (Aggressive) Angiomyxoma

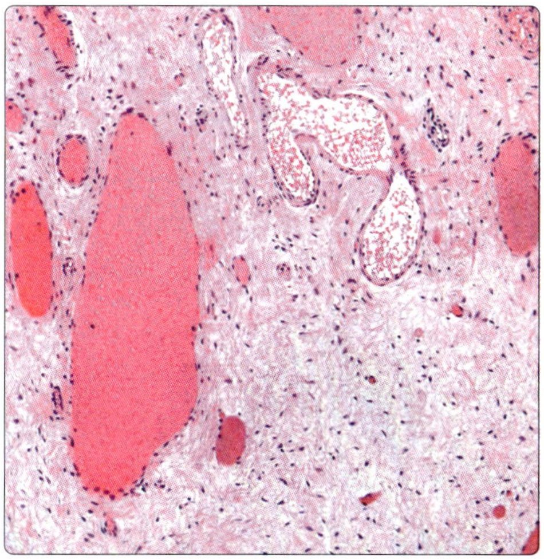

(Left) *In contrast to cellular angiofibroma, angiomyofibroblastoma demonstrates more of an alternating pattern of cellularity with the epithelioid to spindled tumor cells predominantly clustering around capillary vascular channels.* **(Right)** *In contrast to cellular angiofibroma, deep angiomyxoma is usually evenly hypocellular and shows prominent blood vessels that are, on average, larger in caliber. The clinical features of these 2 tumors are also very different.*

Deep (Aggressive) Angiomyxoma

KEY FACTS

TERMINOLOGY

- Hypocellular locally aggressive myxoedematous neoplasm with prominent vessels, typically of deep pelvic tissues

CLINICAL ISSUES

- Vast majority occur in women
- Sites: Vulva, perineum, pelvic cavity
- Deep, slow-growing mass
- Treatment: Surgical excision &/or adjuvant hormone therapy
- Benign, but local recurrences common

MACROSCOPIC

- Usually large (> 10 cm)

MICROSCOPIC

- Overall low cellularity
- Infiltrative growth pattern
- Small spindled to stellate cells
- Prominent myxoedematous stroma rich in collagen fibers
- Numerous blood vessels with sizes ranging from capillaries to thick-walled larger vessels
- Stromal mast cells and extravasated erythrocytes are common

ANCILLARY TESTS

- Immunophenotype: Desmin (+), ER(+), PR(+)
  - Variable SMA; CD34(-)
- Molecular: Various rearrangements involving *HMGA2* (12q13-15)

TOP DIFFERENTIAL DIAGNOSES

- Angiomyofibroblastoma
- Cellular angiofibroma
- Superficial angiomyxoma
- Desmoid fibromatosis
- Leiomyoma

Deep Angiomyxoma

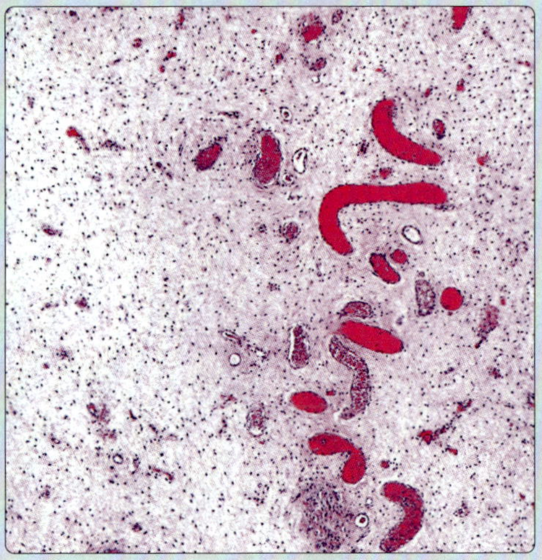

Medium to Large Vessels

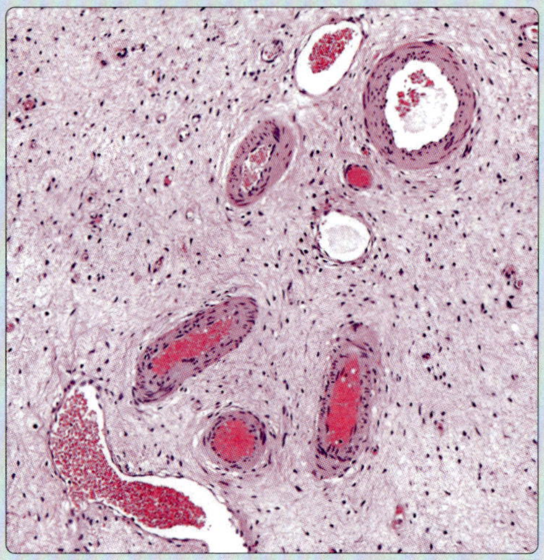

(Left) *Deep angiomyxoma is a locally aggressive genital stromal neoplasm that occurs predominantly in women in the perineopelvic region. This tumor is typically large and deeply located, and it is characterized by a myxoedematous stroma with prominent blood vessels.* **(Right)** *A characteristic finding is the presence of prominent medium- to large-sized blood vessels within the stroma. In some cases, these vessels may also have mature smooth muscle cells radiating away from the vessel wall (not shown).*

Cytologic Features

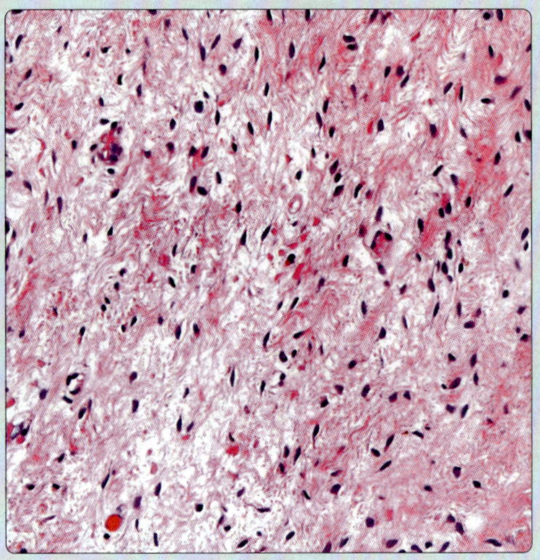

Desmin Expression

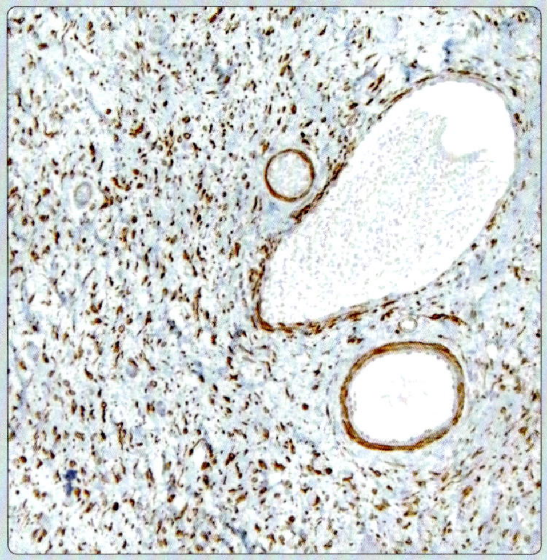

(Left) *Deep angiomyxoma is generally a hypocellular tumor and is composed of small spindled or stellate cells without significant atypia or mitotic activity. Some cases feature areas with a mild to moderate increase in cellularity.* **(Right)** *Desmin is often expressed by the lesional cells in deep angiomyxoma. Smooth muscle actin (SMA) is negative; however, it will highlight any mature smooth muscle cells within the lesion.*

Deep (Aggressive) Angiomyxoma

TERMINOLOGY

Definitions

- Hypocellular locally aggressive myxoedematous neoplasm with prominent vessels, typically of deep pelvic tissues

CLINICAL ISSUES

Epidemiology

- Age
  - Wide range (most common: 20-50 years)
- Sex
  - Vast majority occur in women

Site

- Vulva, perineum, pelvic cavity
  - May simulate Bartholin cyst or inguinal hernia clinically
  - Often infiltrates perirectal or perivaginal soft tissues
- Inguinopelvic or scrotal region in men (very rare)

Presentation

- Deep, slow-growing mass

Treatment

- Surgical excision
  - May be impossible to completely resect due to infiltrative nature of tumor
- Also, may utilize adjuvant hormone therapy, including gonadotrophin-releasing hormone agonists and antiestrogens

Prognosis

- Benign
- Recurrences common (30-40%)
  - Aggressive, complete surgical resection may be associated with lower risk

MACROSCOPIC

General Features

- Variable circumscription
- Lobulated or polypoid mass
- Rubbery, myxoid, or gelatinous cut surface

Size

- Usually large (> 10 cm)

MICROSCOPIC

Histologic Features

- Overall low cellularity
  - May show foci of increased cellularity, particularly in recurrent lesions
- Infiltrative growth pattern
  - May contain adipose tissue &/or small nerve twigs
- Small spindled to stellate cells
  - No significant nuclear atypia or mitotic activity
- Prominent myxoedematous stroma rich in collagen fibers
- Numerous blood vessels with sizes ranging from capillaries to thick-walled larger vessels
  - Some vessels may show perivascular smooth muscle proliferation
- Stromal mast cells and extravasated erythrocytes are common

ANCILLARY TESTS

Immunohistochemistry

- Desmin (+), ER(+), PR(+)
- Variable SMA; CD34(-)
- Keratin (-) , S100 protein (-), myogenin (-)

Genetic Testing

- Various rearrangements involving *HMGA2* (12q13-15)
  - t(8;12) and t(11;12) have been reported

DIFFERENTIAL DIAGNOSIS

Angiomyofibroblastoma

- Well marginated, small, and superficial
- Zones of cellularity and hypocellularity
- Plump epithelioid to spindled cells with enhanced cellularity around prominent capillary vasculature

Cellular Angiofibroma

- Well marginated, superficial
- May be seen in both men and women
- Evenly dispersed small- to medium-sized vessels
  - Perivascular hyalinization may be seen
- CD34(+), ER(+), PR(+), desmin (-)

Superficial Angiomyxoma

- Less common in genital sites
- Usually small and superficial
- Arborizing thin-walled vasculature
- Stromal neutrophils common

Desmoid Fibromatosis

- May show prominent myxoid change
  - Usually contains zones of more conventional fascicular architecture
- Nuclear β-catenin expression in majority of cases
- Desmin (-), ER(-), PR(-)

Leiomyoma

- May show prominent myxoid stromal change
- Smooth muscle cytology
- Diffuse smooth muscle actin (+) and desmin (+)

SELECTED REFERENCES

1. Chen H et al: Clinicopathological features and differential diagnosis of aggressive angiomyxoma of the female pelvis: 5 case reports and literature review. Medicine (Baltimore). 96(20):e6820, 2017
2. Smith HG et al: Selective marginal resections in the management of aggressive angiomyxomas. J Surg Oncol. 114(7):828-832, 2016
3. Sutton BJ et al: Aggressive angiomyxoma. Arch Pathol Lab Med. 136(2):217-21, 2012
4. Bigby SM et al: Aggressive angiomyxoma [corrected] of the female genital tract and pelvis–clinicopathologic features with immunohistochemical analysis. Int J Gynecol Pathol. 30(5):505-13, 2011
5. McCluggage WG et al: HMGA2 is a sensitive but not specific immunohistochemical marker of vulvovaginal aggressive angiomyxoma. Am J Surg Pathol. 34(7):1037-42, 2010
6. McCluggage WG et al: Aggressive angiomyxoma of the vulva: dramatic response to gonadotropin-releasing hormone agonist therapy. Gynecol Oncol. 100(3):623-5, 2006

Low to Mild Cellularity

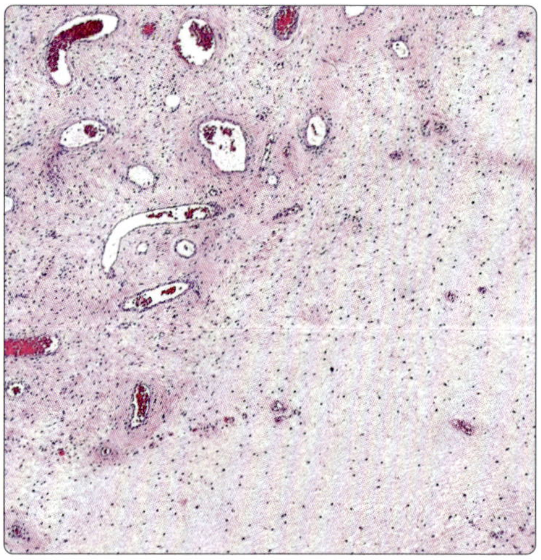

Fat Infiltration

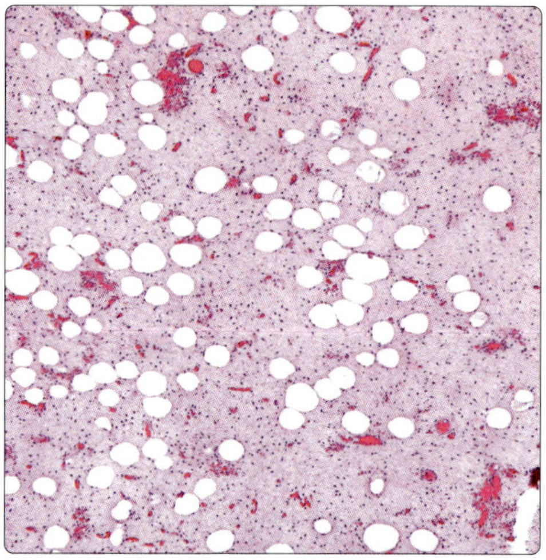

(Left) *Deep angiomyxoma is typically a diffusely hypocellular neoplasm; however, a mild increase in cellularity is not uncommon. On average, recurrent tumors tend to be more cellular.* **(Right)** *Given its infiltrative nature, deep angiomyxoma can show involvement of regional mature adipose tissue. In some areas, the fat may be so prominent as to mimic the pattern of myxoid dermatofibrosarcoma protuberans.*

Entrapment of Nerves

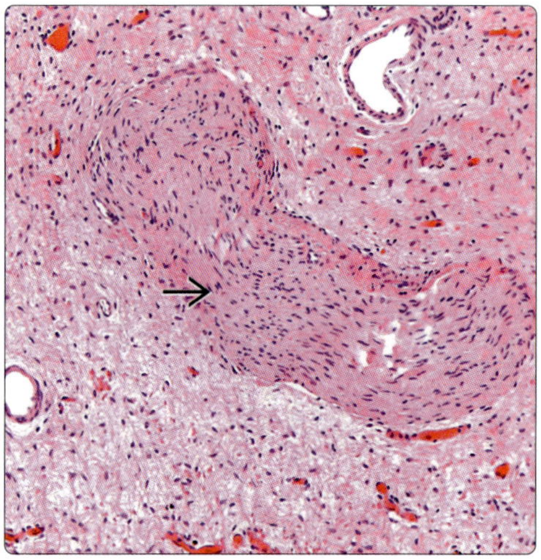

Extravasated Red Blood Cells

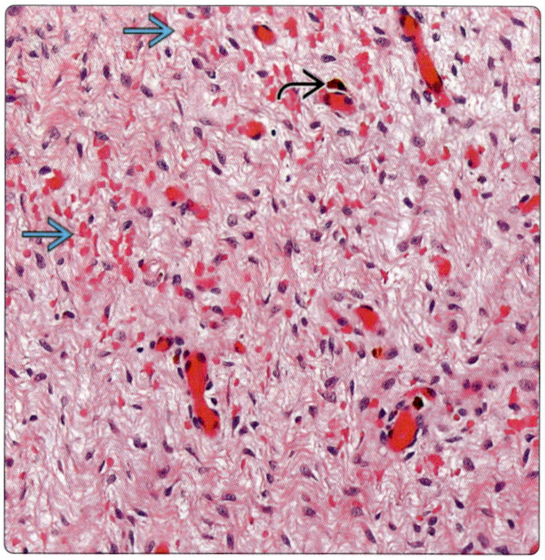

(Left) *Deep angiomyxoma is a locally infiltrative tumor, which is often evidenced by the presence of intratumoral adipose tissue or nerve twigs* →*. Clinically, this tumor often shows involvement of the perivaginal or perirectal soft tissues.* **(Right)** *Given the vascularity of deep angiomyxoma, extravasated red blood cells* → *are a frequent finding, similar to nodular fasciitis. Focal hemosiderin-laden macrophages* ↗ *may be identified as well.*

Smooth Muscle Proliferation

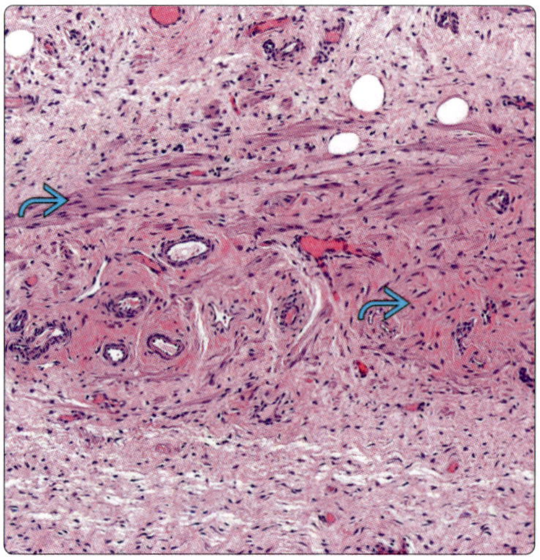

Mast Cells

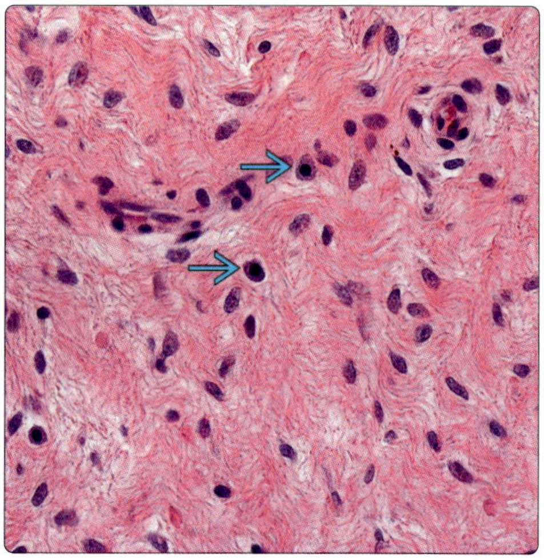

(Left) *A common finding in deep angiomyxoma is the presence of smooth muscle cells* ↗ *proliferating around and near stromal blood vessels. These cells can be highlighted by smooth muscle actin (SMA) as well as desmin.* **(Right)** *Mast cells* → *are frequently identified in deep angiomyxoma and are not specific for the lesion. Scattered lymphocytes can be seen as well.*

Estrogen Receptor (ER) Expression

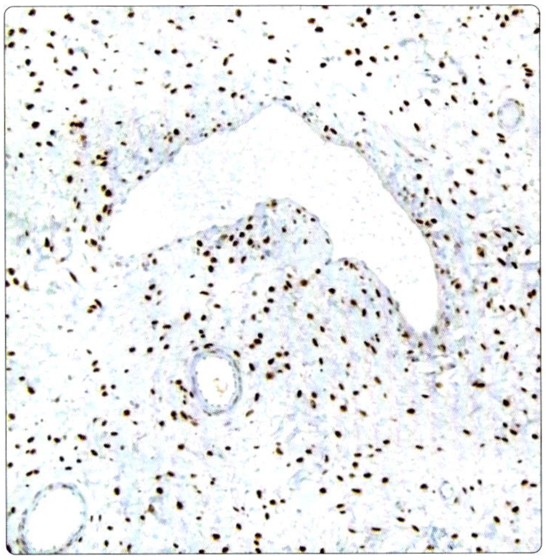

S100 Protein Negativity

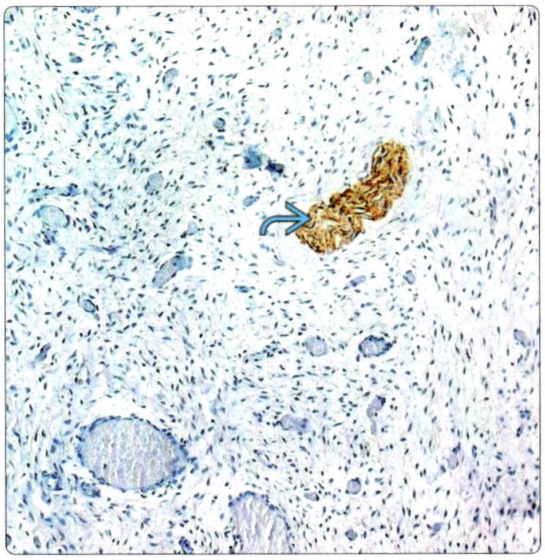

(Left) *Estrogen receptor (ER) is often expressed in the nuclei of lesional cells in deep angiomyxoma. Progesterone receptor (PR) is also positive in most cases.* **(Right)** *Although some areas of deep angiomyxoma can resemble a peripheral nerve sheath tumor, such as neurofibroma, the lesional cells are negative for S100. Note the entrapped nerve twig ➜ serving as an internal positive control for this marker.*

CD34 Negativity

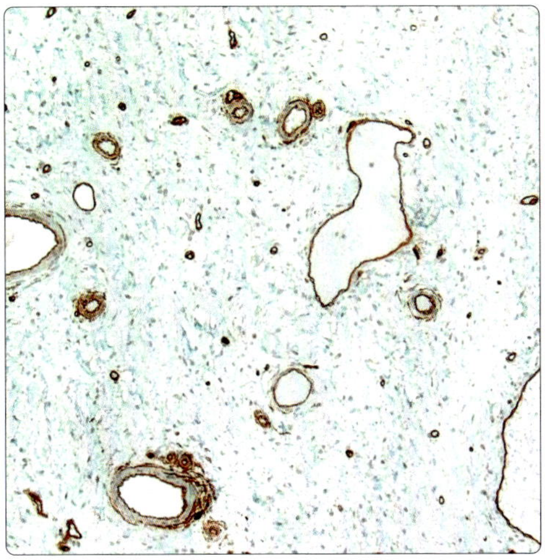

Hypocellularity

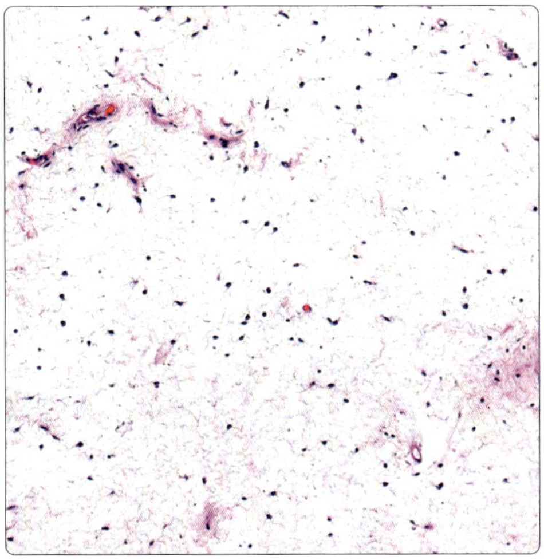

(Left) *CD34 highlights the prominent vascular component of deep angiomyxoma; however, the lesional spindle cells are often negative (or, at most, focally positive).* **(Right)** *Some regions of deep angiomyxoma can show marked hypocellularity, resembling a cutaneous or intramuscular myxoma. However, deep angiomyxoma is localized to the genital region.*

Perivascular Smooth Muscle

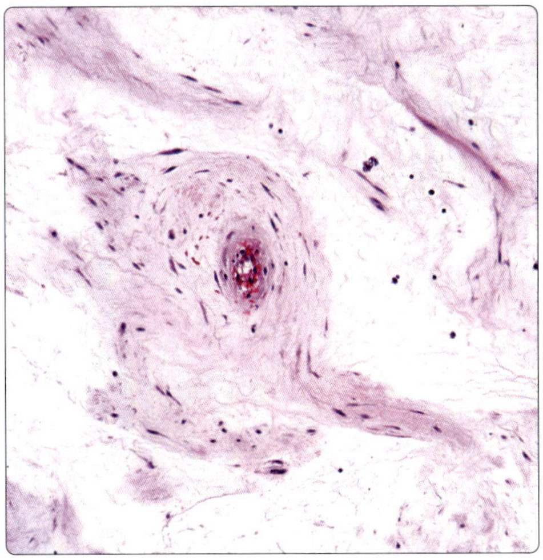

Focal Nuclear Atypia

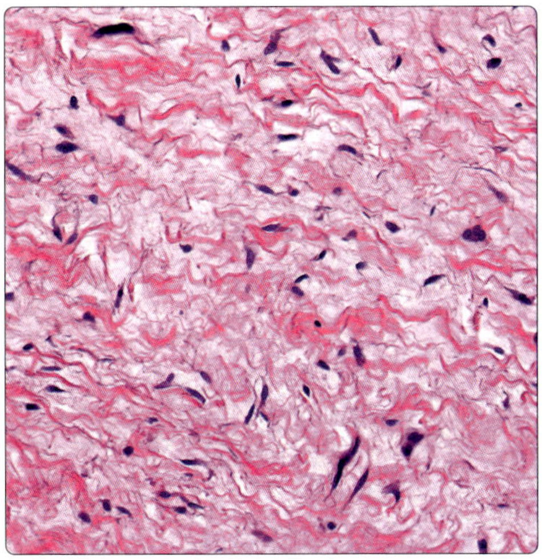

(Left) *This image of deep angiomyxoma shows smooth muscle cells spinning off of a blood vessel that they encircle. This particular case also shows mildly atypical nuclei but is devoid of mitoses.* **(Right)** *Focal nuclear atypia, in the form of hyperchromasia or multinucleation, may be identified in deep angiomyxoma but is generally very rare. This image was taken from a recurrent tumor in the perineum.*

SECTION 14

Tumors of Mesothelial Cells

Benign

Adenomatoid Tumor 590
Multicystic Peritoneal Mesothelioma 592
Well-Differentiated Papillary Mesothelioma 594

Malignant

Malignant Mesothelioma 598

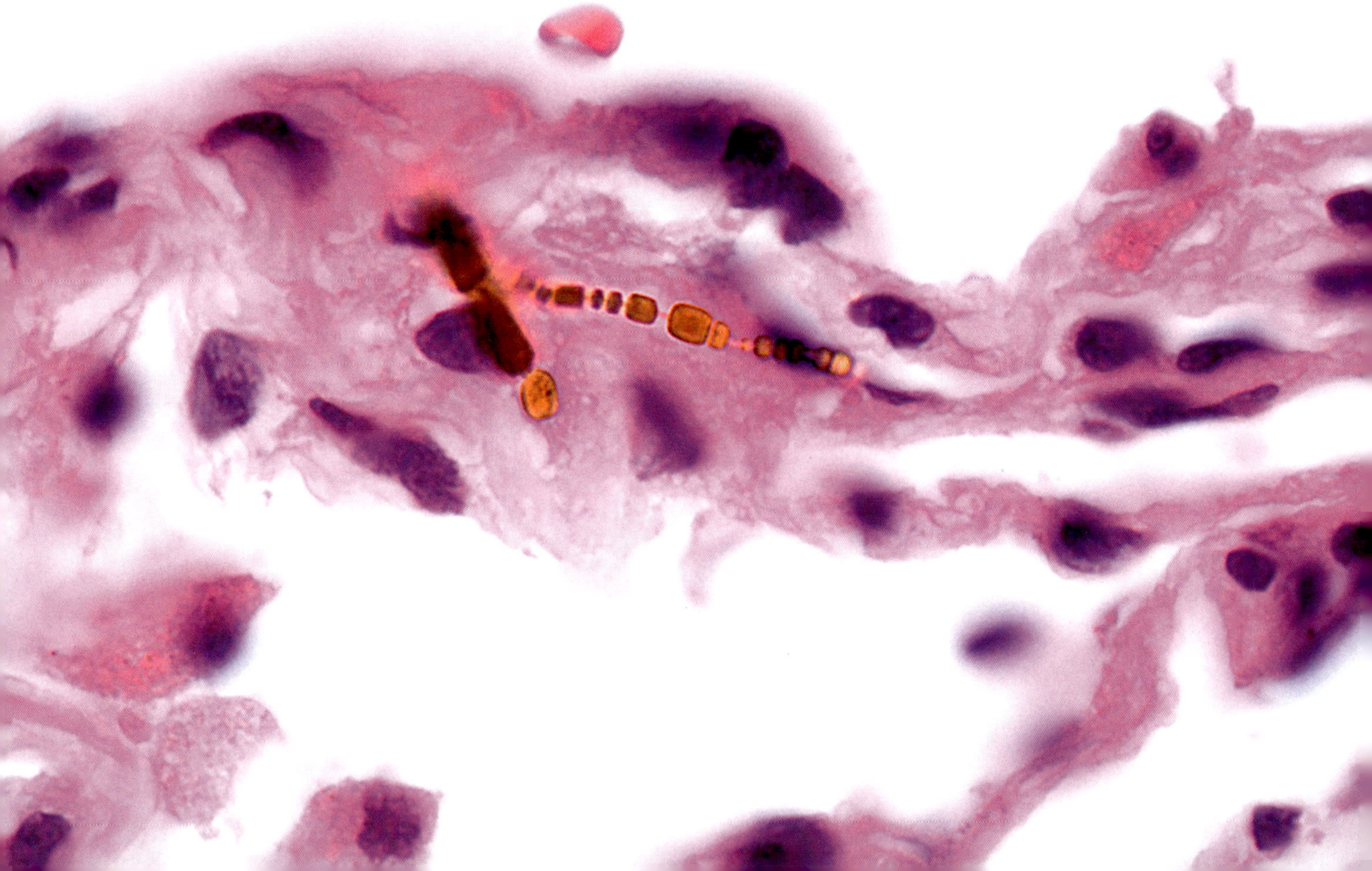

Adenomatoid Tumor

KEY FACTS

TERMINOLOGY

- Benign, localized proliferation of mesothelial cells

CLINICAL ISSUES

- Young to middle-aged adults
- Occurs in both males and females
    - Epididymis, spermatic cord, uterus, fallopian tube, adrenal gland, others
- Painless, firm mass
- Treatment: Simple surgical excision
- Benign

MACROSCOPIC

- Usually < 2 cm

MICROSCOPIC

- Well circumscribed but may show peripheral, infiltrative growth
- Several architectural patterns in varying concentrations and distributions
    - Tubular, gland-like, cords, nests
- Epithelioid or flattened, cytologically bland mesothelial cells
- Fibrous stroma

ANCILLARY TESTS

- Keratin (+), EMA(+)
- Calretinin (+), CK5/6(+), WT1(+), D2-40(+)

TOP DIFFERENTIAL DIAGNOSES

- Metastatic adenocarcinoma
- Well-differentiated papillary mesothelioma
- Multicystic peritoneal mesothelioma
- Malignant mesothelioma
- Lymphangioma

Adenomatoid Tumor

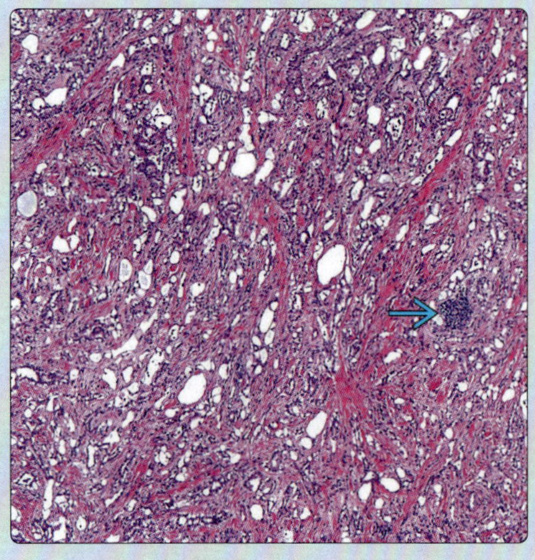

Cytoplasmic "Bridging"

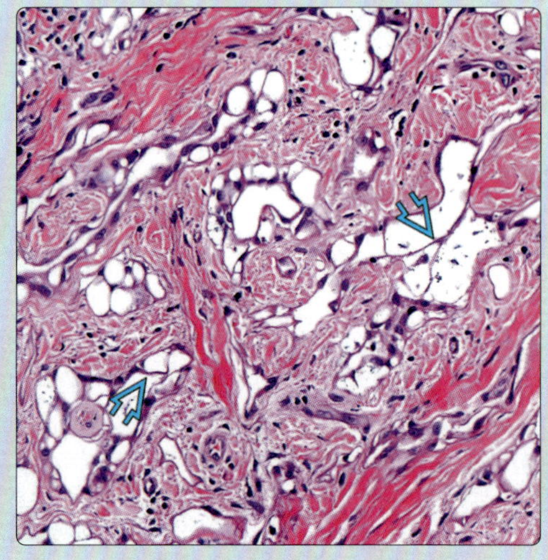

(Left) *Adenomatoid tumor is a benign proliferation of mesothelial cells that is often discovered incidentally. It is characterized by a variety of structural patterns, including tubular, pseudoglandular, angiomatoid, cord, and nest formation. Lymphoid aggregates* → *may be present in some cases.* **(Right)** *Cytoplasmic "bridging"* ⇒*, or the presence of very thin cytoplasmic extensions between cells, is a unique and fairly consistent finding in an adenomatoid tumor.*

Cytoplasmic Vacuolization

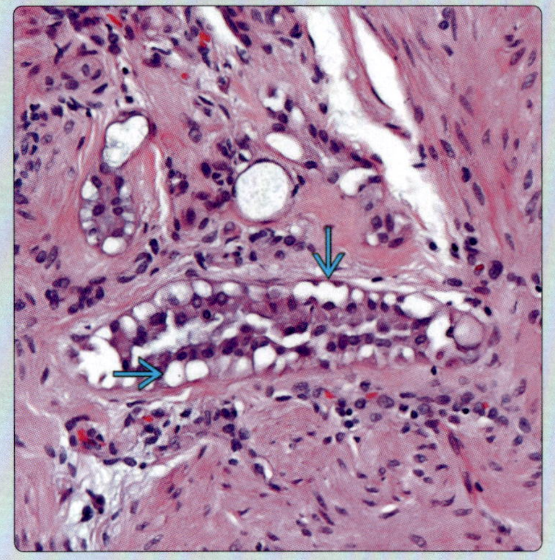

Smooth Muscle Bundles

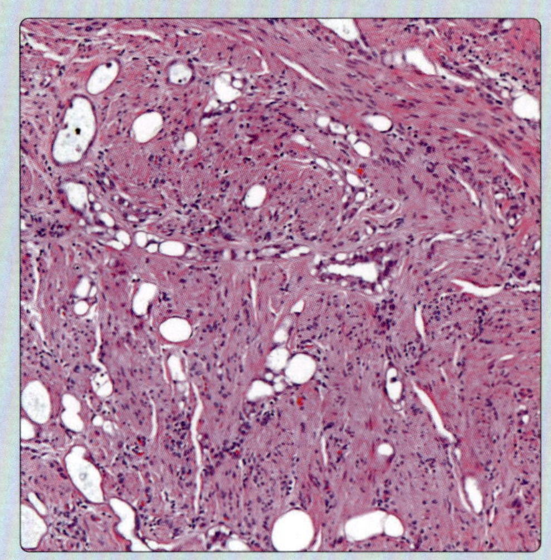

(Left) *Cytoplasmic vacuolization* → *is a common cytologic feature of an adenomatoid tumor.* **(Right)** *In some cases of adenomatoid tumor, bundles of mature smooth muscle can be identified between the tubular structures, as depicted in this image. Given that adenomatoid tumors often occur in tissues that contain smooth muscle, these bundles likely represent normal nonlesional tissue.*

Adenomatoid Tumor

TERMINOLOGY

Definitions

- Benign, localized proliferation of mesothelial cells

CLINICAL ISSUES

Epidemiology

- Incidence
  - Uncommon
- Age
  - Young to middle-aged adults
    - Rare < 20 years
- Sex
  - Occurs in both males and females

Site

- In males
  - Epididymis, spermatic cord
  - Testis (tunica albuginea, body of testis)
  - Prostate
- In females
  - Uterus or fallopian tube
  - Occasionally in ovary
- In either sex
  - Adrenal gland
  - Mesentery, pancreas
  - Pleura, mediastinum
  - Lymph node
- Usually solitary; rarely multiple

Presentation

- Painless, firm mass
  - Scrotal tumors may cause hydrocele
- Often discovered incidentally

Treatment

- Simple surgical excision

Prognosis

- Benign
- Local recurrence rare
- No reports of malignant transformation

MACROSCOPIC

General Features

- Well circumscribed
- Smooth, firm, tan-yellow cut surface
- May rarely show cystic change

Size

- Usually < 2 cm

MICROSCOPIC

Histologic Features

- Well circumscribed but may show peripheral, infiltrative growth
- Several architectural patterns in varying concentrations and distributions
  - Dilated gland-like tubules
  - Solid nests
  - Thin or thick cords
  - Angiomatoid growth
- Cytologically bland mesothelial cells
  - May be plump and epithelioid or small and flattened
  - May show vacuolated cytoplasm or have signet ring morphology
  - Desquamated cells may be present within dilated spaces
- Fibrous stroma
  - May contain scattered lymphoid aggregates or subtle lymphoid infiltrate
  - Can contain smooth muscle bundles
- Rare infarction with necrosis, calcification, or cystic change
- Mitoses rare

ANCILLARY TESTS

Immunohistochemistry

- Keratin (+), EMA(+)
- Mesothelial: Calretinin (+), CK5/6(+), WT1(+), D2-40(+)

Genetic Testing

- *TRAF7* gene mutations

DIFFERENTIAL DIAGNOSIS

Metastatic Adenocarcinoma

- Usually shows nuclear pleomorphism and mitotic activity
- History of prior carcinoma often present
- Absence of expression of mesothelial immunohistochemical markers
- Expression of specific epithelial markers (e.g., colon, prostate)

Well-Differentiated Papillary Mesothelioma

- Papillary architecture
- Can involve peritoneum and omentum

Multicystic Peritoneal Mesothelioma

- Usually involves peritoneal surface
- Larger cysts but histologic features can overlap with adenomatoid tumor

Malignant Mesothelioma

- Larger, more diffuse, or multiple lesions
- Infiltrates adjacent tissues
- Nuclear atypia, mitoses, necrosis variably present

Lymphangioma

- Spaces contain lymphatic fluid
- D2-40(+), keratin (-)

SELECTED REFERENCES

1. Goode B et al: Adenomatoid tumors of the male and female genital tract are defined by TRAF7 mutations that drive aberrant NF-kB pathway activation. Mod Pathol. 31(4):660-673, 2018
2. Terada T: An immunohistochemical study of adenomatoid tumors of the uterus and fallopian tube. Appl Immunohistochem Mol Morphol. 20(2):173-6, 2012
3. Wachter DL et al: Adenomatoid tumors of the female and male genital tract. A comparative clinicopathologic and immunohistochemical analysis of 47 cases emphasizing their site-specific morphologic diversity. Virchows Arch. 458(5):593-602, 2011
4. Amin W et al: Adenomatoid tumor of testis. Clin Med Pathol. 2:17-22, 2009
5. Sangoi AR et al: Adenomatoid tumors of the female and male genital tracts: a clinicopathological and immunohistochemical study of 44 cases. Mod Pathol. 22(9):1228-35, 2009

Multicystic Peritoneal Mesothelioma

KEY FACTS

TERMINOLOGY

- Definition: Benign multicystic proliferation originating from peritoneal mesothelium
- Synonym: Multilocular peritoneal inclusion cyst

CLINICAL ISSUES

- Predominantly in 2nd-6th decades
- More common in females
- Mostly arise on visceral peritoneum
  - Serosal surfaces of uterus, bladder, rectum
- Many patients have history of prior abdominal surgery, endometriosis, or pelvic inflammatory disease
- May present with vague abdominal pain ± other obstructive symptoms
- Treatment
  - Complete surgical excision, if possible, or debulking
- Benign; rare local recurrences

MACROSCOPIC

- Thin-walled, semitransparent cysts or multicystic mass(es)
  - Conglomerate masses can be well over 5 cm

MICROSCOPIC

- Cystic spaces lined by single layer of cuboidal or flattened mesothelial cells
  - Cysts may contain pale eosinophilic granular fluid
- Loose fibrovascular stroma between cysts

ANCILLARY TESTS

- Mesothelial lining cells
  - Keratin (+), calretinin (+), EMA(+) in lining cells
  - CD31(-), CD34(-)

TOP DIFFERENTIAL DIAGNOSES

- Cystic lymphangioma (lymphatic malformation)
- Malignant mesothelioma
- Adenomatoid tumor

Multicystic Peritoneal Mesothelioma

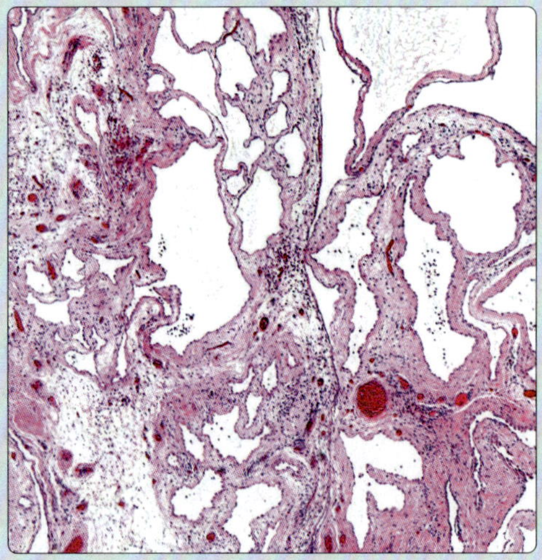

Mesothelial Cell Lining

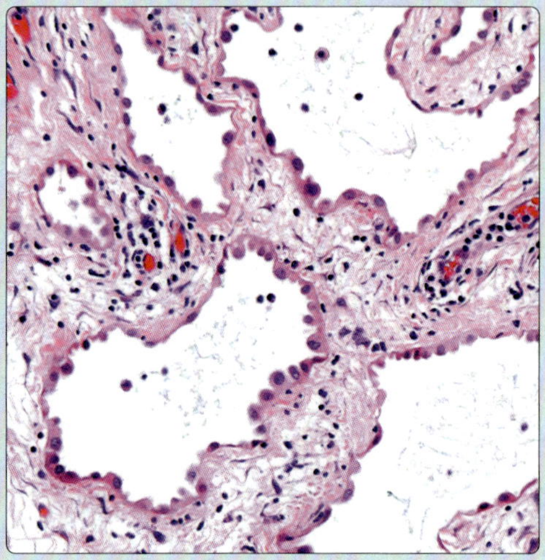

(Left) *Multicystic peritoneal mesothelioma (MPM) generally displays a prominent multicystic appearance at low magnification and can show significant morphologic overlap with a lymphatic malformation.* **(Right)** *Unlike the typically flat endothelial cells that line lymphatic channels, the lining cells of MPM are mesothelial and are often plump and epithelioid. Hobnailing of cells into the cystic spaces is common, and occasionally, focal tufting may be seen.*

Intracystic Fluid

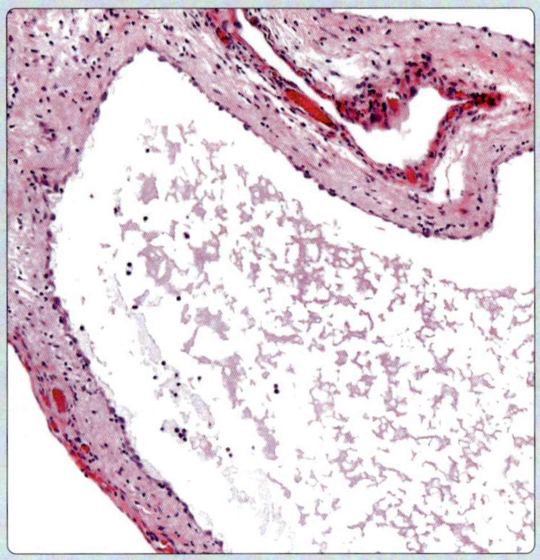

Cytokeratin Expression

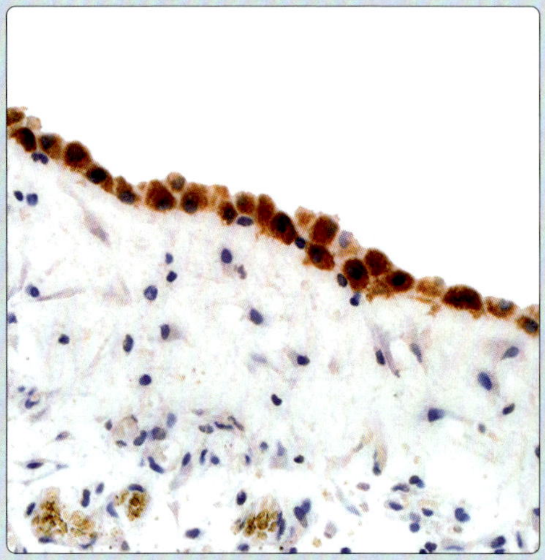

(Left) *Some of the cystic spaces in MPM may contain pale granular eosinophilic fluid with occasional inflammatory cells, similar to lymph seen in cystic lymphangioma (lymphatic malformation).* **(Right)** *Given the mesothelial origin of the lining cells, diffuse expression of CK5/6 (shown) and calretinin is typical in MPM. Endothelial and lymphatic markers, such as CD31, are negative.*

Multicystic Peritoneal Mesothelioma

TERMINOLOGY

Abbreviations

- Multicystic peritoneal mesothelioma (MPM)

Synonyms

- Benign MPM (BMPM)
- Benign cystic mesothelioma
- Multilocular peritoneal inclusion cyst

Definitions

- Benign multicystic proliferation originating from peritoneal mesothelium

CLINICAL ISSUES

Epidemiology

- Incidence
  - Rare
- Age
  - Predominantly in 2nd-6th decades
- Sex
  - More common in females

Site

- Mostly on visceral peritoneum, including surfaces of pelvic organs
  - Uterus, bladder, rectum
  - Rarely involves other viscera, mesentery, omentum
- Can form detached intraperitoneal mass
- Extraperitoneal sites very rare
  - Pericardium, pleura, cesarean section scar

Presentation

- Many patients have history of prior abdominal surgery, endometriosis, or pelvic inflammatory disease
- Vague abdominal pain ± other obstructive symptoms
- May be incidental finding

Treatment

- Complete surgical excision, if possible, or debulking
- Also in situ ablation with sclerosing agents or laser therapy
- Intraperitoneal chemotherapy has been utilized for intractable cases

Prognosis

- Benign
- May recur, or spread, especially if incompletely excised
- Very rare reported cases have been associated with diffuse epithelioid malignant mesothelioma

MACROSCOPIC

General Features

- Thin-walled, semitransparent cysts or multicystic mass(es)
  - Cysts often numerous
    - Contain clear or hemorrhagic fluid

Size

- Conglomerate masses can be well over 5 cm
  - Individual cysts range from 1 mm to > 1 cm

MICROSCOPIC

Histologic Features

- Cystic spaces lined by single layer of cuboidal or flattened mesothelial cells
  - Variable size and number of cysts
    - Often contain pale eosinophilic, granular proteinaceous fluid
  - Uniform, but variably orientated nuclei without cytologic atypia
    - May show bi- or multinucleation
  - Hobnailing, tufting, or small papillations sometimes present
- Loose fibrovascular stroma between cysts
  - May contain lymphocytes &/or occasional lymphoid aggregates
  - Occasionally contains small mesothelial cell clusters, resembling invasive carcinoma
- Rare focal calcifications or hyaline globules
- Occasionally, cases show areas reminiscent of adenomatoid tumor

ANCILLARY TESTS

Immunohistochemistry

- Keratin (+), calretinin (+), EMA(+) in lining cells
- D2-40 (variable)
- CD31(-), CD34(-)

DIFFERENTIAL DIAGNOSIS

Cystic Lymphangioma (Lymphatic Malformation)

- Most common in male children
- Stromal lymphoid aggregates more common
- Smooth muscle may be present around cystic spaces
- Lining cells are CD31(+), CD34(+), D2-40(+) and keratin (-)

Malignant Mesothelioma

- Usually solid or papillary growth, rarely cystic
- Presence of cytologic atypia and mitotic activity
- Stromal invasion

Adenomatoid Tumor

- Well circumscribed, often small
- Pattern of dilated tubules within fibrous stroma
- Cuboidal or flattened mesothelial cell lining
- Generally lacks large cystic spaces of BMPM

SELECTED REFERENCES

1. Rapisarda AMC et al: Benign multicystic mesothelioma and peritoneal inclusion cysts: are they the same clinical and histopathological entities? A systematic review to find an evidence-based management. Arch Gynecol Obstet. ePub, 2018
2. Momeni M et al: Multicystic benign cystic mesothelioma presenting as a pelvic mass. Case Rep Obstet Gynecol. 2014:852583, 2014
3. Elbouhaddouti H et al: Benign cystic mesothelioma of the peritoneum: a case report and literature review. World J Emerg Surg. 8(1):43, 2013
4. Wang TB et al: Diagnosis and treatment of benign multicystic peritoneal mesothelioma. World J Gastroenterol. 19(39):6689-92, 2013
5. Psoinos CM et al: Multicystic peritoneal mesothelioma in an octogenarian: diagnosis, natural history, and treatment. Int J Surg Pathol. 20(1):92-6, 2012

KEY FACTS

TERMINOLOGY

- Well-differentiated papillary mesothelioma (WDPM)
- Synonym: Benign mesothelioma

CLINICAL ISSUES

- Rare
- Incidental finding
- Peritoneal lesions mostly in women
- Pleural lesions show no sex predilection
- Can arise in paratesticular location (tunica vaginalis)
- Solitary or multiple
  - Solitary lesions generally benign
- Some rarely recur after long period as malignant mesothelioma
- Tumors with invasive foci more likely to recur

MACROSCOPIC

- Multiple papillary nodules studding surface of omentum, peritoneum, etc.

MICROSCOPIC

- Well-formed papillary structures
  - Occasional solid nests, tubules, cords
- Uniform cuboidal cells with central, rounded nuclei
- Loose fibrous cores
  - Occasional multinucleated cells in stroma
- Very low mitotic rate
- Invasive foci in some cases

ANCILLARY TESTS

- Positive: Calretinin, CK5/6, WT1, D2-40, pax-8
- Negative: MOC31, BerEP4, desmin, BAP1

TOP DIFFERENTIAL DIAGNOSES

- Malignant mesothelioma
- Mesothelial hyperplasia
- Implants of serous borderline tumor
- Serous carcinoma

Well-Differentiated Papillary Mesothelioma

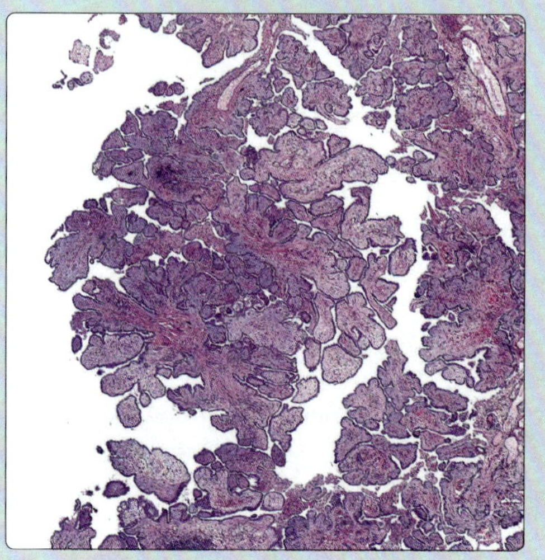

Papillary Architecture

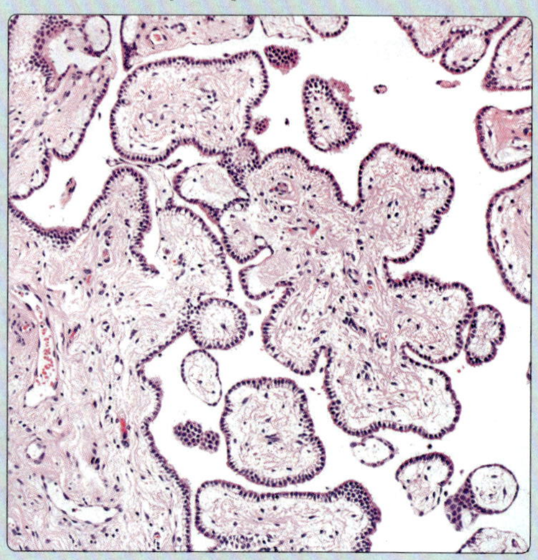

(Left) *Well-differentiated papillary mesothelioma (WDPM) consists of exophytic papillary fronds that arise from mesothelial surfaces as depicted in this scanning-power micrograph. It can be solitary or multifocal and is usually discovered incidentally during surgical operations, most often on the peritoneum in women.* **(Right)** *WDPM is composed of well-formed, branching papillary structures or blunt processes arising from the peritoneal, pleural, or paratesticular mesothelium.*

Fibromyxoid Stroma

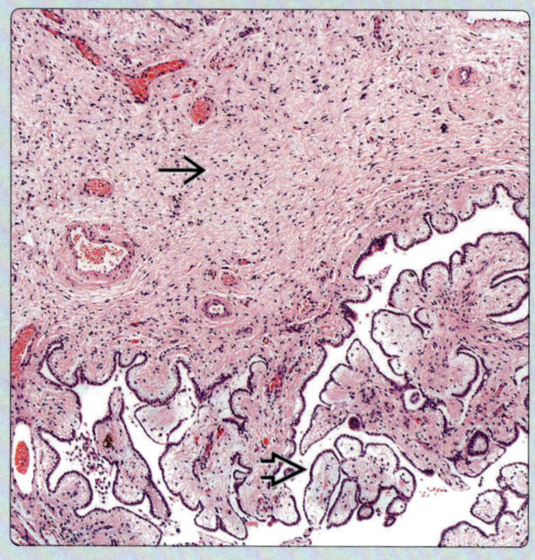

Cytologic Features

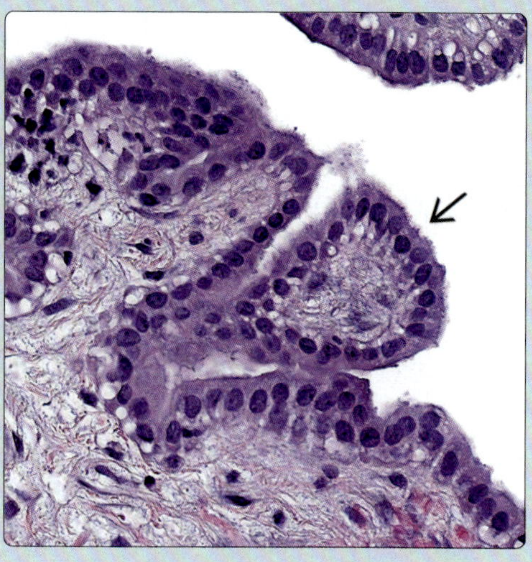

(Left) *Stromal core of WDPM is characterized by loose fibrous or fibromyxoid stroma ➙ with bland fibroblasts and a few blood vessels. Note the uniform papillary structures with simple lining ➩.* **(Right)** *Papillary cores are lined by a single layer of uniform cuboidal cells with eosinophilic cytoplasm, round nuclei with bland cytologic features ➙, and very low mitotic activity.*

Well-Differentiated Papillary Mesothelioma

TERMINOLOGY

Abbreviations

- Well-differentiated papillary mesothelioma (WDPM)

Synonyms

- Benign mesothelioma
- Mesothelioma of low malignant potential

ETIOLOGY/PATHOGENESIS

Neoplasm

- Single familial case with germline *BAP1* mutation

Environmental Exposure

- Some patients have history of asbestos exposure
  - Mostly with pleural tumors

CLINICAL ISSUES

Epidemiology

- Incidence
  - Rare
- Age
  - Predominantly 30-50 years
- Sex
  - Peritoneal lesions arise mostly in women
    - Reproductive age
  - Pleural lesions show no sex predilection

Site

- Peritoneum, omentum, pleura, pericardium
- Paratesticular (tunica vaginalis)

Presentation

- Incidental finding
  - Rarely symptomatic

Treatment

- Surgical excision of localized lesion
- Chemotherapy for multiple or widespread lesions

Prognosis

- Vast majority discovered incidentally; solitary and have excellent prognosis
- Multiple or widespread lesions can be progressive
- Some recur after long period as frank malignant mesothelioma
- Tumors with invasive foci more likely to recur

MACROSCOPIC

General Features

- Multiple papillary nodules studding surface of omentum, peritoneum, etc.

MICROSCOPIC

Histologic Features

- Well-formed papillary structures
  - Lined by single layer of uniform cuboidal cells
    - Central, rounded, benign nuclei
  - Occasional solid nests, tubules, cords
  - Compressive crowding can mimic invasion
- Loose fibrous cores
  - May be myxoid
  - Occasional multinucleated giant cells
- Invasive foci
  - Simple, bland-appearing glands invading papillary stalks
  - Solid foci of higher cytologic grade
- Rare tumors with mixed adenomatoid tumor, cystic mesothelioma, or malignant mesothelioma

ANCILLARY TESTS

Immunohistochemistry

- Positive: Calretinin, CK5/6, WT1, D2-40, pax-8
- Negative: MOC-31, BerEP4, desmin, BAP1 (intact)

DIFFERENTIAL DIAGNOSIS

Malignant Mesothelioma

- Multilayering
- Nuclear atypia, prominent nucleoli, mitoses, necrosis
- Stromal invasion

Mesothelial Hyperplasia

- Can have papillary architecture mimicking WDPM
- Scant amount of fibroconnective tissue in their cores
- Reactive/inflammatory changes in adjacent serosa

Implants of Serous Borderline Tumor

- Complex hierarchical branching papillae
- Micropapillary tufting
- Cytologically bland
- Psammoma bodies

Metastatic or Primary Peritoneal Serous Carcinoma

- Cytologically malignant
- Psammoma bodies
- Positive: pax-8, ER, WT1, MOC-31
- Negative: Calretinin

SELECTED REFERENCES

1. Lee HE et al: BAP1 loss is unusual in well-differentiated papillary mesothelioma and may predict development of malignant mesothelioma. Hum Pathol. 79:168-76, 2018
2. Sun M et al: Well-differentiated papillary mesothelioma: a 17-year single institution experience with a series of 75 cases. Ann Diagn Pathol. 38:43-50, 2018
3. Churg A et al: Well-differentiated papillary mesothelioma with invasive foci. Am J Surg Pathol. 38(7):990-8, 2014
4. Chen X et al: Well-differentiated papillary mesothelioma: a clinicopathological and immunohistochemical study of 18 cases with additional observation. Histopathology. 62(5):805-13, 2013
5. Ribeiro C et al: Well-differentiated papillary mesothelioma: clustering in a Portuguese family with a germline BAP1 mutation. Ann Oncol. 24(8):2147-50, 2013
6. Malpica A et al: Well-differentiated papillary mesothelioma of the female peritoneum: a clinicopathologic study of 26 cases. Am J Surg Pathol. 36(1):117-27, 2012
7. Tolhurst SR et al: Well-differentiated papillary mesothelioma occurring in the tunica vaginalis of the testis with contralateral atypical mesothelial hyperplasia. Urol Oncol. 24(1):36-9, 2006
8. Hoekstra AV et al: Well-differentiated papillary mesothelioma of the peritoneum: a pathological analysis and review of the literature. Gynecol Oncol. 98(1):161-7, 2005
9. Butnor KJ et al: Well-differentiated papillary mesothelioma. Am J Surg Pathol. 25(10):1304-9, 2001
10. Perez-Ordonez B et al: Mesothelial lesions of the paratesticular region. Semin Diagn Pathol. 17(4):294-306, 2000
11. Xiao SY et al: Benign papillary mesothelioma of the tunica vaginalis testis. Arch Pathol Lab Med. 124(1):143-7, 2000

(Left) *WDPM is composed of uniform papillary structures with fibrous cores lined by a simple layer of cytologically benign mesothelial cells.* **(Right)** *High-power micrograph depicts a papilla covered by a single layer of uniform cuboidal mesothelial cells with rounded, central nuclei and eosinophilic cytoplasm →. Note collagen fibers in the papillary core →.*

Papillary Architecture

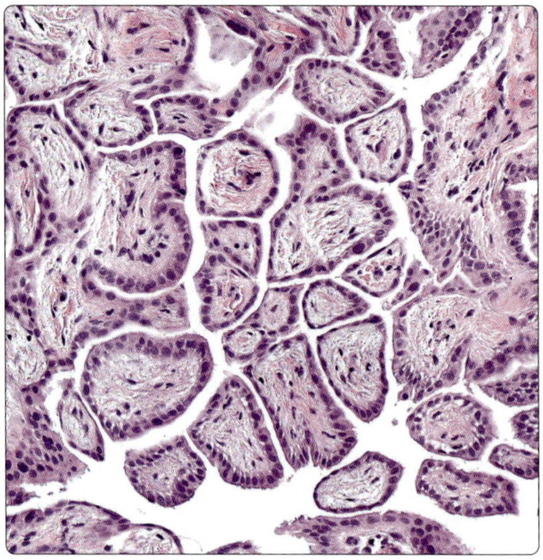

Cytologic Features

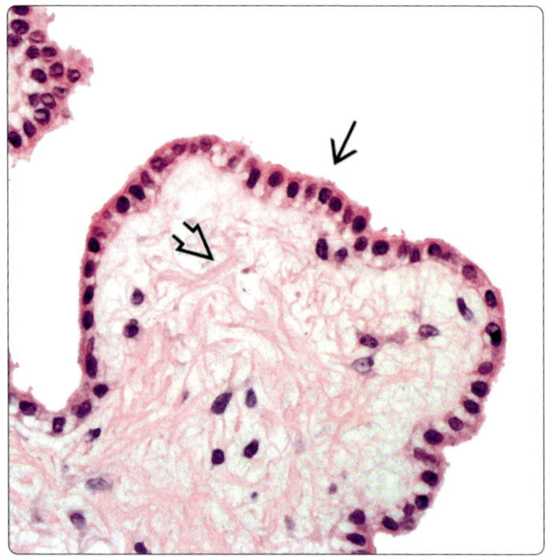

(Left) *Medium-power micrograph shows the simple papillary architecture of WDPM consisting of a broad, central fibrovascular core → and smaller branches → lined by a single layer of cells →.* **(Right)** *Although the papillary structures are usually short and blunt ended, occasionally they can be villiform and pointed →, as illustrated.*

Papillary Architecture

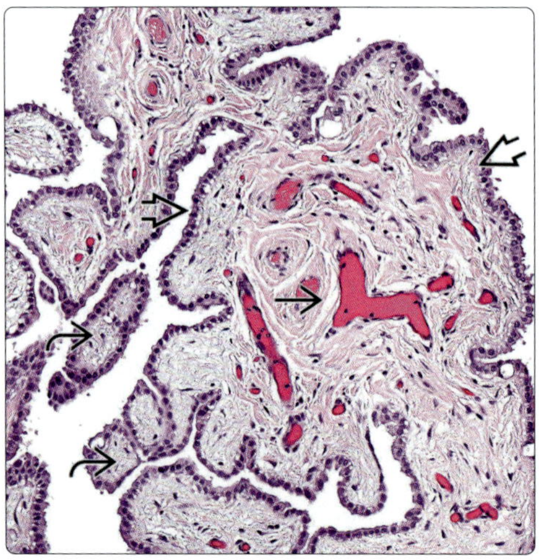

Elongated Papillae

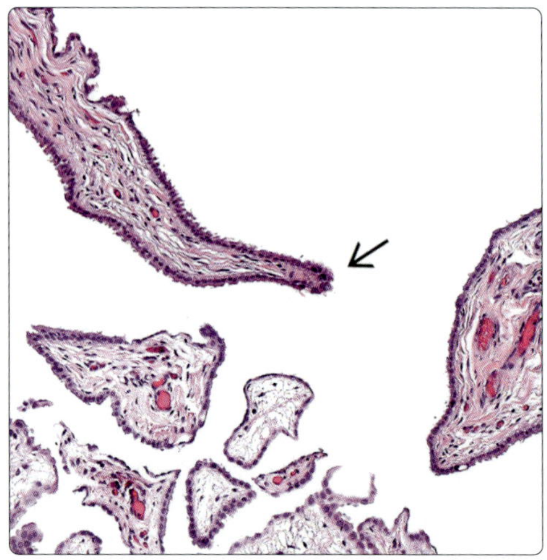

(Left) *Stroma in WDPM frequently contains an abundant myxoid matrix →, rich in proteoglycan, that acquires a pale blue color on hematoxylin and eosin.* **(Right)** *Diffuse, strong, nuclear, and cytoplasmic calretinin expression is present in the lining cells of WDPM →, supportive of mesothelial origin.*

Myxoid Papillary Stroma

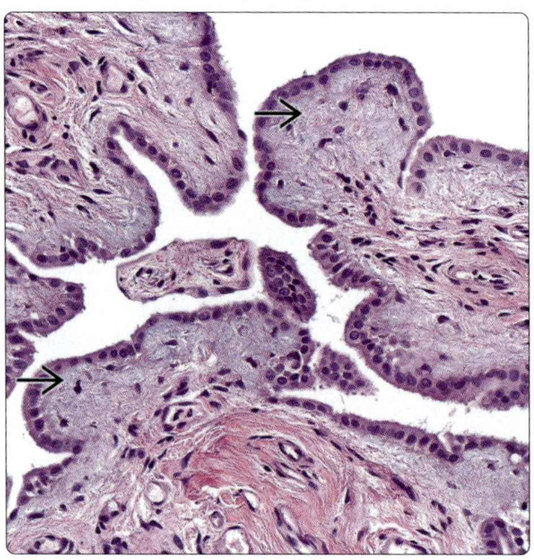

Calretinin

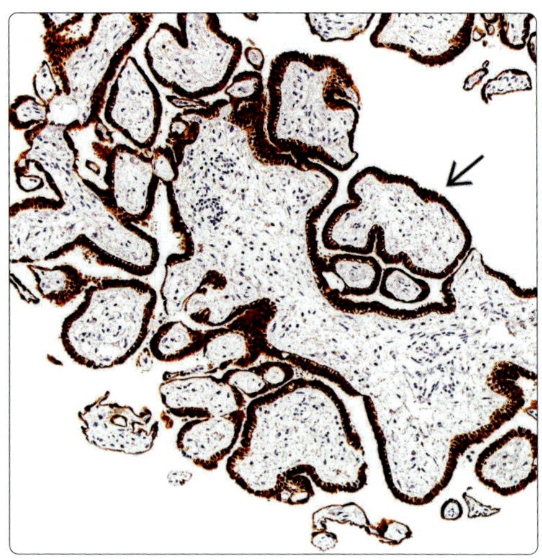

Gross Specimen

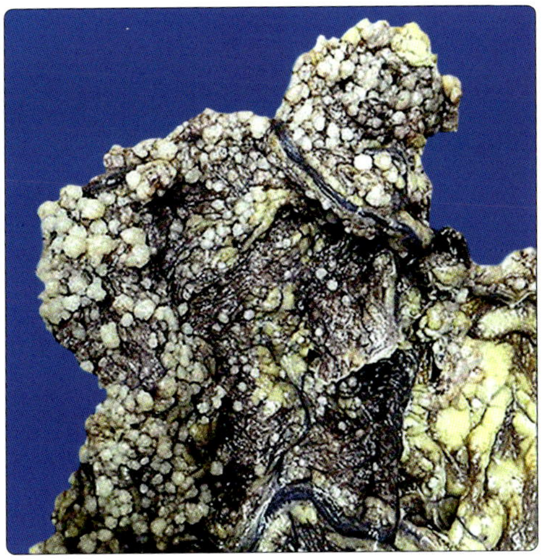

Reactive Fibroblastic Stroma

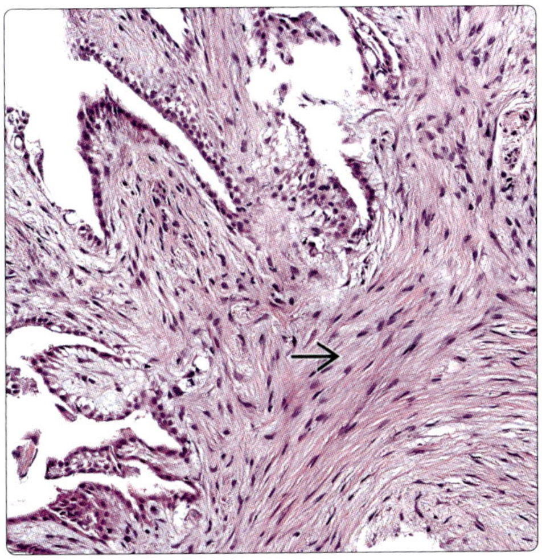

(Left) *Gross appearance of WDPM involving the omentum depicts multiple papillary nodules studding the surface.* **(Right)** *In this example, the stroma is expanded by a reactive proliferation of spindle-shaped fibroblasts arranged in fascicles* → *resembling that of nodular fasciitis.*

Compressive Crowding

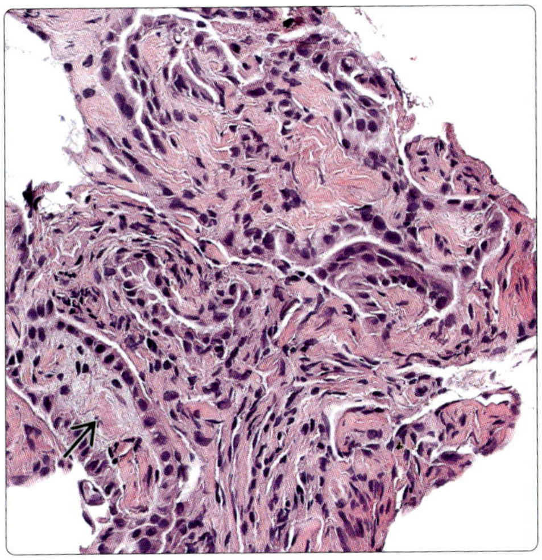

Giant Cells

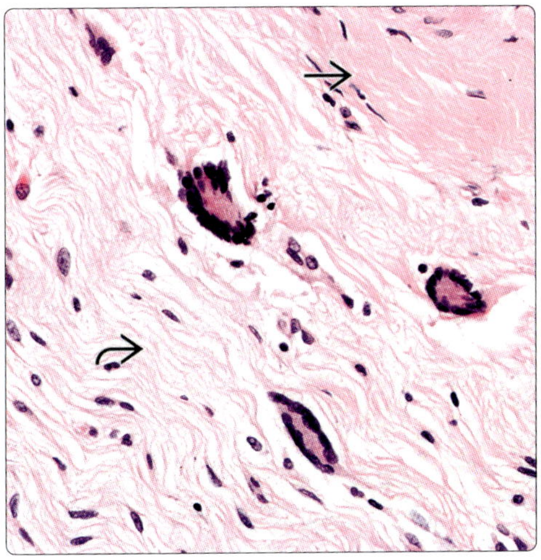

(Left) *Compressive crowding in WDPM represents an artifact of surgical biopsy/excision in which the papillae are squeezed together and can mimic invasive infiltration. Note the intact papilla with fibromyxoid stroma* →*.* **(Right)** *Multinucleated cells are sometimes present within the papillary stroma and base of the lesion. Note both collagenous* → *and more myxoid* ↪ *areas.*

Multiple Invasive Foci

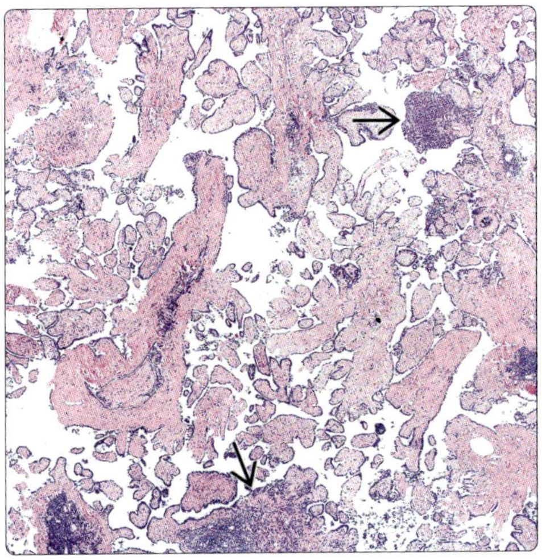

Invasive Foci

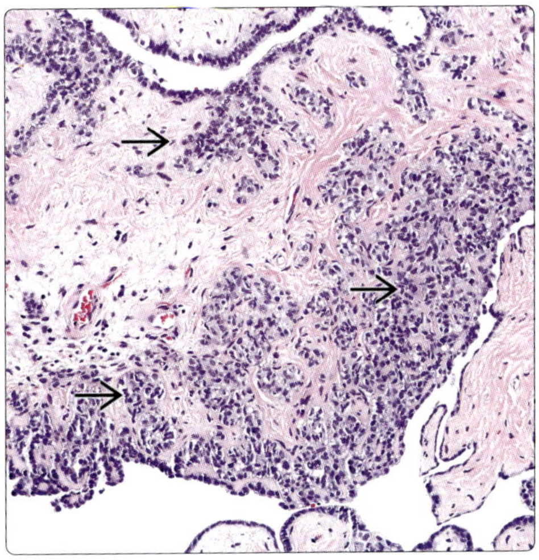

(Left) *Invasive foci are rarely found in WDPM. When present, they consist of simple, bland-appearing glands within the papillary stalks that are often multifocal, as indicated* →*. (Courtesy H. Tazelaar, MD.)* **(Right)** *Invasive foci usually consist of benign-appearing glands* →*. However, rare examples with higher cytologic grade have been reported. Invasive foci, when present, are associated with greater risk for recurrent disease and rarely transformation to life-threatening disease. (Courtesy H. Tazelaar, MD.)*

Malignant Mesothelioma

KEY FACTS

TERMINOLOGY

- Aggressive, malignant tumor of mesothelial cells arising in pleura, peritoneum, or pericardium

ETIOLOGY/PATHOGENESIS

- Asbestos exposure closely linked to development

CLINICAL ISSUES

- Most cases occur > 50 years of age
- M > F
- Treatment: Multimodal therapy more effective than surgery alone
- Overall poor prognosis and high mortality

MACROSCOPIC

- Multiple small nodules, growths, and plaques

MICROSCOPIC

- Epithelioid cytomorphology most common
  - Polygonal dyscohesive cells with eosinophilic cytoplasm
  - Sheet-like, tubular, papillary, glandular, adenomatoid, or mixed patterns
- Sarcomatoid type: Variably pleomorphic spindled cells in sheets and fascicles
  - May contain heterologous elements
- Desmoplastic sarcomatoid type: Prominent stromal fibrosis, hyalinization, sclerosis
- Biphasic type: Mixed epithelioid and sarcomatoid

ANCILLARY TESTS

- Variable mesothelial immunophenotype
  - Use of multistain panel recommended

TOP DIFFERENTIAL DIAGNOSES

- Reactive mesothelial proliferations
- Adenocarcinoma
- Synovial sarcoma
- Solitary fibrous tumor
- Epithelioid hemangioendothelioma

(Left) *Pleural malignant mesothelioma (MM) is generally characterized by patchy or diffuse thickening of the pleura ⇨. The tumor also extends along fissures and septa ⇨.* **(Right)** *Mesothelioma can show a variety of morphologic patterns, including microglandular, tubular, and papillary growth. A stromal reaction may or may not be present, depending upon the site and extent of involvement.*

Malignant Mesothelioma

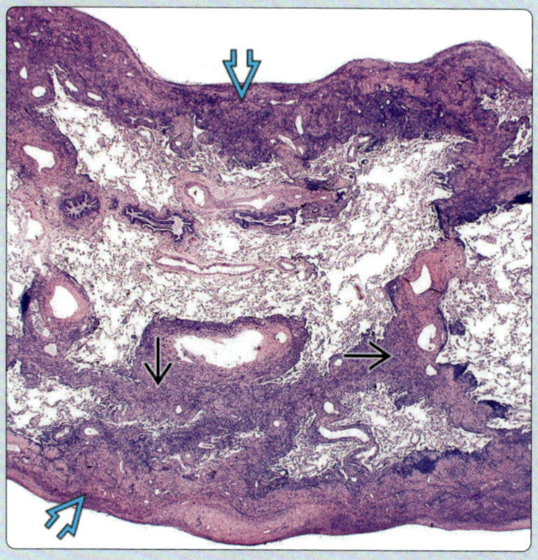

Pattern Variety

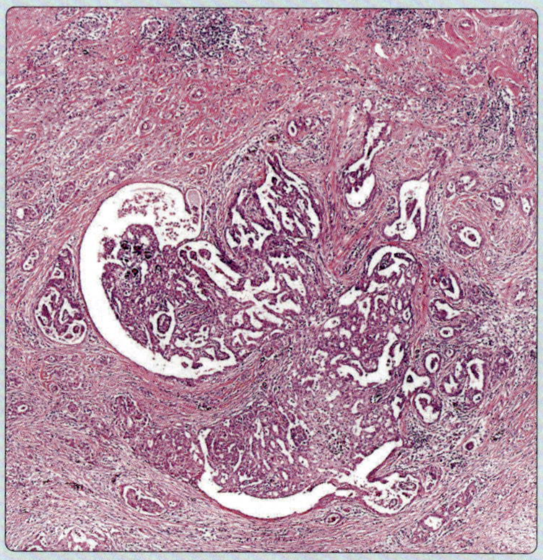

(Left) *Papillary or tubulopapillary growth is common in MM and is often prominent. Small, micropapillary-like clusters may also be seen ⇨ and can sometimes resemble rosette-like structures.* **(Right)** *Invasion of normal soft tissues or structures is typical of MM and is often the best clue to the diagnosis in small biopsies of subtle, well-differentiated tumors. Cytologically, even malignant cells can appear bland.*

Papillary Growth

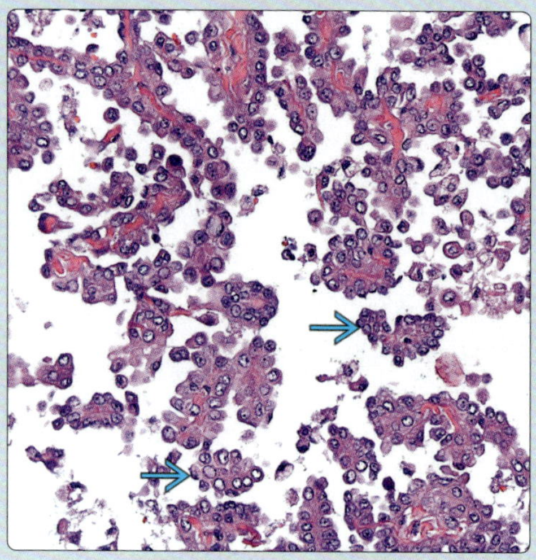

Invasion

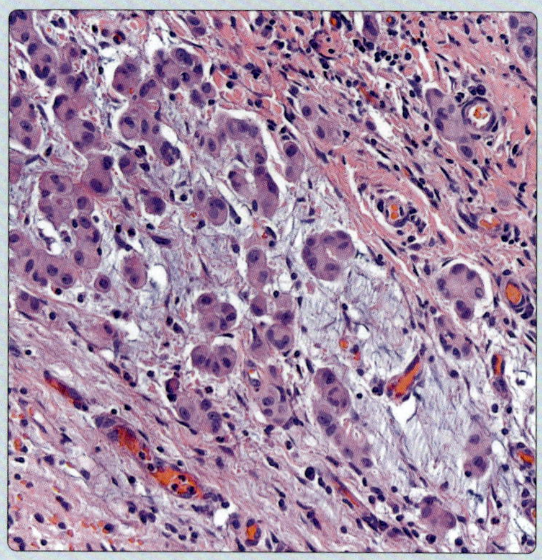

TERMINOLOGY

Abbreviations

- Malignant mesothelioma (MM)

Synonyms

- Diffuse mesothelioma

Definitions

- Aggressive, malignant tumor of mesothelial cells arising in pleura, peritoneum, or pericardium

ETIOLOGY/PATHOGENESIS

Environmental Exposure

- Asbestos
  - Closely linked to development of mesothelioma
  - Occupational exposure
    - Mining, construction, vehicle maintenance, shipbuilding
    - Risk relates to intensity and duration of exposure
  - Amphibole fiber types most carcinogenic
    - Persist in lung ± tissue reaction
    - Crocidolite and amosite have highest risk
    - Longer, thinner fibers more oncogenic
  - Latent period: 15-40 years
- Occasionally, other fiber types implicated (e.g., erionite)

Infectious Agents

- SV40 DNA oncogenic virus
  - Viral sequences found in some mesotheliomas

Radiation Exposure

- Therapy for other cancer (e.g., lymphoma, carcinoma)
- Contrast media (e.g., thorium dioxide)

CLINICAL ISSUES

Epidemiology

- Incidence
  - Geographic variation
    - In USA, ~ 3,000 cases diagnosed per year
    - Higher rates reported in UK, Netherlands, and Australia
    - Lower rates reported in Japan and Central Europe
- Age
  - Most > 50 years
  - Occasional cases at any age
- Sex
  - M > F

Presentation

- Pleural: Dyspnea, chest pain, cough, weight loss
- Peritoneal: Abdominal pain, distension, vague mass

Treatment

- Multimodal therapy more effective than surgery alone
  - Surgery and chemotherapy ± radiotherapy

Prognosis

- Overall poor
  - Median survival: 7 months
  - Mortality rate: 100%
  - Metastases to lung, lymph nodes, liver, other organs
- Histologic features associated with poorer prognosis
  - Nonepithelioid morphology
  - Marked nuclear pleomorphism
  - Loss of p16 by FISH
- Desmoplastic variant of sarcomatoid MM is most aggressive
- Nuclear grading (degree of nuclear atypia and mitotic activity) has been shown to predict overall survival in epithelioid MM

IMAGING

General Features

- Pleural effusion
- Diffuse pleural thickening extending into fissures
- Peritoneal thickening
- Mass lesion

MACROSCOPIC

General Features

- Multiple small nodules, growths, and plaques
  - Rare cases solitary
- May encase lung or abdominal organs
- Firm, white tissue

MICROSCOPIC

Histologic Features

- Usually diffuse, infiltrative
- Epithelioid cytomorphology most common
  - Polygonal or cuboidal dyscohesive cells with eosinophilic cytoplasm
    - Mild nuclear pleomorphism; variable mitoses
  - Variety of morphologic patterns
    - Solid, tubular, papillary, glandular, adenomatoid/microglandular, or mixed patterns
  - Variable stromal collagen and inflammation
    - Occasional myxoid/mucoid change
  - Psammoma bodies may be seen
  - Asbestos bodies may be identified in adjacent lung tissue (pleural mesothelioma)
  - Rare variants: Clear cell, small cell, deciduoid, signet ring, pleomorphic, micropapillary, lymphohistiocytoid, rhabdoid
- Sarcomatoid MM
  - Variably pleomorphic spindled cells in sheets and fascicles
  - Necrosis common
  - May contain heterologous osteosarcoma, rhabdomyosarcoma, chondrosarcoma, or angiosarcoma
  - Desmoplastic variant
    - Prominent stromal fibrosis, hyalinization, sclerosis
    - Storiform architecture common
    - Disorganized, nonuniform growth
    - Usually low cellularity
      - Can show deceptively bland foci
- Some tumors may show mixed epithelioid and sarcomatoid morphology (biphasic)

ANCILLARY TESTS

Immunohistochemistry

- Diffuse pancytokeratin (+)
- Variable mesothelial immunophenotype
  - Panel of expected positive and negative markers strongly recommended
    - Usually positive: Calretinin, CK 5/6, D2-40, WT1, glypican-1, GATA3, CK7, mesothelin, thrombomodulin
    - Usually negative: BER-EP4, MOC31, B72.3, TTF-1, CD34, pax-8
- Loss of nuclear BAP1 favors MM over reactive/atypical mesothelial proliferation
  - Only occurs in ~ 50% of cases, however, and is even much less common in sarcomatoid/desmoplastic MM
- Keratin expression may be only demonstrable marker in sarcomatoid/desmoplastic mesothelioma
  - Use of multiple keratins (e.g., AE1/AE3, CAM 5.2, OSCAR) recommended
  - Pitfall: Submesothelial fibroblasts often express keratin

Molecular Genetics

- *BAP1* gene deletion in majority of cases showing loss of BAP1 expression by IHC
- Deletion of p16 (*CDKN2A*) by FISH in up to 80% of cases of pleural MM and 25% of peritoneal MM
  - Most commonly identified in sarcomatoid MM but also majority of epithelioid and biphasic types
- Rare cases reported of *EWSR1-ATF1*, *FUS-ATF1*, and *EWSR1-YY1* fusions

DIFFERENTIAL DIAGNOSIS

Reactive Mesothelial Proliferations

- Absence of invasion, necrosis
- Usually lacks complicated architectural growth
- Does not form macroscopic lesion or mass
- Retained nuclear BAP1 expression (but also in 50% of MM)

Fibrous Pleurisy

- Can mimic desmoplastic mesothelioma
- Uniform growth of fibroblasts; storiform pattern absent
- No stromal invasion
- Pitfall: Can also show keratin (+)

Adenocarcinoma (Pulmonary)

- Usually positive: BER-EP4, MOC-31, TTF-1
- Usually negative: Calretinin, CK5/6, WT1, glypican-1
- Clinical history and imaging helpful

Adenocarcinoma (Serous Ovarian)

- pax-8(+), ER(+), BER-EP4(+), MOC31(+)
- Calretinin (-)

Synovial Sarcoma

- Highly cellular but monomorphic spindle cell neoplasm
- Can feature epithelial nests or glandular structures
- Spindled cells often keratin (+) but usually focal
- Calretinin (+) and TLE1(+) but also seen in MM
- Demonstration of t(X;18) or *SS18* (SYT) rearrangement most useful

Solitary Fibrous Tumor

- Patternless array of cellular and fibrous areas
- CD34(+), STAT6(+)
- Keratin (-), calretinin (-)

Epithelioid Hemangioendothelioma

- Cords or nests of cells in chondromyxoid stroma
  - Intracytoplasmic vacuoles ("blister cells")
- CD34(+), CD31(+)

Epithelioid Angiosarcoma

- Sheets of atypical cells with prominent nucleoli
- Hemorrhage and necrosis common
- CD34(+), CD31(+), ERG(+)

SELECTED REFERENCES

1. Amatya VJ et al: Glypican-1 immunohistochemistry is a novel marker to differentiate epithelioid mesothelioma from lung adenocarcinoma. Mod Pathol. 31(5):809-15, 2018
2. Brcic L et al: Reproducibility of malignant pleural mesothelioma histopathologic subtyping. Arch Pathol Lab Med. 142(6):747-52, 2018
3. Hjerpe A et al: Cytopathologic diagnosis of epithelioid and mixed-type malignant mesothelioma: ten years of clinical experience in relation to international guidelines. Arch Pathol Lab Med. 142(8):893-901, 2018
4. Husain AN et al: Guidelines for pathologic diagnosis of malignant mesothelioma 2017 update of the consensus statement from the International Mesothelioma Interest Group. Arch Pathol Lab Med. 142(1):89-108, 2018
5. Klebe S et al: Pleural malignant mesothelioma versus pleuropulmonary synovial sarcoma: a clinicopathological study of 22 cases with molecular analysis and survival data. Pathology. 50(6):629-34, 2018
6. Monaco S et al: Recent advances in the diagnosis of malignant mesothelioma: focus on approach in challenging cases and in limited tissue and cytologic samples. Adv Anat Pathol. 25(1):24-30, 2018
7. Pelosi G et al: Pathologic grading of malignant pleural mesothelioma: an evidence-based proposal. J Thorac Oncol. 13(11):1750-61, 2018
8. Pillappa R et al: Loss of BAP1 Expression in Atypical Mesothelial Proliferations Helps to Predict Malignant Mesothelioma. Am J Surg Pathol. 42(2):256-63, 2018
9. Rosen LE et al: Nuclear grade and necrosis predict prognosis in malignant epithelioid pleural mesothelioma: a multi-institutional study. Mod Pathol. 31(4):598-606, 2018
10. Tandon RT et al: Immunohistochemistry in peritoneal mesothelioma: a single-center experience of 244 cases. Arch Pathol Lab Med. 142(2):236-42, 2018
11. Vivero M et al: Clinicopathologic and genetic characteristics of young patients with pleural diffuse malignant mesothelioma. Mod Pathol. 31(1):122-31, 2018
12. Berg KB et al: GATA3 immunohistochemistry for distinguishing sarcomatoid and desmoplastic mesothelioma from sarcomatoid carcinoma of the lung. Am J Surg Pathol. 41(9):1221-5, 2017
13. Desmeules P et al: A subset of malignant mesotheliomas in young adults are associated with recurrent EWSR1/FUS-ATF1 fusions. Am J Surg Pathol. 41(7):980-8, 2017
14. Hwang HC et al: BAP1 immunohistochemistry and p16 fish in the diagnosis of sarcomatous and desmoplastic mesotheliomas. Am J Surg Pathol. 40(5):714-8, 2016
15. Hwang HC et al: Utility of BAP1 immunohistochemistry and p16 (CDKN2A) FISH in the diagnosis of malignant mesothelioma in effusion cytology specimens. Am J Surg Pathol. 40(1):120-6, 2016
16. Cigognetti M et al: BAP1 (BRCA1-associated protein 1) is a highly specific marker for differentiating mesothelioma from reactive mesothelial proliferations. Mod Pathol. 28(8):1043-57, 2015
17. Pavlisko EN et al: Sarcomatoid Peritoneal mesothelioma: clinicopathologic correlation of 13 cases. Am J Surg Pathol. 39(11):1568-75, 2015
18. Panagopoulos I et al: RNA sequencing identifies fusion of the EWSR1 and YY1 genes in mesothelioma with t(14;22)(q32;q12). Genes Chromosomes Cancer. 52(8):733-40, 2013
19. Betta PG et al: Immunohistochemistry and molecular diagnostics of pleural malignant mesothelioma. Arch Pathol Lab Med. 136(3):253-61, 2012
20. Klebe S et al: Sarcomatoid mesothelioma: a clinical-pathologic correlation of 326 cases. Mod Pathol. 23(3):470-9, 2010

Invasion

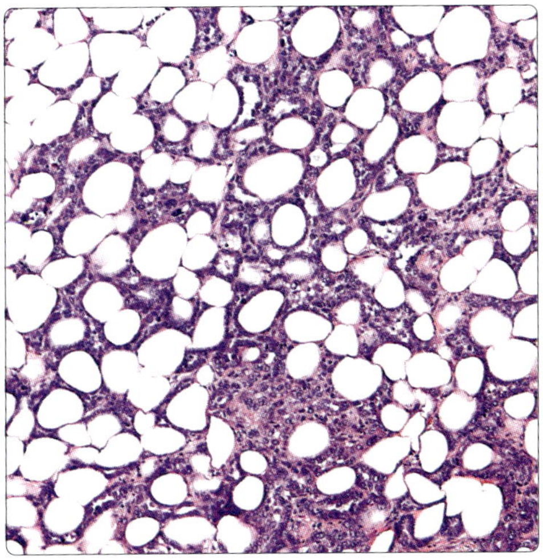

Malignant Mesothelioma

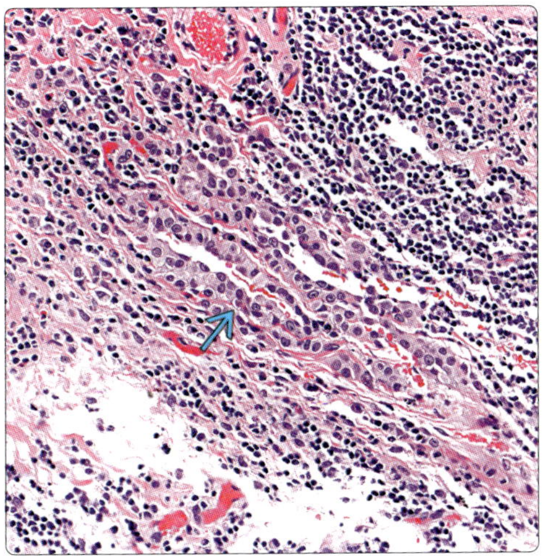

(Left) *Clear-cut invasion of subpleural or subperitoneal soft tissues by atypical mesothelial cells is essentially diagnostic of malignancy. This H&E shows infiltrating tubular structures within the adipose tissue of the chest wall.* **(Right)** *H&E shows ill-defined, invasive, glandular formations* → *in a paratesticular mesothelioma. Note the absence of a desmoplastic stromal reaction in this field.*

Glandular Pattern

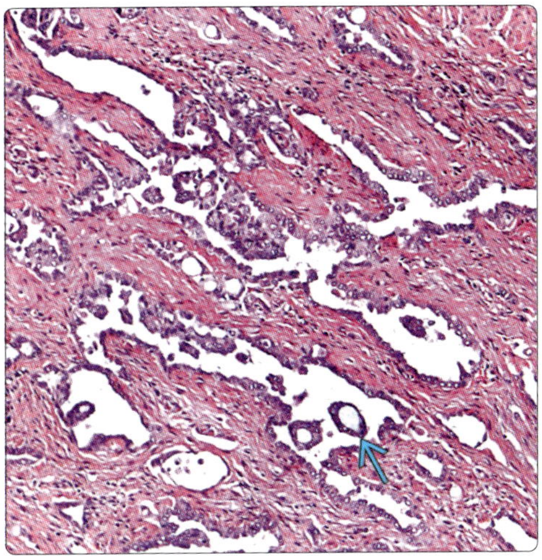

Solid and Papillary Growth

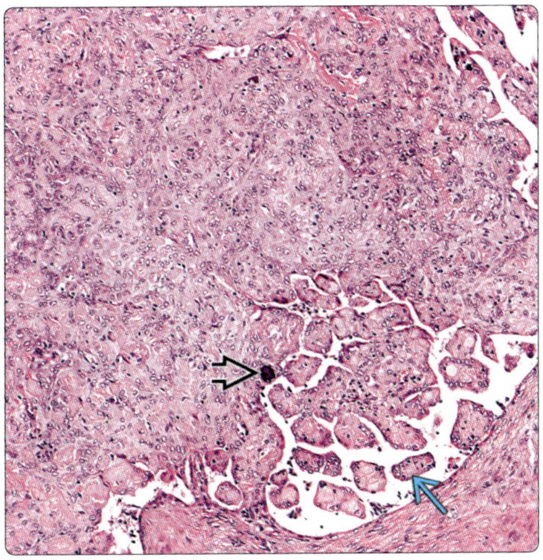

(Left) *H&E of a peritoneal MM shows an irregular, infiltrating, gland-like morphology in the muscularis propria of the large bowel, mimicking adenocarcinoma. Note also the foci of tubular* → *morphology.* **(Right)** *H&E shows MM with a mixture of solid sheets of epithelioid cells and papillae with fibrous cores* →*. Note the small psammoma body* ⇒*.*

Solid and Papillary Growth

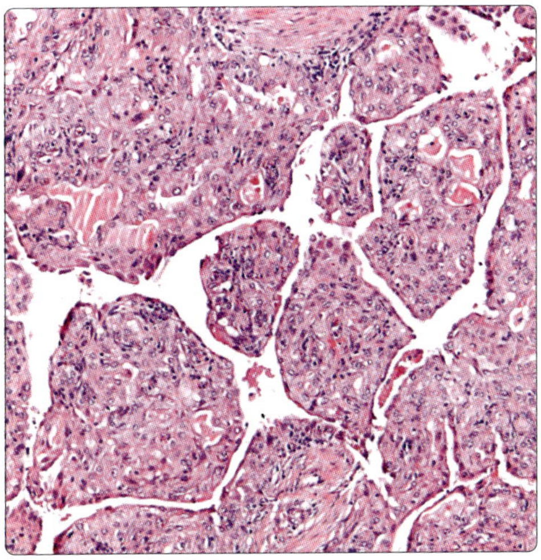

Adenomatoid Pattern

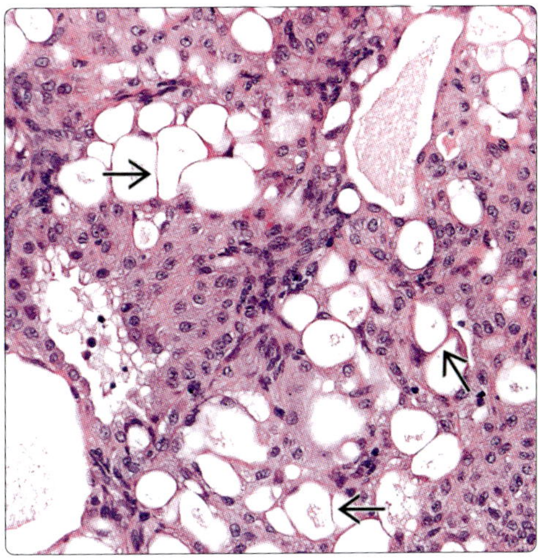

(Left) *The papillary structures in this case of MM were filled with solid sheets of neoplastic mesothelial cells.* **(Right)** *Another type of growth in MM is a microcystic pattern with areas of cytoplasmic "bridging"* →*. This pattern resembles that of an adenomatoid tumor. Clinically, the presentations of these 2 lesions are very different.*

(Left) *An epithelioid cellular morphology is quite common in MM. This H&E shows sheets of polygonal cells and a sprinkling of lymphocytes.* **(Right)** *Some cases of mesothelioma contain a myxoid or mucoid stroma, which rarely may be very prominent and mimic mucinous adenocarcinoma. Tumor cells exist singly or form clusters or loose aggregates and appear to float freely.*

Epithelioid Mesothelioma

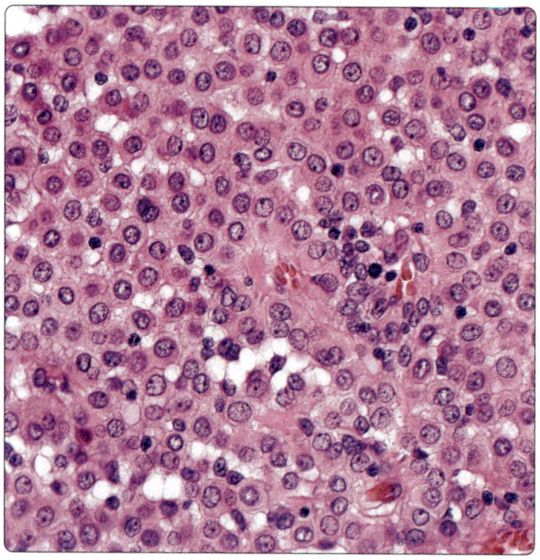

Myxoid Stroma

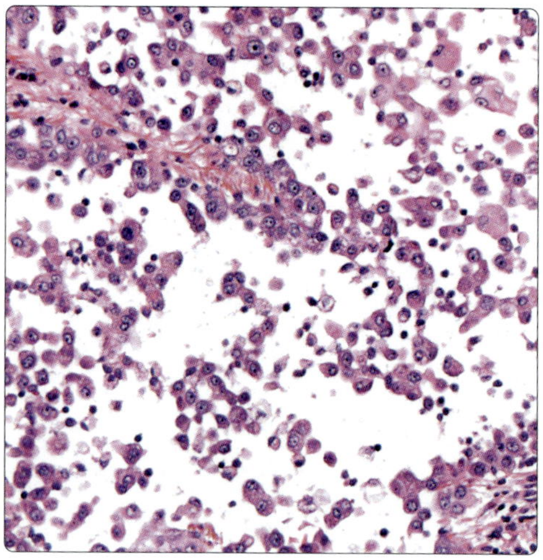

(Left) *The rare deciduoid variant of mesothelioma is characterized by diffuse sheets of large polygonal cells with abundant pale or deep eosinophilic cytoplasm, resembling decidual cells.* **(Right)** *Psammoma bodies ➔ may be identified in MM, particularly cases with a papillary architecture.*

Epithelioid Cells

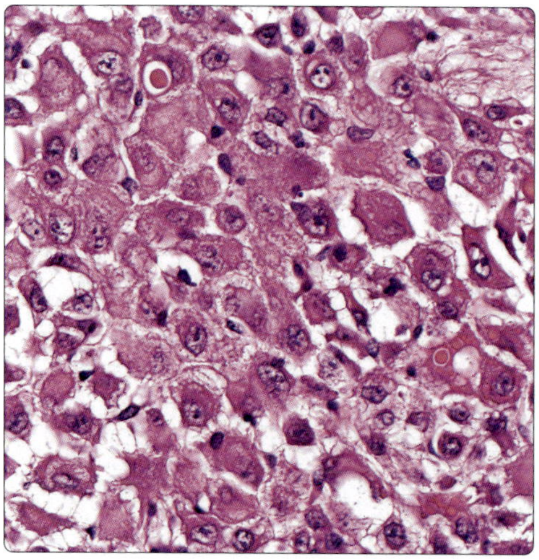

Psammoma Bodies

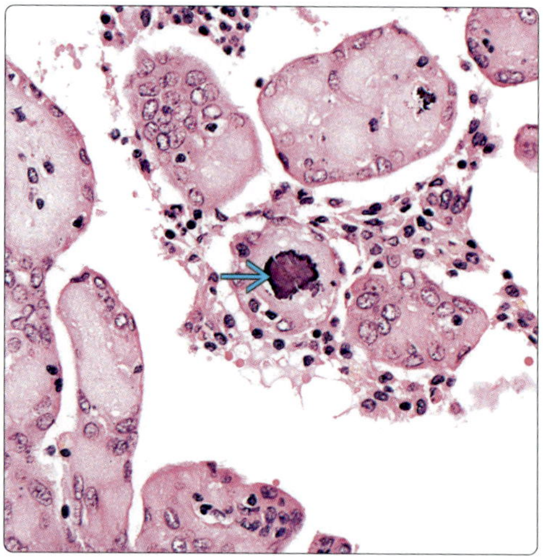

(Left) *Sarcomatoid mesothelioma is characterized by sheets and fascicles of spindled or pleomorphic tumor cells as depicted. Some tumors are biphasic and also contain an epithelioid component.* **(Right)** *Heterologous elements may be identified in sarcomatoid mesothelioma and usually appear as rhabdomyosarcomatous, osteosarcomatous ➔, or chondrosarcomatous foci.*

Sarcomatoid Mesothelioma

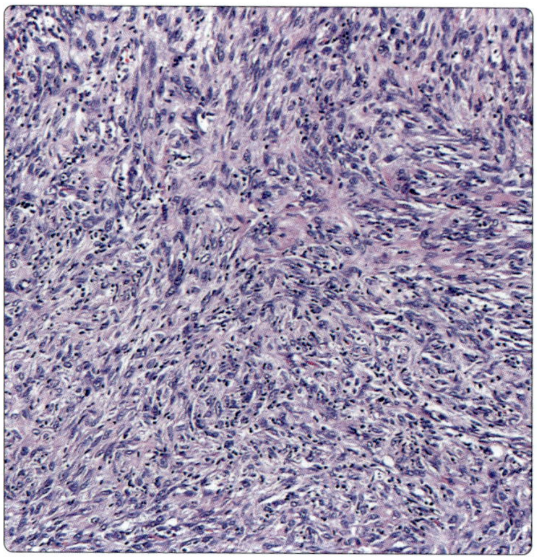

Heterologous Osteosarcoma

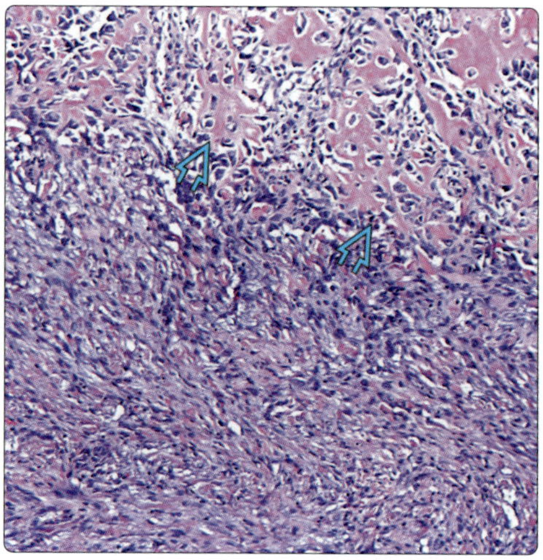

Desmoplastic Mesothelioma

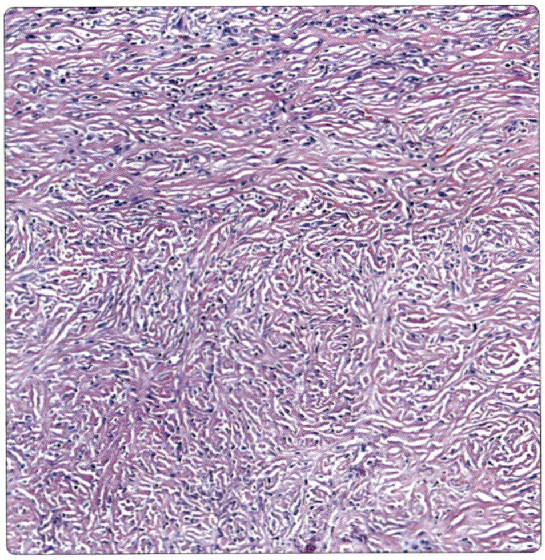

Desmoplastic Mesothelioma

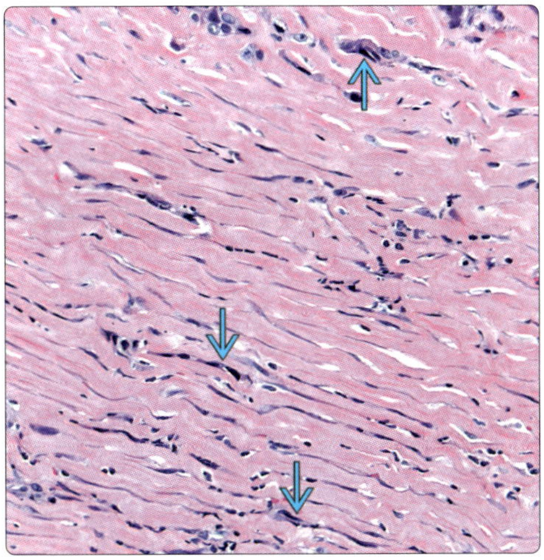

(Left) *The desmoplastic variant of sarcomatoid mesothelioma shows scattered atypical cells amongst abundant collagen or sclerosis. Areas of storiform growth may also be seen. If not considered, this variant may be mistaken for a benign, reactive fibroblastic process.* **(Right)** *Despite the prominent hyalinization/sclerosis and overall hypocellularity of desmoplastic mesothelioma, there is often at least focal nuclear atypia* → *and hyperchromasia that should raise concern for this diagnosis.*

Lymphohistiocytoid Mesothelioma

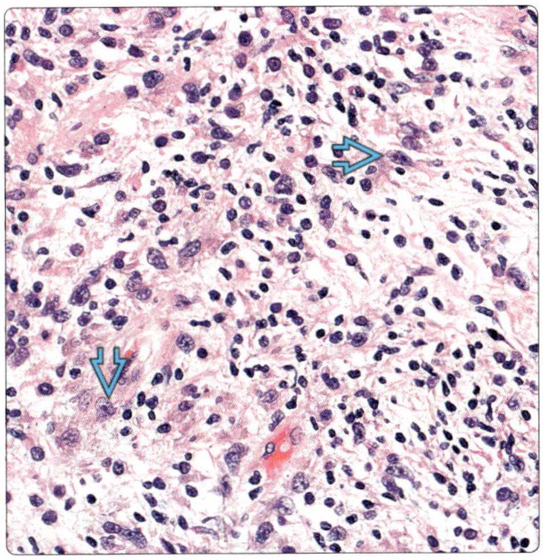

Cytokeratin Expression

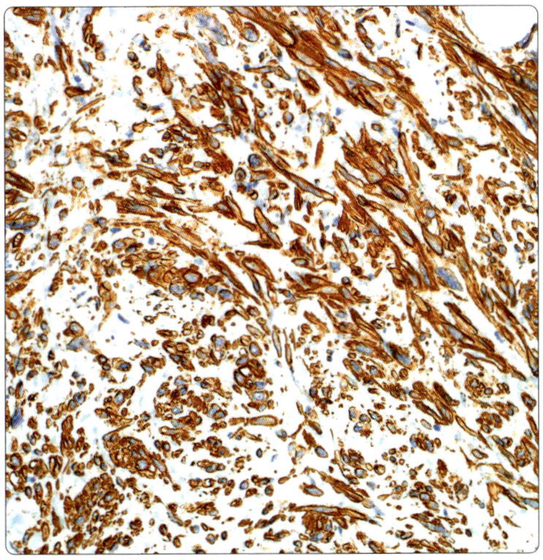

(Left) *H&E of the rare lymphohistiocytoid mesothelioma shows mixed chronic inflammatory cells obscuring scattered malignant mesothelial cells* ⇨*, which may resemble histiocytes. The inflammatory infiltrate is typically dense, and the overall pattern may be similar to thymoma.* **(Right)** *Cytokeratin AE1/AE3 shows diffuse expression in most cases of MM, regardless of its morphology. Other more specific markers are generally required to confirm the diagnosis.*

Electron Microscopy

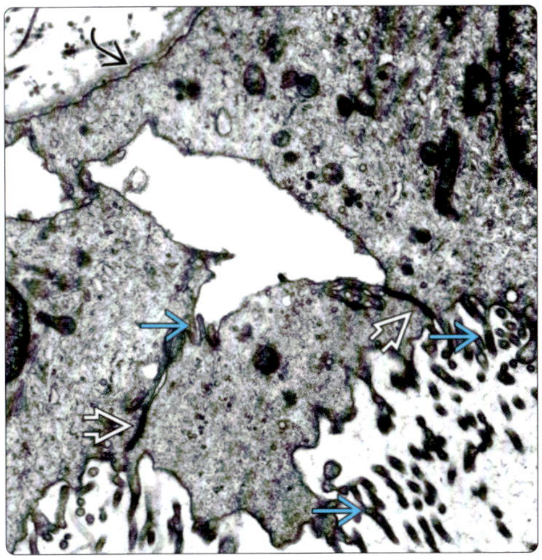

Malignant Mesothelioma

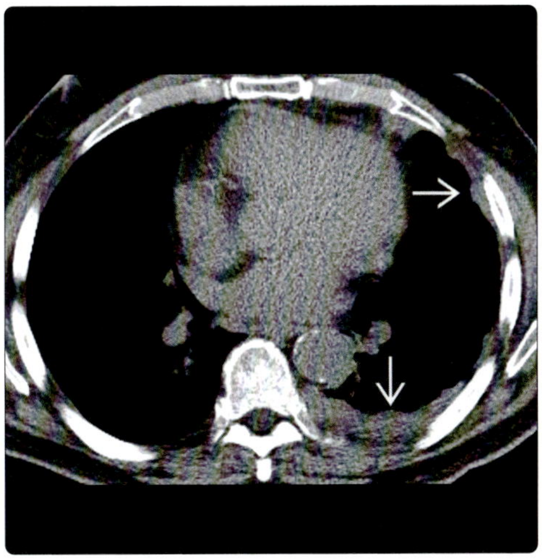

(Left) *Transmission electron microscopy high-power image of mesothelioma cells exhibits the classic features of zonula adherens junctions* ➡ *joining otherwise separated cell surfaces on which are microvilli of various lengths* →*. Cells are oriented on the basal lamina* ⇨*.* **(Right)** *Unenhanced CT of the chest shows typical increased thickness of the pleura* ➡ *from MM. It will frequently have a multifocal appearance, as in this case.*

SECTION 15

Hematopoietic Tumors in Soft Tissue

Solitary Extramedullary Plasmacytoma 606
Myeloid Sarcoma 608
Lymphoma of Soft Tissue 610

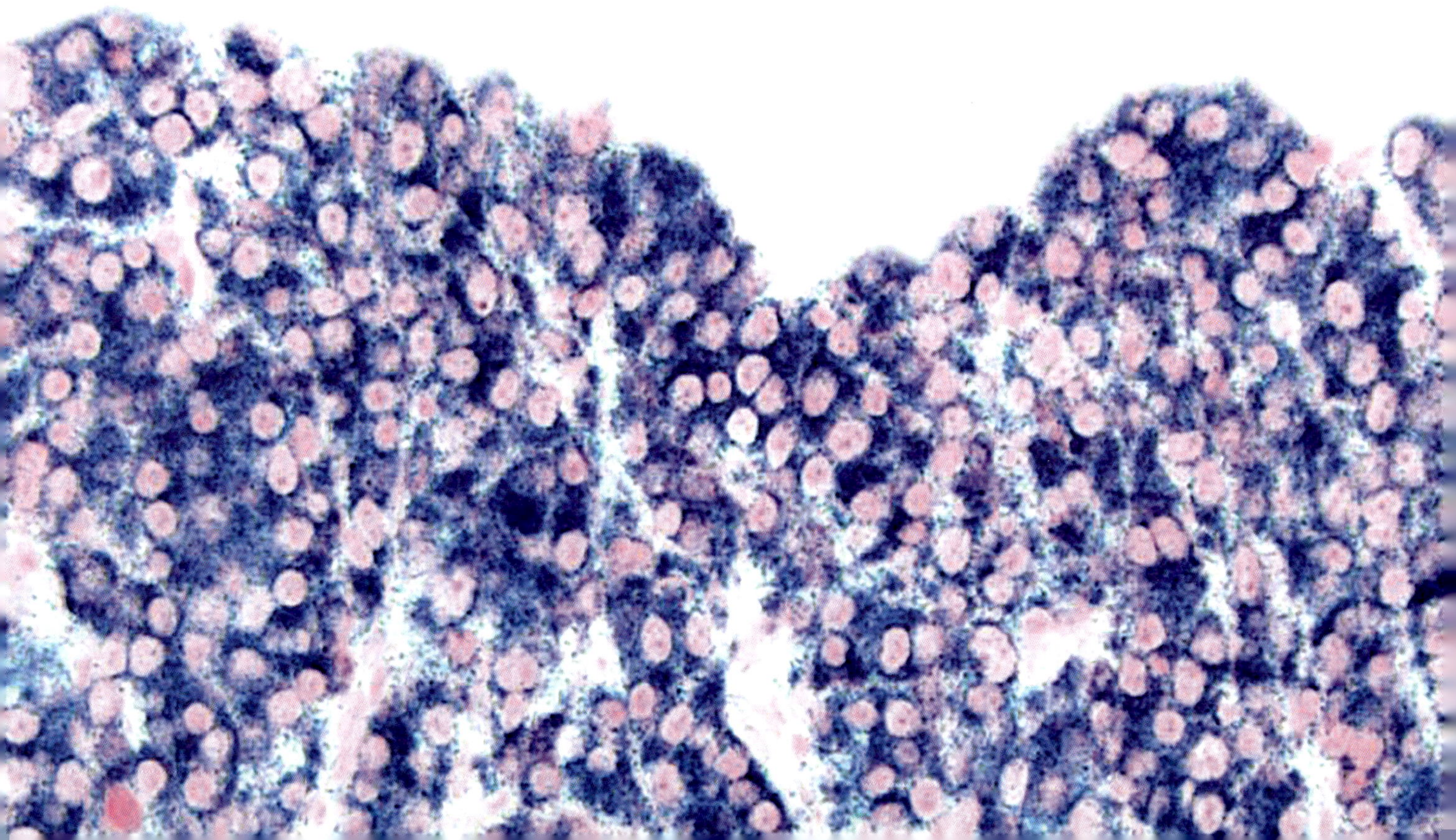

Solitary Extramedullary Plasmacytoma

KEY FACTS

TERMINOLOGY

- Mass-forming proliferation of clonal (neoplastic) plasma cells arising outside of bone marrow
  - Signs or diagnostic features of multiple myeloma must be absent

CLINICAL ISSUES

- Usually older adults (median age: 58 years)
  - 2:1 male predominance
- Head and neck most common site overall
  - Upper aerodigestive tract, including sinonasal cavity, sinuses, and oropharynx
- Symptoms related to location of mass
- Treatment: Radiation therapy; surgical excision in some cases
- Low risk of local recurrence following radiation (up to 7%)
- Risk of progression to myeloma (10-30% at 10 years)

IMAGING

- No lytic lesions in skeleton

MICROSCOPIC

- Sheets and nests of variably differentiated plasma cells
  - Nuclear atypia varies with grade of tumor

ANCILLARY TESTS

- CD138(+), keratin (-), S100 protein (-), CD20(-)
- Shows λ- or κ-light chain restriction by in situ hybridization

TOP DIFFERENTIAL DIAGNOSES

- Myoepithelioma of soft tissue
- Metastatic carcinoma
- Multiple myeloma
- Epithelioid sarcoma
- Malignant melanoma

Solitary Extramedullary Plasmacytoma

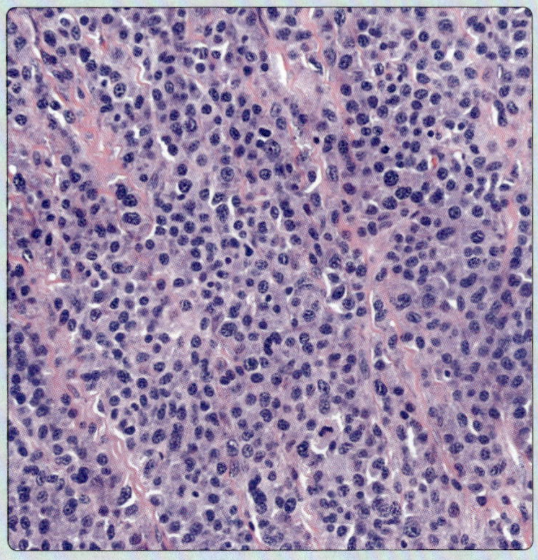

Plasma Cells

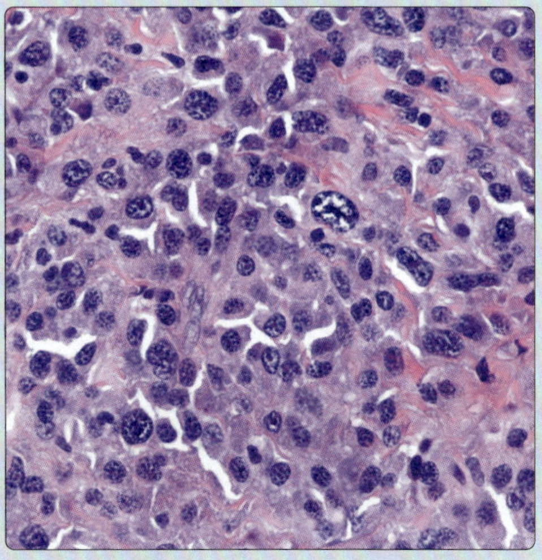

(Left) *Solid extramedullary plasmacytoma (SEP) is characterized by a clonal proliferation of plasma cells occurring outside of the bone marrow. Also, by definition, no clinical evidence of multiple myeloma can be present.* **(Right)** *In general, the degree of nuclear atypia depends upon the grade of the tumor; however, in most cases, the lesional cells are easily identified as plasma cells if attention is paid to cytologic features (eccentric nuclei with "clockface" chromatin).*

Nests and Sheets

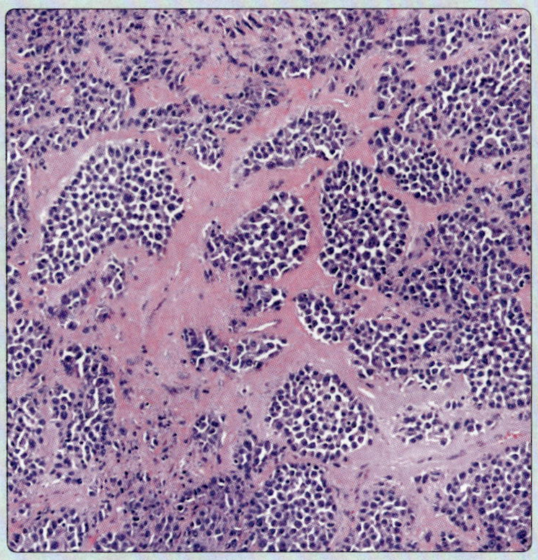

In Situ Hybridization

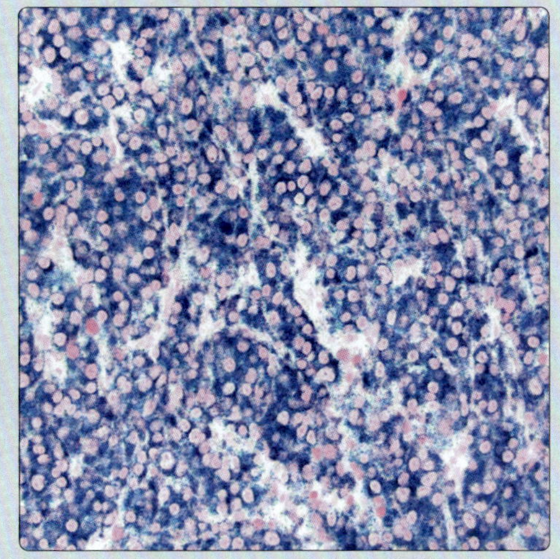

(Left) *The lesional cells of SEP form diffuse sheets and nests within a variable collagenous stroma. In some cases, foci of stromal sclerosis may impart an appearance similar to carcinoma or myoepithelioma.* **(Right)** *In situ hybridization studies are usually utilized to demonstrate light chain restriction in SEP. This particular case shows κ restriction (blue).*

TERMINOLOGY

Abbreviations

- Solitary extramedullary plasmacytoma (SEP)

Synonyms

- Solitary extraosseous plasmacytoma

Definitions

- Mass-forming proliferation of clonal (neoplastic) plasma cells arising outside of bone marrow
- Signs or diagnostic features of multiple myeloma must be absent
  - Including no evidence of anemia, hypercalcemia, renal insufficiency, or lytic bone lesions

CLINICAL ISSUES

Epidemiology

- Incidence
  - Rare (3% of all plasma cell neoplasms)
- Age
  - Usually older adults (median age: 58 years)
- Sex
  - 2:1 male predominance

Site

- Head and neck most common overall
  - Upper aerodigestive tract, including sinonasal cavity, sinuses, and oropharynx
    - May spread to regional lymph nodes (15% of cases)
- Also gastrointestinal tract, skin, soft tissue, liver, central nervous system, lung
- Does not involve bone

Presentation

- Symptoms related to location of mass
  - Epistaxis and nasal-obstructive symptoms in upper airway tumors
- Minority of patients have small M-protein (usually IgA)

Treatment

- Radiation therapy
- Complete surgical excision in some cases
  - Incomplete excisions followed by radiation

Prognosis

- Overall good prognosis
  - Head and neck location and size < 5 cm may be good prognostic factors
- Low risk of local recurrence following radiation (up to 7%)
- Risk of progression to myeloma (10-30% at 10 years)

IMAGING

MR and Bone Scan

- No lytic lesions in skeleton

MACROSCOPIC

Size

- Variable range

MICROSCOPIC

Histologic Features

- Sheets and nests of variably differentiated plasma cells
  - Eccentric nuclei, presence of perinuclear hof, classic clockface chromatin pattern
    - Nuclear atypia varies with grade of tumor
  - Variable mitotic rate
- Stroma may show sclerotic areas

ANCILLARY TESTS

Immunohistochemistry

- CD138(+)
- Keratin (-), S100 protein (-), CD20(-)

In Situ Hybridization

- Shows λ- or κ-light chain restriction

DIFFERENTIAL DIAGNOSIS

Myoepithelioma of Soft Tissue

- Tumor cells may be plasmacytoid with eosinophilic cytoplasm
- Myxoid stroma common; often prominent
- Keratin (+), EMA(+), S100 protein (+)

Metastatic Carcinoma

- Clinical history of primary tumor often present
- Keratin (+)
- Pitfall: CD138(+) in some types of carcinoma

Multiple Myeloma

- Median age older than in SEP
- > 1 lesion present
- Lytic skeletal lesions common
- Presence of 10% or more clonal plasma cells in bone marrow

Epithelioid Sarcoma

- Sheets of epithelioid tumor cells, often with foci of central necrosis
- Keratin (+); CD34 (variable); loss of nuclear INI1

Malignant Melanoma

- Clinical history of primary tumor may or may not be present
- Often marked nuclear atypia, mitotic activity, and necrosis
- S100 protein (+)
- 1 or more melanocytic markers (HMB-45, MART-1, etc.) often present
- May show focal CD138(+)

SELECTED REFERENCES

1. Ghodke K et al: A retrospective study of correlation of morphologic patterns, MIB1 proliferation index, and survival analysis in 134 cases of plasmacytoma. Ann Diagn Pathol. 19(3):117-23, 2015
2. Comfere NI et al: Cutaneous extramedullary plasmacytoma: clinical, prognostic, and interphase cytogenetic analysis. Am J Dermatopathol. 35(3):357-63, 2013
3. Gerry D et al: Epidemiologic evidence of superior outcomes for extramedullary plasmacytoma of the head and neck. Otolaryngol Head Neck Surg. 148(6):974-81, 2013
4. Kilciksiz S et al: A review for solitary plasmacytoma of bone and extramedullary plasmacytoma. ScientificWorldJournal. 2012:895765, 2012

Myeloid Sarcoma

KEY FACTS

TERMINOLOGY

- Tumoral mass of myeloid blasts ± maturation occurring outside of bone marrow
- Synonyms: Granulocytic sarcoma, chloroma

CLINICAL ISSUES

- Wide age range (children to older adults)
- Skin, bone, lymph node, testis most common sites
- Solitary mass
  - May arise de novo or concurrently with acute myeloid leukemia, myeloproliferative neoplasm, or myelodysplastic syndrome
- Prognosis does not seem to be influenced by age, sex, site, histologic features, immunophenotype, or cytogenetic findings

MICROSCOPIC

- Diffuse, sheet-like growth that effaces normal tissue architecture
- Uniform, medium-sized cells with little cytoplasm
  - Round to oval nucleus with prominent nucleolus
  - Cytoplasm may contain eosinophilic granules
  - May show monoblastic, monocytic, myelomonocytic morphologies depending on origin

ANCILLARY TESTS

- CD43(+), lysozyme (+), CD45(+), CD34 (variable)
- Myeloid differentiation: Myeloperoxidase (+), CD117(+)
- Monocytic differentiation: CD68(+), CD13(+)
- CD3(-), CD20(-), keratin (-), S100(-), desmin (-)
- Molecular: Chromosomal aberrations detected in ~ 50% of cases

TOP DIFFERENTIAL DIAGNOSES

- Lymphoma
- Poorly differentiated carcinoma or melanoma
- Various small round blue cell tumors
- Epithelioid angiosarcoma

(Left) *Myeloid sarcoma (a.k.a. granulocytic sarcoma) is an extramedullary tumoral mass of myeloid blasts ± evidence of maturation. Histologically, it is composed of diffuse sheets of uniform cells that efface normal tissue architecture.* **(Right)** *The lesional cells of myeloid sarcoma are uniform myeloblasts with fine chromatin and variably prominent nucleoli. Taken together, this appearance is often morphologically indistinguishable from lymphoma.*

Myeloid Sarcoma

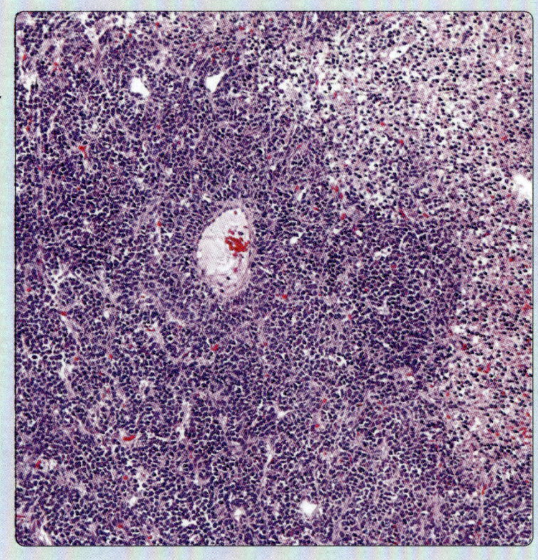

Uniform Myeloblasts

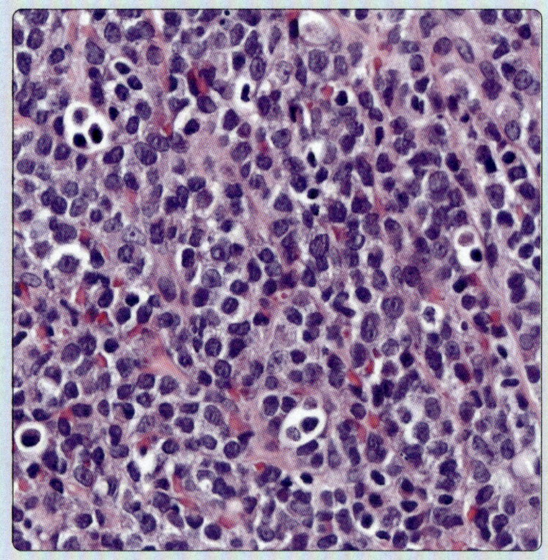

(Left) *Some cases of myeloid sarcoma show larger cells with very prominent nucleoli. The differential diagnosis in these cases naturally includes poorly differentiated carcinoma and melanoma but also sarcomas, such as epithelioid angiosarcoma.* **(Right)** *Myelocytes with eosinophilic cytoplasm may be present in some cases of myeloid sarcoma and can be a helpful clue to suggest myeloid origin. Immunohistochemistry, however, is diagnostic.*

Larger Nucleoli

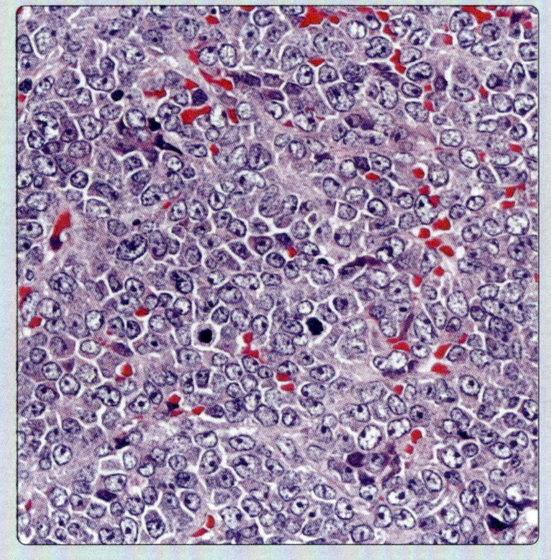

Eosinophilic Myelocytes

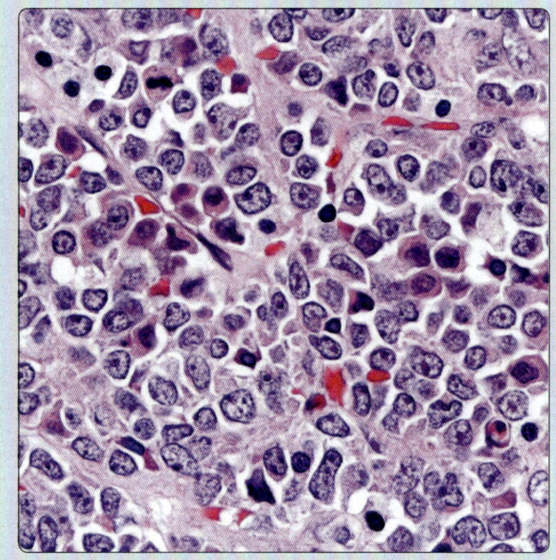

TERMINOLOGY

Synonyms

- Granulocytic sarcoma
- Extramedullary myeloid tumor
- Chloroma

Definitions

- Tumoral mass of myeloid blasts ± maturation occurring outside of bone marrow

CLINICAL ISSUES

Epidemiology

- Incidence
  - Rare
- Age
  - Wide range (children to older adults)
- Sex
  - Slight male predominance

Site

- Can occur anywhere
  - Skin, bone, lymph node, testis most common

Presentation

- Solitary mass
  - < 10% of cases are multifocal
- May arise de novo or concurrently with acute myeloid leukemia, myeloproliferative neoplasm, or myelodysplastic syndrome

Treatment

- Chemotherapy
- Possibly surgical excision for isolated lesions without previous or current evidence of hematogenous disease

Prognosis

- Does not seem to be influenced by age, sex, site, histologic features, immunophenotype, or cytogenetic findings
- Isolated extramedullary tumors without concomitant hematologic disease may fare better
  - Rare reports of isolated tumors in patients who never develop hematogenous disease

MACROSCOPIC

Size

- Varies

MICROSCOPIC

Histologic Features

- Diffuse, sheet-like growth that effaces normal tissue architecture
- Uniform, medium-sized cells with little cytoplasm
  - Round to oval nucleus with prominent nucleolus
  - Cytoplasm may contain eosinophilic granules
- May contain larger cells with more abundant cytoplasm
- Differentiating tumors show > 10% neutrophils
- Necrosis is rare
- May show monoblastic, monocytic, myelomonocytic morphologies depending on origin

ANCILLARY TESTS

Immunohistochemistry

- CD43(+), lysozyme (+), CD45(+), CD34 (variable)
- Myeloid differentiation: Myeloperoxidase (+), CD117(+)
- Monocytic differentiation: CD68(+), CD13(+)
- CD3(-), CD20(-), CD79a(-), keratin (-), S100(-), desmin (-)

Molecular Genetics

- Chromosomal abnormalities detected in ~ 50% of cases
  - t(8;21)(q22;q22) and inv(16) are recurrent aberrations
  - Trisomy 8, monosomy 16, many others
  - Some show *NPM1* mutations

DIFFERENTIAL DIAGNOSIS

Lymphoma

- B cell, T cell, or NK cell
- Can show significant morphologic overlap
- May present without leukemic manifestations
- Specific B-, T-, or NK-cell immunophenotypes

Poorly Differentiated Carcinoma

- Shows more cohesive growth pattern
- Keratin (+)

Malignant Melanoma

- May have small round cell morphology
- S100(+), HMB45(+), MART-1(+)
- Necrosis common

Various Small Round Blue Cell Tumors

- Particularly in children
- Includes alveolar rhabdomyosarcoma, neuroblastoma, extrarenal rhabdoid tumor, Ewing sarcoma
- Immunohistochemistry must be utilized
- Molecular analysis may be helpful

Epithelioid Angiosarcoma

- CD31(+), ERG(+), CD34(+)
- Sheets and clusters of epithelioid cells with macronucleoli

SELECTED REFERENCES

1. Almond LM et al: Myeloid sarcoma: presentation, diagnosis, and treatment. Clin Lymphoma Myeloma Leuk. 17(5):263-267, 2017
2. Seifert RP et al: A practical approach to diagnose soft tissue myeloid sarcoma preceding or coinciding with acute myeloid leukemia. Ann Diagn Pathol. 18(4):253-260, 2014
3. Campidelli C et al: Myeloid sarcoma: extramedullary manifestation of myeloid disorders. Am J Clin Pathol. 132(3):426-37, 2009
4. Alexiev BA et al: Myeloid sarcomas: a histologic, immunohistochemical, and cytogenetic study. Diagn Pathol. 2:42, 2007
5. Pileri SA et al: Myeloid sarcoma: clinico-pathologic, phenotypic and cytogenetic analysis of 92 adult patients. Leukemia. 21(2):340-50, 2007
6. Breccia M et al: Clinico-pathological characteristics of myeloid sarcoma at diagnosis and during follow-up: report of 12 cases from a single institution. Leuk Res. 28(11):1165-9, 2004

Lymphoma of Soft Tissue

KEY FACTS

TERMINOLOGY

- Group of malignant lymphoid proliferations that arise in soft tissue as primary site without evidence of lymph node or skin involvement

CLINICAL ISSUES

- True primary soft tissue lymphoma is rare
  - Soft tissue manifestation/deposit of systemic lymphoma more common
- Most common in extremities, particularly leg
- Usually older adults
- Treatment: Chemotherapy &/or radiotherapy
  - Surgery not indicated
- Prognosis depends upon type of lymphoma

MICROSCOPIC

- Depends upon type of lymphoma
  - Diffuse large B-cell lymphoma (most common overall)
  - Also precursor lymphoblastic lymphoma, anaplastic large cell lymphoma, small cell lymphomas, others

ANCILLARY TESTS

- Most CD45/LCA(+)
- ~ 80-85% of primary soft tissue lymphoid neoplasms originate from B cells and therefore express B-cell markers (e.g., CD19, CD20, CD79a)
- Anaplastic large cell lymphoma: CD30(+), ALK (variable)
- Flow cytometry is useful adjunct to immunohistochemistry

TOP DIFFERENTIAL DIAGNOSES

- Poorly differentiated synovial sarcoma
- Ewing sarcoma
- Malignant melanoma
- Myeloid sarcoma
- Merkel cell carcinoma

Lymphoma

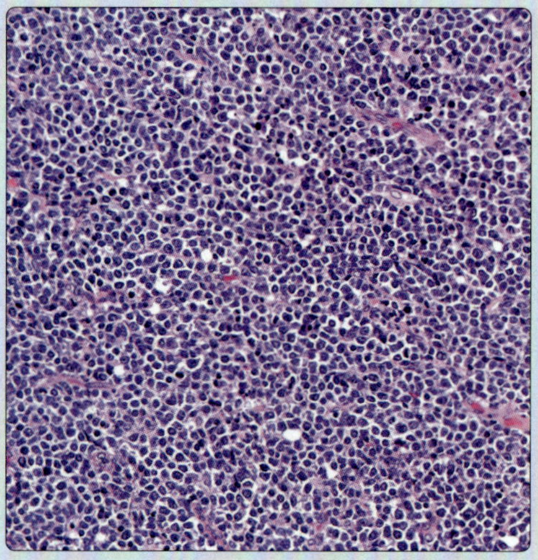

Muscle Infiltration

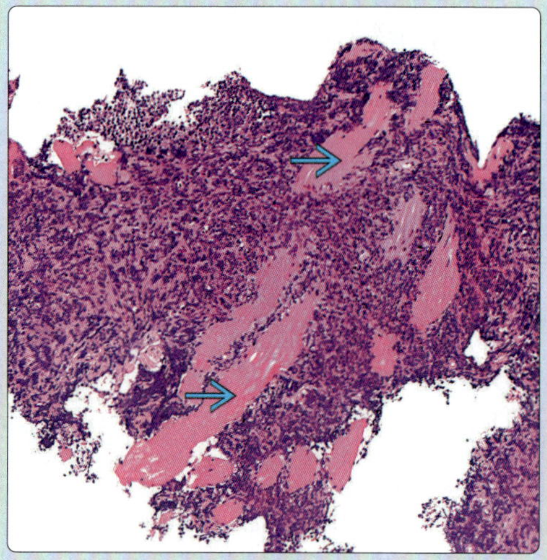

(Left) *Lymphoma characteristically grows in diffuse sheets of dyscohesive atypical lymphoid cells. The degree of atypia and mitotic activity vary depending upon whether the lymphoma is low or high grade.* **(Right)** *When lymphoma arises in or near muscle, it often shows diffuse infiltration between the muscle fibers ➙, splaying them apart. This pattern of infiltration may be referred to as checkerboard.*

High-Grade Lymphoma

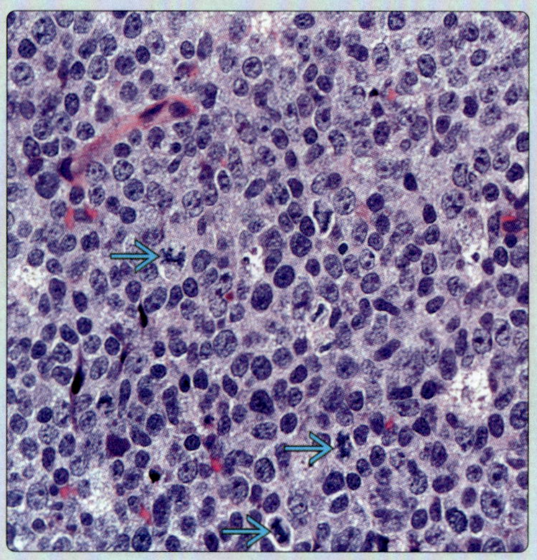

Anaplastic Large Cell Lymphoma

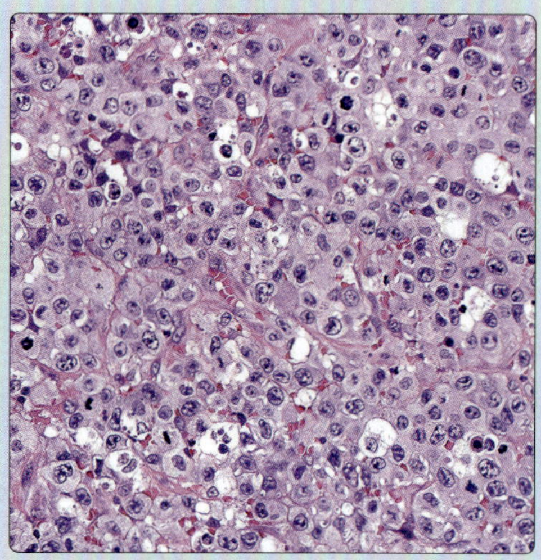

(Left) *This high-grade B-cell lymphoma of the proximal thigh shows diffuse sheets of markedly atypical lymphocytes with numerous mitotic figures ➙.* **(Right)** *Anaplastic large cell lymphoma is composed of sheets of malignant polygonal cells. In soft tissue sites, this tumor can be easily mistaken for carcinoma, melanoma, or some form of pleomorphic or round cell sarcoma.*

TERMINOLOGY

Definitions

- Group of malignant lymphoid proliferations that arise in soft tissue as primary site without evidence of lymph node or skin involvement

CLINICAL ISSUES

Epidemiology

- Incidence
  - True primary soft tissue lymphoma is rare
  - Soft tissue manifestation/deposit of systemic lymphoma more common
- Age
  - Usually older adults
    - Lymphoblastic lymphomas more common in children and young adults

Site

- Most common in extremities, particularly leg

Presentation

- Suddenly enlarging mass
  - Systemic symptoms may be present

Treatment

- Chemotherapy &/or radiotherapy
- Surgical excision not indicated

Prognosis

- Depends upon type of lymphoma
  - Diffuse large B-cell lymphoma of soft tissue is often highly aggressive

MICROSCOPIC

Histologic Features

- Depends upon type of lymphoma
  - Diffuse large B-cell lymphoma (most common overall)
    - Diffuse sheets of medium-to-large malignant lymphoid cells
      - May resemble poorly differentiated carcinoma or melanoma
    - Mitotic figures usually abundant
    - Necrosis common
    - Heterogeneous population of smaller lymphoid cells may be intermixed
  - Lymphoblastic lymphoma/leukemia
    - Diffuse sheets of small primitive lymphocytes
      - May resemble various small round blue cell tumors, e.g., Ewing sarcoma, neuroblastoma, alveolar rhabdomyosarcoma
  - Anaplastic large cell lymphoma
    - Diffuse sheets of large epithelioid lymphoid cells
      - May resemble poorly differentiated carcinoma or melanoma
      - May rarely show "mesenchymal" features, such as myxoid stroma
- Other types include Burkitt lymphoma, follicular lymphoma, extranodal NK-/T-cell lymphoma, and various small cell lymphomas

ANCILLARY TESTS

Immunohistochemistry

- Most CD45/LCA(+)
  - May be (-) in precursor B-cell lymphoma, which is often TdT(+)
- ~ 80-85% of primary soft tissue lymphoid neoplasms originate from B cells
  - CD20, CD79-α, others
  - Additional markers (e.g., CD5, CD10) useful for further classification
- T-cell lymphomas
  - CD2, CD3, CD4, CD7, CD8, others
- Anaplastic large cell lymphoma
  - CD30(+), ALK (variable)

Flow Cytometry

- Useful adjunct to immunohistochemistry

DIFFERENTIAL DIAGNOSIS

Poorly Differentiated Synovial Sarcoma

- May show small round blue cell tumor morphology
- Focal keratin (+) and EMA(+) in some cases
- TLE1(+), CD45(-)
- t(X;18) involving *SS18* (SYT) gene

Malignant Melanoma

- Patient may or may not have past history
- S100 protein(+), SOX10(+) in vast majority of cases
- HMB-45(+), MART-1(+), other melanocytic markers
  - May be (-) in some cases

Ewing Sarcoma

- FLI-1(+), CD45(-), TdT(-)
- CD99(+)
  - Can also be expressed in precursor lymphoblastic lymphomas and anaplastic large cell lymphoma
- t(11;22) and other translocations involving *EWSR1* gene

Merkel Cell Carcinoma

- CK20(+) in perinuclear dot-like pattern
- Synaptophysin (+), chromogranin (+)

Myeloid Sarcoma

- Often history of previous or active acute myeloid leukemia
- Eosinophilic myelocytes may be interspersed
- CD117(+), CD34(+), myeloperoxidase (+) in many cases

SELECTED REFERENCES

1. Gupta P et al: Primary cutaneous non-Hodgkin's lymphoma, clinically mimicking a soft tissue sarcoma. Cytojournal. 15:2, 2018
2. Derenzini E et al: Non-hodgkin lymphomas presenting as soft tissue masses: a single center experience and meta-analysis of the published series. Clin Lymphoma Myeloma Leuk. 13(3):258-65, 2013
3. Knowles B et al: Extra-nodal lymphoma presenting as a mimic of soft-tissue sarcoma. ANZ J Surg. 73(1-2):26-30, 2003
4. Salamao DR et al: Lymphoma in soft tissue: a clinicopathologic study of 19 cases. Hum Pathol. 27(3):253-7, 1996
5. Lanham GR et al: Malignant lymphoma. A study of 75 cases presenting in soft tissue. Am J Surg Pathol. 13(1):1-10, 1989
6. Travis WD et al: Primary extranodal soft tissue lymphoma of the extremities. Am J Surg Pathol. 11(5):359-66, 1987

SECTION 16

Tumors of Uncertain Differentiation

Benign

Intramuscular Myxoma 614
Juxtaarticular Myxoma 618
Superficial Angiomyxoma 620
Acral Fibromyxoma 624
Pleomorphic Hyalinizing Angiectatic Tumor 626
Aneurysmal Bone Cyst of Soft Tissue 630
Ectopic Hamartomatous Thymoma 632

Intermediate (Locally Aggressive)

Hemosiderotic Fibrolipomatous Tumor 634

Intermediate (Rarely Metastasizing)

Atypical Fibroxanthoma 636
Angiomatoid Fibrous Histiocytoma 642
Ossifying Fibromyxoid Tumor 650
Myoepithelioma of Soft Tissue 656
Phosphaturic Mesenchymal Tumor 664

Malignant

Synovial Sarcoma 666
Epithelioid Sarcoma 678
Alveolar Soft Part Sarcoma 684
Clear Cell Sarcoma 688
Perivascular Epithelioid Cell Tumor (PEComa) 692
Desmoplastic Small Round Cell Tumor 700
Extraskeletal Ewing Sarcoma 706
Extraskeletal Myxoid Chondrosarcoma 712
Extrarenal Rhabdoid Tumor 716
Intimal Sarcoma 720

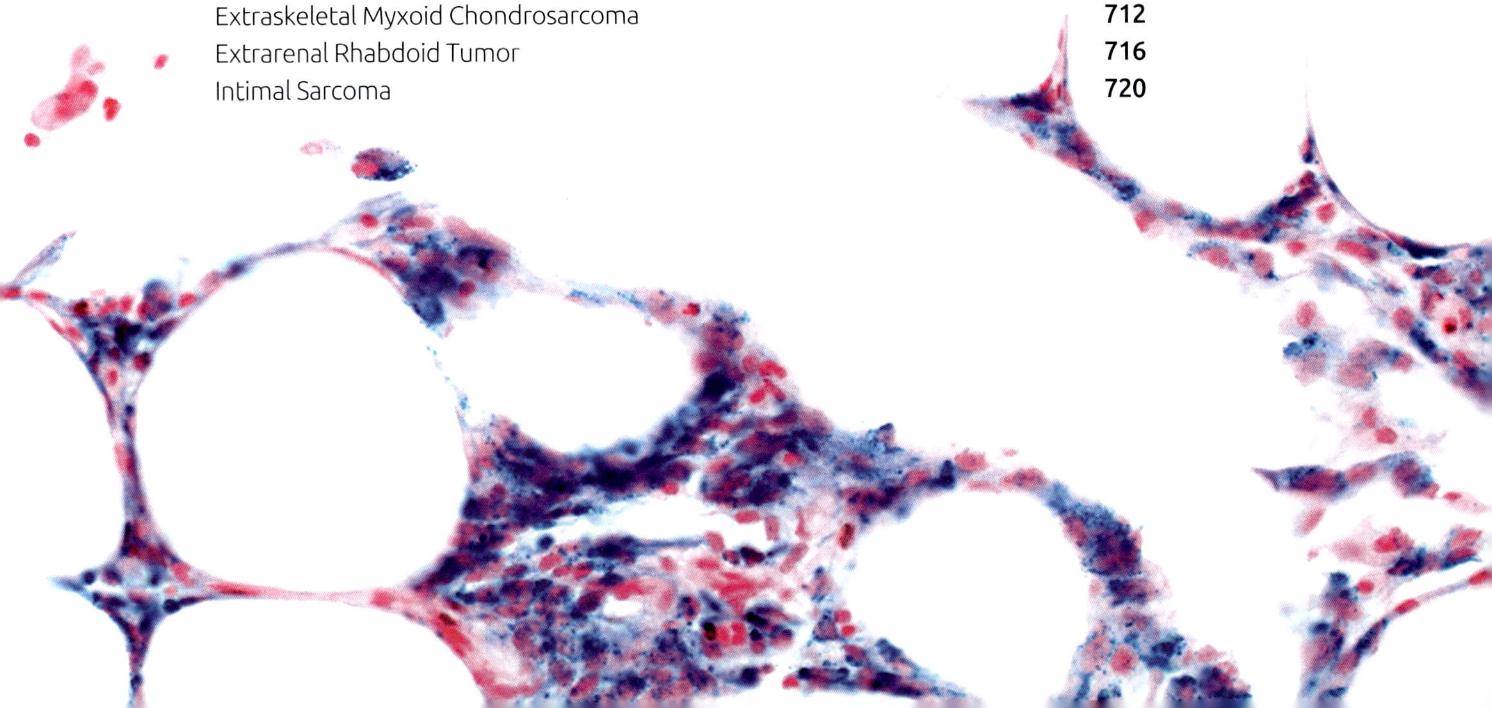

Intramuscular Myxoma

KEY FACTS

TERMINOLOGY

- Benign mesenchymal neoplasm arising within muscle and composed of bland spindled cells within abundant myxoid and hypovascular matrix

CLINICAL ISSUES

- Usually adults (most common 40-70 years)
- Female predilection
- Usually large muscles of thigh, buttock, shoulder, upper arm
- Arise sporadically or within context of Mazabraud syndrome
- Treatment: Simple surgical excision
- Does not recur if excised completely

MACROSCOPIC

- Lobulated, gelatinous cut surface
- Most < 10 cm in greatest dimension

MICROSCOPIC

- Often shows peripheral infiltration of skeletal muscle fibers (sometimes checkerboard pattern)
- Overall uniform, hypocellular, haphazard proliferation of small spindled to stellate cells
- Abundant extracellular myxoid matrix
- Vasculature is characteristically sparse
- Mitoses very rare; no necrosis
- Morphologic variant: Cellular myxoma

ANCILLARY TESTS

- Molecular: Activating missense mutations in codon 201 of *GNAS* gene

TOP DIFFERENTIAL DIAGNOSES

- Myxofibrosarcoma (low grade)
- Low-grade fibromyxoid sarcoma
- Benign peripheral nerve sheath tumors
- Myxoid liposarcoma

Intramuscular Myxoma

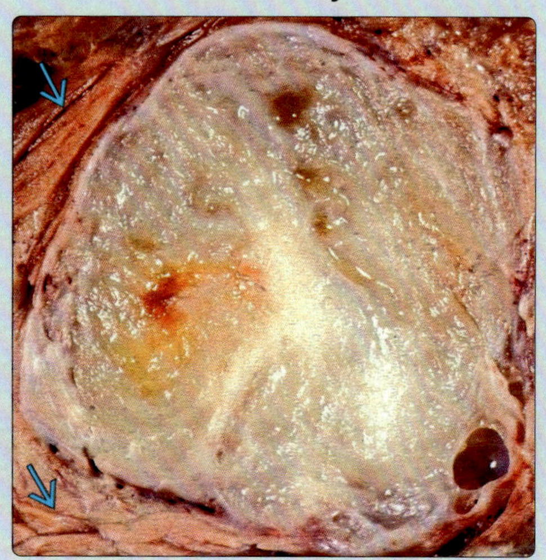

Low-Power Appearance

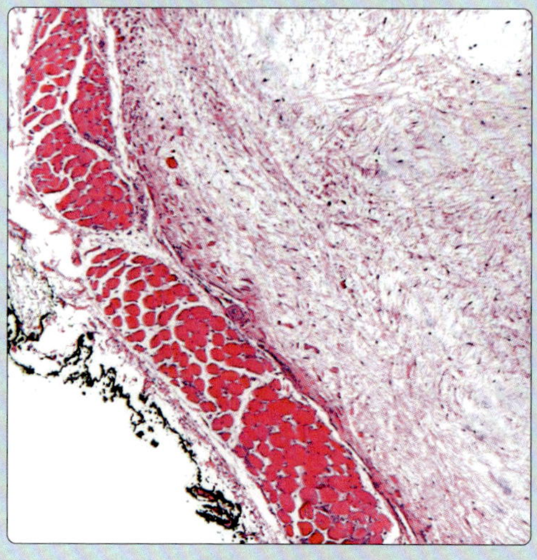

(Left) *Intramuscular myxoma presents as a circumscribed and lobulated mass, most commonly within large muscles, typically showing a gray-white, glistening, or gelatinous cut surface. Note the smooth interface with surrounding skeletal muscle* ➔. **(Right)** *At low power, intramuscular myxoma is characterized by an abundant myxoid matrix and is generally diffusely hypocellular and hypovascular. The interface with adjacent skeletal muscle may be sharp and distinct (as shown) or irregular and infiltrative-appearing.*

Infiltrative Appearance Common

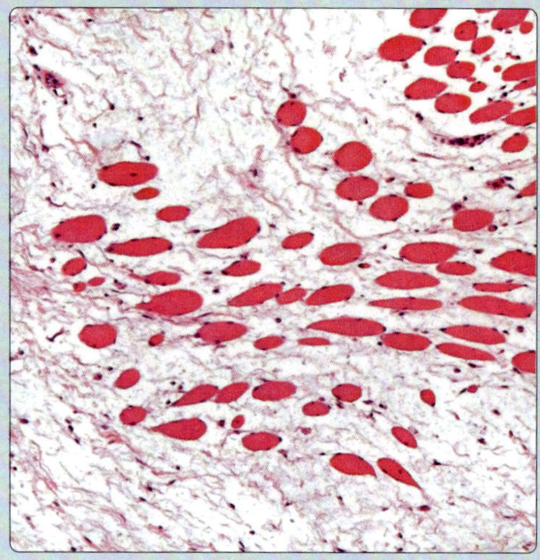

Hypocellular and Cytologically Bland

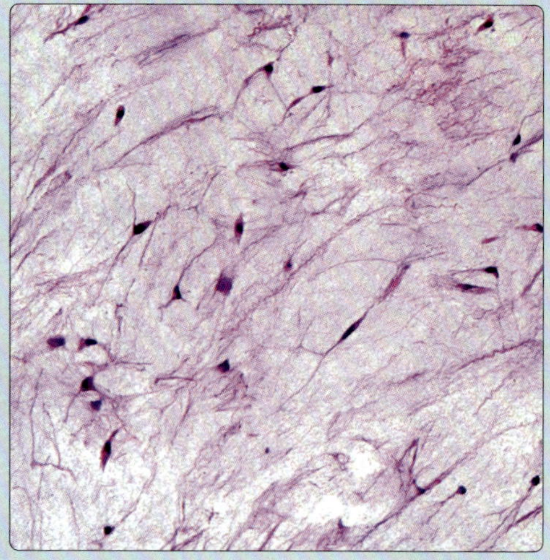

(Left) *Infiltration of tumor cells between bundles of skeletal muscle is a common finding at the periphery of intramuscular myxoma. Not infrequently, the lesional cells grow between individual muscle fibers, imparting a checkerboard appearance.* **(Right)** *The lesional cells of intramuscular myxoma are characteristically small, spindled to stellate in shape, and show small amounts of eosinophilic cytoplasm. Nuclei are often small, dark, and bland. Mitoses are very rare.*

Intramuscular Myxoma

TERMINOLOGY

Definitions

- Benign mesenchymal neoplasm arising within muscle and composed of bland spindled cells within abundant myxoid and hypovascular matrix

CLINICAL ISSUES

Epidemiology

- Age
  - Usually adults (most common 40-70 years)
- Sex
  - Female predilection

Site

- Usually large muscles
  - Thigh (most common)
  - Also buttock, shoulder, upper arm, rarely others

Presentation

- Slow-growing, solitary, painless mass
- Most are sporadic
  - Subset arise in association with fibrous dysplasia (Mazabraud syndrome)
    - Multiple myxomas may be seen
    - Often arise in same anatomic region as fibrous dysplasia lesion(s)

Treatment

- Simple surgical excision

Prognosis

- Typically does not recur if excised completely
  - Local recurrence very rare even if incompletely excised
- No significant prognostic difference between cellular and conventional types
- Does not metastasize or show malignant transformation

MACROSCOPIC

General Features

- Appears well circumscribed
  - May show subtle infiltration of adjacent skeletal muscle on closer inspection
- Lobulated, gelatinous cut surface
- Cystic spaces may be present

Size

- Most < 10 cm in greatest dimension
  - Can measure up to 20 cm

MICROSCOPIC

Histologic Features

- Often shows peripheral infiltration of skeletal muscle fibers (sometimes checkerboard pattern)
- Overall uniform, hypocellular, haphazard proliferation of small spindled to stellate cells
  - Small, bland, oval nuclei ± inconspicuous nucleoli
  - Tapered, eosinophilic, fibrillary cytoplasm
- Abundant extracellular myxoid matrix
  - May appear "frothy" &/or contain microcystic spaces
- Vasculature is characteristically sparse and inconspicuous
- Areas with finely fibrillar stromal collagen may be seen
- Vacuolated macrophages may be present
- Mitoses very rare; no necrosis

Morphologic Variant

- Cellular myxoma
  - Focal to diffuse areas of increased cellularity and vascularity
  - Cytologically identical to noncellular tumors
    - Very rare mitoses; no necrosis
  - Stroma often more collagenous

ANCILLARY TESTS

Immunohistochemistry

- Variable CD34(+), variable SMA(+)
- Negative for S100 protein, desmin, EMA, MUC4, claudin-1

Genetic Testing

- Activating missense mutations in codon 201 of *GNAS* gene
  - Detected in both cellular and noncellular forms, in both sporadic tumors, and those occurring in Mazabraud syndrome

DIFFERENTIAL DIAGNOSIS

Low-Grade Myxofibrosarcoma

- Usually older adults and elderly
- More often superficial (subcutis) than deep
- Usually contains tumor cells with nuclear atypia and pleomorphism, at least focally
- Vascularity more pronounced (curvilinear vessels)

Low-Grade Fibromyxoid Sarcoma

- Alternating myxoid and collagenous zones
  - Vascularity often more pronounced in myxoid areas
- MUC4(+)
- Characteristic t(7;16) with *FUS-CREB3L2*

Benign Peripheral Nerve Sheath Tumors

- Includes neurofibroma, perineurioma, and hybrid nerve sheath tumor
  - All can feature myxoid stroma
- S100 protein (+) in neurofibroma
- EMA(+) &/or claudin-1 (+) in perineurioma
- Admixed S100 protein (+) and EMA/claudin-1 (+) cells in hybrid nerve sheath tumor

Myxoid Liposarcoma

- Characteristic plexiform chicken-wire vasculature
- Uni- and multivacuolated lipoblasts often present
- Characteristic t(12;16) with *FUS-DDIT3* fusion

SELECTED REFERENCES

1. Rachidi S et al: Intramuscular myxoma of the paraspinal muscles: a case report and systematic review of the literature. Oncol Lett. 11(1):466-470, 2016
2. Delaney D et al: GNAS1 mutations occur more commonly than previously thought in intramuscular myxoma. Mod Pathol. 22(5):718-24, 2009
3. Nielsen GP et al: Intramuscular myxoma: a clinicopathologic study of 51 cases with emphasis on hypercellular and hypervascular variants. Am J Surg Pathol. 22(10):1222-7, 1998

(Left) *Some of the tumor cells in intramuscular myxoma are slightly larger and more ovoid and show somewhat darker eosinophilic cytoplasm ⇨. Nuclei are often eccentric.* **(Right)** *Rare tumor cells in intramuscular myxoma, particularly those that are stellate in shape, may somewhat resemble the "floret-like" cells that are seen in other tumors, such as pleomorphic lipoma and myxofibrosarcoma. The latter, in particular, should always be thoroughly excluded.*

Cytologic Features

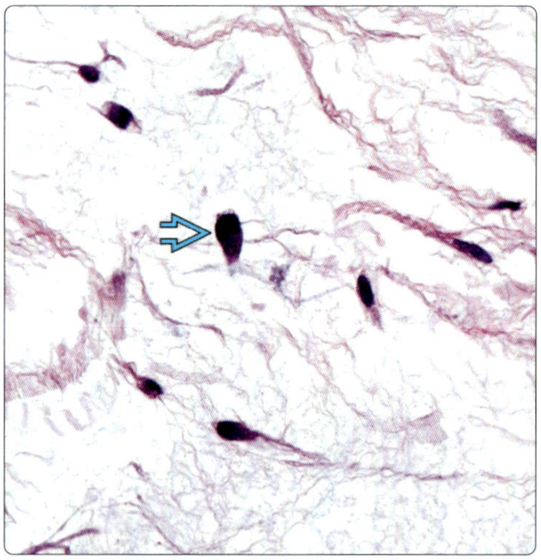

Rare Tumor Cells

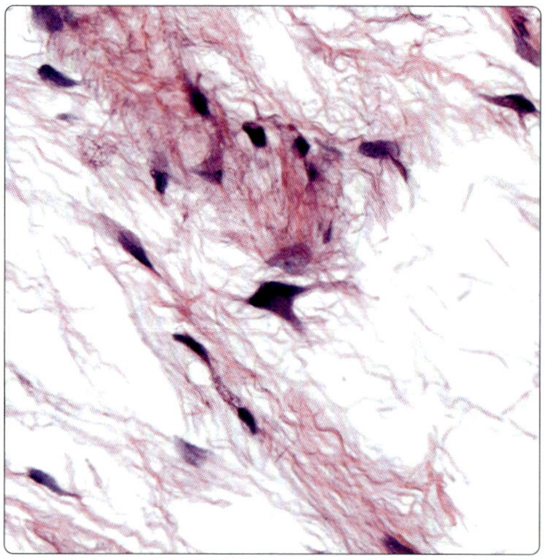

(Left) *Occasionally, small histiocytes with foamy, vacuolated cytoplasm may be encountered in intramuscular myxoma. These cells should not be confused for lipoblasts.* **(Right)** *A frothy or bubbly quality to the myxoid matrix may be seen in intramuscular myxoma. This finding may simulate lipoblastic differentiation.*

Foamy Histiocytes

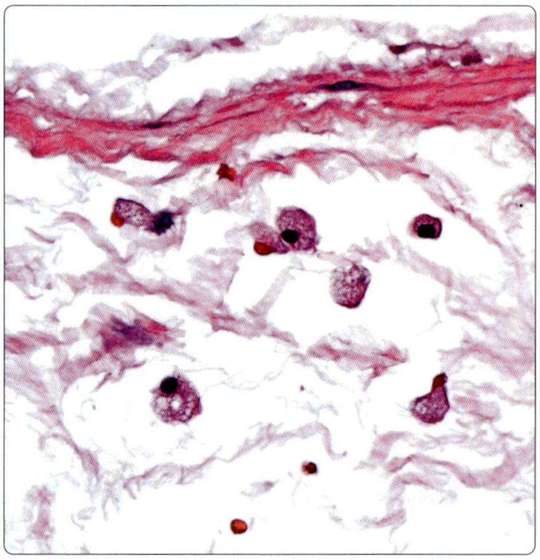

Frothy Myxoid Matrix

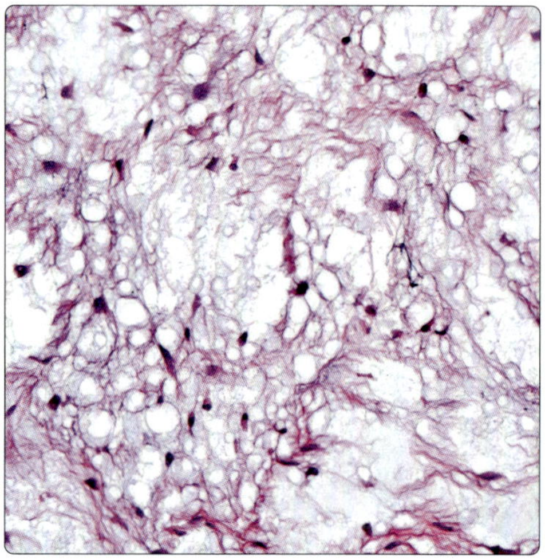

(Left) *Given its highly myxoid nature, slide preparations of an intramuscular myxoma may contain large globs of mucoid material, as shown in this image. This finding is particularly common in frozen section preparations.* **(Right)** *Cystic change is not uncommon in intramuscular myxoma and may be grossly evident in some cases. This finding is encountered more frequently in cellular forms of intramuscular myxoma as well as in the unrelated juxtaarticular myxoma.*

Abundant Mucoid Material

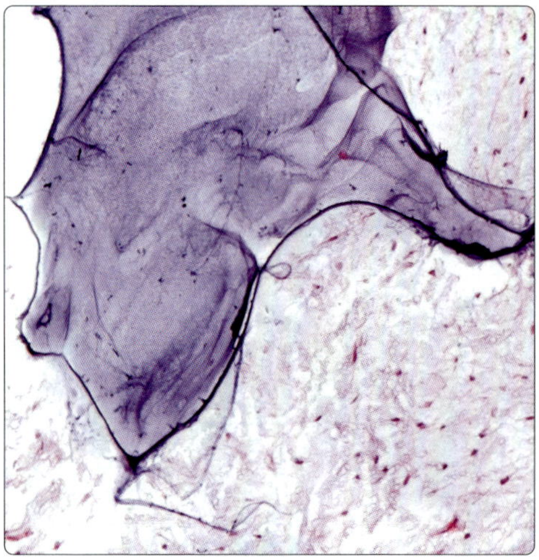

Cystic Change

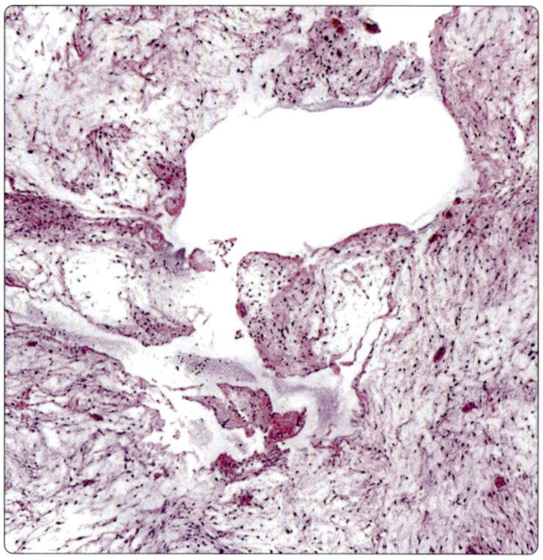

Variable Fine Stromal Collagen

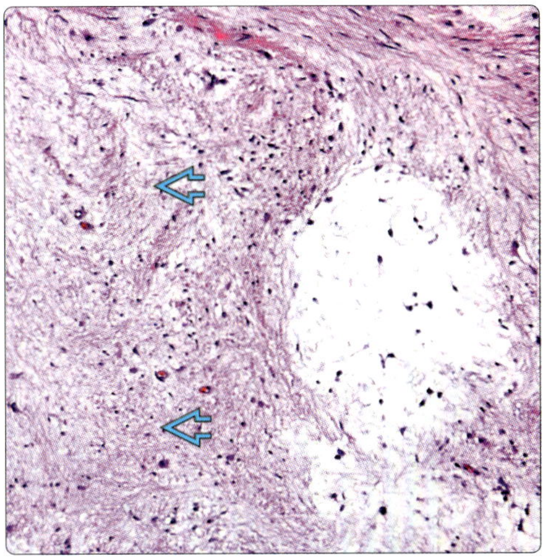

Increased Collagen

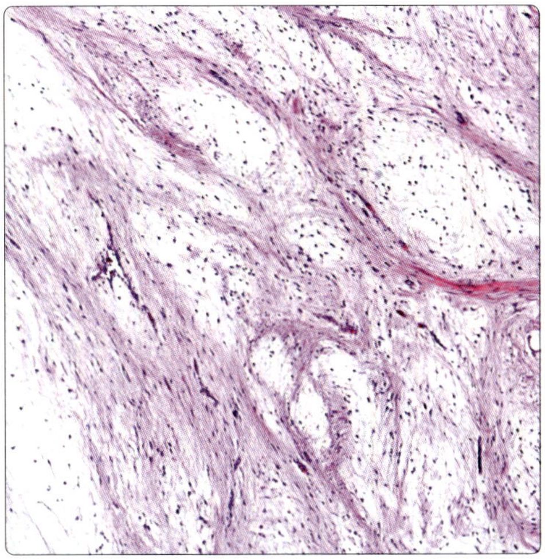

(Left) *Although the abundant myxoid matrix often dominates the histologic picture, areas containing fine, fibrillary stromal collagen* ⇨ *may also be seen in intramuscular myxoma. Large bundled collagen fibers are uncommon.* **(Right)** *Increased stromal collagen may be seen around the periphery, as in this image, and may impart a vague nodular appearance.*

Cellular Intramuscular Myxoma

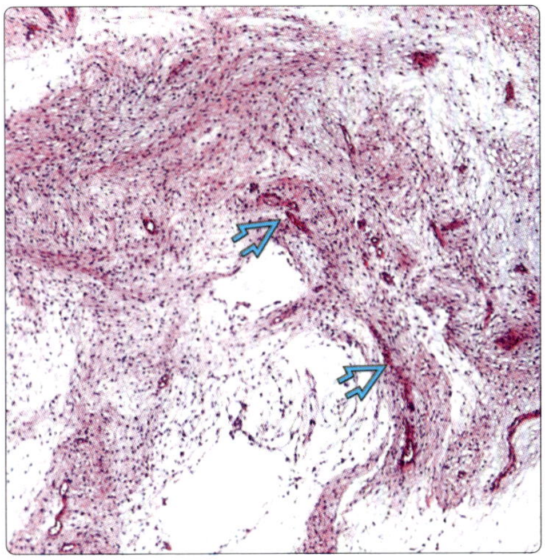

Cellular Intramuscular Myxoma

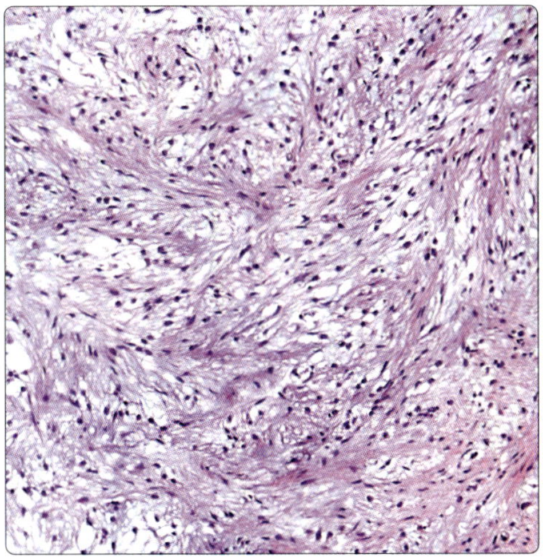

(Left) *Cellular examples of intramuscular myxoma are characterized by regions of increased cellularity with an often concomitant increase in the prominence of stromal collagen and blood vessels* ⇨. *Cellular areas may be focal or comprise most of a given tumor.* **(Right)** *Cellular intramuscular myxoma often shows slightly more architectural organization of the tumor cells compared with typical forms. As a rule, low-grade fibromyxoid sarcoma should always be excluded before a diagnosis of cellular myxoma is made.*

Cellular Intramuscular Myxoma

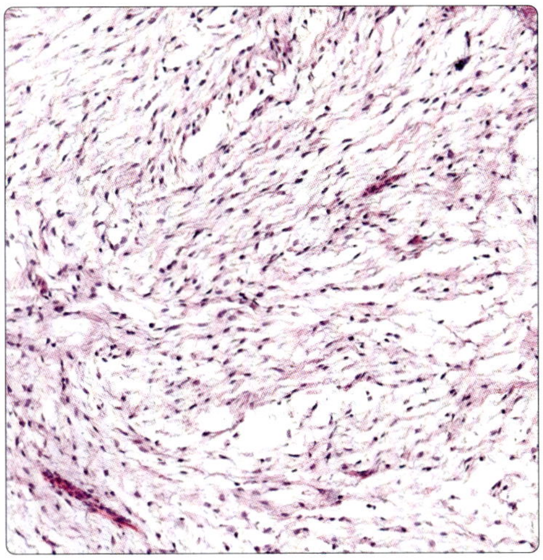

Cellular Intramuscular Myxoma

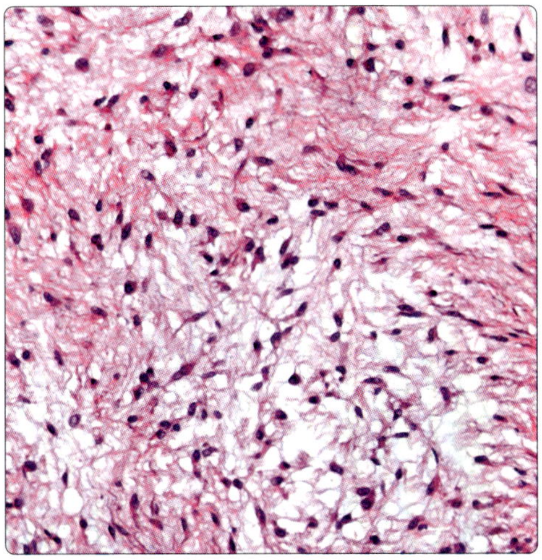

(Left) *Cellular intramuscular myxoma generally lacks the haphazard or patternless growth of tumor cells that characterize conventional cases.* **(Right)** *Importantly, the tumor cells in cellular intramuscular myxoma are still very bland and cytologically identical to cells in conventional tumors. Mitotic figures are very rare.*

Juxtaarticular Myxoma

KEY FACTS

TERMINOLOGY

- Benign lesion occurring in region of large joints that is histologically similar to cellular intramuscular myxoma

CLINICAL ISSUES

- Usually adults (predominantly 20-50 years)
- 90% occur around knee joint
- Benign; local recurrence in 30%

MACROSCOPIC

- Myxoid, gelatinous cut surface
- Cystic areas common
- Mean size: 3.5 cm

MICROSCOPIC

- Peripheral borders often ill defined with infiltration of adjacent tissue
- Histologically very similar to cellular intramuscular myxoma
  - Proliferation of bland spindle or stellate cells
  - Mitotic figures rare or absent
  - Hypovascular myxoid stroma
  - Areas of increased cellularity common
- Cystic, ganglion-like spaces present in many cases

ANCILLARY TESTS

- Variable CD34 and SMA
- Negative for S100 protein, MUC4
- Genetics: Lacks mutations of *GNAS* gene

TOP DIFFERENTIAL DIAGNOSES

- Intramuscular myxoma
- Myxofibrosarcoma (low grade)
- Low-grade fibromyxoid sarcoma
- Deep (aggressive) angiomyxoma
- Superficial angiomyxoma
- Myxoid neurofibroma

Juxtaarticular Myxoma

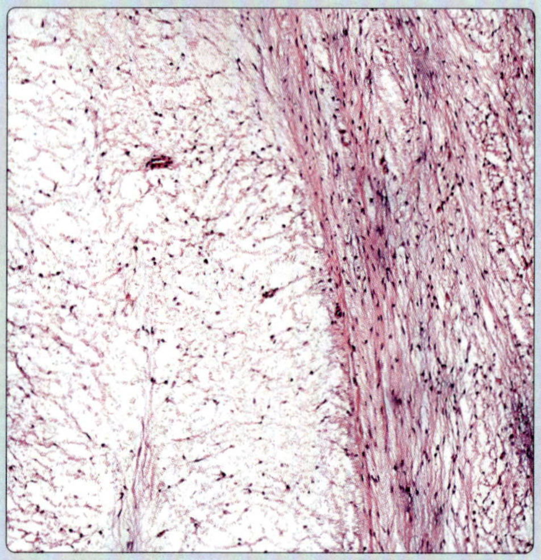

Cystic Spaces

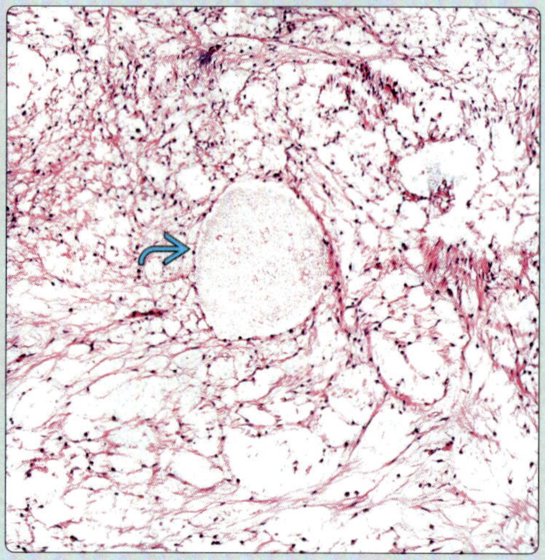

(Left) *Juxtaarticular myxoma (JAM) is histologically similar to the cellular form of intramuscular myxoma and contains areas showing low cellularity (left) and higher cellularity (right). The cells are embedded in patternless distributions within stroma that is myxoid and hypovascular.* **(Right)** *Stromal cysts can be a prominent feature ➡ of JAM. In some cases, large ganglion-like spaces are present. The hypovascularity of the myxoid matrix is also notable.*

Increased Cellularity

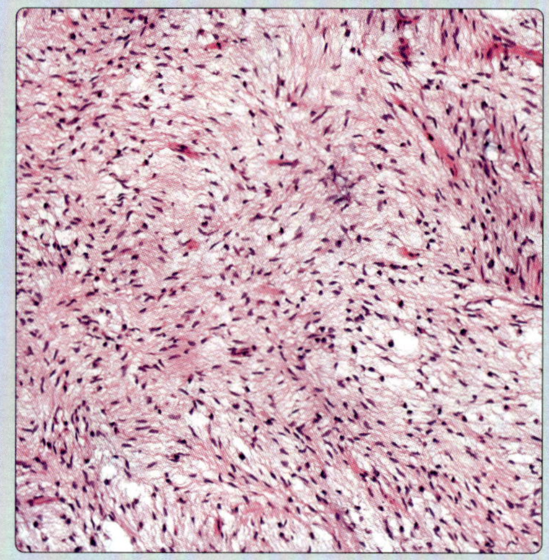

Hypovascular Stroma

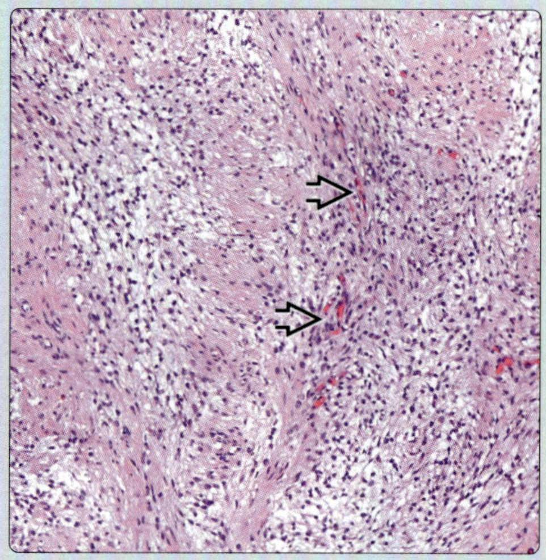

(Left) *Despite the increased cellularity, the cells of JAM are cytologically bland, and mitotic activity is characteristically low or absent. The stroma is typically myxoid or myxocollagenous.* **(Right)** *Unlike many low-grade myxoid sarcomas, the stroma in JAM is characteristically hypovascular. Note the rare scattered small blood vessels ➡ in this image.*

Juxtaarticular Myxoma

TERMINOLOGY

Abbreviations

- Juxtaarticular myxoma (JAM)

Definitions

- Benign lesion occurring in region of large joints that is histologically similar to cellular intramuscular myxoma

ETIOLOGY/PATHOGENESIS

Environmental Exposure

- Lesions have been associated with trauma
- May also occur adjacent to osteoarthritic joint

CLINICAL ISSUES

Epidemiology

- Age
  - Usually adults (predominantly 20-50 years)
- Sex
  - M > F

Site

- Occurs adjacent to large joints
  - 90% occur around knee joint
  - Also shoulder, elbow, ankle, and hip
- Can involve periarticular tendons, ligaments, joint capsules, muscles, and subcutis

Presentation

- Painful or painless mass
  - Lesion duration varies

Prognosis

- Local recurrence in ~ 30%
- No reports of malignant transformation

MACROSCOPIC

General Features

- Myxoid, gelatinous cut surface
- Cystic areas common

Size

- Varies from < 1 cm to > 10 cm
  - Mean size: 3.5 cm

MICROSCOPIC

Histologic Features

- Peripheral borders often ill defined with infiltration of adjacent tissue
- Histologically very similar to cellular intramuscular myxoma
  - Proliferation of spindle or stellate fibroblast-like cells
    - Cytologically bland
    - Mitotic figures rare or absent
  - Hypovascular myxoid stroma
  - Areas of increased cellularity common
- Cystic, ganglion-like spaces present in many cases
  - Lined by fibrin or collagen
- Other findings
  - Hemorrhage with hemosiderin deposition
  - Fibrin deposition
  - Variable mild chronic inflammatory cell infiltrate
  - Reactive fibroblastic proliferation

ANCILLARY TESTS

Immunohistochemistry

- Similar immunoprofile to intramuscular myxoma
  - Variable expression of CD34 and SMA
  - Negative for S100 protein, MUC4

Genetic Testing

- Lack mutations of *GNAS* gene typically found in intramuscular myxoma
  - Therefore, genetically distinct from intramuscular myxoma

DIFFERENTIAL DIAGNOSIS

Intramuscular Myxoma

- Most common in large muscles of lower limb
- Many contain mutations of *GNAS* gene

Myxofibrosarcoma (Low Grade)

- Often subcutaneous location in older/elderly patients
- Multinodular growth
- Atypical, hyperchromatic nuclei
- Prominent "curvilinear" vasculature in most cases

Low-Grade Fibromyxoid Sarcoma

- Admixed fibrous and myxoid zones
  - Myxoid zones more cellular than in JAM
- MUC4(+)
- Characteristic t(7;16) or t(11;16)

Deep (Aggressive) Angiomyxoma

- Adult women
- Deep soft tissues of vulvovaginal region
- Numerous vessels of varying sizes

Superficial Angiomyxoma

- Trunk, head and neck, or vulvovaginal sites
- Prominent vasculature
- Can have neutrophilic infiltrate
- May contain admixed epithelial structures

Myxoid Neurofibroma

- Buckled, elongated nuclei
- S100 protein (+)

SELECTED REFERENCES

1. Ye ZX et al: Juxta-articular myxoma of the temporomandibular joint. J Craniofac Surg. 26(8):e695-6, 2015
2. Wakely Jr PE et al: The cytopathology of soft tissue mxyomas: ganglia, juxta-articular myxoid lesions, and intramuscular myxoma. Am J Clin Pathol. 123(6):858-65, 2005
3. Okamoto S et al: Juxta-articular myxoma and intramuscular myxoma are two distinct entities. Activating Gs alpha mutation at Arg 201 codon does not occur in juxta-articular myxoma. Virchows Arch. 440(1):12-5, 2002
4. Allen PW: Myxoma is not a single entity: a review of the concept of myxoma. Ann Diagn Pathol. 4(2):99-123, 2000
5. Sciot R et al: Clonal chromosomal changes in juxta-articular myxoma. Virchows Arch. 434(2):177-80, 1999
6. Meis JM et al: Juxta-articular myxoma: a clinical and pathologic study of 65 cases. Hum Pathol. 23(6):639-46, 1992

Superficial Angiomyxoma

KEY FACTS

TERMINOLOGY
- Synonym: Cutaneous myxoma
- Benign, cutaneous myxoid lesion, sometimes associated with Carney complex

CLINICAL ISSUES
- Mean age: 3rd-5th decades
- Trunk, head and neck, lower extremities, and genital area
- Ear canal, eyelid, nipple common sites in Carney complex
- Benign but local recurrence in 30-40% if incompletely excised

MACROSCOPIC
- Typically small (up to 5 cm)
- Multinodular gelatinous cut surface with thin fibrous septa

MICROSCOPIC
- Dermal nodule, sometimes extending to subcutis
- Multiple vague lobules divided by thin fibrous septa
- Hypocellular spindle and stellate cells in abundant myxoid background
- Arborizing/plexiform thin-walled vessels
- Neutrophils present in subset of cases
- Entrapped benign epithelial elements in up to 25%

ANCILLARY TESTS
- CD34(+); S100 protein (-)

TOP DIFFERENTIAL DIAGNOSES
- Digital mucous cyst
- Cutaneous focal mucinosis
- Dermal nerve sheath myxoma
- Myxoid neurofibroma
- Superficial acral (digital) fibromyxoma
- Deep (aggressive) angiomyxoma
- Myxoid liposarcoma
- Low-grade myxofibrosarcoma
- Low-grade fibromyxoid sarcoma

Superficial Angiomyxoma

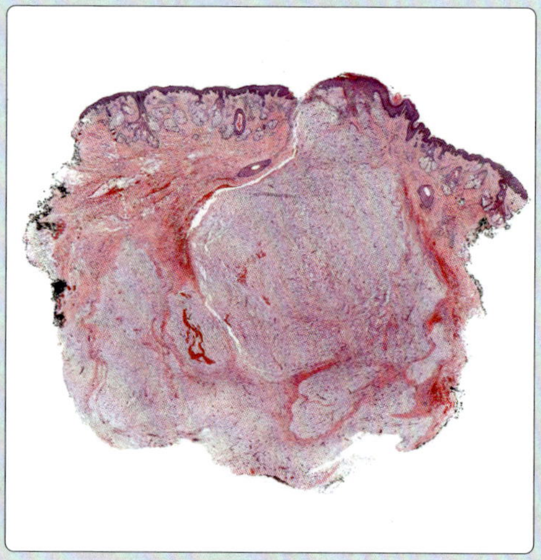

Plexiform Vessels

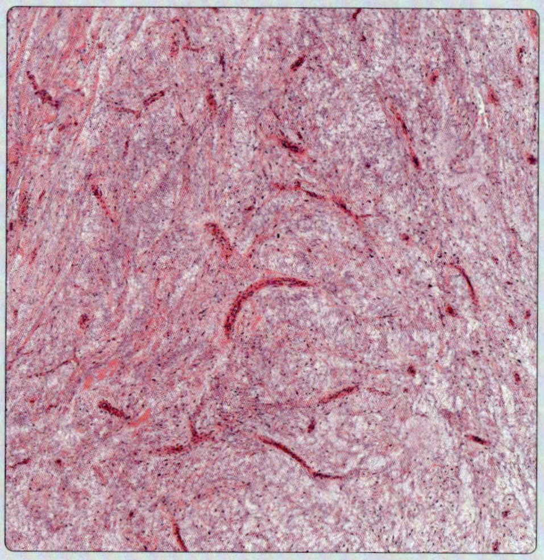

(Left) *In this example of superficial angiomyxoma, multiple hypocellular myxoid lobules in the dermis are divided by thin fibrous septa.* **(Right)** *As seen here, the branching thin vessels may be quite striking in superficial angiomyxoma; however, they are usually not as thin or delicate as the vessels of myxoid liposarcoma.*

Bland Spindle and Stellate Cells

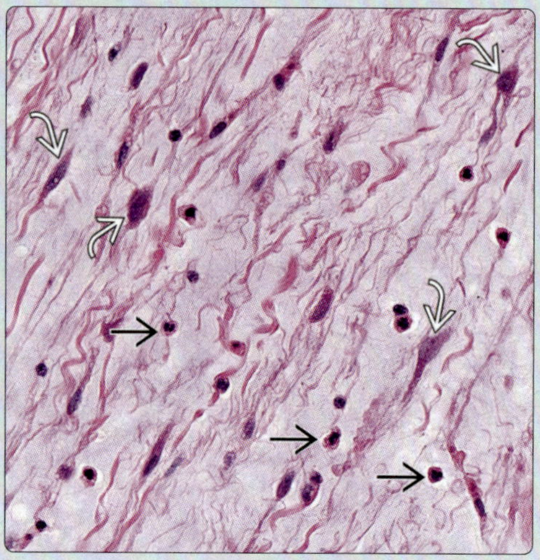

CD34 Expression

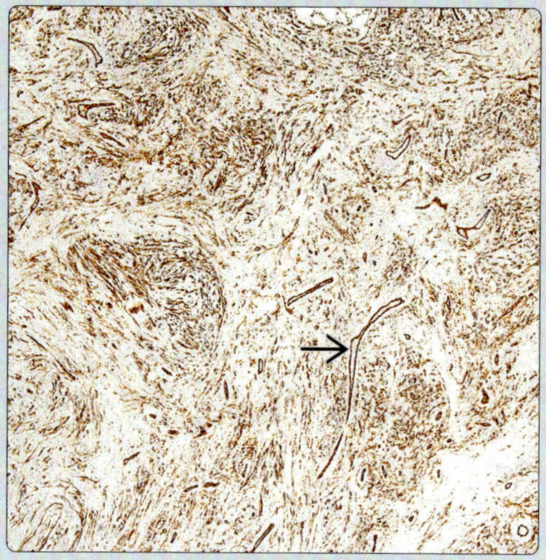

(Left) *Bland spindle and stellate cells* ➡ *with eosinophilic cytoplasm are arranged in a myxoid background in superficial angiomyxoma. A variable amount of collagen fibers may be present. Scattered neutrophils are also characteristically seen* →. **(Right)** *There is strong expression of CD34 within spindle and stellate cells. Note also the prominent vasculature* →.

TERMINOLOGY

Synonyms

- Cutaneous myxoma

Definitions

- Benign myxoid lesion of skin, sometimes associated with Carney complex

CLINICAL ISSUES

Epidemiology

- Age
  - Any age but mostly in middle-aged adults (mean: 20-40 years)

Site

- Trunk, head/neck, lower extremities, genital region
- Ear canal, eyelid, nipple common sites in Carney complex

Presentation

- Incidental, painless papule/nodule or polyp
  - Clinically similar to skin tag, neurofibroma, or cyst

Treatment

- Local excision with follow-up

Prognosis

- Benign but local recurrence in 30-40% if incompletely excised (median time to recurrence: 12 months)
- No metastatic potential

MACROSCOPIC

General Features

- Usually solitary
  - Often multiple in Carney complex
- Multinodular gelatinous cut surface with thin fibrous septa
- May be poorly circumscribed
- May contain cysts with keratin debris

Size

- Typically small (up to 5 cm)

MICROSCOPIC

Histologic Features

- Dermal nodule, sometimes extending to subcutis
- Multiple vague lobules divided by thin fibrous septa
- Hypocellular spindle/stellate cells in myxoid background
  - Bland, round/reniform nuclei, sometimes with nuclear vacuoles
  - Often bi- or multinucleated
  - Mitoses rare
  - Perinuclear protruding "belly" of eosinophilic cytoplasm
- Arborizing/plexiform thin-walled vessels often prominent
- Scattered mixed inflammatory cells, especially neutrophils
  - Neutrophils absent in other dermal myxoid tumors
- Entrapped benign epithelial elements in up to 25%
  - Follicular/"epidermoid" cysts, often with keratin debris
- May have overlying basaloid proliferation in epidermis
  - Can mimic basal cell carcinoma

ANCILLARY TESTS

Immunohistochemistry

- CD34(+); occasionally focal SMA or desmin
- S100 protein, keratin, ER, PR (-)

DIFFERENTIAL DIAGNOSIS

Digital Mucous Cyst

- Typically on dorsum of fingers near nail
- May show mucin-/myxoid-filled pseudocyst &/or noncystic loose myxoid change in dermis
- Lacks plexiform vessels and neutrophils; not multilobular

Cutaneous Focal Mucinosis

- Small papule; usually limited to mid-/upper dermis
- Similar histology but vasculature usually less pronounced

Dermal Nerve Sheath Myxoma

- Strikingly lobular architecture
- Spindle cells arranged in whorled chains/cords
- Strongly SOX10 and S100 protein (+)

Myxoid Neurofibroma

- Buckled, elongated nuclei; minimal cytoplasm
- SOX10 and S100 protein (+)

Superficial Acral (Digital) Fibromyxoma

- Acral sites, especially fingers; often periungual
- More cellularity and more fibrous background
- May show loss of *RB1*/13q abnormalities

Deep (Aggressive) Angiomyxoma

- Large, deep pelvic/perineal mass, usually in females
- Different vascular pattern: Vessels vary in size

Myxoid Liposarcoma

- Large, deep mass; very rare in dermis/subcutis
- Also has plexiform vessels but usually more thin/delicate
- Uniform, round/oval cells with minimal cytoplasm
- Uni- and bivacuolated lipoblasts usually present
- Characteristic gene fusions: *FUS-DDIT3* or *EWSR1-DDIT3*

Low-Grade Myxofibrosarcoma

- Always has at least focal nuclear atypia/pleomorphism
- Spindle cells aggregate near long "curvilinear" vessels

Low-Grade Fibromyxoid Sarcoma

- Usually large/deep, rarely may be small/superficial
- Varying cellularity with hypo- and hypercellular areas
- Alternating fibrous and myxoid background
- Bland spindle cells with minimal cytoplasm; MUC4(+)
- Characteristic translocations: *FUS-CREB3L2* and others

SELECTED REFERENCES

1. Aberdein G et al: Mohs micrographic surgery for the treatment of superficial angiomyxoma. Dermatol Surg. 42(8):1014-6, 2016
2. Calonje E et al: Superficial angiomyxoma: clinicopathologic analysis of a series of distinctive but poorly recognized cutaneous tumors with tendency for recurrence. Am J Surg Pathol. 23(8):910-7, 1999
3. Carney JA: Carney complex: the complex of myxomas, spotty pigmentation, endocrine overactivity, and schwannomas. Semin Dermatol. 14(2):90-8, 1995
4. Allen PW et al: Superficial angiomyxomas with and without epithelial components. Report of 30 tumors in 28 patients. Am J Surg Pathol. 12(7):519-30, 1988

(**Left**) *Superficial angiomyxoma is a dermal hypocellular myxoid nodule. In this example, the tumor has infiltrative borders and lacks fibrous septa.* (**Right**) *Bland spindle and stellate cells are scattered in a pale myxoid background with elongated thin vessels. Vessels are often prominent but do not always display branching/plexiform arrangement.*

Myxoid Dermal Nodule

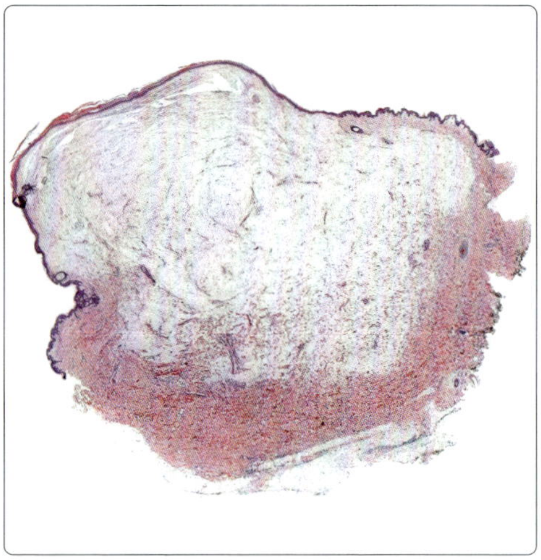

Vasculature

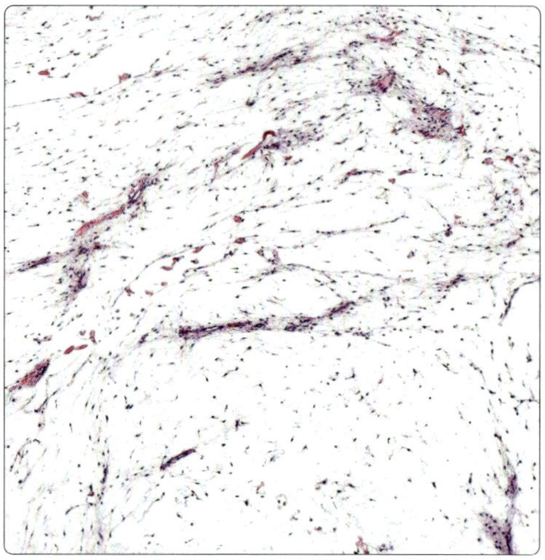

(**Left**) *The branching vessels and hypocellular myxoid background can bear vague resemblance to myxoid liposarcoma.* (**Right**) *A hypocellular proliferation of bland spindle and stellate cells are scattered in a pale myxoid background. Some cases of superficial angiomyxoma have very little collagen, as seen here.*

Branching Vessels

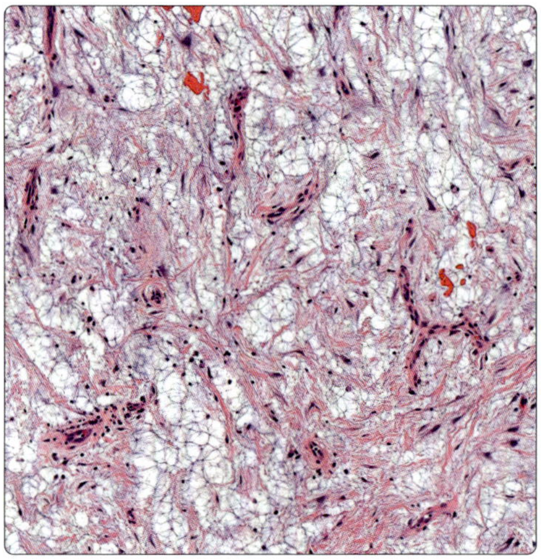

Hypocellularity

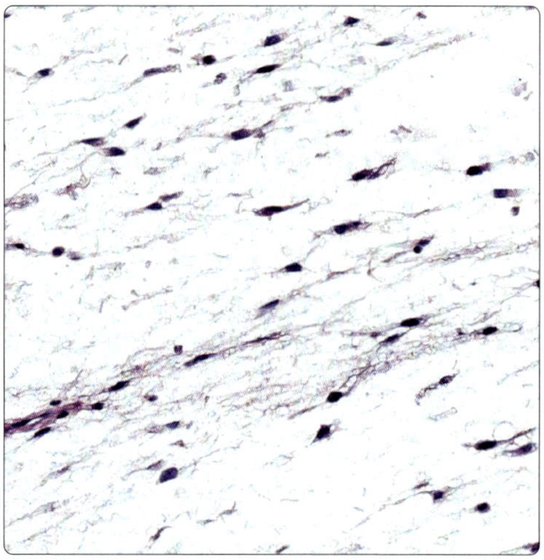

(**Left**) *Superficial angiomyxoma is composed of a hypocellular proliferation of spindle to stellate cells with bland nuclei lacking atypia or significant mitotic activity. The background contains a variable amount of blue mucin.* (**Right**) *The spindle cells of superficial angiomyxoma often have reniform nuclei and an adjacent globular "belly" of eosinophilic cytoplasm* ➙.

Bland Nuclei

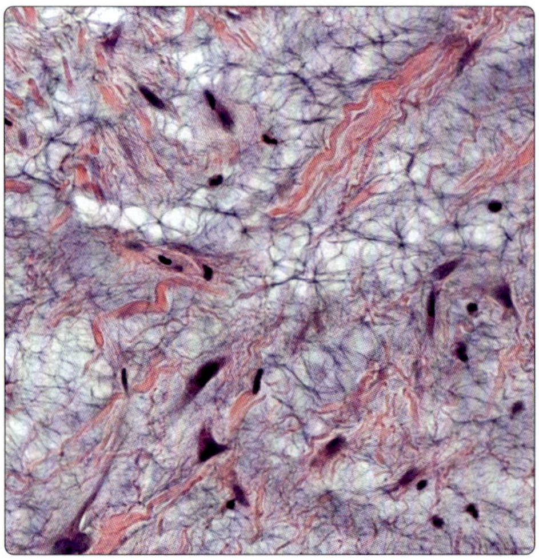

"Bellies" of Eosinophilic Cytoplasm

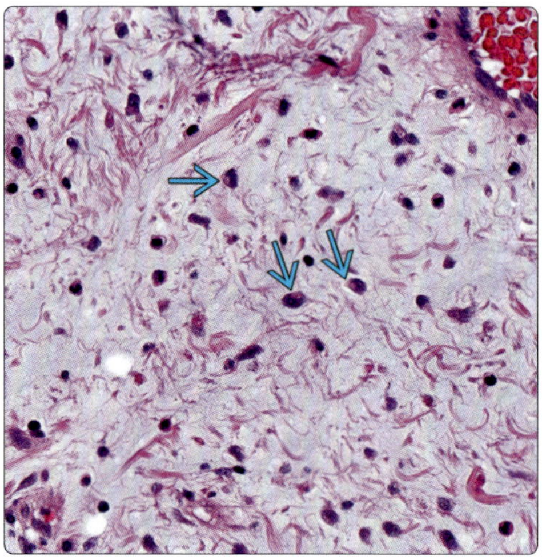

Scattered Neutrophils

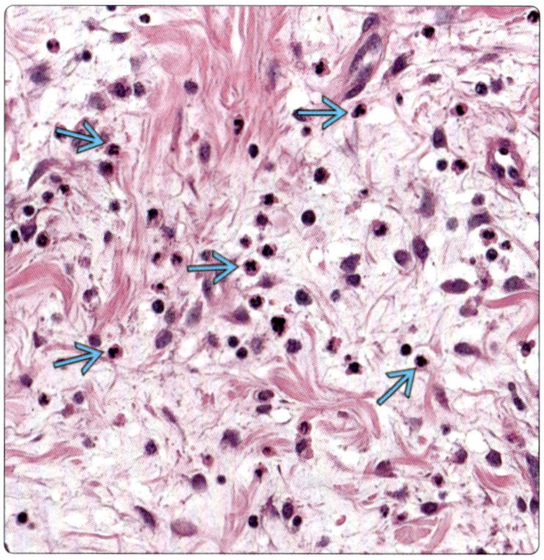

Entrapped Epithelial Elements

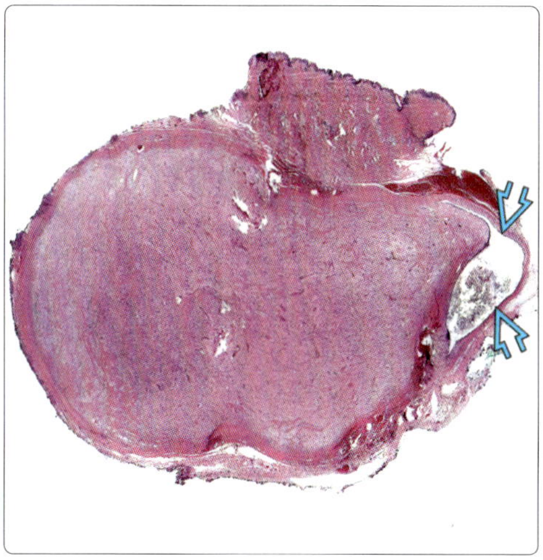

(Left) *Unlike most other cutaneous myxoid neoplasms, superficial angiomyxoma often contains scattered neutrophils* ➙. **(Right)** *A cystically dilated sweat duct* ➙ *is entrapped at the edge of this superficial angiomyxoma. Entrapped benign epithelial elements are seen in up to 25% of cases.*

Entrapped Cystic Sweat Duct

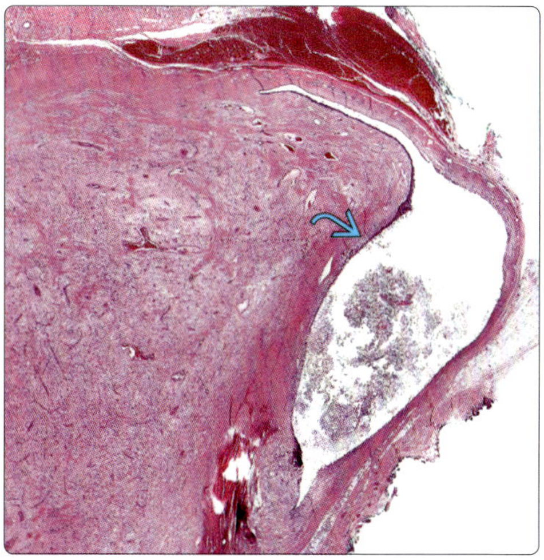

Entrapped Sweat Duct Elements

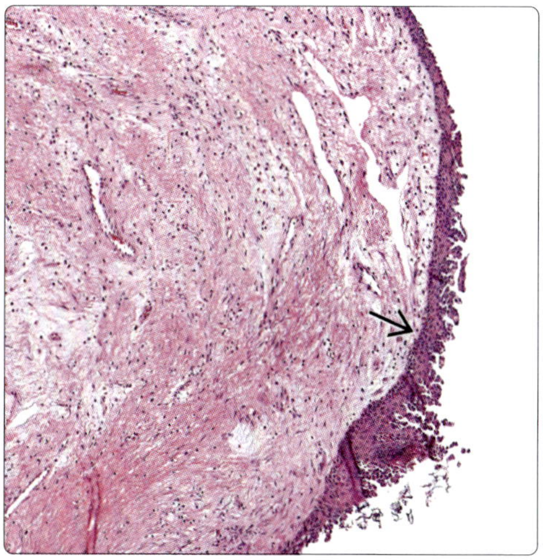

(Left) *A cystically dilated sweat ductal structure* ➙ *is entrapped at the periphery of this superficial angiomyxoma.* **(Right)** *The lining* ➙ *of this entrapped cystic duct alternates between keratinocytes and apocrine cells. There is fibrosis within the adjacent lesion.*

Entrapped Follicular Cyst

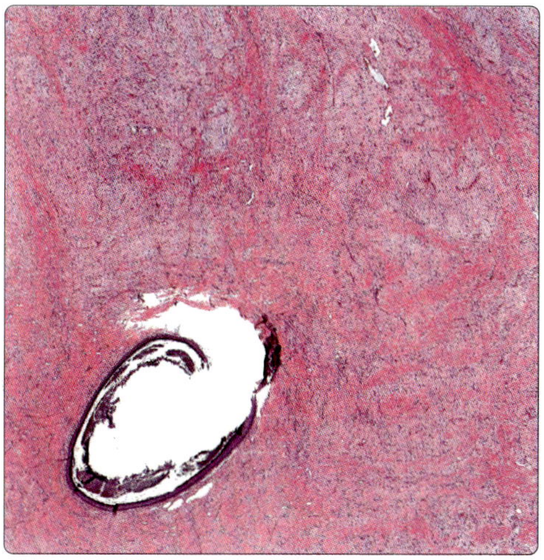

Entrapped Follicular Cyst

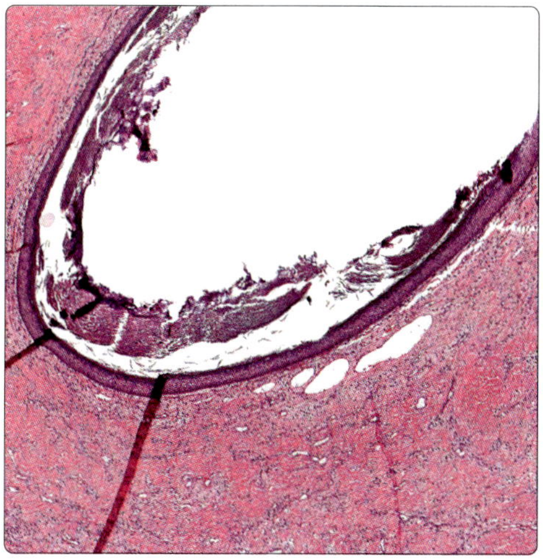

(Left) *Entrapped cystic epithelial structures similar to follicular cysts (so-called epidermal inclusion cysts) may be present.* **(Right)** *The lining of this entrapped cyst is composed of benign keratinocytes similar to the lining of a typical follicular cyst. Fibrosis may be prominent in some superficial angiomyxomas, as seen here.*

Acral Fibromyxoma

KEY FACTS

TERMINOLOGY

- Synonyms: Digital fibromyxoma, cellular digital fibroma
- Benign fibroblastic neoplasm that occurs in hands and feet, particularly nail bed region

CLINICAL ISSUES

- Most common > 40 years
- Male predilection
- Vast majority arise fingers and toes
  - Particularly in or near nail bed
- Solitary, slowly growing, and often longstanding lesion
- Treatment: Complete excision
- Excellent prognosis
- Low rate of recurrence, usually related to incomplete excision

MACROSCOPIC

- Usually < 5 cm (median: 1.5 cm)

MICROSCOPIC

- Moderately cellular proliferation of spindled to stellate fibroblastic cells in randomly arranged, loose fascicles or storiform arrays
- Nuclear atypia minimal to absent
- Rare mitoses; no necrosis
- Variable myxoid, myxocollagenous, or collagenous stroma

ANCILLARY TESTS

- CD34(+)
- Loss of nuclear RB1 expression
- Negative for S100 protein, desmin, keratin, claudin-1, MUC4, STAT6

TOP DIFFERENTIAL DIAGNOSES

- Dermatofibroma (fibrous histiocytoma)
- Perineurioma
- Dermatofibrosarcoma protuberans
- Myxoid neurofibroma

Acral Fibromyxoma

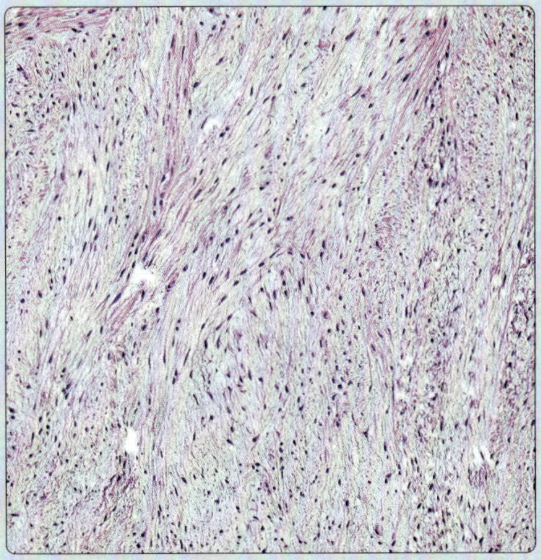

Stromal Collagen

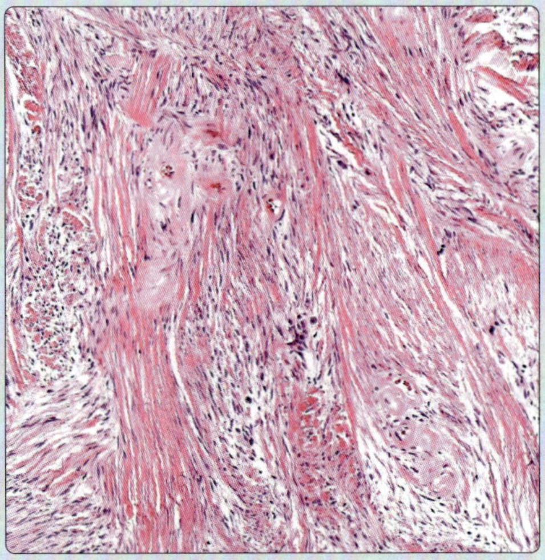

(Left) *Acral fibromyxoma (AF), also referred to as digital fibromyxoma, is a benign fibroblastic tumor that shows a marked predilection for the fingers and toes, particularly the nail bed region. Histologically, it is characterized by bland, spindled, and stellate cells arranged in random, loose fascicles and storiform arrays within a variable myxoid to fibrous stroma.* **(Right)** *Some areas of AF feature prominent stromal collagen, as depicted.*

Loose Storiform Growth

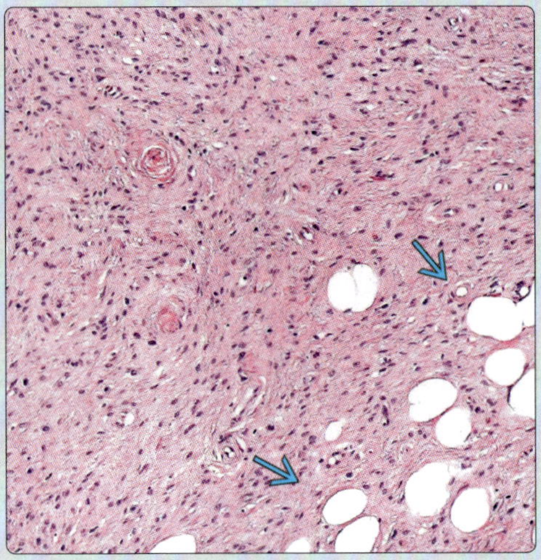

CD34 Expression

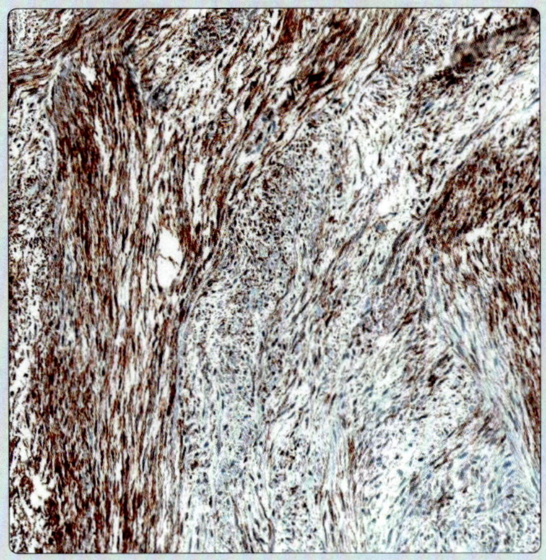

(Left) *AF may also demonstrate a loose arrangement of cells in a more vascularized stroma, somewhat resembling perineurioma. Despite its usual dermal origin, in some cases, AF shows superficial extension into subcutaneous fat ⇨.* **(Right)** *CD34 expression is seen in most cases of AF, but the extent of this positivity varies. Focal EMA and SMA may also be seen in rare cases. S100 protein, claudin-1, desmin, and keratins are negative.*

TERMINOLOGY

Abbreviations

- Acral fibromyxoma (AF)

Synonyms

- Superficial AF
- Digital fibromyxoma
- Cellular digital fibroma

Definitions

- Benign fibroblastic neoplasm that occurs in hands and feet, particularly nail bed region

CLINICAL ISSUES

Epidemiology

- Age
  - Wide range
    - Most common in patients > 40 years
- Sex
  - Male predilection

Site

- Almost exclusively hands and feet
  - Vast majority in fingers and toes
    - Particularly subungual or periungual region (nail bed)
- Extremely rare in nonacral sites

Presentation

- Solitary, slowly growing, and often longstanding lesion
  - Associated with pain in up to 40-50% of cases
- Superficial, dermal based

Treatment

- Complete excision

Prognosis

- Excellent prognosis
- Recurrences have been reported in up to 22%
  - Usually related to incomplete excision
- No reported case of metastasis or progression

MACROSCOPIC

General Features

- May appear dome-shaped, polypoid, or verrucoid
- Overlying mucosa intact or ulcerated
- Rare tumors can erode underlying bone

Size

- Usually < 5 cm (median: 1.5 cm)

MICROSCOPIC

Histologic Features

- Nodular, lobular, or irregular/infiltrative growth
  - Superficial involvement of subcutis and fat in some tumors
- Moderately cellular proliferation of spindled to stellate fibroblastic cells in randomly arranged, loose fascicles or storiform arrays
  - Nuclear atypia generally minimal to absent
    - Rare cases with scattered pleomorphic nuclei
  - Occasional multinucleated cells
  - Rare cases with increased cellularity
- Variable myxoid, myxocollagenous, or collagenous stroma
- Small blood vessels common
- Mast cells common
- Rare mitoses; no necrosis

ANCILLARY TESTS

Immunohistochemistry

- CD34(+)
- Loss of nuclear RB1 expression
- Occasional focal reactivity for EMA or SMA
- Generally negative for S100 protein, desmin, keratin, claudin-1, MUC4, STAT6

In Situ Hybridization

- *RB1* gene deletion by FISH

DIFFERENTIAL DIAGNOSIS

Dermatofibroma (Fibrous Histiocytoma)

- Peripheral collagen trapping
- Chronic inflammation, foamy histiocytes common
- Generally negative for CD34 and EMA

Perineurioma

- Can show morphologic overlap with AF
- Whorled (perivascular) growth pattern often prominent
- Claudin-1 (+), EMA(+), variable CD34(+)

Dermatofibrosarcoma Protuberans

- Prominent infiltration of subcutaneous fat
- Characteristic prominent storiform growth pattern
- Homogeneous CD34(+)
- t(17;22) with *COL1A1-PDGFB* fusion

Myxoid Neurofibroma

- Elongated, wrinkled or buckled nuclei
- Loose fascicular or storiform growth uncommon
- S100 protein (+), variable CD34(+)

Superficial Angiomyxoma

- Lobular growth
- Blood vessels with slightly fibrosed walls
- Prominent myxoid stroma with perivascular neutrophils

Solitary Fibrous Tumor

- Acral extremity involvement very rare
- CD34(+), STAT6(+)
- Retained nuclear RB1 expression

SELECTED REFERENCES

1. Agaimy A et al: Superficial acral fibromyxoma: clinicopathological, immunohistochemical, and molecular study of 11 cases highlighting frequent Rb1 loss/deletions. Hum Pathol. 60:192-198, 2017
2. Cullen D et al: Superficial acral fibromyxoma: report of 13 cases with new immunohistochemical findings. Am J Dermatopathol. 39(1):14-22, 2017
3. Hollmann TJ et al: Digital fibromyxoma (superficial acral fibromyxoma): a detailed characterization of 124 cases. Am J Surg Pathol. 36(6):789-98, 2012
4. Al-Daraji WI et al: Superficial acral fibromyxoma: a clinicopathological analysis of 32 tumors including 4 in the heel. J Cutan Pathol. 35(11):1020-6, 2008
5. Fetsch JF et al: Superficial acral fibromyxoma: a clinicopathologic and immunohistochemical analysis of 37 cases of a distinctive soft tissue tumor with a predilection for the fingers and toes. Hum Pathol. 32(7):704-14, 2001

Pleomorphic Hyalinizing Angiectatic Tumor

KEY FACTS

TERMINOLOGY

- Locally recurring but nonmetastasizing mesenchymal neoplasm characterized by atypical spindled cells amidst clusters of dilated, hyalinized vascular spaces
    - Possible pathogenetic relationship exists with other entities: Hemosiderotic fibrolipomatous tumor (HFLT) and myxoinflammatory fibroblastic sarcoma

CLINICAL ISSUES

- Median age: 51 years
- Usually lower leg, ankle, or foot
- Slow-growing, subcutaneous mass
- Treatment: Complete surgical excision
- Local recurrence in 30-50% of cases
    - May rarely progress to frank myxoid sarcoma
- No metastases reported

MACROSCOPIC

- Usually poorly circumscribed

MICROSCOPIC

- Unencapsulated
- Variably cellular, pleomorphic spindle cell proliferation
    - Intracytoplasmic hemosiderin
    - Intranuclear pseudoinclusions common
- Clusters of ectatic, thin-walled, hyalinized blood vessels
- Inflammatory infiltrate common
- Mitoses rare to absent and no necrosis
- Most cases show peripheral areas resembling HFLT
    - Infiltrative, bland, spindled cells with hemosiderin

ANCILLARY TESTS

- CD34(+) in most cases; S100 protein (-)

TOP DIFFERENTIAL DIAGNOSES

- Schwannoma
- HFLT
- Undifferentiated pleomorphic sarcoma

Pleomorphic Hyalinizing Angiectatic Tumor

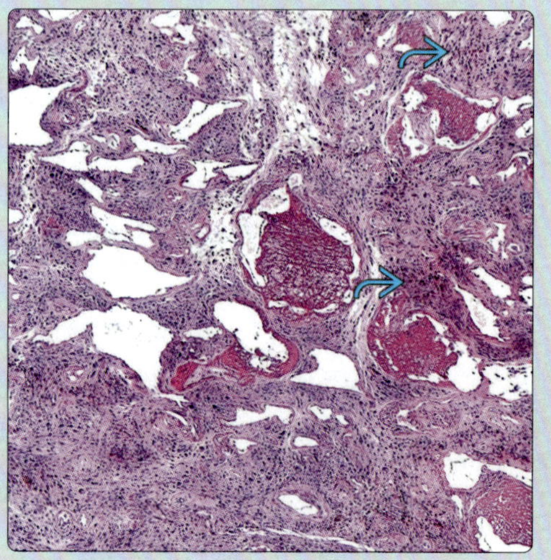

Characteristic Vessels and Pleomorphism

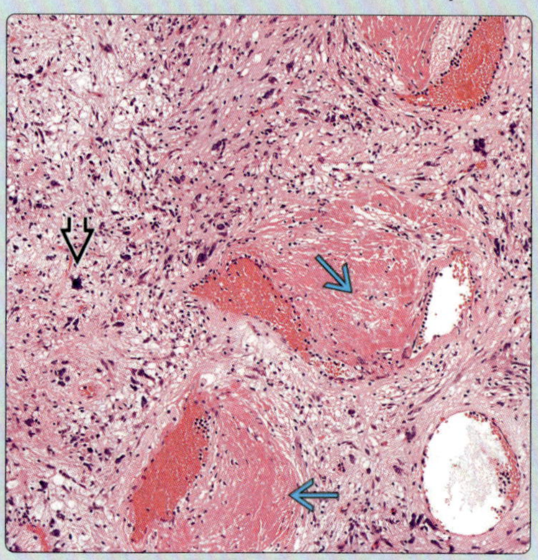

(Left) *Pleomorphic hyalinizing angiectatic tumor (PHAT) is a distinctive, locally recurring but nonmetastasizing soft tissue neoplasm with an unusual predilection for the distal lower extremity. Classic cases feature a variably cellular, pleomorphic spindle cell proliferation, hemosiderin pigment, and dilated, thin-walled blood vessels with fibrinoid change and hyalinization.* **(Right)** *Classic PHAT features pleomorphic spindled cells and ectatic vessels with fibrinoid change, hyalinization, or thrombosis.*

Hemosiderin and Inflammatory Cells

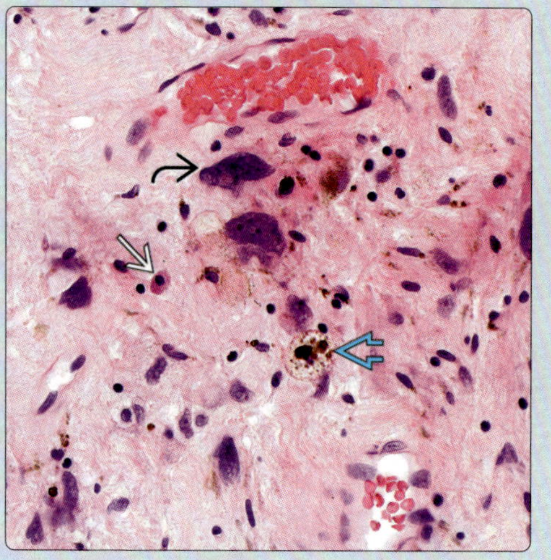

HFLT-Like Areas (Early Pleomorphic Hyalinizing Angiectatic Tumor)

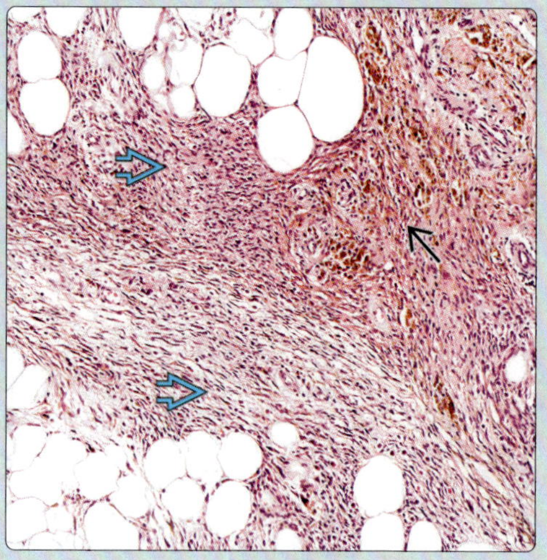

(Left) *High-power H&E of PHAT shows characteristic hyperchromatic, pleomorphic nuclei as well as hemosiderin pigment and chronic inflammatory cells, including mast cells and lymphocytes.* **(Right)** *A bland, infiltrative spindle cell proliferation with hemosiderin is commonly seen at the periphery of PHAT and is generally considered a precursor lesion (early PHAT). It resembles (or is likely identical to) hemosiderotic fibrolipomatous tumor (HFLT).*

Pleomorphic Hyalinizing Angiectatic Tumor

TERMINOLOGY

Abbreviations

- Pleomorphic hyalinizing angiectatic tumor (PHAT)

Definitions

- Locally recurring but nonmetastasizing mesenchymal neoplasm characterized by atypical spindled cells amidst clusters of dilated, hyalinized vascular spaces
  - Possible pathogenetic relationship exists between PHAT, hemosiderotic fibrolipomatous tumor (HFLT), and myxoinflammatory fibroblastic sarcoma (MIFS)
    - Hybrid tumors: HFLT/PHAT or PHAT/MIFS (rare)
    - Current data suggests that HFLT and PHAT are related lesions, whereas PHAT and classic MIFS are not
      - Hybrid PHAT/MIFS cases likely represent PHAT with sarcomatous progression rather than classic MIFS

CLINICAL ISSUES

Epidemiology

- Age
  - Wide range: 10-80 years (median: 51 years)
- Sex
  - Slight female predominance

Site

- Usually lower leg, ankle, or foot
- Rarely thigh or other sites

Presentation

- Slow-growing, often painless mass
  - Usually subcutaneous; rarely deep

Treatment

- Complete surgical excision
- Reexcision of local recurrences

Prognosis

- Local recurrence in 30-50% of cases
  - Rare cases progress to frank myxoid sarcoma
- No metastases reported in PHAT or HFLT/PHAT

MACROSCOPIC

General Features

- Usually poorly circumscribed
- Tan-gray to dark brown or red

Size

- Wide range (median: 6 cm)

MICROSCOPIC

Histologic Features

- Unencapsulated
- Variably cellular proliferation of spindle cells
  - Nuclear hyperchromasia and pleomorphism common
  - Prominent intranuclear cytoplasmic inclusions
  - Intracytoplasmic hemosiderin pigment
    - May be abundant and striking in some cases
  - Mitoses rare to absent
- Clusters of ectatic, thin-walled blood vessels
  - Fibrinoid and hyaline material in vessel walls
- Hyalinized to myxoid stroma
  - Inflammatory infiltrate common
    - Particularly mast cells
- Necrosis absent
- Most cases show peripheral areas resembling HFLT
  - Infiltrative, bland, spindled cells associated with hemosiderin
  - Appears to represent precursor lesion of PHAT
- Rare cases progress to frank myxoid sarcoma
  - Increased cellularity and mitotic activity
  - May resemble MIFS

ANCILLARY TESTS

Immunohistochemistry

- CD34(+) in most cases
- S100 protein, keratin, desmin (-)

Molecular Genetics

- *TGFBR3* &/or *MGEA5* gene rearrangements reported in PHAT and HFLT

DIFFERENTIAL DIAGNOSIS

Schwannoma

- Encapsulated
- Occurs at variety of sites beyond lower extremity
- Verocay body formation in many
- Areas with degenerative/ancient changes may resemble PHAT
- Strong, diffuse S100 protein (+); CD34(-)

Hemosiderotic Fibrolipomatous Tumor

- Appears to be histogenetically related to PHAT
  - Tumors often show hybrid features of HFLT and PHAT
- Lacks large, dilated vessels with fibrinoid material
- Prominent adipose tissue component

Undifferentiated Pleomorphic Sarcoma

- May contain areas with large, hyalinized vessels
- Usually large, deeply situated mass; necrosis common
- High cellularity and nuclear grade; atypical mitoses

Myxoinflammatory Fibroblastic Sarcoma

- Classically, mixture of myxoid, hyalinized, and inflammatory zones
- Large, ganglion-like cells, virocyte-like macronucleoli; pseudolipoblasts

SELECTED REFERENCES

1. Boland JM et al: Hemosiderotic fibrolipomatous tumor, pleomorphic hyalinizing angiectatic tumor, and myxoinflammatory fibroblastic sarcoma: related or not? Adv Anat Pathol. 24(5):268-77, 2017
2. Carter JM et al: TGFBR3 and MGEA5 rearrangements in pleomorphic hyalinizing angiectatic tumors and the spectrum of related neoplasms. Am J Surg Pathol. 38(9):1182-992, 2014
3. Illueca C et al: Pleomorphic hyalinizing angiectatic tumor: a report of 3 new cases, 1 with sarcomatous myxofibrosarcoma component and another with unreported soft tissue palpebral location. Appl Immunohistochem Mol Morphol. 20(1):96-101, 2012
4. Folpe AL et al: Pleomorphic hyalinizing angiectatic tumor: analysis of 41 cases supporting evolution from a distinctive precursor lesion. Am J Surg Pathol. 28(11):1417-25, 2004

(Left) *This PHAT is partially circumscribed* *but focally extends into fat* *. An infiltrative peripheral border is common in this tumor. The tumor is reddish-brown due to a combination of old and recent hemorrhage.* **(Right)** *The characteristic ectatic or dilated vasculature is generally conspicuous in PHAT; however, in more cellular or solid tumors, these vessels may be only focally prominent. Note the fibrinoid change* *and hyalinization apparent even at low power.*

Gross Specimen

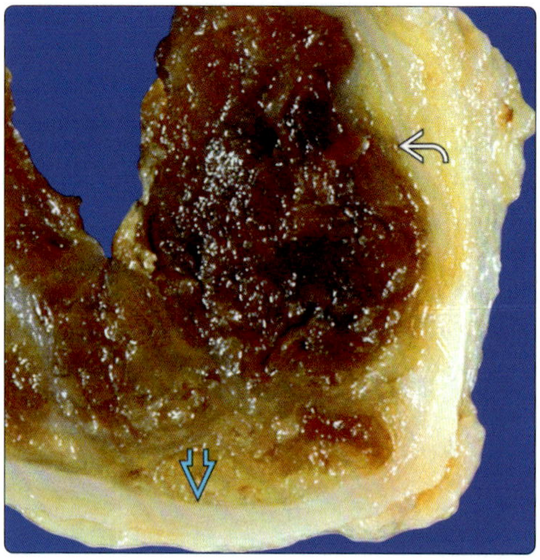

Prominent Ectatic Vasculature

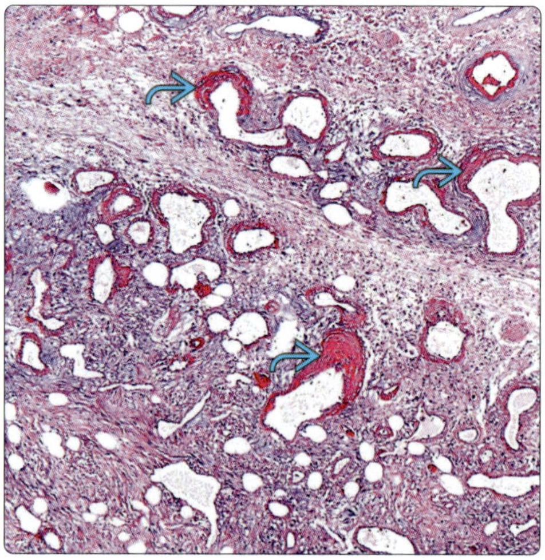

(Left) *Thrombosis* *within vessels is relatively common in PHAT. Focal intraluminal papillary endothelial hyperplasia or recanalization may also be seen in some cases.* **(Right)** *In this PHAT, there are aggregates of angiectatic blood vessels with hyalinized walls that have fused* *. This resembles the vascular changes in ancient schwannoma.*

Partial Thrombosis and Hemosiderin

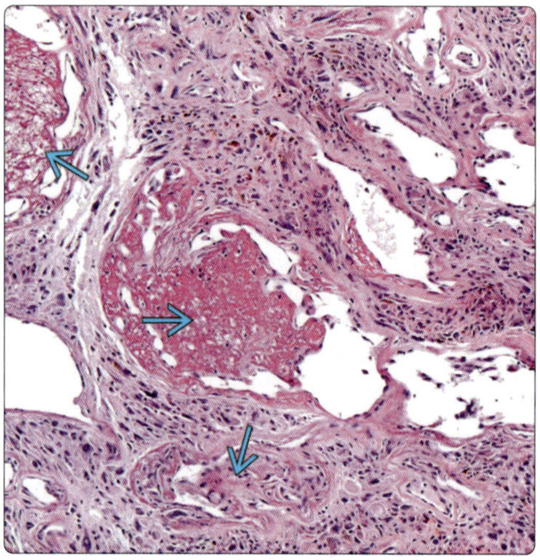

Clusters of Hyalinized Vessels

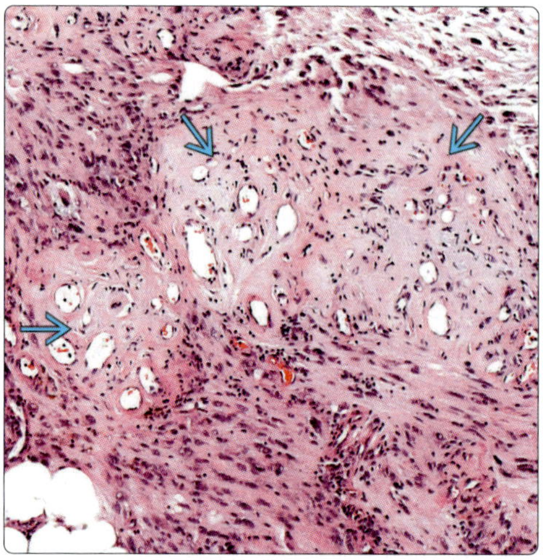

(Left) *This case of PHAT features predominantly large, thrombosed vascular spaces* *separated by cellular fibrous tissue* *. The lesion infiltrates subcutaneous fat at the periphery* *.* **(Right)** *PHAT often shows an infiltrative periphery with tumor cells infiltrating between mature adipocytes* *, as shown in this H&E. These peripheral areas typically show features of HFLT (early PHAT).*

Prominent Thrombosed Vasculature

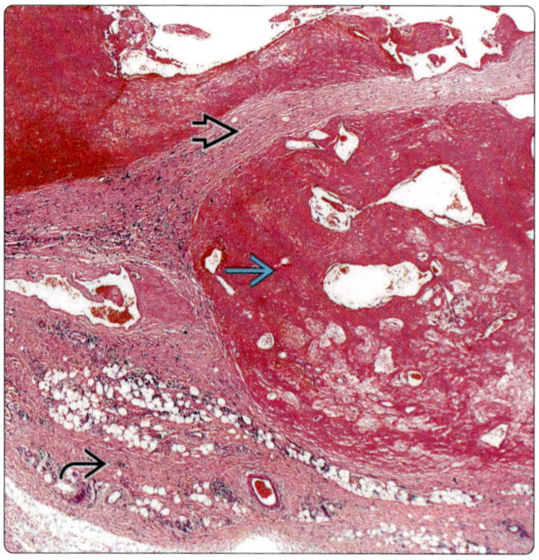

Infiltrative Border

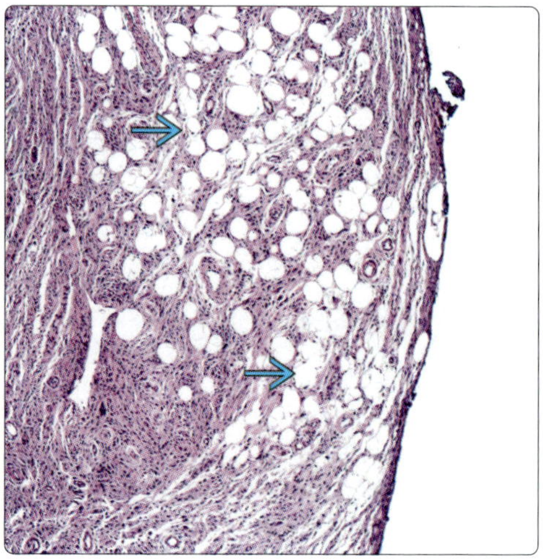

Nuclear Pseudoinclusions

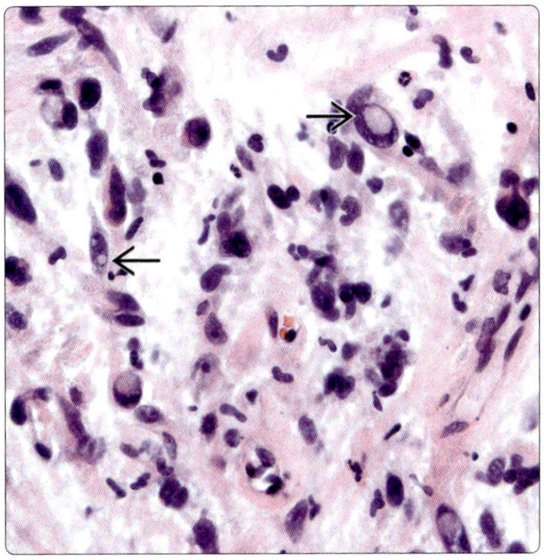

Hemosiderin

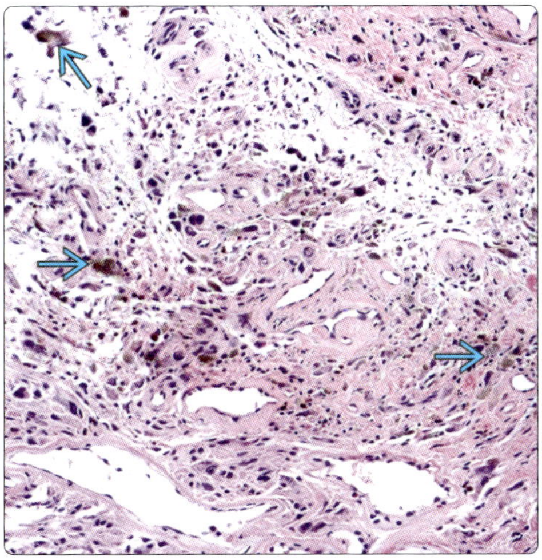

(Left) *Intranuclear pseudoinclusions → are common in PHAT and may appear pale or deeply eosinophilic depending upon the color of the cytoplasm of the cell.* **(Right)** *Intracytoplasmic hemosiderin → is common in PHAT but varies widely in amount and distribution. Some cases feature extensive hemosiderin readily apparent at low magnification, and others require a histochemical stain in order for iron to fully appreciate them.*

Rare Mitotic Figures

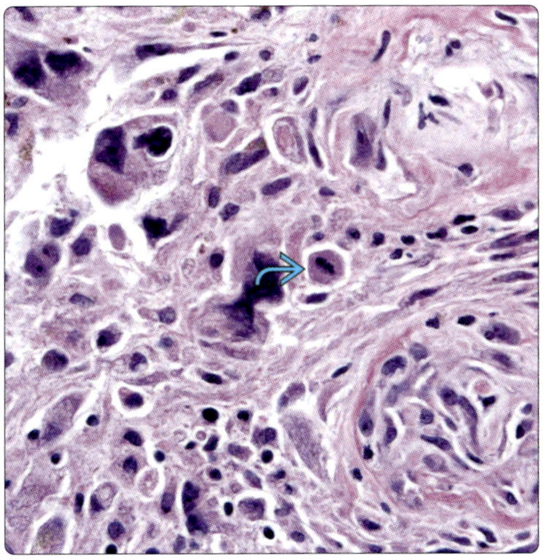

Minimally Pleomorphic Areas

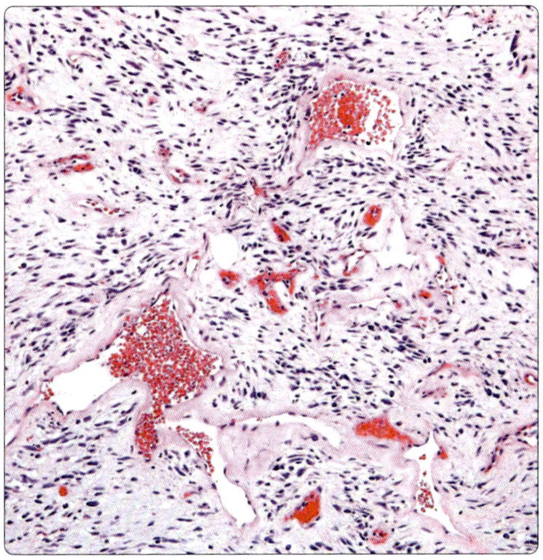

(Left) *Mitoses → are rare in PHAT. More than an occasional mitotic figure should raise concerns for a true pleomorphic sarcoma. Very rare cases have been reported of PHAT recurring as frank sarcoma with abundant mitoses and necrosis.* **(Right)** *Although characteristic of classic PHAT, pleomorphic nuclei may be subtle or absent in some areas, as depicted here.*

Solid/Cellular Areas

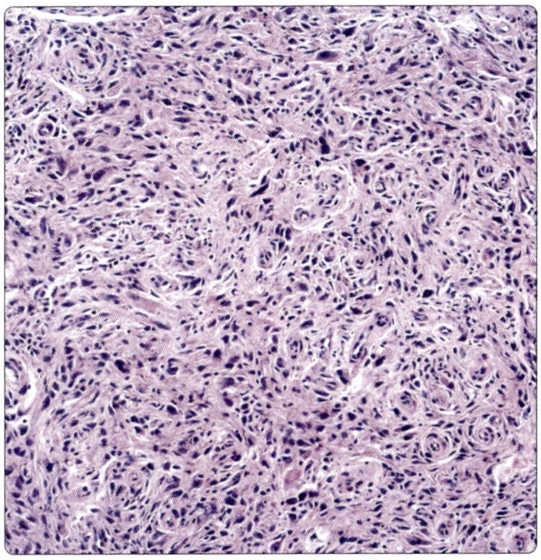

Myxoid Areas

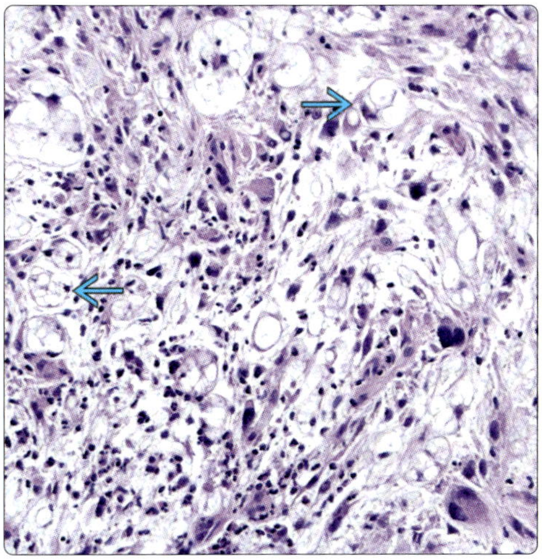

(Left) *Solid areas of PHAT with an absent ectatic vasculature may be easily confused for frank sarcoma; however, the cytologic features are identical to those in more conventional areas, and mitotic figures remain sparse or absent.* **(Right)** *Myxoid stroma is uncommon in PHAT. This unusual case also shows areas somewhat reminiscent of myxoinflammatory fibroblastic sarcoma or myxofibrosarcoma, including pseudolipoblasts →. This rare phenomenon likely represents sarcomatous progression in PHAT.*

Aneurysmal Bone Cyst of Soft Tissue

KEY FACTS

TERMINOLOGY

- Benign, primary soft tissue counterpart of intraosseous aneurysmal bone cyst (ABC)

CLINICAL ISSUES

- Very rare
- Range: 7-57 years (median: 29 years)
- 2:1 = F:M
- Deep soft tissues of upper extremity, shoulder, and thigh
- Usually no history of trauma reported
- Treatment: Complete surgical excision
- Benign; excellent prognosis

IMAGING

- Oval-shaped, variably ossified soft tissue mass
- Intralesional septations and fluid levels

MACROSCOPIC

- Range: 2-9 cm (median: 5.2 cm)

MICROSCOPIC

- Well circumscribed, noninfiltrative
- Histologically identical to intraosseous ABC
  - Variable-sized cystic spaces filled with blood
  - Cystic walls and septa composed of cytologically bland spindled cells
  - Clusters of osteoclast-like giant cells common
  - Immature (woven) bone common in septa and around periphery of lesion

ANCILLARY TESTS

- Molecular: Various rearrangements involving *USP6* (17p13)

TOP DIFFERENTIAL DIAGNOSES

- Myositis ossificans
- Nodular fasciitis
- Giant cell tumor of soft tissue
- Extraskeletal osteosarcoma

Aneurysmal Bone Cyst of Soft Tissue

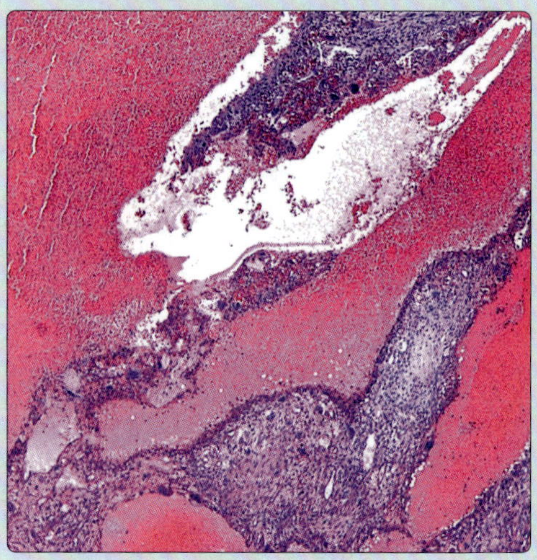

Peripheral Bone Formation

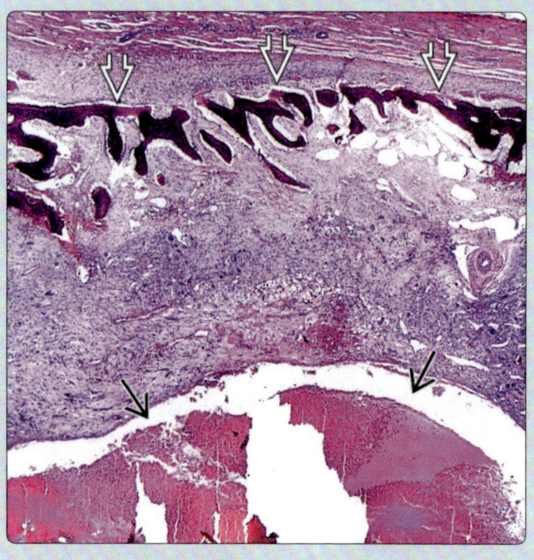

(Left) *Soft tissue ABC is a form of ABC that occurs exclusively in soft tissue sites without bony involvement. It is morphologically nearly identical to intraosseous ABC, and at low power, it shows a multicystic, hemorrhagic lesion with variably cellular septa, as depicted.* **(Right)** *A peripheral rim of immature or mature bone ⇨ is a frequent feature of soft tissue ABC. This finding can lead to histologic, clinical, and radiologic confusion with myositis ossificans. Note the centralized hemorrhagic cavity ➡.*

Classic Features

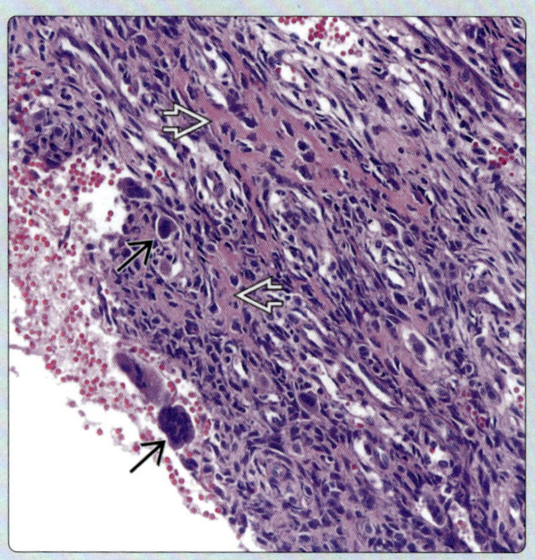

Loose Fibromyxoid Stroma

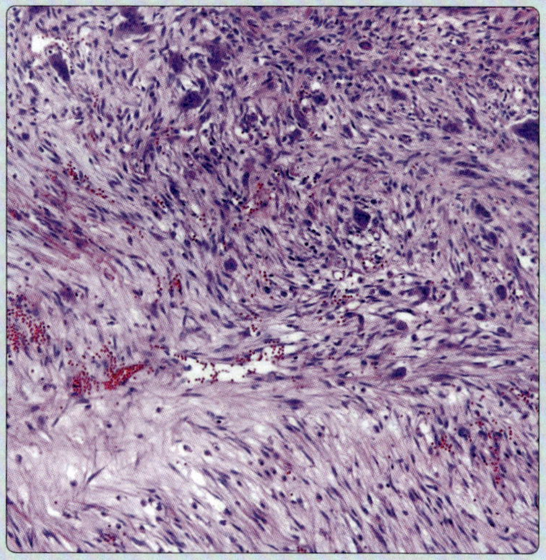

(Left) *The septa and cyst walls of soft tissue ABC are composed of bland spindled fibroblastic cells admixed with scattered, osteoclast-like giant cells ➡ and foci of immature (woven) bone formation ⇨. A mild chronic inflammatory infiltrate may also be present in some cases.* **(Right)** *The stroma in soft tissue ABC is characteristically loose and fibromyxoid in quality, imparting a reactive appearance. This morphology is similar to what is seen in early forms of nodular fasciitis.*

TERMINOLOGY

Abbreviations

- Ectopic hamartomatous thymoma (EHT)

Synonyms

- Branchial anlage mixed tumor

Definitions

- Rare benign tumor composed of spindle, epithelial, and adipose tissue elements that occurs mainly in lower neck region

ETIOLOGY/PATHOGENESIS

Developmental Anomaly

- Suggested derivation from sequestered branchial epithelium
- Possible origin from thymic anlage remnants

CLINICAL ISSUES

Epidemiology

- Incidence
  - Very rare
- Age
  - Adults (median: 40 years)
- Sex
  - Male predominance (4:1)

Site

- Subcutaneous tissue of lower neck, supraclavicular, or suprasternal region
  - May also arise subfascially

Presentation

- Painless, slowly enlarging mass, often of long duration
  - Clinical presentation and diagnostic imaging may suggest malignancy

Treatment

- Conservative surgical excision

Prognosis

- Benign
- Local recurrence is very rare if completely excised
- Does not metastasize
  - Very rare cases of carcinoma arising in EHT have been reported in literature

MACROSCOPIC

General Features

- Well circumscribed, lobulated
- Tan-white to yellow, firm cut surface

Size

- Usually 2-8 cm (average: 5 cm)

MICROSCOPIC

Histologic Features

- Well circumscribed, unencapsulated
- Haphazard admixture of spindle cells, epithelial cells, and mature adipose tissue in varying proportions
  - Spindle cells
    - Sheets, short fascicles, or storiform arrays
      - Variable cellularity
    - Bland, elongated, sometimes tapering nuclei
  - Epithelial cells
    - Solid, cystic, or glandular components
    - Squamous elements are usually predominant
      - May show keratinization
    - Epithelial-lined cysts are seen focally in many cases
  - Mature adipose tissue
    - May be relatively abundant
- Generally low mitotic rate
- Subtle stromal lymphoid infiltrate may be present

ANCILLARY TESTS

Immunohistochemistry

- Diffuse keratin (+) in both epithelial and spindle cells
  - Includes low- and high-molecular-weight keratins
- Variable CD34(+) and SMA(+) in spindle cells
- S100 protein (-), desmin (-), STAT6(-), and pax-8(-)

DIFFERENTIAL DIAGNOSIS

Pleomorphic Adenoma

- Salivary gland origin
- Chondromyxoid stroma &/or cartilaginous differentiation
- Spindle cells are keratin (+), S100(+), EMA(+), CD34(-)
- *PLAG1* gene rearrangements

Synovial Sarcoma (Biphasic)

- Squamous nests and intratumoral adipose tissue uncommon
- Keratin (+) in spindled tumor cells is usually patchy or focal
- Nuclear TLE1(+), CD34(-)
- Characteristic t(X;18) involving *SS18* (SYT)

Sarcomatoid Carcinoma

- Usually overtly cytologically malignant
- Mitoses and necrosis common

Solitary Fibrous Tumor

- Lacks epithelial elements
- STAT6(+)
- Keratins (-)

SELECTED REFERENCES

1. Sato K et al: Ectopic hamartomatous thymoma: a review of the literature with report of new cases and proposal of a new name: biphenotypic branchioma. Head Neck Pathol. 12(2):202-9 2017
2. Weissferdt A et al: Ectopic hamartomatous thymoma-new insights into a challenging entity: a clinicopathologic and immunohistochemical study of 9 cases. Am J Surg Pathol. 40(11):1571-1576, 2016
3. Jing H et al: Ectopic hamartomatous thymoma: report of a case and review of literature. Int J Clin Exp Pathol. 8(9):11776-84, 2015
4. Liang PI et al: Ectopic hamartomatous thymoma is distinct from lipomatous pleomorphic adenoma in lacking PLAG1 aberration. Histopathology. 62(3):518-22, 2013
5. Kushida Y et al: Ectopic hamartomatous thymoma: a case report with immunohistochemical study and review of the literature. J Cutan Pathol. 33(5):369-72, 2006
6. Fetsch JF et al: Ectopic hamartomatous thymoma: a clinicopathologic and immunohistochemical analysis of 21 cases with data supporting reclassification as a branchial anlage mixed tumor. Am J Surg Pathol. 28(10):1360-70, 2004

Hemosiderotic Fibrolipomatous Tumor

KEY FACTS

TERMINOLOGY

- Synonym: Hemosiderotic fibrohistiocytic lipomatous lesion
- Locally aggressive but nonmetastasizing neoplasm featuring mixture of mature adipose tissue, bland spindled cells, abundant hemosiderin, and chronic inflammatory cells
  - Possible pathogenetic relationship exists with other entities: Pleomorphic hyalinizing angiectatic tumor (PHAT) and myxoinflammatory fibroblastic sarcoma (MIFS)

CLINICAL ISSUES

- Most common: 40-60 years
- Marked female predominance
- Predominantly affects distal extremities
  - Particularly foot or ankle
- Treatment: Complete surgical excision
- Local recurrence in up to 50%
- No metastases

MICROSCOPIC

- Unencapsulated
- Lobules of mature adipose tissue with loose fascicles of bland spindled cells in septal, perilobular, or periadipocytic arrangement
- Hemosiderin always present and often abundant
- Mitoses absent to scarce

ANCILLARY TESTS

- CD34(+)
- Keratins, EMA, S100 protein, SMA, desmin (-)
- Molecular: t(1;10)(p22;q24) involving rearrangements of *TGFBR3* &/or *MGEA5*

TOP DIFFERENTIAL DIAGNOSES

- Spindle cell lipoma
- PHAT
- MIFS
- Dermatofibrosarcoma protuberans

Hemosiderotic Fibrolipomatous Tumor

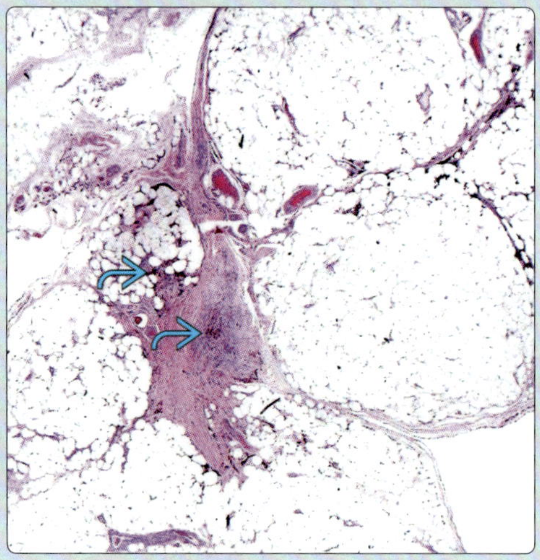

Prominent Hemosiderin

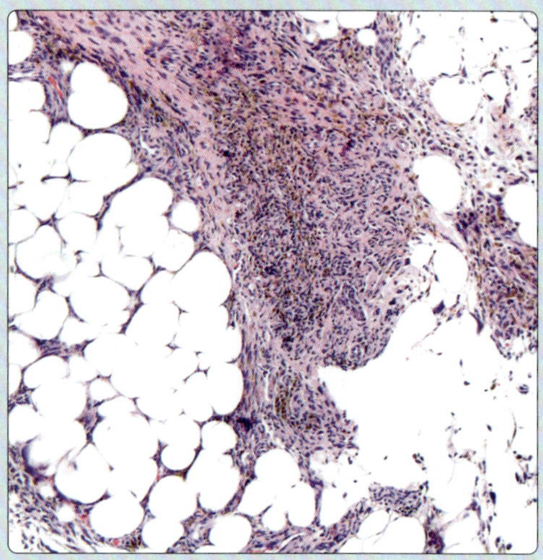

(Left) *Hemosiderotic fibrolipomatous tumor (HFLT) features lobules of mature adipose tissue admixed with variably cellular fascicles of spindle cells, often along septa and around or within lobules. This appearance may resemble a reactive, rather than neoplastic, process. Hemosiderin ↗ is often prominent and appreciable even at low power.* **(Right)** *Hemosiderin deposition is a characteristic feature of HFLT and is usually quite prominent. Note also the irregular septal and perilobular growth around the mature adipose tissue.*

Bland Spindle Cells

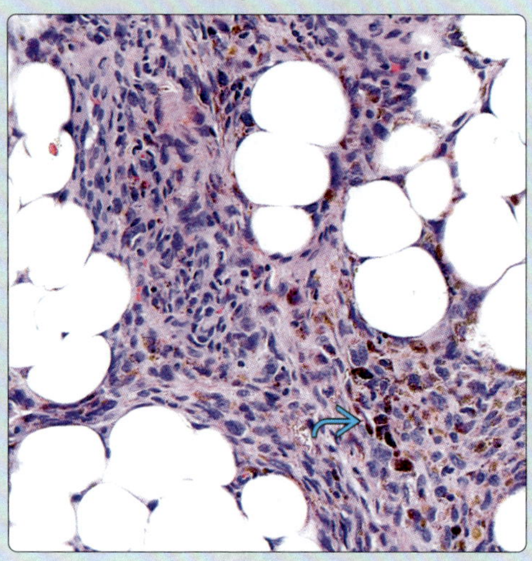

Occasional Multinucleated Giant Cells

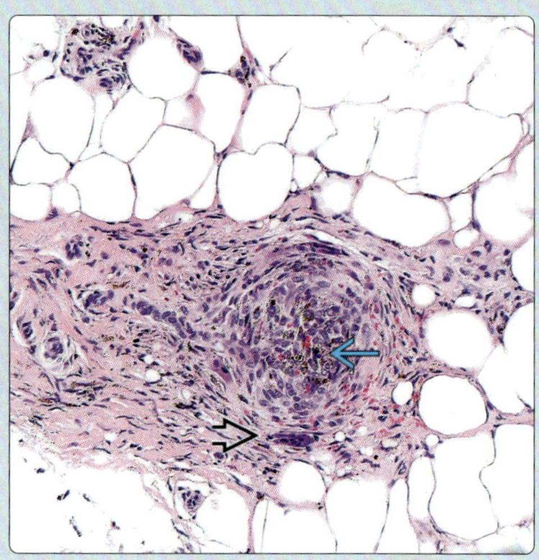

(Left) *In general, tumor cells in HFLT are cytologically banal; however, occasional enlarged or pleomorphic hyperchromatic nuclei (similar to what is seen in pleomorphic hyalinizing angiectatic tumor) may be seen in some cases. Mitoses are absent. Note the hemosiderin ↗.* **(Right)** *Multinucleated giant cells may be seen in HFLT and are often of the osteoclastic variety ⇨. Note also the hemosiderin pigment →.*

TERMINOLOGY

Abbreviations

- Hemosiderotic fibrolipomatous tumor (HFLT)

Synonyms

- Hemosiderotic fibrohistiocytic lipomatous lesion

Definitions

- Locally aggressive but nonmetastasizing neoplasm featuring mixture of mature adipose tissue, bland spindled cells, abundant hemosiderin, and chronic inflammatory cells
  - Possible pathogenetic relationship exists between HFLT, pleomorphic hyalinizing angiectatic tumor (PHAT), and myxoinflammatory fibroblastic sarcoma (MIFS)
    - "Hybrid" tumors: HFLT with PHAT or HFLT with MIFS
    - Current data suggests that HFLT and PHAT are related lesions, whereas HFLT and classic MIFS are not
      - Hybrid HFLT/MIFS cases likely represent HFLT with sarcomatous progression rather than classic MIFS

CLINICAL ISSUES

Epidemiology

- Age
  - Most common: 40-60 years
- Sex
  - Marked female predominance

Site

- Predominantly distal extremities (particularly foot or ankle)
- Less frequent: Calf, cheek, thigh

Presentation

- Slow-growing subcutaneous mass

Treatment

- Complete surgical excision

Prognosis

- Local recurrence in up to 50%
  - Often related to incomplete excision
- No metastases reported

MACROSCOPIC

General Features

- Poorly defined fatty proliferation
- Dark yellow-brown cut surface

Size

- Wide size range (average: 7.7 cm)

MICROSCOPIC

Histologic Features

- Unencapsulated
- Subcutaneous lobules of homogeneous fat
- Loose fascicles of spindled cells in septal, perilobular, or periadipocytic arrangement
  - Cytologically bland; usually no significant pleomorphism
  - Mitoses absent to scarce
- Hemosiderin always present and often abundant
  - May be seen in spindle cells or histiocytes
- Occasional osteoclast-type multinucleated giant cells
- Chronic inflammatory cells, including lymphocytes, foamy histiocytes, plasma cells, and mast cells
- Focal features suggestive of PHAT or MIFS may be present
  - PHAT: Scattered pleomorphic nuclei with pseudoinclusions; ectatic hyalinized blood vessels
  - MIFS: Larger atypical cells with prominent macronucleoli in variable myxoid stroma

ANCILLARY TESTS

Immunohistochemistry

- CD34(+)
- Keratins, EMA, S100 protein, SMA, desmin (-)

Molecular Genetics

- t(1;10)(p22;q24) with rearrangements of *TGFBR3* &/or *MGEA5*
- To date, no *BRAF* mutations reported in pure HFLT or hybrid HFLT/MIFS

DIFFERENTIAL DIAGNOSIS

Spindle Cell Lipoma

- Most common in neck, shoulder, upper back
- Bundles of "ropey" collagen
- Lacks abundant hemosiderin

Pleomorphic Hyalinizing Angiectatic Tumor

- Likely related to HFLT
- Variable cellular, solid proliferation of pleomorphic spindle cells with nuclear pseudoinclusions
- Characteristic clusters of ectatic hyalinized vessels

Myxoinflammatory Fibroblastic Sarcoma

- Classically, mixture of myxoid, hyalinized, and inflammatory zones
- Large ganglion-like cells, virocyte-like macronucleoli; pseudolipoblasts
- Cases reported of HFLT with areas resembling MIFS
  - Likely represent HFLT with sarcomatous progression, unrelated to classic MIFS

Dermatofibrosarcoma Protuberans

- Usually prominent storiform growth pattern
- Lacks abundant inflammation and hemosiderin
- t(17;22) with *COL1A1-PDGFRB* fusion

SELECTED REFERENCES

1. Boland JM et al: Hemosiderotic fibrolipomatous tumor, pleomorphic hyalinizing angiectatic tumor, and myxoinflammatory fibroblastic sarcoma: related or not? Adv Anat Pathol. 24(5):268-277, 2017
2. Kao YC et al: Recurrent BRAF gene rearrangements in myxoinflammatory fibroblastic sarcomas, but not hemosiderotic fibrolipomatous tumors. Am J Surg Pathol. 41(11):1456-1465, 2017
3. Zreik RT et al: TGFBR3 and MGEA5 rearrangements are much more common in "hybrid" hemosiderotic fibrolipomatous tumor-myxoinflammatory fibroblastic sarcomas than in classical myxoinflammatory fibroblastic sarcomas: a morphological and fluorescence in situ hybridization study. Hum Pathol. 53:14-24, 2016
4. Browne TJ et al: Haemosiderotic fibrolipomatous tumour (so-called haemosiderotic fibrohistiocytic lipomatous tumour): analysis of 13 new cases in support of a distinct entity. Histopathology. 48(4):453-61, 2006
5. Marshall-Taylor C et al: Hemosiderotic fibrohistiocytic lipomatous lesion: ten cases of a previously undescribed fatty lesion of the foot/ankle. Mod Pathol. 13(11):1192-9, 2000

Atypical Fibroxanthoma

KEY FACTS

TERMINOLOGY

- Atypical fibroxanthoma (AFX)
- Strictly defined, dermal-based mesenchymal neoplasm showing no specific lineage of differentiation
  - Should be negative for markers of melanocytic (i.e., S100, SOX10, melan-A), epithelial (i.e., cytokeratins and p63), and vascular (i.e., CD34, ERG) differentiation
  - Not allowed: Invasion into deep subcutaneous tissue and beyond, tumor necrosis, lymphovascular invasion, and perineurial involvement
  - Can only be diagnosed on complete excision (diagnosis of exclusion)

CLINICAL ISSUES

- Mass lesion, may be ulcerated or bleeding
- Often rapidly growing tumor in head and neck region of elderly adult
- Rate of local recurrence is low (< 10% reported)

MICROSCOPIC

- Highly atypical and pleomorphic dermal-based proliferation of spindled to epithelioid-appearing cells
- Scattered large, bizarre-appearing, multinucleated cells often seen
- Variants include spindle cell, clear cell, granular, others
- Numerous mitoses, including highly atypical forms

ANCILLARY TESTS

- IHC is essential to exclude other, more specific diagnoses
- Negative for cytokeratins (especially high-molecular-weight cytokeratins), p63, and melanocytic, myogenic, and vascular markers

TOP DIFFERENTIAL DIAGNOSES

- Sarcomatoid carcinoma
- Spindle cell melanoma
- Pleomorphic dermal sarcoma
- Leiomyosarcoma and other sarcomas

Atypical Fibroxanthoma

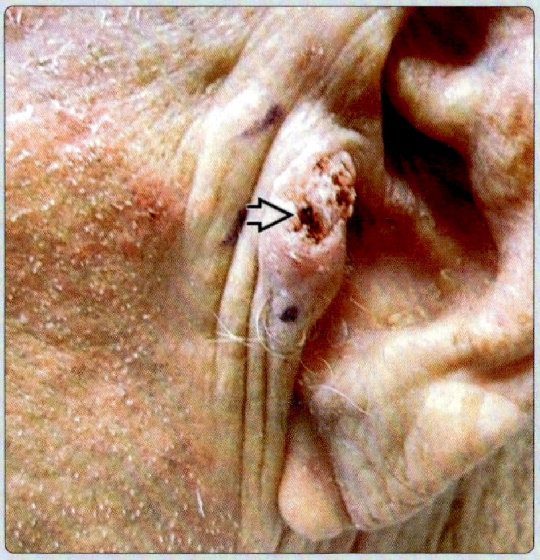

Atypical Fibroxanthoma at Low Magnification

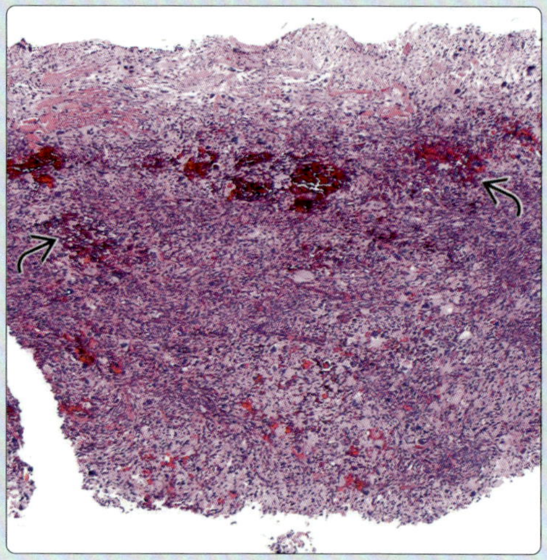

(Left) *Clinical photograph shows an atypical fibroxanthoma (AFX) on the ear of an elderly patient. Note that the surface is ulcerated and shows focal serum crust ➔.* **(Right)** *Histologic section of AFX at low magnification shows a large, dermal-based, nodular to sheet-like collection of atypical tumor cells with diffuse overlying ulceration. The dermis shows several congested dilated vessels and hemorrhage ➔.*

Atypical Fibroxanthoma at High Magnification

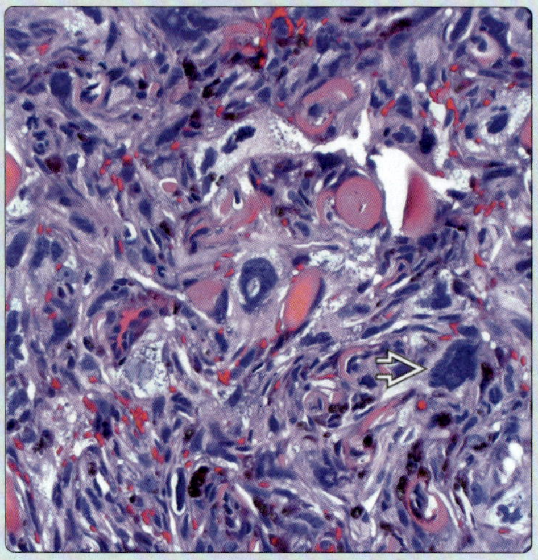

CD10 Immunohistochemical Stain in Atypical Fibroxanthoma

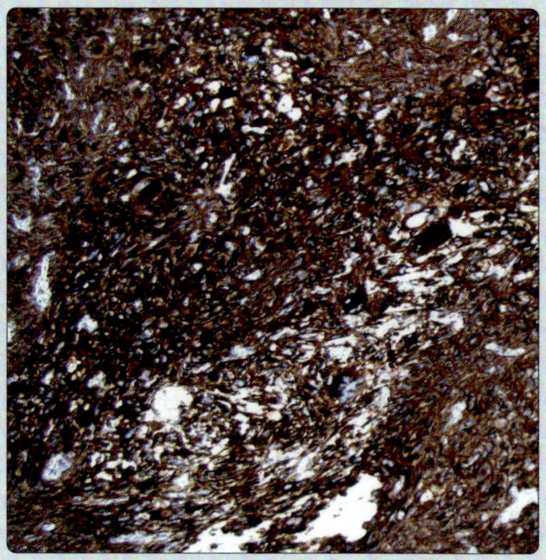

(Left) *High magnification of AFX shows a proliferation of markedly atypical and pleomorphic-appearing, spindled and large, bizarre-appearing, multinucleated ➔ tumor giant cells.* **(Right)** *CD10 shows very strong and diffuse staining in most cases of AFX. Although this is a nonspecific marker, in junction with negative staining for all of the more specific markers, it supports the diagnosis of AFX.*

TERMINOLOGY

Abbreviations

- Atypical fibroxanthoma (AFX)

Definitions

- Strictly defined, dermal-based mesenchymal neoplasm showing no specific lineage of differentiation
  - Should be negative for markers of melanocytic (i.e., S100, SOX10, melan-A), epithelial (i.e., cytokeratins and p63), and vascular (i.e., CD31, ERG) differentiation
  - Not allowed: Invasion into deep subcutaneous tissue or beyond, tumor necrosis, lymphovascular invasion, or perineurial involvement (features which are compatible with pleomorphic dermal sarcoma)
  - Can only be diagnosed on complete excision (diagnosis of exclusion)

ETIOLOGY/PATHOGENESIS

Environmental Exposure

- Likely related to UV exposure, as most cases occur in elderly patients in sun-damaged skin
- Some cases reported following radiation therapy

CLINICAL ISSUES

Epidemiology

- Age
  - Typically occurs in elderly patients
  - Rare cases in children with xeroderma pigmentosum or Li-Fraumeni syndrome
- Sex
  - May have slight male predominance

Site

- Head and neck in general is most commonly affected area
  - Scalp is most common location
- Uncommonly occurs on trunk or extremities

Presentation

- Skin nodule, asymptomatic in most cases
  - Often rapidly growing lesion
  - Dermal based nodule
  - Often shows overlying ulceration or crusting

Treatment

- Complete and wide surgical excision is typically pursued
  - Mohs surgery is also effective

Prognosis

- Very good in most cases
- Progressive lesion; does not regress without treatment
- Rate of local recurrence is low (< 10% reported)
- Vast majority of cases do not metastasize
  - Cases with more than minimal superficial involvement of subcutis are considered pleomorphic sarcoma and have metastatic potential

MACROSCOPIC

General Features

- Large, nodular, unencapsulated, dermal-based tumor

Size

- < 2 cm in greatest dimension in most cases

MICROSCOPIC

Histologic Features

- Nodular, dermal-based proliferation of atypical, pleomorphic spindled and epithelioid-shaped cells
  - Cells are markedly enlarged and often bizarre appearing
  - Show atypical, hyperchromatic-staining nuclei
    - Irregular nuclear borders and prominent nucleoli
  - Cytoplasm of tumor cells is abundant, eosinophilic, and sometimes foamy/vacuolated appearing
  - Variants include spindle cell, clear cell, granular, chondroid, and osteoid
- May show limited superficial pushing extension into subcutis but nothing deeper
- No tumor necrosis, lymphovascular invasion, or perineurial involvement
- Scattered large, bizarre-appearing, multinucleated giant cells typically present
- Numerous mitoses, including highly atypical forms, usually easily found
- No evidence of associated/overlying carcinoma or melanoma in situ
  - Often separated from epidermis by thin grenz zone

ANCILLARY TESTS

Immunohistochemistry

- IHC is key in confirming diagnosis
  - Essential to exclude other, more specific diagnoses
- Negative for S100, SOX10, melanocytic markers, cytokeratins (especially high-molecular-weight cytokeratins), p63, p40, SMA, desmin, myogenin, CD31, CD34, ERG
  - Focal/weak SMA expression or granular CD31 positivity (in histiocytes) may be seen
- Positive for nonspecific markers, including CD10 (usually very strong and diffuse), CD68 (may be focal/weak), CD99, and vimentin

DIFFERENTIAL DIAGNOSIS

Sarcomatoid Carcinoma

- Typically squamous cell carcinoma (SCC), but poorly differentiated adnexal carcinomas and metastatic carcinomas should also be considered
- Positive: High-molecular-weight cytokeratins (CK5/6, CK903/34βE12), p63, and p40 (especially primary cutaneous tumors)
  - May or may not show staining for pancytokeratin, AE1/AE3, EMA, and CAM5.2 (low-molecular-weight cytokeratin)

Pleomorphic, Spindle Cell, and Desmoplastic Melanoma

- Overlying junctional component/melanoma in situ is present in majority of cases (> 70%)
- Positive: S100 and SOX10; ± MART-1/melan-A, HMB-45, tyrosinase, and MITF

Immunohistochemistry Table

Antibody	Reactivity	Staining Pattern	Comment
CD10	Positive	Cell membrane & cytoplasm	Usually strongly and diffusely positive
CD68	Positive	Cell membrane & cytoplasm	Usually positive, may be weak/focal
CK-PAN	Negative		Positive control staining of epidermis and adnexal structures
CK-HMW-NOS	Negative		Positive control staining of epidermis and adnexal structures
p63	Negative		Rare cases reportedly positive; must be CK negative
S100	Negative		Entrapped dendritic cells positive
Melan-A	Negative		Junctional melanocytes serve as positive control
HMB-45	Negative		Junctional melanocytes serve as positive control
Desmin	Negative		
CD34	Negative		Highlights stromal vessels
CD31	Negative		Highlights stromal vessels
Actin-sm	Equivocal	Cytoplasmic	May be weakly positive in some cases, likely indicating myofibroblastic differentiation
MITF	Equivocal	Nuclear	Rare cases may be weakly/focally positive
CD99	Equivocal	Cell membrane & cytoplasm	Some cases positive, but often weak or negative

- S100 and SOX10 often only positive markers in spindle cell and desmoplastic melanoma
- Scattered S100-positive dendritic cells are present in AFX, may be numerous in some cases, and should not be misinterpreted as melanoma

Pleomorphic Dermal Sarcoma

- Contains features incompatible with diagnosis of AFX
  - Tumor necrosis, deep subcutaneous invasion (or beyond), lymphovascular invasion, perineural involvement
- Often shows clinical and histologic overlap with AFX

Leiomyosarcoma

- Proliferation of atypical spindle cells with elongated, blunt-ended, or cigar-shaped nuclei
- Cells show abundant, eosinophilic-staining cytoplasm and perinuclear vacuoles
- Positive: MSA, SMA, desmin (although up to 30% can be negative)

Other Sarcomas

- Much less likely considerations (but differential may include both primary and metastatic sarcomas)
- Angiosarcoma: Irregular, anastomosing vascular spaces; CD31 and CD34 positive
- Malignant peripheral nerve sheath tumor (MPNST)
  - Usually deep-seated lesions but can rarely involve dermis
  - S100 positive in 50-70% of cases, usually focal/weak, may show CD56 and nestin positive
- Fibrosarcoma (FS)
  - Usually arises in dermatofibrosarcoma protuberans (DFSP) in dermis or superficial subcutis
  - Prominent herringbone pattern in FS areas, storiforming in DFSP areas

SELECTED REFERENCES

1. Gaiser T et al: MYC gene amplification is a rare event in atypical fibroxanthoma and pleomorphic dermal sarcoma. Oncotarget. 9(30):21182-9, 2018
2. Griewank KG et al: Atypical fibroxanthoma and pleomorphic dermal sarcoma harbor frequent NOTCH1/2 and FAT1 mutations and similar DNA copy number alteration profiles. Mod Pathol. 31(3):418-28, 2018
3. Helbig D et al: Immunohistochemical expression of melanocytic and myofibroblastic markers and their molecular correlation in atypical fibroxanthomas and pleomorphic dermal sarcomas. J Cutan Pathol. 45(12):880-5, 2018
4. Polcz MM et al: Atypical fibroxanthoma management: recurrence, metastasis and disease-specific death. Australas J Dermatol. 59(1):10-25, 2018
5. Tolkachjov SN et al: Atypical fibroxanthoma: systematic review and meta-analysis of treatment with Mohs micrographic surgery or excision. J Am Acad Dermatol. 79(5):929-34.e6, 2018
6. Nguyen CM et al: Clear cell atypical fibroxanthoma: a case report and review of the literature. J Cutan Pathol. 43(6):538-42, 2016
7. Lai K et al: Genomic analysis of atypical fibroxanthoma. PLoS One. 12(11):e0188272, 2017
8. Henderson SA et al: p40 is more specific than p63 for the distinction of atypical fibroxanthoma from other cutaneous spindle cell malignancies. Am J Surg Pathol. 38(8):1102-10, 2014
9. Tongdee E et al: Keloidal atypical fibroxanthoma: case and review of the literature. Case Rep Dermatol. 8(2):156-63, 2016
10. Lee SM et al: Atypical fibroxanthoma arising in a young patient with Li-Fraumeni syndrome. J Cutan Pathol. 41(3):303-7, 2014
11. Tallon B et al: MITF positivity in atypical fibroxanthoma: a diagnostic pitfall. Am J Dermatopathol. 36(11):888-91, 2014
12. Thum C et al: Atypical fibroxanthoma with pseudoangiomatous features: a histological and immunohistochemical mimic of cutaneous angiosarcoma. Ann Diagn Pathol. 17(6):502-7, 2013
13. Kanner WA et al: CD10, p63 and CD99 expression in the differential diagnosis of atypical fibroxanthoma, spindle cell squamous cell carcinoma and desmoplastic melanoma. J Cutan Pathol. 37(7):744-50, 2010
14. Mirza B et al: Atypical fibroxanthoma: a clinicopathological study of 89 cases. Australas J Dermatol. 46(4):235-8, 2005

Overlying Ulceration in Atypical Fibroxanthoma

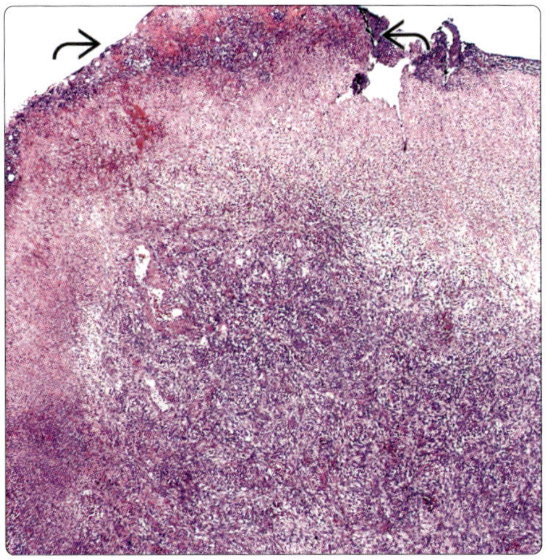

Spindle Cell Variant of Atypical Fibroxanthoma

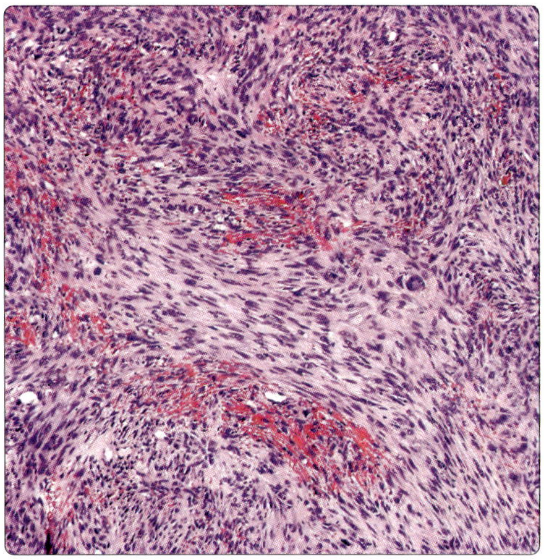

(Left) *Histologic section of AFX at low magnification shows a large, dermal-based, nodular to sheet-like collection of atypical tumor cells with overlying ulceration and dense serum crust with cellular debris.* **(Right)** *Intermediate-power examination of a spindle cell variant of AFX shows a proliferation of atypical, hyperchromatic-staining spindle cells forming dense, short fascicles.*

Multinucleated Tumor Cells

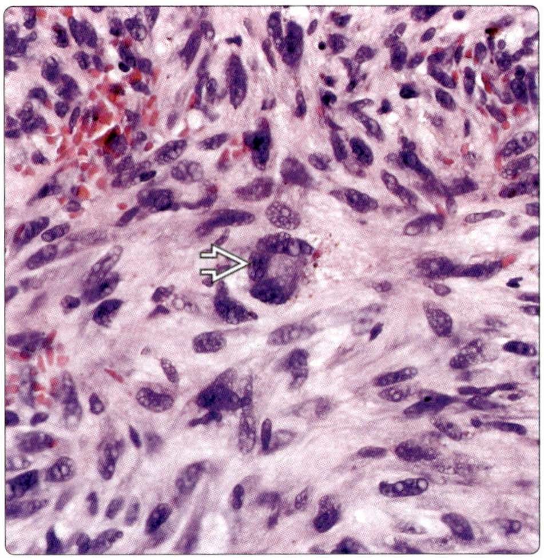

Atypical Mitoses

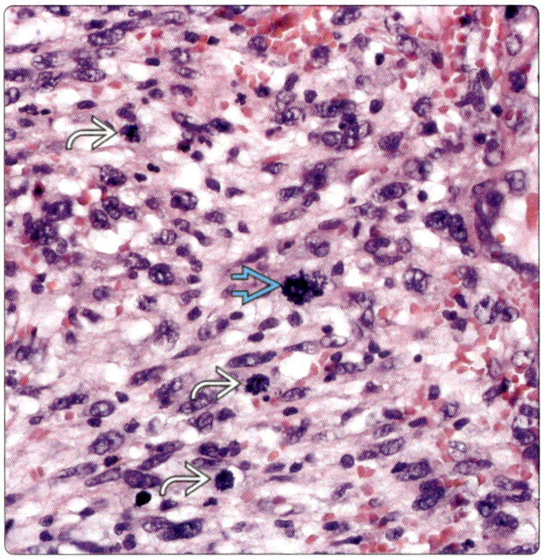

(Left) *High magnification of the same case shows a proliferation of highly atypical and pleomorphic-appearing, spindled and focally multinucleated tumor cells.* **(Right)** *High magnification of another example of AFX shows highly atypical cells with numerous mitoses, including frankly atypical forms.*

Superficial Atypical Fibroxanthoma

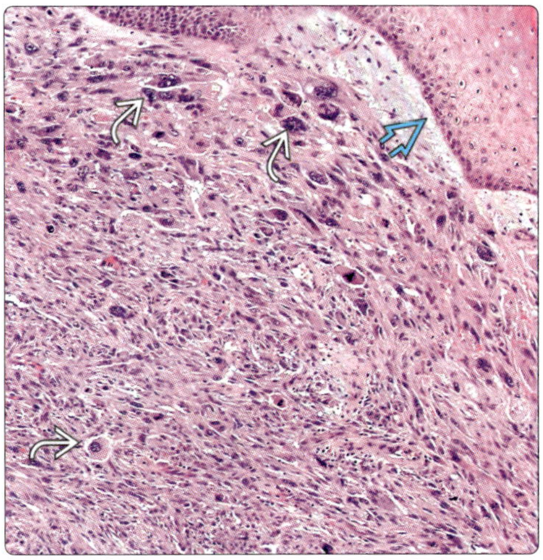

Granular Cell Variant of Atypical Fibroxanthoma

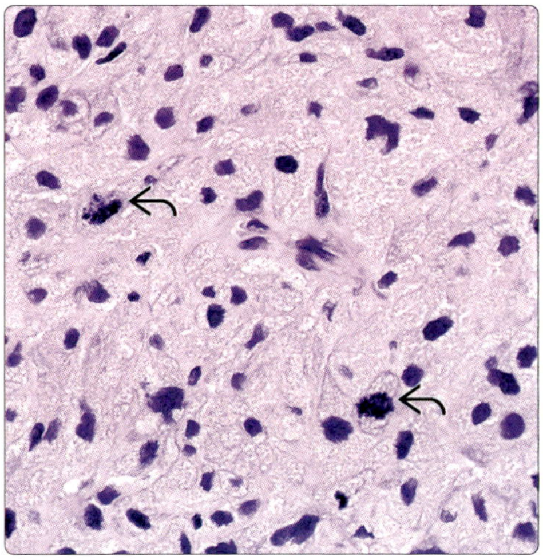

(Left) *Histologic examination of the superficial portion of an AFX shows a proliferation of markedly atypical, spindled and epithelioid-shaped cells with numerous large, multinucleated tumor cells. The tumor closely abuts, but does not involve, the overlying epidermis.* **(Right)** *High magnification of an example of a rare granular cell variant of AFX shows large, bizarre-appearing histiocytoid cells containing abundant granular cytoplasm, similar to a malignant granular cell tumor. Mitoses are easily found.*

Clear Cell Atypical Fibroxanthoma at Low Magnification

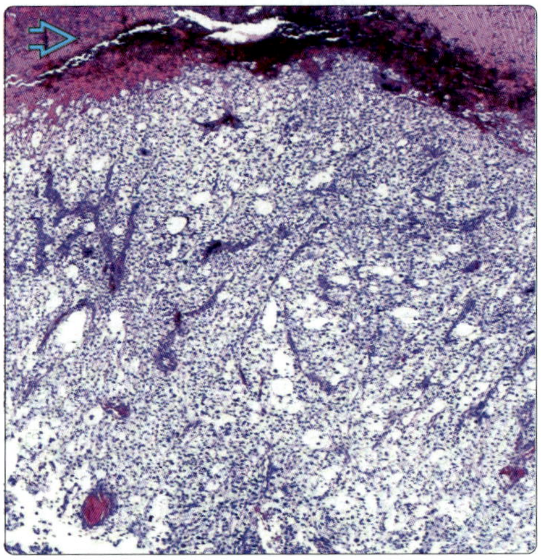

Clear Cell Variant of Atypical Fibroxanthoma at High Magnification

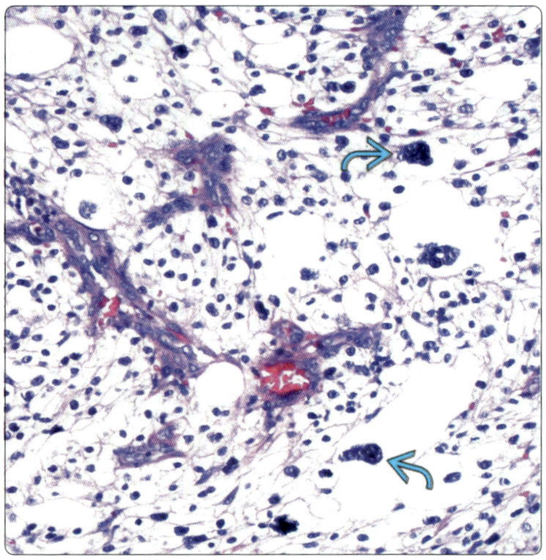

(Left) *Clear cell AFX is a rare variant of AFX, which can be confused with other malignant clear cell tumors. This example shows diffuse overlying ulceration with dense serum crust* ⇒. **(Right)** *This is a rare clear cell variant of AFX, which shows a proliferation of large, atypical, clear-staining cells with multiple bizarre-appearing, hyperchromatic-staining nuclei* ↷.

Keratin Expression in Atypical Fibroxanthoma

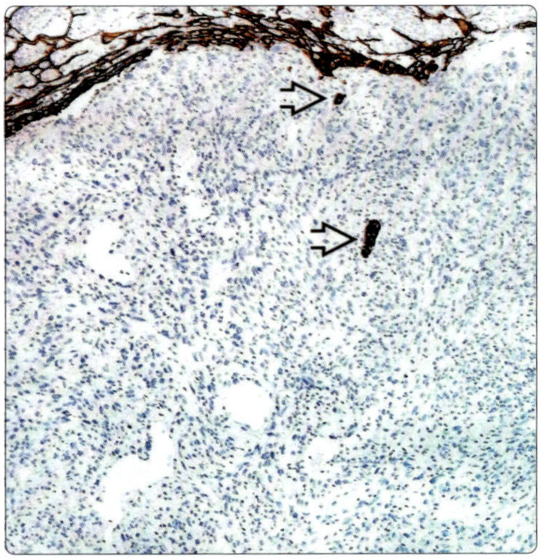

S100 Expression in Atypical Fibroxanthoma

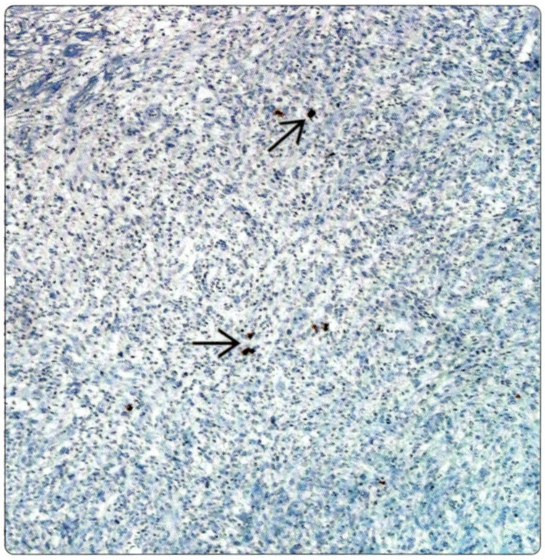

(Left) *High-molecular-weight cytokeratin immunohistochemical stain shows positivity within the epidermis and adnexal ducts* ⇒ *but is negative within the tumor cells.* **(Right)** *S100 IHC shows no staining of the tumor cells but highlights a few scattered small intradermal dendritic cells* →.

Focal SMA Expression in Atypical Fibroxanthoma

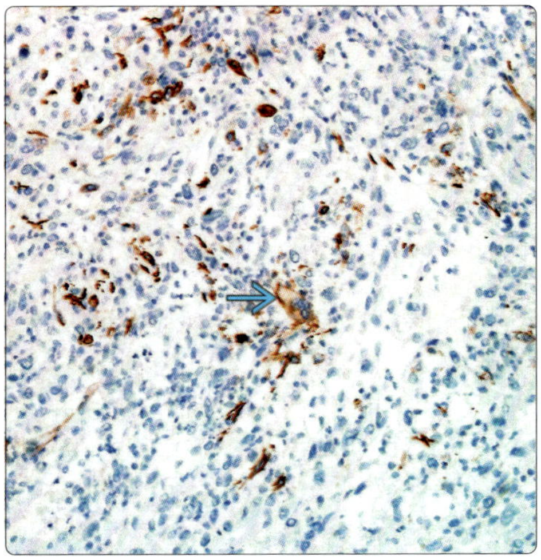

CD68 Expression in Atypical Fibroxanthoma

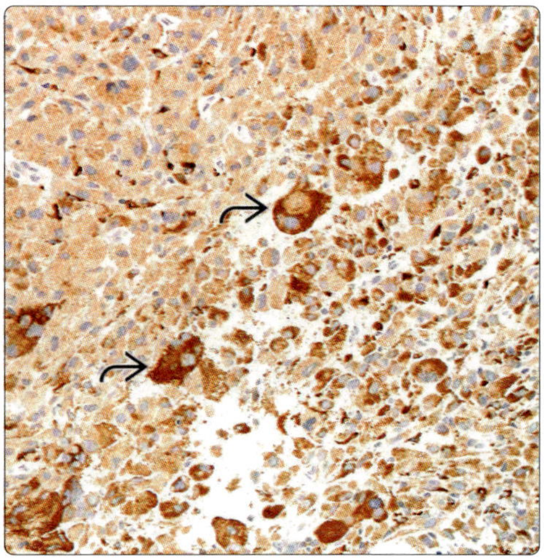

(Left) *SMA stain shows scattered positive cytoplasmic staining* → *in a few of the large cells, likely indicating myofibroblastic differentiation.* **(Right)** *CD68 is a nonspecific marker but is typically positive in AFX. This example shows moderate to strong cytoplasmic staining of most of the tumor cells, especially the large multinucleated tumor giant cells* ↷.

DDx: Melanoma

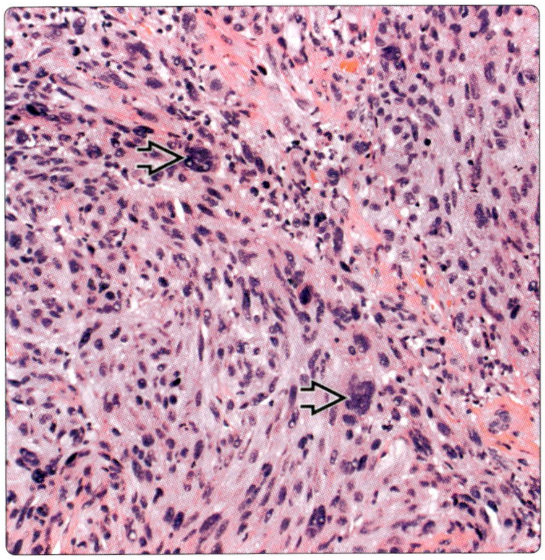

DDx: Melanoma With S100 Positivity

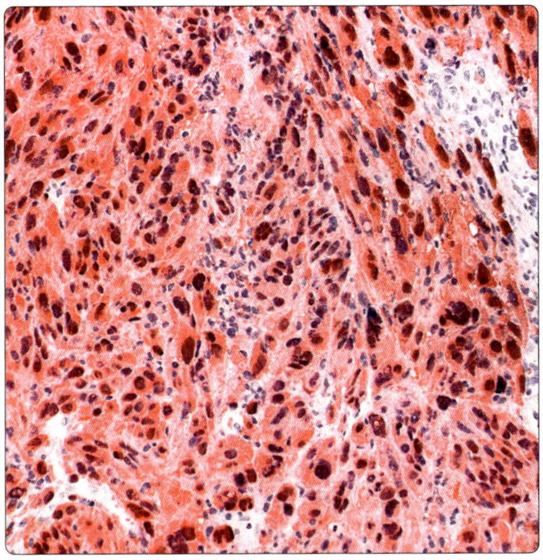

(Left) *Melanoma should always be considered in the differential diagnosis with AFX, especially spindle cell/desmoplastic and metastatic melanomas, which can lack epidermal attachments, be amelanotic, and show striking atypia and pleomorphism, including multinucleated tumor giant cells ➲ similar to AFX.* **(Right)** *S100 IHC shows diffuse, strong nuclear and cytoplasmic staining in a pleomorphic melanoma. This finding would exclude the possibility of AFX.*

DDx: Poorly Differentiated Squamous Cell Carcinoma

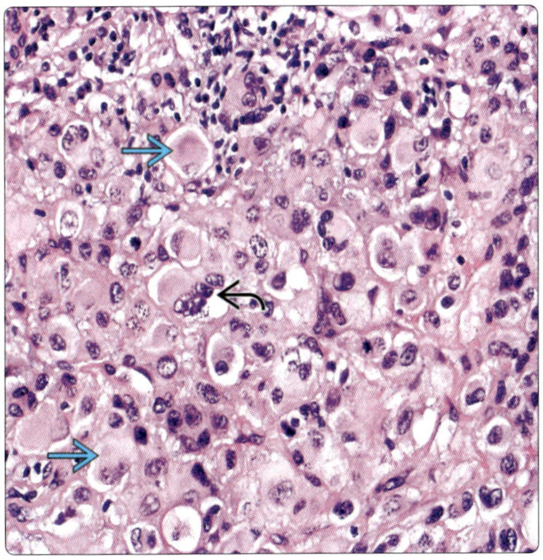

DDx: Squamous Cell Carcinoma and p63 Staining

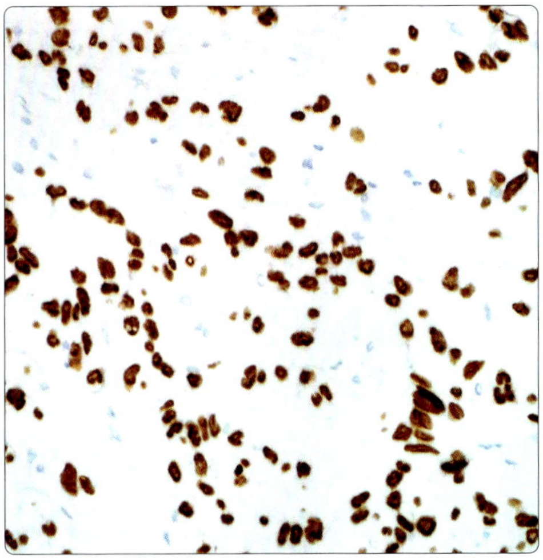

(Left) *This is a poorly differentiated squamous cell carcinoma (SCC) composed of enlarged, markedly atypical epithelioid cells with abundant, pale to eosinophilic-staining cytoplasm ➲. Scattered pleomorphic multinucleated tumor cells ➲ can be seen in some cases of SCC.* **(Right)** *This is a high-magnification view of a p63 stain in a poorly differentiated SCC. High-molecular-weight cytokeratin and p63 are the most sensitive markers for poorly differentiated and spindle cell SCC and are typically negative in AFX.*

DDx: Leiomyosarcoma

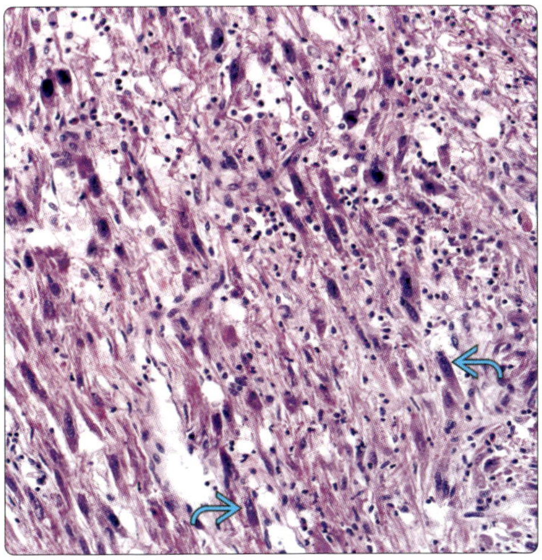

DDx: Leiomyosarcoma Showing Desmin Staining

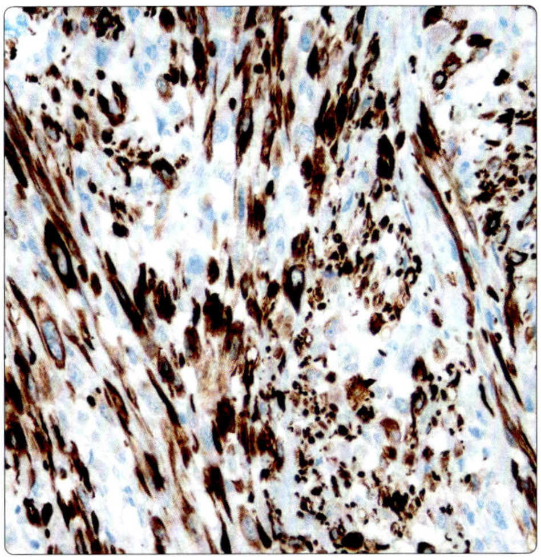

(Left) *Leiomyosarcoma is composed of large, atypical, spindle-shaped cells with oval to elongated, cigar-shaped nuclei ➲ and abundant, eosinophilic-staining cytoplasm.* **(Right)** *Desmin immunostain shows strong cytoplasmic labeling in this leiomyosarcoma. Most cases are positive for both SMA and desmin, although up to 30% of cases can be desmin negative.*

Angiomatoid Fibrous Histiocytoma

KEY FACTS

TERMINOLOGY

- Distinctive, rarely metastasizing mesenchymal neoplasm composed of nodules and sheets of spindled and histiocytoid cells
  - Often demonstrates pseudoangiomatous spaces and peripheral lymphoplasmacytic cuff

CLINICAL ISSUES

- Predominantly children and young adults
- Most often arises in superficial extremities
- Constitutional symptoms in subset (e.g., fever, malaise, anemia)
- Treatment: Wide local excision with follow-up
- ≤ 15% recur locally
- Rare cases metastasize (< 5%)

MICROSCOPIC

- Fibrous pseudocapsule with lymphoplasmacytic cuff (80% of cases)
- Sheets, nodules, and aggregates of ovoid to spindled cells
- Most cells are cytologically bland with vesicular nuclei; mitoses infrequent
  - Scattered cells with nuclear hyperchromasia and pleomorphism are common
- Variably sized, blood-filled pseudovascular spaces in majority of cases

ANCILLARY TESTS

- Desmin (+) in 50-60% of cases
- ALK (+) by IHC common
- Variable, nonspecific expression of EMA, CD68, CD99, SMA
- Molecular: t(2:22) with *EWSR1-CREB1* fusion most common

TOP DIFFERENTIAL DIAGNOSES

- Aneurysmal variant of fibrous histiocytoma
- Nodal metastasis
- Follicular dendritic cell sarcoma
- Granulomatous lesions

Angiomatoid Fibrous Histiocytoma

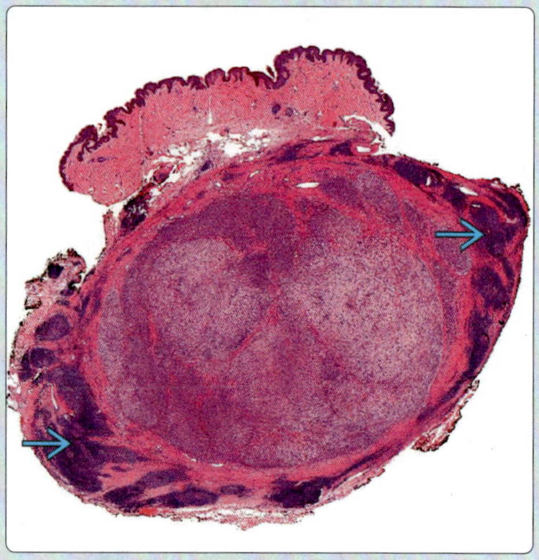

Nodular/Lobular Growth

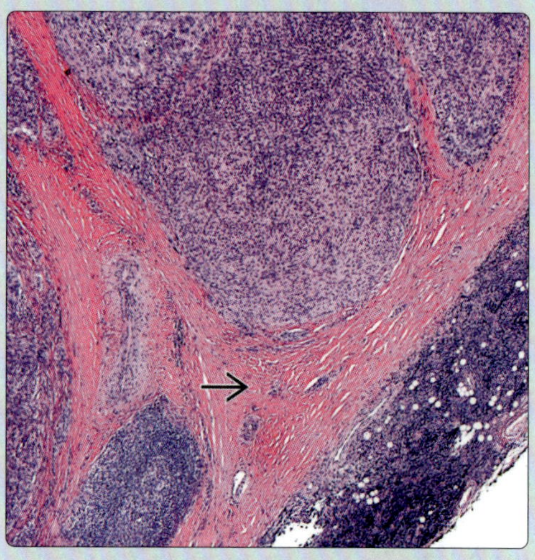

(Left) *Angiomatoid fibrous histiocytoma (AFH) most commonly occurs in the subcutaneous tissue or deep dermis of the extremities. Most examples demonstrate a fibrous pseudocapsule associated with a patchy chronic inflammatory infiltrate ➡. The overall pattern may mimic a lymph node metastasis.* **(Right)** *Many cases of AFH show a multinodular or lobular growth pattern. The fibrous septa are extensions of the characteristic fibrous pseudocapsule ➡ surrounding the tumor.*

Lymphoplasmacytic Cuff

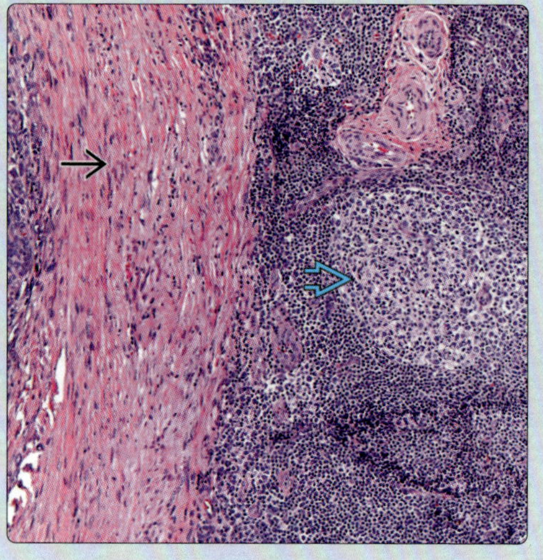

Lymphoplasmacytic Cuff

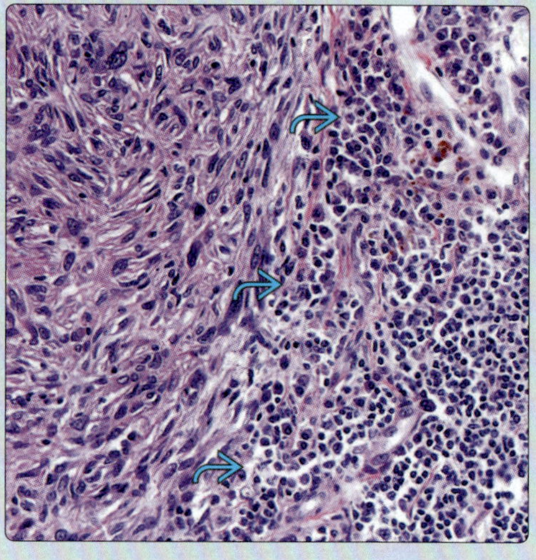

(Left) *The majority of cases of AFH have a lymphoplasmacytic cuff of varying extent and thickness in and around the pseudocapsule ➡. Reactive germinal centers ➡ may also be seen, further simulating the appearance of a lymph node containing metastatic tumor.* **(Right)** *The chronic inflammatory infiltrate ➡ that makes up the characteristic peripheral cuff of AFH is composed of a mixture of nonclonal B- and T-lymphocytes and polytypic plasma cells.*

TERMINOLOGY

Abbreviations

- Angiomatoid fibrous histiocytoma (AFH)

Synonyms

- Angiomatoid malignant fibrous histiocytoma
  - Term "malignant" removed due to relatively indolent clinical behavior (2013 WHO classification)

Definitions

- Distinctive, rarely metastasizing mesenchymal neoplasm composed of nodules and sheets of spindled and histiocytoid cells
  - Often demonstrates pseudoangiomatous spaces and peripheral lymphoplasmacytic cuff

ETIOLOGY/PATHOGENESIS

Lineage Uncertain

- Postulated nodal fibroblastic reticulum cell differentiation
- Myoid, myofibroblastic, endothelial, or histiocytic differentiation not proven

CLINICAL ISSUES

Epidemiology

- Incidence
  - Rare
- Age
  - Predominantly children and young adults
  - Rare in adults > 40 years
    - More likely to arise in extrasomatic locations
- Sex
  - Slight female predilection

Site

- Most common in superficial extremities (deep dermis and subcutis)
  - Rarely arise in deep soft tissue
- Also trunk and head/neck, including scalp
- Rare extrasomatic cases reported in lung, bone, mediastinum, retroperitoneum, brain, ovary, and vulva

Presentation

- Slowly growing, painless mass
  - Rapid growth uncommon and likely attributable to intratumoral hemorrhage
- Constitutional symptoms in subset (e.g., fever, malaise, anemia)
  - May be more common in extrasomatic tumors
  - Possibly related to tumoral cytokine production

Treatment

- Wide surgical excision
- Radiotherapy and chemotherapy may be indicated for rare metastatic or unresectable tumors
- Indefinite long-term clinical follow-up recommended

Prognosis

- Majority of lesions are clinically indolent
- Regional recurrence rate up to 15%
  - Higher rate reported in extrasomatic tumors (up to 33%)
  - May be related to site (difficulty of excision) and tumors showing infiltrative margins
- Rare metastasis (< 5% of reported cases)
  - Most frequently to regional lymph nodes
  - Very rare reports of death due to late distant metastases
- At present, no firm morphologic or clinical indicators of behavior

MACROSCOPIC

General Features

- Well circumscribed
- Lobulated or multinodular
- Blood-filled cystic cavities may be apparent grossly

Size

- Usually small (2-4 cm)

MICROSCOPIC

Histologic Features

- Uni- or multinodular growth
- Fibrous pseudocapsule
  - Contains patchy, dense peripheral lymphoplasmacytic cuff in up to 80%
- Sheets, nodules, and aggregates of ovoid to spindled cells
  - Variety of patterns: Loose swirling, storiform, short fascicles
- Majority of cells are cytologically bland with vesicular nuclei
  - Scattered cells with conspicuous nuclear pleomorphism or atypia are common and likely degenerative
  - Minority of cases show diffuse nuclear pleomorphism
- Fibrosclerotic to myxoid stroma
- Mitotic figures usually infrequent
  - Rare cases may show conspicuous mitotic activity or isolated atypical mitoses
- Variably sized, blood-filled pseudoangiomatous spaces in majority of cases
  - Lined by tumor cells, not endothelial cells
  - Scattered osteoclast-like giant cells common near these areas
- Stromal chronic inflammatory infiltrate may be present
  - May contain variable number of eosinophils
- Less common and exceptional features
  - Myxoid/reticular, clear cell, epithelioid, small cell, and focal palisading patterns
  - Rhabdoid morphology, pulmonary edema-like foci, hyalinized vessels, hemangioendothelioma-like foci

ANCILLARY TESTS

Immunohistochemistry

- Desmin (+) in 50-60% of cases
  - Varies from focal to diffuse cytoplasmic
  - Dendritic process-like staining in many cases
  - Scattered desmin (+) cells may be present within peripheral lymphoid proliferation
- ALK (+) in majority of cases, often with moderate to strong staining
- Variable and nonspecific expression of EMA, CD68, CD99, SMA, calponin
- Negative for myogenin, MyoD1, CD31, and S100 protein

- Isolated reports of focal CD34, CD21, and keratin expression

Molecular Genetics

- 3 characteristic chromosomal translocations identified
  - t(2:22)(q33:q12); *EWSR1-CREB1*
    - Most common overall (90% of cases)
  - t(12:22)(q13:q12); *EWSR1-ATF1*
    - More common in extrasomatic cases of AFH
  - t(12:16)(q13:p11); *FUS-ATF1*
    - Infrequent
- *EWSR1-ATF1* and *EWSR1-CREB1* also identified in clear cell sarcoma of soft tissue and malignant gastrointestinal neuroectodermal tumor

DIFFERENTIAL DIAGNOSIS

Aneurysmal Fibrous Histiocytoma

- Morphologic variant of benign fibrous histiocytoma (dermatofibroma)
- Dermal localization, often with overlying epidermal changes
- No pseudocapsule or lymphoplasmacytic cuff
- Peripheral collagen trapping often present
- Mixed cell population, including chronic inflammatory cells, siderophages, and giant cells
- Desmin (-)

Undifferentiated Pleomorphic Sarcoma (Malignant Fibrous Histiocytoma)

- Older age group
- Mostly large, deeply located masses
- Often profound nuclear atypia
- Atypical mitoses and tumor necrosis are common

Nodal Metastasis

- Metastatic melanoma in particular can mimic AFH
- Arises in regions populated by lymph nodes
- True nodal architecture present
  - Subcapsular and medullary sinuses
- History of malignancy may or may not be present

Follicular Dendritic Cell Sarcoma

- Most arise in lymph nodes
- Infiltrating lymphocytes are common
- CD21(+), CD23(+), CD35(+), EMA(+)
- Desmin (-)

Granulomatous Lesions

- Lack solid growth pattern of AFH
  - Granulomas are usually dispersed and discrete or irregular and confluent
- Large granulomas often show central necrosis and lack cystic hemorrhage
- May contain foreign body-type giant cells
- Predisposing factors may be noted clinically (exposure to infectious agents, etc.)
- CD68(+), CD168(+); desmin (-)

Rhabdomyosarcoma

- May be confused with AFH due to age and desmin (+)
- Morphologic appearance depends upon specific subtype
- Myogenin (+), MyoD1(+)

Kaposi Sarcoma (Nodular)

- May involve lymph nodes
- Predisposing factors often present (AIDS history)
- Moderately cellular neoplasm of spindled endothelial cells
- CD34(+), CD31(+), D2-40 (podoplanin) (+), HHV8(+)
- Desmin (-)

Spindle Cell Hemangioma

- Distal extremities, particularly acral
- No pseudocapsule or lymphoplasmacytic cuff
- Resembles cavernous hemangioma with cellular septa composed of spindle cells
- CD31(+), CD34(+), SMA(+)
- Desmin (-)

Intranodal Palisaded Myofibroblastoma

- Occurs in lymph nodes, predominantly in inguinal region in male patients
- Fascicles of spindle cells with nuclear palisading and amianthoid fibers characteristic
- SMA(+); desmin (-)

Nodular Fasciitis

- Lacks thick fibrous pseudocapsule and lymphoplasmacytic cuff
- Spindle and stellate myofibroblasts with tissue culture appearance
- SMA(+); desmin (-) (rarely focal)
- *MYH9-USP6* fusion

SELECTED REFERENCES

1. Cheah AL et al: ALK expression in angiomatoid fibrous histiocytoma: a potential diagnostic pitfall. Am J Surg Pathol. 43(1):93-101, 2019
2. Zaccarini DJ et al: TLE-1-positive angiomatoid fibrous histiocytoma mimicking synovial sarcoma. Appl Immunohistochem Mol Morphol. 27(1):e1-e4, 2019
3. Saito K et al: Angiomatoid fibrous histiocytoma: a series of seven cases including genetically confirmed aggressive cases and a literature review. BMC Musculoskelet Disord. 18(1):31, 2017
4. Justin Wong SB et al: Angiomatoid fibrous histiocytoma with prominent myxoid stroma: a case report and review of the literature. Am J Dermatopathol. 37(8):623-31, 2015
5. Shi H et al: Clinicopathological features of angiomatoid fibrous histiocytoma: a series of 21 cases with variant morphology. Int J Clin Exp Pathol. 8(1):772-8, 2015
6. Thway K et al: Angiomatoid fibrous histiocytoma: comparison of fluorescence in situ hybridization and reverse transcription polymerase chain reaction as adjunct diagnostic modalities. Ann Diagn Pathol. 19(3):137-42, 2015
7. Bohman SL et al: Angiomatoid fibrous histiocytoma: an expansion of the clinical and histological spectrum. Pathology. 46(3):199-204, 2014
8. Kao YC et al: Angiomatoid fibrous histiocytoma: clinicopathological and molecular characterisation with emphasis on variant histomorphology. J Clin Pathol. 67(3):210-5, 2014
9. Schaefer IM et al: Myxoid variant of so-called angiomatoid "malignant fibrous histiocytoma": clinicopathologic characterization in a series of 21 cases. Am J Surg Pathol. 38(6):816-23, 2014
10. Chen G et al: Angiomatoid fibrous histiocytoma: unusual sites and unusual morphology. Mod Pathol. 24(12):1560-70, 2011
11. Matsumura T et al: Angiomatoid fibrous histiocytoma including cases with pleomorphic features analysed by fluorescence in situ hybridisation. J Clin Pathol. 63(2):124-8, 2010
12. Thway K: Angiomatoid fibrous histiocytoma: a review with recent genetic findings. Arch Pathol Lab Med. 132(2):273-7, 2008
13. Fanburg-Smith JC et al: Angiomatoid "malignant" fibrous histiocytoma: a clinicopathologic study of 158 cases and further exploration of the myoid phenotype. Hum Pathol. 30(11):1336-43, 1999
14. Costa MJ et al: Angiomatoid malignant fibrous histiocytoma. A follow-up study of 108 cases with evaluation of possible histologic predictors of outcome. Am J Surg Pathol. 14(12):1126-32, 1990

Bland Nuclear Features

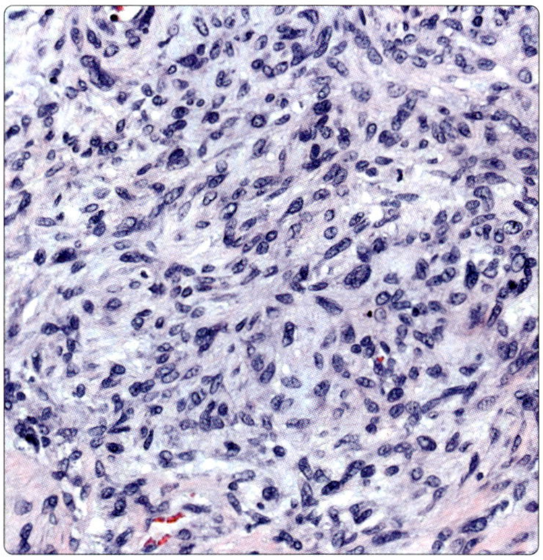

Mitoses Uncommon

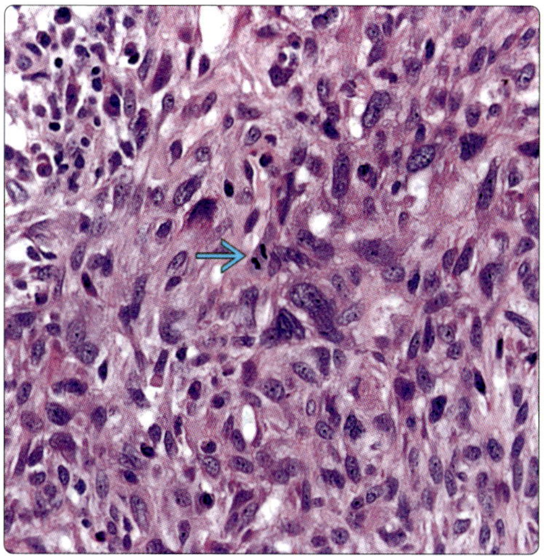

(Left) *In a typical case of AFH, the tumor cells are spindled to ovoid with generally bland nuclei containing pale or vesicular chromatin with small nucleoli and showing minimal to mild pleomorphism. They often appear histiocytoid. The overall cellularity varies widely from case to case.* **(Right)** *The mitotic rate in AFH is generally low, and mitotic figures → are often small and difficult to find. In rare cases, they are more numerous, but this does not appear to affect prognosis. In exceptional cases, atypical mitotic figures may be identified.*

Focal Nuclear Atypia

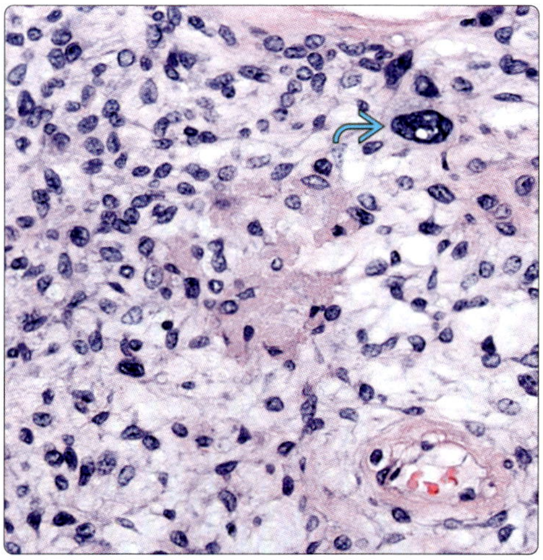

Marked Nuclear Atypia

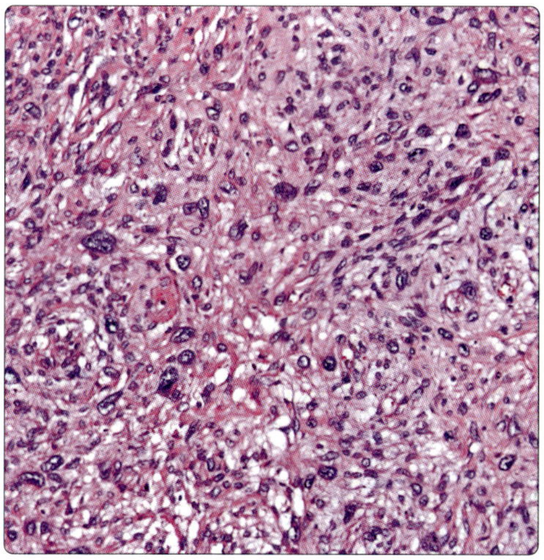

(Left) *It is common for AFH to contain scattered tumor cells ↪ with nuclear enlargement, hyperchromasia, and pleomorphism. Intranuclear pseudoinclusions may be identified. These changes are likely degenerative in nature.* **(Right)** *In some cases, pleomorphic tumor cells are more prominent in number and distribution. Coupled together with an increase in cellularity, these cases may be misdiagnosed as an undifferentiated pleomorphic sarcoma. Notably, however, mitotic activity is disproportionately low.*

Nuclear Grooves

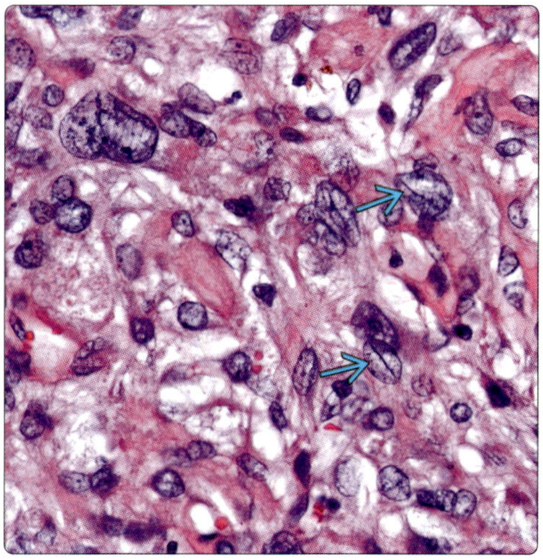

Pseudovascular Spaces

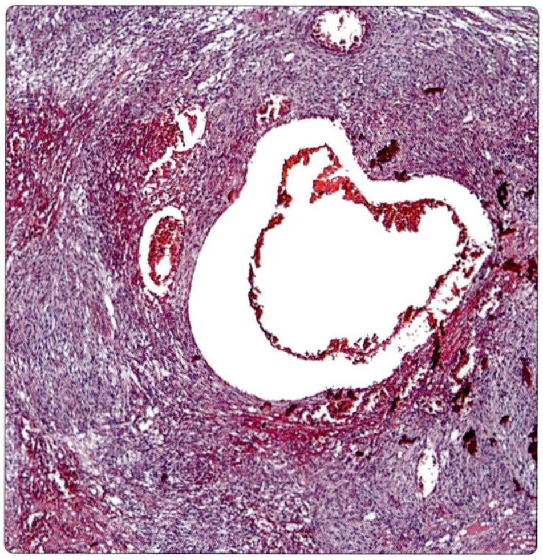

(Left) *Nuclear irregularity with the presence of grooves → or folds is not an uncommon finding in AFH and may even be quite prominent in rare cases.* **(Right)** *Most cases of AFH show at least focal hemorrhage and often the formation of dilated blood-filled spaces, similar to what is seen in the unrelated aneurysmal fibrous histiocytoma. These spaces may predominate in rare cases, clinically and pathologically simulating a hematoma. Thorough histologic examination is required in these cases.*

(Left) *The dilated vascular spaces seen in AFH are not true vessels or cysts, as they lack endothelial and epithelial linings, respectively, but rather are lined by tumor cells. Osteoclast-like giant cells* ➩ *are commonly identified near these spaces and, very rarely, may be numerous.* **(Right)** *Osteoclast-like giant cells* → *are generally infrequent in AFH and may be sparsely scattered throughout the tumor; however, when present, they are most typically identified adjacent to or near hemorrhagic foci and pseudovascular spaces.*

Pseudovascular Space Lining

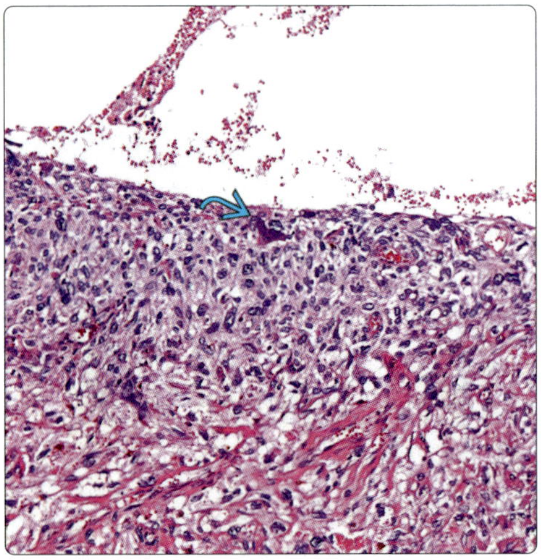

Osteoclast-Like Giant Cells

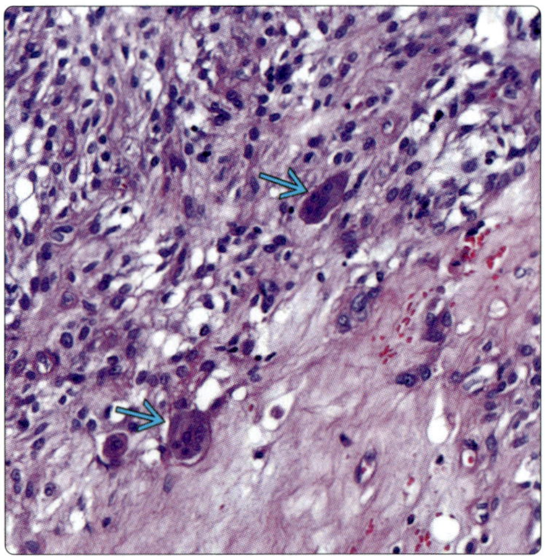

(Left) *Hemosiderin pigment* → *is a common finding in AFH and varies in distribution from case to case. It is most commonly seen around regions of hemorrhage and pseudovascular space formation and may be seen in the stroma or within the cytoplasm of the tumor cells.* **(Right)** *The overall growth pattern of AFH varies widely from one tumor to the next, as does the cellularity. Tumor cells may form sheets, short fascicles, loose storiform arrays, or a variety of other unusual patterns.*

Hemosiderin

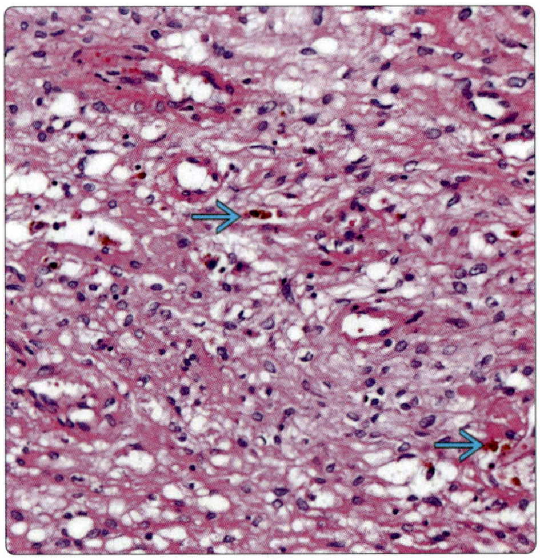

Variable Architecture

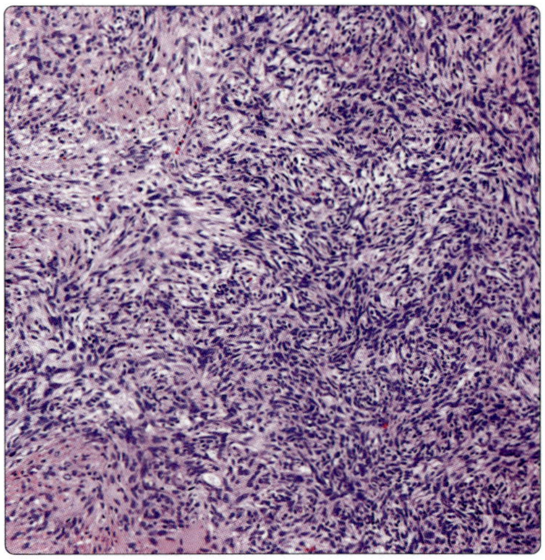

(Left) *The growth pattern in this AFH shows a mixture of short irregular fascicles and a vague, loose storiform architecture. It also contained regions of prominent myxoid stromal change (not shown).* **(Right)** *Myxoid stromal change is uncommon in AFH, and when present, varies from focal to diffuse in extent. Even when these changes are diffuse, other typical pathologic features of AFH, such as the characteristic pseudocapsule and inflammatory cuff, can usually be identified to aid in a correct diagnosis.*

Loose Storiform Growth

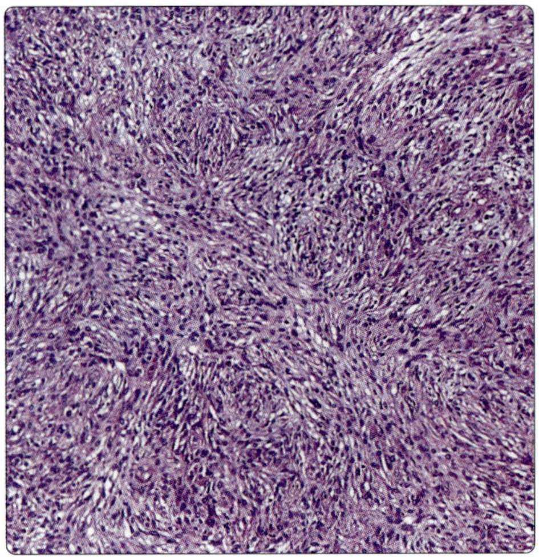

Myxoid Stromal Change

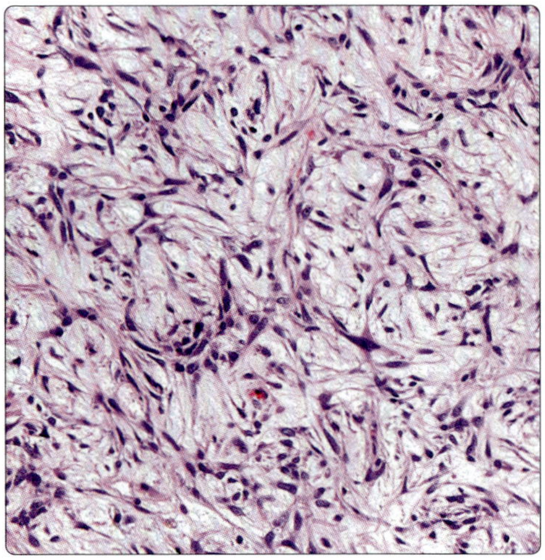

Myxoid/Reticulated Pattern

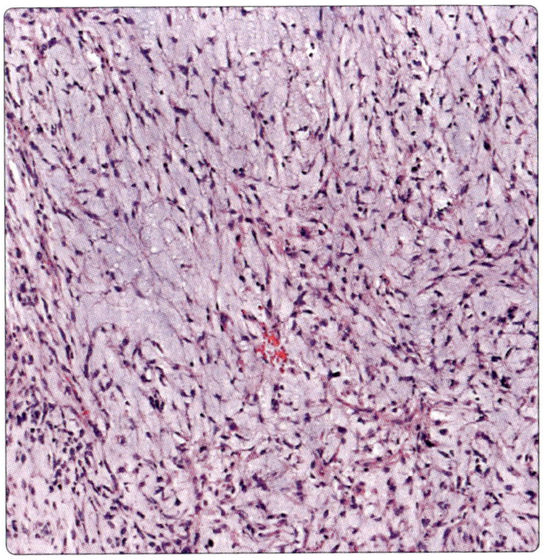

Pulmonary Edema-Like Pattern

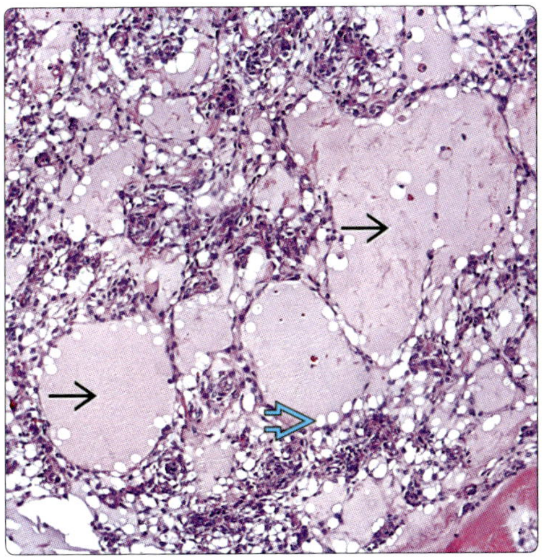

(Left) *In some examples of myxoid AFH, the tumor cells are small, spindled to stellate, and form an interconnecting, reticulated growth pattern. This morphology may cause confusion with a variety of other myxoid neoplasms, particularly extraskeletal myxoid chondrosarcoma.* **(Right)** *Variably dilated, cyst-like foci* ➙ *containing homogeneous eosinophilic material may be seen in AFH. This appearance is reminiscent of edema filling pulmonary alveoli. Scattered vacuolar forms are also seen at the periphery* ➩.

Prominent Vasculature

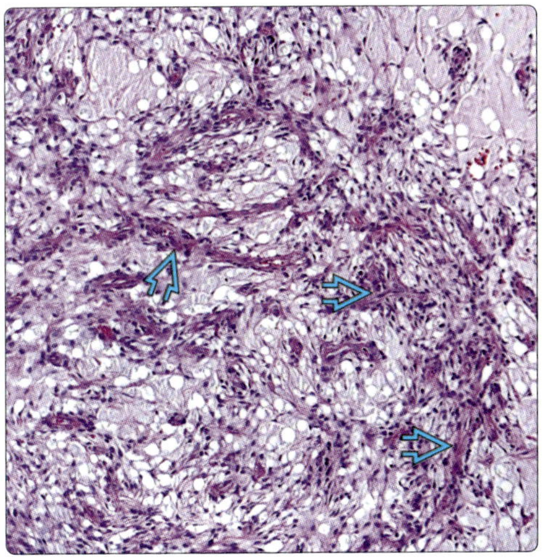

Stromal Hyalinization

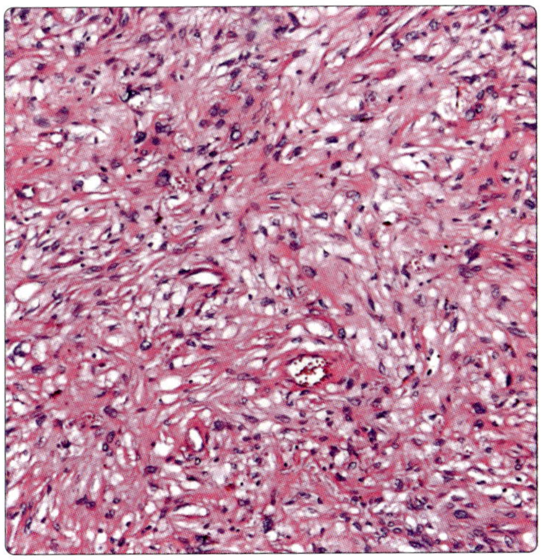

(Left) *A rare finding in some cases of myxoid AFH are thin-walled branching vessels* ➩ *with a curvilinear appearance similar to that seen in low-grade fibromyxoid sarcoma and myxofibrosarcoma. Other, more typical areas of AFH may be present and should be sought out.* **(Right)** *AFH may show regions of stromal hyalinization or hypocellularity, which can vary from focal to extensive. Chronic inflammatory cells are often identified within the stroma, as is hemosiderin.*

Stromal Sclerosis

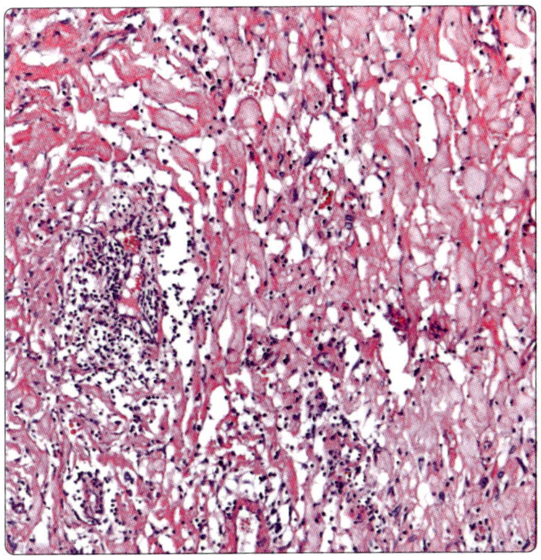

Hemangioendothelioma-Like Foci

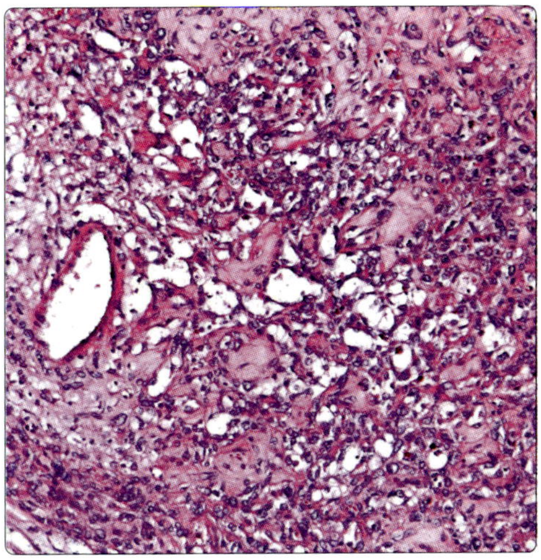

(Left) *In extreme cases, extensive stromal sclerosis may lead to diagnostic difficulties. In particular, tissue-separation artifact may lead to an appearance suggestive of a vascular neoplasm or even a nonneoplastic sclerosing process.* **(Right)** *This unusual case of AFH shows foci containing irregular stromal clefts between tumor cells, imparting a hemangioendothelioma-like appearance. Erythrocytes may be seen within these clefts, furthering mimicking a vascular lesion.*

Whorled Perineurioma-Like Growth

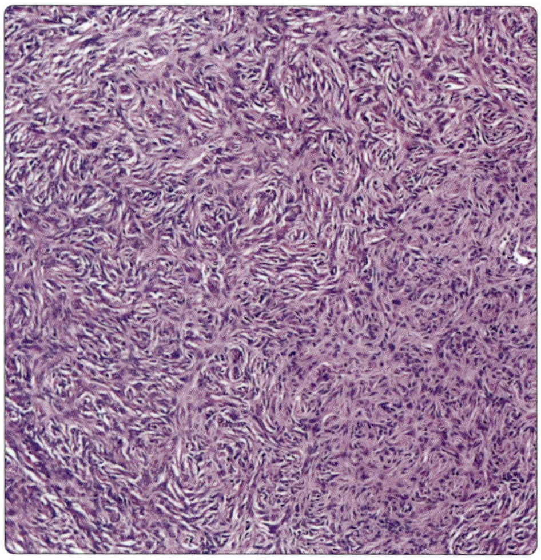

Stromal Inflammation

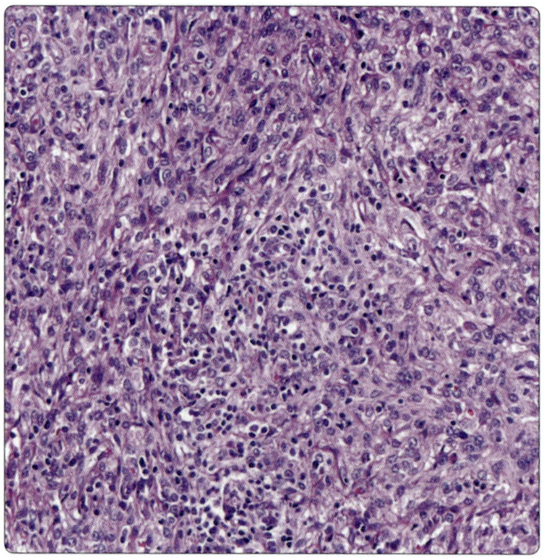

(Left) *Occasional cases of AFH demonstrate areas of tight whorling or storiform growth, mimicking soft tissue perineurioma. Immunohistochemical expression of EMA in AFH may further confound the issue.* **(Right)** *A mixed chronic inflammatory infiltrate is usually present to some degree in AFH; however, it varies from subtle to prominent. Most of the constituent inflammatory cells are lymphocytes and plasma cells, but eosinophils may also be present.*

Stromal Eosinophils

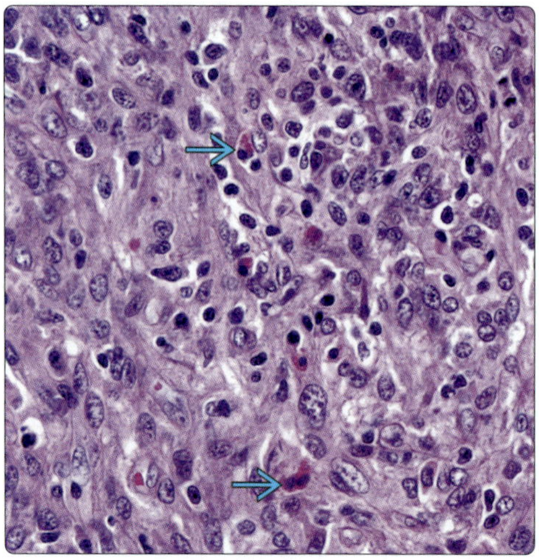

Small Cell Morphology

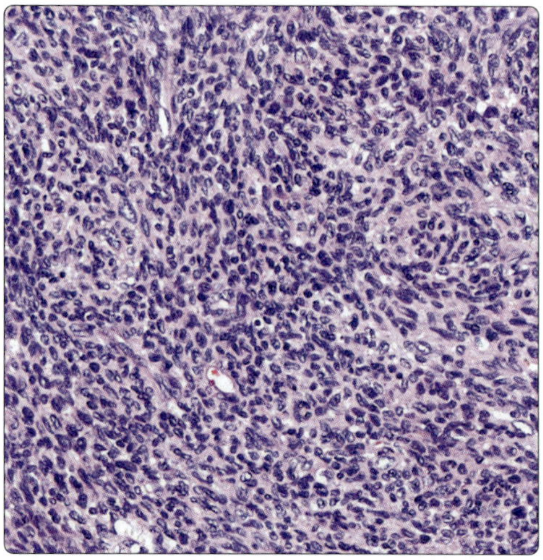

(Left) *Eosinophils* ➡ *are not a common finding in AFH and are usually sparsely distributed, but in very rare cases they can be surprisingly abundant.* **(Right)** *Small cell morphology may also be seen and is characterized by tumor cells with minimal cytoplasm and increased nuclear density. When nuclear monomorphism is prominent, this morphology may resemble Ewing sarcoma, a major pitfall given that the tumor may both express CD99 and show EWSR1 gene fusions.*

Fascicular Growth

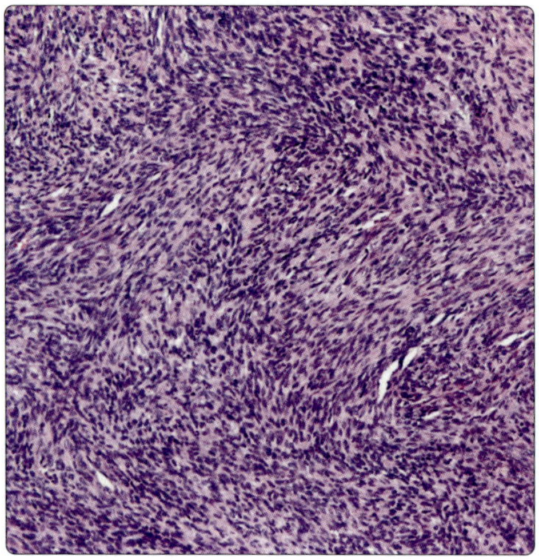

Rare Vascular Hyalinization

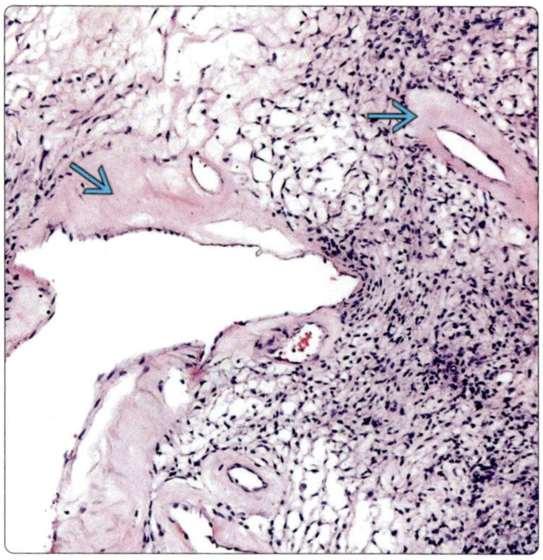

(Left) *A conspicuous short fascicular growth pattern may rarely be seen in AFH and, in combination with small cell morphology and nuclear monomorphism, may resemble other more aggressive tumors, such as synovial sarcoma.* **(Right)** *Focal vascular hyalinization* ➡ *may be seen in some cases of AFH and can simulate the Antoni B zones of schwannoma. In some reported cases, this finding has been associated with focal nuclear palisading, further mimicking schwannoma.*

Carcinoma-Like Morphology

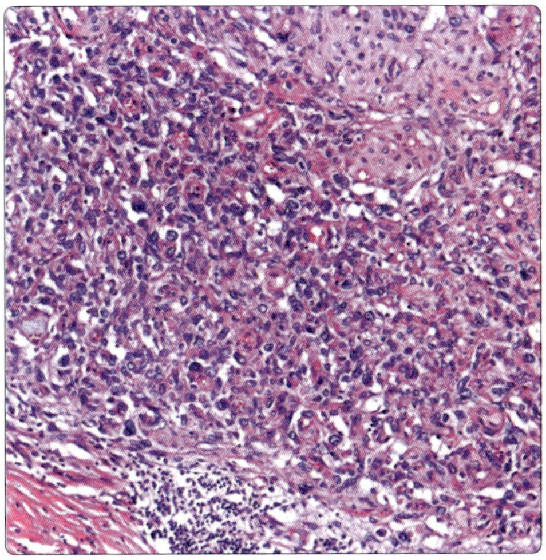

Rhabdoid-Like Morphology

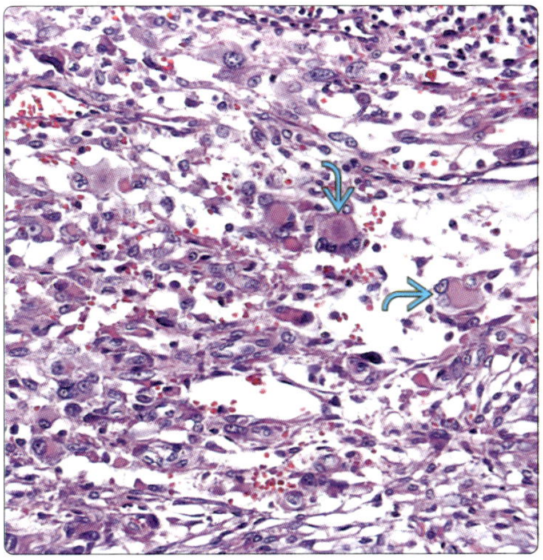

(Left) *This image shows AFH with sheet-like areas of larger eosinophilic tumor cells with diffuse pleomorphism, somewhat mimicking a poorly differentiated carcinoma. A background of stromal sclerosis or fibromyxoid change can also complicate the issue.* **(Right)** *Epithelioid tumor cells with glassy, eosinophilic cytoplasm and eccentric nuclei, resembling rhabdomyoblasts, are a rare finding in AFH. Given the usual age of the patient, care should be taken to avoid a misdiagnosis of rhabdomyosarcoma.*

Hyaline Eosinophilic Globules

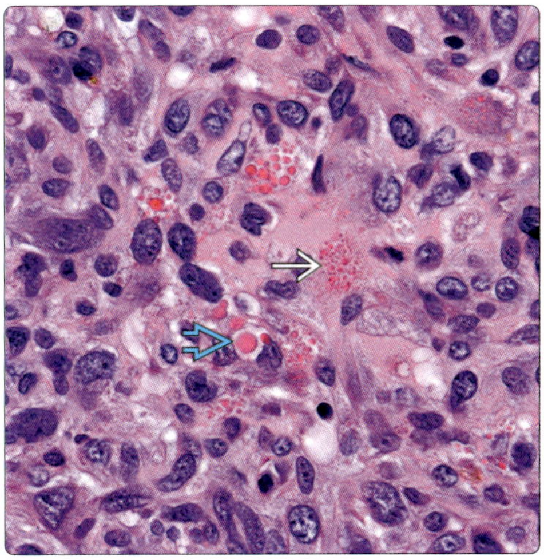

Predominantly Cystic Tumors

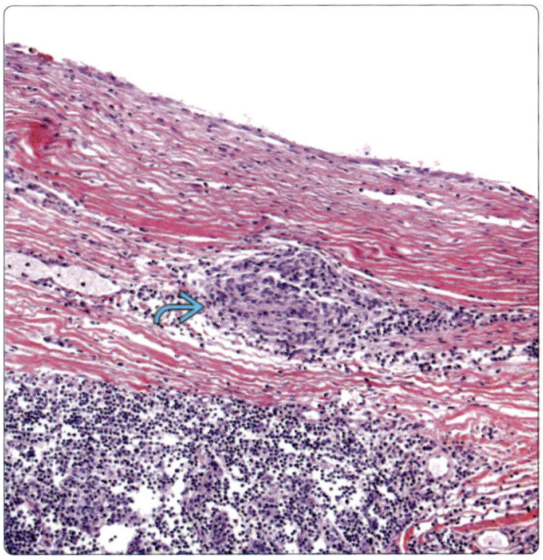

(Left) *Intracytoplasmic eosinophilic globules are a rare finding in AFH and vary from tiny clusters to larger, pale globs. The latter form resembles the hyaline globules seen in Kaposi sarcoma.* **(Right)** *Some cases of AFH are extensively cystic and appear to be a large blood cyst with a collagenous fibrous pseudocapsule, thus closely mimicking a hematoma. Close inspection of the fibrous rind and inflammatory infiltrate often reveals small nodules of diagnostic tumor cells.*

Desmin Expression

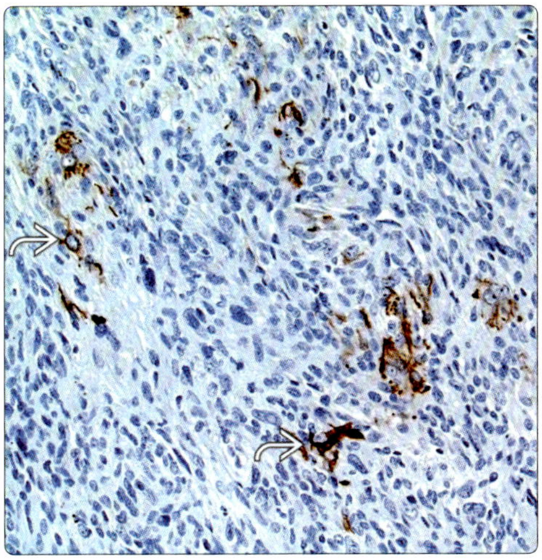

ALK Expression

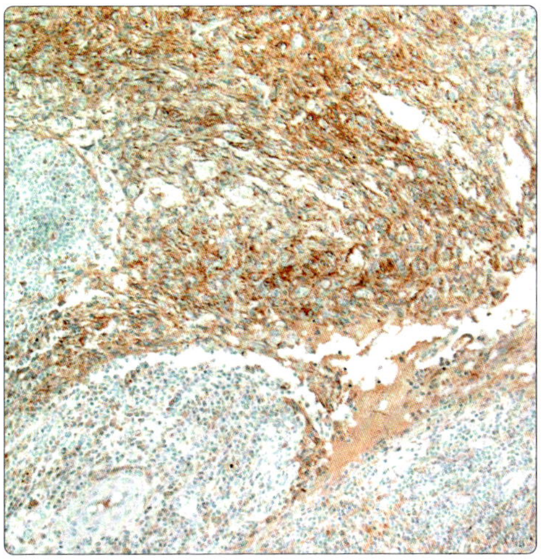

(Left) *Approximately half of cases of AFH show expression of desmin within tumor cells, which varies from focal to extensive, and often shows areas of stellate, dendritic process-like staining. Isolated desmin (+) cells may be identified in the peripheral lymphoplasmacytic infiltrate as well.* **(Right)** *ALK expression by IHC has been recently reported as a common finding in angiomatoid fibrous histiocytoma and may lead to misdiagnosis as IMT, particularly on small biopsy. Notably, rearrangements of the ALK gene are absent.*

Ossifying Fibromyxoid Tumor

KEY FACTS

TERMINOLOGY

- Distinctive mesenchymal neoplasm of intermediate malignant potential arising predominantly in superficial soft tissues and featuring uniform, bland, round to ovoid cells embedded in fibromyxoid stroma, often with incomplete, peripheral shell of bone

CLINICAL ISSUES

- Wide age range (mean: 50 years)
  - ~ 2:1 male predominance
- Extremities (particularly lower), trunk, head/neck
  - Usually originates in subcutaneous tissue
- Slow-growing, often longstanding, painless mass
- Treatment: Complete surgical excision
- Overall good prognosis for most tumors with conventional histologic features
  - Rare, histologically malignant forms show increased risk of local recurrence and metastatic disease

MICROSCOPIC

- Pseudocapsule with metaplastic bone in 75% of cases
- Low to moderately cellular proliferation of uniform, oval to round tumor cells in cords, nests, clusters, or sheets
  - Bland nuclear features
  - Mitoses are rare (< 2 figures per 50 HPF)
- Variable myxoid, fibromyxoid, or hyalinized stroma
- Absence of necrosis and vascular invasion
- Malignant forms show severe nuclear atypia or high cellularity with increased mitotic activity

ANCILLARY TESTS

- S100 protein (+); variable desmin (+)
- Molecular: Rearrangements of 6p21 involving *PHF1*

TOP DIFFERENTIAL DIAGNOSES

- Schwannoma (epithelioid variant)
- Myoepithelioma of soft tissue
- Extraskeletal myxoid chondrosarcoma

Ossifying Fibromyxoid Tumor

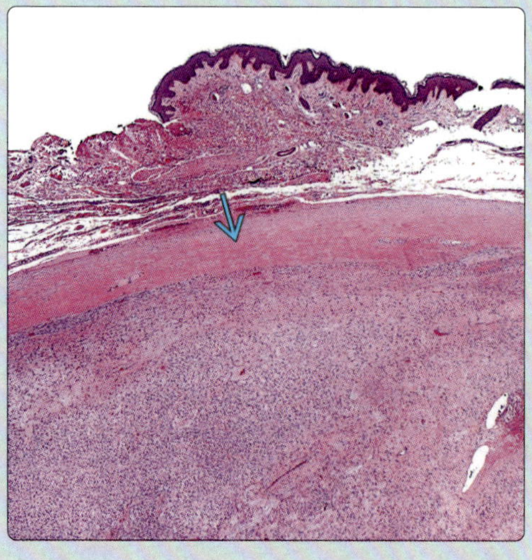

Metaplastic Bone

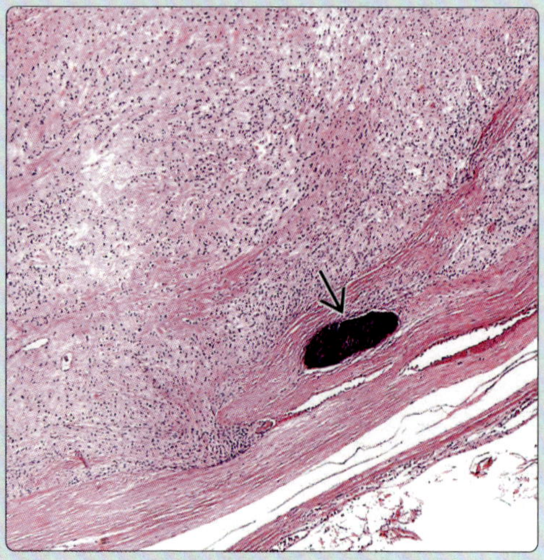

***(Left)** Ossifying fibromyxoid tumor (OFMT) is a distinctive, rarely metastasizing mesenchymal neoplasm that most commonly arises in subcutaneous tissue, as depicted, and usually features a thick, fibrous pseudocapsule* ➡*. **(Right)** Metaplastic bone formation* ➡ *is seen in the majority of cases of OFMT, typically at the periphery within the fibrous pseudocapsule but occasionally within the intratumoral fibrous septa. It may be focal, partial, or extensively present.*

Growth Patterns

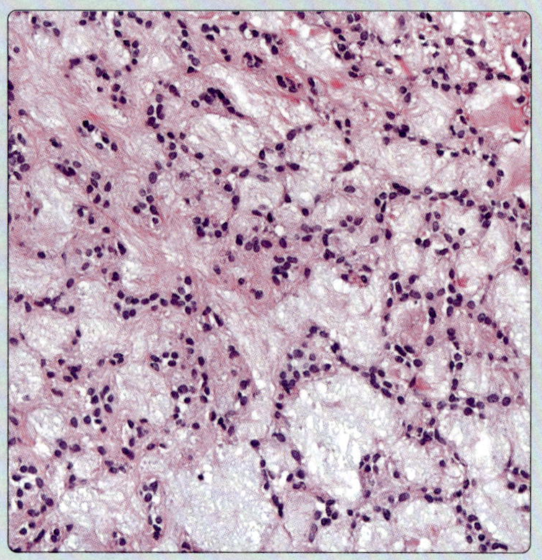

S100 Protein Expression

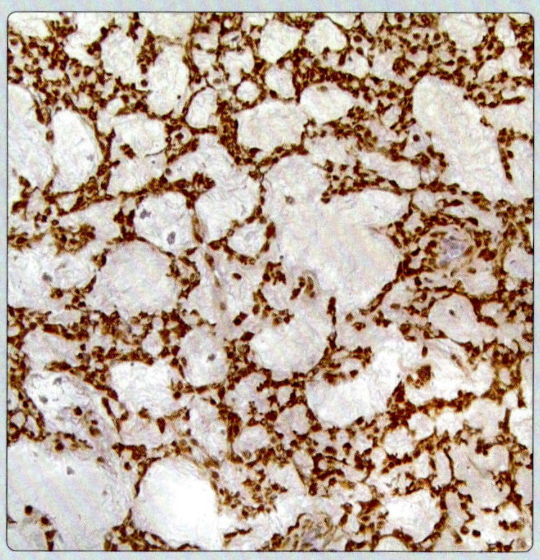

***(Left)** Tumor cells in OFMT are typically small, uniform, and bland and are arranged in a variety of patterns, including branching cords, trabeculae, nests, clusters, or loose sheets. The stroma has a fine, fibrillary fibromyxoid quality. **(Right)** S100 protein expression is seen in most (but not all) cases of OFMT and typically shows both nuclear and cytoplasmic staining. Positivity is often diffuse but can occasionally be patchy.*

TERMINOLOGY

Abbreviations

- Ossifying fibromyxoid tumor (OFMT)

Synonyms

- OFMT of soft parts

Definitions

- Distinctive mesenchymal neoplasm of intermediate malignant potential arising predominantly in superficial soft tissues and featuring uniform, bland, round to ovoid cells embedded in fibromyxoid stroma, often with incomplete, peripheral shell of bone
  - Characterized by recurrent rearrangements of *PHF1* in 50-80% of cases

ETIOLOGY/PATHOGENESIS

Specific Differentiation Unproven

- Various lineages suggested
  - Neural (Schwann cell), chondroid, myoepithelial, osteogenic

CLINICAL ISSUES

Epidemiology

- Incidence
  - Rare
- Age
  - Wide range (mean: 50 years)
    - Rare < 20 years
- Sex
  - ~ 2:1 male predominance

Site

- Extremities most common (particularly lower)
- Also head/neck region and trunk
- Rarely other sites

Presentation

- Slow-growing, often longstanding, painless mass
- Solitary subcutaneous mass
  - Rarely involves skin or deep soft tissues

Treatment

- Complete surgical excision
- Reexcision with negative margins for tumors with atypical or malignant features
- Indefinite long-term clinical follow-up warranted for all cases of OFMT

Prognosis

- Overall good prognosis for conventional OFMT
  - Most are clinically benign
  - Infrequent local recurrence
  - Very rare metastases (< 5% of cases)
- Atypical OFMT shows increased risk of local recurrence
  - Tumors may recur many years after primary surgery
- Malignant OFMT shows increased risk of aggressive local recurrence and metastatic disease
  - Metastases often to lung or other soft tissue sites

IMAGING

Specimen Radiographic Findings

- Partial rim of bone around tumor in many cases

MACROSCOPIC

General Features

- Well-circumscribed, lobular or multinodular mass
- Most show peripheral fibrous pseudocapsule ± bone
  - Bone, if present, may be identifiable grossly
- Firm or rubbery, tan-white or gray cut surface

Size

- Usually < 5 cm (mean: 4 cm)
  - Can grow quite large (> 15 cm)

MICROSCOPIC

Histologic Features

- Most show lobulated or nodular growth
  - May show formation of peripheral satellite nodules
- Peripheral fibrous pseudocapsule common, often with intratumoral septal extensions
  - Incomplete/partial rim of metaplastic bone (often lamellar) in 75% of cases
    - Ossification may extend inward along septa
    - Occasional cartilage component
- Low to moderately cellular proliferation of uniform, oval to round tumor cells in cords, nests, clusters, or sheets
  - Oval to rounded, bland nuclei ± small pinpoint nucleoli
  - Pale eosinophilic cytoplasm
  - Mitoses are rare (< 2 figures per 50 HPF)
  - Rare spindled cytomorphology, fascicular growth
- Variable myxoid, fibromyxoid, or hyalinized stroma
- Occasional cystic change
- Absence of necrosis and vascular invasion

Malignant Ossifying Fibromyxoid Tumor

- Per published criteria of Folpe and Weiss
  - High nuclear grade **or**
  - High cellularity with > 2 mitoses per 50 HPF
    - Overlapping nuclei with loss of intercellular matrix in at least one 4x microscopic field
- Areas with malignant histologic features often associated with areas of conventional OFMT
  - However, malignant OFMT may arise in pure form or in recurrence of conventional/atypical OFMT
- Necrosis, vascular invasion, infiltrative growth more common in malignant OFMT
- Atypical OFMT deviates from conventional OFMT but does not reach criteria for malignant OFMT

ANCILLARY TESTS

Immunohistochemistry

- S100 protein (+) in majority
  - Less frequent expression in malignant OFMT
- Desmin (+) in up to 40%
- Occasional focal expression of keratin, EMA, SMA
- Focal MUC4(+) in minor subset

- Nuclear INI1 expression lost in some but not all tumor cells (mosaic pattern)

Molecular Genetics

- Rearrangements of 6p21 involving *PHF1* (50-80% of reported cases)
  - *EP400-PHF1* fusion most commonly reported
  - *MEAF6-PHF1*, *EPC1-PHF1*, and *ZC3H7B-BCOR* fusions also reported
- *PHF1* rearrangements identified in all forms (conventional, atypical, and malignant) of OFMT
- 2 additional fusions reported: *CREBBP-BCORL1* and *KDM2A-WWTR1*

DIFFERENTIAL DIAGNOSIS

Schwannoma (Epithelioid Variant)

- Can show close morphologic overlap with OFMT
- May contain areas of conventional schwannoma histology
- Generally lacks metaplastic bone formation
- Strong diffuse S100 protein (+); desmin (-)
- No rearrangements of *PHF1*

Myoepithelioma of Soft Tissue

- Wider range of morphologic patterns
- Keratin (+) and S100 protein (+) in many cases
- Variably (+) for SMA, desmin, GFAP, calponin
- *EWSR1* rearrangements in some tumors
- No rearrangements of *PHF1*

Extraskeletal Myxoid Chondrosarcoma

- Large mass arising in deep soft tissues
- Lacks pseudocapsule and peripheral metaplastic bone formation
- Prominent myxoid stroma
- S100 protein (+), often focal/weak
- *NR4A3* gene rearrangements

Extraskeletal Osteosarcoma

- Arises in deep soft tissues
- Marked nuclear atypia and pleomorphism common
- Atypical mitoses and necrosis
- Neoplastic bone formation is often centralized rather than peripheral

Epithelioid Malignant Peripheral Nerve Sheath Tumor

- Origin from large nerve may be demonstrated
- Prominent macronucleoli characteristic
- Lacks metaplastic bone formation
- Desmin (-)
- No rearrangements of *PHF1*

Sclerosing Epithelioid Fibrosarcoma

- Occurs in deep soft tissues
- Matrix usually densely sclerotic rather than myxoid or fibromyxoid
- Clear cell morphology is common
- Negative for S100 protein and desmin
- MUC4(+)
  - However, of limited utility given MUC4(+) in subset of OFMT
- *EWSR1* and *CREB3L1* rearrangements predominate

Low-Grade Fibromyxoid Sarcoma

- Spindle cells usually predominate; occasional epithelioid cytomorphology
- Negative for S100 protein and desmin
- MUC4(+)
  - However, of limited utility given MUC4(+) in subset of OFMT
- Most cases show t(7;16) with *FUS-CREB3L2* fusion

Glomus Tumor

- Uniform epithelioid cells arranged around prominent blood vessels
- Generally lacks metaplastic bone formation
- SMA(+)
- S100 protein (-)
- No rearrangements of *PHF1*

SELECTED REFERENCES

1. Velasco IA et al: Ossifying fibromyxoid tumor of soft parts in head and neck: case report and literature review. Diagn Pathol. 13(1):21, 2018
2. Dantey K et al: Ossifying fibromyxoid tumor: a study of 6 cases of atypical and malignant variants. Hum Pathol. 60:174-9, 2017
3. Kao YC et al: Expanding the molecular signature of ossifying fibromyxoid tumors with two novel gene fusions: CREBBP-BCORL1 and KDM2A-WWTR1. Genes Chromosomes Cancer. 56(1):42-50, 2017
4. Bakiratharajan D et al: Ossifying fibromyxoid tumor: an update. Arch Pathol Lab Med. 140(4):371-5, 2016
5. Schneider N et al: Ossifying fibromyxoid tumor: morphology, genetics, and differential diagnosis. Ann Diagn Pathol. 20:52-8, 2016
6. Atanaskova Mesinkovska N et al: Ossifying fibromyxoid tumor: a clinicopathologic analysis of 26 subcutaneous tumors with emphasis on differential diagnosis and prognostic factors. J Cutan Pathol. 42(9):622-31, 2015
7. Antonescu CR et al: Novel ZC3H7B-BCOR, MEAF6-PHF1, and EPC1-PHF1 fusions in ossifying fibromyxoid tumors–molecular characterization shows genetic overlap with endometrial stromal sarcoma. Genes Chromosomes Cancer. 53(2):183-93, 2014
8. Asirvatham JR et al: Ossifying fibromyxoid tumor of the breast mimicking fibroadenoma: a case report and differential diagnoses. Arch Pathol Lab Med. 138(8):1098-100, 2014
9. Endo M et al: Ossifying fibromyxoid tumor presenting EP400-PHF1 fusion gene. Hum Pathol. 44(11):2603-8, 2013
10. Graham RP et al: PHF1 rearrangements in ossifying fibromyxoid tumors of soft parts: a fluorescence in situ hybridization study of 41 cases with emphasis on the malignant variant. Am J Surg Pathol. 37(11):1751-5, 2013
11. Gebre-Medhin S et al: Recurrent rearrangement of the PHF1 gene in ossifying fibromyxoid tumors. Am J Pathol. 181(3):1069-77, 2012
12. Graham RP et al: Ossifying fibromyxoid tumor of soft parts: a clinicopathologic, proteomic, and genomic study. Am J Surg Pathol. 35(11):1615-25, 2011
13. Miettinen M et al: Ossifying fibromyxoid tumor of soft parts–a clinicopathologic and immunohistochemical study of 104 cases with long-term follow-up and a critical review of the literature. Am J Surg Pathol. 32(7):996-1005, 2008
14. Folpe AL et al: Ossifying fibromyxoid tumor of soft parts: a clinicopathologic study of 70 cases with emphasis on atypical and malignant variants. Am J Surg Pathol. 27(4):421-31, 2003
15. Zámecník M et al: Ossifying fibromyxoid tumor of soft parts: a report of 17 cases with emphasis on unusual histological features. Ann Diagn Pathol. 1(2):73-81, 1997
16. Kilpatrick SE et al: Atypical and malignant variants of ossifying fibromyxoid tumor. Clinicopathologic analysis of six cases. Am J Surg Pathol. 19(9):1039-46, 1995
17. Fisher C et al: Ossifying fibromyxoid tumor of soft parts with stromal cyst formation and ribosome-lamella complexes. Ultrastruct Pathol. 18(6):593-600, 1994
18. Schofield JB et al: Ossifying fibromyxoid tumour of soft parts: immunohistochemical and ultrastructural analysis. Histopathology. 22(2):101-12, 1993
19. Enzinger FM et al: Ossifying fibromyxoid tumor of soft parts. A clinicopathological analysis of 59 cases. Am J Surg Pathol. 13(10):817-27, 1989

Lobular, Fibromyxoid Appearance

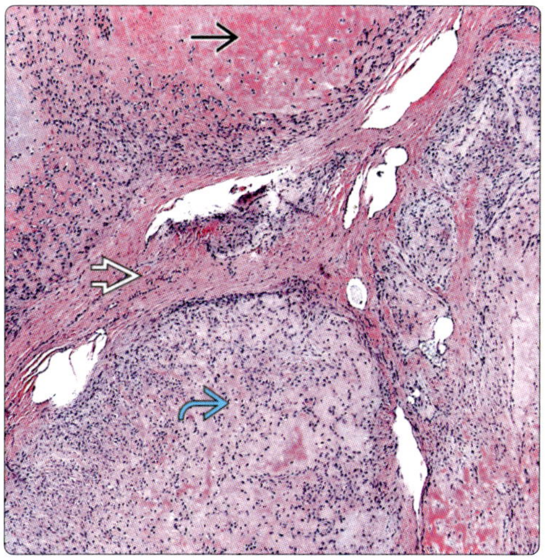

Prominent Bone Formation

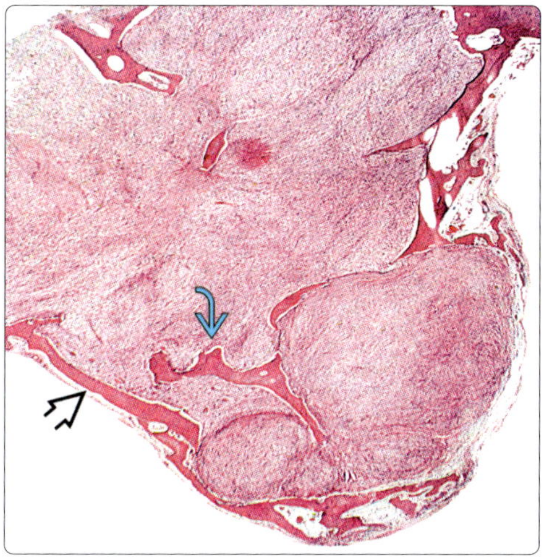

(Left) *Multilobular growth is common in OFMT, with lobules separated by fibrous septa →. The stroma shows variable composition ranging from myxoid to fibromyxoid → to hyalinized →.* **(Right)** *H&E shows an OFMT with an extensive rim of mature bone → with septal extensions → into the tumor mass. This degree of bone formation is often first noticeable during gross examination and sectioning.*

Satellite Nodules

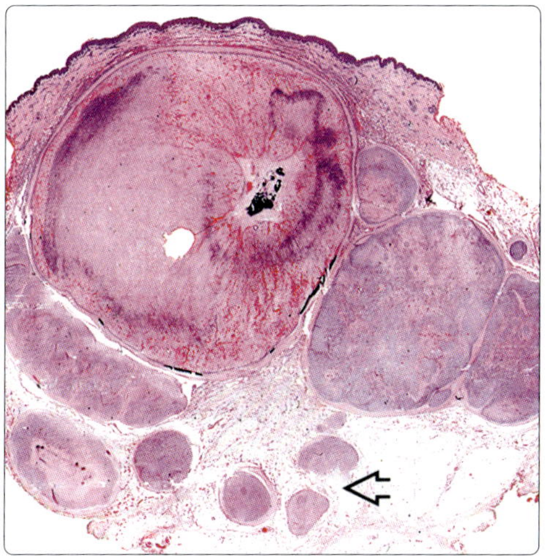

Microcystic Change

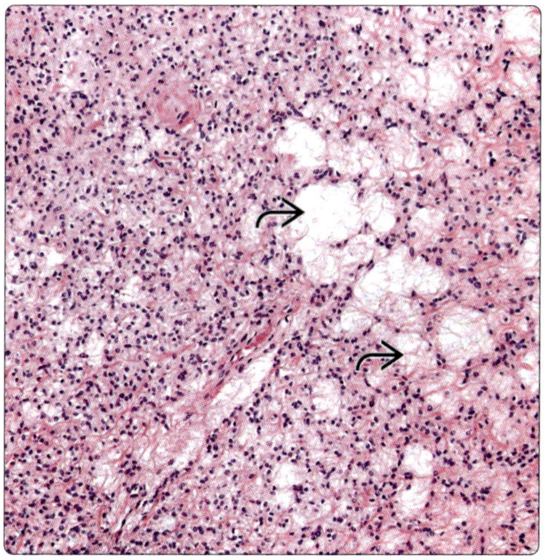

(Left) *Some cases of OFMT feature a distinctly multinodular or plexiform growth, as depicted here. There are also several smaller extracapsular satellite nodules extending into the subcutaneous fat →.* **(Right)** *Formation of stromal microcysts → is common in OFMT. These foci may be of a fibrous, fibromyxoid, or myxoid quality.*

Bland Cytology

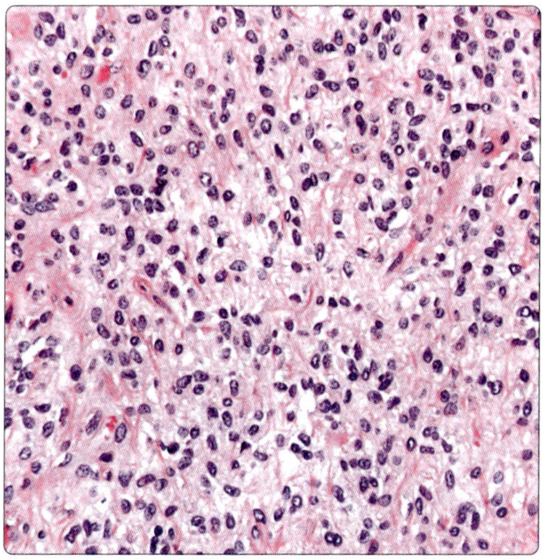

Increased Cellularity

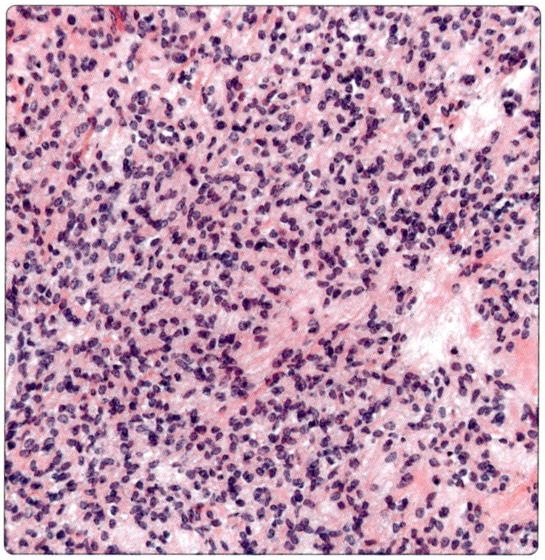

(Left) *The lesional cells of OFMT are typically monomorphic and contain small, round to ovoid, bland nuclei ± small pinpoint nucleoli. Cellularity is generally low, and mitotic figures are typically sparse to absent.* **(Right)** *Areas of moderately increased cellularity, as shown here, are not uncommon in OFMT and have no prognostic significance. Note the lack of cytologic atypia. In contrast, malignant OFMT often feature highly cellular areas with conspicuous mitotic activity or severe nuclear atypia.*

Myxoid Matrix

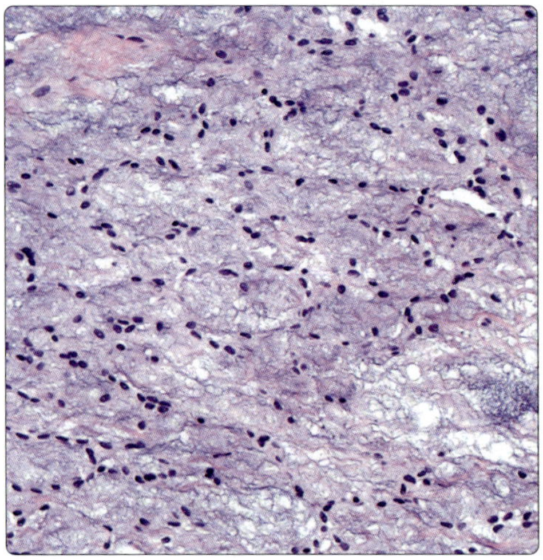

Hyalinized Matrix

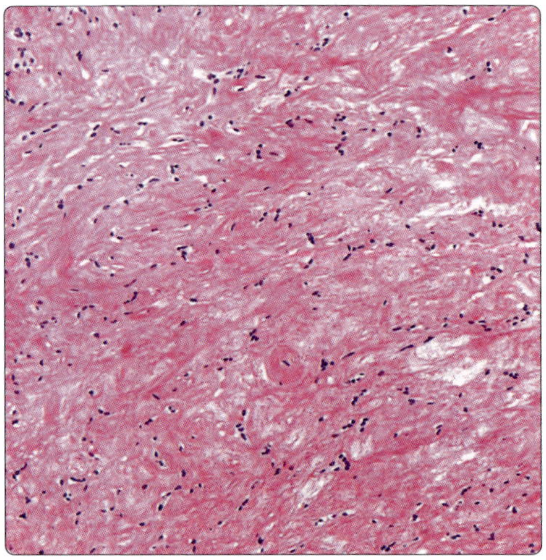

(Left) *Areas with a prominent myxoid stroma may be seen in OFMT. When a myxoid morphology is prominent and diffuse, other tumors, such as extraskeletal myxoid chondrosarcoma and myoepithelioma, must be excluded.* **(Right)** *Prominent fibrous zones may be seen in OFMT, as shown here. Some longstanding tumors may show extensive hyalinization and overall paucicellularity.*

Hyalinized Stroma

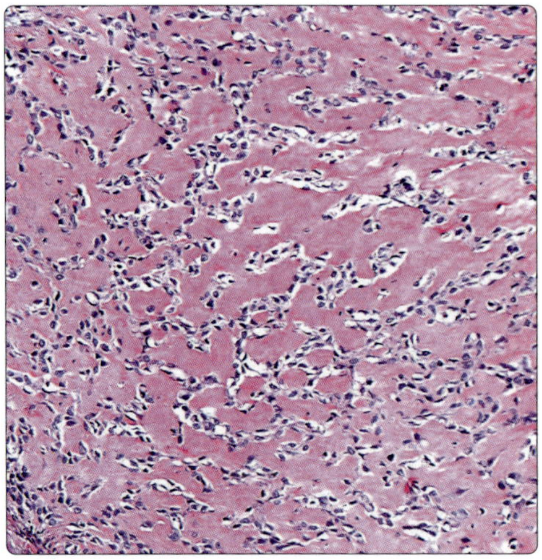

Spindle Cells

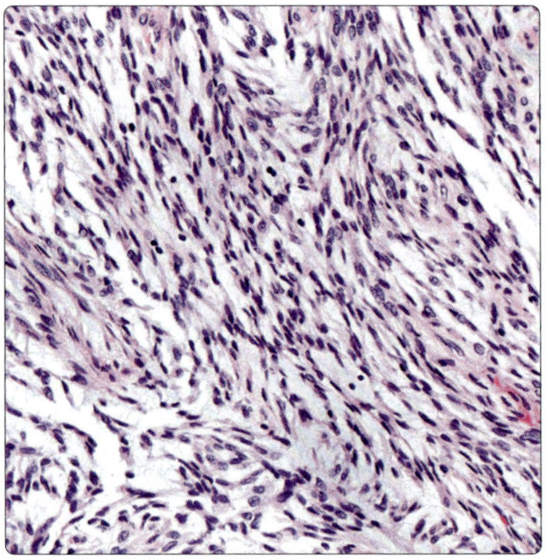

(Left) *This case of OFMT features densely hyalinized or sclerotic stroma, as depicted here. Note the retained branching cord pattern that is commonly seen in this tumor.* **(Right)** *Tumor cells occasionally adopt a spindled cytomorphology in OFMT; however, it is rarely a prominent or diffuse change. Cellular fascicles with mitotic activity have also been reported in histologically malignant forms of OFMT.*

Clear Cell Morphology

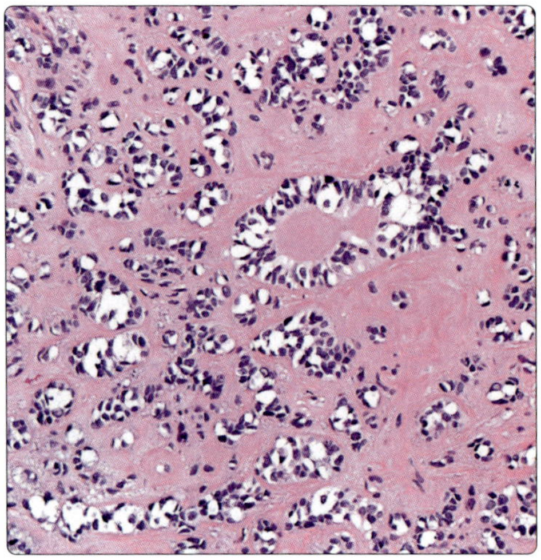

Hyalinized Foci

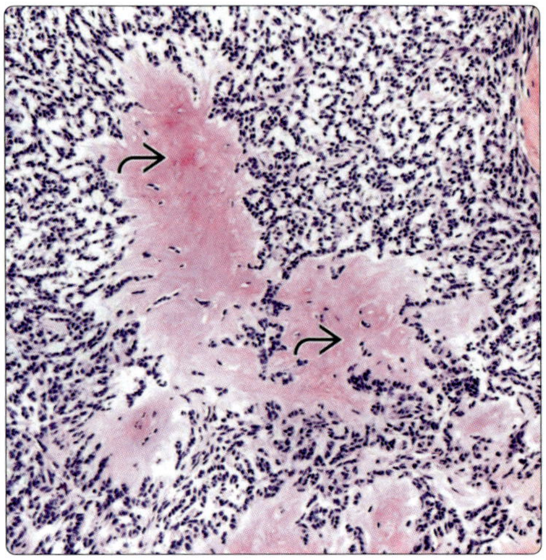

(Left) *Clear cell change is an uncommon finding in OFMT and can vary from focal and inconspicuous to prominent.* **(Right)** *Vague hyalinized nodules ➔ are sometimes noted in cases of otherwise conventional OFMT. These foci are somewhat similar to the rosette-like structures seen in some schwannoma variants and in low-grade fibromyxoid sarcoma; however, the latter structures often show a condensed peripheral rim of tumor cells.*

Desmin Expression

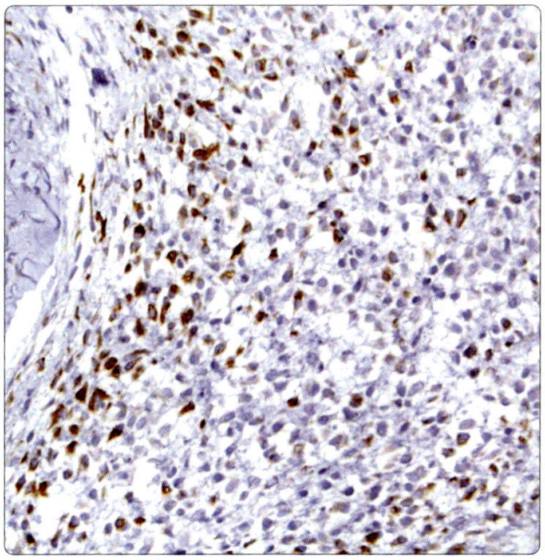

Malignant Ossifying Fibromyxoid Tumor

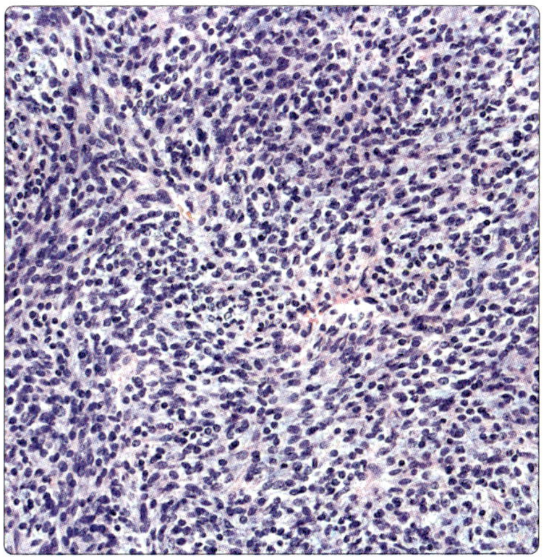

(Left) *Desmin expression is seen in up to 50% of cases of OFMT. Unlike S100 protein, desmin expression is often limited to focal or patchy positivity, as depicted.* **(Right)** *Per criteria set forth by Folpe and Weiss, histologic features of malignancy in OFMT include either high nuclear grade or high cellularity with > 2 mitoses per 50 HPF. As depicted here, areas of high cellularity feature prominent nuclear overlapping and loss of intercellular matrix/stroma. Mitoses were numerous in this case.*

Malignant Ossifying Fibromyxoid Tumor

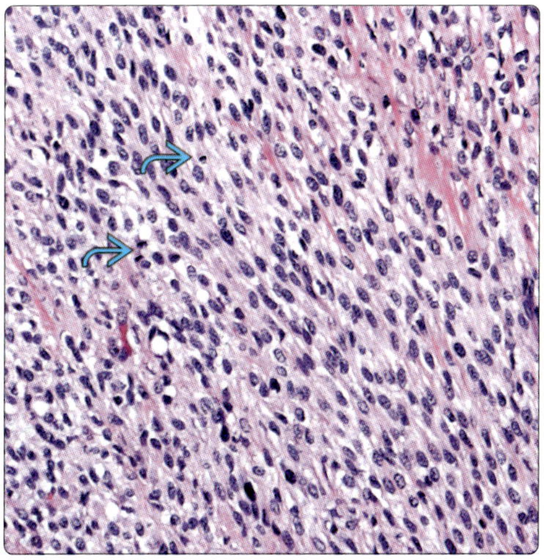

Malignant Ossifying Fibromyxoid Tumor

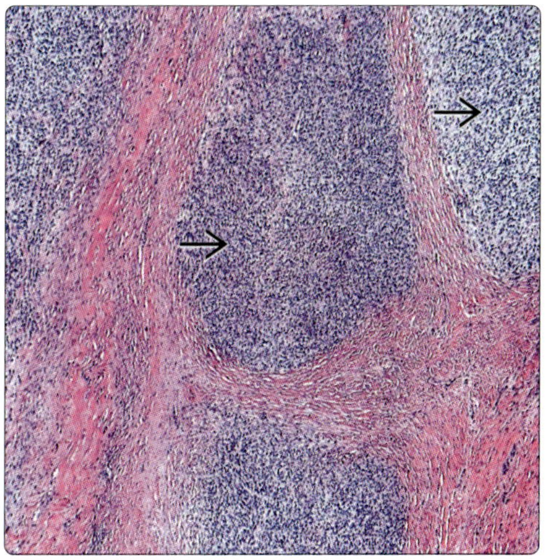

(Left) *Mitoses ⮫ are generally sparse or absent in typical cases of OFMT; however, tumors with ≥ 2 mitoses per 50 HPF show an increased risk for local recurrence and, if associated with high cellularity, are probably best considered as having malignant potential (malignant OFMT).* **(Right)** *Malignant forms of OFMT often retain the lobular configuration of conventional OFMT; however, note the markedly increased cellularity ⇒ evident here even at low power.*

Sclerosing Epithelioid Fibrosarcoma-Like Foci

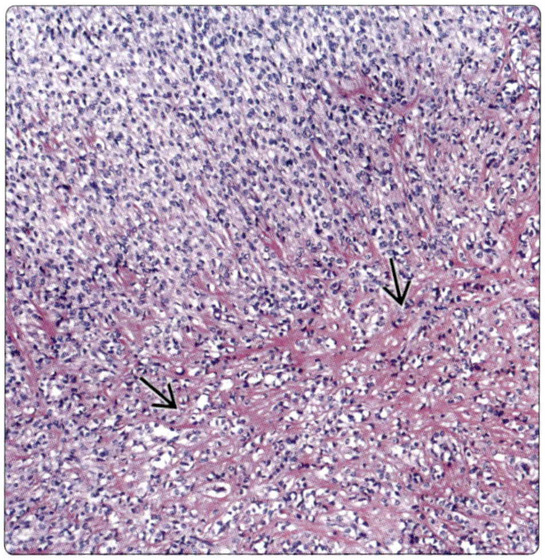

Lung Metastasis

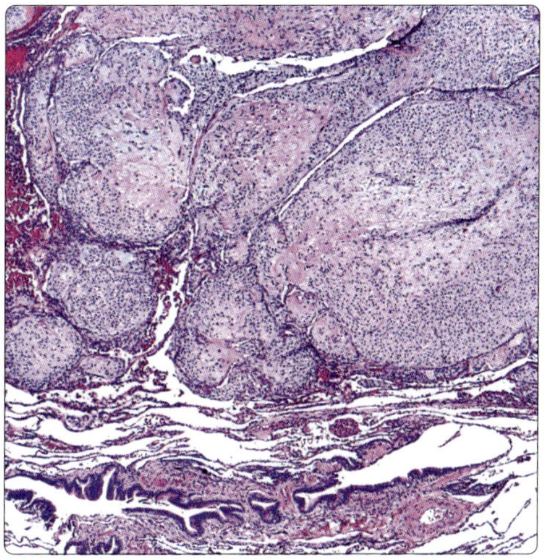

(Left) *Some cases of malignant OFMT contain areas of sclerotic stroma ⇒ with variable clear cell change resembling sclerosing epithelioid fibrosarcoma.* **(Right)** *Malignant OFMT may metastasize to the lung (as shown here) or other soft tissue sites. Notably, metastases often closely resemble the primary tumor morphologically. Bone formation may be particularly prominent in some metastases.*

Myoepithelioma of Soft Tissue

KEY FACTS

TERMINOLOGY

- Soft tissue neoplasm composed exclusively or predominantly of cells demonstrating myoepithelial phenotype
- Synonyms: Parachordoma, mixed tumor

CLINICAL ISSUES

- Wide age range (median: 40 years)
  - Significant number of cases (20%) arise in children
- Most common in limbs and limb girdles (lower > upper)
- Treatment: Complete surgical excision
- Most neoplasms are benign; may locally recur (20%)
- Histologically malignant examples behave aggressively (metastases in up to 50%)

MACROSCOPIC

- Wide size range (mean: 4-6 cm)

MICROSCOPIC

- Well-demarcated, nodular or lobular growth
- Epithelioid, spindled, plasmacytoid, or clear cells
- Cells arranged in nests, cords, sheets, clusters, or singly
- Chondromyxoid to collagenous/hyalinized stroma
- Moderate to severe nuclear atypia in malignant cases
- Variants: Parachordoma, mixed tumor, syncytial

ANCILLARY TESTS

- Variable myoepithelial immunophenotype
- Molecular: Rearrangement of *EWSR1* gene (22q12) in ~ 50% of cases

TOP DIFFERENTIAL DIAGNOSES

- Extraskeletal myxoid chondrosarcoma
- Soft tissue chondroma
- Ossifying fibromyxoid tumor
- Epithelioid malignant peripheral nerve sheath tumor
- Metastatic carcinoma/melanoma

Myoepithelioma of Soft Tissue

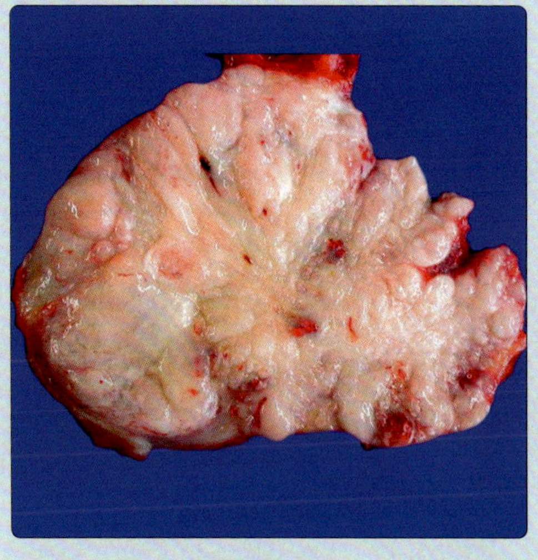

Myoepithelioma of Soft Tissue

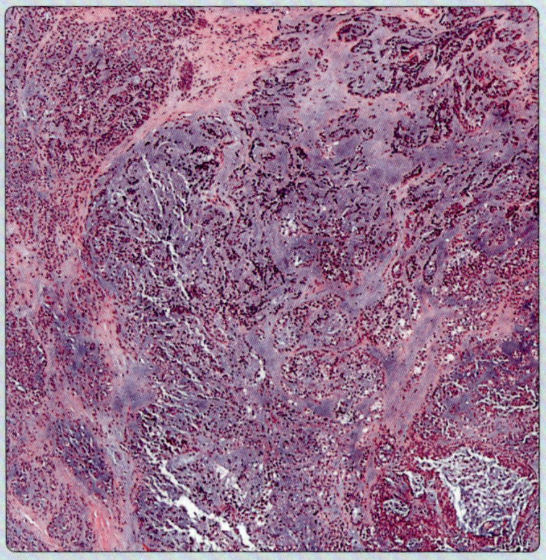

(Left) *Soft tissue myoepithelioma may arise in subcutaneous or deep soft tissue sites and is usually well circumscribed and nodular with a variably firm, gelatinous, fibrotic, or fleshy cut surface.* **(Right)** *Myoepithelioma is a heterogeneous neoplasm and has a broad morphologic spectrum. It shares many histologic patterns with myoepithelioma of salivary gland origin.*

Myxoid Matrix

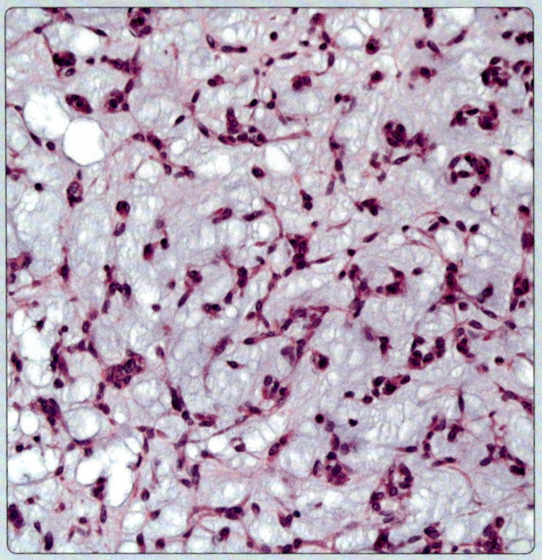

Myoepithelial Immunophenotype

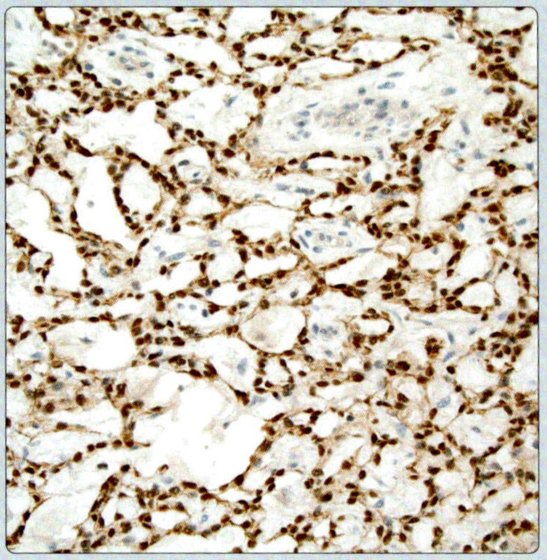

(Left) *A myxoid matrix is very common in myoepithelioma and is often quite prominent. The lesional cells have eosinophilic cytoplasm, vary from epithelioid to spindled in shape, and may form a variety of architectural patterns.* **(Right)** *Most myoepitheliomas express S100 protein (shown), calponin, and epithelial markers, such as pankeratin and EMA. Other markers, such as GFAP, SMA, and p63, are variably positive.*

TERMINOLOGY

Synonyms

- Parachordoma
- Mixed tumor
- Ectomesenchymal chondromyxoid tumor (of tongue)
- Myoepithelial carcinoma (malignant myoepithelioma)

Definitions

- Soft tissue neoplasm composed exclusively or predominantly of cells demonstrating myoepithelial phenotype
  - May also contain evidence of ductal differentiation (mixed tumor)
  - May contain population of larger epithelioid cells with heavily vacuolated cytoplasm (parachordoma)
  - Tumors with diffuse, moderate to severe nuclear atypia classified as malignant myoepithelioma (myoepithelial carcinoma)

CLINICAL ISSUES

Epidemiology

- Incidence
  - Rare
- Age
  - Wide range (median: 40 years)
    - Significant number of cases (20%) arise in children < 10 years old
      - Higher incidence of malignancy (myoepithelial carcinoma) in this age group

Site

- Most common in limbs and limb girdles (lower > upper)
  - Also trunk and head/neck region
- Subcutaneous and deep soft tissue
  - Occasionally in skin
  - Rarely in bone and viscera

Presentation

- Painless, often palpable mass

Treatment

- Complete surgical excision

Prognosis

- Most neoplasms behave in benign fashion
  - Conventional, benign-appearing neoplasms recur in 20% of cases and rarely metastasize
- Histologically malignant examples behave aggressively
  - Recur and metastasize in up to 50% of cases
  - Metastatic sites: Lung, bone, soft tissue, lymph nodes

MACROSCOPIC

General Features

- Usually well circumscribed and nodular
- Firm, fleshy, or gelatinous cut surface

Size

- Wide range (mean: 4-6 cm)

MICROSCOPIC

Histologic Features

- Well-demarcated, nodular or lobular growth
- Epithelioid, spindled, plasmacytoid, or clear cells
  - Minimal nuclear pleomorphism; vesicular nuclei; small nucleoli
  - Few mitoses are usually present (< 2 mitoses per 10 HPF)
- Significant architectural heterogeneity
  - Cells arranged in nests, cords, sheets, clusters, or singly
- Usually prominent chondromyxoid to collagenous/hyalinized stroma
- Minority of cases (10%) show foci of cartilaginous or osseous metaplasia
  - Adipocytic or squamous elements rare
- Malignant myoepithelioma (myoepithelial carcinoma)
  - Diffuse, moderate to severe nuclear atypia appears to be most reliable criterion
    - Nuclear pleomorphism, vesicular or coarse chromatin, and prominent nucleoli
    - Often associated with high mitotic rate and coagulative necrosis
  - Tend to be larger tumors and show more infiltrative margins
  - In children, tumors may contain undifferentiated round cell component
  - May contain areas of more conventional, benign-appearing morphology

Morphologic Variants

- Parachordoma
  - Contains population of larger epithelioid cells with prominent cytoplasmic vacuolization
  - Similar features to conventional myoepithelioma
- Mixed tumor
  - Contain foci of epithelial (ductal) differentiation
  - Similar features to conventional myoepithelioma
- Cutaneous syncytial myoepithelioma
  - Small, dermal-based lesions
  - Solid, sheet-like proliferation of ovoid to spindled cells with pale eosinophilic, syncytial cytoplasm
  - No nuclear atypia; mitoses rare to absent
  - Adipocytic metaplasia &/or lymphoplasmacytic inflammation may be seen

ANCILLARY TESTS

Immunohistochemistry

- Variable myoepithelial immunophenotype
- Loss of nuclear INI1 in many cases of myoepithelial carcinoma

Molecular Genetics

- Rearrangement of *EWSR1* gene (22q12) in ~ 50% of cases
  - Reported gene partners: *POU5F1* (6p21), *PBX1* (1q23), *ZNF44* (19q13), others
- Subset show *FUS* rearrangements (*FUS-KLF17* fusion most common)
- *PLAG1* gene rearrangements identified in myoepitheliomas with ductal differentiation (mixed tumor)
  - Similar to pleomorphic adenoma (benign mixed tumor) of salivary gland

Immunohistochemistry Table

Antibody	Reactivity	Staining Pattern	Comment
S100	Positive	Nuclear & cytoplasmic	Positive in most cases (90%)
CK-PAN	Positive	Cytoplasmic	Positive in most cases (90%); often negative in cutaneous syncytial type
Calponin	Positive	Cytoplasmic	Positive in most cases (80%)
EMA	Positive	Cell membrane and cytoplasm	Positive in most cases (60%)
GFAP	Positive	Cytoplasmic	Positive in 50% of cases
Actin-sm	Positive	Cytoplasmic	Positive in 50% of cases
CD34	Negative		
Brachyury	Negative		
p63	Equivocal	Nuclear	Positive in some cases (30-45%)
Desmin	Equivocal	Cytoplasmic	Positive in some cases (15%)
INI1	Equivocal	Nuclear	Loss of nuclear INI1 in some cases of myoepithelial carcinoma

DIFFERENTIAL DIAGNOSIS

Extraskeletal Myxoid Chondrosarcoma

- Can show striking morphologic overlap with myoepithelioma
- Lacks strong, diffuse keratin and EMA expression
- Variable S100 protein (+), often focal
- *NR4A3* (9q22) gene rearrangements characteristic
  - Most common fusion partner is *EWSR1*
- Tumors with rhabdoid features may show loss of INI1

Soft Tissue Chondroma

- Most common in acral locations
- Nodules of well-developed cartilage
- No expression of epithelial markers

Ossifying Fibromyxoid Tumor

- Can show morphologic overlap with myoepithelioma
- Majority show incomplete peripheral rim of bone
- S100 protein (+) in most cases; desmin (+) in 50%
- No expression of epithelial markers (or at most focal)
- *PHF1* (6p21) gene rearrangements in majority

Epithelioid Malignant Peripheral Nerve Sheath Tumor

- Sheets and nodules of large epithelioid cells with prominent macronucleoli, often in myxoid stroma
- May contain areas of more conventional spindle cell MPNST
- Demonstration of origin from nerve is helpful
- Strong, diffuse S100 protein (+)
- Lacks expression of epithelial markers (or at most focal positivity)
- Lacks *EWSR1* gene rearrangements

Schwannoma (Epithelioid Variant)

- Small, epithelioid Schwann cells with bland nuclei within myxoid or fibrillary stroma
- Strong, diffuse S100 protein (+)
- No expression of epithelial markers

Metastatic Carcinoma/Melanoma

- Clinical history of primary tumor often present
- Chondromyxoid stroma rare in both entities
- Expression of epithelial markers (and absence of other myoepithelial markers) in carcinoma
  - TTF-1, pax-8, CDX-2, etc. in carcinomas from various sites
- Expression of melanocytic markers in melanoma

Epithelioid Sarcoma

- Myxoid stroma uncommon but described
- Proximal-type epithelioid sarcoma show rhabdoid morphology with prominent nucleoli
- Strong expression of epithelial markers; CD34(+) in 50%
- S100 protein (-)
- Complete loss of nuclear INI1 common
- Lacks *EWSR1* gene rearrangements

Chordoma

- In soft tissues sites, more likely to be metastasis from bone tumor than soft tissue primary
- Multivacuolated "physaliferous" cells
- Keratin (+), EMA(+), S100 protein (+), brachyury (+)

Myxofibrosarcoma (Epithelioid Variant)

- Eosinophilic epithelioid tumor cells in background of conventional myxofibrosarcoma
- No expression of S100 protein and epithelial markers

SELECTED REFERENCES

1. Kravtsov O et al: Myoepithelioma of soft tissue: a cytological-pathological correlation with literature review. Ann Diagn Pathol. 27:14-7, 2017
2. Jo VY et al: Myoepithelial neoplasms of soft tissue: an updated review of the clinicopathologic, immunophenotypic, and genetic features. Head Neck Pathol. 9(1):32-8, 2015
3. Jo VY et al: Cutaneous syncytial myoepithelioma: clinicopathologic characterization in a series of 38 cases. Am J Surg Pathol. 37(5):710-8, 2013
4. Antonescu CR et al: EWSR1-POU5F1 fusion in soft tissue myoepithelial tumors. A molecular analysis of sixty-six cases, including soft tissue, bone, and visceral lesions, showing common involvement of the EWSR1 gene. Genes Chromosomes Cancer. 49(12):1114-24, 2010
5. Gleason BC et al: Myoepithelial carcinoma of soft tissue in children: an aggressive neoplasm analyzed in a series of 29 cases. Am J Surg Pathol. 31(12):1813-24, 2007
6. Hornick JL et al: Myoepithelial tumors of soft tissue: a clinicopathologic and immunohistochemical study of 101 cases with evaluation of prognostic parameters. Am J Surg Pathol. 27(9):1183-96, 2003

Epithelioid Cells

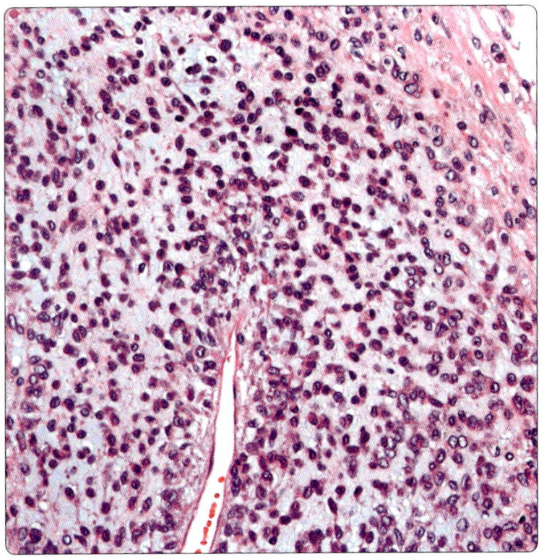

Corded Growth

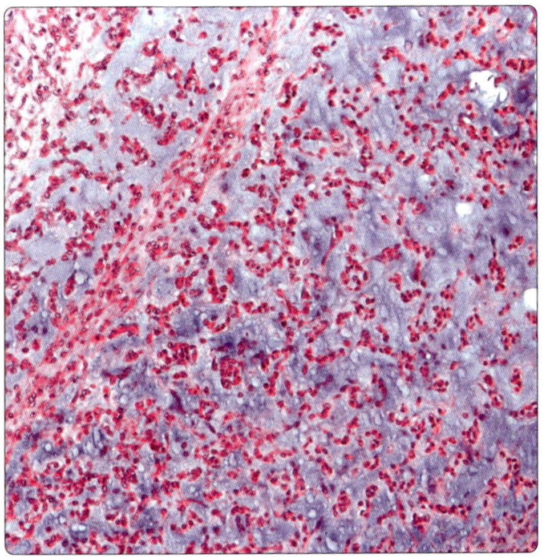

(Left) *H&E of myoepithelioma shows predominantly epithelioid cells in a prominent myxoid matrix. Nuclei are relatively uniform and vesicular and may or may not show small nucleoli. Mitotic activity is low or absent.* **(Right)** *Cords or thin trabeculae of cells is a common pattern in myoepithelioma. These cords may interconnect or appear separated from one another.*

Reticular Pattern

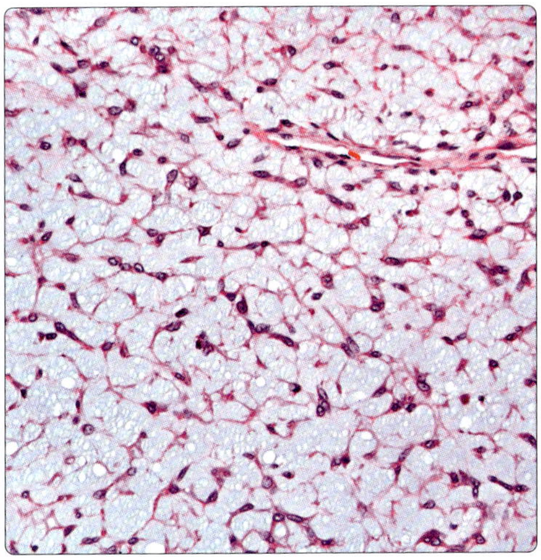

Micronodular Pattern

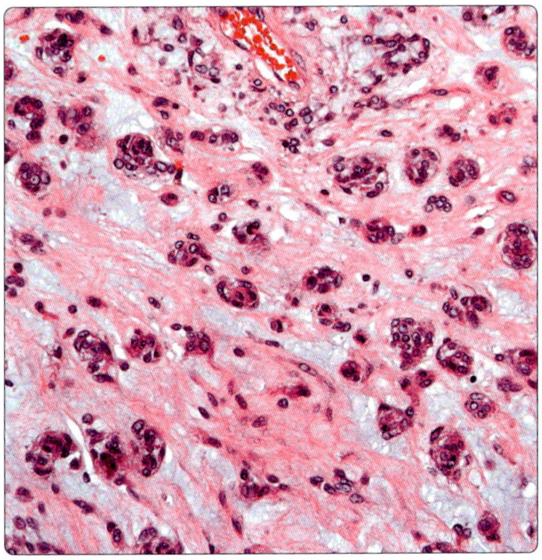

(Left) *Myoepithelioma can show a finely reticular pattern of growth in highly myxoid tumors. Tumors with a prominent collagenous or hyalinized/sclerotic matrix may also show this morphology.* **(Right)** *The lesional cells may form small nests or aggregates and impart an overall micronodular appearance. The background stroma is variably myxoid and collagenous.*

Variable Cellularity

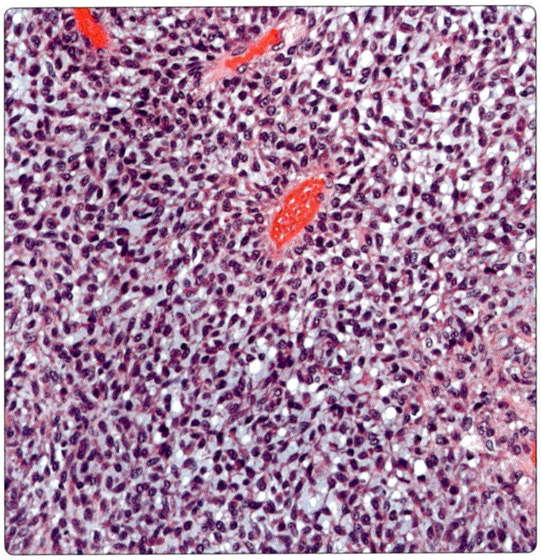

Spindled Morphology

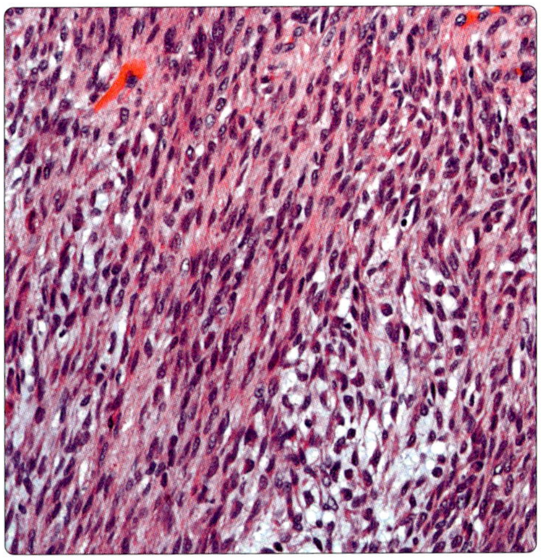

(Left) *H&E shows hypercellularity and density in a myoepithelioma. This finding does not correlate with malignant potential; however, malignant myoepitheliomas are often more cellular than benign types. Importantly, there is no significant nuclear atypia or increased mitotic rate.* **(Right)** *Spindled myoepithelial cells may form loose or tight fascicles and may raise the possibility of a smooth muscle, neural, or myofibroblastic neoplasm.*

Myoepithelioma of Soft Tissue

(**Left**) *Variably sized, solid nests within a loose or dense collagenous stroma characterize occasional cases of myoepithelioma. Areas of intratumoral hemorrhage are seen →.* (**Right**) *Regardless of whether the cells in myoepithelioma are epithelioid or spindled, the nuclei are minimally atypical and relatively uniform. Nucleoli → are often present but should be small and inconspicuous.*

Nodular or Nested Growth

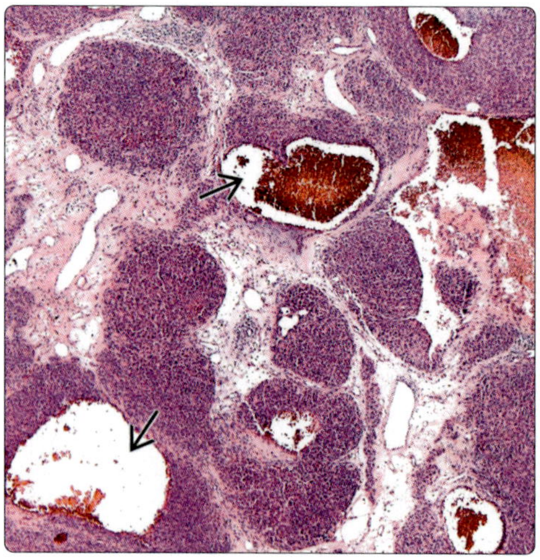

Monomorphic Cytology

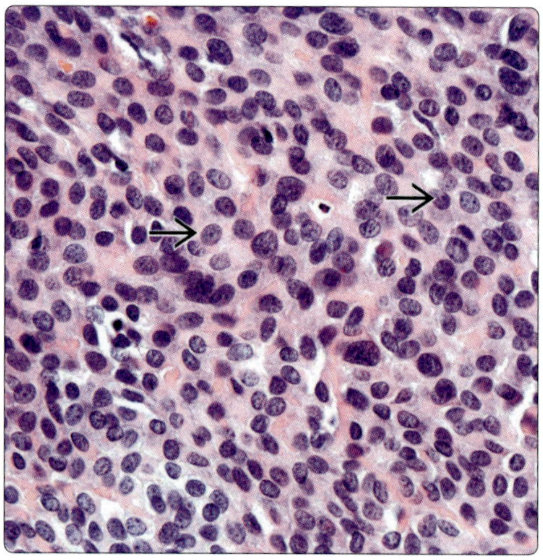

(**Left**) *Clear cell change → is not uncommon in myoepithelioma and may be prominent in some cases. Rarely is a tumor composed entirely of clear cells.* (**Right**) *H&E of myoepithelioma shows sheets of epithelioid cells, many of which show cytoplasmic clearing. Clear cell change in a soft tissue neoplasm should always raise the possibility of a myoepithelial neoplasm.*

Clear Cell Change

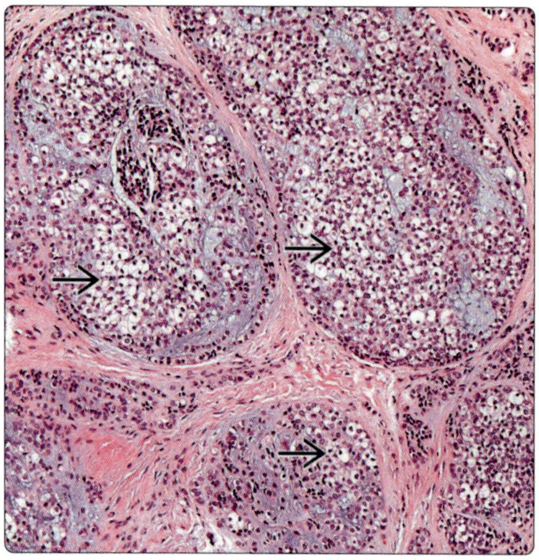

Clear Cell Change

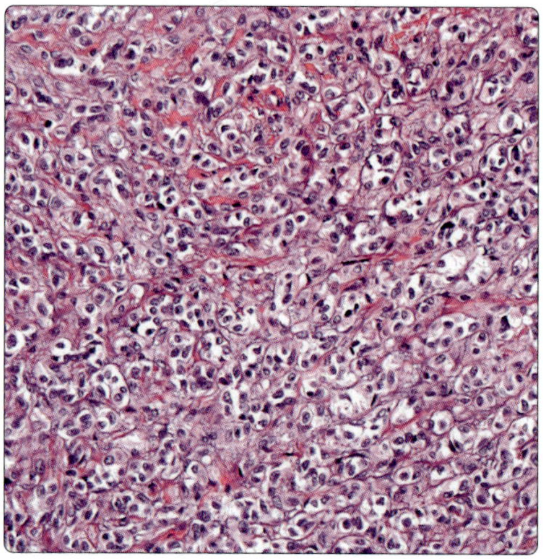

(**Left**) *Some cases of myoepithelioma contain a stroma that is less myxoid and more collagenous and may even be diffusely hyalinized. Lesional myoepithelial cells → are arranged in a variety of patterns, including cords or trabeculae, similar to predominantly myxoid examples.* (**Right**) *In some hyalinized myoepitheliomas, irregular nests and cords of cells show central cellular loss or dyscohesion → resembling vascular spaces.*

Hyalinized Stroma

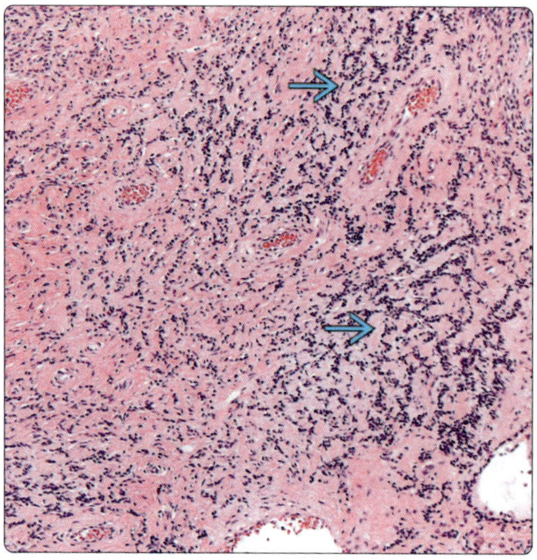

Pseudovascular Spaces

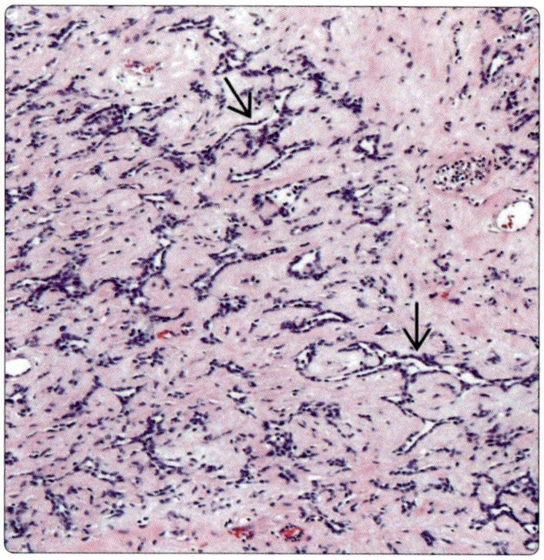

Aggregates of Clear Cells

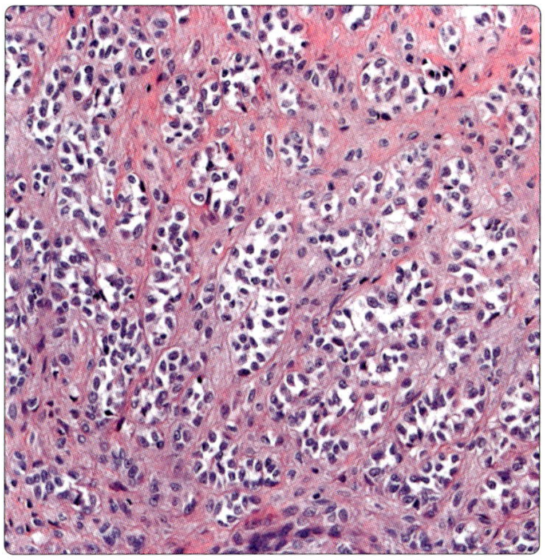

Storiform Architecture

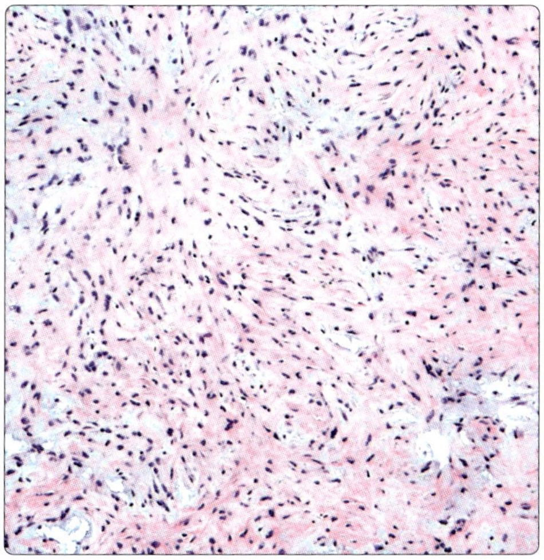

(Left) *This myoepithelioma contained prominent stromal collagen and shows nests and aggregates of neoplastic cells demonstrating abundant clear cytoplasm, thus, raising the possibility of a metastatic clear cell carcinoma.* **(Right)** *Spindled myoepithelial cells in a collagenous stroma may occasionally adopt a loose storiform architecture. The area depicted somewhat resembles a perineurioma.*

Hypocellularity

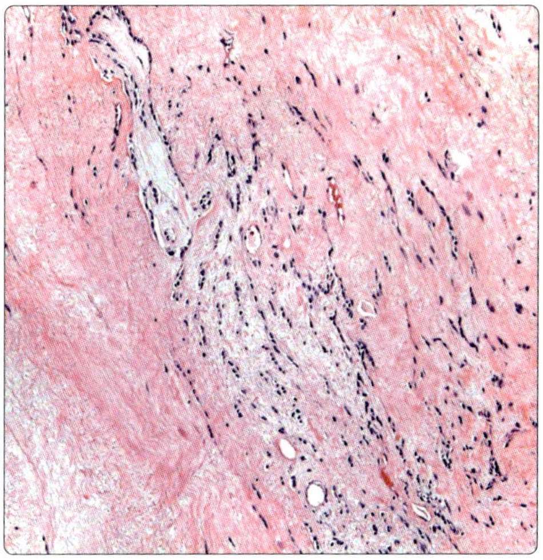

Plasmacytoid Cytomorphology

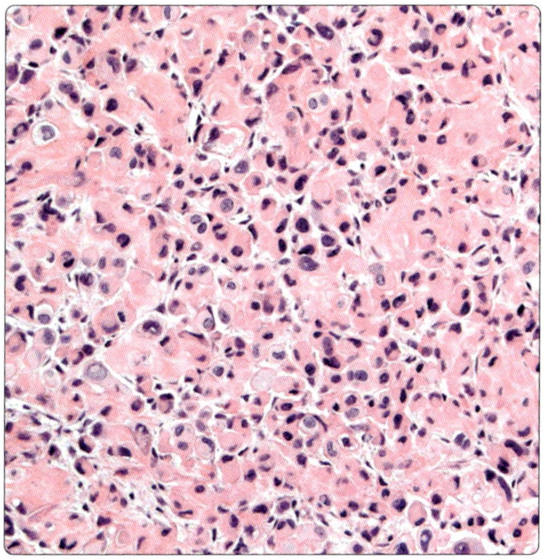

(Left) *This example of myoepithelioma shows diffuse stromal hyalinization and relatively low cellularity overall. Scattered cords and small aggregates of neoplastic myoepithelial cells are evident in scattered patches.* **(Right)** *A plasmacytoid morphology is not uncommon in soft tissue myoepithelioma and may be the predominant cytomorphology in some cases. The cells may form nests, sheets, or cords in a myxoid or collagenous stroma.*

Plasmacytoid Cytomorphology

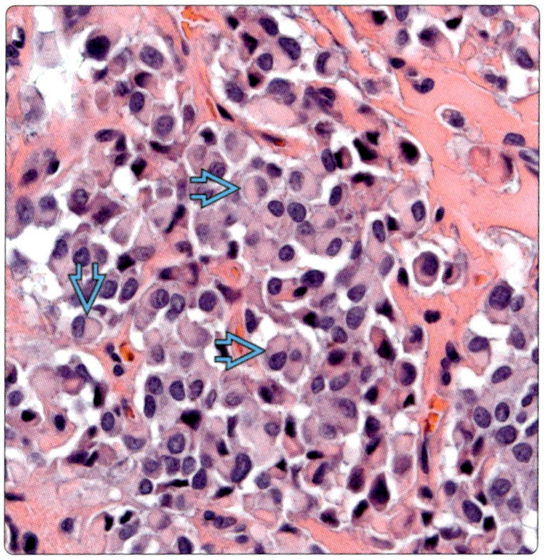

Osteoid-Like Hyalinization

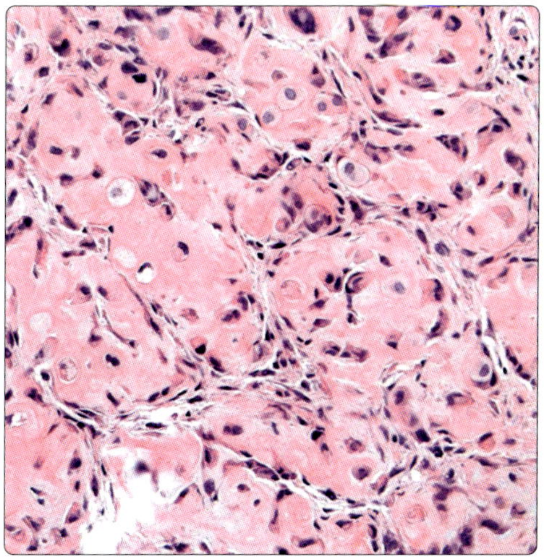

(Left) *Plasmacytoid myoepithelial cells are characterized by eccentric nuclei with tiny nucleoli and an eosinophilic intracytoplasmic inclusion ⇨. Some larger cells may resemble rhabdoid cells.* **(Right)** *This soft tissue myoepithelioma shows loose aggregates of plasmacytoid myoepithelial cells within a dense, osteoid-like sclerotic matrix reminiscent of osteosarcoma.*

Sclerotic Matrix

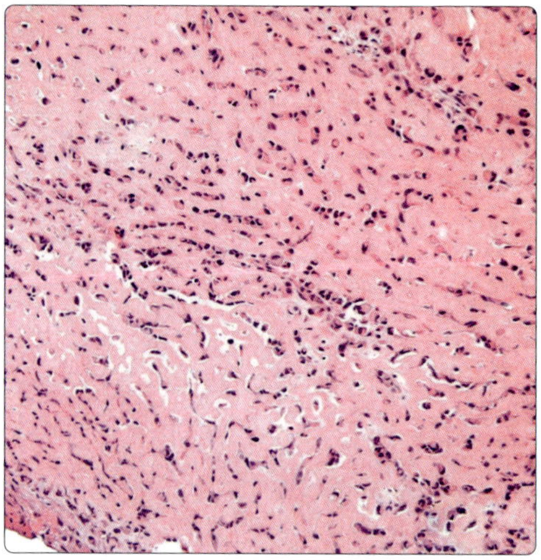

Epithelioid Cell Nests

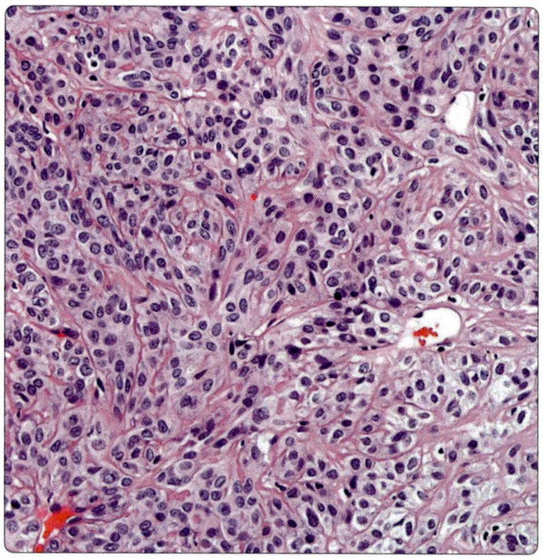

(Left) *This myoepithelioma is composed of cords and aggregates of plasmacytoid myoepithelial cells within a densely sclerotic stroma resembling infiltrating lobular carcinoma of the breast.* **(Right)** *This myoepithelioma is composed of dense nests and aggregates of plump epithelioid and plasmacytoid cells, some of which show clear cytoplasm (bottom right).*

Parachordoma Morphology

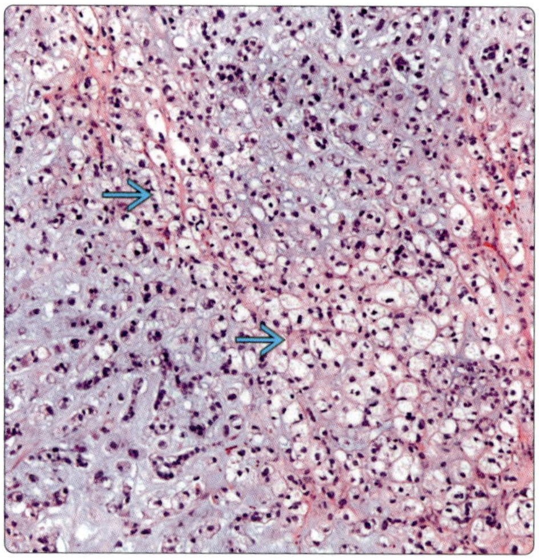

Epithelial Differentiation

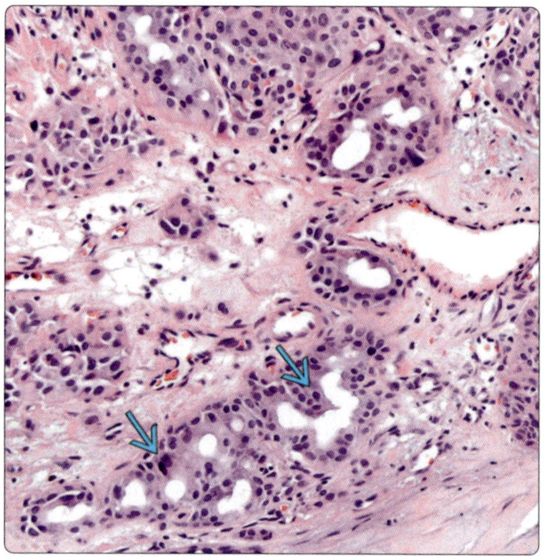

(Left) *Some variants of soft tissue myoepithelioma show a population of larger epithelioid cells with heavily vacuolated cytoplasm ➙ reminiscent of physaliferous cells. These tumors are sometimes referred to as parachordoma but are currently considered a morphologic variant of myoepithelioma.* **(Right)** *Approximately 10% of cases of soft tissue myoepithelioma show evidence of epithelial differentiation, usually in the form of ductular structures ➙. These tumors are also referred to as mixed tumors.*

Cutaneous Syncytial Myoepithelioma

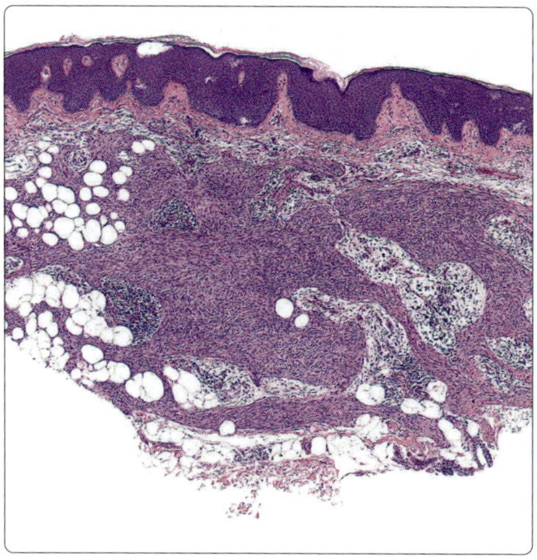

Scattered Atypical Nuclei

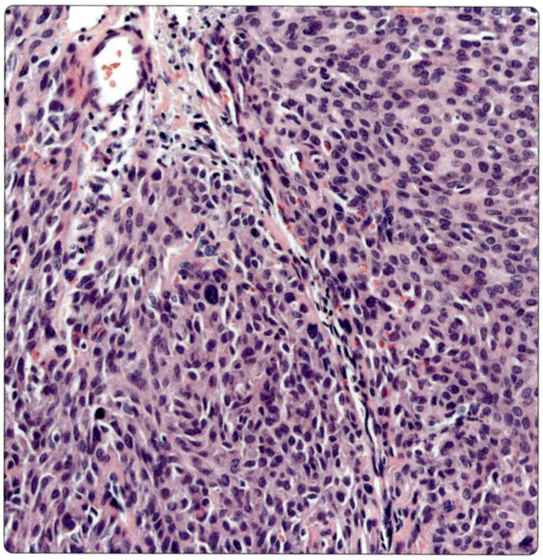

(Left) *This case of cutaneous myoepithelioma is composed predominantly of spindle-shaped tumor cells with a syncytial growth pattern. Note the focal adipocytic metaplasia and scattered chronic inflammatory cells.* **(Right)** *Scattered, enlarged, hyperchromatic nuclei, in an otherwise conventional soft tissue myoepithelioma, does not imply aggressive behavior. In contrast, diffuse nuclear atypia, particularly with prominent nucleoli, correlates well.*

Malignant Myoepithelioma

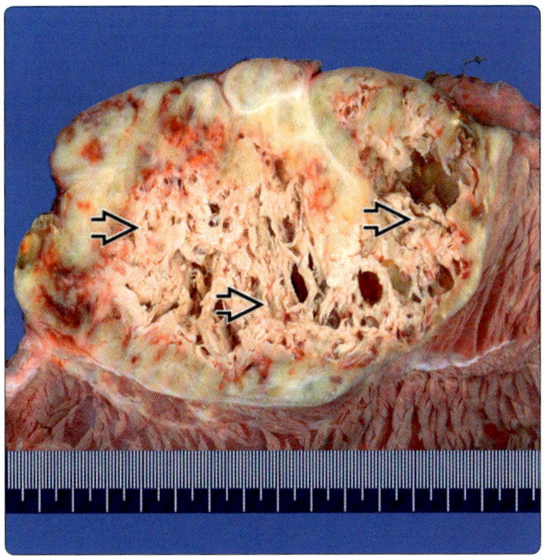

Nuclear Atypia and Mitoses

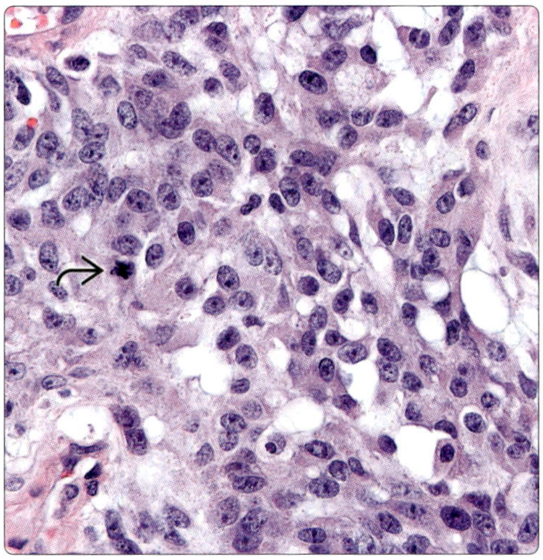

(Left) *A rare case of malignant myoepithelioma of deep soft tissues with gray-white cut surfaces and extensive areas of tumor necrosis* ➩ *is shown.* **(Right)** *This case of clinically malignant and metastatic myoepithelioma shows diffuse nuclear atypia in the form of coarse chromatin and prominent nucleoli. Mitotic figures* ➩ *are also increased in the tumor.*

Rhabdoid Morphology

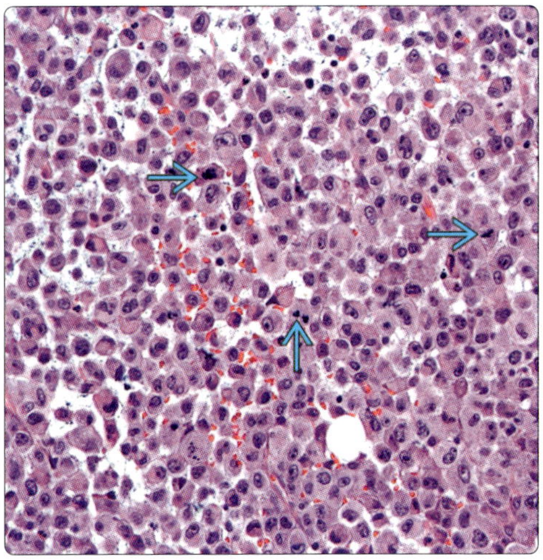

Necrosis

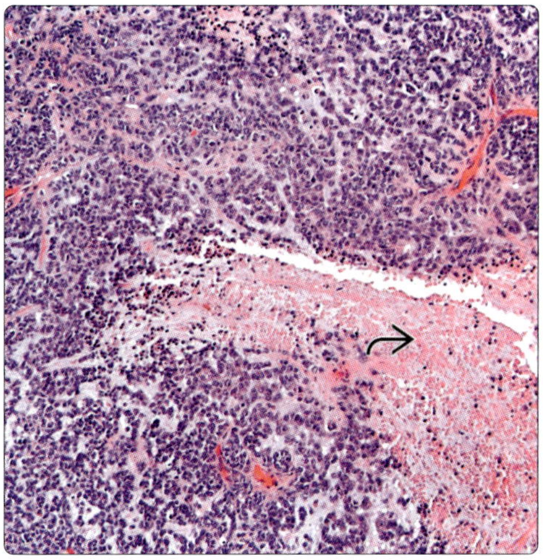

(Left) *This malignant myoepithelioma with a predominant plasmacytoid morphology shows prominent nucleoli imparting a rhabdoid appearance. Note the mitotic figures* ➩*. A subset of malignant cases show loss of nuclear INI1 similar to epithelioid sarcoma and other rhabdoid tumors.* **(Right)** *Coagulative necrosis* ➩ *is a common feature of malignant myoepithelioma.*

Malignant Myoepithelioma

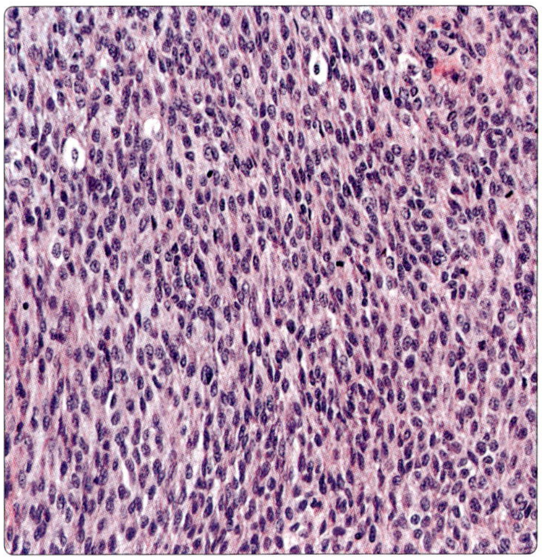

Undifferentiated Morphology

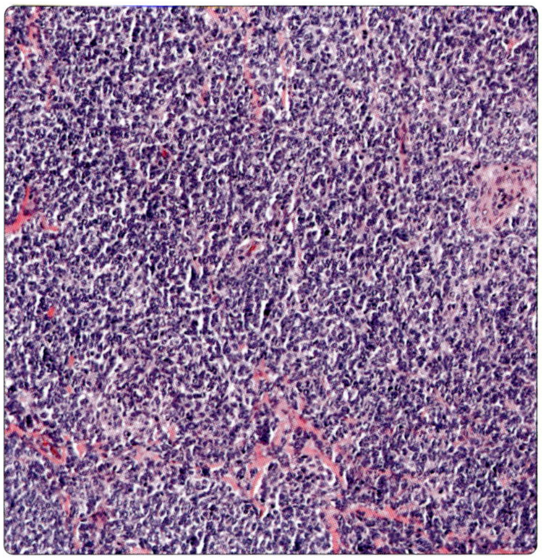

(Left) *Malignant forms of myoepithelioma are often more cellular than benign types, and the mitotic rate is typically elevated. Coagulative necrosis is also not uncommon. Diffuse nuclear atypia, however, correlates best with malignant potential.* **(Right)** *An undifferentiated round cell component may be seen in some cases of malignant myoepithelioma, as depicted, particularly in those that occur in children.*

Phosphaturic Mesenchymal Tumor

KEY FACTS

TERMINOLOGY

- Rare distinctive mesenchymal neoplasm of soft tissue and bone that is often associated in most cases with tumor-induced osteomalacia

CLINICAL ISSUES

- Most common in middle-aged adults
- Predilection for extremities, particularly thigh and foot
  - Also bony sites
- Most patients have symptoms related to osteomalacia
  - Labs: Hypophosphatemia, hyperphosphaturia, normocalcemia
  - Some patients have no clinical or laboratory evidence of osteomalacia
- Treatment: Complete surgical excision
  - Tumor-induced osteomalacia often resolves following resection of tumor
- Most are clinically benign
  - Local recurrence common
- Rare malignant PMT can metastasize and cause death

MICROSCOPIC

- Loose arrays of spindled to stellate cells
- Chondromyxoid or hyalinized matrix with characteristic granular, flocculent calcification
- Well-developed stromal capillary vasculature
- Osteoclast-like multinucleated giant cells common

ANCILLARY TESTS

- Detection of FGF23 mRNA or expression by immunohistochemistry
- ERG(+), SATB2(+), CD56(+)
- *FN1-FGFR1* gene fusion in 40-50% of cases

TOP DIFFERENTIAL DIAGNOSES

- Solitary fibrous tumor
- Soft tissue chondroma
- Mesenchymal chondrosarcoma

Phosphaturic Mesenchymal Tumor

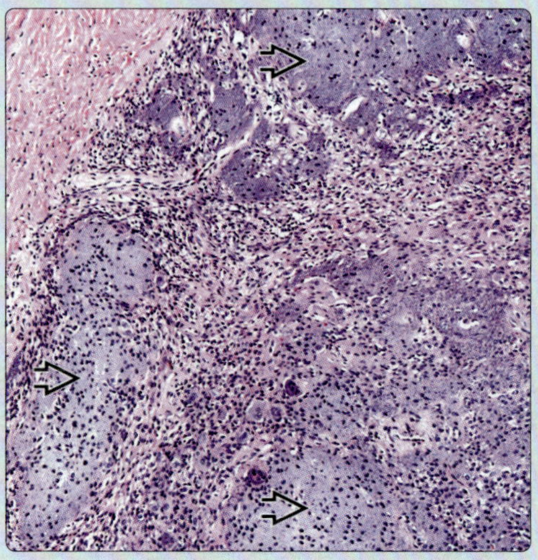

Bland Cytologic Features

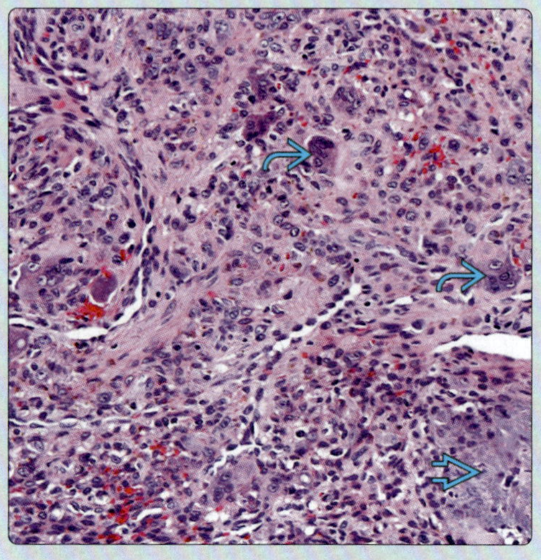

(Left) *Phosphaturic mesenchymal tumor (PMT) is a rare neoplasm of soft tissue and bone that is associated in most cases with clinical features of osteomalacia. A characteristic finding is variable-sized deposits ➩ of amorphous, lightly basophilic calcification.* **(Right)** *The lesional cells of PMT are spindled to stellate and usually cytologically bland; however, rare malignant cases do occur. Osteoclast-like giant cells ➩ are common. Note the deposit ➩ of granular calcification.*

Distinctive Calcification

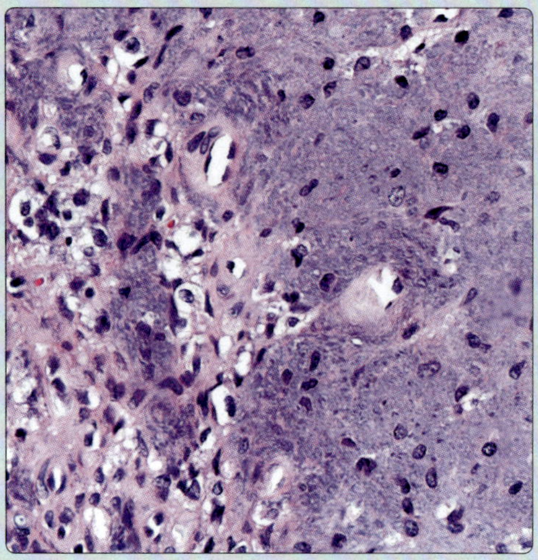

Vascular Stroma

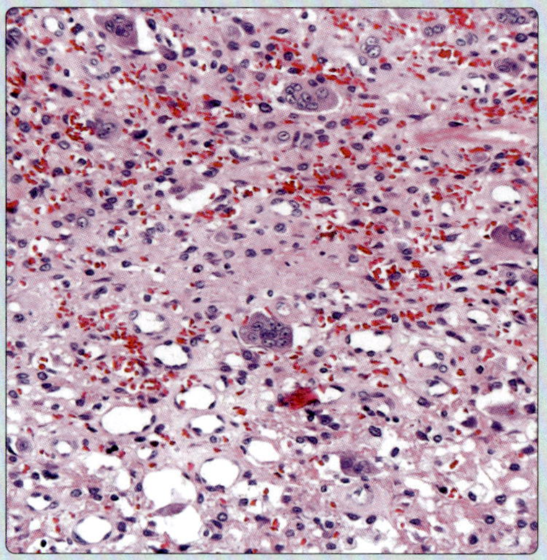

(Left) *The distinctive and characteristic foci of calcification in PMT appear lightly basophilic and granular or flocculent in quality. Sometimes it is referred to as "grungy" calcification.* **(Right)** *The stroma in PMT is often quite vascular, and dilated capillaries or larger channels are usually readily evident and may even impart a hemangioma-like appearance. Larger, ectatic, "staghorn" vessels are also not uncommon.*

TERMINOLOGY

Abbreviations

- Phosphaturic mesenchymal tumor (PMT)

Synonyms

- PMT mixed connective tissue variant

Definitions

- Rare distinctive mesenchymal neoplasm of soft tissue and bone that is often associated with tumor-induced osteomalacia

CLINICAL ISSUES

Epidemiology

- Incidence
  - Very rare
- Age
  - Wide range (middle-aged adults most common)
- Sex
  - Male = female

Site

- Predilection for extremities, particularly thigh and foot, but can occur at any soft tissue site
  - Superficial or deep soft tissues
  - May arise in acral locations
- Occurs with roughly equal frequency in bony sites
- Also sinonasal tract

Presentation

- Most patients have symptoms related to osteomalacia
  - Pain, stress fractures
- Labs: Hypophosphatemia, hyperphosphaturia, normocalcemia
  - Related to oversecretion of fibroblastic growth factor-23 (FGF23)
    - Inhibits phosphate reabsorption by proximal renal tubules
- Some patients have no clinical or laboratory evidence of osteomalacia

Treatment

- Complete surgical excision

Prognosis

- Most are clinically benign
  - Rare malignant PMT can metastasize and cause death
- Local recurrence common
  - Clinically malignant tumors most commonly arise within setting of local recurrence; often repeated
- Tumor-induced osteomalacia often resolves following resection of tumor

MACROSCOPIC

Size

- Mean: 3.9 cm

MICROSCOPIC

Histologic Features

- Usually well circumscribed
- Loose arrays of spindled to stellate cells, often of low cellularity
  - Bland nuclei without atypia
  - Mitoses rare
- Chondromyxoid "smudgy" or hyalinized matrix
  - Characteristic granular, flocculent, "grungy" calcification
  - May show areas resembling osteoid or cartilage
- Well-developed, stromal capillary vasculature
  - Larger, ectatic, "staghorn" vessels common
- Osteoclast-like multinucleated giant cells common
- Adipose tissue, microcystic change, hemorrhage may be present
- No necrosis
- Rare cases can show features similar to chondromyxoid fibroma, giant cell reparative granuloma, or sinonasal glomangiopericytoma
- Malignant PMT
  - Usually shows increased cellularity with high nuclear grade and frequent mitoses (> 5 per 10 HPF)

ANCILLARY TESTS

Immunohistochemistry

- FGF23(+) in most tumors
- ERG(+), SATB2(+), CD56(+)
- CD34(-), STAT6(-), S100(-), desmin (-), keratin (-), DOG1(-)

Molecular Genetics

- Detection of FGF23 mRNA in lesional cells
  - Supports diagnosis within appropriate histologic and clinical setting
- *FN1-FGFR1* gene fusion in 40-50% of cases
  - *FGFR1* rearrangement detectable by FISH

DIFFERENTIAL DIAGNOSIS

Solitary Fibrous Tumor

- Lacks characteristic "grungy" calcified matrix of PMT
- STAT6(+), CD34(+)

Soft Tissue Chondroma

- Most common in fingers and hand
- May be calcified and contain giant cells
- Lacks bland spindle cells and adipose tissue, as seen in PMT

Mesenchymal Chondrosarcoma

- Sheets of malignant small round cells with admixed islands of cartilage
- Lacks characteristic "grungy" calcified matrix of PMT
- Recurrent *HEY1-NCOA2* gene arrangement

SELECTED REFERENCES

1. Agaimy A et al: Phosphaturic mesenchymal tumors: clinicopathologic, immunohistochemical and molecular analysis of 22 cases expanding their morphologic and immunophenotypic spectrum. Am J Surg Pathol. 41(10):1371-80, 2017
2. Lee JC et al: Characterization of FN1-FGFR1 and novel FN1-FGF1 fusion genes in a large series of phosphaturic mesenchymal tumors. Mod Pathol. 29(11):1335-46, 2016
3. Bahrami A et al: RT-PCR analysis for FGF23 using paraffin sections in the diagnosis of phosphaturic mesenchymal tumors with and without known tumor induced osteomalacia. Am J Surg Pathol. 33(9):1348-54, 2009
4. Folpe AL et al: Most osteomalacia-associated mesenchymal tumors are a single histopathologic entity: an analysis of 32 cases and a comprehensive review of the literature. Am J Surg Pathol. 28(1):1-30, 2004

Synovial Sarcoma

KEY FACTS

TERMINOLOGY

- Malignant mesenchymal spindle cell neoplasm with variable epithelial differentiation, including gland formation, and characterized by specific chromosomal translocation t(X;18)(p11;q11)

CLINICAL ISSUES

- Most common in young adults
- Most arise in deep soft tissues of extremities
  - Most common near joints (particularly knee)
- Also head/neck, trunk, many other sites
- Treatment: Complete surgical resection with negative margins
- Adjuvant therapy in some cases
- Local recurrence common
- Metastasis in up to 50% of cases
- Unfavorable prognostic factors
  - High stage, age > 40 years, poorly differentiated histology

MICROSCOPIC

- Predominantly monophasic or biphasic morphologies
- Dense cellular sheets or vague fascicles of uniform spindle cells without significant pleomorphism
- Stromal calcifications, prominent vasculature in some
- Biphasic tumors also contain epithelial structures
- Subset show poorly differentiated areas

ANCILLARY TESTS

- Keratin (+), EMA(+), usually focal/patchy
- Strong, diffuse nuclear TLE-1(+)
- CD56(+), CD99(+)
- CD34, SMA, desmin, synaptophysin, TTF-1 (-)
- Molecular: Characteristic t(X;18)(p11;q11)

TOP DIFFERENTIAL DIAGNOSES

- Malignant peripheral nerve sheath tumor
- Fibrosarcomatous dermatofibrosarcoma protuberans
- Solitary fibrous tumor

(Left) *Macroscopically, synovial sarcoma (SS) often appears as a nodular, circumscribed mass located in skeletal muscle beneath the deep fascia ➙. The cut surface varies from tan to white or pink and may display focal hemorrhage ➔ or cystic change.* **(Right)** *Monophasic SS is the most common form of SS and is characterized by an exclusive spindle cell morphology (no epithelial structures). Sheet-like or fascicular growth is typical of this form, and the cells are always cytologically uniform.*

Synovial Sarcoma

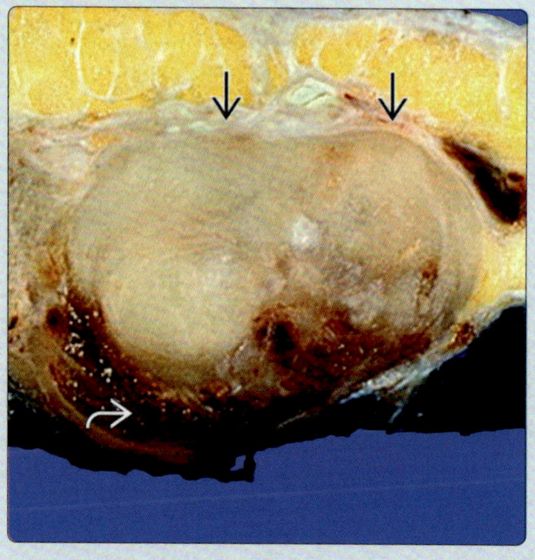

Monophasic Morphology

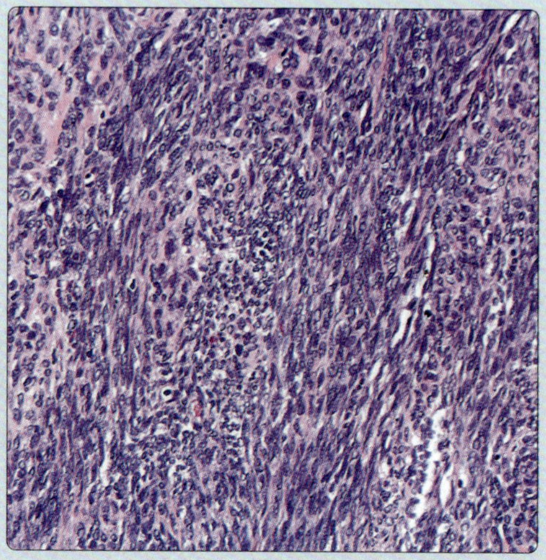

(Left) *Most cases of SS show areas with a high degree of cellularity, which imparts an overall blue or purple color to the tumor tissue at lower magnifications due to the increased nuclear density. Nuclear overlapping is a frequent feature.* **(Right)** *The majority of cases of SS show keratin &/or EMA positivity; however, expression is characteristically focal or patchy, often in a single-cell distribution, as depicted. Diffuse keratin or EMA expression in a spindle cell neoplasm should raise concerns for a different entity.*

High Cellularity

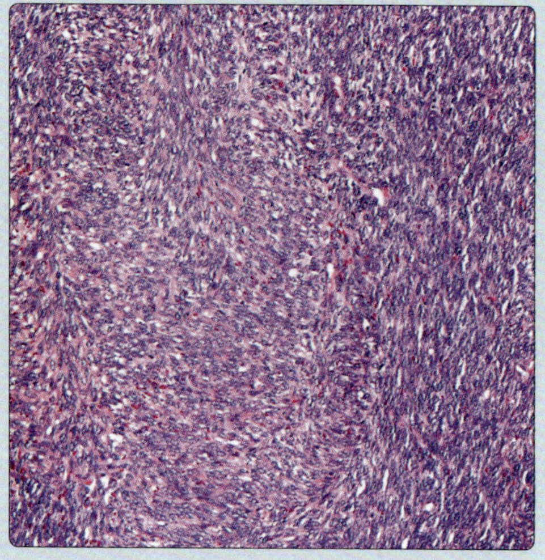

Keratin/EMA Expression

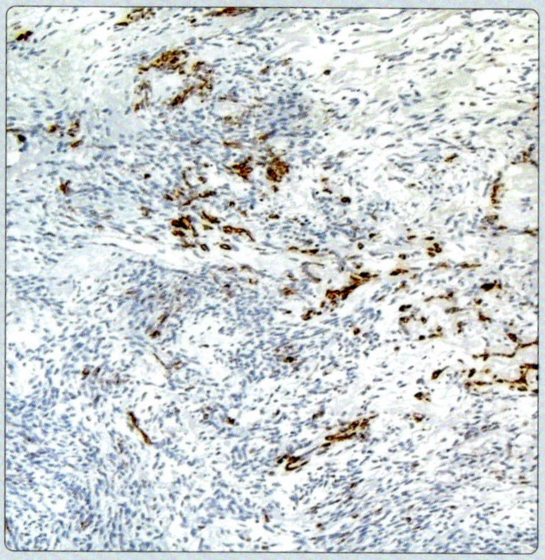

TERMINOLOGY

Abbreviations

- Synovial sarcoma (SS)

Synonyms

- Obsolete terms: Synovial cell sarcoma, malignant synovioma

Definitions

- Malignant mesenchymal spindle cell neoplasm with variable epithelial differentiation, including gland formation, and characterized by specific chromosomal translocation t(X;18)(p11;q11)
  - Despite its name, tumor does not arise from or differentiate toward synovium

CLINICAL ISSUES

Epidemiology

- Incidence
  - 5-10% of all soft tissue sarcomas
- Age
  - Most common in young adults (majority 10-40 years)
    - Rare over 50 years
- Sex
  - Slight male predominance
    - SS of peripheral nerve more common in females

Site

- Most arise in deep soft tissues of extremities
  - Most common near joints (particularly knee)
- Head and neck
  - Parapharynx, oral cavity, tonsil
- Trunk
- Rare subsets
  - Viscera (kidney, pleura, lung, other organs)
  - Retroperitoneum, mediastinum
  - Tumors arising within peripheral nerve
  - Male and female genital tracts
  - Central nervous system, bone

Presentation

- Deeply situated, slowly growing mass
  - Very rare superficial tumors
- 1/2 of cases associated with pain
- History of local trauma sometimes present
- Can be present for long period: 2-20 years

Treatment

- Complete surgical resection with negative margins
  - Usually limb sparing; amputation rarely required
- Resection of recurrences
  - May necessitate radical surgery, including amputation
- Pulmonary metastasectomy for small numbers of surgically accessible metastases
- Role of adjuvant therapy
  - Preoperative irradiation for large or initially unresectable primary tumor
  - Chemotherapy for disseminated disease

Prognosis

- Local recurrence common, especially following incomplete resection
- Metastasis in up to 50% of cases
  - Lung most common site
    - Late metastases can appear after many years
  - Small subset (5-10%) can spread to lymph nodes
- 5-year survival rate (50-85%)
  - Higher rate in children/adolescents
- Prognostic factors
  - Favorable
    - Small tumor size (< 5 cm)
      - Tumors < 1 cm have excellent prognosis
    - Occurrence in childhood
  - Unfavorable
    - Age > 40 years
    - Large tumor size
    - Poorly differentiated histology (> 20% component)
      - More common in elderly patients
    - High stage at presentation
  - Biphasic vs. monophasic morphology has no prognostic relevance

MACROSCOPIC

General Features

- Well circumscribed; can be multinodular
- Soft to firm, tan, gray, yellow, or pink cut surface
- Cystic change not uncommon
- Calcification &/or ossification may be seen

Size

- Usually 3-10 cm
  - Can be minute (< 1 cm) or > 15 cm

MICROSCOPIC

Histologic Features

- Monophasic SS
  - Dense cellular sheets or vague fascicles of uniform spindle cells with scanty cytoplasm
    - Relatively uniform, ovoid, bland nuclei, often overlapping
      - Lack significant pleomorphism
    - Highly variable mitotic rate (from sparse to numerous)
  - Rare herringbone or focal palisaded growth patterns
  - Variable collagenous stroma, often inconspicuous
    - Thickened bundles of "wiry" collagen can be seen
    - Myxoid stromal changes in some tumors (may be prominent)
    - Extensive stromal fibrosis and associated hypocellularity common in irradiated tumors
  - Stromal calcifications are identified in 30% of cases
    - Helpful diagnostic clue
    - May also show metaplastic bone formation
  - Stromal vasculature can be prominent
    - Also, focally "staghorn" or hemangiopericytoma-like
  - Mast cells common (may be prominent in some tumors)
  - Necrosis uncommon
  - Tumors arising within peripheral nerve often strikingly multinodular

- Biphasic SS
  - Contains same spindle cell population as monophasic SS (at least focally)
  - Additionally features epithelial structures
    - Can be focal/subtle or extensive/prominent
    - Glands (well or poorly formed), ducts, nests, and cords
      - Glandular lumina may contain eosinophilic secretions or mucin
      - Epithelial cells show more abundant cytoplasm
    - Rare squamous differentiation or granular cell change
- Poorly differentiated histology
  - Can be seen within monophasic or biphasic SS
    - May be focal or extensive
  - Characterized by hypercellularity, high-grade nuclear features, and increased mitoses
    - Nuclei often show irregular contours and "chunky" chromatin or prominent nucleoli
  - Spindle cell pattern can be highly fascicular
  - Round cell pattern resembles Ewing sarcoma
  - Necrosis more common
- Rare: Rhabdoid cells, clear cell change, rosette-like structures

ANCILLARY TESTS

Immunohistochemistry

- Keratin (+), EMA(+)
  - Characteristic focal/patchy expression in spindled cells
  - Strong expression in epithelial components (biphasic SS)
- Strong, diffuse nuclear TLE1(+)
  - Focal or weak expression is nonspecific
  - Diffuse TLE1 expression also reported in solitary fibrous tumor and biphenotypic sinonasal sarcoma (rare)
- Focal S100 protein (+) &/or SOX10(+) in up to 40% of cases
- CD56(+), CD99(+)
- Calretinin (+) in 40-70% of cases (may be diffuse)
- CD34, SMA, desmin, myogenin, PAX3, synaptophysin, TTF-1, NKX2.2 (-)
- Retention of H3K27me3 in most cases

Molecular Genetics

- Characteristic t(X;18)(p11;q11) in vast majority of tumors
  - One of SSX genes at Xp11 fuses to *SS18* gene (formerly termed SYT) at 18q11
    - May involve *SSX1* (most common), *SSX2*, or *SSX4*
  - Can utilize break-apart FISH for *SS18* (SYT) or RT-PCR for fusion transcripts
- Rare *SS18L1-SSX1* fusion variant reported (not detectable by standard *SS18* FISH)

DIFFERENTIAL DIAGNOSIS

Malignant Peripheral Nerve Sheath Tumor

- Can arise in association with neurofibromatosis type 1
- Nuclei wavy, buckled, or arrowhead-shaped
- Variable CD34(+) common
- Loss of nuclear H3K27me3 by IHC
- Keratin (-)
  - May show focal or weak TLE1(+)
- Lacks *SS18* (SYT) rearrangements

Fibrosarcomatous Dermatofibrosarcoma Protuberans (DFSP)

- Predominantly affects superficial soft tissues
- May be associated with areas of low-grade DFSP
- CD34(+) in some cases (may be patchy or absent)
- Keratin and TLE1 (-)
- Characteristic *COL1A1-PDGFB* fusion

Solitary Fibrous Tumor

- Characteristic dilated, irregular staghorn vasculature
- Stromal collagen usually prominent
- Strong, diffuse CD34(+), STAT6(+); keratin (-)
- Rare tumors can show diffuse TLE1(+)
- Characteristic *NAB2-STAT6* fusion

Ewing Sarcoma

- Can mimic poorly differentiated SS
- Small round cell morphology without spindle cells or epithelial structures
- Diffuse membranous CD99(+); also, NKX2.2(+)
- CD56(-)
- *EWSR1* translocations in vast majority of cases

BCOR-CCNB3 (Ewing-Like) Sarcoma

- Can mimic poorly differentiated SS
- CD99(+), TLE-1 (variable)
- Lacks *SS18* (SYT) rearrangement

Leiomyosarcoma

- Most tumors show prominent eosinophilic cytoplasm
- Nuclear pleomorphism common
- SMA(+), H-caldesmon (+), variable desmin (+)
- Generally keratin and EMA (-)

Biphasic Sinonasal Sarcoma

- Closely resembles monophasic SS
- Some tumors feature rhabdomyoblastic differentiation
- Expression of myogenic markers (SMA, desmin, myogenin)
- PAX3(+); S100 protein (+); SOX10(-)
- Characterized by *PAX3-MAML3* fusion

SELECTED REFERENCES

1. Terra SBSP et al: Mediastinal synovial sarcoma: clinicopathologic analysis of 21 cases with molecular confirmation. Am J Surg Pathol. 42(6):761-766, 2018
2. Chrisinger JSA et al: Synovial sarcoma of peripheral nerves: analysis of 15 cases. Am J Surg Pathol. 41(8):1087-96, 2017
3. El Beaino M et al: Synovial sarcoma: advances in diagnosis and treatment identification of new biologic targets to improve multimodal therapy. Ann Surg Oncol. 24(8):2145-2154, 2017
4. Kao YC et al: BCOR upregulation in a poorly differentiated synovial sarcoma with SS18L1-SSX1 fusion-a pathologic and molecular pitfall. Genes Chromosomes Cancer. 56(4):296-302, 2017
5. Schaefer IM et al: Loss of H3K27 trimethylation distinguishes malignant peripheral nerve sheath tumors from histologic mimics. Mod Pathol. 29(1):4-13, 2016
6. Thway K et al: Synovial sarcoma: defining features and diagnostic evolution. Ann Diagn Pathol. 18(6):369-80, 2014
7. Shi W et al: Long-term treatment outcomes for patients with synovial sarcoma: a 40-year experience at the University of Florida. Am J Clin Oncol. 36(1):83-8, 2013
8. Knösel T et al: TLE1 is a robust diagnostic biomarker for synovial sarcomas and correlates with t(X;18): analysis of 319 cases. Eur J Cancer. 46(6):1170-6, 2010
9. Michal M et al: Minute synovial sarcomas of the hands and feet: a clinicopathologic study of 21 tumors less than 1 cm. Am J Surg Pathol. 30(6):721-6, 2006

Monomorphic Cytology

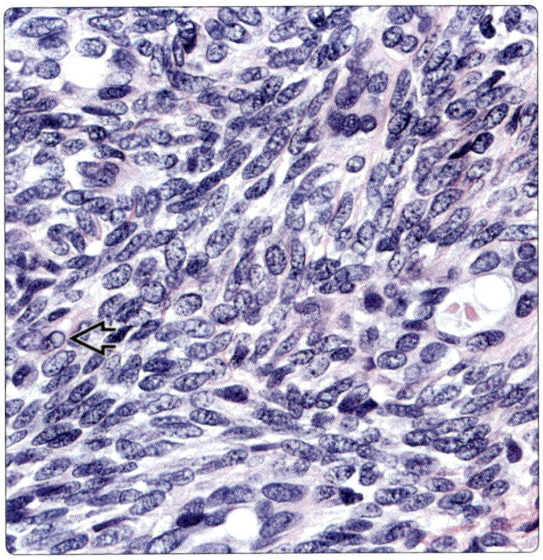

Variations in Cellularity

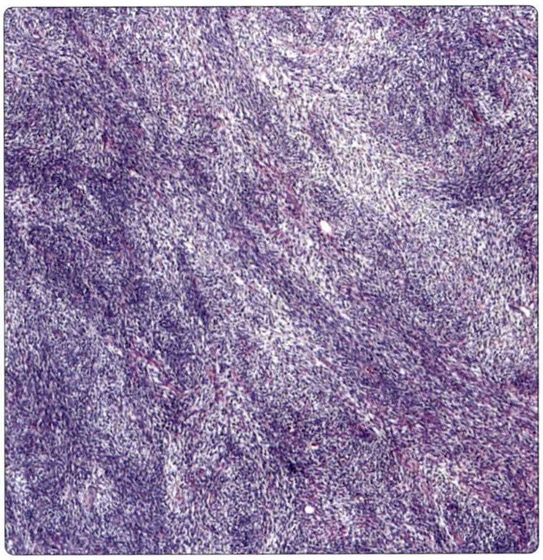

(Left) *Relatively bland, hyperchromatic, and monomorphic nuclei are a constant feature of SS, and significant nuclear pleomorphism in a spindle cell sarcoma should lead to consideration of another diagnosis, such as MPNST. Optically clear nuclear pseudoinclusions ⇨ are common and may be numerous.* **(Right)** *Although many cases of SS are evenly cellular, variations in cellularity may also be seen, as depicted, creating an alternating marbled pattern similar to MPNST.*

Fascicular Growth

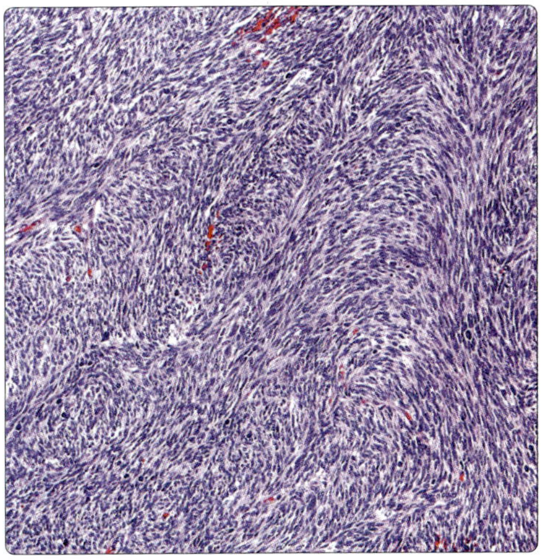

Neural-Like Fascicles

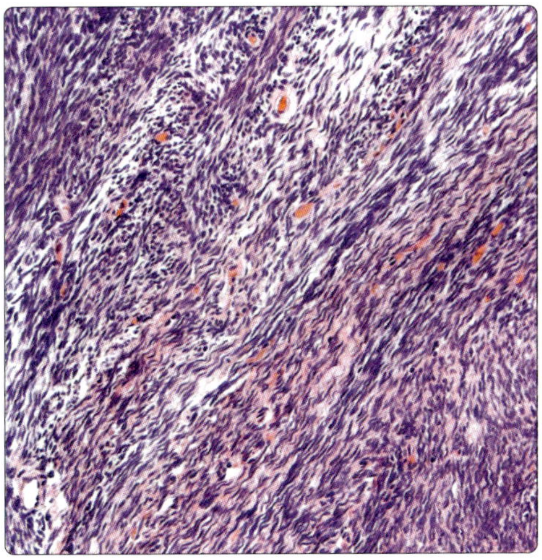

(Left) *Vague or loose fascicular growth is common in SS. In some cases, fascicles are well formed and quite prominent and can even show a focal herringbone pattern of growth, as demonstrated in this H&E.* **(Right)** *On occasion, the spindle cells of monophasic SS may appear highly compressed and with hyperchromatic, wavy nuclei, imparting a neural cytomorphology, as shown. A diagnosis of MPNST should always be considered and excluded in these cases.*

Loose, Hypocellular Areas

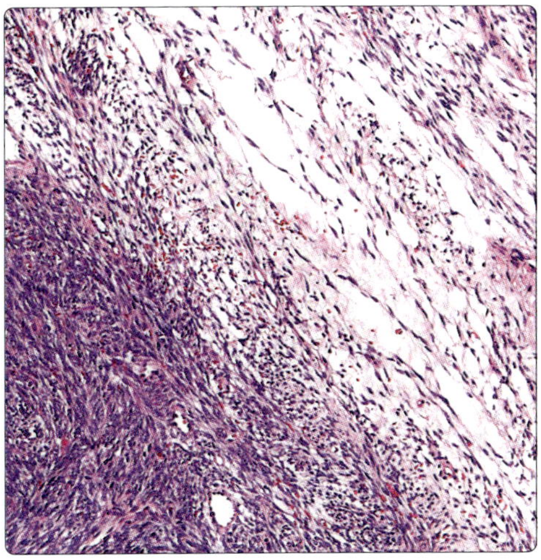

Stromal Calcifications

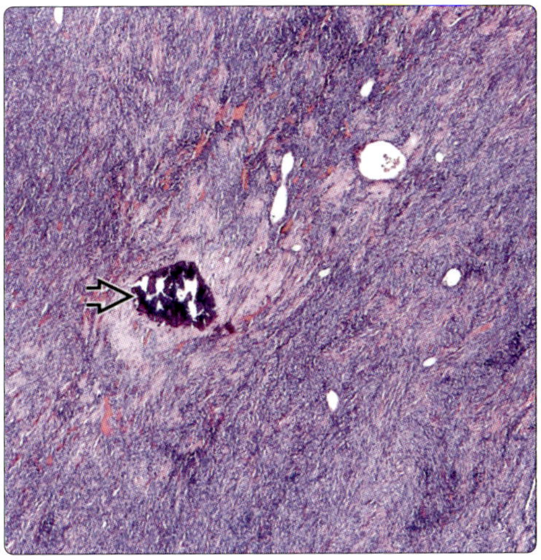

(Left) *Most cases of SS are not diffusely cellular. Some areas are hypocellular secondary to stromal edema, myxoid change, or fibrosis. Familiarity with the entire spectrum of cellularity in SS is important to avoid underdiagnosis.* **(Right)** *Stromal calcifications ⇨ are a characteristic feature of SS and can be seen in up to 30-40% of cases. They are usually unassociated with hemorrhage or evidence of trauma. In helpful contrast, these calcifications are not generally a feature of the morphologically similar MPNST.*

(Left) *Although not always apparent due to the frequent high cellularity of the tumor, a fine eosinophilic collagenous stroma is present in SS. Variably conspicuous, irregular, thin collagen fibers* ➔ *are often described as wiry but can appear as thicker bundles.* **(Right)** *In some cases of SS, the stromal collagen is more prominent and may appear as hyalinized bands, as depicted. Note the presence of stromal calcifications.*

Wiry Stromal Collagen

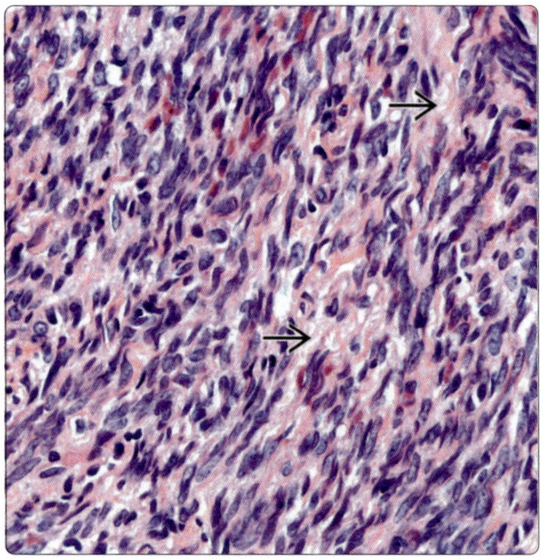

Prominent Stromal Collagen

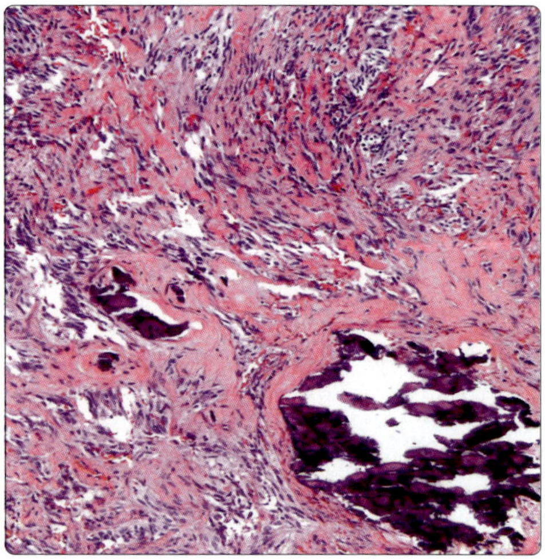

(Left) *Diffuse stromal hyalinization or sclerosis may be seen de novo in rare cases of SS. However, this morphology is much more frequent following radiation therapy or chemotherapy.* **(Right)** *Diffusely hyalinized or fibrotic cases of SS show marked hypocellularity compared to conventional forms and maintain the characteristic cellular monomorphism. A vague fascicular pattern may also be present in these cases.*

Diffuse Hyalinization

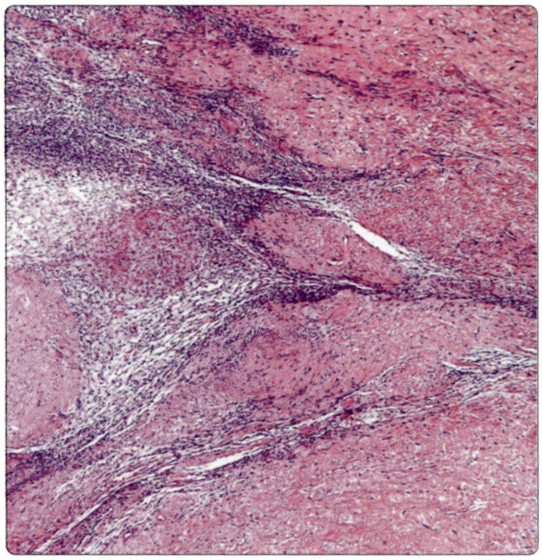

Diffuse Hyalinization

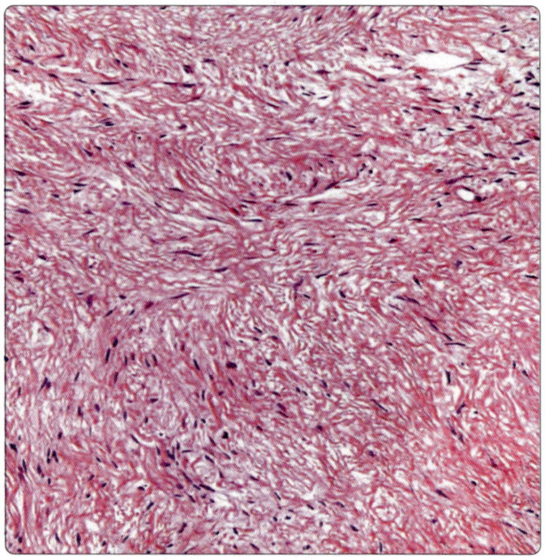

(Left) *Metaplastic bone* ➔ *may be seen in a minority of cases of SS and often shows a mature, lamellar composition with mineralization. This H&E was taken from a pulmonary metastasis of SS following chemotherapy. Note the diffuse fibrosis.* **(Right)** *In rare cases of SS, calcification &/or metaplastic bone formation* ➔ *is extensive and dominates the histologic picture, as shown. The cellularity of this variant is often less than usual and, therefore, may be potentially misdiagnosed as a benign neoplasm.*

Metaplastic Bone Formation

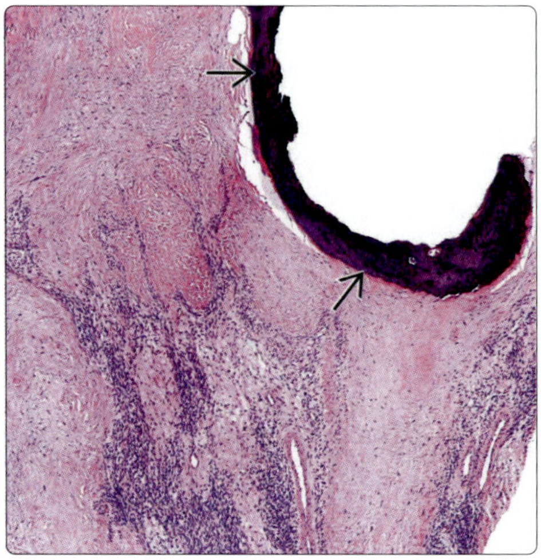

Metaplastic Bone Formation

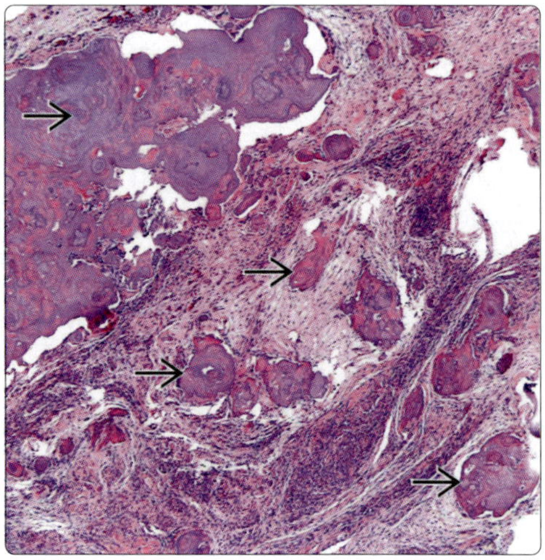

Myxoid Stroma

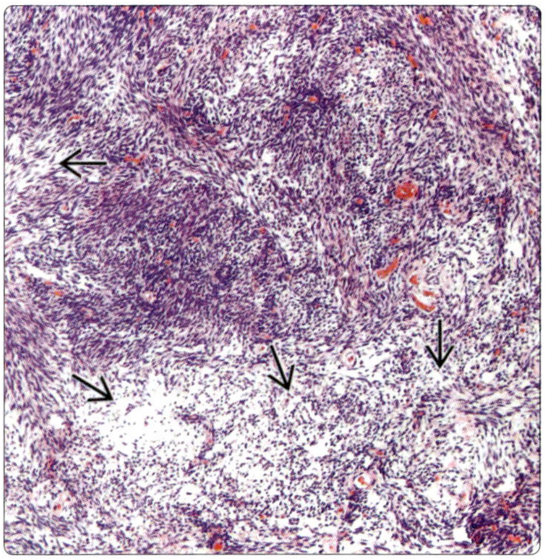

Diffuse Myxoid Stroma

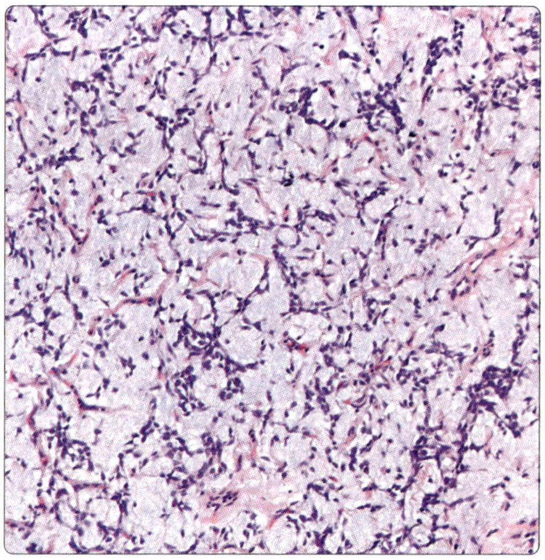

(Left) *Myxoid stroma ⇨ is a relatively common finding in SS but is often minor and overshadowed by more conventional highly cellular areas. The interface between myxoid and nonmyxoid zones may be gradual or abrupt.* **(Right)** *In rare cases of SS, myxoid stroma is diffuse and prominent and may easily lead to confusion with a variety of other myxoid sarcomas. Identification of areas of more typical morphology or utilization of ancillary studies can be very helpful.*

Myxoid Stroma

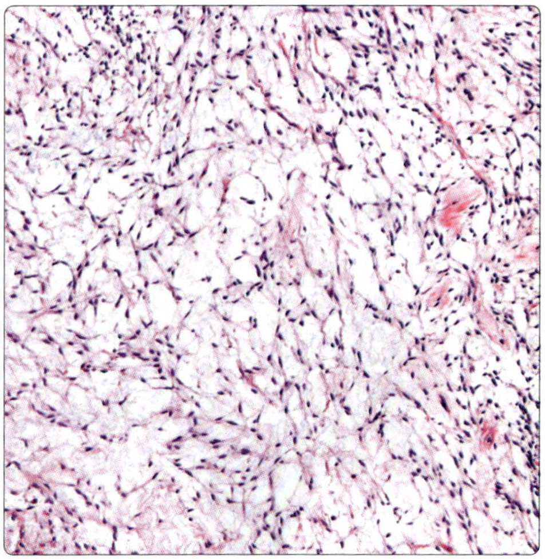

Stromal Vasculature

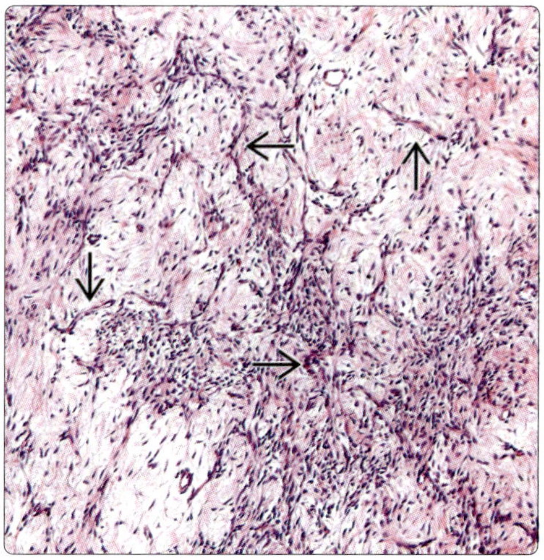

(Left) *The characteristic cellular uniformity or monomorphism of SS is maintained even in highly myxoid areas, as depicted in this H&E. Note the relative blandness of the nuclei, mimicking a low-grade or benign neoplasm.* **(Right)** *Infrequently, some areas of SS may show a more loose, fibromyxoid stroma in which thin-walled blood vessels ⇨ become more prominent. On biopsy, this appearance can lead to confusion with low-grade fibromyxoid sarcoma or myxofibrosarcoma.*

Pleural Synovial Sarcoma

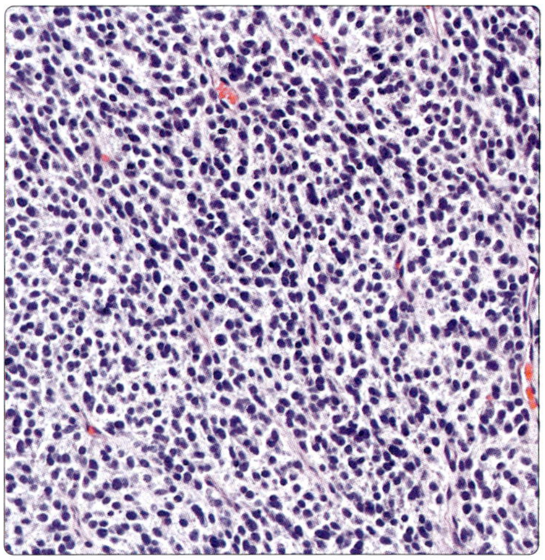

Lung Metastasis

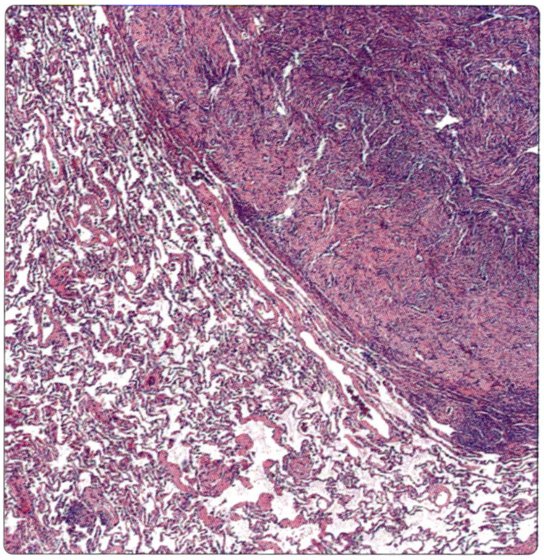

(Left) *This unusual case of SS arising in the pleura shows a prominent myxoid stroma and a more ovoid cytomorphology. Cytologic atypia was mild, and mitoses were not abundant. FISH analysis confirmed the presence of an SS18 (SYT) rearrangement.* **(Right)** *The most common site of metastasis for synovial sarcoma is the lung. Although often histologically similar to the primary tumor, cases of treated/irradiated SS can produce metastatic deposits that are heavily collagenized, resembling pulmonary or subpleural scars.*

(Left) *Nuclear expression of TLE1 has been found to be a highly sensitive marker of SS. It is also relatively specific when the staining is strong and diffuse, as shown. However, solitary fibrous tumor can occasionally show similar positivity. Weak &/or focal expression is nonspecific and may be seen in a variety of other tumors.* **(Right)** *Strong CD56 expression is a common finding in SS. Awareness of this expression is important to avoid confusion with high-grade neuroendocrine carcinoma, particularly in poorly differentiated SS.*

TLE1 Expression

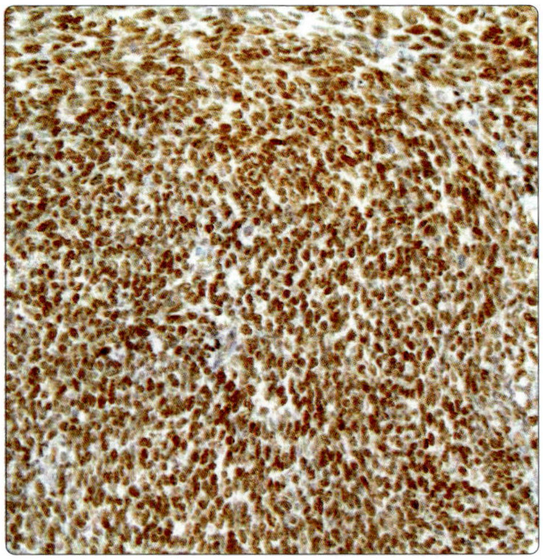

CD56 Expression

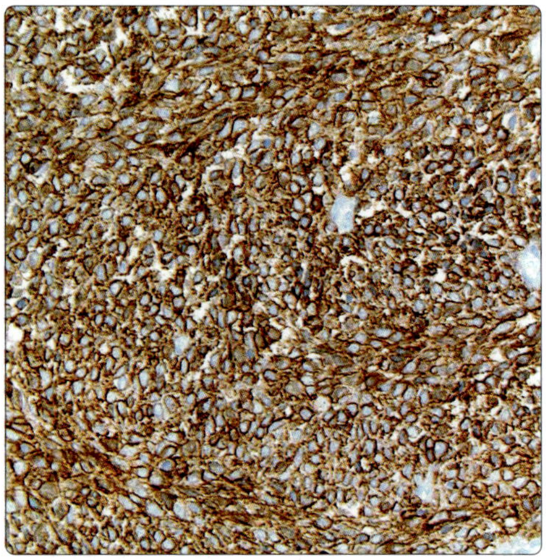

(Left) *CD99 expression is often present in SS. Notably, in poorly differentiated forms with a round cell morphology, membranous expression of this antigen can lead to consideration of Ewing sarcoma. Molecular evaluation is diagnostic in this scenario.* **(Right)** *Mast cells ➜ are a frequent finding in SS; however, the exact number varies widely from tumor to tumor. In some cases, they can be quite prominent, as depicted in this H&E.*

CD99 Expression

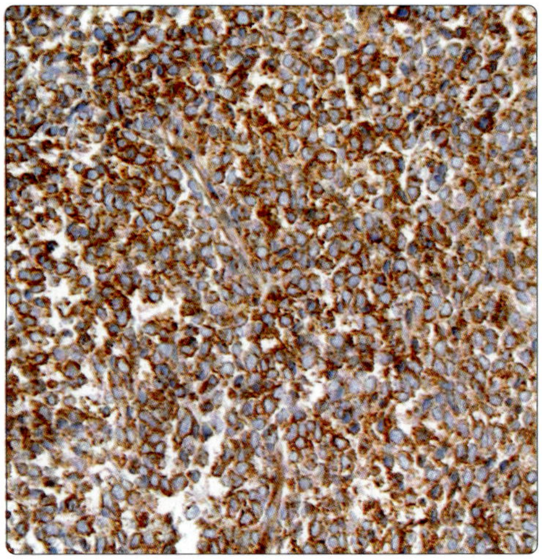

Mast Cells

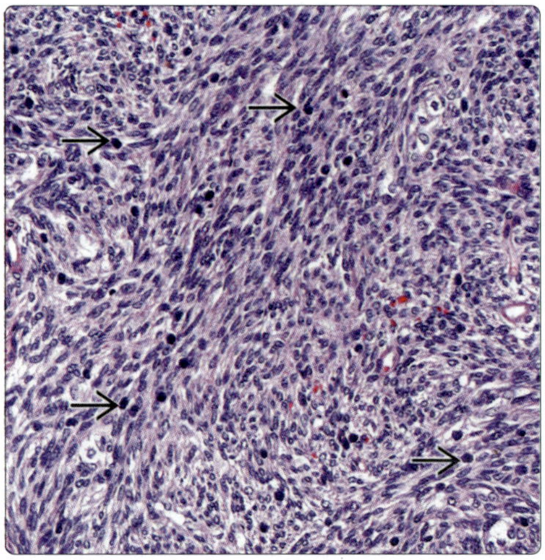

(Left) *Mast cells ➜ may also be noted in hypocellular fibrous or myxoid areas of SS. Given the additional feature of elongated and wavy nuclei, as seen in this H&E, a tumor of neural origin may be considered.* **(Right)** *Hemorrhage may be seen in SS, both grossly and microscopically. In occasional tumors, the presence of extravasated red blood cells among uniform spindled cells can impart an appearance somewhat reminiscent of Kaposi sarcoma.*

Mast Cells

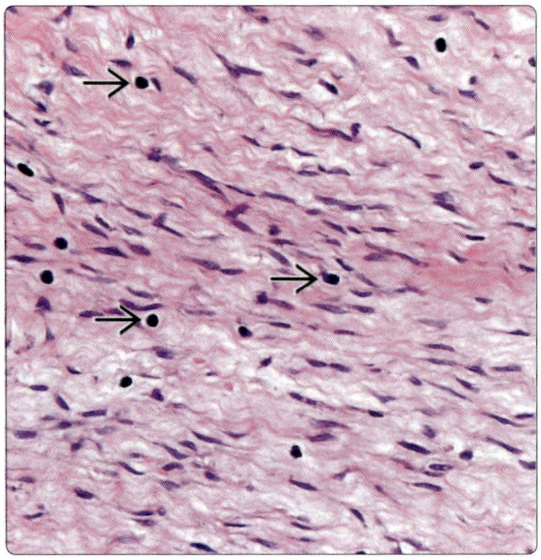

Hemorrhage

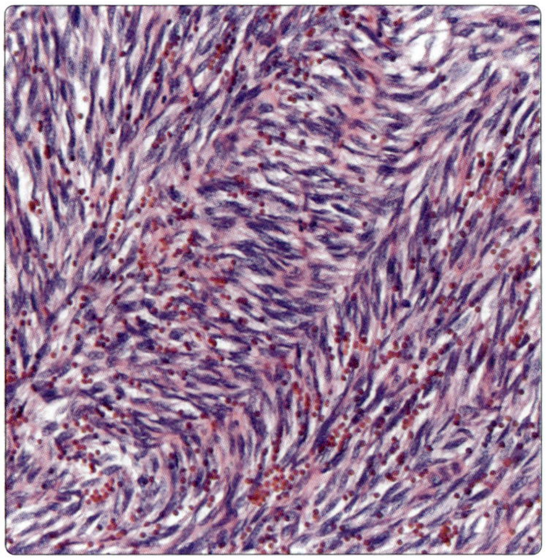

Multinodular Growth

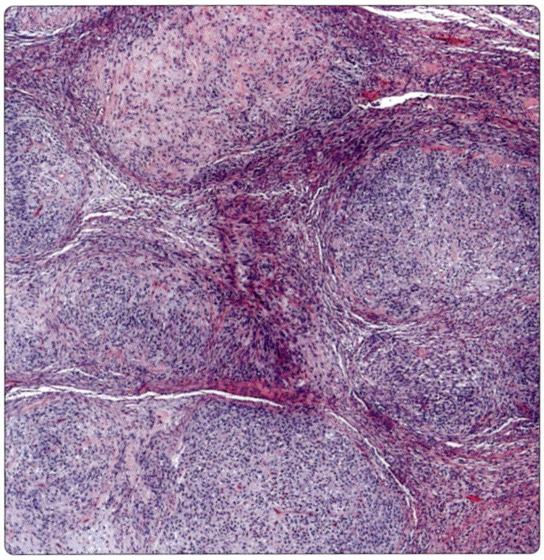

Occasional Whorling Pattern

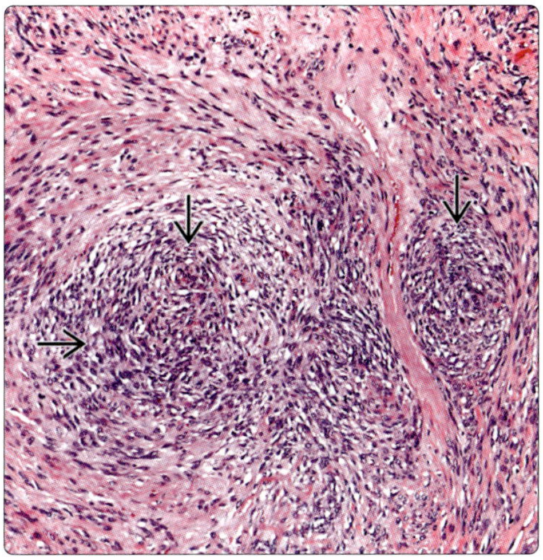

(Left) *A vaguely nodular growth pattern may be seen in rare cases of monophasic SS and may lead to confusion with other entities, including low-grade fibromyxoid sarcoma. A multinodular pattern is also typical of SS arising from the peripheral nerve.* **(Right)** *Whorled foci ➙ are a rare and unusual finding in SS and may be seen in either hypercellular or hypocellular collagenous areas. However, this finding should prompt exclusion of a neural neoplasm, particularly MPNST.*

Biphasic Morphology

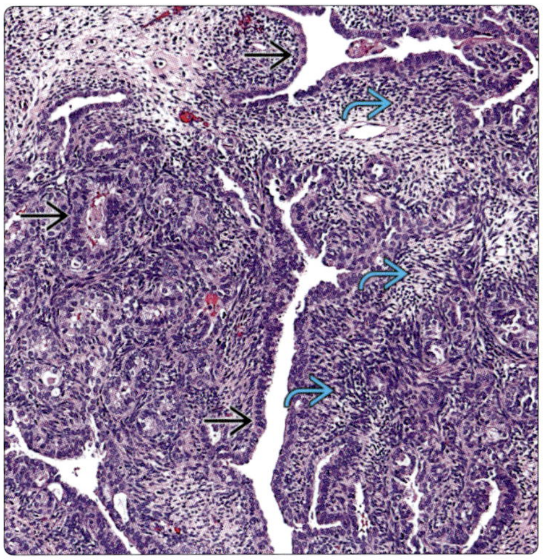

Well-Formed Glands

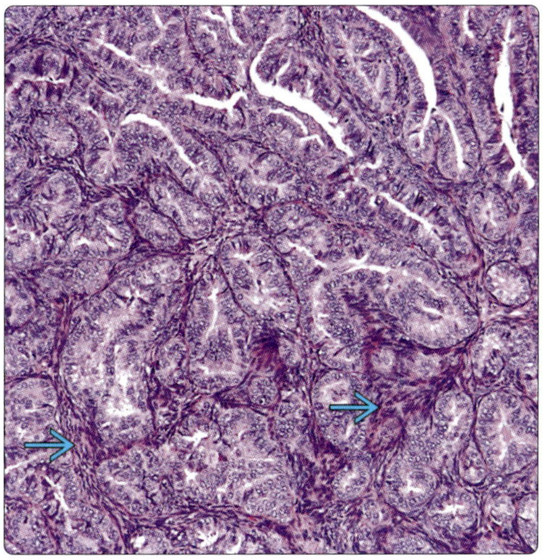

(Left) *Biphasic SS is best conceptualized as a typical monophasic spindled SS but with the formation of epithelial structures, including glands ➙, ducts, or nests. The conventional spindled component ➙ is essentially always present but may be extremely focal.* **(Right)** *The epithelial cells of biphasic SS may be arranged as well-formed glands or ducts, as depicted. This appearance may at first suggest a well- or moderately differentiated adenocarcinoma; however, note the spindle cell component ➙.*

Cystic Glands

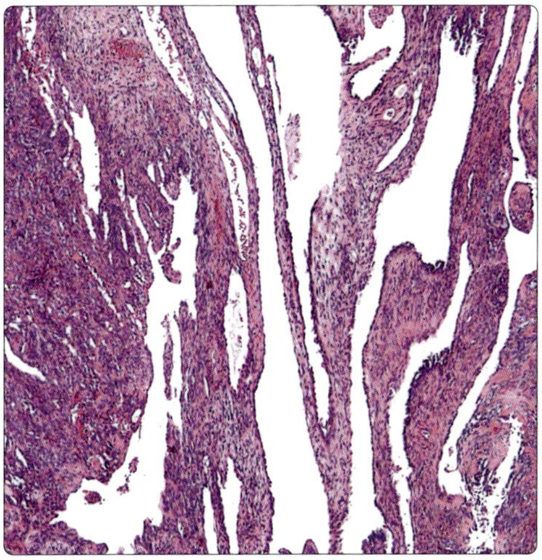

Pseudopapillary Appearance

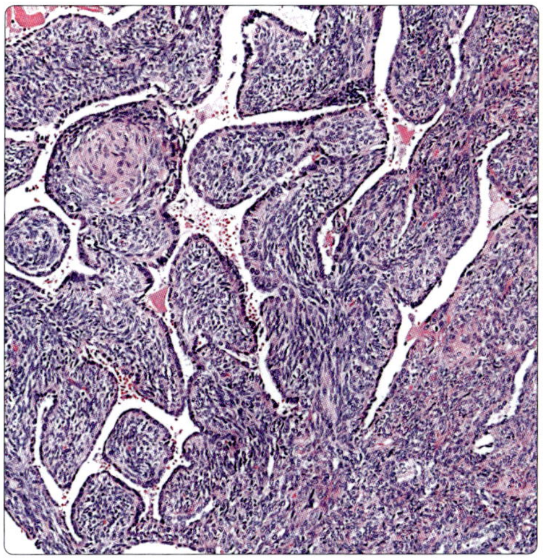

(Left) *Glandular structures in biphasic SS may exhibit cystic change and may become quite prominent in some cases. Larger cysts can often be identified grossly.* **(Right)** *Occasionally, the glandular component of biphasic SS appears ramifying and labyrinthine, creating a pseudopapillary appearance. This pattern can resemble that seen in malignant phyllodes tumor of the breast.*

(Left) *A characteristic finding in biphasic SS is the presence of inspissated eosinophilic secretions ➩ within the glandular or ductular lumina of the tumor. Also note the cytologic features of the epithelial component: Round to oval nuclei without significant pleomorphism.* **(Right)** *Mucin ➩ may also be produced by glands in biphasic SS. This particular case also shows epithelial cells with clear cytoplasm ➩ focally.*

Intraluminal Eosinophilic Secretions

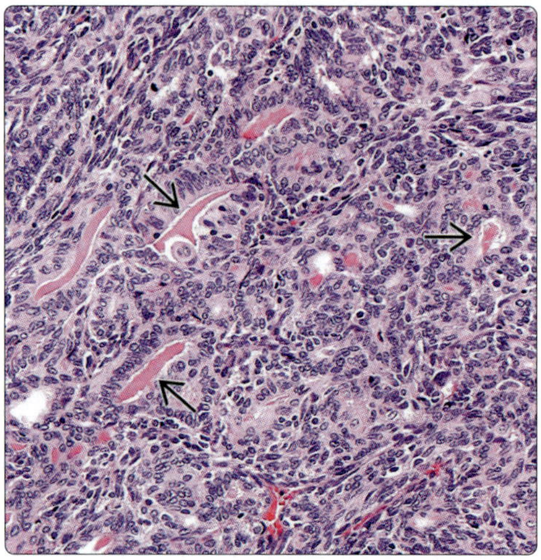

Intraluminal Mucin

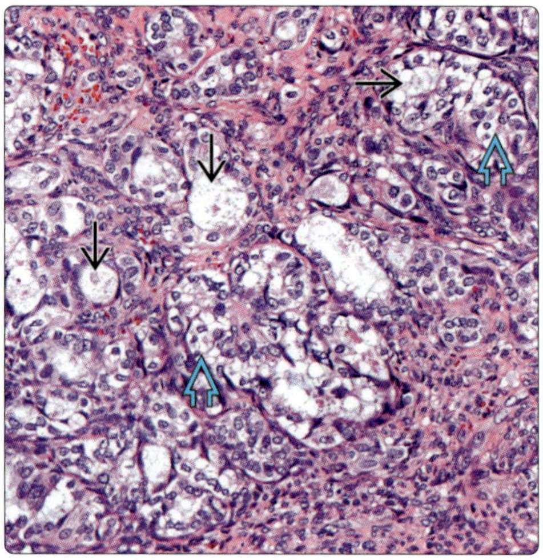

(Left) *The glandular component of biphasic SS may appear highly complex and, in conjunction with the presence of granular eosinophilic secretions ➩ (resembling necrosis), can easily mimic primary or metastatic adenocarcinoma, depending on the site.* **(Right)** *The epithelial component of biphasic SS may comprise the vast majority of a given tumor suggesting the existence of a pure "monophasic epithelial" SS; however, focal spindle cell areas ➩ are essentially always found if carefully sought.*

Adenocarcinoma-Like Morphology

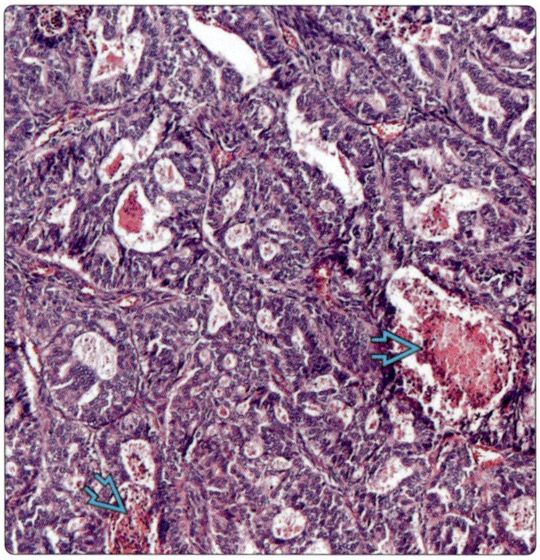

Predominant Biphasic Morphology

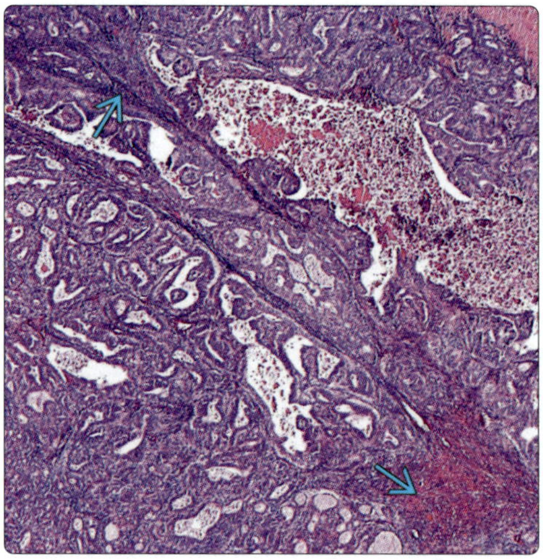

(Left) *Some cases of biphasic SS may show focal myxoid stromal changes ➩ around the glands, mimicking a desmoplastic response to the tumor often seen in many forms of invasive carcinoma.* **(Right)** *Glands may be poorly formed in biphasic SS and appear as distinct, variably sized nests of epithelioid cells, as depicted. Note the presence of eosinophilic secretions ➩, revealing subtle lumina formation.*

Focal Pseudodesmoplastic Stroma

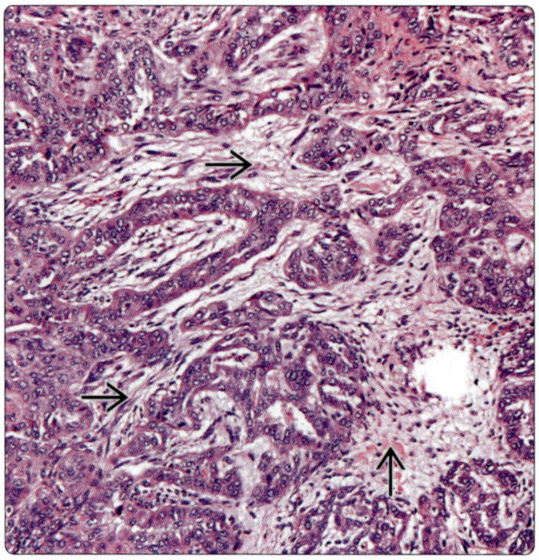

Nests and Poorly Formed Glands

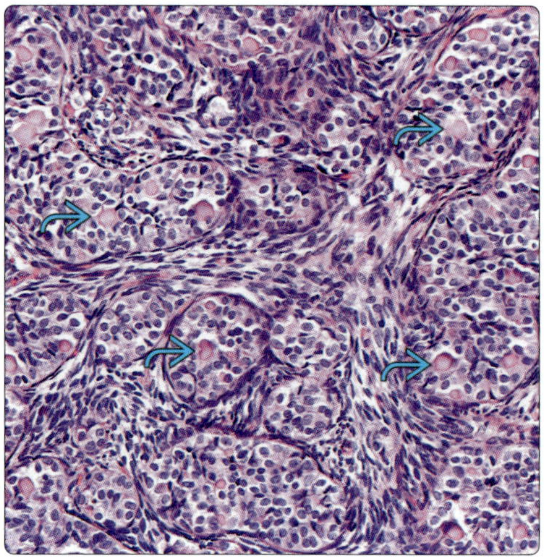

Poorly Formed Epithelial Nests/Cords

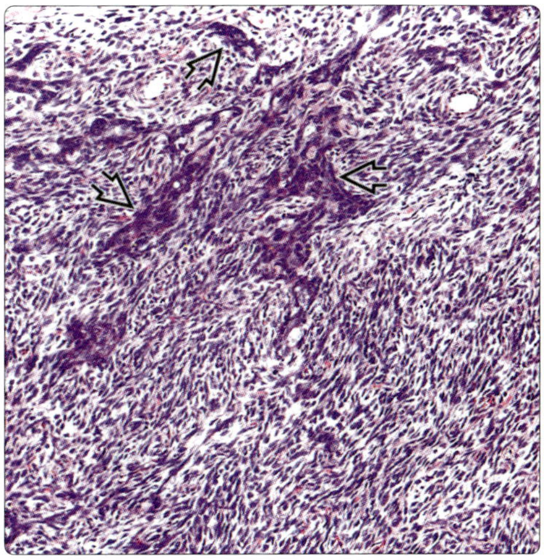

Syncytia-Like Trabecular Morphology

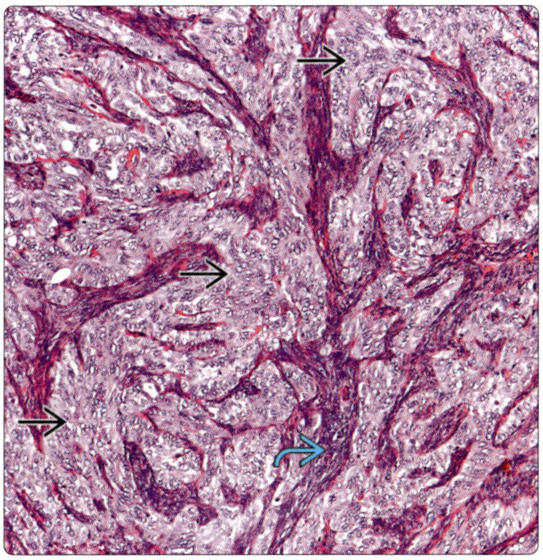

(Left) *In some cases of biphasic SS, the epithelial component is very poorly formed and can appear as irregular nests or cords ⇨ of enlarged tumor cells. These vague structures are often strongly keratin and EMA (+).* **(Right)** *Biphasic SS may contain an extensive epithelial component → that manifests histologically as broad, serpentine trabeculae or sheets of large, pale cells in a syncytia-like arrangement, admixed with a more conventional spindle cell component ↪.*

Subtle Biphasic Component

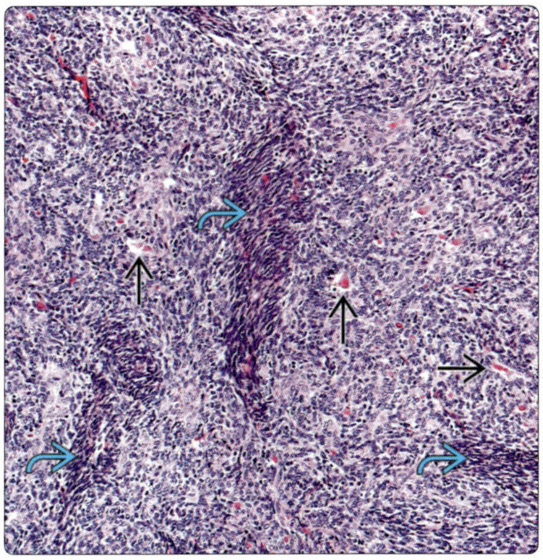

Biphasic With Sclerosis

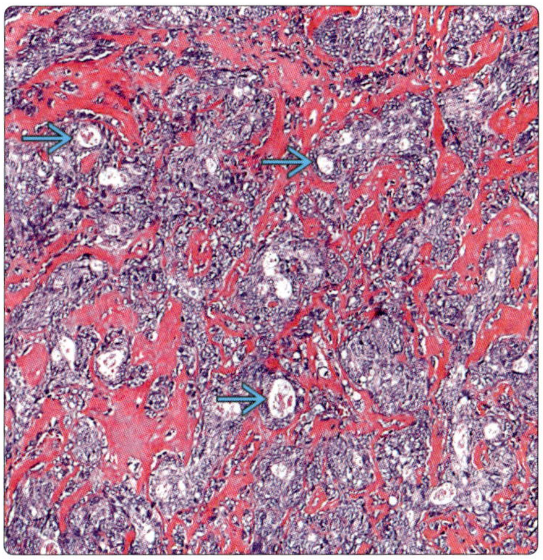

(Left) *At 1st glance, this H&E of SS may appear monophasic; however, closer inspection reveals subtle gland formation (with secretions →) within a very vague and poorly developed epithelial component. Note the focal spindled component ↪.* **(Right)** *This unusual case of biphasic SS showed the characteristic epithelial component → but within a markedly hyalinized/sclerotic stromal matrix.*

Rare Squamous Metaplasia

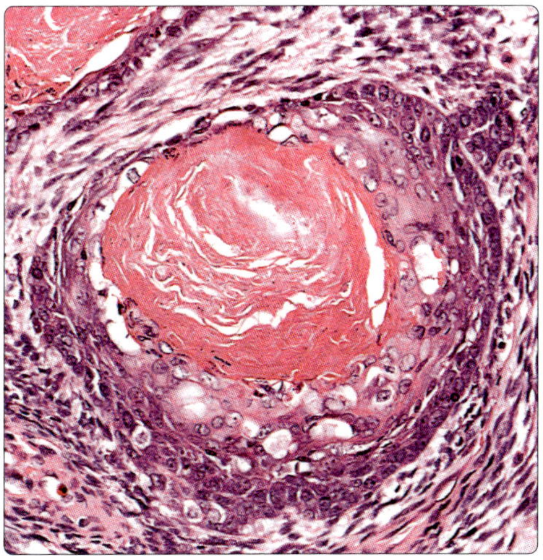

Strong Keratin Expression

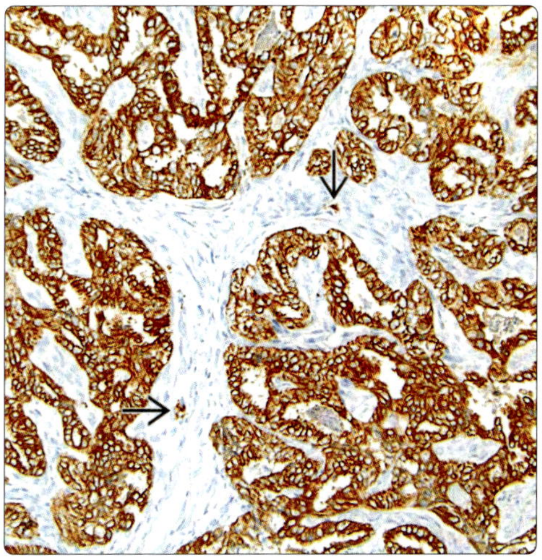

(Left) *Squamous metaplasia with central keratinization is a rare, but well-described finding in the epithelial component of biphasic SS.* **(Right)** *Keratin (shown) and EMA are typically strongly expressed within the epithelial component of biphasic SS, as depicted, similar to conventional epithelial cells. In contrast, the spindle cell component is often focally positive → in a single cell pattern, as is seen in pure monophasic SS.*

(Left) *Poorly differentiated areas may be present within otherwise typical monophasic or biphasic SS and are often hypercellular with abundant mitotic figures ➦. In some cases, the entire tumor is poorly differentiated. The morphology may be spindled/fascicular or round cell.* **(Right)** *Poorly differentiated foci in SS are most readily identified by the presence of severe nuclear atypia, including nuclear enlargement and contour irregularity, and a "chunky" or "clumpy" chromatin ➔ distribution.*

Poorly Differentiated Morphology

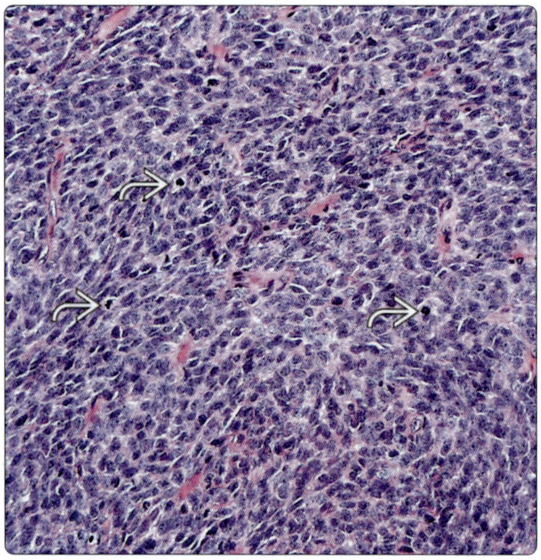

Severe Nuclear Atypia

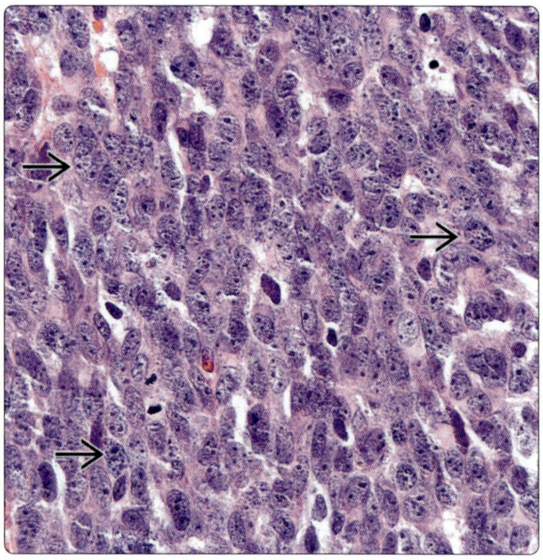

(Left) *Prominent nucleoli ➦ are also a common finding in poorly differentiated SS and can aid in recognition of these higher grade areas.* **(Right)** *Coagulative tumor necrosis ➩ is not a frequent finding in conventional monophasic or biphasic SS; however, it is much more common in poorly differentiated areas, as depicted. The necrosis may be focal or rarely extensive and geographic.*

Prominent Nucleoli

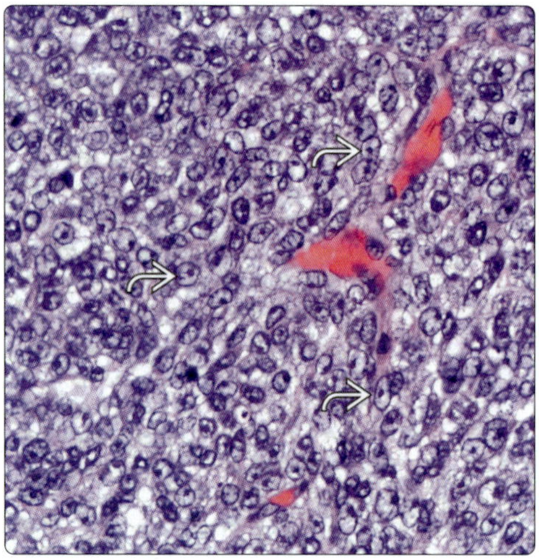

Coagulative Necrosis

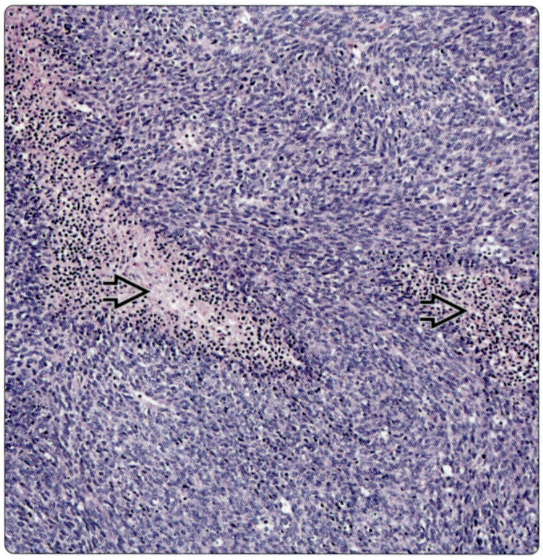

(Left) *Poorly differentiated SS can manifest histologically with a round cell morphology (center) similar to a variety of "round blue cell tumors," including Ewing sarcoma, alveolar rhabdomyosarcoma, and neuroendocrine carcinoma. These round cell areas often "stick out" from more conventional areas ➡ of SS, if present.* **(Right)** *The round cell pattern of poorly differentiated SS can appear as nests and cords within a fibrocollagenous or myxoid stroma, as depicted. Cytologically, these cells differ from those of biphasic SS.*

Round Cell Morphology

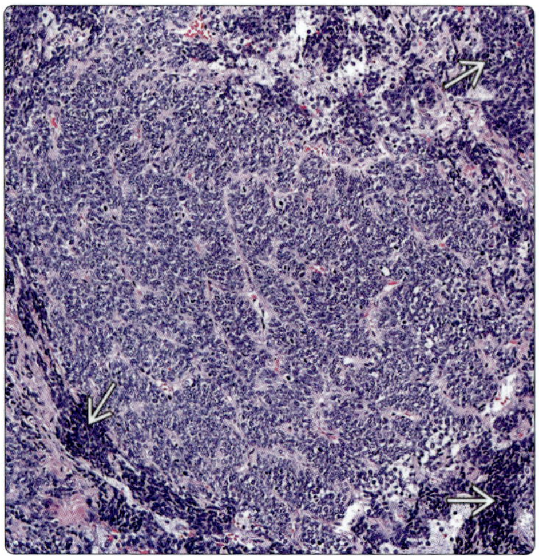

Nested Round Cell Morphology

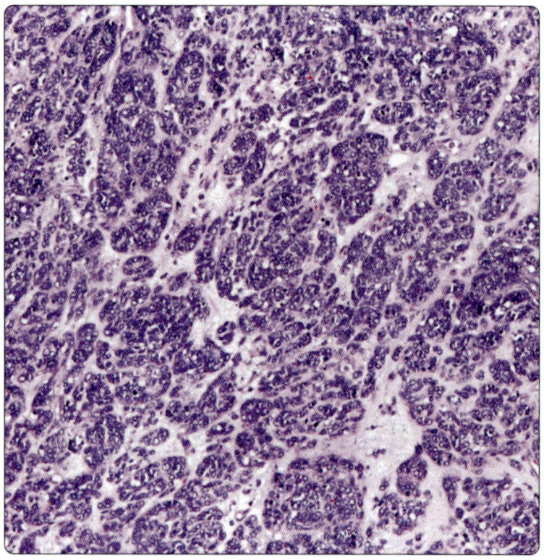

Poorly Differentiated With Sclerosis

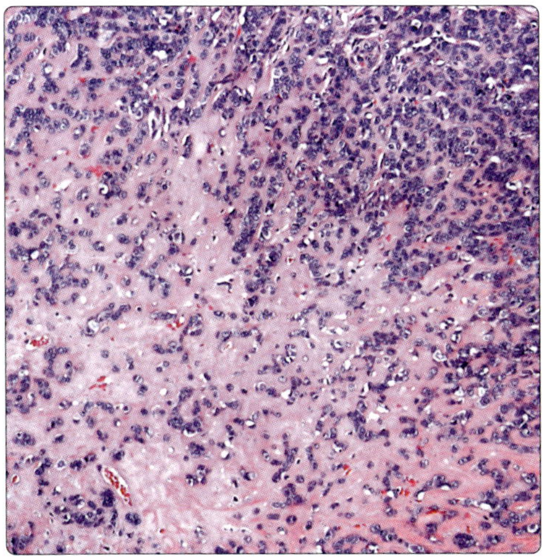

Rhabdoid Cells

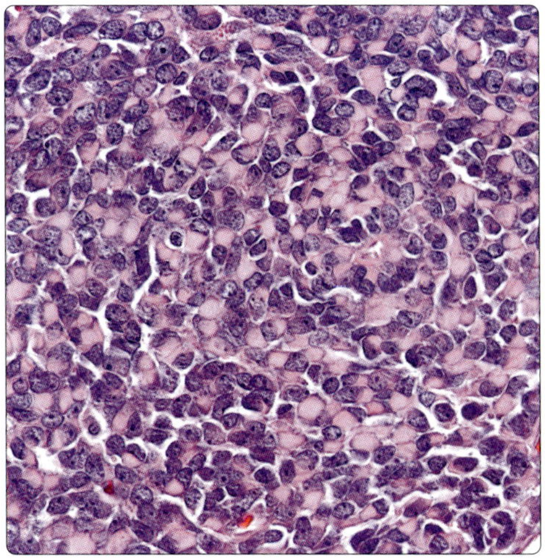

(Left) *Stromal hyalinization may be seen in areas of poorly differentiated SS with round cell morphology, as depicted. In general, however, prominent stromal collagen is more common in conventional SS.* **(Right)** *A distinctive rhabdoid cytomorphology may be identified in some cases of poorly differentiated SS.*

Rare Clear Cell Change

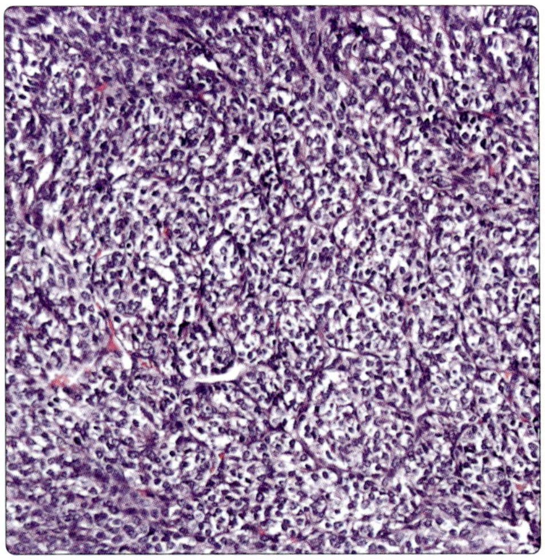

Rare Nuclear Palisading

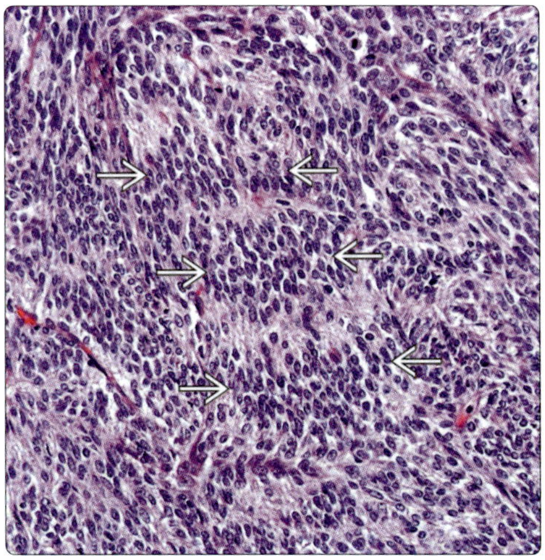

(Left) *H&E shows a rare case of poorly differentiated SS with areas of clear cell change.* **(Right)** *Vague nuclear palisades ➡ may be seen in rare cases of SS (often in poorly differentiated areas); however, in general, the palisades are not as well formed as what is typically seen in some neural tumors.*

Prominent, Ectatic Stromal Vasculature

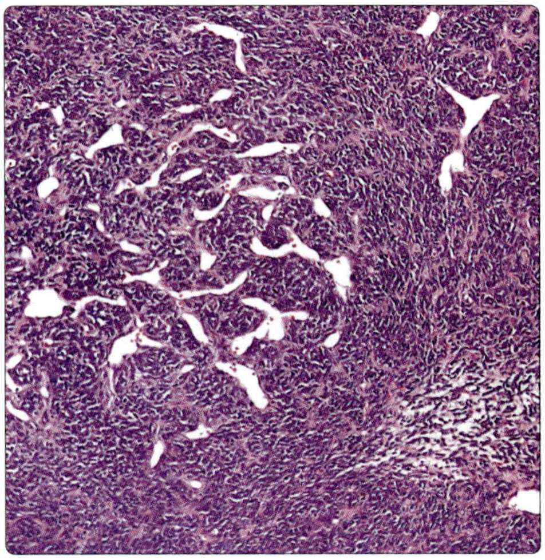

Rare Hemangiopericytoma-Like Pattern

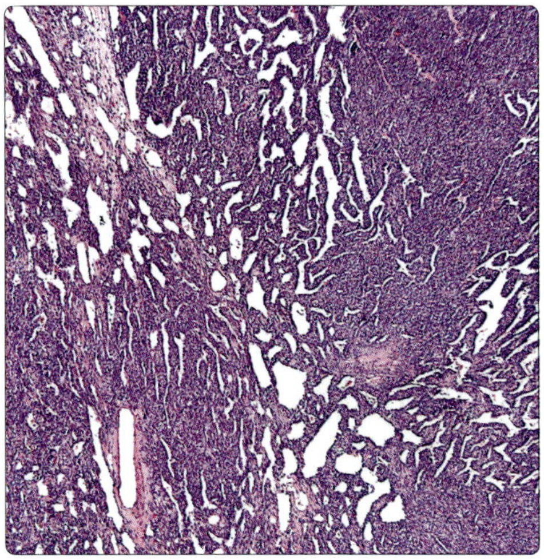

(Left) *Scattered, dilated stromal blood vessels are not uncommon in SS; however, they are more common and often more prominent in poorly differentiated areas. A staghorn appearance may also be present, as depicted.* **(Right)** *Rarely, the vasculature of SS is impressively prominent, as depicted, and can lead to confusion with a cellular solitary fibrous tumor (previously termed hemangiopericytoma).*

Epithelioid Sarcoma

KEY FACTS

TERMINOLOGY

- Distinctive malignant mesenchymal neoplasm that often shows epithelioid cytomorphology and demonstrates evidence of epithelial differentiation
  - Classic ES most commonly affects adolescents and young adults and arises in distal extremities
  - Proximal-type ES tends to affect older age groups (median: 40 years), arises in proximal locations, and is often more clinically aggressive

CLINICAL ISSUES

- Classic ES may appear clinically as nonhealing ulcer
- Clinically aggressive sarcoma
  - High rate of recurrence and metastases
    - Metastases to lymph nodes, lung, and skin

MICROSCOPIC

- Classic ES
  - Nodules with central necrosis (granuloma like)
  - Epithelioid and spindled cells with eosinophilic cytoplasm and uniform, irregular, mildly atypical nuclei
  - Rare predominantly spindled tumors (fibroma-like ES)
- Proximal-type ES
  - Large, cellular nodules of polygonal cells with prominent macronucleoli
  - Rhabdoid morphology common

ANCILLARY TESTS

- Keratin (+); also, CD34(+) in 50%
- Complete loss of nuclear INI1 protein expression
- Molecular: High frequency of *SMARCB1* (*INI1*) deletion (22q11)

TOP DIFFERENTIAL DIAGNOSES

- Granulomatous processes
- Carcinoma or melanoma
- Extrarenal rhabdoid tumor
- Epithelioid angiosarcoma

Epithelioid Sarcoma

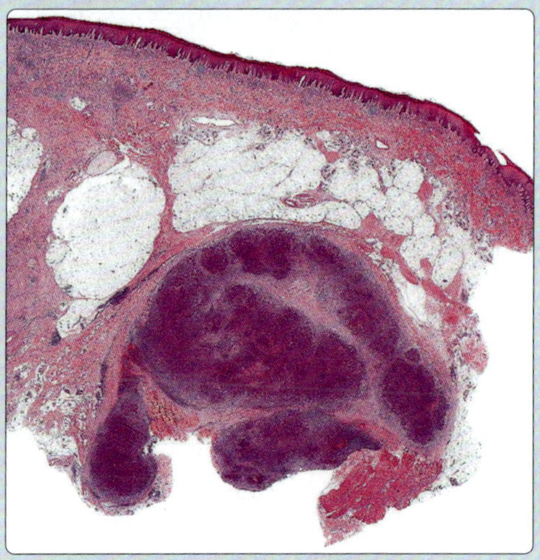

Pseudogranulomatous Morphology

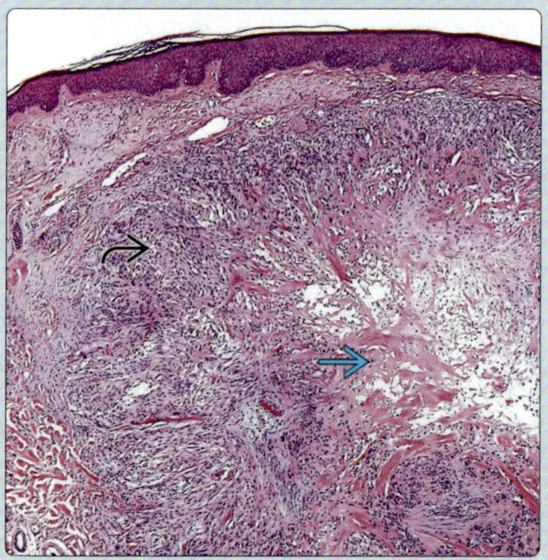

(Left) *Epithelioid sarcoma (ES) is a distinctive malignant mesenchymal neoplasm that classically arises on the distal extremities of adolescents and young adults and shows immunohistochemical evidence of epithelial differentiation. Overlying ulceration, though not shown here, may be present and can lead to clinical misdiagnosis as an infection or chronic reactive process.* **(Right)** *The nodules of ES often contain centralized necrosis, imparting an appearance reminiscent of a true granulomatous process.*

Classic Epithelioid Sarcoma

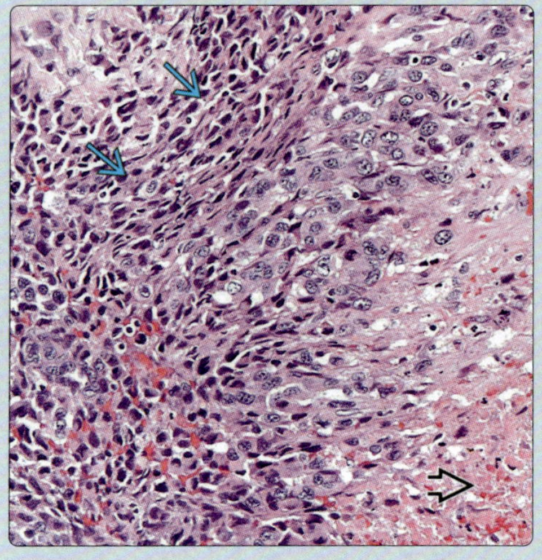

Immunophenotype

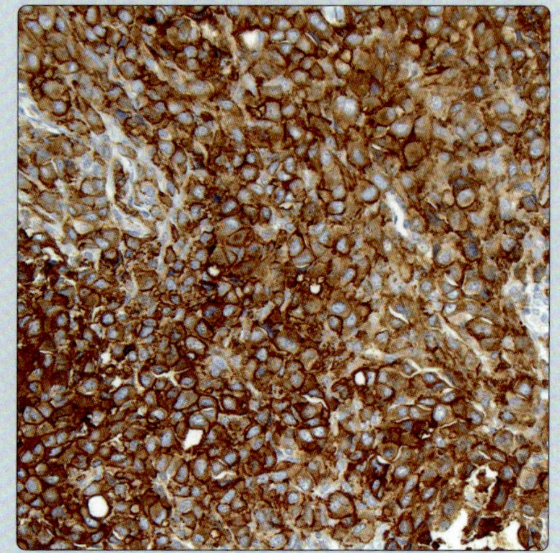

(Left) *The classic type of ES is composed of small- to medium-sized epithelioid cells with eosinophilic cytoplasm. Admixed small spindled cells can also be identified and often appear more conspicuous at the periphery of a nodule. Note the central tumor necrosis.* **(Right)** *ES is notable among most mesenchymal tumors for its expression of epithelial markers, including most keratins and EMA (shown). CD34 is coexpressed in 50% of cases. Complete loss of nuclear INI1 is also characteristic of ES cells.*

TERMINOLOGY

Abbreviations

- Epithelioid sarcoma (ES)

Definitions

- Distinctive malignant mesenchymal neoplasm that often shows epithelioid cytomorphology and demonstrates evidence of epithelial differentiation
  - Classic ES most commonly affects adolescents and young adults and arises in distal extremities
  - Proximal-type ES tends to affect older age groups, arises in proximal locations, and is often more clinically aggressive

CLINICAL ISSUES

Epidemiology

- Incidence
  - Rare
    - Accounts for ~ 1% of all soft tissue sarcomas
    - Classic ES is more common than proximal-type ES
- Age
  - Classic ES
    - Adolescents and young adults (median: 26 years)
  - Proximal-type ES
    - Affects middle-aged to older adults (median: 40 years)
- Sex
  - More frequent in male patients (both types)

Site

- Classic ES
  - Most common in distal extremities, especially hand, wrist, forearm, lower leg
  - Also head and neck, genital sites
- Proximal-type ES
  - Proximal limb girdles
  - Perineum, pelvis, mediastinum
  - Trunk

Presentation

- Classic ES
  - Slow-growing, often painless
  - Indurated dermal or subcutaneous nodule(s)
    - Can appear to track up limb
  - May appear as nonhealing ulcer
    - Can closely mimic infection clinically
    - Raised "sealing wax" margins
- Proximal-type ES
  - Subcutaneous or deep soft tissue mass
  - Can appear and grow more rapidly than classical ES

Treatment

- Wide surgical excision and reexcision
  - Amputation in some cases
- Chemotherapy can be palliative but currently of limited therapeutic benefit
  - Preclinical models suggest possible therapeutic benefit of EGFR-TK, mTOR, and c-MET inhibitors

Prognosis

- Clinically aggressive sarcoma
  - > 70% recur
    - Successive recurrences often extend more proximally in limbs
  - ~ 50% metastasize
    - Lymph nodes and lungs
    - Also skin and other soft tissue sites
  - 5-year survival (70%), 10-year survival (40%)
- Proximal-type ES has worse prognosis
  - Up to 75% metastasize
  - 5-year survival (35-65%)
- Adverse prognostic factors
  - Proximal location
  - Male sex
  - Size > 5 cm
  - Localization to deep soft tissue sites

MACROSCOPIC

General Features

- Uni- or multinodular firm lesion
- Tan/white/gray cut surface
- Hemorrhage and necrosis common in proximal-type ES

Size

- Classic ES: Usually < 5 cm
- Proximal-type ES: Wide range (1-20 cm)

MICROSCOPIC

Histologic Features

- Classic ES
  - Dermal/subcutaneous nodule(s), ± central necrosis
    - Can simulate granulomatous process at low magnification
    - Peripheral infiltration of connective tissue is common
    - Deeply extending lesions often involve and track along tendons/aponeuroses
  - Small- to medium-sized epithelioid cells with eosinophilic cytoplasm
    - Irregular but uniform, mildly atypical nuclei with small nucleoli
    - Admixed cells with spindled morphology common (particularly at periphery)
      - May rarely predominate (termed fibroma-like variant of ES)
      - Can show storiform growth
  - Variable mitotic activity, often low
  - Mixed chronic inflammatory infiltrate common
  - Other findings
    - Densely hyalinized collagenous stroma
    - Rare myxoid change
    - Osteoclast-like giant cells, calcification, metaplastic bone formation
    - Pseudogland formation
    - Pseudovascular morphology
- Proximal-type ES
  - More infiltrative with less-defined peripheral borders
  - Multiple large nodules
  - Large polygonal cells with abundant eosinophilic cytoplasm
    - Rhabdoid morphology common

- Vesicular nuclei with prominent macronucleoli
- Mitoses common
- Necrosis and hemorrhage common

ANCILLARY TESTS

Immunohistochemistry

- High- and low-molecular weight keratins (+), EMA(+), vimentin (+)
  - However, CK5/6(-)
- CD34(+) in 50%
- ERG(+) in 40% of cases; GLUT1(+) in 50% of cases
- Complete loss of nuclear INI1 protein expression
- Negative for CD31, S100 protein, p63, desmin, FLI-1, and PROX1

Molecular Genetics

- High frequency of *SMARCB1* (*INI1*) deletion (22q11)
  - Both classic and proximal-type ES

DIFFERENTIAL DIAGNOSIS

Granulomatous Processes

- Particularly granuloma annulare
- Lacks infiltrative or invasion growth
- Lacks coagulative tumor cell necrosis
- Keratin (-) and EMA(-)
- Retained nuclear INI1 expression

Squamous Cell Carcinoma

- Overlying in situ component may be identifiable
- Prior clinical history may be present
- Usually more pleomorphic than ES
- CK5/6(+) and p63(+)
- CD34(-)
- Retained nuclear INI1 expression

Extrarenal Rhabdoid Tumor

- Can show significant morphologic overlap with proximal-type ES
- Most common in infants and young children
- Keratin(+) but less prominent than in ES
- Consistent loss of nuclear INI1 expression
- Mutation of *SMARCB1* gene

Melanoma

- Junctional component or prior clinical history may be present
- Usually larger, more pleomorphic cells than classic ES
- S100 protein (+), SOX10(+); variable HMB45(+) or MART-1(+)
- Retained nuclear INI1 expression

Epithelioid Angiosarcoma

- Can show significant morphologic overlap with proximal-type ES
- Foci of vasoformation often present at least focally
- CD31(+), CD34(+), FLI1(+)
- May be keratin (+), though usually not diffuse
- Retained nuclear INI1 expression

Pseudomyogenic (Epithelioid Sarcoma-Like) Hemangioendothelioma

- Commonly involves multiple tissue planes
- Predominantly spindled morphology
- Neutrophilic infiltrate characteristic
- Keratin (+), CD31(+)
- CD34(-)
- Retained nuclear INI1 expression

Malignant Myoepithelioma (Myoepithelial Carcinoma)

- Can show morphologic overlap with proximal-type ES
- Myxoid stroma common
- Keratin (+), EMA(+), S100 protein (+)
- Loss of nuclear INI1 expression in subset of cases

Cellular Fibrous Histiocytoma (Dermatofibroma)

- Can show morphologic overlap with predominantly spindled forms of ES
- Keratin (-)
- Retained nuclear INI1 expression

SELECTED REFERENCES

1. Kohashi K et al: SWI/SNF chromatin-remodeling complex status in SMARCB1/INI1-preserved epithelioid sarcoma. Am J Surg Pathol. 42(3):312-8, 2018
2. Alikhan MB et al: Primary epithelioid sarcoma of the kidney and adrenal gland: report of 2 cases with immunohistochemical and molecular cytogenetic studies. Hum Pathol. 61:158-63, 2017
3. Thway K et al: Epithelioid sarcoma: diagnostic features and genetics. Adv Anat Pathol. 23(1):41-9, 2016
4. Coates SJ et al: Epidermotropic metastatic epithelioid sarcoma: a potential diagnostic pitfall. J Cutan Pathol. 41(8):672-6, 2014
5. Folpe AL: Selected topics in the pathology of epithelioid soft tissue tumors. Mod Pathol. 27 Suppl 1:S64-79, 2014
6. Imura Y et al: Combined targeting of mTOR and c-MET signaling pathways for effective management of epithelioid sarcoma. Mol Cancer. 13:185, 2014
7. Stockman DL et al: ERG and FLI1 protein expression in epithelioid sarcoma. Mod Pathol. 27(4):496-501, 2014
8. Miettinen M et al: ERG expression in epithelioid sarcoma: a diagnostic pitfall. Am J Surg Pathol. 37(10):1580-5, 2013
9. Sullivan LM et al: Epithelioid sarcoma is associated with a high percentage of SMARCB1 deletions. Mod Pathol. 26(3):385-92, 2013
10. Kosemehmetoglu K et al: Intra-articular epithelioid sarcoma showing mixed classic and proximal-type features: report of 2 cases, with immunohistochemical and molecular cytogenetic INI-1 study. Am J Surg Pathol. 35(6):891-7, 2011
11. Flucke U et al: Myxoid epithelioid sarcoma: a diagnostic challenge. A report on six cases. Histopathology. 57(5):753-9, 2010
12. Armah HB et al: Epithelioid sarcoma. Arch Pathol Lab Med. 133(5):814-9, 2009
13. Chbani L et al: Epithelioid sarcoma: a clinicopathologic and immunohistochemical analysis of 106 cases from the French sarcoma group. Am J Clin Pathol. 131(2):222-7, 2009
14. Hornick JL et al: Loss of INI1 expression is characteristic of both conventional and proximal-type epithelioid sarcoma. Am J Surg Pathol. 33(4):542-50, 2009
15. Jawad MU et al: Prognostic factors for survival in patients with epithelioid sarcoma: 441 cases from the SEER database. Clin Orthop Relat Res. 467(11):2939-48, 2009
16. Orrock JM et al: INI1 and GLUT-1 expression in epithelioid sarcoma and its cutaneous neoplastic and nonneoplastic mimics. Am J Dermatopathol. 31(2):152-6, 2009
17. Miettinen M et al: Epithelioid sarcoma: an immunohistochemical analysis of 112 classical and variant cases and a discussion of the differential diagnosis. Hum Pathol. 30(8):934-42, 1999
18. Guillou L et al: "Proximal-type" epithelioid sarcoma, a distinctive aggressive neoplasm showing rhabdoid features. Clinicopathologic, immunohistochemical, and ultrastructural study of a series. Am J Surg Pathol. 21(2):130-46, 1997

Cytologic Features

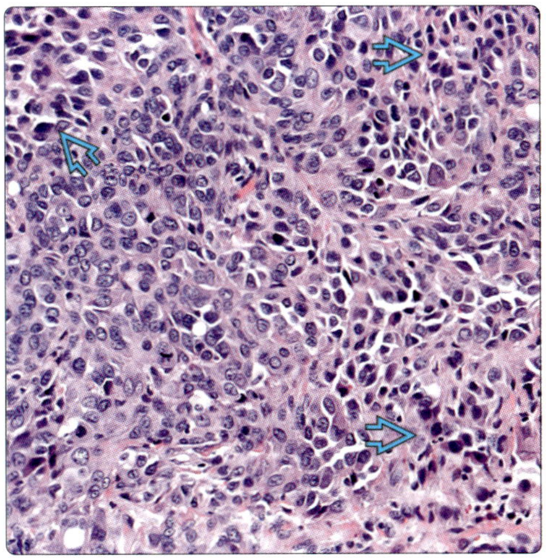

Typical Cytology

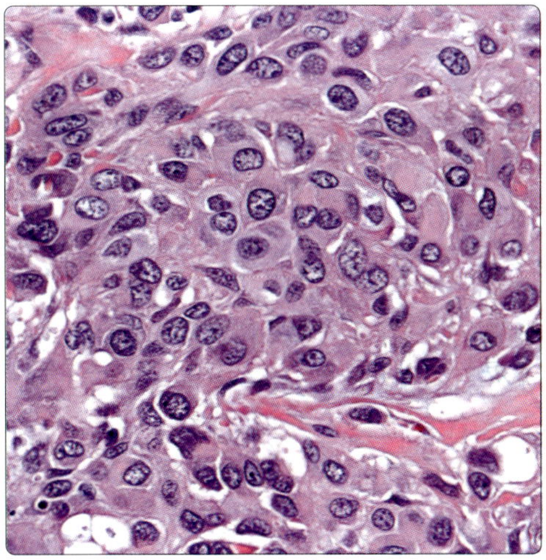

(Left) *The lesional cells of ES show eosinophilic cytoplasm and contain mildly atypical but relatively uniform nuclei. Significant nuclear pleomorphism is very uncommon in this tumor. Note that some cells* ➩ *are compressed and appear to have darker cytoplasm and more hyperchromatic nuclei.* **(Right)** *This high-power image shows typical cytologic features of ES. Mitotic activity varies but is often low in classic forms.*

Spindled Morphology

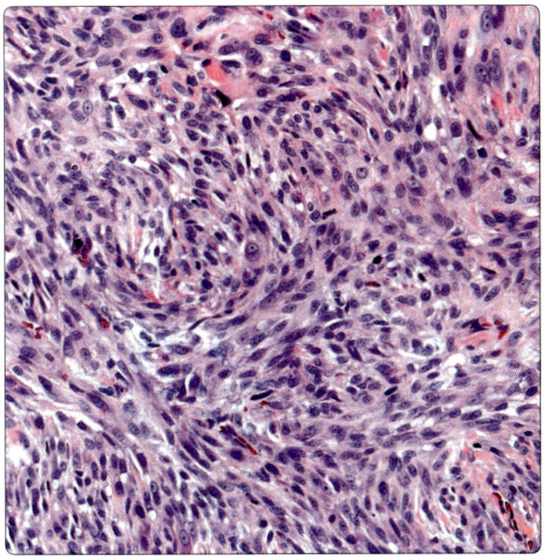

Infiltrative Growth

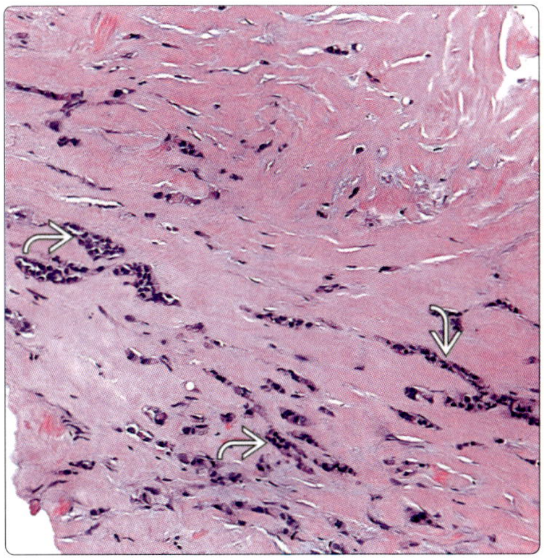

(Left) *Admixed tumor cells with a spindled rather than epithelioid morphology are common in ES. Occasionally, this morphology is more prominent and a vague storiform or fascicular growth pattern may be seen.* **(Right)** *Most cases of ES show infiltrative growth at the periphery of the main tumor mass. Small nests and cords of cells* ➥ *within fibrotic connective tissue, as depicted, can mimic infiltrating carcinoma.*

Stromal Hyalinization/Sclerosis

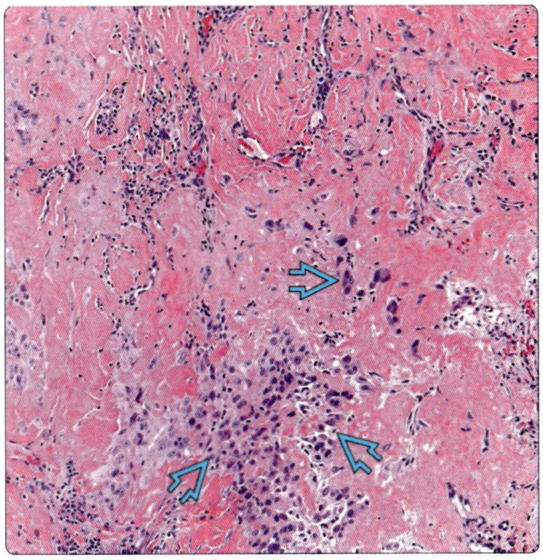

Osteoid-Like Collagen

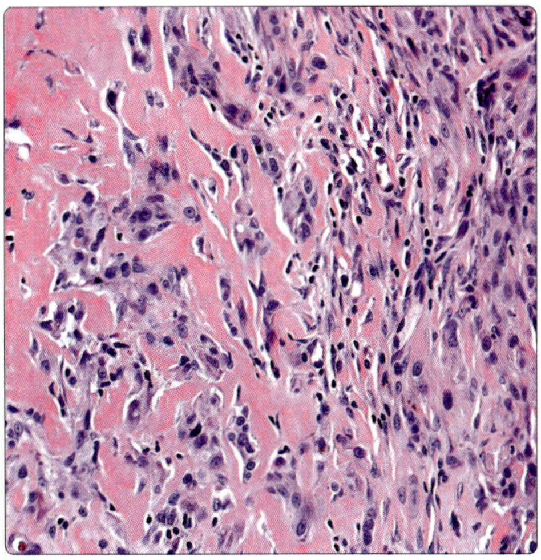

(Left) *Some cases of ES show prominent stromal hyalinization or sclerosis, as depicted. Entrapped tumor cells* ➩ *may appear singly or as irregular clusters, aggregates, or cords.* **(Right)** *Hyalinized stromal collagen may appear as irregular, thickened bundles imparting an appearance reminiscent of osteoid deposition in osteosarcoma.*

(Left) *A mixed chronic inflammatory infiltrate may be seen in ES and rarely can be so prominent as to obscure the underlying neoplasm. Lymphocytes are predominantly seen in this image.* **(Right)** *In contrast to the classic type, the proximal-type variant of ES usually shows a larger, more solid and cellular nodular growth pattern. Clinically, this form of ES generally affects an older age group and arises in proximal locations.*

Chronic Inflammatory Infiltrate

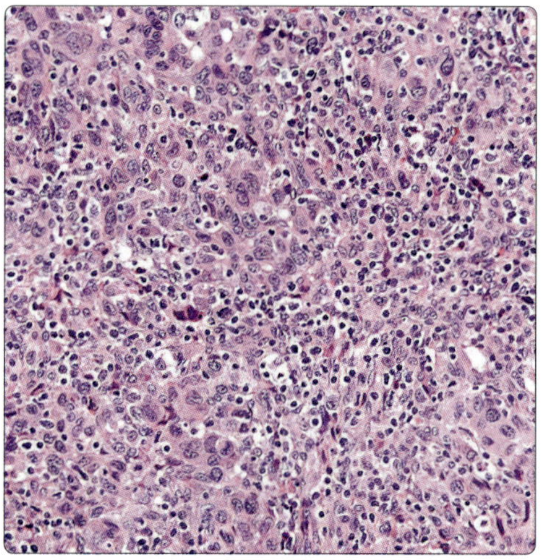

Proximal-Type Epithelioid Sarcoma

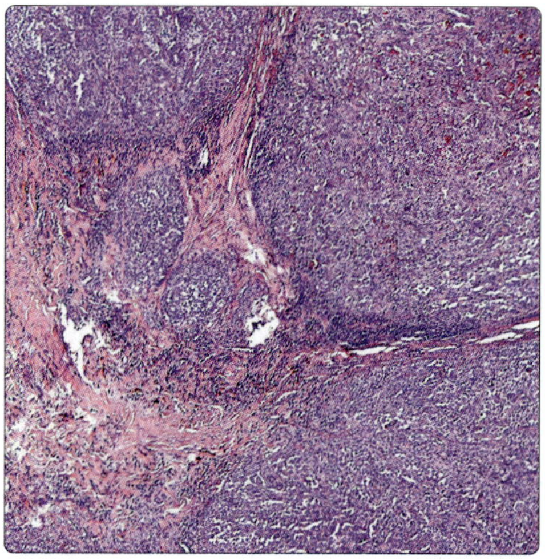

(Left) *The cells of proximal-type ES are larger and plumper than those of classic ES and show more abundant eosinophilic cytoplasm. Vesicular nuclei with prominent macronucleoli are characteristic of this variant and aid in its histologic recognition.* **(Right)** *Rhabdoid cytomorphology, as shown, is not uncommon in proximal-type ES and can lead to significant morphologic overlap with malignant extrarenal rhabdoid tumor; however, the clinical scenarios for these 2 entities are often very different.*

Macronucleoli

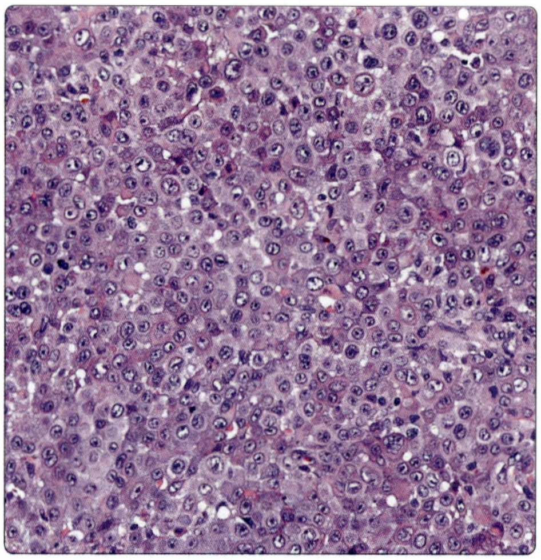

Rhabdoid Cytomorphology

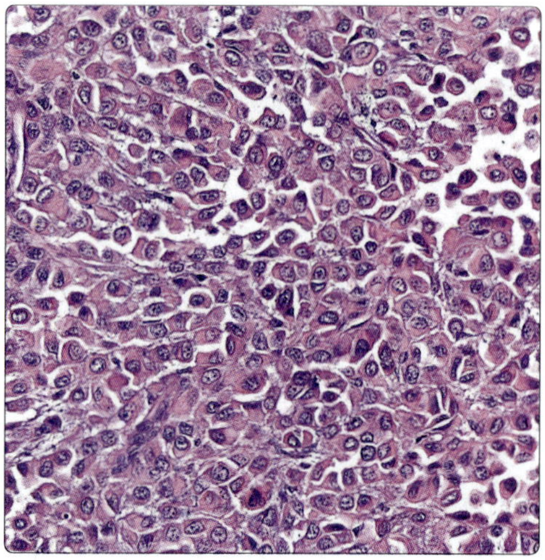

(Left) *Rare cases of ES may contain a population of reactive multinucleated osteoclast-like giant cells* ⇨ *scattered within otherwise typical lesional cells (proximal-type ES in this image). This is usually a focal finding.* **(Right)** *Complete loss of nuclear INI1 protein expression by IHC is characteristic of epithelioid sarcoma and is a helpful feature for supporting the diagnosis. Note that the large cells* → *are negative in this image, whereas the inflammatory cells (bottom left) are positive.*

Osteoclast-Like Giant Cells

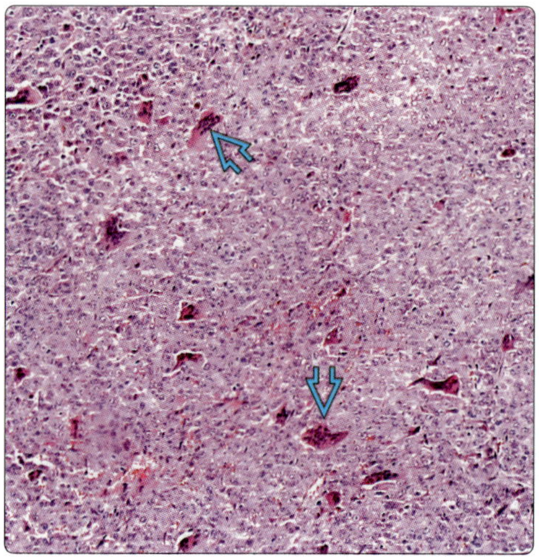

Loss of Nuclear INI1

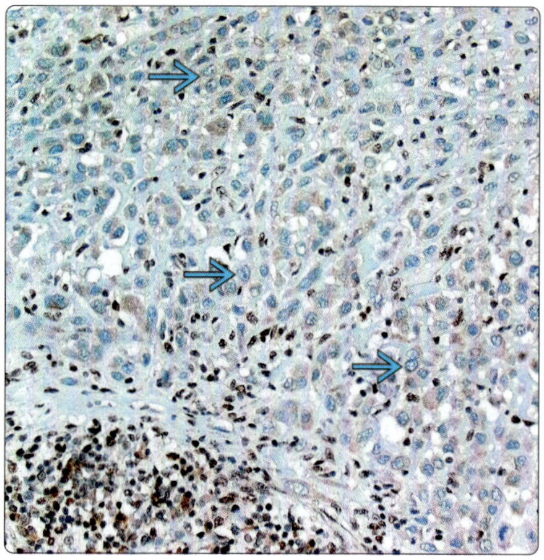

Pseudoglandular Foci

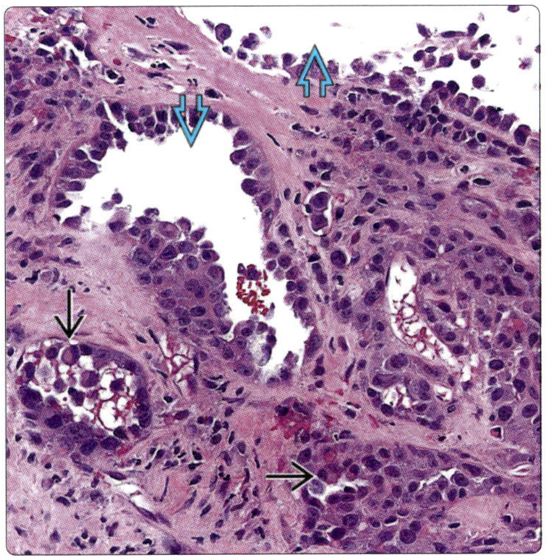

Pseudovascular Morphology

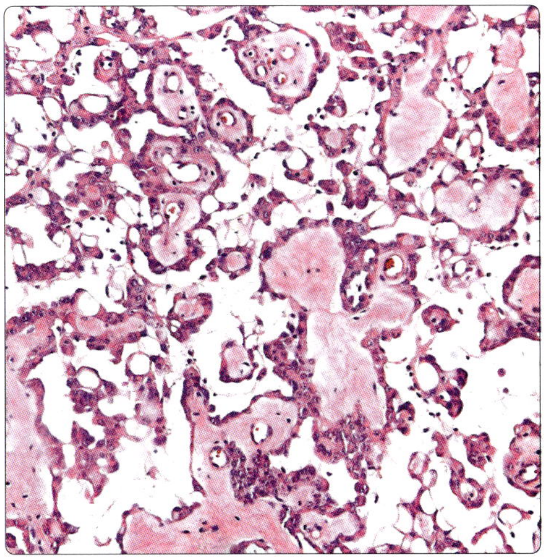

(Left) *Central loss of cellular cohesion → in ES can lead to a pseudoglandular appearance, as depicted. Note the larger lesional cells with prominent nucleoli and scattered rhabdoid forms →, identifying this tumor as a proximal-type ES.* **(Right)** *A loosely dyscohesive, pseudovascular pattern is a rare finding in ES but can resemble angiosarcoma. The absence of CD31 &/or FLI1 expression in ES is helpful in the distinction.*

Myxoid Stroma

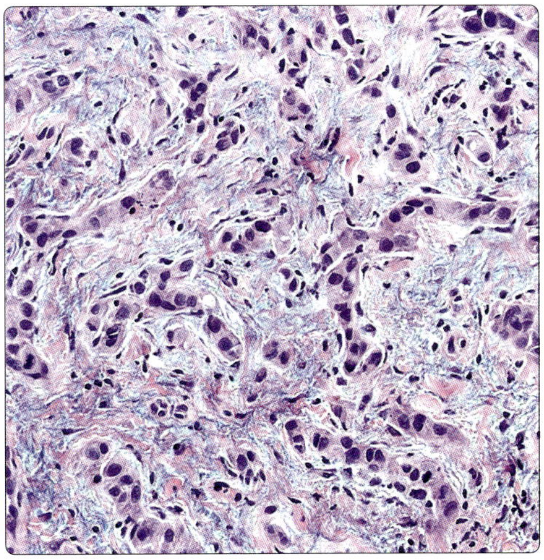

Rare Fibroma-Like Variant

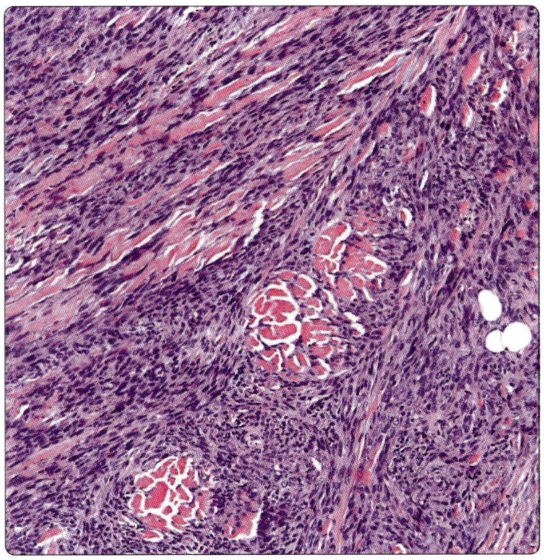

(Left) *Myxoid stromal change is a very rare finding in ES and is usually focal if present. Exceptional cases show diffuse myxoid change.* **(Right)** *Although spindled tumor cells are common in classic ES, rare tumors show a predominant or exclusive spindled morphology. This variant has been described as fibroma-like ES and may lead to consideration of cellular fibrous histiocytoma (cellular dermatofibroma).*

Lymph Node Metastases

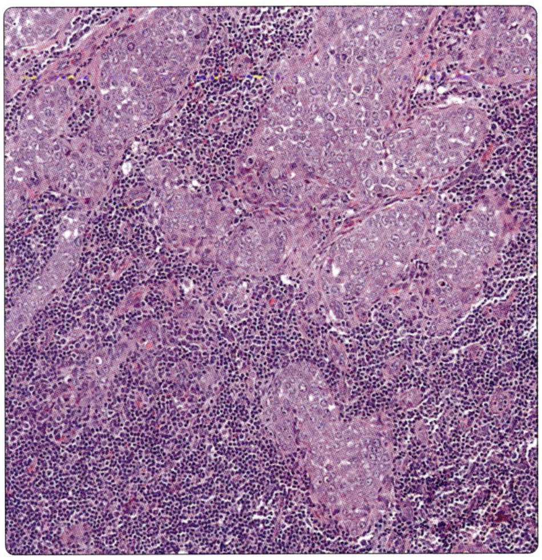

Cutaneous Metastases

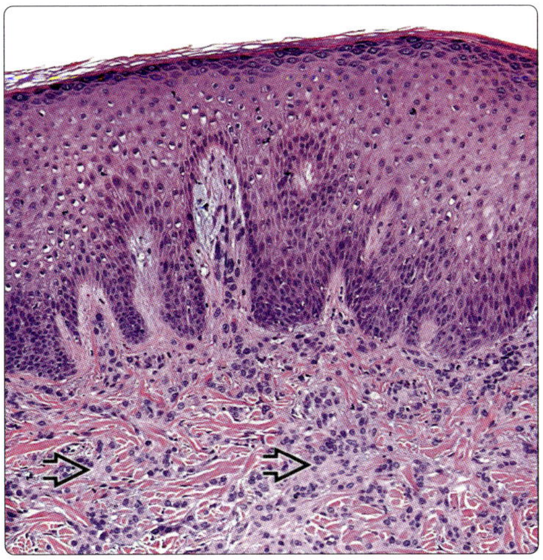

(Left) *ES is one of the few mesenchymal neoplasms that is well known to metastasize to lymph nodes. Spread to the lungs is also common. Overall, metastasis occurs in up to 50% of cases.* **(Right)** *Cutaneous → and soft tissue metastases are not uncommon in ES and may present as small nodules or bumps that do not immediately raise clinical suspicion for malignancy. In some cases, the relatively bland cytologic features may lead to tumor cells getting overlooked.*

Alveolar Soft Part Sarcoma

KEY FACTS

TERMINOLOGY

- Malignant neoplasm composed of large eosinophilic cells in variable pseudoalveolar growth pattern and characterized by specific chromosomal translocation and fusion gene

CLINICAL ISSUES

- Infants, children, and young adults
- Most common in lower extremity (particularly anterior thigh and buttock)
  - Also head and neck (particularly tongue and orbit)
- Slow-growing, painless intramuscular mass
- Treatment: Aggressive surgical resection
- Fully malignant; indefinite long-term follow-up mandatory
  - Late recurrence and metastases (lung, brain) common

MICROSCOPIC

- Prominent compartmentalization
  - Lobules and nests delineated by fibrous septa and sinusoidal blood vessels
- Polygonal tumor cells with eosinophilic, granular cytoplasm
  - Central or eccentric nuclei with prominent nucleoli
- Pseudoalveolar growth pattern (focal or prominent)
  - Some variants show sheet-like growth
- Mitotic rate low; necrosis uncommon

ANCILLARY TESTS

- PAS-D(+) intracytoplasmic crystals in most cases
- Nuclear TFE3(+); negative for S100 and myogenin
- Molecular: der(17)t(X;17)(p11.2;q25) translocation with *ASPSCR1-TFE3* gene fusion

TOP DIFFERENTIAL DIAGNOSES

- Metastatic renal cell carcinoma
- Malignant melanoma
- Paraganglioma
- PEComa
- Granular cell tumor
- Rhabdomyoma

Alveolar Soft Part Sarcoma

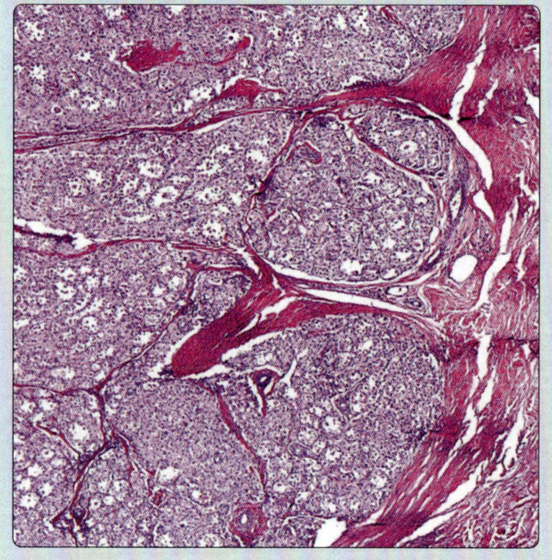

Peripheral Dilated Veins

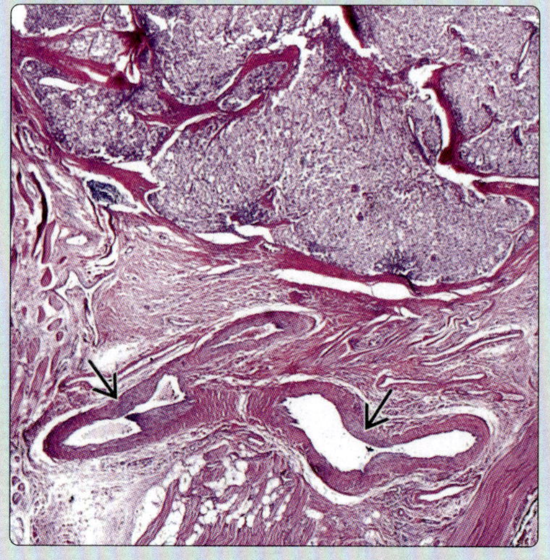

(Left) *Alveolar soft part sarcoma (ASPS) is a rare malignant mesenchymal neoplasm that predominantly affects children and young adults. It is characteristically compartmentalized with variably thick fibrous septa dividing and subdividing lobules of tumor cells.* **(Right)** *Dilated veins ➡ are a common finding at the periphery of ASPS and attest in part to the vascularity of this neoplasm.*

Nested Growth

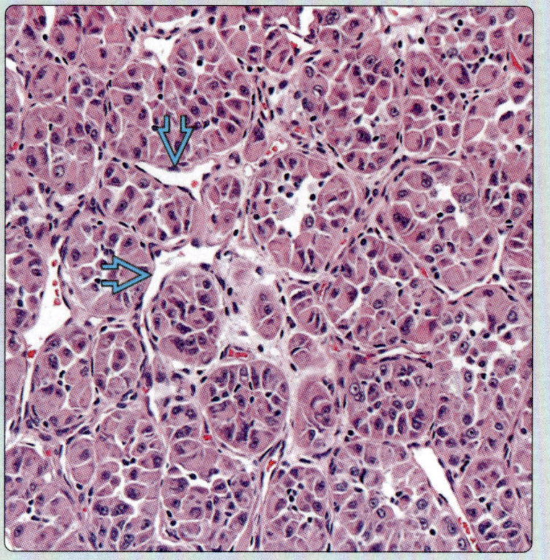

Pseudoalveolar Growth

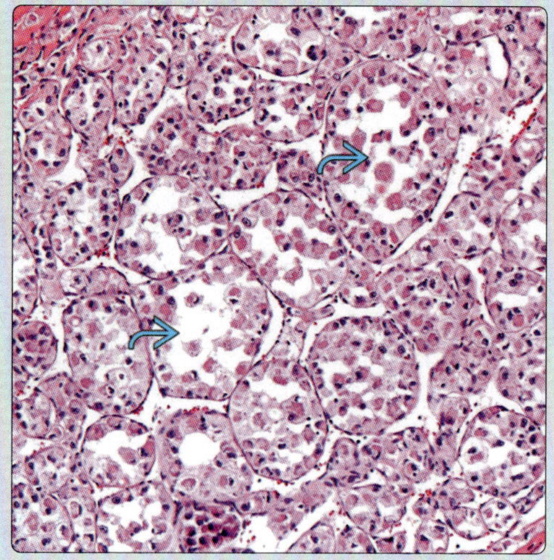

(Left) *A nested growth pattern is commonly seen in ASPS. Conspicuous delicate, thin-walled vascular channels ⇨ are widespread and often readily apparent.* **(Right)** *Central loss of cellular cohesion ↪ within a tumor nest imparts a pseudoalveolar appearance. This morphology can be identified at least focally in most cases and may sometimes be extensive.*

Alveolar Soft Part Sarcoma

TERMINOLOGY

Abbreviations

- Alveolar soft part sarcoma (ASPS)

Definitions

- Malignant neoplasm composed of large eosinophilic cells in variable pseudoalveolar growth pattern and characterized by der(17)t(X;17)(p11;q25) resulting in *ASPSCR1-TFE3* fusion

CLINICAL ISSUES

Epidemiology

- Age
  - Predominantly infants, children, and young adults
- Sex
  - 2:1 = F:M

Site

- Most common in lower extremity (particularly anterior thigh and buttock)
- Head and neck (particularly tongue and orbit)
  - Most common sites in infants and children

Presentation

- Slow-growing, painless intramuscular mass
- Significant proportion of patients (> 50%) have metastases at presentation

Treatment

- Aggressive surgical resection
- Radiation and systemic chemotherapy not shown to be helpful in most studies
- Indefinite, long-term clinical follow-up mandatory

Prognosis

- May have deceptively indolent clinical course initially
- Fully malignant; overall poor prognosis
  - Majority of patients present with high-stage disease
  - Late recurrence and metastases (lung, brain) common
- Most important favorable prognostic parameters
  - Smaller tumor size (< 5 cm), absence of metastases at presentation, younger age at diagnosis (< 10 years)

MACROSCOPIC

Size

- Often 3-10 cm in extremities
- Head and neck cases often smaller (1-3 cm)

MICROSCOPIC

Histologic Features

- Prominent compartmentalization
  - Lobules and nests delineated by fibrous septa
  - Nests separated by sinusoidal vascular channels
- Dilated veins usually present at periphery of mass, often with at least focal involvement by tumor
- Polygonal tumor cells with eosinophilic, granular cytoplasm
  - Central or eccentric nuclei with prominent nucleoli
  - Some cells have clear cytoplasm (may be extensive)
  - Nuclear pleomorphism is rare but may be marked
- Pseudoalveolar growth pattern (focal or prominent)
  - Tumor cell nests with empty centers due to degeneration or loss of cellular cohesion
- Some variants show sheet-like growth
  - Most common morphology in infants and children
- Mitotic rate low; necrosis uncommon

ANCILLARY TESTS

Histochemistry

- PAS(+), diastase-resistant intracytoplasmic crystals in most cases (may be absent)

Immunohistochemistry

- Nuclear TFE3(+); variable desmin (+)
- Negative for vimentin, myogenin, MYOD1, keratin, S100 protein, HMB-45, SMA

Molecular Genetics

- Characteristic der(17)t(X;17)(p11.2;q25) translocation resulting in fusion of *ASPSCR1* (*ASPL*) and *TFE3* genes

DIFFERENTIAL DIAGNOSIS

Metastatic Renal Cell Carcinoma

- Older patients (> 40 years), often with history of renal mass
- Keratin (+), pax-8(+), vimentin (+)
- Subtype of pediatric renal cell carcinoma has similar morphology to ASPS, is TFE3(+), and contains t(X;17)

Malignant Melanoma

- Usually shows significant mitotic activity and necrosis
- S100(+); HMB-45(+); MART-1(+)

Paraganglioma

- Generally more nuclear atypia than ASPS
- Synaptophysin (+); chromogranin (+)

PEComa

- Most tumor cells are spindled and with stringy eosinophilic to clear cytoplasm
- Usual coexpression of SMA and HMB-45 or MART-1
- Rare cases may be TFE3(+)

Granular Cell Tumor

- Cells have distinctly granular, PAS-D(+) cytoplasm
- Diffuse S100 protein (+); TFE3(+) in many cases

Rhabdomyoma

- Lacks pseudoalveolar growth
- Diffuse desmin (+), myogenin (+), MYOD1(+)

SELECTED REFERENCES

1. Flores RJ et al: Alveolar soft part sarcoma in children and young adults: a report of 69 cases. Pediatr Blood Cancer. 65(5):e26953, 2018
2. Schoolmeester JK et al: Alveolar soft part sarcoma of the female genital tract: a morphologic, immunohistochemical, and molecular cytogenetic study of 10 cases with emphasis on its distinction from morphologic mimics. Am J Surg Pathol. 41(5):622-32, 2017
3. Jaber OI et al: Alveolar soft part sarcoma. Arch Pathol Lab Med. 139(11):1459-62, 2015
4. Chamberlain BK et al: Alveolar soft part sarcoma and granular cell tumor: an immunohistochemical comparison study. Hum Pathol. 45(5):1039-44, 2014
5. Cho YJ et al: Alveolar soft part sarcoma: clinical presentation, treatment and outcome in a series of 19 patients. Clin Orthop Surg. 6(1):80-6, 2014
6. Folpe AL et al: Alveolar soft-part sarcoma: a review and update. J Clin Pathol. 59(11):1127-32, 2006

Pseudoalveolar Growth

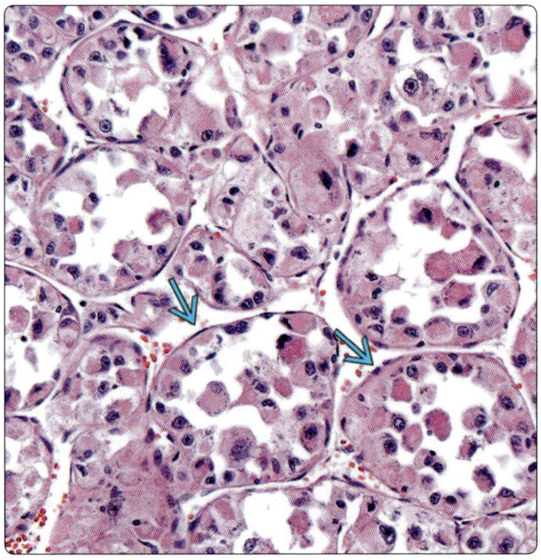

Cytologic Features

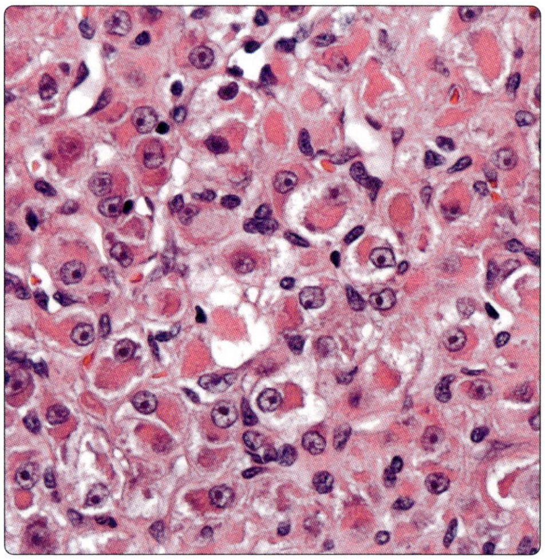

(Left) *Delicate, thin-walled sinusoidal vascular channels separate nests of tumor cells in ASPS. Note the flat, inconspicuous endothelial cell nuclei* ➙. **(Right)** *The tumor cells of ASPS are large, polygonal, and demonstrate eosinophilic cytoplasm. They typically show 1 or more eccentric nuclei with prominent nucleoli.*

Intracytoplasmic Crystals

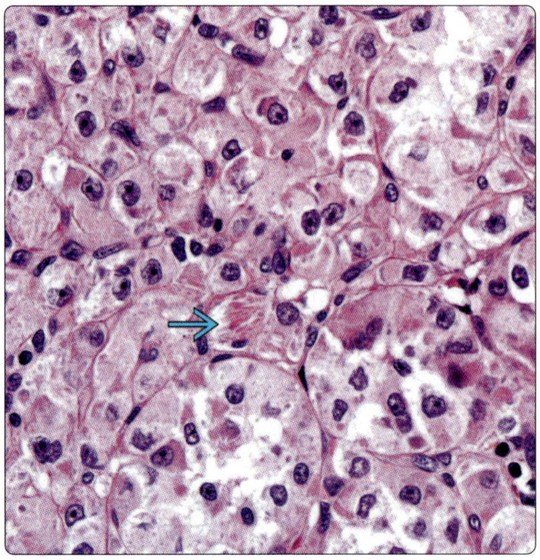

Intracytoplasmic Crystals

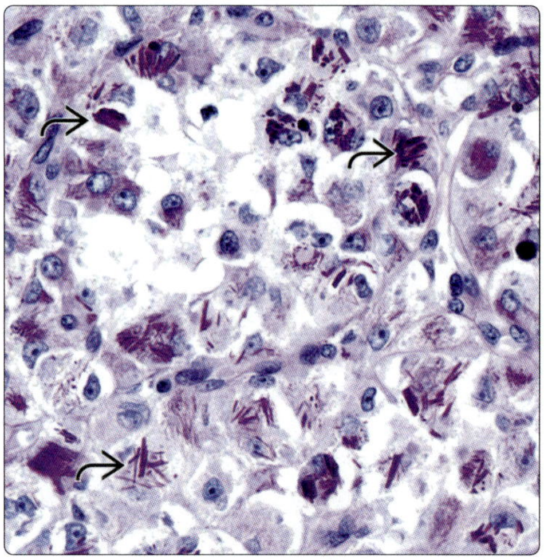

(Left) *The majority of cases of ASPS show an intracytoplasmic accumulation of rod-shaped crystals* ➙. *These crystals vary widely from numerous to focal or may be completely absent.* **(Right)** *A PAS-diastase special stain nicely highlights the intracytoplasmic crystals* ↪ *in ASPS and serves as a useful screening stain. These crystals are known to contain CD147 and monocarboxylate transporter 1 (MCT1).*

Nuclear Notch

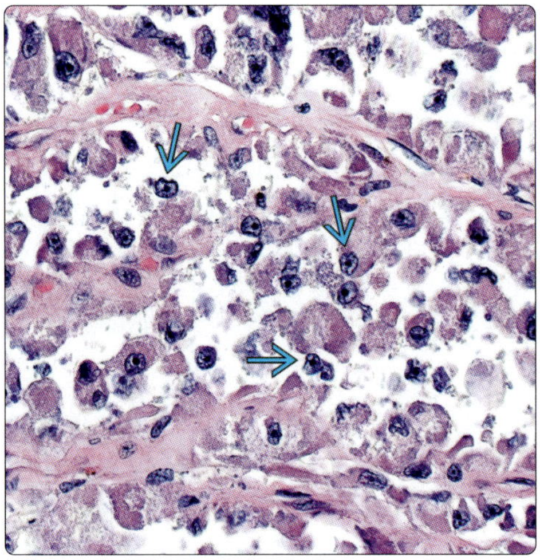

Solid Growth

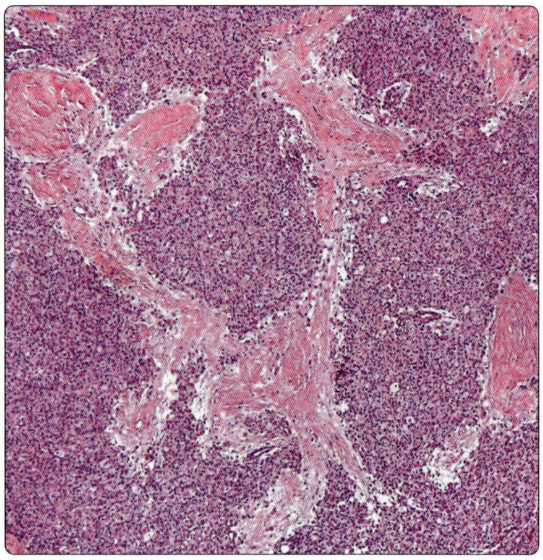

(Left) *An interesting feature of ASPS is the presence of a nuclear indentation or notch* ➙. *This appearance has been colorfully described by some as resembling an apple with a bite taken out of it.* **(Right)** *In the minority of cases, the nested growth is less conspicuous or seemingly absent, imparting a solid morphology. This pattern is particularly common in infants and children in the head and neck region.*

Nuclear and Cytologic Pleomorphism

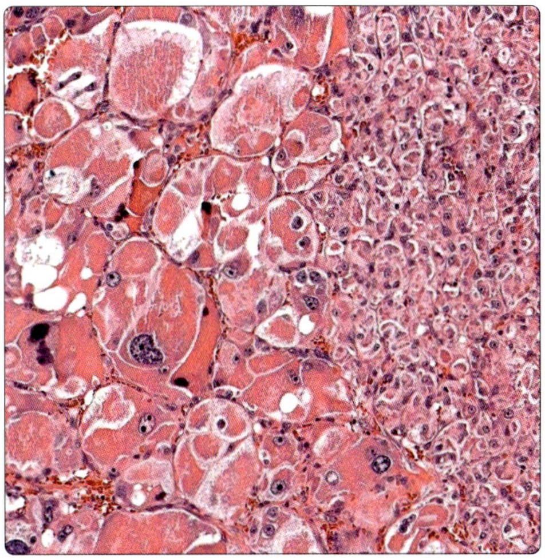

Ectatic "Staghorn" Vessels

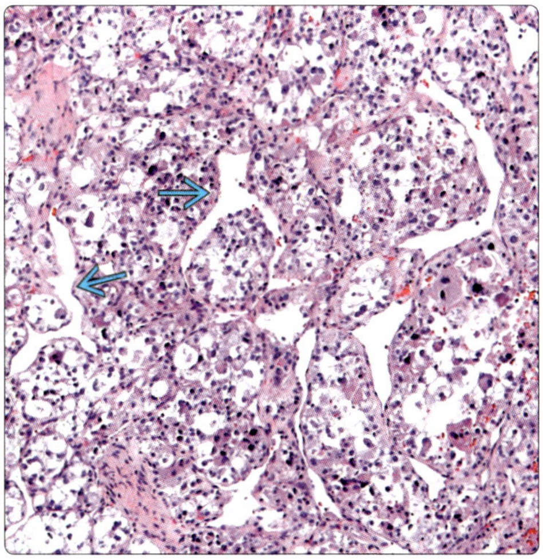

(Left) *Increased cytologic &/or nuclear pleomorphism is uncommon in ASPS but is well described. In rare cases, it can be marked and striking. Most conventional cases show relatively little variation in tumor cell size.* **(Right)** *In addition to smaller sinusoidal vascular channels, large ectatic vessels with a "staghorn" morphology ➔ may also be seen in ASPS and may be quite prominent.*

Granular Cytoplasm

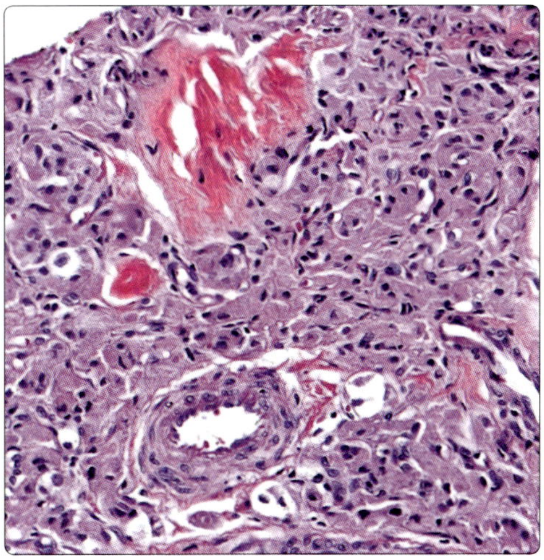

Clear Cell Change

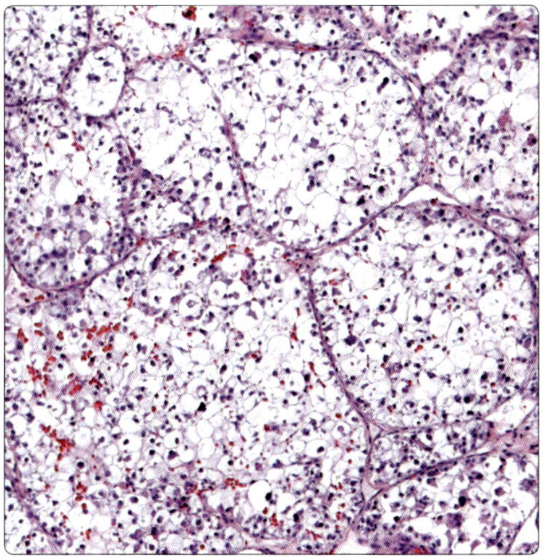

(Left) *In ASPS, the combination of solid sheets or nests of eosinophilic cells with granular cytoplasm may mimic a granular cell tumor. Of note, TFE3 expression can be seen in both tumors. Diffuse S100 protein expression, however, is not a feature of ASPS.* **(Right)** *Degenerative clear cell change may be seen in ASPS and, when extensive, may closely mimic a metastatic carcinoma, particularly clear cell renal cell carcinoma.*

Vascular Invasion

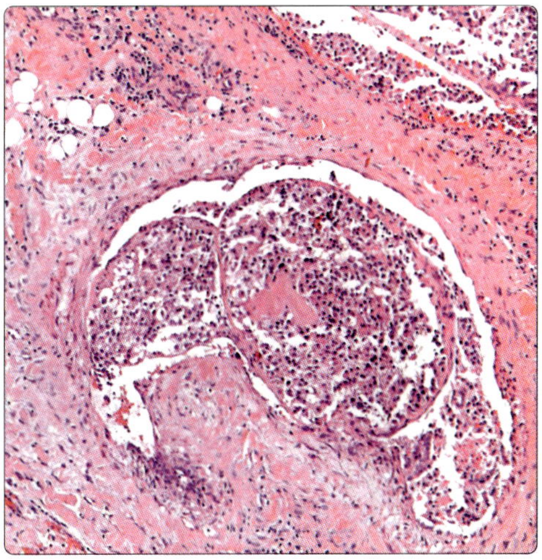

Nuclear TFE3 Expression

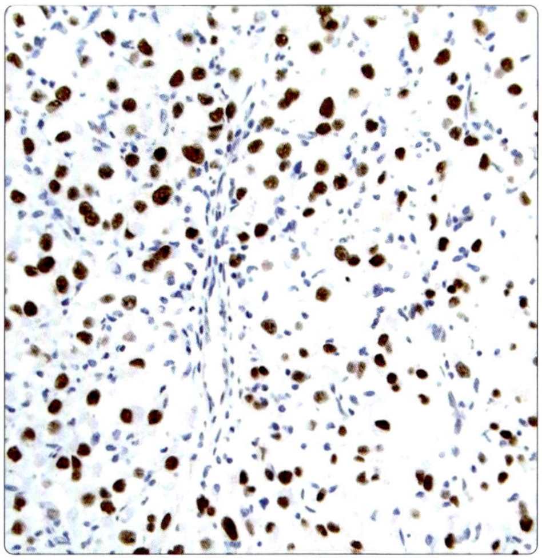

(Left) *Vascular invasion can be identified in the majority of cases of ASPS and is often seen in vessels near the periphery of the tumor mass, as depicted.* **(Right)** *TFE3 often shows strong nuclear expression in ASPS. Although once thought to be relatively specific for ASPS, it has now been reported in several morphologically similar entities (such as granular cell tumor), somewhat limiting its usefulness.*

Clear Cell Sarcoma

KEY FACTS

TERMINOLOGY

- Synonym: Melanoma of soft parts
- Translocation-associated sarcoma of soft tissues showing melanocytic differentiation

CLINICAL ISSUES

- Young adults (3rd-4th decades)
- > 90% arise on extremities, especially feet
- Usually in subcutis or deeper, often involves tendon/aponeurosis
- Poor prognosis but often prolonged clinical course
- Late recurrence or metastasis at 10-20 years is common
- Unlike most sarcomas, lymph node metastases common
- Treatment/prognosis of clear cell sarcoma different than melanoma

MICROSCOPIC

- Uniform, ovoid to spindled cells arranged in nests and fascicles with intervening collagen
- Prominent central nucleoli
- Clear to pale eosinophilic cytoplasm
- Scattered wreath-like multinucleated tumor giant cells

ANCILLARY TESTS

- Essentially identical to melanoma on IHC
    - Positive for S100 protein, SOX10, MART-1, HMB-45
- Molecular: Translocations detected via FISH or RT-PCR
    - t(12;22) with *EWSR1-ATF1* fusion
    - t(2;22) with *EWSR1-CREB1* alternate fusion

TOP DIFFERENTIAL DIAGNOSES

- Metastatic melanoma
- Cellular blue nevus
- Paraganglioma-like dermal melanocytic tumor
- PEComa
- Malignant peripheral nerve sheath tumor
- Monophasic synovial sarcoma

Clear Cell Sarcoma

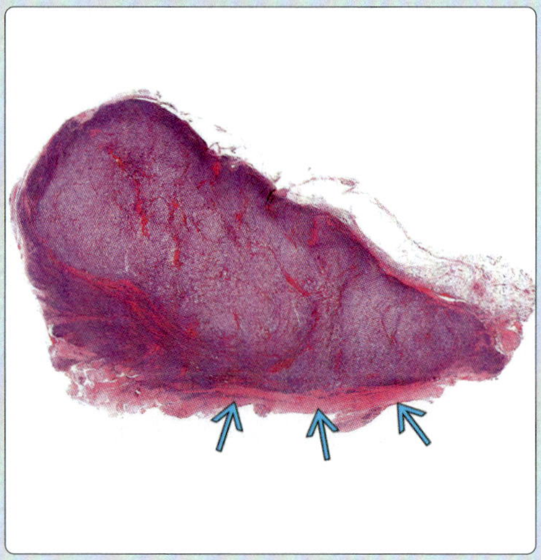

Dermal Involvement

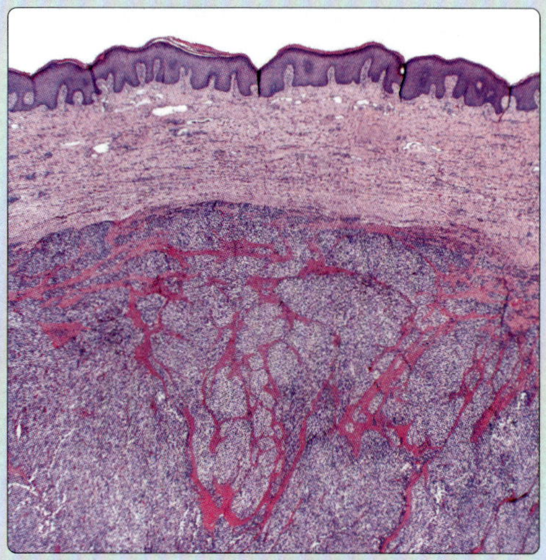

(Left) *Clear cell sarcoma (CCS) of soft tissue often presents as a nodule arising from a tendon or aponeurosis →.* **(Right)** *Nests and large aggregates of tumor cells are divided by thick eosinophilic fibrous septa; this appearance is classic for CCS. Some cases may involve the dermis, as depicted, leading to potential misdiagnosis as melanoma.*

Nested Growth Pattern

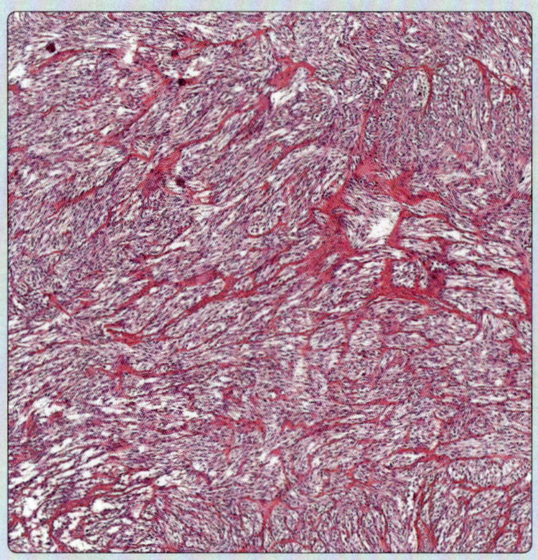

Prominent Nucleoli

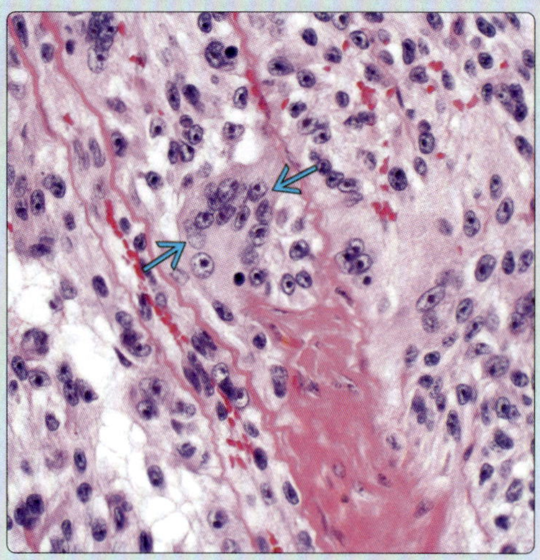

(Left) *Elongated nests and fascicles of clear or pale tumor cells are divided by prominent intervening fibrous septa in CCS, as shown in this H&E.* **(Right)** *Nuclei in CCS are usually relatively uniform, oval/round to spindled in shape, and characteristically feature prominent nucleoli. Wreath-like multinucleated tumor giant cells → with identical nuclear features are also a common finding in CCS.*

TERMINOLOGY

Abbreviations

- Clear cell sarcoma (CCS)

Synonyms

- CCS of tendon and aponeurosis
- Melanoma of soft parts (formerly)

Definitions

- Translocation-associated sarcoma of soft tissues showing melanocytic differentiation
  - Not related to CCS of kidney
  - Probably distinct from malignant gastrointestinal neuroectodermal tumor (GNET) (formerly CCS-like tumor of GI tract)

CLINICAL ISSUES

Epidemiology

- Incidence
  - Rare
- Age
  - Young adults (3rd-4th decades) (median: 39 years)
- Ethnicity
  - 78% Caucasian and 15% African ancestry

Presentation

- Pain in up to 50% of cases
- Usually affects extremities (> 90%)
  - Foot most common site
  - Very uncommon in head, neck, or trunk
- Often attached to tendon or aponeurosis
- Usually in subcutis or deeper, unlike primary cutaneous melanoma
  - Rare cases involve dermis or even epidermis; melanoma must be excluded by molecular testing
- Occasional visceral examples
  - GI tract most common visceral site; must be distinguished from GNET by IHC and other features

Treatment

- Surgical resection is mainstay of treatment
- Usually chemotherapy resistant
- Some may respond to tyrosine kinase inhibitors (crizotinib, sorafenib, sunitinib)
- Rare reported response to PD1 blockade (pembrolizumab) plus radiation

Prognosis

- Poor prognosis, although clinical course often prolonged
  - 5-year survival: 50-67%
  - 10-year survival: 30-33%
  - 20-year survival: 10%
- Late recurrence or metastasis at 10-20 years is common
  - Late metastases more common in patients with multiple local recurrences
    - Local control of tumor is thus important
    - Risk of local recurrence correlates with incomplete initial resection
- Lung most common site of metastasis
- Unlike most sarcomas, lymph node metastasis is common (50%)
  - Role of sentinel lymph node biopsy for CCS still uncertain
- Most important poor prognostic factors
  - Local recurrence
  - Size > 5 cm
  - Necrosis
- Early stage tumors < 2.5 cm associated with 5-year disease-free survival
- Distinction of CCS from melanoma important for treatment and prognosis

MACROSCOPIC

General Features

- Lobulated, gray-white masses, often attached to tendon/aponeurosis
  - Sometimes with dark brown/black melanin deposits

Size

- Usually 2-6 cm (range: 1-15 cm)

MICROSCOPIC

Histologic Features

- Uniform, spindled to ovoid cells arranged in nests and fascicles with intervening collagen
  - Clear to pale eosinophilic cytoplasm
  - Prominent central nucleoli
  - Melanin pigment present in 50% but may be only focal
- As with most translocation sarcomas, nuclei are monotonous not pleomorphic
  - Pleomorphism may be seen in recurrence or metastasis
- Variable mitotic rate (range: 0-43/10 HPF; mean: 4/10 HPF)
- Scattered wreath-like multinucleated tumor giant cells very characteristic finding
- Intervening collagen between nests/fascicles may be delicate or dense/sclerotic (especially if tumor embedded in tendon)

ANCILLARY TESTS

Immunohistochemistry

- Essentially identical to melanoma on IHC
  - Positive for S100 protein, SOX10, MART-1/Melan-A, HMB-45, MITF
  - Sometimes positive for synaptophysin, CD56, CD57, EMA, BCL-2, C-kit, CD34, cytokeratin AE1/AE3 (rare)

Molecular Genetics

- Most cases possess translocations that can be detected by FISH or RT-PCR
  - *EWSR1-ATF1* fusion from t(12;22) (> 90%)
  - *EWSR1-CREB1* alternate fusion from t(2;22) (6%)
- Identical gene fusions found in variety of tumors, including angiomatoid fibrous histiocytoma and GNET
  - Diagnosis of CCS requires combination of clinical, histologic, IHC, and molecular findings
  - As with many tumors, molecular results cannot be used in isolation for diagnosis

DIFFERENTIAL DIAGNOSIS

Metastatic Melanoma

- Similar presentation: Dermal/subcutaneous/deep nodule without epidermal involvement
  - CCS should always be considered in differential diagnosis of skin/soft tissue metastatic melanoma, especially in extremities of young patients who lack known history of primary melanoma
- Immunophenotype may be identical to CCS
  - Positive for S100 protein, SOX10, MART-1/Melan-A, HMB-45, MITF
  - Often CD117(+) (unlike CCS)
- Usually more pleomorphic and mitotically active than CCS
- Often has *BRAF* or *NRAS* mutations (very rare in CCS)
- Lacks *EWSR1-ATF1* and *EWSR1-CREB1* fusions

Cellular Blue Nevus

- Dermal nodule, often with dumbbell-shaped protrusion into subcutis
- Buttocks most common site (50%) but can occur almost anywhere, including extremities
- Clear spindle cells in fascicles/nests divided by dense collagen
  - Usually has areas of typical blue nevus in dermis at periphery of lesion (useful clue)
- May have wreath-like tumor giant cells similar to CCS
- Often more melanin than CCS but may be hypopigmented or amelanotic
- Immunophenotype may be identical to CCS
  - Positive for S100 protein, SOX10, MART-1/Melan-A, HMB-45, MITF
- Cytology is key: Prominent nucleoli lacking, minimal nuclear atypia, low mitotic rate
- Often positive for *GNAQ* mutation (unlike CCS)
- Lacks *EWSR1-ATF1* and *EWSR1-CREB1* fusions

Paraganglioma-Like Dermal Melanocytic Tumor

- Dermal/subcutaneous nodule, usually small and circumscribed
- Cells arranged into packets, nests, cords with intervening collagen
- Spindled or round cells with pale/clear cytoplasm
  - Minimal atypia or mitotic activity
- S100 protein (+), MART-1(+), HMB-45(+)
- Lacks *EWSR1-ATF1* and *EWSR1-CREB1* fusions

PEComa

- Distinctive group of tumors with overlapping smooth muscle and melanocytic differentiation
- Epithelioid or spindle cells with abundant pale/clear often granular cytoplasm
- May be arranged into packets/nests with intervening collagen
- Positive for MART-1 &/or HMB-45 plus SMA &/or desmin
- S100 protein (+) in some but SOX-10(-)
- Lacks *EWSR1-ATF1* and *EWSR1-CREB1* fusions

Malignant Peripheral Nerve Sheath Tumor

- Large sarcoma of deep soft tissue, usually arises from nerve, from neurofibroma, or in neurofibromatosis type 1
  - Dermal involvement very rare
- Relatively uniform spindle cells in fascicles, often herringbone pattern
  - Usually lacks distinct fascicles/nests with intervening collagen seen in CCS
- Immunophenotype easily distinguishes malignant peripheral nerve sheath tumor (MPNST) from CCS
  - Paradoxically, S100 protein (-) or only focally (+) in MPNST
  - Other melanocytic markers (-)
  - H3K27me3 loss in many MPNSTs but also in some CCS
- Lacks *EWSR1-ATF1* and *EWSR1-CREB1* fusions

Monophasic Synovial Sarcoma

- Sarcoma often arising in deep soft tissue of distal extremities (rare in skin)
- Uniform, plump spindle cells in fascicles
- May have brisk mitotic activity, but prominent nucleoli usually absent
- Immunophenotype distinguishes synovial sarcoma (SS) from CCS
  - Keratin (+), EMA(+), TLE-1(+)
    - S100 protein (+) in subset of SS
  - Other melanocytic markers (-)
- Fusions of *SS18* (*SYT*) with *SSX1, SSX2,* or *SSX4* genes
- Lacks *EWSR1-ATF1* and *EWSR1-CREB1* fusions

DIAGNOSTIC CHECKLIST

Clinically Relevant Pathologic Features

- Late recurrence and metastasis
  - Metastasizes to lymph nodes and lungs

Pathologic Interpretation Pearls

- Consider CCS before diagnosing metastatic melanoma in young patient, in extremity, &/or if no known primary melanoma

SELECTED REFERENCES

1. Gonzaga MI et al: The epidemiology and survivorship of clear cell sarcoma: a National Cancer Database (NCDB) review. J Cancer Res Clin Oncol. 144(9):1711-6, 2018
2. Schöffski P et al: Activity and safety of crizotinib in patients with advanced clear-cell sarcoma with MET alterations: European Organization for Research and Treatment of Cancer phase II trial 90101 'CREATE'. Ann Oncol. 28(12):3000-8, 2017
3. Lee HL et al: Prognostic factors associated with clear cell sarcoma in 14 Chinese patients. J Orthop Surg (Hong Kong). 22(2):236-9, 2014
4. Kiuru M et al: Compound clear cell sarcoma misdiagnosed as a Spitz nevus. J Cutan Pathol. 40(11):950-4, 2013
5. Hocar O et al: Clear cell sarcoma (malignant melanoma) of soft parts: a clinicopathologic study of 52 cases. Dermatol Res Pract. 2012:984096, 2012
6. Mir O et al: Objective response to sorafenib in advanced clear-cell sarcoma. Ann Oncol. 23(3):807-9, 2012
7. Hisaoka M et al: Clear cell sarcoma of soft tissue: a clinicopathologic, immunohistochemical, and molecular analysis of 33 cases. Am J Surg Pathol. 32(3):452-60, 2008
8. Garcia JJ et al: Utility of CD117 immunoreactivity in differentiating metastatic melanoma from clear cell sarcoma. Arch Pathol Lab Med. 130(3):343-8, 2006
9. Antonescu CR et al: Molecular diagnosis of clear cell sarcoma: detection of EWS-ATF1 and MITF-M transcripts and histopathological and ultrastructural analysis of 12 cases. J Mol Diagn. 4(1):44-52, 2002
10. Lucas DR et al: Clear cell sarcoma of soft tissues. Mayo Clinic experience with 35 cases. Am J Surg Pathol. 16(12):1197-204, 1992
11. Montgomery E et al: Clear cell sarcoma of tendons and aponeuroses. A clinicopathologic study of 58 cases with analysis of prognostic factors. Int J Surg Pathol. 1:89-100, 1992

Prominent Fibrous Septa

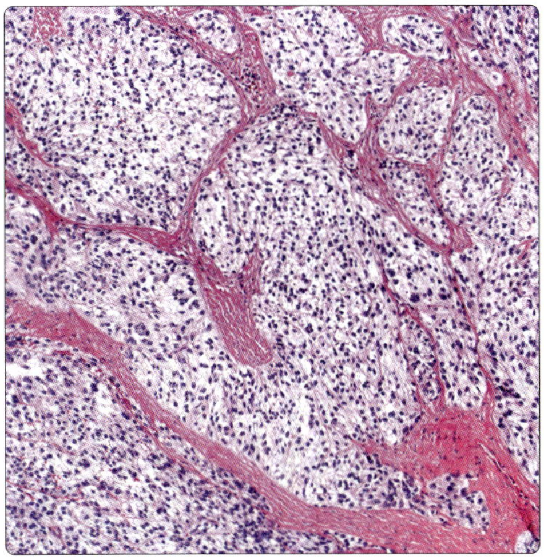

Thin Fibrous Septa

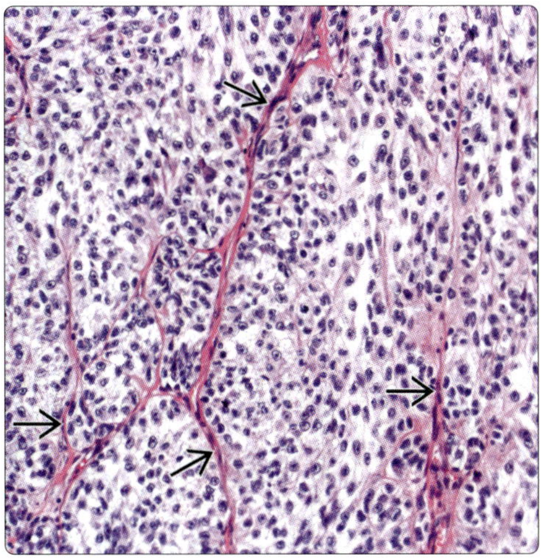

(Left) *Dense fibrous bands divide nests and fascicles of tumor cells in CCS. These septa can be quite prominent in some tumors, as seen in this H&E.* **(Right)** *In areas, the tumor cells have round or oval nuclei and are arranged into nests, packets, or large aggregates. The intervening fibrous septa are sometimes thin and delicate instead of thick and sclerotic →.*

Fascicular Growth

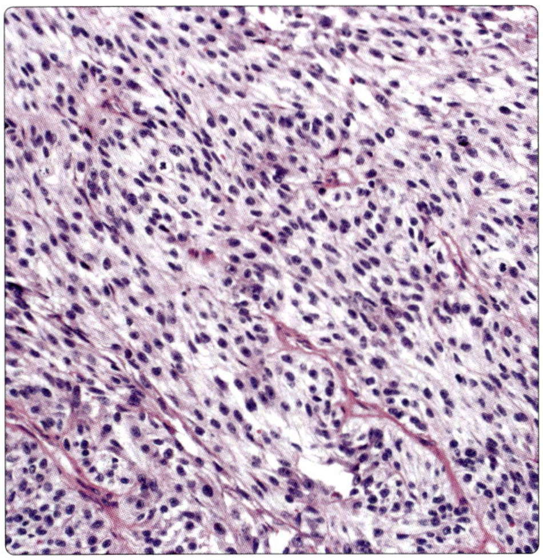

Eosinophilic Cytoplasm

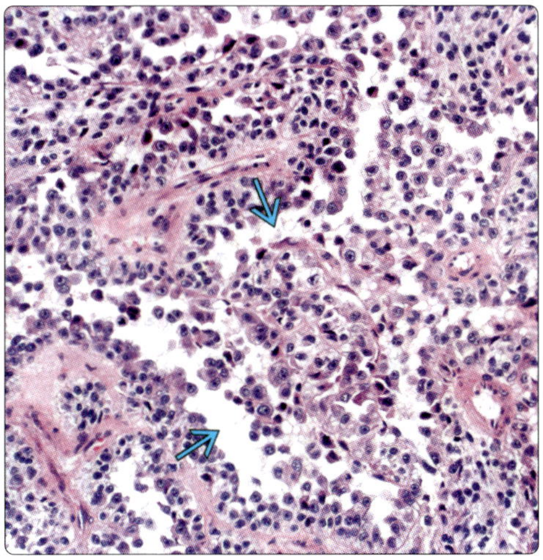

(Left) *When cut longitudinally, the tumor cells have a more spindled appearance and are arranged in long fascicles. Delicate fibrous septa are also present.* **(Right)** *Despite its name, CCS does not always feature clear cells. In many cases, the cells often have pale or eosinophilic cytoplasm, as depicted. Areas of dyscohesion → may be seen imparting a pseudoalveolar pattern.*

Tumor Giant Cells

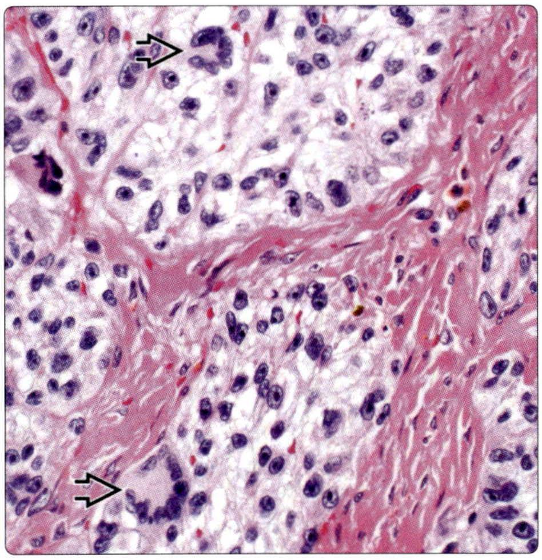

Less Prominent Nucleoli

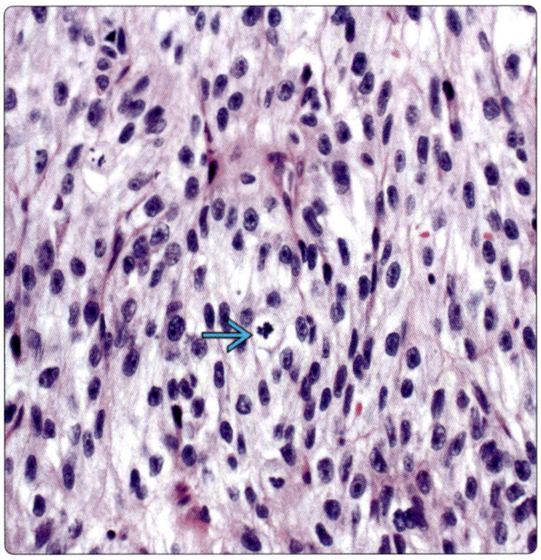

(Left) *In this H&E of CCS, the tumor cells have clear to pale eosinophilic cytoplasm and nuclei that contain prominent nucleoli but lack pleomorphism. Wreath-like multinucleated tumor giant cells → are also seen and are a helpful diagnostic feature of this tumor.* **(Right)** *Spindled pale tumor cells in this area of CCS have mostly small indistinct nucleoli. The classic large prominent nucleoli are not present in all cases. Mitoses are often seen →.*

Perivascular Epithelioid Cell Tumor (PEComa)

KEY FACTS

TERMINOLOGY

- Distinctive mesenchymal neoplasm arising from perivascular epithelioid cells that usually demonstrates combined myomelanocytic immunophenotype
  - PEComa family includes other defined clinical subtypes that arise in specific organs
    - Angiomyolipoma (AML), clear cell sugar tumor (CCST), lymphangioleiomyomatosis (LAM)

ETIOLOGY/PATHOGENESIS

- Deletions of *TSC2* gene with activation of mTOR pathway
- AML, CCST, and LAM associated with tuberous sclerosis complex
  - Most other PEComas are sporadic

CLINICAL ISSUES

- Wide age range (median: 45 years)
- Marked female predominance
- Overall good prognosis
- Clinically malignant tumors exists but are uncommon
  - Criteria have been proposed for assessing risk

MICROSCOPIC

- Nests, trabeculae, or sheets of epithelioid to spindled cells with clear to eosinophilic cytoplasm
- Association with walls of larger vessels in many cases
- Malignant tumors often feature prominent nuclear atypia, pleomorphism, and mitotic activity
- Variants: Sclerosing PEComa, fibroma-like PEComa

ANCILLARY TESTS

- Variable expression of SMA, desmin, melanocytic markers
- Subset of cases show nuclear TFE3(+)

TOP DIFFERENTIAL DIAGNOSES

- Leiomyosarcoma or leiomyoma
- Carcinoma or melanoma
- Clear cell sarcoma
- Alveolar soft part sarcoma

PEComa

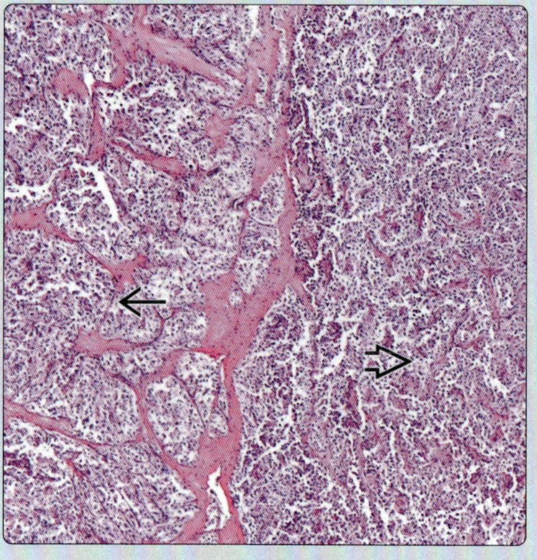

Epithelioid Cells

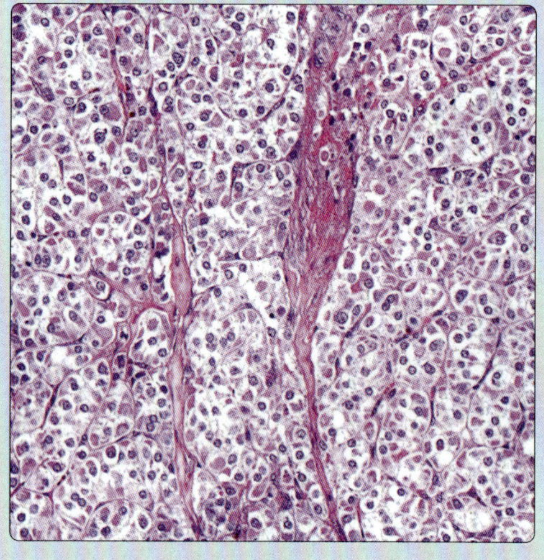

(Left) *The term perivascular epithelioid cell tumor (PEComa) identifies a family of related neoplasms that includes entities such as angiomyolipoma (AML) and lymphangioleiomyomatosis (LAM). PEComas, other than AML and LAM, arise in a variety of soft tissue and visceral sites and often show a nested architecture at low power, which may be well formed → or more subtle ⇨.* **(Right)** *PEComa is most commonly composed of epithelioid cells with variable eosinophilic to clear cytoplasm.*

Spindle Cells

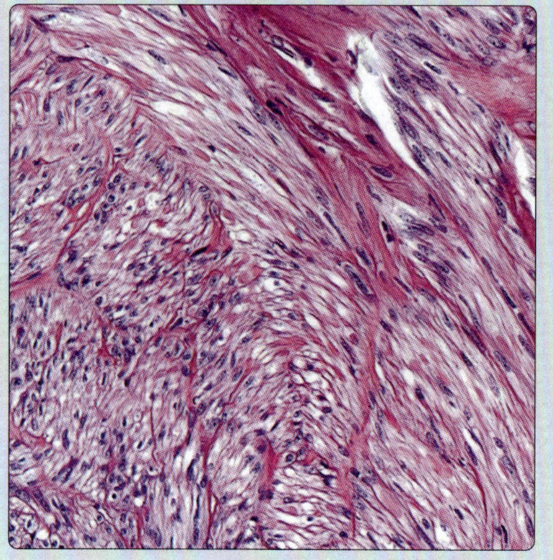

Myomelanocytic Immunophenotype

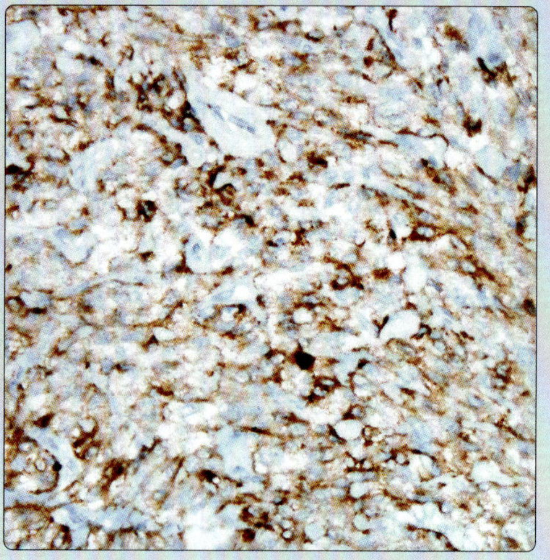

(Left) *Spindled tumor cells are common in PEComa but are overall less frequent than epithelioid cells. They are arranged in bundles and fascicles and show variable eosinophilic to clear cytoplasm. Note the resemblance to smooth muscle cells.* **(Right)** *PEComa characteristically shows a combined myomelanocytic immunophenotype and shows variable expression of a variety of myoid and melanocytic markers (particularly SMA and HMB-45). HMB-45 expression is seen here.*

Perivascular Epithelioid Cell Tumor (PEComa)

TERMINOLOGY

Abbreviations

- Perivascular epithelioid cell tumor (PEComa)

Synonyms

- Clear cell myomelanocytic tumor
- Primary extrapulmonary sugar tumor
- Extrarenal epithelioid angiomyolipoma (AML)
- Abdominopelvic sarcoma of perivascular epithelioid cells

Definitions

- Distinctive mesenchymal neoplasm arising from perivascular epithelioid cells that usually demonstrates combined myomelanocytic immunophenotype
  - PEComa family includes defined clinical subtypes that arise in specific organs
    - AML (kidney and liver)
    - Clear cell sugar tumor (CCST) (lung)
    - Lymphangioleiomyomatosis (LAM) (lung)

ETIOLOGY/PATHOGENESIS

Genetics

- Frequent deletions of *TSC2* gene with activation of mTOR pathway
- AML, CCST, and LAM show association with tuberous sclerosis complex (TSC)
  - Most other PEComas are sporadic
    - Subset associated with *TFE3* rearrangements/fusions

CLINICAL ISSUES

Epidemiology

- Incidence
  - Rare
- Age
  - Wide range (median: 45 years)
- Sex
  - Marked female predominance

Site

- May arise in almost any site
  - Retroperitoneum, abdomen, pelvis
  - Uterus, GI tract
  - Kidney, liver (AML)
  - Lung (CCST, LAM)
  - Uncommon in extremities, bone, skin

Presentation

- Usually painless mass
- Site-specific symptoms
  - Vaginal bleeding with uterine tumors
  - Obstructive symptoms or hematochezia with GI tumors
- May present with signs/symptoms of TSC, if affected
  - e.g., seizures, developmental delay, behavioral problems

Treatment

- Complete surgical excision
- Indefinite, long-term clinical follow-up recommended
- mTOR inhibitors (e.g., sirolimus) may have efficacy in malignant PEComa

Prognosis

- Overall good prognosis
  - Clinically malignant tumors exists but are uncommon
    - Generally aggressive sarcomas
    - Metastases to lung, liver, lymph nodes, bone
- Criteria have been proposed for assessing risk for malignant behavior (Folpe criteria)
  - High-risk features
    - Size > 5 cm
    - High nuclear grade and cellularity, readily identifiable mitotic figures
    - Infiltrative growth, necrosis, vascular invasion
  - Risk categories
    - Likely benign
      - Size < 5 cm and < 2 high-risk features
    - Uncertain malignant potential
      - Size ≥ 5 cm with no other high-risk features or
      - Nuclear pleomorphism/multinucleated giant cells only
    - Malignant
      - ≥ 2 high-risk features

MACROSCOPIC

General Features

- Well-demarcated, firm mass
- Fleshy or fibrous cut surface

Size

- Wide range (average: 6 cm)

MICROSCOPIC

Histologic Features

- Nests, trabeculae, or sheets of epithelioid to spindled cells
  - Clear to granular, lightly eosinophilic cytoplasm
    - Cytoplasm sometimes described as moth-eaten or stringy
    - Some larger epithelioid cells may appear spider-like
  - Round to oval nuclei with small nucleoli
    - Limited pleomorphism may be seen
- Thin-walled capillary vessels between nests of tumor cells
- Association with walls of larger vessels often present, at least focally
  - Cells appear to radiate outward from lumen
- Perivascular hyalinization not common
- Multinucleated giant cells in some cases
- Intracytoplasmic melanin pigment in some cases
- *TFE3*-rearranged PEComa
  - Epithelioid cells with clear cytoplasm
  - Distinctive nested or alveolar growth pattern
- Malignant PEComa
  - Proposed predictive criteria exist (Folpe)
  - Most cases of malignant PEComa show overtly malignant features
    - Marked cellularity with prominent nuclear pleomorphism/atypia and abundant mitoses
    - Also, infiltrative growth, necrosis, vascular invasion
- Unique features of specific clinical subtypes
  - AML often contains component of mature adipose tissue

- LAM of lung features cystic spaces associated with bundles of spindled cells
  - Localized tumors (lymphangiomyoma) show prominent pericytic growth

Morphologic Variants

- Sclerosing PEComa
  - Not associated with tuberous sclerosis
  - Prominent densely collagenous stroma
  - Cords, nests, and trabeculae of epithelioid cells
  - Most common in retroperitoneum
- Fibroma-like PEComa
  - Affects patients with tuberous sclerosis
  - Bland spindled to stellate cells within abundant collagenous stroma
  - Epithelioid cells rare or absent

ANCILLARY TESTS

Immunohistochemistry

- Classic combined myomelanocytic immunophenotype
  - SMA(+), desmin (+), caldesmon (+)
    - SMA is most sensitive
  - HMB-45(+), MART-1/melan-A (+), MITF(+)
    - HMB-45 is most sensitive
- Overall expression pattern is highly variable
  - Most tumors do not express all myomelanocytic antigens
  - Occasional tumors lack expression of either myoid markers or melanocytic markers
- Subset of cases show nuclear TFE3(+)
  - These tumors often have negative myoid markers
- Focal S100 protein (+) or CD117(+) in minority of cases
- Keratin, CD34, myogenin, DOG1 (-)

Molecular Genetics

- Subset lacking *TSC2* mutations show *TFE3* gene fusions
  - Suggests different pathogenesis for some types of PEComa
  - *SFPQ-TFE3* fusion most common
    - *DVL2-TFE3* and *NONO-TFE3* fusions rare

DIFFERENTIAL DIAGNOSIS

Leiomyosarcoma (and Leiomyoma)

- Can show morphologic overlap with spindle cell-predominant PEComa
- Perpendicularly oriented fascicles and bundles of spindled cells with brightly eosinophilic cytoplasm and blunt-ended nuclei
- Perivascular hyalinization &/or stromal sclerosis uncommon
- HMB-45, MART-1, MITF (-)

Carcinoma

- Particularly renal cell, adrenocortical, hepatocellular
- Lacks particular association with vessel walls
- Usually strong expression of epithelial antigens (keratin, EMA)
- May express markers of specific differentiation (pax-8, Hep-Par1, etc.)
- Myoid and melanocytic markers (-)

Melanoma

- Previous clinical history may be present
- Marked cytologic atypia with prominent nucleoli common
- Most show strong, diffuse S100 protein (+)
- Usually myoid markers (-)

Clear Cell Sarcoma

- Most common in distal extremities of young adults
- Nests of uniform cells with clear to pale eosinophilic cytoplasm and uniform nuclei with single large nucleolus
- May feature multinucleated giant cells
- S100 protein, HMB-45, MART-1 (+)
- SMA and desmin (-)
- t(12;22) with *EWSR1-ATF1* (most common)

Alveolar Soft Part Sarcoma

- Deep soft tissue of extremities in young adults
- Head/neck region in children
- Nests of large eosinophilic or clear epithelioid cells with variable central loss of cellular cohesion
  - Spindle cells absent
- Nuclear TFE3(+)
- Focal expression of SMA or desmin in some cases
- HMB-45, MART-1, MITF (-)
- t(X;17) with *ASPSCR1-TFE3* fusion

Granular Cell Tumor

- Diffuse cytoplasmic granularity
- Strongly S100 protein (+)
- Myoid and melanocytic markers (-)
- TFE3(+) in majority of cases

SELECTED REFERENCES

1. Bennett JA et al: Uterine PEComas: a morphologic, immunohistochemical, and molecular analysis of 32 tumors. Am J Surg Pathol. 42(10):1370-83, 2018
2. Larque AB et al: Fibroma-like PEComa: a tuberous sclerosis complex-related lesion. Am J Surg Pathol. 42(4):500-5, 2018
3. Maloney N et al: Expanding the histomorphologic spectrum of TFE3 rearranged PEComas. Hum Pathol. 82:125-30, 2018
4. McGregor SM et al: Melanotic PEComa of the sinonasal mucosa with NONO-TFE3 fusion: an elusive mimic of sinonasal melanoma. Am J Surg Pathol. 41(5):717-22, 2017
5. Agaram NP et al: Dichotomy of genetic abnormalities in PEComas with therapeutic implications. Am J Surg Pathol. 39(6):813-25, 2015
6. Schoolmeester JK et al: TFE3 translocation-associated perivascular epithelioid cell neoplasm (PEComa) of the gynecologic tract: morphology, immunophenotype, differential diagnosis. Am J Surg Pathol. 39(3):394-404, 2015
7. Shen Q et al: Perivascular epithelioid cell tumor (PEComa) with TFE3 gene rearrangement: clinicopathological, immunohistochemical, and molecular features. Virchows Arch. 465(5):607-13, 2014
8. Doyle LA et al: PEComa of the gastrointestinal tract: clinicopathologic study of 35 cases with evaluation of prognostic parameters. Am J Surg Pathol. 37(12):1769-82, 2013
9. Bleeker JS et al: "Malignant" perivascular epithelioid cell neoplasm: risk stratification and treatment strategies. Sarcoma. 2012:541626, 2012
10. Folpe AL et al: Perivascular epithelioid cell neoplasms: pathology and pathogenesis. Hum Pathol. 41(1):1-15, 2010
11. Hornick JL et al: Sclerosing PEComa: clinicopathologic analysis of a distinctive variant with a predilection for the retroperitoneum. Am J Surg Pathol. 32(4):493-501, 2008
12. Folpe AL et al: Perivascular epithelioid cell neoplasms of soft tissue and gynecologic origin: a clinicopathologic study of 26 cases and review of the literature. Am J Surg Pathol. 29(12):1558-75, 2005

Cytologic Features

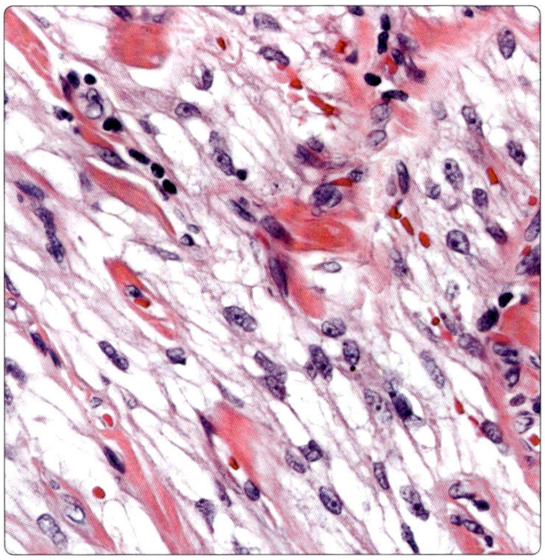

Nested Growth

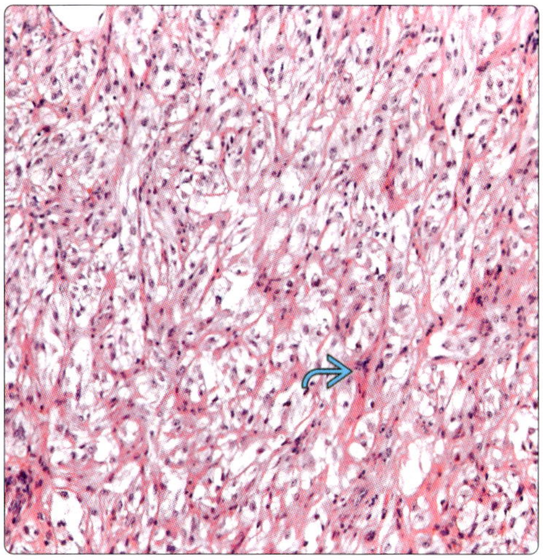

(Left) *Nuclei in PEComa are generally round to ovoid and contain small nucleoli. Note that the cytoplasm often varies from eosinophilic to clear and may show a "frayed" quality that has been described as stringy or moth-eaten.* **(Right)** *Nested growth of tumor cells is common in PEComa, but trabecular and sheet-like patterns may also be seen. Nests are often demarcated by variably prominent, thin-walled capillary channels, similar to that seen in renal cell carcinoma.*

Clear Cells

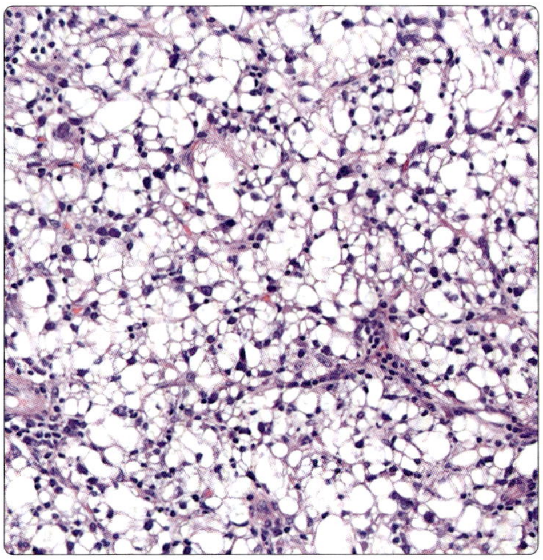

Spider Cells

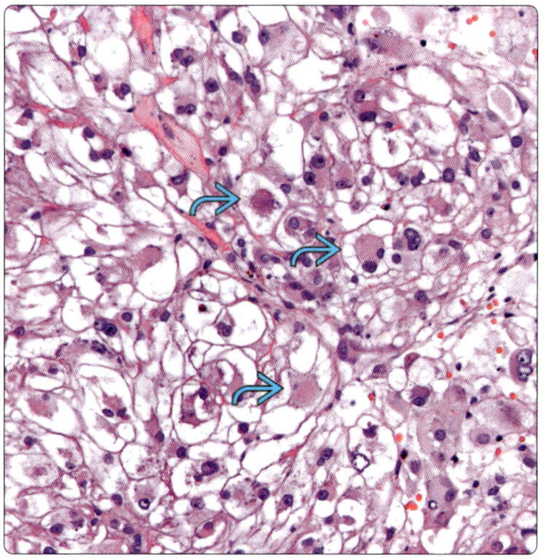

(Left) *Tumor cells with abundant clear cytoplasm may be diffuse and prominent in some cases of PEComa, as depicted. Note the vague nested architecture with intervening capillaries. This appearance can mimic clear cell renal cell carcinoma.* **(Right)** *Some larger epithelioid tumor cells in PEComa may show centralized cytoplasmic retraction, similar to the "spider cells" seen in adult-type rhabdomyoma.*

Pale Granular Cells

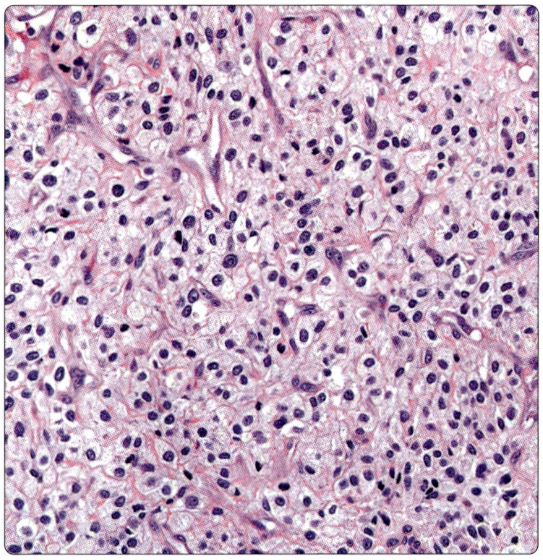

Eosinophilic Granular Cells

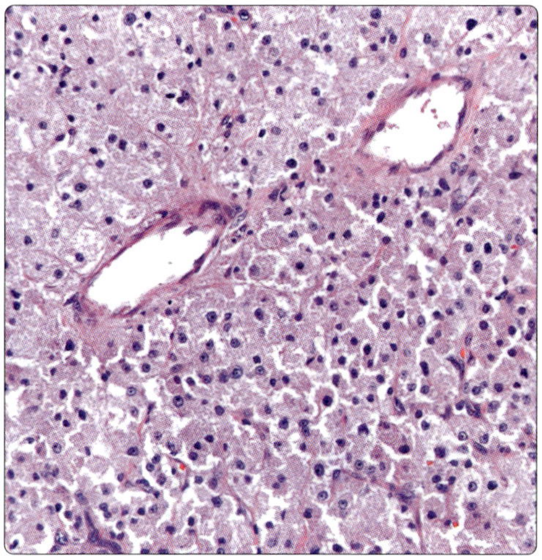

(Left) *PEComa may contain epithelioid tumor cells with pale, eosinophilic and finely granular cytoplasm, reminiscent of histiocytes or possibly even an adrenocortical neoplasm.* **(Right)** *Finely granular cytoplasm with more distinctive eosinophilia may be encountered in PEComa, reminiscent of granular cell tumor. This tumor arose in the uterus.*

(Left) *A prominent alveolar growth pattern, as depicted, is seen in a subset of PEComa. These particular tumors are more likely to harbor TFE3 gene fusions and show nuclear TFE3 immunoreactivity. Note the resemblance to alveolar soft part sarcoma, another tumor with TFE3 gene fusion.* **(Right)** *This PEComa shows predominantly smaller epithelioid cells with exclusively eosinophilic cytoplasm. In visceral organs, this morphology may lead to confusion with carcinoma.*

Prominent Alveolar Growth

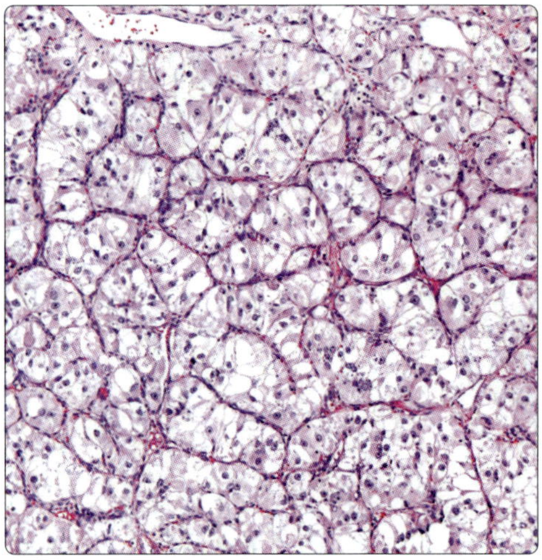

Eosinophilic Epithelioid Cells

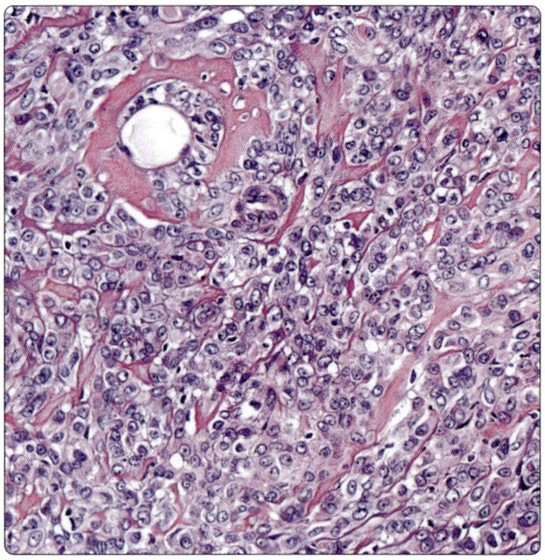

(Left) *Trabecular growth may be conspicuous in PEComa, although areas with a nested pattern are usually also present.* **(Right)** *Multinucleated tumor giant cells ➡ are focally present in some cases of PEComa, and they can adopt a variety of cytomorphologies, including wreath-like, Touton, osteoclastic, and Langhans. The presence of these cells does not appear to affect behavior unless there are other atypical features (mitoses, significant nuclear atypia, etc.).*

Trabecular Pattern

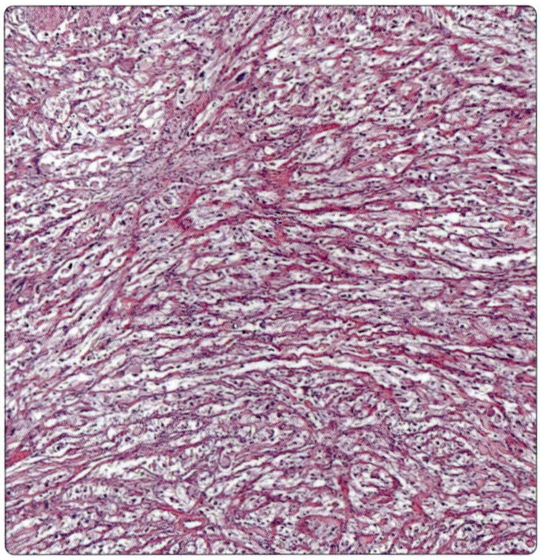

Multinucleated Giant Cells

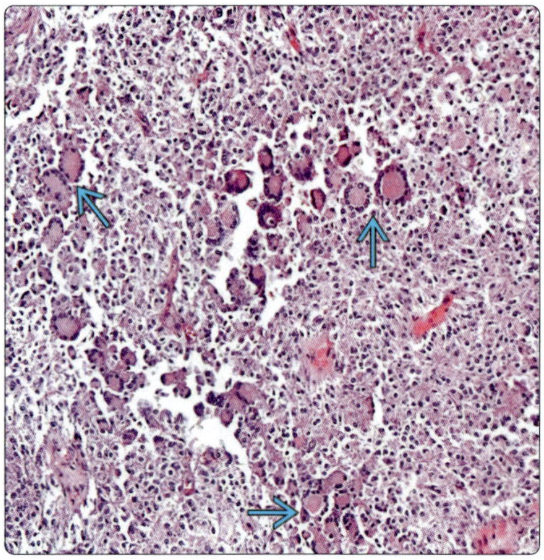

(Left) *Perivascular hyalinization ↪ or sclerosis is not uncommon in PEComa and may be prominent and extensive in some cases, as shown in this H&E.* **(Right)** *An interesting finding seen in many cases of PEComa is the association of tumor cells with blood vessel walls, often with a outward-radiating arrangement ↪. This finding is particularly evident in renal PEComa (AML).*

Perivascular Hyalinization

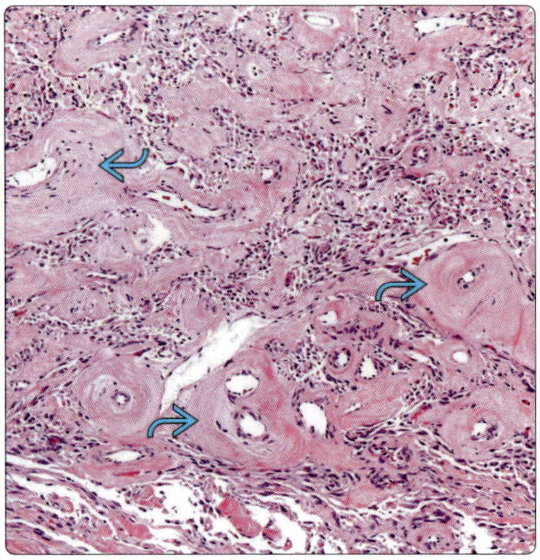

Vessel Wall Association

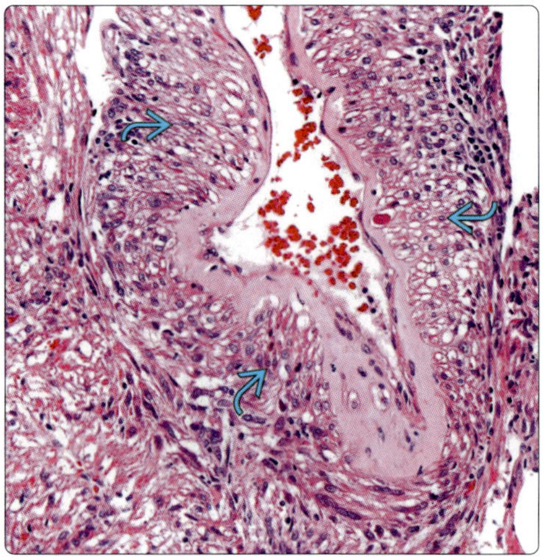

Stromal Hyalinization

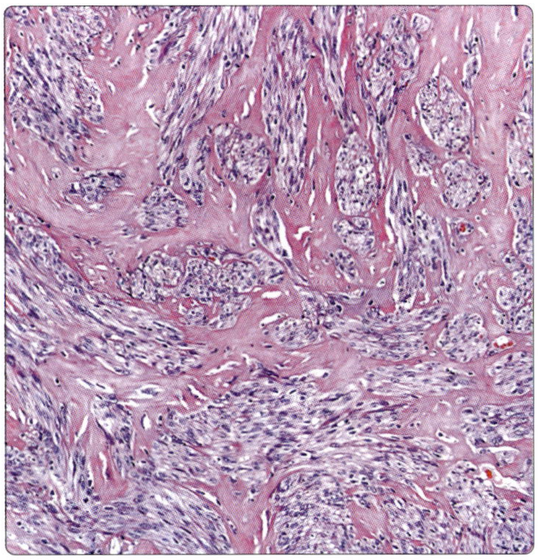

Stromal Sclerosis

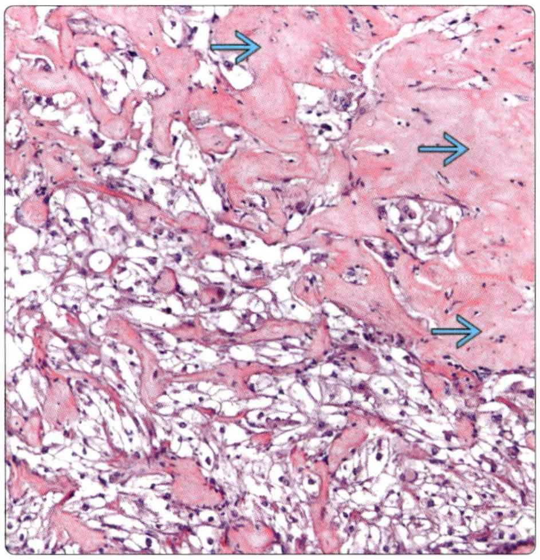

(Left) *Although thin fibrous septa are not uncommon between nests of tumor cells in PEComa, more extensive seams and bands of glassy hyalinized collagen may be present in some cases.* **(Right)** *In this case of PEComa, paucicellular areas of dense sclerosis* ➔ *are seen adjacent to more conventional areas featuring tumor cells with prominent clear cytoplasm.*

Sclerosing PEComa

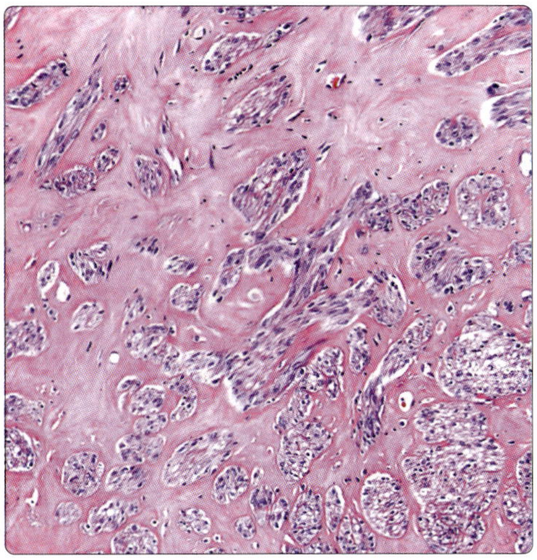

Sclerosing PEComa

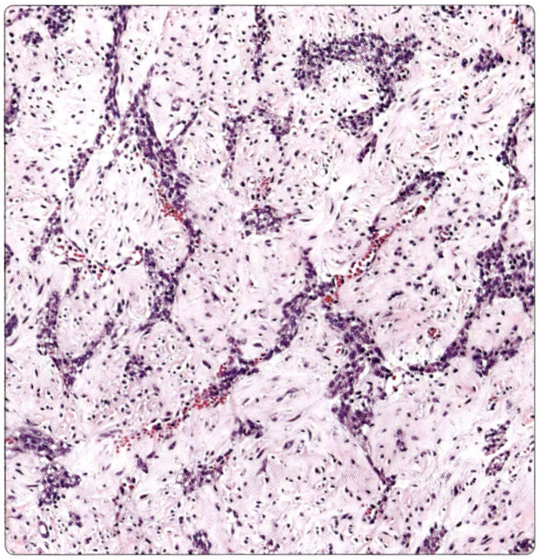

(Left) *Sclerosing PEComa is a morphologic variant characterized by a prominent, densely hyalinized or sclerotic stroma. Tumor cells may appear in small nests, cords, clusters, or even singly.* **(Right)** *This case of sclerosing PEComa shows thin anastomosing cords of epithelioid tumor cells within an abundant collagenous stroma. This particular variant is most frequent in the retroperitoneum, particularly near the kidneys.*

Myoid Marker Expression

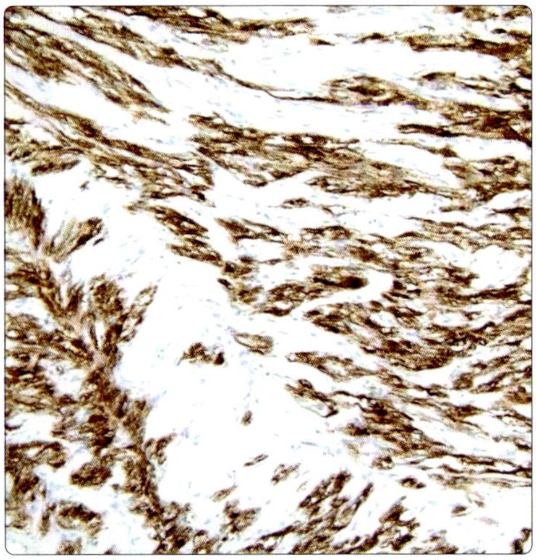

Cutaneous PEComa

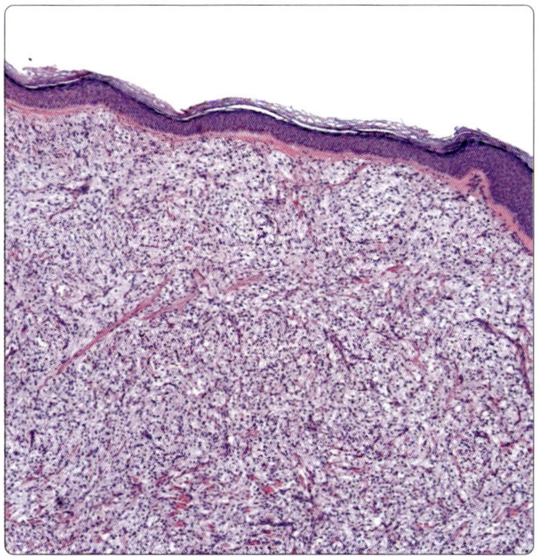

(Left) *SMA expression (shown) is seen in most cases of PEComa. Other myoid markers (such as MSA, desmin, and caldesmon) are usually less consistently expressed. Rare cases are completely negative for all of these markers.* **(Right)** *Although rare, PEComa may also arise in the skin, as depicted. Although similar in many respects to more deeply situated and visceral tumors, cutaneous PEComa does not appear to harbor TFE3 gene fusions or express nuclear TFE3.*

(Left) *Clear cytoplasm is usually prominent in cases of cutaneous PEComa, as shown. Note the dermal collagen fibers →.* **(Right)** *Primary renal PEComa (better known as AML) contains spindled tumor cells similar to those of other forms of PEComa; however, it also usually contains mature adipose tissue → and shows a more conspicuous association with intratumoral blood vessels →. Epithelioid variants also exist.*

Cutaneous PEComa

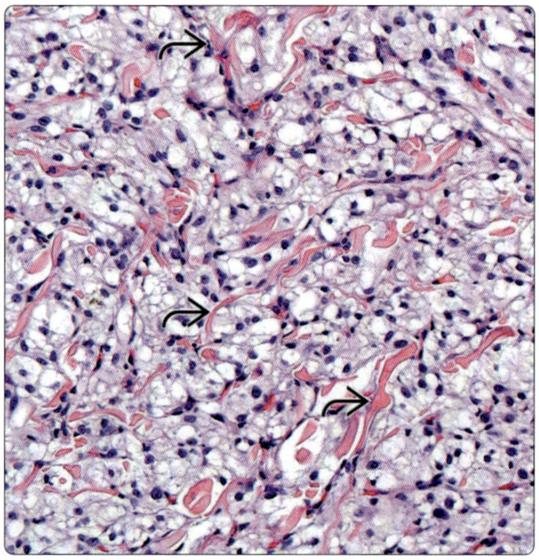

Angiomyolipoma

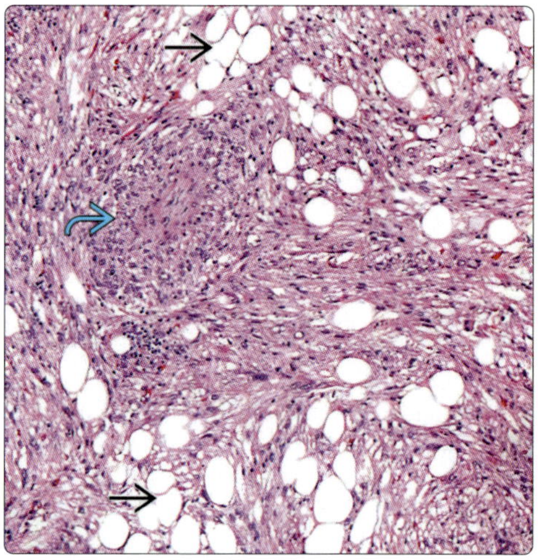

(Left) *Pulmonary LAM is a form of PEComa that affects female patients almost exclusively and features bundles → of uniform, spindled myomelanocytic cells, often associated with prominent cystic spaces.* **(Right)** *Rare, localized forms of LAM (known as lymphangiomyoma) may arise outside of the lungs, mainly within the retroperitoneum or mediastinum, and often in association with large lymphatic ducts or lymph nodes.*

Lymphangioleiomyomatosis

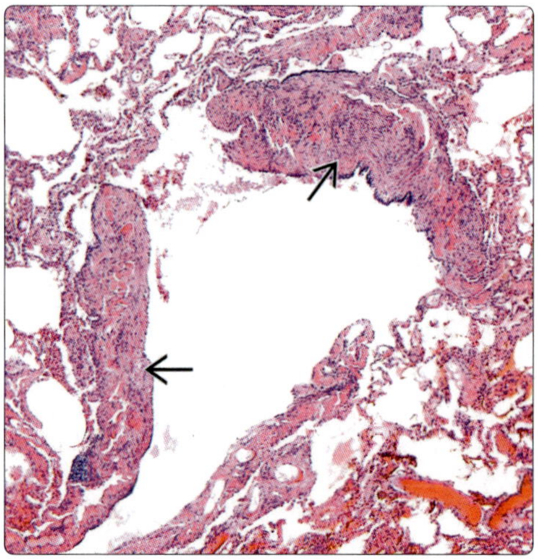

Lymphangiomyoma

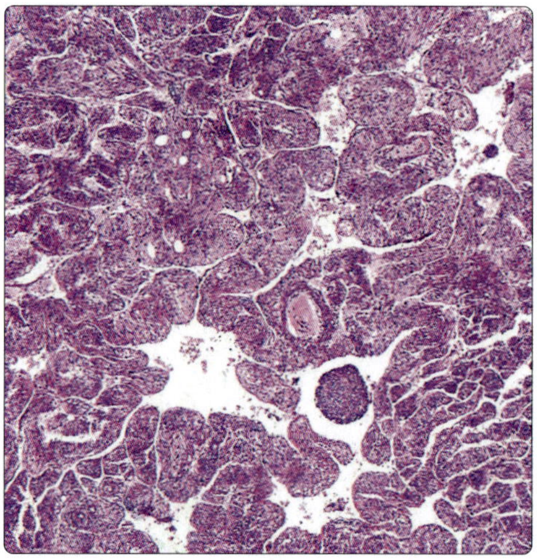

(Left) *Lymphangiomyoma features bundles of uniformed, spindled cells arranged around endothelial-lined channels →, creating a pericytic growth pattern. Scattered lymphocytes &/or lymphoid aggregates are common. Dilated spaces → containing lymphatic fluid are also frequently seen.* **(Right)** *Clinically malignant PEComa is uncommon but is generally aggressive. Criteria have been proposed for risk assessment that include tumor size as well as significant nuclear atypia (shown), among other features.*

Lymphangiomyoma

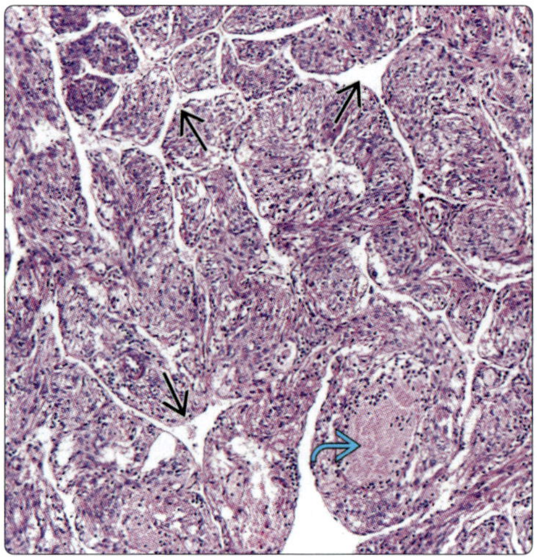

Malignant PEComa

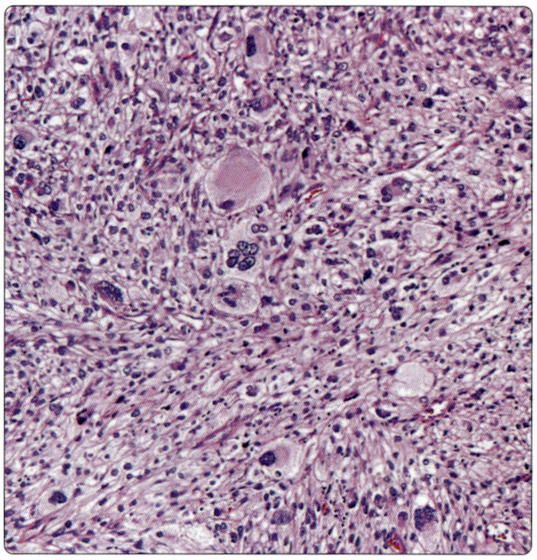

Cellular Malignant PEComa

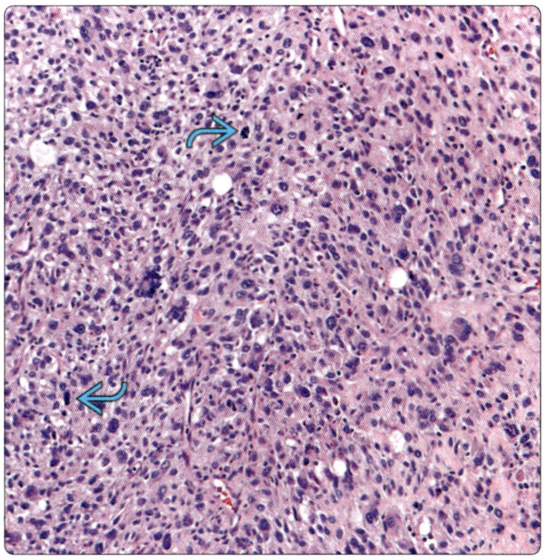

Vessel Wall Association

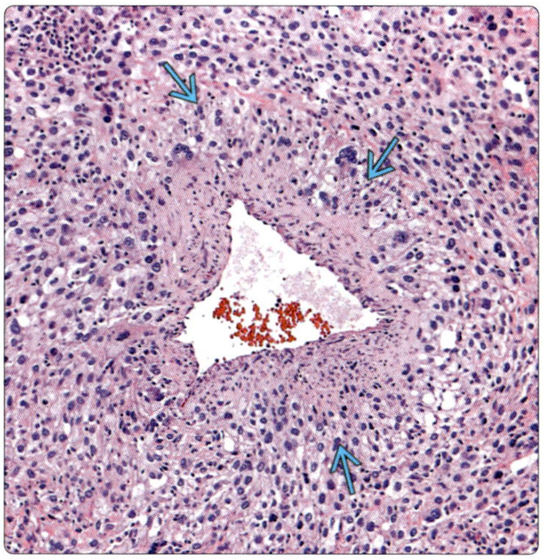

(Left) *Malignant PEComa usually features significant nuclear atypia and pleomorphism, and mitotic figures ↪ are often readily identified, including atypical forms.* **(Right)** *The characteristic finding of vessel wall involvement in typical PEComa can also be seen in malignant forms, as depicted. Note the radial arrangement of tumor cells →.*

Clear Cell Malignant PEComa

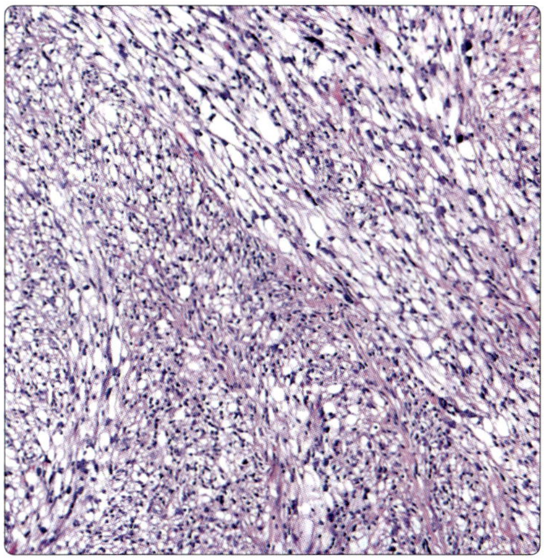

Coagulative Necrosis

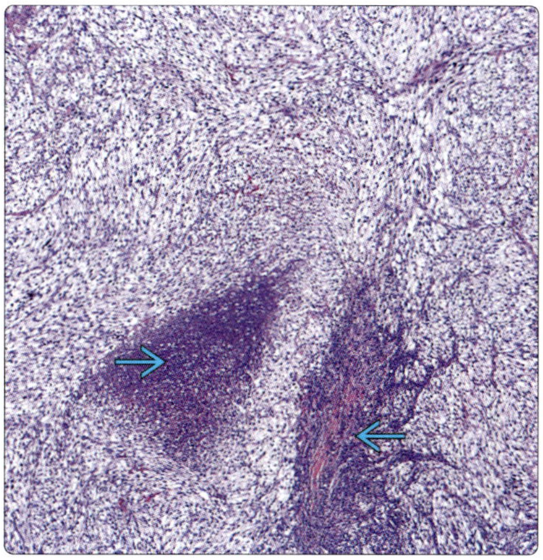

(Left) *Malignant PEComa can show features of any form of typical PEComa, including a diffuse clear cell morphology. This large tumor contained numerous mitoses and diffuse nuclear atypia.* **(Right)** *Coagulative necrosis → is rare in PEComa but is more frequently seen in malignant forms. Vascular invasion and infiltrative growth are also atypical findings and should be considered when assessing risk of malignant behavior.*

Spindle Cell Malignant PEComa

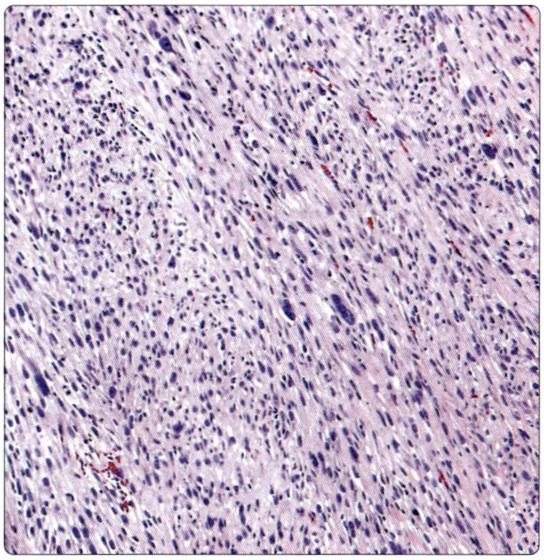

Deceptively Bland Malignant PEComa

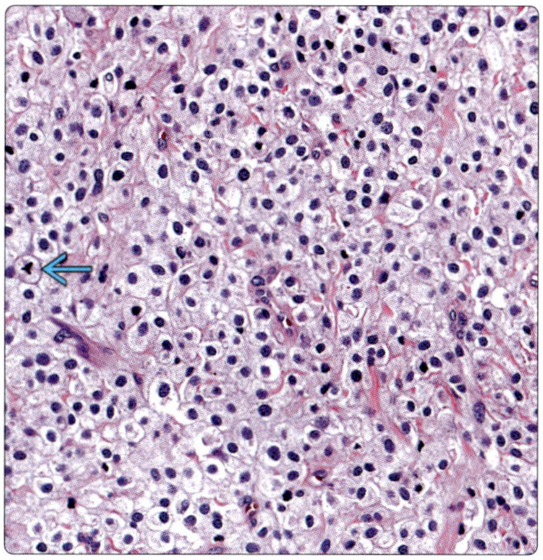

(Left) *Malignant PEComa may also contain areas showing a fascicular, spindled morphology and may be difficult to distinguish from leiomyosarcoma.* **(Right)** *This PEComa from the thigh demonstrates mostly relatively uniform, pale, granular tumor cells, suggesting benignity; however, mitoses were abundant, including atypical forms →. Areas of increased nuclear atypia were present very focally. This tumor metastasized to the mediastinum 2 years after initial complete resection.*

Desmoplastic Small Round Cell Tumor

KEY FACTS

TERMINOLOGY

- Malignant mesenchymal neoplasm of polyphenotypic differentiation composed of primitive cells embedded in abundant desmoplastic stroma

CLINICAL ISSUES

- Usually children and young adults (median age: 20 years)
  - Strong male predilection
- Abdominal cavity most common site
  - Peritoneum, retroperitoneum, omentum, mesentery
- Treatment: Multimodality therapy with surgery/chemotherapy
- Overall poor prognosis

MACROSCOPIC

- Bulky, diffuse multinodular or solitary
- Wide range, usually large (often > 10 cm)

MICROSCOPIC

- Nests, sheets, and trabeculae of small undifferentiated cells
- Characteristic abundant desmoplastic fibrous stroma
- Mitoses and necrosis common
- Other findings: Rosette-like structures, tubule/gland formation, clear cell change

ANCILLARY TESTS

- Polyphenotypic differentiation, with keratin (+), desmin (+), NSE(+)
  - Key finding: Perinuclear dot-like desmin expression
- Molecular: Characteristic recurrent t(11;22)(p13;q12) involving *EWSR1* and *WT1* genes

TOP DIFFERENTIAL DIAGNOSES

- Ewing sarcoma
- Alveolar rhabdomyosarcoma
- Neuroendocrine carcinoma

Desmoplastic Small Round Cell Tumor

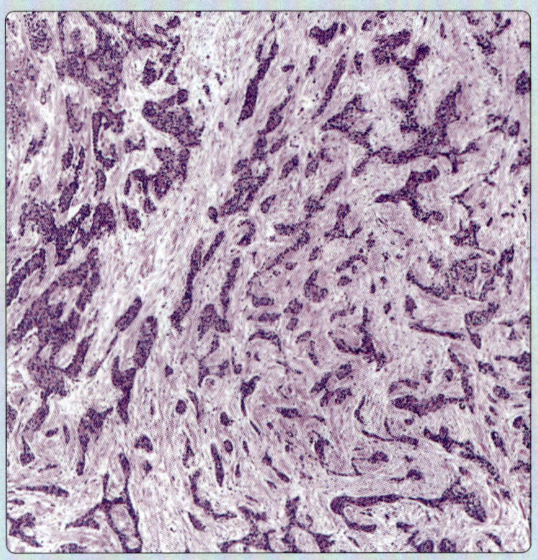

Undifferentiated Cells

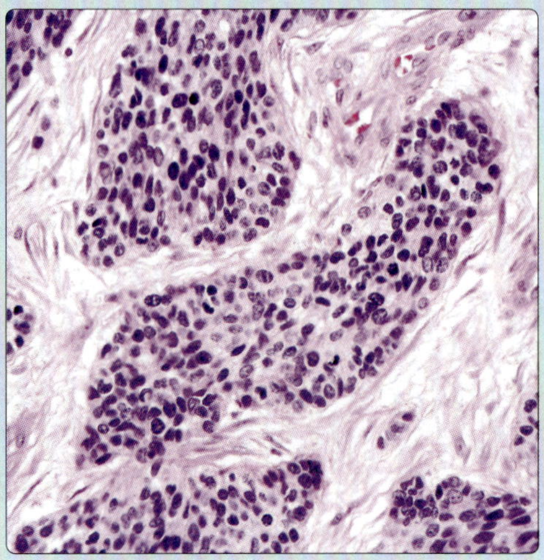

(Left) *Desmoplastic small round cell tumor (DSRCT) is an aggressive malignant neoplasm that most commonly affects children and young adults, particularly males. Morphologically, it is characterized by nests, sheets, and cords of relatively monomorphic cells in a prominent desmoplastic fibrous stroma.* **(Right)** *The lesional cells of DSRCT are generally small, relatively monomorphic, and appear undifferentiated. Nucleoli are inconspicuous and mitoses are common.*

Desmin Expression

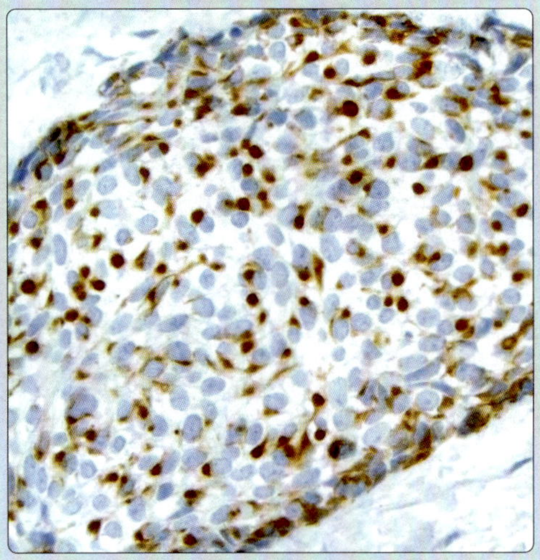

Keratin Expression

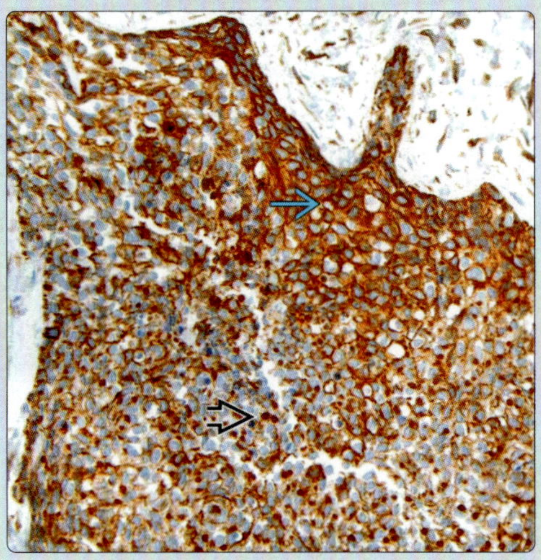

(Left) *Diffuse desmin expression is common in DSRCT and characteristically manifests as dot-like staining adjacent to the nucleus. Diffuse cytoplasmic expression may also be seen in this tumor.* **(Right)** *Cytokeratins are usually strongly expressed in DSRCT and vary in pattern from diffuse cytoplasmic* → *to perinuclear dot-like* ⇨ *(less common). A similar pattern of reactivity is seen with vimentin.*

Desmoplastic Small Round Cell Tumor

TERMINOLOGY

Abbreviations

- Desmoplastic small round cell tumor (DSRCT)

Synonyms

- DSRCT with divergent differentiation
- Polyphenotypic small round cell tumor
- Intraabdominal DSRCT

Definitions

- Malignant mesenchymal neoplasm of polyphenotypic differentiation composed of primitive cells embedded in abundant desmoplastic stroma

CLINICAL ISSUES

Epidemiology

- Incidence
  - Rare
- Age
  - Usually children and young adults (median: 20 years)
    - Occasionally older adults
- Sex
  - Strong male predilection

Site

- Abdominal cavity most common
  - Peritoneum, retroperitoneum, pelvis, omentum, mesentery
- Sporadic involvement of extraabdominal sites, including paratesticular region, thoracic cavity, and many others

Presentation

- Abdominal distention, pain, weight loss, obstructive symptoms
- Diffuse serosal involvement by multiple tumor nodules common

Treatment

- Multimodality therapy, including surgical resection/debulkment and chemotherapy

Prognosis

- Overall poor prognosis
  - Nearly uniformly fatal
  - Median survival: 24 months
- Frequent local recurrence; occasionally metastasizes

MACROSCOPIC

General Features

- Large, bulky, multinodular or solitary
- Firm tan-white homogeneous cut surface
- Foci of necrosis &/or hemorrhage

Size

- Wide range, usually large (often > 10 cm)

MICROSCOPIC

Histologic Features

- Nests of small undifferentiated cells within abundant desmoplastic fibrous stroma
- Desmoplastic stroma is characteristic
  - Fibroblasts/myofibroblasts within loose extracellular matrix or collagen
  - May show myxoid change or hyalinization
  - Variably prominent stromal vascularity
- Variety of architectural configurations
  - Nests (individual or confluent), sheets, cords, trabeculae, organoid, others
    - Central necrosis and cystic change common; may occasionally be diffuse
- Small, relatively monomorphic, round to oval cells with scant eosinophilic cytoplasm
  - Small hyperchromatic nuclei with inconspicuous nucleoli
    - Nuclear pleomorphism may be present (focal or diffuse) in some cases
  - Mitotic figures often numerous
  - Cells may be epithelioid with more abundant cytoplasm
    - Also cytoplasm may be vacuolated or show clear cell change
  - Intracytoplasmic paranuclear hyaline inclusions in some tumors
  - Focal cytoplasmic spindling rare
- Rare focal epithelial differentiation: Rosette-like structures, tubule/gland formation, papillary areas

ANCILLARY TESTS

Immunohistochemistry

- Polyphenotypic differentiation (see table)
- Key finding: Perinuclear dot-like desmin expression
- Nuclear WT1 expression only seen with antibodies directed against carboxy (C) terminus of WT1

Molecular Genetics

- Characteristic recurrent t(11;22)(p13;q12) involving *EWSR1* and *WT1* genes
  - Rare isolated reports of *EWSR1-ERG* and *EWSR1-FLI1* fusions
    - Appear to be hybrid tumors with features of DSRCT and Ewing sarcoma

DIFFERENTIAL DIAGNOSIS

Extraskeletal Ewing Sarcoma

- Lacks prominent desmoplastic stroma
- Strong, membranous CD99(+)
  - Variety of other small blue cell tumors, such as DSRCT, can show patchy cytoplasmic positivity
- Negative for desmin, EMA, and WT1
- FLI-1(+); may show focal keratin (+)
- *EWSR1* translocation in most cases
  - Most commonly t(11;22)(q24;q12) involving *EWSR1* and *FLI1*
    - Distinct from t(11;22)(p13;q12) of DSRCT, which involves *WT1* instead of *FLI1*

Alveolar Rhabdomyosarcoma

- Nests with central dyscohesion and divided by fibrous septa
- Lacks prominent desmoplastic stroma
- May contain multinucleated (wreath-like) giant cells
- Diffuse desmin (+), myogenin (+), MYOD1(+)
- May show focal keratin (+)

Immunohistochemistry Table

Antibody	Reactivity	Staining Pattern	Comment
AE1/AE3	Positive	Cytoplasmic	May also show perinuclear dot-like staining
Desmin	Positive	Dot positivity	Cytoplasmic expression also common
Vimentin	Positive	Cytoplasmic	May also show perinuclear dot-like staining
EMA	Positive	Cell membrane	
NSE	Positive	Cytoplasmic	Very nonspecific marker
Actin-sm	Negative	Cytoplasmic	Expressed in stromal myofibroblasts but not tumor cells
Synaptophysin	Negative	Cytoplasmic	Rare focal positivity
CD56	Negative		
Myogenin	Negative		
MYOD1	Negative		
WT1	Equivocal	Nuclear	Selective carboxy-terminus immunoreactivity only
CD99	Equivocal	Cell membrane and cytoplasm	Usually cytoplasmic, if present; rarely membranous
NB84	Equivocal	Cytoplasmic	Usually focal, if present

- Characteristic t(2;13) or t(1;13) involving *FOXO1*

Metastatic Neuroendocrine Carcinoma

- Clinical history of primary tumor
- Lacks prominent desmoplastic stroma separating tumor cell nests
- Has distinctive smudged or salt and pepper chromatin pattern
- Synaptophysin (+), chromogranin (+), CD56(+)
- Negative for desmin and WT1
- Can show perinuclear dot-like expression of keratins

Extrarenal Rhabdoid Tumor

- Affects infants and children
- Sheets of epithelioid cells with prominent rhabdoid differentiation
  - Rhabdoid morphology may be less prominent in small cell variant
- Desmin (-)
- Loss of nuclear INI1 by immunohistochemistry

Malignant Lymphoma

- Dyscohesive pattern of growth without striking desmoplasia
- Expresses hematolymphoid markers (e.g., CD45, CD3, CD20, CD30, CD43)
- Negative for keratin, desmin, nuclear WT1
- Lymphoblastic lymphoma in children and adolescents shows nuclear positivity for TdT and is positive for CD99

Neuroblastoma

- Most diagnosed < 5 years of age
- NB84(+)
- Negative for desmin and keratins
- Lacks *EWSR1* translocation

SELECTED REFERENCES

1. Stiles ZE et al: Desmoplastic small round cell tumor: a nationwide study of a rare sarcoma. J Surg Oncol. 117(8):1759-67, 2018
2. Subbiah V et al: Multimodality treatment of desmoplastic small round cell tumor: chemotherapy and complete cytoreductive surgery improve patient survival. Clin Cancer Res. 24(19):4865-73, 2018
3. Mohamed M et al: Desmoplastic small round cell tumor: evaluation of reverse transcription-polymerase chain reaction and fluorescence in situ hybridization as ancillary molecular diagnostic techniques. Virchows Arch. 471(5):631-40, 2017
4. de Alava E et al: Birth and evolution of the desmoplastic small round-cell tumor. Semin Diagn Pathol. 33(5):254-61, 2016
5. Thway K et al: Desmoplastic small round cell tumor: pathology, genetics, and potential therapeutic strategies. Int J Surg Pathol. 24(8):672-84, 2016
6. Arnold MA et al: Diagnostic pitfalls of differentiating desmoplastic small round cell tumor (DSRCT) from Wilms tumor (WT): overlapping morphologic and immunohistochemical features. Am J Surg Pathol. 38(9):1220-6, 2014
7. Wong HH et al: Desmoplastic small round cell tumour: characteristics and prognostic factors of 41 patients and review of the literature. Clin Sarcoma Res. 3(1):14, 2013
8. Dufresne A et al: Desmoplastic small round cell tumor: current management and recent findings. Sarcoma. 2012:714986, 2012
9. Jordan AH et al: Management of desmoplastic small round-cell tumors in children and young adults. J Pediatr Hematol Oncol. 34 Suppl 2:S73-5, 2012
10. Bono F et al: Desmoplastic small cell tumor with bizarre giant nuclei. Int J Surg Pathol. 19(6):843-6, 2011
11. Yin WH et al: Desmoplastic small round cell tumor of the submandibular gland--a rare but distinctive primary salivary gland neoplasm. Hum Pathol. 41(3):438-42, 2010
12. Saab R et al: Desmoplastic small round cell tumor in childhood: the St. Jude Children's Research Hospital experience. Pediatr Blood Cancer. 49(3):274-9, 2007
13. Chang F: Desmoplastic small round cell tumors: cytologic, histologic, and immunohistochemical features. Arch Pathol Lab Med. 130(5):728-32, 2006
14. Lae ME et al: Desmoplastic small round cell tumor: a clinicopathologic, immunohistochemical, and molecular study of 32 tumors. Am J Surg Pathol. 26(7):823-35, 2002
15. Ordóñez NG: Desmoplastic small round cell tumor: I: a histopathologic study of 39 cases with emphasis on unusual histological patterns. Am J Surg Pathol. 22(11):1303-13, 1998
16. Ordóñez NG: Desmoplastic small round cell tumor: II: an ultrastructural and immunohistochemical study with emphasis on new immunohistochemical markers. Am J Surg Pathol. 22(11):1314-27, 1998
17. Gerald WL et al: Intra-abdominal desmoplastic small round-cell tumor. Report of 19 cases of a distinctive type of high-grade polyphenotypic malignancy affecting young individuals. Am J Surg Pathol. 15(6):499-513, 1991

Variably Sized Nests

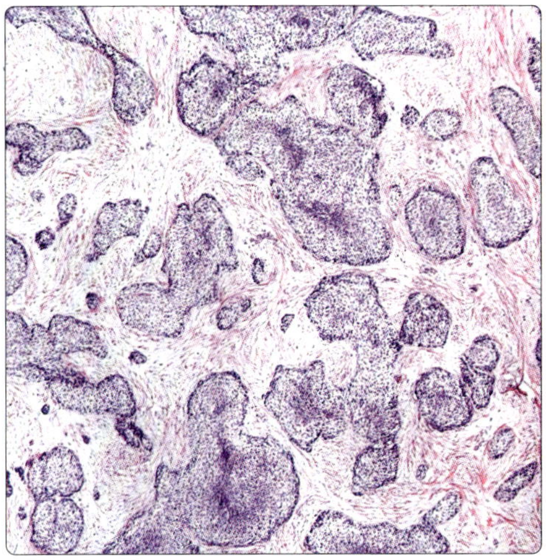

Infiltrative Areas

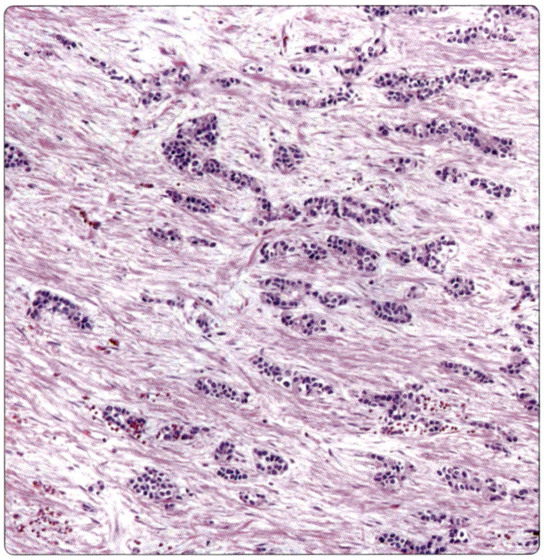

(Left) *Although the exact pattern varies from case to case, most examples of DSRCT show nests of varying sizes and shapes. Note the desmoplastic background stroma that is characteristic of this tumor.* **(Right)** *In some areas of DSRCT, particularly at the periphery, the tumor cells may adopt a less cellular and corded morphologic pattern that resembles infiltrating carcinoma.*

Clear Cell Change

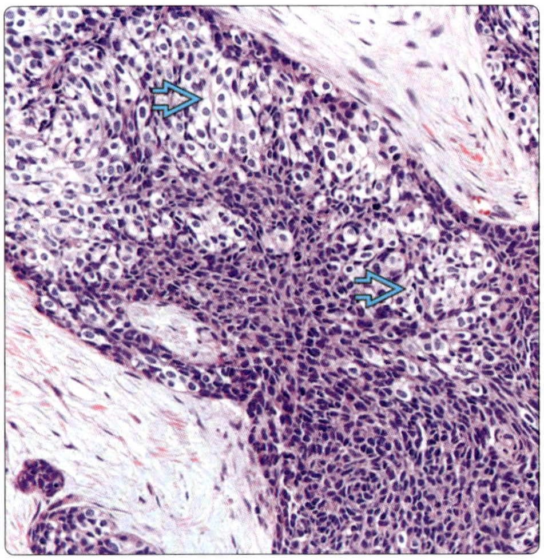

Central Necrosis

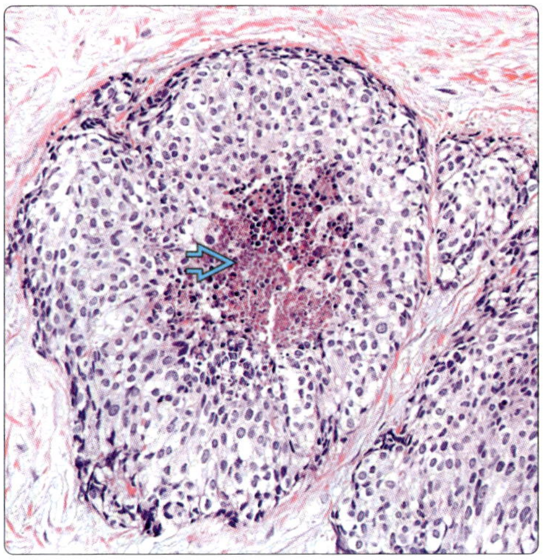

(Left) *Tumor cells with cytoplasmic clearing are seen in some cases of DSRCT and may be focal or extensive. Vacuolated cytoplasm or a signet ring-like cytologic appearance may also be seen in some tumors.* **(Right)** *Larger nests in DSRCT often show central necrosis. Rarely, a tumor may show extensive, zonal coagulative necrosis with scattered islands of viable cells.*

Desmoplastic Fibrous Stroma

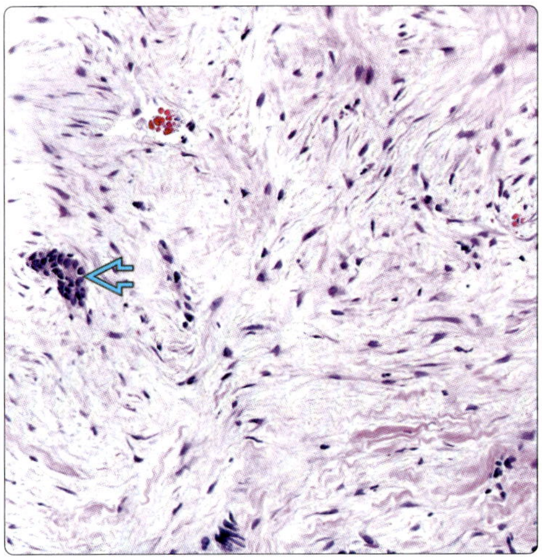

Collagenous Stroma

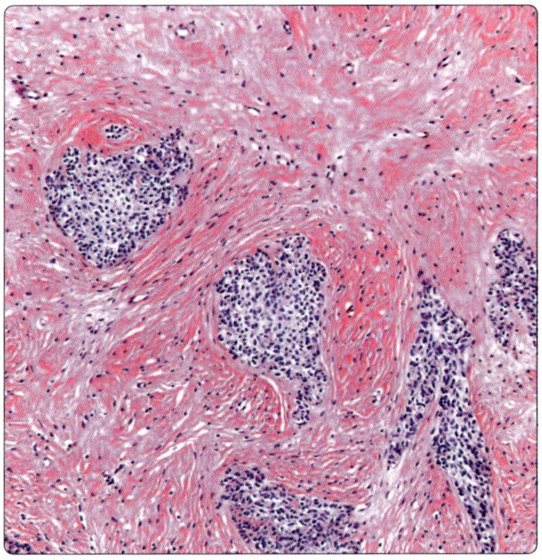

(Left) *The desmoplastic fibrous stroma of DSRCT is composed of spindled fibroblasts and myofibroblasts within a loose extracellular matrix. It characteristically surrounds and separates tumor cell nests.* **(Right)** *The stroma of DSRCT may occasionally appear less desmoplastic and more fibrous and collagenous, as depicted.*

(Left) *The fibrous stroma of DSRCT often contains a large number of blood vessels ranging in size from capillaries to larger channels. Of note, complex capillary proliferations ⇨ may be identified in some cases.* (Right) *Rarely, cases of DSRCT with collagenous stroma may show foci of dense hyalinization, as depicted.*

Stromal Vasculature

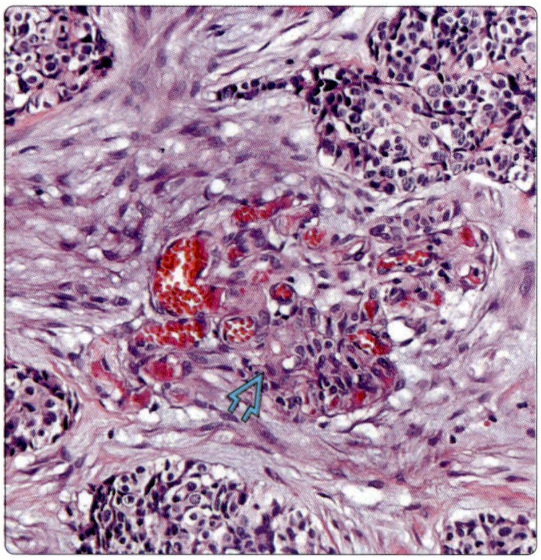

Focal Stromal Hyalinization

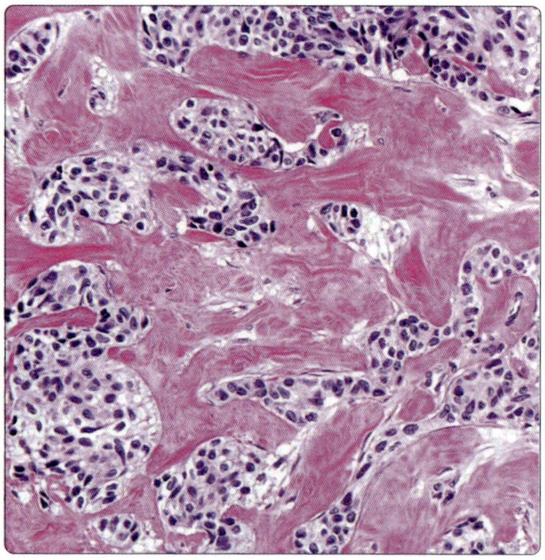

(Left) *Larger nests with areas of confluency may be seen in DSRCT, although it is usually not a prominent feature. This morphology may suggest a poorly differentiated carcinoma. Note the 2 foci ⇨ of centralized coagulative necrosis.* (Right) *Nuclear molding is not generally a feature of DSRCT but may be seen in rare cases. Neuroendocrine carcinoma should be excluded; however, in this image, the desmoplastic stroma provides a clue to the diagnosis of DSRCT.*

Large Confluent Nests

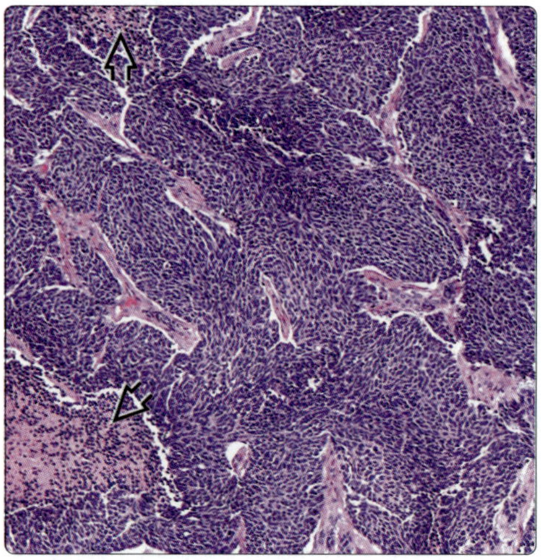

Occasional Nuclear Molding

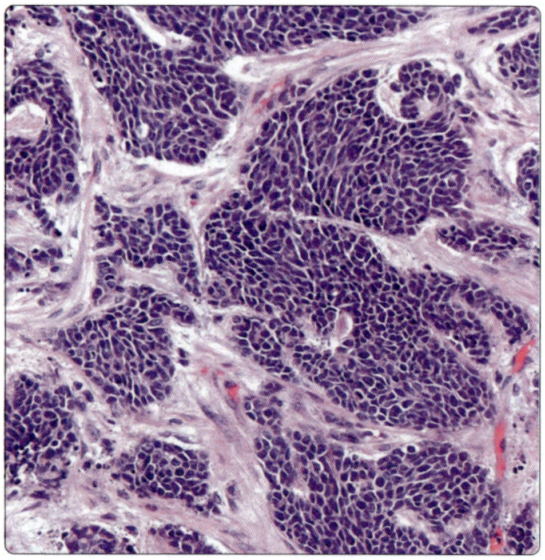

(Left) *Not uncommonly, some of the tumor cells in DSRCT may contain paranuclear eosinophilic hyaline inclusions → reminiscent of rhabdoid cells. This is often a focal finding.* (Right) *Epithelial architectural arrangements → such as a glandular or tubular appearance are an uncommon finding in DSRCT and are often focal if present.*

Intracytoplasmic Hyaline Inclusions

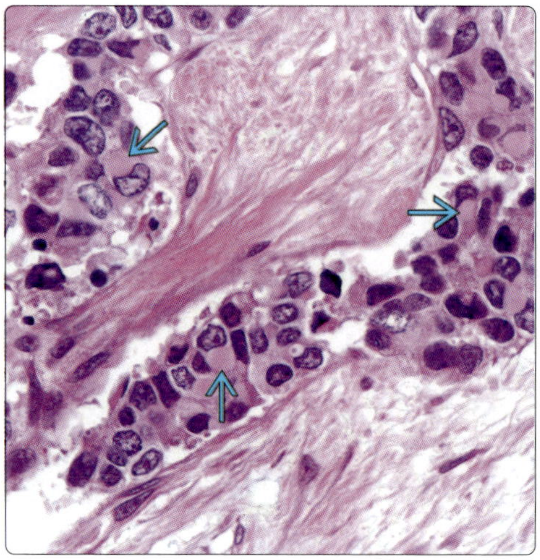

Epithelial Architectures

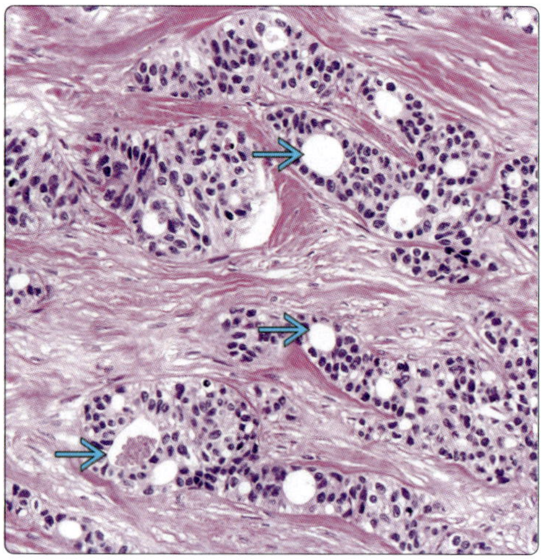

Abundant Cytoplasm

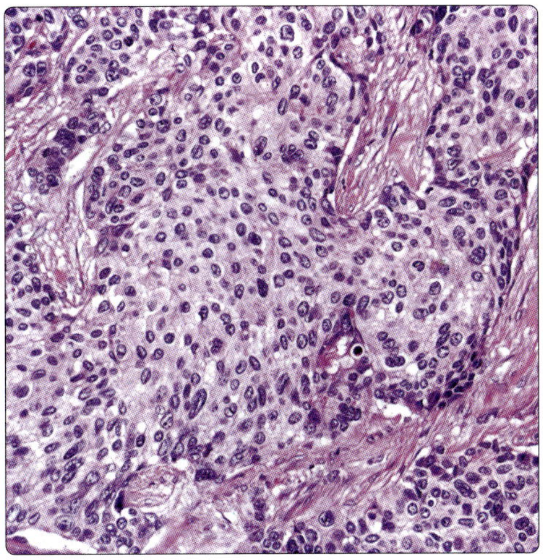

Dense Nested Growth

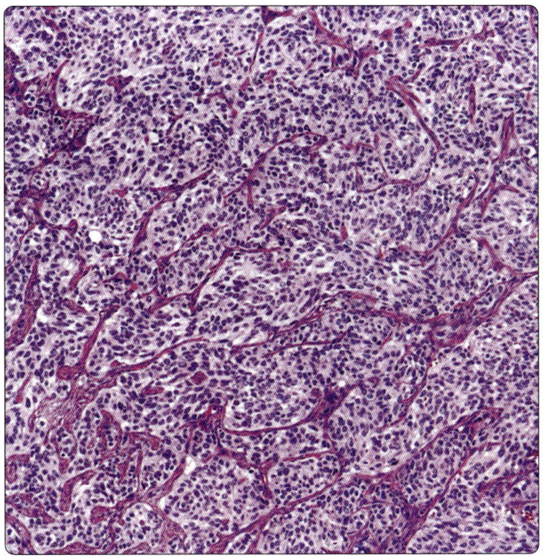

(Left) *The tumor cells of DSRCT generally contain scant eosinophilic cytoplasm; however, in some cases it is more abundant and prominent, as depicted. Confusion with carcinoma is more likely in this setting.* **(Right)** *A rare finding in DSRCT with larger tumor cells is the presence of tightly nested growth with scant stroma and fibrovascular septa. This morphology may closely mimic urothelial carcinoma or the zellballen pattern of paraganglioma.*

Rare Rosette Pattern

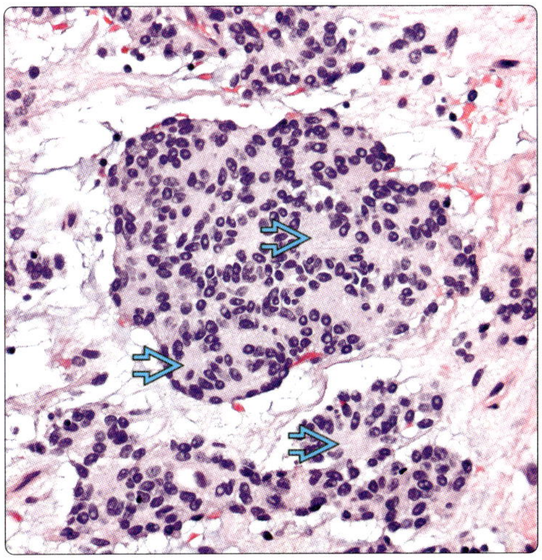

Rare Nuclear Pleomorphism

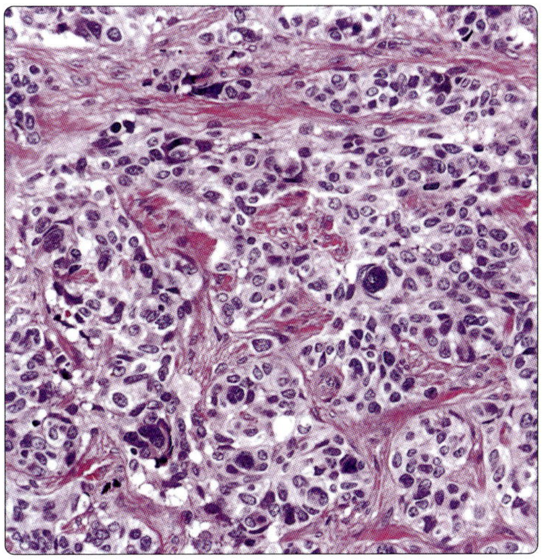

(Left) *This image shows a rosette pattern in DSRCT. This morphology is focal, when present, and is overall a rare finding.* **(Right)** *Nuclei in DSRCT are generally uniform in most cases; however, some cases show scattered nuclear atypia in the form of enlargement and pleomorphism, as shown. This finding is often focal and inconspicuous but may rarely be diffuse and prominent.*

Rare Bizarre Atypia

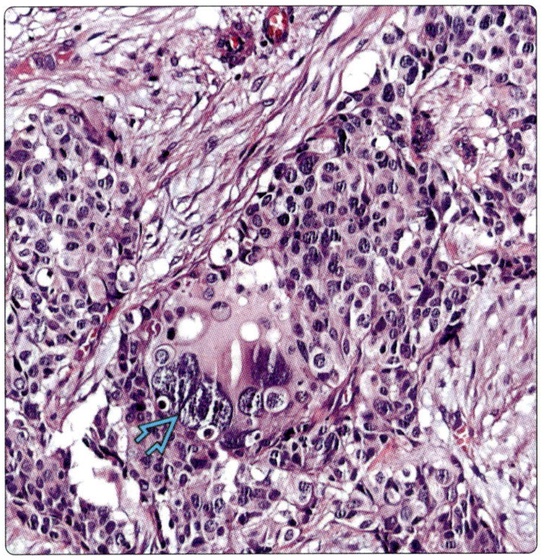

Submesothelial Fibroblasts

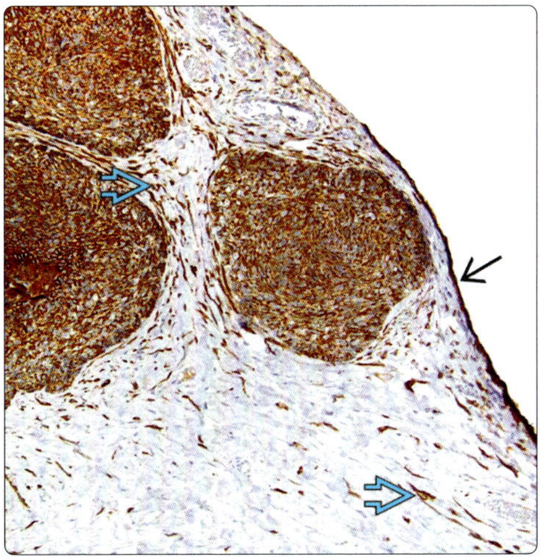

(Left) *Frankly bizarre nuclear atypia is an exceptionally rare, but reported, finding in DSRCT.* **(Right)** *Many cases of DSRCT arise near a peritoneal surface, as evidenced by a mesothelial lining in this image from a cytokeratin AE1/AE3 immunostain. Note that spindled submesothelial fibroblasts also stain for keratin.*

Extraskeletal Ewing Sarcoma

KEY FACTS

TERMINOLOGY

- Malignant small round blue cell neoplasm of bone and soft tissue characterized by specific *EWSR1* mutations
- Ewing sarcoma (ES) and primitive neuroectodermal tumor (PNET) represent continuous morphologic spectrum

CLINICAL ISSUES

- Children, adolescents, and young adults
- Aggressive with propensity for early metastases
- 10-year survival
  - Localized disease at presentation: 67%
  - Metastatic disease at presentation: 28%

MICROSCOPIC

- Sheets of densely packed cells with round, uniform nuclei
- Scant, glycogen-rich cytoplasm with indistinct cell membranes
- Homer Wright rosettes may be seen (PNET)

ANCILLARY TESTS

- CD99(+), characteristically strong, diffuse, and membranous
- Nuclear FLI-1(+)
- Myogenin, BCOR, TdT, CD45, CD56, WT1 (-)
- Molecular: Multiple balanced translocations and fusions involving *EWSR1* gene on chromosome 22
  - Most fusion transcripts are *EWSR1-FLI1* (90-95%) and *EWSR1-ERG* (5-10%)

TOP DIFFERENTIAL DIAGNOSES

- Alveolar rhabdomyosarcoma
- Poorly differentiated synovial sarcoma
- Undifferentiated sarcoma with *CIC-DUX4* translocation
- *BCOR-CCNB3* fusion-positive sarcoma
- Desmoplastic small round cell tumor
- Neuroblastoma
- Lymphoma

Ewing Sarcoma

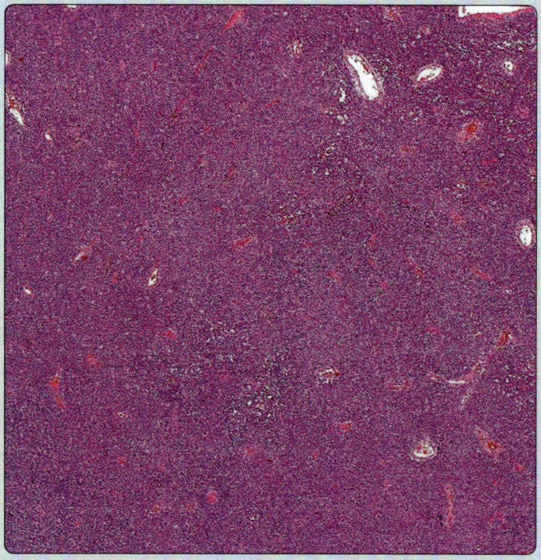

Cellular, Uniform Morphology

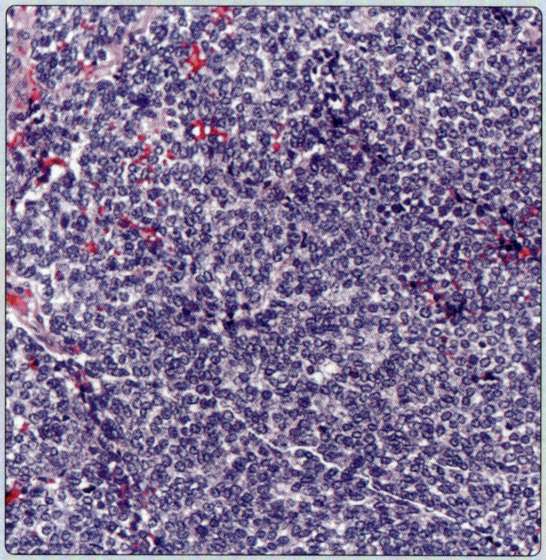

(Left) *Ewing sarcoma (ES) is a highly cellular, high-grade sarcoma with a dense, solid to sheet-like distribution of cells, as depicted. Most tumors are diagnosed on small biopsy prior to treatment with chemotherapy, and large, preserved sections, as shown, are uncommon.* **(Right)** *Tumor cells in ES are generally very uniform, and overlapping of nuclei is quite common. Chromatin is finely and evenly distributed, and nucleoli are small, if present.*

Clear Cytoplasm Common

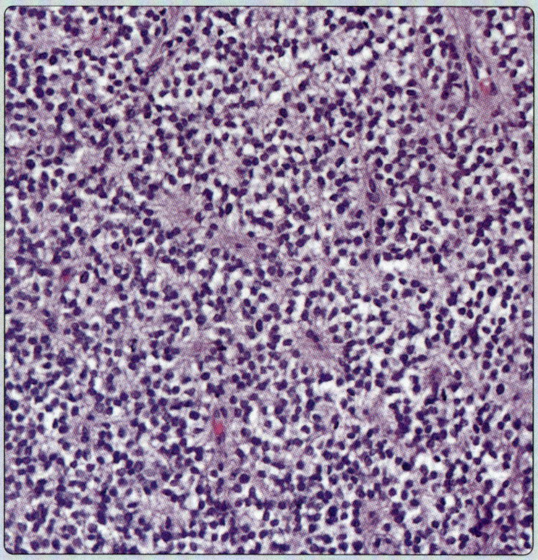

Diffuse, Membranous CD99 Expression

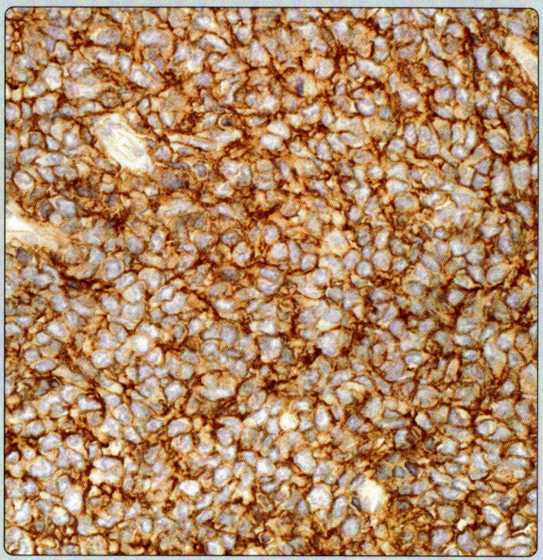

(Left) *Accumulation of intracytoplasmic glycogen is common in ES and results in a conspicuous clear cell appearance. This morphology may be focal, patchy, or diffuse in any given tumor.* **(Right)** *ES characteristically shows strong, diffuse membranous staining for CD99 (MIC2), as shown. Once thought to be specific for ES, CD99 has since been well described in many other small round blue cell tumors; however, expression is usually weak or focal in these other entities.*

TERMINOLOGY

Abbreviations

- Ewing sarcoma (ES)

Synonyms

- Primitive neuroectodermal tumor (PNET)
- Askin tumor

Definitions

- Malignant small round blue cell neoplasm of bone and soft tissue characterized by specific *EWSR1* mutations
- ES and PNET represent continuous morphologic spectrum
  - Overlapping morphologic features, immunophenotype, and molecular/genetic alterations
  - PNET displays morphologic evidence of neuronal differentiation
- Askin tumor refers to ES/PNET of chest wall or thoracopulmonary region

CLINICAL ISSUES

Epidemiology

- Incidence
  - Rare
- Age
  - Children, adolescents, and young adults (median: 15 years)
  - Peak incidence in 2nd decade of life
- Sex
  - Slight male predominance (M:F ratio = 1.4:1.0)
- Ethnicity
  - More common in Caucasians
  - Very rare in Africans and African Americans

Site

- Trunk (lung, mediastinum, paravertebral region)
- Extremities (deep soft tissues)
  - Primary bone tumor can extend into and present in soft tissue
- Head and neck
- Retroperitoneum

Presentation

- Painful or swelling at site of involvement
- Constitutional symptoms (fever, anemia, leukocytosis) often seen

Treatment

- Multimodality therapy
  - Chemotherapy is typically initial treatment of choice
  - Surgical resection of residual tumor
  - Radiation therapy or combined radiation and surgical resection for select cases

Prognosis

- Aggressive with propensity for early metastases
  - Lungs, bone, and bone marrow are most frequent sites of metastasis
  - Most predictive prognostic factor
    - 10-year survival for localized disease at presentation: 67%
    - 10-year survival for metastatic disease at presentation: 28%
- Prognostic factors associated with decreased survival
  - Metastatic disease at presentation
  - Axial tumor location
  - Tumor size > 10 cm
  - Patient age > 19 years

MACROSCOPIC

General Features

- Tan to gray, friable cut surfaces
- Hemorrhage and necrosis common
- May display cystic change with necrotic, semiliquid contents

Size

- Variable, up to 20 cm

MICROSCOPIC

Histologic Features

- Sheets of densely packed cells with round, uniform nuclei
- Dispersed fine chromatin and inconspicuous nucleoli
- Scant cytoplasm with indistinct cell membranes
  - Can be clear due to glycogen content
- Neuroectodermal differentiation (Homer Wright rosettes) may be seen in PNET
  - Central fibrillary core without lumen
- Rarely have focal spindled morphology
- Minimal intercellular collagen or reticulin
- Rare myxoid change with microcyst formation may be seen
- Necrosis frequently seen with perivascular preservation of tumor cells
- Rare morphologic variants
  - Atypical (large cell) variant
    - Larger, vesicular nuclei with irregular nuclear contours
    - Conspicuous nucleoli
    - Pleomorphism and spindling
  - Adamantinoma-like variant occurs mostly in bone
  - Sclerosing and clear cell variants described

ANCILLARY TESTS

Histochemistry

- PAS(+) intracytoplasmic glycogen
- Reticulin (-)
  - Staining pattern: Minimal or no intercellular reticulin except around blood vessels

Immunohistochemistry

- CD99(+), characteristically strong, diffuse, and membranous
  - Weak, patchy, or focal expression should lead to consideration of other diagnoses
- Nuclear FLI-1(+)
- NKX2.2(+)
- Focal expression of keratin, CD117, or S100 protein in 25-30% of cases
- Very rare focal desmin expression reported
- Myogenin, MYOD1, BCOR, TdT, CD56, WT1, CD45, TLE1, SMA (-)

Molecular Genetics

- Multiple balanced translocations and fusions involving *EWSR1* gene on chromosome 22
  - *EWSR1* rearrangements detectable by RT-PCR and break-apart FISH probes
- Most common translocation: t(11;22)(q24;q12), *EWSR1-FLI1* fusion
  - Type 1 fusion: Exons 1-7 of *EWSR1* to exons 6-9 of *FLI1*
    - Most common (60-65% of cases)
  - Type 2 fusion: Exons 1-7 of *EWSR1* fuse to exons 6-9 of *FLI1*
- 2nd most common translocation: t(21;22)(q12;q12), *EWSR1-ERG* fusion (5-10%)
- Less common *EWSR1* variant translocations (< 1%)
  - ETS family
    - t(2;22)(q33;q12), *EWSR1-FEV* fusion
    - t(7;22)(p22;q12), *EWSR1-ETV1* fusion
    - t(17;22)(q12;q12), *EWSR1-ETV4* (E1AF) fusion
  - Non-ETS family
    - t(2;22)(q31;q12), *EWSR1-SP3* fusion
    - t(6;22)(p21;q12), *EWSR1-POU5F1* fusion
    - t(20;22)(q13;q12), *EWSR1-NFATC2* fusion
    - t(4;22)(q31;q12), *EWSR1-SMARCA5* fusion
- Genetic changes do not correlate with site or morphology

DIFFERENTIAL DIAGNOSIS

Alveolar Rhabdomyosarcoma

- Nests of small cells separated by variable-sized fibrous septa
- Multinucleated "wreath" cells
- Diffuse desmin (+)
- Nuclear myogenin (+)
- *FOXO1* gene fusions with *PAX3* or *PAX7*

Poorly Differentiated Synovial Sarcoma

- Nuclei less regular, appear to overlap
- May be spindled or have spindled component
- Strong, diffuse nuclear TLE1(+)
- *SS18* gene fusions

Desmoplastic Small Round Cell Tumor

- Usually intraabdominal, rarely other sites
- Nests of cells in cellular fibrous or desmoplastic stroma
- Polyphenotypic
  - Expresses keratin, desmin, and neural markers
- CD99(-) in most cases
- WT1(+) (carboxy-terminus only)
- *EWSR1-WT1* gene fusion

Undifferentiated Sarcoma With *CIC-DUX4* Translocation

- Nuclear WT1(+)
- Variable CD99(+)
- Lacks *EWSR1* rearrangements

BCOR-CCNB3 Fusion-Positive Sarcoma

- Heterogeneous morphology (round to spindled cells)
- Myxoid matrix common
- CCNB3(+) by IHC
- Lacks *EWSR1* rearrangements

Neuroblastoma

- Usually < 4 years of age
- Associated with sympathetic ganglia
- Sheets of neuroblasts, variable ganglionic differentiation
- NB84(+); CD99(-)
- Lacks specific translocations of ES

Lymphoma

- Involvement of lymphoid tissue
  - Lymph node, spleen
- Immunoreactivity with lymphoid markers
- Pitfall: Strong CD99(+) common in lymphoblastic lymphomas

Extraskeletal Mesenchymal Chondrosarcoma

- Often prominent pericytomatous growth pattern
- Focal chondroid formation (can be sparse)
- Recurrent *HEY1-NCOA2* fusion

Small Cell Carcinoma

- Usually older adults
- Nuclear molding, scanty cytoplasm
- Diffuse keratin (+), often dot-like
- CD56(+), nuclear TTF-1(+)
- CD99(-) in majority of cases
- Lacks specific fusion genes

SELECTED REFERENCES

1. Kao YC et al: BCOR-CCNB3 fusion positive sarcomas: a clinicopathologic and molecular analysis of 36 cases with comparison to morphologic spectrum and clinical behavior of other round cell sarcomas. Am J Surg Pathol. 42(5):604-15, 2018
2. Antonescu CR et al: Sarcomas with CIC-rearrangements are a distinct pathologic entity with aggressive outcome: a clinicopathologic and molecular study of 115 cases. Am J Surg Pathol. 41(7):941-9, 2017
3. Hamilton SN et al: Long-term outcomes and complications in pediatric Ewing sarcoma. Am J Clin Oncol. 40(4):423-28, 2017
4. Yoshida A et al: CIC-rearranged sarcomas: a study of 20 cases and comparisons with Ewing sarcomas. Am J Surg Pathol. 40(3):313-23, 2016
5. Duchman KR et al: Prognostic factors for survival in patients with Ewing's sarcoma using the surveillance, epidemiology, and end results (SEER) program database. Cancer Epidemiol. 39(2):189-95, 2015
6. Pan HY et al: Prognostic factors and patterns of relapse in Ewing sarcoma patients treated with chemotherapy and R0 resection. Int J Radiat Oncol Biol Phys. 92(2):349-57, 2015
7. Tomazou EM et al: Epigenome mapping reveals distinct modes of gene regulation and widespread enhancer reprogramming by the oncogenic fusion protein EWS-FLI1. Cell Rep. 10(7):1082-95, 2015
8. Brasme JF et al: Time to diagnosis of Ewing tumors in children and adolescents is not associated with metastasis or survival: a prospective multicenter study of 436 patients. J Clin Oncol. 32(18):1935-40, 2014
9. Crompton BD et al: The genomic landscape of pediatric Ewing sarcoma. Cancer Discov. 4(11):1326-41, 2014
10. Fisher C: The diversity of soft tissue tumours with EWSR1 gene rearrangements: a review. Histopathology. 64(1):134-50, 2014
11. Warren M et al: Integrated multimodal genetic testing of Ewing sarcoma--a single-institution experience. Hum Pathol. 44(10):2010-9, 2013
12. Llombart-Bosch A et al: Histological heterogeneity of Ewing's sarcoma/PNET: an immunohistochemical analysis of 415 genetically confirmed cases with clinical support. Virchows Arch. 455(5):397-411, 2009
13. Machado I et al: Molecular diagnosis of Ewing sarcoma family of tumors: a comparative analysis of 560 cases with FISH and RT-PCR. Diagn Mol Pathol. 18(4):189-99, 2009
14. Jambhekar NA et al: Comparative analysis of routine histology, immunohistochemistry, reverse transcriptase polymerase chain reaction, and fluorescence in situ hybridization in diagnosis of Ewing family of tumors. Arch Pathol Lab Med. 130(12):1813-8, 2006
15. Lucas DR et al: Ewing sarcoma vs lymphoblastic lymphoma. A comparative immunohistochemical study. Am J Clin Pathol. 115(1):11-7, 2001

Cytologic Features

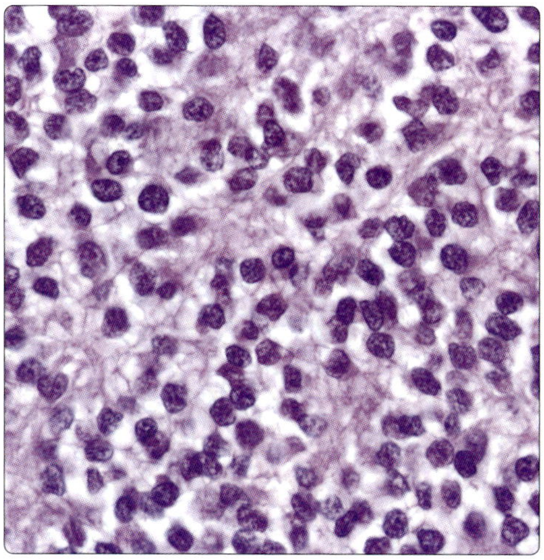

Admixed Clear Cells

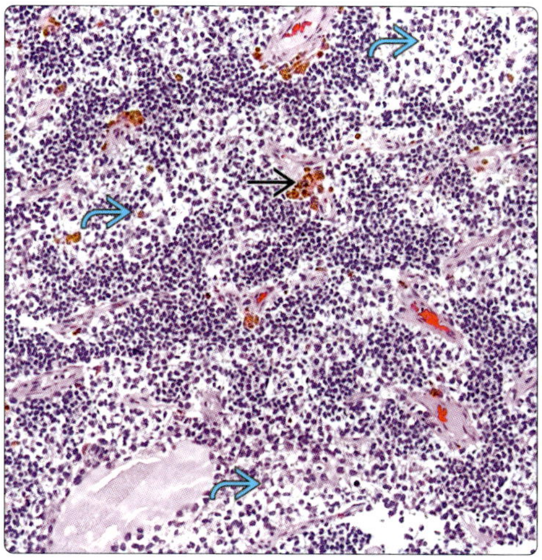

(Left) *Nuclei in ES are generally small, round, and relatively uniform. Nucleoli are small, if present. Occasional cases show scattered cells with more prominent nucleoli.* **(Right)** *Clear tumor cells → are admixed with more conventional small cells in this case of ES. Hemosiderin pigment → is also present and associated with stromal vessels.*

"Dark" Cells

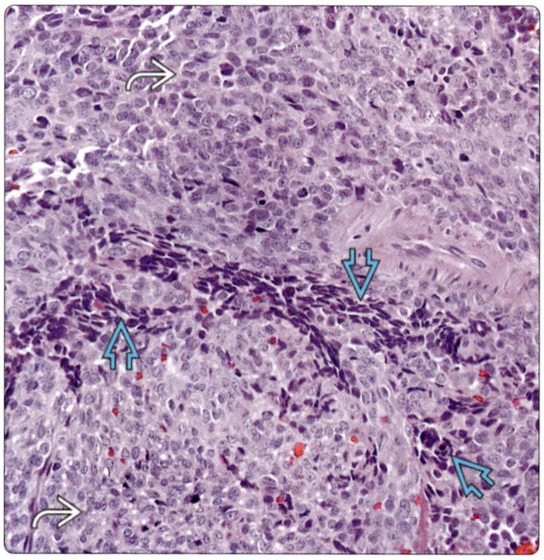

Degenerating Cells

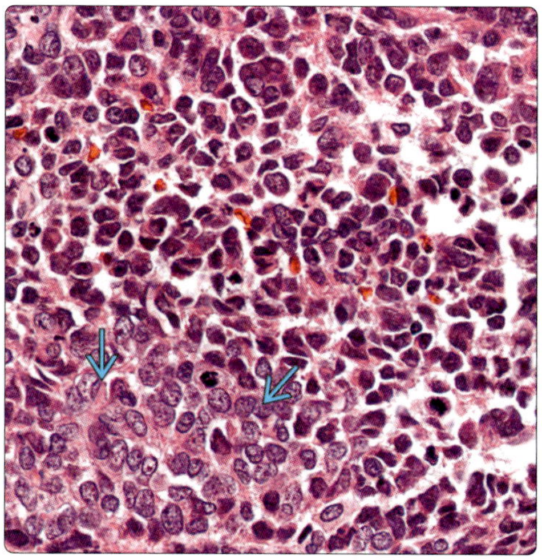

(Left) *An admixed population of degenerating tumor cells with smaller, hyperchromatic, and angulated nuclei → may be seen in many cases of ES and have been referred to as "dark" cells. Note the contrast with the more conventional tumor cells →.* **(Right)** *This case of ES is beginning to undergo degeneration with a number of apoptotic bodies and cells with smaller, angulated hyperchromatic nuclei ("dark" cells). Note the distinct population of more viable tumor cells → in this H&E.*

Vague Lobular Growth

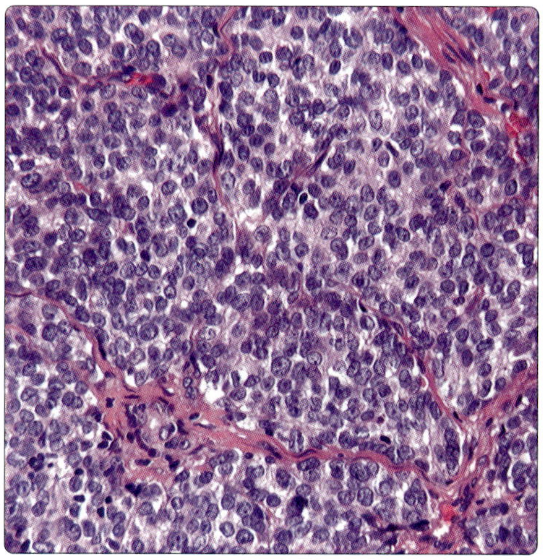

Prominent Lobulated Growth

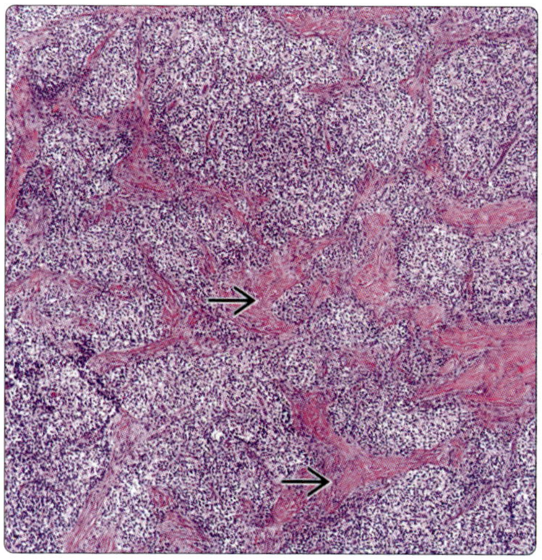

(Left) *A vaguely lobular appearance with focal, thin fibrovascular septa can be appreciated in this case of ES. Note the monotonous cell population and small, round, uniform nuclei.* **(Right)** *This case of ES features a more prominent lobulated pattern of growth with large nests and sheets of clear tumor cells separated by thickened fibrocollagenous septa →.*

(Left) *Some cases of ES feature conspicuous morphologic evidence of neuroectodermal differentiation in the form of scattered true rosettes. These tumors have also been described as primitive neuroectodermal tumors (PNETs).* **(Right)** *The true rosettes of ES (PNET) are formed by tumor cells arranged around a core of fibrillary material without formation of a central lumen. Cell boundaries are indistinct. These structures are also known as Homer Wright rosettes.*

Neuroectodermal Differentiation

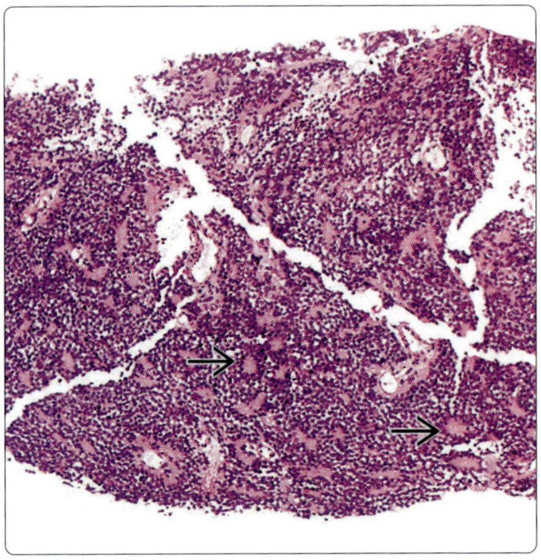

True Rosette Formation

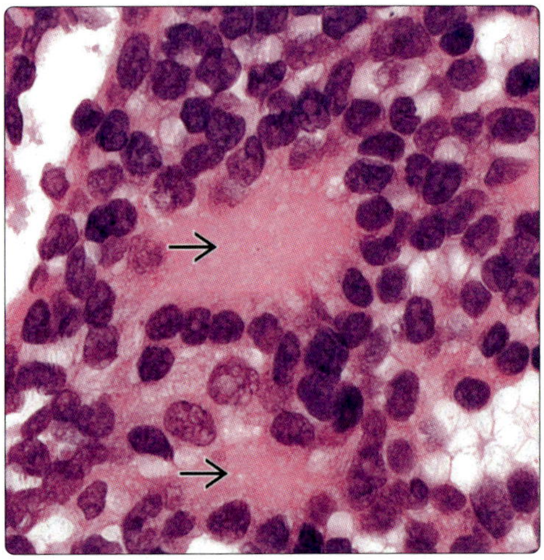

(Left) *Occasional cases of ES contain tumor cells that are larger, show greater nuclear irregularity, and often feature prominent nucleoli. This variant is known as atypical or large cell ES.* **(Right)** *Coagulative necrosis is common in ES and is often geographic in distribution. A common finding is the presence of perivascular tumor cell preservation ("peritheliomatous growth") with degeneration and death of surrounding cells.*

Large Cell (Atypical) Variant

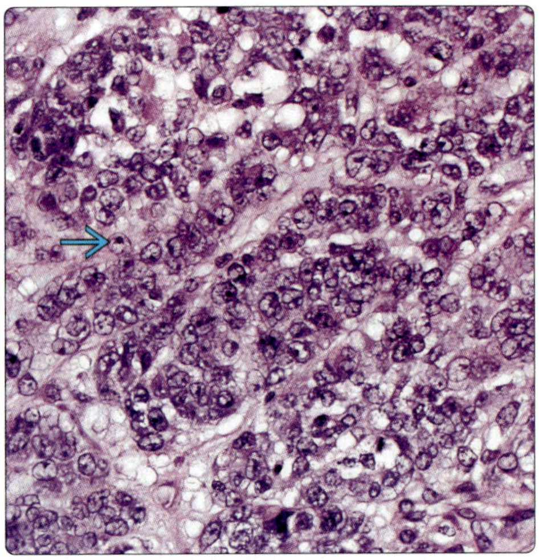

Coagulative Necrosis

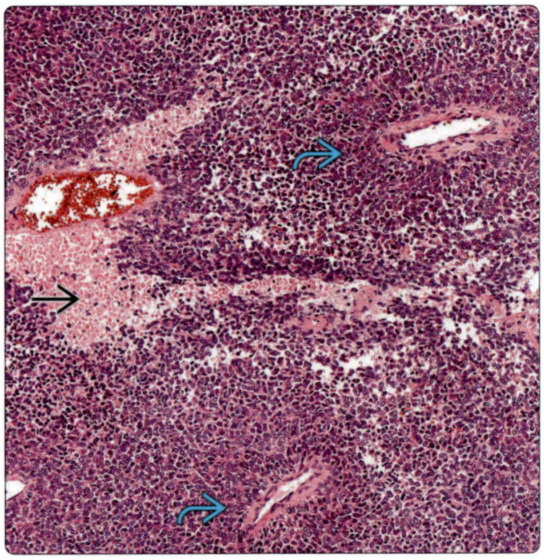

(Left) *Focal spindle cell morphology is a rare finding in ES. In this H&E, spindled tumor cells within an area of myxoid stromal changes (also rare) merge with more typical round cells. Spindling is more frequently seen in the large cell (atypical) variant.* **(Right)** *Focal keratin expression can be seen in up to 25-30% of cases of ES, often in a dot-like pattern. Other morphologically similar entities, such as desmoplastic small round cell tumor and poorly differentiated synovial sarcoma, should be carefully excluded.*

Focal Spindled Cytomorphology

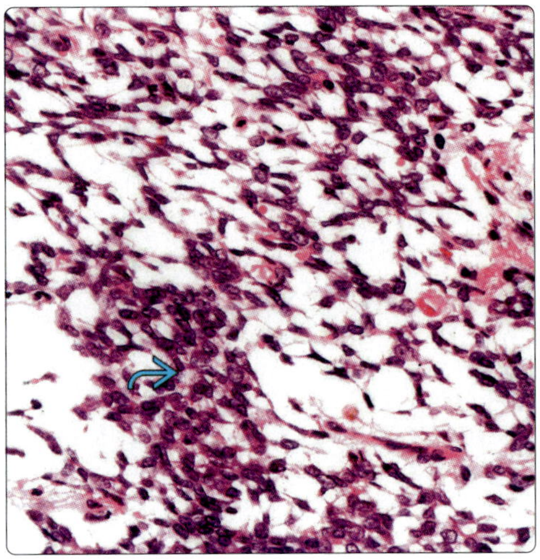

Focal Keratin Expression

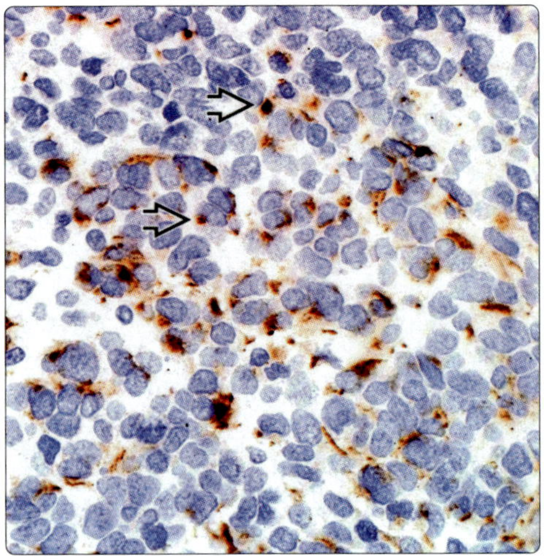

Treated Ewing Sarcoma

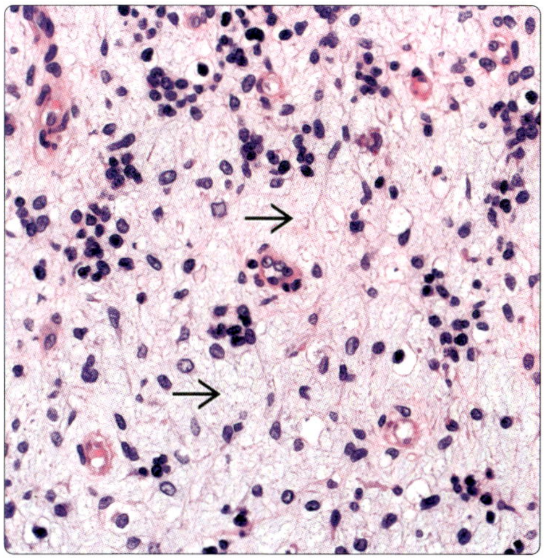

Superficial Ewing Sarcoma

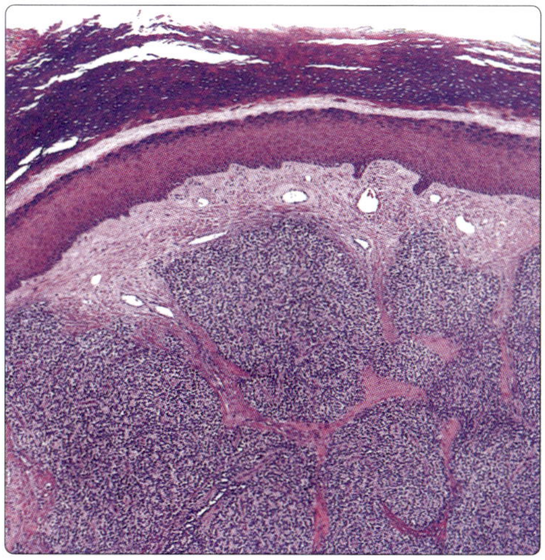

(Left) *After chemotherapy, there is often shrinkage and loss of tumor cells with prominent edema ➔ &/or fibrosis of the stroma. Large areas of necrosis are also common after therapy.* **(Right)** *Rare cases of ES arise superficially in the dermis. Most are well demarcated and many appear encapsulated. Rosette formation is also common. This group of ES shows an overall better prognosis than conventional deep tumors.*

Cytoplasmic Glycogen

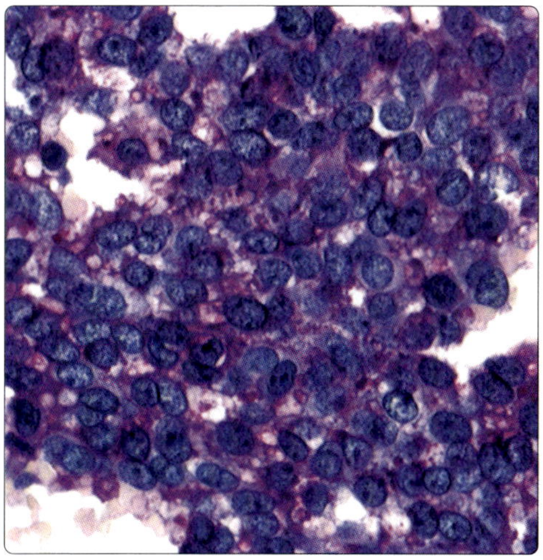

Absence of Reticulin Staining

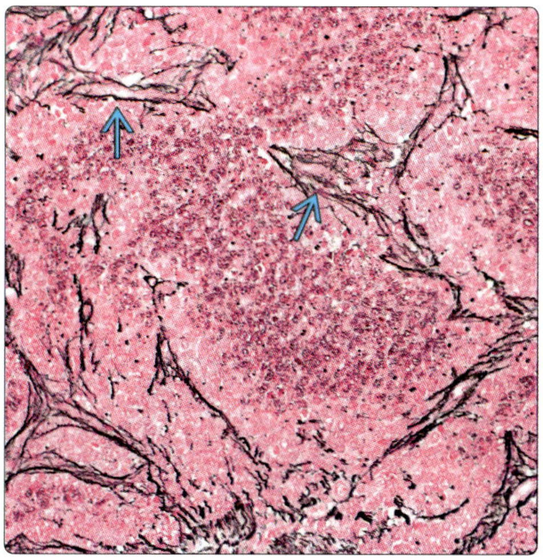

(Left) *Intracytoplasmic glycogen in ES can be demonstrated by a periodic acid-Schiff (PAS) stain and is removed by pretreatment with diastase. Glycogen appears granular and brightly pink or magenta.* **(Right)** *Reticulin fibers are seen around blood vessels ➔ and between tumor lobules in ES; however, these fibers are absent between neoplastic cells. By contrast, reticulin often surrounds small groups of cells in the morphologically similar, poorly differentiated synovial sarcoma.*

Characteristic Translocation

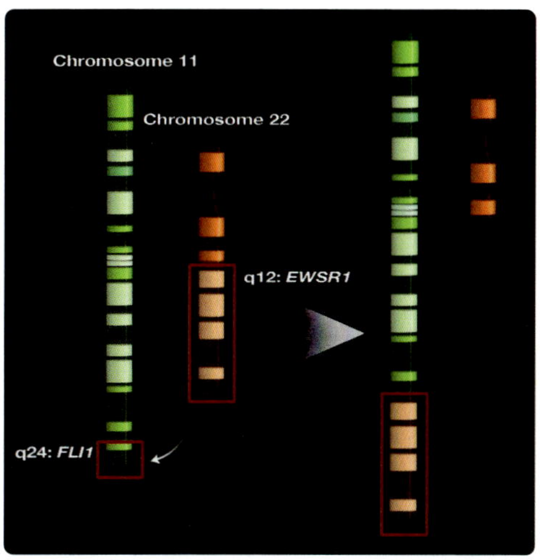

FISH Analysis for *EWSR1*

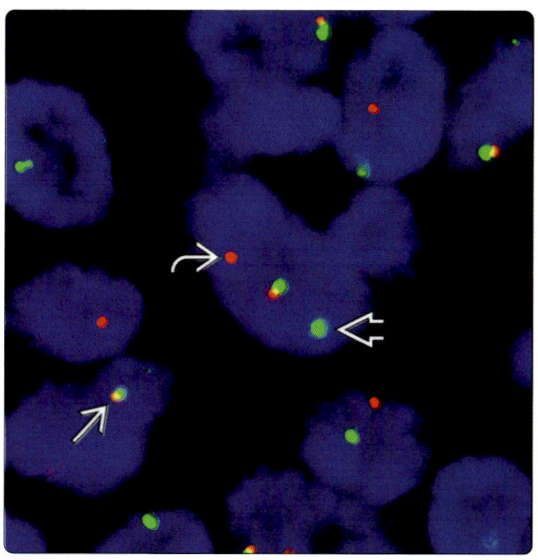

(Left) *This graphic depicts the t(11;22)(q24;q12) translocation between the carboxy-terminal domain of FLI1 (11q24) and the EWSR1 gene aminoterminal domain (22q12), resulting in an EWSR1-FLI1 fusion gene.* **(Right)** *In this fluorescence in situ hybridization (FISH) preparation, dual color break-apart probes are used for the EWSR1 gene on chromosome 22. In the nucleus of a tumor cell, split red ➔ and green ➔ signals, instead of a fused yellow one ➔, indicate a translocation involving EWSR1.*

Extraskeletal Myxoid Chondrosarcoma

KEY FACTS

TERMINOLOGY

- Soft tissue or bone sarcoma of uncertain differentiation with abundant myxoid matrix, multilobular architecture, uniform cells in cords, clusters and fine networks, and *NR4A3* rearrangement

CLINICAL ISSUES

- Median age: 50 years
- 2:1 male predominance
- Lower extremity most common
- Often prolonged clinical course
- High rate of local and distant recurrence
- Poor response to chemotherapy
- Tumors with variant *NR4A3* translocations higher grade, more aggressive

MACROSCOPIC

- Gelatinous lobules separated by thick, fibrous septa
- Cystic areas, hemorrhage, and necrosis common

MICROSCOPIC

- Abundant myxoid matrix; hyaline cartilage absent
- Cells interconnect to form cords, clusters, or fine networks
- Cellular variant with minimal myxoid matrix and epithelioid &/or rhabdoid cells

ANCILLARY TESTS

- S100(+) but variable and inconsistent
- Cytogenetics, t(9;22)(q22;q12.2) most common
- Break-apart FISH for *EWSR1* or *NR4A3*

TOP DIFFERENTIAL DIAGNOSES

- Chordoma
- Myoepithelioma/myoepithelial carcinoma
- Soft tissue chondroma
- Myxofibrosarcoma (epithelioid variant)
- Epithelioid gastrointestinal stromal tumor
- Myxoid mesothelioma
- Chordoid meningioma

Extraskeletal Myxoid Chondrosarcoma

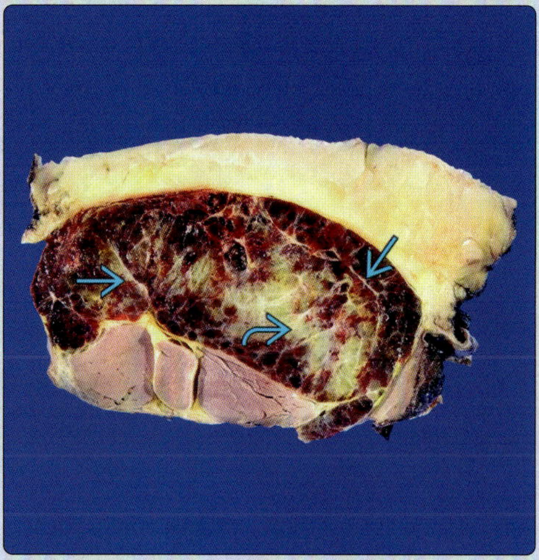

Lobular Architecture and Hemorrhage

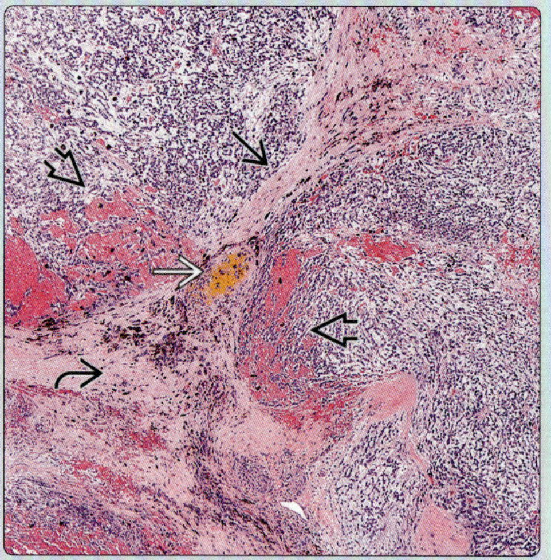

(Left) *Grossly, EMC usually forms a large, well-demarcated mass as illustrated by this thigh tumor. The cut surface has a well-defined, lobular architecture with fibrous septa* → *and gelatinous lobules* →*. This tumor also has extensive intralesional hemorrhage.* **(Right)** *This low-power H&E highlights the lobular growth pattern of EMC, defined by thick, fibrous septa* →*. Areas of acute hemorrhage* →*, hemosiderosis* →*, and scar* → *are common, as are necrosis and cyst formation (not shown).*

Uniform Interconnecting Cells

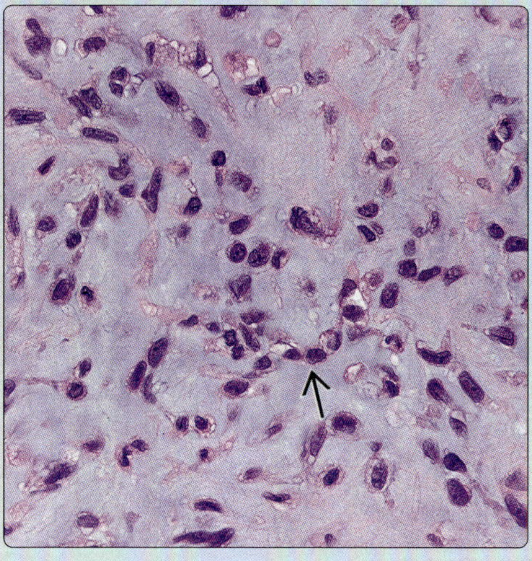

***EWSR1* Break-Apart FISH**

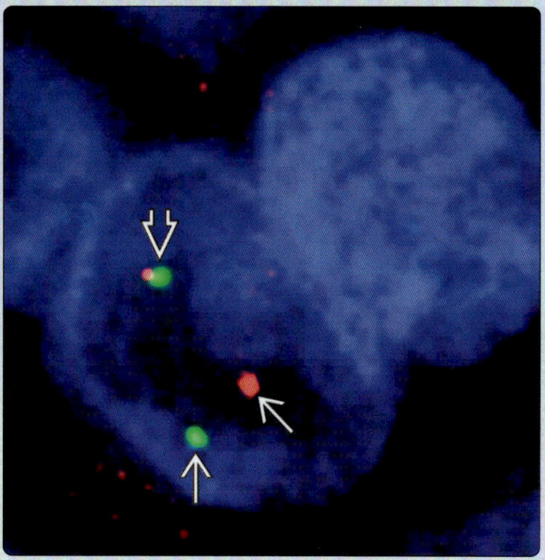

(Left) *Conventional EMC is typically composed of uniform cells with round to oval nuclei and wisps of eosinophilic cytoplasm that interconnect* → *with each other.* **(Right)** *Break-apart FISH for EWSR1 is a useful diagnostic test for EMC. This immunofluorescence image depicts a normal allele with fused red and green signals* → *and a broken apart allele* →*. Although sensitive, it will miss tumors with variant NR4A3 fusions.*

TERMINOLOGY

Abbreviations

- Extraskeletal myxoid chondrosarcoma (EMC)

Synonyms

- Chordoid sarcoma

Definitions

- Soft tissue or bone sarcoma of uncertain differentiation with abundant myxoid matrix, multilobular architecture, uniform cells in cords, clusters and fine networks, and *NR4A3* rearrangement

CLINICAL ISSUES

Epidemiology

- Rare: < 3% of soft tissue sarcomas
- Median age: 50 years (range: 5-90 years); rare in children; M:F = 2:1

Site

- Extremities; lower extremity most common
- Rare in abdomen, pelvis, head and neck, cranium, pleura
- Rare primary bone tumors

Presentation

- Deep soft tissue mass
- Pulmonary metastases at presentation in 13%

Treatment

- Wide local excision; poor response to chemotherapy

Prognosis

- Local recurrence rate (30-50%)
- Metastases (35-45%), usually pulmonary
- Often prolonged clinical course
- Tumors with variant *NR4A3* translocations more aggressive

MACROSCOPIC

General Features

- Well demarcated; contained by pseudocapsule
- Gelatinous lobules separated by fibrous septa
- Cystic areas, hemorrhage, and necrosis common

Size

- Usually large; median: 7 cm; range: 1-30 cm

MICROSCOPIC

Histologic Features

- Conventional EMC
  - Multilobular architecture, fibrous septa, abundant myxoid matrix
  - Uniform cells with eosinophilic cytoplasm and round to spindle-shaped nuclei arranged in cords, clusters, or fine networks and low mitotic rate
  - Necrosis, hemorrhage, and hemosiderosis common
- Cellular/poorly differentiated EMC
  - Densely cellular, often with little myxoid matrix
  - Large epithelioid &/or rhabdoid cells
  - Nonmyxoid spindle cell areas (dedifferentiation)

ANCILLARY TESTS

Immunohistochemistry

- S100(+) but variable and inconsistent
- Minority of cases cytokeratin &/or EMA (+)
- Loss of INI1 (SNF5) in tumors with rhabdoid features
- Neuroendocrine marker expression in some

In Situ Hybridization

- Break-apart FISH for *NR4A3* rearrangement

Genetic Testing

- t(9;22)(q22;q12.2) most common; t(9;17)(q22;q11.2) and other variants
- *EWSR1-NR4A3* fusion in majority; variant *NR4A3* fusions (*TFG*, *TCF12*, *TAF15*, *FUS*) in high-grade and rhabdoid EMCs

Electron Microscopy

- Intracisternal bundles of parallel microtubules

DIFFERENTIAL DIAGNOSIS

Chordoma

- Larger cells with more abundant cytoplasm and physaliferous cells
- Cytokeratin (+), EMA(+), S100(+), brachyury (+)
- Affects sacrum, clivus, vertebral bodies

Myoepithelioma/Myoepithelial Carcinoma

- Cords of cells in myxoid matrix, benign or malignant
- Variable expression of cytokeratin, S100, p63, SMA
- Can show *EWSR1* rearrangement

Soft Tissue Chondroma

- Lobular myxoid architecture and interconnecting cells
- True hyaline cartilage, often heavily calcified
- Predilection for hands and feet

Myxofibrosarcoma (Epithelioid Variant)

- High-grade pleomorphic cells
- Prominent curvilinear blood vessels
- Usually admixed with conventional myxofibrosarcoma

Epithelioid Gastrointestinal Stromal Tumor

- May have abundant myxoid matrix and cell cords
- CD117(+) and DOG1(+)

Myxoid Mesothelioma

- Epithelioid mesothelioma with abundant myxoid matrix
- Cytokeratin (+), calretinin (+), WT1(+)
- Pleural/peritoneal tumor

Chordoid Meningioma

- Usually admixed with conventional meningioma
- EMA(+)

SELECTED REFERENCES

1. Agaram NP et al: Extraskeletal myxoid chondrosarcoma with non-EWSR1-NR4A3 variant fusions correlate with rhabdoid phenotype and high-grade morphology. Hum Pathol. 45(5):1084-91, 2014
2. Meis-Kindblom JM et al: Extraskeletal myxoid chondrosarcoma: a reappraisal of its morphologic spectrum and prognostic factors based on 117 cases. Am J Surg Pathol. 23(6):636-50, 1999

(Left) *Spindle cell differentiation is common in EMC, and the amount varies from case to case. Note the interconnecting pattern of spindle cells with abundant eosinophilic cytoplasm and low-grade, elongated nuclei forming cords and fine networks.* **(Right)** *Axial T2-weighted MR discloses a large, deep-seated EMC of the thigh with heterogeneous, hyperintense signal and well-defined, lobular architecture.*

Spindle Cells

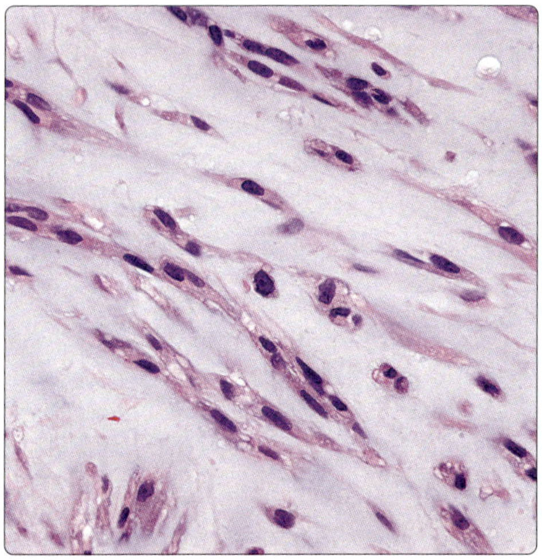

Lobular Pattern on MR

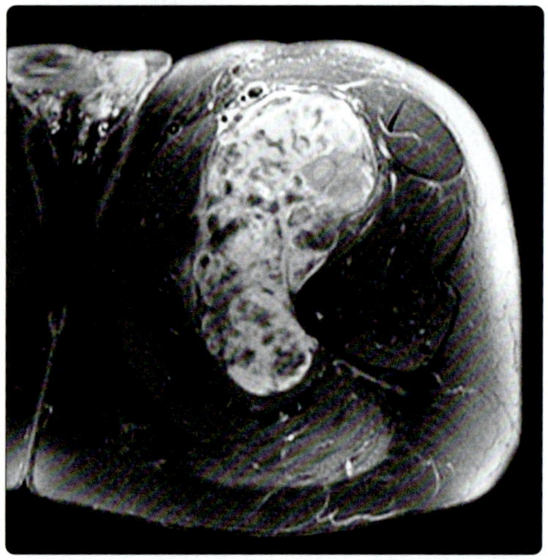

(Left) *Grossly, EMC has a very well-defined, lobular architecture consisting of gelatinous, yellow lobules* → *separated by fibrous septa. Intralesional hemorrhage* ↗ *is common.* **(Right)** *This scanning-power H&E highlights the well-defined, lobular architecture and abundant pale blue myxoid matrix in EMC.*

Lobular Architecture and Hemorrhage

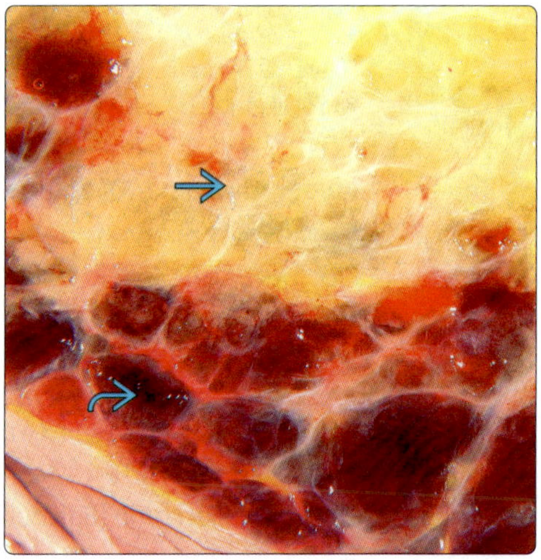

Lobular Architecture

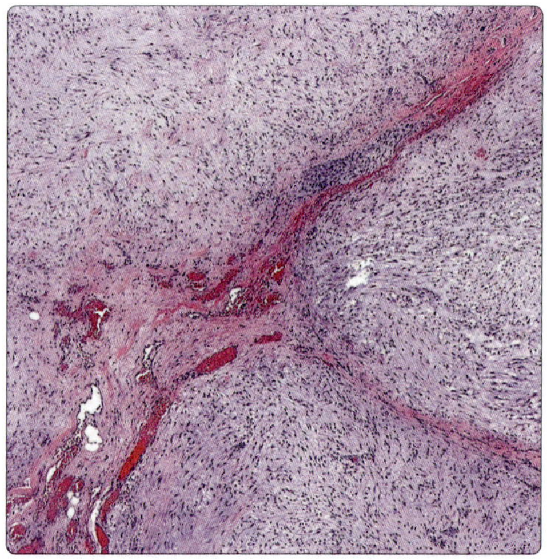

(Left) *EMC has a lobular architecture defined by thick, fibrous septa* → *that divide it into myxoid lobules containing cords of interconnecting uniform cells.* **(Right)** *Grossly, most EMCs form large, demarcated tumors with a well-defined, lobular pattern created by thick, fibrous septa* → *that divide it into gelatinous lobules* ↗*. Necrosis* ⇉*, intratumoral hemorrhage, and cyst formation are often present, as shown.*

Fibrous Septum

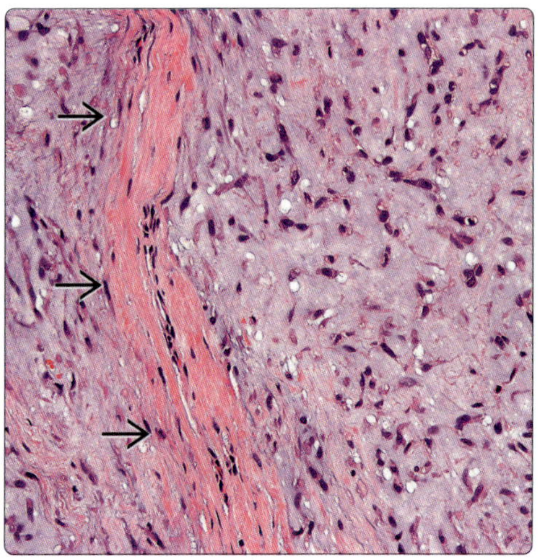

Cystic Areas, Necrosis, and Hemorrhage

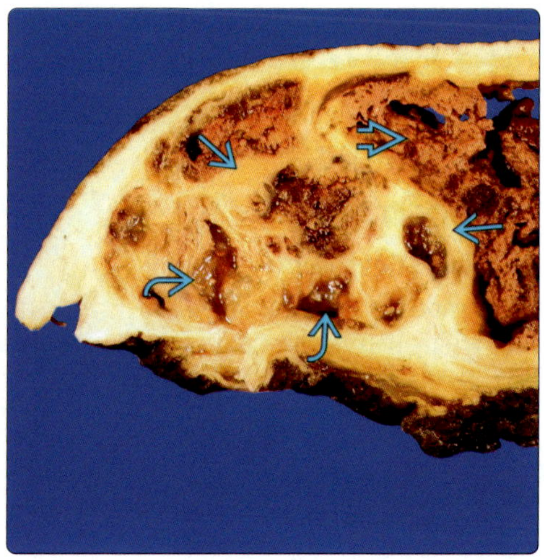

Cell Clusters

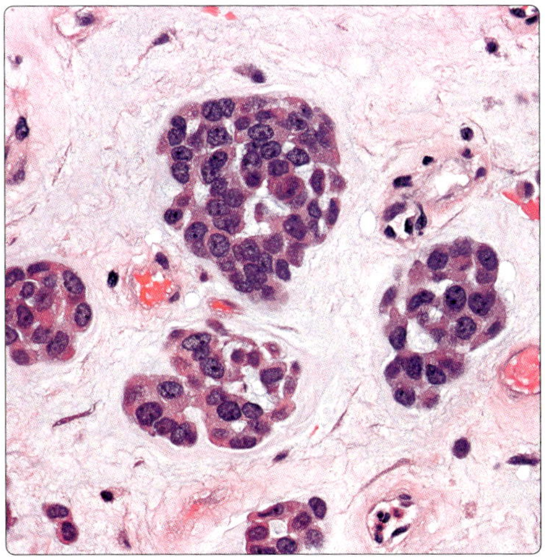

Complex Cohesive Structures

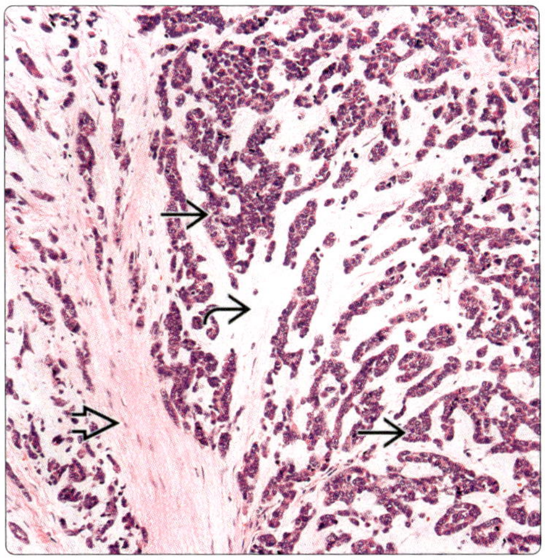

(Left) *The neoplastic cells in EMC can form rounded, cohesive clusters. Note the epithelioid cytology with densely eosinophilic cytoplasm and abundant pale blue myxoid matrix.* **(Right)** *The neoplastic cells in EMC interconnect to form cords, clusters, and more complex structures →, as shown within a background of myxoid matrix ↪. True hyaline cartilage is virtually never seen. Note the thick, fibrous band ⇨.*

Complex Reticular Pattern

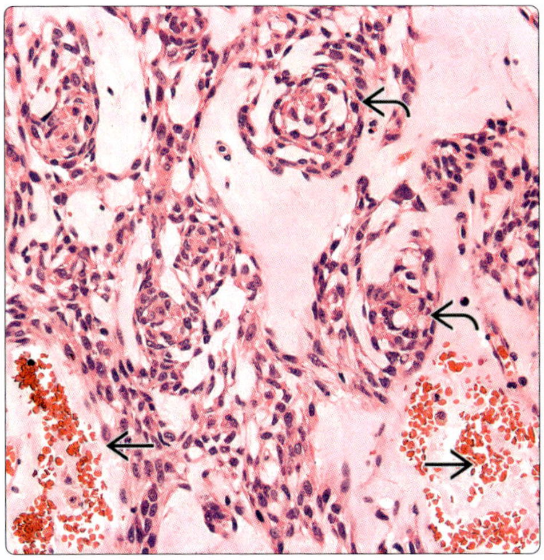

Cellular Extraskeletal Myxoid Chondrosarcoma With Large Epithelioid Cells

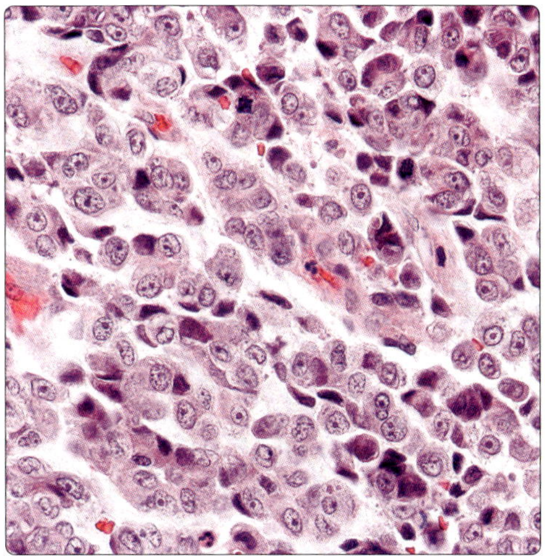

(Left) *This EMC has a complex reticular architecture characterized by cohesive arrays of epithelioid and spindle cells forming cribriform and whorling ↪ patterns. Note the acute hemorrhage →.* **(Right)** *Cellular EMC is characterized by sheets of cells with little or no intervening matrix. These tumors often have large, epithelioid cells with vesicular nuclei, prominent nucleoli, and brisk mitotic activity. Histologic grade is regarded as a prognostic variable in EMC.*

Rhabdoid Cells

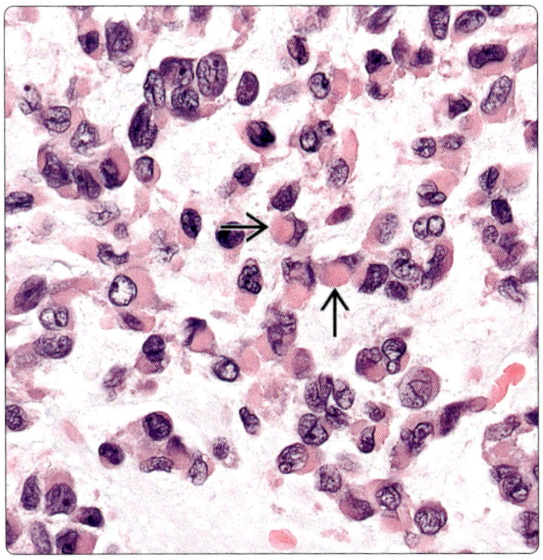

Ultrastructure

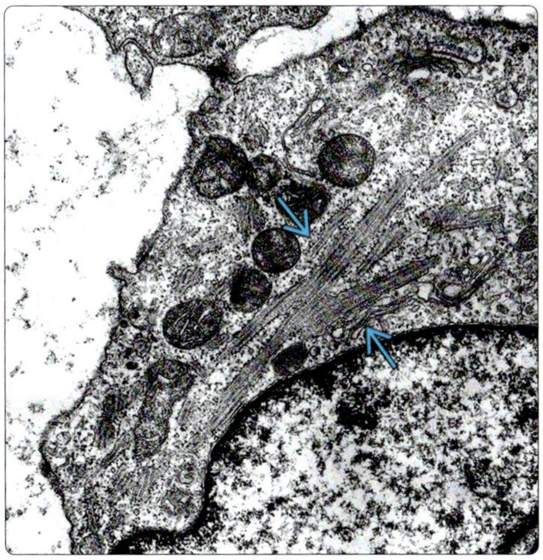

(Left) *Rhabdoid cells with eccentric, eosinophilic cytoplasm and perinuclear hyalin globules → can be found in EMC. As in rhabdoid tumor, these cells are negative for SNF5 (INI1). Rhabdoid EMCs often have variant NR4A3 fusions.* **(Right)** *Electron micrograph depicts parallel bundles of microtubules → within the cisternal compartment of an EMC, a highly characteristic feature found only in a minority of cases. Rhabdoid cells in EMC (not shown) have perinuclear whorls of intermediate filaments.*

Extrarenal Rhabdoid Tumor

KEY FACTS

TERMINOLOGY

- Highly malignant neoplasm composed of cells with rhabdoid morphology and characterized by alterations in *SMARCB1/INI1* gene
  - No other line of cellular differentiation can be present

ETIOLOGY/PATHOGENESIS

- Familial cases are often associated with germline mutations of *SMARCB1/INI1* gene

CLINICAL ISSUES

- Affects infants and young children
- Deep soft tissues in axial locations
  - Paraspinal, retroperitoneum, perineum, others
- Rapidly growing mass
- Treatment: Chemotherapy/radiation followed by resection
  - Genetic testing is recommended to evaluate for germline *SMARCB1* alterations
- Dismal prognosis
  - Frequent local recurrence and metastasis

MICROSCOPIC

- Sheets of characteristic polygonal rhabdoid cells
- MItotic figures and necrosis common
- Some cases show predominant component of undifferentiated small round cells

ANCILLARY TESTS

- Keratin (+), EMA(+), vimentin (+)
- Loss of nuclear INI1 expression characteristic
- CD99(+) in 50% of cases
- Molecular: Chromosome 22q11.2 monosomy or deletions (involving *SMARCB1/hSN5/INI1* gene)

TOP DIFFERENTIAL DIAGNOSES

- Epithelioid sarcoma
- Carcinoma or melanoma
- Rhabdomyosarcoma

Extrarenal Rhabdoid Tumor

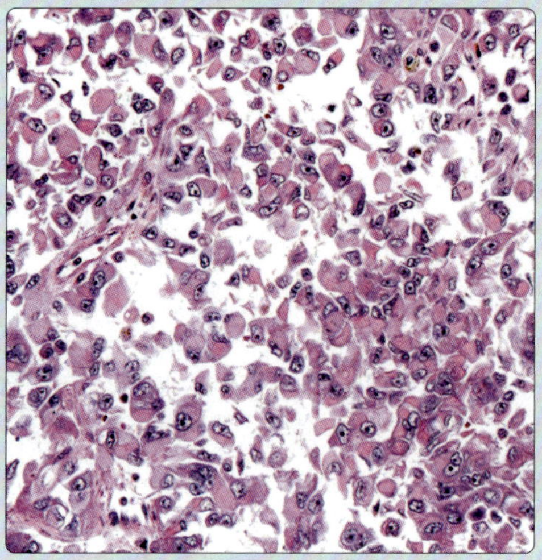

Rhabdoid Cells

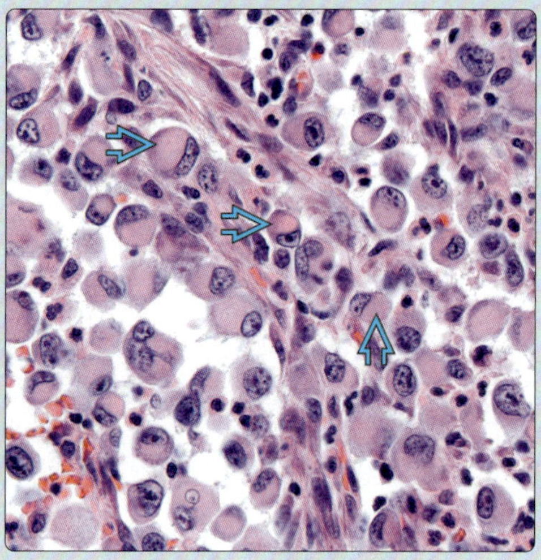

(Left) *Extrarenal rhabdoid tumor (ERT) of soft tissue is a highly aggressive malignancy that usually affects infants and young children and has a uniformly dismal prognosis. It is composed of variably cohesive sheets of polygonal cells with a rhabdoid morphology.* **(Right)** *Rhabdoid cells are characteristic of ERT but can be seen in a variety of other, unrelated tumors. Cytologically, they feature large, eccentric vesicular nuclei with prominent nucleoli and a glassy, eosinophilic cytoplasmic inclusion.*

Keratin Expression

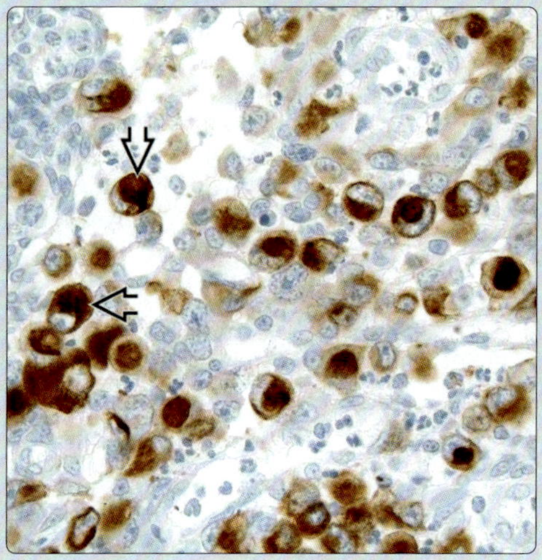

Loss of Nuclear INI1 Expression

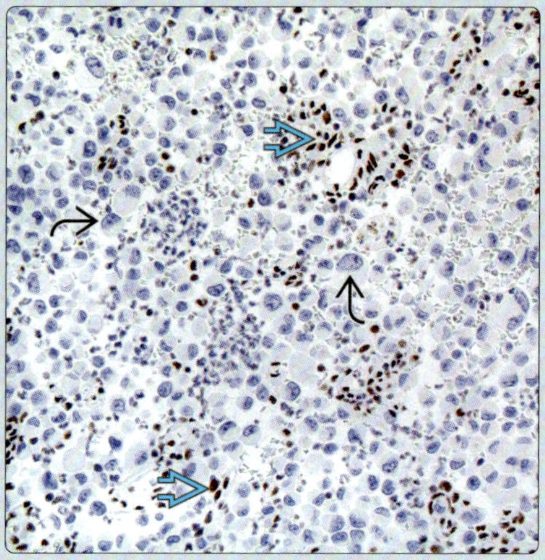

(Left) *Keratin (especially CK8 and CK18) and vimentin are commonly expressed in ERT and show cytoplasmic staining with accentuation in the paranuclear inclusion (contains aggregates of intermediate filaments).* **(Right)** *Loss of nuclear expression of INI1 is a characteristic feature of ERT; however, other tumors (such as epithelioid sarcoma) are known to show loss as well. Note the negative tumor cell nuclei amidst the positive stromal and endothelial cell nuclei.*

TERMINOLOGY

Abbreviations

- Extrarenal rhabdoid tumor (ERT)

Synonyms

- Malignant rhabdoid tumor
- Atypical teratoid/rhabdoid tumor (term for similar neoplasm occurring in central nervous system)

Definitions

- Highly malignant neoplasm composed of cells with rhabdoid morphology and characterized by alterations in *SMARCB1/INI1* gene
- No other line of cellular differentiation can be present (i.e., diagnosis of exclusion)
  - Specific tumor types that are known to occasionally exhibit rhabdoid cytomorphology
    - Carcinoma, melanoma
    - Epithelioid sarcoma, desmoplastic small round cell tumor, epithelioid malignant peripheral nerve sheath tumor
    - Mesothelioma, extraskeletal myxoid chondrosarcoma, rhabdomyosarcoma
    - Myoepithelial tumors, gastrointestinal stromal tumor, synovial sarcoma

ETIOLOGY/PATHOGENESIS

Genetic Factors

- Most are sporadic
- Familial cases are often associated with germline mutations of *SMARCB1/INI1* gene
  - May present with multiple rhabdoid tumors
  - Increased incidence of schwannomatosis in this group
- Genetic testing is recommended for all patients who develop ERT to evaluate for germline *SMARCB1* alterations
- Rare cases show retained *SMARCB1* expression but mutation &/or loss of *SMARCA4* (*BRG1*) gene

CLINICAL ISSUES

Epidemiology

- Incidence
  - Very rare
- Age
  - Infants and young children
    - May be congenital
  - Very rarely in adults

Site

- Deep soft tissues in axial locations
  - Paravertebral, neck, retroperitoneum, perineum, abdominopelvic cavities
- Also extremities, particularly thigh
- Viscera
  - Liver, GI tract, bladder, thymus, heart
- Cutaneous lesions also described

Presentation

- Rapidly growing mass
- Large tumors may ulcerate overlying skin
- May present with multiple cutaneous nodules

Treatment

- Multiagent chemotherapy regimen and radiotherapy followed by complete surgical resection, if feasible
- Genetic testing is recommended to evaluate for germline *SMARCB1* alterations

Prognosis

- Very poor
  - 5-year survival rate: 15-20%
- Frequent local recurrence and metastasis

MACROSCOPIC

General Features

- Multinodular, nonencapsulated, poorly circumscribed
- Pale or tan, with hemorrhage and necrosis

Size

- Often > 5 cm

MICROSCOPIC

Histologic Features

- Infiltrative peripheral borders
- Characteristic polygonal rhabdoid cells of varying sizes
  - Large eccentric, vesicular nuclei with prominent nucleoli
  - Variably abundant eosinophilic cytoplasm
    - Often contains glassy paranuclear intracytoplasmic inclusion (aggregates of intermediate filaments)
  - Mitotic figures are frequent
- Growth patterns: Cellular sheets or solid trabeculae
  - Cellular dyscohesion common
    - Pseudopapillary pattern may be seen
- Necrosis common
- Some cases show predominant component of undifferentiated small round cells
  - Characteristic rhabdoid cells may be focal or inconspicuous
- Other findings: Epithelioid change, spindled morphology, myxoid stroma, osteoclast-like giant cells

ANCILLARY TESTS

Histochemistry

- Cytoplasmic inclusions are PAS(+), diastase resistant

Immunohistochemistry

- Keratin (+), EMA(+), vimentin (+)
  - Most often low molecular weight keratins (CK8, CK18)
    - Often localized to paranuclear inclusions
- CD99(+) or synaptophysin (+) in 50% of cases, often patchy
- Loss of nuclear INI1 expression (negative nuclear staining)
  - Highly characteristic but not specific
- Also SALL4(+)
- May show focal expression of S100 protein or actins
- Negative for desmin, HMB-45, MART-1, CD31, CD34, myogenin

Molecular Genetics

- Chromosome 22q11.2 monosomy or deletions
  - Site of *SMARCB1/hSN5/INI1* tumor suppressor gene, which often shows homozygous deletion or mutation
    - Gene product is INI1 (BAF47)

- Translocations with 1p, 6p, 11p, or 18q
- 46,X,t(X;22;11)(q13;q11.2;q14.2) reported in one case
- Rare cases show retained *SMARCB1* expression but mutation &/or loss of *SMARCA4* (*BRG1*) gene

DIFFERENTIAL DIAGNOSIS

Epithelioid Sarcoma

- Affects older age group than ERT
- Multinodular growth pattern
- Proximal variant can show marked morphologic overlap with ERT
  - Prominent rhabdoid cells
- Keratin (+); CD34(+) in 50% of cases
- Loss of nuclear INI1 in 80-93% of cases

Metastatic Melanoma

- History of melanoma may be present
- Cells may show rhabdoid morphology
- S100 protein (+) in almost all cases
- HMB-45, Melan-A positivity in many cases (may be focal)
- Retention of nuclear INI1

Carcinoma

- Some high-grade carcinomas may show focal or predominant rhabdoid morphology
- Usually organ based
  - Can be metastatic in soft issue, but primary site is usually evident
- More conventional, nonrhabdoid morphology usually present
  - Expression of specific site markers (TTF-1, PSA, pax-8, etc.)
- Retention of nuclear INI1
  - Some GI tract carcinomas with rhabdoid morphology may lose INI1 expression

Rhabdomyosarcoma

- Desmin (+), myogenin (+), myoD1(+)
- Focal keratin (+) may be seen in alveolar rhabdomyosarcoma
- Retention of nuclear INI1

Ewing Sarcoma

- Can be morphologically similar to small cell variant of ERT
- Strong, membranous CD99(+)
- May be keratin (+)
- Retention of nuclear INI1
- *EWSR1* gene translocations in most cases

Myoepithelioma

- Can have rhabdoid cytoplasmic morphology
  - Often prominent nucleoli in myoepithelial carcinoma
- Myoepithelial marker expression
  - S100 protein, SMA, GFAP, calponin
- Retention of nuclear INI1
  - Loss of INI1 may be seen in myoepithelial carcinoma

Epithelioid Malignant Peripheral Nerve Sheath Tumor

- Prominent nucleoli; may show rhabdoid morphology
- Diffuse S100 protein (+); keratin (-)
- Loss of nuclear INI1 in 50% of cases

Extraskeletal Myxoid Chondrosarcoma

- Affects older age group than ERT
- Most common in extremities
- May show focal rhabdoid morphology in cellular or poorly differentiated cases
- Often prominent myxoid stroma
- Keratin (-)
- Retention of nuclear INI1
- *NR4A3* gene translocations characteristic

Desmoplastic Small Round Cell Tumor

- Characteristic abundant desmoplastic fibrous stroma
- May show focal rhabdoid morphology
- Keratin (+), desmin (+)
- Retention of nuclear INI1

SELECTED REFERENCES

1. Ginat DT et al: Disseminated malignant rhabdoid tumor of the head and neck. Head Neck Pathol. 11(2):224-7, 2017
2. Huang SC et al: Secondary EWSR1 gene abnormalities in SMARCB1-deficient tumors with 22q11-12 regional deletions: potential pitfalls in interpreting EWSR1 FISH results. Genes Chromosomes Cancer. 55(10):767-76, 2016
3. Agaimy A et al: SMARCB1 (INI1)-negative rhabdoid carcinomas of the gastrointestinal tract: clinicopathologic and molecular study of a highly aggressive variant with literature review. Am J Surg Pathol. 38(7):910-20, 2014
4. Bahrami A et al: SMARCB1 deletion by a complex three-way chromosomal translocation in an extrarenal malignant rhabdoid tumor. Cancer Genet. 207(9):437-40, 2014
5. Margol AS et al: Pathology and diagnosis of SMARCB1-deficient tumors. Cancer Genet. 207(9):358-64, 2014
6. Chakrapani AL et al: Congenital extrarenal malignant rhabdoid tumor in an infant with distal 22q11.2 deletion syndrome: the importance of SMARCB1. Am J Dermatopathol. 34(6):e77-80, 2012
7. Rizzo D et al: SMARCB1 deficiency in tumors from the peripheral nervous system: a link between schwannomas and rhabdoid tumors? Am J Surg Pathol. 36(7):964-72, 2012
8. Eaton KW et al: Spectrum of SMARCB1/INI1 mutations in familial and sporadic rhabdoid tumors. Pediatr Blood Cancer. 56(1):7-15, 2011
9. Schneppenheim R et al: Germline nonsense mutation and somatic inactivation of SMARCA4/BRG1 in a family with rhabdoid tumor predisposition syndrome. Am J Hum Genet. 86(2):279-84, 2010
10. Argenta PA et al: Proximal-type epithelioid sarcoma vs. malignant rhabdoid tumor of the vulva: a case report, review of the literature, and an argument for consolidation. Gynecol Oncol. 107(1):130-5, 2007
11. Kohashi K et al: Highly aggressive behavior of malignant rhabdoid tumor: a special reference to SMARCB1/INI1 gene alterations using molecular genetic analysis including quantitative real-time PCR. J Cancer Res Clin Oncol. 133(11):817-24, 2007
12. Biegel JA: Molecular genetics of atypical teratoid/rhabdoid tumor. Neurosurg Focus. 20(1):E11, 2006
13. Izumi T et al: Prognostic significance of dysadherin expression in epithelioid sarcoma and its diagnostic utility in distinguishing epithelioid sarcoma from malignant rhabdoid tumor. Mod Pathol. 19(6):820-31, 2006
14. Oda Y et al: Extrarenal rhabdoid tumors of soft tissue: clinicopathological and molecular genetic review and distinction from other soft-tissue sarcomas with rhabdoid features. Pathol Int. 56(6):287-95, 2006
15. Tekkök IH et al: Primary malignant rhabdoid tumor of the central nervous system–a comprehensive review. J Neurooncol. 73(3):241-52, 2005
16. Higashino K et al: Malignant rhabdoid tumor shows a unique neural differentiation as distinct from neuroblastoma. Cancer Sci. 94(1):37-42, 2003
17. Duvdevani M et al: Pure rhabdoid tumor of the bladder. J Urol. 166(6):2337, 2001
18. Ogino S et al: Malignant rhabdoid tumor: a phenotype? An entity?–A controversy revisited. Adv Anat Pathol. 7(3):181-90, 2000
19. White FV et al: Congenital disseminated malignant rhabdoid tumor: a distinct clinicopathologic entity demonstrating abnormalities of chromosome 22q11. Am J Surg Pathol. 23(3):249-56, 1999
20. Fanburg-Smith JC et al: Extrarenal rhabdoid tumors of soft tissue: a clinicopathologic and immunohistochemical study of 18 cases. Ann Diagn Pathol. 2(6):351-62, 1998
21. Wick MR et al: Malignant rhabdoid tumors: a clinicopathologic review and conceptual discussion. Semin Diagn Pathol. 12(3):233-48, 1995

Cellular Dyscohesion

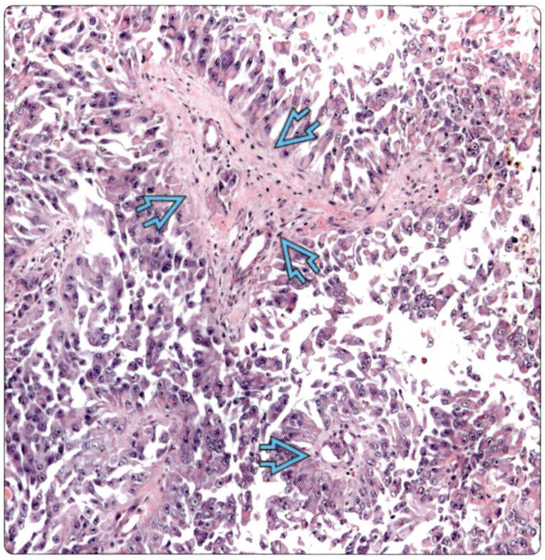

Small Rhabdoid Cell Morphology

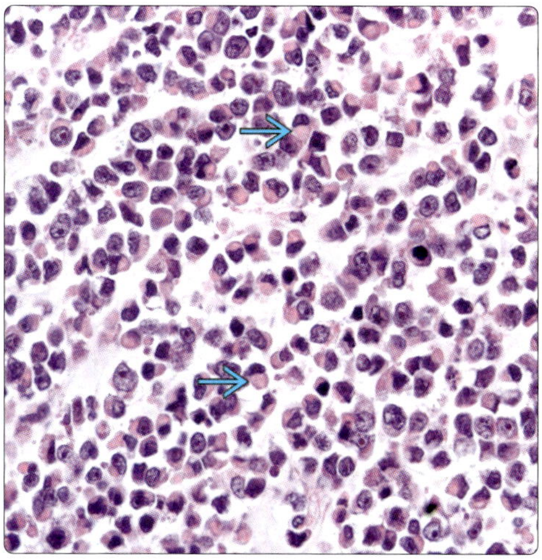

(Left) *Loss of cellular cohesion is common in ERT and may impart a pseudopapillary pattern around blood vessels. Other areas show solid, dense sheets or trabeculae of rhabdoid cells.* **(Right)** *In some cases of ERT, the rhabdoid cells are smaller and less plump; however, they still show eccentric nuclei with prominent nucleoli and intracytoplasmic eosinophilic inclusions. Confusion with a hematopoietic neoplasm is possible with this morphology.*

Large Epithelioid Cell Morphology

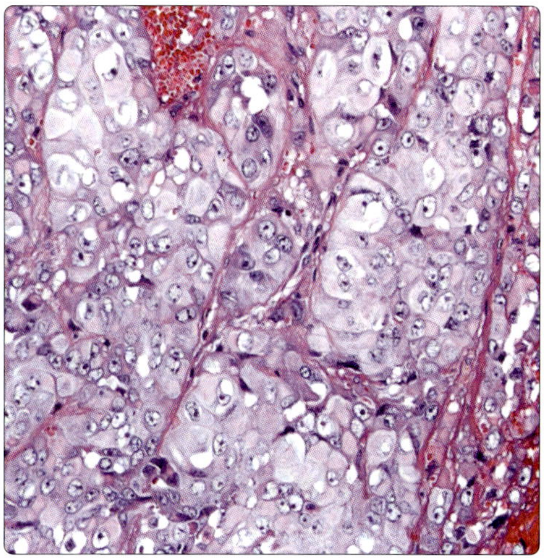

Myxoid Stromal Change

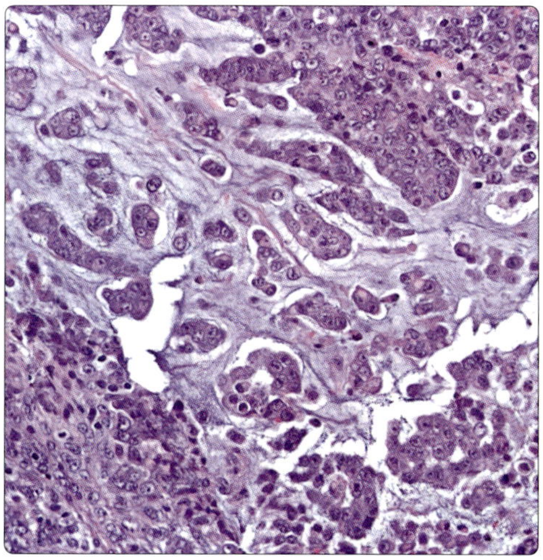

(Left) *A large, epithelioid cell morphology may be present in ERT and mimic a poorly differentiated carcinoma. Intracytoplasmic inclusions are also more difficult to identify. However, prominent nucleoli are easily identified.* **(Right)** *Myxoid stromal changes are uncommonly seen in ERT and are generally focal, if present.*

Stromal Hyalinization

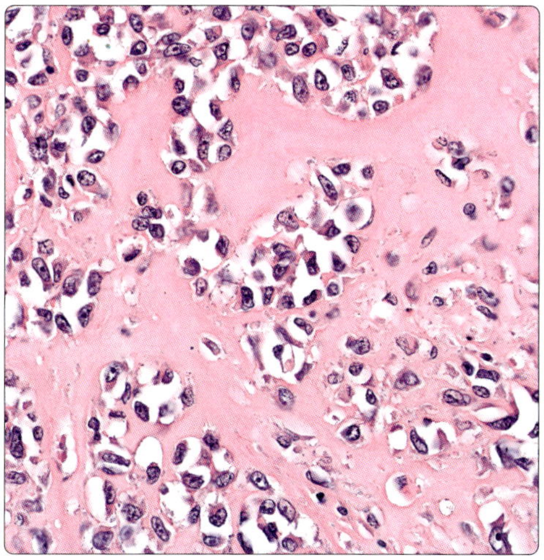

Undifferentiated Small Round Cells

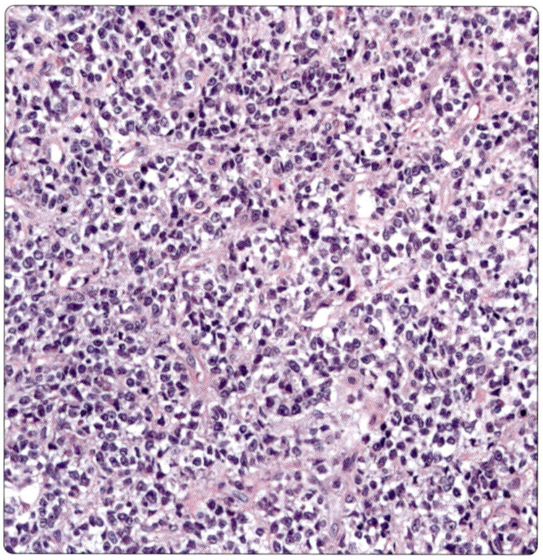

(Left) *Stromal hyalinization may be seen in ERT, imparting a sclerotic/nested appearance to the tumor and potentially leading to confusion with other sclerosing tumors. Areas of typical morphology are often present elsewhere.* **(Right)** *Some cases of ERT show a predominant component of small undifferentiated cells and few classic rhabdoid cells. Awareness of this morphology is important to avoid confusion with a variety of other small round blue cell tumors, such as Ewing sarcoma.*

Intimal Sarcoma

KEY FACTS

TERMINOLOGY

- Malignant mesenchymal neoplasm arising within lumina of large blood vessels

CLINICAL ISSUES

- Pulmonary trunk or pulmonary artery
- Descending thoracic or lower abdominal aorta
- Variety of symptoms due to vascular occlusion by tumor
  - Pulmonic tumors: Recurrent pulmonary embolism
  - Aortic tumors: Systemic embolic symptoms
    - Claudication of legs
    - Abdominal pain (superior mesenteric artery occlusion)
    - Ruptured aortic aneurysm at site of tumor
- Often not discovered until autopsy
- Poor prognosis; 80% mortality at 12 months

MACROSCOPIC

- Intravascular mass adherent to vessel wall, often polypoid
- May grossly mimic thrombus

MICROSCOPIC

- Usually poorly differentiated spindle cells, but wide range of features
  - May be epithelioid
- Cellularity, atypia/pleomorphism, and mitotic activity vary
- Myxoid background common
- Specific differentiation sometimes present
  - Rhabdomyosarcoma
  - Osteosarcoma
  - Angiosarcoma

TOP DIFFERENTIAL DIAGNOSES

- Cardiac (atrial) myxoma
- Primary cardiac sarcomas
- Leiomyosarcoma
- Epithelioid hemangioendothelioma
- Metastatic carcinoma
- Metastatic melanoma

Intimal Sarcoma of Pulmonary Artery

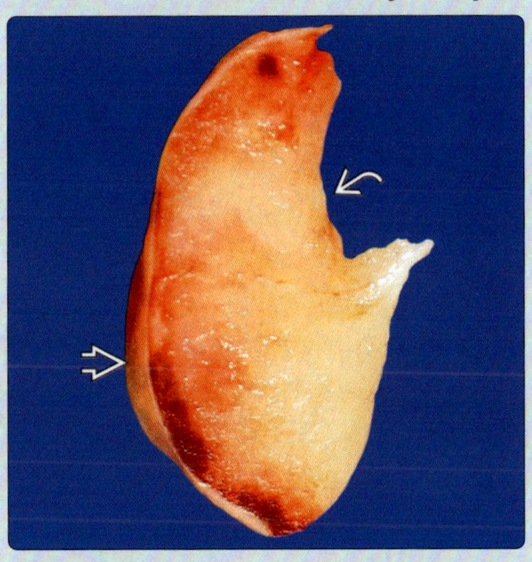

Plaque-Like Intravascular Growth

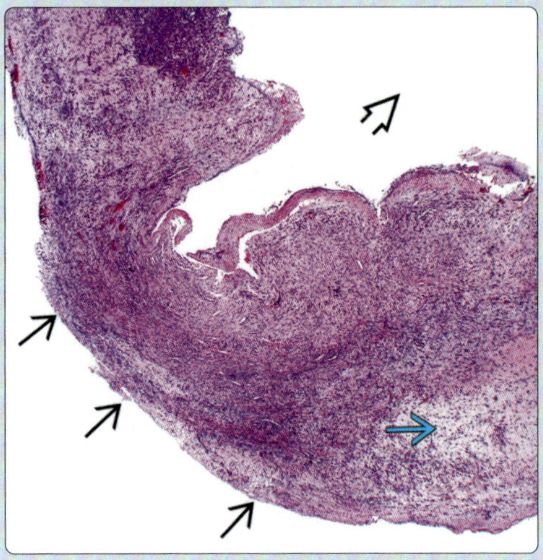

(Left) *This pulmonary artery intimal sarcoma adheres to the vessel wall and extends along a large part of its circumference filling much of the arterial lumen. The tumor has a gelatinous cut surface.* **(Right)** *Intimal sarcoma often forms an intravascular plaque that adheres to and conforms to the vessel wall (not present in this image) similar to atherosclerosis (side adherent to vessel wall and lumen). There are alternating areas of cellularity, and foci of myxoid background change are apparent.*

Myxoid and Hypocellular

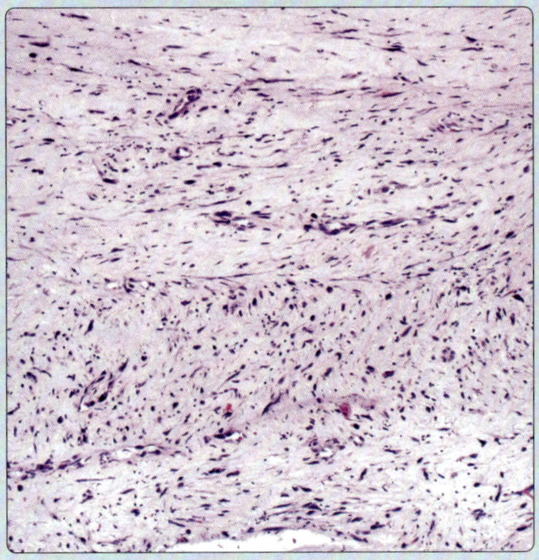

Atypical Epithelioid Cells

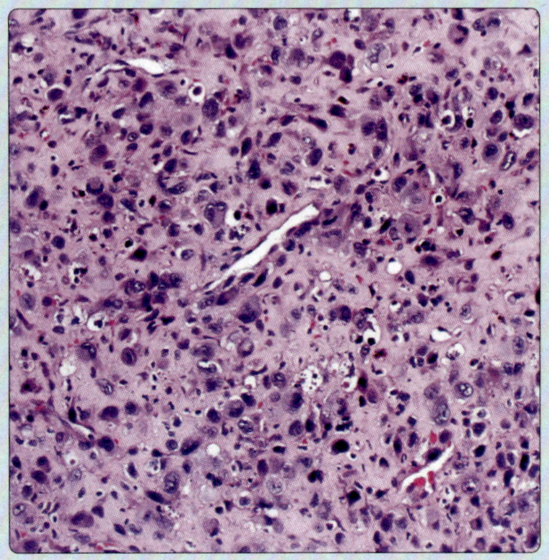

(Left) *Some areas of intimal sarcoma are relatively hypocellular with hyperchromatic atypical spindle cells set in a myxoid background. The appearance in these areas is somewhat similar to myxofibrosarcoma.* **(Right)** *Other foci are more cellular and display strikingly atypical epithelioid cells.*

TERMINOLOGY

Definitions

- Malignant mesenchymal neoplasm arising within lumina of large blood vessels

ETIOLOGY/PATHOGENESIS

Environmental Exposure

- Rare association with Dacron prosthetic graft

CLINICAL ISSUES

Epidemiology

- Incidence
  - Rare
- Age
  - Older adults

Site

- Pulmonary trunk or pulmonary artery
  - Can extend to pulmonary valve or right ventricle
  - Direct invasion or metastasis to lung parenchyma
  - Extrathoracic metastasis less common: Skin, brain, lymph nodes, kidneys
- Descending thoracic or lower abdominal aorta
  - Distant metastasis common: Bone, liver, peritoneum, mesenteric nodes

Presentation

- Variety of symptoms due to vascular occlusion by tumor
  - Pulmonic tumors: Recurrent pulmonary embolism
    - Rarely, acute myocardial infarction
  - Aortic tumors: Systemic embolic symptoms
    - Claudication of legs
    - Abdominal pain (superior mesenteric artery occlusion)
    - Ruptured aortic aneurysm at site of tumor
- Often not discovered until autopsy

Treatment

- Surgical removal when possible
- Chemotherapy for inoperable or disseminated disease

Prognosis

- Poor; 80% mortality at 12 months
  - Survival shorter for aortic (5-9 months) vs. pulmonary (13-18 months) tumors

MACROSCOPIC

General Features

- Intravascular mass adherent to vessel wall, often polypoid
  - Extends along vessel
  - May grossly mimic thrombus
  - In aorta, may resemble aneurysm or atherosclerosis
- Myxoid, hemorrhagic, fibrous, or ossified areas

MICROSCOPIC

Histologic Features

- Usually poorly differentiated spindle cells, but wide range of features
  - May be epithelioid
- Cellularity, atypia/pleomorphism, and mitotic activity vary
- Myxoid background common
- May have fascicular pattern resembling leiomyosarcoma
- Specific differentiation sometimes present
  - Rhabdomyosarcoma
  - Osteosarcoma
  - Angiosarcoma

ANCILLARY TESTS

Immunohistochemistry

- Variable SMA(+); may show focal desmin (+)
- Endothelial markers usually negative (unless angiosarcomatous differentiation is present)
- Nuclear MDM2(+) in up to 70% of cases

Genetic Testing

- Amplification/gains of *MDM2*, *PDGFRA*, *EGFR* common

DIFFERENTIAL DIAGNOSIS

Cardiac (Atrial) Myxoma

- Pedunculated lesion mostly in left atrium
- Arises from interatrial septum
- Bland spindle cells
- Myxoid stroma

Primary Cardiac Sarcomas

- Similar histologic features as intimal sarcoma
- Arising within heart rather than great vessels
  - Debatable if undifferentiated cardiac sarcoma should be classified as intimal sarcoma

Leiomyosarcoma

- Arise from media of large veins rather than within lumina
- Fascicles of spindle cells with stringy eosinophilic cytoplasm
- Usually stronger and more diffuse SMA and desmin expression

Epithelioid Hemangioendothelioma

- Often angiocentric: Fills lumen, expanding vessel (usually vein), and infiltrates adjacent tissue
- Aorta or pulmonary artery uncommon sites
- Cords of epithelioid cells with intracytoplasmic vacuoles containing erythrocytes ("blister" cells)
- Expresses endothelial markers (CD31, CD34, ERG)
- Often keratin (+)

Metastatic Carcinoma or Melanoma

- Primary site elsewhere
- Express markers for carcinoma (keratins, EMA, p63/p40, TTF-1, etc.) or melanoma (S100, SOX10, MART-1, HMB-45)

SELECTED REFERENCES

1. Maleszewski JJ et al: Do "intimal" sarcomas of the heart exist? Am J Surg Pathol. 38(8):1158-9, 2014
2. Neuville A et al: Intimal sarcoma is the most frequent primary cardiac sarcoma: clinicopathologic and molecular retrospective analysis of 100 primary cardiac sarcomas. Am J Surg Pathol. 38(4):461-9, 2014
3. Dewaele B et al: Coactivated platelet-derived growth factor receptor {alpha} and epidermal growth factor receptor are potential therapeutic targets in intimal sarcoma. Cancer Res. 70(18):7304-14, 2010
4. Sebenik M et al: Undifferentiated intimal sarcoma of large systemic blood vessels: report of 14 cases with immunohistochemical profile and review of the literature. Am J Surg Pathol. 29(9):1184-93, 2005

SECTION 17

Undifferentiated/Unclassified Sarcomas

Undifferentiated Pleomorphic Sarcoma 724

Undifferentiated Round Cell Sarcoma With *CIC-DUX4* Translocation 728

BCOR-CCNB3 Fusion-Positive Sarcoma 734

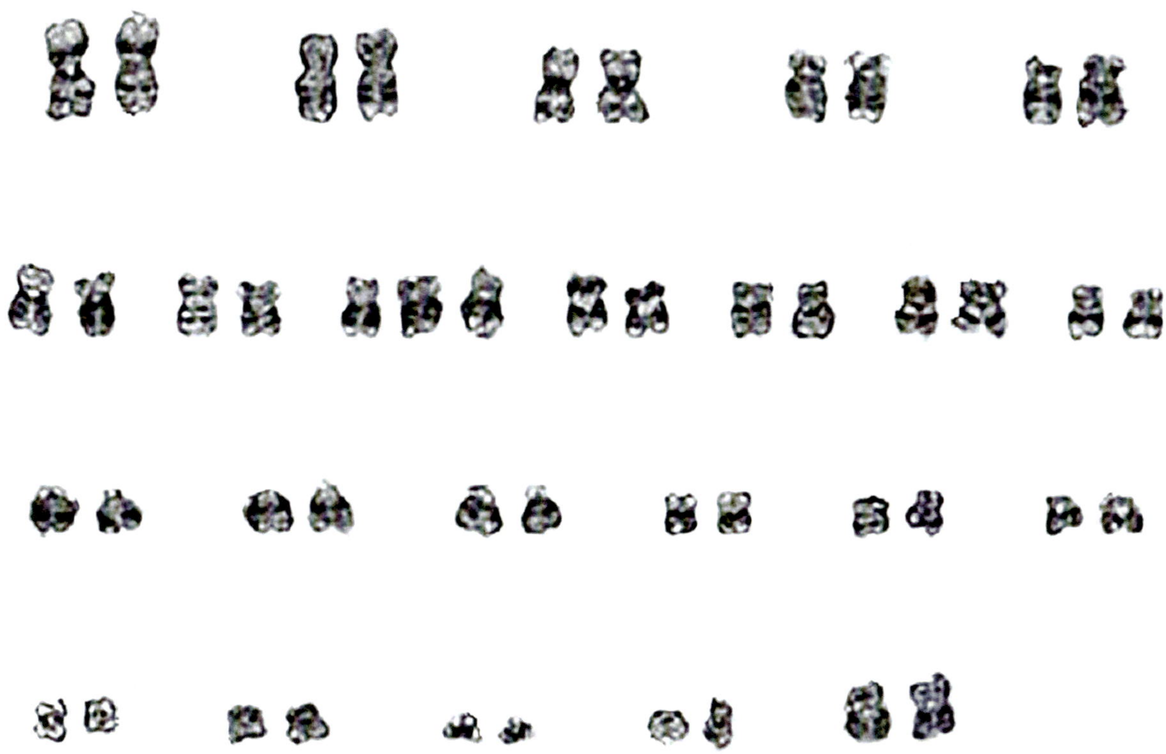

Undifferentiated Pleomorphic Sarcoma

KEY FACTS

TERMINOLOGY

- High-grade sarcoma composed of pleomorphic spindle and polygonal cells and showing no other identifiable line of differentiation
  - Essentially diagnosis of exclusion
- Synonym: Malignant fibrous histiocytoma

CLINICAL ISSUES

- Usually older and elderly adults (50-70 years)
- Most arise in deep soft tissues of extremities (thigh common)
- Treatment: Complete surgical resection with margins
- Fully malignant; usually high grade
  - Local recurrence in up to 30%; distant metastasis in up to 50%

MACROSCOPIC

- Usually large (most 5-15 cm)

MICROSCOPIC

- Storiform, fascicular, or patternless arrangement of highly atypical spindled &/or polygonal cells
  - Marked nuclear pleomorphism in most cases
  - Abundant mitoses, often abnormal, and necrosis
- May contain chronic inflammatory infiltrate or osteoclast-like giant cells
- No discernible microscopic evidence of any specific form of differentiation (e.g., lipoblasts, bone formation)

ANCILLARY TESTS

- Immunohistochemistry used to exclude other diagnoses
- Molecular: Complex and nonspecific cytogenetic abnormalities

TOP DIFFERENTIAL DIAGNOSES

- Dedifferentiated liposarcoma
- Other high-grade pleomorphic sarcomas
- Carcinoma, melanoma, lymphoma

Undifferentiated Pleomorphic Sarcoma | **Undifferentiated Pleomorphic Sarcoma**

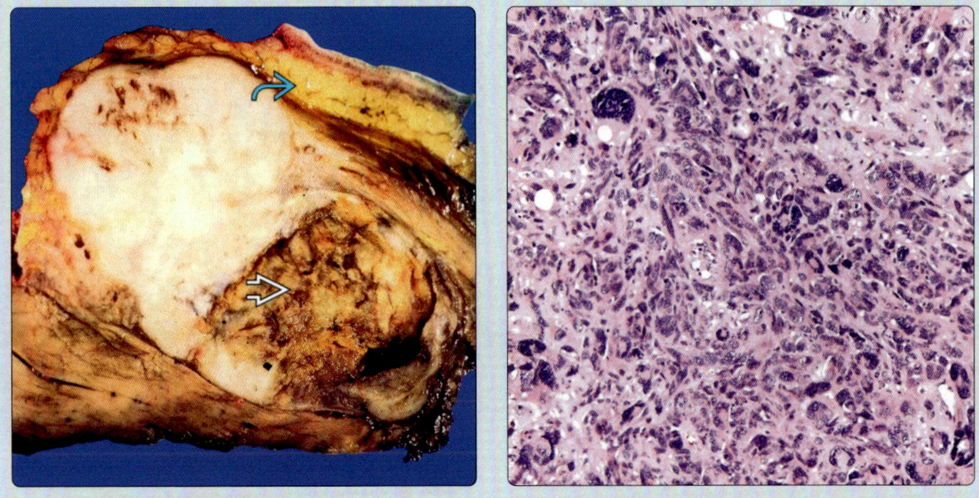

(Left) *Gross photograph of undifferentiated pleomorphic sarcoma (UPS) shows a lobulated, tan-white mass within skeletal muscle and focally abutting the subcutis* ➚*. Necrosis is a prominent feature* ➨. **(Right)** *Most cases of UPS show markedly atypical cytologic features with marked nuclear enlargement, hyperchromasia, and pleomorphism. Mitotic figures are also easily identified, and tumor necrosis is common.*

Extreme Atypia | **Variable Growth Patterns**

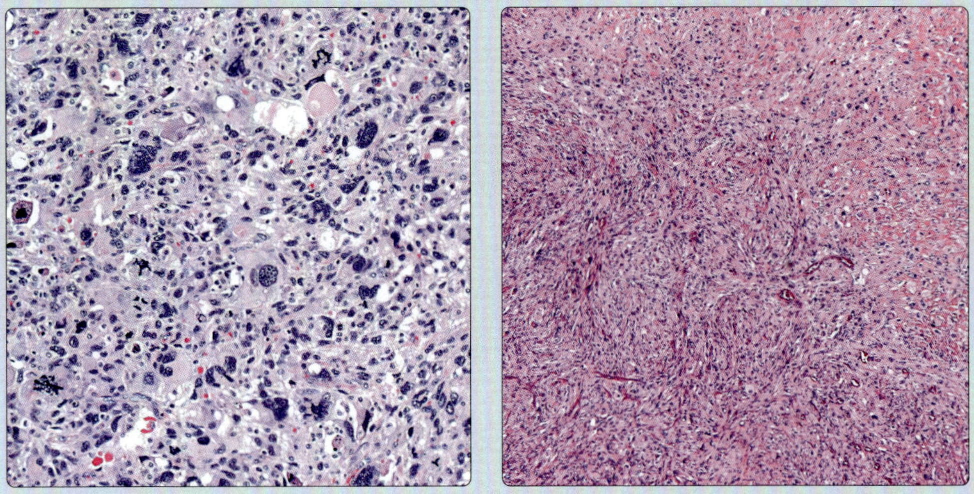

(Left) *Extreme nuclear and cytologic atypia are not uncommon in UPS. The bizarre cells are often significantly enlarged and show anaplastic nuclear configurations and extremely deranged mitotic figures.* **(Right)** *The patterns of growth in UPS vary from case to case, but most show a mixture of storiform and short, fascicular architectures. The stroma is generally collagenous but is often difficult to appreciate due to the high cellularity of the tumor.*

TERMINOLOGY

Abbreviations

- Undifferentiated pleomorphic sarcoma (UPS)

Synonyms

- Malignant fibrous histiocytoma

Definitions

- High-grade sarcoma composed of pleomorphic spindle and polygonal cells and showing no other identifiable line of differentiation
  - Essentially diagnosis of exclusion

CLINICAL ISSUES

Epidemiology

- Age
  - Most occur in older and elderly adults (50-70 years)
    - Very rare in adolescents and young adults
- Sex
  - 2:1 male predominance

Site

- Most arise in deep soft tissues of extremities (subfascial)
  - Lower limb (thigh) most common
  - Minority arise in subcutaneous tissue (superficially)
- May also arise on trunk

Presentation

- Enlarging, painless mass
  - Patient may have history of radiation to area

Treatment

- Complete surgical resection with margins
- Adjuvant radiation therapy

Prognosis

- Fully malignant; usually high grade
  - ~ 50% 5-year survival
- Local recurrence in up to 30% of cases
- Distant metastasis in up to 50% of cases
  - Minority of patients have metastases at time of presentation
- Superficial tumors have better prognosis than deep ones

MACROSCOPIC

General Features

- Generally circumscribed; multilobulated
- Heterogeneous cut surface with gray-tan firm and fleshy areas
- Necrosis and hemorrhage are common and may be extensive

Size

- Usually large (most 5-15 cm)

MICROSCOPIC

Histologic Features

- Storiform, fascicular, or patternless arrangement of highly atypical spindled &/or polygonal cells
  - Eosinophilic or amphophilic cytoplasm
  - Marked nuclear pleomorphism in most cases
    - Bizarre nuclei &/or multinucleation common
    - Abundant mitoses, often with abnormal forms
- Coagulative necrosis is common and may be abundant
- Collagenous stroma that may be focally myxoid or sclerotic
- Chronic inflammatory cells common, including lymphocytes and histiocytes
  - May rarely show prominent neutrophilic infiltrate
- May contain osteoclast-like giant cells
- No discernible microscopic evidence of any specific form of differentiation (e.g., lipoblasts, bone formation, epithelial structures)

ANCILLARY TESTS

Immunohistochemistry

- No diffuse expression of keratins, S100 protein, CD31, CD34, CD68, CD163, desmin, SMA, CD45, CD30
  - Focal SMA, CD34, keratin, EMA (+) may occur and is likely nonspecific
    - SMA expression is usually wispy (myofibroblastic staining pattern)
  - CD68, CD163, CD31, MiTF highlight intratumoral histiocytes
- Myogenin, MYOD1, p63, ERG (-)
- Main purpose of immunohistochemistry is to exclude other diagnoses

Molecular Genetics

- Complex and nonspecific cytogenetic abnormalities

DIFFERENTIAL DIAGNOSIS

Dedifferentiated Liposarcoma

- Relatively common in extremities and retroperitoneum
  - True UPS very rare in retroperitoneum
- May have component of well-differentiated liposarcoma
- *MDM2* amplification by FISH
- MDM2(+), CDK4(+) by immunohistochemistry

Other High-Grade Pleomorphic Sarcomas

- Often contain areas indistinguishable from UPS
- Mainly myxofibrosarcoma, leiomyosarcoma, rhabdomyosarcoma, pleomorphic liposarcoma, extraskeletal osteosarcoma, angiosarcoma, malignant peripheral nerve sheath tumor
  - Thorough sampling and careful scrutiny is necessary to identify characteristic histologic findings that support these other diagnoses
- Immunohistochemistry often necessary in pleomorphic leiomyosarcoma, rhabdomyosarcoma, and angiosarcoma

Carcinoma, Melanoma, Lymphoma

- Can be excluded through immunohistochemistry and often clinical history

SELECTED REFERENCES

1. Le Guellec S et al: Are peripheral purely undifferentiated pleomorphic sarcomas with MDM2 amplification dedifferentiated liposarcomas? Am J Surg Pathol. 38(3):293-304, 2014
2. Fletcher CD et al: Clinicopathologic re-evaluation of 100 malignant fibrous histiocytomas: prognostic relevance of subclassification. J Clin Oncol. 19(12):3045-50, 2001

(Left) *A loose or vague storiform growth pattern is common in UPS and is seen in the majority of cases, at least focally.* **(Right)** *Formation of short, irregular fascicles by tumor cells is common in UPS; however, long fascicles are less frequent and should at least raise the possibility of other entities, such as malignant peripheral nerve sheath tumor, synovial sarcoma, or adult-type fibrosarcoma.*

Storiform Growth

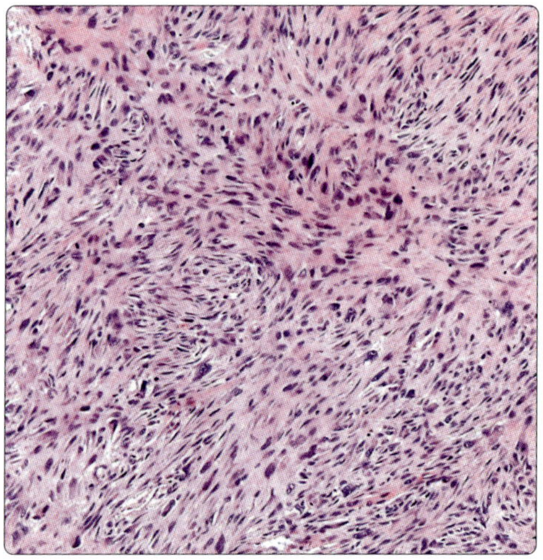

Fascicular Growth

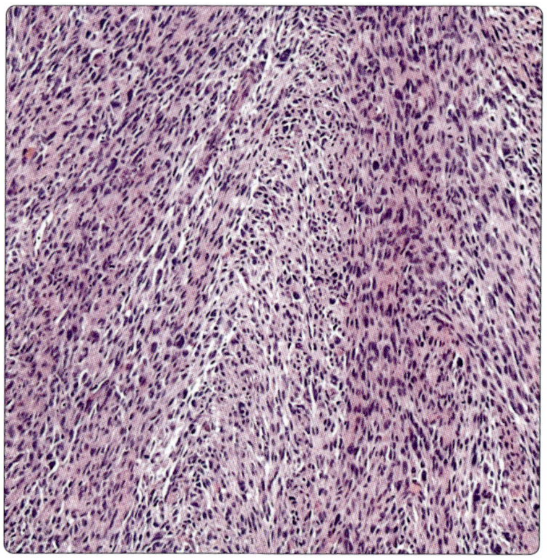

(Left) *Some cases of UPS may show focal or extensive stromal collagen and sclerosis. This finding is more common following neoadjuvant therapy but may be seen in untreated tumors as well.* **(Right)** *Coagulative tumor necrosis is very common in UPS and ranges from multiple small pockets to large zones. In some cases, nearly the entire tumor may be necrotic.*

Stromal Sclerosis

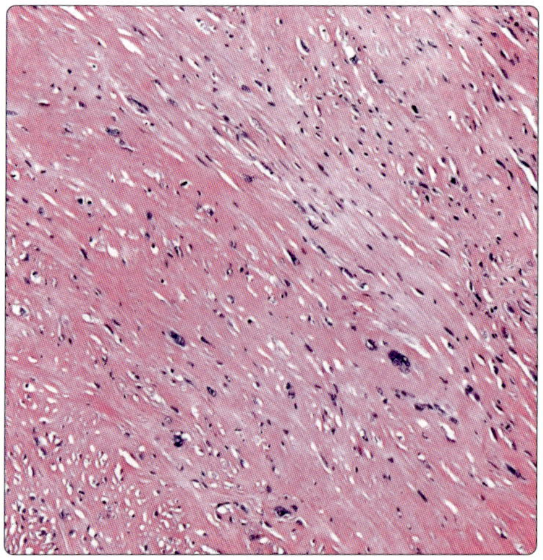

Coagulative Necrosis

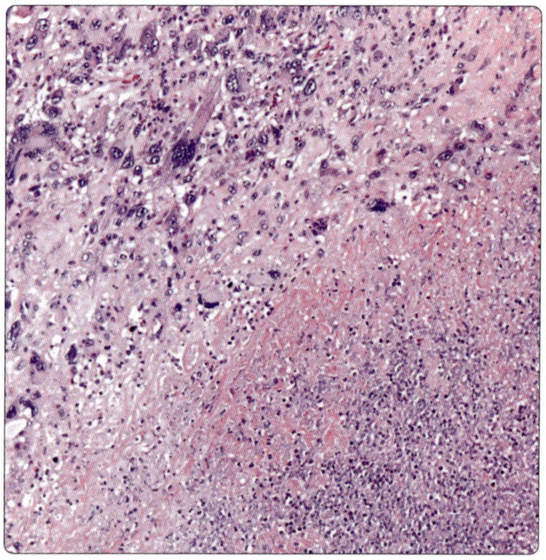

(Left) *A chronic inflammatory infiltrate is not uncommon in UPS and often consists of lymphocytes. This infiltrate is usually mild or inconspicuous, but in occasional cases, it can be marked (shown).* **(Right)** *A prominent neutrophilic infiltrate associated with foamy histiocytes ➡ is a feature of rare cases of UPS, particularly of the retroperitoneum. However, in this location, a dedifferentiated liposarcoma is far more likely and should always be thoroughly excluded first.*

Chronic Inflammation

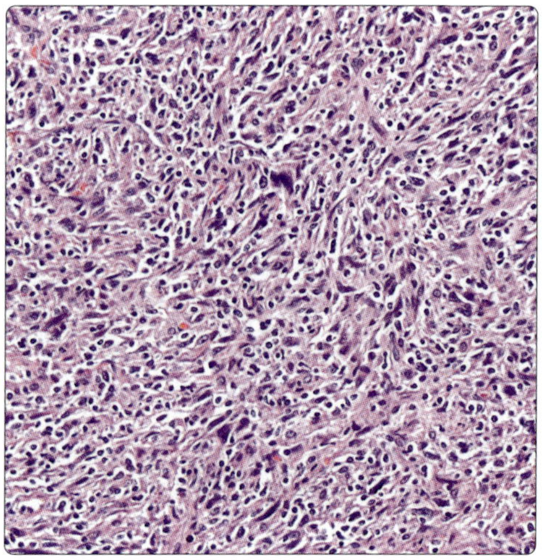

Neutrophils and Foamy Histiocytes

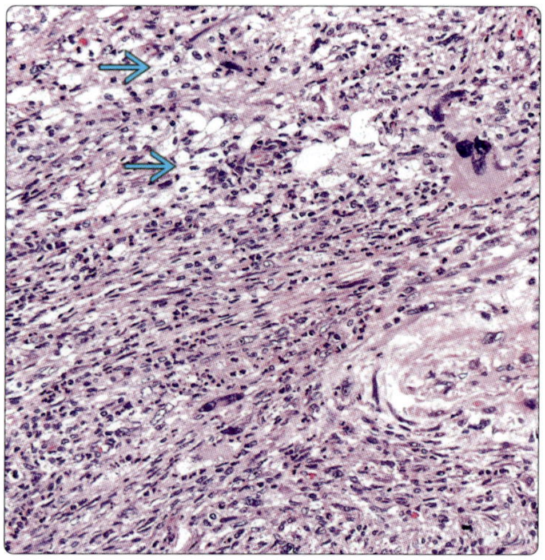

Osteoclast-Like Giant Cells

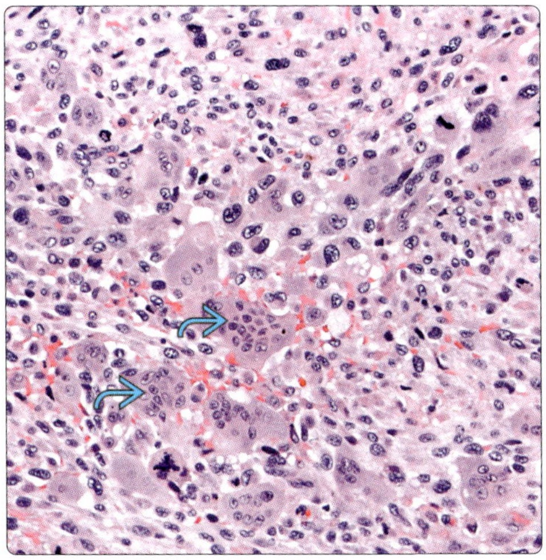

Focal Myxoid Stroma

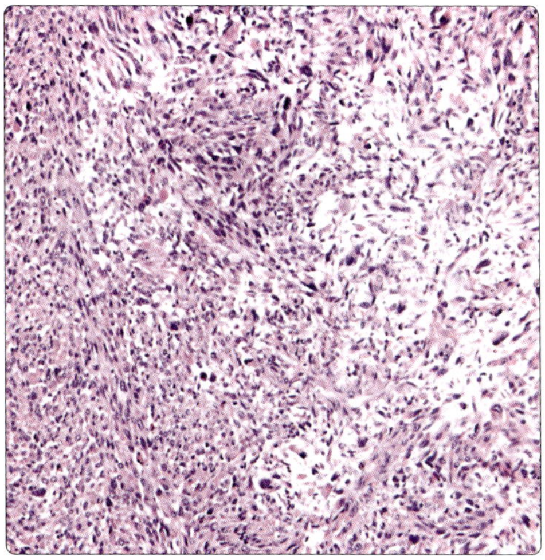

(Left) *Osteoclast-like multinucleated giant cells may be seen in UPS and are occasionally numerous. These cells are often also a feature of extraskeletal osteosarcoma, which should always be excluded.* **(Right)** *Focal myxoid stromal change may be seen in UPS and is not immediately diagnostic of myxofibrosarcoma. However, if the myxoid change is diffuse or shows more typical features of myxofibrosarcoma, the latter diagnosis is more appropriate.*

Skeletal Muscle Infiltration

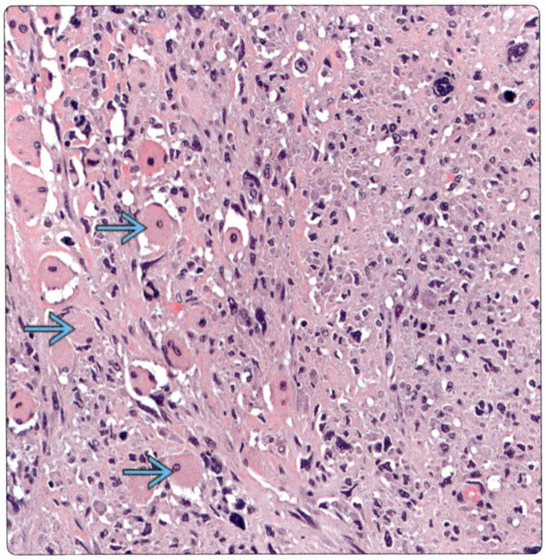

Epithelioid Cells

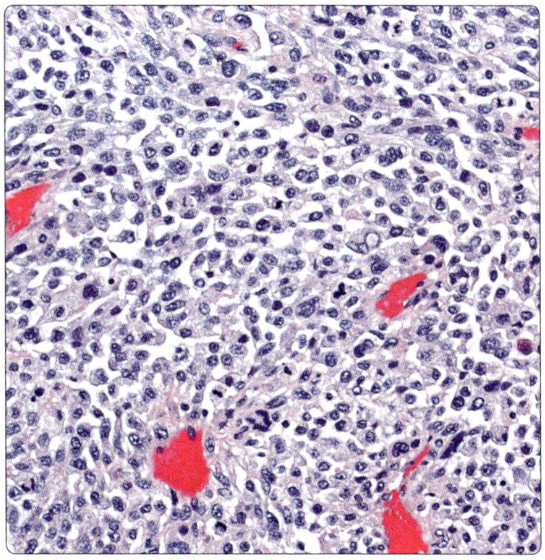

(Left) *Given that UPS shows a predilection for subfascial sites, it is not uncommon to see infiltrated skeletal myocytes at or near the periphery of the tumor. These otherwise mature-appearing cells should not be used as evidence for diagnosing pleomorphic rhabdomyosarcoma.* **(Right)** *An epithelioid cytomorphology may be seen in UPS; however, it is often focal. Rare cases may show prominent epithelioid change and warrant consideration of carcinoma and melanoma.*

CD31 Expression in Histiocytes

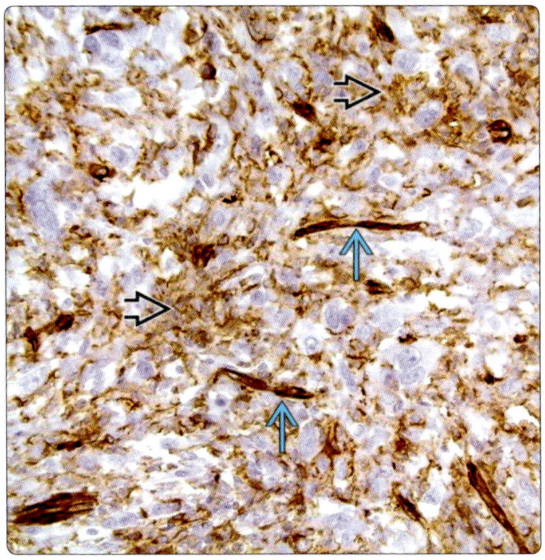

Postradiation Sarcoma

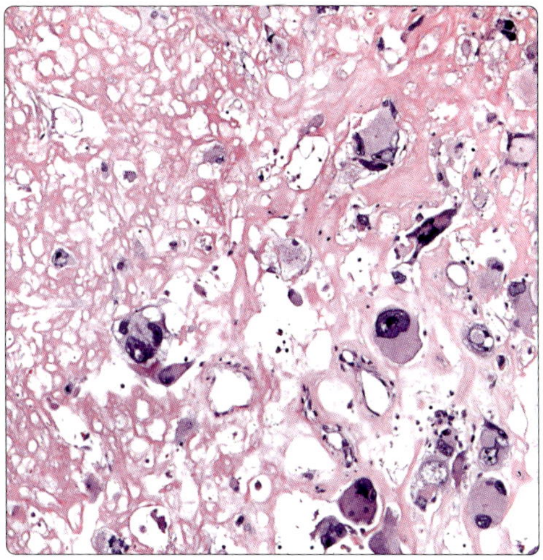

(Left) *CD31 often shows a faint, granular expression pattern in histiocytes and is not indicative of endothelial differentiation in a pleomorphic sarcoma (angiosarcoma). In contrast, note the strong, sharp CD31 expression by endothelial cells of intratumoral vessels.* **(Right)** *Bizarre atypia is not a specific feature of UPS and may be seen in just about any high-grade sarcoma treated with neoadjuvant therapy. Note the hypocellular, microcystic, and sclerotic stroma, further evidence of treatment effect.*

Undifferentiated Round Cell Sarcoma With *CIC-DUX4* Translocation

KEY FACTS

TERMINOLOGY

- Highly aggressive translocation-associated round cell sarcoma
- Oncogenic fusion of *CIC* and *DUX4*

CLINICAL ISSUES

- Age: children and young adults; range: 6-62 years
- Rapidly enlarging, deep or superficial soft tissue mass
- High metastatic rate
- Most patients die of disease within 2 years

MACROSCOPIC

- Large, bulky, necrotizing mass

MICROSCOPIC

- Sheets of closely spaced small round cells
  - Coarse chromatin with prominent nucleoli
  - Brisk mitotic activity
  - Focal cytoplasmic clearing
- Geographic necrosis
  - Perivascular preservation in necrotic areas
- Focal myxoid matrix
- Focal cord-like arrangement of cells

ANCILLARY TESTS

- Cytogenetics/molecular
  - t(4;19)(q35;q13.1) or t(10;19)(q26.3;q13) translocation
  - *CIC* rearrangement (FISH)
  - *CIC-DUX4* fusion (FISH or RT-PCR)

TOP DIFFERENTIAL DIAGNOSES

- Extraskeletal Ewing sarcoma
- Malignant peripheral nerve sheath tumor
- Synovial sarcoma (poorly differentiated)
- Alveolar rhabdomyosarcoma
- Other undifferentiated round cell sarcomas

CIC-DUX4 Sarcoma

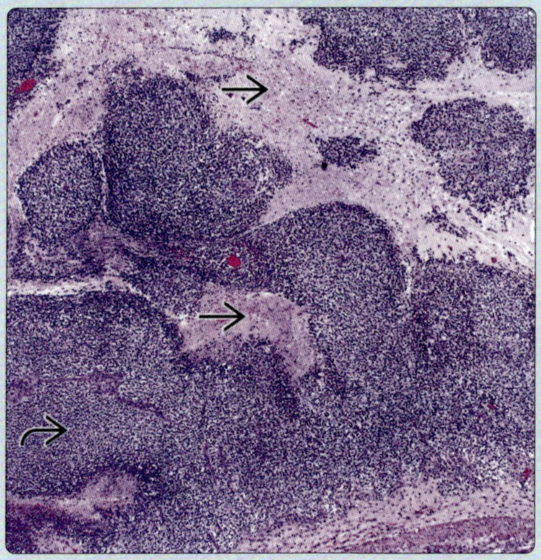

Cytologic Features

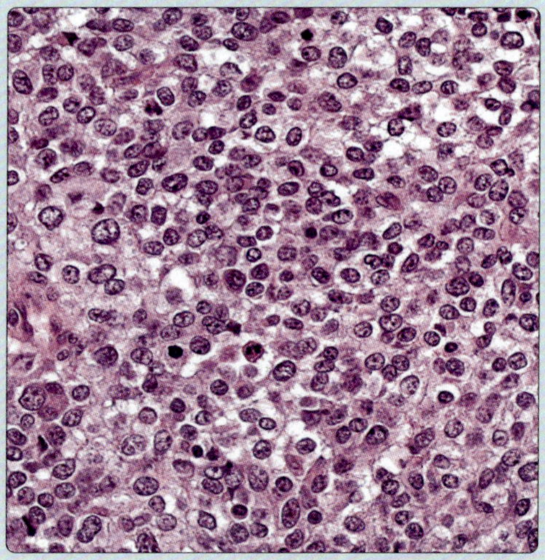

(Left) *CIC-DUX4 sarcoma is a necrotizing round cell tumor with distinctive histological features. Most tumors have extensive areas of geographic necrosis ➔ and sheets of closely spaced small round cells ➔, as depicted in this low-power micrograph.* **(Right)** *Although often referred to as Ewing-like, the cells of CIC-DUX4 sarcoma are more pleomorphic and hyperchromatic than those of Ewing sarcoma, containing coarse chromatin, prominent nucleoli, and ill-defined, eosinophilic, or clear cytoplasm.*

Myxoid Matrix

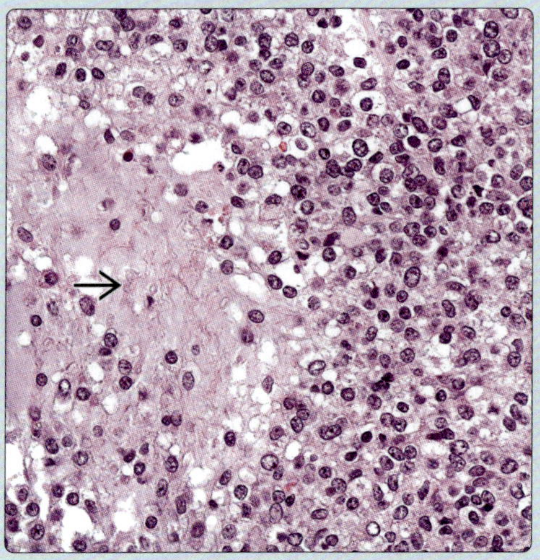

Simple Karyotype: t(4;19) and Trisomy 8

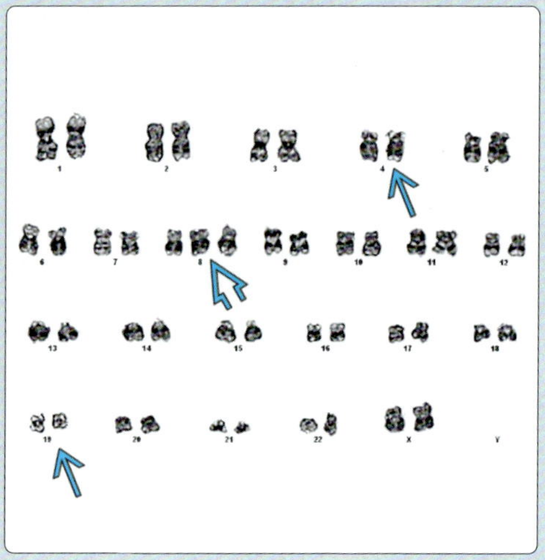

(Left) *Although often sparse, extracellular myxoid matrix is present in most tumors. It usually presents as a small area of pale blue, hyalinized or fine fibrillary material ➔.* **(Right)** *CIC-DUX4 sarcoma is a translocation-associated sarcoma that often has a simple karyotype. The only cytogenetic aberrations in this tumor are its pathognomonic t(4;19) ➔ and trisomy 8 ➔, which is frequently present, as depicted.*

TERMINOLOGY

Synonyms

- *CIC*-rearranged sarcoma, Ewing-like sarcoma

Definitions

- Highly aggressive, translocation-associated round cell sarcoma
- No specific line of differentiation
- Oncogenic fusion of *CIC* and *DUX4*

ETIOLOGY/PATHOGENESIS

CIC-DUX4 Functions as Transcription Factor

- Upregulates expression of *ETV1*, *ETV4*, and *ETV5*

MYC Amplification

- Majority of cases

CLINICAL ISSUES

Epidemiology

- Incidence
  - Rare; < 150 reported cases
    - ~ 2/3 of *EWSR1*-negative small blue round cell sarcomas
- Age
  - Children and young adults mostly
    - Range: 6-62 years

Site

- Extremities and trunk most common
- Other sites: Pelvis, retroperitoneum, head and neck, pleura, bone, brain, visceral organs

Presentation

- Rapidly enlarging mass
- Deep or superficial soft tissue
- Metastatic disease often present at presentation

Treatment

- Wide surgical excision or amputation
- May show initial response to chemotherapy
  - Often acquires chemoresistance
- Radiation for local control and palliation
- Best therapeutic strategy poorly defined

Prognosis

- Very poor
  - 43% 5-year overall survival
    - Most die of disease within 2 years
- High metastatic rate
  - Lungs most common
    - Other sites: Brain, soft tissue, bone

IMAGING

General Features

- Large, lobulated, heterogeneous soft tissue mass
  - Usually deep seated
  - Secondary bone invasion in some cases

MACROSCOPIC

General Features

- Large, bulky mass
- Fleshy cut surface
- Geographic necrosis and hemorrhage

MICROSCOPIC

Histologic Features

- Sheets of closely spaced small round cells
  - Moderate nuclear pleomorphism
  - Coarse chromatin with prominent nucleoli
  - Indistinct cytoplasm
    - Focal cytoplasmic clearing
      - With sharp cell borders
  - High mitotic rate
  - Spindle-shaped, epithelioid &/or rhabdoid cells in some
- Geographic necrosis common
  - Perivascular preservation in necrotic areas
- Myxoid matrix in most
  - Variable amount, usually focal
- Focal cord-like arrangement of cells

ANCILLARY TESTS

Immunohistochemistry

- Mostly useful for ruling out other neoplasms
- WT1(+) and ETV4(+)
  - Useful for distinguishing *CIC*-rearranged from Ewing sarcoma

Cytogenetics

- t(4;19)(q35;q13.1)
  - t(10;19)(q26.3;q13) variant translocation
- Simple karyotype in most tumors
  - Complex karyotype post treatment
- Trisomy 8 frequent

Molecular Genetics

- *CIC* rearrangement by FISH
- *CIC-DUX4* fusion by RT-PCR or FISH
- Array-based DNA-methylation analysis

DIFFERENTIAL DIAGNOSIS

Extraskeletal Ewing Sarcoma

- More uniform nuclear size
- Softer chromatin
- Smaller nucleoli
- Cytoplasmic clearing common
- CD99 diffuse membrane positivity
- *EWSR1* translocation

Malignant Peripheral Nerve Sheath Tumor

- Can mimic round cell sarcoma
- Geographic necrosis common
- Spindle cells common
- Often associated with nerve or neurofibromatosis type 1 (NF1) syndrome
- S100(+) in 60% but often focal

Immunohistochemistry Table

Antibody	Reactivity	Staining Pattern	Comment
CD99	Positive	Cell membrane & cytoplasm	Focal in most, sometimes diffuse
WT1	Positive	Nuclear	> 90%
ETV4	Positive	Nuclear	> 90%
FLI-1	Positive	Nuclear	Usually strong, diffuse
ERG	Positive	Nuclear	Variable expression
CK-PAN	Equivocal	Cytoplasmic	Rarely focally positive
S100	Equivocal	Nuclear & cytoplasmic	Rarely focally positive
Desmin	Equivocal	Cytoplasmic	Rarely focally positive
Myogenin	Negative	Nuclear	
TLE1	Negative	Nuclear	
INI1	Positive	Nuclear	Retained expression

Synovial Sarcoma (Poorly Differentiated)

- Can mimic round cell sarcoma
- Softer ("blastoid") chromatin
- Strong, diffuse nuclear TLE1(+)
- Usually cytokeratin (+), EMA(+), CD99(+)
- *SS18-SSX1*, *SS18-SSX2*, or *SS18-SSX4* fusion

Alveolar Rhabdomyosarcoma

- Small round cell sarcoma
- Alveolar growth pattern in most cases
- Rhabdomyoblasts can be scarce
- Multinucleated cells often present
- Diffuse desmin (+) and nuclear myogenin (+)
- *PAX3-FOXO1* or *PAX7-FOXO1* fusion

Other Undifferentiated Round Cell Sarcomas

- *BCOR-CCNB3* sarcoma
  - Involves bone > soft tissue
  - Either round cell or spindle cell morphology
  - *BCOR-CCNB3* fusion transcript
- *CIC-FOXO4* sarcoma
  - Very rare round cell soft tissue sarcoma
  - Abundant desmoplastic stroma
  - CD99(+)

DIAGNOSTIC CHECKLIST

Clinically Relevant Pathologic Features

- Rapidly enlarging soft tissue mass
- Affects both children and adults
- High metastatic potential
  - Often present at time of diagnosis
- Poor or unsustained response to chemotherapy

Pathologic Interpretation Pearls

- Closely spaced small round cells
- Geographic zones of necrosis
- Coarse chromatin, prominent nucleoli, moderate pleomorphism
- Clear cell areas; focal myxoid matrix
- WT1(+) and ETV4(+) by IHC
- Molecular confirmation required for diagnosis

SELECTED REFERENCES

1. Koelsche C et al: Array-based DNA-methylation profiling in sarcomas with small blue round cell histology provides valuable diagnostic information. Mod Pathol. 31(8):1246-56, 2018
2. Renzi S et al: Ewing-like sarcoma: an emerging family of round cell sarcomas. J Cell Physiol. ePub, 2018
3. Antonescu CR et al: Sarcomas With CIC-rearrangements are a distinct pathologic entity with aggressive outcome: a clinicopathologic and molecular study of 115 cases. Am J Surg Pathol. 41(7):941-9, 2017
4. Maghrebi H et al: Round cell sarcoma of the colon with CIC rearrangement. BMC Res Notes. 10(1):582, 2017
5. Hung YP et al: Evaluation of ETV4 and WT1 expression in CIC-rearranged sarcomas and histologic mimics. Mod Pathol. 29(11):1324-34, 2016
6. Le Guellec S et al: ETV4 is a useful marker for the diagnosis of CIC-rearranged undifferentiated round-cell sarcomas: a study of 127 cases including mimicking lesions. Mod Pathol. 29(12):1523-31, 2016
7. Bielle F et al: Unusual primary cerebral localization of a CIC-DUX4 translocation tumor of the Ewing sarcoma family. Acta Neuropathol. 128(2):309-11, 2014
8. Puls F et al: BCOR-CCNB3 (Ewing-like) sarcoma: a clinicopathologic analysis of 10 cases, in comparison with conventional Ewing sarcoma. Am J Surg Pathol. 38(10):1307-18, 2014
9. Smith SC et al: CIC-DUX sarcomas demonstrate frequent MYC amplification and ETS-family transcription factor expression. Mod Pathol. 28(1):57-68, 2014
10. Solomon DA et al: Clinicopathologic features of a second patient with Ewing-like sarcoma harboring CIC-FOXO4 gene fusion. Am J Surg Pathol. 38(12):1724-5, 2014
11. Specht K et al: Distinct transcriptional signature and immunoprofile of CIC-DUX4 fusion-positive round cell tumors compared to EWSR1-rearranged Ewing sarcomas: further evidence toward distinct pathologic entities. Genes Chromosomes Cancer. 53(7):622-33, 2014
12. Sugita S et al: A novel CIC-FOXO4 gene fusion in undifferentiated small round cell sarcoma: a genetically distinct variant of Ewing-like sarcoma. Am J Surg Pathol. 38(11):1571-6, 2014
13. Choi EY et al: Undifferentiated small round cell sarcoma with t(4;19)(q35;q13.1) CIC-DUX4 fusion: a novel highly aggressive soft tissue tumor with distinctive histopathology. Am J Surg Pathol. 37(9):1379-86, 2013
14. Graham C et al: The CIC-DUX4 fusion transcript is present in a subgroup of pediatric primitive round cell sarcomas. Hum Pathol. 43(2):180-9, 2012
15. Italiano A et al: High prevalence of CIC fusion with double-homeobox (DUX4) transcription factors in EWSR1-negative undifferentiated small blue round cell sarcomas. Genes Chromosomes Cancer. 51(3):207-18, 2012
16. Kawamura-Saito M et al: Fusion between CIC and DUX4 up-regulates PEA3 family genes in Ewing-like sarcomas with t(4;19)(q35;q13) translocation. Hum Mol Genet. 15(13):2125-37, 2006
17. Richkind KE et al: t(4;19)(q35;q13.1): a recurrent change in primitive mesenchymal tumors? Cancer Genet Cytogenet. 87(1):71-4, 1996

MR

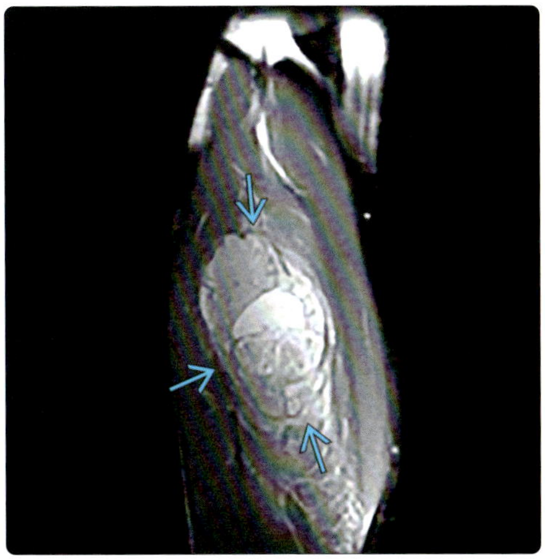

Calf Mass

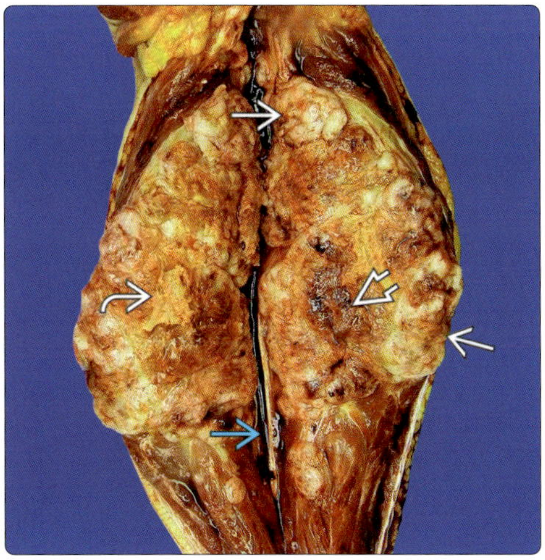

(Left) *On MR, CIC-DUX4 sarcoma usually presents as a large, heterogeneous, lobulated, deep-seated soft tissue mass, as depicted by this 11-cm calf mass in a 29-year-old woman.* **(Right)** *In the amputation specimen, the tumor has been bivalved to display the cut surface, which shows a multinodular mass containing fleshy, necrotic, and hemorrhagic areas. Note the entrapped sciatic nerve.*

Gross Appearance

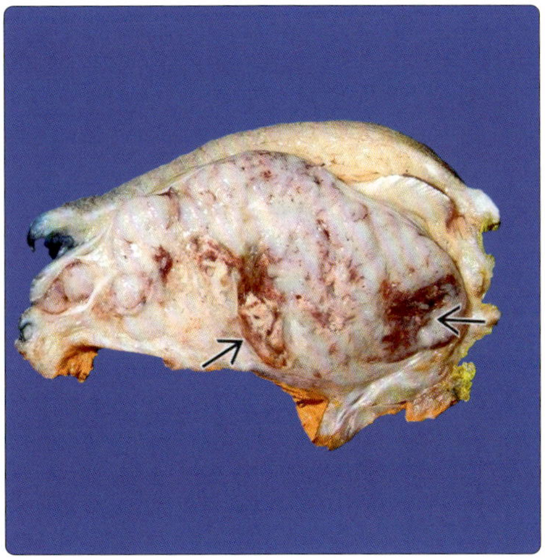

Gross Appearance

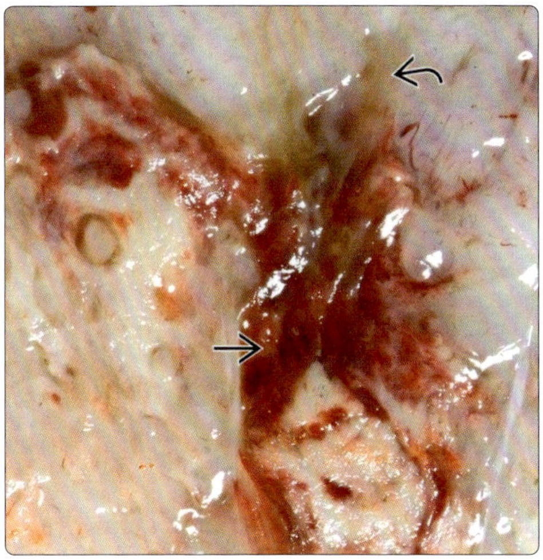

(Left) *This gross specimen is from an inguinal soft tissue metastasis from a primary popliteal CIC-DUX4 sarcoma in a 40-year-old man. The cut surface depicts a bulky, white, fleshy soft tissue tumor with geographic areas of hemorrhagic necrosis.* **(Right)** *This gross photograph shows an irregular zone of hemorrhagic necrosis. Note the tan, gelatinous area that corresponds to extracellular myxoid matrix of the tumor.*

Amputation Specimen

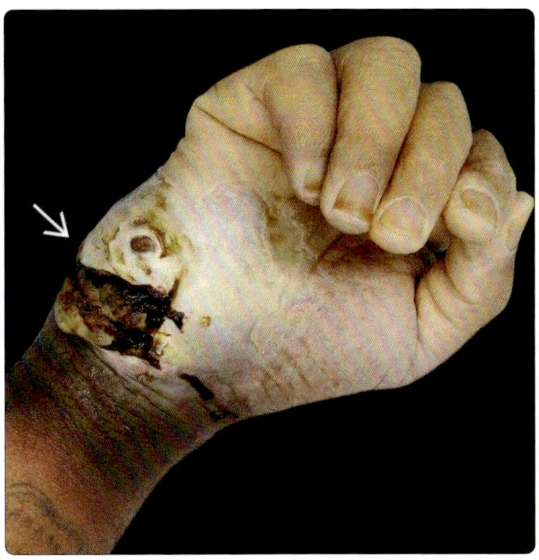

Shoulder Mass

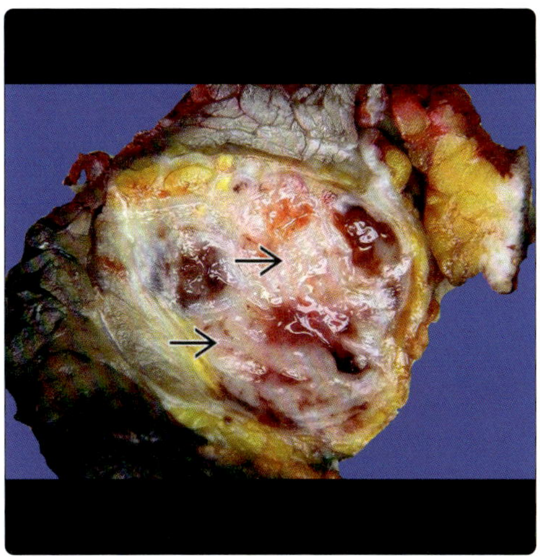

(Left) *This patient had an above-elbow amputation for a painful, locally aggressive CIC-DUX4 sarcoma of the wrist. The tumor ulcerated the skin, invaded and destroyed the underling bones, and spread proximally throughout the forearm (not shown).* **(Right)** *This bulky shoulder mass, initially misdiagnosed as a poorly differentiated synovial sarcoma, was treated with neoadjuvant chemotherapy. It showed no histologic response to therapy, which is noted grossly by an extensive white, fleshy viable tumor.*

Undifferentiated Round Cell Sarcoma With *CIC-DUX4* Translocation

(Left) *The cells in CIC-DUX4 sarcoma are uniform in size and shape with coarse chromatin, irregular nuclear membranes, prominent nucleoli, and pale, eosinophilic to clear cytoplasm. The mitotic rate is high.* **(Right)** *Areas containing cells with clear cytoplasm and sharply defined cell membranes are found in most tumors. The clearing is due to glycogen accumulation. Such areas mimic Ewing sarcoma. However, the nuclear chromatin in CIC-DUX4 sarcoma is coarser than in Ewing sarcoma.*

Cytologic Features

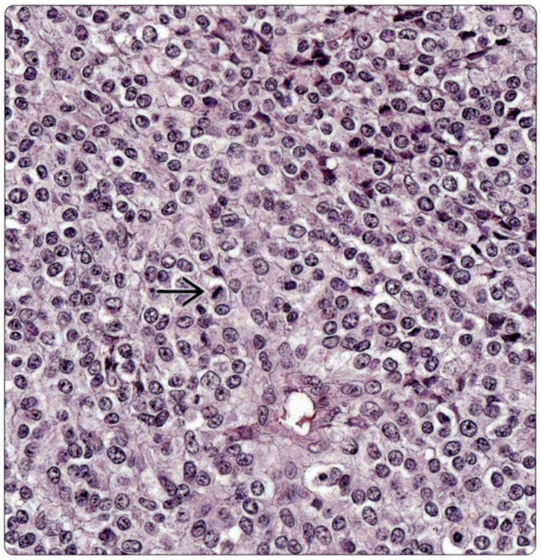

Clear Cells

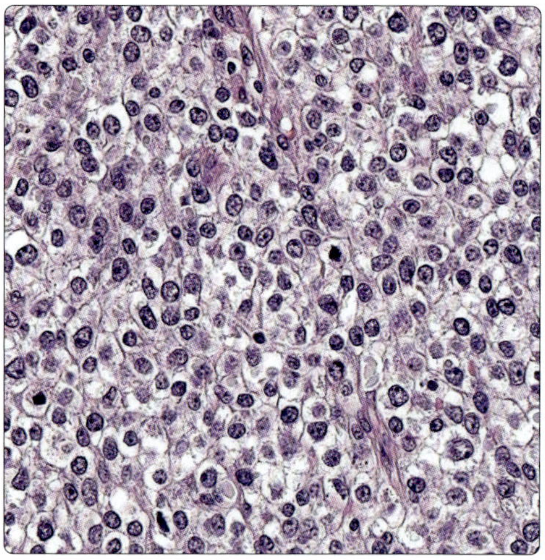

(Left) *Scanning-power view shows large geographic zones of necrosis in between nodules and garlands of viable tumor, a typical pattern in CIC-DUX4 sarcoma.* **(Right)** *Large geographic areas of necrosis and hemorrhagic necrosis alternating with viable neoplasm is a typical low-power pattern in CIC-DUX4 sarcoma, as depicted. Note the areas of perivascular preservation.*

***CIC-DUX4* Sarcoma**

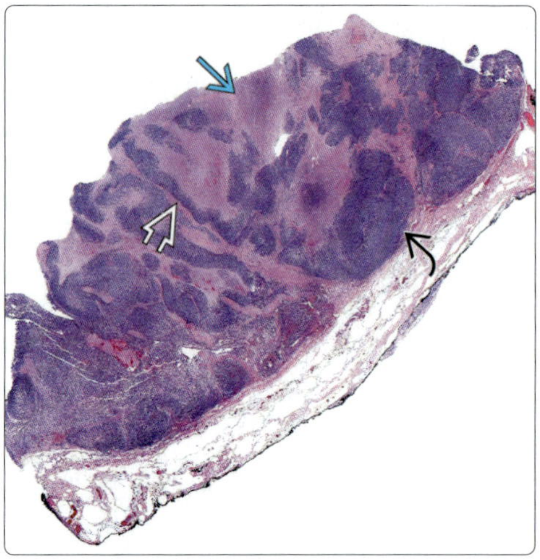

Geographic Necrosis

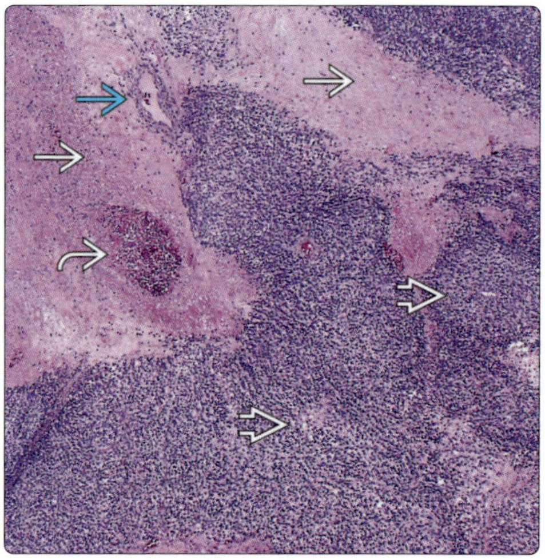

(Left) *This medium-power micrograph illustrates the interface between viable neoplasm and coagulation tumor necrosis. In the necrotic area, one can still make out individual necrotic cells.* **(Right)** *Although nonspecific, perivascular preservation of viable neoplastic cells is a common finding in CIC-DUX4 sarcoma. This H&E depicts a medium-sized blood vessel surrounded by a cuff of viable round cells within an area of necrosis.*

Necrosis

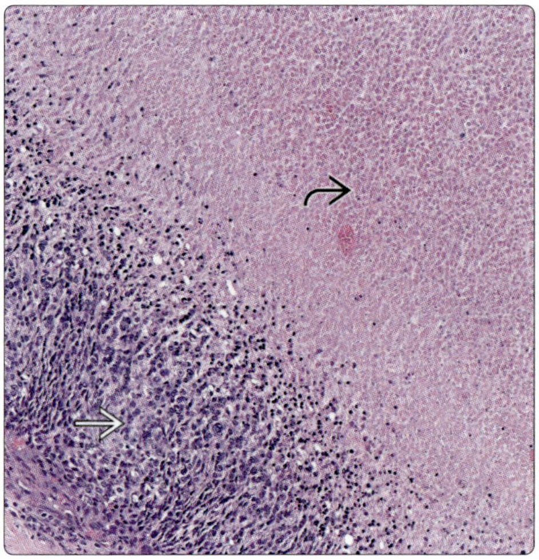

Perivascular Preservation

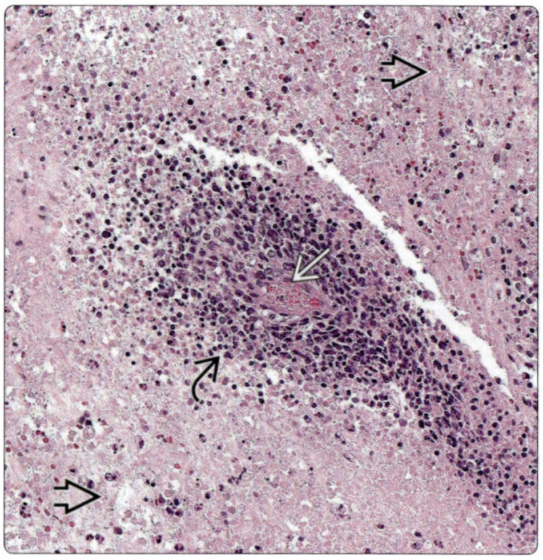

Undifferentiated Round Cell Sarcoma With *CIC-DUX4* Translocation

Myxoid Matrix and Nuclear Pleomorphism

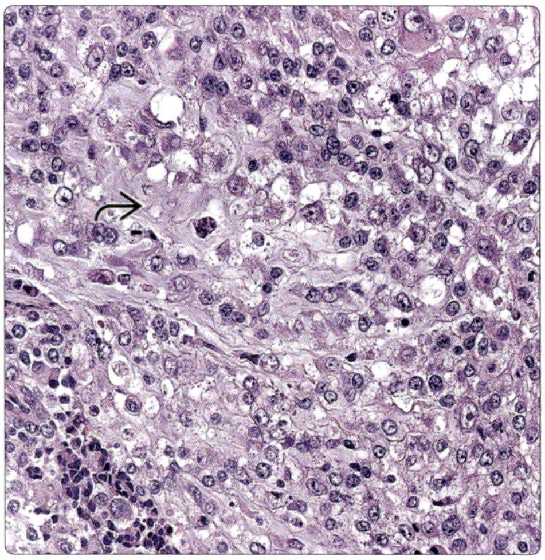

Multinodular Architecture

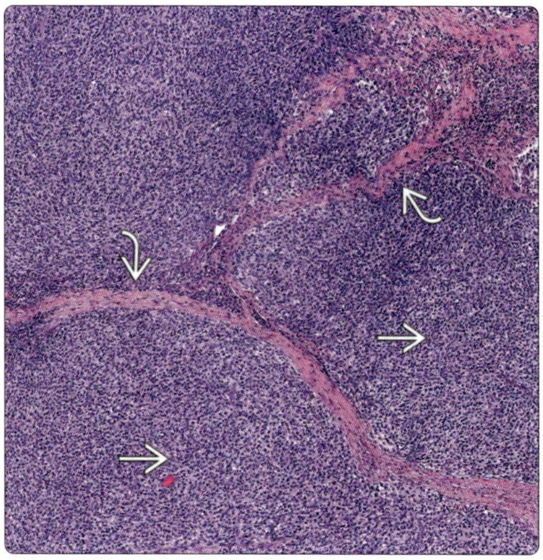

(Left) *This high-power H&E illustrates malignant round cells with moderate nuclear pleomorphism admixed with pale blue myxoid matrix ⮫ in a CIC-DUX4 sarcoma. The nuclei are generally more pleomorphic than those of Ewing sarcoma.* **(Right)** *This low-power H&E highlights the nodular architecture of a CIC-DUX4 sarcoma consisting of sheets of closely spaced round cells ➡ divided by fibrous septa ⮫.*

Cell Cords

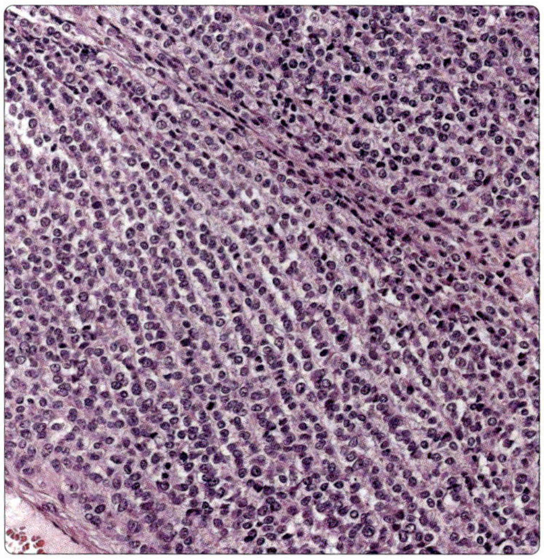

CD99 Expression

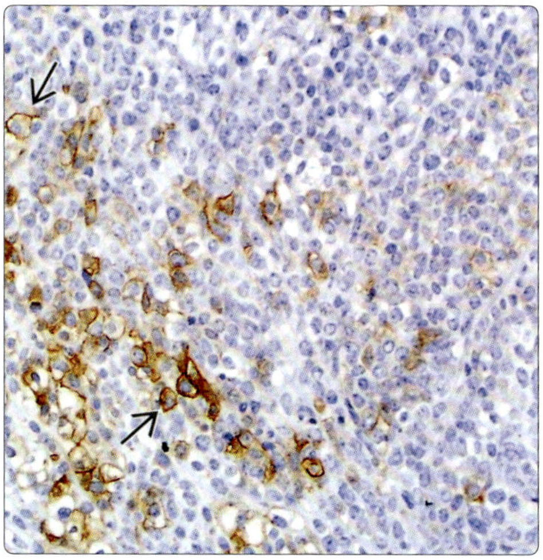

(Left) *Cords of round cells arranged in parallel, single-file rows are present focally in many CIC-DUX4 sarcomas, as illustrated.* **(Right)** *CIC-DUX4 sarcoma is undifferentiated and has no specific immunohistochemical marker. CD99 is frequently positive and usually shows only focal staining, as illustrated. However, it can sometimes be diffuse. Note the cytoplasmic membrane pattern →.*

WT1 Expression

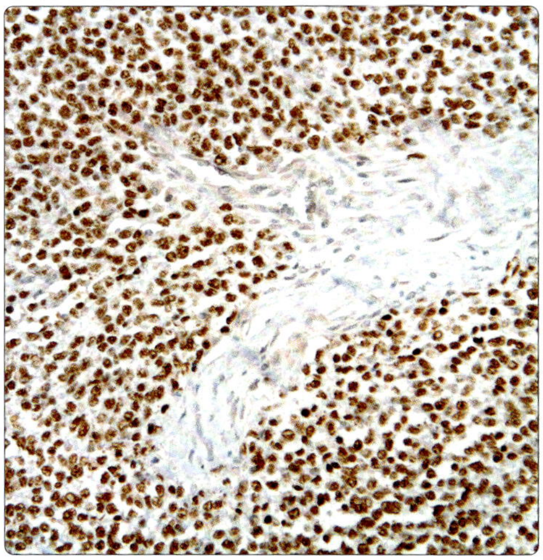

CIC Rearrangement

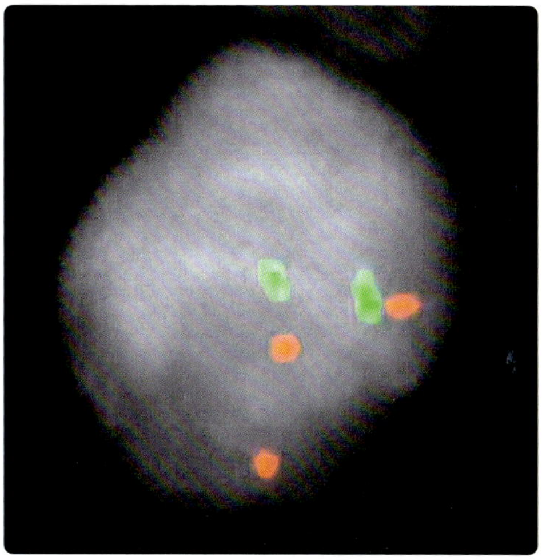

(Left) *CIC-DUX4 sarcoma shows diffuse nuclear staining for WT1 in most tumors (95%), which is useful for distinguishing it from Ewing sarcoma (0%). Similar results for ETV4 staining have also been reported.* **(Right)** *CIC gene rearrangement can be detected by FISH. The green probe, which marks the centromere of chromosome 19, shows the normal 2 homologs. The red probe that spans the CIC gene indicates an extra (3rd) signal, indicating gene rearrangement.*

BCOR-CCNB3 Fusion-Positive Sarcoma

KEY FACTS

TERMINOLOGY

- Translocation-associated, undifferentiated round to spindle cell sarcoma arising in bone or soft tissue with *BCOR-CCNB3* gene fusion

CLINICAL ISSUES

- Median age in 2nd decade (range: 0-44 years)
- Male predominance (75%)
- Various bone and soft tissue locations
- Favorable clinical response to chemotherapy
- 77% 5-year survival rate

MICROSCOPIC

- Solid sheets of closely spaced, small, round to plump spindle cells
- Fascicles of elongated spindle cells in some tumors
- Variable amounts of myxoid matrix (50% of tumors)
- Dense collagenous matrix in some
- Small concentric whorls in some
- Uniform, monomorphic small round cells
- Hyperchromatic or finely dispersed chromatin
- Mitotic activity highly variable

ANCILLARY TESTS

- CCNB3(+) in almost all tumors
- BCOR(+) in almost all tumors (less specific than CCNB3)
- CD99(+) in 60-90%
- SATB2(+) in 80%
- TLE1(+) in 75%
- *BCOR-CCNB3* fusion created by X-chromosomal paracentric inversion
- Dual-fusion FISH required due to X-chromosomal inversion

TOP DIFFERENTIAL DIAGNOSES

- Ewing sarcoma
- *CIC-DUX4* sarcoma
- Poorly differentiated synovial sarcoma
- Small cell osteosarcoma

(Left) *Scanning-power view of BCOR-CCNB3 sarcoma depicts sheets of closely spaced small round cells and an area of geographic necrosis.* **(Right)** *CT scan taken from a 5-year-old boy shows a large (9.8-cm) soft tissue tumor involving the left chest with heterogeneous signal due to tumor necrosis. BCOR-CCNB3 more often presents as a primary bone tumor than a soft tissue tumor.*

BCOR-CCNB3 Sarcoma

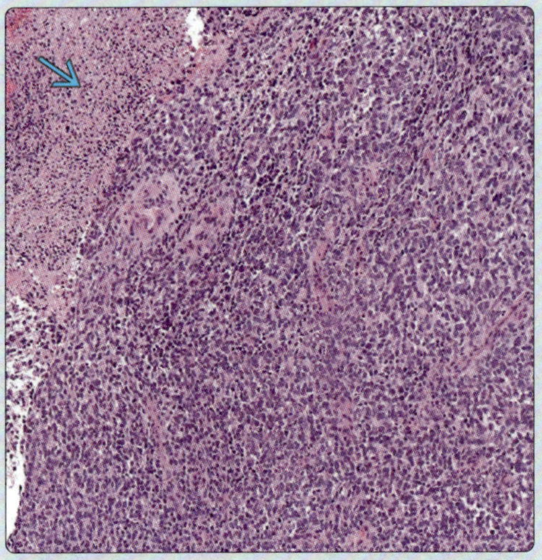

CT Scan

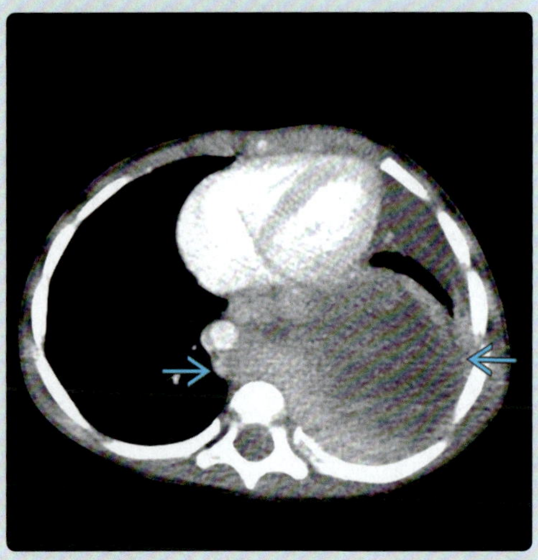

(Left) *High-power H&E highlights the cytologic features of BCOR-CCNB3 sarcoma, consisting of sheets of closely spaced small cells with round to oval nuclei with dispersed nuclear chromatin, smooth nuclear membranes, and pinpoint nucleoli and scant, ill-defined cytoplasm.* **(Right)** *In some BCOR-CCNB3 sarcomas, the nuclei have fine "powdery" nuclear chromatin and well-defined nuclear membranes mimicking poorly differentiated synovial sarcoma. (Courtesy W.-S. Li, MD.)*

Small Round Cells

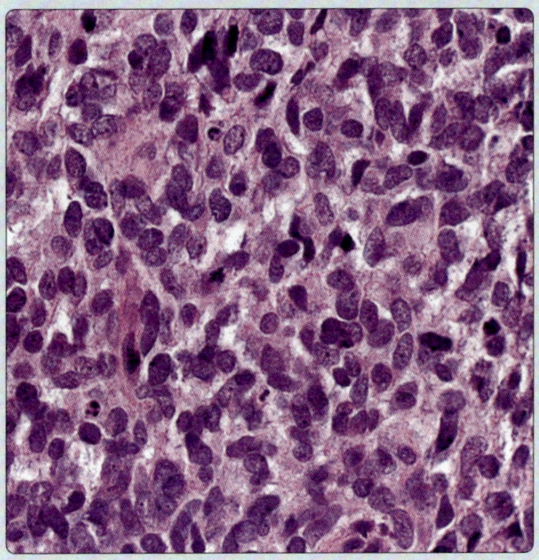

Soft Chromatin Mimicking Synovial Sarcoma

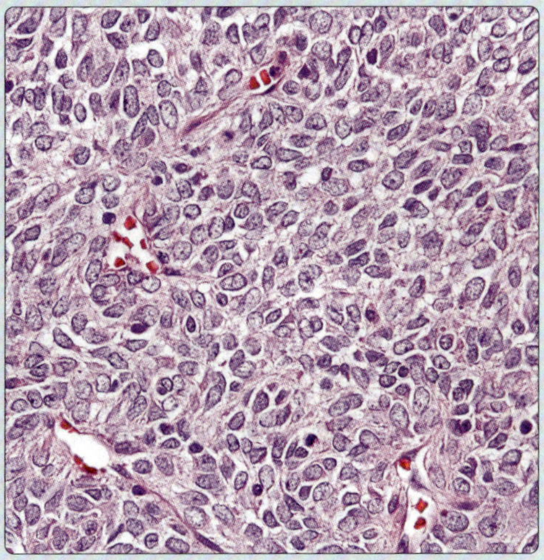

TERMINOLOGY

Abbreviations

- *BCOR-CCNB3* sarcoma

Synonyms

- *BCOR*-rearranged sarcoma, undifferentiated round/spindle cell sarcoma, Ewing-like sarcoma

Definitions

- Translocation-associated, undifferentiated round to spindle cell sarcoma arising in bone or soft tissue with *BCOR-CCNB3* gene fusion
  - Alternate *BCOR*-rearrangements: *BCOR-MAML3* and *ZC3H7B-BCOR*

CLINICAL ISSUES

Epidemiology

- Incidence
  - Rare
    - ~ 120 reported cases
    - Represents ~ 15% of undifferentiated unclassified sarcomas
- Age
  - Adolescents and young adults
    - Median age in 2nd decade (range: 0-44 years)
    - Rare congenital tumors
- Sex
  - Male predominance (75%)

Site

- Various bone and soft tissue locations
  - 60% are primary bone tumors

Presentation

- Pain and swelling

Treatment

- Wide local excision
- Chemotherapy
  - Favorable clinical response
- Radiotherapy

Prognosis

- Most tumors are localized at time of diagnosis
- 77% 5-year survival; 68% disease-free survival

MACROSCOPIC

General Features

- Destructive osteolytic bone tumors
- Circumscribed or ill-defined soft tissue tumors
  - Multinodular architecture
  - Necrosis and hemorrhage in 1/2 of tumors

Size

- Average size: 10 cm (range: 2-25 cm)

MICROSCOPIC

Histologic Features

- Solid sheets of closely spaced, small, round to plump spindle cells (80% of tumors)
- Fascicles of elongated spindle cells (20% of tumors)
  - Long fascicles with slit-like spaces and hemorrhage in some
- Variable amounts of myxoid matrix (50% of tumors)
- Rich capillary vascular stroma
  - May have gaping or thin-walled, branching (pericytomatous) vessels
- Necrosis present to varying degrees in ~ 1/2 of tumors
- Dense collagenous matrix in some
  - Hypocellular fibrotic areas some tumors
- Small concentric whorls in some tumors
- Focal osteoid in rare tumors

Cytologic Features

- Uniform, monomorphic small round cells
  - Scant, ill-defined eosinophilic cytoplasm
  - Round, oval or angulated nuclei
  - Hyperchromatic or finely dispersed chromatin
  - Inconspicuous nucleoli
  - Smooth nuclear contours
  - Round cells may be admixed with minor population of spindle cells
- Spindle cells
  - Plump spindle cells in short fascicles
  - Elongated spindle cells in some tumors
  - Most often mixed with round cells
    - Pure spindle cell population in some tumors
- Mitotic activity highly variable
  - Average number: 6-8 mitotic figures per 10 HPF (range: 1-25)

ANCILLARY TESTS

Immunohistochemistry

- CCNB3(+) in almost all tumors
- BCOR(+) in almost all tumors
  - Less specific than CCNB3
- CD99(+) in 60-90%
  - More heterogeneous staining distribution compared to Ewing sarcoma
  - Can stain with membranous; cytoplasmic; or perinuclear, dot-like patterns
- SATB2(+) in 80%
- TLE1(+) in 75%
- pax-8(+) 50%
- NKX2.2(+) in 25%
- EMA rarely (+)
- Negative markers include: ETV4, WT1, SMA, desmin, cytokeratin, S100 protein, and BCL-2

Cytogenetics

- *BCOR-CCNB3* fusion created by X-chromosomal paracentric inversion

In Situ Hybridization

- Dual-fusion FISH required due to X-chromosomal inversion

PCR

- Useful when fusion transcript is known

DIFFERENTIAL DIAGNOSIS

Ewing Sarcoma

- Spindle cells very uncommon
- Myxoid matrix not present
- More often CD99(+) and NKX2.2(+)
- *EWSR1* rearrangement by FISH
- *EWSR1-FLI1, EWSR1-ERG, EWSR1-FEV, EWSR1-ETV1*, EWSR1-ETV4, and rare fusions involving *FUS*

Undifferentiated Sarcoma With *CIC-DUX4* Translocation

- Overlapping morphologic features with *BCOR-CCNB3* sarcoma
- ETV4(+), WT1(+), BCOR(-), and CCNB3(-) by immunohistochemistry
- *CIC* rearrangement by FISH
- *CIC-DUX4* or *CIC-DUX4L1* fusions

Undifferentiated Round or Spindle Cell Sarcomas

- All diagnoses of exclusion
- No specific immunohistochemical or molecular signature

Poorly Differentiated Synovial Sarcoma

- Soft or "powdery" chromatin mimics *BCOR-CCNB3* sarcoma
- Immunohistochemical overlap with *BCOR-CCNB3* sarcoma
  - BCOR(+), TLE1(+), EMA(+), CD99(+), SATB2(+)
- *SS18* (SYT) rearrangement by FISH
- *SS18-SSX* fusions

Malignant Peripheral Nerve Sheath Tumor

- Alternating hyper-/hypocellular marbled architecture sometimes seen in *BCOR-CCNB3* sarcoma
- S100 protein (+) &/or SOX10(+) in most, though often patchy/focal
- Diffuse loss of nuclear H3K27me3 by immunohistochemistry

Solitary Fibrous Tumor

- Can show morphologic overlap with *BCOR-CCNB3* sarcoma
  - Areas of stromal fibrosis
  - Pericytomatous vascular pattern
- STAT6(+)

Vascular Neoplasms

- Spindle cell-rich morphology with blood-filled, slit-like spaces can mimic *BCOR-CCNB3*
- CD31(+), CD34(+), ERG(+)
- HHV-8(+) in Kaposi sarcoma

Small Cell Osteosarcoma

- *BCOR-CCNB3* sarcoma can rarely produce osteoid and is often SATB2(+)
- Lacks *BCOR-CCNB3* fusion

DIAGNOSTIC CHECKLIST

Clinically Relevant Pathologic Features

- Primary bone or soft tissue round or spindle cell sarcoma in adolescent or young adult patient
- Usually localized at time of diagnosis
- Responsive to chemotherapy
- Relatively favorable prognosis (77% 5-year survival rate)

Pathologic Interpretation Pearls

- Heterogeneous morphology with round &/or spindle cells and variable myxoid stroma
- CCNB3(+) by immunohistochemistry
- Molecular confirmation for definitive diagnosis

SELECTED REFERENCES

1. Miettinen M et al: New fusion sarcomas histopathology and clinical significance of selected entities. Hum Pathol. ePub, 2019
2. Anderson WJ et al: Immunohistochemical correlates of recurrent genetic alterations in sarcomas. Genes Chromosomes Cancer. 58(2):111-23, 2018
3. Machado I et al: Review with novel markers facilitates precise categorization of 41 cases of diagnostically challenging, "undifferentiated small round cell tumors". A clinicopathologic, immunophenotypic and molecular analysis. Ann Diagn Pathol. 34:1-12, 2018
4. Alfaro-Cervello C et al: Congenital undifferentiated sarcoma associated to BCOR-CCNB3 gene fusion. Pathol Res Pract. 213(11):1435-9, 2017
5. Argani P et al: Primary renal sarcomas with BCOR-CCNB3 gene fusion: a report of 2 cases showing histologic overlap with clear cell sarcoma of kidney, suggesting further link between BCOR-related sarcomas of the kidney and soft tissues. Am J Surg Pathol. 41(12):1702-12, 2017
6. Creytens D: SATB2 and TLE1 expression in BCOR-CCNB3 (Ewing-like) sarcoma, mimicking small cell osteosarcoma and poorly differentiated synovial sarcoma. Appl Immunohistochem Mol Morphol. ePub, 2017
7. Le Loarer F et al: Update on families of round cell sarcomas other than classical Ewing sarcomas. Surg Pathol Clin. 10(3):587-620, 2017
8. Ludwig K et al: BCOR-CCNB3 undifferentiated sarcoma-does immunohistochemistry help in the identification? Pediatr Dev Pathol. 20(4):321-9, 2017
9. Ludwig K et al: BCOR-CCNB3 undifferentiated sarcoma-does immunohistochemistry help in the identification? Pediatr Dev Pathol. 20(4):321-9, 2017
10. Matsuyama A et al: Clinicopathologic diversity of undifferentiated sarcoma with BCOR-CCNB3 fusion: analysis of 11 cases with a reappraisal of the utility of immunohistochemistry for BCOR and CCNB3. Am J Surg Pathol. 41(12):1713-21, 2017
11. Yamada Y et al: Histological and immunohistochemical characteristics of undifferentiated small round cell sarcomas associated with CIC-DUX4 and BCOR-CCNB3 fusion genes. Virchows Arch. 470(4):373-80, 2017
12. Hung YP et al: Evaluation of ETV4 and WT1 expression in CIC-rearranged sarcomas and histologic mimics. Mod Pathol. 29(11):1324-34, 2016
13. Kao YC et al: BCOR overexpression is a highly sensitive marker in round cell sarcomas with BCOR genetic abnormalities. Am J Surg Pathol. 40(12):1670-8, 2016
14. Li WS et al: BCOR-CCNB3-positive soft tissue sarcoma with round-cell and spindle-cell histology: a series of four cases highlighting the pitfall of mimicking poorly differentiated synovial sarcoma. Histopathology. 69(5):792-801, 2016
15. Machado I et al: Defining Ewing and Ewing-like small round cell tumors (SRCT): the need for molecular techniques in their categorization and differential diagnosis. A study of 200 cases. Ann Diagn Pathol. 22:25-32, 2016
16. Specht K et al: Novel BCOR-MAML3 and ZC3H7B-BCOR gene fusions in undifferentiated small blue round cell sarcomas. Am J Surg Pathol. 40(4):433-42, 2016
17. Peters TL et al: BCOR-CCNB3 fusions are frequent in undifferentiated sarcomas of male children. Mod Pathol. 28(4):575-86, 2015
18. Cohen-Gogo S et al: Ewing-like sarcomas with BCOR-CCNB3 fusion transcript: a clinical, radiological and pathological retrospective study from the Soci√©t√© Fran√ßaise des Cancers de L'Enfant. Pediatr Blood Cancer. 61(12):2191-8, 2014
19. Puls F et al: BCOR-CCNB3 (Ewing-like) sarcoma: a clinicopathologic analysis of 10 cases, in comparison with conventional Ewing sarcoma. Am J Surg Pathol. 38(10):1307-18, 2014

Spindle Cells

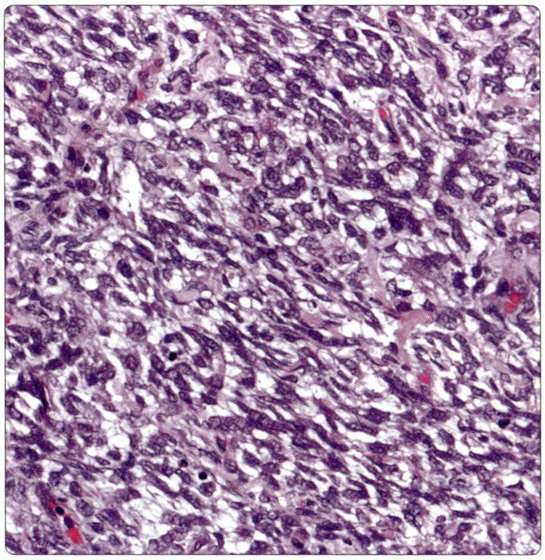

Pericytomatous Vessels and Myxoid Matrix

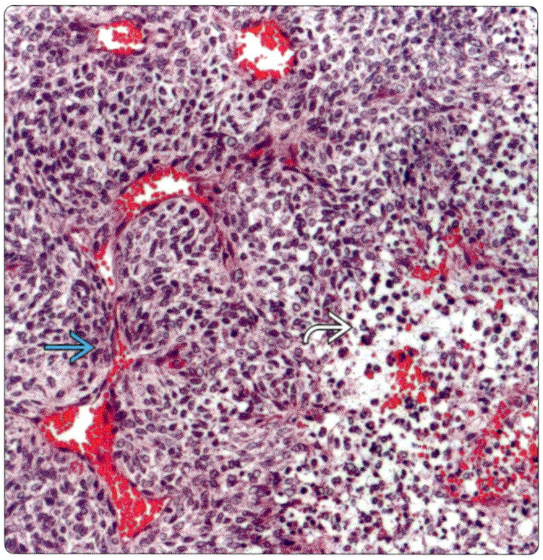

(Left) *The microscopic features of BCOR-CCNB3 sarcoma are heterogeneous. In some tumors, prominent areas composed of spindle cells arranged in fascicles are present, as depicted in this medium-power micrograph. (Courtesy A. Matsuyama, MD.)* **(Right)** *Some BCOR-CCNB3 sarcomas display a prominent pericytomatous vascular pattern consisting of thin-walled, branching vessels ➙. This micrograph also depicts cellular dyscohesion and pale blue myxoid matrix in an area of necrosis ➦.*

Spindle Cells and Myxoid Stroma

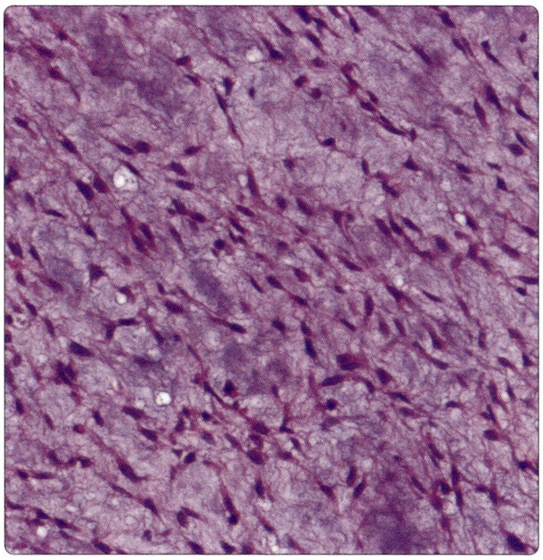

Whorling Pattern

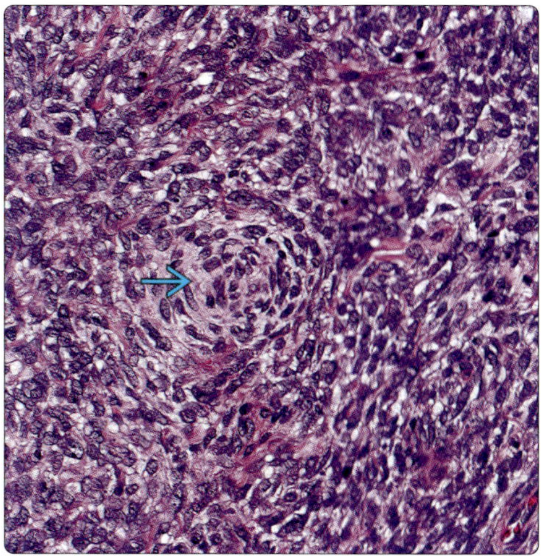

(Left) *The heterogeneous morphologic spectrum of BCOR-CCNB3 sarcomas includes tumors with prominent pale blue myxoid stroma and spindle cells with eosinophilic cytoplasm arranged in a reticulated fascicular pattern, as depicted. (Courtesy W.-S. Li, MD.)* **(Right)** *Small foci of cellular whorling can be found in some tumors, as highlighted in this high-power micrograph that shows spindle cells arranged in a concentric spiral pattern ➙. (Courtesy A. Matsuyama, MD.)*

Lobular Configuration

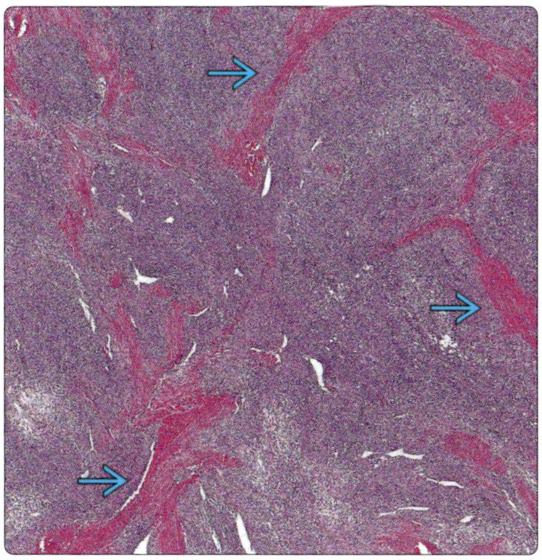

CCNB3 Immunohistochemistry

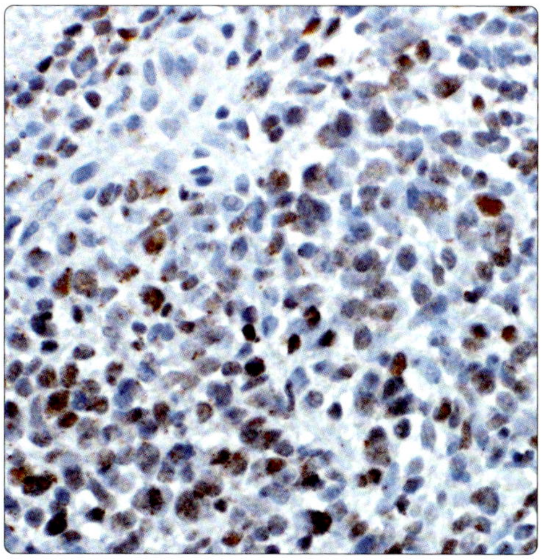

(Left) *BCOR-CCNB3 sarcomas often have a lobular architecture highlighted by solid cellular areas surrounded by fibrous septa ➙. (Courtesy A. Matsuyama, MD.)* **(Right)** *Immunohistochemistry for CCNB3 is highly sensitive and specific for BCOR-CCNB3 sarcoma, as depicted by strong nuclear staining in this case.*

SECTION 18

Mesenchymal Tumors of Gastrointestinal Tract

Benign Neural Gastrointestinal Polyps	740
Gastrointestinal Stromal Tumor	744
Gastrointestinal Schwannoma	760
Gastrointestinal Smooth Muscle Neoplasms	762
Inflammatory Fibroid Polyp	766
Gangliocytic Paraganglioma	770
Plexiform Fibromyxoma	772
Malignant Gastrointestinal Neuroectodermal Tumor	776

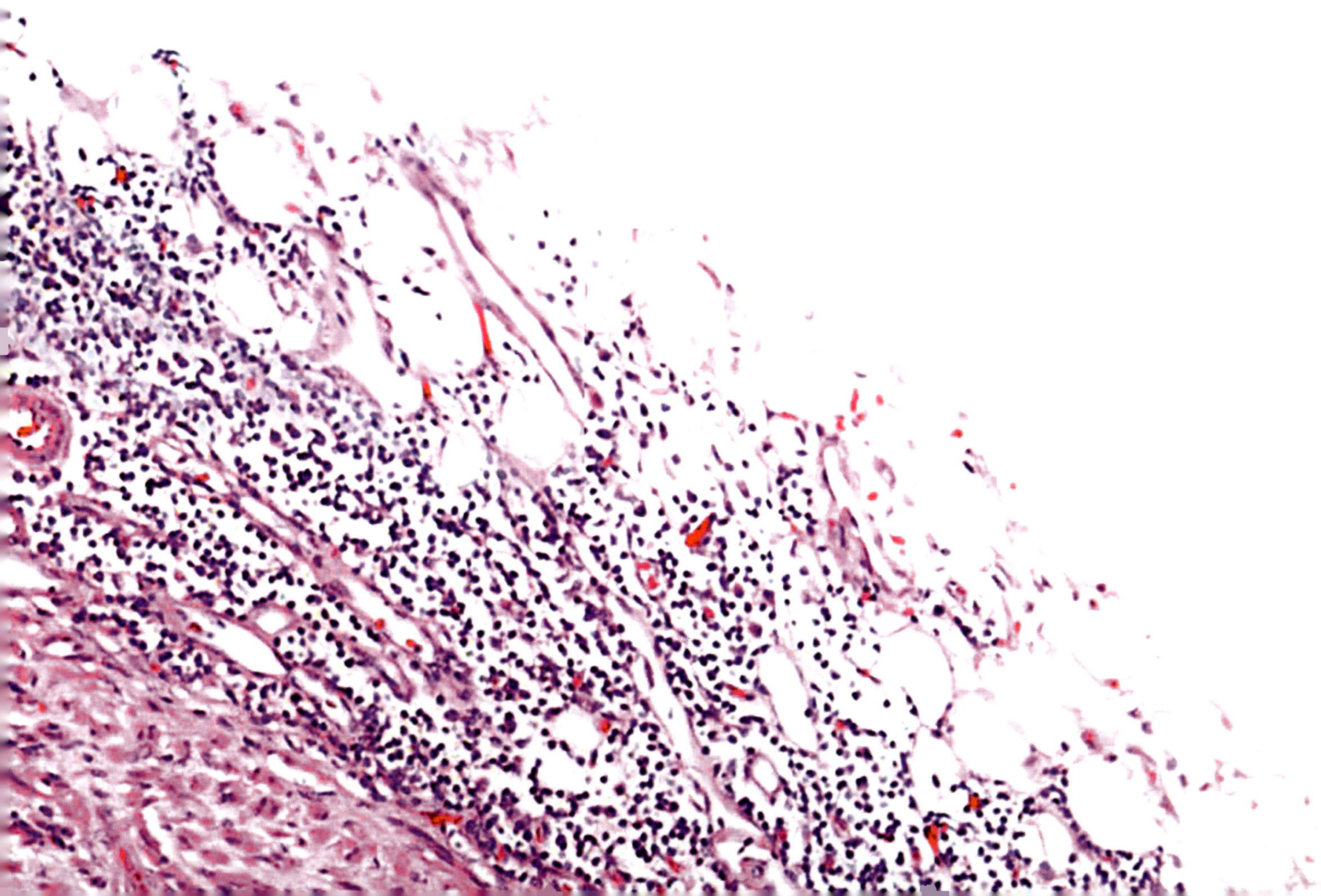

Benign Neural Gastrointestinal Polyps

KEY FACTS

TERMINOLOGY

- Benign neural proliferations that present as polypoid growths in GI tract
  - Schwann cell hamartoma, ganglioneuroma, perineurioma, granular cell tumor

CLINICAL ISSUES

- Wide age range (most common in adults)
- Most arise in colon
  - Esophagus most common GI site for granular cell tumor
- Small, asymptomatic polyps or nodules discovered endoscopically
- Most are solitary and sporadic
  - Multiple ganglioneuromas often associated with various syndromes
- Treatment: Polypectomy
- Benign

MICROSCOPIC

- Schwann cell hamartoma, ganglioneuroma, and perineurioma all show uniform, bland spindled cells proliferating between and around crypts of colonic lamina propria
  - Ganglioneuroma also has ganglion cells
- Granular cell tumor shows large, polygonal cells with abundant granular, eosinophilic cytoplasm and small nuclei

ANCILLARY TESTS

- S100 protein (+) in Schwann cell hamartoma, ganglioneuroma, granular cell tumor
- EMA(+), claudin-1 (+), GLUT1(+) in perineurioma
- All keratin (-), SMA(-), desmin (-), CD117(-), CD34(-)

TOP DIFFERENTIAL DIAGNOSES

- Submucosal leiomyoma
- Inflammatory fibroid polyp
- Neurofibroma

Schwann Cell Hamartoma

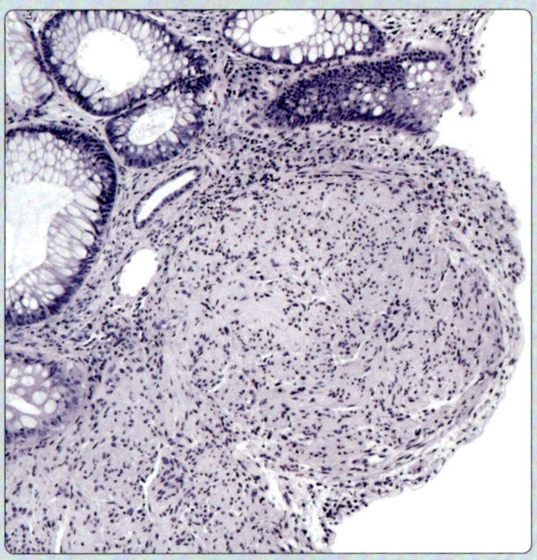

Schwann Cells

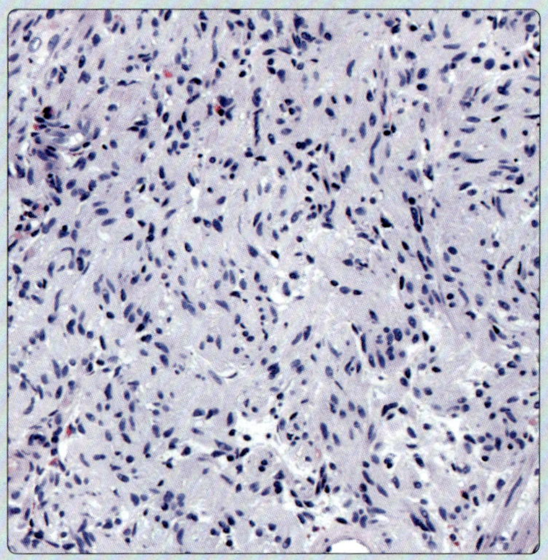

(Left) *Schwann cell hamartoma is a benign neural proliferation that usually arises in the lamina propria of the colon or rectum. It can be nodular and well demarcated or irregular and poorly circumscribed.* **(Right)** *Schwann cell hamartoma is composed of a variably cellular proliferation of spindled Schwann cells. Nuclei are usually small, elongated, and bland, but occasionally larger nuclei are evident. Small areas lacking nuclei are common, but true Verocay body formation is not seen.*

Subtle Proliferation

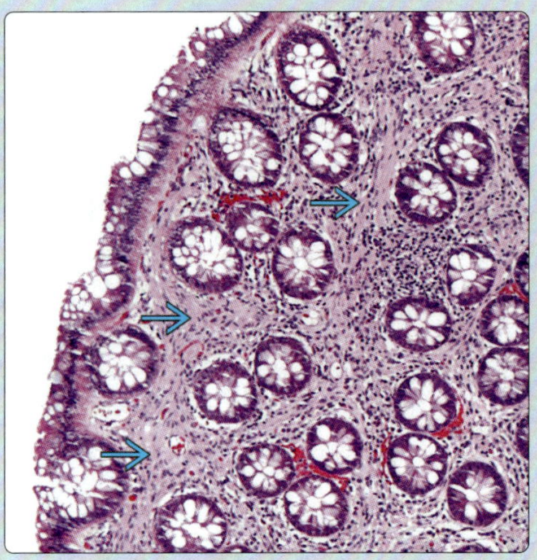

S100 Expression in Schwann Cell Hamartoma

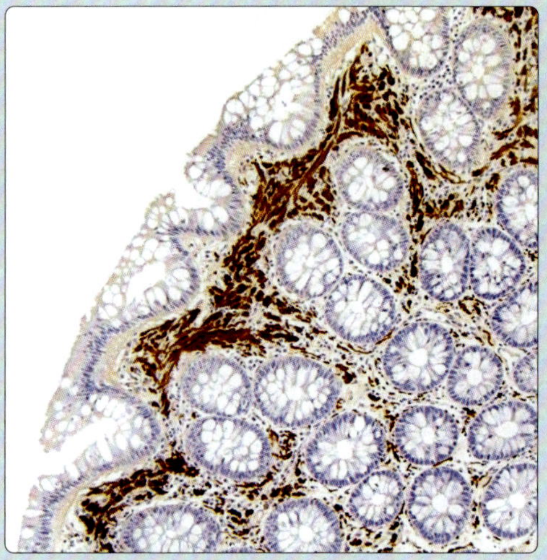

(Left) *Schwann cell hamartoma may lack nodularity and appear to subtly infiltrate the lamina propria as small, elongated groups → of eosinophilic spindle cells. This morphology may be easily overlooked as fibrosis.* **(Right)** *All Schwann cell hamartomas strongly express S100 protein, consistent with their cellular origin. This image highlights a more irregular and subtly infiltrative example.*

TERMINOLOGY

Definitions

- Benign neural proliferations that present as polypoid growths in GI tract
  - Schwann cell hamartoma
  - Ganglioneuroma
  - Perineurioma
  - Granular cell tumor

CLINICAL ISSUES

Epidemiology

- Incidence
  - Uncommon
- Age
  - Wide range (most common in adults)

Site

- Most arise in large bowel
- Esophagus most common GI site for granular cell tumor

Presentation

- Small asymptomatic polyps or nodules discovered endoscopically
- Most are solitary and sporadic
  - Multiple ganglioneuromas may indicate presence of genetic syndrome, such as multiple endocrine neoplasia type 2B (MEN 2B), neurofibromatosis type 1, familial adenomatous polyposis, or Cowden syndrome

Treatment

- Polypectomy

Prognosis

- Benign
- Solitary polyps do not recur if completely removed

MICROSCOPIC

Histologic Features

- Schwann cell hamartoma
  - Poorly delineated or nodular; most confined to mucosa
  - Cellular proliferation of relatively uniform spindle cells with bland nuclei
    - Cells proliferate between and around crypts of colonic lamina propria, pushing them apart
    - Generally no palisading or whorling architectures
- Ganglioneuroma
  - Uniform, bland spindled cells proliferating between crypts of lamina propria
    - Essentially indistinguishable from Schwann cell hamartoma
  - Presence of ganglion cells necessary for diagnosis
    - May be sparse or numerous and clustered
  - May rarely have diffuse growth pattern and arise deeper than mucosa (associated with genetic syndromes)
- Perineurioma
  - Uniform, pale spindle cells with indistinct cell borders and bland, often pale nuclei
  - Cells proliferate between and around crypts of colonic lamina propria, splaying them apart
    - May show circumferential whorling around crypts
    - Some cases extend into superficial submucosa
  - Entrapped crypts often have serrated architecture
    - May show features of hyperplastic polyp or sessile serrated polyp/adenoma
- Granular cell tumor
  - Usually based in submucosa (colon) or lamina propria (esophagus)
  - Large, polygonal cells with abundant granular, eosinophilic cytoplasm and small, bland nuclei
  - Small nests and sheets separated by fibrous septa
  - May incite overlying reactive pseudoepitheliomatous hyperplasia in esophagus

ANCILLARY TESTS

Immunohistochemistry

- S100 protein (+) and SOX10(+) in Schwann cell hamartoma, ganglioneuroma, granular cell tumor
- EMA(+), claudin-1 (+), GLUT1(+) in perineurioma
- All keratin (-), SMA(-), desmin (-), CD117(-), CD34(-)

DIFFERENTIAL DIAGNOSIS

Submucosal Leiomyoma

- Based in submucosa (arise from muscularis mucosa)
- Bundles and fascicles of plump, eosinophilic spindled cells with blunted nuclei
- SMA(+), desmin (+), S100 protein (-)

Gastrointestinal Stromal Tumor

- Arises only in muscularis propria
- CD117(+), DOG1(+), S100 protein (-)

Inflammatory Fibroid Polyp

- Often based in submucosa
- CD34(+), S100 protein (-)
- Bland, hypocellular spindle cell proliferation with chronic inflammatory infiltrate, particularly eosinophils

Neurofibroma

- Very rare in GI tract
- Not composed entirely of Schwann cells
- Usually plexiform and associated with neurofibromatosis type 1

Mucosal Neuroma

- Most arise on tongue or lips (rare in GI tract)
- Highly associated with MEN 2B
- Hyperplastic bundles of nerve fibers; axons common

SELECTED REFERENCES

1. van Wyk AC et al: Colonic perineurioma (benign fibroblastic polyp): case report and review of the literature. Diagn Pathol. 13(1):16, 2018
2. An S et al: Granular cell tumor of the gastrointestinal tract: histologic and immunohistochemical analysis of 98 cases. Hum Pathol. 46(6):813-9, 2015
3. Rittershaus AC et al: Benign gastrointestinal mesenchymal BUMPS: a brief review of some spindle cell polyps with published names. Arch Pathol Lab Med. 135(10):1311-9, 2011
4. Singhi AD et al: Colorectal granular cell tumor: a clinicopathologic study of 26 cases. Am J Surg Pathol. 34(8):1186-92, 2010
5. Gibson JA et al: Mucosal Schwann cell "hamartoma": clinicopathologic study of 26 neural colorectal polyps distinct from neurofibromas and mucosal neuromas. Am J Surg Pathol. 33(5):781-7, 2009
6. Hornick JL et al: Intestinal perineuriomas: clinicopathologic definition of a new anatomic subset in a series of 10 cases. Am J Surg Pathol. 29(7):859-65, 2005

(Left) *Polypoid ganglioneuroma of the colon may occur in both children and adults and is histologically similar to Schwann cell hamartoma except for the presence of admixed ganglion cells →, which vary in number.* **(Right)** *Ganglion cells may be difficult to find in some cases of ganglioneuroma, and the overall morphology of the lesion may be indistinguishable from Schwann cell hamartoma. Careful searching and cutting of deeper levels often reveals at least 1 ganglion cell in a true ganglioneuroma.*

Ganglioneuroma

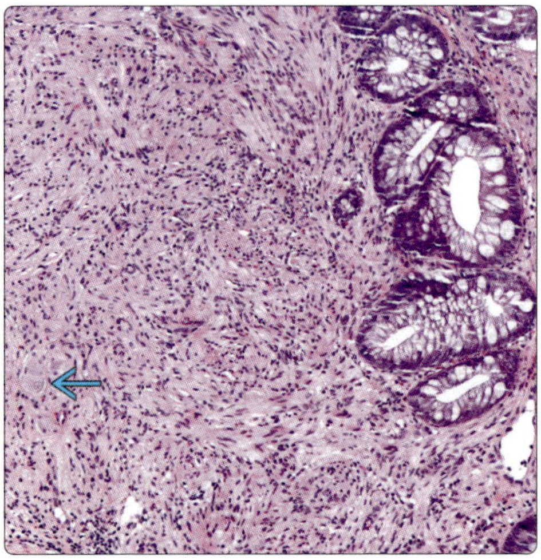

Schwann Cell Component

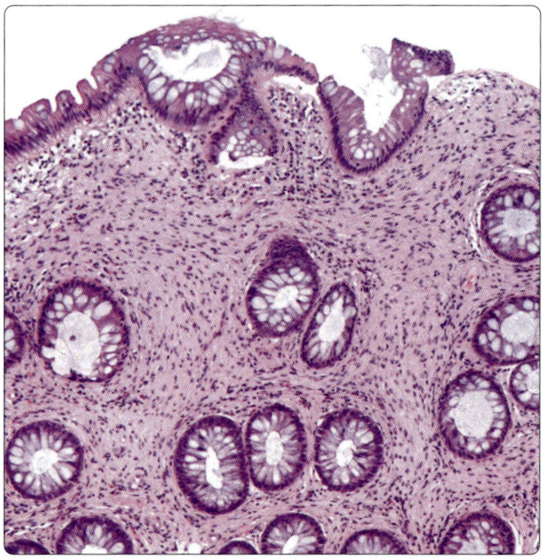

(Left) *In some cases of ganglioneuroma, the ganglion cells are quite numerous and form clusters and loose aggregates. They are easily identified by their large nuclei with prominent nucleoli →.* **(Right)** *Intestinal perineurioma → is a small neural proliferation that may bear some resemblance to Schwann cell hamartoma; however, there are several key histologic differences. For one, they are commonly identified along with serrated lesions, particularly a hyperplastic polyp → or sessile serrated adenoma/polyp.*

Ganglion Cells

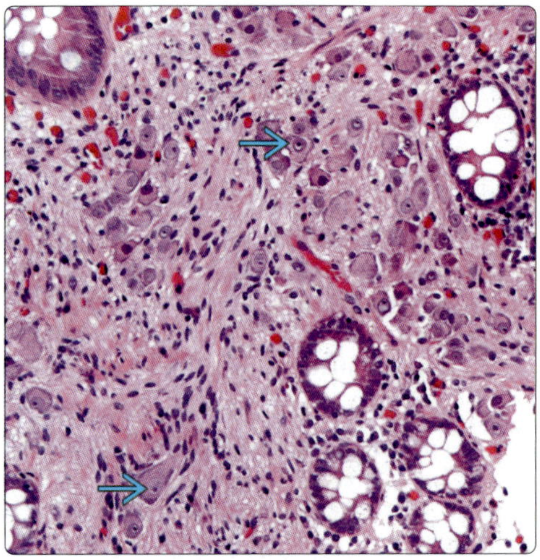

Perineurioma

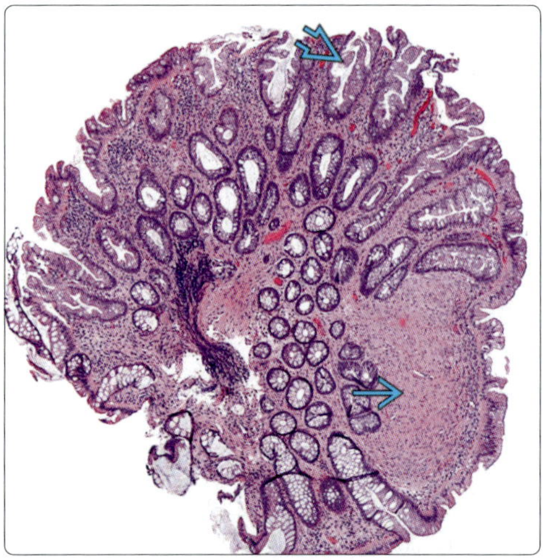

(Left) *Perineurioma often proliferates between and around the colonic crypts, splaying them apart. Many cases also characteristically show a concentric "onion-skin" pattern of growth around the crypts.* **(Right)** *The cells of perineurioma are palely eosinophilic and have very indistinct cell borders, often leading to the appearance of small pale nuclei "floating in a sea" of pink stroma. Note the compressed, but normal overlying lamina propria →.*

Perineurioma

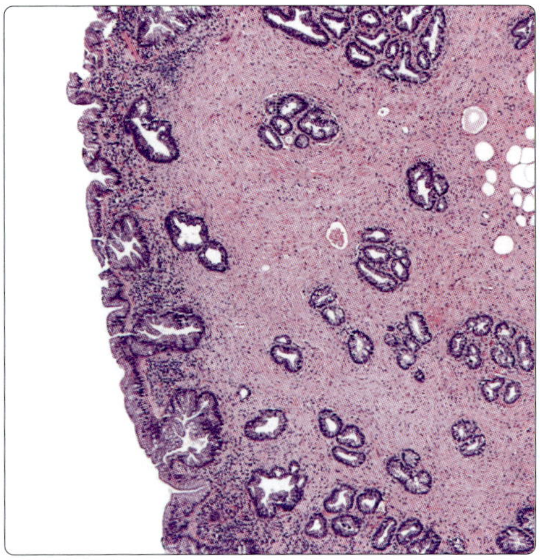

Perineurioma

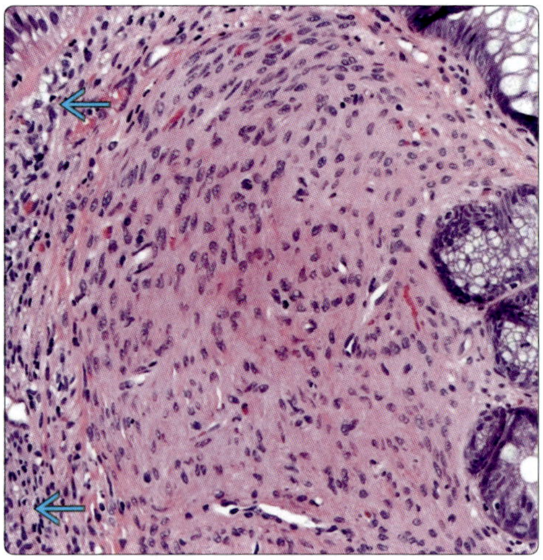

Nuclear Vacuoles

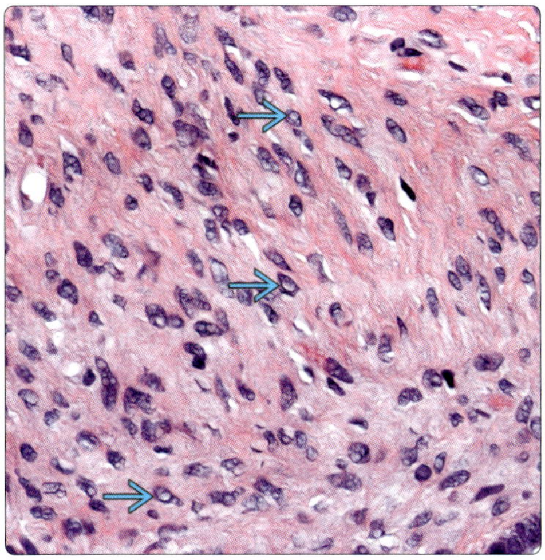

Perineurial Markers

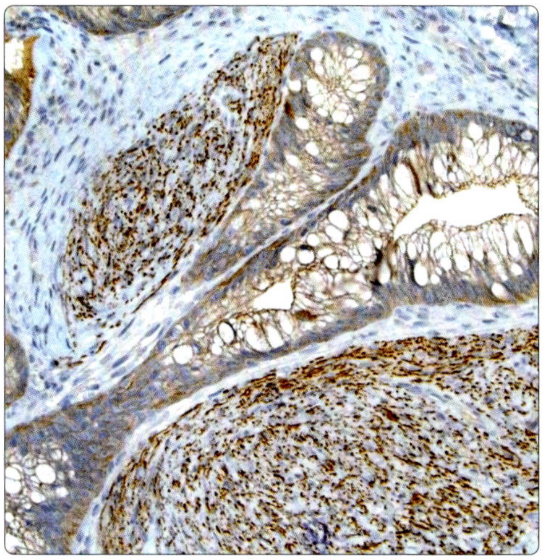

(Left) *The nuclei of perineurioma are often small, irregular, and pale and usually show conspicuous nuclear vacuoles → or pseudoinclusions. Note the absence of distinct cytoplasmic borders.* **(Right)** *Similar to their cutaneous and soft tissue counterparts, intestinal perineuriomas express markers such as EMA, claudin-1 (shown), and GLUT-1. They are negative for S100 protein, helping to distinguish them from Schwann cell hamartoma and ganglioneuroma.*

Granular Cell Tumor

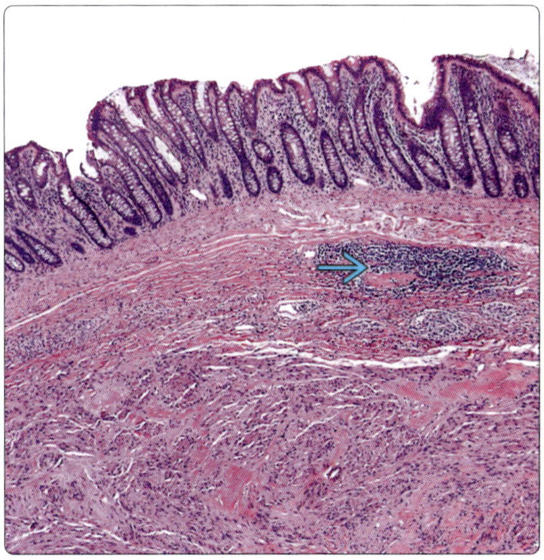

Nests and Sheets

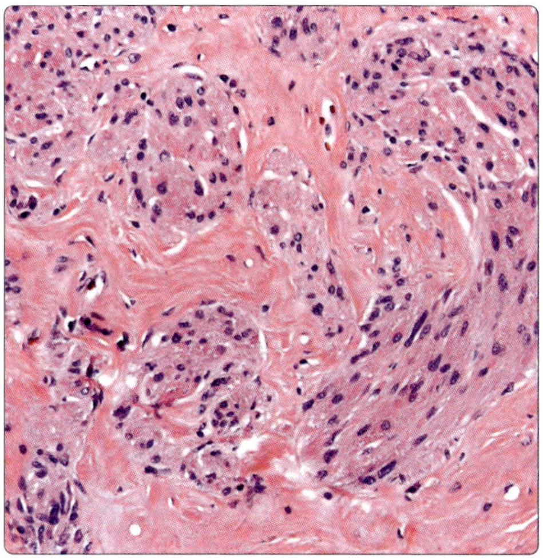

(Left) *Granular cell tumor of the GI tract is histologically similar to its counterparts found elsewhere. Although many are small, some may be > 1 cm in size. Peripheral lymphoid aggregates → and focal calcifications may also be seen at low power.* **(Right)** *Granular cell tumor is composed of nests and sheets of polygonal to spindled cells with abundant granular, eosinophilic cytoplasm. Nuclei are often small and bland but may be mildly enlarged. Mitoses are absent.*

Esophageal Granular Cell Tumor

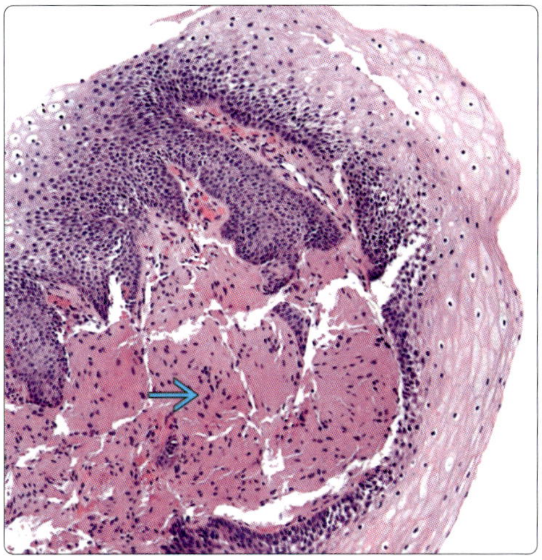

Smooth Muscle Resemblance

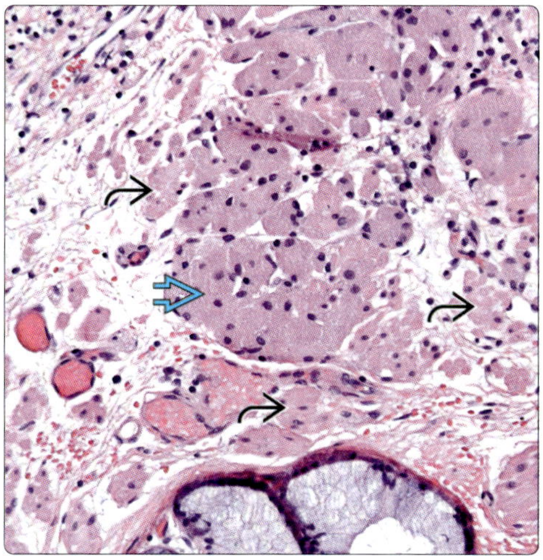

(Left) *The esophagus is the most common site for granular cell tumor within the tubular GI tract. It often presents as a small nodule endoscopically and may be easily overlooked on a superficial biopsy. Note the prominent eosinophilia → of the subepithelial region, indicating the presence of a granular cell tumor.* **(Right)** *The cells → of an esophageal granular cell tumor may resemble small bundles of smooth muscle fibers → from the muscularis mucosa cut in cross section; however, the former are often larger and granular.*

Gastrointestinal Stromal Tumor

KEY FACTS

TERMINOLOGY

- Histologically versatile, spindled or epithelioid mesenchymal neoplasm thought to arise from or differentiate toward interstitial cells of Cajal (ICC)

ETIOLOGY/PATHOGENESIS

- Most are sporadic
- Some associated with clinical syndromes
  - Carney triad, Carney-Stratakis, NF1, GIST

CLINICAL ISSUES

- Most common primary mesenchymal neoplasm of GI tract
- Usually older adults (median age: 60 years)
- Stomach and small bowel most common sites
- Treatment: Complete surgical resection, regardless of site
  - Chemotherapy (imatinib, others) for advanced GIST
- Risk of malignant behavior currently assessed by observing anatomic site, size, and mitotic rate
  - Also, molecular prognostication for GISTs

MICROSCOPIC

- Extremely broad and variable morphologic spectrum
- Tumors are spindled, epithelioid, or mixed type
- Succinate dehydrogenase (SDH)-deficient GIST is distinctive subtype

ANCILLARY TESTS

- Characteristic CD117 and DOG1 (+)
- CD34(+) in majority (75%)
- Loss of SDHB in SDH-deficient GIST
- Molecular: *KIT* or *PDGFRA* mutations in majority (85-90%)

TOP DIFFERENTIAL DIAGNOSES

- GI smooth muscle neoplasms
- GI schwannoma
- Solitary fibrous tumor
- Carcinoma or melanoma
- Malignant GI neuroectodermal tumor

Gastrointestinal Stromal Tumor

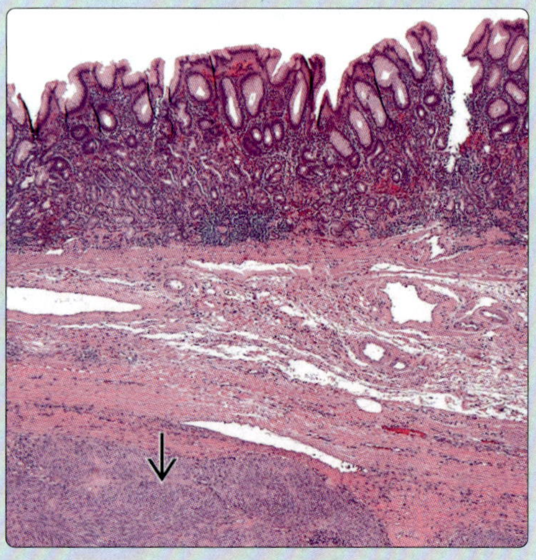

Spindle Cell Morphology

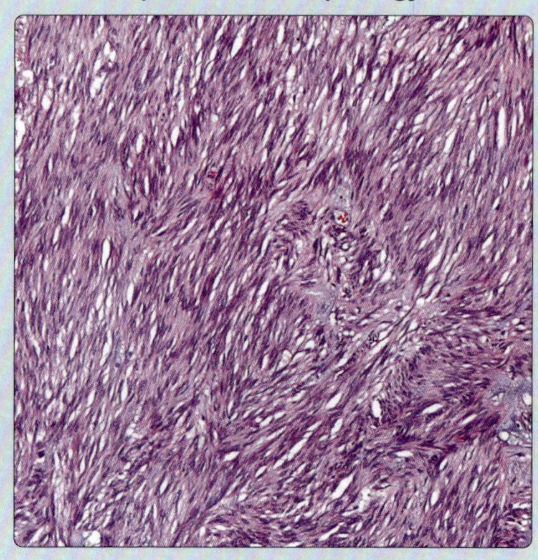

(Left) *Gastrointestinal stromal tumor (GIST) is the most common primary mesenchymal neoplasm of the GI tract. As shown in this low-power H&E, GIST ⇨ arises from within the muscularis propria. It can arise at any location in the GI tract but is most commonly seen in the stomach (shown) or small bowel.* **(Right)** *Most GISTs contain spindled cells, which are generally cytologically low grade and uniform. Cellularity varies.*

Epithelioid Morphology

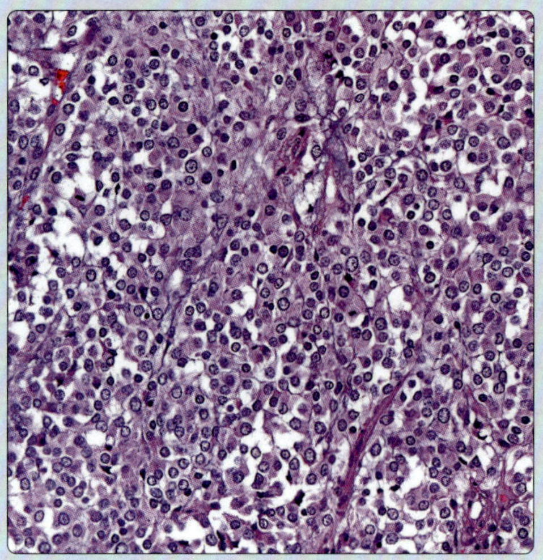

Immunophenotype

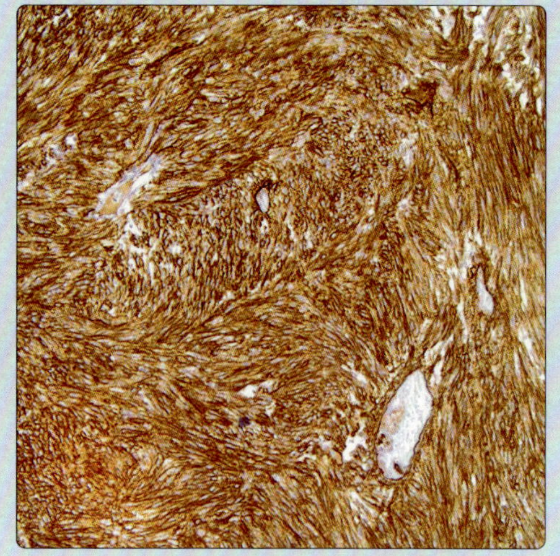

(Left) *A minority of GISTs demonstrate an epithelioid, rather than spindled, morphology, as shown. Nuclear pleomorphism is uncommon in GIST, overall, but is more frequent in tumors with an epithelioid morphology. Occasional tumors feature a mixture of spindled and epithelioid cells.* **(Right)** *CD117 (C-kit) and DOG1 are highly sensitive and specific markers for GIST, particularly when diffusely expressed. CD34 (shown) is also positive in up to 75% of cases and is also diffusely expressed.*

TERMINOLOGY

Abbreviations

- Gastrointestinal stromal tumor (GIST)

Synonyms

- GI stromal sarcoma
- Leiomyoblastoma
- GI autonomic nerve tumor

Definitions

- Histologically versatile, spindled or epithelioid mesenchymal neoplasm thought to arise from or differentiate toward interstitial cells of Cajal (ICC)

ETIOLOGY/PATHOGENESIS

Subset Associated With Various Clinical Syndromes

- Carney triad
  - Gastric GIST, paraganglioma, and pulmonary chondroma
  - Noninherited
  - Lacks mutations in *KIT*, *PDGFRA*, and succinate dehydrogenase (SDH) complex
- Carney-Stratakis syndrome
  - Familial paraganglioma and GIST
  - Autosomal dominant with incomplete penetrance
  - Germline inactivating mutations in SDH complex
- Familial GIST syndrome
  - Autosomal dominant
  - Multiple GISTs, often throughout GI tract (most commonly small bowel)
  - Hyperpigmentation of skin; mast cell disorders
  - Germline *KIT* or *PDGFRA* mutations
- Neurofibromatosis type 1 (NF1)
  - Increased risk of GIST (particularly in small bowel)
  - May have multiple primary tumors; often associated with ICC hyperplasia
  - Somatic inactivating *NF1* mutations of wild-type allele
  - Lacks *KIT* and *PDGFRA* mutations

CLINICAL ISSUES

Epidemiology

- Incidence
  - Most common primary mesenchymal neoplasm of GI tract
  - Minute (< 1 cm), clinically silent lesions ("micro-GIST") are seemingly common
    - Potentially present in up to 35% of general population
- Age
  - Usually older adults (median: 60 years); tumors rare in children and young adults
    - Syndromic tumors often affect young age groups, including children
- Sex
  - Female predominance in SDH-deficient GIST

Site

- Stomach most common site (60%)
  - Site of all SDH-deficient GIST
- Small bowel (30-35%)
  - Particularly jejunum and ileum
  - Preferred site of origin for NF1-associated GIST
- Colorectum (< 5%)
- Esophagus and appendix (rare)
- Primary extraintestinal (mesentery, omentum) is rare
  - Possibility of metastases/direct spread from GI tract must be excluded
- Retroperitoneal tumors most commonly arise around or near pancreas
  - Vast majority arise from stomach or small bowel, however

Presentation

- GI bleeding (most common)
- Abdominal pain, obstructive symptoms
- May be incidentally discovered
  - During surgery, imaging studies, or endoscopy
- Can present with other signs/features of clinical syndrome (e.g., NF1)

Treatment

- Complete surgical resection, regardless of site, if possible
- Chemotherapy [tyrosine kinase inhibitors (TKIs)] for advanced GIST (unresectable or metastatic)
  - 1st-line therapy: Imatinib mesylate (Gleevec)
  - Additional approved therapies for use within setting of imatinib resistance (primary or secondary)
    - Approved 2nd (sunitinib) and 3rd lines (regorafenib)
  - Additional drugs in development
  - SDH-deficient GIST often resistant to imatinib
    - May show better response to 2nd- and 3rd-line drugs
    - Reports of IGF1R overexpression suggest potential role for IGF1R and VEGFR inhibitor therapy
- Genetic testing and long-term clinical follow-up for all patients with SDH-deficient GIST

Prognosis

- Risk of malignant behavior currently assessed by observing anatomic site, size, and mitotic rate of tumor
  - Site is important factor
    - Small intestinal, colorectal, and esophageal GIST more likely to be clinically aggressive than gastric GIST
  - Size < 2 cm always associated with very low risk
    - Micro-GISTs (< 1 cm) are essentially invariably benign
  - This system does not predict behavior of SDH-deficient GISTs
    - Overall indolent clinical course despite metastatic potential and poor imatinib response
- Molecular prognostication for GISTs
  - Can assist in predicting tumor response to TKI therapy
  - Molecular analysis not indicated in all cases
    - Best reserved for patients with advanced (unresectable &/or metastatic) disease or disease refractory to treatment
- Metastases to liver (most common) or other intraabdominal sites (e.g., ovary)
  - Very rarely to extraabdominal sites (e.g., lung)
  - Lymph node metastases characteristic of SDH-deficient GIST
- Dedifferentiated GIST follows highly aggressive clinical course
- Up to 1/3 of patients with GIST may develop subsequent, non-GIST tumor

- Includes carcinomas, hematologic malignancies

MACROSCOPIC

General Features

- Usually well-marginated lesions with their epicenter in muscularis propria
  - May lead to overlying surface ulceration
- Often fleshy cut surface
- Variable cystic change, hemorrhage, necrosis
- Rarely multinodular peritoneal growth

Size

- Wide range (millimeters to > 30 cm)
  - Median: 5 cm
  - Subcentimeter tumors known as GIST tumorlets or micro-GISTs

MICROSCOPIC

Histologic Features

- Extremely broad and variable morphologic spectrum
- Site, size, and mitotic rate of each tumor should be noted for purposes of risk assessment
  - Mitotic rate traditionally expressed in terms of 50 HPF
- Tumors show spindled, epithelioid, or mixed-type morphology
  - Spindle cell GIST (most common; 70% of cases)
    - Uniform fusiform cells arranged in sheets, fascicles, bundles, or whorls
      - Relatively monomorphic nuclei; marked pleomorphism is very rare
      - Fine chromatin with inconspicuous nucleoli
      - Pale fibrillary eosinophilic cytoplasm
      - Paranuclear vacuoles common in gastric tumors
    - Occasional nuclear palisading
    - Fibrocollagenous to myxoid stroma
      - May show diffuse myxoid change or prominent stromal hyalinization/sclerosis
    - Skeinoid fibers common in small bowel GIST
      - Coarse, wire-like, haphazardly arranged collagen bundles
    - Aggressive tumors are often hypercellular
  - Epithelioid GIST (20% of cases)
    - Uniform, rounded cells arranged in sheets, nests, or clusters
      - Cells may appear epithelioid, plasmacytoid, rhabdoid
      - Variable eosinophilic to clear cytoplasm
    - Relatively monomorphic nuclei in many cases
    - Subset of tumors show prominent nuclear pleomorphism and multinucleation
      - Mitoses often sparse or absent, however
    - Cytoplasmic vacuolization in some cases; may be prominent (signet ring cell-like or lipoblast-like)
    - Fibrous to myxoid stroma
      - Myxoid, epithelioid GIST more likely to harbor *PDGFRA* mutation or be associated with SDH-deficiency
    - Aggressive tumors often hypercellular
- Stromal lymphocytic infiltrate may be present; occasionally brisk
- Inconspicuous stromal vasculature
  - Occasional larger, ectatic "staghorn" vessels
- Calcification or chondroosseous metaplasia in occasional tumors
- Coagulative tumor necrosis uncommon
  - Most common in aggressive tumors
  - Perivascular tumor cell preservation in background of geographic necrosis (peritheliomatous growth)
- Posttherapy GIST
  - Hypo- or paucicellularity
  - Stromal fibrosis, hyalinization, myxoid change, necrosis
  - Occasional increased nuclear pleomorphism
  - Can lose CD117 expression
  - Histologic response does not appear to correlate well with clinical response
- Rare rhabdomyoblastic differentiation reported in progressive tumors, often following years of therapy

Dedifferentiated Gastrointestinal Stromal Tumor

- Rare
- Defined as conventional GIST (usually spindled type) with abrupt transition to high-grade pleomorphic (dedifferentiated) areas
  - Dedifferentiated areas lose CD117 and DOG1 (and often CD34) and feature abundant mitoses and necrosis
    - Anomalous keratin &/or desmin expression may be seen
- May occur in de novo or following chronic imatinib therapy

Succinate Dehydrogenase-Deficient Gastrointestinal Stromal Tumor

- Characteristic multinodular and plexiform growth within muscularis propria of stomach
- Epithelioid morphology predominates
- Regional lymph node metastases in up to 30% of cases
- Strong CD117(+) and DOG1(+) despite absence of *KIT* and *PDGFRA* mutations
- SDHB IHC useful in morphologically suggestive cases

ANCILLARY TESTS

Immunohistochemistry

- Characteristic CD117(+), often diffuse
  - a.k.a. KIT or C-kit
  - Cytoplasmic or membranous expression (occasionally dot-like)
  - Negative in 5% of cases (usually epithelioid gastric GIST with *PDGFRA* mutations)
- DOG1(+), often diffuse, cytoplasmic, membranous
  - Similar sensitivity and specificity as CD117
  - Expressed in ~ 30-60% of CD117(-) GIST
    - Therefore, useful 2nd-line diagnostic marker
- Very rare cases (< 3%) are CD117 and DOG1 (-)
- CD34(+) in majority (75%)
- Minor subset are SMA(+) &/or caldesmon (+); can be diffuse
  - Often small bowel GIST
- Markers for SDH-deficient GIST
  - Loss of cytoplasmic SDHB expression in tumors with mutations in *SDHA*, *SDHB*, *SDHC*, or *SDHD*
  - Loss of both SDHB and SDHA expression seen only in tumors with *SDHA* mutations

  - Also, recent reports indicate overexpression of IGFR1 in this subtype
- Generally keratin, S100 protein, desmin, HMB-45, melan-A, STAT5, MDM2 (-)
  - Rare focal positivity for these markers in sporadic GIST
  - S100 protein (+) reported in up to 35% of NF1-associated GISTs

Molecular Genetics

- Most tumors (85-90%) harbor *KIT* or *PDGFRA* oncogenic activating mutations
  - *KIT* mutations in majority (80-85%)
    - Exon 11 (most common), 9, 13, 17, or 8
  - *PDGFRA* mutations
    - Most common in stomach or omentum
    - Exon 8 (most common), 12, or 14
    - D842V associated with resistance to imatinib
  - *KIT* and *PDGFRA* mutations are mutually exclusive
- Wild-type GIST (10-15% of tumors)
  - Defined as GIST that lacks *KIT* and *PDGFRA* mutations
  - Most cases (90%) of pediatric GIST
  - SDH-deficient GIST
    - Harbor mutations in 25% of cases
      - *SDHA* > *SDHB* > > *SDHC* and *SDHD*
  - Also those associated with NF1 or *BRAF* (V600E) mutations

DIFFERENTIAL DIAGNOSIS

Gastrointestinal Smooth Muscle Neoplasms

- Leiomyoma
  - Most common in esophagus (mural mass) or colorectum (polyp)
  - Low cellularity; brightly eosinophilic spindled cells with blunt-ended nuclei
  - Strongly SMA(+), desmin (+)
  - CD117 and DOG1 (-)
- Leiomyosarcoma
  - Nuclear pleomorphism and mitotic activity common
  - Perpendicularly oriented fascicles of brightly eosinophilic spindled cells
  - Subset contains myxoid stroma
  - SMA(+); variable desmin (+)
  - CD117 and DOG1 (-)

Gastrointestinal Schwannoma

- Microtrabecular architecture common
- Characteristic patchy peripheral lymphoid cuff
- Strong, diffuse S100 protein (+)
- CD117 and DOG1 (-)

Inflammatory Fibroid Polyp

- Originates in submucosa (usually gastric antrum or intestines)
- Bland spindled cells, often with at least focal "whorling" growth around blood vessels
- Conspicuous inflammatory component, particularly eosinophils
- CD34(+)
- CD117 and DOG1 (-)
- Harbors *PDGFRA* mutations but no *KIT* mutations

Solitary Fibrous Tumor

- Usually extrinsic to GI tract
- Prominent ectatic, "staghorn" vasculature
- CD34 and STAT6 (+)
- CD117 and DOG1 (-)
- *NAB2-STAT6* fusion

Desmoid Fibromatosis

- Epicenter in mesentery with extension into muscularis propria
  - Some mesenteric tumors associated with Gardner syndrome
- More common in younger adults
- Poorly marginated with highly infiltrative growth pattern
- Abundant stromal collagen with characteristic thin-walled blood vessels
- SMA(+), often wispy/patchy expression
- Usually CD117, CD34, and DOG1 (-)
- No *KIT* or *PDGFRA* mutations

Poorly Differentiated Carcinoma

- Morphologic overlap with pleomorphic epithelioid GIST
  - Particularly epithelioid GIST with vacuoles (signet ring-like)
- Mitotic figures common
- Keratin and EMA(+)
- CD117 and CD34 (-)
- DOG1 expression seen in gastric carcinomas; rare in colorectal carcinoma

Melanoma

- Morphologic overlap with pleomorphic epithelioid GIST
  - However, melanoma often shows greater atypia and mitotic activity
- May have prior history of melanoma
  - Metastases to GI tract tend to affect small bowel
    - Can involve mucosal lymphatics
- Strong S100 protein (+)
- Variable expression of melanocytic markers
- Variable CD117(+)
  - Usually CD34 and DOG1 (-)

Malignant Gastrointestinal Neuroectodermal Tumor

- Very rare but most frequently arise in small bowel
- Scattered osteoclast-like multinucleated giant cells common
- Strong S100 protein (+)
- Usually CD117 and DOG1 (-)
- *EWSR1* rearrangements

Plexiform Fibromyxoma

- Essentially always involves gastric antrum
- Characteristic multinodular, plexiform growth with myxoid stroma
- SMA(+)
- CD117, DOG1, CD34 (-)

SELECTED REFERENCES

1. Miettinen M et al: GIST manifesting as a retroperitoneal tumor: clinicopathologic immunohistochemical, and molecular genetic study of 112 cases. Am J Surg Pathol. 41(5):577-85, 2017

Risk Stratification for GISTs (Untreated With Imatinib)

Size	Mitoses/50 HPF	Risk of Aggressive Behavior
Gastric GISTs		
≤ 2 cm	≤ 5	Very low
> 2 and ≤ 5 cm	≤ 5	Low
> 5 and ≤ 10 cm	≤ 5	Intermediate
> 10 cm	≤ 5	Intermediate
≤ 2 cm	> 5	Low
> 2 and ≤ 5 cm	> 5	Intermediate
> 5 and ≤ 10 cm	> 5	High
> 10 cm	> 5	High
Any size	> 10	High
Small Bowel GISTs		
≤ 2 cm	≤ 5	Very low
> 2 and ≤ 5 cm	≤ 5	Low
> 5 and ≤ 10 cm	≤ 5	Intermediate
≤ 2 cm	> 5	Intermediate
> 2 and ≤ 10 cm	> 5	High
> 10 cm	Any mitotic rate	High
Any size	> 10	High

Note: Small bowel schematic can be applied to other nongastric sites (e.g., esophagus, colorectum); GIST = gastrointestinal stromal tumor.

Molecular Prognostication for GISTs

Mutation	Most Common Site	Response to Imatinib Therapy	Comment
KIT exon 11 mutation	All sites	Excellent	Deletions associated with worse outcome (vs. insertions and substitutions)
KIT exon 9 mutation	Small and large intestines	Limited unless higher dosage is used	Sunitinib shows efficacy in setting of imatinib resistance
KIT exon 13 or 17 mutation	Small bowel	Partial	Rare
PDGFRA exon 18	Stomach	Poor	D842V (most common exon 18 mutation) results in total imatinib resistance
PDGFRA exon 12 or 14 mutation	Stomach	Variable	Most respond to imatinib
SDHA, SDHB, SDHC, SDHD mutations	Stomach	Poor or resistant	Most follow indolent clinical course
BRAF V600E mutant	Small bowel	Poor or resistant	
NF1-associated GIST	Small bowel	Poor or resistant	Better overall outcome

GIST = gastrointestinal stromal tumor.

2. Mason EF et al: Conventional risk stratification fails to predict progression of succinate dehydrogenase-deficient gastrointestinal stromal tumors: a clinicopathologic study of 76 cases. Am J Surg Pathol. 40(12):1616-21, 2016
3. Patil DT et al: Utility of BRAF V600E mutation-specific immunohistochemistry in detecting BRAF V600E-mutated gastrointestinal stromal tumors. Am J Clin Pathol. 144(5):782-9, 2015
4. Miettinen M et al: Succinate dehydrogenase deficient gastrointestinal stromal tumors (GISTs) - a review. Int J Biochem Cell Biol. 53:514-9, 2014
5. Antonescu CR et al: Dedifferentiation in gastrointestinal stromal tumor to an anaplastic KIT-negative phenotype: a diagnostic pitfall: morphologic and molecular characterization of 8 cases occurring either de novo or after imatinib therapy. Am J Surg Pathol. 37(3):385-92, 2013
6. Doyle LA et al: Loss of succinate dehydrogenase subunit B (SDHB) expression is limited to a distinctive subset of gastric wild-type gastrointestinal stromal tumours: a comprehensive genotype-phenotype correlation study. Histopathology. 61(5):801-9, 2012
7. Joensuu H: Risk stratification of patients diagnosed with gastrointestinal stromal tumor. Hum Pathol. 39(10):1411-9, 2008
8. Miettinen M et al: Gastrointestinal stromal tumors of the jejunum and ileum: a clinicopathologic, immunohistochemical, and molecular genetic study of 906 cases before imatinib with long-term follow-up. Am J Surg Pathol. 30(4):477-89, 2006
9. Miettinen M et al: Gastrointestinal stromal tumors of the stomach: a clinicopathologic, immunohistochemical, and molecular genetic study of 1765 cases with long-term follow-up. Am J Surg Pathol. 29(1):52-68, 2005

Gross Appearance

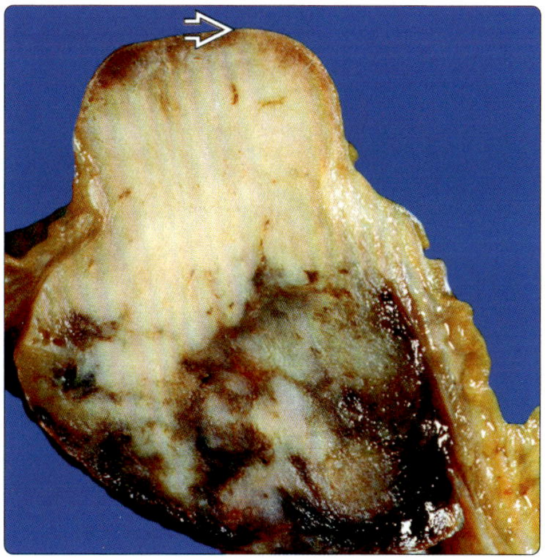

Radiologic Imaging of Gastrointestinal Stromal Tumor

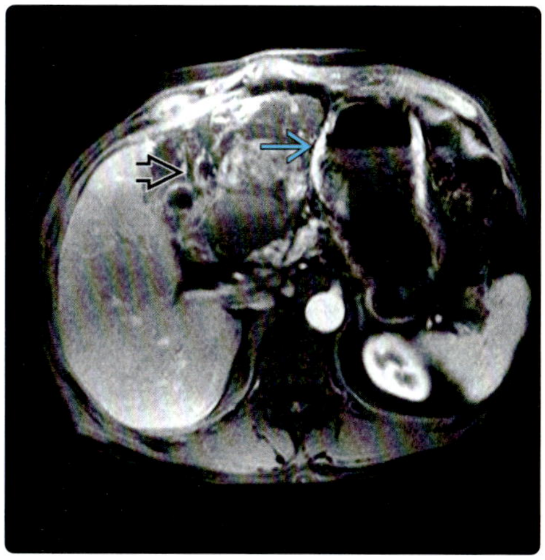

(Left) *This gross photograph shows a small intestinal GIST. The bulk of the tumor is in the muscularis propria, but the lesion has extended into the submucosa and was diagnosed by mucosal biopsy. Note the overlying mucosa* ➡, *which is eroded in places.* **(Right)** *This axial radiologic image shows a large GIST arising in association with the gastric wall* ➡ *and showing local compression of the liver* ➡.

Origin From Muscularis Propria

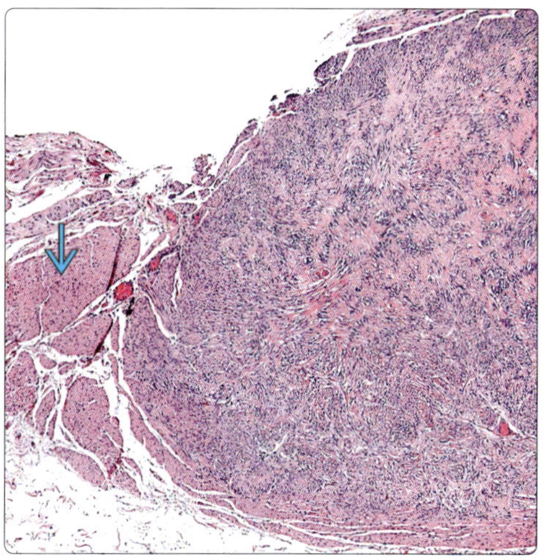

Microgastrointestinal Stromal Tumor

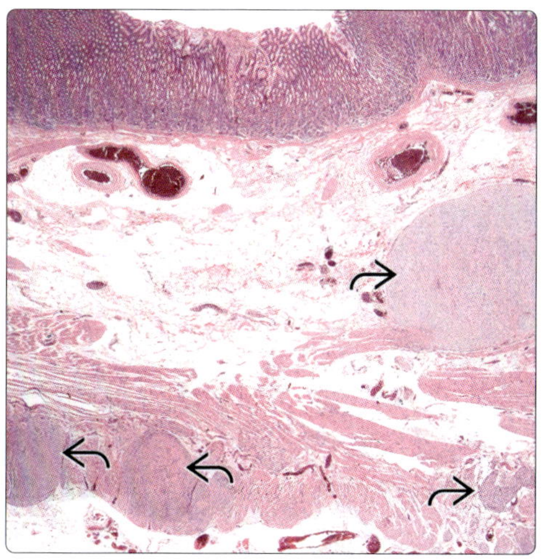

(Left) *GIST arises from within the muscularis propria* ➡. *Smaller tumors may be completely confined, as depicted, but larger tumors often grow outward into the submucosa &/or the serosa.* **(Right)** *Several tiny micro-GISTs or "seedling" GISTs can be seen* ➡ *near the gastroesophageal junction in this resection specimen. These were found incidentally in a resection performed for a separate gastric carcinoma. These tiny lesions are not uncommon and do not imply familial GIST syndrome.*

CD34 in Microgastrointestinal Stromal Tumor

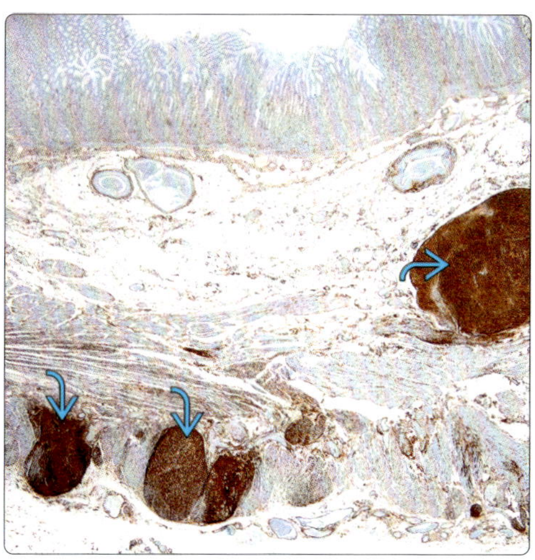

Liver Metastasis

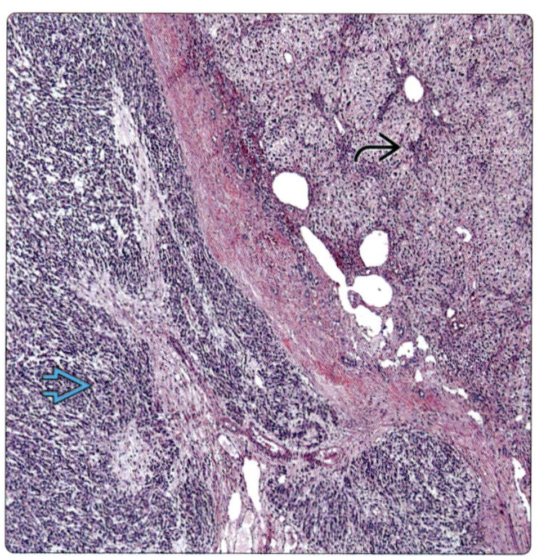

(Left) *CD34 shows prominent staining in micro-GISTs* ➡ *similar to what is seen in the larger, more clinically significant versions. These micro-GISTs are relatively common in all populations, particularly if sought out in resection or autopsy specimens.* **(Right)** *The liver* ➡ *is the most common site of metastasis for malignant GIST* ➡. *Intraabdominal spread may also be seen. Metastatic disease outside of the abdomen is extremely rare.*

(Left) *DOG1 is a newer marker for GIST and can be used as a 2nd-line marker to support a diagnosis of GIST in which CD117 is negative. The sensitivity, specificity, and expression pattern are all similar to CD117.* **(Right)** *CD117 expression is typically diffuse in GIST. Normal mast cells in adjacent tissue serve as a nice internal positive control. Of note, it is important to recognize that some non-GIST tumors, such as leiomyoma, can contain scattered mast cells. These tumors lack diffuse CD117 positivity, however.*

DOG1 Expression

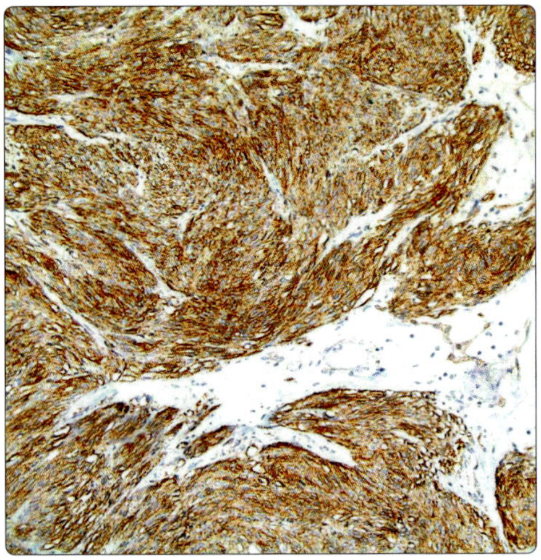

CD117 and Mast Cells

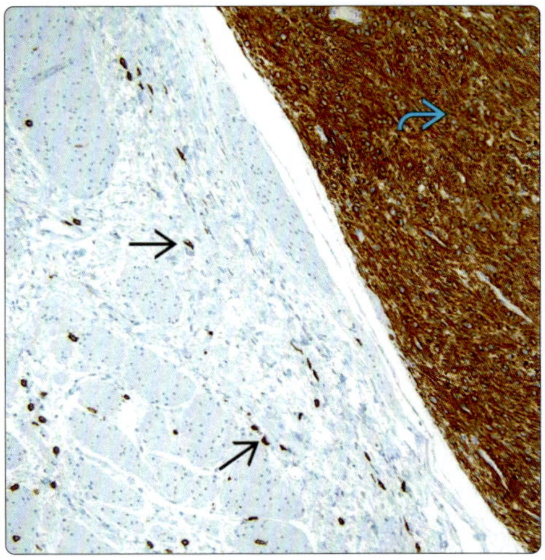

(Left) *GISTs most frequently demonstrate a spindled tumor cell morphology. Cellularity varies from case to case and sometimes from field to field. The morphologic spectrum of these tumors is quite broad.* **(Right)** *Spindled tumor cells in GIST are arranged in sheets, fascicles, or bundles and generally show monomorphic cytologic features. Prominent nuclear pleomorphism is very rare in spindled GIST.*

Spindled Gastrointestinal Stromal Tumor

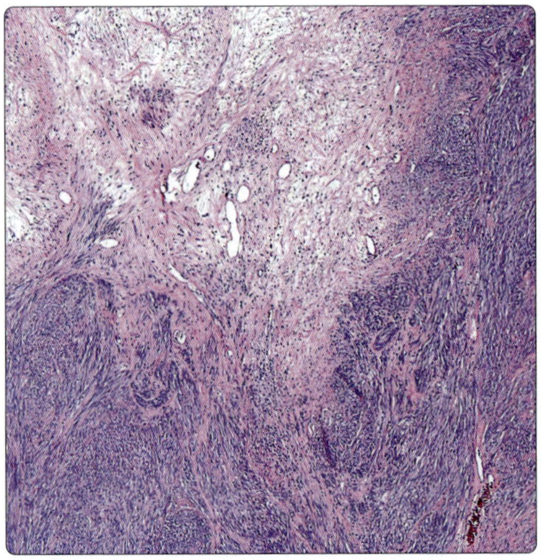

Uniform Spindle Cells

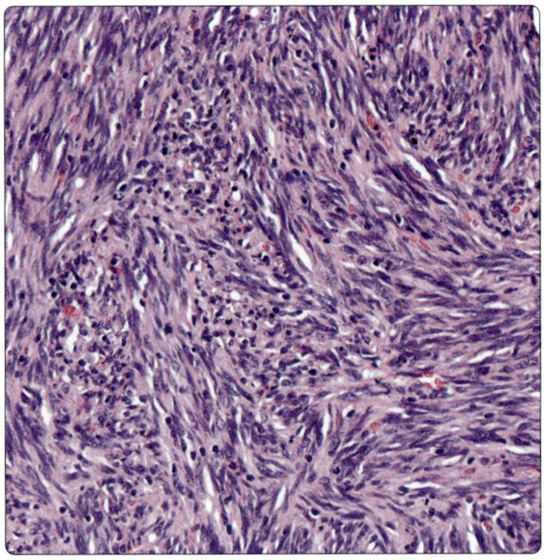

(Left) *Myxoid foci are common in GIST and may be prominent in occasional cases.* **(Right)** *A subtle intratumoral lymphocytic infiltrate is common in GIST and may occasionally be brisk. Lymphocytes can sometime be difficult to distinguish from mitotic figures. Note also the bland, uniform, elongated nuclei characteristic of most low-grade spindled tumors.*

Myxoid Stroma

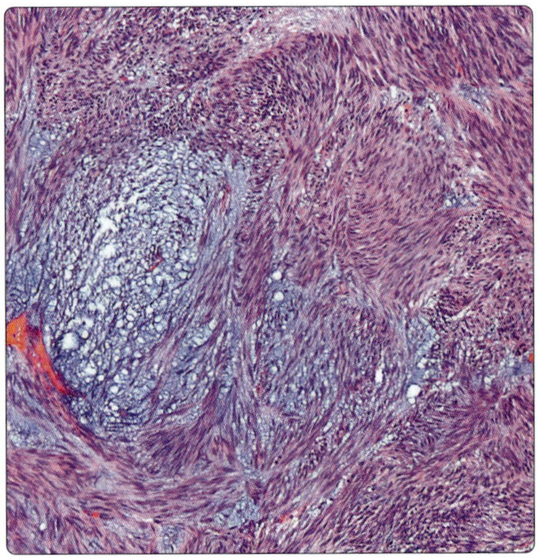

Lymphocytes

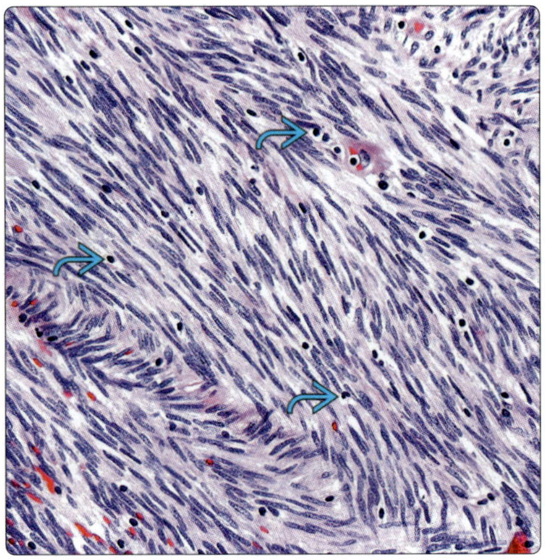

Paranuclear Vacuoles

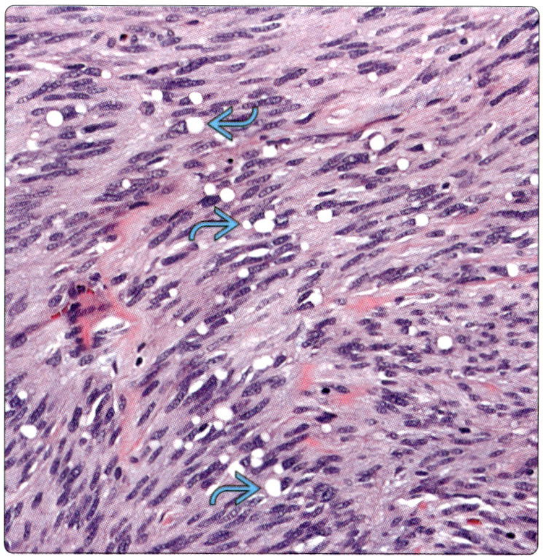

Abundant Vacuoles

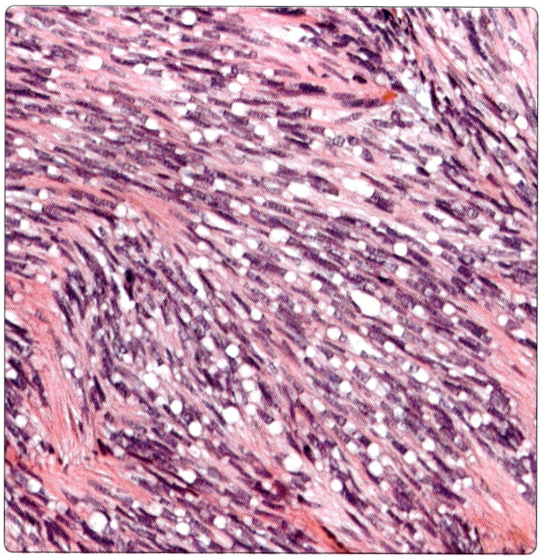

(Left) *Tumor cells in GIST may contain paranuclear vacuoles* ➦*, similar to what is seen in some smooth muscle neoplasms. This finding is particularly common in GIST arising in the stomach.* **(Right)** *This gastric GIST featured numerous spindled tumor cells with paranuclear vacuoles diffusely present throughout the tumor.*

Rare Prominently Myxoid Gastrointestinal Stromal Tumor

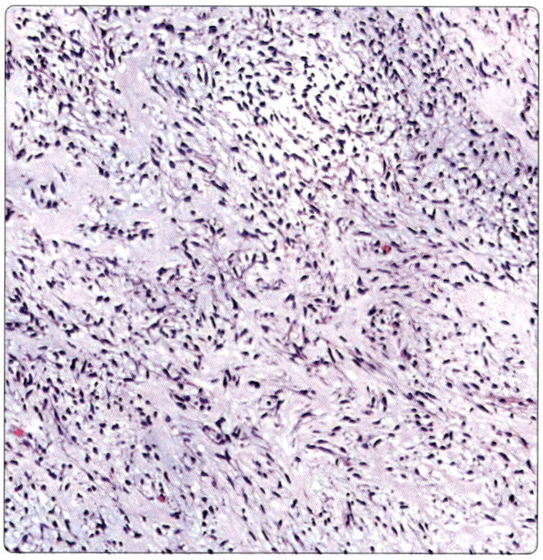

Stromal Hyalinization

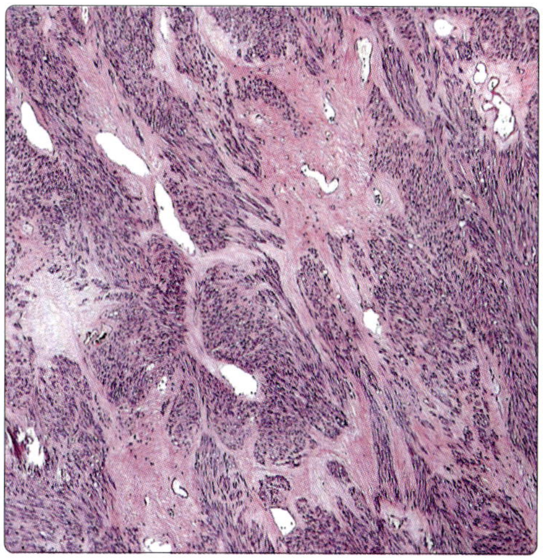

(Left) *Myxoid stroma is not uncommon in GIST but is usually focal or patchy. Rare cases show diffuse, prominent myxoid change, as depicted.* **(Right)** *Stromal hyalinization is seen in many GISTs but varies widely in extent. Not uncommonly, hyalinization appears to form septa dividing sheets and nests of spindled tumor cells and imparting a lobular appearance.*

Hyalinizing Gastrointestinal Stromal Tumor

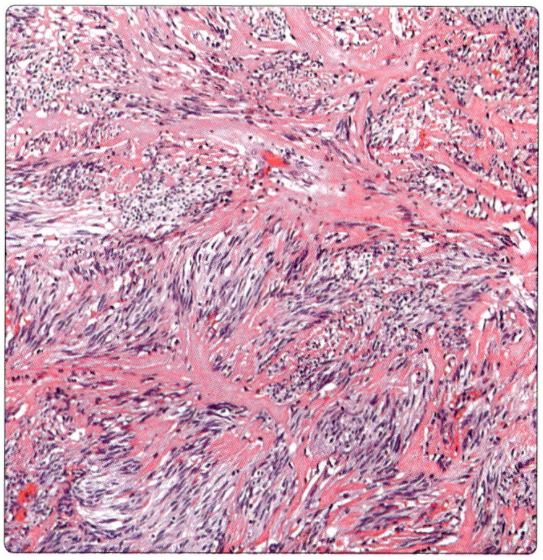

Sclerosis

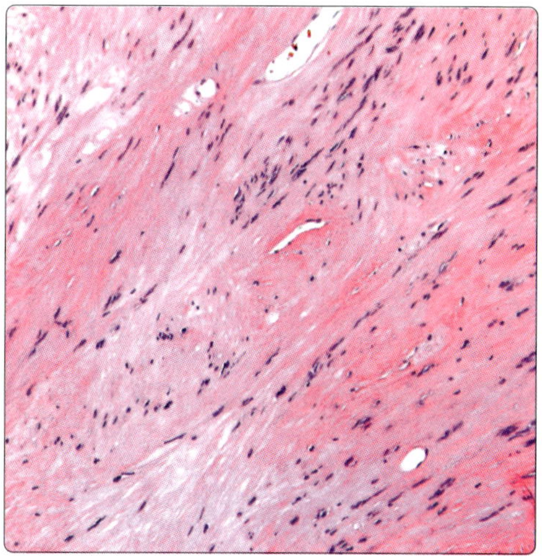

(Left) *The morphologic appearance of nests and bundles of spindled cells within a hyalinized stroma raises the possibility of a smooth muscle tumor or PEComa. IHC often makes this distinction easy.* **(Right)** *Diffuse stromal hyalinization or sclerosis with concomitant paucicellularity is uncommon in untreated GIST and may lead to consideration of leiomyoma.*

(Left) *Increased stromal collagen without overt hyalinization, as depicted, is seen in some GISTs and can impart an appearance suggestive of smooth muscle.* **(Right)** *Degenerative changes in GIST include mainly fibrosis, hemorrhage, hemosiderin deposition, and architectural disruptions. As seen in this H&E, the tissue can appear to tear apart and is associated with myxoedematous stroma and hemorrhage.*

Stromal Collagen

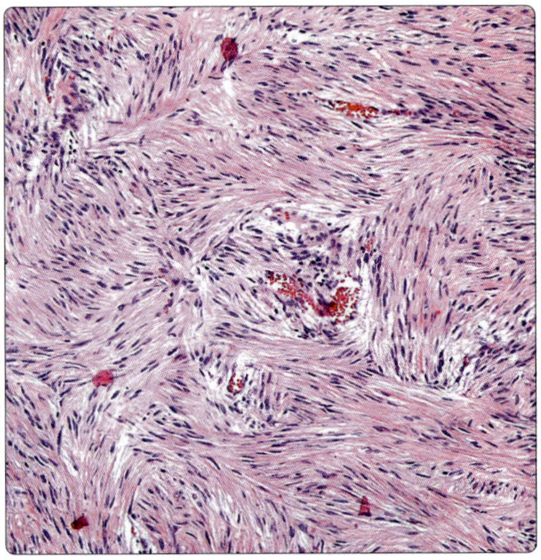

Degenerative Changes

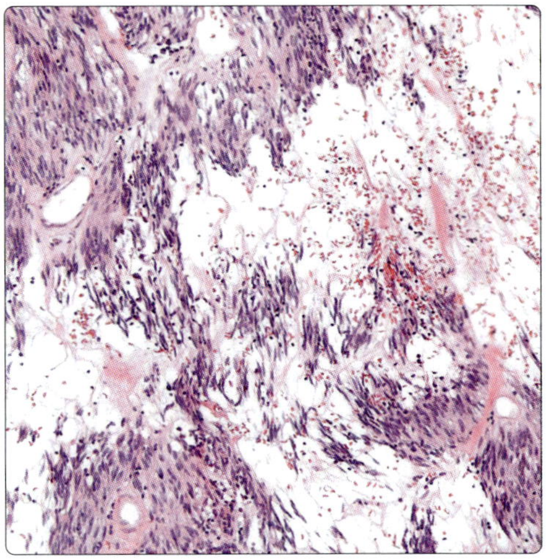

(Left) *Hemorrhage may be seen in GIST and may even be evident at the time of gross examination. Cellular spindled tumors with hemorrhage can mimic Kaposi sarcoma, which can also express CD34 and CD117.* **(Right)** *This H&E shows a focus of chunky calcification →. Calcification is uncommon in GIST and, in the stomach, is more likely to be seen in mural leiomyomas.*

Intratumoral Hemorrhage

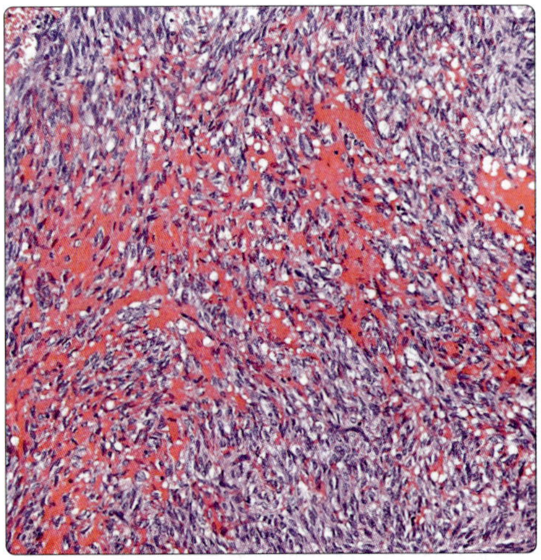

Calcifications

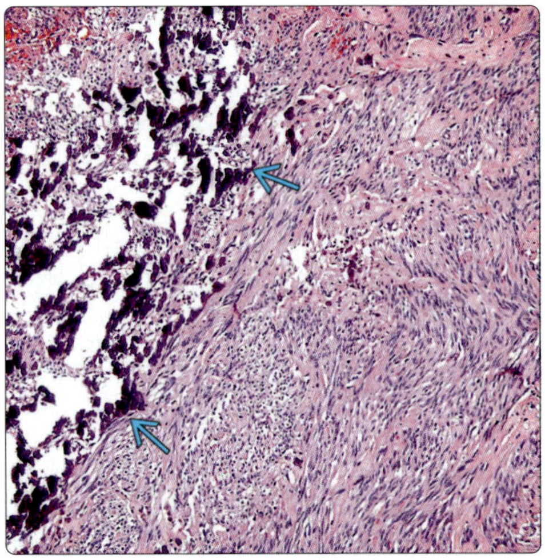

(Left) *Perivascular hyalinization ↪ is seen in some cases of GIST and is often associated with other degenerative features, such as myxoedematous stroma and architectural disruption. Rare cases can show striking, diffusely hyalinized vessels.* **(Right)** *Stromal blood vessels are generally small and inconspicuous in GIST; however, occasional tumors feature larger, ectatic vessels, as depicted. Some may even show irregular shapes (staghorn) similar to solitary fibrous tumor.*

Hyalinized Blood Vessels

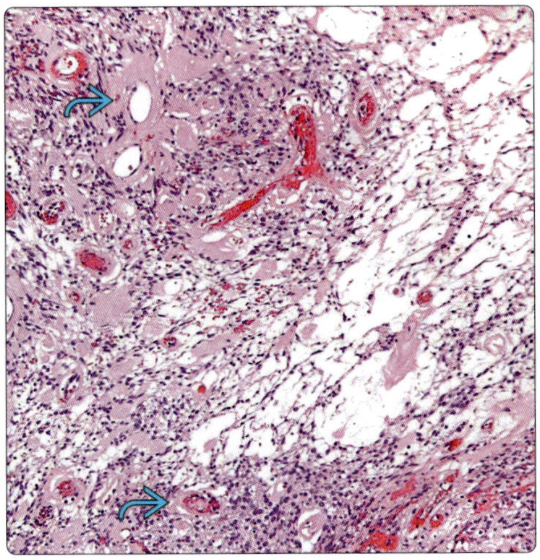

Ectatic Blood Vessels

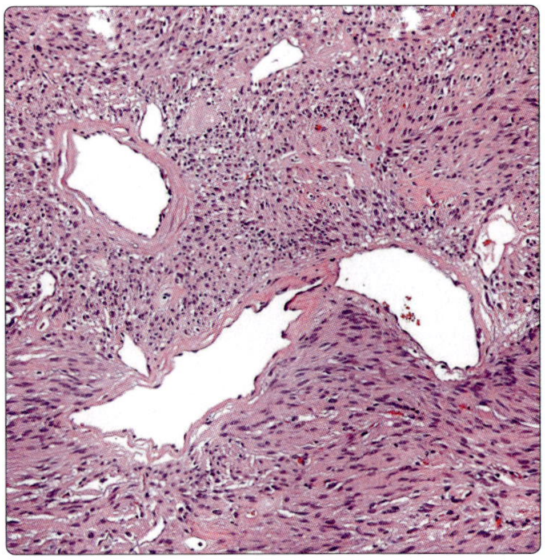

Nuclear Palisading

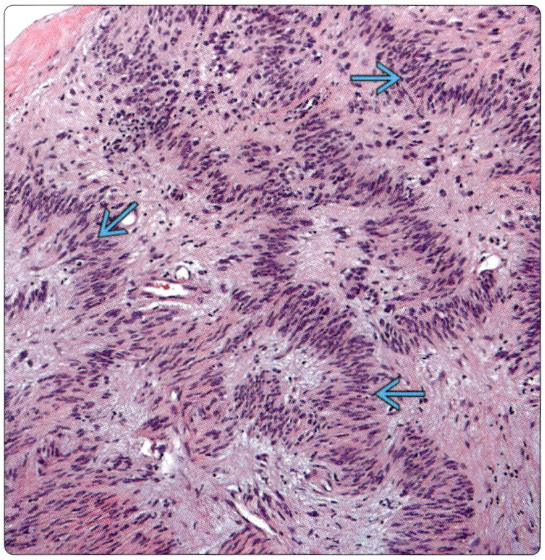

Small Bowel Gastrointestinal Stromal Tumor

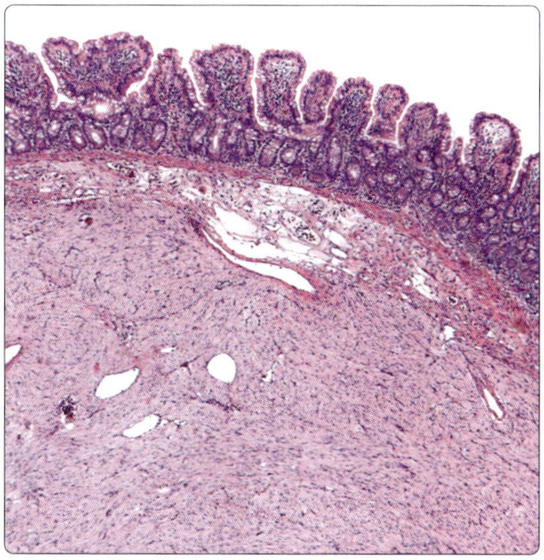

(Left) *Nuclear palisading may be seen in spindled GIST. Interestingly, palisading is more common in GIST than in other primary spindle cell neoplasms of the GI tract, including schwannoma.* **(Right)** *After the stomach, the small bowel is the 2nd most common site for GIST. The jejunum and ileum are preferentially affected. This site is also the most common site for GIST arising within the context of NF1.*

Discrete Vascular Network

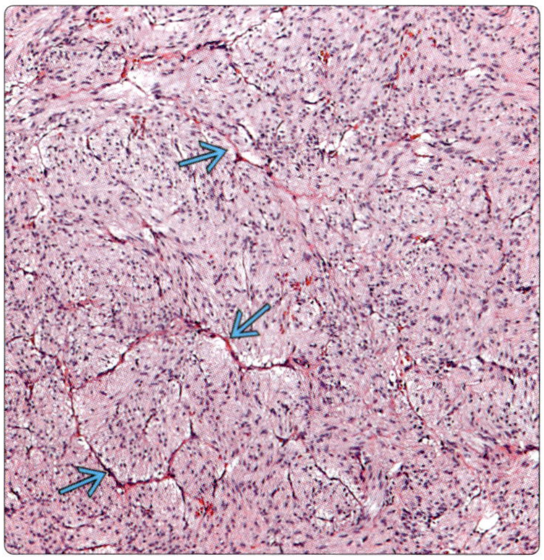

Skeinoid Fibers

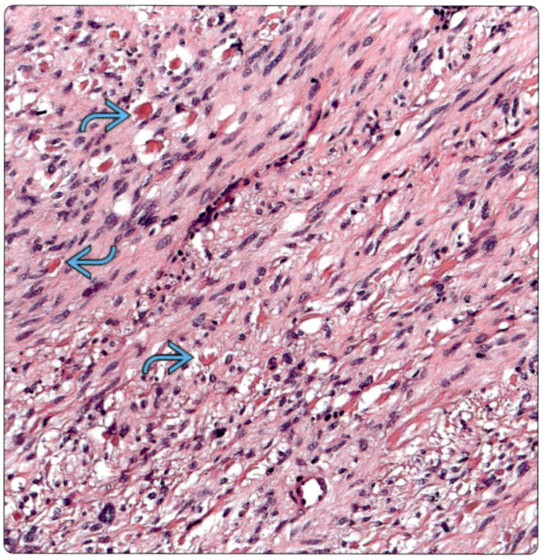

(Left) *This neurofibromatosis type 1 (NF1)-associated GIST arose within the small bowel and showed in areas a distinctive compartmentalized pattern demarcated by thin capillary channels. Occasional GISTs can feature a prominent nested growth pattern.* **(Right)** *Skeinoid fibers are well described in GIST and consist of thick ropy matrix deposited between tumor cells. They are most commonly seen in small bowel tumors but have been described in other GI sites.*

Prominent Skeinoid Fibers

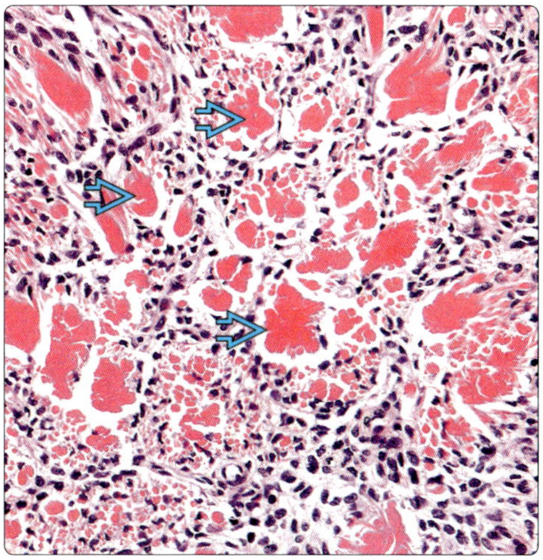

Fascicular Growth

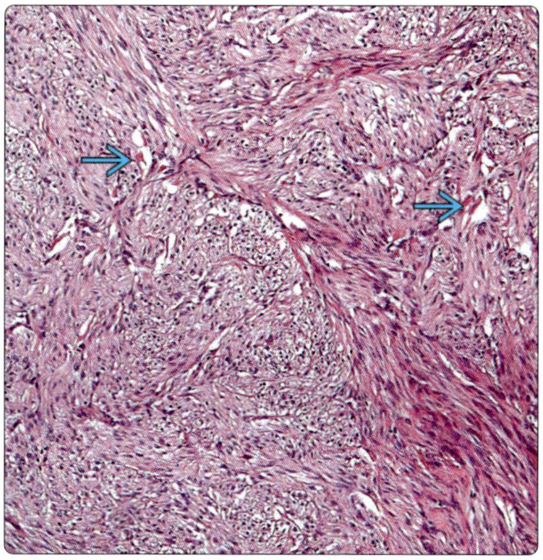

(Left) *This GIST features prominent skeinoid fibers. These fibers are principally found in small bowel GISTs, where they are associated with a favorable outcome.* **(Right)** *This more cellular area of an NF1-associated small bowel GIST shows fascicular growth, resembling a smooth muscle neoplasm. Note the focal skeinoid fibers.*

(Left) *Risk of aggressive behavior in GIST is assessed primarily by evaluating the combination of site, size, and mitotic activity of a given tumor. Although cellularity is not a defined factor in stratifying GIST, most malignant cases show a marked increased in overall cellularity, as depicted.* **(Right)** *Hypercellularity is a common finding in high-risk GIST and portends a strong likelihood of identifying a high mitotic count in a tumor.*

Malignant Gastrointestinal Stromal Tumor

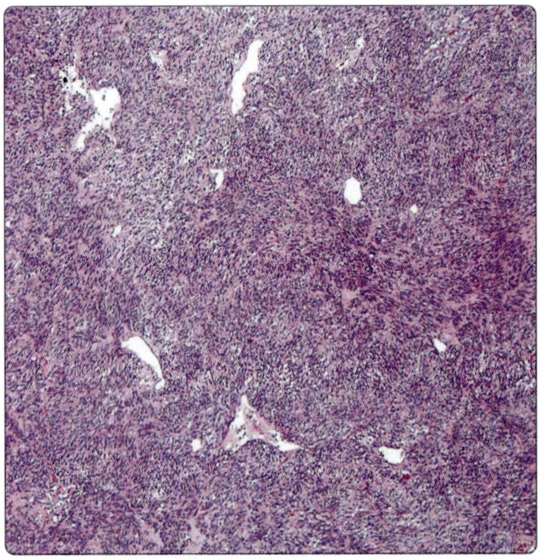

Hypercellularity

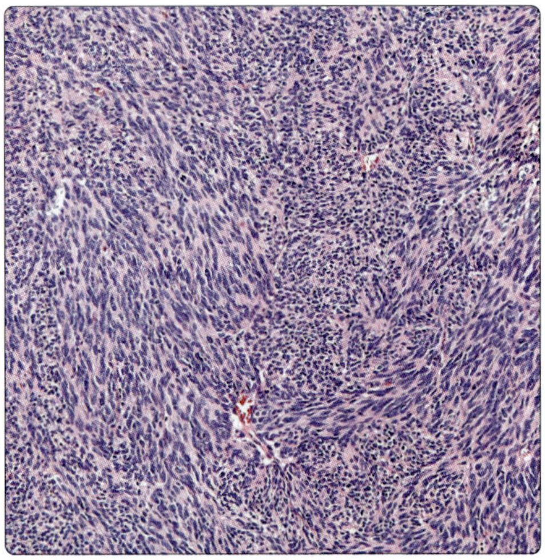

(Left) *Fascicular growth is often more pronounced in malignant GIST and may even show a herringbone architectural pattern, as depicted.* **(Right)** *Myxoid change can also be seen in malignant GIST and may be extensive in rare cases, as shown in this example. This tumor contained abundant mitoses and showed diffuse CD117 and DOG1 expression.*

Prominent Fascicular Growth

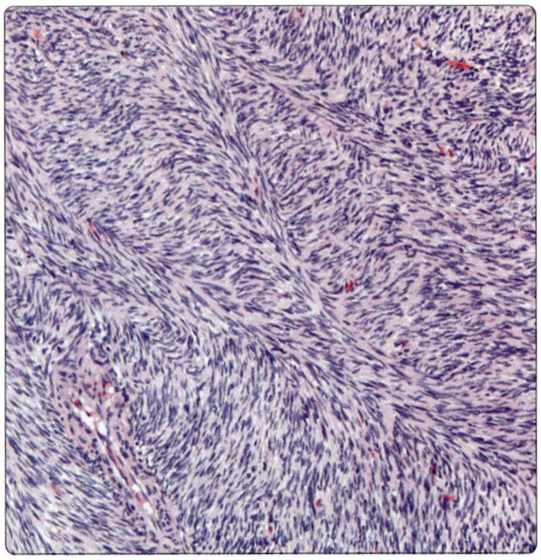

Myxoid Change in Malignant Gastrointestinal Stromal Tumor

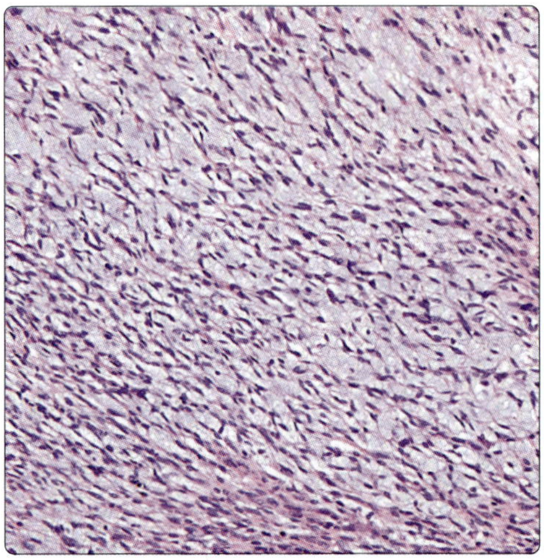

(Left) *This malignant GIST showed prominent nuclear palisading. Note the overall high cellularity and mitotic activity* ➡. **(Right)** *Significant nuclear pleomorphism is very uncommon in an untreated spindle cell GIST; however, this finding may be present in resection specimens following imatinib therapy. As a general rule, any spindle cell neoplasm with pleomorphism in the GI tract should lead to consideration of many other entities (e.g., leiomyosarcoma) before GIST.*

Nuclear Palisading in Malignant Gastrointestinal Stromal Tumor

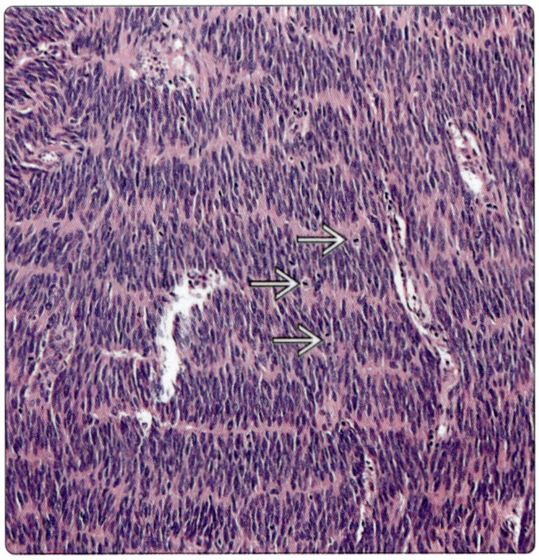

Nuclear Pleomorphism in Spindled Gastrointestinal Stromal Tumor

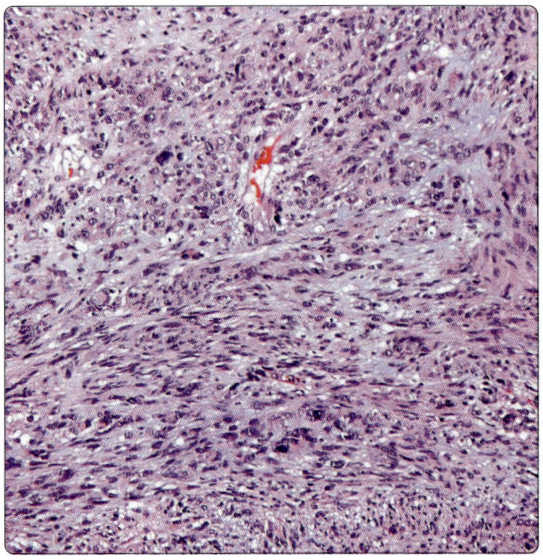

Necrosis

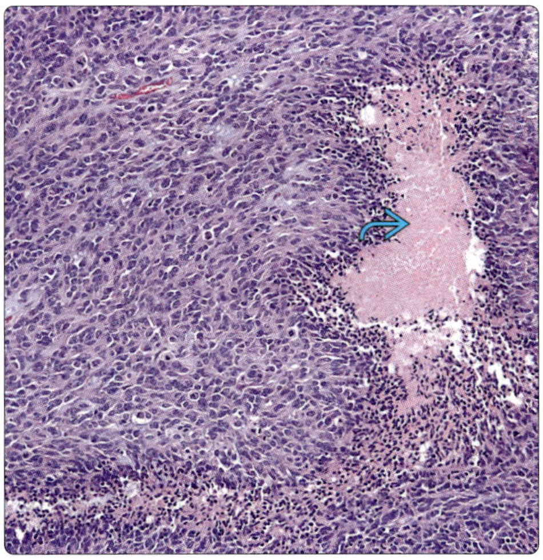

Geographic Necrosis

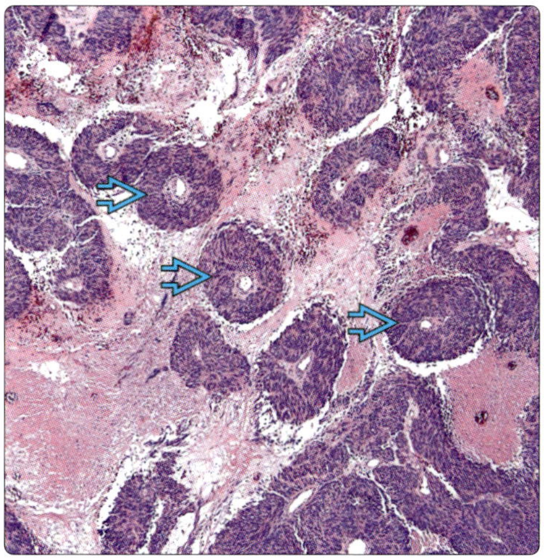

(Left) *Necrosis is generally uncommon in GIST and may be associated with a poorer prognosis in high-risk tumors. Necrosis can also be seen in the setting of ischemia/degeneration or following imatinib therapy.* **(Right)** *Geographic necrosis in GIST is often associated with retained viability of perivascular tumor cells (peritheliomatous pattern). This morphology is also classically associated with Ewing sarcoma and malignant peripheral nerve sheath tumor.*

Unusual Pseudopapillary Appearance

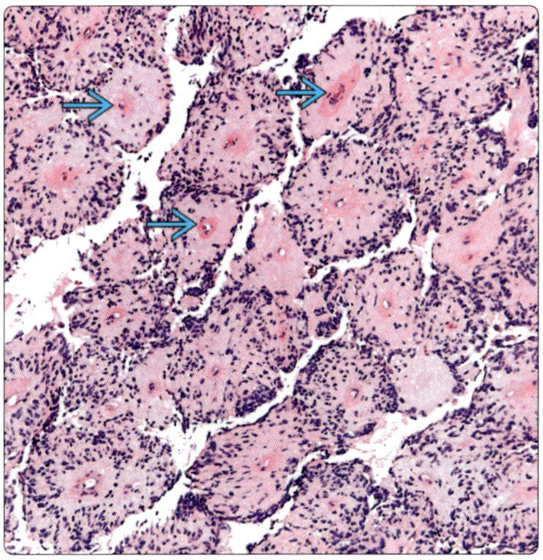

Highly Cystic Gastrointestinal Stromal Tumor

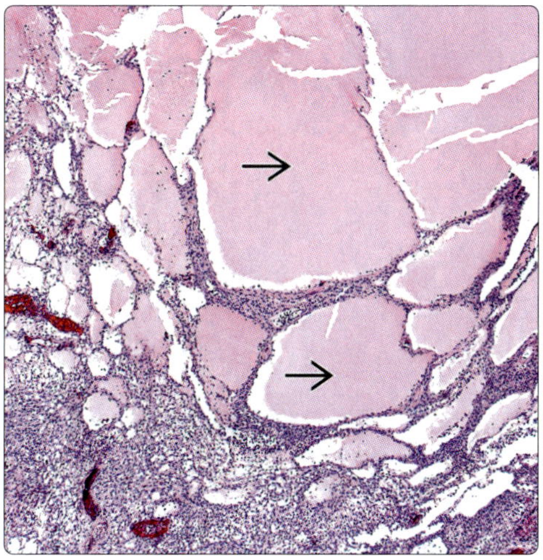

(Left) *This unusual GIST showed areas of cellular degeneration and dyscohesion around hyalinized stromal vessels, creating a pseudopapillary appearance.* **(Right)** *This case of GIST showed abundant cystic and microcystic changes, resembling schwannoma as well as other neoplasms.*

Posttherapy Gastrointestinal Stromal Tumor

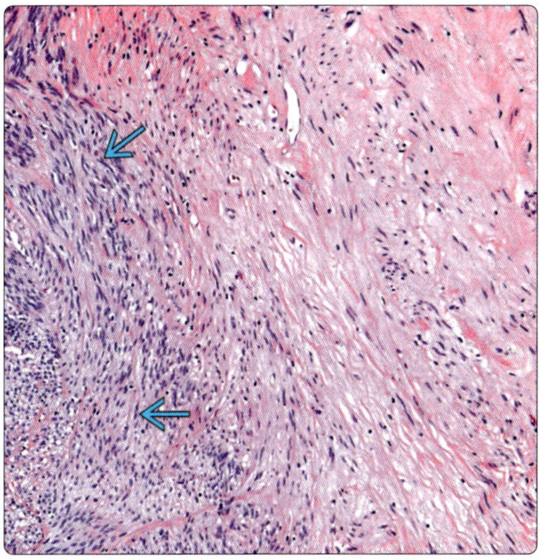

Rare Rhabdomyoblastic Differentiation

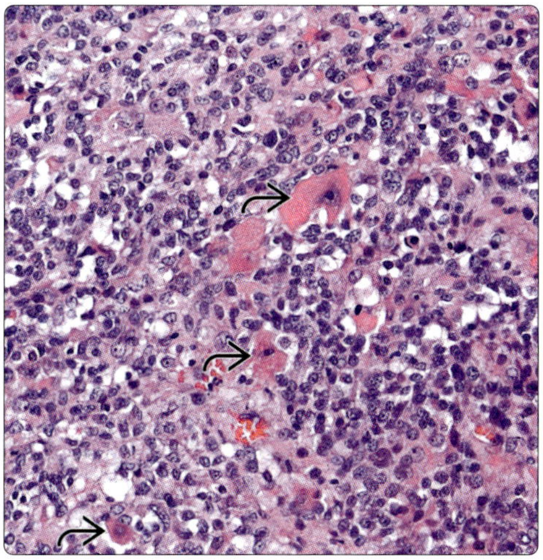

(Left) *Following therapy with imatinib, GIST may show a variety of changes, including fibrosis, myxoid change, or necrosis. Areas of residual viable tumor are almost always seen in resection specimens, however.* **(Right)** *Rare progressive GISTs, often after years of therapy, have been reported to show areas of rhabdomyoblastic differentiation, which can be highlighted with desmin &/or myogenin immunostains. These areas may also closely resemble pleomorphic rhabdomyosarcoma.*

(Left) *An epithelioid morphology is less common than a spindled morphology in GIST, but awareness is very important due to the potential for confusion with carcinoma and melanoma. Cells may form nests, clusters, or sheets.* **(Right)** *Epithelioid tumor cells in GIST feature variable eosinophilic* → *to clear* ↷ *cytoplasm. Cytoplasmic borders are distinct in some tumors, but inapparent in others, and can appear syncytial.*

Epithelioid Gastrointestinal Stromal Tumor

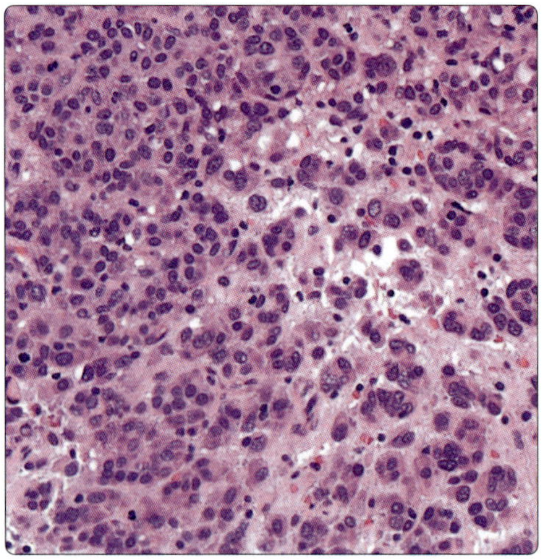

Eosinophilic to Clear Cytoplasm

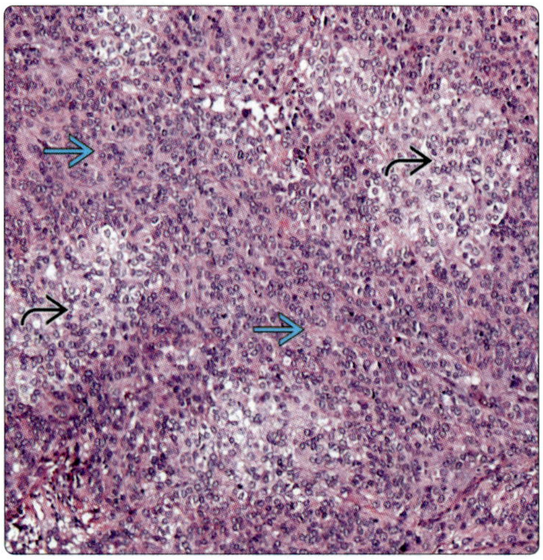

(Left) *GIST may feature distinctly epithelioid cells with sharp, prominent cytoplasmic borders and peripheral cytoplasmic retraction, creating a halo-like* ↷ *effect around nuclei.* **(Right)** *Myxoid stromal changes are more common in epithelioid than spindled GIST. In the stomach, myxoid epithelioid tumors are more likely to harbor PDGFRA than KIT mutations.*

Prominent Epithelioid Morphology

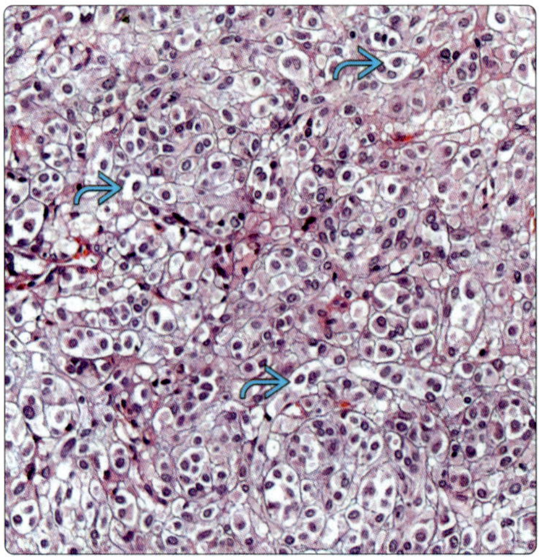

Myxoid Stroma

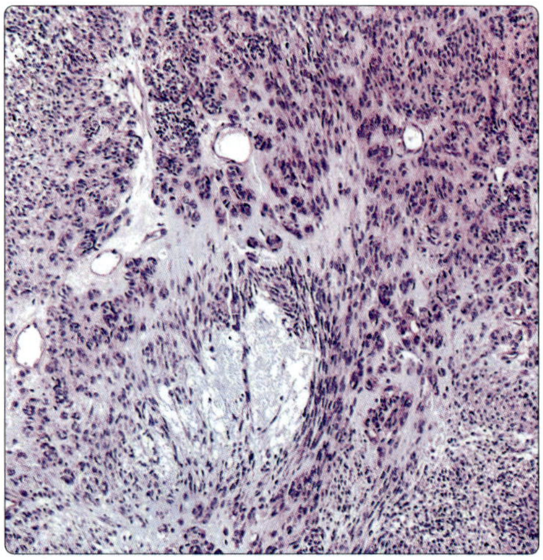

(Left) *Paranuclear vacuoles may be seen in epithelioid GIST as with spindled GIST. Notably, vacuoles in epithelioid cells tend to produce a signet ring-like appearance, which can lead to a significant misdiagnosis of adenocarcinoma.* **(Right)** *Larger, more prominent vacuolizations in epithelioid GIST can impart a morphologic appearance reminiscent of lipoblastic differentiation, as depicted.*

Signet Ring-Like Vacuolizations

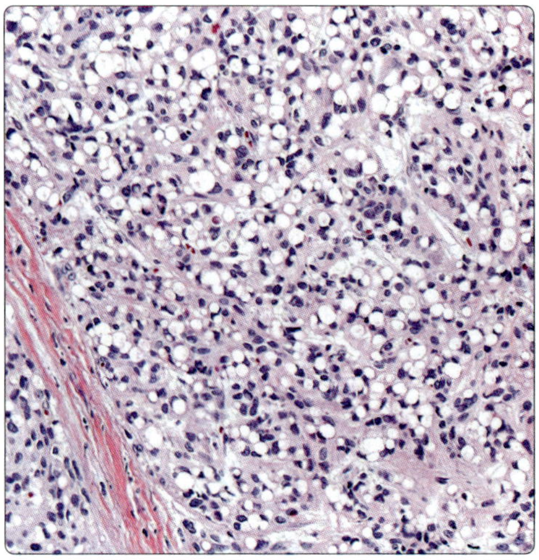

Pseudolipoblastic Appearance

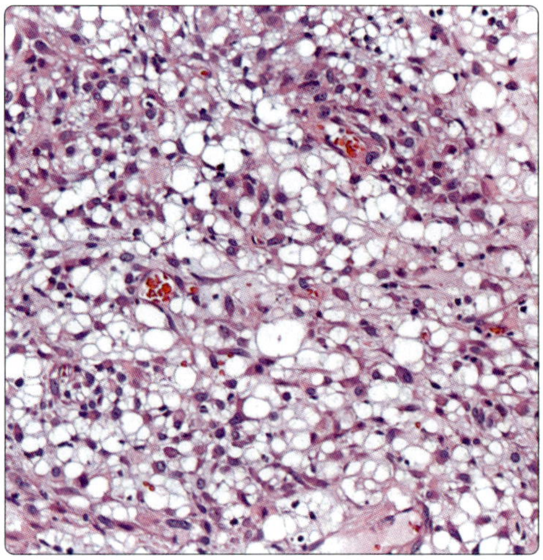

Sclerosing Epithelioid Gastrointestinal Stromal Tumor

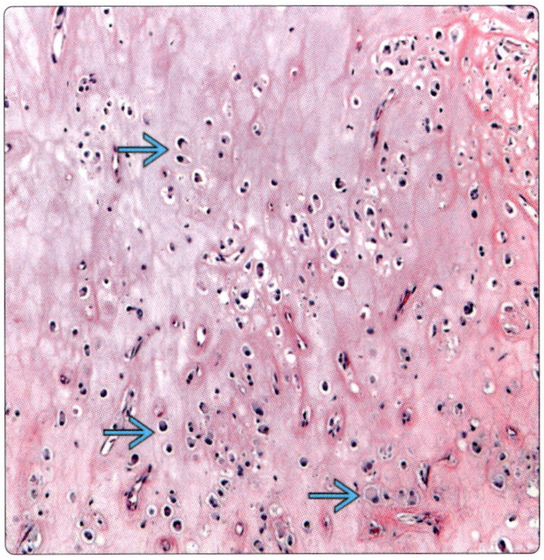

Multinucleated Tumor Cells

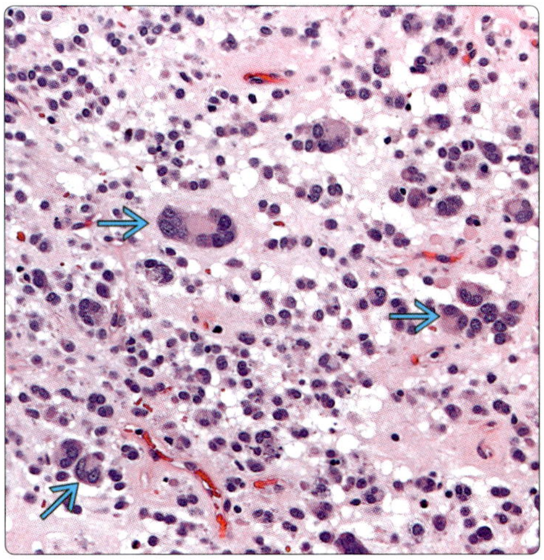

(Left) *Prominent hyalinized or sclerotic stroma may be seen in epithelioid GIST. Individual tumor cells* → *and small clusters of cells may resemble plasma cells or even osteoblasts.* **(Right)** *Scattered bi- or multinucleated tumor cells* → *are relatively common in epithelioid GIST.*

Pleomorphic Epithelioid Gastrointestinal Stromal Tumor

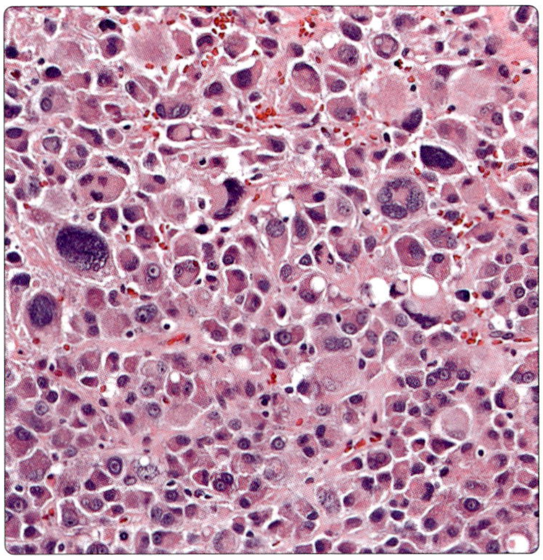

Retraction Artifact

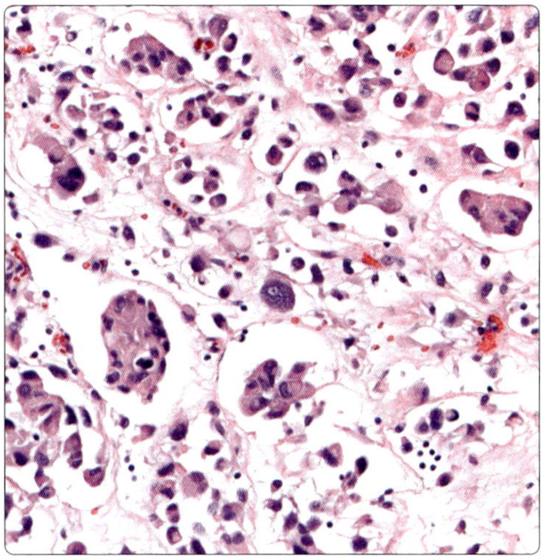

(Left) *Nuclear pleomorphism and multinucleation may be quite prominent in some cases of epithelioid GIST. Interestingly, mitotic figures in these tumors are often rare to absent. On a small biopsy, there is significant risk of confusion with melanoma or carcinoma.* **(Right)** *This particularly unfriendly case of pleomorphic epithelioid GIST showed areas with significant retraction space artifact, simulating lymphatic space invasion. Note, however, the lack of an endothelial lining to the spaces.*

Rhabdoid Morphology

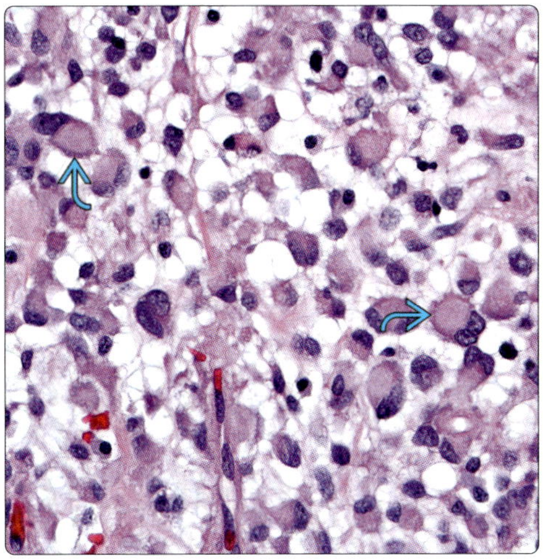

Plasmacytoid Morphology

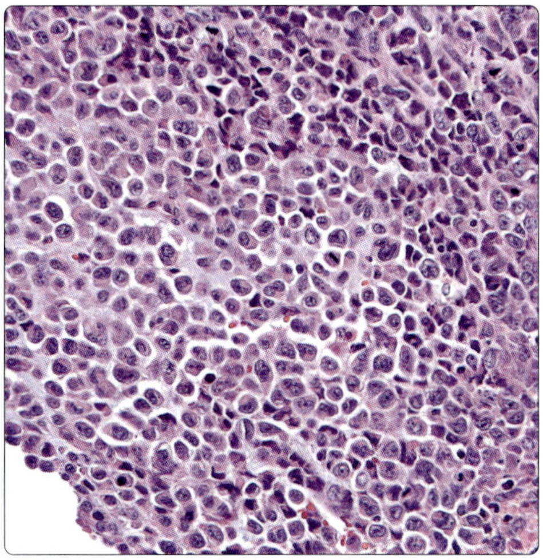

(Left) *Occasional tumor cells in epithelioid GIST may feature a rhabdoid morphology* ↗ *characterized by glassy eosinophilic cytoplasm associated with eccentric enlarged nuclei.* **(Right)** *This case of malignant epithelioid GIST featured dense sheets of tumor cells with a decidedly plasmacytoid morphology.*

(Left) *This case of GIST arose from the muscularis propria of the esophagus and initially presented as a large mediastinal mass. It shows a distinctive growth pattern composed of variably sized nodules of tumor cells within a hypocellular myxocollagenous stroma. Some areas also showed dense stromal hyalinization.* **(Right)** *Similar to spindled forms, epithelioid GISTs with a high risk for malignant behavior often show a marked increased in cellularity with a concomitant marked increased in mitotic activity.*

Distinct Nodular Growth

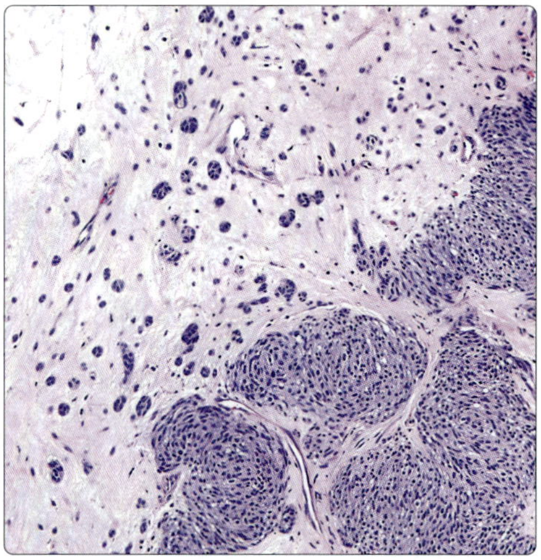

Malignant Epithelioid Gastrointestinal Stromal Tumor

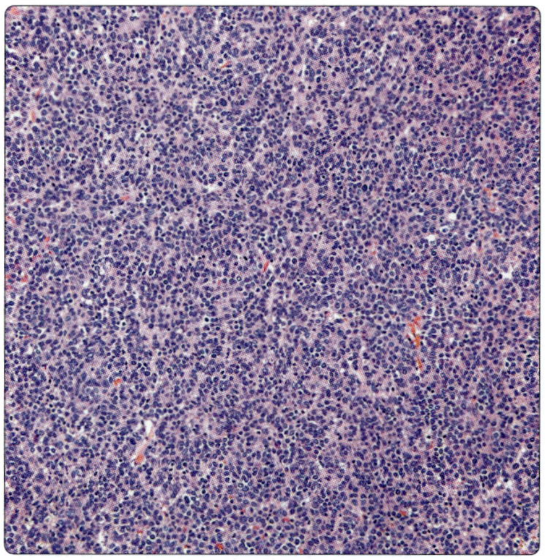

(Left) *Malignant epithelioid GIST can show a variety of growth patterns similar to low-risk GIST; however, hypercellularity is often a feature.* **(Right)** *As suggested by the markedly increased cellularity, the high mitotic rate ⇨ of this epithelioid GIST assists in classifying it as having a high risk of aggressive/malignant behavior. Size and anatomic location are also usually important in this endeavor.*

Hypercellularity

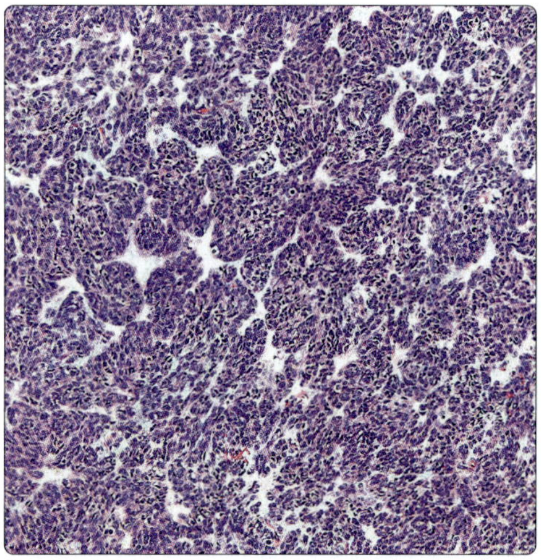

Abundant Mitoses

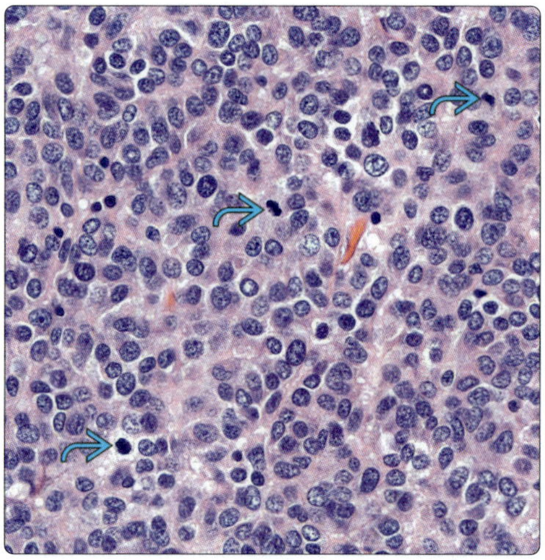

(Left) *This case of malignant epithelioid GIST showed focal areas of corded growth within a fibrous stroma, mimicking an infiltrating lobular carcinoma or a variety of sclerosing sarcomas.* **(Right)** *Some GISTs show a mixture of spindled ⇨ and epithelioid ⇨ morphologies. This clinically malignant tumor shows an abrupt transition between the 2 components.*

Corded Growth

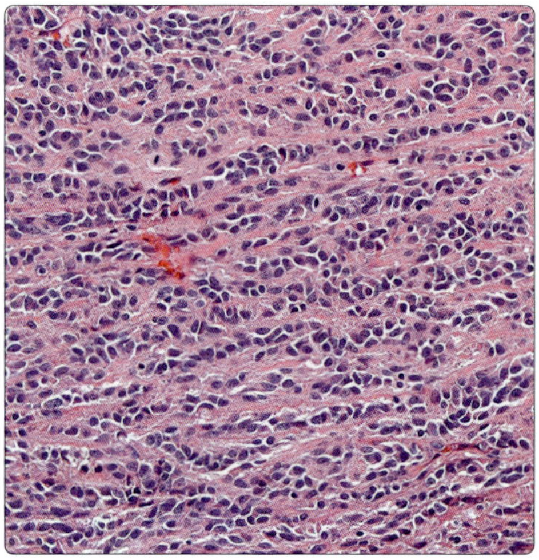

Mixed-Type Gastrointestinal Stromal Tumor

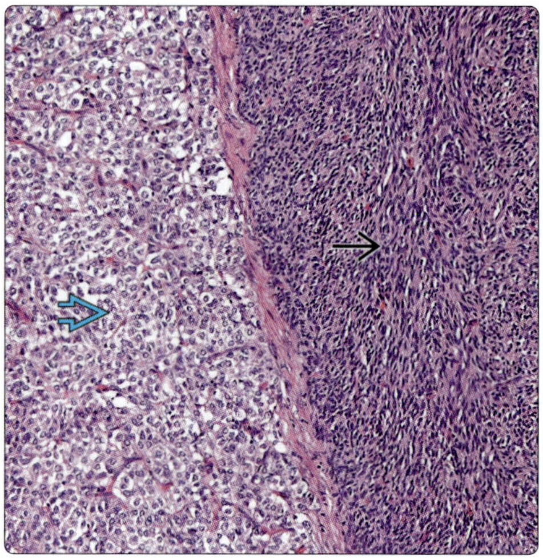

Dedifferentiated Gastrointestinal Stromal Tumor

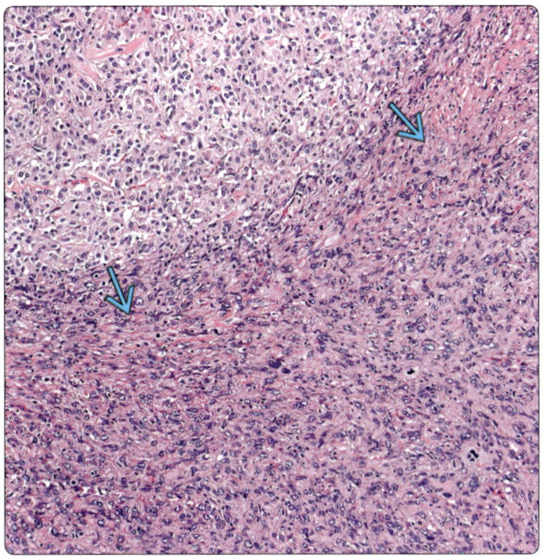

Dedifferentiated Gastrointestinal Stromal Tumor

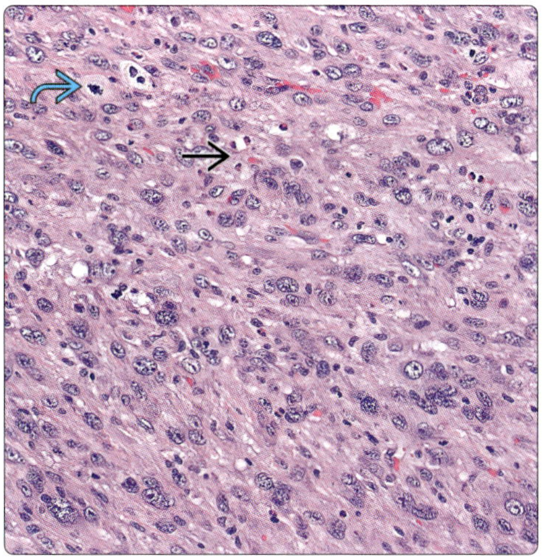

(Left) *Dedifferentiated GIST is rare and is defined as morphologically conventional GIST with abrupt transition to high-grade pleomorphic areas ⇨ lacking CD117 &/or DOG1 expression. The dedifferentiated areas usually show abundant mitoses and necrosis.* **(Right)** *The sarcomatous areas of dedifferentiated GIST often show a nonspecific high-grade morphology; however, prominent nucleoli, mitotic figures ↗, and inflammatory infiltrates → are all common.*

Succinate Dehydrogenase-Deficient Gastrointestinal Stromal Tumor

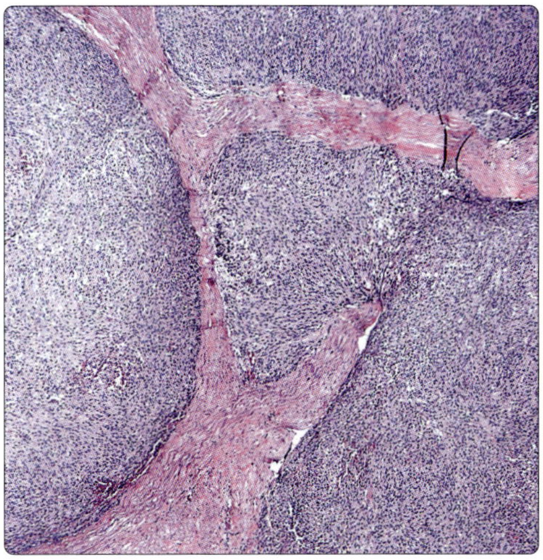

Epithelioid Predominant

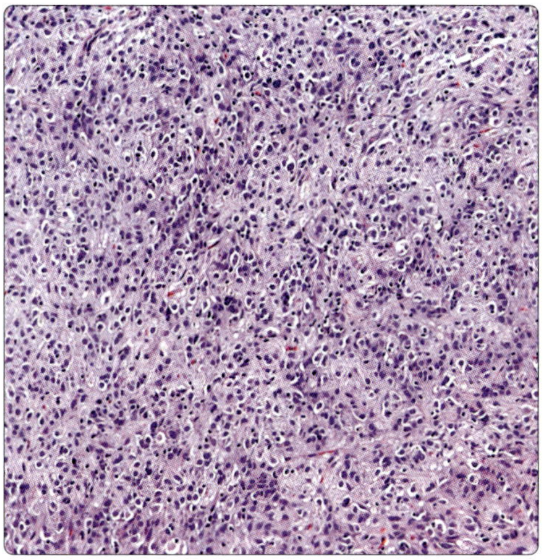

(Left) *Succinate dehydrogenase (SDH)-deficient GIST is a distinctive clinicopathologic subtype that shows several unique features, including a characteristic multinodular and plexiform growth pattern within the muscularis propria of the stomach.* **(Right)** *An epithelioid tumor cell morphology predominates in SDH-deficient GIST, although a mixture of spindled and epithelioid cells can also be seen. Myxoid stroma can also be seen.*

SDHB Immunohistochemistry

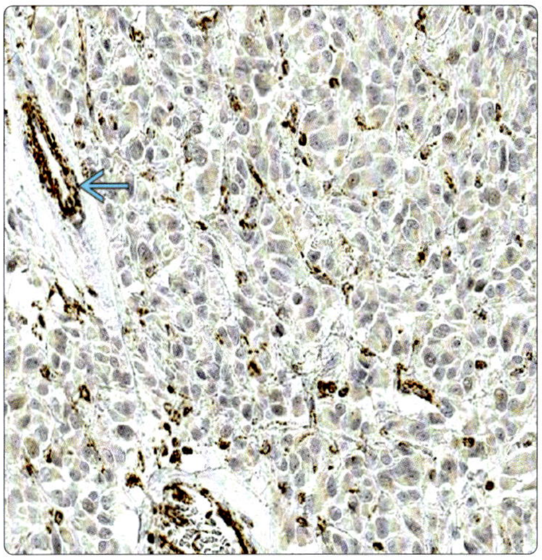

Lymph Node Metastases

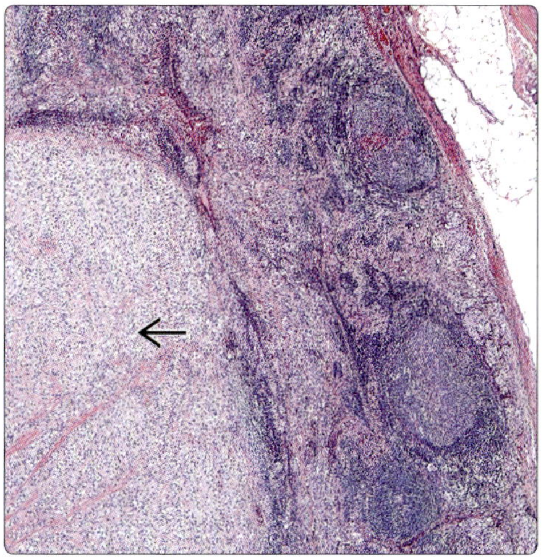

(Left) *Loss of granular cytoplasmic SDHB expression is highly useful in the diagnosis of SDH-deficient GIST. Note the positive internal control (endothelial cells ⇨), which should always be present when evaluating this stain.* **(Right)** *SDH-deficient GIST shows a notable tendency for lymph node metastases →, which may be identified and removed along with the resected tumor. Despite this apparent aggressive behavior, these tumors are often relatively clinically indolent.*

Gastrointestinal Schwannoma

KEY FACTS

TERMINOLOGY

- Benign peripheral nerve sheath tumor composed predominantly of Schwann cells and arising directly within tubular gastrointestinal tract

CLINICAL ISSUES

- Affects predominantly middle-aged and older adults
- Overall female predominance
- Majority arise in stomach
- Often incidentally discovered
- Treatment: Simple surgical excision is curative
- Excellent prognosis

MACROSCOPIC

- Tumor is centered in muscularis propria but can grow to fill submucosa
- Usually < 10 cm (median: 4.5)

MICROSCOPIC

- Well circumscribed but encapsulated
- Characteristic patchy peripheral lymphoid cuff in 90%
- Predominantly interlacing bundles, fascicles, and microtrabeculae of banal spindled cells
  - Mild nuclear atypia with scattered, degenerative, "ancient" nuclei may be seen
  - Mitotic rate low to absent
- Nuclear palisading, hyalinized vessels, Verocay body formation all rare to absent

ANCILLARY TESTS

- S100 protein (+), SOX10 (+), GFAP(+)
- SMA(-), desmin (-), CD117(-), DOG1(-)

TOP DIFFERENTIAL DIAGNOSES

- Gastrointestinal stromal tumor
- Leiomyoma
- Neurofibroma

(Left) *Although it bears similarities to cellular schwannoma of the soft tissues, gastrointestinal (GI) schwannoma is distinctive in that it is unencapsulated and generally shows an absence of hyalinized vessels and well-formed Verocay bodies.* **(Right)** *A diagnostically useful (though not completely pathognomonic) feature of GI schwannoma is the presence of a patchy lymphoid cuff around the periphery of the tumor. Lymphoid aggregates can also be seen within the lesion.*

Gastrointestinal Schwannoma

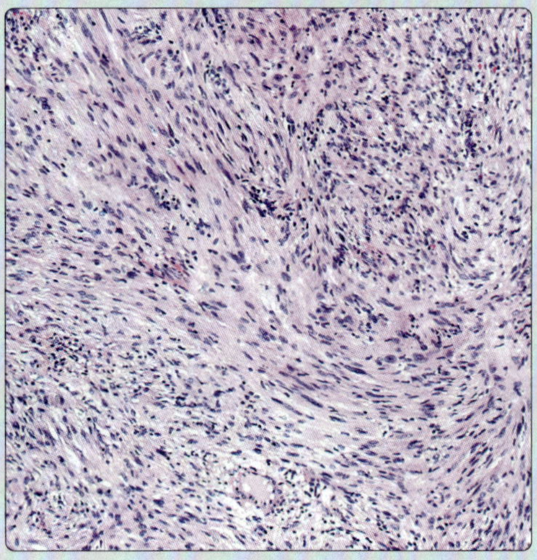

Patchy, Peripheral Lymphoid Cuff

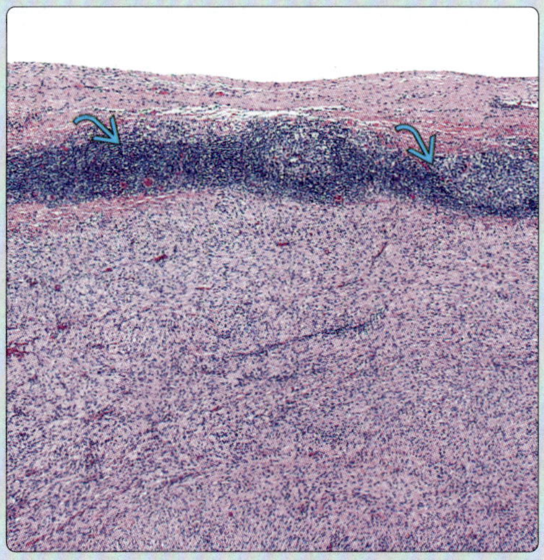

(Left) *An interesting feature of many cases of GI schwannoma is a microtrabecular growth pattern identified by distinct, small linear clusters and cords of tumor cells. This architecture is often seen in addition to more typical fascicular and whorled growth patterns. Note also the lymphocytic infiltrate, another common finding in this tumor.* **(Right)** *Like conventional schwannoma of soft tissue, GI schwannoma classically shows strong and diffuse expression of S100 protein.*

Microtrabecular Growth Pattern

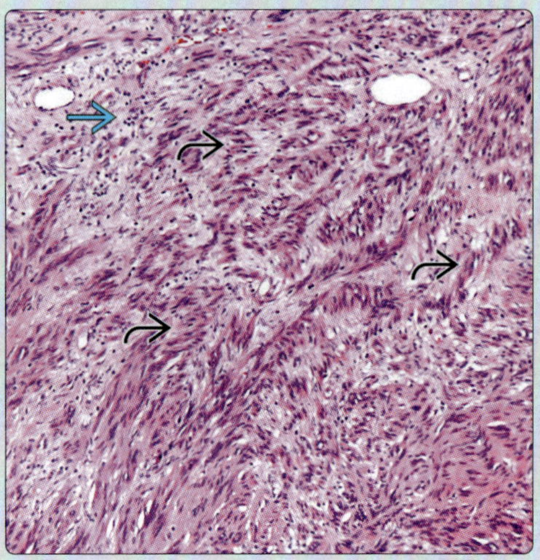

S100 Protein Expression

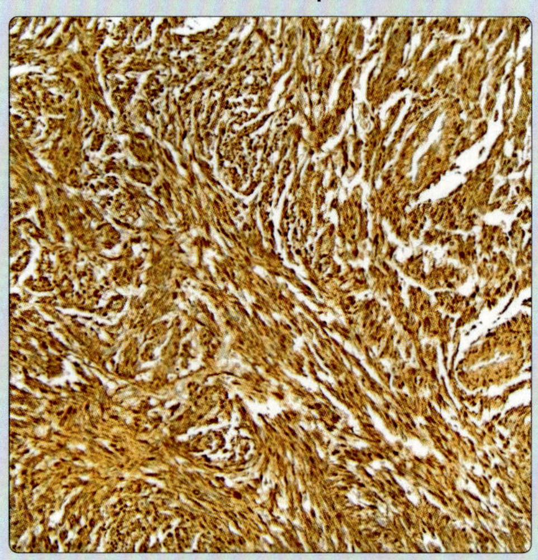

TERMINOLOGY

Definitions

- Benign peripheral nerve sheath tumor composed predominantly of Schwann cells and arising directly within tubular gastrointestinal (GI) tract

ETIOLOGY/PATHOGENESIS

Genetics

- Most analyzed cases lack alteration of *NF2* gene
  - In contrast to conventional, non-GI schwannoma

CLINICAL ISSUES

Epidemiology

- Incidence
  - Rare
    - Greatly outnumbered by gastrointestinal stromal tumor (GIST) in GI tract
- Age
  - Predominantly middle-aged and older adults
- Sex
  - Overall female predominance
    - 4:1 in stomach (largest series)

Site

- Majority arise in stomach
- Less frequent in small intestine, colorectum, and esophagus

Presentation

- Often incidentally discovered
- Can cause bleeding, discomfort, &/or obstructive symptoms
- Association with neurofibromatosis exceptionally rare

Treatment

- Simple surgical excision is curative

Prognosis

- Excellent
- No recurrences or metastases reported

MACROSCOPIC

General Features

- Well-circumscribed, firm mass
  - Overlying ulceration of mucosa in 1/2 of cases
- Tan/gray to yellow/white cut surface
- Tumor is centered in muscularis propria but can grow to fill submucosa

Size

- Usually < 10 cm (median: 4.5)

MICROSCOPIC

Histologic Features

- Well circumscribed but encapsulated
  - Tumor cells can appear to infiltrate between fibers of muscularis propria
  - Characteristic patchy peripheral lymphoid cuff in most cases (90%)
    - May contain reactive germinal centers
- Predominantly interlacing bundles, fascicles, and microtrabeculae of banal spindled cells
  - Moderate cellularity
  - Mild nuclear atypia with scattered, degenerative, "ancient" nuclei may be seen
  - Mitotic rate low to absent
- Stromal lymphocytic infiltrate (± plasma cells) common
- In contrast to conventional soft tissue schwannoma, some features of GI schwannoma are rare to absent
  - Nuclear palisading, hyalinized vessels, foamy histiocytes, well-formed Verocay bodies
- Finely collagenous to myxoid stroma
- Occasional tumors (usually intestinal) can show morphologic patterns of conventional non-GI schwannoma
  - Epithelioid, plexiform, pseudoglandular, microcystic/reticular

ANCILLARY TESTS

Immunohistochemistry

- Strong, diffuse S100 protein (+), SOX10(+)
- Variable GFAP(+)
- May rarely express cytokeratin AE1/AE3
- Usually SMA(-), desmin (-), CD117(-), DOG1(-), HMB-45(-)

DIFFERENTIAL DIAGNOSIS

Gastrointestinal Stromal Tumor

- Much more common than GI schwannoma
- Generally lacks peripheral lymphoid cuff
- CD117(+), DOG1(+), CD34(+), S100 protein (-)
- *KIT* or *PDGFRA* mutations in most cases

Leiomyoma

- Prominent cytologic eosinophilia
- Generally lacks peripheral lymphoid cuff
- SMA(+), desmin (+), S100 protein (-)

Neurofibroma

- Usually plexiform type in GI tract
- Lacks fascicular and microtrabecular growth patterns
- Less cellular than GI schwannoma

Hybrid Nerve Sheath Tumor

- Can arise within GI tract but very rare
- Few reported cases have been schwannoma/perineurioma
  - Lacks peripheral lymphoid cuff and microtrabecular architecture of GI schwannoma
  - Expression of S100 protein and perineurial cell markers (EMA, claudin-1)

SELECTED REFERENCES

1. Hu BG et al: Gastric schwannoma: a tumor must be included in differential diagnoses of gastric submucosal tumors. Case Rep Gastrointest Med. 2017:9615359, 2017
2. Mohanty SK et al: Gastric GIST or gastric schwannoma-a diagnostic dilemma in a young female. Int J Surg Case Rep. 28:60-64, 2016
3. Tao K et al: Clinicopathologic features of gastric schwannoma: 8-year experience at a single institution in china. Medicine (Baltimore). 94(45):e1970, 2015
4. Voltaggio L et al: Gastrointestinal tract spindle cell lesions-just like real estate, it's all about location. Mod Pathol. 28 Suppl 1:S47-66, 2015
5. Voltaggio L et al: Gastric schwannoma: a clinicopathologic study of 51 cases and critical review of the literature. Hum Pathol. 43(5):650-9, 2012

Gastrointestinal Smooth Muscle Neoplasms

KEY FACTS

TERMINOLOGY

- Leiomyoma (LM)
- Leiomyosarcoma (LMS)
- Mesenchymal tumors in GI tract composed of smooth muscle cells
  - Benign (LM) or malignant (LMS)
  - May arise as small polyp from muscularis mucosa (superficial LM) or as mural mass from muscularis propria

CLINICAL ISSUES

- General male predominance (~ 2.5:1)
- Superficial LM presents as asymptomatic polyp, usually in colorectum
- Mural LM most common in esophagus; also, stomach
- Excellent prognosis in superficial and mural LMs
- Generally poor prognosis for LMS at any GI site

MACROSCOPIC

- Superficial LM is usually 1-5 mm
- Mural LM several cm or larger

MICROSCOPIC

- All show smooth muscle cytologic features (prominent cytoplasmic eosinophilia, oval blunted nuclei)
  - Nuclear pleomorphism, mitoses, necrosis in LMS

ANCILLARY TESTS

- SMA(+), desmin (+) in all types of LM
- Desmin may be focal or negative in LMS
- Negative for CD117, DOG1, CD34, S100 protein

TOP DIFFERENTIAL DIAGNOSES

- Gastrointestinal stromal tumor
- Gastrointestinal schwannoma
- Inflammatory fibroid polyp
- LMS (extrinsic to GI tract)

Superficial (Polypoid) Leiomyoma

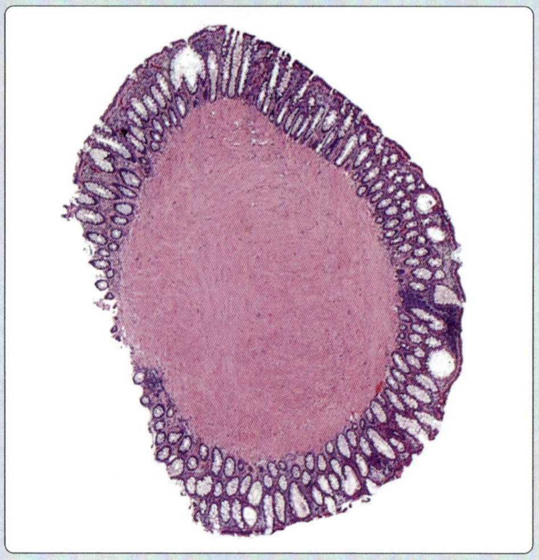

Superficial Leiomyoma

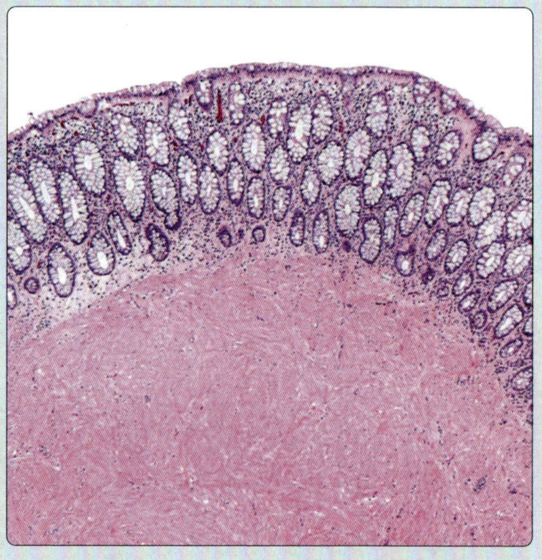

(Left) *Leiomyoma (LM) of the GI tract most commonly arises from the muscularis mucosa and appears as a small polyp, most frequently in the sigmoid or rectum. All show a well-circumscribed contour and appear as an eosinophilic nodule at low power.* **(Right)** *Superficial LM usually shows a sharp demarcation from the overlying mucosa; however, it is not uncommon to see small strands or fascicles of tumor cells extending into the base of the mucosa.*

Smooth Muscle Cytology

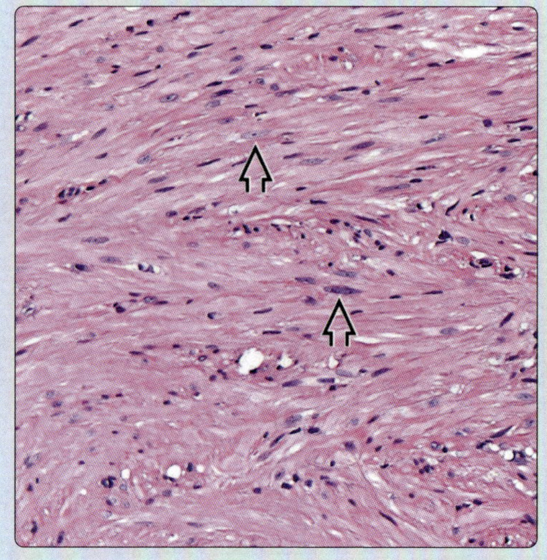

Smooth Muscle Actin (SMA) Expression

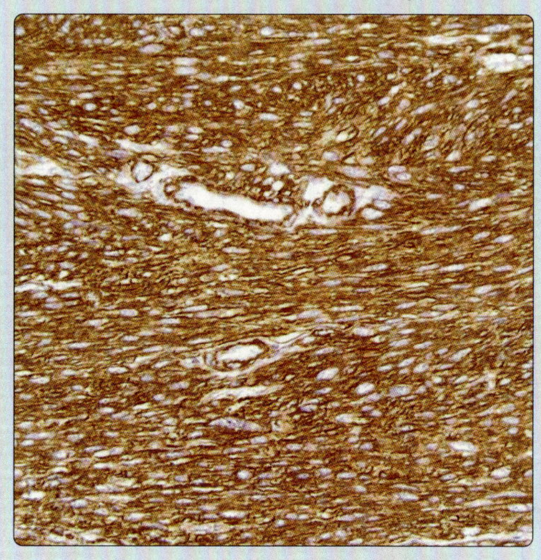

(Left) *As is the case in sites throughout the body, LM (both superficial and mural types) is composed of spindled cells with mature smooth muscle differentiation (prominent eosinophilic cytoplasm and oval cigar-shaped nuclei ⇨). The overall cellularity is generally low.* **(Right)** *Expression of diffuse SMA (shown) and desmin is characteristic of LM. Note, however, that desmin expression may be focal or absent in leiomyosarcoma (LMS).*

TERMINOLOGY

Abbreviations

- Leiomyoma (LM)
- Leiomyosarcoma (LMS)

Synonyms

- Mural leiomyoma (deep leiomyoma)

Definitions

- Mesenchymal tumors in GI tract composed of smooth muscle cells
  - Benign (LM) or malignant (LMS)
  - May arise as small polyp from muscularis mucosa (superficial LM) or as mural mass from muscularis propria

CLINICAL ISSUES

Epidemiology

- Incidence
  - Generally uncommon overall
    - Superficial LM is more common than mural LM
  - Varies depending on site in GI tract
    - Mural LM is most common mesenchymal tumor in esophagus
    - Superficial LM most frequent in sigmoid colon and rectum
    - LMS very rare, regardless of GI tract site
      - Secondary GI tract involvement by LMS from other primary site (e.g., retroperitoneum, uterus) must always be excluded
- Age
  - Median of 62 years in superficial LM
  - 30-50 years most common in mural LM
  - Most patients with LMS over age 50
- Sex
  - General male predominance (~ 2.5:1)

Site

- Superficial LM usually arises in colorectum
- Mural LM most common in esophagus (particularly distal, near gastroesophageal junction)
  - Also arise in stomach
  - Rarely anorectum, duodenum
- LMS may arise in colon (particularly right side), esophagus, stomach, duodenum

Presentation

- Superficial LM is usually asymptomatic (detected on screening endoscopy)
  - Small, nonspecific polyp
- Mural esophageal LM may present with dysphagia or be incidental discovery on imaging
  - Small, microscopic ("seedling") mural LM may be discovered incidentally on resection for unrelated tumor
- GI bleeding, abdominal pain, obstruction in rare deep colonic tumors (mural LM/LMS)

Treatment

- Polypectomy for small, superficial lesions
- Simple excision (enucleation) for mural LM
- Complete surgical resection for LMS

Prognosis

- Excellent prognosis in superficial and mural LM
  - All benign with no risk of malignant degeneration
- Generally poor prognosis for LMS at any GI site
  - Polypoid intraluminal LMS may have better prognosis

IMAGING

General Features

- Mural LM is often misconstrued as gastrointestinal stromal tumor on imaging
- Large esophageal LM may bulge externally and be confused clinically for primary tumor of posterior mediastinum

MACROSCOPIC

General Features

- Firm, fibrous, tan-white cut surface
  - LMS additionally often features necrosis, hemorrhage, &/or surface ulceration
- LM is generally a well-circumscribed mass
  - Esophageal LM may show lobulations or serpiginous contours

Size

- Superficial LM is usually 1-5 mm
- Esophageal mural LM has median of 5 cm
  - Microscopic "seedling" mural LM
  - Some cases > 10 cm
- LMS tends to be much larger on average than mural LM

MICROSCOPIC

Histologic Features

- Superficial (polypoid) LM
  - Arises from muscularis mucosa
    - Cells often peripherally merge with adjacent normal smooth muscle
  - Small, well circumscribed, nodular
  - Usually of low cellularity
  - Composed of uniform spindled smooth muscle cells
    - Prominent eosinophilic cytoplasm, bland oval (cigar-shaped) nuclei
    - Very rare cases with isolated bizarre nuclear atypia ("symplastic LM")
    - Eosinophilic intracytoplasmic globules common
    - Mitoses and necrosis absent
  - Scattered intratumoral mast cells may be present
- Mural (deep) LM
  - Arises from muscularis propria
  - Well circumscribed or rounded
    - Esophageal tumors may be more lobular or show serpentine borders
  - Composed of uniform, bland, spindled smooth muscle cells
  - Calcification and other degenerative changes (e.g., edema) may be seen
  - Intratumoral mast cells &/or interstitial cells of Cajal (ICC) may be present
    - May lead to diagnostic confusion when using immunohistochemistry

- LMS
  - Usually large, invasive, destructive tumors
    - Surface ulceration common
  - Morphologically similar to LMS elsewhere
    - Nuclear pleomorphism and necrosis common
    - Mitoses often numerous and include atypical forms

ANCILLARY TESTS

Immunohistochemistry

- Diffuse cytoplasmic SMA(+), desmin (+), h-caldesmon (+) in all types of LM
  - Desmin (+) less frequent in LMS (40-50% of cases)
- Negative for CD117 (KIT), DOG1, CD34, S100 protein, keratin
  - Pitfalls
    - Intratumoral mast cells express CD117
    - Intratumoral ICCs, if present, may express CD117 and DOG1
      - Seen in mural (deep) LM, not superficial LM

DIFFERENTIAL DIAGNOSIS

Gastrointestinal Stromal Tumor

- Arises from muscularis propria, not muscularis mucosa
- Most common in stomach; rare in esophagus and colorectum
- May show spindled &/or epithelioid morphologies
  - Often much more cellular than LM
- Strong, diffuse CD117(+) &/or DOG1(+)
- Majority are CD34(+)
- Occasional tumors express SMA or H-caldesmon
- Generally negative for S100 protein, keratin, and desmin
- Majority show *KIT* or *PDGFRA* mutation

Gastrointestinal Schwannoma

- Most common in stomach
- Arises in muscularis propria but often grows into submucosa
- Lacks prominent cytoplasmic eosinophilia of LM
- Patchy, peripheral lymphoid cuff common
- Strong S100 protein (+)
- Generally negative for SMA and desmin

Mucosal Schwann Cell Hamartoma

- Small, bland spindle cell proliferation within superficial mucosa
- Strong S100 protein (+)
- Negative for SMA and desmin

Inflammatory Fibroid Polyp

- Arise in submucosa
- Most common in stomach (particularly antrum) and small intestine
- Lacks prominent cytoplasmic eosinophilia of LM
- Prominent chronic inflammatory infiltrate (particularly eosinophils)
- CD34(+)
- Negative for SMA and desmin
- *PDGFRA* mutations

Mucosal Perineurioma

- Presents as small mucosal polyp
- Often associated with serrated lesion (hyperplastic polyp, serrated adenoma)
- Grows in between and around crypts in mucosa
- Lacks prominent cytoplasmic eosinophilia of LM
- EMA(+), claudin-1 (+)
- Negative for SMA and desmin

Leiomyosarcoma (Extrinsic to GI Tract)

- Must always be excluded before diagnosing primary GI tract LMS
- Most often from retroperitoneum or gynecologic tract (e.g., uterus)
- Histologic and immunohistochemical features are identical

Granular Cell Tumor

- Polygonal to spindled cells with prominent granular cytoplasm
- Strong S100 protein (+)
- Negative for SMA and desmin

SELECTED REFERENCES

1. Lopes CV et al: Differential diagnosis of mesenchymal neoplasms of the digestive tract by cell block and immunohistochemistry. Cytopathology. ePub, 2018
2. Voltaggio L et al: Gastrointestinal tract spindle cell lesions-just like real estate, it's all about location. Mod Pathol. 28 Suppl 1:S47-66, 2015
3. Deshpande A et al: Leiomyoma of the gastrointestinal tract with interstitial cells of Cajal: a mimic of gastrointestinal stromal tumor. Am J Surg Pathol. 38(1):72-7, 2014
4. Hechtman JF et al: Corpora amylacea in gastrointestinal leiomyomas: a clinical, light microscopic, ultrastructural and immunohistochemical study with comparison to hyaline globules. J Clin Pathol. 66(11):951-5, 2013
5. Rittershaus AC et al: Benign gastrointestinal mesenchymal BUMPS: a brief review of some spindle cell polyps with published names. Arch Pathol Lab Med. 135(10):1311-9, 2011
6. Abraham SC: Distinguishing gastrointestinal stromal tumors from their mimics: an update. Adv Anat Pathol. 14(3):178-88, 2007
7. Abraham SC et al: "Seedling" mesenchymal tumors (gastrointestinal stromal tumors and leiomyomas) are common incidental tumors of the esophagogastric junction. Am J Surg Pathol. 31(11):1629-35, 2007
8. Agaimy A et al: True smooth muscle neoplasms of the gastrointestinal tract: morphological spectrum and classification in a series of 85 cases from a single institute. Langenbecks Arch Surg. 392(1):75-81, 2007
9. Matsukuma S et al: Endoscopically resected colorectal leiomyomas often containing eosinophilic globules. Histopathology. 45(3):302-3, 2004
10. Miettinen M et al: Gastrointestinal stromal tumors, intramural leiomyomas, and leiomyosarcomas in the duodenum: a clinicopathologic, immunohistochemical, and molecular genetic study of 167 cases. Am J Surg Pathol. 27(5):625-41, 2003
11. Miettinen M et al: Gastrointestinal stromal tumors, intramural leiomyomas, and leiomyosarcomas in the rectum and anus: a clinicopathologic, immunohistochemical, and molecular genetic study of 144 cases. Am J Surg Pathol. 25(9):1121-33, 2001
12. Miettinen M et al: Gastrointestinal stromal tumors and leiomyosarcomas in the colon: a clinicopathologic, immunohistochemical, and molecular genetic study of 44 cases. Am J Surg Pathol. 24(10):1339-52, 2000
13. Miettinen M et al: Esophageal stromal tumors: a clinicopathologic, immunohistochemical, and molecular genetic study of 17 cases and comparison with esophageal leiomyomas and leiomyosarcomas. Am J Surg Pathol. 24(2):211-22, 2000

Mural Leiomyoma

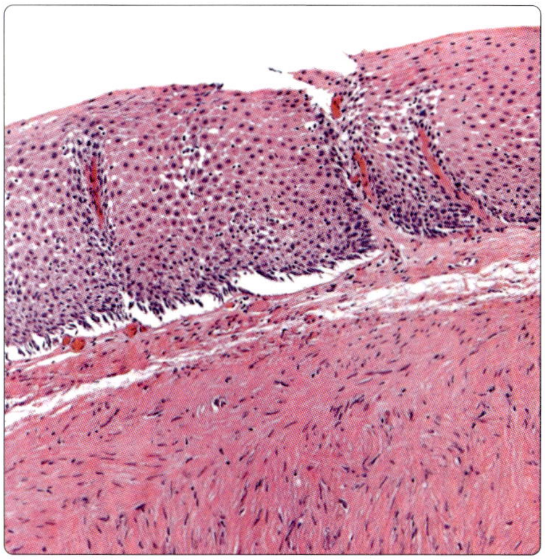

Calcifications

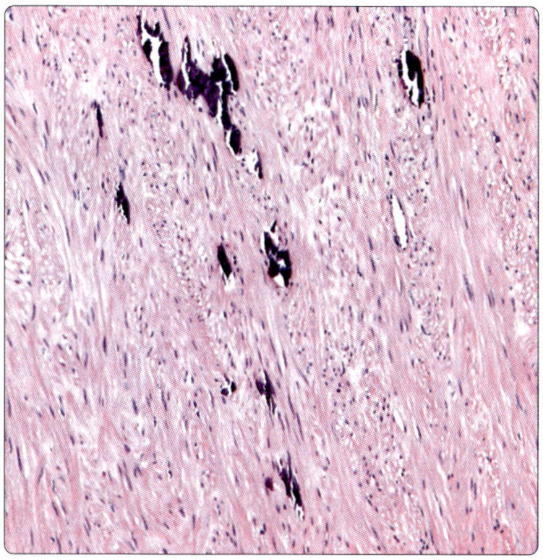

(Left) *Mural LM is histologically identical to superficial LM; however, it arises from the muscularis propria rather than the muscularis mucosa and therefore is often much larger. It most commonly arises in the esophagus (shown), and the overlying epithelium can show features suggestive of reflux esophagitis.* **(Right)** *Calcifications are common in mural leiomyoma.*

Hyaline Globules

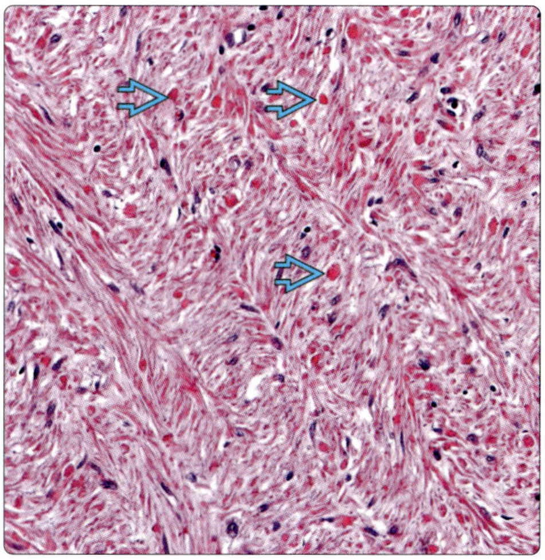

Leiomyosarcoma of GI Tract

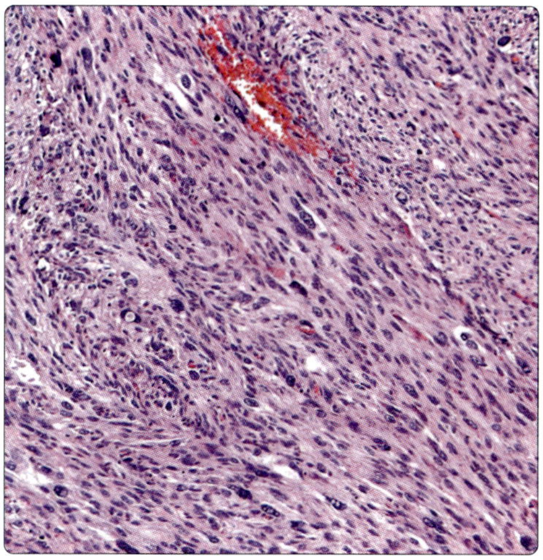

(Left) *Hyaline globules are relatively common in all forms of GI leiomyoma and can be focal or abundant. They are likely a form of cellular degeneration.* **(Right)** *Primary LMS of the GI tract is very rare, and secondary involvement from an external primary (such as from the retroperitoneum or uterus) should always be excluded. Histologically, GI LMS is indistinguishable from LMS at other sites and usually features overt nuclear pleomorphism and atypia, at least focally.*

Leiomyosarcoma of GI Tract

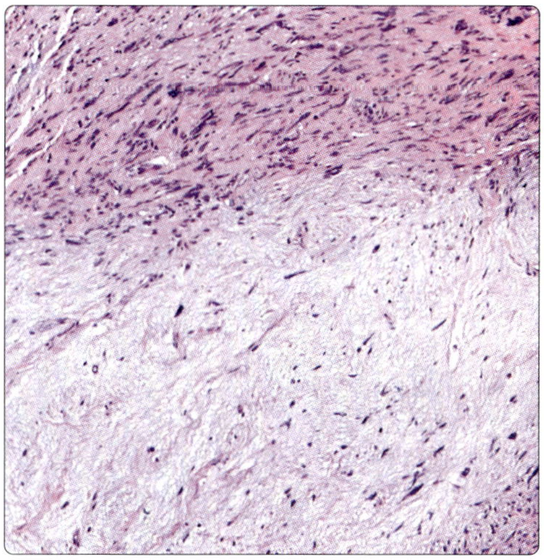

Leiomyosarcoma of GI Tract

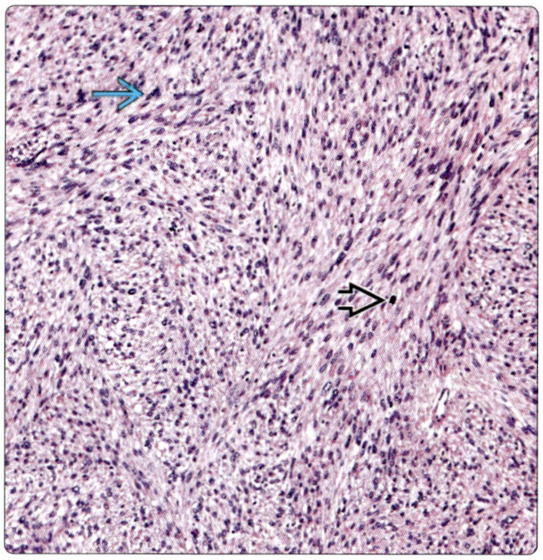

(Left) *As can be seen in tumors from other sites/organs, myxoid change is a feature in some cases of GI LMS and may lead to consideration of a gastrointestinal stromal tumor (GIST). Note, however, that nuclear pleomorphism is rare in spindled GISTs.* **(Right)** *Some cases of GI LMS are well differentiated and show only mild or focal nuclear pleomorphism. Identification of mitoses and observation of aggressive, infiltrative growth is helpful.*

Inflammatory Fibroid Polyp

KEY FACTS

TERMINOLOGY

- Distinctive benign fibroblastic neoplasm of gastrointestinal tract characterized by bland, spindled to stellate cells and admixed chronic inflammatory cells within prominent vascularized stroma

CLINICAL ISSUES

- Most common in older adults (mean: 60 years)
- Stomach (particularly antrum) is most common site overall
  - Also arises in small intestine and colorectum
- Nonspecific abdominal pain or asymptomatic
- Small intestinal tumors often cause intussusception
- Treatment: Simple excision
- Excellent prognosis

MACROSCOPIC

- Solitary sessile or polypoid submucosal growth
- Most 1-5 cm in size

MICROSCOPIC

- Loose, haphazard proliferation of bland, spindled to stellate cells within prominent vascularized stroma
  - Perivascular or periglandular orientation of tumor cells ("onion-skin") in most cases
- Loose collagenous to myxoid stroma
- Multinucleated stromal giant cells in minority of cases
- Mixed chronic inflammatory infiltrate in all cases
  - Eosinophils typically prominent but may be sparse

ANCILLARY TESTS

- CD34(+)
- CD117, DOG1, S100, EMA, keratin, ALK1 (-)
- Molecular: *PDGFRA* mutations in majority of cases

TOP DIFFERENTIAL DIAGNOSES

- Gastrointestinal stromal tumor
- Inflammatory myofibroblastic tumor
- Perineurioma

Inflammatory Fibroid Polyp

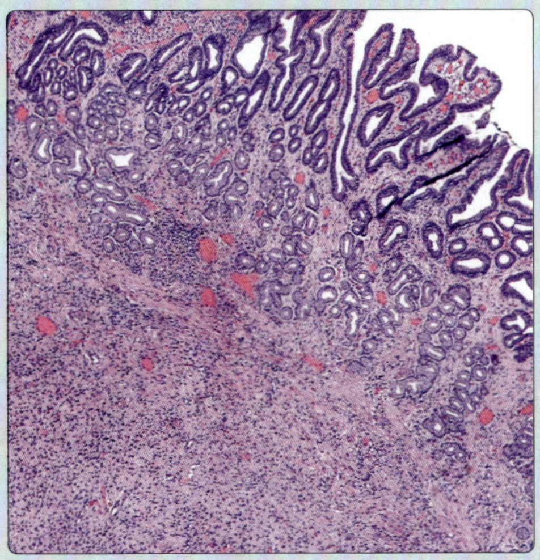

Inflammatory Fibroid Polyp

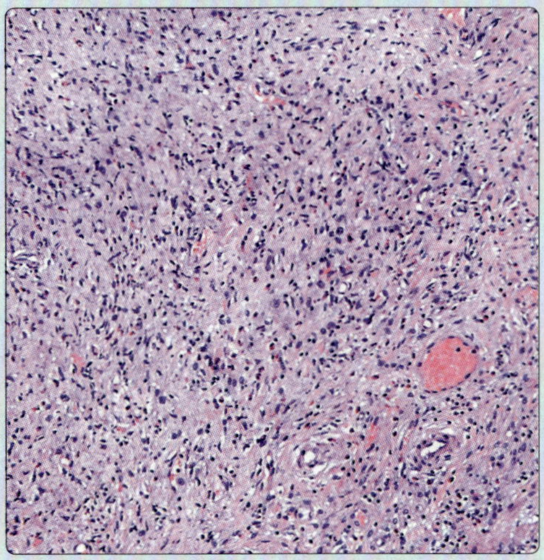

(Left) *Inflammatory fibroid polyp (IFP) is a distinctive benign mesenchymal neoplasm of the gastrointestinal tract that occurs predominantly in the stomach, large bowel, and small intestine. As shown in this H&E, IFP arises in the submucosa but often extends into the overlying mucosa.* **(Right)** *The typical case of IFP is composed of a haphazard arrangement of cytologically bland, spindled and stellate fibroblastic cells within a variable fibromyxoid and vascularized stroma.*

Onion-Skin Pattern

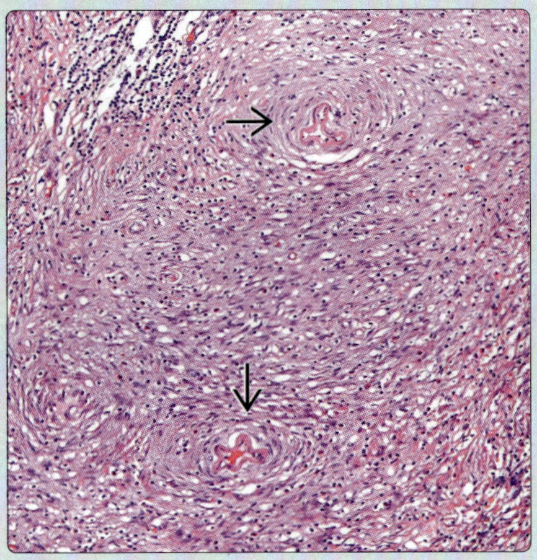

Eosinophils

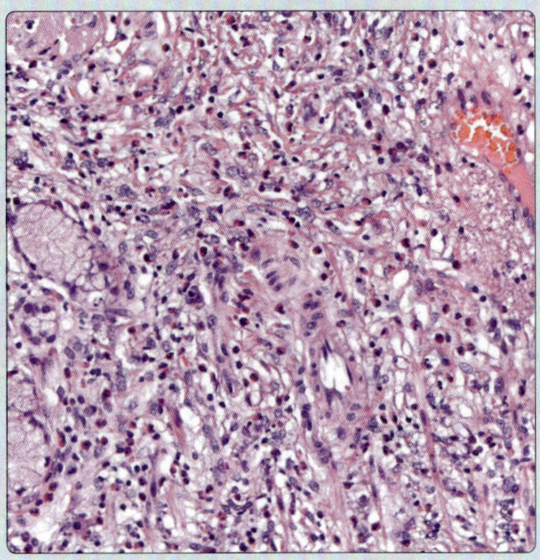

(Left) *A characteristic finding seen in most cases of IFP is a concentric onion-skin arrangement ➩ of tumor cells around stromal blood vessels &/or mucosal glands; however, this finding may be subtle or entirely absent in some cases.* **(Right)** *A mixed chronic inflammatory infiltrate is present in all cases of IFP but varies in prominence. Eosinophils are often the most noticeable type of cell and can be numerous; however, lymphocytes, plasma cells, and mast cells are also often seen.*

TERMINOLOGY

Abbreviations

- Inflammatory fibroid polyp (IFP)

Synonyms

- Vanek tumor

Definitions

- Distinctive benign fibroblastic proliferation of gastrointestinal tract characterized by bland, spindled to stellate cells and admixed chronic inflammatory cells within prominent vascularized stroma

CLINICAL ISSUES

Epidemiology

- Incidence
  - Rare
- Age
  - Most common in older adults (mean: 60 years)
- Sex
  - Female predominance

Site

- Stomach is most common site overall
  - Particularly gastric antrum
- Also arises in small intestine and colorectum
- Very rare cases reported in esophagus, appendix, anus

Presentation

- Nonspecific abdominal pain or asymptomatic
- Can be incidental finding discovered on endoscopy
  - For routine screening or for other diseases (e.g., inflammatory bowel disease)
- May present with obstructive symptoms related to intussusception
  - Particularly small bowel tumors

Treatment

- Simple excision or polypectomy

Prognosis

- Excellent
- No significant risk of recurrence
- No malignant potential

MACROSCOPIC

General Features

- Solitary sessile or polypoid growth
  - Overlying surface ulceration in 1/3 of cases
- Arises from submucosa

Size

- Most 1-5 cm

MICROSCOPIC

Histologic Features

- Well marginated and submucosal based but can involve overlying mucosa
- Loose, haphazard proliferation of bland, spindled to stellate cells within prominent vascularized stroma
  - Variable cellularity
  - Perivascular or periglandular orientation of tumor cells ("onion-skin") in most cases
  - Short fascicular growth seen in some cases
- Multinucleated stromal giant cells in minority of cases
- Loose collagenous to myxoid stroma
  - Can be hyalinized
- Mixed chronic inflammatory infiltrate in all cases
  - Eosinophils typically prominent but may be sparse
  - Lymphoid aggregates common
- Mitoses rare to absent; no necrosis
- Background gastric mucosa often shows features of chronic gastritis
  - Concomitant *Helicobacter pylori* infection not uncommon (up to 1/2 of cases in one large series)

ANCILLARY TESTS

Immunohistochemistry

- CD34(+) in majority
- Occasional cases show focal SMA(+), desmin (+)
- CD117, DOG1, S100, EMA, keratin, ALK1 (-)

Molecular Genetics

- Activating *PDGFRA* mutations in majority of cases
  - Exon 18 mutations most common in stomach
  - Exon 12 mutations most common in small intestine

DIFFERENTIAL DIAGNOSIS

Gastrointestinal Stromal Tumor

- CD117(+), DOG1(+), CD34(+)
- Most contain *KIT* mutations
- *PDGFRA*-mutant gastrointestinal stromal tumor much less common than *KIT* mutants and often shows epithelioid morphology

Inflammatory Myofibroblastic Tumor

- Most common in children, adolescents, and young adults
- Arises externally to gastrointestinal tract (i.e., mesentery)
- ALK1(+) in majority of cases

Perineurioma

- Lamellar, storiform, and whorled growth common
- EMA(+), claudin-1 (+), variable CD34(+)
- Lacks *PDGFRA* mutations

SELECTED REFERENCES

1. Voltaggio L et al: Polypoid stromal lesions of the intestines. Histopathology. 66(1):88-101, 2015
2. Albuquerque A et al: Evaluation of clinico-pathological features and Helicobacter pylori infection in gastric inflammatory fibroid polyps. Virchows Arch. 465(6):643-7, 2014
3. Liu TC et al: Inflammatory fibroid polyps of the gastrointestinal tract: spectrum of clinical, morphologic, and immunohistochemistry features. Am J Surg Pathol. 37(4):586-92, 2013
4. Daum O et al: Comparison of morphological, immunohistochemical, and molecular genetic features of inflammatory fibroid polyps (Vanek's tumors). Virchows Arch. 456(5):491-7, 2010
5. Lasota J et al: Gain-of-function PDGFRA mutations, earlier reported in gastrointestinal stromal tumors, are common in small intestinal inflammatory fibroid polyps. A study of 60 cases. Mod Pathol. 22(8):1049-56, 2009

(Left) *Although IFP arises in the submucosa and is relatively well marginated, variable extension into the overlying mucosa is not uncommon. Tumor cells often grow around clusters of mucosal glands* ➡*, as shown here.* **(Right)** *Fragments or strips of overrun smooth muscle fibers* ➡ *of the muscularis mucosa may be seen in cases of IFP with mucosal extension. Note the entrapped mucosal glands* ⇨*.*

Mucosal Extension

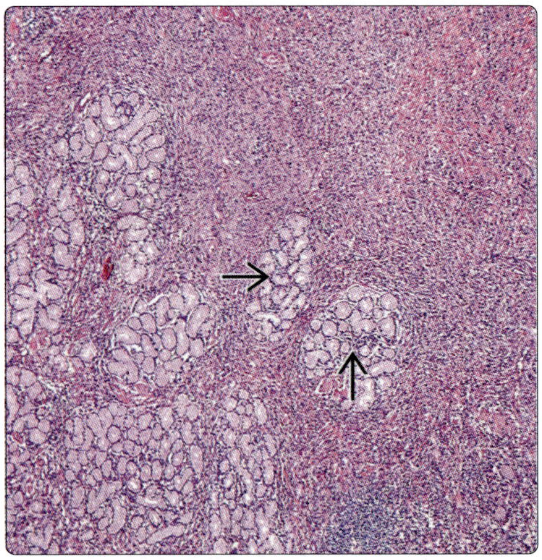

Entrapped Muscularis Mucosa

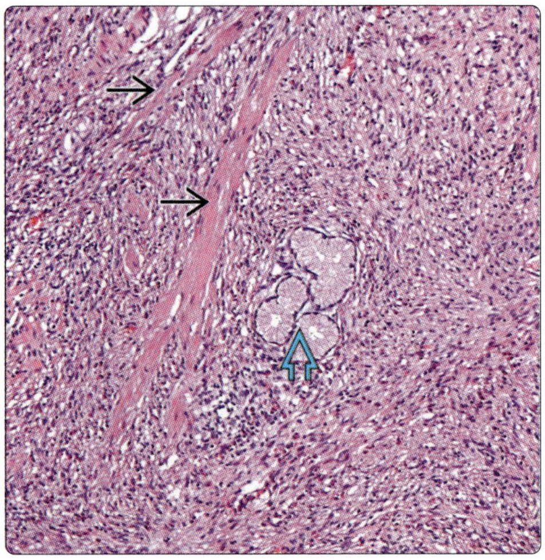

(Left) *The most common gastrointestinal tract location for IFP to arise in is the stomach (particularly the antrum); however, it also occurs in the small intestine and large intestine (shown). Note how the tumor cells grow through and around mucosal crypts. Although not obvious at low power, eosinophils were abundant in this case.* **(Right)** *Stromal lymphocytes are a common finding in IFP, as are large mucosal and submucosal lymphoid aggregates* ⇨*.*

Colonic Inflammatory Fibroid Polyp

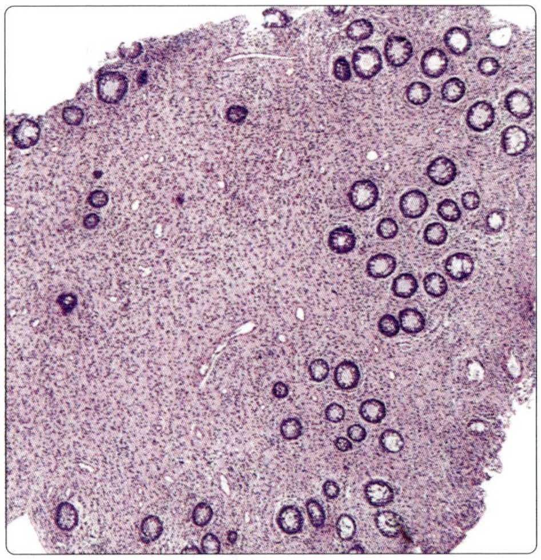

Lymphoid Aggregates

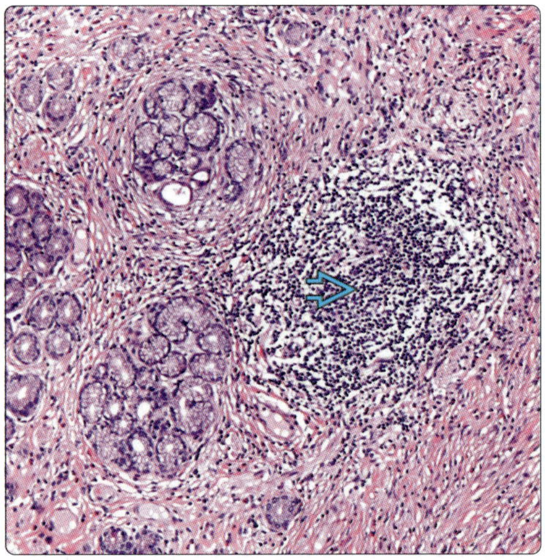

(Left) *Multinucleated stromal giant cells* ➡ *are seen in ~ 1/3 of cases of IFP. Note the perivascular "onion-skin" growth* ↪ *in this H&E.* **(Right)** *The stroma in IFP varies from loose and collagenous to myxoid or edematous. Thin collagen bundles may be prominent in some cases, as depicted in this H&E.*

Multinucleated Giant Cells

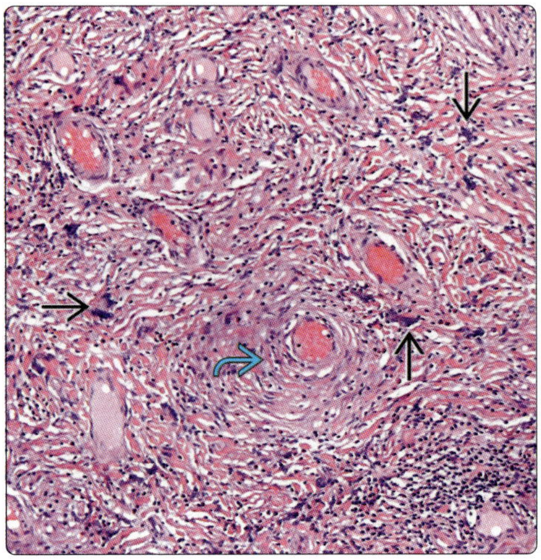

Stromal Collagen

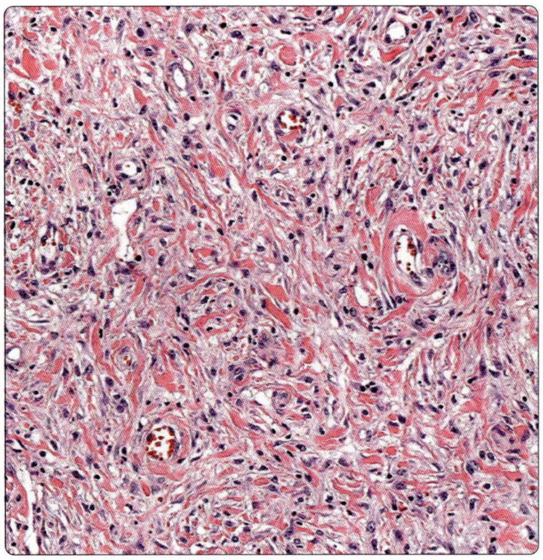

Hypocellular Tumors

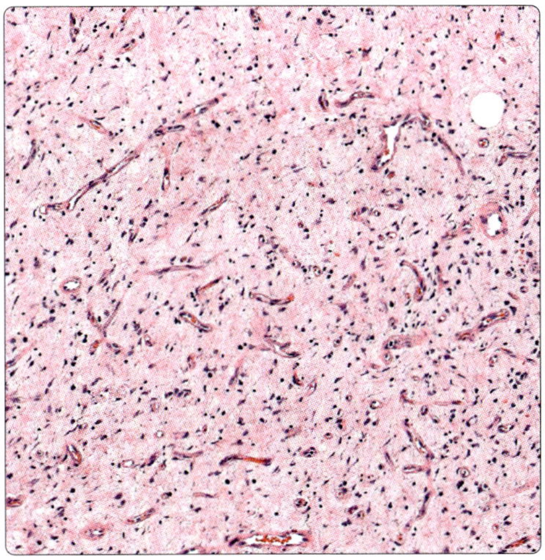

Mast Cells

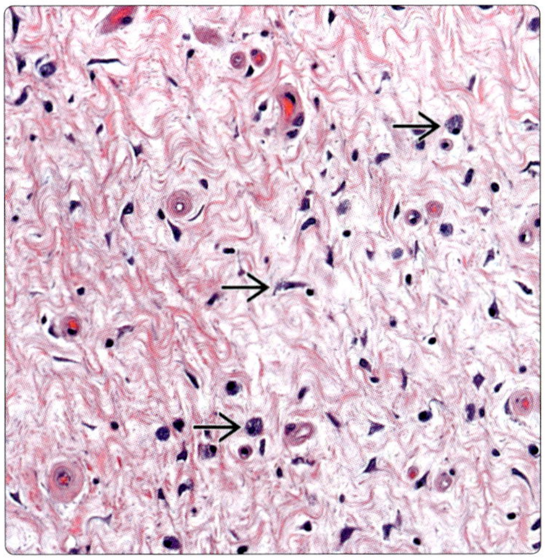

(Left) *Some cases of IFP are paucicellular and can be prominently hyalinized. The vascularized stroma is often better appreciated in these examples. Of note, eosinophils may be less conspicuous in cases of IFP with stromal hyalinization.* **(Right)** *Although the eosinophil is the most recognized type of inflammatory cell associated with IFP, other types of cells are commonly present, including lymphocytes, plasma cells, and mast cells* ➞*. Neutrophils are not generally a feature of IFP.*

Short Fascicular Growth

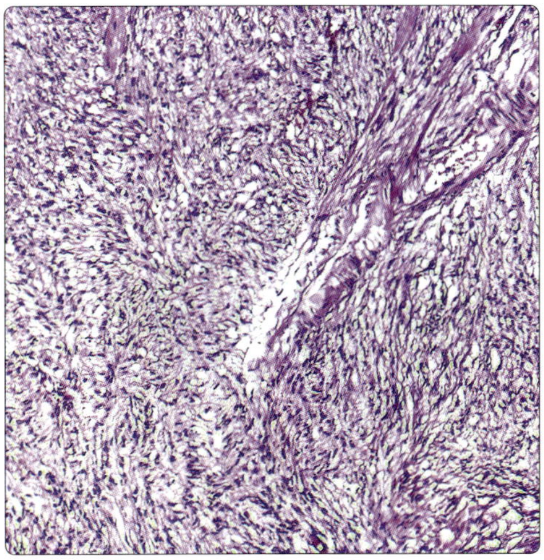

Vascularized Stroma

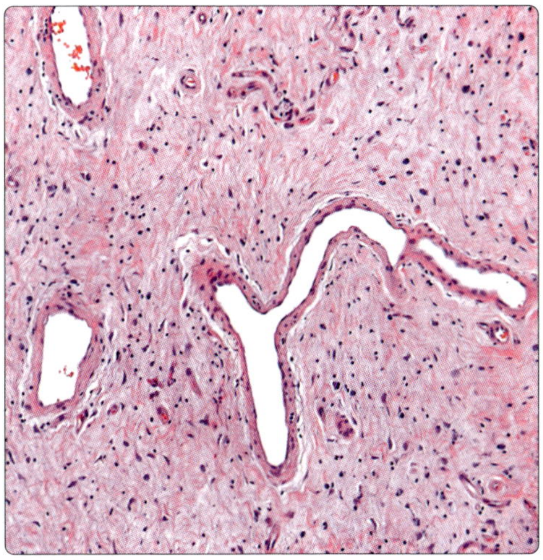

(Left) *A more organized, short, fascicular or bundled pattern of growth can be seen in some cases of IFP and may lead to morphologic confusion with gastrointestinal stromal tumor (GIST) or neural tumors. Expression of CD34 in IFP can also lead to confusion with GIST; however, IFP is CD117 and DOG1 negative.* **(Right)** *A vascularized stroma is a typical feature of IFP but varies in prominence. Vessels range from small capillaries to larger, thin-walled vessels.*

Myxoid Stroma

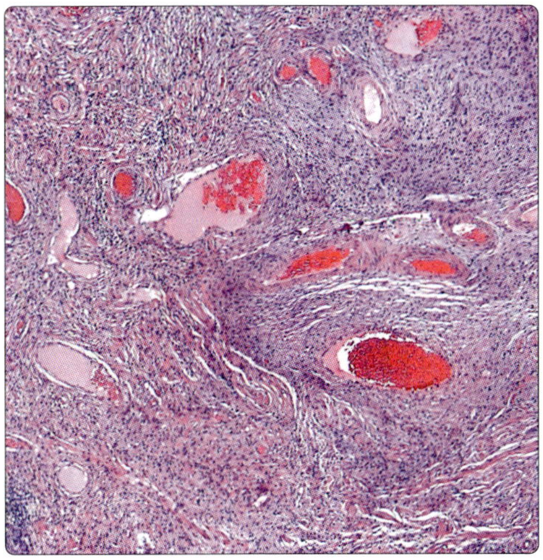

Myxoid Stroma

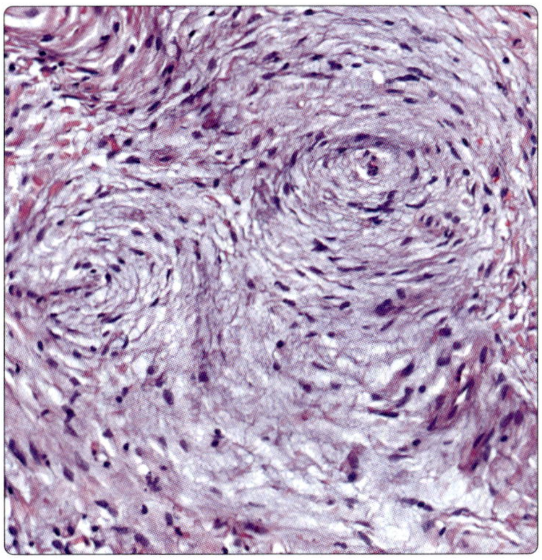

(Left) *H&E shows an IFP with areas of loose collagenous stroma (left) admixed with areas of prominent myxoid stroma (right). Some cases are entirely myxoid. Note the prominent stromal vasculature in this H&E.* **(Right)** *Even in areas of myxoid stroma, other classic features of IFP, including "onion-skin" growth (shown) and a mixed inflammatory cell infiltrate, can be identified.*

Gangliocytic Paraganglioma

KEY FACTS

TERMINOLOGY

- Rare, usually benign, neoplasm composed of 3 distinct cellular components (neuroendocrine, schwannian, and ganglion cell) showing marked predilection for duodenum

CLINICAL ISSUES

- Wide age range (median: 50-55 years)
- Arises in duodenum almost exclusively
- Obstructive biliary symptoms common
- Treatment: Complete surgical excision
- Usually benign with great prognosis
- Rare cases may spread to local lymph nodes

MACROSCOPIC

- Pedunculated or sessile mass
- Often small (1-3 cm)

MICROSCOPIC

- Expansile or infiltrative
- 3 main cellular components in varying proportions
  - Epithelial (neuroendocrine), schwannian, ganglion cells
    - Epithelial component may resemble carcinoid tumor
- Low mitotic activity

ANCILLARY TESTS

- Keratin (+), synaptophysin (+), chromogranin (+) in epithelial component
- S100 protein (+) in spindled Schwann cell component
- Synaptophysin (+), NSE(+) in ganglion cells

TOP DIFFERENTIAL DIAGNOSES

- Carcinoid tumor
- Gastrointestinal stromal tumor (spindled)
- Paraganglioma (conventional)

(Left) *Gangliocytic paraganglioma (GPG) is an unusual neoplasm that shows a striking predilection for the duodenum, particularly in the 2nd part near the ampulla of Vater. Tumors arise in the submucosa but may extend to involve the mucosa or muscular propria.* **(Right)** *The epithelial component of GPG is composed of nests and trabeculae of neuroendocrine cells and is often the most prominent of the 3 components. The morphology may closely resemble a carcinoid tumor.*

Gangliocytic Paraganglioma

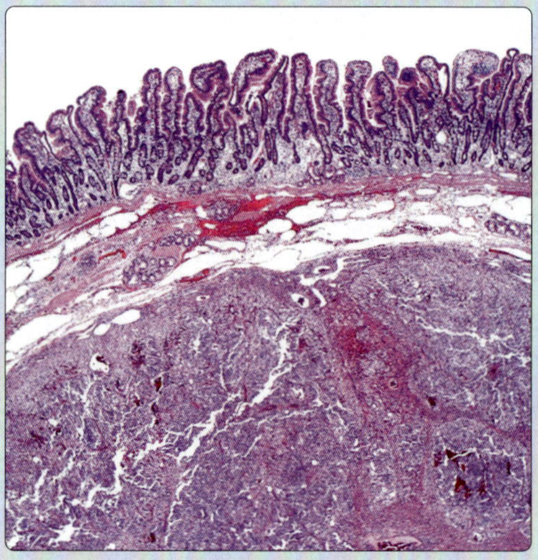

Neuroendocrine Cell Component

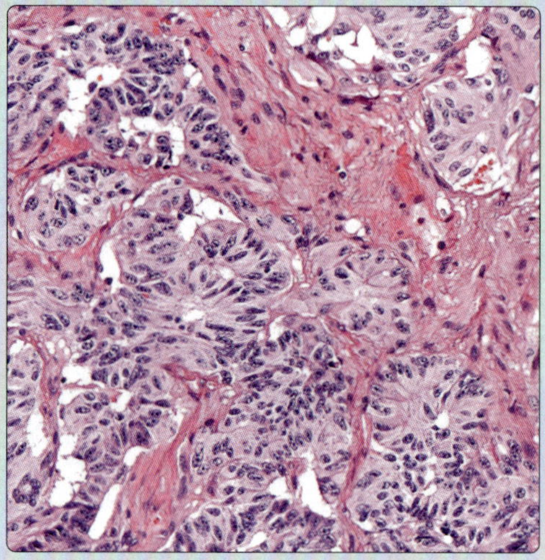

(Left) *The stromal component ➡ of GPG is composed of bland spindled cells with abundant eosinophilic cytoplasm that show evidence of schwannian differentiation, particularly strong S100 protein expression.* **(Right)** *Ganglion cells ➡ may be seen within GPG either singly or in aggregates, and they characteristically show prominent nucleoli. Although they are well developed in many cases, in some tumors, they can be difficult to visualize.*

Spindled Schwann Cell Component

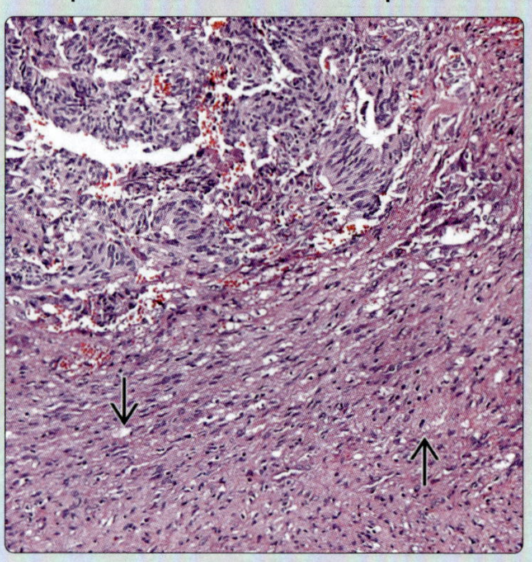

Ganglion Cells

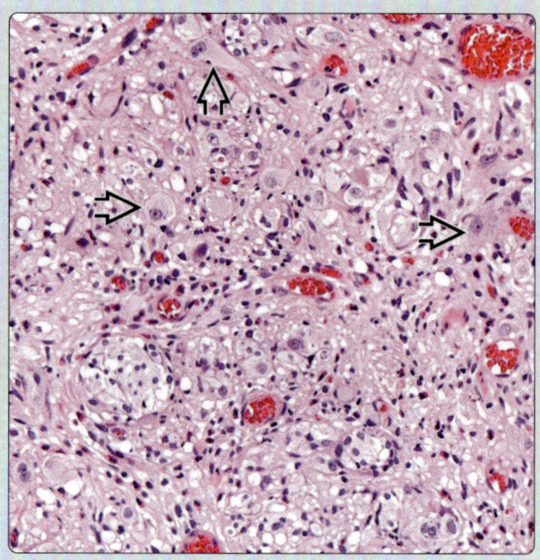

TERMINOLOGY

Abbreviations

- Gangliocytic paraganglioma (GPG)

Synonyms

- Duodenal ganglioneuroma

Definitions

- Rare, usually benign neoplasm composed of 3 distinct cellular components (neuroendocrine, schwannian, and ganglion cell) showing marked predilection for duodenum

CLINICAL ISSUES

Epidemiology

- Incidence
  - Rare
    - Comprise up to 25% of ampullary/periampullary neuroendocrine neoplasms
- Age
  - Wide range (median: 50-55 years)

Site

- Arises in duodenum almost exclusively
  - Usually 2nd portion, around ampulla of Vater
- Very rarely in other sites such as jejunum, stomach, appendix, lung
  - Of note, paraganglioma of cauda equina often shows histologic similarities to GPG

Presentation

- Obstructive biliary symptoms common
- May be asymptomatic

Treatment

- Complete surgical excision
- Local lymph node dissection may be warranted

Prognosis

- Usually benign with great prognosis
- Some cases may spread to local lymph nodes
  - Mostly tumors > 2 cm
  - Generally does not affect prognosis

MACROSCOPIC

General Features

- Pedunculated or sessile mass
- May show ulceration of overlying mucosa

Size

- Often small (1-3 cm)
- Very rare cases > 10 cm

MICROSCOPIC

Histologic Features

- Expansile or infiltrative appearance
  - Arises in submucosa and may involve muscularis propria
  - Admixed smooth muscle fibers of muscularis may be seen within tumor
- 3 main components in varying proportions
  - Epithelial (neuroendocrine)
    - Often most prevalent of 3 components
    - Epithelioid to spindled cells with eosinophilic to amphophilic cytoplasm
      - Uniform ovoid nuclei
    - Arranged in nests ("zellballen" configuration), trabeculae/ribbons, or pseudoglandular structures (often focal)
      - May closely resemble carcinoid tumor
  - Schwannian
    - Short fascicles and sheets of spindled cells
    - May surround epithelial nests, similar to sustentacular cells
  - Ganglion cells
    - Singly or in clusters; uni- or multinucleated
- Rare psammoma bodies
- Mitotic activity low to absent
- No necrosis

ANCILLARY TESTS

Immunohistochemistry

- Keratin (+), synaptophysin (+), chromogranin (+) in epithelial component
- S100 protein (+) in spindled Schwann cell component
  - Also highlights sustentacular cells, if present
- Synaptophysin (+), NSE(+) in ganglion cells

DIFFERENTIAL DIAGNOSIS

Carcinoid Tumor

- Keratin (+), synaptophysin (+), chromogranin (+)
- Lacks spindled S100 protein (+) schwannian component
- Lacks ganglion cells

Gastrointestinal Stromal Tumor (Spindled)

- Originates in muscularis propria
- Diffuse CD117(+), DOG1(+) in lesional cells
- Lacks spindled S100 protein (+) schwannian component
- Lacks ganglion cells

Paraganglioma (Conventional)

- Commonly arise along sympathetic nerve trunk
- Synaptophysin (+), chromogranin (+)
- Lacks spindled S100 protein (+) schwannian component
- Negative for keratins

SELECTED REFERENCES

1. Cathcart SJ et al: Duodenal gangliocytic paraganglioma with lymph node metastases: a case report and comparative review of 31 cases. World J Clin Cases. 5(6):222-233, 2017
2. Park HK et al: Duodenal aangliocytic paraganglioma with lymph node metastasis. Arch Pathol Lab Med. 140(1):94-8, 2016
3. Loftus TJ et al: Duodenal gangliocytic paraganglioma: a case report and literature review. Int J Surg Case Rep. 8C:5-8, 2015
4. Rowsell C et al: Gangliocytic paraganglioma: a rare case with metastases of all 3 elements to liver and lymph nodes. Ann Diagn Pathol. 15(6):467-71, 2011
5. Witkiewicz A et al: Gangliocytic paraganglioma: case report and review of the literature. J Gastrointest Surg. 11(10):1351-4, 2007
6. Plaza JA et al: Duodenal gangliocytic paraganglioma: a radiological-pathological correlation. Ann Diagn Pathol. 9(3):143-7, 2005
7. Hironaka M et al: Pulmonary gangliocytic paraganglioma: case report and comparative immunohistochemical study of related neuroendocrine neoplasms. Am J Surg Pathol. 25(5):688-93, 2001

Plexiform Fibromyxoma

KEY FACTS

TERMINOLOGY

- Distinctive, presumably benign mesenchymal spindle cell neoplasm of stomach that exhibits multinodular and plexiform growth and abundant myxoid to fibromyxoid matrix
- Synonym: Plexiform angiomyxoid myofibroblastic tumor

CLINICAL ISSUES

- Very rare disease
- Age range: 7-75 years (mean: 43 years)
- Arises in stomach (specifically antrum)
- Treatment: Complete surgical excision
- No recurrences or metastases reported

MACROSCOPIC

- Arises in submucosa &/or muscularis propria
- Overlying mucosal ulceration often present
- Size range: 1.9-15.0 cm (mean: 6.3 cm)

MICROSCOPIC

- Characteristic infiltrative, multinodular, plexiform growth pattern
- Small, bland spindled cells within abundant myxoid, fibromyxoid, or collagenous matrix
- Prominent arborizing capillary vascular network
- Mitoses sparse to absent

ANCILLARY TESTS

- SMA(+), often diffuse
- Occasional focal expression of desmin, caldesmon, CD10
- Negative for CD117, DOG1, S100 protein, CD34, keratin

TOP DIFFERENTIAL DIAGNOSES

- Gastrointestinal stromal tumor
- Leiomyoma
- Inflammatory fibroid polyp
- Plexiform neurofibroma

Plexiform Fibromyxoma

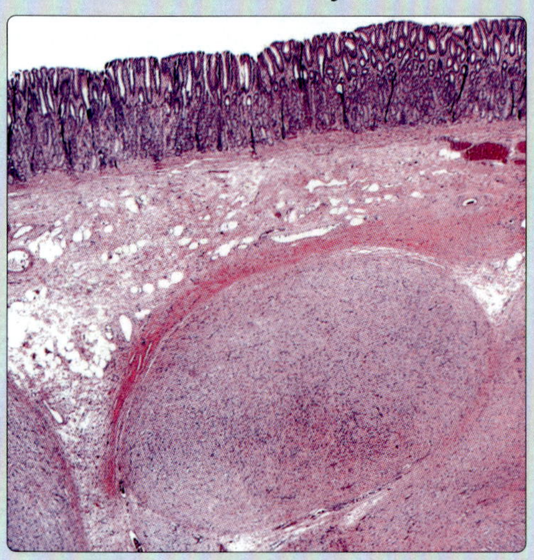

Multinodular, Plexiform Growth

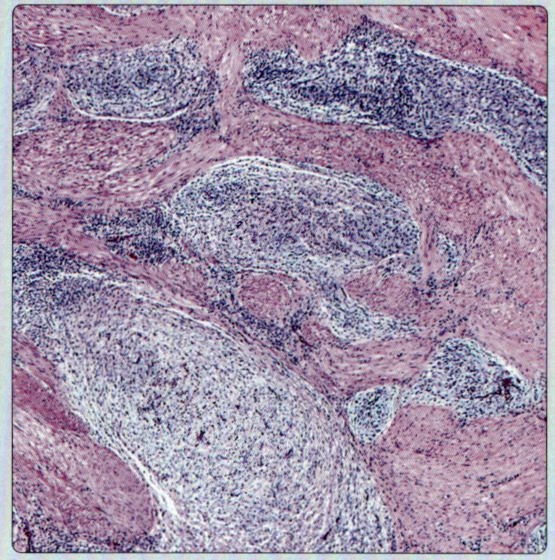

(Left) *Plexiform fibromyxoma (PFM) is a very rare but distinctive gastric mesenchymal neoplasm. As its name implies, the growth pattern of the tumor is characteristically plexiform and multinodular, and involvement of the muscularis propria and submucosa is common.* **(Right)** *In most cases of PFM, the irregular nodules of the tumor often show a more pronounced plexiform growth pattern within the muscularis propria than in the submucosa or serosa (if involved).*

Prominent Stromal Vasculature

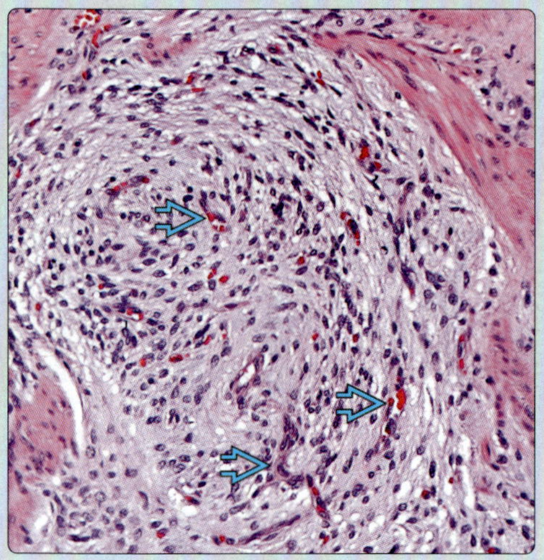

SMA Expression

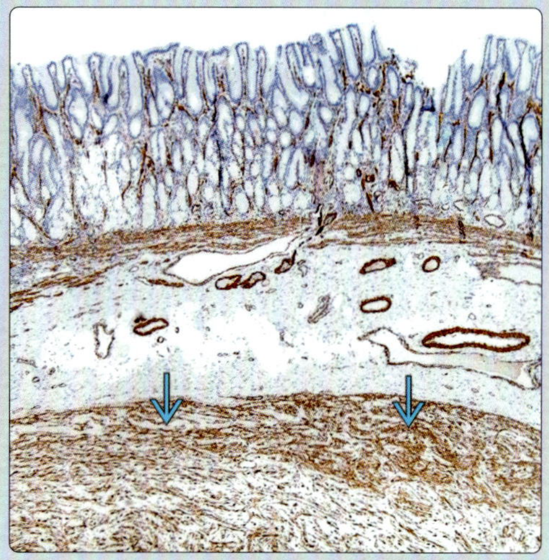

(Left) *The matrix of PFM is typically myxoid or fibromyxoid, and the lesional spindle cells are cytologically bland. The stromal vasculature is often prominent and is composed of mostly small, thin-walled capillary channels ➡; however, larger ectatic vessels can also be seen.* **(Right)** *Although still a matter of discussion, the lesional cells of PFM appear to be either myofibroblasts or modified smooth muscle cells. Accordingly, SMA expression is routinely expressed by tumor cells ➡ to a variable degree.*

TERMINOLOGY

Abbreviations

- Plexiform fibromyxoma (PFM)

Synonyms

- Plexiform angiomyxoid myofibroblastic tumor
- Plexiform angiomyxoid tumor

Definitions

- Distinctive, presumably benign mesenchymal spindle cell neoplasm of stomach that exhibits multinodular and plexiform growth and abundant myxoid to fibromyxoid matrix

CLINICAL ISSUES

Epidemiology

- Incidence
  - Very rare
- Age
  - Range: 7-75 years (mean: 43 years)

Site

- Arises in stomach
  - Specifically, gastric antrum in all reported case series
    - May involve pylorus and can extend to duodenal bulb

Presentation

- Variable: Abdominal pain, nausea/vomiting, weight loss, obstructive symptoms
- Hematemesis &/or anemia in ulcerated tumors

Treatment

- Complete surgical excision

Prognosis

- No recurrences or metastases reported

MACROSCOPIC

General Features

- Arises in muscularis propria and often extends into submucosa (and mucosa)
  - Larger tumors may show extragastric (serosal) extension
- Overlying mucosal ulceration often present and may be extensive
- Multinodular, firm or gelatinous, white to brown-red cut surface

Size

- Range: 1.9-15.0 cm (mean: 6.3 cm)

MICROSCOPIC

Histologic Features

- Characteristic infiltrative, multinodular, plexiform growth pattern
- Small spindled cells within abundant myxoid, fibromyxoid, or collagenous matrix
  - Variable cellularity but often low
    - More cellular nodules can show focal fascicular growth
  - Oval, bland nuclei with inconspicuous nucleoli
  - Pale eosinophilic cytoplasm with indistinct cytoplasmic borders
  - Mitoses sparse to absent
- Prominent arborizing capillary vascular network
  - Larger, dilated, thin-walled vessels can be seen
- Mast cell infiltrate common
- Coagulative tumor necrosis absent

ANCILLARY TESTS

Immunohistochemistry

- SMA(+), often diffuse but can be patchy
- Occasional focal expression of desmin, caldesmon, CD10
- Negative for CD117, DOG1, S100 protein, CD34, keratin

Molecular Genetics

- Subset with *MALAT1-GLI1* fusion
- No *KIT* or *PDGFRA* mutations reported

DIFFERENTIAL DIAGNOSIS

Gastrointestinal Stromal Tumor

- Significantly higher incidence than PFM
- Generally lacks plexiform growth
  - Exceptions: Pediatric and SDH-deficient gastrointestinal stromal tumors
- CD117(+), DOG1(+)
- Detectable *KIT* or *PDGFRA* mutations

Leiomyoma

- Generally lack plexiform growth pattern
- Cytologic features of smooth muscle differentiation are conspicuous
- Prominent myxoid matrix uncommon
- Strong diffuse SMA(+), desmin (+)

Inflammatory Fibroid Polyp

- Arises in submucosa (very rarely involves muscularis propria)
- Plexiform growth absent
- CD34(+); SMA(-)

Plexiform Neurofibroma

- S100 protein (+) and SMA(-)
- Most patients show evidence of neurofibromatosis
- Most common in intestines

Inflammatory Myofibroblastic Tumor

- Prominent chronic inflammatory cell infiltrate, particularly plasma cells
- Most common in children and young adults
- ALK(+) in most cases

SELECTED REFERENCES

1. Spans L et al: Recurrent MALAT1-GLI1 oncogenic fusion and GLI1 up-regulation define a subset of plexiform fibromyxoma. J Pathol. 239(3):335-43, 2016
2. Kang Y et al: Plexiform angiomyxoid myofibroblastic tumor of the stomach: report of two cases and review of the literature. Korean J Pathol. 46(3):292-6, 2012
3. Miettinen M et al: Plexiform fibromyxoma: a distinctive benign gastric antral neoplasm not to be confused with a myxoid GIST. Am J Surg Pathol. 33(11):1624-32, 2009
4. Takahashi Y et al: Plexiform angiomyxoid myofibroblastic tumor of the stomach. Am J Surg Pathol. 31(5):724-8, 2007

(Left) *This intermediate-power image shows the classic myxoid nodules of PFM containing bland spindle cells and conspicuous thin-walled vascular channels.* **(Right)** *Similar to a gastrointestinal stromal tumor (GIST), PFM often arises within the muscularis propria, at least in part. However, plexiform growth is generally uncommon in GIST, and this pattern should always raise the possibility of PFM.*

Classic Appearance

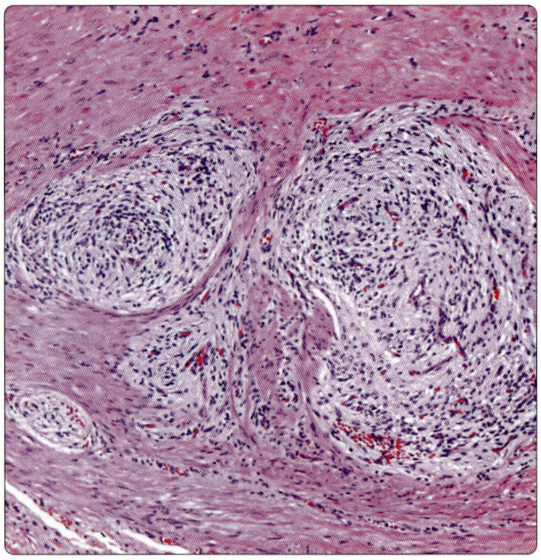

Muscularis Propria Involvement

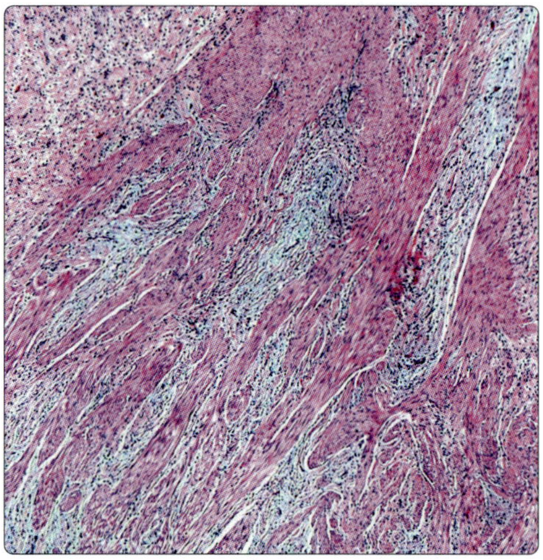

(Left) *Serosal fat involvement by PFM is generally uncommon; however, it can be seen in larger lesions. This image shows the tumor ↷ pushing into adipose tissue. Muscularis propria can be seen to the left.* **(Right)** *Myxoid matrix is common in PFM and, in hypocellular areas, may appear quite prominent.*

Serosal Involvement

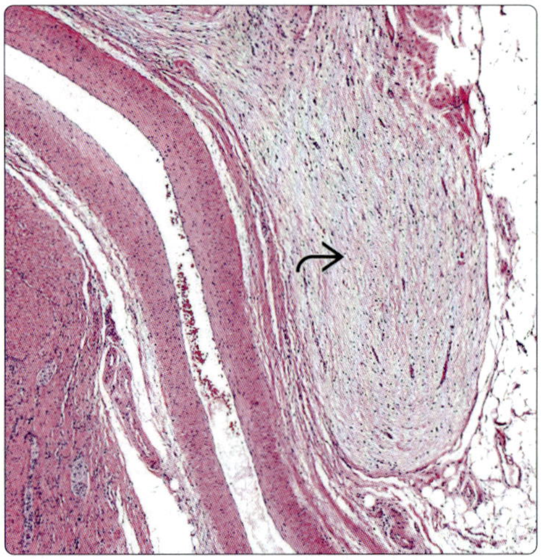

Prominent Myxoid Matrix

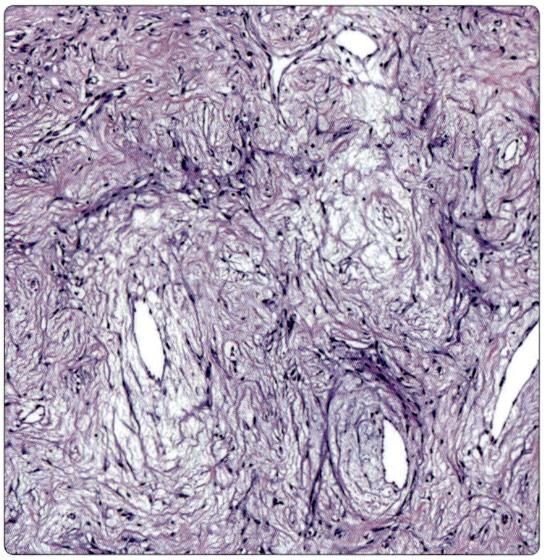

(Left) *A small zone of clearing ⇨ may form around some tumor cells in PFM, reminiscent of lacunae, and, when focally prominent, can impart a clear cell appearance.* **(Right)** *Some cases of PFM can ulcerate the overlying mucosa, introducing a mixed inflammatory infiltrate to the tumor. Granulation tissue can also be present.*

Focal Clear Cell Appearance

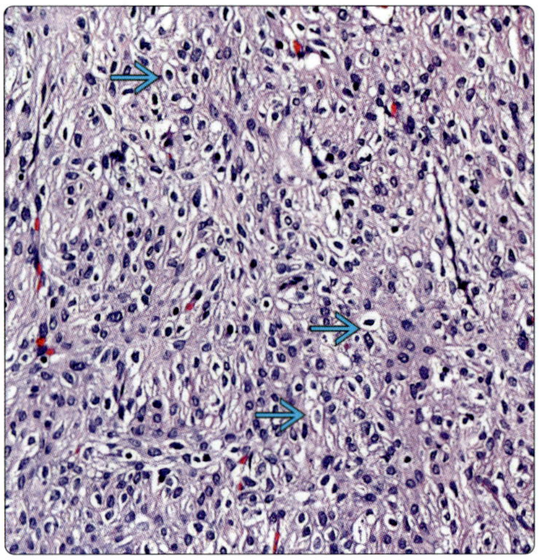

Inflammation

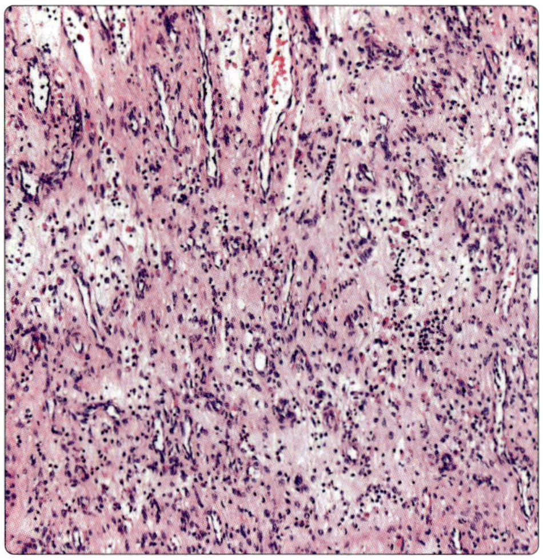

Fibrocollagenous Matrix

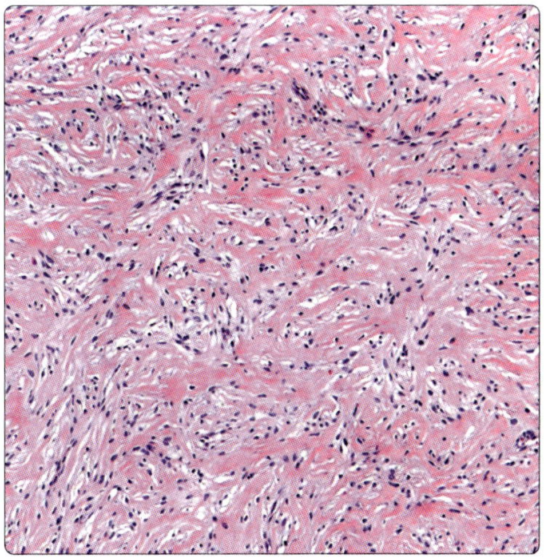

Fibrocollagenous Matrix

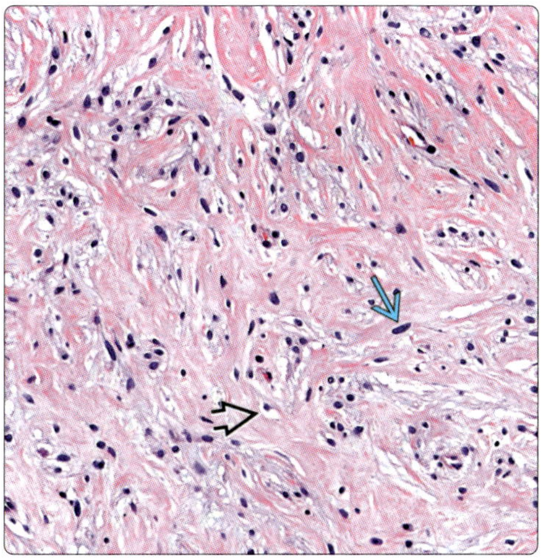

(Left) *Although the matrix in PFM is often myxoid, in some cases it may be fibromyxoid or fibrocollagenous, as depicted.* **(Right)** *This higher power image of PFM shows a nodule with collagenous matrix. The cells are overall bland with at most mild nuclear enlargement →. Note also the lacuna-like small zone ⇨ of clear spacing around some of the tumor cells.*

Increased Cellularity

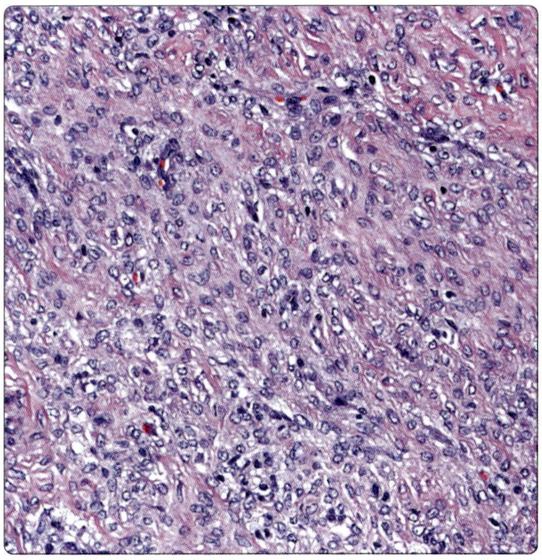

Rare Fascicular Growth

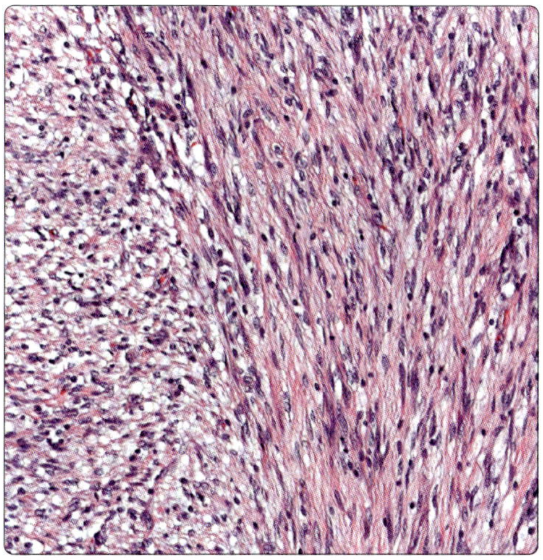

(Left) *Most cases of PFM are relatively hypocellular or paucicellular; however, it is not uncommon for some nodules to show increased cellularity. Note, though, the retention of bland nuclear features and an absence of mitotic activity.* **(Right)** *Areas of increased cellularity may be seen in PFM, and fascicular growth may be a focal finding, as depicted. Note the banal nature of the tumor cells.*

Vascular Involvement

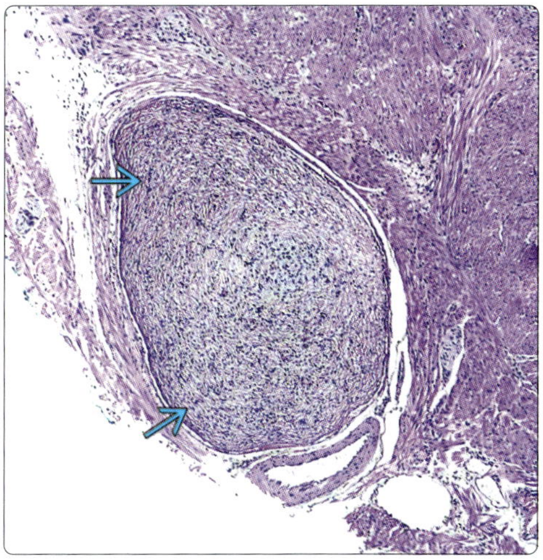

SMA Expression

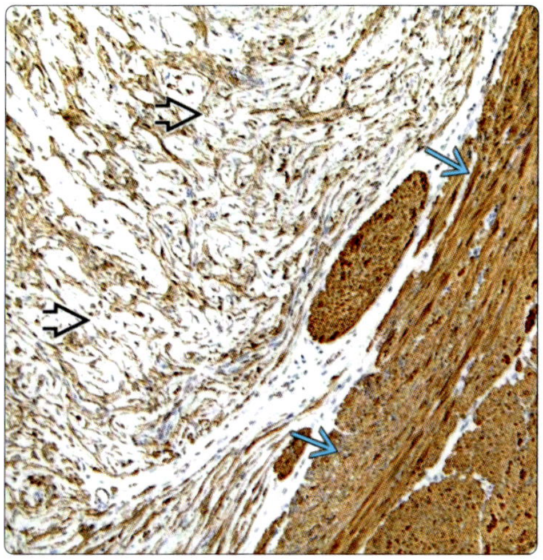

(Left) *Occasional cases of PFM may show focal luminal involvement → of capillaries, lymphatics, or larger muscular-walled veins. This finding does not appear to alter the benign nature of this tumor.* **(Right)** *Expression of SMA is a relatively consistent finding in PFM, though variable in degree. Note the less prominent staining of the tumor cells ⇨ as compared to the smooth muscle cells of the muscularis propria →. CD117 and DOG1 are negative in PFM.*

Malignant Gastrointestinal Neuroectodermal Tumor

KEY FACTS

TERMINOLOGY

- Synonym: Clear cell sarcoma-like tumor of gastrointestinal (GI) tract
- Rare, malignant neoplasm of GI tract showing evidence of primitive neural or neuroectodermal differentiation
  - Melanocytic differentiation absent

CLINICAL ISSUES

- Very rare
- Median age: 36 years
- Most common in small intestine (particularly ileum)
  - Also occurs in stomach and large bowel
- Treatment: Complete surgical resection
- Aggressive clinical course with high mortality rate
  - High rate of local recurrence and metastases (usually to lymph nodes, liver)

MACROSCOPIC

- Mean: 5.5 cm

MICROSCOPIC

- Cellular proliferation of epithelioid, ovoid, or spindled cells forming sheets and nests
  - Pale eosinophilic to amphophilic cytoplasm
  - Relatively uniform, vesicular nuclei with small nucleoli
- Other patterns: Pseudopapillary, pseudoalveolar, fascicular
- Osteoclast-like multinucleated giant cells common

ANCILLARY TESTS

- Diffuse S100 protein (+), SOX10(+)
- Keratin, CD117, SMA, melanocytic markers (-)
- Molecular: *EWSR1* rearrangements with *CREB1* or *ATF1*

TOP DIFFERENTIAL DIAGNOSES

- Gastrointestinal stromal tumor
- Clear cell sarcoma
- Metastatic melanoma
- Malignant peripheral nerve sheath tumor
- Synovial sarcoma (monophasic or poorly differentiated)

Malignant Gastrointestinal Neuroectodermal Tumor

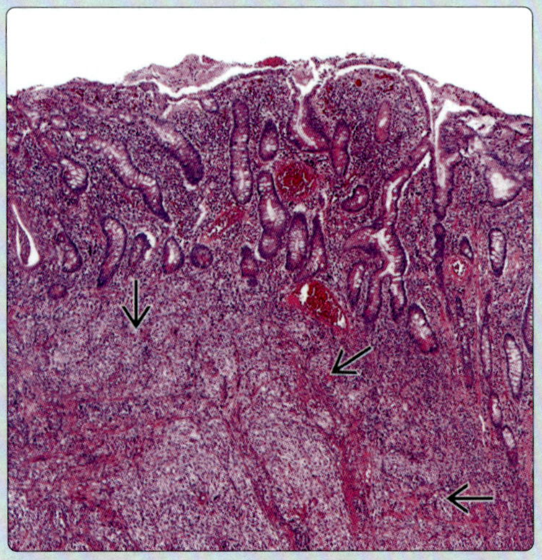

Sheets and Nests

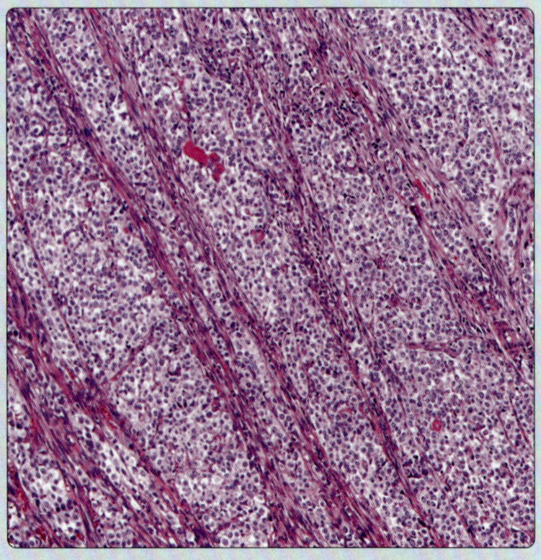

(Left) *Malignant gastrointestinal neuroectodermal tumor (GNET) is a very rare but distinctive neoplasm of the gastrointestinal tract that is usually characterized by an aggressive clinical course. The tumor → primarily involves the submucosa and muscularis propria; however, mucosal involvement is noted in some cases.* **(Right)** *Most cases of GNET are composed of nests and sheets of relatively uniform epithelioid tumor cells with predominantly pale eosinophilic cytoplasm.*

Cytologic Features

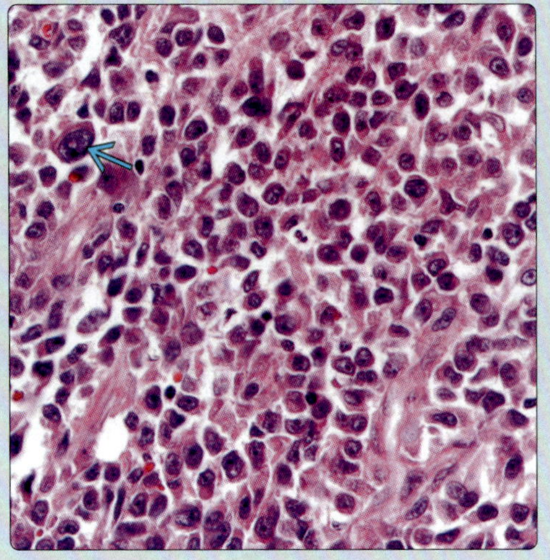

S100 Protein Expression

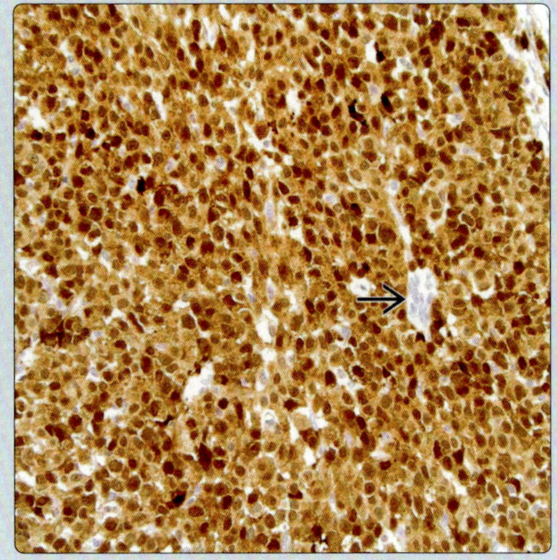

(Left) *Nuclei in GNET are typically round to oval with somewhat irregular contours and often contain small nucleoli; however, in some areas, nucleoli are prominent. Nuclear pseudoinclusions → can also be seen.* **(Right)** *Similar to clear cell sarcoma (CCS) of soft tissue, most cases of GNET display strong, diffuse expression of S100 protein (shown). In contrast to CCS, melanocytic antigens (e.g., HMB-45, Melan-A) are not expressed. Note the osteoclast-like giant cell →, which is negative for S100 but can be highlighted with CD68.*

TERMINOLOGY

Abbreviations

- Gastrointestinal neuroectodermal tumor (GNET)

Synonyms

- Clear cell sarcoma-like tumor of GI tract (CCSLTGT)
- Clear cell sarcoma-like tumor with osteoclast-like giant cells of GI tract

Definitions

- Rare, malignant neoplasm of GI tract showing evidence of primitive neural or neuroectodermal differentiation
  - Melanocytic differentiation absent

ETIOLOGY/PATHOGENESIS

Unknown

- Several reports of GNET/CCSLTGT arising in patients with prior history of neuroblastoma, acute leukemia, hepatoblastoma
  - Potential link to previous radiation therapy

CLINICAL ISSUES

Epidemiology

- Incidence
  - Very rare
- Age
  - Wide range: 10-81 years
  - Median: 36 years
- Sex
  - M = F

Site

- Can arise at any location in GI tract
  - Most common in small intestine (particularly ileum)

Presentation

- Abdominal pain, distention, weight loss, occasional systemic symptoms
- Metastatic disease frequent at initial presentation

Treatment

- Complete surgical resection

Prognosis

- Aggressive clinical course with high mortality rate
- High rate of local recurrence and metastases
  - Metastases most frequently go to regional lymph nodes and liver

MACROSCOPIC

General Features

- Transmural, often ulcerating mass
  - Can also be exophytic/polypoid or circumferential
- Firm, solid, tan to gray-brown cut surface
  - May show foci of hemorrhage or necrosis

Size

- Range: 2.4-15.0 cm
- Mean: 5.5 cm

MICROSCOPIC

Histologic Features

- Tumor generally involves submucosa and muscularis propria
  - May extend into mucosa
- Cellular proliferation of epithelioid, ovoid, or spindled cells forming sheets and nests
  - Pale eosinophilic to amphophilic cytoplasm
    - Variable clear cell morphology (often minor)
  - Relatively uniform, vesicular nuclei with small nucleoli
    - Nuclear pseudoinclusions may be seen
    - Cells with prominent nucleoli or nuclear pleomorphism can be seen
      - Nuclear pleomorphism more common in recurrent/metastatic lesions
- Variety of other architectural growth patterns described
  - Pseudoalveolar
  - Pseudopapillary
  - Trabecular/corded
  - Fascicular
  - Microcystic
  - Formation of rosette-like structures
- Osteoclast-like multinucleated giant cells common
  - Vary widely in number; may be absent
- Variable mitotic rate (mean: 6 mitoses per 10 HPF)
- Tumor necrosis common
  - May be extensive
- Rare findings: Oncocytic cytomorphology, stromal myxoid change

ANCILLARY TESTS

Immunohistochemistry

- Diffuse S100 protein (+), SOX10(+)
- All melanocytic markers (-)

Molecular Genetics

- *EWSR1* gene (22q12) rearrangement in most cases
  - Fusion partners: *CREB1* (2q34) or *ATF1* (12q13)
    - Identical to true clear cell sarcoma of soft tissue

DIFFERENTIAL DIAGNOSIS

Gastrointestinal Stromal Tumor

- Much more common than GNET
- Osteoclast-like giant cells rare
- CD117(+), DOG1(+)
- Also CD34(+)
- *KIT* or *PDGFRA* mutations
- Lacks *EWSR1* rearrangement

Clear Cell Sarcoma

- May be primary to GI tract (rare) or metastasis from soft tissue site
- Can be morphologically indistinguishable from GNET
- Macronucleoli common
- Expression of melanocytic markers (HMB-45, Melan-A, etc.)
  - Key distinguishing feature from GNET
- Identical *EWSR1* rearrangements as seen in GNET

Immunohistochemistry

Antibody	Reactivity	Staining Pattern	Comment
S100	Positive	Nuclear & cytoplasmic	Strong, diffuse expression
SOX10	Positive	Nuclear	Strong, diffuse expression
HMB-45	Negative		
Melan-A	Negative		Also MART-1 negative
Tyrosinase	Negative		
MITF	Negative		
CD68	Negative		Highlights osteoclast-like giant cells only
CK-PAN	Negative		
CD99	Negative		
GFAP	Negative		
CD117	Negative		
DOG1	Negative		
CD34	Negative		
Desmin	Negative		
Myogenin	Negative		
Actin-sm	Negative		
CD56	Equivocal	Cell membrane	Variable expression (70% of cases)
Synaptophysin	Equivocal	Cytoplasmic	Variable expression (50% of cases)
NB84	Equivocal	Cytoplasmic	Variable (50% of cases)

- Ultrastructural examination (electron microscopy) may be helpful
  - True melanosomes present in clear cell sarcoma

Metastatic Melanoma

- Clinical history of previous melanoma may be present
  - Intestinal metastases can present as multiple nodules
- Can show close morphologic overlap with GNET
  - However, nuclear atypia is usually more prominent in melanoma
- Evidence of melanocytic differentiation
  - Melanin pigment, expression of melanocytic markers by IHC
- Lacks *EWSR1* rearrangement

Alveolar Rhabdomyosarcoma

- May show some morphologic overlap (nests, pseudoalveolar growth) with GNET
- Desmin (+), myogenin (+)
- S100 protein (-)
- Characteristic t(2;13) or t(1;13)
- Lacks *EWSR1* rearrangement

Malignant Peripheral Nerve Sheath Tumor

- Alternating cellularity (marbled pattern) with perivascular cellularity in classic cases
- Diffuse S100 protein (+) in epithelioid malignant peripheral nerve sheath tumor (MPNST)
  - Can be challenging to distinguish from GNET
  - Lacks osteoclast-like giant cells
- S100 protein (+) in 60% of spindle cell MPNST
  - Characteristically focal/patchy rather than diffuse
- Lacks *EWSR1* rearrangement

Synovial Sarcoma (Monophasic or Poorly Differentiated)

- Very rare in GI tract
- Keratin (+) &/or EMA(+), often focal or patchy
- Strong, diffuse nuclear TLE1
- Minority show focal S100 protein (+)
  - Diffuse expression is not feature
- Characteristic t(X;18) involving *SS18* (SYT)
- Lacks *EWSR1* rearrangements

SELECTED REFERENCES

1. Green C et al: Clear cell sarcoma of the gastrointestinal tract and malignant gastrointestinal neuroectodermal tumour: distinct or related entities? A review. Pathology. 50(5):490-8, 2018
2. Libertini M et al: Clear cell sarcoma-like tumor of the gastrointestinal tract: clinical outcome and pathologic features of a molecularly characterized tertiary center case series. Anticancer Res. 38(3):1479-83, 2018
3. Boland JM et al: Oncocytic variant of malignant gastrointestinal neuroectodermal tumor: a potential diagnostic pitfall. Hum Pathol. 57:13-6, 2016
4. Wang J et al: Clear cell sarcoma-like tumor of the gastrointestinal tract: an evolving entity. Arch Pathol Lab Med. 139(3):407-12, 2015
5. Kong J et al: Malignant gastrointestinal neuroectodermal tumor: a case report and review of the literature. Oncol Lett. 8(6):2687-290, 2014
6. Thway K et al: Clear cell sarcoma-like tumor of the gastrointestinal tract, presenting as a second malignancy after childhood hepatoblastoma. Case Rep Med. 2014:984369, 2014
7. Stockman DL et al: Malignant gastrointestinal neuroectodermal tumor: clinicopathologic, immunohistochemical, ultrastructural, and molecular analysis of 16 cases with a reappraisal of clear cell sarcoma-like tumors of the gastrointestinal tract. Am J Surg Pathol. 36(6):857-68, 2012
8. Kosemehmetoglu K et al: Clear cell sarcoma of tendons and aponeuroses, and osteoclast-rich tumour of the gastrointestinal tract with features resembling clear cell sarcoma of soft parts: a review and update. J Clin Pathol. 63(5):416-23, 2010
9. Friedrichs N et al: Clear cell sarcoma-like tumor with osteoclast-like giant cells in the small bowel: further evidence for a new tumor entity. Int J Surg Pathol. 13(4):313-8, 2005

Osteoclast-Like Giant Cells

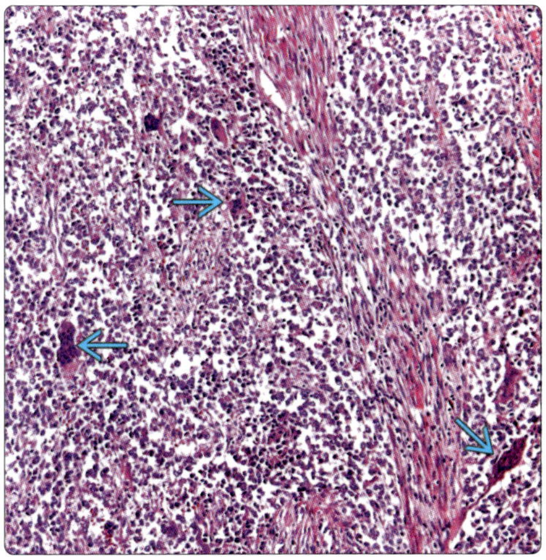

Clear Cell Change

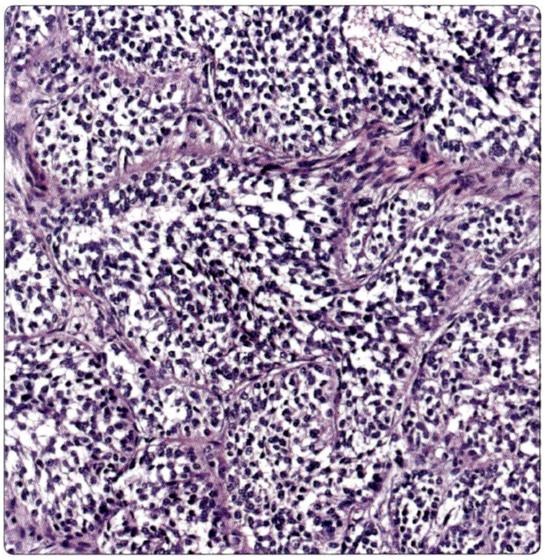

(Left) *Osteoclast-like giant cells are seen in ~ 50% of cases of GNET and are a helpful clue to the diagnosis when present. Metastatic clear cell sarcoma and melanoma, however, may feature these giant cells as well and therefore must always be considered and excluded.* **(Right)** *Cytoplasmic clearing may be seen in GNET but is generally not a prominent finding.*

Pseudoalveolar Growth

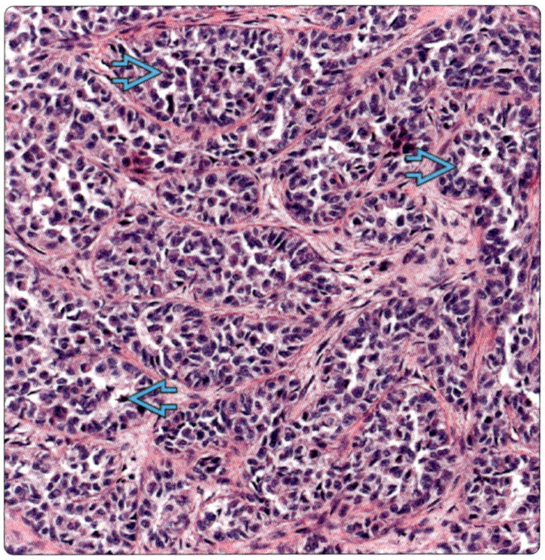

Pseudopapillary Growth

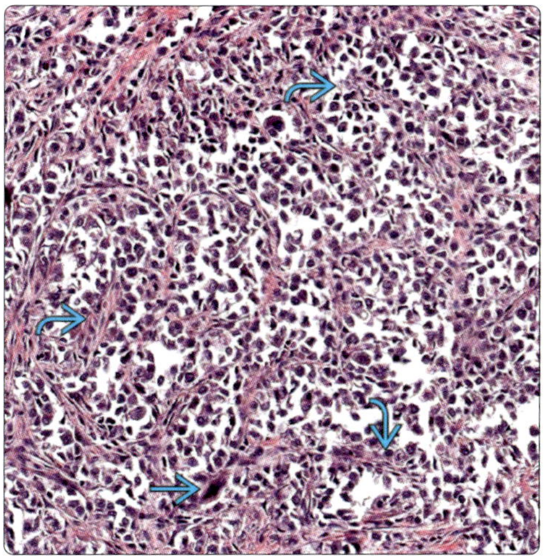

(Left) *A pseudoalveolar pattern may manifest in GNET, created by nests of tumor cells with central loss of cellular cohesion. This appearance is similar to what is seen in alveolar rhabdomyosarcoma.* **(Right)** *This H&E shows an area of GNET with prominent cellular dyscohesion, rendering the vasculature more prominent and imparting a vague pseudopapillary pattern. Note the larger osteoclast-like giant cell.*

Trabecular/Corded Growth

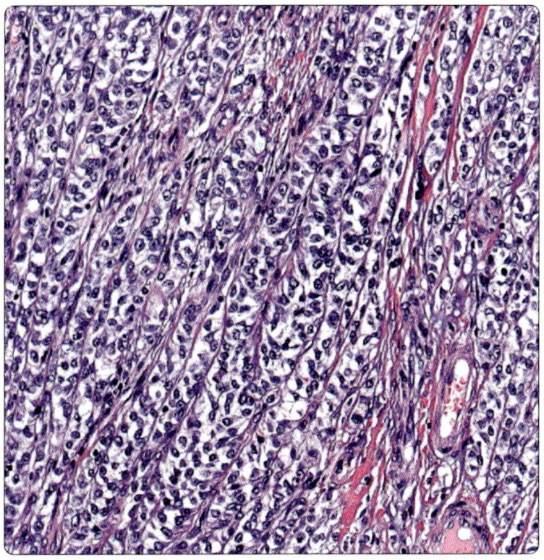

Fascicular Spindle Cell Morphology

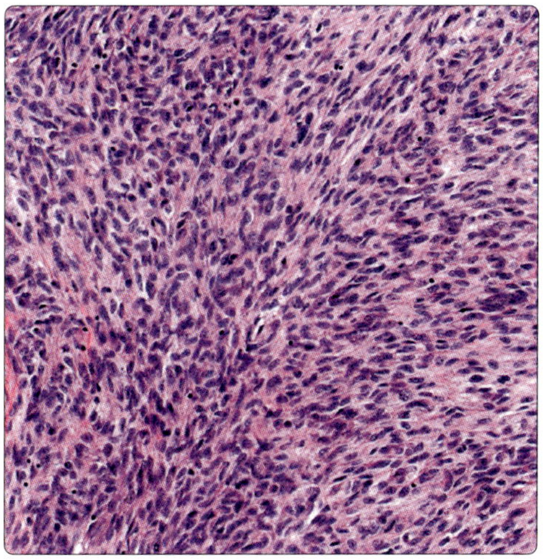

(Left) *A compressed trabecular or corded growth pattern may also be seen in GNET, as depicted. Although not shown here, microcystic foci and rosette-like structures have also been reported in this tumor.* **(Right)** *Although most tumor cells in GNET are epithelioid, spindled cells can also often be identified, at least focally. In some tumors, areas of fascicular growth can be appreciated, as depicted.*

SECTION 19

Other Entities

Benign

Amyloidoma 782
Ganglion Cyst 784
Tumoral Calcinosis 786
Idiopathic Tumefactive Fibroinflammatory Lesions 788
Cardiac Myxoma 792
Cardiac Fibroma 796
Congenital Granular Cell Epulis 798
Nasopharyngeal Angiofibroma 800
Sinonasal Glomangiopericytoma 804
Ectopic Meningioma 810
Glial Heterotopia 812

Intermediate

Paraganglioma 814
Peripheral Hemangioblastoma 822
Melanotic Neuroectodermal Tumor of Infancy 824
Ependymoma of Soft Tissue 826

Malignant

Metastatic Tumors to Soft Tissue Sites 828
Neuroblastoma and Ganglioneuroblastoma 832
Extraaxial Soft Tissue Chordoma 842
Undifferentiated Embryonal Sarcoma of Liver 844
Primary Pulmonary Myxoid Sarcoma 846
Biphenotypic Sinonasal Sarcoma 850
Spindle Epithelial Tumor With Thymus-Like Differentiation 854
Low-Grade Endometrial Stromal Sarcoma 856

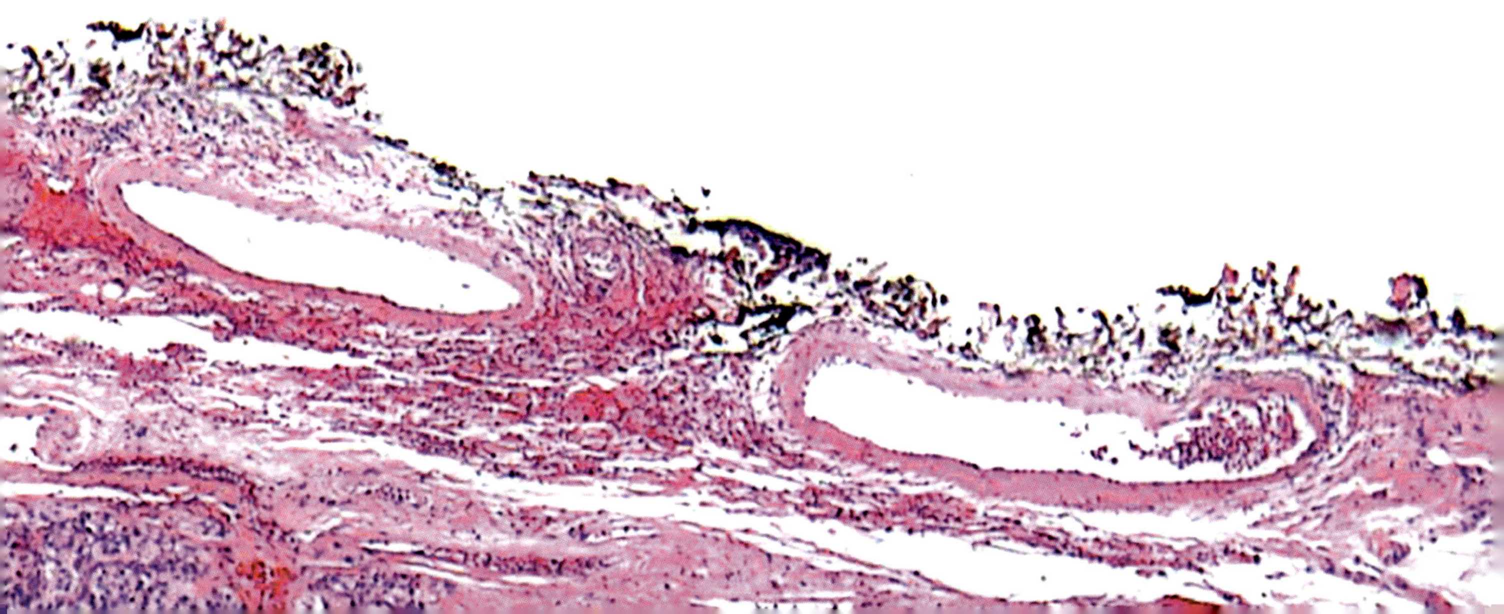

Amyloidoma

KEY FACTS

TERMINOLOGY

- Solitary, localized, tumor-like deposit of amyloid

ETIOLOGY/PATHOGENESIS

- Idiopathic
- Related to underlying hematologic disease (myeloma, lymphoplasmacytic lymphoma)
- Long-term hemodialysis
- Chronic inflammatory or infectious disease

CLINICAL ISSUES

- May occur in essentially any site
- Treated by excision
- Prognosis related to underlying disease, if present

MACROSCOPIC

- Pale waxy cut surface

MICROSCOPIC

- Amorphous acellular eosinophilic material in lobules and sheets
- Adjacent lymphoplasmacytic infiltrate
- Multinucleated foreign body-type giant cells
- Vessel walls often involved

ANCILLARY TESTS

- Congo red (+)
  - Apple green birefringent areas in polarized light

TOP DIFFERENTIAL DIAGNOSES

- Elastofibroma
- Collagen
- Tophaceous gout
- Fibrin deposits
- Tumoral calcinosis

(Left) *Amyloid appears histologically as acellular, amorphous eosinophilic material in well-delineated lobules and sheets. A patchy lymphoplasmacytic infiltrate ➡ is often present, and a peripheral multinucleated foreign body giant cell reaction ➡ may also be seen.* **(Right)** *Amyloid deposits are essentially acellular and may involve vessel walls, surrounding connective tissue, or both.*

Amyloidoma

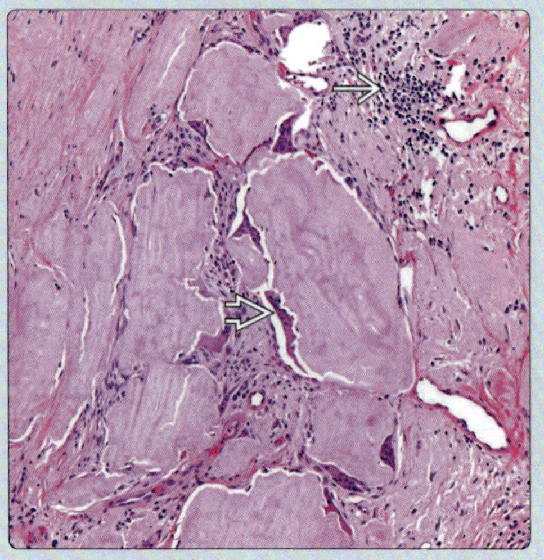

Amyloid

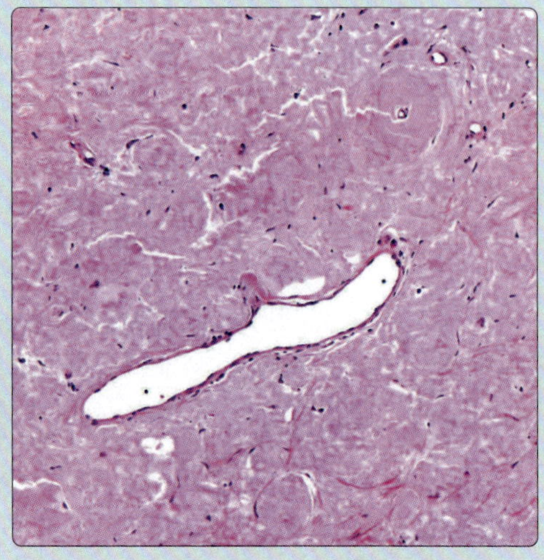

(Left) *A Congo red stain highlights amyloid deposits with a prominent red-orange coloration. Care must be taken, however, as Congo red can also stain collagen, albeit somewhat less intensely.* **(Right)** *Under polarized light, amyloid deposits stained with Congo red show a characteristic apple green birefringence ➡. Other colors, such as yellow and orange, may be seen as well but are nonspecific.*

Congo Red Stain

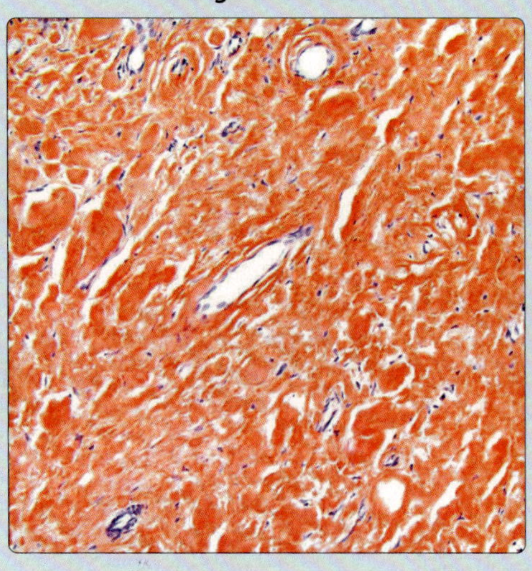

Polarized Congo Red

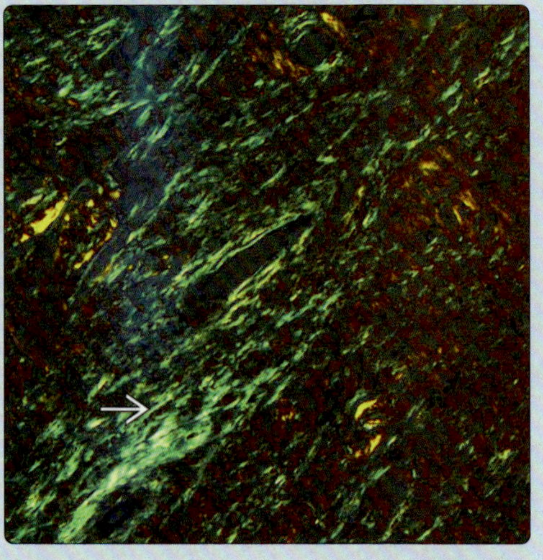

TERMINOLOGY

Synonyms

- Tumoral amyloidosis

Definitions

- Solitary, localized tumor-like deposit of amyloid

ETIOLOGY/PATHOGENESIS

Idiopathic

- No associated disease

Immunocytic Dyscrasias

- Plasma cell myeloma, lymphoplasmacytic lymphoma
- Usually AL (light chain) type of amyloid
  - Overall most common type of amyloid in localized tumors

Long-Term Hemodialysis

- β2-microglobulin type of amyloid

Chronic Inflammatory or Infectious Disease

- Rheumatoid arthritis
- Osteomyelitis
- Tuberculosis
- AA type of amyloid (associated with serum amyloid A protein)

CLINICAL ISSUES

Epidemiology

- Incidence
  - Rare
- Age
  - Usually older adults
- Sex
  - Male or female

Site

- Extremities, trunk, head and neck region
- Mediastinum, retroperitoneum
- Bone, lung, bladder, gastrointestinal tract, and nervous system also reported

Presentation

- Solitary, painless mass
  - Rarely multifocal
- May have symptoms related to underlying hematologic, inflammatory, or infectious disease

Treatment

- Surgical excision

Prognosis

- Relates to prognosis of underlying condition (myeloma, etc.)

MACROSCOPIC

General Features

- Lobulated firm mass
- Pale, waxy cut surface

MICROSCOPIC

Histologic Features

- Amorphous, acellular, eosinophilic material in lobules and sheets
- Vessel walls often involved
- Plasma cell and lymphocytic infiltrate
- Multinucleated foreign body-type giant cells
- Calcification or metaplastic bone/cartilage may be present

ANCILLARY TESTS

Histochemistry

- Congo red (+)
  - Prominent red-orange staining
- PAS-diastase (+)
- Crystal violet (+)

Electron Microscopy

- Nonbranching fibrils 7-10 nm in diameter

DIFFERENTIAL DIAGNOSIS

Elastofibroma

- Scapular location
- Elastic stain shows fragmented and globular fibers
- Congo red (-)

Collagen

- Appears Congo red (+)
  - Less intense staining than amyloid
  - Difficult cases can be evaluated for amyloid by mass spectrometry
- Associated with fibroblasts
- Parallel orientation

Tophaceous Gout

- Amorphous eosinophilic material associated with multinucleated giant cells
- Congo red (-)
- Contains needle-shaped crystals that polarize

Tumoral Calcinosis

- Associated with fibroblastic proliferation
- Prominent basophilic calcification

Fibrin

- Fibrillary &/or grainy appearance
- Associated red cells and neutrophils
- Congo red (-)

SELECTED REFERENCES

1. Clark TC et al: Bilateral multifocal lower extremity localized soft tissue amyloidomas: case report with ultrasonographic characterization. Skeletal Radiol. 46(12):1783-1789, 2017
2. Pasternak S et al: Soft tissue amyloidoma of the extremities: report of a case and review of the literature. Am J Dermatopathol. 29(2):152-5, 2007
3. Bardin RL et al: Soft tissue amyloidoma of the extremities: a case report and review of the literature. Arch Pathol Lab Med. 128(11):1270-3, 2004
4. Sidoni A et al: Amyloid tumours in the soft tissues of the legs. Case report and review of the literature. Virchows Arch. 432(6):563-6, 1998
5. Krishnan J et al: Tumoral presentation of amyloidosis (amyloidomas) in soft tissues. A report of 14 cases. Am J Clin Pathol. 100(2):135-44, 1993

Ganglion Cyst

KEY FACTS

TERMINOLOGY

- Presumably nonneoplastic cystic formation often associated with tendon sheath or joint capsule

ETIOLOGY/PATHOGENESIS

- Formation may be related to degeneration of fibroconnective and meniscal tissue

CLINICAL ISSUES

- Most common tumor of hand and wrist
- Usually 25-45 years of age
- More common in women
- Dorsal surface of wrist is most common site
- History of trauma may be present
- Treated by aspiration or surgical excision
- Benign; excellent prognosis
    - Rare recurrences

MACROSCOPIC

- Usually attached to tendon sheath or joint capsule
- Soft, cystic, superficial mass
- Often fragmented when surgically excised

MICROSCOPIC

- Uni- or multiloculated cystic areas lined by dense collagenous rind
    - Cysts often filled with mucoid fluid
        - No epithelial lining
- Myxoid stromal changes
- No significant nuclear atypia or mitoses

TOP DIFFERENTIAL DIAGNOSES

- Myxoma
- Myxofibrosarcoma (low grade)
- Neurofibroma

Uni- and Multiloculated Cysts

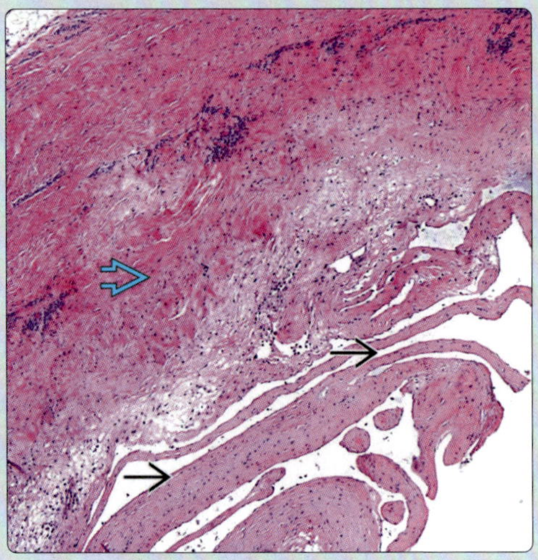

Nonepithelial Lining

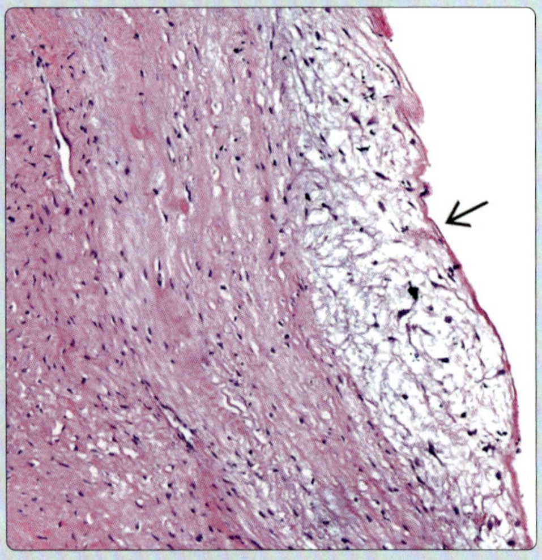

(Left) *Ganglion cysts are uni- or multiloculated cystic growths that classically arise in the dorsal wrist. Note the cyst walls →. These cysts are often surrounded by a thick fibrous lining or capsule ⇨.* **(Right)** *The cystic spaces are not true cysts as they lack an epithelial lining →. The adjacent connective tissue contains bland fibroblasts and generally appears histologically innocuous.*

Reactive Changes

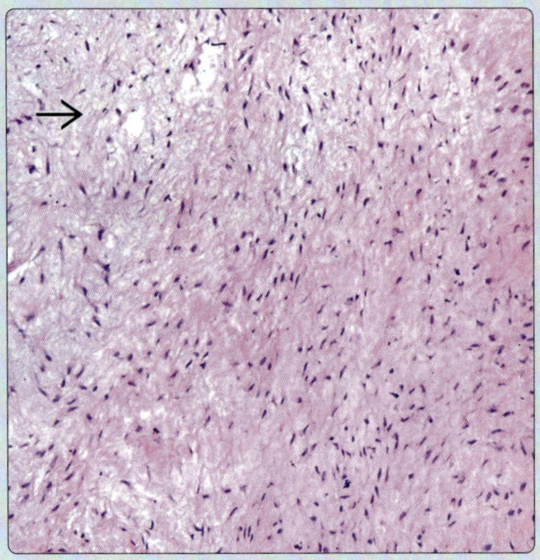

Myxoid Material

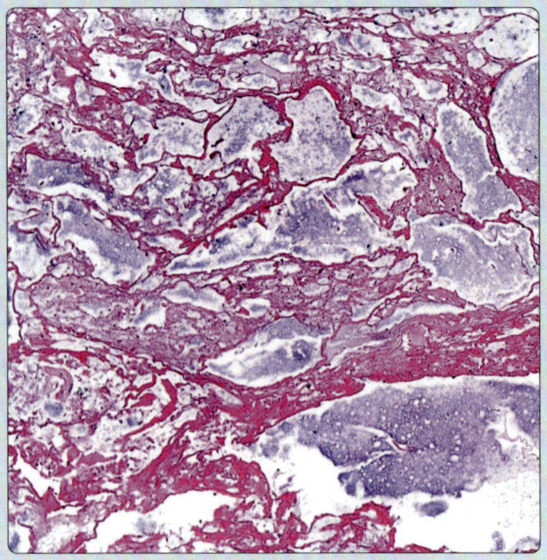

(Left) *The connective tissue between the cysts often shows a variable degree of reactive change, and foci of subtle myxoid change, resembling myxoma →, are common.* **(Right)** *The material within the cysts is usually clear and gelatinous grossly but appears myxoid histologically. In some cases it can also spill into the surrounding connective tissue (shown), occasionally inciting a reactive myofibroblastic or vascular proliferation.*

Ganglion Cyst

TERMINOLOGY

Synonyms

- Ganglion

Definitions

- Presumably nonneoplastic cystic formation often associated with tendon sheath or joint capsule

ETIOLOGY/PATHOGENESIS

Nonneoplastic

- Exact etiology uncertain
- Formation may be related to degeneration of fibroconnective and meniscal tissue

CLINICAL ISSUES

Epidemiology

- Incidence
  - Common
    - Most common tumor of hand and wrist
- Age
  - Usually 25-45 years
    - Can be seen in pediatric population
- Sex
  - More common in women

Site

- Dorsal surface of wrist (most common)
- Less likely foot, toes, knee, hip, and volar surface of wrist
- May arise in bone (intraosseous ganglion) or rarely involve nerve (intraneural ganglion)

Presentation

- Soft, cystic, superficial mass
- Main be painful or tender (50% of cases)
- History of trauma may be present

Treatment

- Surgical approaches
  - Surgical excision
  - Nonoperative approach by aspiration of fluid

Prognosis

- Excellent
- Benign
- Higher risk of recurrence reported in pediatric population

MACROSCOPIC

General Features

- Usually attached to tendon sheath or joint capsule
- No communication with joint space
- Small cysts often contain clear, sticky fluid
- Often excised in fragments

Size

- Usually < 3 cm

MICROSCOPIC

Histologic Features

- Cystic areas lined by dense collagenous rind
  - No true epithelial lining
  - Cysts are uni- or multiloculated and may be filled with mucoid fluid
- Myxoid stromal changes adjacent to cysts
  - Extension of mucoid fluid into surrounding tissue may incite reactive myofibroblastic or vascular proliferation
- No significant nuclear atypia
- No significant mitotic activity

DIFFERENTIAL DIAGNOSIS

Myxoma

- Absence of thick-walled cystic structures
- Not common in dorsal wrist

Myxofibrosarcoma (Low Grade)

- Multinodular, subcutaneous neoplasm
  - Evidence of infiltrative growth
- Often extensively myxoid with at least focal nuclear atypia
- Patient age often > 50 years
- Usually > 3 cm

Neurofibroma

- Generally lacks cystic spaces with mucoid material
- S100(+)

DIAGNOSTIC CHECKLIST

Clinically Relevant Pathologic Features

- Small, superficial fluctuant mass
- Most common in dorsal wrist
- May also arise in bone (intraosseous ganglion)

Pathologic Interpretation Pearls

- Thick-walled cystic structures containing mucoid material
- Often fragmented when surgically excised
- No nuclear hyperchromasia or pleomorphism

SELECTED REFERENCES

1. Meyerson J et al: Pediatric ganglion cysts: a retrospective review. Hand (N Y). 1558944717751195, 2018
2. Crawford C et al: Arthroscopic versus open excision of dorsal ganglion cysts: a systematic review. J Hand Surg Eur Vol. 1753193417734428, 2017
3. Wilson TJ et al: Intraneural ganglion cysts: a predictable method to their madness. Ann Phys Rehabil Med. 60(6):414-415, 2017
4. Kim JP et al: Arthroscopic excision of dorsal wrist ganglion: factors related to recurrence and postoperative residual pain. Arthroscopy. 29(6):1019-24, 2013
5. Sakamoto A et al: Intraosseous Ganglia: a series of 17 treated cases. Biomed Res Int. 2013:462730, 2013
6. Simon Cypel TK et al: Ganglion cyst in children: reviewing treatment and recurrence rates. Can J Plast Surg. 19(2):53-5, 2011
7. Casal D et al: Paresthesia and hypesthesia in the dorsum of the foot as the presenting complaints of a ganglion cyst of the foot. Clin Anat. 23(5):606-10, 2010
8. Schajowicz F et al: Juxta-articular bone cysts (intra-osseous ganglia): a clinicopathological study of eighty-eight cases. J Bone Joint Surg Br. 61(1):107-16, 1979

Tumoral Calcinosis

KEY FACTS

TERMINOLOGY

- Tumor-like deposits of calcium hydroxyapatite in periarticular soft tissues

ETIOLOGY/PATHOGENESIS

- 3 forms: Sporadic/idiopathic, familial, and secondary

CLINICAL ISSUES

- Usually < 20 years of age
- Firm, painless subcutaneous mass
- Subcutis around large joints
  - Hip, elbow, and shoulder most common
- Attached to underlying fascia or tendons
- Treatment: Surgical excision for sporadic/idiopathic and familial forms
  - Treatment of underlying systemic condition is often necessary in secondary forms

MACROSCOPIC

- Firm, rubbery, multiloculated cystic mass containing milky fluid or semisolid gritty material

MICROSCOPIC

- Morphology is same regardless of form (sporadic, familial, secondary)
- Variably calcified amorphous granular material (hydroxyapatite crystals) within cystic spaces
- Cystic spaces separated by thick fibrous septa
  - Lined by histiocytes and variable number of multinucleated giant cells

TOP DIFFERENTIAL DIAGNOSES

- Calcified soft tissue chondroma
- Milk alkali syndrome
- Tophaceous gout
- Tophaceous pseudogout

Multiloculated Cystic Pattern

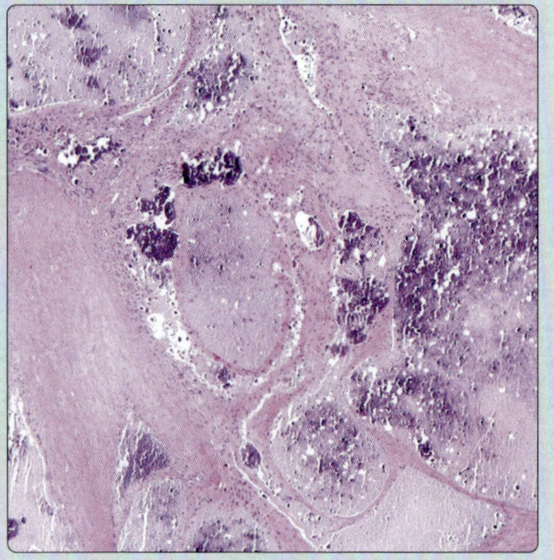

Calcification

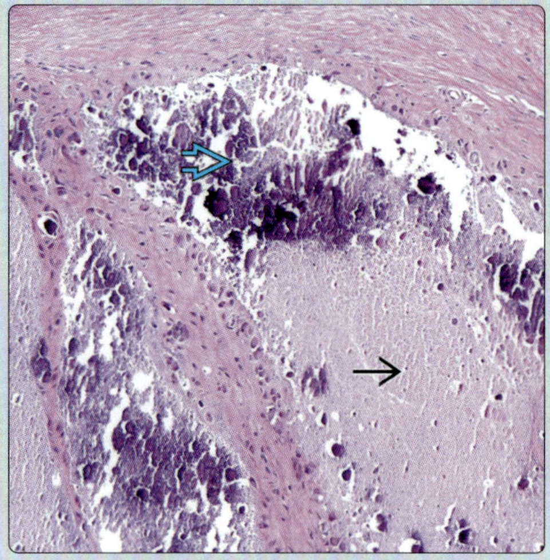

(Left) *Tumoral calcinosis is characterized by multiple variably sized cystic spaces containing amorphous granular material and divided by thick fibrous septa. The overall degree of calcification varies based upon the duration of the lesion.* **(Right)** *The calcium apatite crystals of tumoral calcinosis appear as amorphous eosinophilic granular material → within the cystic spaces. Superimposed basophilic calcification ⇨ often varies from cyst to cyst and ranges from heavy involvement to absent.*

Multinucleated Giant Cells

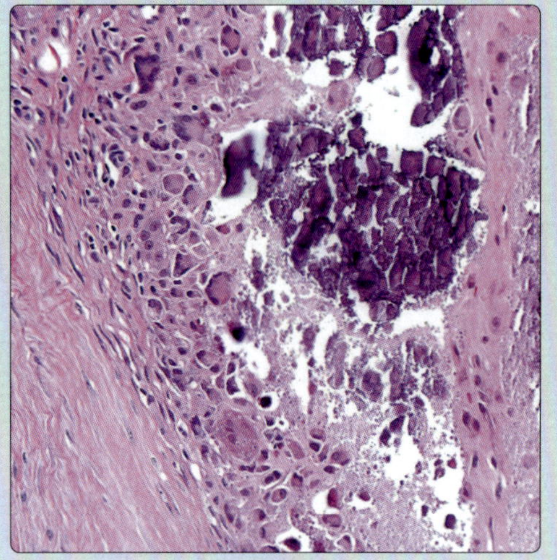

Psammoma Body-Like Calcification

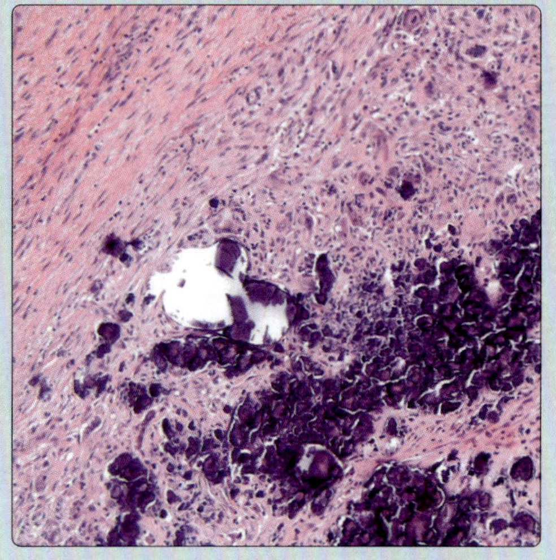

(Left) *Histiocytes and multinucleated giant cells are commonly identified in association with calcium apatite crystals in active tumoral calcinosis.* **(Right)** *In more longstanding cases of tumoral calcinosis, cystic spaces may be absent and only calcified aggregates remain within hyalinized fibrous tissue. Occasionally, the calcium deposits are rounded and lamellated (shown), resembling psammoma bodies or possibly even parasitic ova.*

TERMINOLOGY

Synonyms

- Lipid calcinosis, tumoral lipocalcinosis
- Calcifying collagenolysis, calcifying bursitis
- Hip stone disease

Definitions

- Tumor-like deposits of calcium hydroxyapatite in periarticular soft tissues

ETIOLOGY/PATHOGENESIS

Three Forms

- Sporadic/idiopathic (most common)
- Familial
  - Autosomal recessive
  - Hyperphosphatemic type: Mutations in *GALNT3*, *FGF23*, or *KL* genes
  - Normophosphatemic type: Mutations in *SAMD9* gene
- Secondary
  - Presence of underlying disorder (e.g., chronic renal failure) that promotes ectopic calcification

CLINICAL ISSUES

Epidemiology

- Age
  - Most cases < 20 years (rarely over 50 years)
- Ethnicity
  - Familial form more common in African Americans

Site

- Subcutis around large joints
  - Hip, elbow, and shoulder most common
- May be multiple
- Subset of similar lesions in acral extremities (tumoral calcinosis-like lesions)
  - Some associated with trauma or scleroderma

Presentation

- Firm, painless, subcutaneous mass
  - Attached to underlying fascia and tendons
  - Unrelated to bone and joint
  - Rarely ulcerates overlying skin
- In secondary forms, may show symptoms related to underlying disease

Treatment

- Surgical excision for sporadic/idiopathic and familial forms
- Medical treatment of underlying systemic condition is often necessary in secondary forms

Prognosis

- Benign
- Familial forms may recur
- Secondary forms depend upon treatment of underlying systemic condition

IMAGING

General Features

- Rounded nodules of dense periarticular calcification
- Radiolucent septations
- May see fluid levels in some nodules

MACROSCOPIC

General Features

- Firm, rubbery, multiloculated cystic mass
- Cystic spaces contain milky white-yellow fluid or semisolid, gritty material

Size

- Ranges from several mm up to 30 cm

MICROSCOPIC

Histologic Features

- Morphology is same regardless of form (sporadic, familial, secondary)
- Amorphous granular material (hydroxyapatite crystals) within cystic spaces
  - Variable degrees of chunky basophilic calcification
- Cystic spaces separated by thick fibrous septa
  - Lined by histiocytes and variable number of multinucleated giant cells
- May have psammoma body-like calcospherites
- Early lesions may show fibrohistiocytic proliferation without calcification, and late lesions may be entirely calcified

DIFFERENTIAL DIAGNOSIS

Calcified Soft Tissue Chondroma

- Usually distal extremities (hands and feet)
- Component of hyaline cartilage

Milk Alkali Syndrome

- Clinical history
- Hypercalcemia

Tophaceous Gout

- Polarizable, negatively birefringent needle-shaped crystals
- Usually lack degree of calcification seen in tumoral calcinosis
- Deposits appear amorphous and eosinophilic

Tophaceous Pseudogout

- Polarizable, positively birefringent, rhomboid-shaped calcium pyrophosphate crystals
- Deposits appear basophilic (calcium)
- Incites fibroblastic rather than histocytic response

SELECTED REFERENCES

1. Banshelkikar SN et al: Idiopathic tumoral calcinosis with unusual presentation-case report with review of literature. J Orthop Case Rep. 4(3):59-62, 2014
2. Fathi I et al: Review of tumoral calcinosis: a rare clinico-pathological entity. World J Clin Cases. 2(9):409-14, 2014
3. Chaabane S et al: Idiopathic tumoral calcinosis. Acta Orthop Belg. 74(6):837-45, 2008
4. Laskin WB et al: Calcareous lesions of the distal extremities resembling tumoral calcinosis (tumoral calcinosislike lesions): clinicopathologic study of 43 cases emphasizing a pathogenesis-based approach to classification. Am J Surg Pathol. 31(1):15-25, 2007
5. Möckel G et al: Tumoral calcinosis revisited: pathophysiology and treatment. Rheumatol Int. 25(1):55-9, 2005

Idiopathic Tumefactive Fibroinflammatory Lesions

KEY FACTS

TERMINOLOGY

- Group of mass-forming inflammatory disorders of uncertain etiology characterized by fibrosclerosis and variable chronic inflammatory infiltrate
  - Sclerosing mesenteritis, idiopathic retroperitoneal fibrosis (IRF), and IgG4-related sclerosing disease (IgG4-SD)

ETIOLOGY/PATHOGENESIS

- Uncertain/unknown

CLINICAL ISSUES

- Middle-aged to elderly adults
  - Male predominance in IRF and IgG4-SD
- IgG4-SD commonly shows visceral organ involvement
- Urinary obstructive symptoms common in IRF
- Serum IgG4 levels often elevated in IgG4-SD
- Treatment: Surgical excision for sclerosing mediastinitis
  - Long-term corticosteroid therapy for IRF and IgG4-SD
- Benign, nonneoplastic; good overall prognosis

MICROSCOPIC

- Sclerosing mesenteritis and IRF
  - Abundant fibrosis with chronic inflammatory infiltrate
  - Fat necrosis common in sclerosing mesenteritis
- IgG4-SD
  - Storiform fibrosis, prominent lymphoplasmacytic infiltrate, obliterative phlebitis, native tissue atrophy

ANCILLARY TESTS

- Elevated numbers of IgG4(+) plasma cells or increased IgG4:IgG ratio can support diagnosis of IgG4-SD

TOP DIFFERENTIAL DIAGNOSES

- Inflammatory myofibroblastic tumor
- Lymphoma
- Well-differentiated liposarcoma (sclerosing type)

Fibroinflammatory Process

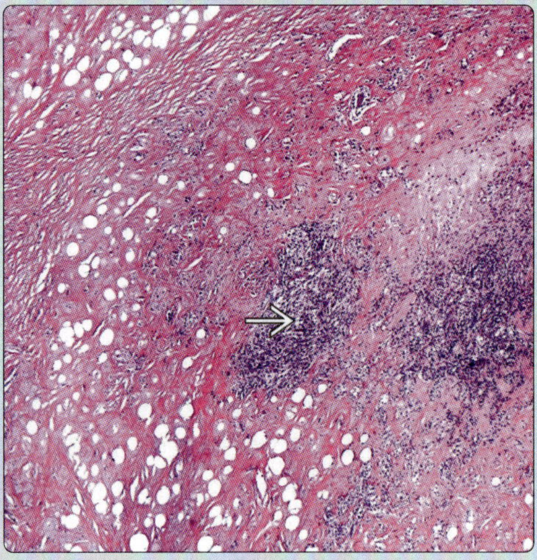

Chronic Inflammatory Infiltrate

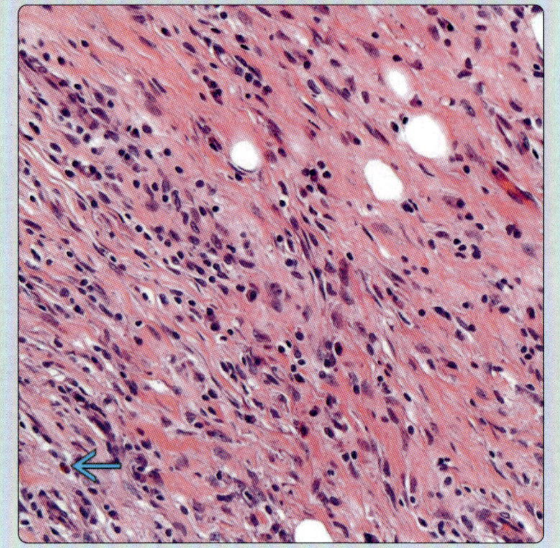

(Left) *Sclerosing mesenteritis and idiopathic retroperitoneal fibrosis (IRF) are histologically similar. Both are characterized by fibrosclerosis of region adipose and connective tissue with a variable prominent chronic inflammatory infiltrate* ➡. **(Right)** *Chronic inflammatory cells are typical of the tumoral fibroinflammatory diseases and usually consist of mainly lymphocytes and plasma cells; the latter is usually more prominent in a true IgG4-related disease. Eosinophils* → *may also be seen.*

Fat Necrosis

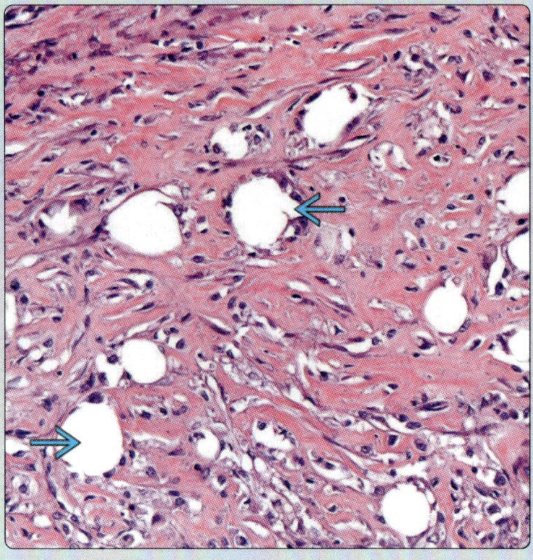

Germinal Centers

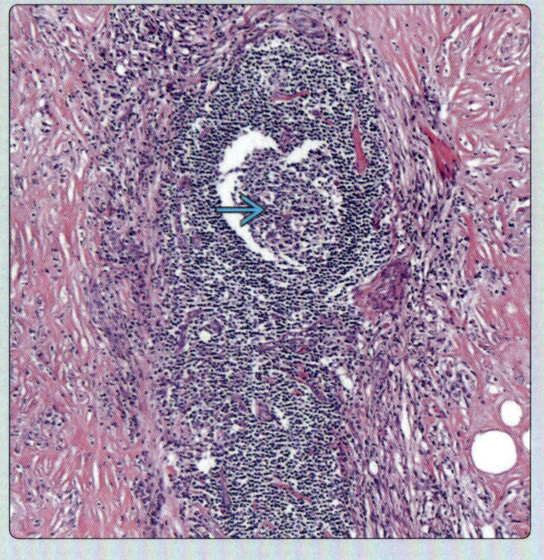

(Left) *Fat necrosis is a common finding in sclerosing mesenteritis but may be seen in other disorders. It is identified by eosinophilic to clear/foamy histiocytes associated with adipocytes* →. **(Right)** *A few germinal centers* → *may be seen in sclerosing mesenteritis and IRF; however, they are often much more numerous in an IgG4-related process.*

TERMINOLOGY

Abbreviations

- IgG4-related sclerosing disease (IgG4-SD)
- Idiopathic retroperitoneal fibrosis (IRF)

Synonyms

- Idiopathic tumoral fibroinflammatory disorders
- Mesenteric lipodystrophy, mesenteric panniculitis, or retractile mesenteritis (sclerosing mesenteritis)
- Ormond disease (IRF)

Definitions

- Group of mass-forming inflammatory disorders of uncertain etiology characterized by fibrosclerosis and variable chronic inflammatory infiltrate
  - Sclerosing mesenteritis
  - IRF
  - IgG4-SD
    - Systemic fibrosing disorder + visceral involvement and variably elevated serum IgG4

ETIOLOGY/PATHOGENESIS

Uncertain Etiology

- IgG4-SD may be related to autoimmune, infection (e.g., *Helicobacter pylori*), or allergy/hypersensitivity
  - Specific trigger unknown
- Subset of cases of sclerosing mesenteritis and primary IRF are related to IgG4-SD
  - Secondary retroperitoneal fibrosis can occur from radiotherapy, certain drugs (e.g., methysergide), and certain tumors (e.g., lymphoma)

CLINICAL ISSUES

Epidemiology

- Incidence
  - Sclerosing mesenteritis is most common of idiopathic fibroinflammatory disorders
- Age
  - Middle-aged to elderly adults
- Sex
  - Male predominance in IRF and IgG4-SD

Site

- Mesentery or retroperitoneum (sclerosing mesenteritis and IRF, respectively)
- IgG4-SD
  - Pancreas, liver/biliary tract, orbit, salivary gland, lung, other visceral organs
  - Skin, central nervous system, lymph nodes, retroperitoneum

Presentation

- Usually slow-growing masses
- Sclerosing mesenteritis
  - Abdominal pain
  - May be detected incidentally
    - Solitary or multiple mesenteric masses or diffuse thickening of mesentery
  - Cases with coexistence of visceral organ involvement suggests IgG4-SD (rare)
- IRF
  - Abdominal or back pain
  - Urinary obstructive symptoms; possible acute renal failure
  - Elevated C-reactive protein level and erythrocyte sedimentation rate common
  - Cases with coexistence of visceral organ involvement suggests IgG4-SD
- IgG4-SD
  - Symptoms depend upon sites involved
    - Organ involvement common and characteristic
  - Fever, constitutional symptoms uncommon
  - Serum IgG4 levels often elevated
    - May be low or normal following resection of tumoral mass

Treatment

- Sclerosing mesenteritis
  - Simple surgical excision
- IRF
  - Long-term corticosteroid therapy
  - Ureteral stenting
- IgG4-SD
  - Long-term corticosteroid therapy

Prognosis

- Benign, nonneoplastic
- Good overall; treatments generally effective
- Rare reported cases complicated by development of lymphoma

MACROSCOPIC

General Features

- Hard, tan-white tissue + gritty cut surface

Size

- Wide range (nodules/masses can be > 10 cm)

MICROSCOPIC

Histologic Features

- Sclerosing mesenteritis
  - Hypocellular + abundant fibrosis
  - Chronic inflammatory infiltrate
    - Mainly lymphocytes and histiocytes
    - Occasional lymphoid aggregates
  - Fat necrosis may be prominent
  - May show calcification
- IRF
  - Similar to sclerosing mesenteritis
    - Abundant fibrosis or sclerosis + chronic inflammatory infiltrate
- IgG4-SD
  - Storiform fibrosis characteristic
    - Extraparenchymal extension common
  - Prominent lymphoplasmacytic infiltrate
    - Often abundant lymphoid aggregates
    - May show increased eosinophils
  - May show inflammation and destructive of large veins and venules (obliterative phlebitis)
  - Atrophy &/or destruction of native tissue

ANCILLARY TESTS

Immunohistochemistry

- IgG4-SD
  - In general, elevated numbers of IgG4(+) plasma cells can support diagnosis
    - Minimum of 30-40 IgG4(+) plasma cells per HPF
    - IgG4 plasma cells comprise > 40% of total IgG plasma cells (> 0.4:1.0 ratio)
- Sclerosing mesenteritis and IRF
  - Immunohistochemistry best used to exclude other diagnoses (e.g., carcinoma, lymphoma)
  - Subset may be related to IgG4-SD [show elevated IgG4(+) plasma cells or increased IgG4:total IgG ratio]

DIFFERENTIAL DIAGNOSIS

Inflammatory Myofibroblastic Tumor

- Most common in children, adolescents, and young adults
- Generally well circumscribed
- More cellular with fascicles of plump myofibroblasts
- Absence of obliterative phlebitis and lack of abundant lymphoid aggregates
- Most cases have few IgG4(+) plasma cells
- ALK(+) in 50-60% of cases

Lymphoma

- Clonal B-cell lymphoid population
  - Immunohistochemistry can be very helpful
- Stromal sclerosis uncommon in lymphoma
  - Exception: Rare cases of follicular lymphoma
- Most lymphomas lack plasma cell population

Well-Differentiated Liposarcoma (Sclerosing Type)

- Can show histologic overlap with IRF
- Atypical, pleomorphic stromal "smudge" cells are characteristic of well-differentiated liposarcoma

Reactive Nonlesional Fibroblastic Proliferation

- Different clinical presentation from sclerosing mesenteritis, IRF, and IgG4-SD
- Mixed acute and chronic inflammation ± granulation tissue formation
- May be related to prior surgical procedure or secondary to unsampled carcinoma

Fibrosing (Sclerosing) Mediastinitis

- Related to chronic *Histoplasma* infection
- May show histologic overlap with IgG4-SD
  - Occasional cases show increased numbers of IgG4(+) plasma cells

Desmoid Fibromatosis

- Generally young adults
- Usually more cellular with long, "sweeping" fascicles of myofibroblastic cells
- Negligible inflammatory infiltrate
- Nuclear β-catenin (+) in 70% of cases

Gastrointestinal Stromal Tumor

- More cellular but variety of architectures and morphologies
- Stromal sclerosis uncommon
- CD117(+), DOG1(+), CD34(+)

Extranodal Rosai-Dorfman Disease

- Most cases lack diffuse sclerosis
- Large histiocytes with emperipolesis
  - S100 protein (+)

SELECTED REFERENCES

1. Martorana D et al: A large-scale genetic analysis reveals an autoimmune origin of idiopathic retroperitoneal fibrosis. J Allergy Clin Immunol. 142(5):1662-65, 2018
2. Sulieman I et al: IgG4-related disease mimicking pancreatic cancer: case report and review of the literature. Int J Surg Case Rep. 50:100-5, 2018
3. Tzou M et al: Retroperitoneal fibrosis. Vasc Med. 19(5):407-14, 2014
4. Khosroshahi A et al: Rethinking Ormond's disease: "idiopathic" retroperitoneal fibrosis in the era of IgG4-related disease. Medicine (Baltimore). 92(2):82-91, 2013
5. Cheuk W et al: Lymphadenopathy of IgG4-related disease: an underdiagnosed and overdiagnosed entity. Semin Diagn Pathol. 29(4):226-34, 2012
6. Divatia M et al: IgG4-related sclerosing disease, an emerging entity: a review of a multi-system disease. Yonsei Med J. 53(1):15-34, 2012
7. Grimm KE et al: Histopathological findings in 29 lymph node biopsies with increased IgG4 plasma cells. Mod Pathol. 25(3):480-91, 2012
8. Saab ST et al: IgG4 plasma cells in inflammatory myofibroblastic tumor: inflammatory marker or pathogenic link? Mod Pathol. 24(4):606-12, 2011
9. Cheuk W et al: IgG4-related sclerosing disease: a critical appraisal of an evolving clinicopathologic entity. Adv Anat Pathol. 17(5):303-32, 2010
10. Geyer JT et al: Chronic sclerosing sialadenitis (Küttner tumor) is an IgG4-associated disease. Am J Surg Pathol. 34(2):202-10, 2010
11. Inoue D et al: Immunoglobulin G4-related lung disease: CT findings with pathologic correlations. Radiology. 251(1):260-70, 2009
12. Vega J et al: Treatment of idiopathic retroperitoneal fibrosis with colchicine and steroids: a case series. Am J Kidney Dis. 53(4):628-37, 2009
13. Yamamoto H et al: Inflammatory myofibroblastic tumor versus IgG4-related sclerosing disease and inflammatory pseudotumor: a comparative clinicopathologic study. Am J Surg Pathol 33: 1330-40, 2009
14. Zen Y et al: Retroperitoneal fibrosis: a clinicopathologic study with respect to immunoglobulin G4. Am J Surg Pathol. 33(12):1833-9, 2009
15. Chen TS et al: Are tumefactive lesions classified as sclerosing mesenteritis a subset of IgG4-related sclerosing disorders? J Clin Pathol. 61(10):1093-7, 2008
16. Cheuk W et al: Lymphadenopathy of IgG4-related sclerosing disease. Am J Surg Pathol. 32(5):671-81, 2008
17. Akram S et al: Sclerosing mesenteritis: clinical features, treatment, and outcome in ninety-two patients. Clin Gastroenterol Hepatol. 5(5):589-96; quiz 523-4, 2007
18. Björnsson E et al: Immunoglobulin G4 associated cholangitis: description of an emerging clinical entity based on review of the literature. Hepatology. 45(6):1547-54, 2007
19. Zhang L et al: IgG4-positive plasma cell infiltration in the diagnosis of autoimmune pancreatitis. Mod Pathol. 20(1):23-8, 2007
20. Kitagawa S et al: Abundant IgG4-positive plasma cell infiltration characterizes chronic sclerosing sialadenitis (Küttner's tumor). Am J Surg Pathol. 29(6):783-91, 2005
21. Zen Y et al: IgG4-positive plasma cells in inflammatory pseudotumor (plasma cell granuloma) of the lung. Hum Pathol. 36(7):710-7, 2005
22. Abraham SC et al: Pancreaticoduodenectomy (Whipple resections) in patients without malignancy: are they all 'chronic pancreatitis'? Am J Surg Pathol. 27(1):110-20, 2003
23. Montgomery E et al: Beta-catenin immunohistochemistry separates mesenteric fibromatosis from gastrointestinal stromal tumor and sclerosing mesenteritis. Am J Surg Pathol. 26(10):1296-301, 2002
24. Emory TS et al: Sclerosing mesenteritis, mesenteric panniculitis and mesenteric lipodystrophy: a single entity? Am J Surg Pathol. 21(4):392-8, 1997

Dense Collagen

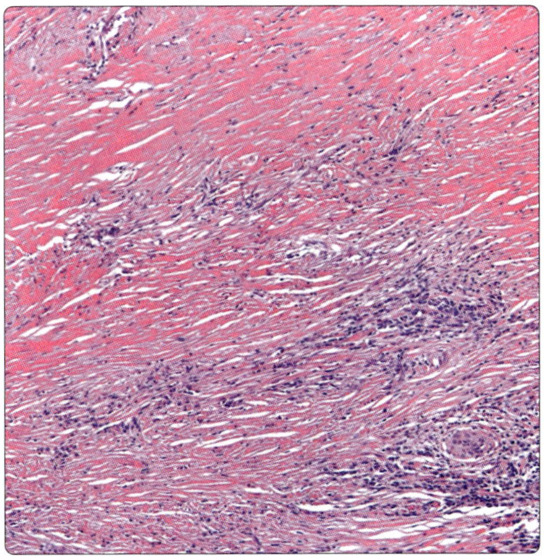

Calcification

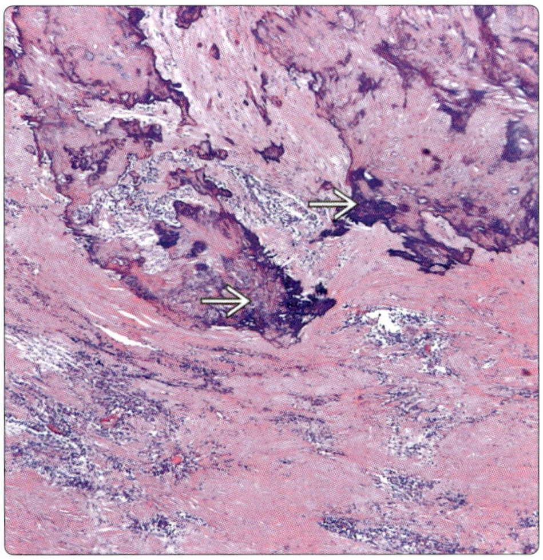

(Left) *Dense or sclerotic collagen is a consistent finding in the tumoral fibroinflammatory diseases and may be patchy or extensive.* **(Right)** *Calcification ➡ may be seen in some cases of sclerosing mesenteritis or IRF, particularly in longstanding lesions. The presence of this feature is often readily noticed during gross sectioning of the specimen.*

IgG4-Related Sclerosing Disease

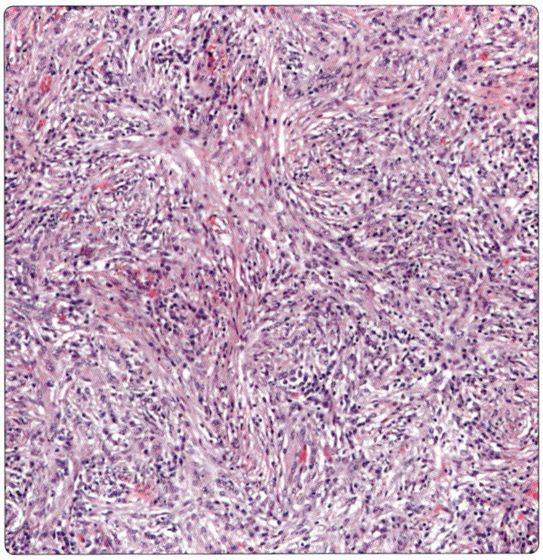

IgG4-Related Sclerosing Disease

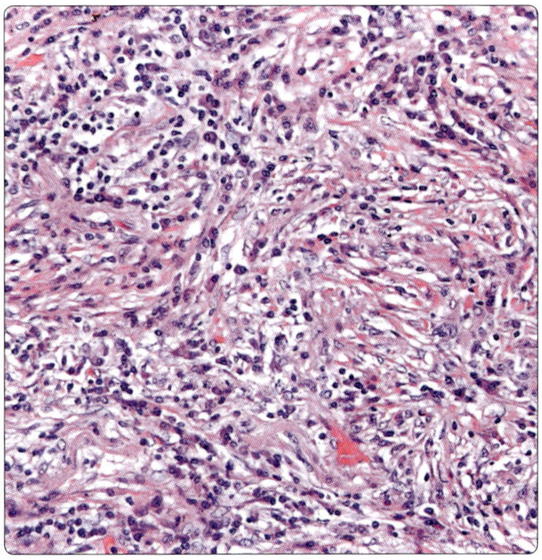

(Left) *Fibrosis with a storiform or loose-swirling pattern is characteristic of IgG4-related sclerosing disease. This image is of the disease affecting the lung in a 52-year-old man.* **(Right)** *A lymphoplasmacytic infiltrate is often prominent in IgG4-related sclerosing disease, and plasma cells are usually plentiful. Eosinophils may also be increased.*

Phlebitis

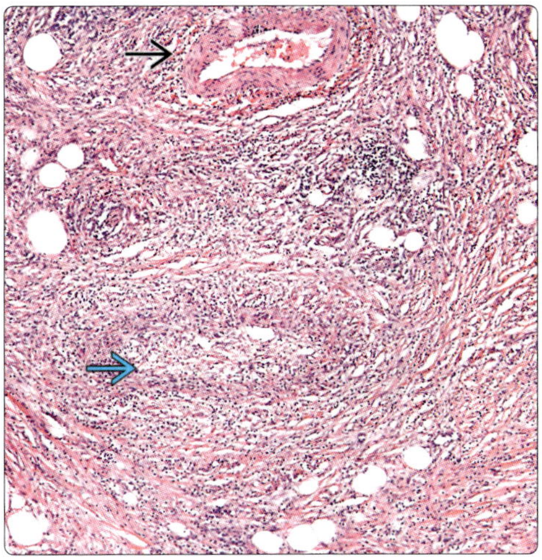

IgG4(+) Plasma Cells

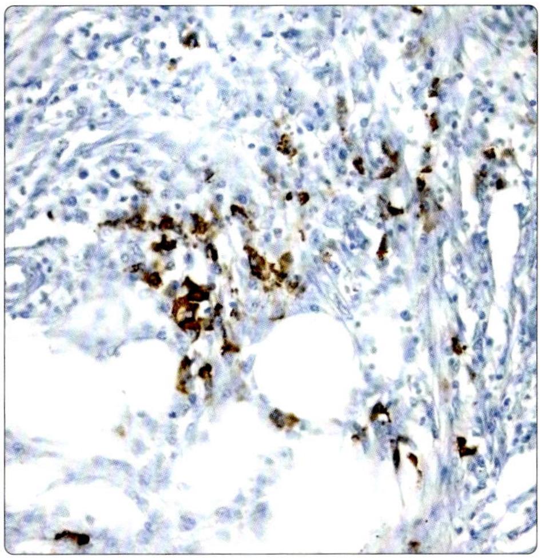

(Left) *This H&E shows inflammation and destruction of a vein ➡ (lymphocytic or obliterative phlebitis) within the setting of IgG4-related sclerosing disease. Note the normal artery ➡. A mild form of this finding may be seen focally in rare cases of sclerosing mesenteritis and IRF.* **(Right)** *Quantification of IgG4(+) plasma cells or the ratio of IgG4(+):IgG(+) plasma cells is often a helpful method for supporting a diagnosis of IgG4-related sclerosing disease.*

Cardiac Myxoma

KEY FACTS

TERMINOLOGY

- Benign myxoid neoplasm that occurs specifically in heart and is of uncertain etiology

CLINICAL ISSUES

- Most common tumor of heart overall
- Most cases are sporadic; rarely familial
- Usually left atrium (most common) or right atrium
- Symptoms at presentation depend upon site of origin
  - Often valvular obstruction
- Surgical excision is generally curative; recurrences rare
- Systemic or pulmonary embolization may occur, depending on site of origin

MACROSCOPIC

- Soft, gelatinous mass

MICROSCOPIC

- Generally hypocellular with abundant myxoid stroma
- Cells are spindled or stellate and often associated with capillaries in concentric onion-skin or sheath-like arrangement
- Hemorrhage and degenerative changes are common
- Mitoses uncommon

ANCILLARY TESTS

- Immunophenotype
  - CD34(+), CD31(+), vimentin (+)
  - Variably positive for calretinin, desmin, SMA, S100
  - Negative for keratin, CD117
- Molecular
  - Rearrangements of 12p1 and 17p1
  - *PRKAR1A* gene (17q24) mutations occur in cases associated with Carney complex

TOP DIFFERENTIAL DIAGNOSES

- Myxofibrosarcoma

(Left) *Cardiac myxoma ➡ is the most common tumor of the heart and frequently arises from the interatrial wall of the left atrium. Cardiac muscle ⇨ is usually identified in histologic sections near the base of the myxoma.* **(Right)** *Cardiac myxoma classically shows an abundant eosinophilic myxoid matrix containing small spindled, polygonal, or stellate cells in various architectures, including singly and in cords.*

Cardiac Myxoma

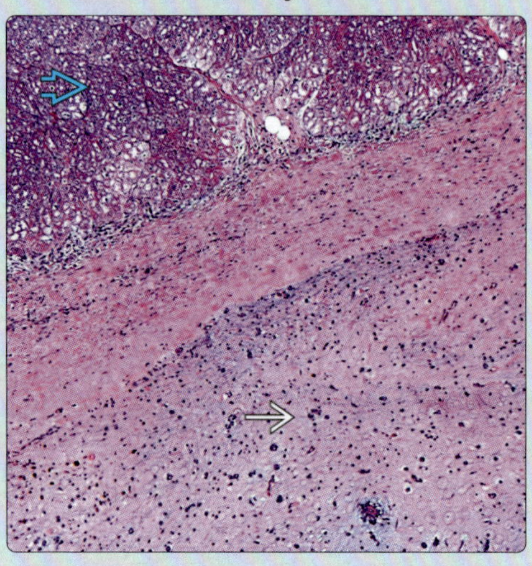

Myxoid Stroma

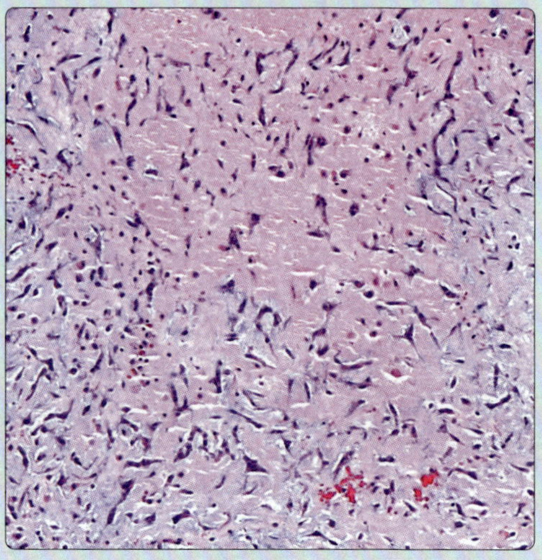

(Left) *The constituent cells of cardiac myxoma generally show small hyperchromatic nuclei, which may number from 1 to several. Significant nuclear atypia is not a feature of this tumor. Mitoses are generally rare but may be more prominent in cellular foci.* **(Right)** *Among other growth patterns, a distinct perivascular orientation of tumor cells is common in cardiac myxoma. In this image, the cells adopt a loose, concentric arrangement.*

Myxoma Cells

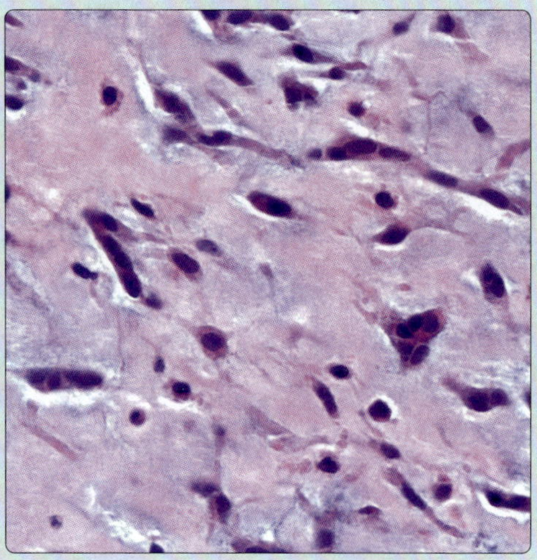

Perivascular Organization

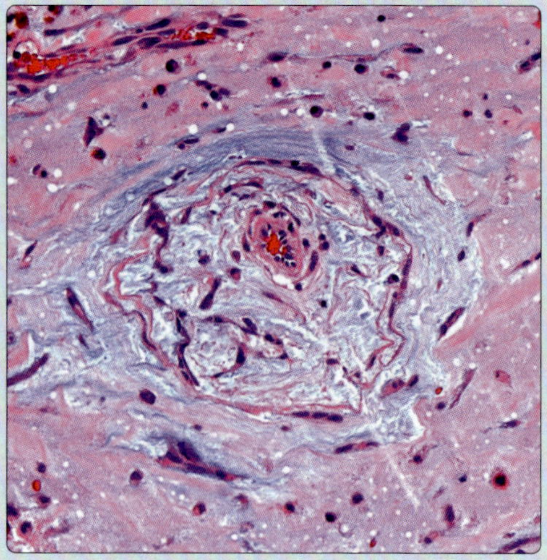

TERMINOLOGY

Definitions

- Benign myxoid neoplasm that occurs specifically in heart and is of uncertain etiology

CLINICAL ISSUES

Epidemiology

- Incidence
  - Most common tumor of heart
  - Most cases are sporadic
    - Rare cases are familial and may present as part of syndrome (including Carney complex)
- Age
  - All ages (most common: 30-60 years)
- Sex
  - 2:1 female predominance

Site

- Usually left atrium (70% of cases) or right atrium
  - Often at or near foramen ovale
  - Usually attached by narrow pedicle
- Rare locations: Left ventricle, right ventricle, and valves
- Syndromic examples are more likely to be multiple and occur in unusual intracardiac locations

Presentation

- Up to 20% of cases are asymptomatic at time of diagnosis
- Symptomatic cases depend upon site of origin
  - Left atrium
    - Symptoms of mitral valve obstruction
    - May also send tumor emboli into systemic circulation, which may result in myocardial infarction, stroke, or peripheral infarction
  - Right atrium
    - Symptoms related to tricuspid valve obstruction
    - May send tumor emboli to lungs

Treatment

- Surgical excision of myxoma with portion of interatrial septum or surrounding tissue

Prognosis

- Recurrences are rare
  - Higher risk in familial and syndromic cases
- Systemic or pulmonary embolization may occur
  - Tumors with irregular/papillary/villous outer contour have increased risk

IMAGING

Ultrasonographic Findings

- Usually detected on echocardiography

MACROSCOPIC

General Features

- Soft, gelatinous mass
- Smooth or irregular/papillary/villous outer contour

Size

- 0.1-10.0 cm (average: 5 cm)

MICROSCOPIC

Histologic Features

- Luminal surface may be smooth or irregular/papillary/villous
- Generally hypocellular with abundant myxoid stroma
  - Luminal and subluminal cellularity may be seen
- Cells have eosinophilic cytoplasm and are spindled, stellate, or polygonal
  - 1 or more small hyperchromatic nuclei
  - Often associated with capillaries in concentric onion-skin or sheath-like arrangement
- Hemorrhage and degenerative changes are common
  - Hemosiderin deposition, fibrosis, chronic inflammation, macrophages
  - Calcification, extramedullary hematopoiesis, and metaplastic bone formation are less common
- Mitoses uncommon
  - Both normal and atypical figures may be seen in cellular regions
- Very rare findings
  - Mucinous glandular differentiation, thymic rests

ANCILLARY TESTS

Immunohistochemistry

- CD34(+), CD31(+), vimentin (+)
- Negative for keratin, CD117
- Loss of PRKAR1-α protein expression
- Variable expression of calretinin, desmin, SMA, S100
- Rare epithelial elements express keratins, EMA, CK7, and CEA and may also show neuroendocrine differentiation

Molecular Genetics

- Rearrangements of 12p1 and 17p1
- *PRKAR1A* gene (17q24) mutations occur in cases associated with Carney complex

DIFFERENTIAL DIAGNOSIS

Myxofibrosarcoma

- Much rarer in heart than cardiac myxoma
- Often prominent nuclear atypia and often numerous mitotic figures
- Invasive growth with involvement of pedicle/cardiac muscle

SELECTED REFERENCES

1. Wang JG et al: Clinicopathologic features and outcomes of primary cardiac tumors: a 16-year-experience with 212 patients at a Chinese medical center. Cardiovasc Pathol. 33:45-54, 2018
2. Nath D et al: Immunohistochemical characterization of glandular elements in glandular cardiac myxoma: study of six cases. Indian J Pathol Microbiol. 60(3):319-23, 2017
3. Maleszewski JJ et al: PRKAR1A in the development of cardiac myxoma: a study of 110 cases including isolated and syndromic tumors. Am J Surg Pathol. 38(8):1079-87, 2014
4. Zhang M et al: Cardiac myxoma with glandular elements: a clinicopathological and immunohistochemical study of five new cases with an emphasis on differential diagnosis. Pathol Res Pract. 210(1):55-8, 2014
5. Swartz MF et al: Atrial myxomas: pathologic types, tumor location, and presenting symptoms. J Card Surg. 21(4):435-40, 2006
6. Pucci A et al: Histopathologic and clinical characterization of cardiac myxoma: review of 53 cases from a single institution. Am Heart J. 140(1):134-8, 2000

(Left) *A tight perivascular growth pattern* → *with increased cellularity (often referred to as "cuffing") is commonly seen in cardiac myxoma. The degree of cellularity may be striking in some cases.* **(Right)** *Although tumor cells in cardiac myxoma most often occur singly or in small groups, a relatively delicate anastomosing corded growth pattern may also be seen.*

Perivascular Organization

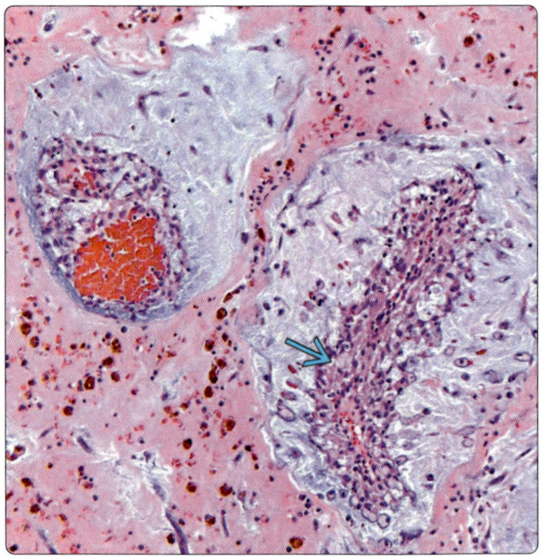

Corded Growth

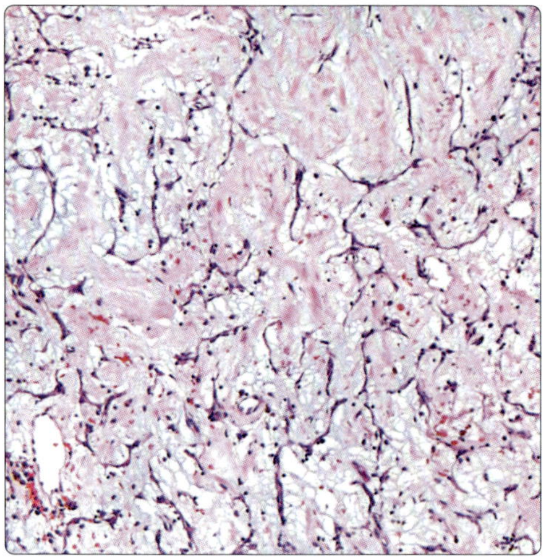

(Left) *Hemorrhage is common in cardiac myxoma and is hardly surprising given the vascularity of this tumor. Hemosiderin deposition* → *is also easily identified in most cases, even away from areas of hemorrhage.* **(Right)** *In many cases of cardiac myxoma, thrombus formation can be identified grossly on the surface of the tumor. Thrombi* → *may also be identified within the tumor in dilated vessels.*

Hemorrhage and Hemosiderin

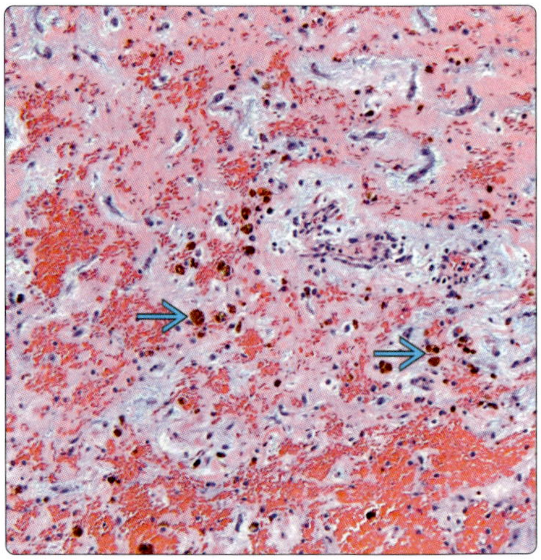

Thrombus Formation

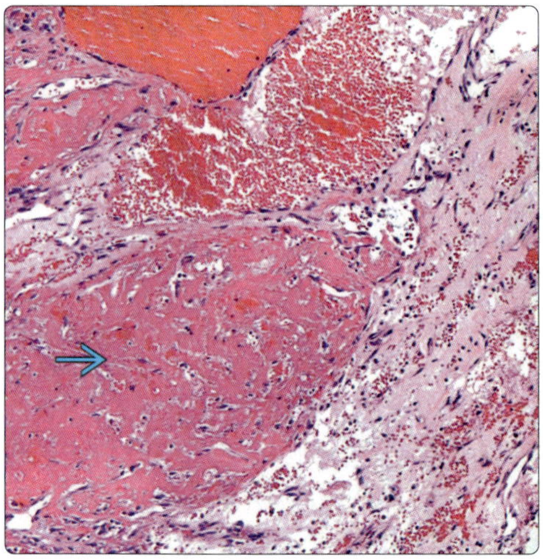

(Left) *In some cases of cardiac myxoma, a collection of thick-walled and often tortuous blood vessels can be identified, particularly near the base/pedicle of the tumor.* **(Right)** *A chronic inflammatory infiltrate is quite common in cardiac myxoma and usually consists of lymphocytes, plasma cells, and histiocytes. Neutrophils may also be identified and in some cases might possibly represent an overlying, coexisting infection.*

Thick-Walled Vessels

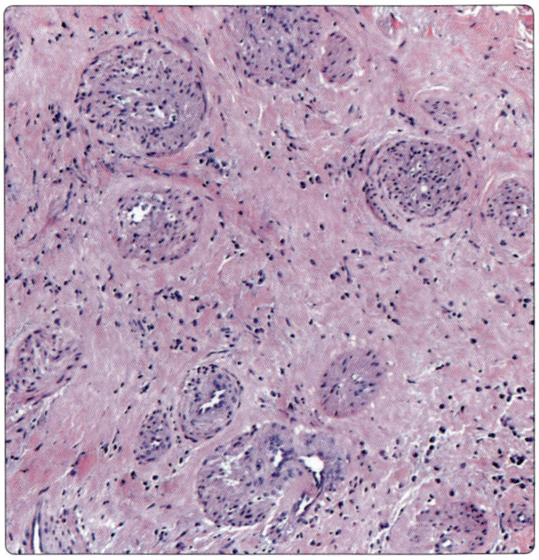

Inflammatory Infiltrate

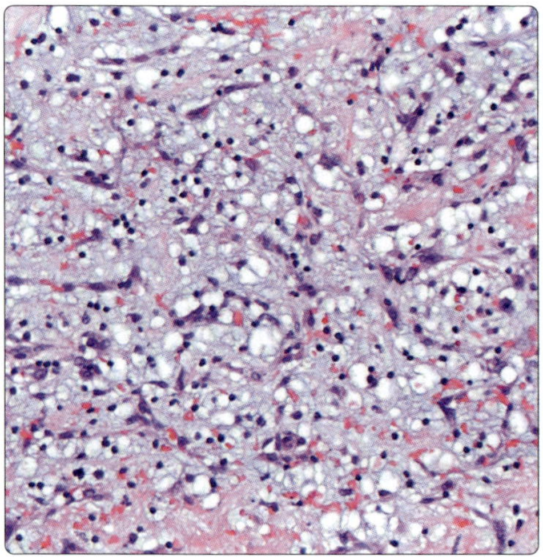

Calcification

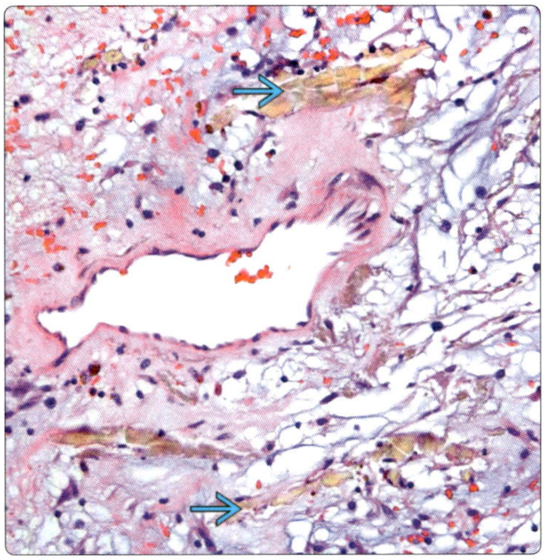

Smooth Luminal Contour

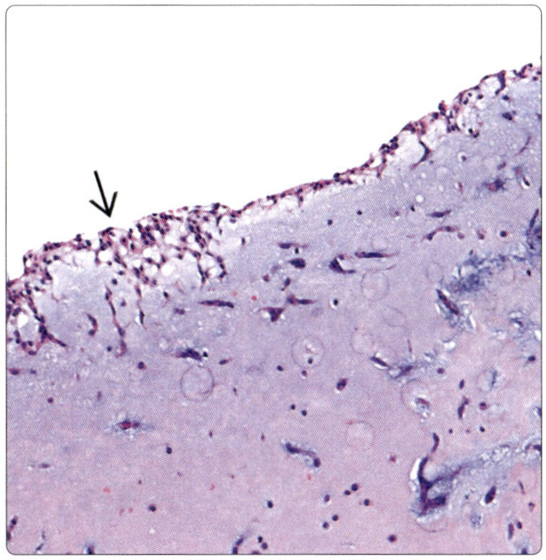

(Left) *Stromal calcification* → *may be seen in some cases of cardiac myxoma, particularly tumors localized to the right atrium. Foci of calcification superimposed upon elastic fibers have been referred to as Gamna-Gandy bodies.* **(Right)** *In most cases of cardiac myxoma, the outer/luminal surface is smooth and regular, both macro- and microscopically. This surface is often lined by tumor cells, which may show focal increases in cellularity* →, *reminiscent of synovial lining.*

Papillary/Villous Configuration

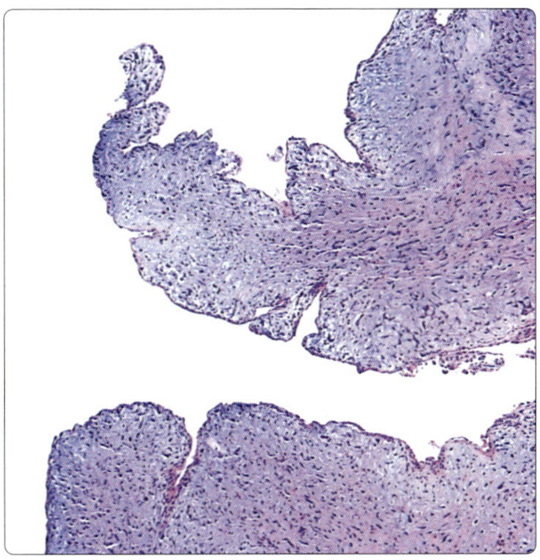

Increased Surface Cellularity

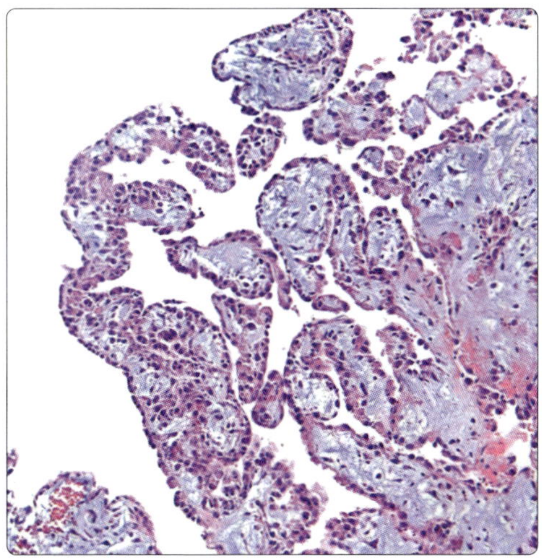

(Left) *Less commonly, a cardiac myxoma may show an irregular papillary or villous luminal configuration, which can also be appreciated grossly. This variant has a higher risk of shedding tumor emboli due to its relative friability.* **(Right)** *Increased surface cellularity may be seen in papillary/villous forms of cardiac myxoma and can be alarming. The tumor cells are also often more rounded and plump, as depicted.*

Mitotic Figures

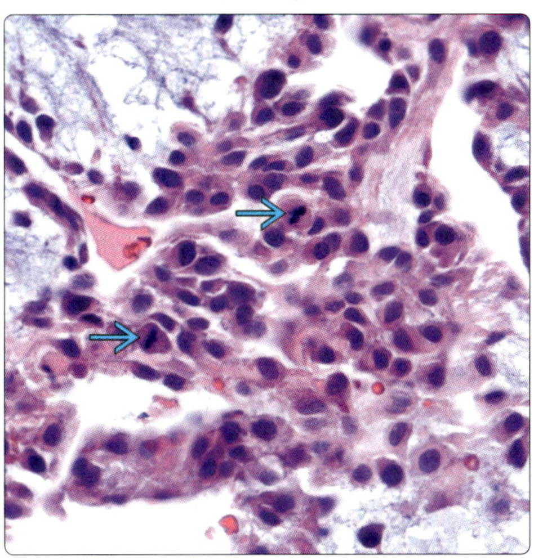

Glandular Myxoma

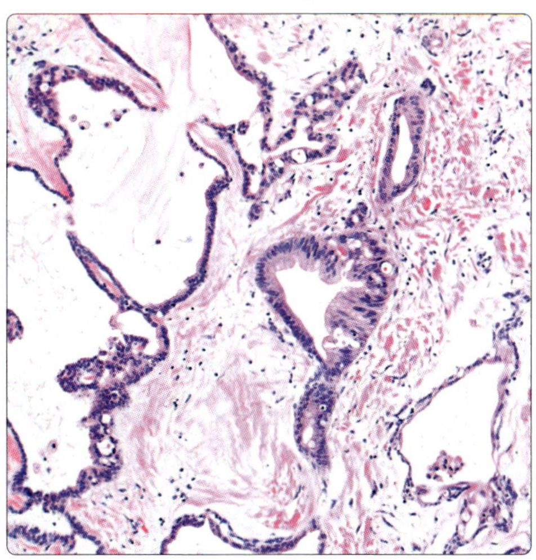

(Left) *In areas of increased cellularity, mitotic figures* → *(including atypical forms) may be identified in cardiac myxoma.* **(Right)** *Rare cases of cardiac myxoma contain glandular elements, as depicted. Note that no cellular anaplasia, mitotic activity, or necrosis is present. Most reported cases have shown CK7 expression in these elements, while markers such as CK20 and TTF-1 are negative.*

Cardiac Fibroma

KEY FACTS

TERMINOLOGY

- Benign cardiac neoplasm composed of fibroblasts and occurring predominantly in childhood

ETIOLOGY/PATHOGENESIS

- Most are sporadic
- May occur as feature of Gorlin (nevoid basal cell carcinoma) syndrome

CLINICAL ISSUES

- 2nd most common primary pediatric heart tumor
- Most cases (80%) occur in children
- Primarily ventricular septum or free wall of left ventricle
- May be asymptomatic or present with heart murmur, arrhythmia, symptoms of congestive heart failure, or as sudden death
- Treatment: Surgical excision

IMAGING

- Often detected on echocardiogram or MR

MACROSCOPIC

- Usually 3-8 cm

MICROSCOPIC

- Often mildly infiltrative border with normal cardiac tissue
- Spindle cells in irregular, loose fascicles
- Edematous or myxoid matrix containing collagen and elastic fibers
- Bland nuclear cytology and rare-to-no mitotic figures
- May show foci of extramedullary hematopoiesis, chronic inflammation, or calcification

ANCILLARY TESTS

- Immunophenotype: SMA(+), desmin (-), S100 protein (-)
- *PTCH1* gene (9q22) abnormalities (deletion/translocations)

TOP DIFFERENTIAL DIAGNOSES

- Inflammatory myofibroblastic tumor
- Atrial myxoma

Cardiac Fibroma

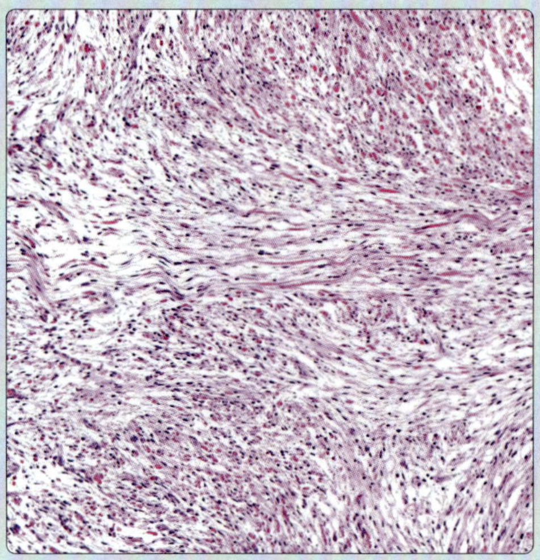

Infiltrative Border

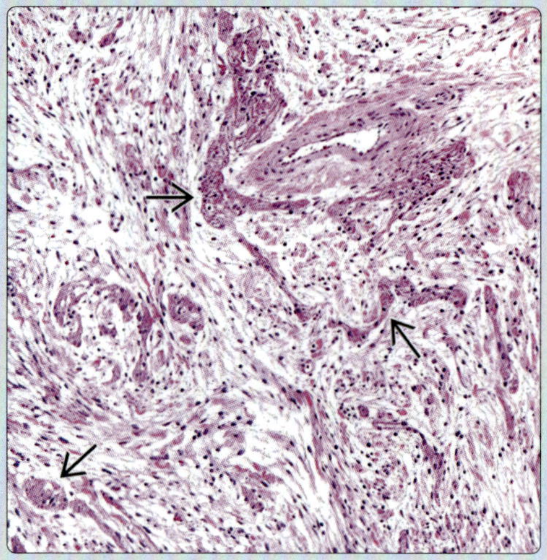

(Left) *Cardiac fibroma is the 2nd most common primary pediatric heart tumor and is most frequently encountered in the ventricular wall or septum during the 1st year of life. Histologically, it is characterized by loose fascicles of fibroblastic spindled cells.* **(Right)** *In cardiac fibroma, there is often evidence of focal infiltration at the peripheral interface with the normal heart. Note the irregular clusters of cardiac myocytes ➙ between tumor cells.*

Bland Cytology

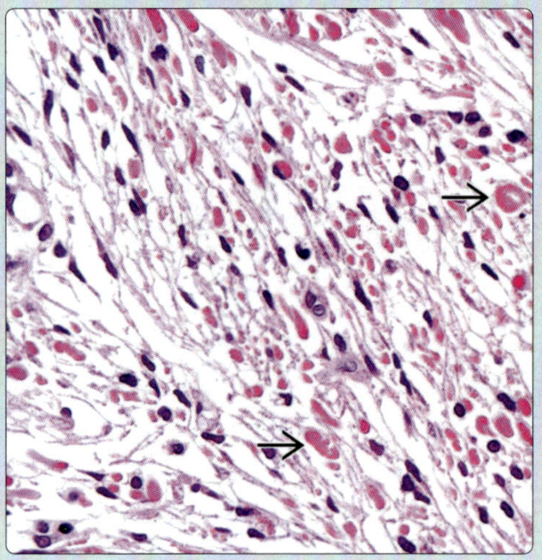

Extramedullary Hematopoiesis

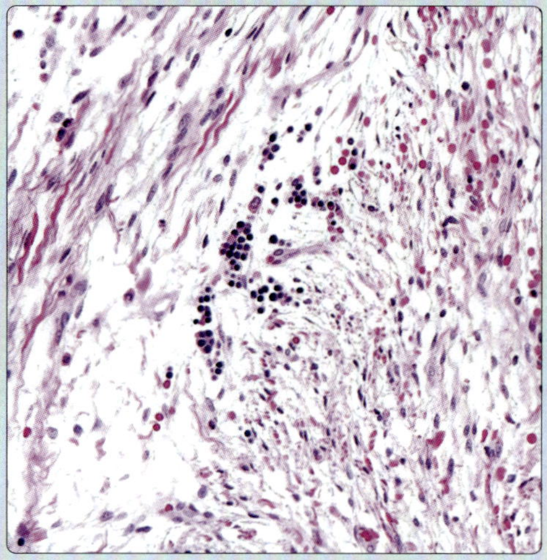

(Left) *The cytologic features of cardiac fibroma are uniformly bland, and there is often a conspicuous component of stromal collagen ➙ and small, irregular elastic fibers. Mitotic figures are rare to absent in most cases.* **(Right)** *In some cases of cardiac fibroma, particularly in patients younger than 5 months, foci of extramedullary hematopoiesis are seen. Calcification and chronic inflammation may also be seen in rare cases.*

TERMINOLOGY

Definitions

- Benign cardiac neoplasm composed of fibroblasts

ETIOLOGY/PATHOGENESIS

Genetics

- Most are sporadic
- May occur as feature of Gorlin (nevoid basal cell carcinoma) syndrome
  - Autosomal dominant inheritance
  - Other features: Basal cell carcinoma, skeletal abnormalities, jaw cysts, ovarian fibromas, medulloblastoma, cataracts
- *PTCH1* (tumor suppressor) gene on 9q22 appears to play role in pathogenesis
  - Identified in both syndromic and sporadic cases

CLINICAL ISSUES

Epidemiology

- Incidence
  - 2nd most common primary pediatric heart tumor
- Age
  - Most cases (80%) occur in children
    - Particularly 1st year of life
  - Rare cases in young adults

Site

- Primarily ventricular septum or free wall of left ventricle
- Less commonly free wall of right ventricle

Presentation

- May be asymptomatic or present with heart murmur, arrhythmia, or symptoms of congestive heart failure
  - Also sudden death
- Usually solitary lesions

Treatment

- Surgical excision
- Reports of heart transplant being performed for large, unresectable tumors

Prognosis

- Benign
- Surgical removal often relieves symptoms

IMAGING

General Features

- Intramural growth
- Often detected on echocardiogram or MR

MACROSCOPIC

General Features

- Well demarcated
- Firm, tan/gray/white cut surface

Size

- Usually 3-8 cm

MICROSCOPIC

Histologic Features

- Often mildly infiltrative border with normal cardiac tissue
  - Unencapsulated
- Spindle cells in irregular, loose fascicles
- Edematous or myxoid matrix containing collagen and elastic fibers
- Bland nuclear cytology
- Mitotic figures rare
- May show foci of extramedullary hematopoiesis or chronic inflammation
- Focal calcification in 25% of cases

ANCILLARY TESTS

Immunohistochemistry

- SMA(+)
- Desmin (-), CD34(-), S100 protein (-)

Genetic Testing

- *PTCH1* gene (9q22) abnormalities
  - Loss/deletion
  - Translocations reported include t(1;9)(q32;q22) and t(1;9;5)(q24;q22;q22)

DIFFERENTIAL DIAGNOSIS

Inflammatory Myofibroblastic Tumor

- Very rare in heart
- Usually endocardial or polypoid growth
- Inflammatory cells (both acute and chronic) are usually abundant

Atrial Myxoma

- Rarely occur in cardiac ventricles
- Very different morphologic appearance

Papillary Fibroelastoma

- Most commonly arise from cardiac valves
- Prominent papillary fronds with collagen- and elastin-rich cores
- Fronds lined by plump endothelial cells

SELECTED REFERENCES

1. Humez S et al: [Cardiac fibroma: a rare cause of sudden child death.] Ann Pathol. 35(5):445-8, 2015
2. Zhang Q et al: Somatic copy number losses on chromosome 9q21.33q22.33 encompassing the PTCH1 loci associated with cardiac fibroma. Cancer Genet. 208(12):615-20, 2015
3. Chu ZG et al: Cardiac fibromas in the adult. J Card Surg. 29(2):159-62, 2014
4. Cronin B et al: Cardiac fibroma presenting as sudden unexpected death in an adolescent. Forensic Sci Med Pathol. 10(4):647-50, 2014
5. Kumar N et al: Primary cardiac tumours in a paediatric population: an experience from a tertiary centre with a review of literature. Afr J Paediatr Surg. 11(1):44-7, 2014
6. Tao TY et al: Pediatric cardiac tumors: clinical and imaging features. Radiographics. 34(4):1031-46, 2014
7. Piazza N et al: Primary cardiac tumours: eighteen years of surgical experience on 21 patients. Can J Cardiol. 20(14):1443-8, 2004
8. Ferguson HL et al: Infant cardiac fibroma with clonal t(1;9)(q32;q22) and review of benign fibrous tissue cytogenetics. Cancer Genet Cytogenet. 87(1):34-7, 1996

Congenital Granular Cell Epulis

KEY FACTS

TERMINOLOGY

- Rare, benign lesion of uncertain histogenesis that most commonly arises in newborn girls and is composed of large, granular cells

CLINICAL ISSUES

- Exclusively newborn infants
- Marked female predominance (10:1)
- Maxillary alveolar ridge most common site
- Enlarging gingival growth while in utero
- Most cases are solitary and polypoid
- No reported associations with syndromes or genetic anomalies
- Treatment: Conservative excision
- Benign

MACROSCOPIC

- Well circumscribed
- Usually 1-2 cm

MICROSCOPIC

- Overlying squamous mucosa is thinned/attenuated or ulcerated
- Nests, sheets, and cords of polygonal to ovoid cells with abundant granular cytoplasm and distinct cell membranes
- Small nuclei with vesicular to stippled chromatin and often small nucleoli
- Prominent stromal capillary network

ANCILLARY TESTS

- Negative for S100 protein, CD68, keratins, CD34, SMA, desmin, calponin

TOP DIFFERENTIAL DIAGNOSES

- Granular cell tumor
- Adult-type rhabdomyoma
- Alveolar soft part sarcoma
- Lobular capillary hemangioma (pyogenic granuloma)

(Left) *Congenital granular cell epulis (CGCE) is a rare but distinctive lesion that arises along the maxillary or mandibular alveolar ridges in newborns, particularly girls. These lesions are well circumscribed and commonly show thinning of the overlying squamous epithelium ➡.* **(Right)** *CGCE is composed of nests and sheets of polygonal to ovoid cells with granular cytoplasm. Stromal vessels are prominent ➡, and a chronic inflammatory infiltrate ⇨ may be seen.*

Congenital Granular Cell Epulis

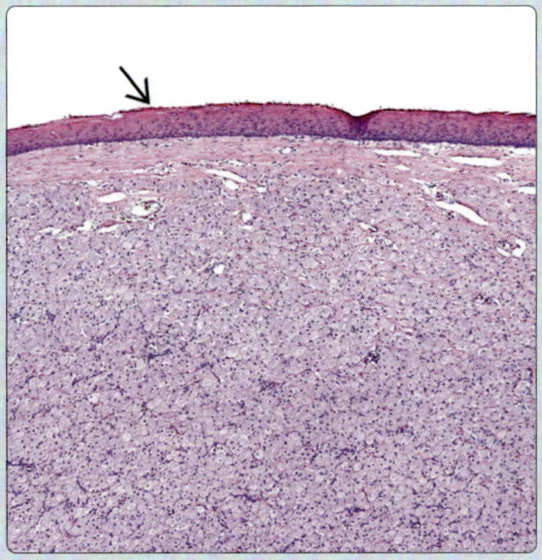

Nests and Sheets

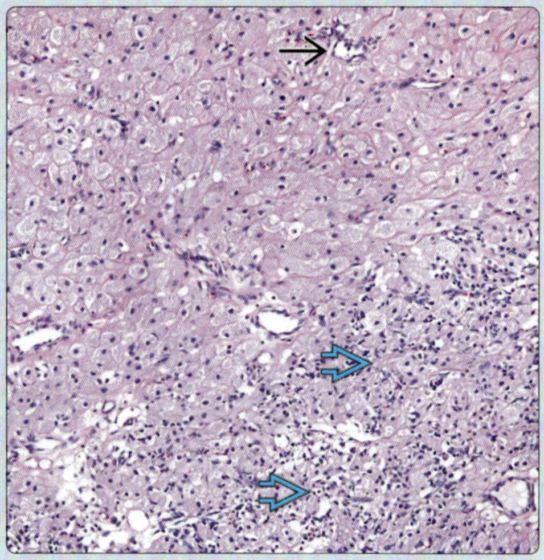

(Left) *The lesional cells of CGCE demonstrate prominent granular cytoplasm and sharp cytoplasmic borders. Nuclei are often slightly irregular in contour with vesicular to stippled chromatin and small nucleoli.* **(Right)** *Some cases of CGCE show zones of fibrosis or other uncommon findings, such as spindled cells and odontogenic epithelial rests. Note the ectatic (sometimes "staghorn") stromal vessels ➡, a relatively common finding in CGCE, at least focally.*

Granular Cells

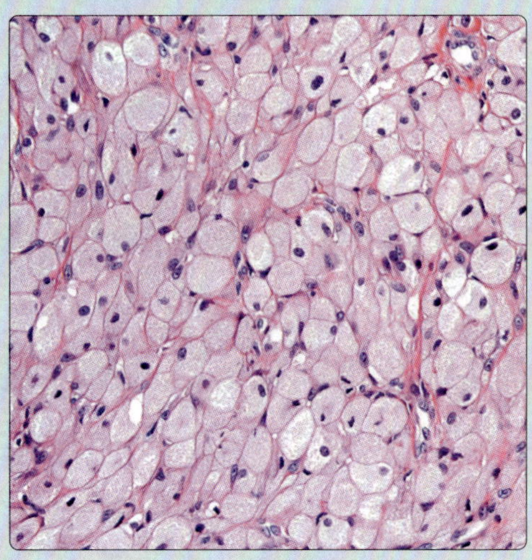

Fibrosis

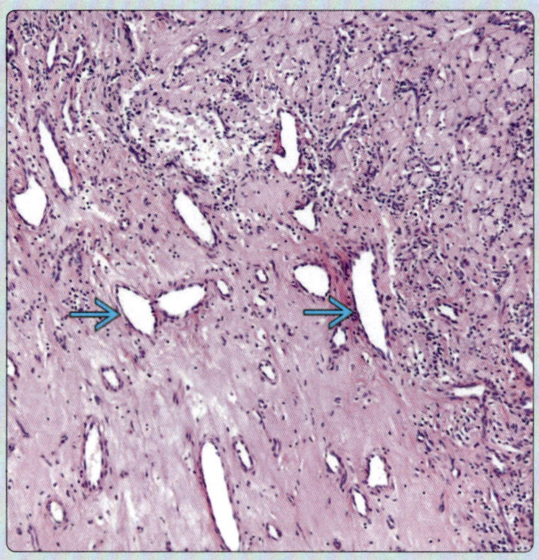

Congenital Granular Cell Epulis

TERMINOLOGY

Synonyms

- Congenital epulis of newborn
- Congenital granular cell tumor
- Granular cell fibroblastoma

Definitions

- Rare, benign lesion of uncertain histogenesis that most commonly arises in newborn girls and is composed of large, granular cells

CLINICAL ISSUES

Epidemiology

- Incidence
  - Rare
- Age
  - Exclusively newborn infants
- Sex
  - Marked female predominance (10:1)

Site

- Dental alveolar ridge
  - Maxilla more common than mandible

Presentation

- Can be diagnosed prenatally by ultrasound
- Enlarging growth while in utero
  - Growth is rapid during 3rd trimester and ceases after birth
- Most cases are solitary and polypoid
  - Up to 10% may be multiple
- Bone and teeth are not involved
- No reported associations with syndromes or genetic anomalies

Treatment

- Conservative excision
- Rare cases may regress spontaneously

Prognosis

- Benign
- Local recurrence very rare; no malignant transformation

MACROSCOPIC

General Features

- Well circumscribed
- Overlying mucosa intact or ulcerated

Size

- Usually 1-2 cm
  - Rare, larger examples reported

MICROSCOPIC

Histologic Features

- Overlying squamous mucosa is thinned/attenuated or ulcerated
- Nests, sheets, and cords of polygonal to ovoid cells with abundant granular cytoplasm and distinct cell membranes
  - Cytoplasmic hyaline globules usually absent
- Small nuclei with vesicular to stippled chromatin and often small nucleoli
- Mitoses absent
- Prominent stromal capillary network
  - May be associated with lymphocytic infiltrate
  - Some vessels may be large and ectatic with staghorn appearance
- Uncommon findings: Spindle cell morphology, fibrotic zones, odontogenic epithelial rests

ANCILLARY TESTS

Immunohistochemistry

- Negative for S100 protein, CD68, keratins, CD34, SMA, desmin, calponin

DIFFERENTIAL DIAGNOSIS

Granular Cell Tumor

- Occurs mainly in adults
- Wide distribution but common in tongue
- Overlying squamous epithelium often shows pseudoepitheliomatous hyperplasia
- Large nest and sheet-like growth patterns typical
- Small nerve involvement is commonly identified
- Diffuse S100 protein expression (schwannian)

Adult-Type Rhabdomyoma

- Most common in older adults, particularly men
- Large polygonal cells with prominent eosinophilic cytoplasm
- Desmin (+), myogenin (+)

Alveolar Soft Part Sarcoma

- Rare < 3 years of age
- Large, deeply situated tumors
- Prominent lobularity
- PAS-D(+) intracytoplasmic crystals in most cases

Lobular Capillary Hemangioma (Pyogenic Granuloma)

- Prominent lobulated vascular component (hemangioma)
- Lacks granular cells
- Surface ulceration common

SELECTED REFERENCES

1. Kumar RM et al: Congenital epulis of the newborn. J Oral Maxillofac Pathol. 19(3):407, 2015
2. Conrad R et al: Congenital granular cell epulis. Arch Pathol Lab Med. 138(1):128-31, 2014
3. Garg S et al: Congenital epulis: from birth to childhood. Turk J Pediatr. 56(1):97-9, 2014
4. Saki N et al: Multiple congenital epulis in alveolar ridges of maxilla and mandible in a newborn: a rare case report. Case Rep Otolaryngol. 2014:606985, 2014
5. Yee J: Congenital epulis in a newborn. Minn Med. 97(5):39, 2014
6. Bhatia SK et al: Spontaneous regression of a congenital epulis in a newborn. J Clin Pediatr Dent. 37(3):297-9, 2013
7. Prigkos AC et al: Spindle cell epulis in an 8-month-old child: a histologic variant of congenital granular cell epulis? Head Neck Pathol. 6(4):467-70, 2012
8. Childers EL et al: Congenital epulis of the newborn: 10 new cases of a rare oral tumor. Ann Diagn Pathol. 15(3):157-61, 2011

Nasopharyngeal Angiofibroma

KEY FACTS

TERMINOLOGY

- Benign, highly cellular, and richly vascularized mesenchymal neoplasm arising in nasopharynx in male patients
- Associated with familial adenomatous polyposis

CLINICAL ISSUES

- Most arise in patients < 25 years
- Occurs exclusively in male patients
- Arises in nasopharynx
- Recurrent, spontaneous epistaxis is common presentation
- Often shows locally aggressive growth
- Overall good prognosis

IMAGING

- Anterior bowing of posterior wall of maxillary sinus with posterior displacement of pterygoid plates (Holman-Miller sign)
- Angiography identifies feeding vessel(s) and allows for presurgical embolization
    - Tumor blush is characteristic

MICROSCOPIC

- Scattered, variably sized vessels within prominent fibrocollagenous stroma
    - Stroma composed of plump spindle, angular, or stellate-shaped cells
- Mitotic figures rare

ANCILLARY TESTS

- Stromal cells are androgen receptor (+) and nuclear β-catenin (+)
    - SMA, desmin, and CD34 (-)

TOP DIFFERENTIAL DIAGNOSES

- Lobular capillary hemangioma (pyogenic granuloma)
- Solitary fibrous tumor
- Sinonasal glomangiopericytoma
- Desmoid fibromatosis
- Antrochoanal polyp

(Left) *Nasopharyngeal angiofibroma (NPA) is a rare mesenchymal neoplasm of the male nasopharynx that is classically composed of irregularly scattered, variably sized blood vessels within a fibrocollagenous stroma.* **(Right)** *NPA contains numerous vessels of various calibers, some with smooth muscle, set in a heavily collagenized stroma. The stroma varies in cellularity but is often relatively hypocellular.*

Nasopharyngeal Angiofibroma

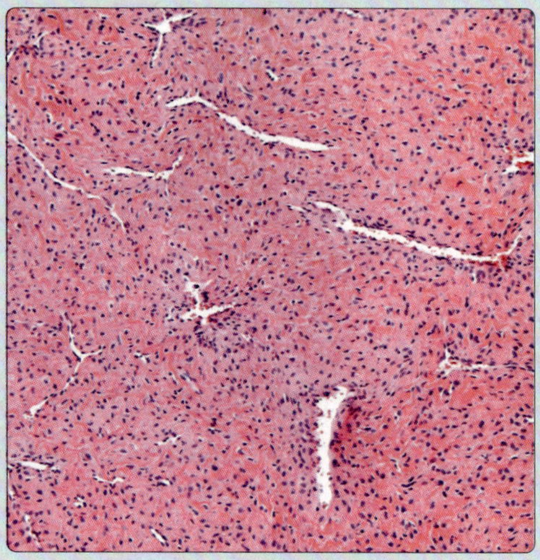

Characteristic Vasculature

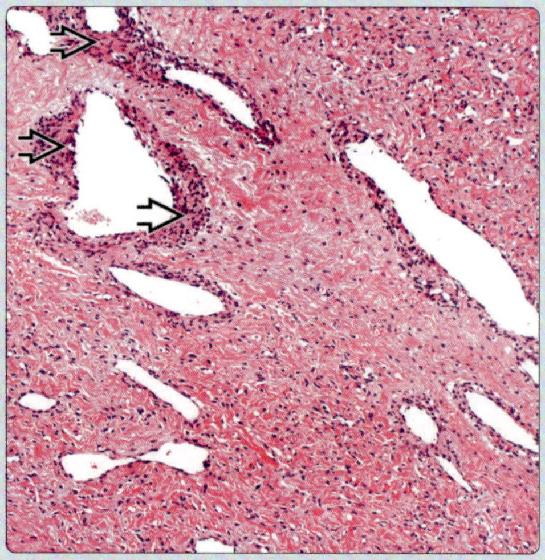

(Left) *The lesional cells of NPA have plump, ovoid nuclei and indistinct cell margins. The cells are randomly oriented within a fibrous stroma that contains scattered mast cells and lymphocytes.* **(Right)** *Increased collagen deposition is often seen in NPAs of a long duration. Note how the vessels are compressed and narrowed in this image. In some cases, they appear slit-like.*

Cytologic Features

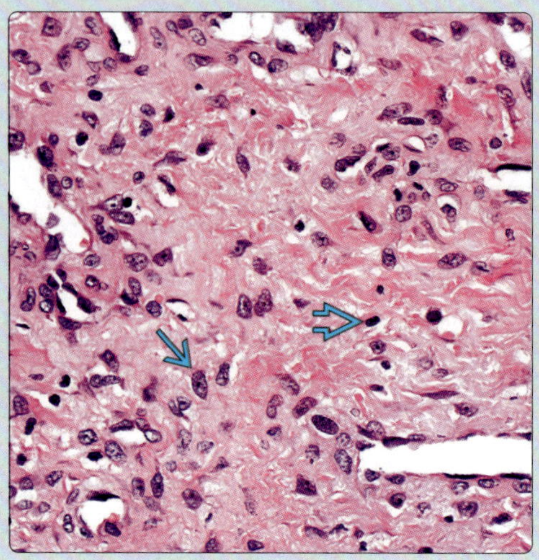

Increased Stromal Collagen

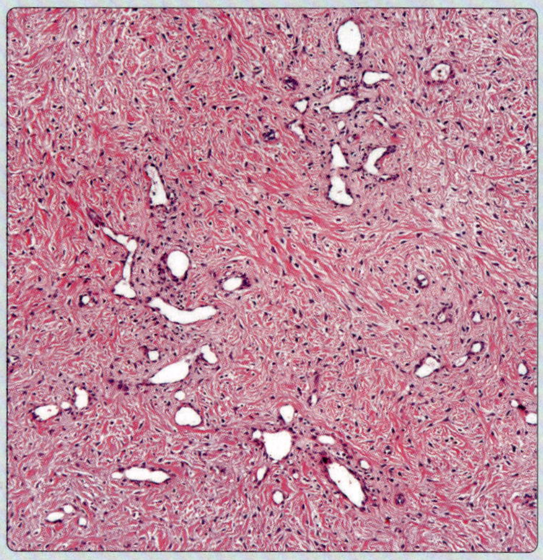

Nasopharyngeal Angiofibroma

TERMINOLOGY

Abbreviations

- Nasopharyngeal angiofibroma (NPA)

Synonyms

- Juvenile NPA
- Angiofibroma

Definitions

- Benign, richly vascularized mesenchymal neoplasm arising in nasopharynx in male patients

ETIOLOGY/PATHOGENESIS

Hormonal

- Testosterone-dependent growth

Genetic

- Association with familial adenomatous polyposis

CLINICAL ISSUES

Epidemiology

- Incidence
  - Rare
- Age
  - Most arise in patients < 25 years
    - Peak incidence: 10-20 years
  - Rare cases in older adults
    - Supports notion of avoiding term juvenile NPA
- Sex
  - Occurs exclusively in male patients
    - If diagnosed in female patients, studies of sex chromosomes required to confirm gender

Site

- Arises in nasopharynx
  - Usually affects posterolateral region
- May expand to involve surrounding structures (30% of cases)
  - Anterior: Nasal cavity and maxillary sinus via roof of nasopharynx
  - Lateral: Temporal and infratemporal fossae via pterygomaxillary fissure, resulting in cheek or intraoral buccal mass
  - Posterior: Middle cranial fossa
  - Superior: Pterygopalatine fossa and orbit via inferior and superior orbital fissures resulting in proptosis
  - Medial: Contralateral side

Presentation

- Symptoms often present for 12-24 months (nonspecific presentation)
- Recurrent, spontaneous epistaxis
- Nasal obstruction
- Nasal discharge
- Facial deformity (proptosis), exophthalmia, diplopia
- Rhinolalia, sinusitis
- Otitis media, tinnitus, deafness
- Headaches
- Rarely, anosmia or pain

Natural History

- Often shows locally aggressive growth
- Potential for facial deformity if allowed to grow

Treatment

- Surgical resection is treatment of choice
  - Definitive resection is frequently associated with significant morbidity
- Biopsy is contraindicated due to potential fatal exsanguination
- Selective angiography preoperatively allows embolization with sclerosing agent or cryotherapy
- Nonsurgical medical management (preoperative hormone therapy) is option
  - Not as popular as other modalities
    - Giving estrogen to pubertal male patients is undesirable
- Radiation may be used to manage large, intracranial, or recurrent tumors

Prognosis

- Overall good prognosis
  - Very low mortality rate (1%)
- Benign, but locally aggressive neoplasm
  - Recurrences in ~ 20% of patients
    - Often related to incomplete excision
    - Usually develop within 2 years of diagnosis
    - Commonly extend intracranially

IMAGING

General Features

- Best diagnostic clue
  - Anterior bowing of posterior wall of maxillary sinus with posterior displacement of pterygoid plates (Holman-Miller sign)
- Location
  - Nasopharynx with extension into surrounding structures
- Angiography identifies feeding vessel(s) and allows for presurgical embolization
  - Tumor blush is characteristic

CT Findings

- Allows for accurate determination of size and extent
- Enhancement is different from adjacent muscle, accentuated with contrast
- Bony margins may be eroded

MACROSCOPIC

General Features

- Sessile or lobulated
- Can be polypoid or pedunculated
- Red, gray-tan cut surface

Size

- Most are 3-5 cm (mean: 4 cm)
- Rare cases are much larger

MICROSCOPIC

Histologic Features

- Unencapsulated

- Submucosal proliferation of vascular channels within fibrocollagenous stroma
  - Many variably sized, disorganized vessels
    - Varying thickness of vessel wall with patchy muscle content
      - Focal, pad-like smooth muscle thickenings within vessel walls
    - Vessels are mostly thin walled, slit-like ("staghorn")
    - Range from capillary size to large, dilated vessels
    - Endothelial cells may be plump but are usually attenuated
  - Fibrocollagenous stroma consists of plump spindle or stellate-shaped cells
    - Stromal cells may be angulated, multinucleated, and pleomorphic
    - Variable amounts of fine and coarse collagen fibers
    - Myxoid degeneration is common (especially in embolized specimens)
      - Embolization material may be present within vessel
    - As stroma increases, vascular compression results in virtually nonexistent lumina
      - Central areas may lack vessels
    - Elastic tissue is not identified within stroma
    - Hormone-treated cases show increased collagenization of stroma with fewer but thicker walled vessels
- Mitotic figures are sparse
- Mast cells are common
- Sarcomatous transformation is exceedingly uncommon event
  - Develops following massive doses of radiation

ANCILLARY TESTS

Histochemistry

- Reticulin shows positive black staining around stromal cells and blood vessels
- Elastic van Gieson highlights elastic tissue within vessel walls

Immunohistochemistry

- Stromal cells
  - Androgen receptor (+)
  - Nuclear β-catenin (+)
  - SMA, desmin, and CD34 (-)

DIFFERENTIAL DIAGNOSIS

Lobular Capillary Hemangioma (Pyogenic Granuloma)

- Usually in nasal cavity (vs. nasopharynx)
- Blood vessels are more organized
  - Lobular growth with central "feeder" vessels
- Often ulcerated and inflamed

Solitary Fibrous Tumor

- Striking ectatic "staghorn" vasculature
- CD34(+), STAT6(+)

Sinonasal Glomangiopericytoma

- Affects older adults
- Ovoid to spindled tumor cells
- Hyalinized vessels frequently present
- SMA(+)
- Nuclear β-catenin (+)

Desmoid Fibromatosis

- Usually contain long, "streaming" fascicles of tumor cells
- Does not express androgen/testosterone receptors
- Nuclear β-catenin (+) in 70%

Antrochoanal Polyp

- Arise in maxillary sinus
- Heavy stromal fibrosis but usually lacks characteristic vascular pattern of NPA

SELECTED REFERENCES

1. Jones JW et al: Differential gene expression and pathway analysis in juvenile nasopharyngeal angiofibroma using RNA sequencing. Otolaryngol Head Neck Surg. 194599818769879, 2018
2. Sánchez-Romero C et al: Nasopharyngeal angiofibroma: a clinical, histopathological and immunohistochemical study of 42 cases with emphasis on stromal features. Head Neck Pathol. 12(1):52-61, 2018
3. Agaimy A et al: CTNNB1 (β-catenin)-altered neoplasia: a review focusing on soft tissue neoplasms and parenchymal lesions of uncertain histogenesis. Adv Anat Pathol. 23(1):1-12, 2016
4. Renkonen S et al: Tenascin-C, GLUT-1, and syndecan-2 expression in juvenile nasopharyngeal angiofibroma: correlations to vessel density and tumor stage. Head Neck. 35(7):1036-42, 2013
5. Wang JJ et al: Endoglin (CD105) expression on microvessel endothelial cells in juvenile nasopharyngeal angiofibroma: tissue microarray analysis and association with prognostic significance. Head Neck. 35(12):1719-25, 2013
6. Yi Z et al: Nasopharyngeal angiofibroma: a concise classification system and appropriate treatment options. Am J Otolaryngol. 34(2):133-41, 2013
7. Silveira SM et al: Tumor microenvironmental genomic alterations in juvenile nasopharyngeal angiofibroma. Head Neck. 34(4):485-92, 2012
8. Blount A et al: Juvenile nasopharyngeal angiofibroma. Otolaryngol Clin North Am. 44(4):989-1004, ix, 2011
9. Renkonen S et al: Stem cell-related proteins C-KIT, C-MYC and BMI-1 in juvenile nasopharyngeal angiofibroma–do they have a role? Virchows Arch. 458(2):189-95, 2011
10. Zhang M et al: Biological distinctions between juvenile nasopharyngeal angiofibroma and vascular malformation: an immunohistochemical study. Acta Histochem. 113(6):626-30, 2011
11. Sun XC et al: Analysis of risk factors associated with recurrence of nasopharyngeal angiofibroma. J Otolaryngol Head Neck Surg. 39(1):56-61, 2010
12. Bleier BS et al: Current management of juvenile nasopharyngeal angiofibroma: a tertiary center experience 1999-2007. Am J Rhinol Allergy. 23(3):328-30, 2009
13. Carrillo JF et al: Juvenile nasopharyngeal angiofibroma: clinical factors associated with recurrence, and proposal of a staging system. J Surg Oncol. 98(2):75-80, 2008
14. Coutinho-Camillo CM et al: Genetic alterations in juvenile nasopharyngeal angiofibromas. Head Neck. 30(3):390-400, 2008
15. Glad H et al: Juvenile nasopharyngeal angiofibromas in Denmark 1981-2003: diagnosis, incidence, and treatment. Acta Otolaryngol. 127(3):292-9, 2007
16. Tyagi I et al: Staging and surgical approaches in large juvenile angiofibroma–study of 95 cases. Int J Pediatr Otorhinolaryngol. 70(9):1619-27, 2006
17. Thompson LDR et al: Tumours of the nasopharynx: nasopharyngeal angiofibroma. In Barnes EL et al: Pathology and Genetics of Head and Neck Tumours. World Health Organization Classification of Tumours. Lyon: IARC Press. 102-3, 2005
18. Fletcher CD: Distinctive soft tissue tumors of the head and neck. Mod Pathol. 15(3):324-30, 2002
19. Lee JT et al: The role of radiation in the treatment of advanced juvenile angiofibroma. Laryngoscope. 112(7 Pt 1):1213-20, 2002
20. Coffin CM et al: Fibroblastic-myofibroblastic tumors in children and adolescents: a clinicopathologic study of 108 examples in 103 patients. Pediatr Pathol. 11(4):569-88, 1991
21. Makek MS et al: Malignant transformation of a nasopharyngeal angiofibroma. Laryngoscope. 99(10 Pt 1):1088-92, 1989

Embolization Material

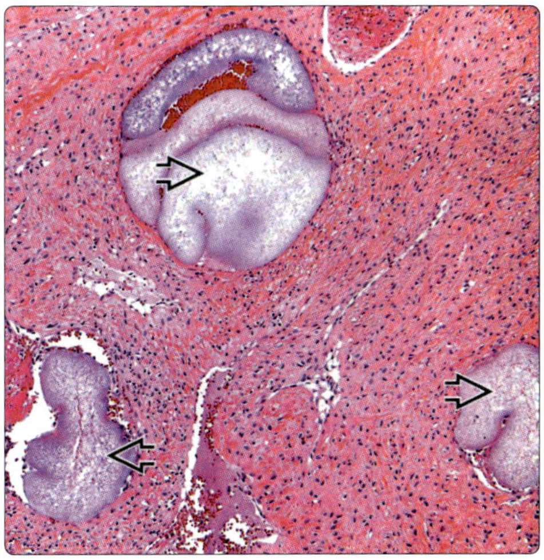

Marked Stromal Collagen

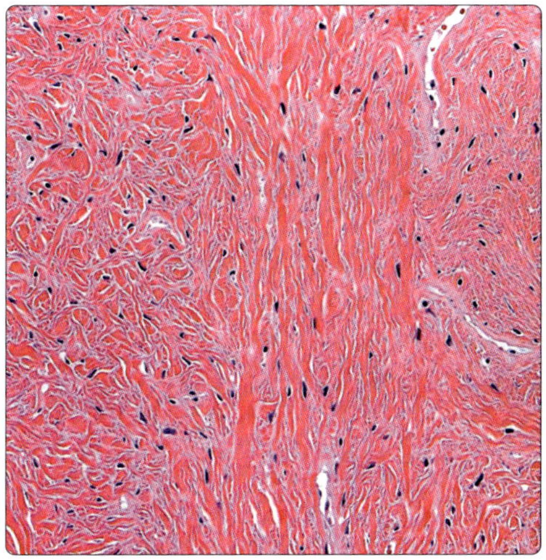

(Left) *Cases of NPA preoperatively treated by embolization prior to surgical resection show embolization material ➔ within blood vessels.* **(Right)** *Longstanding cases of NPA and those treated with hormonal therapy often show increased stromal collagen and fewer vessels, as depicted.*

Scattered Atypical Cells

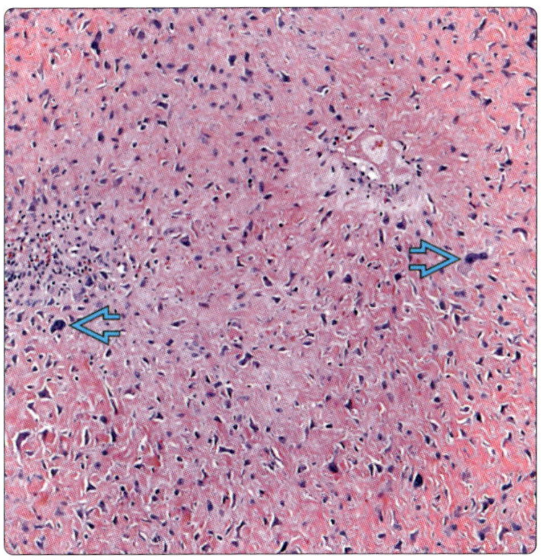

Perivascular Smooth Muscle

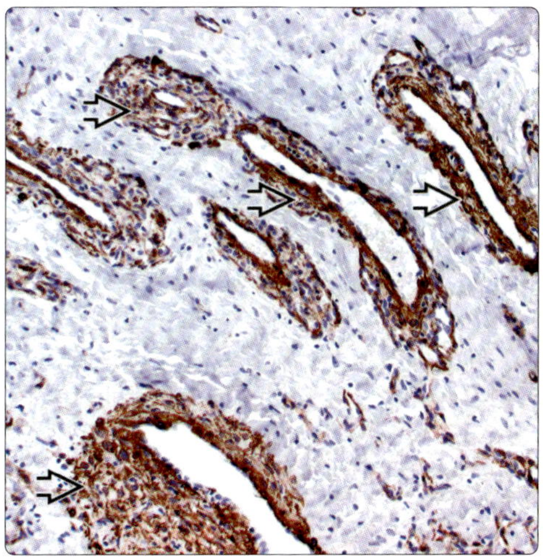

(Left) *Occasional cases of NPA contain scattered cells with nuclear atypia ➔ or multinucleation. This finding does not affect the prognosis.* **(Right)** *Muscle specific actin (shown) and smooth muscle actin (SMA) highlight the smooth muscle walls around vessels ➔ in NPA. The variable intensity of the reaction helps to demonstrate the variable amounts of smooth muscle associated with the vessels. Note that the stromal cells are negative.*

Nuclear β-Catenin Expression

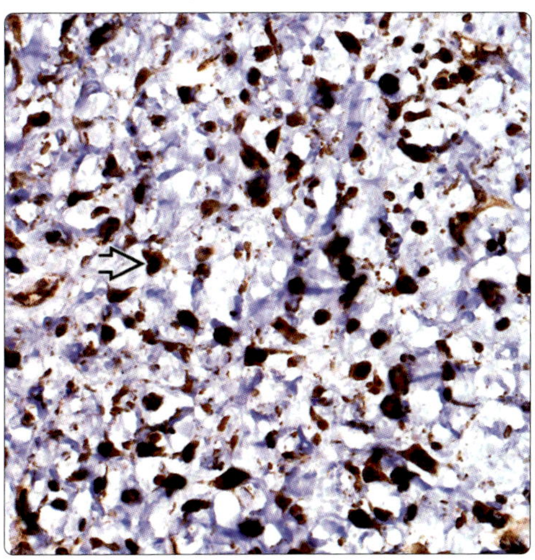

Nasopharyngeal Angiofibroma

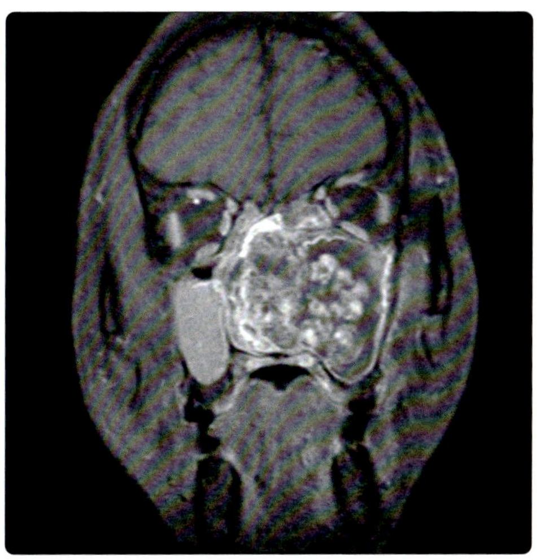

(Left) *Immunohistochemistry for β-catenin shows strong, diffuse positivity in nuclei ➔ in the majority of the lesional cells of NPA. The nonfascicular architecture, nuclear features, vascular pattern, and absence of SMA in lesional cells allow distinction from desmoid fibromatosis.* **(Right)** *MR of NPA shows intracranial extension of a large, destructive, hyperintense mass in the nasopharynx. The bone has been remodeled and pushed aside.*

Sinonasal Glomangiopericytoma

KEY FACTS

TERMINOLOGY

- Distinctive mesenchymal neoplasm of sinonasal cavity demonstrating pericytic (perivascular) myoid phenotype
- Synonym: Sinonasal-type hemangiopericytoma

ETIOLOGY/PATHOGENESIS

- Mutational activation of β-catenin involved in pathogenesis

CLINICAL ISSUES

- 75% of cases occur in 6th-8th decades
- Slight female predilection
- Most frequently arises in nasal cavity
- Unilateral polypoid intranasal mass
- Complete surgical excision
- Benign; ~ 1/3 will recur/persist

MACROSCOPIC

- Mean size: 3.5 cm (range: 1.5-8.0 cm)

MICROSCOPIC

- Composed of uniform, syncytial sheets and fascicles of round to spindle-shaped cells intimately associated with vascular component
  - Perivascular hyalinization common
- Stroma often scant but may be myxoid or loose and edematous
- Chronic inflammatory cells common

ANCILLARY TESTS

- Smooth muscle actin (+), nuclear β-catenin (+)
- Desmin, CD34, S100 protein, keratin (-)

TOP DIFFERENTIAL DIAGNOSES

- Phosphaturic mesenchymal tumor
- Solitary fibrous tumor
- Nasopharyngeal angiofibroma
- Lobular capillary hemangioma
- Myoepithelioma

Sinonasal Glomangiopericytoma

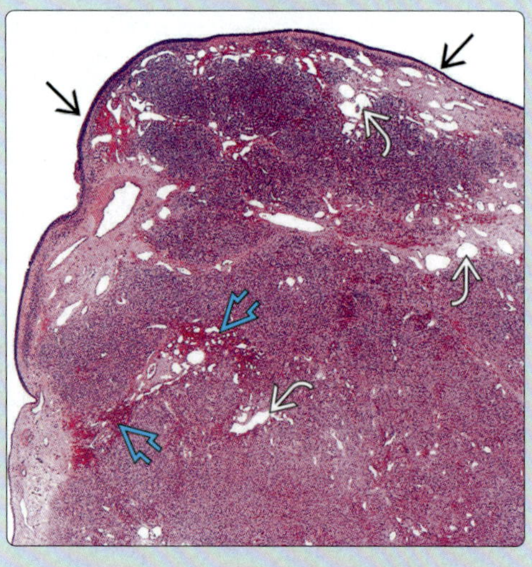

Characteristic Vasculature

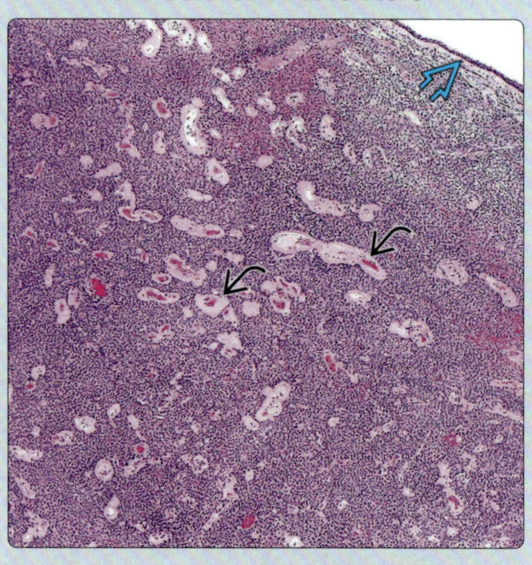

(Left) *Low-power H&E of sinonasal glomangiopericytoma (GPC) shows an intact surface and a subepithelial mesenchymal neoplastic proliferation with prominent vascularity and extravasated blood. Normal regional subepithelial structures are also effaced.* **(Right)** *A characteristic feature of sinonasal GPC is the presence of prominent perivascular hyalinization. This histologic feature is seen in up to 90% of tumors. Note the overlying intact surface (schneiderian) epithelium.*

Cytologic Features

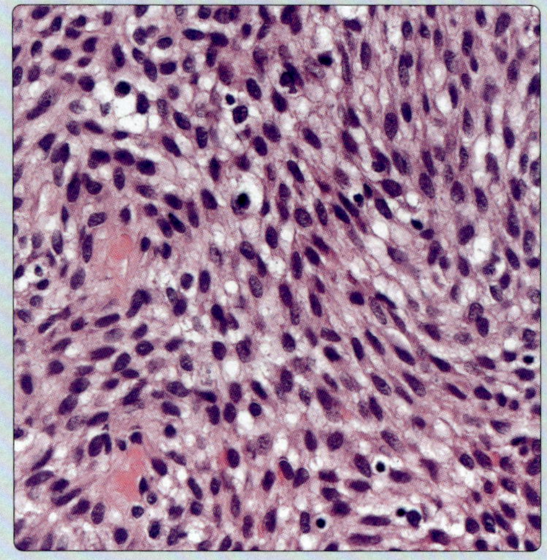

Smooth Muscle Actin Expression

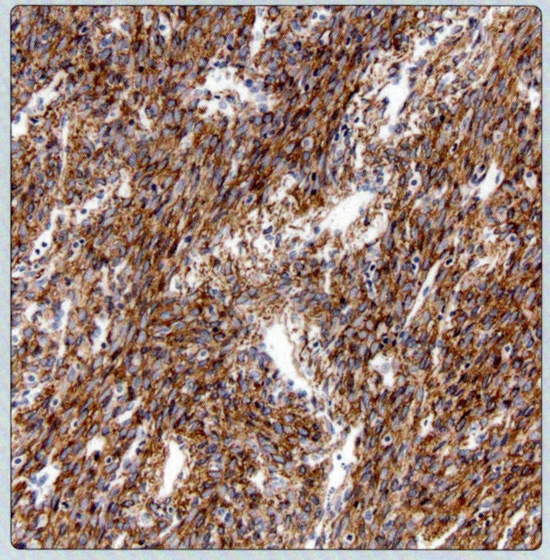

(Left) *Sinonasal GPC is composed of cytologically bland to ovoid spindle cells with oval nuclei containing even chromatin and small nucleoli. The cytoplasm is eosinophilic and finely vacuolated with indistinct cell borders imparting a syncytial appearance.* **(Right)** *The cells of sinonasal GPC are true pericytic cells, and they demonstrate a myoid phenotype both ultrastructurally and immunophenotypically. Diffuse SMA expression (shown) is characteristic.*

TERMINOLOGY

Abbreviations

- Glomangiopericytoma (GPC)

Synonyms

- Sinonasal-type hemangiopericytoma
- Hemangiopericytoma-like tumor of sinonasal cavity

Definitions

- Distinctive mesenchymal neoplasm of sinonasal cavity demonstrating pericytic (perivascular) myoid phenotype

ETIOLOGY/PATHOGENESIS

Genetics

- Mutational activation of β-catenin involved in pathogenesis

CLINICAL ISSUES

Epidemiology

- Incidence
  - Rare
    - Accounts for < 0.5% of sinonasal neoplasms
- Age
  - Wide range (5-86 years)
    - 75% of cases occur in 6th-8th decades
- Sex
  - Slight female predilection

Site

- Most frequently arises in nasal cavity
  - Often have concomitant paranasal sinus involvement
  - Right and left side equally affected
- Rarely arise primarily in paranasal sinuses

Presentation

- Unilateral polypoid intranasal mass
- Nasal obstruction, epistaxis
- Congestion, sinusitis, &/or difficulty breathing

Treatment

- Complete surgical excision
- Radiation therapy is of unproven value

Prognosis

- Excellent overall 5-year survival (> 90%)
- ~ 1/3 will recur/persist (range: 18-44%)
  - Recurrences can occur after many years
    - Mean interval to 1st recurrence is ~ 6.5 years (range: 1.0-17.5 years)
    - Long-term follow-up warranted

IMAGING

Radiographic Findings

- Opacification filling nasal cavity ± adjacent sinuses
- Bone erosion or sclerosis can be seen
- Concomitant sinusitis not uncommon

MACROSCOPIC

General Features

- Often removed piecemeal
- If resected intact, appears as polypoid solid mass with tan hemorrhagic cut surface
- Surface mucosa typically intact

Size

- Mean: 3.5 cm (range: 1.5-8.0 cm)

MICROSCOPIC

Histologic Features

- Subepithelial, well-demarcated but unencapsulated, cellular mesenchymal proliferation
  - Surface (schneiderian) mucosa usually intact but may be eroded or show squamous metaplasia
  - Usually efface but may surround submucosal minor salivary glands
- Composed of uniform, closely packed sheets of round to spindle-shaped cells intimately associated with vascular component
  - Vascular channels are variable in size, ranging from capillaries to patulous "staghorn" vessels
    - Prominent perivascular hyalinization is characteristic and seen in up to 90% of cases
  - Neoplastic cells have uniform, oval to round nuclei
    - Nuclear chromatin is typically homogeneous or vesicular with 1 or more small nucleoli
    - Cytoplasm is lightly eosinophilic and indiscrete, resulting in syncytial appearance
      - Focal areas composed of clear cells may be seen
    - Rare mitoses and mild nuclear pleomorphism may be identified
- Stroma is typically scant but may be myxoid or loose and edematous
  - Stromal edema may result in hypocellular zones with residual smaller cellular lobules
- Most tumors have solid or fascicular growth, but mixed growth patterns are common
  - Whorled growth patterns can be seen in up to 10% of cases
  - Also occasional nuclear palisading
- Chronic inflammatory cells are invariably present
  - Particularly eosinophils and mast cells
- Extravasated red blood cells are usually present
- Scattered tumor giant cells (~ 5%) may be present
  - Likely represent degenerative phenomenon
  - Consist of agglomerated tumor cells

ANCILLARY TESTS

Immunohistochemistry

- Vast majority demonstrate myoid phenotype with actin positivity
  - Smooth muscle actin (+) (80-100%)
  - Muscle specific actin (+) (77-100%)
- Nuclear β-catenin (+)
- Desmin, keratin, and C-kit (CD117) (-)
- Usually CD34 and S100 protein (-)

DIFFERENTIAL DIAGNOSIS

Phosphaturic Mesenchymal Tumor

- Sinonasal examples can show significant morphologic overlap with sinonasal GPC
- Often associated with clinical evidence of osteomalacia
- Overexpression of fibroblast growth factor 23 (FGF23)

Solitary Fibrous Tumor

- Also previously known as hemangiopericytoma
- Prominent ectatic "staghorn" vasculature
- Stromal collagen often prominent
- Uniform CD34(+)
- SMA and MSA (-)

Nasopharyngeal Angiofibroma

- Majority occur in adolescent males
- Arise in posterior nasal cavity with extension into nasopharynx
  - Often involve nasal cavity, sinuses, and skull base when they enlarge
- Evenly spaced spindled and stellate tumor cells
- Stromal collagen prominent
- Nuclear β-catenin (+) in stromal cells
  - Some cases occur in patients with familial adenomatosis polyposis (FAP)

Lobular Capillary Hemangioma (Pyogenic Granuloma)

- Composed of vascular lobules arranged in fibrovascular stroma
- Lobules contain small, slit-like vascular channels emanating from larger central "feeder" vessels
- Absence of sheet-like growth
- Surface erosion is frequent

Myoepithelioma

- Myxoid stroma common
- Keratin (+) &/or S100 protein (+) common
- Can also expression SMA, GFAP, calponin, desmin, p63

Sinonasal Smooth Muscle Neoplasms

- Rare
- Tumor cells arranged in bundled fascicles
- Abundant fibrillary eosinophilic cytoplasm
- Blunt-ended, cigar-shaped, oval nuclei
- SMA(+), desmin (+)

Schwannoma

- Nuclear palisading much more frequent than in sinonasal GPC
- Diffuse S100 protein (+)
- SMA(-)

Glomus Tumor

- Extremely rare in sinonasal sites
- Rounded tumor cells with central round nucleus, eosinophilic cytoplasm, and prominent cell borders
- Spindled morphology uncommon and usually focal, if present
- SMA(+)

DIAGNOSTIC CHECKLIST

Clinically Relevant Pathologic Features

- Localization to sinonasal cavity
- Bland spindle and rounded cells associated with prominent vascular component
- Low mitotic rate
- Myoid immunophenotype (SMA and MSA)

Pathologic Interpretation Pearls

- Features that can lead to misdiagnosis
  - Lack of awareness of this unique sinonasal tumor
  - Multinodularity secondary to edema or degenerative changes
  - Multinucleated tumor giant cells
  - Whorled growth pattern &/or nuclear palisading

SELECTED REFERENCES

1. Suzuki Y et al: β-catenin (CTNNB1) mutation and LEF1 expression in sinonasal glomangiopericytoma (sinonasal-type hemangiopericytoma). Virchows Arch. ePub, 2018
2. Park ES et al: Characteristics and prognosis of glomangiopericytomas: a systematic review. Head Neck. 39(9):1897-1909, 2017
3. Asimakopoulos P et al: Sinonasal glomangiopericytoma: Is anything new? Ear Nose Throat J. 95(2):E1-5, 2016
4. Lasota J et al: Nuclear expression and gain-of-function β-catenin mutation in glomangiopericytoma (sinonasal-type hemangiopericytoma): insight into pathogenesis and a diagnostic marker. Mod Pathol. 28(5):715-20, 2014
5. Duval M et al: Systematic review of treatment and prognosis of sinonasal hemangiopericytoma. Head Neck. 35(8):1205-10, 2013
6. Brandwein-Gensler M et al: Striking pathology gold: a singular experience with daily reverberations: sinonasal hemangiopericytoma (glomangiopericytoma) and oncogenic osteomalacia. Head Neck Pathol. 6(1):64-74, 2012
7. Dandekar M et al: Sinonasal glomangiopericytoma: case report with emphasis on the differential diagnosis. Arch Pathol Lab Med. 134(10):1444-9, 2010
8. Hofmann V et al: Sinonasal hemangiopericytoma. Rev Laryngol Otol Rhinol (Bord). 131(4-5):313-5, 2010
9. Lin SH et al: Diagnosis and treatment of sinonasal hemangiopericytoma: three case reports and review of the literature. J Otolaryngol. 35(2):141-3, 2006
10. Kuo FY et al: Sinonasal hemangiopericytoma-like tumor with true pericytic myoid differentiation: a clinicopathologic and immunohistochemical study of five cases. Head Neck. 27(2):124-9, 2005
11. Li XQ et al: Intranasal pericytic tumors (glomus tumor and sinonasal hemangiopericytoma-like tumor): report of two cases with review of the literature. Pathol Int. 53(5):303-8, 2003
12. Thompson LD et al: Sinonasal-type hemangiopericytoma: a clinicopathologic and immunophenotypic analysis of 104 cases showing perivascular myoid differentiation. Am J Surg Pathol. 27(6):737-49, 2003
13. Tse LL et al: Sinonasal haemangiopericytoma-like tumour: a sinonasal glomus tumour or a haemangiopericytoma? Histopathology. 40(6):510-7, 2002
14. Watanabe K et al: True hemangiopericytoma of the nasal cavity. Arch Pathol Lab Med. 125(5):686-90, 2001
15. Catalano PJ et al: Sinonasal hemangiopericytomas: a clinicopathologic and immunohistochemical study of seven cases. Head Neck. 18(1):42-53, 1996
16. Thiringer JK et al: Sinonasal hemangiopericytoma: case report and literature review. Skull Base Surg. 5(3):185-90, 1995
17. el-Naggar AK et al: Sinonasal hemangiopericytomas. A clinicopathologic and DNA content study. Arch Otolaryngol Head Neck Surg. 118(2):134-7, 1992
18. Eichhorn JH et al: Sinonasal hemangiopericytoma. A reassessment with electron microscopy, immunohistochemistry, and long-term follow-up. Am J Surg Pathol. 14(9):856-66, 1990
19. Batsakis JG et al: Hemangiopericytoma of the nasal cavity: electron-optic study and clinical correlations. J Laryngol Otol. 97(4):361-8, 1983
20. Compagno J: Hemangiopericytoma-like tumors of the nasal cavity: a comparison with hemangiopericytoma of soft tissues. Laryngoscope. 88(3):460-9, 1978
21. Compagno J et al: Hemangiopericytoma-like intranasal tumors. A clinicopathologic study of 23 cases. Am J Clin Pathol. 66(4):672-83, 1976

Prominent Vasculature

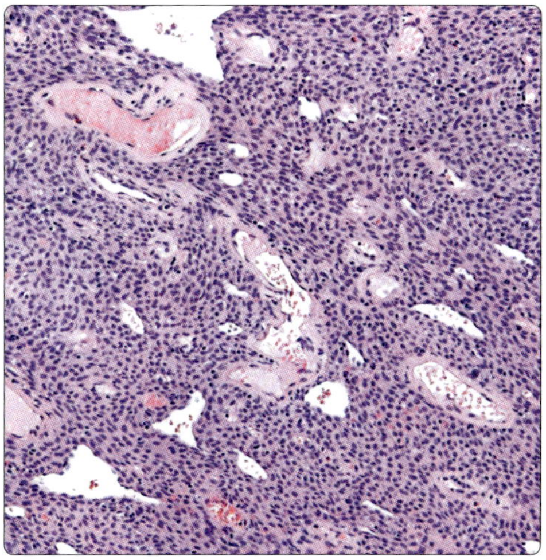

Perivascular Hyalinization

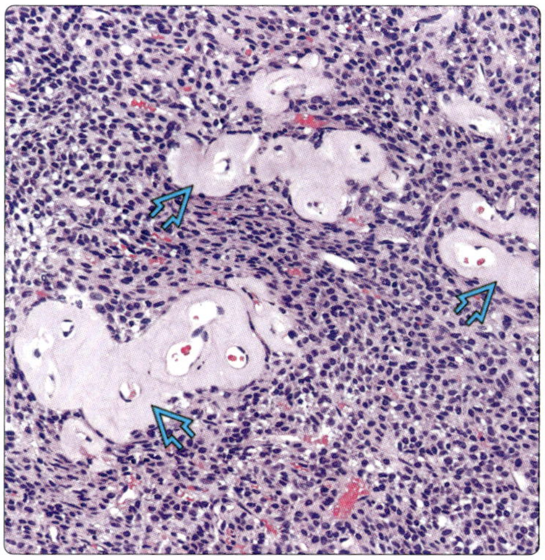

(Left) *The stromal vasculature of sinonasal GPC is characteristic of the tumor. The vessels range from small capillaries to larger, dilated and "staghorn" vessels similar to what is seen in solitary fibrous tumor.* **(Right)** *H&E shows the characteristic perivascular hyalinization* ⇨ *seen in most cases of sinonasal GPC. It manifests as a sharply demarcated zone of homogeneous and paucicellular eosinophilic collagen surrounding capillaries.*

Nonhyalinized Blood Vessels

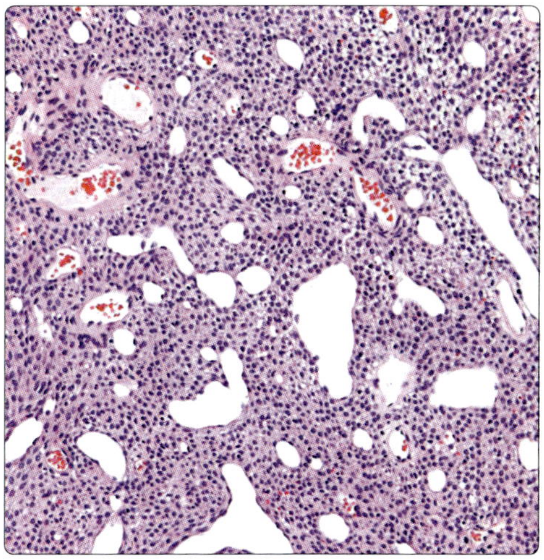

Hypovascular Areas

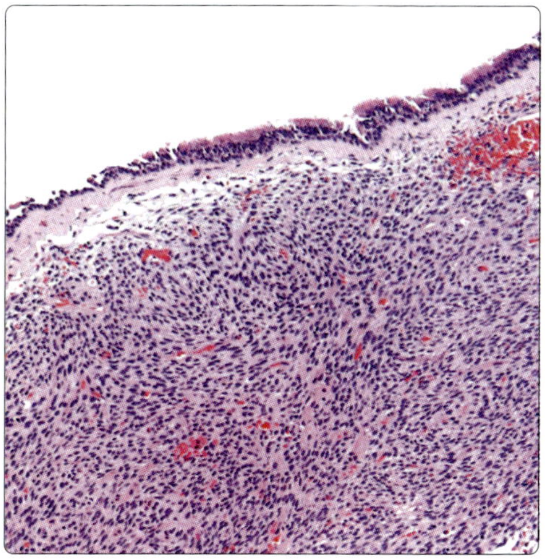

(Left) *In the minority of cases of sinonasal GPC, perivascular hyalinization is focal or absent. Therefore, the absence of this otherwise characteristic finding does not exclude the diagnosis.* **(Right)** *Although the vasculature of sinonasal GPC is a characteristic feature of the tumor, blood vessels may be absent in some fields, as shown. This absence may potentially lead to diagnostic problems on small biopsy.*

Fascicular Growth

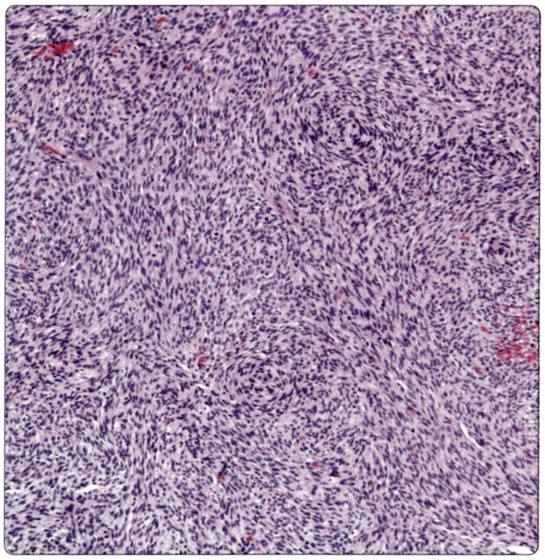

Inflammatory Infiltrate

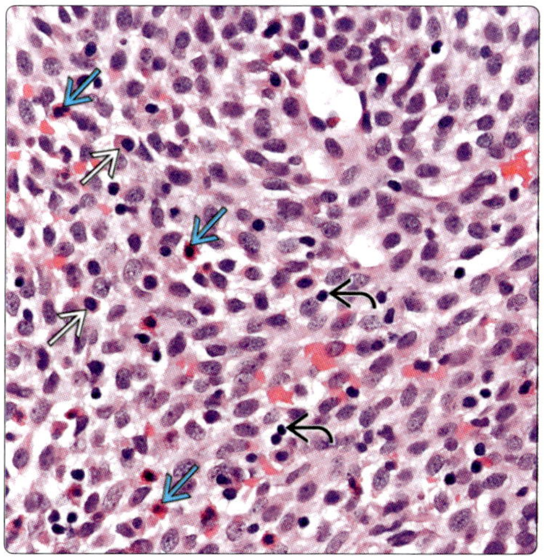

(Left) *The most common growth patterns in sinonasal GPC are sheet-like and fascicular (shown), and a mixture of patterns in a given tumor is common. The latter may naturally raise concerns for sarcoma if the pathologist is unaware of this entity.* **(Right)** *A chronic inflammatory infiltrate is invariably present in sinonasal GPC and usually consists of a mixture of eosinophils* → *and mast cells, but neutrophils, plasma cells* ➡*, and lymphocytes* ↗ *may also be seen.*

(Left) *In addition to a spindled morphology, tumor cells in sinonasal GPC may show a round or oval cytomorphology, similar to glomus tumor. This morphology varies in extent but is often not prominent.* (Right) *The round cell areas in sinonasal GPC may resemble glomus tumors but lack the prominent cell borders seen in the latter entity.*

Rounded Cellular Morphology

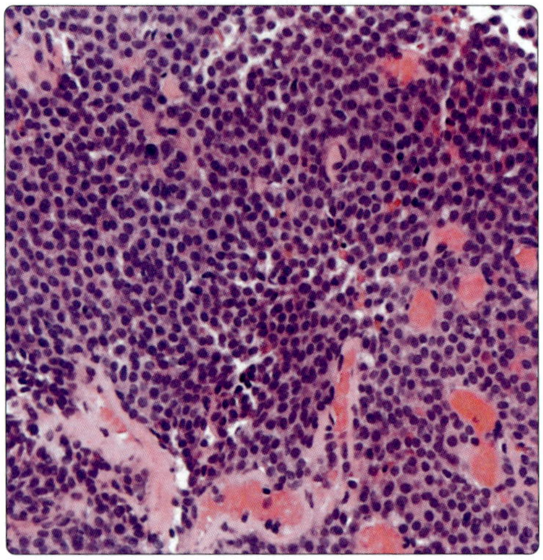

Rounded Cellular Morphology

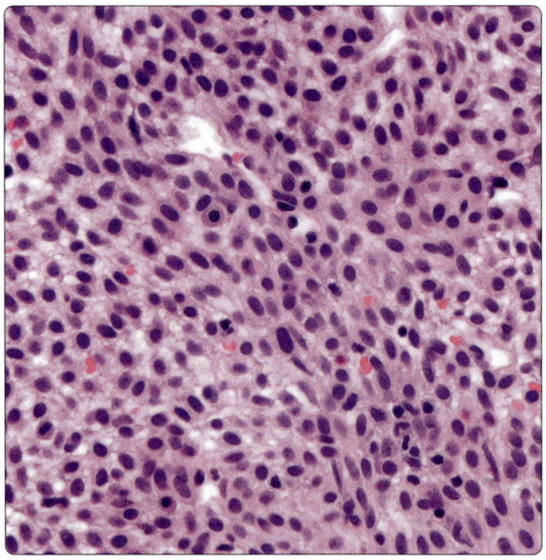

(Left) *Sinonasal GPC usually contains minimal stroma, predominantly consisting of only mesenchymal cells and vessels. Focal areas of stromal edema ⇒ or myxoid change can often be seen, however.* (Right) *Extensive stromal edema may be seen in sinonasal GPC and is usually more prominent at the periphery. The stromal edema in this example imparts a reticular appearance in the paucicellular region and multinodularity ⇒ in the preserved cellular zones.*

Stromal Changes

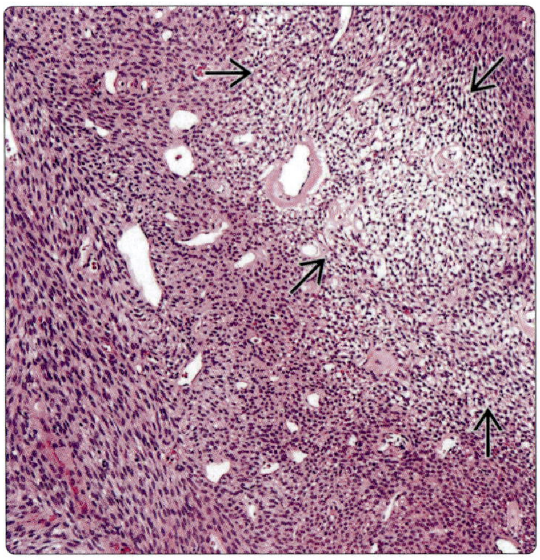

Stromal Edema

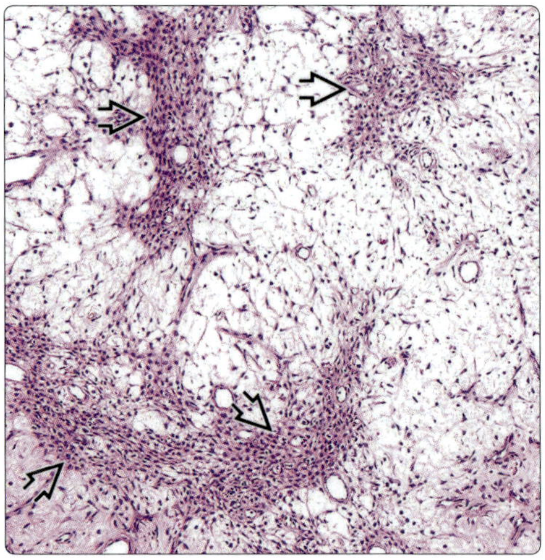

(Left) *Some cases of sinonasal GPC show large zones of loose, edematous matrix and can suggest an inflammatory or allergic polyp. Residual islands ⇒ of tumor cells within these paucicellular areas are diagnostic.* (Right) *Although focal myxoid stromal change is not uncommon in sinonasal GPC, rare cases show prominent myxoid stroma, as depicted.*

Extensive Stromal Edema

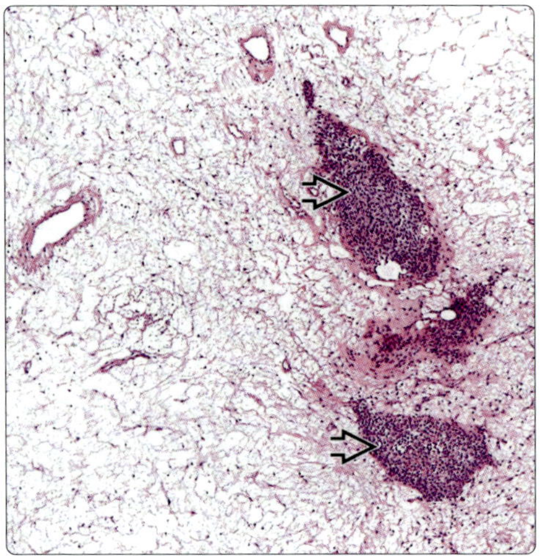

Myxoid Stroma

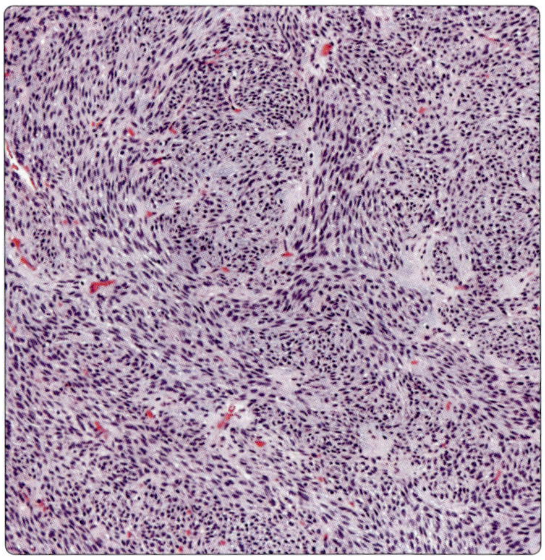

Architectural Whorling

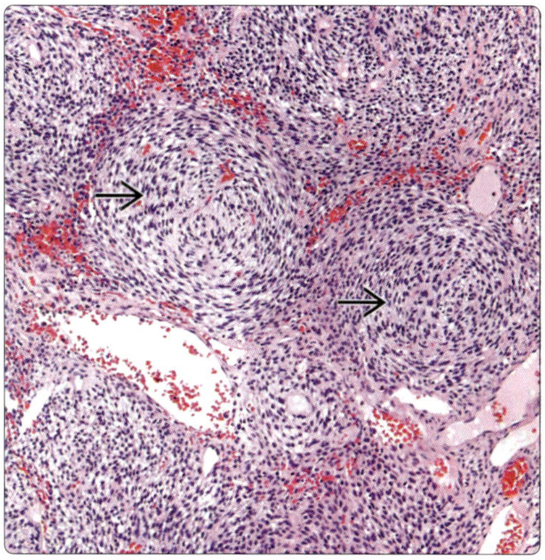

Rare Nuclear Palisading

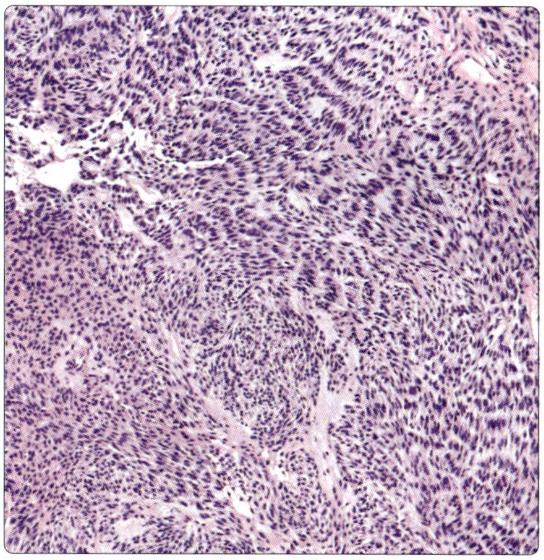

(Left) *This case of a sinonasal GPC shows a prominent whorled or meningothelial-like growth pattern ➜. This pattern can be seen in up to 10% of cases and is usually limited in extent when present.* **(Right)** *Nuclear palisading is a rare finding in sinonasal GPC but can lead to diagnostic confusion with other tumors (particularly those of nerve sheath origin).*

Focal Clear Cell Change

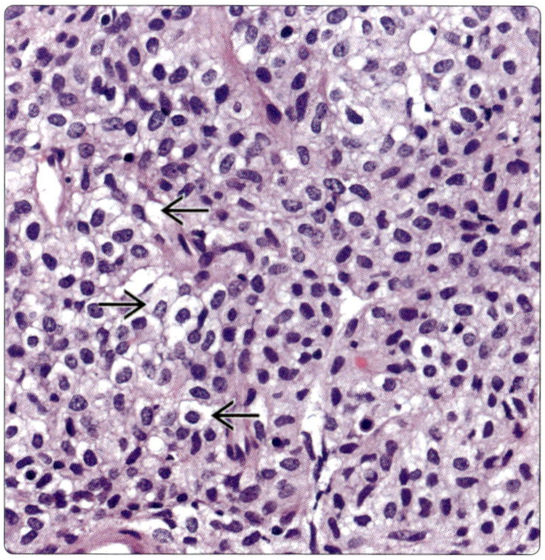

Multinucleated Cells

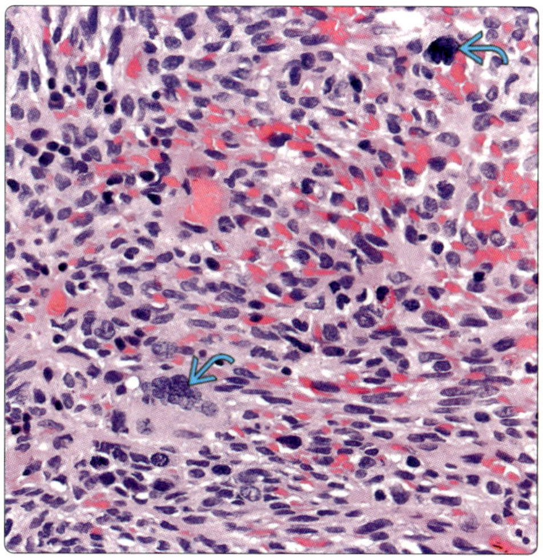

(Left) *H&E shows a focus of rounded tumor cells with clear cytoplasm ➜. Clear cytoplasm can be seen in many sinonasal GPCs, but it is usually only focal and rarely is extensive.* **(Right)** *Multinucleated tumor giant cells ➜ can be seen in up to 5% of cases of sinonasal GPC and likely represent a degenerative change. Note the extravasated blood, which is typical of sinonasal GPC and seen in almost all tumors.*

Desmin, S100, CD34 Negativity

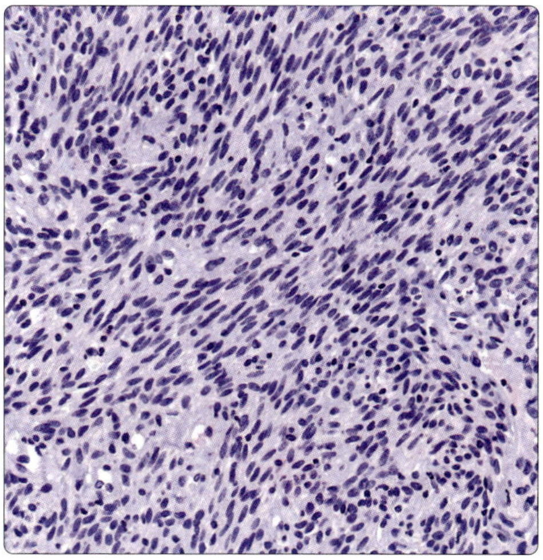

Imaging Features

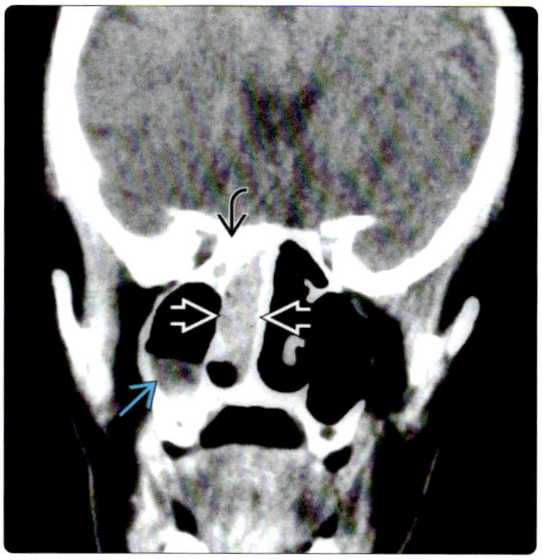

(Left) *While SMA and MSA expression is present in most cases of sinonasal GPC, desmin (shown), keratin, CD34, and S100 protein are negative. The latter 2 antigens, however, may be weakly and focally expressed in some tumors.* **(Right)** *Coronal CT scan shows a sinonasal GPC filling the right nasal cavity ➜ with bone erosion and extension into the adjacent ethmoid sinus ➜. The right maxillary sinus has associated sinusitis ➜.*

Ectopic Meningioma

KEY FACTS

TERMINOLOGY

- Meningothelial neoplasm occurring outside of cranial vault and spinal column
  - Soft tissue extension from intracranial or intraspinal tumor are excluded from definition

CLINICAL ISSUES

- Rare
- Most common in children and young adults
- Usually occurs in head and neck region
  - Skin and subcutis of scalp
  - Sinonasal tract
- Treatment: Complete surgical excision, if possible
- Overall prognosis depends upon grade of tumor and completeness of resection
  - Similar to CNS meningiomas
- Meningothelial hamartoma is benign; recurrences rare

MICROSCOPIC

- Often infiltrative into surrounding tissues
- Morphologic spectrum similar to CNS tumors
  - Meningothelial, fibrous, psammomatous, transitional morphologies
- Meningothelial hamartoma variant: Slit-like pseudovascular spaces lined by meningothelial cells; variable meningothelial nodules

ANCILLARY TESTS

- Positive: EMA, progesterone receptor
- Variable: Claudin-1, S100 protein, p63
- Negative: Chromogranin, synaptophysin, CD31, SMA

TOP DIFFERENTIAL DIAGNOSES

- Primary meningioma of CNS
- Cellular neurothekeoma
- Plexiform fibrohistiocytic tumor

Ectopic Meningioma

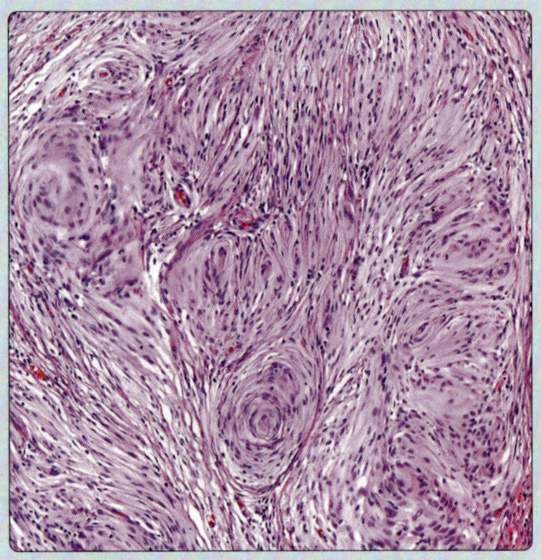

Whorls and Nodules

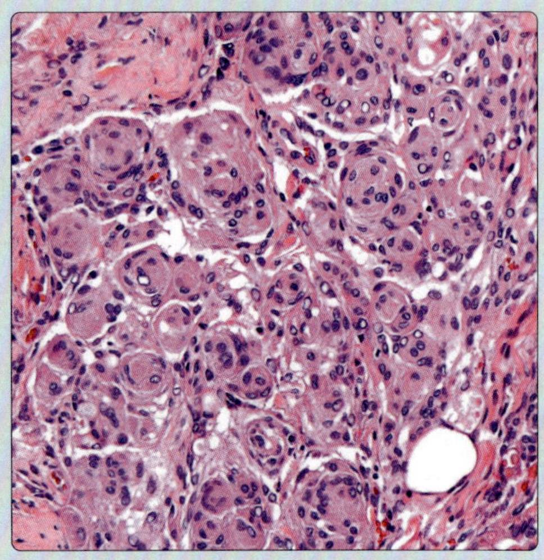

(Left) *Ectopic meningioma shows a similar morphologic spectrum to intracranial/intraspinal tumors. The meningothelial or transitional form is most common. Architectural whorling and small nest/nodule formation are characteristic.* **(Right)** *Extensive nested or nodular growth may mimic a cellular neurothekeoma or even paraganglioma, depending on the site. Immunohistochemistry is valuable in the distinction.*

Infiltrative Growth

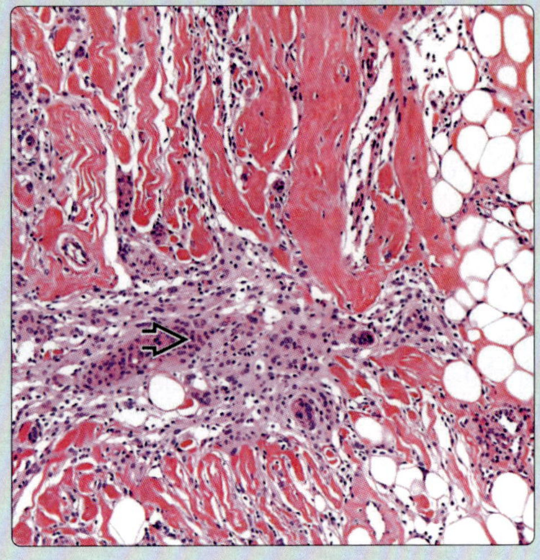

Meningothelial Hamartoma

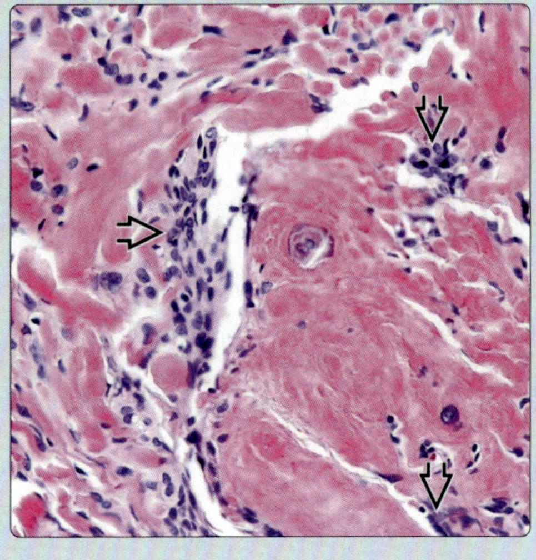

(Left) *Ectopic meningioma ⇨ typically shows infiltrative growth within the surrounding soft tissues, as evidence in this H&E by the admixed collagen bundles and mature adipose tissue.* **(Right)** *Meningothelial hamartoma is a variant of ectopic meningioma that classically occurs in infants around the posterior scalp. Histologically, it shows collagenous stroma with slit-like vascular spaces lined by meningothelial cells ⇨.*

Ectopic Meningioma

TERMINOLOGY

Synonyms

- Cutaneous meningioma, meningothelial choristoma, extracranial meningioma

Definitions

- Meningothelial proliferation or neoplasm occurring outside of cranial vault and spinal column
  - Soft tissue extension from intracranial or intraspinal tumor are not included in definition
  - Meningothelial hamartoma is distinctive, benign clinical variant

ETIOLOGY/PATHOGENESIS

Unknown

- Various hypotheses, including ectopic arachnoid cap cells, displaced meningothelial cells, others

CLINICAL ISSUES

Epidemiology

- Incidence
  - Rare
- Age
  - Wide range reported (most common in children and young adults)
    - Meningothelial hamartoma usually in neonates/infants

Site

- Most common in head and neck region
  - Skin and subcutis of scalp, paravertebral areas
    - Meningothelial hamartoma most common in posterior scalp
  - Sinonasal tract
  - Rarely in other sites, including orbit (unassociated with optic nerve dural sheath), skull, facial bones, oropharynx

Presentation

- Varies widely depending upon site of origin
  - Skin/subcutis
    - Often painless, slow-growing mass
    - May be mistaken for skin tag or epidermal cyst
  - Sinonasal tract
    - Nasal obstruction, discharge, epistaxis

Treatment

- Complete surgical excision

Prognosis

- Similar to CNS tumors
  - Overall prognosis depends upon grade of tumor and completeness of resection
    - Recurrences not uncommon
    - Distant metastases in rare malignant (anaplastic) meningiomas
- Meningothelial hamartoma is benign, and recurrences are rare

MACROSCOPIC

General Features

- Usually tan-white-gray, rubbery mass
- May infiltrate bone

Size

- Range: 1-8 cm (mean: 3.5 cm)

MICROSCOPIC

Histologic Features

- Often infiltrative into surrounding tissues
- Morphologic spectrum similar to CNS tumors
  - Meningothelial (most common)
    - Syncytial lobules of neoplastic cells without distinct borders
    - Whorled architecture
    - Round, regular nuclei with even nuclear chromatin and small nucleoli
    - Pale intranuclear cytoplasmic inclusions
  - Variant morphologies: Transitional, fibroblastic, psammomatoid, atypical, others
- Meningothelial hamartoma variant
  - Slit-like pseudovascular spaces lined by meningothelial cells
  - Small to large clusters of meningothelial cells

ANCILLARY TESTS

Immunohistochemistry

- Positive: EMA, progesterone receptor
- Variable: Claudin-1, S100 protein, p63
- Negative: Chromogranin, synaptophysin, CD31, SMA

DIFFERENTIAL DIAGNOSIS

Primary Meningioma of Central Nervous System

- May grow out into (or metastasize to) extracranial/extraspinal soft tissues
  - Must always be excluded through imaging

Cellular Neurothekeoma

- May show morphological overlap with meningioma
- Head, neck, upper extremity of young adults
- Prominent micronodular growth
- NKI/C3(+); MITF(+); EMA(-); S100 protein (-)

Plexiform Fibrohistiocytic Tumor

- Usually mixture of spindled fibroblastic cells and histiocytoid nodules
  - Multinucleated giant cells common
- Plexiform growth pattern
- SMA(+), EMA(-)

SELECTED REFERENCES

1. Jaiswal P et al: Primary type I cutaneous meningioma of the scalp: cytohistological and immunohistochemical features of a rare neoplasm. Asian J Neurosurg. 13(1):110-112, 2018
2. Lee DH et al: Extracranial meningioma presenting as an eyebrow mass. J Craniofac Surg. 28(4):e305-e307, 2017
3. Miedema JR et al: Cutaneous meningioma. Arch Pathol Lab Med. 136(2):208-11, 2012

Glial Heterotopia

KEY FACTS

TERMINOLOGY

- Mature, heterotopic neuroglial tissue arising as mass outside of cranial cavity
- Synonyms: Nasal glial heterotopia, nasal glioma

ETIOLOGY/PATHOGENESIS

- Congenital, nonhereditary malformation

CLINICAL ISSUES

- Very rare
- Most common in newborns
- Occurs most frequently in nasal area
  - Dorsum of nose, nasal cavity
    - Nasal cavity lesions may present with obstructive symptoms
- Treatment: Simple surgical excision
- Benign, nonneoplastic

MACROSCOPIC

- Firm, smooth, well-circumscribed mass
- Usually 1-3 cm (can reach 7 cm)

MICROSCOPIC

- Nonencapsulated
- Variably sized nests of mature glial tissue within vascularized connective tissue
  - Evenly distributed astrocytes within fine neurofibrillary matrix
- Lacks mitoses

ANCILLARY TESTS

- GFAP(+), S100 protein (+)

TOP DIFFERENTIAL DIAGNOSES

- True encephalocele
- Neurofibroma
- Meningothelial hamartoma

Glial Heterotopia

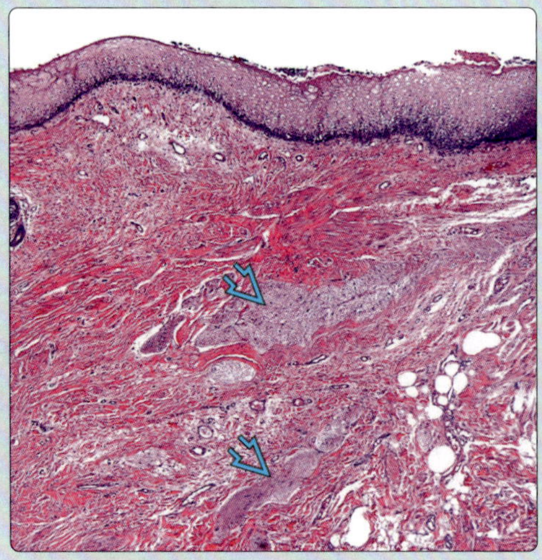

Mature Glial Tissue

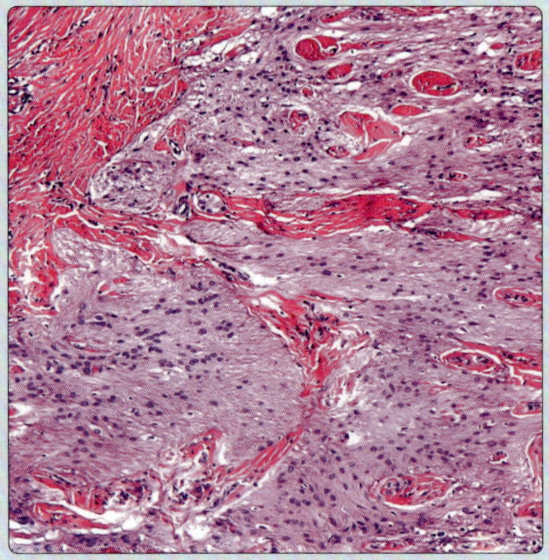

(Left) *Heterotopic glial tissue is most commonly seen in the region of the nose and nasal cavity and is characterized by nests of mature glial tissue within a vascularized connective tissue stroma.* **(Right)** *The glial tissue resembles that of the central nervous system; however, neurons are often rare. The size of the nests varies from small and well formed to large and confluent.*

Fine Fibrillary Matrix

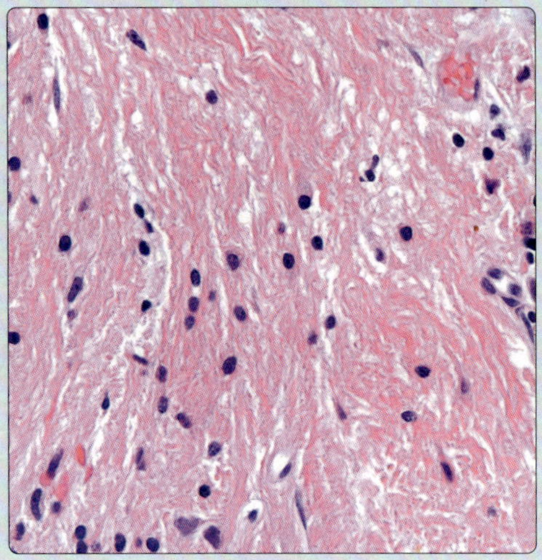

Rare Eccrine Hyperplasia

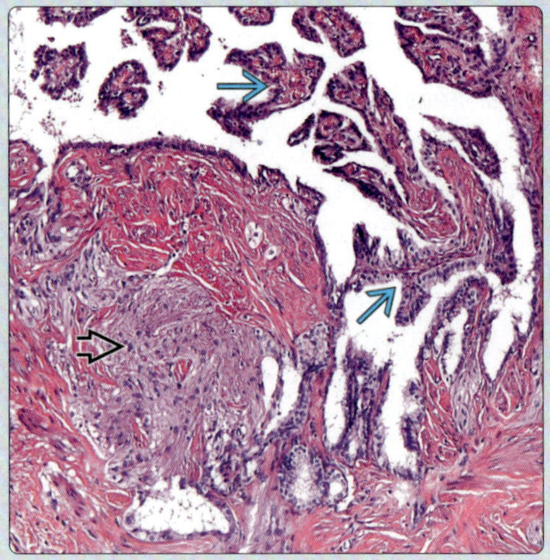

(Left) *Mature glial tissue is evidenced by the presence of astrocytes and other cells lightly distributed within a fine fibrillary matrix. Thin or thick bundles of collagen are not present.* **(Right)** *Rare cases of cutaneous glial heterotopia of the nose may show an associated hyperplasia of eccrine sweat glands. Note the focus of mature glial tissue.*

TERMINOLOGY

Synonyms

- Nasal glial heterotopia
- Heterotopic glial tissue
- Nasal glioma

Definitions

- Mature, heterotopic neuroglial tissue arising as mass outside of cranial cavity

ETIOLOGY/PATHOGENESIS

Developmental Anomaly

- Congenital, nonhereditary malformation
- Anterior displacement of mature neuroglial tissue without intracranial connection

CLINICAL ISSUES

Epidemiology

- Incidence
  - Very rare
    - Rarely associated with other brain or systemic anomalies
- Age
  - Most common in newborns
    - Usually identified at birth or within first 2 years of life
  - Very rare cases reported in adults
- Sex
  - M = F

Site

- Nasal area
  - Bridge of nose is most common site (60% of cases)
  - Nasal cavity (30%)
    - Can be attached to septum
- May rarely occur in other sites such as tongue, pharynx, tonsil, orbit, palate

Presentation

- Extranasal
  - Smooth, subcutaneous mass on dorsum of nose
- Intranasal
  - Nasal obstruction or deformity
  - No intracranial component or bony defect
    - If present, encephalocoele is more likely
- Rare parapharyngeal lesions may present with airway obstruction

Treatment

- Simple surgical excision

Prognosis

- Benign; nonneoplastic
- Local recurrence (up to 30%) with incomplete excision

MACROSCOPIC

General Features

- Firm, smooth, well-circumscribed mass
- Intranasal lesions are smooth and polypoid

Size

- Usually 1-3 cm (can reach 7 cm)

MICROSCOPIC

Histologic Features

- Nonencapsulated; often poorly defined borders
- Variably sized nests of mature glial tissue within vascularized connective tissue
  - Evenly distributed astrocytes within fine, neurofibrillary matrix
    - Larger gemistocytes may be seen
    - Neurons are often absent
  - May contain choroid plexus, ependyma, or retinal epithelium
- Lacks mitoses
- Focal calcification may be seen
- Rarely may be associated with proliferation of eccrine ducts
- In older patients, lesions may be more fibrotic or collagenous
- Isolated case report of tumor showing combined glial and meningothelial features ("gliomeningeal heterotopia")

ANCILLARY TESTS

Immunohistochemistry

- GFAP(+), S100 protein (+)
- Negative for EMA, CD34, SMA, desmin

DIFFERENTIAL DIAGNOSIS

True Encephalocele

- Histologically indistinguishable
- Shows connection with brain
  - Requires imaging studies

Neurofibroma

- Wide distribution
- Spindled cells with wavy, buckled, tapered nuclei
- Collagenous rather than fibrillary stroma

Meningothelial Hamartoma

- Most common in posterior scalp
- Meningothelial-lined, slit-like spaces and small meningothelial clusters
- Fibrocollagenous stroma
- EMA(+), S100 protein (-)

SELECTED REFERENCES

1. Schauer A et al: Unusual case of combined gliomeningeal heterotopia on the nose of an infant. Am J Dermatopathol. 40(7): 515-8, 2018
2. Riffaud L et al: Glial heterotopia of the face. J Pediatr Surg. 43(12):e1-3, 2008
3. Ma KH et al: Nasal glioma. Hong Kong Med J. 12(6):477-9, 2006
4. Chen CY et al: Parapharyngeal neuroglial heterotopia presenting as a growing single locular cyst: MR imaging findings. AJNR Am J Neuroradiol. 26(1):96-9, 2005
5. Penner CR et al: Nasal glial heterotopia: a clinicopathologic and immunophenotypic analysis of 10 cases with a review of the literature. Ann Diagn Pathol. 7(6):354-9, 2003
6. Cerdá-Nicolás M et al: Nasal glioma or nasal glial heterotopia? Morphological, immunohistochemical and ultrastructural study of two cases. Clin Neuropathol. 21(2):66-71, 2002
7. Jartti PH et al: MR of a nasal glioma in a young infant. Acta Radiol. 43(2):141-3, 2002

Paraganglioma

KEY FACTS

TERMINOLOGY

- Distinctive tumor of neural crest origin that arises from paraganglia at specified locations
- Pheochromocytoma is paraganglioma (PG) arising exclusively within medulla of adrenal gland

ETIOLOGY/PATHOGENESIS

- May be sporadic or arise within setting of various hereditary tumor syndromes

CLINICAL ISSUES

- Usually affects adults (but overall wide age range)
- Head and neck (particularly carotid body), mediastinum, retroperitoneum, bladder, other sites
- May be solitary, bilateral, or multicentric
- Treatment: Complete surgical excision
- Most are clinically benign but may recur
- Malignant behavior in specific subset
    - Associated with germline *SDHB* mutations

MICROSCOPIC

- Characteristic zellballen growth of tumor cells within highly vascularized fibrous stroma
- Epithelioid or polygonal tumor cells with eosinophilic, basophilic, or amphophilic, finely granular cytoplasm
- Sustentacular cells often present (but not always)
- Sinusoidal vascular pattern common, often prominent
- Variant: Sclerosing PG

ANCILLARY TESTS

- Synaptophysin (+), chromogranin (+), CD56(+)
- Sustentacular cells are S100 protein (+), SOX10(+)
- Keratin (-), SMA(-), desmin (-), TFE3(-)
- Molecular: Significant subset harbors *SDH* mutations

TOP DIFFERENTIAL DIAGNOSES

- Alveolar soft part sarcoma
- Carcinoid tumor
- Carcinoma or melanoma

Paraganglioma

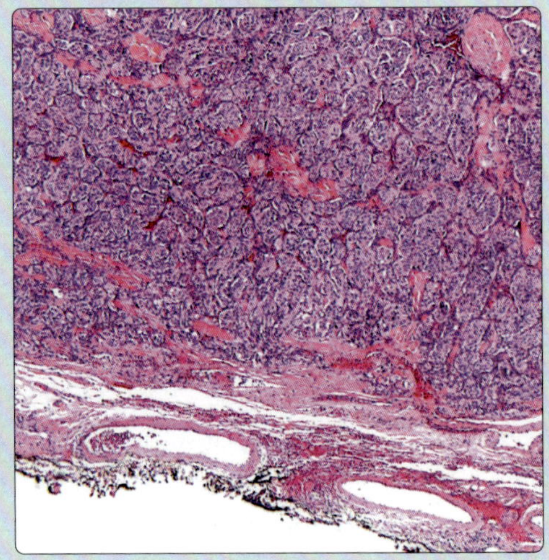

Characteristic Zellballen Pattern

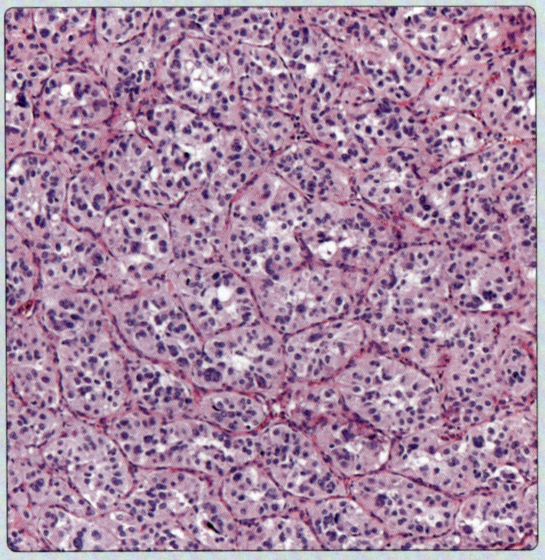

(Left) *Paraganglioma (PG) is a well-circumscribed neuroendocrine neoplasm that arises from parasympathetic paraganglia in the neck (particularly carotid body) and within thoracoabdominal sites along the sympathetic chain. PG arising in the adrenal gland is usually referred to as a pheochromocytoma.* **(Right)** *The zellballen pattern of PG features rounded nests of tumor cells within a vascularized fibrous stroma. This growth pattern is not well developed in all tumors, however, and may be absent.*

Cytologic Features

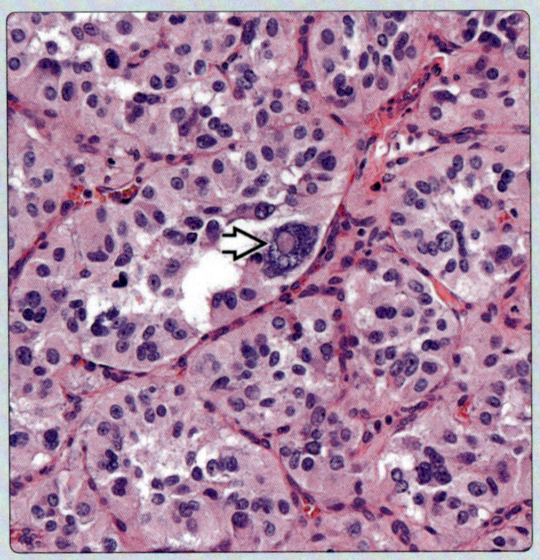

Prominent Vasculature

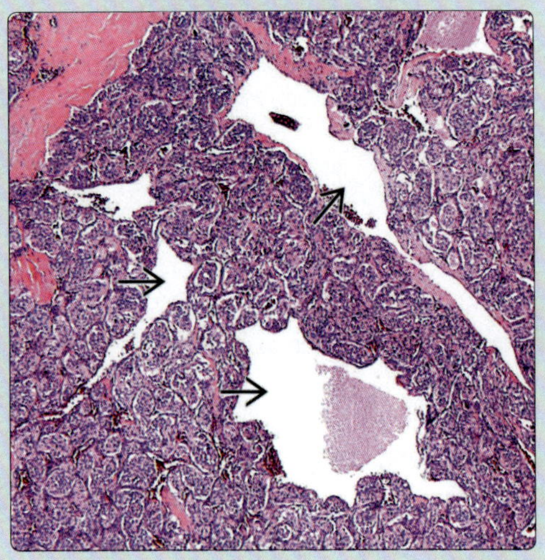

(Left) *The tumor cells of PG often contain finely granular, eosinophilic cytoplasm and regular, centralized nuclei that may or may not show nucleoli. Intranuclear pseudoinclusions ⇨ are common, as are scattered nuclei with enlargement and pleomorphism.* **(Right)** *PG characteristically contains a conspicuous stromal vasculature. The vessels are often compressed and sinusoidal, but larger ectatic or "staghorn" vessels ⇨ can also be seen, as depicted in this H&E.*

TERMINOLOGY

Abbreviations

- Paraganglioma (PG)

Synonyms

- Chemodectoma
- Glomus tympanicum (middle ear) and glomus jugulare (jugular foramen of temporal bone)
  - These tumors are PGs and are not related to soft tissue glomus tumor
- Extraadrenal PG

Definitions

- Distinctive tumor of neural crest origin that arises from paraganglia at specified locations and often demonstrates characteristic nested zellballen growth pattern
  - Parasympathetic paraganglia in head and neck
    - Usually nonfunctional
  - Sympathetic paraganglia of abdomen, pelvis, and thorax
    - Usually functional
- Pheochromocytoma is PG that arises from within medulla of adrenal gland

ETIOLOGY/PATHOGENESIS

Genetics

- May be sporadic or arise within setting of various hereditary tumor syndromes
  - Hereditary PG-pheochromocytoma syndrome
    - Germline mutations in *SDH* (succinate dehydrogenase) gene subunits
  - Multiple endocrine neoplasia type 2 (MEN2) syndrome
    - Germline mutations in *RET* gene
  - von Hippel-Lindau syndrome
    - Germline mutations in *VHL* gene
  - Neurofibromatosis type 1
    - Germline mutations in *NF1* gene
  - Carney-Stratakis syndrome
    - Germline mutations in *SDH* gene subunits
    - Features gastric gastrointestinal stromal tumor (GIST) and multicentric PG
  - Carney triad
    - Features GIST, PG, and pulmonary chondroma
    - Exact genetic mechanism unclear

CLINICAL ISSUES

Epidemiology

- Incidence
  - Rare
- Age
  - Usually adults (but overall wide age range)
    - Tumors associated with hereditary syndromes often affect younger age group
- Sex
  - M = F overall
    - Female predominance reported in sclerosing PG and in PG arising in patients who live in high-altitude habitats

Site

- Head and neck (most common extraadrenal location)
  - Majority arise in carotid body
    - More common in high-altitude habitat
  - Also jugular bulb, middle ear, vagus nerve
- Mediastinum (aorticopulmonary)
- Retroperitoneum (from aorticosympathetic paraganglia or organ of Zuckerkandl)
- May also arise in bladder, heart, other organs

Presentation

- Often painless mass
- May be solitary, bilateral, or multicentric
- Head and neck PG may be associated with features of cranial nerve palsies
- Thoracoabdominal PG often associated with symptoms/signs attributable to catecholamine production
  - Hypertension, palpitations, headache, tachycardia, sweating

Treatment

- Complete surgical excision
  - Preoperative embolization may be utilized
- Radiotherapy may be utilized in larger, unresectable tumors
- Recommendation: All patients with PG should be evaluated for possible hereditary syndromes (particularly those found to be SDH deficient)

Prognosis

- Most are clinically benign but may recur
- Malignant behavior in specific subset
  - Metastasize to lymph nodes, lung, bone
  - Significantly increased risk in PG with germline *SDHB* mutations

MACROSCOPIC

General Features

- Well-demarcated mass
- Pink-tan to pink and dark red cut surface

Size

- Usually < 5 cm

MICROSCOPIC

Histologic Features

- Well circumscribed
- Characteristic rounded, nested, or compartmentalized growth pattern of tumor cells within highly vascularized fibrous stroma
  - Termed zellballen
  - Often best developed in carotid body tumors
  - Tumor cells may also grow in sheets, trabeculae, or pseudopapillary arrangements
- Epithelioid or polygonal tumor cells with eosinophilic, basophilic, or amphophilic, finely granular cytoplasm
  - Centralized nuclei ± nucleoli
    - May contain nuclear pseudoinclusions
    - Nuclear pleomorphism not uncommon and often focal
  - Clear cell change may be present

  - May be prominent and resemble lipoblastic differentiation
- Intracytoplasmic pigment (lipofuscin, neuromelanin) or eosinophilic globules in occasional cases
- Tumor cells may show spindled morphology
- Mitotic figures rare
- Spindled to stellate sustentacular cells at periphery of nests
  - Can be absent
- Sinusoidal vascular pattern common, often prominent
  - May show extensive hemorrhage or vascular congestion
- Variably prominent fibrous stroma/septa
- Clinically malignant tumors generally histologically indistinguishable from clinically benign tumors
  - However, malignant PG is more likely to show overall worrisome features (marked nuclear pleomorphism, mitotic activity, necrosis, and vascular invasion)
- Rare retroperitoneal extraadrenal PG can contain component of ganglioneuroma

Morphologic Variant

- Sclerosing PG
  - Prominent, diffuse stromal fibrosis
  - Most common in head and neck

ANCILLARY TESTS

Immunohistochemistry

- Synaptophysin (+), chromogranin (+), CD56(+)
- Sustentacular cells (if present) are S100 protein (+) and SOX10(+)
- Keratin (-), SMA (-), desmin (-), TFE3(-)
- Loss of SDHB protein expression (if PG contains germline *SDH* mutations)
  - Specific mutation (*SDHA, SDHB, SDHC, SDHD*) should be confirmed by mutation analysis

Genetic Testing

- Significant subset of PG harbors *SDH* mutations (*SDHA, SDHB, SDHC*, or *SDHD*)
  - *SDHD* mutation most common in head/neck PG
  - *SDHB* mutation most common in thoracoabdominal PG
- Very rare *SDHAF2* gene mutations in head/neck PG

DIFFERENTIAL DIAGNOSIS

Alveolar Soft Part Sarcoma

- Usually located in deep soft tissues
- Large polygonal cells with abundant eosinophilic cytoplasm
- Synaptophysin (-), chromogranin (-), S100 protein (-)
- Nuclear TFE3(+)
- t(X;17)(p11;q25), with *ASPSCR1-TFE3* fusion

Carcinoid Tumor

- Speckled salt and pepper chromatin pattern
- Keratin (+), synaptophysin (+)
- Sustentacular cells absent

Primary or Metastatic Carcinoma

- Particularly renal cell or adrenocortical in abdomen
- Keratin (+)
- Coexisting or prior renal/adrenal mass

Metastatic Melanoma

- Previous clinical history may or may not be present
- S100 protein (+)
- Expression of melanocytic markers (HMB-45, MART-1, etc.)

Gastrointestinal Stromal Tumor (SDH-Deficient Type)

- Arises in muscular wall of stomach
- Loss of SDHB by immunohistochemistry
- CD117(+), DOG1(+)
- Synaptophysin (-), chromogranin (-)

SELECTED REFERENCES

1. Cho YY et al: A clinical prediction model to estimate the metastatic potential of pheochromocytoma/paraganglioma: ASES score. Surgery. ePub, 2018
2. Fite JJ et al: Paraganglioma: Cytomorphologic features, radiologic and clinical findings in 12 cases. Diagn Cytopathol. 46(6):473-81, 2018
3. Turchini J et al: Pathology and genetics of phaeochromocytoma and paraganglioma. Histopathology. 72(1):97-105, 2018
4. Udager AM et al: The utility of SDHB and FH immunohistochemistry in patients evaluated for hereditary paraganglioma-pheochromocytoma syndromes. Hum Pathol. 71:47-54, 2017
5. Amato B et al: Surgical resection of carotid body paragangliomas: 10 years of experience. Am J Surg. 207(2):293-8, 2014
6. Santi R et al: Sclerosing paraganglioma of the carotid body: a potential pitfall of malignancy. Head Neck Pathol. 9(2):300-4, 2014
7. Fishbein L et al: Inherited mutations in pheochromocytoma and paraganglioma: why all patients should be offered genetic testing. Ann Surg Oncol. 20(5):1444-50, 2013
8. Galan SR et al: Genetics and molecular pathogenesis of pheochromocytoma and paraganglioma. Clin Endocrinol (Oxf). 78(2):165-75, 2013
9. Jimenez C et al: Current and future treatments for malignant pheochromocytoma and sympathetic paraganglioma. Curr Oncol Rep. 15(4):356-71, 2013
10. Letouzé E et al: SDH mutations establish a hypermethylator phenotype in paraganglioma. Cancer Cell. 23(6):739-52, 2013
11. Mason EF et al: Identification of succinate dehydrogenase-deficient bladder paragangliomas. Am J Surg Pathol. 37(10):1612-8, 2013
12. Rattenberry E et al: A comprehensive next generation sequencing-based genetic testing strategy to improve diagnosis of inherited pheochromocytoma and paraganglioma. J Clin Endocrinol Metab. 98(7):E1248-56, 2013
13. Barletta JA et al: Succinate dehydrogenase-deficient tumors: diagnostic advances and clinical implications. Adv Anat Pathol. 19(4):193-203, 2012
14. Castelblanco E et al: Thyroid paraganglioma. Report of 3 cases and description of an immunohistochemical profile useful in the differential diagnosis with medullary thyroid carcinoma, based on complementary DNA array results. Hum Pathol. 43(7):1103-12, 2012
15. Mazzaglia PJ: Hereditary pheochromocytoma and paraganglioma. J Surg Oncol. 106(5):580-5, 2012
16. van Hulsteijn LT et al: Risk of malignant paraganglioma in SDHB-mutation and SDHD-mutation carriers: a systematic review and meta-analysis. J Med Genet. 49(12):768-76, 2012
17. King KS et al: Metastatic pheochromocytoma/paraganglioma related to primary tumor development in childhood or adolescence: significant link to SDHB mutations. J Clin Oncol. 29(31):4137-42, 2011
18. Singhi AD et al: Peripancreatic paraganglioma: a potential diagnostic challenge in cytopathology and surgical pathology. Am J Surg Pathol. 35(10):1498-504, 2011
19. Gill AJ et al: Immunohistochemistry for SDHB triages genetic testing of SDHB, SDHC, and SDHD in paraganglioma-pheochromocytoma syndromes. Hum Pathol. 41(6):805-14, 2010
20. Sangoi AR et al: A tissue microarray-based comparative analysis of novel and traditional immunohistochemical markers in the distinction between adrenal cortical lesions and pheochromocytoma. Am J Surg Pathol. 34(3):423-32, 2010
21. Petri BJ et al: Phaeochromocytomas and sympathetic paragangliomas. Br J Surg. 96(12):1381-92, 2009
22. Plaza JA et al: Sclerosing paraganglioma: report of 19 cases of an unusual variant of neuroendocrine tumor that may be mistaken for an aggressive malignant neoplasm. Am J Surg Pathol. 30(1):7-12, 2006
23. Wasserman PG et al: Paragangliomas: classification, pathology, and differential diagnosis. Otolaryngol Clin North Am. 34(5):845-62, v-vi, 2001

Paraganglia

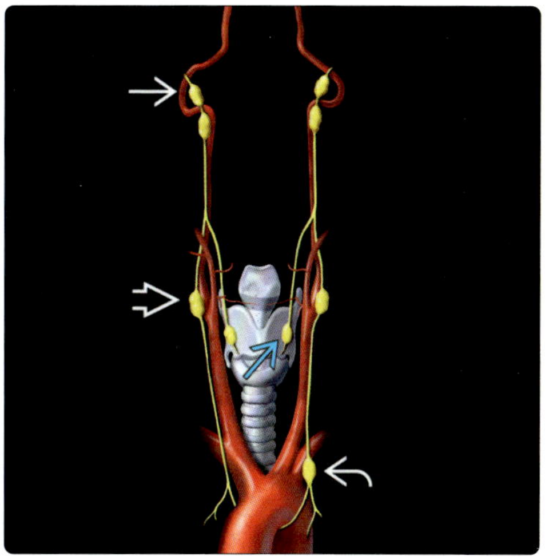

Paraganglia

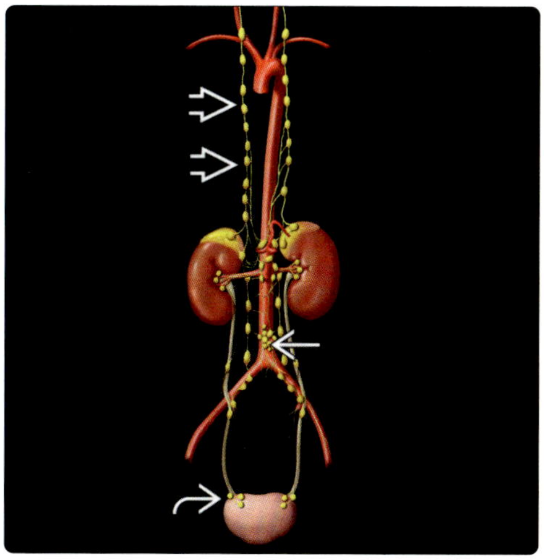

(Left) *Graphic shows the location of paraganglia in the head, neck, and upper thorax associated with arteries or cranial nerves. They include aortic ➔ and carotid ➔ bodies, jugulotympanic ➔, and laryngeal ➔ paraganglia.* **(Right)** *Graphic shows aorticosympathetic paraganglia in thorax and abdomen. These are associated with the sympathetic chain ➔ and arterial plexuses and include the adrenal medulla and organ of Zuckerkandl ➔. Paraganglia in the bladder ➔ can be the site of PG.*

Carotid Body

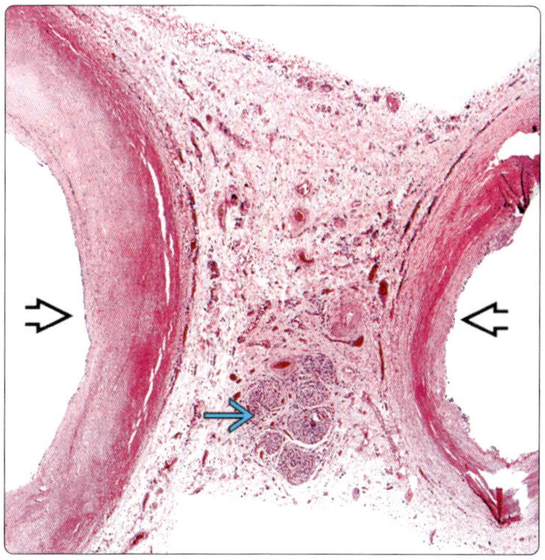

Carotid Body

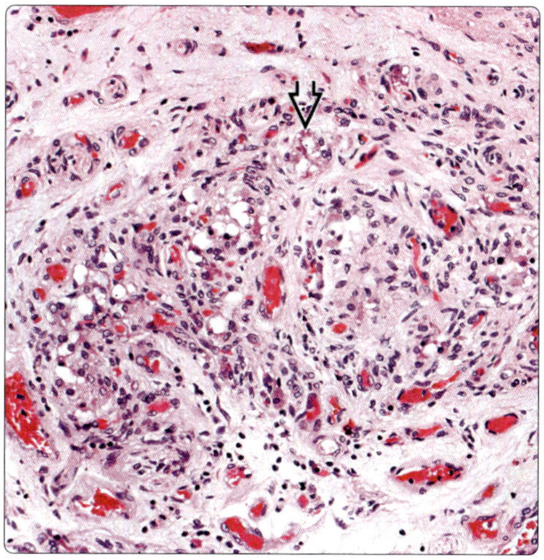

(Left) *Low-power H&E shows a normal carotid body ➔ in connective tissue at the bifurcation of the carotid artery ➔ in the neck. This structure represents an aggregate of chemoreceptor tissue that is not encapsulated.* **(Right)** *Higher magnification of a carotid body shows nested or organoid appearance with small nests of chief cells ➔ intimately admixed with thin-walled blood vessels. Note the absence of nuclear pleomorphism.*

Variable Nested Growth

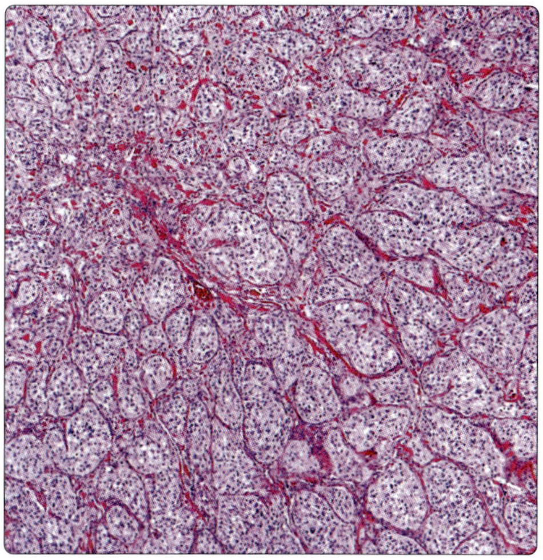

Trabecular Growth

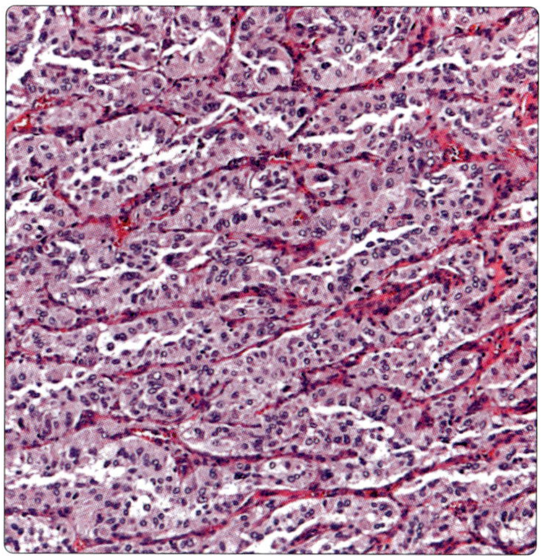

(Left) *The small, nested, organoid or zellballen growth that is characteristic of PG varies somewhat from case to case. The pattern is often well developed in head/neck PG but may be less noticeable or even absent in other sites. Note the larger and less rounded nests in the lower right as compared to the smaller, rounder nests in the upper left.* **(Right)** *Trabecular growth may be seen in PG, as shown in this H&E.*

(Left) *The combination of artifactual clefting and a sinusoidal vasculature can impart a focal morphologic appearance that mimics carcinoid tumor, as depicted. Unlike the latter tumor, however, PG is negative for keratins.* **(Right)** *Occasional cases of PG may show formation of pseudorosettes with tumor cells oriented around small blood vessels* → *. This morphology is more frequently seen in PG of the cauda equina, where it can resemble myxopapillary ependymoma.*

Focal Carcinoid-Like Morphology

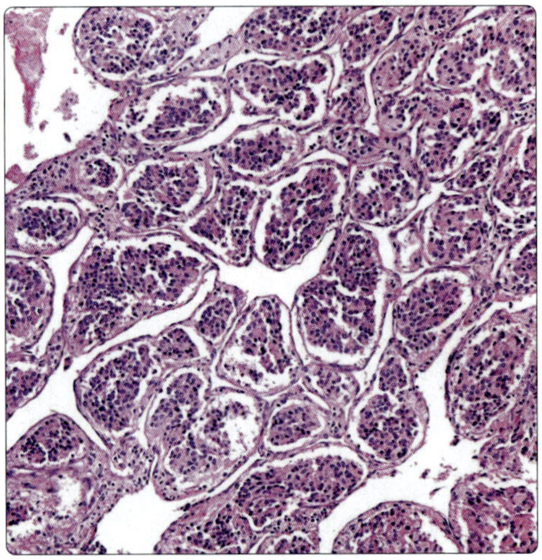

Pseudorosette Pattern

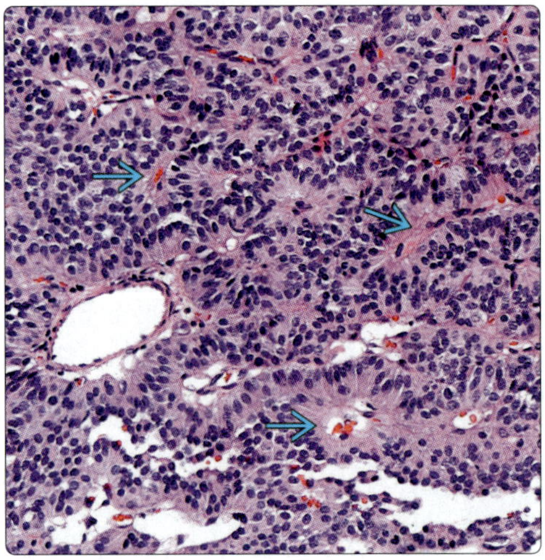

(Left) *Nuclear pleomorphism &/or multinucleation* → *is common as a focal finding in PG, but it may be more extensive and prominent in some tumors. This finding has no prognostic significance in isolation. Note the nested zellballen pattern in this H&E.* **(Right)** *Nuclear pleomorphism may be striking in some cases of PG; however, its presence does not appear to directly predict behavior.*

Nuclear Pleomorphism

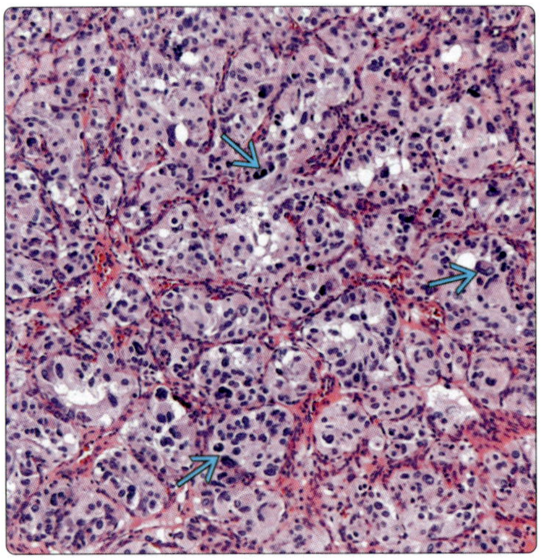

Nuclear Pleomorphism

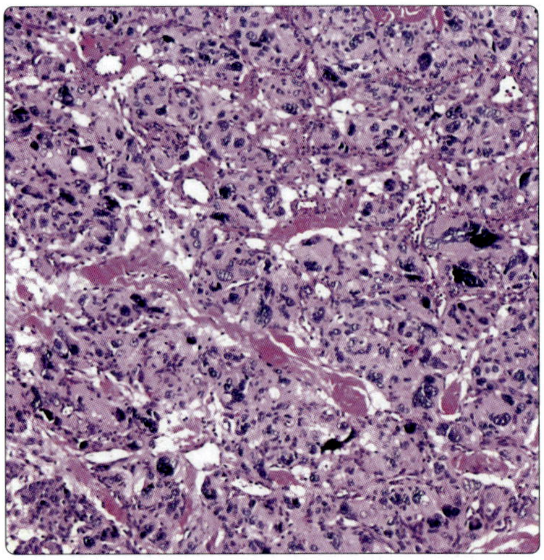

(Left) *Nuclear pseudoinclusions* → *are frequently identified in PG and are formed by projections of eosinophilic cytoplasm into the nucleus.* **(Right)** *Although many examples of PG are composed of tumor cells with eosinophilic cytoplasm, some tumors show prominent basophilic cytoplasm, as depicted. This finding is most characteristic of pheochromocytoma (adrenal PG) but can also be seen in extraadrenal sites.*

Nuclear Pseudoinclusions

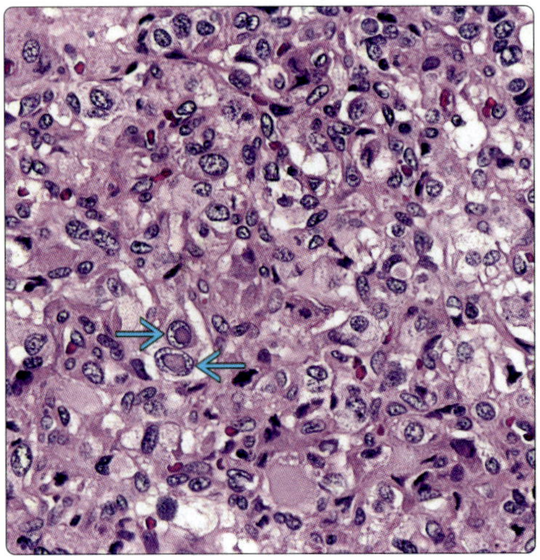

Basophilic Cytoplasm

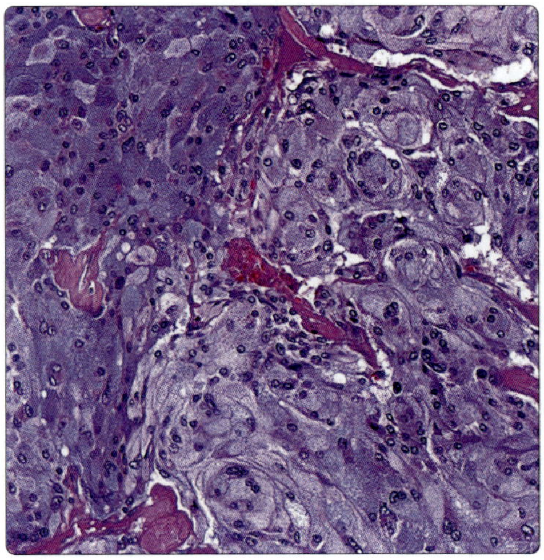

Basophilic Cytoplasm

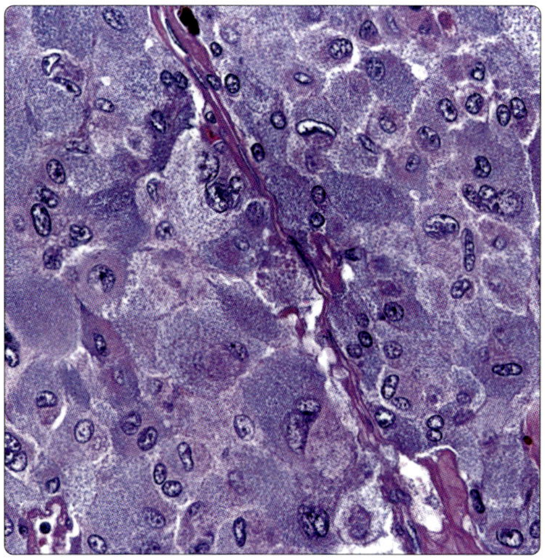

Basophilia and Nuclear Pleomorphism

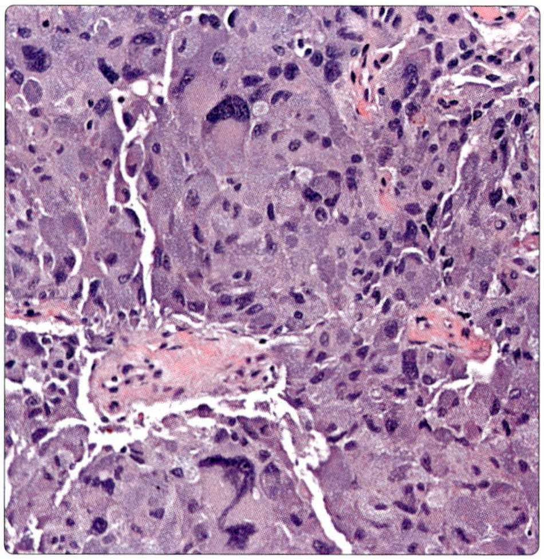

(Left) *Basophilic tumor cells in PG often show a more prominent granular quality to the cytoplasm than eosinophilic tumor cells.* **(Right)** *Similar to their predominantly eosinophilic counterparts, PG with basophilic tumor cells can also show nuclear pleomorphism &/or multinucleation.*

Granular Cytoplasm

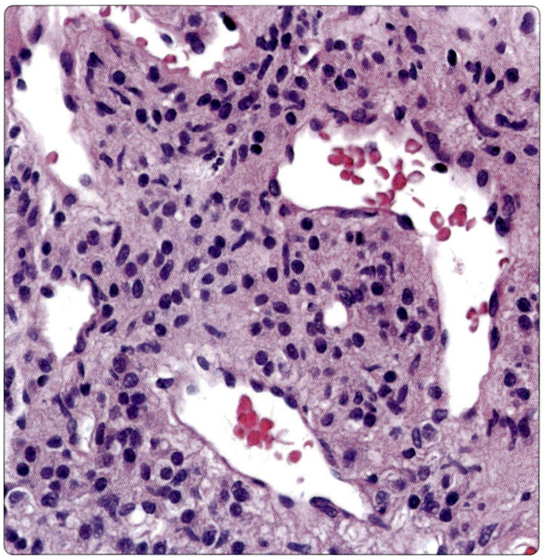

Vacuolated Cells

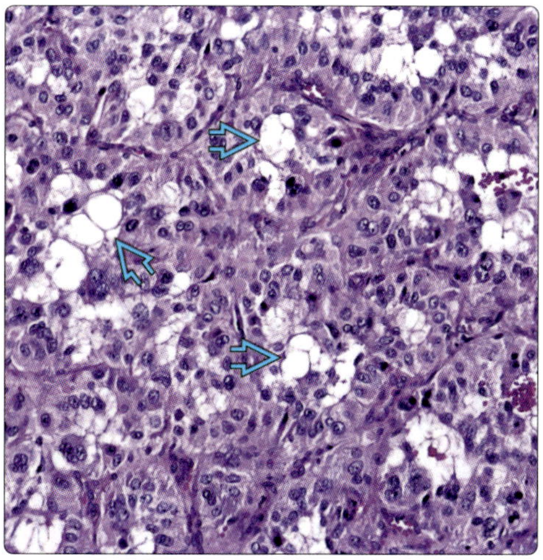

(Left) *Granular eosinophilic cytoplasm is an occasional finding in PG and may somewhat resemble a soft tissue granular cell tumor. This tumor arose in the mediastinum.* **(Right)** *Clear cell change due to cytoplasmic vacuolization ⇨ is a common finding in PG and may be focal, patchy, or, rarely, diffuse.*

Clear Cell Change

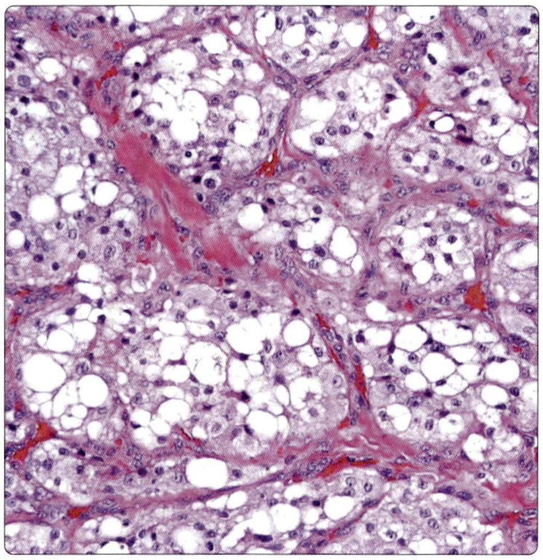

Sheet-Like Growth

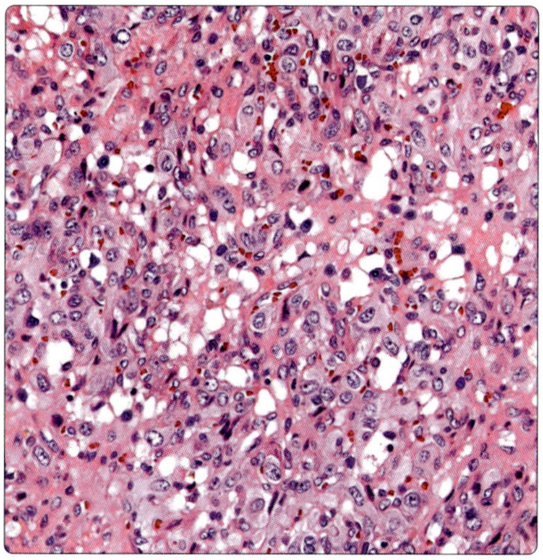

(Left) *Intracytoplasmic vacuolizations may be quite prominent in some cases of PG and can lend a bubbly appearance to the cell, sometimes suggesting lipoblastic differentiation.* **(Right)** *Although nested or organoid growth is more common in PG, some tumors can show areas with sheet-like growth, as depicted. Note the vacuolated tumor cells.*

(**Left**) *Tumor cells in PG may show an accumulation of dark intracytoplasmic pigment (often neuromelanin). Rarely, it can be diffuse and prominent and obscure the underlying tumor. Lipofuscin and hemosiderin can also be seen in PG.* (**Right**) *Most tumor cells in PG are polygonal or epithelioid; however, a spindled morphology can also be seen focally, as depicted.*

Intracytoplasmic Pigment

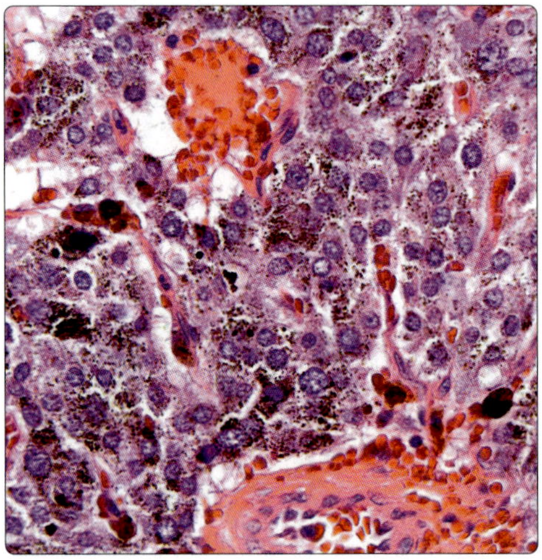

Spindle Cell Morphology

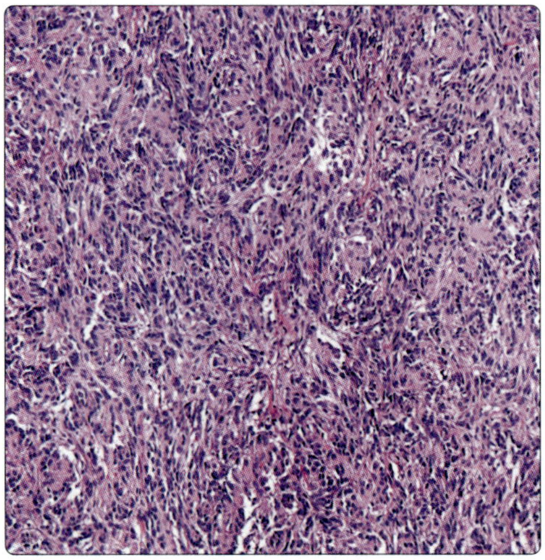

(**Left**) *Given the vascular nature of PG, hemorrhage is not an uncommon histologic finding. In the setting of extensive intratumoral hemorrhage, a vascular neoplasm may even be considered.* (**Right**) *Vascular congestion is common in PG and may lead to the formation of large dilated spaces ➔ filled with proteinaceous fluid and blood.*

Hemorrhage

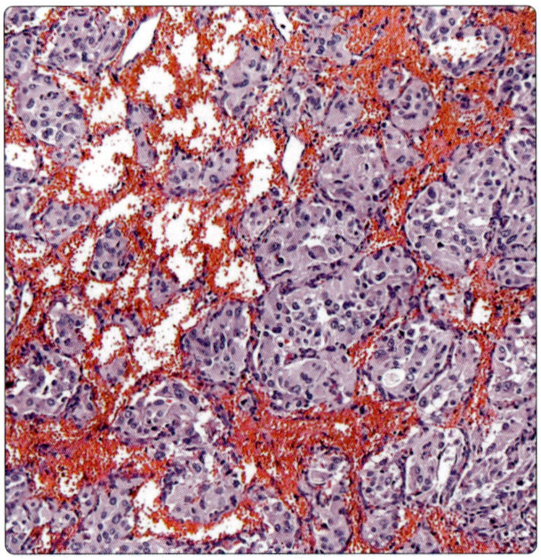

Vascular Congestion

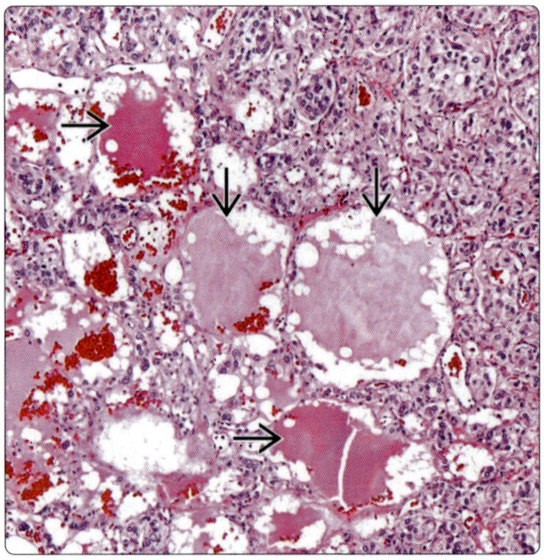

(**Left**) *Centralized areas with loose, edematous stroma ↪ can be seen within otherwise typical PG. Note the micronodular appearance that results.* (**Right**) *Scattered dilated, irregular ("staghorn") blood vessels are not uncommon in PG. In some cases, they can be numerous and prominent in areas, closely resembling solitary fibrous tumor at low power, as depicted.*

Stromal Edema

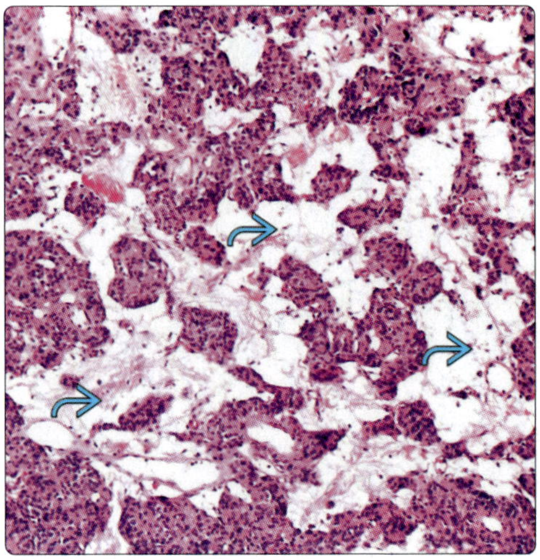

Hemangiopericytoma-Like Vasculature

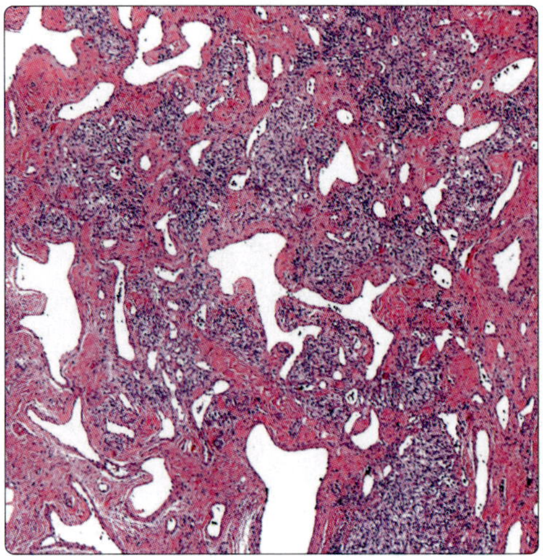

Lobular Growth

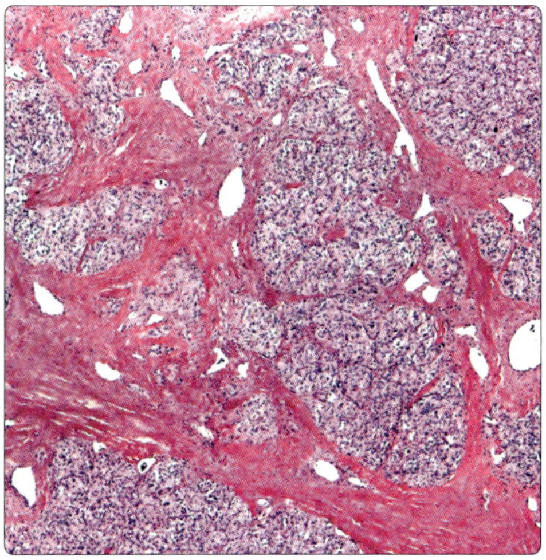

Sclerosing Paraganglioma

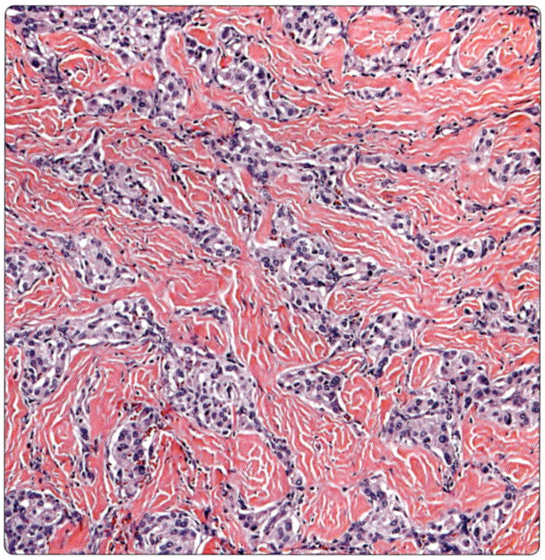

(Left) *Some cases of PG show a lobulated growth pattern with thick fibrous septa, as depicted, particularly near the tumor periphery. This morphology can lead to consideration of alveolar soft part sarcoma.* **(Right)** *The sclerosing variant of PG is characterized by irregularly compressed nests of tumor cells within a prominent fibrocollagenous stroma, as shown. This variant appears to be most common in the head and neck region. Smaller foci of stromal fibrosis may also be seen in otherwise conventional PG.*

Composite Paraganglioma-Ganglioneuroma

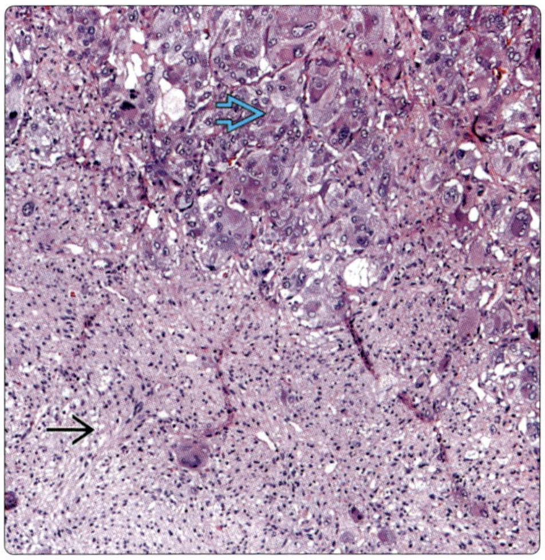

Neuroendocrine Marker Expression

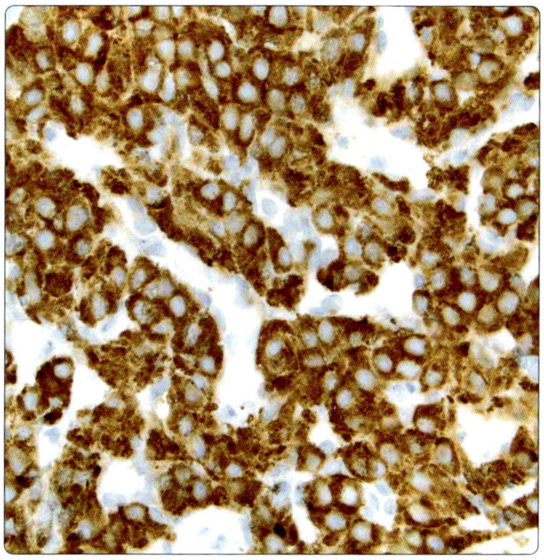

(Left) *Rare cases of pheochromocytoma* ⇨ *(adrenal PG) arise in association with ganglioneuroma* ⇨*. This event is even rarer in extraadrenal PG but has been reported in the retroperitoneum.* **(Right)** *Tumor cells in PG typically show diffuse expression of neuroendocrine markers, including synaptophysin (shown), chromogranin, and CD56. Unlike carcinoid tumors, keratins are negative in PG.*

Sustentacular Cells

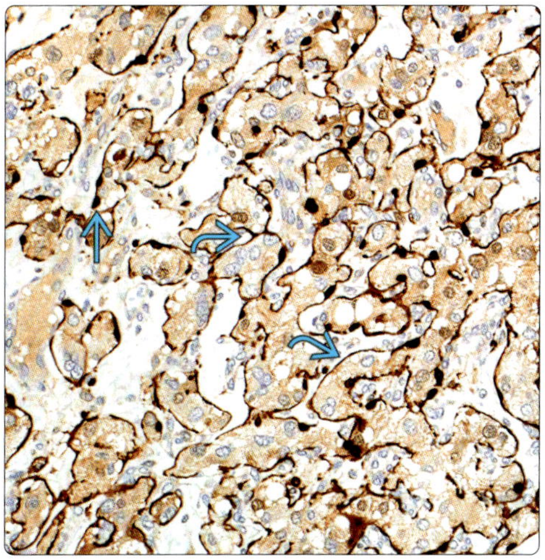

Sustentacular Cells

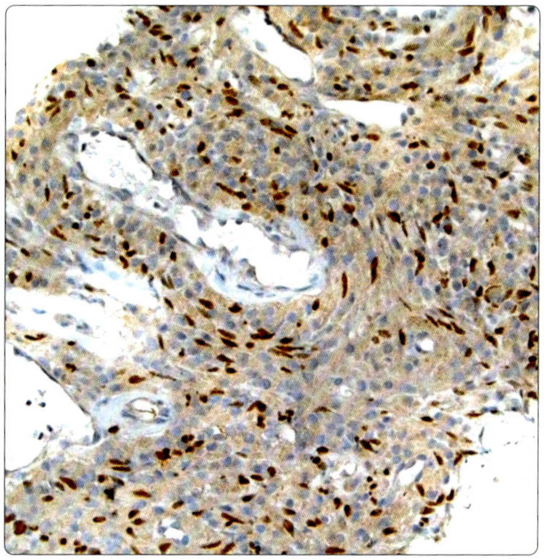

(Left) *Sustentacular cells, or modified Schwann cells that surround nests and aggregates of tumor cells in PG, are best visualized on an S100 protein immunostain. Note the characteristic thin, delicate cytoplasmic processes* ↪ *and nuclei* ⇨ *of these cells. These cells are not present in all cases, however.* **(Right)** *SOX10, a nuclear marker of neural crest origin, is expressed by sustentacular cells in PG and may be used as an alternative to S100 protein.*

Peripheral Hemangioblastoma

KEY FACTS

TERMINOLOGY

- True hemangioblastoma (HB) arising in locations outside CNS
  - Uncertain cellular origin

ETIOLOGY/PATHOGENESIS

- Associated with von Hippel-Lindau (VHL) syndrome

CLINICAL ISSUES

- Very rare
- Median age: 56.5 years
- Most frequently arise in spinal nerve roots (extradural)
  - Also visceral organs (rare)
- Patients may show other features or tumors of VHL
- Treatment: Complete surgical excision
- True local recurrence or distant metastasis has yet to be documented
- Genetic testing for VHL should be performed for all patients

MICROSCOPIC

- Morphologically very similar to CNS HB
  - However, peripheral HB lacks prominent cystic growth
- Well-circumscribed, often lobular growth pattern
- Mixture of spindled cells and larger, polygonal cells ± prominent cytoplasmic vacuolization
- Rich, delicate, ramifying capillary vascular network between cells

ANCILLARY TESTS

- Inhibin (+); variable S100 protein (+)
- Keratin (-), SMA(-), CD34(-), CD31(-), synaptophysin (-)

TOP DIFFERENTIAL DIAGNOSES

- Solitary fibrous tumor
- Metastatic renal cell carcinoma
- Well-differentiated liposarcoma
- PEComa
- Paraganglioma

(Left) *Peripheral hemangioblastoma (HB) is a very rare form of HB that occurs outside of the CNS. It is a highly vascularized neoplasm and features vessels ranging from interconnecting, thin-walled capillary channels to larger, ectatic vessels.* **(Right)** *A mixture of spindled and polygonal cells comprise most cases of HB. A prominent, blood-filled capillary vascular network is often easily appreciated, as depicted.*

Peripheral Hemangioblastoma

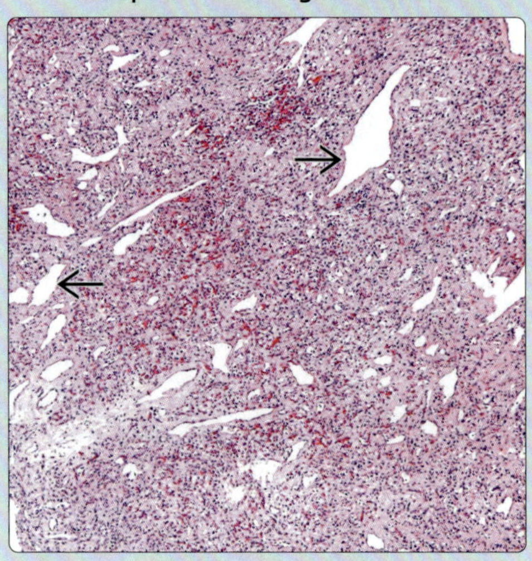

2 Cell Populations

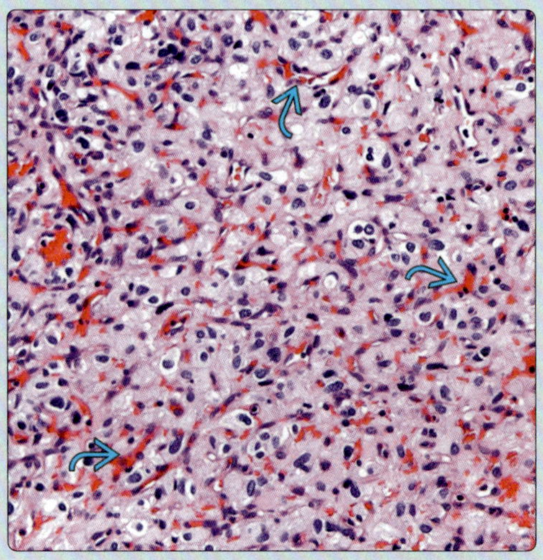

(Left) *Some of the larger polygonal cells in HB may show numerous cytoplasmic vacuolizations and closely resemble multivacuolated lipoblasts; however, the vacuoles in HB generally do not indent or scallop the nucleus. This finding is characteristic of HB and helps establish the diagnosis.* **(Right)** *Scattered tumor cell nuclei showing hyperchromasia and pleomorphism are not uncommon in HB and in some cases may be focally prominent.*

Vacuolated Cells

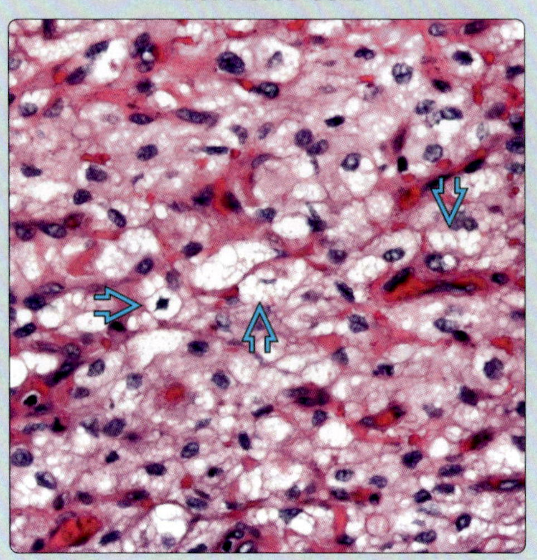

Focal Nuclear Pleomorphism

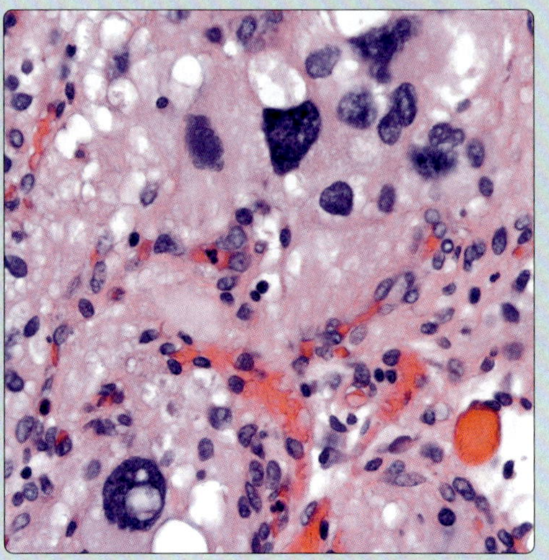

TERMINOLOGY

Abbreviations

- Hemangioblastoma (HB)

Synonyms

- Capillary HB
- Extraneuraxial HB

Definitions

- True HB arising in locations outside CNS
  - Uncertain cellular origin

ETIOLOGY/PATHOGENESIS

Genetics

- Associated with von Hippel-Lindau (VHL) syndrome
  - Similar to CNS HB

CLINICAL ISSUES

Epidemiology

- Incidence
  - Very rare
- Age
  - Median: 56.5 years

Site

- Most frequently arise in spinal nerve roots (extradural)
  - Cervical, thoracic, lumbosacral
    - Can present as mediastinal, retroperitoneal, or pelvic mass
- Visceral organs (rare)
  - Kidney, intestines, liver, adrenal gland
- Extremities (very rare)

Presentation

- Usually solitary mass
  - Rare multifocality, mainly within setting of VHL
- Site-specific symptoms
  - Extremity weakness or numbness, hematuria, etc.
- Patients may show other features or tumors of VHL

Treatment

- Complete surgical excision
- Genetic testing for VHL should be performed for all patients with peripheral (and CNS) HB

Prognosis

- True local recurrence or distant metastasis has yet to be documented
  - Persistent local disease in cases with incomplete excision

MACROSCOPIC

General Features

- Well-circumscribed, solid mass
- Yellow, tan-gray, or red-brown cut surface

Size

- Median: 4 cm (range: 1.3-15.0 cm)

MICROSCOPIC

Histologic Features

- Well-circumscribed, often lobular growth pattern
- Morphologically very similar to CNS HB
  - However, peripheral HB (PHB) lacks prominent cystic growth
- Mixture of 2 cell populations
  - Spindle cells with scant pale eosinophilic cytoplasm
    - Irregular, vesicular, or hyperchromatic nuclei with small nucleoli
  - Large polygonal cells with hypervacuolated eosinophilic or clear cytoplasm
    - These cells may be focal or absent in areas
- Nuclear pleomorphism may be present
- Rich, delicate, capillary vascular network between cells
  - Larger, ectatic, or "staghorn" vessels not uncommon
- Loose-to-dense collagenous stroma, may be focally myxoid
- Mitotic activity low to absent
- Necrosis absent

ANCILLARY TESTS

Immunohistochemistry

- Spindled and polygonal cells
  - Inhibin (+) in nearly all cases
  - Variable S100 protein (+)
- Only vascular endothelial cells are CD31(+), CD34(+)
- Variable GLUT1(+) in endothelial cells
- Keratin (-), EMA(-), SMA(-), desmin (-), synaptophysin (-), chromogranin (-), GFAP(-), HMB-45(-)

DIFFERENTIAL DIAGNOSIS

Solitary Fibrous Tumor

- Lacks vacuolated cells
- Diffuse CD34(+)

Metastatic Renal Cell Carcinoma

- History of current or prior renal mass
- Keratin (+), EMA(+)

Well-Differentiated Liposarcoma

- True lipoblasts are often less vacuolated than cells of HB and more commonly show nuclear scalloping
- *MDM2* gene amplification

PEComa

- Lacks prominent cytoplasmic vacuolization
- SMA(+), HMB-45(+), MART-1(+)

Paraganglioma

- May show morphologic overlap with PHB
- Synaptophysin (+), chromogranin (+)
- S100 protein (+) but only in sustentacular cells

SELECTED REFERENCES

1. Bisceglia M et al: Extraneuraxial hemangioblastoma: clinicopathologic features and review of the literature. Adv Anat Pathol. ePub, 2017
2. Doyle LA et al: Peripheral hemangioblastoma: clinicopathologic characterization in a series of 22 cases. Am J Surg Pathol. 38(1):119-27, 2014
3. Nonaka D et al: Extraneural hemangioblastoma: a report of 5 cases. Am J Surg Pathol. 31(10):1545-51, 2007

Melanotic Neuroectodermal Tumor of Infancy

KEY FACTS

TERMINOLOGY

- Rare, fast-growing, pigmented neoplasm, likely of neural crest origin

CLINICAL ISSUES

- Most present in 1st year of life (> 90%)
- Most involve craniofacial sites, particularly maxilla
- Rapidly enlarging, painless, expansile mass
- Treatment: Complete local excision
- Benign to intermediate clinical course
    - Recurrence rate: 10-15%
    - Metastatic spread in < 5%
- Age at diagnosis is prognostic factor
    - Shorter disease-free survival in patients < 2 months

MACROSCOPIC

- Usually 2-6 cm

MICROSCOPIC

- Irregular nests, cords, and alveolar spaces within fibrocollagenous stroma
    - Nests/spaces are lined by large epithelioid cells containing melanin granules
    - Clusters of small round neuroblastic cells often located centrally within nests/spaces
- Mitoses are rare

ANCILLARY TESTS

- Large epithelioid cells: Keratin (+), HMB-45(+), synaptophysin (variable), S100 protein (-)
- Neuroblastic cells: Synaptophysin (+), keratin (-), S100(-)
- All cells desmin (-)

TOP DIFFERENTIAL DIAGNOSES

- Desmoplastic small round cell tumor
- Alveolar rhabdomyosarcoma
- Neuroblastoma

Melanotic Neuroectodermal Tumor of Infancy

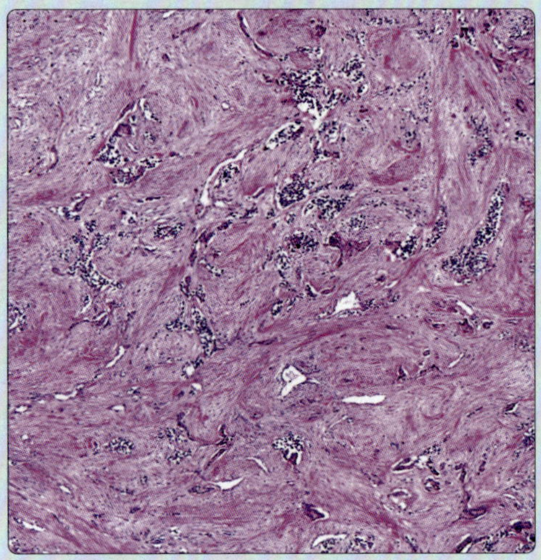

Biphasic Morphology

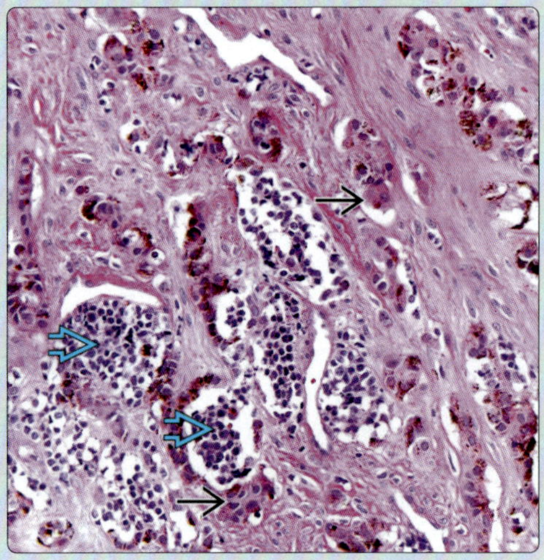

(Left) *Melanotic neuroectodermal tumor of infancy (MNTI) is a rare, rapidly growing neuroectodermal neoplasm that usually affects infants and most commonly involves the jaw. The classic case shows irregular nests, cords, and alveolar spaces within a prominent fibrocollagenous stroma.* **(Right)** *A biphasic morphology is observed in MNTI, composed of larger eosinophilic cells ➙ and smaller, more primitive cells ➙. Melanin pigment is often conspicuous in the larger cells.*

Melanin Pigment

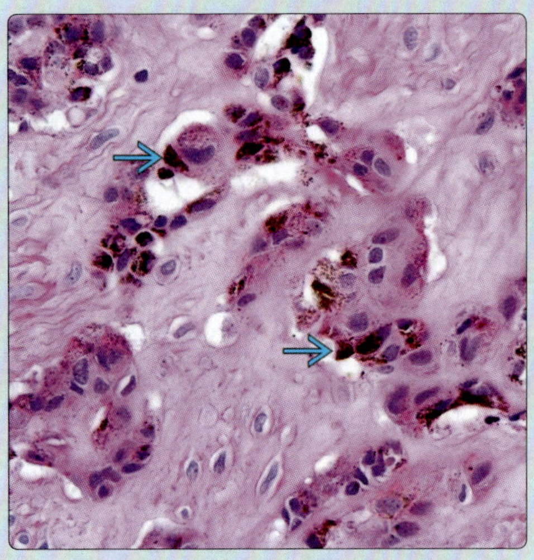

Primitive Neuroblastic Cells

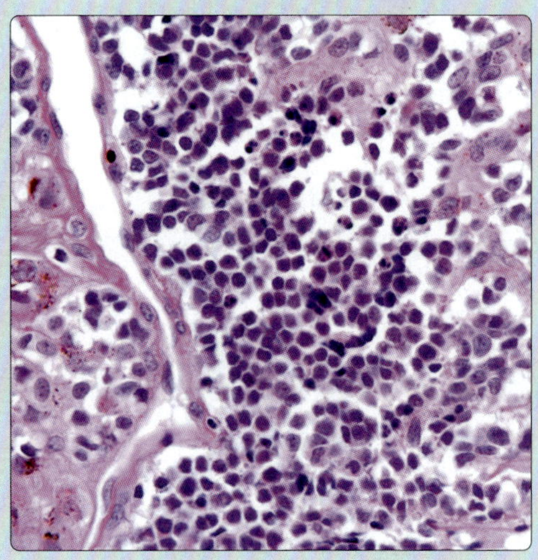

(Left) *The larger eosinophilic cells characteristically contain melanin pigment ➙, which may be abundant. They routinely express keratin and HMB-45, but S100 protein is negative. Synaptophysin is variably positive.* **(Right)** *The smaller, more primitive neuroblastic cells resemble the constituent cells of other small round blue cell tumors, such as neuroblastoma. These cells express synaptophysin and are negative for keratin, S100 protein, and desmin.*

Melanotic Neuroectodermal Tumor of Infancy

TERMINOLOGY

Abbreviations

- Melanotic neuroectodermal tumor of infancy(MNTI)

Synonyms

- Retinal anlage tumor
- Melanotic progonoma
- Melanotic ameloblastoma

Definitions

- Rare, fast-growing, pigmented neoplasm, likely of neural crest origin

CLINICAL ISSUES

Epidemiology

- Incidence
  - Rare
- Age
  - Most present in 1st year of life (> 90%)

Site

- Most involve craniofacial sites
  - Upper and lower jaw
    - Maxilla (69%)
    - Mandible (6%)
  - Skull (11%)
- Unusual sites reported
  - Epididymis, mediastinum, brain, skin, soft tissue

Presentation

- Rapidly enlarging, painless, expansile mass
  - Intact overlying mucosa, often with bluish discoloration
- Erosion into adjacent bone

Laboratory Tests

- Elevated urinary vanillylmandelic acid may be present

Treatment

- Complete local excision

Prognosis

- Benign to intermediate clinical course
  - Recurrence rate: 10-15%
  - Metastatic spread reported in < 5%
- Age at diagnosis is prognostic factor
  - Shorter disease-free survival in patients < 2 months of age
  - Minimal risk of recurrence in patients > 4.5 months
- No morphologic features predict aggressive behavior

MACROSCOPIC

General Features

- Firm, well circumscribed
- Gray to blue-black cut surface

Size

- Usually 2-6 cm (median: 3.5 cm)

MICROSCOPIC

Histologic Features

- Irregular nests, cords, and alveolar spaces within fibrocollagenous stroma
  - Nests/spaces are lined by large epithelioid cells with round vesicular nuclei
    - Abundant pale eosinophilic cytoplasm containing melanin granules
  - Clusters of small round neuroblastic cells often located centrally within nests/spaces
    - Small round hyperchromatic nuclei and scant cytoplasm
    - May be present without larger epithelioid cells
    - Rarely, may be associated with glial tissue
  - Thick-walled capillaries within stroma
  - Mitoses are rare

ANCILLARY TESTS

Immunohistochemistry

- Large epithelioid cells: Keratin (+), HMB-45(+), synaptophysin (variable), S100 (-)
- Neuroblastic cells: Synaptophysin (+), keratin (-), S100(-)
- All cells desmin (-)

DIFFERENTIAL DIAGNOSIS

Desmoplastic Small Round Cell Tumor

- Rare in jaw and in infants
- Nests of small cells within prominent desmoplastic stroma
- Keratin (+), desmin (+)
- *EWSR1-WT1* gene fusion

Alveolar Rhabdomyosarcoma

- Nests of poorly differentiated small hyperchromatic cells separated by fibrous septa
- Desmin (+), myogenin (+), keratin (-), HMB-45(-)
- *FOXO1* gene rearrangements

Neuroblastoma

- Sheets and lobules of small round hyperchromatic cells
- Absence of large cell component with intracytoplasmic melanin pigment
- NB84(+), keratin (-), HMB-45(-)

Malignant Melanoma

- S100 protein (+), HMB-45(+), MART-1(+), keratin (-)
- Usually overtly malignant cytology with numerous mitoses

SELECTED REFERENCES

1. Moreau A et al: Melanotic neuroectodermal tumor of infancy (MNTI) of the head and neck: a French multicenter study. J Craniomaxillofac Surg. 46(2):201-206, 2018
2. Rachidi S et al: Melanotic neuroectodermal tumor of infancy: a systematic review. J Oral Maxillofac Surg. 73(10):1946-56, 2015
3. Camuzard O et al: Melanotic neuroectodermal tumor of infancy: case report and review of the literature. Rev Laryngol Otol Rhinol (Bord). 132(3):173-6, 2011
4. Chaudhary A et al: Melanotic neuroectodermal tumor of infancy: 2 decades of clinical experience with 18 patients. J Oral Maxillofac Surg. 67(1):47-51, 2009
5. Kruse-Losler B et al: Melanotic neuroectodermal tumor of infancy: systematic review of the literature and presentation of a case. Oral Surg Oral Med Oral Pathol Oral Radiol Endod. 102:204-16, 2006

Ependymoma of Soft Tissue

KEY FACTS

TERMINOLOGY

- Ependymal neoplasm arising outside of CNS

CLINICAL ISSUES

- Wide age range (most common in children and young adults)
- Most commonly arises in subcutaneous tissue dorsal to sacrum and coccyx
- Slow-growing, longstanding masses
- Treatment: Complete surgical excision
  - Long-term clinical follow-up recommended
- Protracted clinical course
  - Local recurrences common
  - Up to 25% metastasize to regional lymph nodes or lung

MACROSCOPIC

- Lobulated, myxoid masses ± hemorrhage

MICROSCOPIC

- Most are well-marginated lesions
- Usually resemble myxopapillary ependymoma
  - Pseudopapillary architecture
  - Abundant perivascular and intercellular myxoid matrix
  - Perivascular pseudorosettes may be present
- May also form cellular sheets of epithelioid cells

ANCILLARY TESTS

- GFAP, S100, CD99, and CD56 (+)
- Keratin (+) in most cases, at least focally
- EMA, synaptophysin, and PLAP (-)

TOP DIFFERENTIAL DIAGNOSES

- Chordoma
- Schwannoma

Soft Tissue Ependymoma

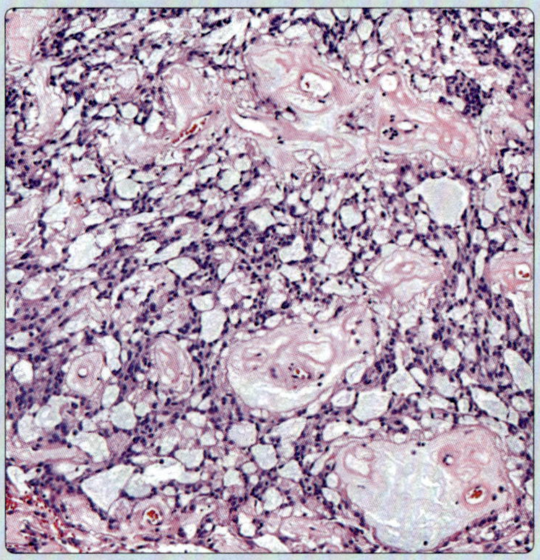

Myxopapillary Pattern

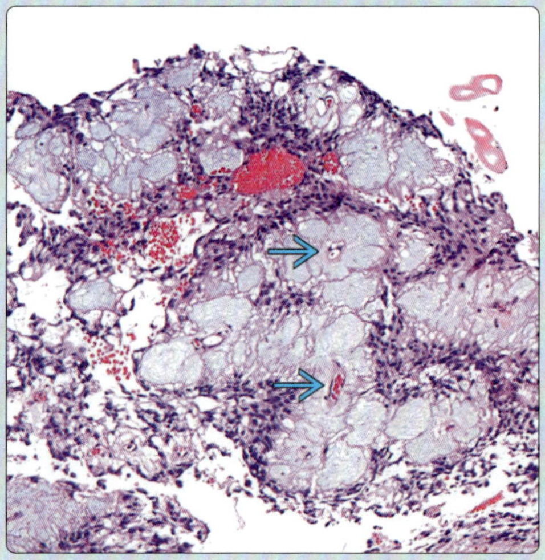

(Left) *Ependymoma of soft tissue is very rare compared to its counterpart in the CNS. Most cases arise in the dorsal subcutaneous tissue overlying the sacrum and coccyx and demonstrate the morphologic appearance of a myxopapillary ependymoma. A microcystic pattern (shown) is common.* **(Right)** *These tumors are often heavily myxoid and show formation of pseudopapillae around a centralized fibrovascular core ➔ secondary to degenerative changes.*

Hyalinization

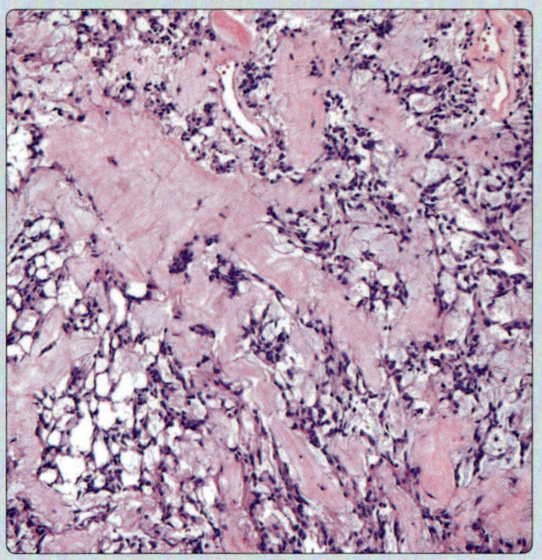

Cytologic Features

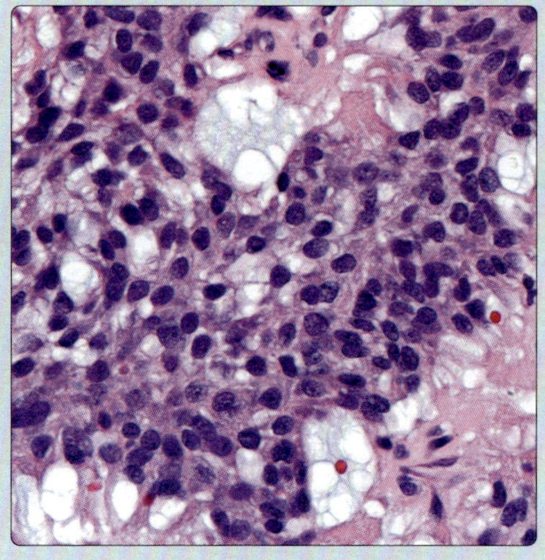

(Left) *In addition to extensive myxoid changes, ependymoma of soft tissue may show stromal hyalinization. Note the prominent microcystic morphology.* **(Right)** *Cytologically, the cells of ependymoma usually contain ovoid or elongated nuclei with a finely granular, evenly distributed chromatin pattern and inconspicuous nucleoli. Mitotic activity is often low.*

TERMINOLOGY

Synonyms

- Extraspinal ependymoma, sacrococcygeal ependymoma

Definitions

- Ependymal neoplasm arising outside of CNS

ETIOLOGY/PATHOGENESIS

Subcutaneous Sacrococcygeal Ependymomas

- Believed to arise from coccygeal medullary vestige

Presacral Ependymomas

- Believed to arise from extradural remnants of filum terminale
- Anterior soft tissue extension from cauda equina primary tumor

Ependymomas of Ovary and Mediastinum

- Germ cell origin postulated

CLINICAL ISSUES

Epidemiology

- Incidence
  - Rare
- Age
  - Wide range; most common in children and young adults

Site

- Subcutaneous tissue dorsal to sacrum and coccyx (most common)
  - Can be mistaken clinically for teratoma, pilonidal cyst, or sweat gland tumors
- Anterior to sacrum and posterior to rectum (presacral region)
  - May be soft tissue extension of cauda equina primary tumor

Presentation

- Slow-growing, longstanding masses
- Dorsal subcutaneous tumors may be associated with spina bifida

Treatment

- Complete surgical excision
- Radiation may be indicated for residual or inoperable disease
- Long-term clinical follow-up recommended

Prognosis

- Protracted clinical course
  - Local recurrences common
  - Up to 25% metastasize to regional lymph nodes or lung
    - Distant metastases usually occur late in clinical course

MACROSCOPIC

General Features

- Lobulated, myxoid masses ± hemorrhage

Size

- Wide range (usually < 10 cm)

MICROSCOPIC

Histologic Features

- Most are well-marginated lesions
- Usually resemble myxopapillary ependymoma
  - Pseudopapillary architecture
  - Abundant perivascular and intercellular myxoid matrix
    - Microcystic change common
  - Ovoid to elongated nuclei with evenly distributed, finely granular chromatin
  - Perivascular pseudorosettes may be present in more cellular, compact areas
  - Hemorrhage common
- May also form cellular sheets of epithelioid cells
- Low mitotic rate
  - Rare atypical mitotic figures

ANCILLARY TESTS

Immunohistochemistry

- GFAP, S100, CD99, and CD56 (+)
- Keratin (+) in most cases, at least focally
- EMA, synaptophysin, TTF-1, PLAP, and brachyury (-)

DIFFERENTIAL DIAGNOSIS

Chordoma

- Sacrococcygeal
- Usually arises in bone with soft tissue extension
- Contains uni- and multivacuolated (physaliferous) cells
- Inconspicuous vascularity
- CK(+), EMA(+), brachyury (+), S100 protein (+), GFAP(-)

Schwannoma

- Wide anatomic distribution
- Spindle cell lesions with variable hypercellular (Antoni A) and hypocellular myxoid (Antoni B) zones
  - Also often hyalinized vessels, hemosiderin deposition, foam cells, and lymphocytes
- Pseudorosettes generally absent
- Diffuse, strong S100(+)

SELECTED REFERENCES

1. Shelekhova KV et al: Myxopapillary ependymoma of lumbar soft tissue: a case report with gene expression evaluation. Int J Surg Pathol. 1066896917748195, 2017
2. Lamzabi I et al: Immunophenotype of myxopapillary ependymomas. Appl Immunohistochem Mol Morphol. 21(6):485-9, 2013
3. Lee KJ et al: Subcutaneous sacrococcygeal myxopapillary ependymoma in asian female: a case report. J Clin Med Res. 4(1):61-3, 2012
4. Hussein SA et al: Cytokeratin positivity in myxopapillary ependymoma--a potential diagnostic pitfall. Diagn Pathol. 3:40, 2008
5. Ma YT et al: Case report: primary subcutaneous sacrococcygeal ependymoma: a case report and review of the literature. Br J Radiol. 79(941):445-7, 2006
6. Takano T et al: Primary ependymoma of the ovary: a case report and literature review. Int J Gynecol Cancer. 15(6):1138-41, 2005
7. King P et al: Soft tissue ependymoma: a report of three cases. Histopathology. 22(4):394-6, 1993
8. Helwig EB et al: Subcutaneous sacrococcygeal myxopapillary ependymoma. A clinicopathologic study of 32 cases. Am J Clin Pathol. 81(2):156-61, 1984
9. Estrozi B et al: Myxopapillary ependymoma of the posterior mediastinum. Ann Diagn Pathol. 10(5):283-7, 2006

Metastatic Tumors to Soft Tissue Sites

KEY FACTS

TERMINOLOGY

- Nonnodal somatic soft tissue deposits of nonmesenchymal visceral, extrasomatic, or cutaneous primary tumors

CLINICAL ISSUES

- Sites: Extremity, back, abdominal wall, others
- Localized soft tissue mass; may be painful
  - Often clinical or radiologic evidence of primary disease elsewhere (e.g., lung, colon)
  - Soft tissue mass can be initial manifestation of disease (up to 25% of cases)
  - In up to 15% of cases, no known primary tumor can be detected
- Treatment individualized according to primary neoplasm and clinical stage
- Generally poor prognosis due to high clinical stage of disease

MICROSCOPIC

- Histologic features vary according to primary tumor
  - Adenocarcinoma, squamous cell carcinoma, neuroendocrine carcinoma, sarcomatoid carcinoma
  - Metastatic melanoma
  - Metastatic sarcoma

ANCILLARY TESTS

- Diffuse cytokeratin (+) in most cases of carcinoma
  - Lineage markers often helpful (e.g., TTF-1, CDX2, pax-8)
- S100 protein (+), SOX10(+) in melanoma

TOP DIFFERENTIAL DIAGNOSES

- Undifferentiated pleomorphic sarcoma
- Malignant peripheral nerve sheath tumor
- Myoepithelial carcinoma
- Clear cell sarcoma

Metastatic Carcinoma

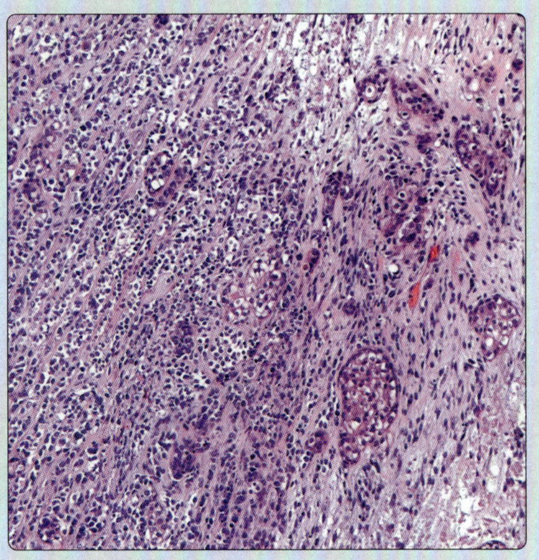

Sarcomatoid Carcinoma

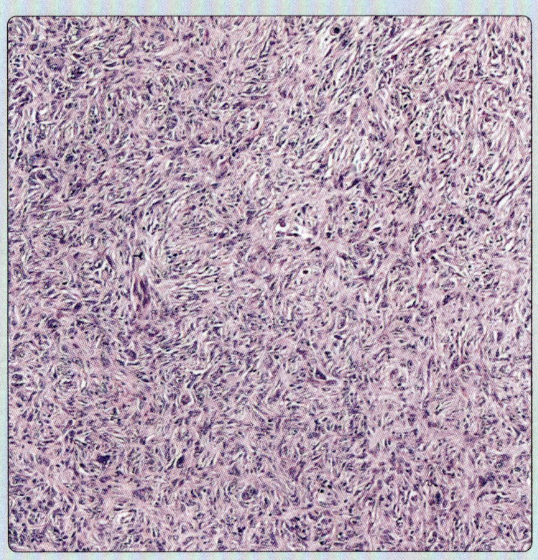

(Left) *Carcinoma metastatic to soft tissue sites is most easily recognized when tumor cells form clear epithelial structures, such as cohesive nests, glands, or tubules. However, in poorly differentiated metastases, histologic confusion with sarcoma is possible.* **(Right)** *Sarcomatoid (or spindle cell) carcinoma often lacks formation of cohesive epithelial structures and can closely mimic a spindle cell sarcoma. Sheets of highly pleomorphic cells can likewise mimic a high-grade pleomorphic sarcoma.*

Metastatic Melanoma

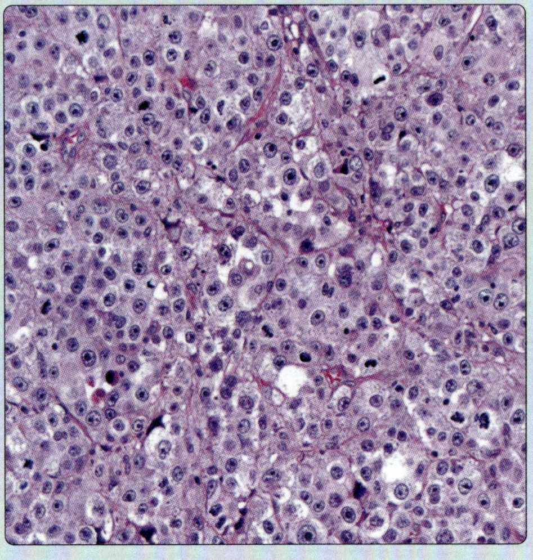

Rhabdoid Melanoma

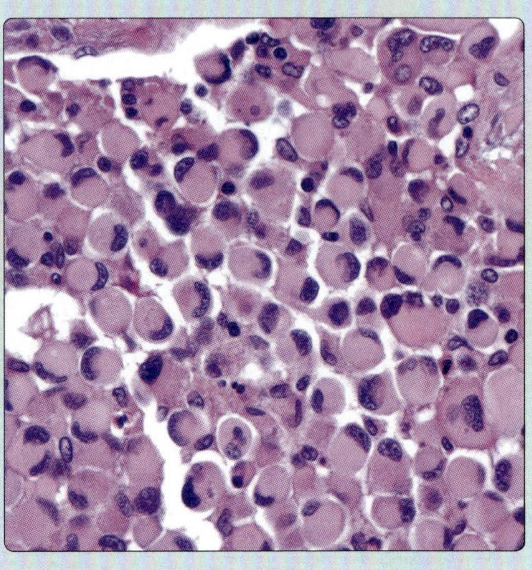

(Left) *Metastatic melanoma must always be considered when evaluating a soft tissue mass. Most cases are epithelioid with prominent nucleoli, as depicted, but some cases can show a spindled morphology. Sarcomas with similar morphology include clear cells sarcoma, epithelioid sarcoma, and epithelioid angiosarcoma.* **(Right)** *Rhabdoid cytologic change in metastatic melanoma can lead to confusion with extrarenal rhabdoid tumor, epithelioid rhabdomyosarcoma, epithelioid MPNST, malignant myoepithelioma, and others.*

TERMINOLOGY

Definitions

- Nonnodal somatic soft tissue deposits of nonmesenchymal visceral, extrasomatic, or cutaneous primary tumors
  - Hematopoietic neoplasms not included

CLINICAL ISSUES

Epidemiology

- Rare

Site

- Extremity
- Back, abdominal wall, chest wall
- Occasionally other sites

Presentation

- Localized soft tissue mass; may be painful
  - Often clinical or radiologic evidence of primary disease elsewhere (e.g., lung, colon)
    - Previous or concurrent nodal or bony metastases may also be present
  - Soft tissue mass can be initial manifestation of disease (up to 25% of cases)
  - In up to 15% of cases, no known primary tumor can be detected

Treatment

- Individualized according to primary neoplasm and clinical stage
- Lesion may be resected de novo if easily accessible
  - Often due to clinical misdiagnosis as mesenchymal neoplasm

Prognosis

- Generally poor, due to high clinical stage of disease

MICROSCOPIC

Histologic Features

- Metastatic carcinoma
  - Lung, skin, kidney, breast, uterus/ovary, GI tract, others
  - Specific morphology depends on specific type of carcinoma
    - Adenocarcinoma
      - Nests, sheets, or cords of malignant epithelioid cells
      - May show gland formation, mucin production, or cribriform architecture
    - Squamous cell
      - Nests and sheets of eosinophilic cells ± keratin production
    - Neuroendocrine
      - Usually nests and sheets of epithelioid cells with limited cytoplasm
      - Also acinar, trabecular, micronodular patterns
      - Small cell carcinoma often shows nuclear molding, prominent apoptosis
    - Sarcomatoid
      - Atypical spindled cells in sheets or vague fascicles
      - Myxoid zones in some cases
  - Desmoplastic, inflammatory, or sclerosing stromal response can be present
- Metastatic melanoma
  - Sheets of epithelioid cells most common
  - Marked nuclear atypia common, including macronucleoli
  - Melanin pigment, if present, is helpful feature
  - Variants: Spindle cell, balloon cell, others
- Metastatic sarcoma
  - Highly variable; depends on type of sarcoma
- Other primaries reported
  - Seminoma, carcinosarcoma, neuroblastoma, teratoma, malignant gastrointestinal stromal tumor

ANCILLARY TESTS

Immunohistochemistry

- Diffuse cytokeratin (+) in most cases of carcinoma
  - Expression may be focal or even absent in poorly differentiated or undifferentiated tumors
  - Squamous cell carcinoma usually p63(+) and p40(+)
- Synaptophysin, chromogranin, CD56 in neuroendocrine carcinomas
- Lineage markers often helpful (e.g., TTF-1, CDX2, pax-8)
- S100 protein (+), SOX10(+) in melanoma
  - Variable expression of melanocytic markers

DIFFERENTIAL DIAGNOSIS

Undifferentiated Pleomorphic Sarcoma

- Keratin, S100 protein, and almost all other markers (-)
- Usually severe nuclear pleomorphism, including bizarre atypia

Malignant Peripheral Nerve Sheath Tumor

- Highly atypical spindled cells in sheets and fascicles; necrosis common
- Heterologous epithelial elements very rare
- Keratins (-); limited S100 protein expression (focal to negative)
  - Caveat: Epithelioid MPNST shows diffuse S100 protein
    - Can closely mimic melanoma

Myoepithelial Carcinoma

- Can be difficult to distinguish from metastatic carcinoma
  - Presence of primary tumor elsewhere favors carcinoma
- Variable expression of keratins, S100, SMA, GFAP, calponin, others

Clear Cell Sarcoma

- Often challenging to distinguish from metastatic melanoma
- Deep mass; lacks overlying junctional component
- Characteristic *EWSR1* translocations (usually *EWSR1-ATF1*)

SELECTED REFERENCES

1. Sammon J et al: Magnetic resonance imaging appearance of soft-tissue metastases: our experience at an orthopedic oncology center. Skeletal Radiol. 46(4):513-521, 2017
2. Plaza JA et al: Metastases to soft tissue: a review of 118 cases over a 30-year period. Cancer. 112(1):193-203, 2008
3. Damron TA et al: Distant soft tissue metastases: a series of 30 new patients and 91 cases from the literature. Ann Surg Oncol. 7(7):526-34, 2000
4. Lodding P et al: Metastases of malignant melanoma simulating soft tissue sarcoma. A clinico-pathological, light- and electron microscopic and immunohistochemical study of 21 cases. Virchows Arch A Pathol Anat Histopathol. 417(5):377-88, 1990

(Left) *This case of metastatic sarcomatoid squamous cell carcinoma of the lung features a prominent myxoid and spindle cell morphology, leading to consideration of MPNST. Note the focal tumor cell nest with clear cell change .* **(Right)** *Metastatic neuroendocrine carcinoma can closely mimic a variety of mesenchymal tumors, including myoepithelioma, ossifying fibromyxoid tumor, desmoplastic small round cell tumor, and Ewing sarcoma. Immunohistochemistry is often required in these cases.*

Sarcomatoid Squamous Cell Carcinoma

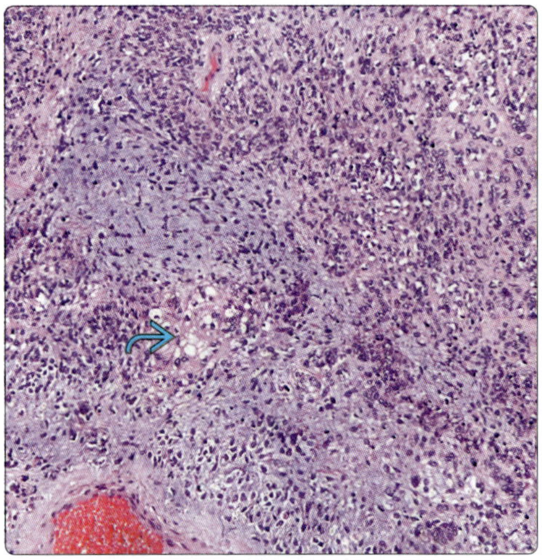

Neuroendocrine Carcinoma

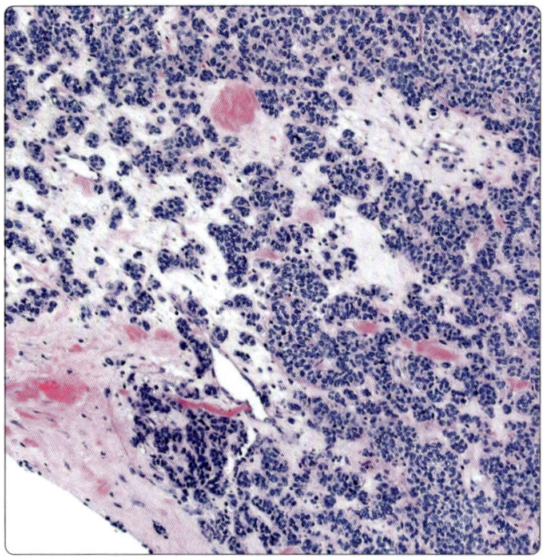

(Left) *Metastatic hepatocellular carcinoma to soft tissue locations is very rare but can morphologically resemble mesenchymal tumors, such as alveolar soft part sarcoma and granular cell tumor.* **(Right)** *This case of metastatic ductal breast carcinoma to the proximal thigh features well-developed epithelial structures but also contains a population of osteoclast-like multinucleated giant cells . The latter finding is more common in bony metastases.*

Hepatocellular Carcinoma

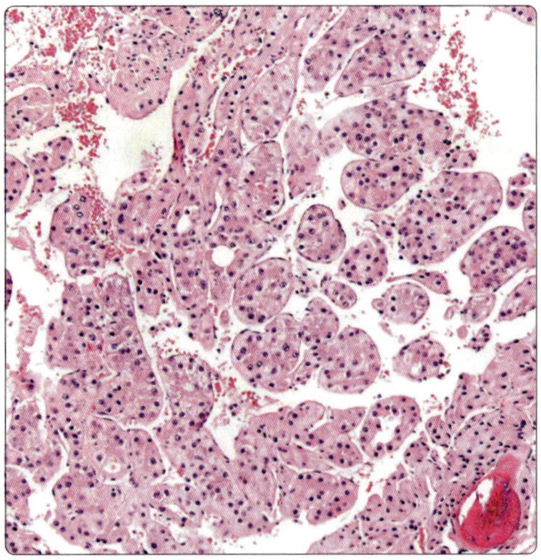

Metastatic Breast Carcinoma

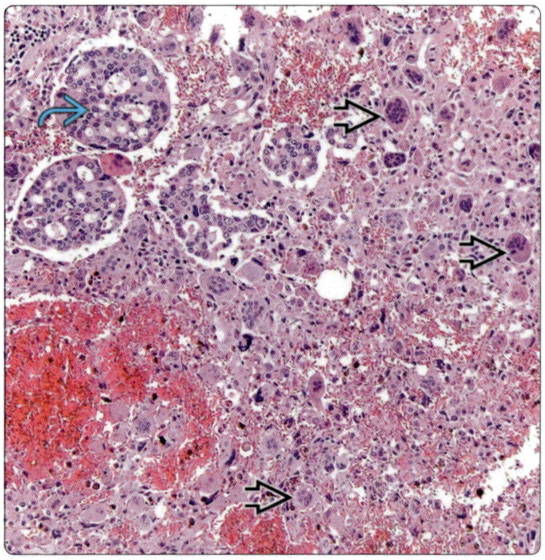

(Left) *Low-power H&E of sarcomatoid squamous cell sarcoma shows a diffuse spindle cell proliferation, indistinguishable from a spindle cell sarcoma, such as MPNST. Immunostains revealed diffuse keratin and P63 expression by the lesional cells.* **(Right)** *Tumor cells in sarcomatoid carcinoma may show more abundant eosinophilic cytoplasm, mimicking a smooth muscle neoplasm, particularly leiomyosarcoma.*

Sarcomatoid Carcinoma

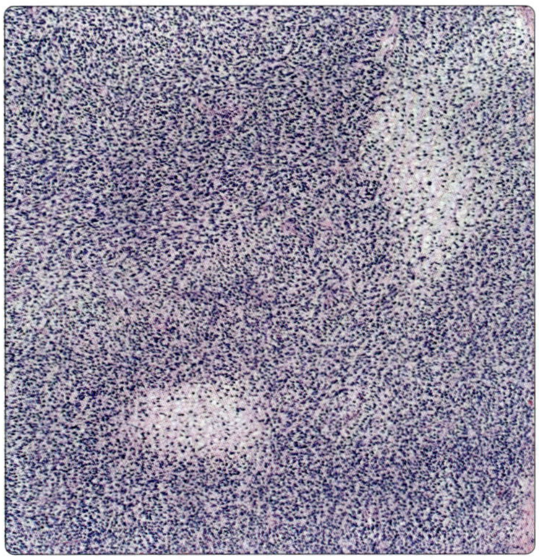

Spindled Eosinophilic Tumor Cells

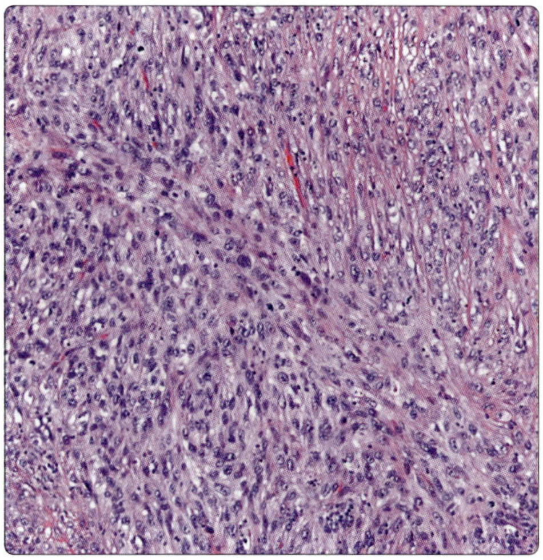

Edematous Zones With Necrosis

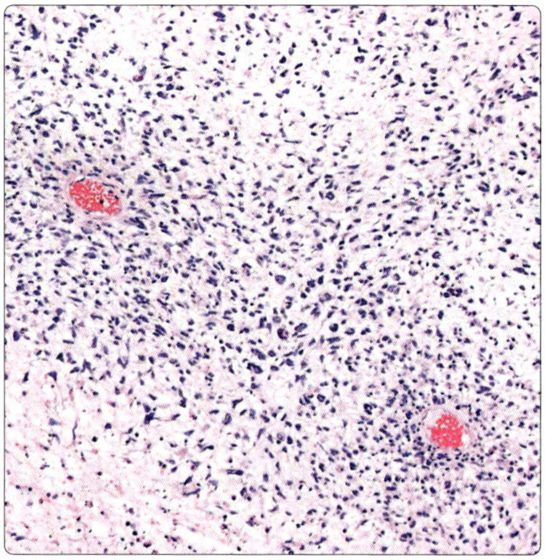

Large Epithelioid Cells in Melanoma

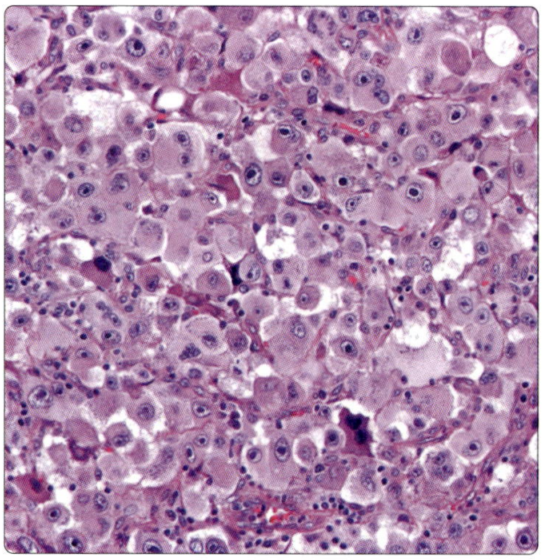

(Left) *This sarcomatoid carcinoma contains zones of small pleomorphic cells arranged around small vessels. A focus of coagulative can be seen in the lower left.* **(Right)** *The combination of voluminous eosinophilic cytoplasm and macronucleoli in metastatic melanoma can lead to confusion with solid-type alveolar soft part sarcoma.*

Balloon Cell Melanoma

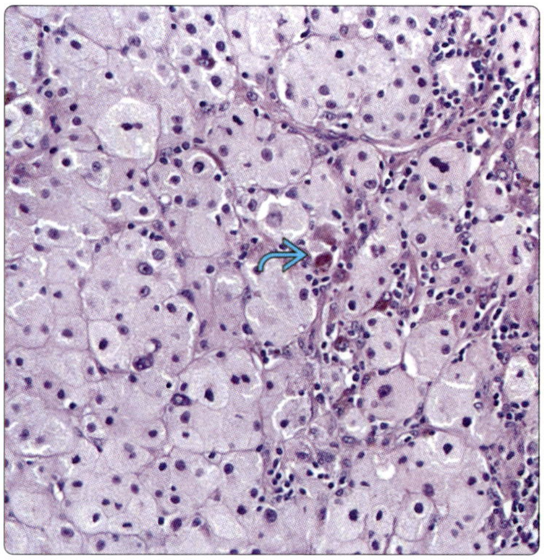

Spindled Melanoma With Giant Cells

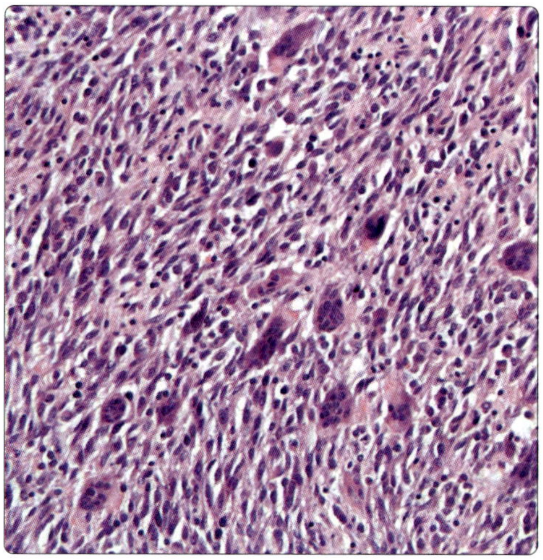

(Left) *Some cases of melanoma show focal to diffuse granular cell change, mimicking a granular cell tumor. Note the presence of melanin pigment ⮫, a helpful diagnostic clue.* **(Right)** *Rare cases of melanoma can feature a component of osteoclast-like multinucleated giant cells. This example also showed a conspicuous spindled morphology.*

Metastatic Seminoma

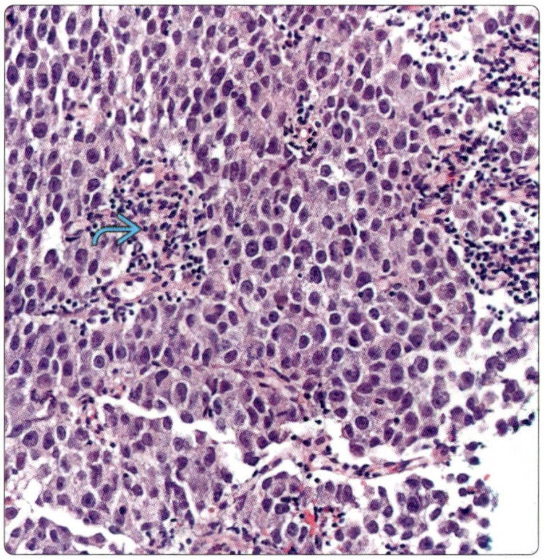

CD117 Expression in Seminoma

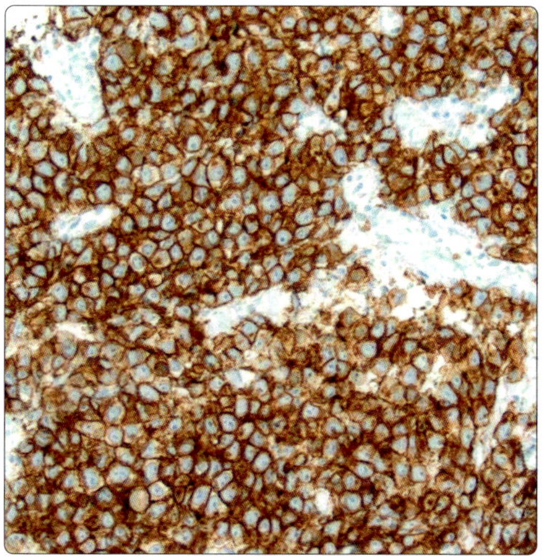

(Left) *Metastatic germ cell tumors, particularly seminoma, can be easily misdiagnosed if not considered in the differential diagnosis. Seminoma, pictured here, generally shows epithelioid tumor cells with prominent nucleoli and a fibrovascular stroma containing lymphocytes ⮫.* **(Right)** *Most cases of seminoma are negative for keratins, but they do express markers, such as CD117 (shown), OCT 3/4, D2-40, SALL4, and PLAP.*

Neuroblastoma and Ganglioneuroblastoma

KEY FACTS

TERMINOLOGY

- Malignant tumor derived from pluripotent sympathetic cells

ETIOLOGY/PATHOGENESIS

- Majority of cases sporadic
- Autosomal dominant familial cases have been reported

CLINICAL ISSUES

- Most common malignancy in infants < 12 months of age
- 90% diagnosed by 5 years of age
- Follows distribution of sympathetic ganglia
- ~ 2/3 have metastases at presentation
- Elevated urine catecholamines in 95%

MICROSCOPIC

- International Neuroblastoma Pathology Committee Classification
  - Undifferentiated neuroblastoma (NB)
  - Poorly differentiated NB
  - Differentiating NB
  - Nodular GNB and intermixed GNB
- Mitotic-karyorrhectic index (MKI)

ANCILLARY TESTS

- Immunoreactive for neural markers: NB84, NSE, synaptophysin, chromogranin
- Strong nuclear GATA3(+)
- S100(+) in schwannian stroma
- Molecular aberrations (*MYCN*, *ALK*, *ATRX*) well described

TOP DIFFERENTIAL DIAGNOSES

- Alveolar rhabdomyosarcoma (ARMS)
- Ewing sarcoma/primitive neuroectodermal tumor (PNET)
- Translocation-associated undifferentiated sarcomas
  - CIC-DUX4 and BCOR-CCNB3
- Lymphoma
- Ganglioneuroma

Neuroblastoma

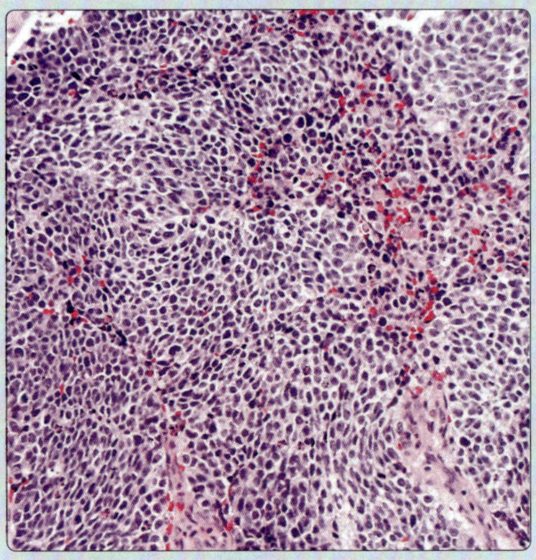

Poorly Differentiated Neuroblastoma

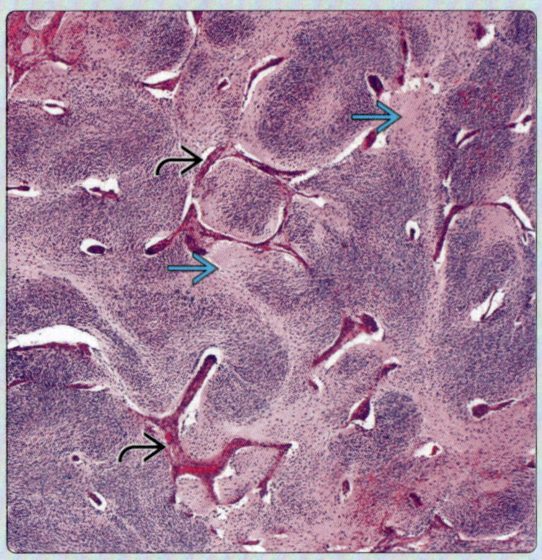

(Left) *The typical appearance of an undifferentiated neuroblastoma (NB) is a small round cell tumor without histologic differentiation. IHC is generally required to make the diagnosis and to exclude other neoplasms.* **(Right)** *This low-power view of a poorly differentiated NB shows thin septa of schwannian stroma ⮫. Pale, eosinophilic neuropil ⇨ is seen in places between the nodules or nests of NB cells.*

Intermixed Ganglioneuroblastoma

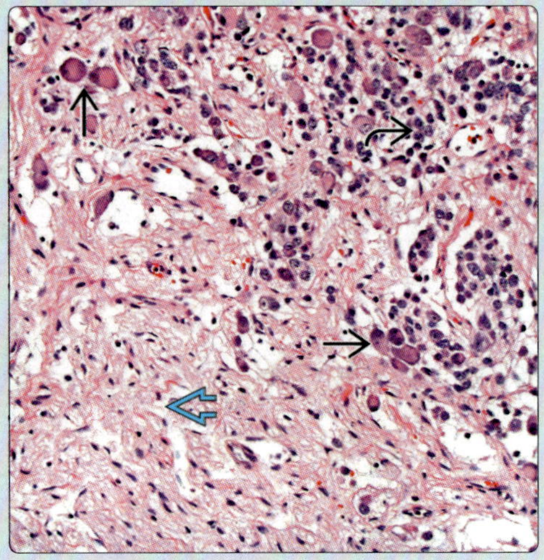

NB84 Expression

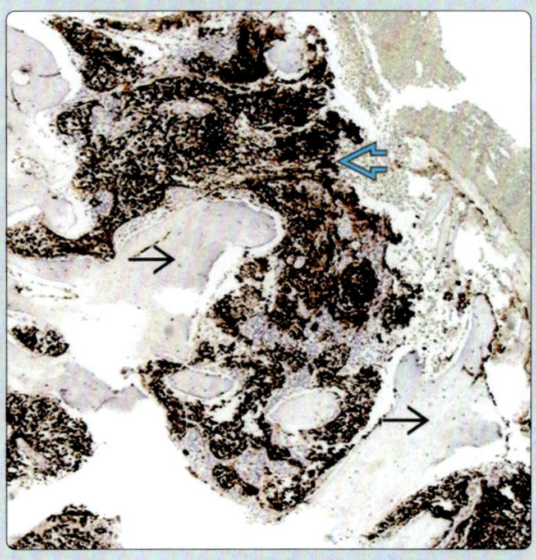

(Left) *A typical intermixed ganglioneuroblastoma (GNB) is seen in this H&E. The tumor is composed of a mixture of maturing ganglion cells →, neuroblasts ⮫, and abundant schwannian stroma ⇨.* **(Right)** *In this bone marrow trephine specimen, there is diffuse immunoreactivity for NB antigen (NB84) in metastatic deposits of NB ⇨ that extend between bony trabeculae →. This marker is not entirely specific, however, and may be seen focally in other small round blue cell tumors.*

TERMINOLOGY

Abbreviations

- Neuroblastoma (NB)
- Ganglioneuroblastoma (GNB)

Synonyms

- Schwannian stroma-poor neuroblastic tumor (NB)
- Schwannian stroma-rich neuroblastic tumor (GNB)

Definitions

- Malignant tumor derived from pluripotent sympathetic cells
- Maturational spectrum of neuroblastic tumors
  - NB is least differentiated
  - GNB is moderately differentiated
  - Ganglioneuroma (GN) is well differentiated, benign

ETIOLOGY/PATHOGENESIS

Developmental Anomaly

- Derived from primordial neural crest cells
  - During fetal development, these cells migrate along neuraxis to adrenal medulla and sympathetic ganglia
- Majority of cases sporadic
  - Some autosomal dominant familial cases have been reported

CLINICAL ISSUES

Epidemiology

- Incidence
  - ~ 650 new cases per year in USA
  - 3rd most common malignant tumor in children
  - Most common extracranial solid tumor in first 2 years of life
  - Most common malignancy in infants < 12 months of age
- Age
  - 40% of patients diagnosed by 2 years (median age: 17 months)
  - 90% diagnosed by 5 years
  - ~ 25% are congenital with some detected prenatally on ultrasound
- Sex
  - Slight male predominance
- Ethnicity
  - More common in white infants

Site

- Follows distribution of sympathetic ganglia
  - Paramidline from base of skull to pelvis
  - Most common sites: Abdomen, retroperitoneum, and posterior mediastinum
- Adrenal medulla
- Dorsal root ganglia
- Sites of metastasis: Bone, lymph nodes, liver, and skin

Presentation

- Depends on age of patient, location of tumor, and associated clinical syndromes
- Most have nonspecific symptoms
  - Fever, weight loss, diarrhea, anemia, hypertension
- Fetuses may have hydrops
- Palpable mass in ~ 1/2
- ~ 2/3 have metastases at presentation
- "Blueberry muffin" baby
  - Blue-red, cutaneous masses in infants
- Paraneoplastic myoclonus-opsoclonus-ataxia syndrome
  - Rapid, alternating eye movements and myoclonic movements of extremities
  - Associated with more favorable prognosis
  - Resolves with tumor eradication but many will have permanent neurologic deficits
- Other associated syndromes
  - Myasthenia gravis, Beckwith-Wiedemann syndrome, Cushing syndrome, neurofibromatosis, fetal hydantoin syndrome, Hirschsprung disease

Laboratory Tests

- Urine catecholamines (elevated in 95% of patients with NB)
  - Epinephrine, norepinephrine
  - Homovanillic acid (HVA), vanillylmandelic acid (VMA)
    - VMA:HVA ratio > 1.5 associated with better prognosis
  - May not be elevated in undifferentiated tumors
- Associated with worse clinical outcome
  - Lactate dehydrogenase > 1,500 IU/L
  - Ferritin > 142 ng/mL
  - Neuron-specific enolase (NSE) > 100 ng/mL

Natural History

- 1-2% will spontaneously regress
  - Most in children < age 1 year
- NB can metastasize widely via lymphatics and vessels

Treatment

- Low risk
  - Surgery or observation alone
- Intermediate risk
  - Surgery and adjuvant chemotherapy
- High risk
  - Chemotherapy
  - Delayed tumor resection
  - Radiation of primary site
  - Myeloablative chemotherapy with stem cell recovery

Prognosis

- Favorable prognostic factors
  - Age < 1.5 years at diagnosis
  - Favorable histology
  - Stage 1, 2, or 4S
    - Related to location of tumor
  - No *MYCN* amplification
  - Hyperdiploidy
  - No loss of 1p or 11q
  - High expression of TrKA and TrKC
  - Normal serum ferritin, NSE, and LDH
  - Urinary VMA:HVA ratio > 1.5

IMAGING

General Features

- Extensive radiographic evaluation is required to determine extent of disease and identify metastatic foci
- Calcifications often seen in central portion of tumor

Bone Scan

- Radiolabeled metaiodobenzylguanidine (MIBG) incorporates into catecholamine-secreting cells and can detect NB

MACROSCOPIC

General Features

- **NB**
  - Fine, membranous capsules
  - Cut surface is soft, fleshy, often with hemorrhage and necrosis
- **GNB**
  - Cut surface is firm, gray-white
  - Nodular GNB must have grossly visible, usually hemorrhagic nodules
  - Intermixed GNB can look like NB or GN depending on extent of differentiation

Size

- Average: 6- to 8-cm diameter

MICROSCOPIC

Histologic Features

- Variable tumor composition depending on degree of differentiation/maturation
  - Neuroblasts: Small round blue cells with minimal cytoplasm
  - Homer Wright pseudorosettes: Neuroblasts forming ring around central core of fibrillary cytoplasmic processes
  - Ganglionic differentiation
    - Cells enlarge
    - Increased eosinophilic or amphophilic cytoplasm
    - Nuclear chromatin pattern becomes vesicular
    - Must have synchronous differentiation of cytoplasm and nucleus
  - Neuropil characterized by fibrillar eosinophilic matrix
  - Schwannian stroma appears as thin septa composed of bland spindle cells
- Mitotic-karyorrhectic index (MKI) calculated in neuroblastic component
  - Count of number of cells undergoing mitosis or karyorrhexis, per 5,000 cells
    - Can be estimated
    - Cannot use bone marrow to calculate MKI
  - Low: < 100 cells per 5,000
  - Intermediate: 100-200 cells per 5,000
  - High: > 200 cells per 5,000

International Neuroblastoma Pathology Committee Classification

- Note: Do not classify posttreatment resections
  - "NB with treatment effect" is sufficient
  - May classify metastatic disease if resection/biopsy is pretreatment
- **Undifferentiated NB**
  - No ganglionic differentiation
  - No neuropil and no or minimal schwannian stroma
  - Often requires IHC for accurate diagnosis
- **Poorly differentiated NB**
  - < 5% of tumor cells showing ganglionic differentiation
  - Neuropil background
  - No or minimal schwannian stroma
- **Differentiating NB**
  - > 5% of tumor cells showing ganglionic differentiation
  - Usually more abundant neuropil
  - Usually more prominent schwannian stroma (must be < 50%)
- **Nodular GNB**
  - Grossly identifiable nodules will be NB
  - Abrupt demarcation between stroma-poor NB and stroma-rich component
  - Fibrous pseudocapsule often seen surrounding NB component
  - > 50% schwannian stroma
- **Intermixed GNB**
  - Microscopic nests of NB within schwannian stroma
  - > 50% schwannian stroma

ANCILLARY TESTS

Immunohistochemistry

- NB84(+) in almost all NBs
  - Not entirely specific; occasionally positive in other small round cell tumors (often focally)
- Strong nuclear GATA3(+)
- NSE
  - Most sensitive but least specific
  - Found at least focally even in very undifferentiated NBs
- S100 protein (+) in schwannian stroma
- Also, frequently synaptophysin, chromogranin, CD56 (+)
- Newer markers: PHOX2B(+) and HuC/D(+)

Genetic Testing

- *MYCN*
  - Amplification is associated with worse prognosis
  - Usually seen in advanced disease
- *ALK* mutation &/or gene amplification
  - Associated with advanced disease
  - Alterations seen in both sporadic and hereditary cases
- *ATRX* inactivating mutations
  - More frequent in children > 12 years of age
  - Worse prognosis

DIFFERENTIAL DIAGNOSIS

Alveolar Rhabdomyosarcoma

- More marked alveolar pattern except in solid variant
- More pleomorphism
- Cells have more abundant cytoplasm than NB
- Diffuse desmin (+) and myogenin (+)
- Characteristic t(1;13) or t(2;13) with *FOXO1* fusions

Ewing Sarcoma/Primitive Neuroectodermal Tumor

- Usually in older patients than those with NB
- CD99(+) with diffuse membranous immunoreactivity
- Specific gene fusions, most commonly *EWSR1-FLI1*

Translocation-Associated Undifferentiated Sarcomas

- Molecular testing required for definitive diagnosis
  - CIC-DUX4 sarcoma
  - BCOR-CCNB3 sarcoma
    - CCNB3(+) by IHC also helpful

Favorable vs. Unfavorable Histology in Neuroblastic Tumors

Classification	Subclass	MKI	Age at Diagnosis	Histologic Category
Neuroblastoma (NB)	Undifferentiated	Any	Any	Unfavorable
	Poorly differentiated	High	Any	Unfavorable
		Low or intermediate	> 1.5 years	Unfavorable
			< 1.5 years	Favorable
	Differentiating	High	Any	Unfavorable
		Intermediate	> 1.5 years	Unfavorable
			< 1.5 years	Favorable
		Low	> 5.0 years	Unfavorable
			< 5.0 years	Favorable
Ganglioneuroblastoma (GNB)	Nodular	**	**	Unfavorable or favorable
	Intermixed	N/A	Any	Favorable
Ganglioneuroma (GN)	Mature or maturing	N/A	Any	Favorable

***The determination of favorable vs. unfavorable histology in nodular GNB is based on the NB component. MKI = mitotic-karyorrhectic index; N/A = not applicable.*

Prognosis Based on *MYCN* Amplification and Histology

MYCN Amplification	Favorable Histology	Unfavorable Histology
Nonamplified	Excellent prognosis	Poor prognosis
Amplified	Rare	Extremely poor prognosis

Neuroblastoma Staging System

Stage	Definition
1	Localized tumor; complete gross resection; ipsilateral nodes negative
2A	Localized tumor; incomplete gross resection; nonadherent ipsilateral nodes negative
2B	Localized tumor ± complete gross resection; nonadherent ipsilateral nodes negative
3	Unresectable tumor that crosses midline ± positive nodes; or localized tumor with positive contralateral nodes; or midline tumor with bilateral extension (includes nodal involvement)
4	Distant metastases to nodes, bone, bone marrow, liver, skin, &/or other organs (except as defined for stage 4S)
4S	Localized primary tumor (stage 1 or 2) with metastases limited to skin, liver, &/or bone marrow (infants < 1 year old)

Lymphoma

- NSE, synaptophysin, and chromogranin (-)
- Has confirmatory lymphoid markers
  - CD45, CD3, CD20
  - TdT in lymphoblastic lymphoma

Maturing Ganglioneuroma

- Differs from intermixed GNB in having single ganglion cells instead of nests of cells within schwannian stroma

SELECTED REFERENCES

1. Machado I et al: Review with novel markers facilitates precise categorization of 41 cases of diagnostically challenging, "undifferentiated small round cell tumors". A clinicopathologic, immunophenotypic and molecular analysis. Ann Diagn Pathol. 34:1-12, 2018
2. Takemoto J et al: HuC/D expression in small round cell tumors and neuroendocrine tumors: a useful tool for distinguishing neuroblastoma from childhood small round cell tumors. Hum Pathol. ePub, 2018
3. Hung YP et al: PHOX2B reliably distinguishes neuroblastoma among small round blue cell tumors. Histopathology. 71(5):786-94, 2017
4. Wiles AB et al: GATA3 is a reliable marker for neuroblastoma in limited samples, including FNA cell blocks, core biopsies, and touch imprints. Cancer Cytopathol. 125(12):940-6, 2017
5. Bresler SC et al: ALK mutations confer differential oncogenic activation and sensitivity to ALK inhibition therapy in neuroblastoma. Cancer Cell. 26(5):682-94, 2014
6. Vo KT et al: Clinical, biologic, and prognostic differences on the basis of primary tumor site in neuroblastoma: a report from the international neuroblastoma risk group project. J Clin Oncol. 32(28):3169-76, 2014
7. Wang LL et al: Neuroblastoma of undifferentiated subtype, prognostic significance of prominent nucleolar formation, and MYC/MYCN protein expression: a report from the Children's Oncology Group. Cancer. 119(20):3718-26, 2013

(Left) *Graphic shows the anatomic extent of the sympathetic chain* ➡ *(including adrenal gland) from the cervical region through the mediastinum and abdomen to the inferior pelvis. NB can arise anywhere along the sympathetic chain.* **(Right)** *Coronal T2-weighted MR in a patient with GNB shows a mildly hyperintense posterior mediastinal mass* ➡ *with no abnormality in the adjacent osseous marrow signal.*

Sympathetic Chain

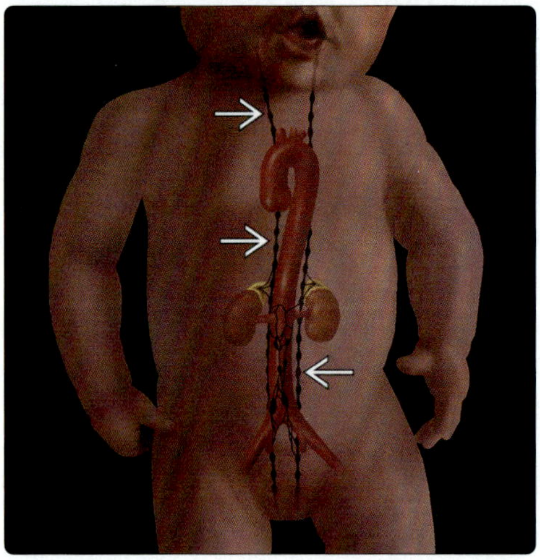

MR of Ganglioneuroblastoma

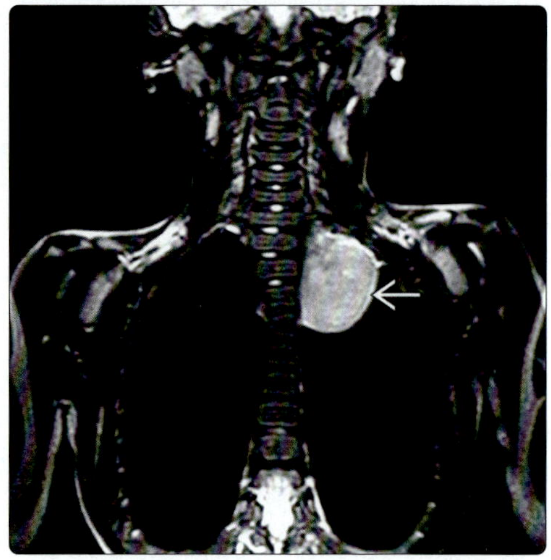

(Left) *Gross photograph of NB shows a large, circumscribed mass* ➡ *arising from the adrenal gland and compressing the upper pole of the subjacent kidney* ➡*. NB is often grossly hemorrhagic with areas of necrosis and calcification seen on sectioning the specimen.* **(Right)** *Coronal T2-weighted MR shows an NB* ➡ *of the left adrenal gland with an area of central necrosis* ➡*.*

Adrenal Neuroblastoma

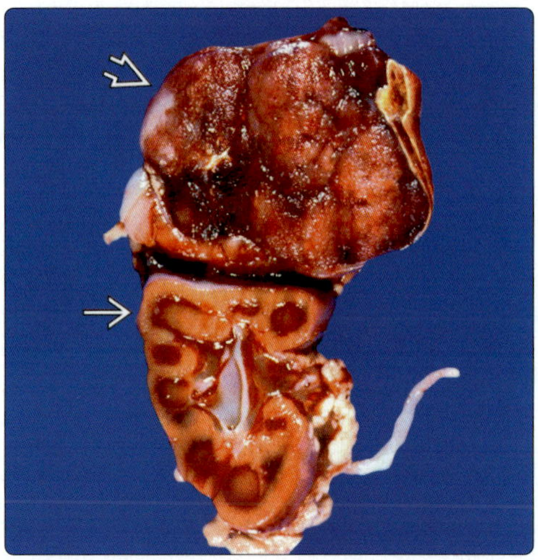

MR of Adrenal Neuroblastoma

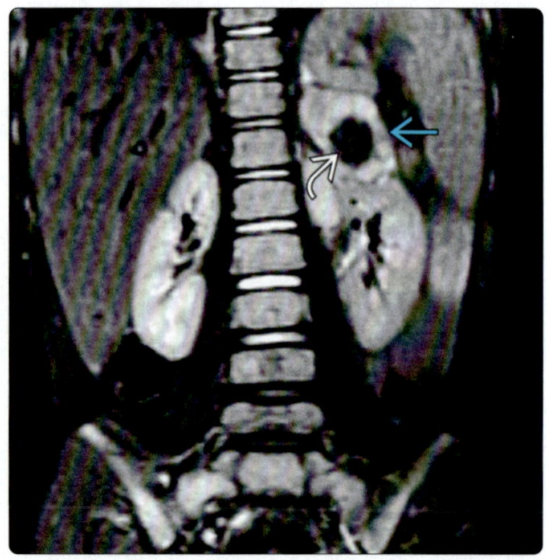

(Left) *This whole liver specimen shows diffuse involvement and extensive replacement by multiple deposits of metastatic NB. There are several foci of hemorrhage.* **(Right)** *Axial T2-weighted MR shows a left adrenal mass* ➡*, which proved to be an NB. It was widely metastatic; the liver was filled with multiple high-signal nodular lesions* ➡ *with little normal remaining hepatic parenchyma.*

Metastatic Neuroblastoma

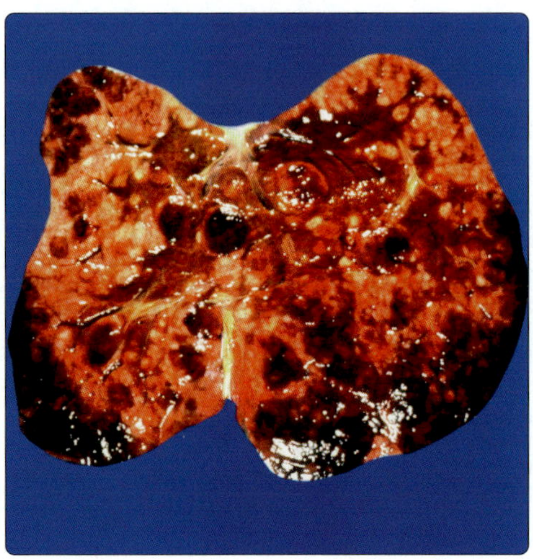

MR of Metastatic Neuroblastoma

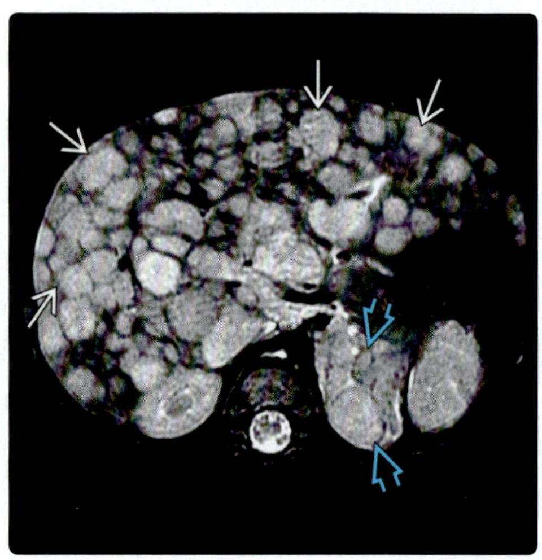

Undifferentiated Neuroblastoma

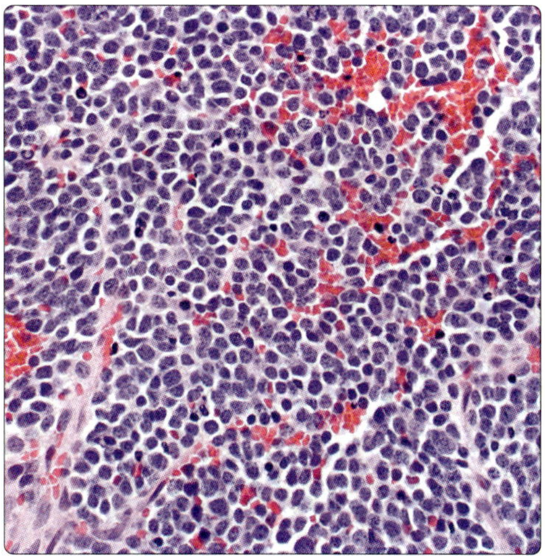

Cytologic Features

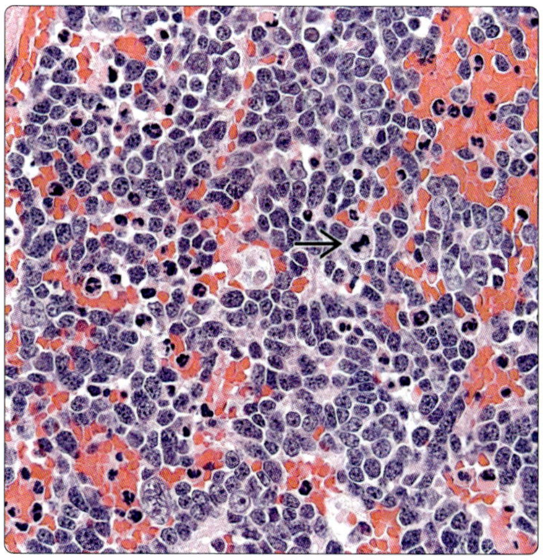

(Left) *In undifferentiated NB, the cells have scant cytoplasm and rounded, deeply staining nuclei. On H&E, this morphology could be easily mistaken for Ewing sarcoma, alveolar rhabdomyosarcoma, or lymphoma.* **(Right)** *Tumor cells in undifferentiated NB show scant cytoplasm and feature relatively monomorphic nuclei. Areas of nuclear molding may be seen. Mitoses → and apoptotic cells are common.*

Apoptosis and Necrosis

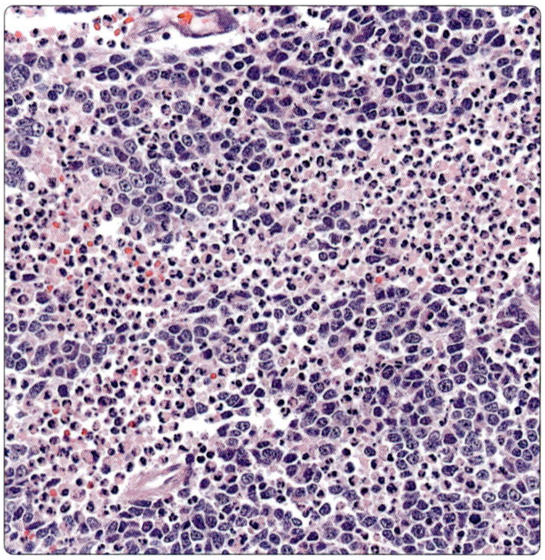

Poorly Differentiated Neuroblastoma

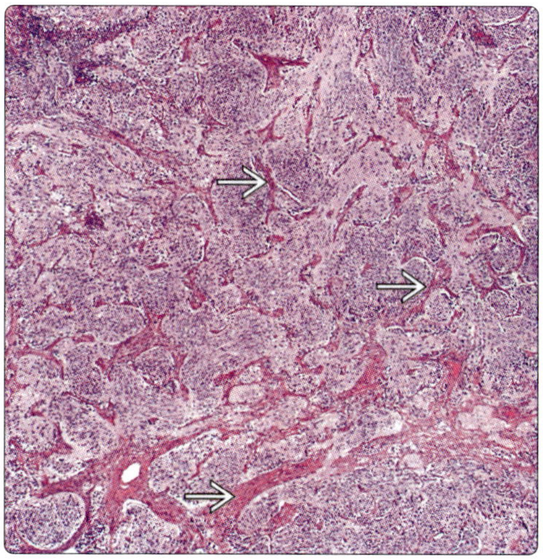

(Left) *Apoptotic and necrotic cells are common in undifferentiated NB. Necrosis often varies from focal and patchy to diffuse and geographic.* **(Right)** *H&E shows the typical low-power appearance of a poorly differentiated NB. Small strips of schwannian stroma → separate the neuroblasts and neuropil, imparting a nested or multinodular appearance.*

Neuropil

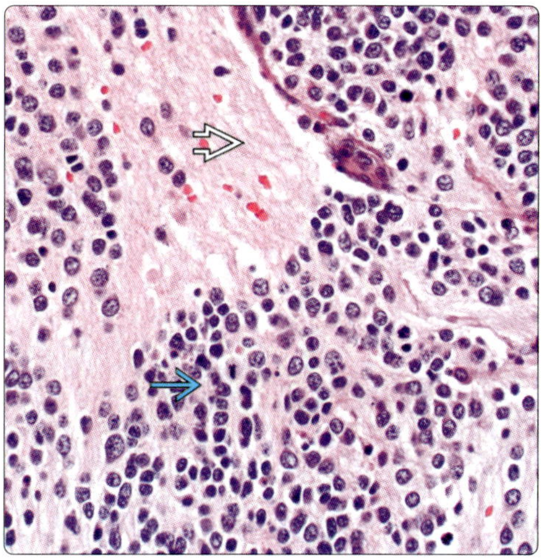

True Rosette Formation

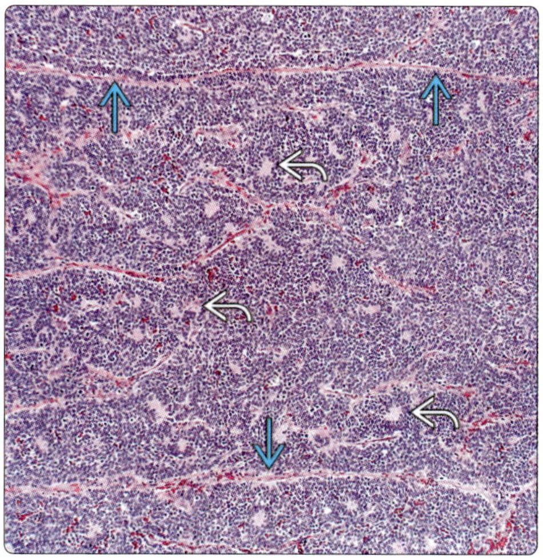

(Left) *This poorly differentiated NB shows sheets of small round cells → in aggregates within a background of neuropil →. The neuropil is composed of a dense tangle of fibrillary, eosinophilic cytoplasmic processes.* **(Right)** *This poorly differentiated NB shows scattered rosettes ↩, an early sign of differentiation. Also seen are thin bands of schwannian stroma →.*

(Left) *Homer Wright rosettes are composed of neuroblasts surrounding a central core of neurites (cytoplasmic processes) without a central lumen. These can be found in varying numbers in poorly differentiated NB but are not wholly specific.* **(Right)** *Schwannian stroma in an NB is often present as thin septa composed of spindled cells, sometimes with wavy nuclei. The Schwann cell component can be demonstrated by IHC for S100 protein.*

Homer Wright Rosettes

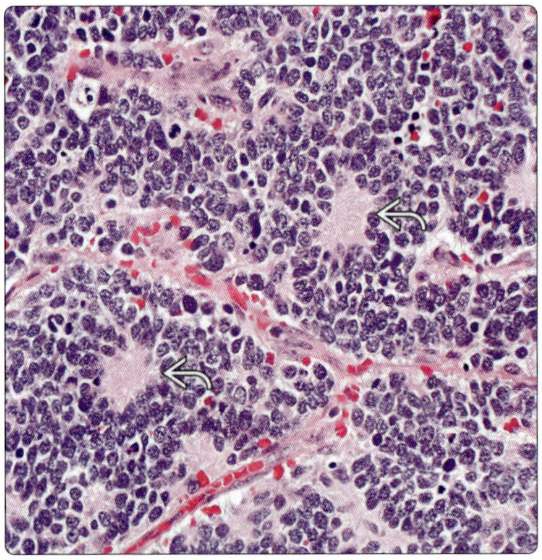

Subtle Schwannian Stroma

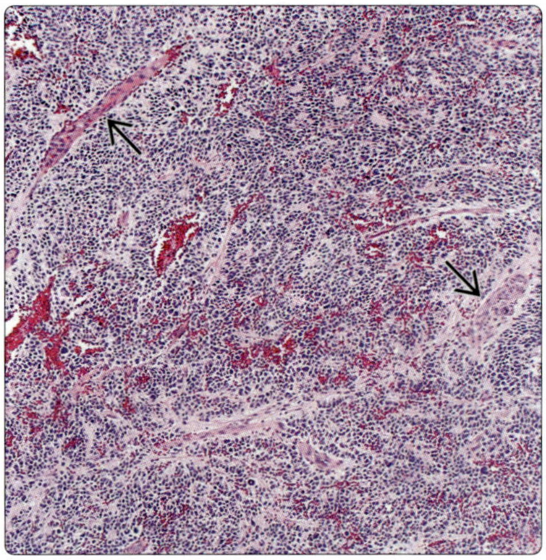

(Left) *NBs are commonly hemorrhagic with areas of necrosis. These changes can also be seen after treatment. NBs that have undergone treatment should not be classified in the International Neuroblastoma Pathology Committee system.* **(Right)** *This is an example of differentiating NB, in which > 5% of the neuroblasts show differentiation with increased cytoplasm and vesicular nuclei.*

Hemorrhage and Necrosis

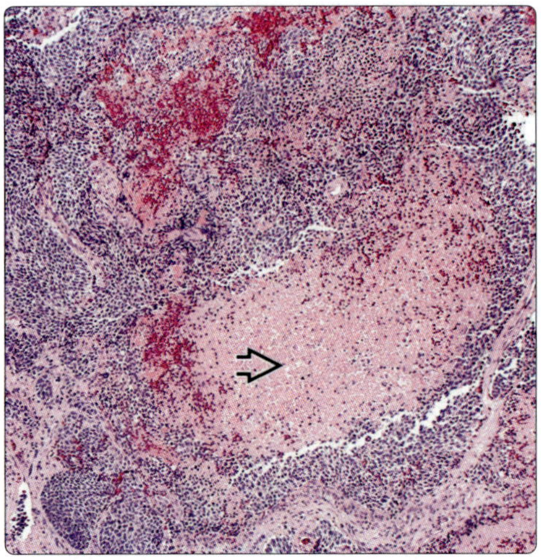

Differentiating Neuroblastoma

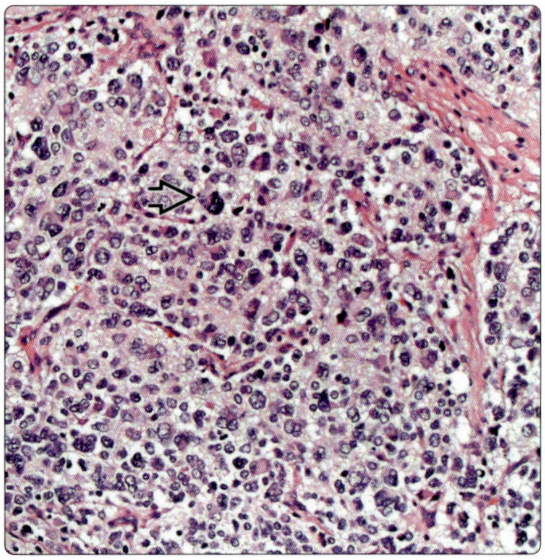

(Left) *Differentiating neuroblasts are characterized by an increased amount of eosinophilic cytoplasm, an eccentrically placed nucleus, and vesicular chromatin.* **(Right)** *The mitotic-karyorrhectic index (MKI) is determined by counting the number of mitoses and karyorrhectic cells per 5,000 tumor cells. An estimated result is usually considered acceptable, as counting 5,000 cells can be tedious. MKI counts should be averaged over the entire tumor and not assessed in only the worst-looking areas.*

Differentiating Neuroblasts

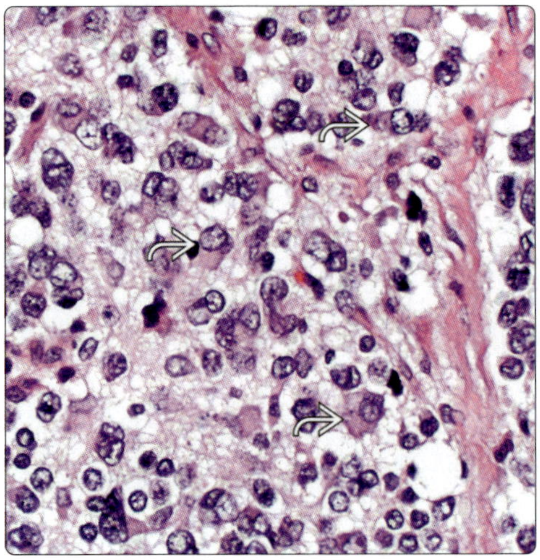

Mitotic-Karyorrhectic Index

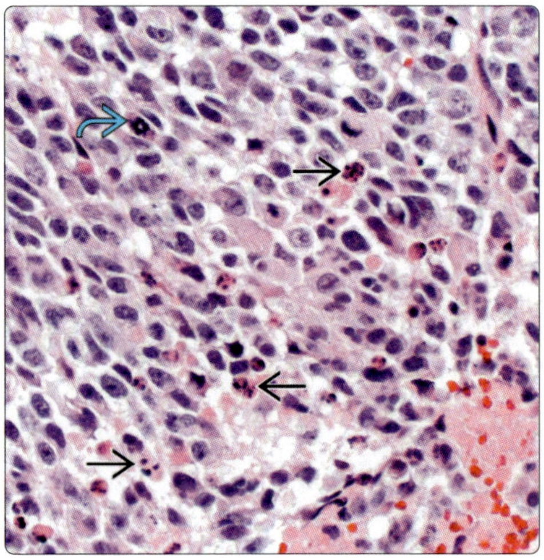

Intermediate Mitotic-Karyorrhectic Index Tumor

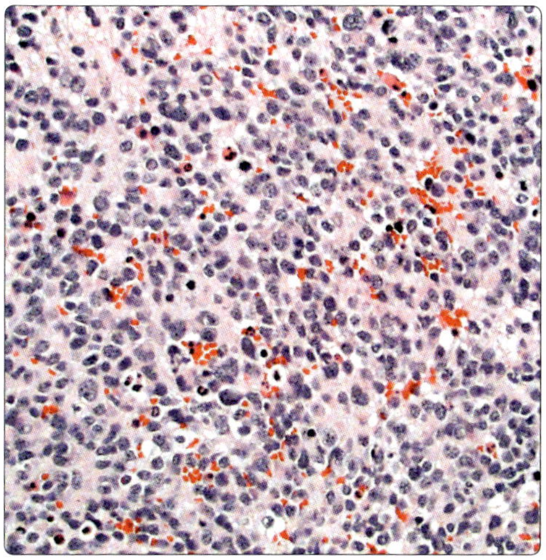

Bony Metastasis in Neuroblastoma

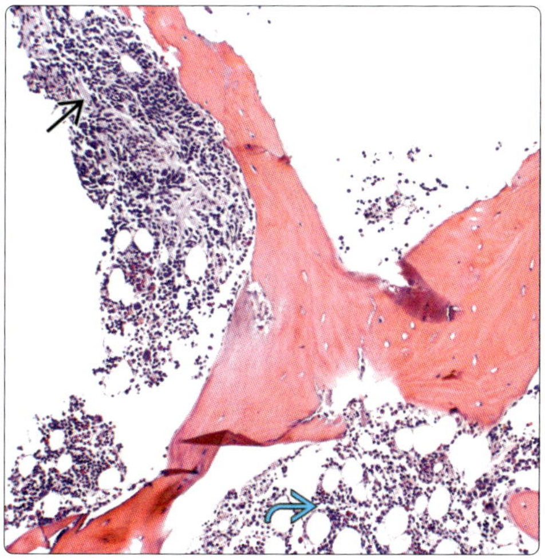

(Left) *This is an example of a poorly differentiated NB, which has an intermediate MKI.* **(Right)** *This core biopsy specimen of bone marrow shows normal marrow in the lower part of the field and a focus of metastatic NB in the upper part. Notice how the architecture changes in the focus of metastatic tumor.*

Focus of Metastatic Neuroblastoma

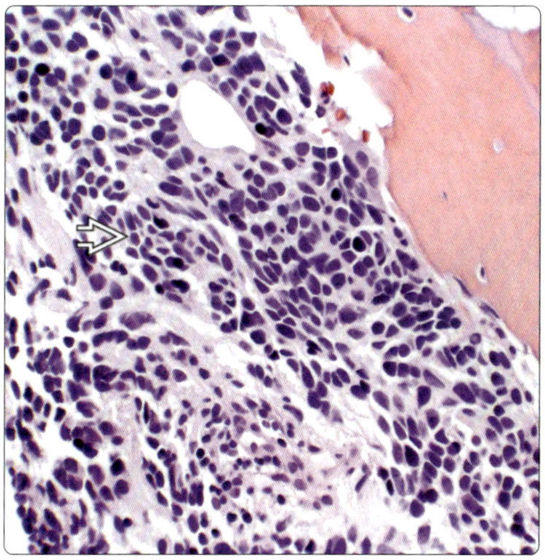

NSE Expression

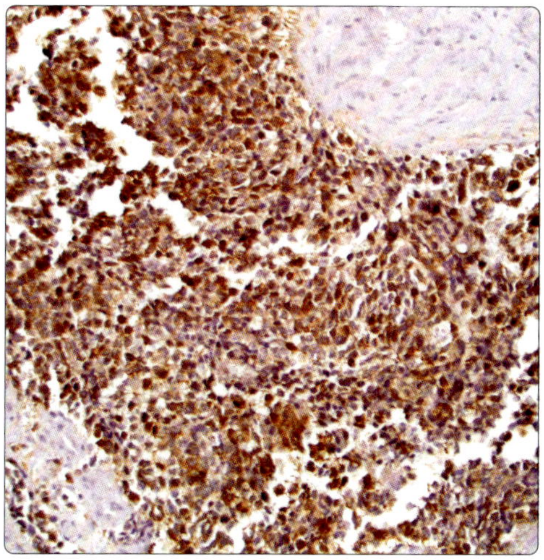

(Left) *This is a focus of metastatic NB in a core biopsy specimen of bone. The marrow has been extensively replaced by sheets of metastatic small round cell tumor and shows no areas with normal trilineage hematopoiesis.* **(Right)** *Immunohistochemical staining for NSE shows strong, diffuse cytoplasmic staining in NB. NSE is a sensitive marker for NB, and although very nonspecific, it can usefully be included in a panel of antibodies in the differential diagnosis with other small round cell tumors.*

Neurofilament Protein

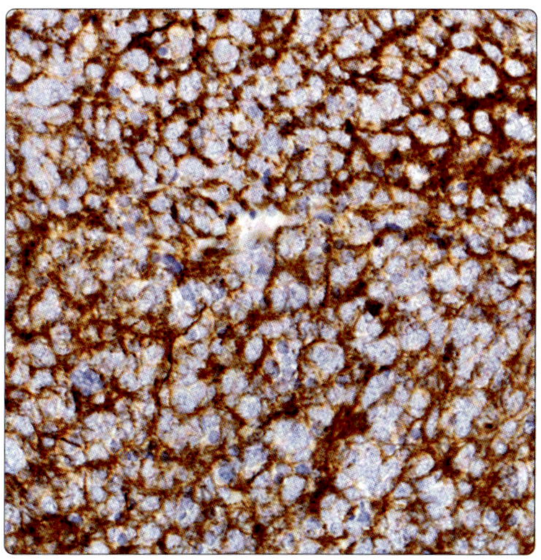

Amplification of MYCN

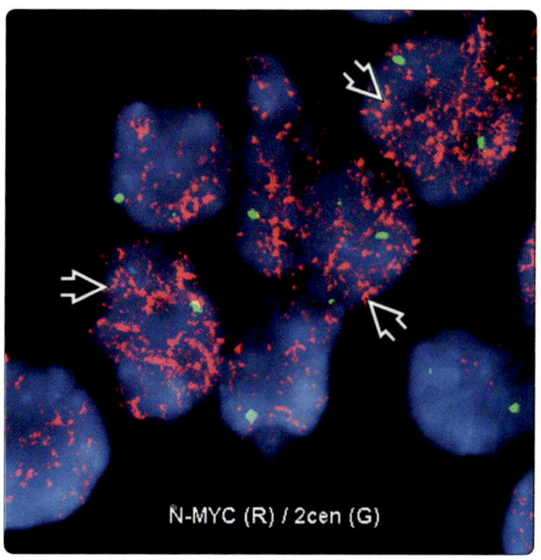

(Left) *Neurofilament protein is demonstrable, diffusely or focally, in cytoplasm of 70% of NBs. It is negative in most Ewing sarcomas.* **(Right)** *Fluorescence in situ hybridization (FISH) of this NB shows marked amplification of MYCN demonstrated by numerous red dots. This finding predicts poor prognosis, although the amount of amplification does not relate to outcome. (Courtesy L. McGavran, PhD, and K. Swisshelm, PhD.)*

(Left) *Gross photograph of GNB from the mediastinum depicts a tumor with a tan, firm cut surface, but the gross appearance of GNB depends on how much of the tumor is neuroblastic.* **(Right)** *This is the typical look of a nodular GNB on cut surface. The hemorrhagic nodule in the center* ↪ *is stroma-poor NB, whereas the tan, fleshy rim* ⇨ *is either ganglioneuroma (GN) or intermixed GNB. The diagnosis of nodular GNB requires grossly visible nodules.*

Ganglioneuroblastoma

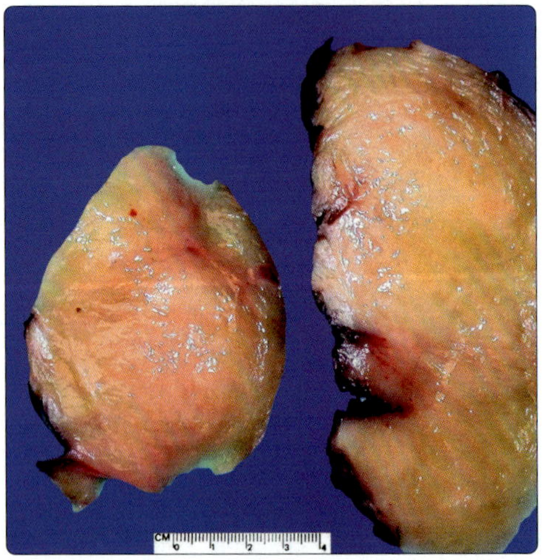

Nodular Ganglioneuroblastoma

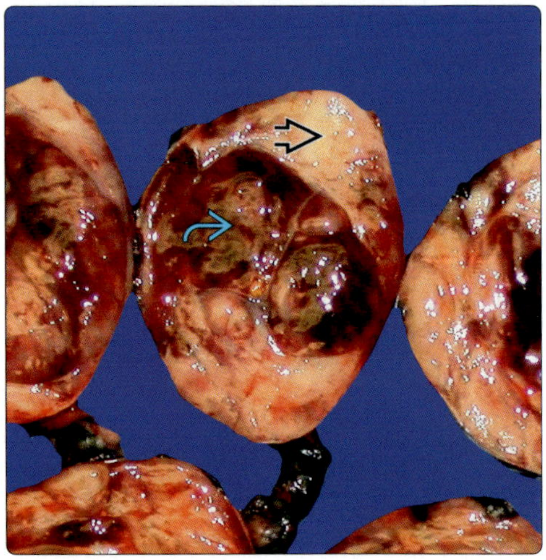

(Left) *This nodular GNB shows the pushing border between the stroma-poor NB component* ↪ *and the GN component* →*. There is often a fibrous pseudocapsule between the 2 components. Even with this histologic picture, a grossly visible nodule is required to diagnose nodular GNB.* **(Right)** *In intermixed GNB, the nests of NB can vary in size and maturation of neuroblasts. Here, a larger nest of immature neuroblasts is seen* →*.*

Nodular Ganglioneuroblastoma

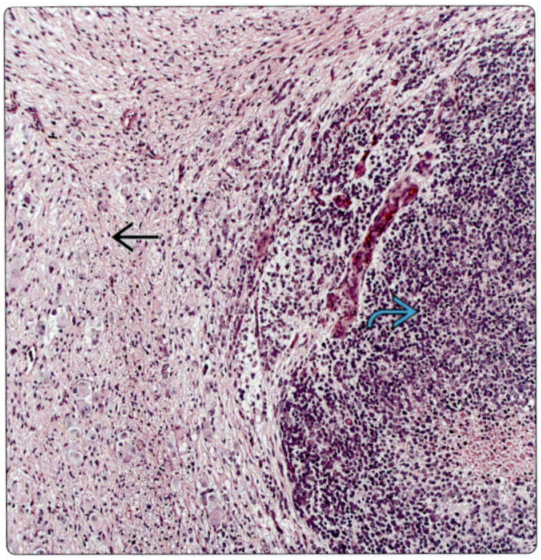

Intermixed Ganglioneuroblastoma

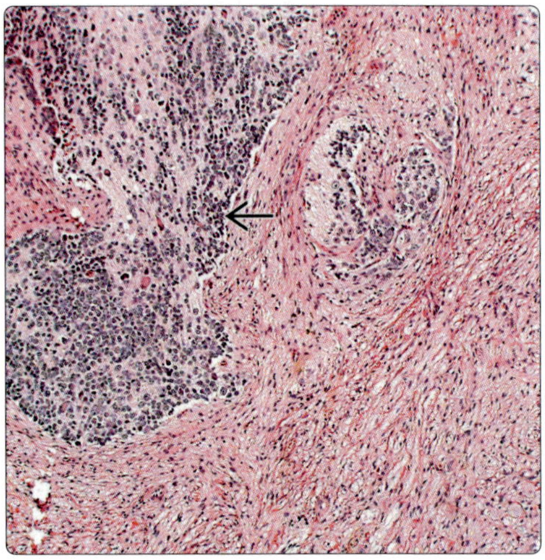

(Left) *To diagnose intermixed GNB, at least 50% of the tumor must be composed of schwannian stroma. This is characterized by spindled, wavy cells in bundles of varying cellularity. The Schwann cells lack nuclear atypia and demonstrate nuclear immunoreactivity for S100 protein.* **(Right)** *This intermixed GNB shows well-defined nests* ↪ *of maturing neuroblasts, ganglion cells, and neuropil within a schwannian stroma* →*.*

Schwannian Stroma in Intermixed Ganglioneuroblastoma

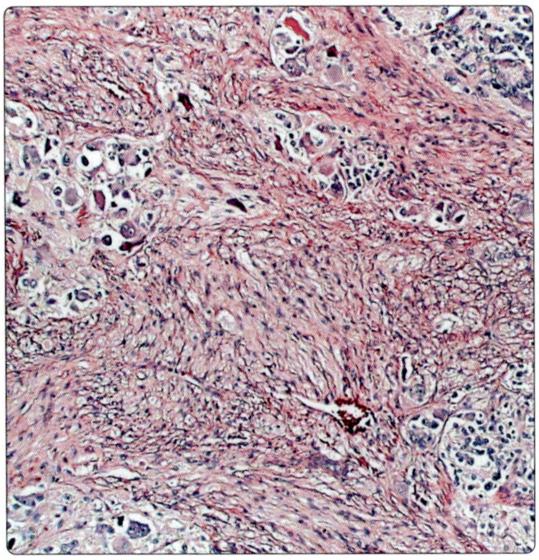

Nested Growth

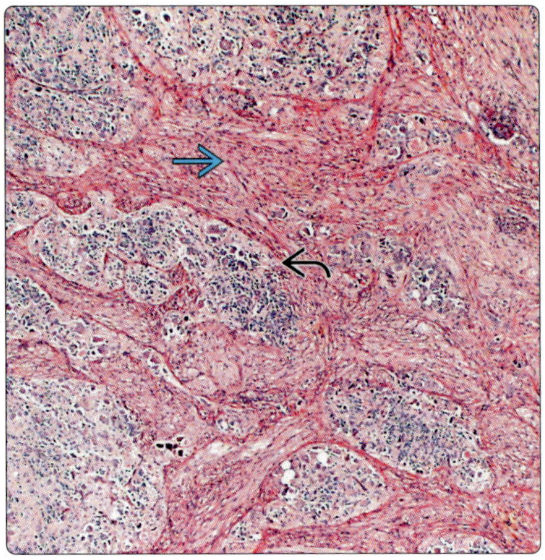

Clusters of Ganglion Cells

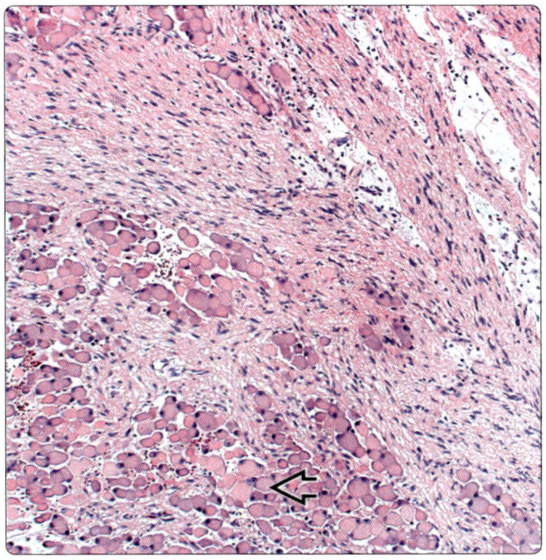

Mature Ganglion Cells

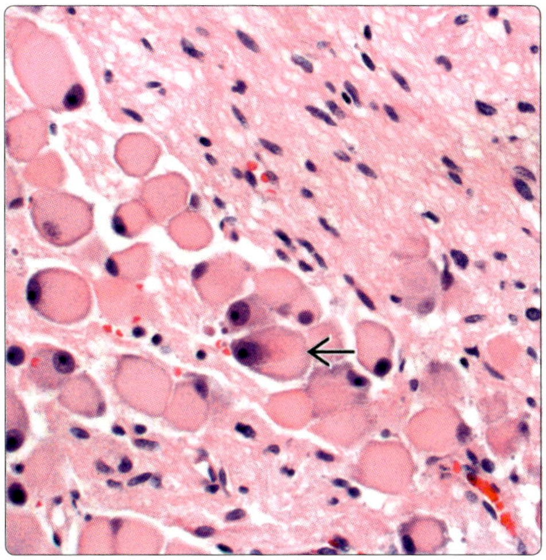

(Left) *The neuroblastomatous component of this intermixed GNB is predominantly mature (or nearly mature) ganglion cells ⇨. The ganglion cells are present in clusters in this tumor, differing from the pattern in maturing GN in which they are present as single cells.* **(Right)** *Mature ganglion cells → are characterized by abundant eosinophilic to amphophilic cytoplasm, eccentric nuclei, and prominent nucleoli. Nissl substance may or may not be present.*

Intermixed Ganglioneuroblastoma

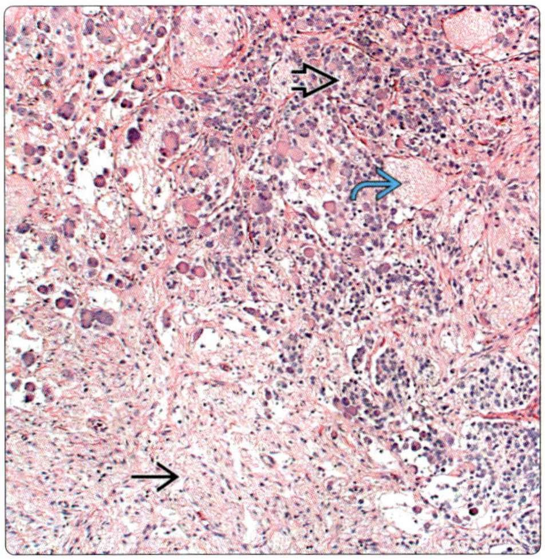

Neuroblasts and Ganglion Cells

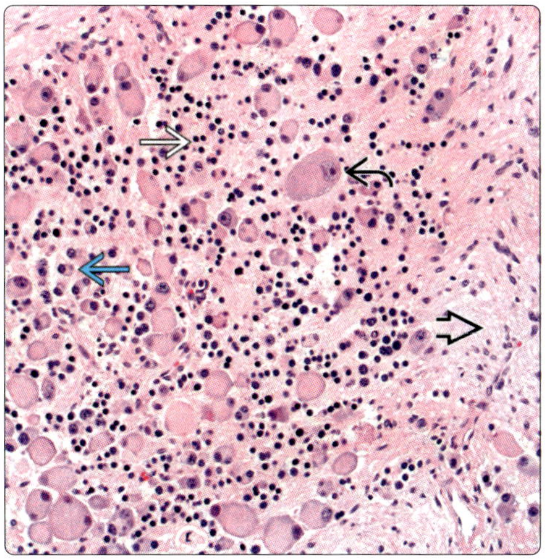

(Left) *This low-magnification field of intermixed GNB shows clusters of maturing neuroblasts and ganglion cells ⇨, foci of neuropil ↱, and areas of schwannian stroma →.* **(Right)** *Higher magnification of intermixed GNB shows details of neuroblasts ➡, maturing neuroblasts →, and ganglion cells ↩ blending into the schwannian stroma ⇨.*

Prominent Schwannian Stroma

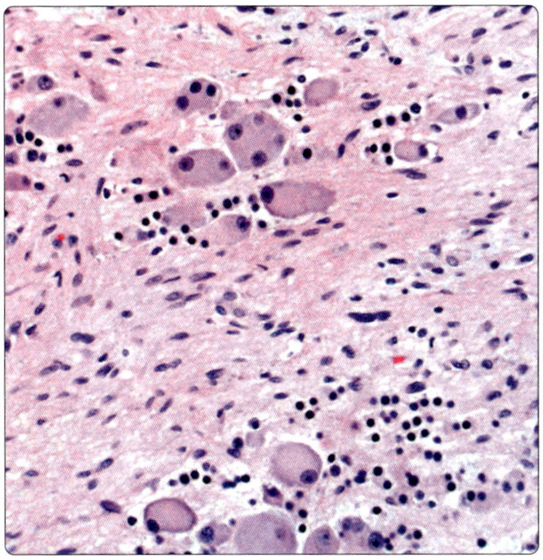

Neurofibroma-Like Areas

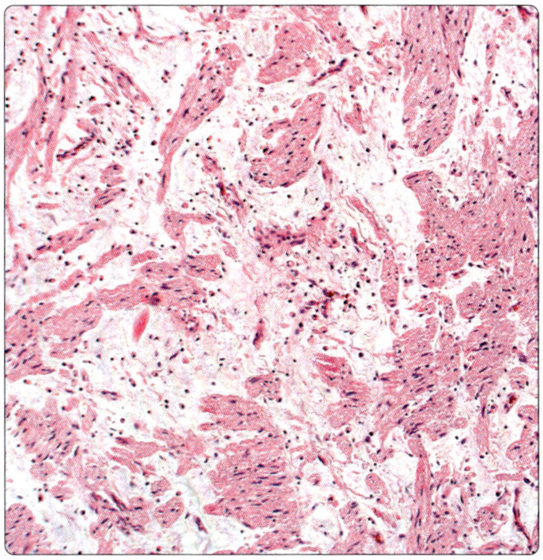

(Left) *This section from an intermixed GNB could be mistaken for a maturing GN. In maturing GN, the tumor is predominantly composed of schwannian stroma, and individual neuroblastic cells merge into the schwannian stroma instead of forming distinct nests.* **(Right)** *This field of an intermixed GNB could be mistaken for neurofibroma (spindled wavy cells in a myxoid background) or mature GN. Adequate sampling, generally 1 section per cm of tumor, is required to make an accurate diagnosis.*

Extraaxial Soft Tissue Chordoma

KEY FACTS

TERMINOLOGY

- True chordoma arising in soft tissue without evidence of skeletal origin

CLINICAL ISSUES

- Very rare (< 30 cases in literature)
- Usually adults
- Acral sites (~ 50%)
  - Remainder in proximal extremity or trunk
- Subcutaneous or deep mass, usually slowly growing
- Majority behave indolently
  - Local recurrence &/or distant metastasis (lung or intraabdominal) in subset (20-30%)

MACROSCOPIC

- Multilobulated, circumscribed mass
- Gelatinous cut surface

MICROSCOPIC

- Histologic features identical to skeletal (axial) chordoma
- Multinodular with fibrous septa
- Epithelioid or spindle cells in cords/nests set in myxoid background
- Pale eosinophilic or clear cytoplasm with vacuoles
- Characteristic physaliferous cells may be present

ANCILLARY TESTS

- Strong nuclear brachyury (+)
  - Present in essentially 100% of cases (defining criterion for diagnosis)
- Usually also keratin (+), EMA(+), S100 protein (+)

TOP DIFFERENTIAL DIAGNOSES

- Myoepithelioma of soft tissue
- Extraskeletal myxoid chondrosarcoma
- Metastatic or primary cutaneous mucinous carcinoma
- Soft tissue metastasis from axial chordoma

Multinodular Growth

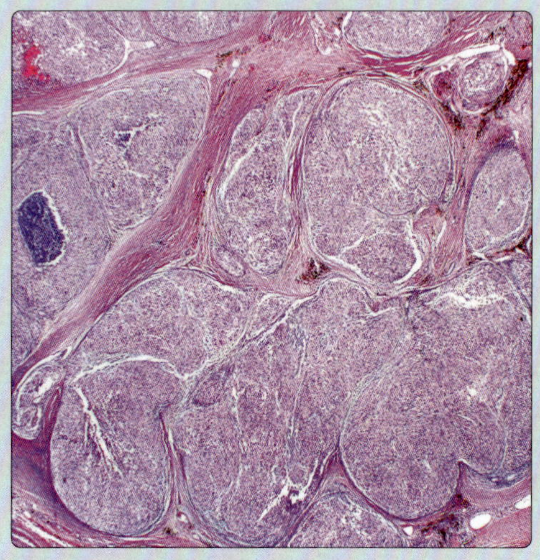

Cords Within Myxoid Matrix

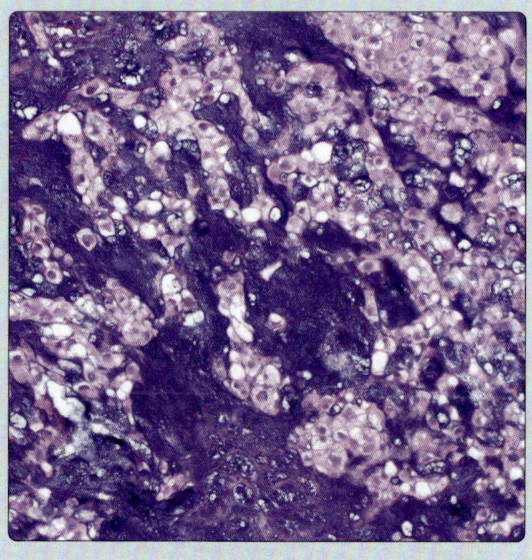

(Left) *Similar to its primary skeletal counterpart, extraaxial soft tissue chordoma typically shows a multinodular growth pattern with intervening fibrous septa similar to conventional chordoma. This case gave rise to a lung metastasis that had a strikingly similar architecture.* **(Right)** *Epithelioid tumor cells with pale vacuolated cytoplasm form cords, chains, and nests set within a blue myxoid matrix in chordoma.*

Physaliferous Cells

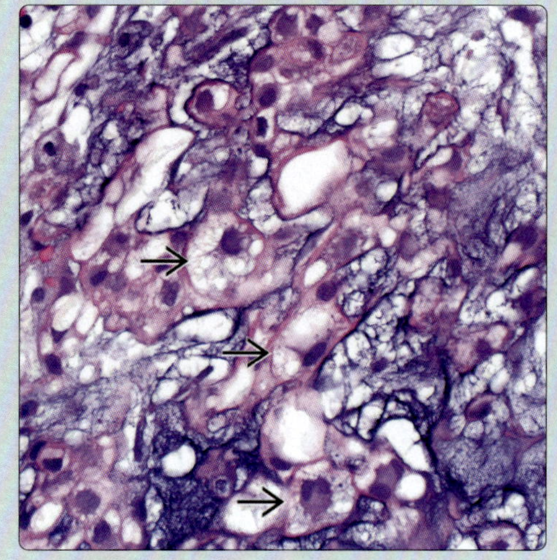

Nuclear Atypia

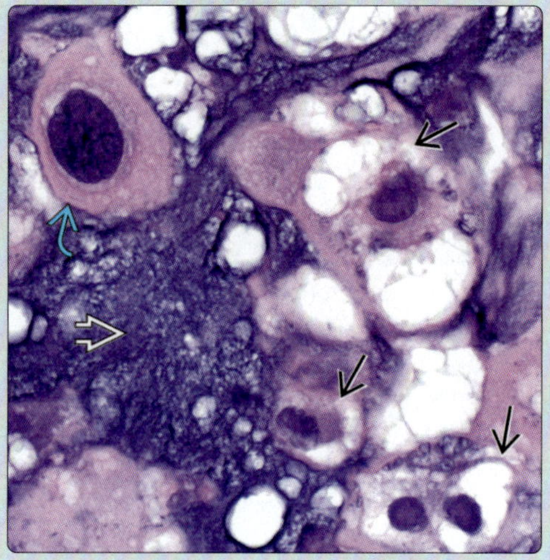

(Left) *Tumor cells with bubbly vacuolated cytoplasm (physaliferous cells) ➔ are a characteristic finding in chordoma; however, they are not always present and are not required for the diagnosis.* **(Right)** *High-power H&E shows physaliferous cells ➔ with multiple cytoplasmic vacuoles set within an abundant blue myxoid matrix ➔. Nuclear atypia and pleomorphism ➔ may be present.*

Extraaxial Soft Tissue Chordoma

TERMINOLOGY

Definitions

- True chordoma arising in soft tissue without evidence of skeletal origin

CLINICAL ISSUES

Epidemiology

- Incidence
  - Very rare (< 30 cases in literature)
- Age
  - Usually adults
- Sex
  - M > F

Site

- Most cases occur in soft tissue near bone or joints
  - Acral sites (~ 50%)
  - Remainder in proximal extremity or trunk

Presentation

- Subcutaneous or deep mass, usually slowly growing
  - Clinically resemble benign cyst (when small, subcutaneous, distal) or sarcoma (when large, deep, proximal)

Treatment

- Complete excision with free margins
- Chemotherapy has been attempted for metastatic lesions

Prognosis

- Majority behave indolently
- Local recurrence &/or distant metastasis (lung or intraabdominal) in subset (20-30%)
  - Larger proximally located tumors may have higher risk of aggressive behavior

IMAGING

Radiographic Findings

- Small tumors: Circumscribed nodules
- Large tumors: Circumscribed, multilobulated masses with heterogeneous enhancement

MACROSCOPIC

General Features

- Multilobulated, circumscribed mass
- Gelatinous cut surface
- May have hemorrhage or necrosis

MICROSCOPIC

Histologic Features

- Histologically identical to skeletal (axial) chordoma
- Multinodular with fibrous septa
- Epithelioid or spindle cells in cords/nests set in myxoid background
- Pale eosinophilic or clear cytoplasm with vacuoles
  - Characteristic physaliferous cells may be present
- Nuclear atypia usually mild but can be focally moderate to severe
- Usually low cellularity but can be hypercellular
- Tumor cells may wrap around each other
- May have rhabdoid cytology
- Cartilaginous matrix may be present focally

ANCILLARY TESTS

Immunohistochemistry

- Strong nuclear brachyury (+)
  - Present in essentially 100% of cases (defining criterion for diagnosis)
  - Only marker that can reliably distinguish chordoma from myoepithelioma
- Usually also keratin (+), EMA(+), and S100 protein (+)
- Nuclear SMARCB1/INI1 retained in few cases tested to date (subset of pediatric axial chordomas show SMARCB1/INI1 loss)

DIFFERENTIAL DIAGNOSIS

Myoepithelioma of Soft Tissue

- May show morphologic overlap with chordoma
- Usually keratin (+), EMA(+), and S100 protein (+); other myoepithelial markers variable
- Brachyury (-) (key distinguishing feature)
- Obsolete synonyms for myoepithelioma: Parachordoma, chordoma periphericum, peripheral chordoma, chordoid tumor
  - Older literature often incorrectly equated these with true soft tissue chordomas

Extraskeletal Myxoid Chondrosarcoma

- May have similar histologic features to chordoma
- EMA(+) in subset; S100 protein and keratins usually (-) or only focally (+)
- Brachyury (-)
- Characteristic translocations usually detectable, including t(9;22) and variants

Metastatic or Primary Cutaneous Mucinous Carcinoma

- Known primary site elsewhere in some cases
- Usually has larger nests of tumor cells floating in mucin pools
- Keratin (+); may coexpress other more specific lineage markers
- Brachyury (-)

Soft Tissue Metastasis From Axial Chordoma

- Uncommon scenario that can be excluded by clinical history &/or imaging studies

SELECTED REFERENCES

1. Righi A et al: Extra-axial chordoma: a clinicopathologic analysis of six cases. Virchows Arch. 472(6):1015-1020, 2018
2. Lauer SR et al: Soft tissue chordomas: a clinicopathologic analysis of 11 cases. Am J Surg Pathol. 37(5):719-26, 2013
3. Suzuki H et al: Extra-axial soft tissue chordoma of wrist. Pathol Res Pract. 207(5):327-31, 2011
4. Tirabosco R et al: Brachyury expression in extra-axial skeletal and soft tissue chordomas: a marker that distinguishes chordoma from mixed tumor/myoepithelioma/parachordoma in soft tissue. Am J Surg Pathol. 32(4):572-80, 2008

Undifferentiated Embryonal Sarcoma of Liver

KEY FACTS

TERMINOLOGY

- Malignant, primitive neoplasm of liver, often with evidence of partial divergent differentiation

CLINICAL ISSUES

- Usually < 20 years (most common: 6-10 years)
- Occurs in liver
- Abdominal swelling and pain
- Treatment: Complete surgical resection, often with chemotherapy
  - Much improved 5-year survival rate with combination therapy (surgery, neoadjuvant and adjuvant therapy)
- Local recurrence is common; metastases rare

MACROSCOPIC

- Well-demarcated mass; variegated cut surface with solid, cystic, and gelatinous areas
- Often large (> 10 cm)

MICROSCOPIC

- Spindled, ovoid, and stellate cells with granular or bubbly eosinophilic cytoplasm
  - Cellularity varies from loose to compact
  - Marked nuclear pleomorphism and hyperchromasia
  - Multinucleation and bizarre atypia
- Usually prominent myxoid stroma
- Clusters of variably sized eosinophilic globules common
- Mitoses usually numerous
- Hemorrhage and coagulative necrosis common

ANCILLARY TESTS

- Globules are PAS(+), diastase resistant
- CD31(-), CD34(-), myogenin (-), S100 protein (-), CD117(-), HMB-45(-)

TOP DIFFERENTIAL DIAGNOSES

- Embryonal rhabdomyosarcoma

(Left) *Undifferentiated embryonal sarcoma of the liver (UESL) is a primitive malignant neoplasm that most commonly occurs in childhood. Most cases show a prominent myxoid stroma, and cellularity varies from low and dispersed* ⇨ *to highly compact* ⇨*. Hemorrhage and necrosis are common.* **(Right)** *Nuclear pleomorphism and hyperchromasia are consistent features of UESL, at least focally. In many tumors, multinucleated forms and bizarre atypia are present, as depicted.*

Undifferentiated Embryonal Sarcoma

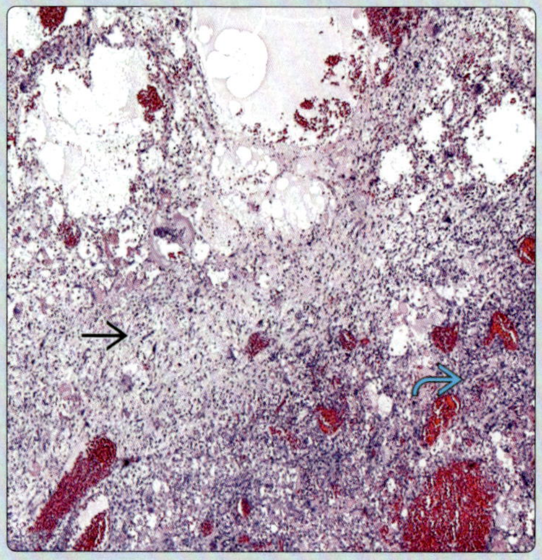

Marked Nuclear Atypia

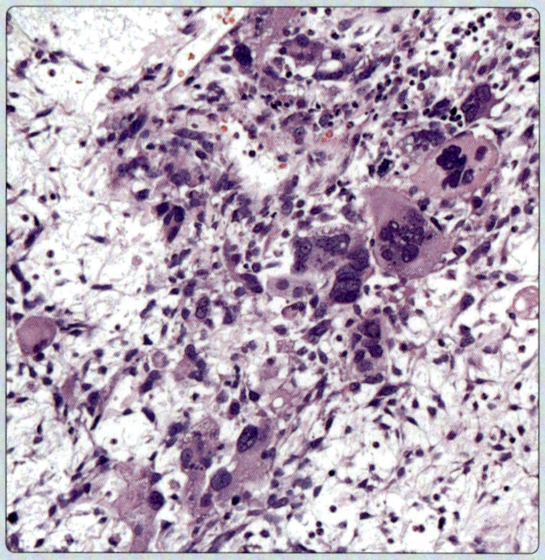

(Left) *Eosinophilic globules* ⇨ *of varying shapes and sizes are common in UESL. They may be intracytoplasmic or found extracellularly, and they are PAS(+), diastase resistant.* **(Right)** *Entrapment of residual normal biliary ductules* ⇨ *or hepatic parenchyma* ⇨ *can be seen in UESL, particularly near the periphery of the tumor.*

Eosinophilic Globules

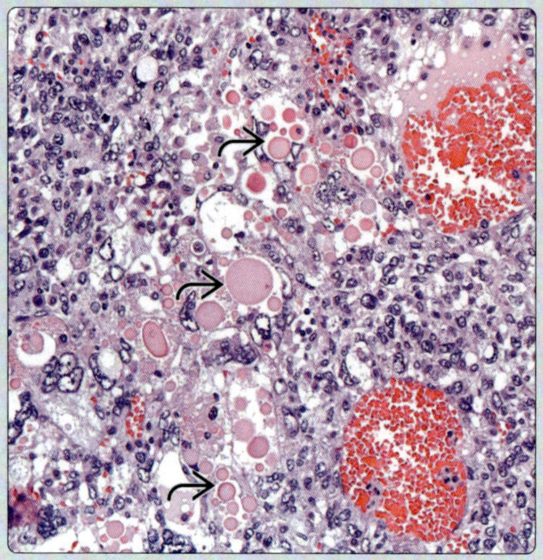

Entrapment of Hepatobiliary Elements

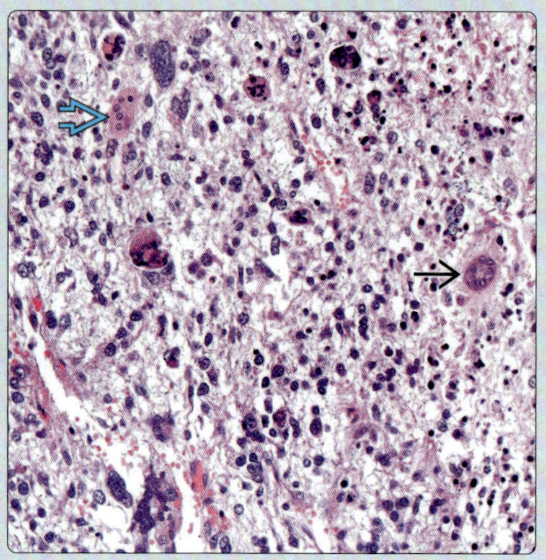

TERMINOLOGY

Abbreviations

- Undifferentiated embryonal sarcoma of liver (UESL)

Synonyms

- Embryonal sarcoma

Definitions

- Malignant, primitive neoplasm of liver, often with evidence of partial divergent differentiation

ETIOLOGY/PATHOGENESIS

Unknown

- May rarely occur in association with mesenchymal hamartoma of liver
  - Both contain chromosome 19 abnormalities

CLINICAL ISSUES

Epidemiology

- Incidence
  - Rare
- Age
  - Usually < 20 years (most commonly 6-10 years)
    - Very rare cases in adults

Site

- Exclusive to liver
  - More common in right lobe

Presentation

- Abdominal swelling and pain
- Large mass
  - May or may not be palpable
- Possible fever &/or weight loss
- Normal serum α-fetoprotein levels

Treatment

- Multimodal therapy ideal
  - Complete surgical resection
  - Chemotherapy &/or radiation
- Transplantation may be considered in unresectable cases

Prognosis

- Markedly improved survival in recent years (> 70%) with combination therapy (surgery, neoadjuvant and adjuvant chemotherapy, and radiation)
- Local recurrence is common
- Rare metastases

MACROSCOPIC

General Features

- Well demarcated, partially encapsulated
- Variegated cut surface with solid, cystic, and gelatinous areas
  - Hemorrhage, necrosis common

Size

- Wide range (often large, > 10 cm)

MICROSCOPIC

Histologic Features

- May show partial pseudocapsule formation
  - Entrapped biliary ductules and hepatocytes often entrapped near tumor periphery
    - Tumor cells may involve sinusoids
- Spindled, ovoid, and stellate cells with granular or bubbly eosinophilic cytoplasm
  - Cellularity varies from loose to compact
    - May rarely show formation of cellular fascicles or storiform arrays
  - Marked nuclear pleomorphism and hyperchromasia
  - Multinucleation and bizarre atypia
- Usually prominent myxoid stroma
  - May be fibrous or focally hyalinized
- Clusters of variably sized eosinophilic globules common
  - Intracytoplasmic or extracellular
- Mitoses usually numerous
- Hemorrhage and coagulative necrosis common
- Extramedullary hematopoiesis may be present

ANCILLARY TESTS

Histochemistry

- Globules are PAS(+), diastase resistant

Immunohistochemistry

- Vimentin (+), α-1-antitrypsin (+)
- Variable, focal expression of glypican-3, keratins, SMA, desmin, CD68, and others
  - Evidence of partial divergent differentiation
- CD31(-), CD34(-), myogenin (-), S100 protein (-), CD117(-), HMB-45(-)

DIFFERENTIAL DIAGNOSIS

Embryonal Rhabdomyosarcoma

- Usually biliary tree; rare in liver
- Rhabdomyoblasts often present, at least focally
- Desmin, myogenin, MYOD1 (+)

Sarcomatoid Carcinoma

- Usually adults
- Often more extensive keratin (+)

Mesenchymal Hamartoma

- Most occur < 3 years of age
- Absence of marked cytologic atypia
- Rare reports of UESL arising in mesenchymal hamartoma

SELECTED REFERENCES

1. Shi Y et al: Characteristics and outcomes in children with undifferentiated embryonal sarcoma of the liver: a report from the National Cancer Database. Pediatr Blood Cancer. 64(4), 2017
2. Putra J et al: Undifferentiated embryonal sarcoma of the liver: a concise review. Arch Pathol Lab Med. 139(2):269-73, 2015
3. Shehata BM et al: Undifferentiated embryonal sarcoma of the liver is associated with mesenchymal hamartoma and multiple chromosomal abnormalities: a review of eleven cases. Pediatr Dev Pathol. 14(2):111-6, 2011
4. Zheng JM et al: Primary and recurrent embryonal sarcoma of the liver: clinicopathological and immunohistochemical analysis. Histopathology. 51(2):195-203, 2007

Primary Pulmonary Myxoid Sarcoma

KEY FACTS

TERMINOLOGY

- Low-grade translocation-associated sarcoma, exclusively occurring in lung, adjacent to or within bronchus, composed of abundant myxoid matrix with reticulated cords, clusters, or sheets of epithelioid to spindle cells

CLINICAL ISSUES

- Rare: 23 reported cases
- Mean age: 45 years
- 2:1 female predominance
- Most patients alive with no evidence of disease
- 3 reports of metastasis

MACROSCOPIC

- Well circumscribed
- Partially encapsulated
- Frequently forms endobronchial mass
- Mean size: 4.9 cm

MICROSCOPIC

- Related to bronchus
- Abundant myxoid matrix
- Epithelioid to spindle cells with low-level nuclear pleomorphism
- Prominent reticulated cytoarchitecture
  - Interconnecting cord and strands of cells
- Solid sheets of cells
- Peripheral rind of fibrosis
- Patchy chronic inflammation

ANCILLARY TESTS

- *EWSR1* rearrangement by FISH
- *EWSR1-CREB1* fusion by RT-PCR

TOP DIFFERENTIAL DIAGNOSES

- Angiomatoid fibrous histiocytoma
- Extraskeletal myxoid chondrosarcoma
- Myoepithelioma

(Left) *Primary pulmonary myxoid sarcoma (PPMS) typically presents as a well-circumscribed, lobular mass. It is typically associated with a bronchus* ⇨ *and often forms an endobronchial mass. It is often surrounded by a thick rind of fibrosis* ↪*. However, focal pulmonary parenchymal infiltration may be present.* **(Right)** *The dominant histological pattern in PPMS is a reticulated or net-like pattern formed by interconnecting cords of cells* ⇨ *within abundant pale blue myxoid matrix* ↪*.*

Primary Pulmonary Myxoid Sarcoma

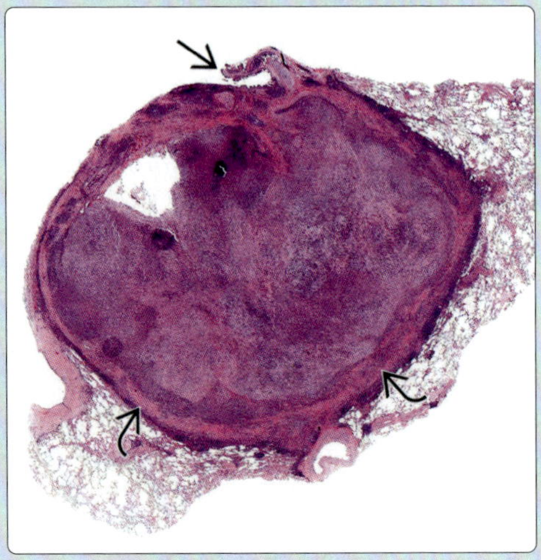

Architectural Features

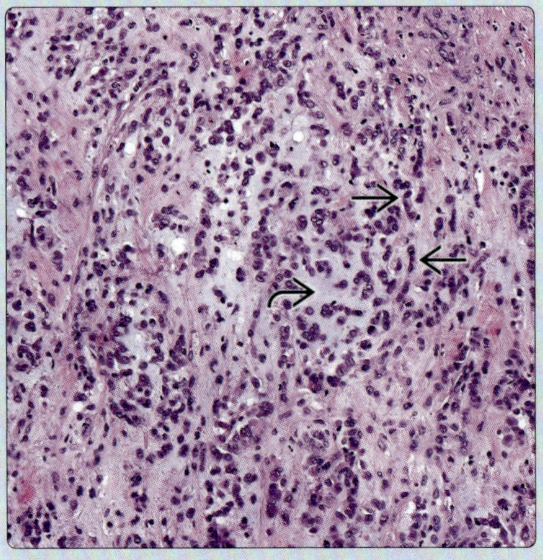

(Left) *This medium-power micrograph highlights the reticulated pattern composed of cords* ⇨ *and clusters* ↪ *of epithelioid cells with abundant eosinophilic cytoplasm within a myxoid stroma* ⇘*.* **(Right)** *EWSR1 break-apart FISH can confirm the diagnosis of PPMS since EWSR1-CREB1 translocations can be detected in most tumors. This FISH assay shows 1 normal, intact allele with fused red and green signals* ➡ *adjacent to 2 abnormal, separated, red and green signals* ↪ *within single cells. (Courtesy S. Smith, MD.)*

Reticulated Pattern

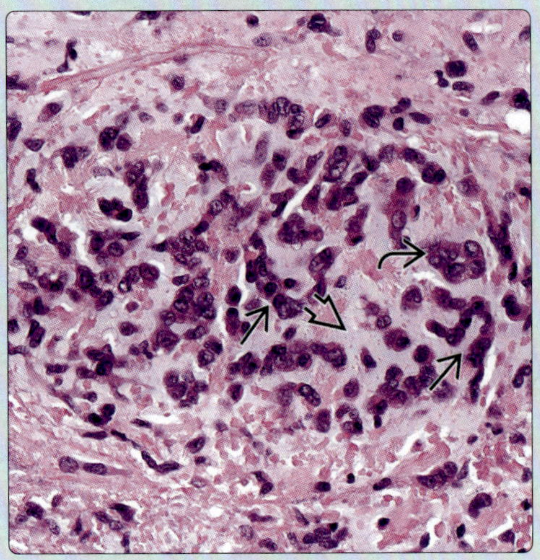

***EWSR1* Rearrangement**

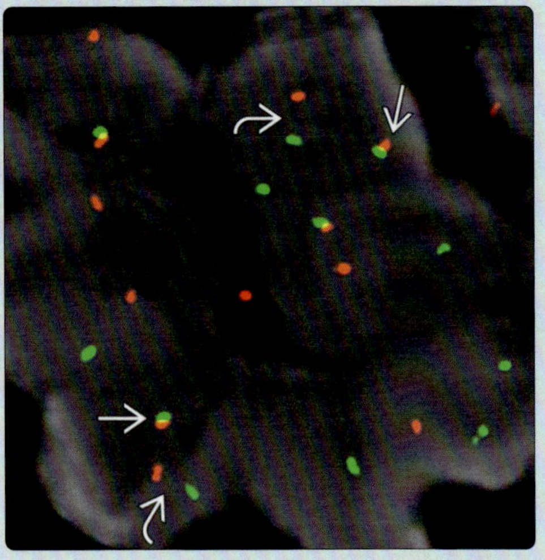

TERMINOLOGY

Abbreviations

- Primary pulmonary myxoid sarcoma (PPMS)

Synonyms

- Malignant myxoid endobronchial tumor

Definitions

- Low-grade translocation-associated sarcoma, exclusively occurring in lung, adjacent to or within bronchus, composed of abundant myxoid matrix with reticulated cords, clusters, or sheets of epithelioid to spindle cells
  - Characterized by *EWSR1-CREB1* fusion

CLINICAL ISSUES

Epidemiology

- Incidence
  - Rare: 23 reported cases
- Age
  - Mean: 45 years (median: 30 years)
  - Range: 27-80 years
- Sex
  - 2:1 female predominance

Presentation

- Cough
- Hemoptysis
- Fever
- Weight loss

Treatment

- Complete surgical resection

Prognosis

- Very good
  - Most patients alive with no evidence of disease
- 3 reports of metastasis
  - Brain
    - May not be true PPMS
  - Kidney
  - Contralateral lung

MACROSCOPIC

General Features

- Well circumscribed
  - Partially encapsulated
  - Focally infiltrates pulmonary parenchyma
- Most tumors associated with bronchus
  - Frequently forms endobronchial polypoid mass
- Lobular, gelatinous to firm cut surface

Size

- Mean: 4.9 cm
- Range: 1.5-13.0 cm

MICROSCOPIC

Histologic Features

- Related to bronchus
  - Often endobronchial
  - Focally infiltrates pulmonary parenchyma
- Lobular architecture
- Abundant myxoid matrix
- Epithelioid, spindled, and polygonal/stellate cells
  - Vesicular chromatin
  - Mild to moderate nuclear pleomorphism
  - Low mitotic rate in most tumors
- Prominent reticulated cytoarchitecture
  - Interconnecting cord and strands of cells
    - Major component in most tumors
  - Small clusters of cells
  - Individual cells
  - Solid sheets of cells
    - Usually minor component
    - Pericytomatous vascular pattern in some tumors
- Fibrosis
  - Often forming peripheral rind
- Patchy chronic inflammation
  - Lymphoplasmacytic most common
  - Hemosiderophages, xanthoma cells, giant cells, &/or eosinophils common
- Necrosis common
  - Usually focal when present

ANCILLARY TESTS

Immunohistochemistry

- No distinct immunophenotype
- Most helpful for excluding other entities

In Situ Hybridization

- *EWSR1* rearrangement by FISH

PCR

- *EWSR1-CREB1* fusion

DIFFERENTIAL DIAGNOSIS

Angiomatoid Fibrous Histiocytoma

- Endobronchial mass
- Sheets or short fascicles
- Ovoid to spindle cells
- Less myxoid matrix, less reticulated cell pattern
- Dense lymphoplasmacytic infiltrate and fibrous capsule
- Blood-filled spaces may be absent
- Desmin (+)
- *EWSR1-ATF1* or *EWSR1-CREB1*

Extraskeletal Myxoid Chondrosarcoma

- Very rare as primary pulmonary tumor
- Reticulated cell cords
- Epithelioid or spindle cells
- Rhabdoid cells in some tumors
- Abundant myxoid matrix
  - Alcian blue (+) but not abolished by hyaluronidase (unlike PPMS)
- Necrosis common
- *NR4A3-EWSR1* or alternate *NR4A3* fusions

Myoepithelioma

- Abundant myxoid matrix
- Reticulated cell cords

Immunohistochemistry

Antibody	Reactivity	Staining Pattern	Comment
Vimentin	Positive	Cytoplasmic	
EMA	Positive	Cell membrane and cytoplasm	Focally &/or weakly positive in subset of tumors
CK-PAN	Negative		
p63	Negative		
Desmin	Negative		
S100	Negative		
CD34	Negative		
Synaptophysin	Negative		
HMB-45	Negative		
Melan-A	Negative		
Actin-sm	Equivocal	Cytoplasmic	Only 1 positive tumor reported
CD56	Equivocal		Only 1 positive tumor reported
Chromogranin-A	Equivocal		Only 1 positive tumor reported

- Plasmacytoid cells
- Fascicles of spindle cells
- Variable expression of keratins, S100, SMA, p63
- *EWSR1-ZNF444*, *EWSR1-PBX1*, or *EWSR1-POU5F1* fusions

Myxofibrosarcoma

- Very rare as primary pulmonary tumor
- Abundant myxoid matrix
- Lacks reticulated cell cords
- Nuclear pleomorphism
- Curvilinear, thin-walled vascular pattern

Myxoid Liposarcoma

- Very rare as primary pulmonary tumor
- Abundant myxoid matrix
- Ovoid to spindle cells
- Lipoblasts
- Chicken-wire vascular pattern
- *FUS-DDIT3* or *EWSR1-DDIT3* fusion

Myxoid Leiomyosarcoma

- Very rare as primary pulmonary tumor
- Long fascicles of spindle cells
- Blunt-ended nuclei
- Eosinophilic fibrillary cytoplasm
- SMA(+); variable desmin (+)

DIAGNOSTIC CHECKLIST

Clinically Relevant Pathologic Features

- Mean age: 45 years

Pathologic Interpretation Pearls

- Associated with bronchus
- Usually forms endobronchial mass
- Abundant myxoid matrix
- Interconnecting cords of cell
- Chronic inflammation and fibrosis
- No distinct immunophenotype
- *EWSR1-CREB1* fusion

SELECTED REFERENCES

1. Agaimy A et al: EWSR1-fusion-negative, SMARCB1-deficient primary pulmonary myxoid sarcoma. Pol J Pathol. 68(3):261-7, 2017
2. Kim S et al: Primary pulmonary myxoid sarcoma located in interlobar fissure without parenchymal invasion. Thorac Cancer. 8(5):535-8, 2017
3. Yanagida R et al: Primary pulmonary myxoid sarcoma, a potential mimic of metastatic extraskeletal myxoid chondrosarcoma. Pathology. 49(7):792-94, 2017
4. Fisher C: The diversity of soft tissue tumours with EWSR1 gene rearrangements: a review. Histopathology. 64(1):134-50, 2014
5. Jeon YK et al: Primary pulmonary myxoid sarcomas with EWSR1-CREB1 translocation might originate from primitive peribronchial mesenchymal cells undergoing (myo)fibroblastic differentiation. Virchows Arch. 465(4):453-61, 2014
6. Shen W et al: Primary pulmonary leiomyosarcoma. J Chin Med Assoc. 77(1):49-51, 2014
7. Smith SC et al: At the intersection of primary pulmonary myxoid sarcoma and pulmonary angiomatoid fibrous histiocytoma: observations from three new cases. Histopathology. 65(1):144-6, 2014
8. Matsukuma S et al: Primary pulmonary myxoid sarcoma with EWSR1-CREB1 fusion, resembling extraskeletal myxoid chondrosarcoma: case report with a review of Literature. Pathol Int. 62(12):817-22, 2012
9. Son C et al: Primary Pulmonary myxoid liposarcoma with translocation t(12;16)(q13;p11) in a young female patient: a brief case report. Korean J Pathol. 46(4):392-4, 2012
10. Thway K et al: Tumors with EWSR1-CREB1 and EWSR1-ATF1 fusions: the current status. Am J Surg Pathol. 36(7):e1-e11, 2012
11. Thway K et al: Endobronchial pulmonary angiomatoid fibrous histiocytoma: two cases with EWSR1-CREB1 and EWSR1-ATF1 fusions. Am J Surg Pathol. 36(6):883-8, 2012
12. Zhou Q et al: Extraskeletal myxoid chondrosarcoma in the lung: asymptomatic lung mass with severe anemia. Diagn Pathol. 7:112, 2012
13. Chen G et al: Angiomatoid fibrous histiocytoma: unusual sites and unusual morphology. Mod Pathol. 24(12):1560-70, 2011
14. Hasanoğlu HC et al: A mass of myxofibrosarcoma in the lung. Tuberk Toraks. 59(1):73-6, 2011
15. Thway K et al: Primary pulmonary myxoid sarcoma with EWSR1-CREB1 fusion: a new tumor entity. Am J Surg Pathol. 35(11):1722-32, 2011
16. Kourda J et al: Benign myoepithelioma of the lung - a case report and review of the literature. Cases J. 3(1):25, 2010
17. Inayama Y et al: Low-grade pulmonary myxoid sarcoma of uncertain histogenesis. Pathol Int. 51(3):204-10, 2001
18. Nicholson AG et al: Malignant myxoid endobronchial tumour: a report of two cases with a unique histological pattern. Histopathology. 35(4):313-8, 1999

Primary Pulmonary Myxoid Sarcoma

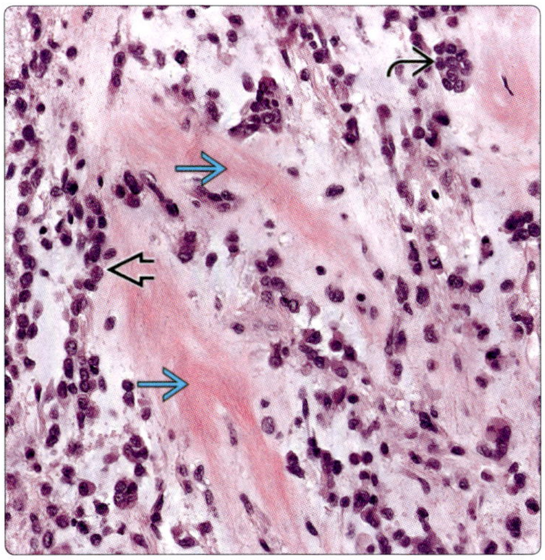

Fibrosis and Chronic Inflammation

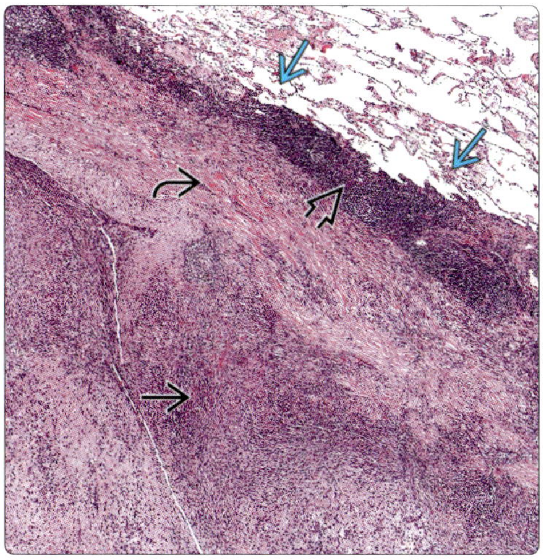

(Left) *This micrograph depicts classic features of PPMS. The neoplastic cells have round to ovoid nuclei and eosinophilic cytoplasm and are arranged in cords ➞, clusters ➞, and single cells. There is abundant pale blue myxoid matrix and bundles of collagen ➞.* **(Right)** *Fibrosis and chronic inflammation are present in most PPMSs. In this example, a neoplastic area ➞ is surrounded by a peripheral rind of dense collagen ➞, which is surrounded by a band of chronic inflammatory cells ➞. Note the sharp interface with adjacent lung ➞.*

Epithelioid Cells

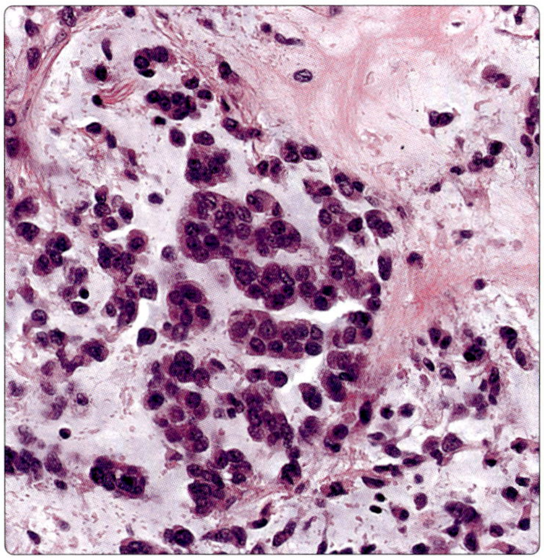

Spindle Cells

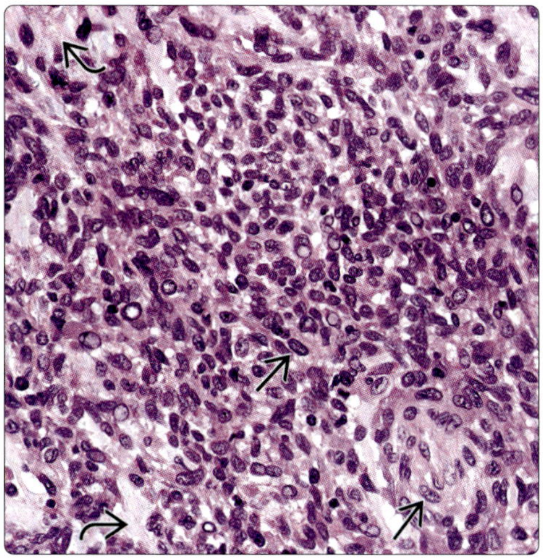

(Left) *The neoplastic cells in PPMS typically have low-grade cytological features and low mitotic activity. They range from epithelioid to spindle and stellate cells. This high-power micrograph depicts clusters of epithelioid cells with round, vesicular nuclei and abundant eosinophilic cytoplasm.* **(Right)** *The neoplastic cells in PPMS are often spindle-shaped with elongated nuclei ➞ and extended tails of eosinophilic cytoplasm. This area has only a small amount of myxoid matrix ➞.*

Solid Area

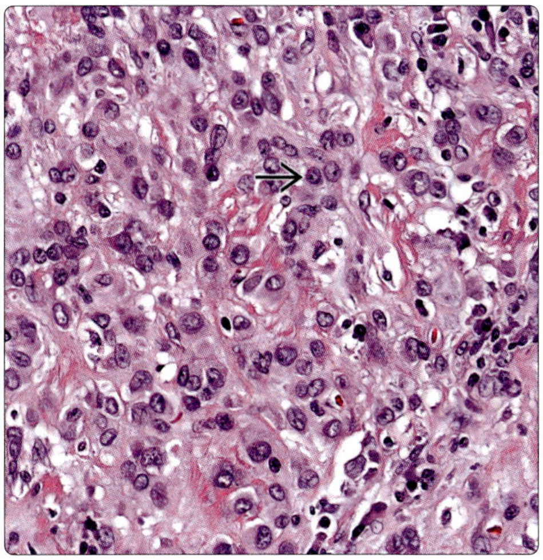

EMA

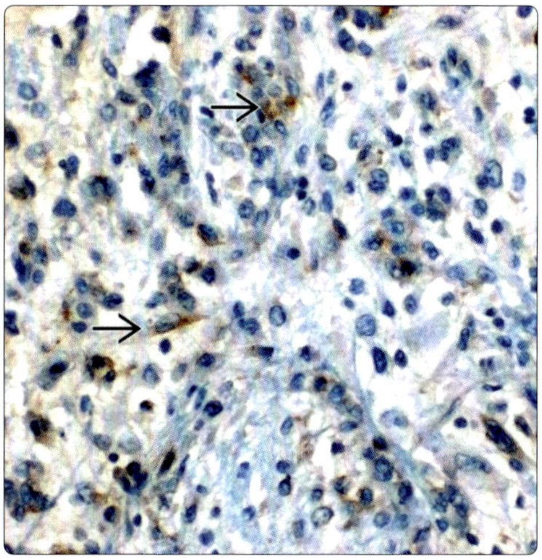

(Left) *Solid areas consisting of closely spaced neoplastic cells with little intervening matrix usually account for a minor component in PPMS. In this case, the cells are large epithelioid cells with abundant cytoplasm and vesicular, round nuclei ➞.* **(Right)** *There is no specific immunohistochemical marker for PPMS, which is negative for most markers other than vimentin. Focal EMA staining ➞, which is often weakly positive, is common. (Courtesy S. Smith, MD.)*

Biphenotypic Sinonasal Sarcoma

KEY FACTS

TERMINOLOGY

- Synonym: Low-grade sinonasal sarcoma with neural and myogenic features
- Definition: Rare, distinctive sarcoma of sinonasal tract that shows neural and myogenic differentiation and is characterized by unique t(2;4) chromosomal translocation

CLINICAL ISSUES

- Middle-aged women most commonly affected
- Most arise in nasal cavity &/or ethmoid sinus
- Present with obstructive symptoms
- Treatment: Complete surgical resection
- Prognosis
  - Local recurrence in 44%
  - No reported cases of metastases or death from disease

MICROSCOPIC

- Poorly circumscribed, unencapsulated, infiltrative
- Highly cellular proliferation of monomorphic spindle cells
  - Fascicular growth with "herringbone" architecture common
  - Uniform, elongated nuclei, often overlapping
- Most cases associated with benign epithelial component
- Rhabdomyoblastic elements in subset
- Mitotic figures, necrosis, hemorrhage rare

ANCILLARY TESTS

- Variable S100 protein (+), SMA(+), MSA(+) in most cases
- Subset contain myogenin (+) cells
- Molecular: Recurrent t(2;4)(q35;q31) resulting in *PAX3-MAML3* fusion

TOP DIFFERENTIAL DIAGNOSES

- Synovial sarcoma
- Malignant peripheral nerve sheath tumor with rhabdomyoblastic differentiation
- Solitary fibrous tumor
- Spindle cell rhabdomyosarcoma

(Left) *Biphenotypic sinonasal sarcoma (SNS) is a distinctive sinonasal tumor that most commonly arises in middle-aged women. The sarcomas are infiltrative and poorly circumscribed spindle cell neoplasms and often contain invaginations of benign surface respiratory epithelium (not shown).* **(Right)** *A fascicular growth pattern is a common feature of biphenotypic SNS, as depicted. A herringbone architecture such as that seen in fibrosarcomatous DFSP and several other sarcomas is also a frequent finding.*

Biphenotypic Sinonasal Sarcoma

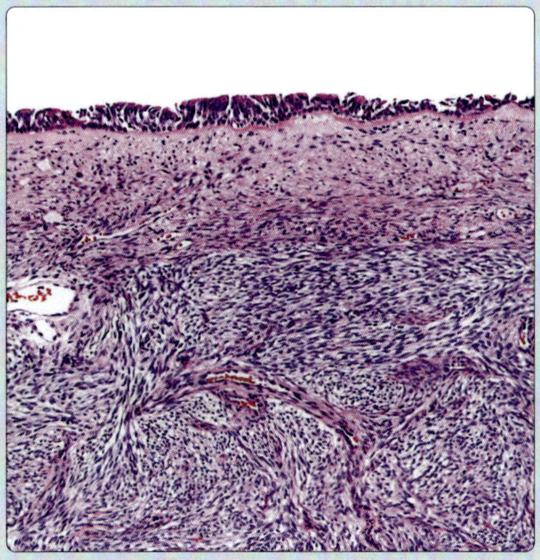

Cellular, Fascicular Growth

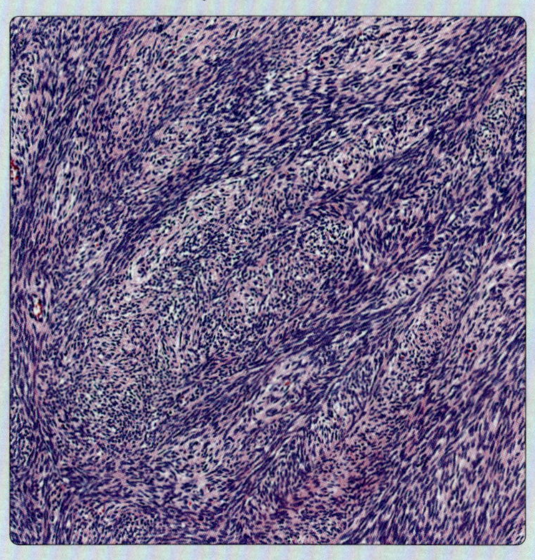

(Left) *The tumor cells of biphenotypic SNS are uniform, elongated, and lack nuclear pleomorphism. A wavy or neural-like cytologic appearance may be evident in some cases. Mitotic activity is typically very low.* **(Right)** *S100 protein expression is characteristic of biphenotypic SNS. Notably, SOX10 expression is absent, which suggests that these tumors may not actually feature partial neural derivation. Vascular elements ➩ are negative for S100 in this image.*

Uniform Cytologic Features

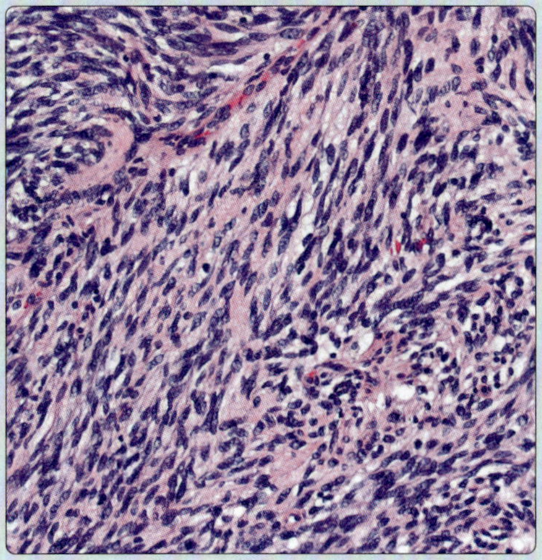

S100 Protein Expression

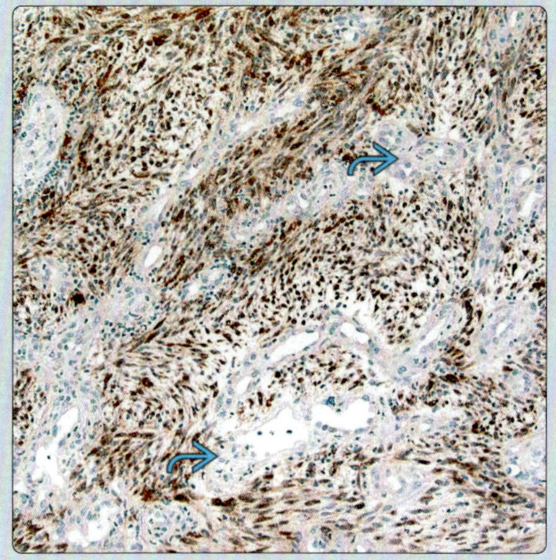

TERMINOLOGY

Abbreviations

- Biphenotypic sinonasal sarcoma (SNS)

Synonyms

- Low-grade sinonasal sarcoma with neural and myogenic features

Definitions

- Rare, distinctive sarcoma of sinonasal tract that shows evidence of neural and myogenic differentiation and is characterized by *PAX3* rearrangements

CLINICAL ISSUES

Epidemiology

- Incidence
  - Rare; incidence likely underestimated due to lack of recognition
- Age
  - Mean: 52 years (range: 24-85 years)
- Sex
  - 3:1 female predominance

Site

- Most arise in nasal cavity &/or ethmoid sinus
  - May extend to involve orbit, cribriform plate, or rarely cranial vault

Presentation

- Obstructive symptoms
- Pain may or may not be present
- No reported associations with neurofibromatosis

Treatment

- Complete surgical resection

Prognosis

- Limited data
  - Local recurrence in 44%
  - No reported cases of metastases or death from disease

MACROSCOPIC

Size

- Often 2-4 cm

MICROSCOPIC

Histologic Features

- Poorly circumscribed, unencapsulated
- Infiltrative growth
- Highly cellular proliferation of monomorphic spindle cells
  - Fascicular growth + herringbone architecture common
  - Uniform, elongated nuclei, often overlapping
    - May appear wavy or buckled
- Delicate stromal collagen present but often inapparent
- Majority of reported cases associated with benign epithelial component
  - Invaginations of surface-type respiratory epithelium
- Focal rhabdomyoblastic elements in subset of cases
- Stromal vasculature may be prominent and appear to be like hemangiopericytoma
- Mitotic figures rare
- Necrosis, hemorrhage, surface ulceration uncommon

ANCILLARY TESTS

Immunohistochemistry

- S100 protein (+), SMA(+), calponin (+), desmin (+/-)
  - Expression may be focal, patchy, or diffuse
- Nuclear β-catenin (+)
- Negative for keratin, SOX10, CD34, TLE1
- Subset of cases feature desmin &/or myogenin (+) cells

Molecular Genetics

- Distinctive recurrent t(2;4)(q35;q31) resulting in *PAX3-MAML3* fusion
- Also, *PAX3-NCOA1* and *PAX3-FOXO1* fusions reported
  - *PAX3-NCOA1* tumors associated with rhabdomyoblastic differentiation

DIFFERENTIAL DIAGNOSIS

Synovial Sarcoma

- May show significant morphologic overlap with biphenotypic SNS
- Keratin (+); TLE1(+); negative for myogenic markers
- Characteristic t(X;18) involving *SS18* (SYT)

Malignant Peripheral Nerve Sheath Tumor With Rhabdomyoblastic Differentiation

- Usually shows variations in cellularity and conspicuous nuclear pleomorphism, mitoses, and necrosis
- May arise from demonstrable nerve or in setting of neurofibromatosis
- Usually negative for SMA and MSA
- Lacks genetic features of biphenotypic SNS

Solitary Fibrous Tumor

- Characteristic ectatic, "staghorn" vasculature
- Thick bands of stromal collagen common
- Diffuse CD34(+), STAT6(+)

Spindle Cell Rhabdomyosarcoma

- Can show significant morphologic overlap with biphenotypic SNS
- Negative for S100 protein
- Lacks genetic features of biphenotypic SNS

SELECTED REFERENCES

1. Kakkar A et al: Biphenotypic sinonasal sarcoma: a series of six cases with evaluation of role of β-catenin immunohistochemistry in differential diagnosis. Ann Diagn Pathol. 33:6-10, 2018
2. Cannon RB et al: Imaging and outcomes for a new entity: low-grade sinonasal sarcoma with neural and myogenic features. J Neurol Surg Rep. 78(1):e15-e19, 2017
3. Huang SC et al: Novel PAX3-NCOA1 Fusions in biphenotypic sinonasal sarcoma with focal rhabdomyoblastic differentiation. Am J Surg Pathol. 40(1):51-9, 2016
4. Rooper LM et al: Biphenotypic sinonasal sarcoma: an expanded immunoprofile including consistent nuclear beta-catenin positivity and absence of SOX10 expression. Hum Pathol. 55:44-50, 2016
5. Wang X et al: Recurrent PAX3-MAML3 fusion in biphenotypic sinonasal sarcoma. Nat Genet. 46(7):666-8, 2014
6. Lewis JT et al: Low-grade sinonasal sarcoma with neural and myogenic features: a clinicopathologic analysis of 28 cases. Am J Surg Pathol. 36(4):517-25, 2012

Surface Epithelial Invaginations

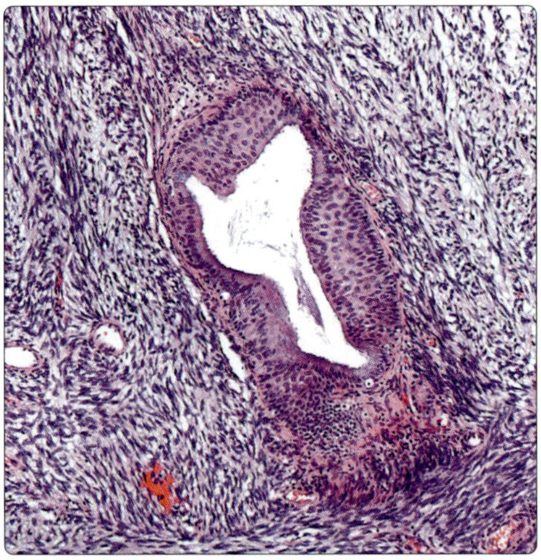

Prominent Sinonasal Epithelium

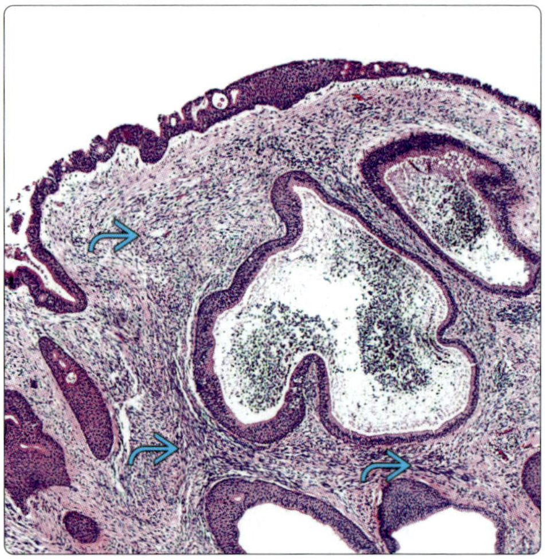

(Left) *A common finding in biphenotypic SNS is the presence of invaginations of surface epithelium within the tumor, at least focally. The appearance may lead to confusion with a biphasic synovial sarcoma.* **(Right)** *Surface sinonasal epithelium may be prominent in tissue samples of biphenotypic sinonasal sarcoma, somewhat overshadowing the actual neoplastic spindle cells.*

Stromal Vasculature

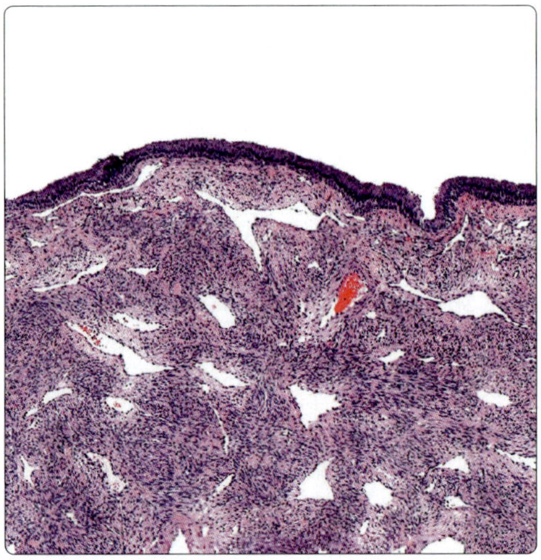

Infiltration of Bone

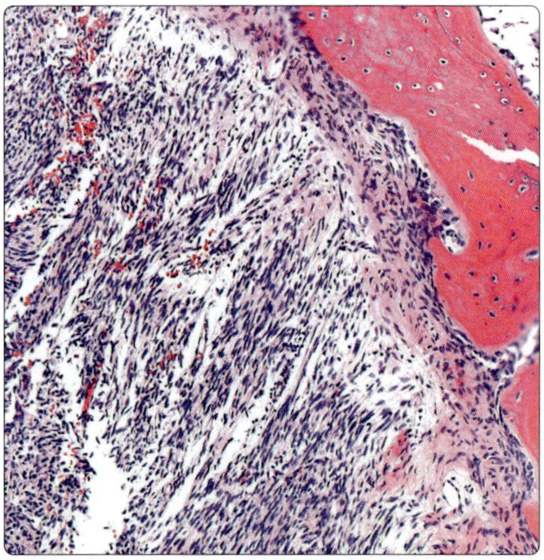

(Left) *A prominent hemangiopericytoma-like vascular pattern, as shown in this image, can be present in a subset of cases of biphenotypic SNS, lending morphologic overlap with solitary fibrous tumor.* **(Right)** *Bone invasion by tumor cells may be seen in up to 20% of cases of biphenotypic SNS. Extension into the orbit is one of the more frequent events.*

Stromal Collagen

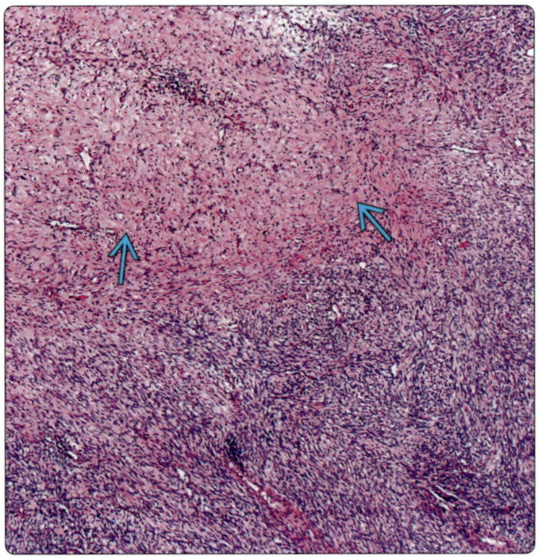

Hemorrhage

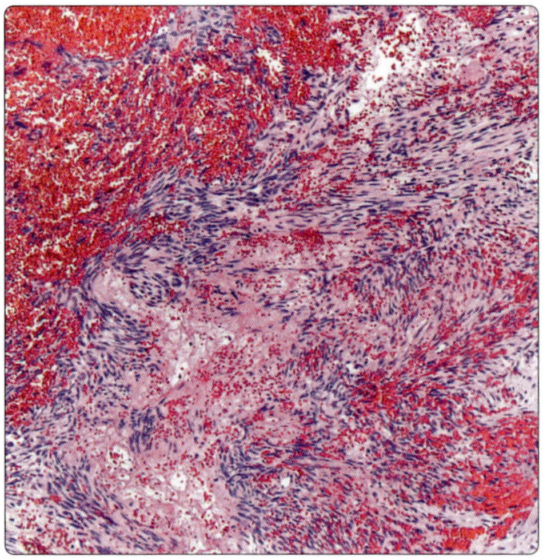

(Left) *Similar to synovial sarcoma, stromal collagen may be difficult to appreciate in cellular examples of biphenotypic SNS. In less cellular zones, however, prominent collagen can resemble a benign fibroblastic neoplasm.* **(Right)** *Stromal hemorrhage (shown) and surface ulceration can be seen in biphenotypic SNS, though neither feature is common. Necrosis is usually absent as well.*

SMA Expression

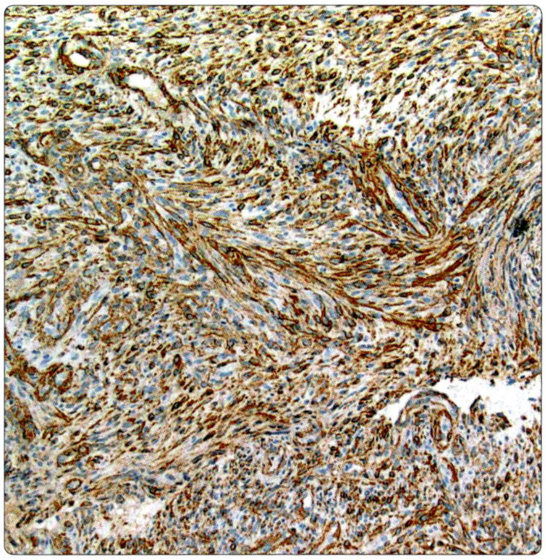

Desmin Expression

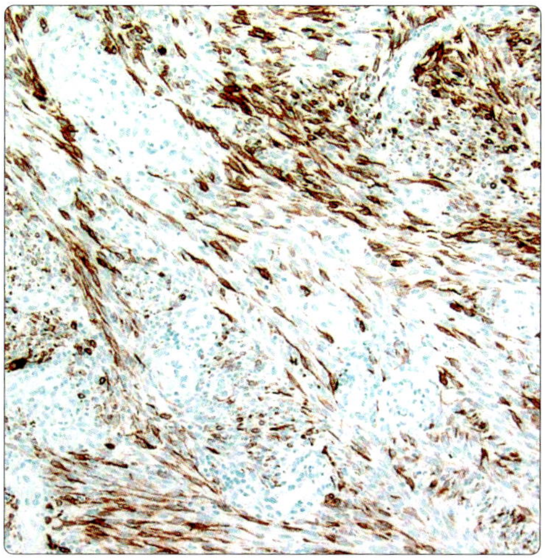

(Left) *SMA expression is characteristic of biphenotypic SNS and is classically coexpressed with S100 protein. This immunophenotype gave rise to the original name for this tumor: Low-grade sinonasal sarcoma with neural and myogenic features.* **(Right)** *Biphenotypic SNS can show expression of desmin in a small subset of cases; however, the positivity is likely to be focal.*

Cytokeratin Immunostain

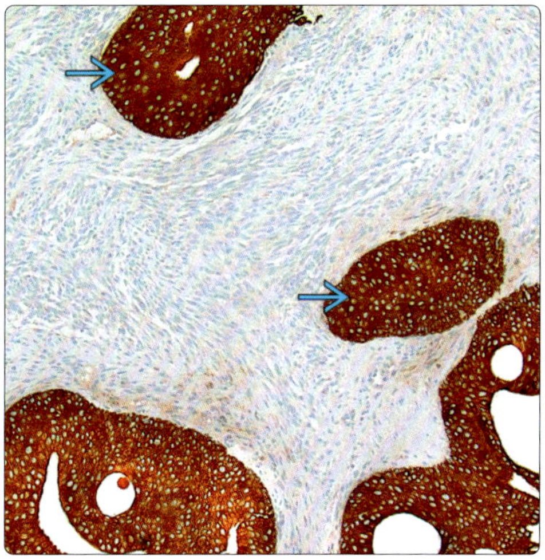

Rhabdomyoblasts

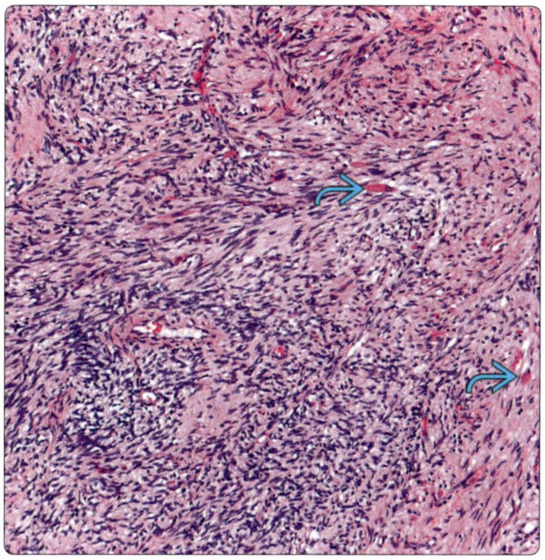

(Left) *Keratin immunostains are negative in the lesional cells of biphenotypic SNS. Entrapped epithelial elements* [arrow] *serve as a prominent internal control.* **(Right)** *A subset of cases of biphenotypic SNS contain rhabdomyoblastic elements* [curved arrow]*. This finding may be related to the presence of a PAX3-NCOA1 gene fusion in these variant tumors.*

Rhabdomyoblasts

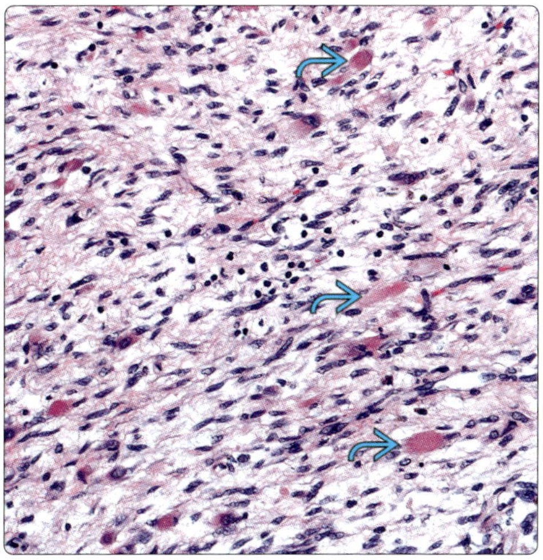

Myogenin Expression

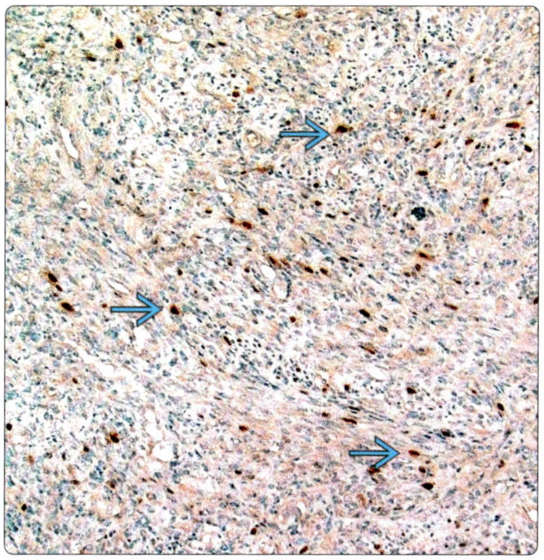

(Left) *Rhabdomyoblastic elements* [curved arrow] *may be focally prominent in biphenotypic SNS and, in conjunction with loose stroma, may resemble embryonal rhabdomyosarcoma.* **(Right)** *Nuclear expression* [arrow] *of myogenin is seen in a subset of cases of biphenotypic SNS and is often focal. Morphologically distinct rhabdomyoblastic elements may or may not be readily identifiable.*

Spindle Epithelial Tumor With Thymus-Like Differentiation

KEY FACTS

TERMINOLOGY

- Spindle epithelial tumor with thymus-like differentiation (SETTLE)
- Low-grade, often biphasic malignant neoplasm showing evidence of primitive thymic differentiation

CLINICAL ISSUES

- Most common in children and young adults (mean: 19 years)
- Affects thyroid or perithyroidal soft tissues
- Often presents as painless, slow-growing neck mass or enlarged thyroid
- Treatment: Complete surgical resection
- Metastases occur in 25% of cases, often after many years
    - Indefinite, long-term clinical follow-up recommended
- Overall reported survival rate 83% at 5 years

MACROSCOPIC

- Range: 1-12 cm (mean: 3.6 cm)

MICROSCOPIC

- Moderately to highly cellular neoplasm, usually with biphasic morphology
    - Fascicles, bands, and sheets of uniform spindled cells
    - Glands, cysts, cords, nests, tubules, or papillary structures
- Oval to round monomorphic nuclei with fine chromatin
- Stromal hyalinization very common
- Mitoses &/or necrosis rare

ANCILLARY TESTS

- Keratin (+), EMA(+), CK7(+) in spindled and epithelial cells
- S100 protein (-), CD34(-), CK20(-), CD5(-), TTF-1(-)

TOP DIFFERENTIAL DIAGNOSES

- Synovial sarcoma
- Solitary fibrous tumor
- Spindle cell carcinoma

Spindle Epithelial Tumor With Thymus-Like Differentiation

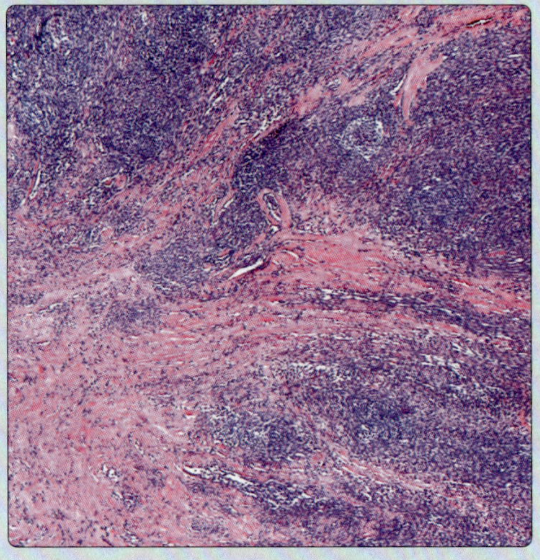

Stromal Sclerosis

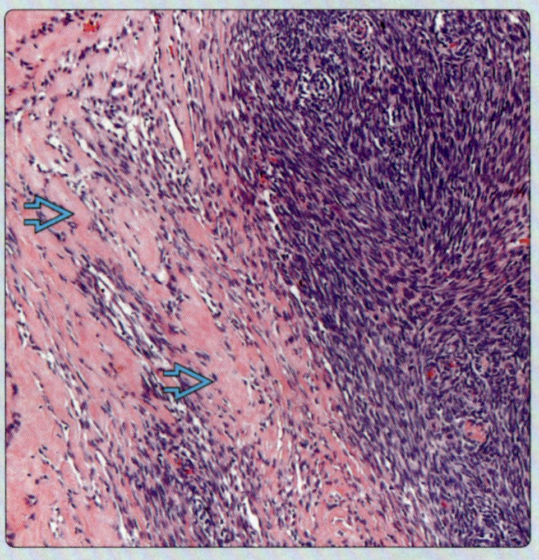

(Left) *Spindle epithelial tumor with thymus-like differentiation (SETTLE) is a low-grade malignancy of the thyroid that generally shows moderate to high cellularity and vague lobules of spindled cells separated by hyalinized fibrous stroma.* **(Right)** *The morphologic appearance of SETTLE is characterized by cellular sheets and fascicles of monomorphic spindle cells, very similar to synovial sarcoma. Of note, stromal sclerosis ⇨ is more common and more abundant in SETTLE.*

Epithelial Structures

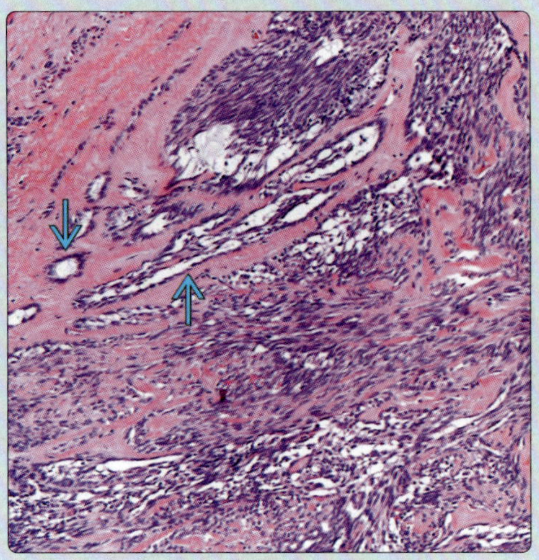

Uniform Cytologic Features

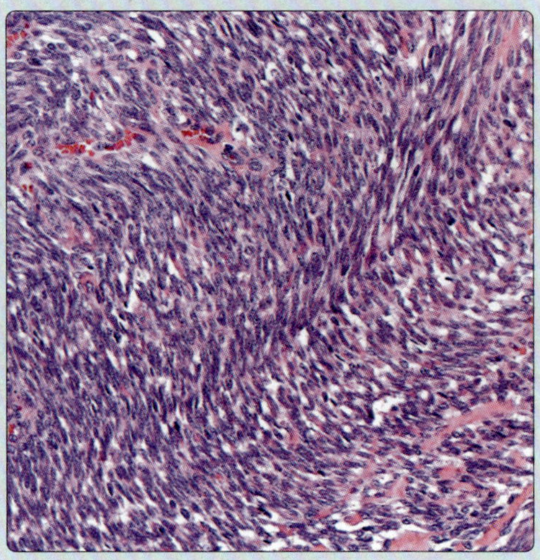

(Left) *The spindled component of SETTLE often blends imperceptibly into epithelial structures ⇨, such as glands, tubules, and papillary structures. Ciliated or mucinous epithelium may also be seen. Squamous metaplasia is rare.* **(Right)** *The tumor cells in SETTLE are cytologically uniform and show round to elongated nuclei with fine chromatin. Mitoses are generally rare.*

TERMINOLOGY

Abbreviations

- Spindle epithelial tumor with thymus-like differentiation (SETTLE)

Definitions

- Low-grade, often biphasic malignant neoplasm showing evidence of primitive thymic differentiation

ETIOLOGY/PATHOGENESIS

Pathogenesis

- Intrathyroidal ectopic thymic tissue
- Remnants of branchial pouches that retained ability to differentiate into thymic-type tumor

CLINICAL ISSUES

Epidemiology

- Incidence
  - Very rare
- Age
  - Most common in children and young adults (mean: 19 years)
    - May be congenital
    - Rarely occurs in adults > 30 years
- Sex
  - Slight male predominance

Site

- Thyroid
  - Right lobe more common (59%)
- Very rarely in soft tissues of neck, adjacent to thyroid

Presentation

- Often painless, slow-growing neck mass or enlarged thyroid
  - Mass may be present for many years before diagnosis is sought
- Usually unilateral; rarely bilateral
- Metastases may be present at time of presentation

Treatment

- Complete surgical resection (partial or complete thyroidectomy)
- Long-term clinical follow-up recommended to monitor for metastatic disease
- Chemotherapy &/or radiotherapy may be utilized in setting of metastatic disease

Prognosis

- Overall reported survival rate: 83% at 5 years
- Metastases occur in 25% of cases, often after many years
  - Rate appears higher with follow-up > 5 years
  - Cervical lymph nodes, lung, mediastinum most common sites

MACROSCOPIC

General Features

- Vaguely lobulated, circumscribed, or infiltrative
- Firm, usually solid, gray-white cut surface

Size

- Range: 1-12 cm (mean: 3.6 cm)

MICROSCOPIC

Histologic Features

- Often peripherally infiltrative
- Moderately to highly cellular
- Most show biphasic morphology
  - Fascicles, bands, and sheets of uniform spindled cells
    - May appear myxoid/reticular
  - Epithelial component
    - Glands, cysts, cords, nests, tubules, or papillary structures
      - May be ciliated, mucinous, or show focal squamous metaplasia
    - Intraluminal necrotic debris rare
  - Rare cases are monophasic
- Oval to round monomorphic nuclei with fine chromatin
- Stromal hyalinization very common
- Mitoses &/or necrosis rare

ANCILLARY TESTS

Immunohistochemistry

- Keratin (+), EMA(+), CK7(+) in both spindled and epithelial cells
  - Diffuse high-molecular-weight keratin and CK7
  - Often focal low-molecular-weight keratin and EMA
- Also CD117(+)
- S100 protein (-), CD34(-), CK20(-), CD5(-), TTF-1(-)
- Usually TLE1(-) [may rarely be (+)]

DIFFERENTIAL DIAGNOSIS

Synovial Sarcoma

- Less elaborate array of epithelial structures than is seen in SETTLE
- Usually less prominent stromal hyalinization than is seen in SETTLE
- Characteristic t(X;18) with *SS18* (SYT) gene arrangement

Solitary Fibrous Tumor

- Patternless growth pattern
- Prominent ectatic staghorn vascular pattern
- CD34(+), STAT6(+)

Spindle Cell Carcinoma

- Usually affects older age group than SETTLE
- Malignant cytologic features, often with mitotic activity

SELECTED REFERENCES

1. Ippolito S et al: Spindle epithelial tumor with thymus-like differentiation (SETTLE): clinical-pathological features, differential pathological diagnosis and therapy. Endocrine. 51(3):402-12, 2016
2. Recondo G Jr et al: Spindle epithelial tumor with thymus-like differentiation: a case report and comprehensive review of the literature and treatment options. Head Neck. 37(5):746-54, 2014
3. Folpe AL et al: Spindle epithelial tumor with thymus-like differentiation: a morphologic, immunohistochemical, and molecular genetic study of 11 cases. Am J Surg Pathol. 33(8):1179-86, 2009
4. Grushka JR et al: Spindle epithelial tumor with thymus-like elements of the thyroid: a multi-institutional case series and review of the literature. J Pediatr Surg. 44(5):944-8, 2009

Low-Grade Endometrial Stromal Sarcoma

KEY FACTS

TERMINOLOGY

- Malignant tumor composed of cells that resemble those of proliferative endometrium

CLINICAL ISSUES

- Peak incidence in 4th-5th decades
- Can present as intraabdominal soft tissue tumor
  - Extends from uterus or arises in endometriosis
- Mass or abdominal distension
- Wide differential diagnosis

MACROSCOPIC

- Often shows worm-like configuration of large vessel involvement

MICROSCOPIC

- Sheets of uniform ovoid cells
- Minimal nuclear atypia
- Minimal cytoplasm
- Plexiform vascular pattern
- Associated endometriosis in some cases
- Focal smooth muscle differentiation in some

ANCILLARY TESTS

- Diffuse CD10(+) in most
- Diffuse ER(+) and PR(+)
- Desmin and SMA are typically focally positive with increased positivity in fibrous or mixed variants
- Molecular: Rearrangements involving *JAZF1*, *SUZ12*, or *PHF1*

TOP DIFFERENTIAL DIAGNOSES

- Synovial sarcoma
- Ewing sarcoma
- Desmoplastic small round cell tumor
- Smooth muscle neoplasm
- Solitary fibrous tumor
- Gastrointestinal stromal tumor

(Left) *At low power, endometrial stromal sarcoma (ESS) is a multilobulated, highly cellular tumor composed of islands of ovoid cells with scant cytoplasm, some in vessels* ➔. **(Right)** *At higher power, the cells of ESS contain bland, vesicular nuclei and small amounts of amphophilic cytoplasm. The mitotic index can be high, although this is not thought to alter prognosis. The stroma here is fibrous, but it can also be myxoid.*

Endometrial Stromal Sarcoma

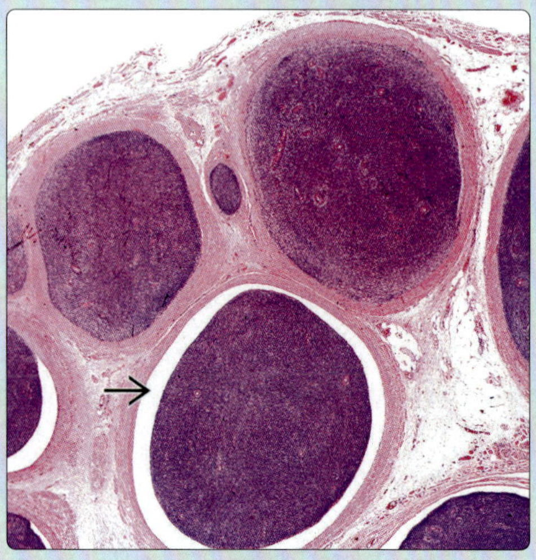

Cytologic Features

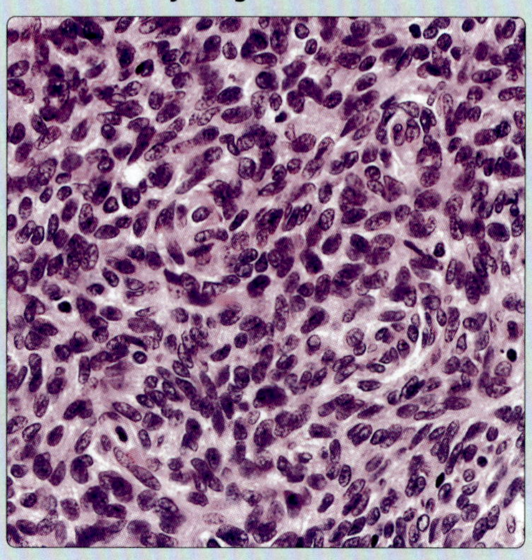

(Left) *Medium-power view of ESS shows the homogeneous appearance of the small spindled cells. Note the numerous curvilinear arterioles that are spread evenly throughout the tumor* ➔. *These thin vessels set ESS apart from smooth muscle tumors, which have thick-walled vessels.* **(Right)** *Lymphovascular space invasion* ➔ *can be found in nearly every case of ESS and can be a helpful feature in differentiating ESS from endometrial stromal nodule and smooth muscle tumors.*

Characteristic Vasculature

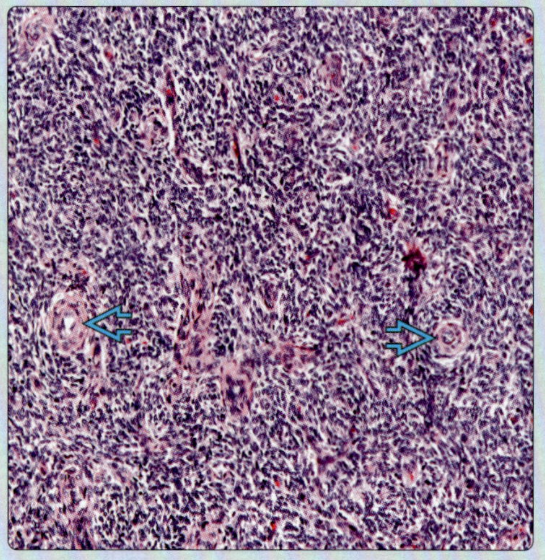

Lymphovascular Invasion

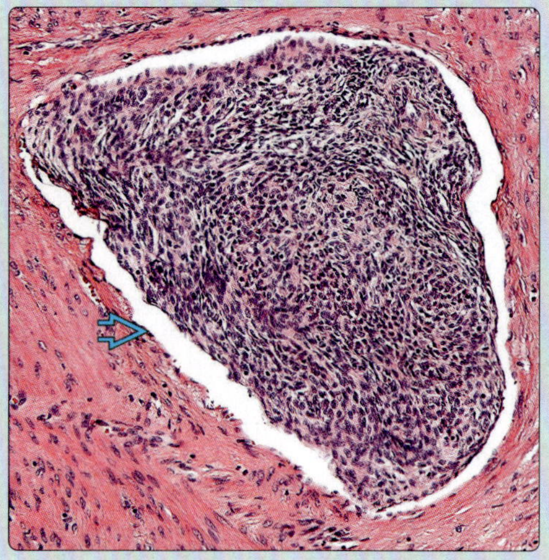

TERMINOLOGY

Abbreviations

- Endometrial stromal sarcoma (ESS)

Synonyms

- Endolymphatic stromal myosis
- Low-grade stromal sarcoma

Definitions

- Malignant mesenchymal tumor composed of cells that resemble those of proliferative endometrium

CLINICAL ISSUES

Epidemiology

- Age
  - Peak incidence in 4th-5th decades

Site

- Most tumors are intrauterine (arise from endometrium)
  - May extend to parametria or abdomen, especially through vascular channels
- Some arise in extrauterine sites, usually associated with endometriosis

Presentation

- Painful or painless intraabdominal mass

Prognosis

- Although tumor is low grade, there may be recurrence in ~ 1/3 of patients
- Distant metastases and death in smaller percentage

MACROSCOPIC

General Features

- Solid, white to yellow cut surface that typically presents as polypoid mass, intramural nodules, or thickened myometrium
- Occasional tumors contain cystic degeneration, hemorrhage, and necrosis
- Tumor often has worm-like configuration of tumor processes in vessels

MICROSCOPIC

Histologic Features

- Monotonous sheets of small cells with ovoid to round nuclei, vesicular chromatin, and scant cytoplasm
  - Cells have minimal nuclear atypia but are typically mitotically active
- Characteristic vascular pattern that recapitulates endometrial spiral arterioles
- Stroma can be focally fibrous or myxoid or may show smooth muscle differentiation
- Small tubules or other sex cord-stromal tumor elements may be present
- Residual or associated endometriosis in some cases, especially extrauterine sites
- Marked nuclear pleomorphism is seen in clinically aggressive, high-grade tumors

ANCILLARY TESTS

Immunohistochemistry

- Diffuse CD10(+) in majority
- Diffuse nuclear ER(+) and PR(+)
- Variable, focal desmin (+) and SMA(+)
  - Often increased expression in fibrous or mixed variants
- H-caldesmon and keratin (-)

Molecular Genetics

- *JAZF1-SUZ12* (formerly *JAZF1*-JJAZ1) fusions most common in low-grade tumors
  - Rearrangements involving *PHF1* less common
- *YWHAE-NUTM2A/B* fusion associated with higher grade tumors

DIFFERENTIAL DIAGNOSIS

Synovial Sarcoma

- Can be biphasic
- Short ovoid nuclei with overlapping nuclei
- CK(+), EMA(+), TLE1(+)
- Characteristic t(X;18) involving *SS18*(*SYT*)

Ewing Sarcoma

- Younger age group
- Sheets of rounded cells
- Diffuse CD99(+) in membranous distribution
- Various rearrangements involving *EWSR1* gene

Desmoplastic Small Round Cell Tumor

- Adolescent age group
- Islands of small cells in desmoplastic stroma
- CK(+), desmin (+), WT1(+)
- Characteristic t(11;22) with *EWSR1-WT1* gene fusion

Endometrial Stromal Nodule

- Histologically identical to ESS but lacks infiltrative borders

Smooth Muscle Neoplasm

- Prominently eosinophilic spindle cells with blunt-ended nuclei
- Diffuse desmin, H-caldesmon, and SMA expression

Solitary Fibrous Tumor

- Variable cellular and fibrous areas with hemangiopericytomatous pattern
- Diffuse CD34(+)

Gastrointestinal Stromal Tumor

- Usually monomorphic spindled or epithelioid cells
- Diffuse CD117(+) &/or DOG1(+)

SELECTED REFERENCES

1. Lee CH et al: Endometrial stromal sarcoma-the new genetic paradigm. Histopathology. 67(1):1-19, 2015
2. Conklin CM et al: Endometrial stromal tumors: the new WHO classification. Adv Anat Pathol. 21(6):383-93, 2014
3. Lee CH et al: Cyclin D1 as a diagnostic immunomarker for endometrial stromal sarcoma with YWHAE-FAM22 rearrangement. Am J Surg Pathol. 36(10):1562-70, 2012
4. Chiang S et al: Frequency of known gene rearrangements in endometrial stromal tumors. Am J Surg Pathol. 35(9):1364-72, 2011
5. Oliva E et al: Endometrial stromal tumors: an update on a group of tumors with a protean phenotype. Adv Anat Pathol. 7(5):257-81, 2000

INDEX

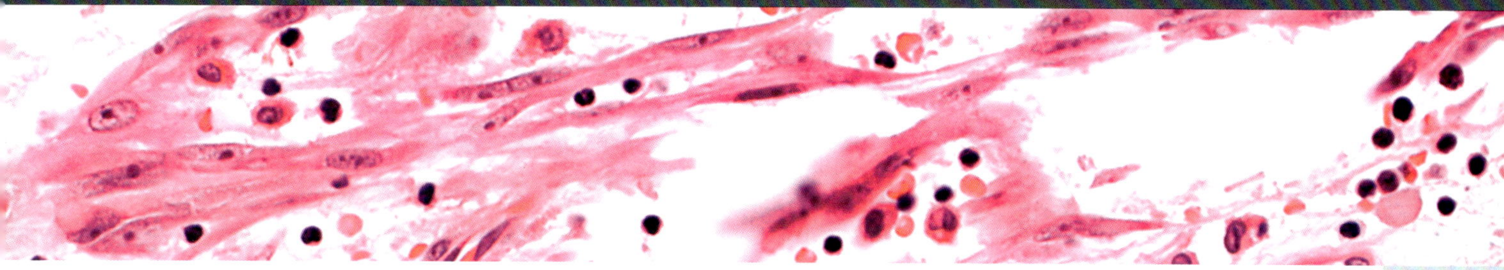

A

Abdominopelvic sarcoma of perivascular epithelioid cells. *See* Perivascular epithelioid cell tumor.
Abrikossoff tumor. *See* Granular cell tumor.
Acquired smooth muscle "hamartoma" of scrotum, smooth muscle hamartoma vs., **333**
Acquired tufted angioma, **436–437**
- diagnostic checklist, **437**
- differential diagnosis, **437**
- Kaposi sarcoma vs., **478**
- kaposiform hemangioendothelioma vs., **455**
- prognosis, **437**
Acquired tufted hemangioma, glomeruloid hemangioma vs., **443**
Acral fibrokeratoma, storiform collagenoma vs., **161**
Acral fibromyxoma, **624–625**
- dermal nerve sheath myxoma vs., **547**
- differential diagnosis, **625**
- inclusion body fibromatosis vs., **251**
- prognosis, **625**
Acral myxoinflammatory fibroblastic sarcoma. *See* Myxoinflammatory fibroblastic sarcoma.
Acroangiodermatitis, Kaposi sarcoma vs., **478**
Adenocarcinoma
- metastatic, adenomatoid tumor vs., **591**
- ovarian serous, malignant mesothelioma vs., **600**
- pulmonary, malignant mesothelioma vs., **600**
Adenomatoid tumor, **590–591**
- differential diagnosis, **591**
- genetic testing, **591**
- multicystic peritoneal mesothelioma vs., **593**
- prognosis, **591**
Adipose tissue, tumors of
- angiolipoma, **56–59**
    diagnostic checklist, **57**
    differential diagnosis, **57**
    prognosis, **57**
- atypical lipomatous tumor/well-differentiated liposarcoma, **88–93**
    differential diagnosis, **90**
    molecular genetics, **90**
    prognosis, **89**
- atypical spindle cell lipomatous tumor, **84–87**
    differential diagnosis, **85**
    molecular genetics, **85**
    prognosis, **85**
- chondroid lipoma, **66–69**
    differential diagnosis, **67**
    genetic testing, **67**
    lipoma vs., **48**
    prognosis, **67**
- dedifferentiated liposarcoma, **94–99**
    differential diagnosis, **96**
    molecular genetics, **96**
    prognosis, **95**
- hibernoma, **74–77**
    differential diagnosis, **75**
    molecular genetics, **75**
    prognosis, **75**
- lipoblastoma, **80–83**
    differential diagnosis, **81**
    molecular genetics, **81**
    prognosis, **81**
- lipoma, **46–51**
    diagnostic checklist, **48**
    differential diagnosis, **48**
    genetic testing, **48**
    prognosis, **47**
    spindle cell, lipoma vs., **48**
- lipomatosis of nerve, **52–53**
    differential diagnosis, **53**
    prognosis, **53**
- myelolipoma, **78–79**
    differential diagnosis, **79**
    molecular genetics, **79**
    prognosis, **79**
- myolipoma, **70–73**
    differential diagnosis, **71**
    prognosis, **71**
- myxoid liposarcoma, **100–105**
    differential diagnosis, **102**
    molecular genetics, **102**
    prognosis, **101**
- pleomorphic liposarcoma, **106–111**
    differential diagnosis, **107–108**
    molecular genetics, **107**
    prognosis, **107**
- spindle cell/pleomorphic lipoma, **60–65**
    differential diagnosis, **62**
    molecular genetics, **61**
    prognosis, **61**
- synovial lipomatosis, **54–55**
    differential diagnosis, **55**
    prognosis, **55**
Adrenocortical adenoma, myelolipoma vs., **79**
Adult-type fibrosarcoma, **214–215**
- differential diagnosis, **215**
- genetic testing, **215**
- prognosis, **215**
- spindle cell rhabdomyosarcoma vs., **394**
Adult-type rhabdomyoma, **372–373**
- cardiac rhabdomyoma vs., **379**

INDEX

- congenital granular cell epulis vs., **799**
- differential diagnosis, **373**
- embryonal rhabdomyosarcoma vs., **382**
- granular cell tumor vs., **542**
- prognosis, **373**

AFH. *See* Angiomatoid fibrous histiocytoma.
AFX. *See* Atypical fibroxanthoma.
Aggressive fibromatosis. *See* Desmoid-type fibromatosis.
ALT/WDLPS. *See* Atypical lipomatous tumor/well-differentiated liposarcoma.
Alveolar rhabdomyosarcoma, **386–391**
- desmoplastic small round cell tumor vs., **701**
- differential diagnosis, **388**
- embryonal rhabdomyosarcoma vs., **382**
- extraskeletal Ewing sarcoma vs., **708**
- malignant gastrointestinal neuroectodermal tumor vs., **778**
- melanotic neuroectodermal tumor of infancy vs., **825**
- neuroblastoma and ganglioneuroblastoma vs., **834**
- pleomorphic rhabdomyosarcoma vs., **401**
- prognosis, **387**
- sclerosing epithelioid fibrosarcoma vs., **234**
- sclerosing rhabdomyosarcoma vs., **397**
- undifferentiated round cell sarcoma with *CIC-DUX4* translocation vs., **729**

Alveolar soft part sarcoma, **684–687**
- adult rhabdomyoma vs., **373**
- alveolar rhabdomyosarcoma vs., **388**
- congenital granular cell epulis vs., **799**
- differential diagnosis, **685**
- granular cell tumor vs., **542**
- molecular genetics, **685**
- paraganglioma vs., **816**
- PEComa vs., **694**
- prognosis, **685**

AMFB. *See* Angiomyofibroblastoma.
Amyloidoma, **782–783**
- differential diagnosis, **783**
- prognosis, **783**

Anaplastic large cell lymphoma
- inflammatory myofibroblastic tumor vs., **198**
- pleomorphic rhabdomyosarcoma vs., **401**

Ancient schwannoma, **510**
Aneurysmal bone cyst of soft tissue, **630–631**
- differential diagnosis, **631**
- molecular genetics, **631**
- myositis ossificans vs., **127**
- prognosis, **631**

Aneurysmal fibrous histiocytoma, angiomatoid fibrous histiocytoma vs., **644**
Angioblastoma
- glomeruloid hemangioma vs., **443**
- of Nakagawa. *See* Acquired tufted angioma.

Angioendothelioma, papillary intralymphatic, **456–457**
- diagnostic checklist, **457**
- differential diagnosis, **457**
- prognosis, **457**
- retiform hemangioendothelioma vs., **459**

Angiofibroma
- cellular, **580–583**
  - angiomyofibroblastoma vs., **577**
  - deep (aggressive) angiomyxoma vs., **585**
  - differential diagnosis, **581**
  - fibroepithelial stromal polyp vs., **575**
  - mammary-type myofibroblastoma vs., **149**
  - prognosis, **581**
  - solitary fibrous tumor vs., **186**
  - spindle cell/pleomorphic lipoma vs., **62**
- giant cell. *See* Solitary fibrous tumor.
- nasopharyngeal, **800–803**
  - differential diagnosis, **802**
  - genetics, **801**
  - prognosis, **801**
  - sinonasal glomangiopericytoma vs., **806**
- pleomorphic fibroma vs., **157**
- of soft tissue, **144–147**
  - differential diagnosis of, **145**
  - lobular capillary hemangioma vs., **421**
  - molecular genetics, **145**
  - solitary fibrous tumor vs., **186**

Angioleiomyoma, **366–367**
- differential diagnosis, **367**
- Epstein-Barr virus-associated smooth muscle tumor vs., **343**
- glomus tumors vs., **354**
- myopericytoma vs., **359**
- prognosis, **367**
- superficial leiomyoma vs., **335**

Angiolipoma, **56–59**
- diagnostic checklist, **57**
- differential diagnosis, **57**
- infiltrating. *See* Angiomatosis.
- intramuscular hemangioma vs., **431**
- prognosis, **57**

Angiolymphoid hyperplasia with eosinophilia. *See* Epithelioid hemangioma.
Angioma
- acquired tufted, **436–437**
  - diagnostic checklist, **437**
  - differential diagnosis, **437**
  - Kaposi sarcoma vs., **478**
  - kaposiform hemangioendothelioma vs., **455**
  - prognosis, **437**
- cherry, sinusoidal hemangioma vs., **441**
- glomeruloid. *See* Glomeruloid hemangioma.
- microcapillary. *See* Microvenular hemangioma.
- tufted
  - congenital hemangioma vs., **414**
  - infantile hemangioma vs., **418**

Angiomatoid fibrous histiocytoma (AFH), **642–649**
- differential diagnosis, **644**
- molecular genetics, **644**
- nodular fasciitis vs., **116**
- primary pulmonary myxoid sarcoma vs., **847**
- prognosis, **643**

Angiomatoid malignant fibrous histiocytoma. *See* Angiomatoid fibrous histiocytoma.
Angiomatosis, **444–445**
- bacillary, **410–411**
  - diagnostic checklist, **411**
  - differential diagnosis, **411**
  - lobular capillary hemangioma vs., **421**

INDEX

prognosis, **411**
- differential diagnosis, **445**
- intramuscular hemangioma vs., **431**
- prognosis, **445**
- systemic. *See* Lymphangioma.

Angiomyofibroblastoma (AMFB), **576–579**
- cellular angiofibroma vs., **581**
- deep (aggressive) angiomyxoma vs., **585**
- differential diagnosis, **577**
- fibroepithelial stromal polyp vs., **575**
- prognosis, **577**

Angiomyofibroblastoma-like tumor, of male genital tract. *See* Cellular angiofibroma.

Angiomyolipoma
- angiolipoma vs., **57**
- extrarenal epithelioid. *See* Perivascular epithelioid cell tumor.
- myolipoma vs., **71**

Angiomyoma. *See* Angioleiomyoma.

Angiomyxoma
- deep (aggressive), **584–587**
  - angiomyofibroblastoma vs., **577**
  - cellular angiofibroma vs., **581**
  - desmoid-type fibromatosis vs., **170**
  - differential diagnosis, **585**
  - fibroepithelial stromal polyp vs., **575**
  - genetic testing, **585**
  - juxtaarticular myxoma vs., **619**
  - prognosis, **585**
  - superficial angiomyxoma vs., **621**
- superficial, **620–623**
  - acral fibromyxoma vs., **625**
  - deep (aggressive) angiomyxoma vs., **585**
  - dermal nerve sheath myxoma vs., **547**
  - differential diagnosis, **621**
  - juxtaarticular myxoma vs., **619**
  - prognosis, **621**

Angiosarcoma, **470–475**
- atypical fibroxanthoma vs., **638**
- dermatofibroma vs., **272**
- differential diagnosis, **472**
- epithelioid
  - epithelioid hemangioendothelioma vs., **468**
  - epithelioid hemangioma vs., **423**
  - epithelioid sarcoma vs., **680**
  - malignant mesothelioma vs., **600**
  - myeloid sarcoma vs., **609**
- giant cell fibroblastoma vs., **261**
- intramuscular hemangioma vs., **431**
- Kaposi sarcoma vs., **478**
- lobular capillary hemangioma vs., **421**
- lymphangioma vs., **448**
- molecular genetics, **472**
- papillary endothelial hyperplasia vs., **409**
- papillary intralymphatic angioendothelioma vs., **457**
- prognosis, **471**
- retiform hemangioendothelioma vs., **459**
- sclerosing rhabdomyosarcoma vs., **397**
- undifferentiated pleomorphic sarcoma vs., **725**
- well-differentiated
  - atypical vascular lesion vs., **453**
  - composite hemangioendothelioma vs., **461**

Antrochoanal polyp, nasopharyngeal angiofibroma vs., **802**

Aponeurotic fibroma, calcifying, **244–247**
- differential diagnosis, **245**
- inclusion body fibromatosis vs., **251**
- prognosis, **245**
- soft tissue chondroma vs., **488**

Arteriovenous hemangioma, sinusoidal hemangioma vs., **441**

Arteriovenous malformation
- papillary endothelial hyperplasia vs., **409**
- sinusoidal hemangioma vs., **441**

ASCLT. *See* Atypical spindle cell lipomatous tumor.

Askin tumor. *See* Extraskeletal Ewing sarcoma.

Atrial myxoma, cardiac fibroma vs., **797**

Atypical decubital fibroplasia. *See* Ischemic fasciitis.

Atypical fibroxanthoma (AFX), **636–641**
- angiosarcoma vs., **472**
- dermatofibroma vs., **272**
- differential diagnosis, **637–638**
- immunohistochemistry, **638**
- pleomorphic fibroma vs., **157**
- prognosis, **637**
- superficial CD34(+) fibroblastic tumor vs., **211**

Atypical intradermal smooth muscle neoplasm, smooth muscle hamartoma vs., **333**

Atypical lipomatous tumor/well-differentiated liposarcoma (ALT/WDLPS), **88–93**
- atypical spindle cell lipomatous tumor vs., **85**
- chondroid lipoma vs., **67**
- differential diagnosis, **90**
- elastofibromas vs., **143**
- hibernoma vs., **75**
- massive localized lymphedema vs., **451**
- molecular genetics, **90**
- myxoid liposarcoma vs., **102**
- pleomorphic liposarcoma vs., **108**
- prognosis, **89**
- spindle cell/pleomorphic lipoma vs., **62**
- synovial lipomatosis vs., **55**

Atypical myxoinflammatory fibroblastic tumor. *See* Myxoinflammatory fibroblastic sarcoma.

Atypical neurofibroma, malignant peripheral nerve sheath tumor vs., **560**

Atypical spindle cell lipoma. *See* Atypical spindle cell lipomatous tumor.

Atypical spindle cell lipomatous tumor (ASCLT), **84–87**
- atypical lipomatous tumor/well-differentiated liposarcoma vs., **90**
- dedifferentiated liposarcoma vs., **96**
- differential diagnosis, **85**
- molecular genetics, **85**
- prognosis, **85**

Atypical teratoid/rhabdoid tumor. *See* Extrarenal rhabdoid tumor.

Atypical vascular lesion, **452–453**
- angiosarcoma vs., **472**
- diagnostic checklist, **453**
- differential diagnosis, **453**

- prognosis, **453**
Atypical vascular proliferation. *See* Atypical vascular lesion.
Atypical vascular proliferation, lymphangioma vs., **448**
AVL. *See* Atypical vascular lesion.
Axial chordoma, soft tissue metastasis from, extraaxial soft tissue chordoma vs., **843**

B

Bacillary angiomatosis (BA), **410–411**
- diagnostic checklist, **411**
- differential diagnosis, **411**
- lobular capillary hemangioma vs., **421**
- prognosis, **411**
Basal cell carcinoma, dermatofibroma vs., **272**
BCOR-CCNB3 (Ewing-like) sarcoma, synovial sarcoma vs., **668**
BCOR-CCNB3 fusion-positive sarcoma
- undifferentiated round cell sarcoma with *CIC-DUX4* translocation vs., **730**
BCOR-CCNB3 fusion-positive sarcoma, **734–737**
- cytogenetics, **735**
- differential diagnosis, **736**
- extraskeletal Ewing sarcoma vs., **708**
- prognosis, **735**
BCOR-CCNB3 sarcoma. *See BCOR-CCNB3* fusion-positive sarcoma.
BCOR-rearranged sarcoma. *See BCOR-CCNB3* fusion-positive sarcoma.
Benign adnexal tumors, glomus tumors vs., **354**
Benign cutaneous biphasic (or plexiform) hybrid tumor of perineurioma, cellular neurothekeoma vs., **291**
Benign cystic mesothelioma. *See* Multicystic peritoneal mesothelioma.
Benign fibrous histiocytoma, fibroma of tendon sheath vs., **136**
Benign lymphangioendothelioma
- atypical vascular lesion vs., **453**
- Kaposi sarcoma vs., **478**
Benign mesothelioma. *See* Well-differentiated papillary mesothelioma.
Benign neural gastrointestinal polyps, **740–743**
- differential diagnosis, **741**
- prognosis, **741**
Biopsy, soft tissue tumors, **22–23**
- specimens, **22–23**
Biphasic sinonasal sarcoma, synovial sarcoma vs., **668**
Biphasic synovial sarcoma, **668**
Biphenotypic sinonasal sarcoma, **850–853**
- differential diagnosis, **851**
- prognosis, **851**
Bizarre parosteal osteochondromatous proliferation, fibroosseous pseudotumor of digit vs., **131**
Blastoma, pleuropulmonary, embryonal rhabdomyosarcoma vs., **382**
Blue nevus
- cellular, clear cell sarcoma vs., **690**
- combined, smooth muscle hamartoma vs., **333**
Botryoid-type embryonal rhabdomyosarcoma, fibroepithelial stromal polyp vs., **575**
Branchial anlage mixed tumor. *See* Ectopic hamartomatous thymoma.
Brown fat, normal, hibernoma vs., **75**

C

Calcifying aponeurotic fibroma, **244–247**
- differential diagnosis, **245**
- inclusion body fibromatosis vs., **251**
- prognosis, **245**
- soft tissue chondroma vs., **488**
Calcifying bursitis. *See* Tumoral calcinosis.
Calcifying collagenolysis. *See* Tumoral calcinosis.
Calcifying fibroma. *See* Calcifying aponeurotic fibroma.
Calcifying fibrous pseudotumor. *See also* Calcifying fibrous tumor.
- desmoplastic fibroblastoma vs., **141**
Calcifying fibrous tumor (CFT), **248–249**
- differential diagnosis, **249**
- prognosis, **249**
Calcinosis, tumoral, **786–787**
- amyloidoma vs., **783**
- differential diagnosis, **787**
- prognosis, **787**
- soft tissue chondroma vs., **488**
Capillary hemangioblastoma. *See* Peripheral hemangioblastoma.
Capillary hemangioma, lobular, **420–421**
- acquired tufted angioma vs., **437**
- angiofibroma of soft tissue vs., **145**
- congenital granular cell epulis vs., **799**
- differential diagnosis, **421**
- glomeruloid hemangioma vs., **443**
- infantile hemangioma vs., **418**
- nasopharyngeal angiofibroma vs., **802**
- prognosis, **421**
- sinonasal glomangiopericytoma vs., **806**
Carcinoid tumor
- gangliocytic paraganglioma vs., **771**
- glomus tumors vs., **354**
- paraganglioma vs., **816**
Carcinoma
- extrarenal rhabdoid tumor vs., **718**
- metastatic
    angiosarcoma vs., **472**
    epithelioid hemangioendothelioma vs., **468**
    histiocytic sarcoma vs., **325**
    intimal sarcoma vs., **721**
    myoepithelioma of soft tissue vs., **656**
    myxofibrosarcoma vs., **218**
    paraganglioma vs., **816**
    pleomorphic rhabdomyosarcoma vs., **401**
    sclerosing epithelioid fibrosarcoma vs., **233**
    sclerosing rhabdomyosarcoma vs., **397**
    solitary extramedullary plasmacytoma vs., **607**
- metastatic renal cell, alveolar soft part sarcoma vs., **685**

INDEX

- myoepithelial. *See also* Myoepithelioma, of soft tissue.
    epithelioid rhabdomyosarcoma vs., **405**
    epithelioid sarcoma vs., **680**
    extraskeletal myxoid chondrosarcoma vs., **713**
    metastatic tumors to soft tissue sites vs., **829**
- neuroendocrine, metastatic, desmoplastic small round cell tumor vs., **702**
- PEComa vs., **694**
- poorly differentiated
    epithelioid rhabdomyosarcoma vs., **405**
    gastrointestinal stromal tumor vs., **747**
    myeloid sarcoma vs., **609**
    pleomorphic liposarcoma vs., **108**
- sarcomatoid
    atypical fibroxanthoma vs., **637**
    ectopic hamartomatous thymoma vs., **633**
    extraskeletal osteosarcoma vs., **498**
    metastatic, follicular dendritic cell sarcoma vs., **327**
    spindle cell rhabdomyosarcoma vs., **394**
    squamous cell, leiomyosarcoma vs., **346**
    undifferentiated embryonal sarcoma of liver vs., **845**
- small cell, extraskeletal Ewing sarcoma vs., **708**
- spindle cell, spindle epithelial tumor with thymus-like differentiation vs., **855**
- undifferentiated, pleomorphic rhabdomyosarcoma vs., **401**
- undifferentiated pleomorphic sarcoma vs., **725**

Cardiac fibroma, **796–797**
- cardiac rhabdomyoma vs., **379**
- differential diagnosis, **797**
- genetics, **797**
- prognosis, **797**

Cardiac myxoma, **792–795**
- differential diagnosis, **793**
- intimal sarcoma vs., **721**
- molecular genetics, **793**
- prognosis, **793**

Cardiac rhabdomyoma, **378–379**
- adult rhabdomyoma vs., **373**
- differential diagnosis, **379**
- genetics, **379**
- prognosis, **379**

Cavernous hemangioma
- lobular capillary hemangioma vs., **421**
- sinusoidal hemangioma vs., **441**
- spindle cell hemangioma vs., **427**

Cavernous lymphangioma. *See* Lymphangioma.

Cellular angiofibroma, **580–583**
- angiomyofibroblastoma vs., **577**
- deep (aggressive) angiomyxoma vs., **585**
- differential diagnosis, **581**
- fibroepithelial stromal polyp vs., **575**
- mammary-type myofibroblastoma vs., **149**
- prognosis, **581**
- solitary fibrous tumor vs., **186**
- spindle cell/pleomorphic lipoma vs., **62**

Cellular blue nevus, clear cell sarcoma vs., **690**

Cellular dermatofibroma
- adult-type fibrosarcoma vs., **215**
- dermatofibrosarcoma protuberans vs., **176**
- Kaposi sarcoma vs., **478**

Cellular digital fibroma. *See* Acral fibromyxoma.

Cellular fibrous histiocytoma
- epithelioid sarcoma vs., **680**
- Kaposi sarcoma vs., **478**
- leiomyosarcoma vs., **346**
- pseudomyogenic hemangioendothelioma vs., **463**

Cellular neurothekeoma, **290–293**
- differential diagnosis, **291**
- ectopic meningioma vs., **811**
- plexiform fibrohistiocytic tumor vs., **317**
- prognosis, **291**

Cellular pseudosarcomatous fibroepithelial stromal polyp. *See* Fibroepithelial stromal polyp.

Cellular schwannoma, **510**
- deep leiomyoma vs., **339**
- ganglioneuroma vs., **551**
- malignant peripheral nerve sheath tumor vs., **560**
- spindle cell rhabdomyosarcoma vs., **394**

Central nervous system, primary meningioma of, ectopic meningioma vs., **811**

Cerebrotendinous xanthomatosis, **295**

CFT. *See* Calcifying fibrous tumor.

Checkerboard skeletal muscle pattern, **30**

Chemodectoma. *See* Paraganglioma.

Cherry angioma, sinusoidal hemangioma vs., **441**

Chloroma. *See* Myeloid sarcoma.

Chondroblastoma, diffuse-type tenosynovial giant cell tumor vs., **286**

Chondroid lipoma, **66–69**
- differential diagnosis, **67**
- epithelioid hemangioendothelioma vs., **468**
- genetic testing, **67**
- lipoma vs., **48**
- prognosis, **67**

Chondroid meningioma, extraskeletal myxoid chondrosarcoma vs., **713**

Chondroid metaplasia, cutaneous mixed tumor with, soft tissue chondroma vs., **488**

Chondroma
- extraskeletal myxoid chondrosarcoma vs., **713**
- juxtaarticular, synovial chondromatosis vs., **493**
- soft tissue, **486–491**
    calcified, tumoral calcinosis vs., **787**
    calcifying aponeurotic fibroma vs., **245**
    chondroid lipoma vs., **67**
    diagnostic checklist, **488**
    differential diagnosis, **487–488**
    extraskeletal myxoid chondrosarcoma vs., **713**
    myoepithelioma of soft tissue vs., **656**
    phosphaturic mesenchymal tumor vs., **665**
    prognosis, **487**
    synovial chondromatosis vs., **493**

Chondromatosis, synovial, **492–495**
- diagnostic checklist, **493**
- differential diagnosis, **493**
- prognosis, **493**
- soft tissue chondroma vs., **487–488**

Chondroosseous tumors
- extraskeletal mesenchymal chondrosarcoma, **500–503**
    differential diagnosis, **502**
    extraskeletal Ewing sarcoma vs., **708**

extraskeletal osteosarcoma vs., **498**
molecular genetics, **501**
prognosis, **501**
- extraskeletal osteosarcoma, **496–499**
aneurysmal bone cyst of soft tissue vs., **631**
diagnostic checklist, **498**
differential diagnosis, **498**
fibroosseous pseudotumor of digit vs., **131**
myositis ossificans vs., **127**
ossifying fibromyxoid tumor vs., **652**
prognosis, **497**
sclerosing epithelioid fibrosarcoma vs., **234**
sclerosing rhabdomyosarcoma vs., **397**
undifferentiated pleomorphic sarcoma vs., **725**
- soft tissue chondroma, **486–491**
calcified, tumoral calcinosis vs., **787**
calcifying aponeurotic fibroma vs., **245**
chondroid lipoma vs., **67**
diagnostic checklist, **488**
differential diagnosis, **487–488**
extraskeletal myxoid chondrosarcoma vs., **713**
myoepithelioma of soft tissue vs., **656**
phosphaturic mesenchymal tumor vs., **665**
prognosis, **487**
synovial chondromatosis vs., **493**
- synovial chondromatosis, **492–495**
diagnostic checklist, **493**
differential diagnosis, **493**
prognosis, **493**
soft tissue chondroma vs., **487–488**

Chondrosarcoma
- extraskeletal mesenchymal, **500–503**
differential diagnosis, **502**
extraskeletal Ewing sarcoma vs., **708**
extraskeletal osteosarcoma vs., **498**
molecular genetics, **501**
prognosis, **501**
- extraskeletal myxoid, **712–715**
chondroid lipoma vs., **67**
differential diagnosis, **713**
epithelioid hemangioendothelioma vs., **468**
extraaxial soft tissue chordoma vs., **843**
extrarenal rhabdoid tumor vs., **718**
extraskeletal mesenchymal chondrosarcoma vs., **502**
genetic testing, **713**
myoepithelioma of soft tissue vs., **656**
myxoid liposarcoma vs., **102**
ossifying fibromyxoid tumor vs., **652**
perineurioma vs., **532**
primary pulmonary myxoid sarcoma vs., **847**
prognosis, **713**
soft tissue chondroma vs., **488**
- mesenchymal, phosphaturic mesenchymal tumor vs., **665**
- synovial, synovial chondromatosis vs., **493**

Chordoid sarcoma. *See* Extraskeletal myxoid chondrosarcoma.

Chordoma
- axial, soft tissue metastasis from, extraaxial soft tissue chordoma vs., **843**
- ependymoma of soft tissue vs., **827**
- extraaxial soft tissue, **842–843**
differential diagnosis, **843**
prognosis, **843**
- myoepithelioma of soft tissue vs., **656**

Chrondroblastoma-like chondroma. *See* Soft tissue chondroma.

CIC-FOXO4 sarcoma, undifferentiated round cell sarcoma with *CIC-DUX4* translocation vs., **730**

CIC-rearranged sarcoma. *See* Undifferentiated round cell sarcoma with *CIC-DUX4* translocation.

Clear cell myomelanocytic tumor. *See* Perivascular epithelioid cell tumor.

Clear cell sarcoma, **688–691**
- diagnostic checklist, **690**
- differential diagnosis, **690**
- epithelioid malignant peripheral nerve sheath tumor vs., **567**
- malignant gastrointestinal neuroectodermal tumor vs., **777–778**
- melanotic schwannoma vs., **557**
- metastatic tumors to soft tissue sites vs., **829**
- molecular genetics, **689**
- PEComa vs., **694**
- prognosis, **689**
- of tendon and aponeurosis, **689**

Clear cell sarcoma-like tumor
- of gastrointestinal tract (CCSLTGT). *See* Malignant gastrointestinal neuroectodermal tumor.
- with osteoclast-like giant cells, of gastrointestinal tract. *See* Malignant gastrointestinal neuroectodermal tumor.

Collagen, amyloidoma vs., **783**

Collagenoma, storiform, **160–161**
- diagnostic checklist, **161**
- differential diagnosis, **161**
- prognosis, **161**

Collagenosis nuchae. *See* Nuchal-type fibroma.

Collagenous fibroma. *See also* Desmoplastic fibroblastoma.
- Gardner fibroma vs., **257**
- nodular fasciitis vs., **116**
- storiform collagenoma vs., **161**

Combined blue nevus, smooth muscle hamartoma vs., **333**

Composite hemangioendothelioma, **460–461**
- differential diagnosis, **461**
- epithelioid hemangioendothelioma vs., **468**
- papillary intralymphatic angioendothelioma vs., **457**
- prognosis, **461**
- retiform hemangioendothelioma vs., **459**

Congenital epulis of newborn. *See* Congenital granular cell epulis.

Congenital fibrosarcoma. *See* Infantile fibrosarcoma.

Congenital granular cell epulis, **798–799**
- differential diagnosis, **799**
- granular cell tumor vs., **542**
- prognosis, **799**

Congenital granular cell tumor. *See* Congenital granular cell epulis.

Congenital hemangioma, **412–415**
- differential diagnosis, **414**

- genetics, **413**
- infantile hemangioma vs., **418**
- prognosis, **413**

Congenital nonprogressive hemangioma. *See* Congenital hemangioma.
Congenital smooth muscle hamartoma. *See* Smooth muscle hamartoma.
Conventional lipoma, myelolipoma vs., **79**
Cranial fasciitis, **115**
Crystal-storing histiocytosis, **314–315**
- adult rhabdomyoma vs., **373**
- differential diagnosis, **315**
- prognosis, **315**

Cutaneous focal mucinosis, superficial angiomyxoma vs., **621**
Cutaneous leiomyoma. *See also* Superficial leiomyoma.
- smooth muscle hamartoma vs., **333**

Cutaneous leiomyosarcoma, smooth muscle hamartoma vs., **333**
Cutaneous lymphangioma, superficial. *See* Lymphangioma.
Cutaneous meningioma. *See* Ectopic meningioma.
Cutaneous mixed tumor, with chondroid metaplasia, soft tissue chondroma vs., **488**
Cutaneous mucinous carcinoma, metastatic or primary
- extraaxial soft tissue chordoma vs., **843**

Cutaneous myxoma. *See also* Superficial angiomyxoma.
- in Carney complex, dermal nerve sheath myxoma vs., **547**

Cutaneous reticulohistiocytosis, generalized, reticulohistiocytoma vs., **301–302**
Cutaneous syncytial myoepithelioma, **657**
Cystic hygroma. *See* Lymphangioma.
Cystic lymphangioma. *See also* Lymphangioma.
- multicystic peritoneal mesothelioma vs., **593**

D

D-TGCT. *See* Diffuse-type tenosynovial giant cell tumor.
Dabska tumor. *See* Papillary intralymphatic angioendothelioma.
DDLPS. *See* Dedifferentiated liposarcoma.
Dedifferentiated liposarcoma (DDLPS), **94–99**
- atypical lipomatous tumor/well-differentiated liposarcoma vs., **90**
- atypical spindle cell lipomatous tumor vs., **85**
- differential diagnosis, **96**
- extraskeletal osteosarcoma vs., **498**
- histiocytic sarcoma vs., **325**
- low-grade morphology, myolipoma vs., **71**
- molecular genetics, **96**
- pleomorphic liposarcoma vs., **107**
- prognosis, **95**
- undifferentiated pleomorphic sarcoma vs., **725**

Deep (aggressive) angiomyxoma, **584–587**
- angiomyofibroblastoma vs., **577**
- cellular angiofibroma vs., **581**
- desmoid-type fibromatosis vs., **170**
- differential diagnosis, **585**
- fibroepithelial stromal polyp vs., **575**
- genetic testing, **585**
- juxtaarticular myxoma vs., **619**
- prognosis, **585**
- superficial angiomyxoma vs., **621**

Deep benign fibrous histiocytoma, **276–277**
- angiofibroma of soft tissue vs., **145**
- dermatofibrosarcoma protuberans vs., **176**
- differential diagnosis, **277**
- prognosis, **277**
- solitary fibrous tumor vs., **186**

Deep granuloma annulare, **304–305**
- differential diagnosis, **305**
- prognosis, **305**
- rheumatoid nodule vs., **307**

Deep leiomyoma, **338–341**
- differential diagnosis, **339**
- prognosis, **339**

Deep lymphangioma. *See* Lymphangioma.
Dendritic cell sarcoma
- follicular, **326–327**
  - angiomatoid fibrous histiocytoma vs., **644**
  - differential diagnosis, **327**
  - extranodal Rosai-Dorfman disease vs., **312**
  - interdigitating dendritic cell sarcoma vs., **329**
  - prognosis, **327**
- interdigitating, **328–329**
  - differential diagnosis, **329**
  - follicular dendritic cell sarcoma vs., **327**
  - prognosis, **329**

Dermal melanocytic nevus, glomus tumors vs., **354**
Dermal nerve sheath myxoma, **546–549**
- cellular neurothekeoma vs., **291**
- differential diagnosis of, **547**
- prognosis, **547**
- superficial angiomyxoma vs., **621**

Dermatofibroma, **270–275**
- acral fibromyxoma vs., **625**
- cellular
  - adult-type fibrosarcoma vs., **215**
  - dermatofibrosarcoma protuberans vs., **176**
  - Kaposi sarcoma vs., **478**
- dermatofibrosarcoma protuberans vs., **176**
- dermatomyofibroma vs., **159**
- diagnostic checklist, **272**
- differential diagnosis, **272**
- epithelioid sarcoma vs., **680**
- giant cell fibroblastoma vs., **261**
- lipidized-type, xanthomas vs., **296**
- localized-type tenosynovial giant cell tumor vs., **280**
- nodular fasciitis vs., **116**
- pleomorphic fibroma vs., **157**
- prognosis, **271**
- solitary (juvenile) xanthogranuloma vs., **299**
- storiform collagenoma vs., **161**

Dermatofibrosarcoma protuberans, **174–183**
- acral fibromyxoma vs., **625**
- atypical spindle cell lipomatous tumor vs., **85**
- deep benign fibrous histiocytoma vs., **277**
- dermatofibroma vs., **272**
- dermatomyofibroma vs., **159**

INDEX

- differential diagnosis, **176**
- fibrosarcomatous, **175**
  - adult-type fibrosarcoma vs., **215**
  - infantile fibrosarcoma vs., **265**
  - spindle cell rhabdomyosarcoma vs., **394**
  - synovial sarcoma vs., **668**
- giant cell fibroblastoma vs., **261**
- hemosiderotic fibrolipomatous tumor vs., **635**
- molecular genetics, **176**
- myxoid
  - dermal nerve sheath myxoma vs., **547**
  - myxoid liposarcoma vs., **102**
- neurofibroma vs., **524**
- perineurioma vs., **532**
- prognosis, **175**
- solitary fibrous tumor vs., **186**
- spindle cell/pleomorphic lipoma vs., **62**

Dermatomyofibroma, **158–159**
- dermatofibrosarcoma protuberans vs., **176**
- differential diagnosis, **159**
- prognosis, **159**
- superficial leiomyoma vs., **335**

Desmoid tumor. *See* Desmoid-type fibromatosis.

Desmoid-type fibromatosis, **168–173**
- adult-type fibrosarcoma vs., **215**
- deep (aggressive) angiomyxoma vs., **585**
- differential diagnosis, **170**
- elastofibromas vs., **143**
- Gardner fibroma vs., **257**
- gastrointestinal stromal tumor vs., **747**
- idiopathic tumefactive fibroinflammatory lesions vs., **790**
- inclusion body fibromatosis vs., **251**
- inflammatory myofibroblastic tumor vs., **198**
- intranodal palisade myofibroblastoma vs., **153**
- leiomyosarcoma vs., **346**
- low-grade fibromyxoid sarcoma vs., **224**
- low-grade myofibroblastic sarcoma vs., **193**
- molecular genetics, **169**
- nasopharyngeal angiofibroma vs., **802**
- nodular fasciitis vs., **116**
- palmar/plantar fibromatosis vs., **167**
- perineurioma vs., **532**
- primary, neuromuscular choristoma vs., **555**
- prognosis, **169**
- spindle cell rhabdomyosarcoma vs., **394**

Desmoplastic fibroblastoma, **140–141**
- differential diagnosis, **141**
- fibroma of tendon sheath vs., **136**
- Gardner fibroma vs., **257**
- nodular fasciitis vs., **116**
- prognosis, **141**

Desmoplastic melanoma
- atypical fibroxanthoma vs., **637–638**
- keloid vs., **163**
- neurofibroma vs., **524**

Desmoplastic small round cell tumor, **700–705**
- alveolar rhabdomyosarcoma vs., **388**
- differential diagnosis, **701–702**
- extrarenal rhabdoid tumor vs., **718**
- extraskeletal Ewing sarcoma vs., **708**
- immunohistochemistry, **702**
- low-grade endometrial stromal sarcoma vs., **857**
- melanotic neuroectodermal tumor of infancy vs., **825**
- molecular genetics, **701**
- prognosis, **701**

Diffuse hemangioma. *See* Angiomatosis.

Diffuse mesothelioma. *See* Malignant mesothelioma.

Diffuse neurofibroma
- dermatofibrosarcoma protuberans vs., **176**
- lipoma vs., **48**

Diffuse-type tenosynovial giant cell tumor (D-TGCT), **284–289**
- differential diagnosis, **286**
- localized-type tenosynovial giant cell tumor vs., **280**
- myxoinflammatory fibroblastic sarcoma vs., **204**
- prognosis, **285**
- synovial lipomatosis vs., **55**

Digital fibromyxoma. *See* Acral fibromyxoma.

Digital fibrous tumor of childhood. *See* Inclusion body fibromatosis.

Digital mucoid cyst
- dermal nerve sheath myxoma vs., **547**
- superficial angiomyxoma vs., **621**

Duodenal ganglioneuroma. *See* Gangliocytic paraganglioma.

Dupuytren contracture. *See* Palmar/plantar fibromatosis.

E

Early scar, microvenular hemangioma vs., **439**

Ectomesenchymal chondromyxoid tumor. *See* Myoepithelioma, of soft tissue.

Ectomesenchymoma, **570–571**
- differential diagnosis, **571**
- embryonal rhabdomyosarcoma vs., **382**
- genetic testing, **571**
- prognosis, **571**

Ectopic hamartomatous thymoma (EHT), **632–633**
- differential diagnosis, **633**
- prognosis, **633**

Ectopic meningioma, **810–811**
- differential diagnosis, **811**
- perineurioma vs., **532**
- prognosis, **811**

EHE. *See* Epithelioid hemangioendothelioma.

EHT. *See* Ectopic hamartomatous thymoma.

Elastofibroma, **142–143**
- amyloidoma vs., **783**
- desmoplastic fibroblastoma vs., **141**
- differential diagnosis, **143**
- Gardner fibroma vs., **257**
- nuchal-type fibroma vs., **165**
- prognosis, **143**

Elastofibroma dorsi. *See* Elastofibroma.

Elastofibromatous change, elastofibromas vs., **143**

Embryonal rhabdomyosarcoma, **380–385**
- alveolar rhabdomyosarcoma vs., **388**
- botryoid-type, fibroepithelial stromal polyp vs., **575**

INDEX

- differential diagnosis, **382**
- fetal rhabdomyoma vs., **375**
- pleomorphic rhabdomyosarcoma vs., **401**
- prognosis, **381**
- proliferative fasciitis/myositis vs., **121**
- spindle cell rhabdomyosarcoma vs., **394**
- undifferentiated embryonal sarcoma of liver vs., **845**

Embryonic fat, lipoma. *See* Hibernoma.
Embryonic lipoma. *See* Lipoblastoma.
EMC. *See* Extraskeletal mesenchymal chondrosarcoma; Extraskeletal myxoid chondrosarcoma.
Encephalocele, true, glial heterotopia vs., **813**
Endolymphatic stromal myosis. *See* Low-grade Endometrial stromal sarcoma.
Endometrial stromal nodule, low-grade endometrial stromal sarcoma vs., **857**
Endometrial stromal sarcoma, low-grade, **856–857**
- differential diagnosis, **857**
- prognosis, **857**

Endothelial hyperplasia, papillary
- angiosarcoma vs., **472**
- diagnostic checklist, **409**
- differential diagnosis, **409**
- prognosis, **409**

Endovascular papillary angioendothelioma. *See* Papillary intralymphatic angioendothelioma.
Eosinophilic granuloma. *See* Langerhans cell histiocytosis.
Ependymoma, of soft tissue, **826–827**
- differential diagnosis, **827**
- prognosis, **827**

Epithelioid angiomatosis. *See* Bacillary angiomatosis.
Epithelioid angiosarcoma
- epithelioid hemangioendothelioma vs., **468**
- epithelioid hemangioma vs., **423**
- epithelioid sarcoma vs., **680**
- malignant mesothelioma vs., **600**
- myeloid sarcoma vs., **609**

Epithelioid cell patterns, **30**
- abundant cytoplasm, **30**
- arranged in cords or trabeculae, **30**
- arranged in nests or lobules, **30**
- associated with adipose tissue, **30**
- associated with prominent stromal vasculature, **30**
- within collagenous, hyalinized or sclerotic stroma, **30**
- minimal/scant cytoplasm, **30**
- within myxoid stroma, **30**

Epithelioid fibrosarcoma, sclerosing, **232–237**
- differential diagnosis, **233–234**
- low-grade fibromyxoid sarcoma vs., **224**
- ossifying fibromyxoid tumor vs., **652**
- prognosis, **233**
- sclerosing rhabdomyosarcoma vs., **397**

Epithelioid fibrous histiocytoma, cellular neurothekeoma vs., **291**
Epithelioid gastrointestinal stromal tumor, extraskeletal myxoid chondrosarcoma vs., **713**
Epithelioid hemangioendothelioma (EHE), **466–469**
- angiosarcoma vs., **472**
- composite hemangioendothelioma vs., **461**
- differential diagnosis, **468**
- epithelioid hemangioma vs., **423**
- intimal sarcoma vs., **721**
- malignant mesothelioma vs., **600**
- molecular genetics, **467**
- prognosis, **467**
- pseudomyogenic hemangioendothelioma, **463**
- spindle cell hemangioma vs., **427**

Epithelioid hemangioma, **422–425**
- differential diagnosis, **423**
- epithelioid hemangioendothelioma vs., **468**
- molecular genetics, **423**
- prognosis, **423**

Epithelioid malignant peripheral nerve sheath tumor, **566–569**
- differential diagnosis, **567**
- extrarenal rhabdoid tumor vs., **718**
- myoepithelioma of soft tissue vs., **656**
- ossifying fibromyxoid tumor vs., **652**
- prognosis, **567**

Epithelioid rhabdomyosarcoma, **404–405**
- differential diagnosis, **405**
- molecular genetics, **405**
- pleomorphic rhabdomyosarcoma vs., **401**
- prognosis, **405**

Epithelioid sarcoma (ES), **678–683**
- angiosarcoma vs., **472**
- classic, **679**
- deep granuloma annulare vs., **305**
- differential diagnosis, **680**
- epithelioid hemangioendothelioma vs., **468**
- epithelioid rhabdomyosarcoma vs., **405**
- extrarenal rhabdoid tumor vs., **718**
- inclusion body fibromatosis vs., **251**
- ischemic fasciitis vs., **125**
- molecular genetics, **680**
- myoepithelioma of soft tissue vs., **656**
- prognosis, **679**
- proximal-type, **679–680**
- pseudomyogenic hemangioendothelioma, **463**
- rheumatoid nodule vs., **307**
- solitary extramedullary plasmacytoma vs., **607**
- superficial CD34(+) fibroblastic tumor vs., **211**

Epithelioid sarcoma-like hemangioendothelioma. *See* Pseudomyogenic hemangioendothelioma.
Epithelioid schwannoma, **510**
- epithelioid malignant peripheral nerve sheath tumor vs., **567**

Epstein-Barr virus-associated smooth muscle tumor, **342–343**
- differential diagnosis, **343**
- prognosis, **343**

Eruptive xanthoma, **295**
Evans tumor. *See* Low-grade fibromyxoid sarcoma.
Ewing-like sarcoma. *See* *BCOR-CCNB3* fusion-positive sarcoma; Undifferentiated round cell sarcoma with *CIC-DUX4* translocation.
Ewing sarcoma
- alveolar rhabdomyosarcoma vs., **388**
- *BCOR-CCNB3* fusion-positive sarcoma vs., **736**
- extrarenal rhabdoid tumor vs., **718**
- extraskeletal, **706–711**
  - desmoplastic small round cell tumor vs., **701**

differential diagnosis, **708**
extraskeletal osteosarcoma vs., **498**
molecular genetics, **708**
prognosis, **707**
undifferentiated round cell sarcoma with *CIC-DUX4* translocation vs., **729**
- extraskeletal mesenchymal chondrosarcoma vs., **502**
- low-grade endometrial stromal sarcoma vs., **857**
- lymphoma of soft tissue vs., **611**
- myxoid liposarcoma vs., **102**
- neuroblastoma and ganglioneuroblastoma vs., **834**
- synovial sarcoma vs., **668**

Extraadrenal paraganglioma. *See* Paraganglioma.
Extraaxial soft tissue chordoma, **842–843**
- differential diagnosis, **843**
- prognosis, **843**

Extracranial meningioma. *See* Ectopic meningioma.
Extramedullary hemopoiesis, myelolipoma vs., **79**
Extramedullary plasmacytoma, solitary, **606–607**
- differential diagnosis, **607**
- prognosis, **607**

Extraneural soft tissue perineurioma. *See* Perineurioma.
Extraneuraxial hemangioblastoma. *See* Peripheral hemangioblastoma.
Extranodal Rosai-Dorfman disease, **310–313**
- differential diagnosis, **312**
- histiocytic sarcoma vs., **325**
- idiopathic tumefactive fibroinflammatory lesions vs., **790**
- Langerhans cell histiocytosis vs., **309**
- prognosis, **311**

Extraosseous plasmacytoma, solitary. *See* Solitary extramedullary plasmacytoma.
Extrarenal epithelioid angiomyolipoma. *See* Perivascular epithelioid cell tumor.
Extrarenal rhabdoid tumor, **716–719**
- alveolar rhabdomyosarcoma vs., **388**
- desmoplastic small round cell tumor vs., **702**
- differential diagnosis, **718**
- epithelioid rhabdomyosarcoma vs., **405**
- epithelioid sarcoma vs., **680**
- molecular genetics, **717–718**
- prognosis, **717**

Extraskeletal chondroma. *See* Soft tissue chondroma.
Extraskeletal Ewing sarcoma, **706–711**. *See also* Ewing sarcoma.
- desmoplastic small round cell tumor vs., **701**
- differential diagnosis, **708**
- extraskeletal osteosarcoma vs., **498**
- molecular genetics, **708**
- prognosis, **707**
- undifferentiated round cell sarcoma with *CIC-DUX4* translocation vs., **729**

Extraskeletal mesenchymal chondrosarcoma, **500–503**
- differential diagnosis, **502**
- extraskeletal Ewing sarcoma vs., **708**
- extraskeletal osteosarcoma vs., **498**
- molecular genetics, **501**
- prognosis, **501**

Extraskeletal myxoid chondrosarcoma, **712–715**
- chondroid lipoma vs., **67**
- differential diagnosis, **713**
- epithelioid hemangioendothelioma vs., **468**
- extraaxial soft tissue chordoma vs., **843**
- extrarenal rhabdoid tumor vs., **718**
- extraskeletal mesenchymal chondrosarcoma vs., **502**
- genetic testing, **713**
- myoepithelioma of soft tissue vs., **656**
- myxoid liposarcoma vs., **102**
- ossifying fibromyxoid tumor vs., **652**
- perineurioma vs., **532**
- primary pulmonary myxoid sarcoma vs., **847**
- prognosis, **713**
- soft tissue chondroma vs., **488**

Extraskeletal osteosarcoma, **496–499**
- aneurysmal bone cyst of soft tissue vs., **631**
- diagnostic checklist, **498**
- differential diagnosis, **498**
- fibroosseous pseudotumor of digit vs., **131**
- myositis ossificans vs., **127**
- ossifying fibromyxoid tumor vs., **652**
- prognosis, **497**
- sclerosing epithelioid fibrosarcoma vs., **234**
- sclerosing rhabdomyosarcoma vs., **397**
- undifferentiated pleomorphic sarcoma vs., **725**

Extraskeletal recurrence of giant cell tumor of bone, giant cell tumor of soft tissue vs., **321**
Extraspinal ependymoma. *See* Ependymoma, of soft tissue.
Extrauterine lipoleiomyoma. *See* Myolipoma.

F

Fasciitis
- ischemic, **124–125**
  differential diagnosis, **125**
  prognosis, **125**
- nodular, **114–119**
  aneurysmal bone cyst of soft tissue vs., **631**
  angiomatoid fibrous histiocytoma vs., **644**
  desmoid-type fibromatosis vs., **170**
  desmoplastic fibroblastoma vs., **141**
  differential diagnosis, **116**
  fibroma of tendon sheath vs., **136**
  fibromatosis colli vs., **255**
  inflammatory myofibroblastic tumor vs., **198**
  ischemic fasciitis vs., **125**
  keloid vs., **163**
  molecular genetics, **116**
  myofibroma and myofibromatosis vs., **363**
  myositis ossificans vs., **127**
  prognosis, **115**
  proliferative fasciitis/myositis vs., **121**
- proliferative fasciitis/myositis, **120–123**
  desmoid-type fibromatosis vs., **170**
  differential diagnosis, **121**
  ischemic fasciitis vs., **125**

myxoinflammatory fibroblastic sarcoma vs., **204**
nodular fasciitis vs., **116**
prognosis, **121**
Fasciitis ossificans. *See* Fibroosseous pseudotumor of digit.
Fatty infiltration of median nerve. *See* Lipomatosis.
FDCS. *See* Follicular dendritic cell sarcoma.
Fédération Nationale des Centres de Lutte Contre le Cancer (FNCLCC), **6**
Fetal lipoma. *See* Hibernoma; Lipoblastoma.
Fetal rhabdomyoma, **374–375**
- differential diagnosis, **375**
- embryonal rhabdomyosarcoma vs., **382**
- genetics, **375**
- genital rhabdomyoma vs., **377**
- prognosis, **375**
- spindle cell rhabdomyosarcoma vs., **394**
FHI. *See* Fibrous hamartoma of infancy.
Fibrin, amyloidoma vs., **783**
Fibroblastic connective tissue nevus, lipofibromatosis vs., **259**
Fibroblastic/myofibroblastic lesions
- adult-type fibrosarcoma, **214–215**
  differential diagnosis, **215**
  genetic testing, **215**
  prognosis, **215**
- angiofibroma of soft tissue, **144–147**
  differential diagnosis of, **145**
  molecular genetics, **145**
- dermatofibrosarcoma protuberans, **174–183**
  differential diagnosis, **176**
  fibrosarcomatous, **175**
  molecular genetics, **176**
  prognosis, **175**
- dermatomyofibroma, **158–159**
  differential diagnosis, **159**
  prognosis, **159**
- desmoid-type fibromatosis, **168–173**
  differential diagnosis, **170**
  molecular genetics, **169**
  prognosis, **169**
- desmoplastic fibroblastoma, **140–141**
  differential diagnosis, **141**
  prognosis, **141**
- elastofibroma, **142–143**
  differential diagnosis, **143**
  nuchal-type fibroma vs., **165**
  prognosis, **143**
- fibroma of tendon sheath, **134–139**
  differential diagnosis, **136**
  prognosis, **135**
- fibroosseous pseudotumor of digit, **130–133**
  differential diagnosis, **131**
- inflammatory myofibroblastic tumor, **196–201**
  differential diagnosis, **198**
  molecular genetics, **197–198**
  prognosis, **197**
- intranodal palisade myofibroblastoma, **152–155**
  differential diagnosis, **153**
  molecular genetics, **153**
  prognosis, **153**
- ischemic fasciitis, **124–125**
  differential diagnosis, **125**
  prognosis, **125**
- keloid, **162–163**
  diagnostic checklist, **163**
  differential diagnosis, **163**
  prognosis, **163**
- low-grade fibromyxoid sarcoma, **222–231**
  differential diagnosis, **224**
  prognosis, **223**
- low-grade myofibroblastic sarcoma, **192–195**
  differential diagnosis, **193**
  prognosis, **193**
- mammary-type myofibroblastoma, **148–151**
  differential diagnosis, **149**
  molecular genetics, **149**
  prognosis, **149**
- myositis ossificans, **126–129**
  differential diagnosis, **127**
  prognosis, **127**
- myxofibrosarcoma, **216–221**
  differential diagnosis, **218**
  prognosis, **217**
- myxoinflammatory fibroblastic sarcoma, **202–209**
  differential diagnosis, **204**
  molecular genetics, **204**
  prognosis, **203**
- nodular fasciitis, **114–119**
  differential diagnosis, **116**
  molecular genetics, **116**
  prognosis, **115**
- nuchal fibrocartilaginous pseudotumor, nuchal-type fibroma vs., **165**
- nuchal-type fibroma, **164–165**
  differential diagnosis, **165**
  prognosis, **165**
- palmar/plantar fibromatosis, **166–167**
  differential diagnosis, **167**
  prognosis, **167**
- pleomorphic fibroma, **156–157**
  diagnostic checklist, **157**
  differential diagnosis, **157**
  prognosis, **157**
- proliferative fasciitis/myositis, **120–123**
  differential diagnosis, **121**
  prognosis, **121**
- sclerosing epithelioid fibrosarcoma, **232–237**
  differential diagnosis, **233–234**
  prognosis, **233**
- solitary fibrous tumor, **184–191**
  differential diagnosis, **186**
  molecular genetics, **186**
  prognosis, **185**
- storiform collagenoma, **160–161**
  diagnostic checklist, **161**
  differential diagnosis, **161**
  prognosis, **161**
- superficial CD34(+) fibroblastic tumor, **210–213**
  differential diagnosis, **211**
  prognosis, **211**

INDEX

Fibroblastic/myofibroblastic tumors, pediatric
- calcifying aponeurotic fibroma, **244–247**
  differential diagnosis, **245**
  prognosis, **245**
- calcifying fibrous tumor, **248–249**
  differential diagnosis, **249**
  prognosis, **249**
- fibromatosis colli, **254–255**
  differential diagnosis, **255**
  prognosis, **255**
- fibrous hamartoma of infancy, **240–243**
  differential diagnosis, **241**
  prognosis, **241**
- Gardner fibroma, **256–257**
  diagnostic checklist, **257**
  differential diagnosis, **257**
  prognosis, **257**
- giant cell fibroblastoma, **260–263**
  differential diagnosis, **261**
  prognosis, **261**
- hyaline fibromatosis syndrome, **252–253**
  differential diagnosis, **253**
  prognosis, **253**
- inclusion body fibromatosis, **250–251**
  differential diagnosis, **251**
  prognosis, **251**
- infantile fibrosarcoma, **264–267**
  differential diagnosis, **265**
  molecular genetics, **265**
  prognosis, **265**
- lipofibromatosis, **258–259**
  calcifying aponeurotic fibroma vs., **245**
  differential diagnosis, **259**
  fibrous hamartoma of infancy vs., **241**
  genetics, **259**
  prognosis, **259**
Fibroblastic sarcoma, myxoinflammatory, **202–209**
- differential diagnosis, **204**
- extranodal Rosai-Dorfman disease vs., **312**
- hemosiderotic fibrolipomatous tumor vs., **635**
- molecular genetics, **204**
- myxofibrosarcoma vs., **218**
- pleomorphic hyalinizing angiectatic tumor vs., **627**
- prognosis, **203**
- superficial CD34(+) fibroblastic tumor vs., **211**
Fibroblastic tumor, superficial CD34(+), myxoinflammatory fibroblastic sarcoma vs., **204**
Fibroblastoma
- desmoplastic
  differential diagnosis, **141**
  fibroma of tendon sheath vs., **136**
  Gardner fibroma vs., **257**
  nodular fasciitis vs., **116**
  prognosis, **141**
- giant cell
  angiosarcoma vs., **472**
  differential diagnosis, **261**
  fibrous hamartoma of infancy vs., **241**
  prognosis, **261**
  spindle cell/pleomorphic lipoma vs., **62**
Fibrocartilaginous pseudotumor, nuchal
- Gardner fibroma vs., **257**
- nuchal-type fibroma vs., **165**
Fibrochondroma. *See* Soft tissue chondroma.
Fibrodysplasia (myositis) ossificans progressiva, hyaline fibromatosis syndrome vs., **253**
Fibroepithelial stromal polyp (FSP), **574–575**
- angiomyofibroblastoma vs., **577**
- differential diagnosis, **575**
- genital rhabdomyoma vs., **377**
- prognosis, **575**
Fibrohistiocytic, histiocytic, and dendritic cell tumors
- crystal-storing histiocytosis, **314–315**
- deep granuloma annulare, **304–305**
- extranodal Rosai-Dorfman disease, **310–313**
- giant cell tumor of soft tissue, **320–323**
- histiocytic sarcoma, **324–325**
- Langerhans cell histiocytosis, **308–309**
- plexiform fibrohistiocytic tumor, **316–319**
- reticulohistiocytoma, **300–303**
- rheumatoid nodule, **306–307**
- solitary (juvenile) xanthogranuloma, **298–299**
Fibrohistiocytic tumor, plexiform, **316–319**
- cellular neurothekeoma vs., **291**
- differential diagnosis, **317**
- ectopic meningioma vs., **811**
- localized-type tenosynovial giant cell tumor vs., **280**
- prognosis, **317**
- xanthomas vs., **296**
Fibroid polyp, inflammatory, **766–769**
- benign neural gastrointestinal polyps vs., **741**
- differential diagnosis, **767**
- gastrointestinal smooth muscle neoplasms vs., **764**
- gastrointestinal stromal tumor vs., **747**
- inflammatory myofibroblastic tumor vs., **198**
- plexiform fibromyxoma vs., **773**
Fibrokeratoma, acral, storiform collagenoma vs., **161**
Fibrolipoma
- elastofibromas vs., **143**
- Gardner fibroma vs., **257**
- nuchal-type fibroma vs., **165**
Fibrolipomatous hamartoma
- of nerve. *See* Lipomatosis.
- neuromuscular choristoma vs., **555**
Fibrolipomatous tumor, hemosiderotic, **634–635**
- differential diagnosis, **635**
- molecular genetics, **635**
- myxoinflammatory fibroblastic sarcoma vs., **204**
- pleomorphic hyalinizing angiectatic tumor vs., **627**
- prognosis, **635**
Fibroma
- cardiac, **796–797**
  cardiac rhabdomyoma vs., **379**
  differential diagnosis, **797**
  genetics, **797**
  prognosis, **797**
- collagenous, storiform collagenoma vs., **161**
- Gardner, **256–257**
  diagnostic checklist, **257**
  differential diagnosis, **257**
  elastofibromas vs., **143**

nuchal-type fibroma vs., **165**
prognosis, **257**
- nuchal-type, **164–165**
differential diagnosis, **165**
elastofibromas vs., **143**
Gardner fibroma vs., **257**
prognosis, **165**
- plaque-like CD34(+) dermal, dermatofibrosarcoma protuberans vs., **176**
- pleomorphic, **156–157**
diagnostic checklist, **157**
differential diagnosis, **157**
prognosis, **157**
storiform collagenoma vs., **161**
- subungual and periungual, storiform collagenoma vs., **161**
- tendon sheath, **134–139**
desmoplastic fibroblastoma vs., **141**
differential diagnosis, **136**
localized-type tenosynovial giant cell tumor vs., **280**
nodular fasciitis vs., **116**
prognosis, **135**
Fibromatosis
- calcifying fibrous tumor vs., **249**
- desmoid-type, **168–173**
adult-type fibrosarcoma vs., **215**
deep (aggressive) angiomyxoma vs., **585**
differential diagnosis, **170**
elastofibromas vs., **143**
Gardner fibroma vs., **257**
gastrointestinal stromal tumor vs., **747**
idiopathic tumefactive fibroinflammatory lesions vs., **790**
inclusion body fibromatosis vs., **251**
inflammatory myofibroblastic tumor vs., **198**
intranodal palisade myofibroblastoma vs., **153**
leiomyosarcoma vs., **346**
low-grade fibromyxoid sarcoma vs., **224**
low-grade myofibroblastic sarcoma vs., **193**
molecular genetics, **169**
nasopharyngeal angiofibroma vs., **802**
nodular fasciitis vs., **116**
palmar/plantar fibromatosis vs., **167**
perineurioma vs., **532**
primary, neuromuscular choristoma vs., **555**
prognosis, **169**
spindle cell rhabdomyosarcoma vs., **394**
- desmoplastic fibroblastoma vs., **141**
- fibromatosis colli vs., **255**
- fibrous hamartoma of infancy vs., **241**
- inclusion body, **250–251**
differential diagnosis, **251**
fibroma of tendon sheath vs., **136**
prognosis, **251**
- myofibroma and myofibromatosis vs., **363**
- palmar/plantar, **166–167**
calcifying aponeurotic fibroma vs., **245**
differential diagnosis, **167**
prognosis, **167**
- plexiform fibrohistiocytic tumor vs., **317**
- superficial
dermatomyofibroma vs., **159**
fibroma of tendon sheath vs., **136**
inclusion body fibromatosis vs., **251**
Fibromatosis colli, **254–255**
- differential diagnosis, **255**
- prognosis, **255**
Fibromyxoid sarcoma, low-grade
- angiofibroma of soft tissue vs., **145**
- desmoid-type fibromatosis vs., **170**
- desmoplastic fibroblastoma vs., **141**
- differential diagnosis, **224**
- intramuscular myxoma vs., **615**
- juxtaarticular myxoma vs., **619**
- myxofibrosarcoma vs., **218**
- myxoid liposarcoma vs., **102**
- ossifying fibromyxoid tumor vs., **652**
- perineurioma vs., **532**
- prognosis, **223**
- sclerosing epithelioid fibrosarcoma vs., **233**
- superficial angiomyxoma vs., **621**
Fibromyxoid sarcoma, low-grade, **222–231**
Fibromyxoid tumor, ossifying, **650–655**
- differential diagnosis, **652**
- extraskeletal osteosarcoma vs., **498**
- fibroosseous pseudotumor vs., **131**
- malignant, **651**
- molecular genetics, **652**
- myoepithelioma of soft tissue vs., **656**
- myositis ossificans vs., **127**
- prognosis, **651**
- sclerosing epithelioid fibrosarcoma vs., **234**
Fibromyxoma
- acral, **624–625**
differential diagnosis, **625**
inclusion body fibromatosis vs., **251**
prognosis, **625**
- plexiform, **772–775**
differential diagnosis, **773**
gastrointestinal stromal tumor vs., **747**
- superficial acral
dermal nerve sheath myxoma vs., **547**
superficial angiomyxoma vs., **621**
Fibroosseous pseudotumor of digit, **130–133**
- differential diagnosis, **131**
- extraskeletal osteosarcoma vs., **498**
Fibrosarcoma
- adult-type, **214–215**
differential diagnosis, **215**
genetic testing, **215**
prognosis, **215**
spindle cell rhabdomyosarcoma vs., **394**
- atypical fibroxanthoma vs., **638**
- fibromyxoid type. *See* Low-grade fibromyxoid sarcoma.
- infantile, **264–267**
differential diagnosis, **265**
embryonal rhabdomyosarcoma vs., **382**
molecular genetics, **265**
myofibroma and myofibromatosis vs., **363**
prognosis, **265**
spindle cell rhabdomyosarcoma vs., **394**

- sclerosing epithelioid, **232–237**
  differential diagnosis, **233–234**
  low-grade fibromyxoid sarcoma vs., **224**
  ossifying fibromyxoid tumor vs., **652**
  prognosis, **233**
  sclerosing rhabdomyosarcoma vs., **397**
Fibrosarcoma-like lipomatous neoplasm. *See* Atypical spindle cell lipomatous tumor.
Fibrosarcomatous dermatofibrosarcoma protuberans, **175**
- adult-type fibrosarcoma vs., **215**
- infantile fibrosarcoma vs., **265**
- spindle cell rhabdomyosarcoma vs., **394**
- synovial sarcoma vs., **668**
Fibrosing (sclerosing) mediastinitis, idiopathic tumefactive fibroinflammatory lesions vs., **790**
Fibrous hamartoma of infancy (FHI), **240–243**
- differential diagnosis, **241**
- lipofibromatosis vs., **259**
- prognosis, **241**
Fibrous histiocytoma, **270–275**
- acral fibromyxoma vs., **625**
- angiomatoid, **642–649**
  differential diagnosis, **644**
  molecular genetics, **644**
  nodular fasciitis vs., **116**
  primary pulmonary myxoid sarcoma vs., **847**
  prognosis, **643**
- cellular
  epithelioid sarcoma vs., **680**
  Kaposi sarcoma vs., **478**
  leiomyosarcoma vs., **346**
  pseudomyogenic hemangioendothelioma vs., **463**
- deep benign, **276–277**
  angiofibroma of soft tissue vs., **145**
  dermatofibrosarcoma protuberans vs., **176**
  differential diagnosis, **277**
  prognosis, **277**
  solitary fibrous tumor vs., **186**
- diagnostic checklist, **272**
- differential diagnosis, **272**
- epithelioid, cellular neurothekeoma vs., **291**
- giant cell fibroblastoma vs., **261**
- granular cell tumor vs., **542**
- nodular fasciitis vs., **116**
- pleomorphic fibroma vs., **157**
- prognosis, **271**
- solitary (juvenile) xanthogranuloma vs., **299**
- xanthomas vs., **296**
Fibrous papule, pleomorphic fibroma vs., **157**
Fibrous pleurisy, malignant mesothelioma vs., **600**
Fibrous scar, desmoid-type fibromatosis vs., **170**
Fibrous tumor
- calcifying, **248–249**
  differential diagnosis, **249**
  prognosis, **249**
- solitary, **184–191**
  acral fibromyxoma vs., **625**
  angiofibroma of soft tissue vs., **145**
  BCOR-CCNB3 fusion-positive sarcoma vs., **736**
  biphenotypic sinonasal sarcoma vs., **851**
  calcifying fibrous tumor vs., **249**
  cellular angiofibroma vs., **581**
  cellular/malignant, extraskeletal mesenchymal chondrosarcoma vs., **502**
  deep benign fibrous histiocytoma vs., **277**
  dermatofibrosarcoma protuberans vs., **176**
  differential diagnosis, **186**
  ectopic hamartomatous thymoma vs., **633**
  gastrointestinal stromal tumor vs., **747**
  low-grade endometrial stromal sarcoma vs., **857**
  malignant mesothelioma vs., **600**
  mammary-type myofibroblastoma vs., **149**
  molecular genetics, **186**
  myopericytoma vs., **359**
  nasopharyngeal angiofibroma vs., **802**
  nuchal-type fibroma vs., **165**
  perineurioma vs., **532**
  peripheral hemangioblastoma vs., **823**
  phosphaturic mesenchymal tumor vs., **665**
  prognosis, **185**
  sinonasal glomangiopericytoma vs., **806**
  spindle cell/pleomorphic lipoma vs., **62**
  spindle epithelial tumor with thymus-like differentiation vs., **855**
  synovial sarcoma vs., **668**
Fibroxanthoma, atypical, **636–641**
- angiosarcoma vs., **472**
- dermatofibroma vs., **272**
- differential diagnosis, **637–638**
- immunohistochemistry, **638**
- pleomorphic fibroma vs., **157**
- prognosis, **637**
- superficial CD34(+) fibroblastic tumor vs., **211**
Focal myositis, **370–371**
- differential diagnosis, **371**
- fibromatosis colli vs., **255**
- prognosis, **371**
Follicular dendritic cell sarcoma (FDCS), **326–327**
- angiomatoid fibrous histiocytoma vs., **644**
- differential diagnosis, **327**
- extranodal Rosai-Dorfman disease vs., **312**
- interdigitating dendritic cell sarcoma vs., **329**
- prognosis, **327**
Follicular dendritic reticulum cell sarcoma. *See* Follicular dendritic cell sarcoma.
Fracture callus, fibroosseous pseudotumor of digit vs., **131**

G

Gangliocytic paraganglioma, **770–771**
- differential diagnosis, **771**
Ganglion cyst, **784–785**
- differential diagnosis, **785**
- prognosis, **785**
Ganglioneuroblastoma, neuroblastoma and, **832–841**
- differential diagnosis, **834–835**
- favorable vs. unfavorable histology in neuroblastic tumors, **835**
- ganglioneuroma vs., **551**

INDEX

- genetic testing, **834**
- intermixed, **834**
- International Neuroblastoma Pathology Committee (INPC) classification, **834**
- neuroblastoma staging system, **835**
- nodular, **834**
- poorly differentiated, **834**
- prognosis, **833**
- prognosis based on *MYCN* amplification and histology, **835**
- undifferentiated, **834**

Ganglioneuroma, **550–553**
- differential diagnosis, **551**
- ectomesenchymoma vs., **571**
- maturing, neuroblastoma and ganglioneuroblastoma vs., **835**
- prognosis, **551**

Gangliorhabdomyosarcoma. *See* Ectomesenchymoma.

Gardner fibroma, **256–257**
- diagnostic checklist, **257**
- differential diagnosis, **257**
- elastofibromas vs., **143**
- nuchal-type fibroma vs., **165**
- prognosis, **257**

Gastrointestinal autonomic nerve tumor. *See* Gastrointestinal stromal tumor.

Gastrointestinal mesenchymal tumors, by location, **27**

Gastrointestinal neuroectodermal tumor, malignant, **776–779**
- differential diagnosis, **777–778**
- gastrointestinal stromal tumor vs., **747**
- immunohistochemistry, **778**
- molecular genetics, **777**

Gastrointestinal schwannoma, **760–761**
- differential diagnosis, **761**
- gastrointestinal smooth muscle neoplasms vs., **764**
- gastrointestinal stromal tumor vs., **747**
- melanotic schwannoma vs., **557**
- prognosis, **761**

Gastrointestinal smooth muscle neoplasms, **762–765**
- differential diagnosis, **764**
- gastrointestinal stromal tumor vs., **747**
- prognosis, **763**

Gastrointestinal stromal sarcoma. *See* Gastrointestinal stromal tumor.

Gastrointestinal stromal tumor
- malignant gastrointestinal neuroectodermal tumor vs., **777**

Gastrointestinal stromal tumor (GIST), **744–759**
- benign neural gastrointestinal polyps vs., **741**
- calcifying fibrous tumor vs., **249**
- deep leiomyoma vs., **339**
- desmoid-type fibromatosis vs., **170**
- differential diagnosis, **747**
- epithelioid, extraskeletal myxoid chondrosarcoma vs., **713**
- gastrointestinal schwannoma vs., **761**
- gastrointestinal smooth muscle neoplasms vs., **764**
- histiocytic sarcoma vs., **325**
- idiopathic tumefactive fibroinflammatory lesions vs., **790**
- inflammatory fibroid polyp vs., **767**
- inflammatory myofibroblastic tumor vs., **198**
- leiomyosarcoma vs., **346**
- low-grade endometrial stromal sarcoma vs., **857**
- malignant gastrointestinal neuroectodermal tumor vs., **777**
- molecular prognostication, **748**
- paraganglioma vs., **816**
- plexiform fibromyxoma vs., **773**
- prognosis, **745–746**
- risk stratification, **748**
- solitary fibrous tumor vs., **186**
- spindled, gangliocytic paraganglioma vs., **771**

GCFB. *See* Giant cell fibroblastoma.

Generalized lymphangioma. *See* Lymphangioma.

Genital rhabdomyoma, **376–377**
- botryoid-type embryonal, fibroepithelial stromal polyp vs., **575**
- differential diagnosis, **377**
- embryonal rhabdomyosarcoma vs., **382**
- fetal rhabdomyoma vs., **375**
- prognosis, **377**

Genital stromal tumors
- angiomyofibroblastoma, **576–579**
  - differential diagnosis, **577**
  - prognosis, **577**
- cellular angiofibroma, **580–583**
  - differential diagnosis, **581**
  - prognosis, **581**
- deep (aggressive) angiomyxoma, **584–587**
  - differential diagnosis, **585**
  - genetic testing, **585**
  - prognosis, **585**
- fibroepithelial stromal polyp, **574–575**
  - differential diagnosis, **575**
  - prognosis, **575**

GH. *See* Glomeruloid hemangioma.

Giant cell angiofibroma. *See* Solitary fibrous tumor.

Giant cell fibroblastoma (GCFB), **260–263**
- angiosarcoma vs., **472**
- differential diagnosis, **261**
- fibrous hamartoma of infancy vs., **241**
- prognosis, **261**
- spindle cell/pleomorphic lipoma vs., **62**

Giant cell reticulohistiocytoma. *See* Reticulohistiocytoma.

Giant cell tumor
- diffuse-type tenosynovial
  - differential diagnosis, **286**
  - localized-type tenosynovial giant cell tumor vs., **280**
  - myxoinflammatory fibroblastic sarcoma vs., **204**
  - prognosis, **285**
  - synovial lipomatosis vs., **55**
- diffuse-type tenosynovial, **284–289**
- localized-type tenosynovial, **278–283**
  - deep benign fibrous histiocytoma vs., **277**
  - differential diagnosis, **280**
  - diffuse-type tenosynovial giant cell tumor vs., **286**
  - fibroma of tendon sheath vs., **136**
  - prognosis, **279**

INDEX

xanthomas vs., **296**
- tenosynovial
  fibroosseous pseudotumor vs., **131**
  giant cell tumor of soft tissue vs., **321**
  malignant, diffuse-type tenosynovial giant cell tumor vs., **286**
  soft tissue chondroma vs., **488**

Giant cell tumor of bone
- extraskeletal recurrence of, giant cell tumor of soft tissue vs., **321**
- localized-type tenosynovial giant cell tumor vs., **280**

Giant cell tumor of soft tissue, **320–323**
- aneurysmal bone cyst of soft tissue vs., **631**
- differential diagnosis, **321**
- diffuse-type tenosynovial giant cell tumor vs., **286**
- extraskeletal osteosarcoma vs., **498**
- fibroosseous pseudotumor vs., **131**
- localized-type tenosynovial giant cell tumor vs., **280**
- plexiform fibrohistiocytic tumor vs., **317**
- prognosis, **321**

GIST. *See* Gastrointestinal stromal tumor.

Glial heterotopia, **812–813**
- differential diagnosis, **813**
- prognosis, **813**

Glomangiomatosis, angiomatosis vs., **445**

Glomangiopericytoma, sinonasal, **804–809**
- diagnostic checklist, **806**
- differential diagnosis, **806**
- genetics, **805**
- nasopharyngeal angiofibroma vs., **802**
- prognosis, **805**

Glomeruloid angioma. *See* Glomeruloid hemangioma.

Glomeruloid hemangioma, **442–443**
- acquired tufted angioma vs., **437**
- diagnostic checklist, **443**
- differential diagnosis, **443**
- prognosis, **443**
- sinusoidal hemangioma vs., **441**

Glomus jugulare. *See* Paraganglioma.

Glomus tumors (and variants), **352–357**
- differential diagnosis, **354**
- myopericytoma vs., **359**
- ossifying fibromyxoid tumor vs., **652**
- prognosis, **353**
- sinonasal glomangiopericytoma vs., **806**

Glomus tympanicum. *See* Paraganglioma.

Gout, tophaceous
- amyloidoma vs., **783**
- tumoral calcinosis vs., **787**

Grading and staging, **6–11**
- additional descriptors (pTNM system), **9**
- anatomic stage/prognostic groups
  retroperitoneum, **9**
  trunk and extremities, **7**
- grading system of French FNCLCC system, **6**
- histologic features evaluated in grading (FNCLCC), **6**
- soft tissue sarcoma staging (pTNM System), for head and neck, **8**
- soft tissue sarcoma staging (TNM System)
  for abdomen and thoracic organs, **8**
  for orbit, **7**
  for retroperitoneum, **7**
  for trunk and extremities, **7**

Granular cell change, reactive, granular cell tumor vs., **542**

Granular cell dermatofibroma, granular cell tumor vs., **542**

Granular cell epulis, congenital, granular cell tumor vs., **542**

Granular cell fibroblastoma. *See* Congenital granular cell epulis.

Granular cell histiocytosis, crystal-storing histiocytosis vs., **315**

Granular cell myoblastoma. *See* Granular cell tumor.

Granular cell schwannoma. *See* Granular cell tumor.

Granular cell tumor, **540–545**
- adult rhabdomyoma vs., **373**
- alveolar soft part sarcoma vs., **685**
- congenital granular cell epulis vs., **799**
- crystal-storing histiocytosis vs., **315**
- differential diagnosis, **542**
- gastrointestinal smooth muscle neoplasms vs., **764**
- hibernoma vs., **75**
- nonneural, granular cell tumor vs., **542**
- PEComa vs., **694**
- prognosis, **541**

Granulocytic sarcoma. *See* Myeloid sarcoma.

Granuloma
- infectious
  deep granuloma annulare vs., **305**
  rheumatoid nodule vs., **307**
- palisading subcutaneous. *See* Deep granuloma annulare.
- pyogenic. *See also* Lobular capillary hemangioma.
  angiofibroma of soft tissue vs., **145**
  antrochoanal, nasopharyngeal angiofibroma vs., **802**
  bacillary angiomatosis vs., **411**
  congenital granular cell epulis vs., **799**
  glomeruloid hemangioma vs., **443**
  infantile hemangioma vs., **418**
  nasopharyngeal angiofibroma vs., **802**
  sinonasal glomangiopericytoma vs., **806**

Granuloma annulare, deep, **304–305**
- differential diagnosis, **305**
- prognosis, **305**

Granulomatous inflammation, Langerhans cell histiocytosis vs., **309**

Granulomatous lesions, angiomatoid fibrous histiocytoma vs., **644**

Granulomatous processes, epithelioid sarcoma vs., **680**

Gross examination, **4–5**
- clinical findings, **4**
- procedure, **4**

H

Hamartoma
- fibrolipomatous
  of nerve. *See* Lipomatosis.
  neuromuscular choristoma vs., **555**
- fibrous hamartoma of infancy, **240–243**
  differential diagnosis, **241**

INDEX

lipofibromatosis vs., **259**
prognosis, **241**
- meningothelial, glial heterotopia vs., **813**
- mucosal Schwann cell, gastrointestinal smooth muscle neoplasms vs., **764**
- smooth muscle, **332–333**
congenital, superficial leiomyoma vs., **335**
differential diagnosis, **333**
prognosis, **333**
superficial leiomyoma vs., **335**

Hamartomatous thymoma, ectopic, **632–633**
- differential diagnosis, **633**
- prognosis, **633**

Hand-Schüller-Christian disease. *See* Langerhans cell histiocytosis.

Hemangioblastoma, peripheral, **822–823**
- differential diagnosis, **823**
- genetics, **823**
- prognosis, **823**

Hemangioendothelioma
- composite, **460–461**
differential diagnosis, **461**
epithelioid hemangioendothelioma vs., **468**
papillary intralymphatic angioendothelioma vs., **457**
prognosis, **461**
retiform hemangioendothelioma vs., **459**
- epithelioid, **466–469**
angiosarcoma vs., **472**
composite hemangioendothelioma vs., **461**
differential diagnosis, **468**
epithelioid hemangioma vs., **423**
intimal sarcoma vs., **721**
malignant mesothelioma vs., **600**
molecular genetics, **467**
prognosis, **467**
pseudomyogenic hemangioendothelioma, **463**
spindle cell hemangioma vs., **427**
- epithelioid sarcoma-like. *See* Pseudomyogenic hemangioendothelioma.
- hobnail. *See* Retiform hemangioendothelioma.
- Kaposiform, **454–455**
acquired tufted angioma vs., **437**
congenital hemangioma vs., **414**
diagnostic checklist, **455**
differential diagnosis, **455**
infantile hemangioma vs., **418**
Kaposi sarcoma vs., **478**
prognosis, **455**
spindle cell hemangioma vs., **427**
- pseudomyogenic, **462–465**
differential diagnosis, **463**
epithelioid hemangioendothelioma vs., **468**
epithelioid sarcoma vs., **680**
molecular genetics, **463**
prognosis, **463**
- retiform, **458–459**
angiosarcoma vs., **472**
composite hemangioendothelioma vs., **461**
diagnostic checklist, **459**
differential diagnosis, **459**
hobnail hemangioma vs., **435**
papillary intralymphatic angioendothelioma vs., **457**
prognosis, **459**

Hemangioma
- acquired tufted, glomeruloid hemangioma vs., **443**
- angioleiomyoma vs., **367**
- angiosarcoma vs., **472**
- arteriovenous, sinusoidal hemangioma vs., **441**
- cavernous, sinusoidal hemangioma vs., **441**
- congenital, **412–415**
differential diagnosis, **414**
genetics, **413**
infantile hemangioma vs., **418**
prognosis, **413**
- diffuse. *See* Angiomatosis.
- epithelioid, **422–425**
differential diagnosis, **423**
epithelioid hemangioendothelioma vs., **468**
molecular genetics, **423**
prognosis, **423**
- glomeruloid, **442–443**
acquired tufted angioma vs., **437**
diagnostic checklist, **443**
differential diagnosis, **443**
prognosis, **443**
sinusoidal hemangioma vs., **441**
- hobnail, **434–435**
atypical vascular lesion vs., **453**
diagnostic checklist, **435**
differential diagnosis, **435**
glomeruloid hemangioma vs., **443**
Kaposi sarcoma vs., **478**
microvenular hemangioma vs., **439**
prognosis, **435**
- infantile, **416–419**
acquired tufted angioma vs., **437**
angiomatosis vs., **445**
congenital hemangioma vs., **414**
differential diagnosis, **418**
genetics, **417**
kaposiform hemangioendothelioma vs., **455**
prognosis, **417**
- intramuscular
angiolipoma vs., **57**
angiomatosis vs., **445**
differential diagnosis, **431**
lipoma vs., **48**
prognosis, **431**
- lobular capillary, **420–421**
acquired tufted angioma vs., **437**
angiofibroma of soft tissue vs., **145**
congenital granular cell epulis vs., **799**
differential diagnosis, **421**
glomeruloid hemangioma vs., **443**
infantile hemangioma vs., **418**
nasopharyngeal angiofibroma vs., **802**
prognosis, **421**
sinonasal glomangiopericytoma vs., **806**
- lymphangioma vs., **448**
- microvenular, **438–439**
diagnostic checklist, **439**
differential diagnosis, **439**

INDEX

hobnail hemangioma vs., **435**
Kaposi sarcoma vs., **478**
prognosis, **439**
- papillary endothelial hyperplasia vs., **409**
- sinusoidal, **440–441**
diagnostic checklist, **441**
differential diagnosis, **441**
prognosis, **441**
- spindle cell, **426–429**
angiolipoma vs., **57**
angiomatoid fibrous histiocytoma vs., **644**
composite hemangioendothelioma vs., **461**
diagnostic checklist, **427**
differential diagnosis, **427**
Kaposi sarcoma vs., **478**
kaposiform hemangioendothelioma vs., **455**
prognosis, **427**
- targetoid hemosiderotic
glomeruloid hemangioma vs., **443**
microvenular hemangioma vs., **439**
Hemangiopericytoma. *See* Solitary fibrous tumor.
Hemangiopericytoma-like tumor of sinonasal cavity. *See* Sinonasal glomangiopericytoma.
Hemangiosarcoma. *See* Angiosarcoma.
Hemarthrosis, diffuse-type tenosynovial giant cell tumor vs., **286**
Hematoma, papillary endothelial hyperplasia vs., **409**
Hematopoietic tumors in soft tissue
- lymphoma of soft tissue, **610–611**
differential diagnosis, **611**
prognosis, **611**
- myeloid sarcoma, **608–609**
differential diagnosis, **609**
molecular genetics, **609**
prognosis, **609**
- solitary extramedullary plasmacytoma, **606–607**
differential diagnosis, **607**
prognosis, **607**
Hemosiderotic fibrohistiocytic lipomatous lesion. *See* Hemosiderotic fibrolipomatous tumor.
Hemosiderotic fibrolipomatous tumor (HFLT), **634–635**
- differential diagnosis, **635**
- molecular genetics, **635**
- myxoinflammatory fibroblastic sarcoma vs., **204**
- pleomorphic hyalinizing angiectatic tumor vs., **627**
- prognosis, **635**
Hemosiderotic hemangioma, targetoid
- glomeruloid hemangioma vs., **443**
- microvenular hemangioma vs., **439**
Hereditary leiomyomatosis and renal cell cancer syndrome (HLRCC), **335**
Heterotopic glial tissue. *See* Glial heterotopia.
HFLT. *See* Hemosiderotic fibrolipomatous tumor.
HH. *See* Hobnail hemangioma.
Hibernoma, **74–77**
- adult rhabdomyoma vs., **373**
- atypical lipomatous tumor/well-differentiated liposarcoma vs., **90**
- differential diagnosis, **75**
- granular cell tumor vs., **542**
- lipoma vs., **48**
- molecular genetics, **75**
- prognosis, **75**
Hip stone disease. *See* Tumoral calcinosis.
Histiocytic proliferations, extranodal Rosai-Dorfman disease vs., **312**
Histiocytic proliferations, miscellaneous, extranodal Rosai-Dorfman disease vs., **312**
Histiocytic sarcoma, **324–325**
- differential diagnosis, **325**
- extranodal Rosai-Dorfman disease vs., **312**
- interdigitating dendritic cell sarcoma vs., **329**
- Langerhans cell histiocytosis vs., **309**
- prognosis, **325**
Histiocytoma
- deep benign fibrous, angiofibroma of soft tissue vs., **145**
- fibrous. *See* Fibrous histiocytoma.
- myxoid malignant fibrous. *See* Myxofibrosarcoma.
Histiocytosis
- crystal-storing, **314–315**
adult rhabdomyoma vs., **373**
differential diagnosis, **315**
prognosis, **315**
- granular cell, crystal-storing histiocytosis vs., **315**
- Langerhans cell, **308–309**
differential diagnosis, **309**
extranodal Rosai-Dorfman disease vs., **312**
prognosis, **309**
reticulohistiocytoma vs., **302**
solitary (juvenile) xanthogranuloma vs., **299**
Histiocytosis X. *See* Langerhans cell histiocytosis.
HLRCC. *See* Hereditary leiomyomatosis and renal cell cancer syndrome.
Hobnail hemangioendothelioma. *See* Retiform hemangioendothelioma.
Hobnail hemangioma, **434–435**
- atypical vascular lesion vs., **453**
- diagnostic checklist, **435**
- differential diagnosis, **435**
- glomeruloid hemangioma vs., **443**
- Kaposi sarcoma vs., **478**
- microvenular hemangioma vs., **439**
- prognosis, **435**
Hodgkin disease, extranodal, myxoinflammatory fibroblastic sarcoma vs., **204**
Hoffa disease, synovial lipomatosis vs., **55**
Hyaline fibromatosis syndrome, **252–253**
- differential diagnosis, **253**
- prognosis, **253**
Hyalinizing spindle cell tumor, with giant rosettes. *See* Low-grade fibromyxoid sarcoma.
Hybrid nerve sheath tumor, **536–539**
- differential diagnosis, **537**
- gastrointestinal schwannoma vs., **761**
- low-grade fibromyxoid sarcoma vs., **224**
- perineurioma vs., **532**
- prognosis, **537**
Hyperlipoproteinemia (Fredrickson) classification, **296**
Hyperplasia, papillary endothelial, **408–409**
- angiosarcoma vs., **472**

INDEX

- diagnostic checklist, **409**
- differential diagnosis, **409**
- prognosis, **409**

Hypertrophic scar
- dermatomyofibroma vs., **159**
- keloid vs., **163**

I

IDCS. *See* Interdigitating dendritic cell sarcoma.

Idiopathic retroperitoneal fibrosis, **789**
- atypical lipomatous tumor/well-differentiated liposarcoma vs., **90**
- desmoid-type fibromatosis vs., **170**

Idiopathic tumefactive fibroinflammatory lesions, **788–791**
- differential diagnosis, **790**
- prognosis, **789**

Idiopathic tumoral fibroinflammatory disorders. *See* Idiopathic tumefactive fibroinflammatory lesions.

IFS. *See* Infantile fibrosarcoma.

IgG4-related sclerosing disease, **789**

Inclusion body fibromatosis, **250–251**
- differential diagnosis, **251**
- fibroma of tendon sheath vs., **136**
- prognosis, **251**

Infantile digital fibroma. *See* Inclusion body fibromatosis.

Infantile digital fibromatosis. *See* Inclusion body fibromatosis.

Infantile fibrosarcoma (IFS), **264–267**
- differential diagnosis, **265**
- embryonal rhabdomyosarcoma vs., **382**
- molecular genetics, **265**
- myofibroma and myofibromatosis vs., **363**
- prognosis, **265**
- spindle cell rhabdomyosarcoma vs., **394**

Infantile hemangioma, **416–419**
- acquired tufted angioma vs., **437**
- angiomatosis vs., **445**
- congenital hemangioma vs., **414**
- differential diagnosis, **418**
- genetics, **417**
- kaposiform hemangioendothelioma vs., **455**
- prognosis, **417**

Infantile/juvenile fibromatosis, nondesmoid type. *See* Fibromatosis.

Infectious granulomas
- deep granuloma annulare vs., **305**
- rheumatoid nodule vs., **307**

Infiltrating angiolipoma. *See* Angiomatosis.

Infiltrating/intramuscular angiolipoma. *See* Intramuscular hemangioma.

Inflammatory fibroid polyp, **766–769**
- benign neural gastrointestinal polyps vs., **741**
- differential diagnosis, **767**
- gastrointestinal smooth muscle neoplasms vs., **764**
- gastrointestinal stromal tumor vs., **747**
- inflammatory myofibroblastic tumor vs., **198**
- plexiform fibromyxoma vs., **773**

Inflammatory fibrosarcoma. *See* Inflammatory myofibroblastic tumor.

Inflammatory myofibroblastic sarcoma. *See* Inflammatory myofibroblastic tumor.

Inflammatory myofibroblastic tumor, **196–201**
- calcifying fibrous tumor vs., **249**
- cardiac fibroma vs., **797**
- desmoid-type fibromatosis vs., **170**
- differential diagnosis, **198**
- focal myositis vs., **371**
- follicular dendritic cell sarcoma vs., **327**
- idiopathic tumefactive fibroinflammatory lesions vs., **790**
- inflammatory fibroid polyp vs., **767**
- leiomyosarcoma vs., **346**
- low-grade myofibroblastic sarcoma vs., **193**
- molecular genetics, **197–198**
- myxoinflammatory fibroblastic sarcoma vs., **204**
- nodular fasciitis vs., **116**
- plexiform fibromyxoma vs., **773**
- prognosis, **197**
- spindle cell rhabdomyosarcoma vs., **394**
- superficial CD34(+) fibroblastic tumor vs., **211**

Inflammatory myxohyaline tumor of distal extremities with virocyte or Reed-Sternberg-like cells. *See* Myxoinflammatory fibroblastic sarcoma.

Inflammatory pseudotumor. *See* Inflammatory myofibroblastic tumor.

Interdigitating dendritic cell sarcoma (IDCS), **328–329**
- differential diagnosis, **329**
- follicular dendritic cell sarcoma vs., **327**
- prognosis, **329**

Interdigitating dendritic reticulum cell sarcoma. *See* Interdigitating dendritic cell sarcoma.

Internal evaluation, gross examination, **4**

Intimal sarcoma, **720–721**
- differential diagnosis, **721**
- genetic testing, **721**
- prognosis, **721**

Intraabdominal DSRCT. *See* Desmoplastic small round cell tumor.

Intraarticular fibroma. *See* Fibroma, tendon sheath.

Intralymphatic angioendothelioma, papillary, retiform hemangioendothelioma vs., **459**

Intramuscular angioma. *See* Intramuscular hemangioma.

Intramuscular hemangioma (IMH), **430–433**
- angiolipoma vs., **57**
- angiomatosis vs., **445**
- differential diagnosis, **431**
- lipoma vs., **48**
- prognosis, **431**

Intramuscular myxoma, **614–617**
- differential diagnosis, **615**
- genetic testing, **615**
- juxtaarticular myxoma vs., **619**
- low-grade fibromyxoid sarcoma vs., **224**
- myxofibrosarcoma vs., **218**
- myxoid liposarcoma vs., **102**
- prognosis, **615**

INDEX

Intranodal palisade myofibroblastoma, **152–155**
- differential diagnosis, **153**
- molecular genetics, **153**
- prognosis, **153**

Intranodal palisaded myofibroblastoma, angiomatoid fibrous histiocytoma vs., **644**
Intravascular angiomatosis. *See* Papillary endothelial hyperplasia.
Intravascular bronchioloalveolar tumor. *See* Epithelioid hemangioendothelioma.
Intravascular papillary endothelial hyperplasia, spindle cell hemangioma vs., **427**
Ischemic fasciitis, **124–125**
- differential diagnosis, **125**
- prognosis, **125**

J

Juvenile aponeurotic fibroma. *See* Calcifying aponeurotic fibroma.
Juvenile hemangioma. *See* Infantile hemangioma.
Juvenile nasopharyngeal angiofibroma. *See* Nasopharyngeal angiofibroma.
Juvenile xanthogranuloma, **298–299**
- differential diagnosis, **299**
- extranodal Rosai-Dorfman disease vs., **312**
- prognosis, **299**
- reticulohistiocytoma vs., **302**
- xanthomas vs., **296**

Juxtaarticular chondroma
- synovial chondromatosis vs., **493**

Juxtaarticular myxoma, **618–619**
- differential diagnosis, **619**
- genetic testing, **619**
- myxofibrosarcoma vs., **218**
- perineurioma vs., **532**
- prognosis, **619**

K

Kaposi sarcoma, **476–483**
- acquired tufted angioma vs., **437**
- angiolipoma vs., **57**
- angiomatoid fibrous histiocytoma vs., **644**
- angiosarcoma vs., **472**
- bacillary angiomatosis vs., **411**
- composite hemangioendothelioma vs., **461**
- dermatofibroma vs., **272**
- differential diagnosis, **478**
- glomeruloid hemangioma vs., **443**
- hobnail hemangioma vs., **435**
- intranodal palisade myofibroblastoma vs., **153**
- kaposiform hemangioendothelioma vs., **455**
- lymphangioma-like, lymphangioma vs., **448**
- microvenular hemangioma vs., **439**
- nodular fasciitis vs., **116**
- papillary intralymphatic angioendothelioma vs., **457**
- prognosis, **477**
- retiform hemangioendothelioma vs., **459**
- spindle cell hemangioma vs., **427**

Kaposiform hemangioendothelioma, **454–455**
- acquired tufted angioma vs., **437**
- congenital hemangioma vs., **414**
- diagnostic checklist, **455**
- differential diagnosis, **455**
- infantile hemangioma vs., **418**
- Kaposi sarcoma vs., **478**
- prognosis, **455**
- spindle cell hemangioma vs., **427**

Keloid, **162–163**
- diagnostic checklist, **163**
- differential diagnosis, **163**
- prognosis, **163**

Kimura disease, epithelioid hemangioma vs., **423**

L

Langerhans cell histiocytosis (LCH), **308–309**
- differential diagnosis, **309**
- extranodal Rosai-Dorfman disease vs., **312**
- prognosis, **309**
- reticulohistiocytoma vs., **302**
- solitary (juvenile) xanthogranuloma vs., **299**

Langerhans cell sarcoma
- interdigitating dendritic cell sarcoma vs., **329**
- Langerhans cell histiocytosis vs., **309**

LCH. *See* Langerhans cell histiocytosis.
Ledderhose disease. *See* Palmar/plantar fibromatosis.
Leiomyoblastoma. *See* Gastrointestinal stromal tumor.
Leiomyoma
- cutaneous
    - smooth muscle hamartoma vs., **333**
- cutis. *See* Superficial leiomyoma.
- deep, **338–341**
    - differential diagnosis, **339**
    - prognosis, **339**
- deep (aggressive) angiomyxoma vs., **585**
- dermatomyofibroma vs., **159**
- desmoid-type fibromatosis vs., **170**
- Epstein-Barr virus-associated smooth muscle tumor vs., **343**
- with fatty metaplasia/degeneration, myolipoma vs., **71**
- ganglioneuroma vs., **551**
- gastrointestinal schwannoma vs., **761**
- gastrointestinal stromal tumor vs., **747**
- granular cell tumor vs., **542**
- leiomyosarcoma vs., **346**
- myofibroma and myofibromatosis vs., **363**
- palmar/plantar fibromatosis vs., **167**
- PEComa vs., **694**
- pilar
    - inclusion body fibromatosis vs., **251**
    - smooth muscle hamartoma vs., **333**
- plexiform fibromyxoma vs., **773**

INDEX

- schwannoma vs., **511**
- submucosal, benign neural gastrointestinal polyps vs., **741**
- superficial, **334–337**
  differential diagnosis, **335**
  prognosis, **335**

Leiomyosarcoma, **344–349**
- adult-type fibrosarcoma vs., **215**
- atypical fibroxanthoma vs., **638**
- cutaneous, smooth muscle hamartoma vs., **333**
- dedifferentiated liposarcoma vs., **96**
- deep leiomyoma vs., **339**
- differential diagnosis, **346**
- Epstein-Barr virus-associated smooth muscle tumor vs., **343**
- gastrointestinal smooth muscle neoplasms vs., **764**
- gastrointestinal stromal tumor vs., **747**
- inflammatory myofibroblastic tumor vs., **198**
- intimal sarcoma vs., **721**
- Kaposi sarcoma vs., **478**
- low-grade myofibroblastic sarcoma vs., **193**
- malignant peripheral nerve sheath tumor vs., **560**
- myxoid, primary pulmonary myxoid sarcoma vs., **848**
- nodular fasciitis vs., **116**
- PEComa vs., **694**
- prognosis, **345**
- spindle cell rhabdomyosarcoma vs., **394**
- superficial, superficial leiomyoma vs., **335**
- synovial sarcoma vs., **668**
- undifferentiated pleomorphic sarcoma vs., **725**

Letterer-Siwe disease. *See* Langerhans cell histiocytosis.

Leukemia, alveolar rhabdomyosarcoma vs., **388**

LGFMS. *See* Low-grade fibromyxoid sarcoma.

LGMS. *See* Low-grade myofibroblastic sarcoma.

Lipid calcinosis. *See* Tumoral calcinosis.

Lipidized-type dermatofibroma, xanthomas vs., **296**

Lipoblastoma, **80–83**
- differential diagnosis, **81**
- fibrous hamartoma of infancy vs., **241**
- hibernoma vs., **75**
- lipofibromatosis vs., **259**
- molecular genetics, **81**
- myxoid liposarcoma vs., **102**
- prognosis, **81**

Lipoblastoma-like tumor of vulva
- lipoblastoma vs., **81**
- myxoid liposarcoma vs., **102**

Lipofibromatosis, **258–259**
- calcifying aponeurotic fibroma vs., **245**
- differential diagnosis, **259**
- genetics, **259**
- infantile fibrosarcoma vs., **265**
- prognosis, **259**

Lipofibromatosis-like neural tumor
- fibrous hamartoma of infancy vs., **241**
- infantile fibrosarcoma vs., **265**
- lipofibromatosis vs., **259**

Lipoid proteinosis, hyaline fibromatosis syndrome vs., **253**

Lipoleiomyoma, extrauterine. *See* Myolipoma.

Lipoma, **46–51**
- angiolipoma vs., **57**
- atypical lipomatous tumor/well-differentiated liposarcoma vs., **90**
- chondroid, **66–69**
  differential diagnosis, **67**
  epithelioid hemangioendothelioma vs., **468**
  genetic testing, **67**
  lipoma vs., **48**
  prognosis, **67**
- diagnostic checklist, **48**
- differential diagnosis, **48**
- of embryonic fat. *See* Hibernoma.
- fetal. *See* Hibernoma.
- genetic testing, **48**
- lipoblastoma vs., **81**
- of nerve, lipomatosis of nerve vs., **53**
- pleomorphic, giant cell fibroblastoma vs., **261**
- prognosis, **47**
- spindle cell, **60–65**
  cellular angiofibroma vs., **581**
  differential diagnosis, **62**
  hemosiderotic fibrolipomatous tumor vs., **635**
  lipoma vs., **48**
  mammary-type myofibroblastoma vs., **149**
  molecular genetics, **61**
  myolipoma vs., **71**
  prognosis, **61**
  solitary fibrous tumor vs., **186**

Lipoma arborescens. *See* Synovial lipomatosis.

Lipomatosis
- of nerve, **52–53**
  differential diagnosis, **53**
  lipofibromatosis vs., **259**
  lipoma vs., **48**
  neuromuscular choristoma vs., **555**
  prognosis, **53**
- synovial, **54–55**
  differential diagnosis, **55**
  prognosis, **55**

Lipomatous tumor/well-differentiated liposarcoma
- atypical, **88–93**
  atypical spindle cell lipomatous tumor vs., **85**
  chondroid lipoma vs., **67**
  differential diagnosis, **90**
  elastofibromas vs., **143**
  hibernoma vs., **75**
  massive localized lymphedema vs., **451**
  molecular genetics, **90**
  myxoid liposarcoma vs., **102**
  pleomorphic liposarcoma vs., **108**
  prognosis, **89**
  spindle cell/pleomorphic lipoma vs., **62**
  synovial lipomatosis vs., **55**
- lipoma vs., **48**
- spindle cell, spindle cell/pleomorphic lipoma vs., **62**

Liposarcoma
- dedifferentiated, **94–99**
  desmoid-type fibromatosis vs., **170**
  differential diagnosis, **96**
  extraskeletal osteosarcoma vs., **498**
  histiocytic sarcoma vs., **325**
  inflammatory myofibroblastic tumor vs., **198**

INDEX

low-grade morphology, myolipoma vs., **71**
malignant peripheral nerve sheath tumor vs., **560**
molecular genetics, **96**
myxofibrosarcoma vs., **218**
prognosis, **95**
solitary fibrous tumor vs., **186**
undifferentiated pleomorphic sarcoma vs., **725**
- myxoid, **100–105**
angiofibroma of soft tissue vs., **145**
atypical lipomatous tumor/well-differentiated liposarcoma vs., **90**
chondroid lipoma vs., **67**
dedifferentiated liposarcoma vs., **96**
differential diagnosis, **102**
hibernoma vs., **75**
intramuscular myxoma vs., **615**
lipoblastoma vs., **81**
lipoma vs., **48**
low-grade fibromyxoid sarcoma vs., **224**
massive localized lymphedema vs., **451**
molecular genetics, **102**
myxofibrosarcoma vs., **218**
pleomorphic liposarcoma vs., **108**
primary pulmonary myxoid sarcoma vs., **848**
prognosis, **101**
spindle cell/pleomorphic lipoma vs., **62**
superficial angiomyxoma vs., **621**
- pleomorphic, **106–111**
dedifferentiated liposarcoma vs., **96**
differential diagnosis, **107–108**
molecular genetics, **107**
myxofibrosarcoma vs., **218**
prognosis, **107**
undifferentiated pleomorphic sarcoma vs., **725**
- well-differentiated, **88–93**
dedifferentiated liposarcoma vs., **96**
differential diagnosis, **90**
elastofibromas vs., **143**
idiopathic tumefactive fibroinflammatory lesions vs., **790**
inflammatory myofibroblastic tumor vs., **198**
ischemic fasciitis vs., **125**
massive localized lymphedema vs., **451**
molecular genetics, **90**
myelolipoma vs., **79**
peripheral hemangioblastoma vs., **823**
prognosis, **89**
synovial lipomatosis vs., **55**

Lobular capillary hemangioma, **420–421**
- acquired tufted angioma vs., **437**
- angiofibroma of soft tissue vs., **145**
- congenital granular cell epulis vs., **799**
- differential diagnosis, **421**
- glomeruloid hemangioma vs., **443**
- infantile hemangioma vs., **418**
- nasopharyngeal angiofibroma vs., **802**
- prognosis, **421**
- sinonasal glomangiopericytoma vs., **806**

Localized fibrous mesothelioma. *See* Solitary fibrous tumor.

Localized hypertrophic neuropathy of limbs. *See* Perineurioma.

Localized lymphedema, massive, **450–451**
- atypical lipomatous tumor/well-differentiated liposarcoma vs., **90**
- differential diagnosis, **451**
- prognosis, **451**

Localized-type tenosynovial giant cell tumor, **278–283**
- deep benign fibrous histiocytoma vs., **277**
- differential diagnosis, **280**
- diffuse-type tenosynovial giant cell tumor vs., **286**
- fibroma of tendon sheath vs., **136**
- prognosis, **279**
- xanthomas vs., **296**

Low-grade endometrial stromal sarcoma, **856–857**
- differential diagnosis, **857**
- prognosis, **857**

Low-grade fibromyxoid sarcoma (LGFMS), **222–231**
- angiofibroma of soft tissue vs., **145**
- desmoid-type fibromatosis vs., **170**
- desmoplastic fibroblastoma vs., **141**
- differential diagnosis, **224**
- intramuscular myxoma vs., **615**
- juxtaarticular myxoma vs., **619**
- myxofibrosarcoma vs., **218**
- myxoid liposarcoma vs., **102**
- ossifying fibromyxoid tumor vs., **652**
- perineurioma vs., **532**
- prognosis, **223**
- sclerosing epithelioid fibrosarcoma vs., **233**
- superficial angiomyxoma vs., **621**

Low-grade myofibroblastic sarcoma, **192–195**
- adult-type fibrosarcoma vs., **215**
- desmoid-type fibromatosis vs., **170**
- differential diagnosis, **193**
- nodular fasciitis vs., **116**
- plexiform fibrohistiocytic tumor vs., **317**
- prognosis, **193**
- spindle cell rhabdomyosarcoma vs., **394**

Low-grade sinonasal sarcoma with neural and myogenic features. *See* Biphenotypic sinonasal sarcoma.

Low-grade stromal sarcoma. *See* Low-grade Endometrial stromal sarcoma.

Lymph node metastasis, intranodal palisade myofibroblastoma vs., **153**

Lymphangiectasia, secondary, lymphangioma vs., **448**

Lymphangioendothelioma, benign
- atypical vascular lesion vs., **453**
- Kaposi sarcoma vs., **478**

Lymphangioma, **446–449**
- adenomatoid tumor vs., **591**
- cystic, multicystic peritoneal mesothelioma vs., **593**
- diagnostic checklist, **448**
- differential diagnosis, **448**
- genetics, **447**
- prognosis, **447**
- progressive
atypical vascular lesion vs., **453**
hobnail hemangioma vs., **435**
Kaposi sarcoma vs., **478**
lymphangioma vs., **448**

INDEX

Lymphangioma circumscriptum. *See also* Lymphangioma.
- atypical vascular lesion vs., **453**

Lymphangioma-like Kaposi sarcoma, lymphangioma vs., **448**
Lymphangiomatosis. *See* Lymphangioma.
Lymphatic malformation. *See* Lymphangioma.
Lymphatic pseudotumor. *See* Massive localized lymphedema.
Lymphedema, massive localized, **450–451**
- atypical lipomatous tumor/well-differentiated liposarcoma vs., **90**
- differential diagnosis, **451**
- prognosis, **451**

Lymphoma
- alveolar rhabdomyosarcoma vs., **388**
- anaplastic large cell
  - inflammatory myofibroblastic tumor vs., **198**
  - pleomorphic rhabdomyosarcoma vs., **401**
- extraskeletal Ewing sarcoma vs., **708**
- focal myositis vs., **371**
- idiopathic tumefactive fibroinflammatory lesions vs., **790**
- malignant, desmoplastic small round cell tumor vs., **702**
- myeloid sarcoma vs., **609**
- neuroblastoma and ganglioneuroblastoma vs., **835**
- non-Hodgkin, histiocytic sarcoma vs., **325**
- sclerosing, sclerosing epithelioid fibrosarcoma vs., **234**
- undifferentiated pleomorphic sarcoma vs., **725**

Lymphoma of soft tissue, **610–611**
- differential diagnosis, **611**
- prognosis, **611**

M

Malakoplakia, crystal-storing histiocytosis vs., **315**
Malignant ectomesenchymoma. *See* Ectomesenchymoma.
Malignant epithelioid schwannoma. *See* Epithelioid malignant peripheral nerve sheath tumor.
Malignant fibrous histiocytoma. *See* Undifferentiated pleomorphic sarcoma.
Malignant gastrointestinal neuroectodermal tumor, **776–779**
- differential diagnosis, **777–778**
- gastrointestinal stromal tumor vs., **747**
- immunohistochemistry, **778**
- molecular genetics, **777**

Malignant hemangioendothelioma. *See* Angiosarcoma.
Malignant lymphoma, desmoplastic small round cell tumor vs., **702**
Malignant melanoma. *See* Melanoma, malignant.
Malignant melanotic schwannian tumor (proposed). *See* Melanotic schwannoma.
Malignant mesothelioma, **598–603**
- adenomatoid tumor vs., **591**
- differential diagnosis, **600**
- molecular genetics, **600**
- multicystic peritoneal mesothelioma vs., **593**
- prognosis, **599**
- well-differentiated papillary mesothelioma vs., **595**

Malignant myoepithelioma, **657**. *See also* Myoepithelioma, of soft tissue.
- epithelioid malignant peripheral nerve sheath tumor vs., **567**

Malignant myxoid endobronchial tumor. *See* Primary pulmonary myxoid sarcoma.
Malignant ossifying fibromyxoid tumor, **651**
Malignant peripheral nerve sheath tumor (MPNST), **558–565**
- adult-type fibrosarcoma vs., **215**
- atypical fibroxanthoma vs., **638**
- *BCOR-CCNB3* fusion-positive sarcoma vs., **736**
- clear cell sarcoma vs., **690**
- dedifferentiated liposarcoma vs., **96**
- differential diagnosis, **560**
- epithelioid, **566–569**
  - differential diagnosis, **567**
  - extrarenal rhabdoid tumor vs., **718**
  - myoepithelioma of soft tissue vs., **656**
  - ossifying fibromyxoid tumor vs., **652**
  - prognosis, **567**
- extraskeletal mesenchymal chondrosarcoma vs., **502**
- extraskeletal osteosarcoma vs., **498**
- genetic predisposition, **559**
- hybrid nerve sheath tumor vs., **537**
- leiomyosarcoma vs., **346**
- malignant gastrointestinal neuroectodermal tumor vs., **778**
- metastatic tumors to soft tissue sites vs., **829**
- myxofibrosarcoma vs., **218**
- neurofibroma vs., **524**
- palmar/plantar fibromatosis vs., **167**
- prognosis, **559**
- with rhabdomyoblastic differentiation
  - biphenotypic sinonasal sarcoma vs., **851**
  - embryonal rhabdomyosarcoma vs., **382**
- schwannoma vs., **511**
- spindle cell rhabdomyosarcoma vs., **393**
- synovial sarcoma vs., **668**
- undifferentiated pleomorphic sarcoma vs., **725**
- undifferentiated round cell sarcoma with *CIC-DUX4* translocation vs., **729**

Malignant rhabdoid tumor. *See* Extrarenal rhabdoid tumor.
Malignant schwannoma. *See* Malignant peripheral nerve sheath tumor.
Malignant synovioma. *See* Synovial sarcoma.
Malignant tenosynovial giant cell tumor, diffuse-type tenosynovial giant cell tumor vs., **286**
Mammary-type myofibroblastoma, **148–151**
- atypical spindle cell lipomatous tumor vs., **85**
- cellular angiofibroma vs., **581**
- differential diagnosis, **149**
- molecular genetics, **149**
- prognosis, **149**
- spindle cell/pleomorphic lipoma vs., **62**

Massive localized lymphedema, **450–451**
- atypical lipomatous tumor/well-differentiated liposarcoma vs., **90**
- differential diagnosis, **451**

INDEX

- prognosis, **451**
Masson tumor. *See* Papillary endothelial hyperplasia.
Mature adipose tissue, ectopic hamartomatous thymoma, **633**
Melanocytic nevus, dermal, glomus tumors vs., **354**
Melanoma
- angiosarcoma vs., **472**
- desmoplastic, keloid vs., **163**
- desmoplastic, neurofibroma vs., **524**
- epithelioid rhabdomyosarcoma vs., **405**
- epithelioid sarcoma vs., **680**
- gastrointestinal stromal tumor vs., **747**
- malignant
  alveolar soft part sarcoma vs., **685**
  epithelioid malignant peripheral nerve sheath tumor vs., **567**
  granular cell tumor vs., **542**
  lymphoma of soft tissue vs., **611**
  malignant peripheral nerve sheath tumor vs., **560**
  melanotic neuroectodermal tumor of infancy vs., **825**
  metastatic, pleomorphic liposarcoma vs., **108**
  myeloid sarcoma vs., **609**
  schwannoma vs., **511**
  solitary extramedullary plasmacytoma vs., **607**
- metastatic
  clear cell sarcoma vs., **690**
  extrarenal rhabdoid tumor vs., **718**
  histiocytic sarcoma vs., **325**
  interdigitating dendritic cell sarcoma vs., **329**
  intimal sarcoma vs., **721**
  malignant gastrointestinal neuroectodermal tumor vs., **778**
  melanotic schwannoma vs., **557**
  myoepithelioma of soft tissue vs., **656**
  paraganglioma vs., **816**
  schwannoma vs., **511**
- myxofibrosarcoma vs., **218**
- osteogenic, extraskeletal osteosarcoma vs., **498**
- PEComa vs., **694**
- pleomorphic, atypical fibroxanthoma vs., **637–638**
- pleomorphic rhabdomyosarcoma vs., **401**
- of soft parts (formerly). *See* Clear cell sarcoma.
- spindle cell
  atypical fibroxanthoma vs., **637–638**
  desmoplastic, dermatofibrosarcoma protuberans vs., **176**
  spindle cell rhabdomyosarcoma vs., **394**
- undifferentiated pleomorphic sarcoma vs., **725**
Melanotic ameloblastoma. *See* Melanotic neuroectodermal tumor of infancy.
Melanotic neuroectodermal tumor of infancy (MNTI), **824–825**
- differential diagnosis, **825**
- prognosis, **825**
Melanotic progonoma. *See* Melanotic neuroectodermal tumor of infancy.
Melanotic schwannoma, **556–557**
- differential diagnosis, **557**
- prognosis, **557**
Meningioma
- chondroid, extraskeletal myxoid chondrosarcoma vs., **713**
- ectopic, **810–811**
  differential diagnosis, **811**
  perineurioma vs., **532**
  prognosis, **811**
Meningothelial choristoma. *See* Ectopic meningioma.
Meningothelial hamartoma, glial heterotopia vs., **813**
Merkel cell carcinoma, lymphoma of soft tissue vs., **611**
Mesenchymal chondrosarcoma
- extraskeletal, **500–503**
  differential diagnosis, **502**
  extraskeletal Ewing sarcoma vs., **708**
  extraskeletal osteosarcoma vs., **498**
  molecular genetics, **501**
  prognosis, **501**
- phosphaturic mesenchymal tumor vs., **665**
Mesenchymal hamartoma, undifferentiated embryonal sarcoma of liver vs., **845**
Mesenchymal tumors
- gastrointestinal, by location, **27**
- involving lymph nodes, **27**
Mesenteric lipodystrophy. *See* Idiopathic tumefactive fibroinflammatory lesions.
Mesenteric panniculitis. *See* Idiopathic tumefactive fibroinflammatory lesions.
Mesenteritis, sclerosing, desmoid-type fibromatosis vs., **170**
Mesodermal stromal polyp. *See* Fibroepithelial stromal polyp.
Mesothelial cells, tumors of
- adenomatoid tumor, **590–591**
  differential diagnosis, **591**
  genetic testing, **591**
  prognosis, **591**
- malignant mesothelioma, **598–603**
  differential diagnosis, **600**
  molecular genetics, **600**
  prognosis, **599**
- multicystic peritoneal mesothelioma, **592–593**
  adenomatoid tumor vs., **591**
  differential diagnosis, **593**
  prognosis, **593**
- well-differentiated papillary mesothelioma, **594–597**
  differential diagnosis, **595**
  prognosis, **595**
Mesothelial hyperplasia, well-differentiated papillary mesothelioma vs., **595**
Mesothelial proliferation, reactive, malignant mesothelioma vs., **600**
Mesothelioma
- localized fibrous. *See* Solitary fibrous tumor.
- of low malignant potential. *See* Well-differentiated papillary mesothelioma.
- malignant, **598–603**
  adenomatoid tumor vs., **591**
  differential diagnosis, **600**
  molecular genetics, **600**
  multicystic peritoneal mesothelioma vs., **593**

INDEX

prognosis, **599**
well-differentiated papillary mesothelioma vs., **595**
- multicystic peritoneal, **592–593**
adenomatoid tumor vs., **591**
differential diagnosis, **593**
prognosis, **593**
- myxoid, extraskeletal myxoid chondrosarcoma vs., **713**
- well-differentiated papillary, **594–597**
adenomatoid tumor vs., **591**
differential diagnosis, **595**
prognosis, **595**

Metastatic adenocarcinoma, adenomatoid tumor vs., **591**
Metastatic carcinoma
- angiosarcoma vs., **472**
- epithelioid hemangioendothelioma vs., **468**
- histiocytic sarcoma vs., **325**
- intimal sarcoma vs., **721**
- myoepithelioma of soft tissue vs., **656**
- myxofibrosarcoma vs., **218**
- paraganglioma vs., **816**
- pleomorphic rhabdomyosarcoma vs., **401**
- sclerosing epithelioid fibrosarcoma vs., **233**
- sclerosing rhabdomyosarcoma vs., **397**
- solitary extramedullary plasmacytoma vs., **607**

Metastatic melanoma
- clear cell sarcoma vs., **690**
- extrarenal rhabdoid tumor vs., **718**
- histiocytic sarcoma vs., **325**
- interdigitating dendritic cell sarcoma vs., **329**
- intimal sarcoma vs., **721**
- malignant gastrointestinal neuroectodermal tumor vs., **778**
- melanotic schwannoma vs., **557**
- myoepithelioma of soft tissue vs., **656**
- paraganglioma vs., **816**
- schwannoma vs., **511**

Metastatic neuroendocrine carcinoma, desmoplastic small round cell tumor vs., **702**
Metastatic or primary cutaneous mucinous carcinoma, extraaxial soft tissue chordoma vs., **843**
Metastatic renal cell carcinoma, alveolar soft part sarcoma vs., **685**
Metastatic sarcomatoid carcinoma, follicular dendritic cell sarcoma vs., **327**
Metastatic tumors, to soft tissue sites, **828–831**
- differential diagnosis, **829**
- prognosis, **829**

Microcapillary angioma. *See* Microvenular hemangioma.
Microcystic/reticular schwannoma, **510**
Microvenular hemangioma (MVH), **438–439**
- diagnostic checklist, **439**
- differential diagnosis, **439**
- hobnail hemangioma vs., **435**
- Kaposi sarcoma vs., **478**
- prognosis, **439**

Milk alkali syndrome, tumoral calcinosis vs., **787**
Mixed tumor, **657**. *See also* Myoepithelioma, of soft tissue.
Molecular features, soft tissue tumors, **18–19**
Monomorphic spindle cell patterns, **28**
Monophasic synovial sarcoma, **667**
- clear cell sarcoma vs., **690**
- malignant peripheral nerve sheath tumor vs., **560**
- palmar/plantar fibromatosis vs., **167**
- solitary fibrous tumor vs., **186**
- spindle cell rhabdomyosarcoma vs., **393**

Monoplastic synovial sarcoma, calcifying aponeurotic fibroma vs., **245**
Mucoid cyst, digital
- dermal nerve sheath myxoma vs., **547**
- superficial angiomyxoma vs., **621**

Mucosal neuroma
- benign neural gastrointestinal polyps vs., **741**
- solitary circumscribed neuroma vs., **507**

Mucosal perineurioma, gastrointestinal smooth muscle neoplasms vs., **764**
Mucosal Schwann cell hamartoma, gastrointestinal smooth muscle neoplasms vs., **764**
Multicentric cutaneous reticulohistiocytosis, reticulohistiocytoma vs., **301–302**
Multicystic peritoneal mesothelioma, **592–593**
- adenomatoid tumor vs., **591**
- differential diagnosis, **593**
- prognosis, **593**

Multilocular peritoneal inclusion cyst. *See* Multicystic peritoneal mesothelioma.
Multiple myeloma, solitary extramedullary plasmacytoma vs., **607**
Mural leiomyoma. *See* Gastrointestinal smooth muscle neoplasms.
Musculoaponeurotic fibromatosis. *See* Desmoid-type fibromatosis.
MVH. *See* Microvenular hemangioma.
Mycobacterial pseudotumor, crystal-storing histiocytosis vs., **315**
Myeloid sarcoma, **608–609**
- differential diagnosis, **609**
- lymphoma of soft tissue vs., **611**
- molecular genetics, **609**
- myelolipoma vs., **79**
- prognosis, **609**

Myelolipoma, **78–79**
- differential diagnosis, **79**
- molecular genetics, **79**
- prognosis, **79**

Myoepithelial carcinoma, **657**. *See also* Myoepithelioma, of soft tissue.
- epithelioid rhabdomyosarcoma vs., **405**
- epithelioid sarcoma vs., **680**
- extraskeletal myxoid chondrosarcoma vs., **713**
- metastatic tumors to soft tissue sites vs., **829**

Myoepithelioma
- extrarenal rhabdoid tumor vs., **718**
- extraskeletal myxoid chondrosarcoma vs., **713**
- malignant, **657**
epithelioid malignant peripheral nerve sheath tumor vs., **567**
- perineurioma vs., **532**
- primary pulmonary myxoid sarcoma vs., **847**
- sinonasal glomangiopericytoma vs., **806**
- of soft tissue, **656–663**
chondroid lipoma vs., **67**

differential diagnosis, **658**
epithelioid hemangioendothelioma vs., **468**
extraaxial soft tissue chordoma vs., **843**
immunohistochemistry, **658**
molecular genetics, **657**
ossifying fibromyxoid tumor vs., **652**
prognosis, **657**
solitary extramedullary plasmacytoma vs., **607**
Myofibroblastic sarcoma, low-grade, **192–195**
- adult-type fibrosarcoma vs., **215**
- desmoid-type fibromatosis vs., **170**
- differential diagnosis, **193**
- nodular fasciitis vs., **116**
- plexiform fibrohistiocytic tumor vs., **317**
- prognosis, **193**
- spindle cell rhabdomyosarcoma vs., **394**
Myofibroblastic tumor, inflammatory, **196–201**
- calcifying fibrous tumor vs., **249**
- cardiac fibroma vs., **797**
- desmoid-type fibromatosis vs., **170**
- differential diagnosis, **198**
- focal myositis vs., **371**
- follicular dendritic cell sarcoma vs., **327**
- idiopathic tumefactive fibroinflammatory lesions vs., **790**
- inflammatory fibroid polyp vs., **767**
- leiomyosarcoma vs., **346**
- low-grade myofibroblastic sarcoma vs., **193**
- molecular genetics, **197–198**
- myxoinflammatory fibroblastic sarcoma vs., **204**
- nodular fasciitis vs., **116**
- plexiform fibromyxoma vs., **773**
- prognosis, **197**
- spindle cell rhabdomyosarcoma vs., **394**
- superficial CD34(+) fibroblastic tumor vs., **211**
Myofibroblastoma, mammary-type
- atypical spindle cell lipomatous tumor vs., **85**
- cellular angiofibroma vs., **581**
- differential diagnosis, **149**
- molecular genetics, **149**
- prognosis, **149**
- spindle cell/pleomorphic lipoma vs., **62**
Myofibroblastoma, mammary-type, **148–151**
Myofibroma, **362–365**
- differential diagnosis, **363**
- infantile fibrosarcoma vs., **265**
- myopericytoma vs., **359**
- nodular fasciitis vs., **116**
- prognosis, **363**
- spindle cell rhabdomyosarcoma vs., **394**
Myofibromatosis, **362–365**
- differential diagnosis, **363**
- infantile, hyaline fibromatosis syndrome vs., **253**
- infantile fibrosarcoma vs., **265**
- prognosis, **363**
Myofibrosarcoma. *See also* Low-grade myofibroblastic sarcoma.
- low-grade, angiofibroma of soft tissue vs., **145**
Myolipoma, **70–73**
- differential diagnosis, **71**
- prognosis, **71**
Myoma, juxtaarticular, perineurioma vs., **532**
Myopericytoma, **358–361**
- angioleiomyoma vs., **367**
- differential diagnosis, **359**
- Epstein-Barr virus-associated smooth muscle tumor vs., **343**
- glomus tumors vs., **354**
- prognosis, **359**
- solitary fibrous tumor vs., **186**
Myositis, focal, **370–371**
- differential diagnosis, **371**
- fibromatosis colli vs., **255**
- prognosis, **371**
Myositis ossificans, **126–129**
- aneurysmal bone cyst of soft tissue vs., **631**
- differential diagnosis, **127**
- extraskeletal osteosarcoma vs., **498**
- fibroosseous pseudotumor of digit vs., **131**
- focal myositis vs., **371**
- nodular fasciitis vs., **116**
- prognosis, **127**
Myxochondroid metaplasia, of plantar foot, soft tissue chondroma vs., **488**
Myxochondroma. *See* Soft tissue chondroma.
Myxofibrosarcoma, **216–221**
- cardiac myxoma vs., **793**
- dedifferentiated liposarcoma vs., **96**
- differential diagnosis, **218**
- epithelial variant, extraskeletal myxoid chondrosarcoma vs., **713**
- giant cell fibroblastoma vs., **261**
- ischemic fasciitis vs., **125**
- low-grade
ganglion cyst vs., **785**
massive localized lymphedema vs., **451**
- low-grade
dermal nerve sheath myxoma vs., **547**
intramuscular myxoma vs., **615**
juxtaarticular myxoma vs., **619**
superficial angiomyxoma vs., **621**
- low-grade fibromyxoid sarcoma vs., **224**
- myoepithelioma of soft tissue vs., **656**
- myxoid liposarcoma vs., **102**
- myxoinflammatory fibroblastic sarcoma vs., **204**
- pleomorphic liposarcoma vs., **108**
- primary pulmonary myxoid sarcoma vs., **848**
- prognosis, **217**
Myxoid chondrosarcoma, extraskeletal, **712–715**
- chondroid lipoma vs., **67**
- differential diagnosis, **713**
- epithelioid hemangioendothelioma vs., **468**
- extraaxial soft tissue chordoma vs., **843**
- extrarenal rhabdoid tumor vs., **718**
- extraskeletal mesenchymal chondrosarcoma vs., **502**
- genetic testing, **713**
- myoepithelioma of soft tissue vs., **656**
- myxoid liposarcoma vs., **102**
- ossifying fibromyxoid tumor vs., **652**
- perineurioma vs., **532**
- primary pulmonary myxoid sarcoma vs., **847**
- prognosis, **713**

- soft tissue chondroma vs., **488**
Myxoid dermatofibrosarcoma protuberans
- dermal nerve sheath myxoma vs., **547**
- myxoid liposarcoma vs., **102**
Myxoid leiomyosarcoma, primary pulmonary myxoid sarcoma vs., **848**
Myxoid liposarcoma (MLPS), **100–105**
- angiofibroma of soft tissue vs., **145**
- atypical lipomatous tumor/well-differentiated liposarcoma vs., **90**
- chondroid lipoma vs., **67**
- dedifferentiated liposarcoma vs., **96**
- differential diagnosis, **102**
- hibernoma vs., **75**
- intramuscular myxoma vs., **615**
- lipoblastoma vs., **81**
- lipoma vs., **48**
- low-grade fibromyxoid sarcoma vs., **224**
- massive localized lymphedema vs., **451**
- molecular genetics, **102**
- myxofibrosarcoma vs., **218**
- pleomorphic liposarcoma vs., **108**
- primary pulmonary myxoid sarcoma vs., **848**
- prognosis, **101**
- spindle cell/pleomorphic lipoma vs., **62**
- superficial angiomyxoma vs., **621**
Myxoid malignant fibrous histiocytoma. *See* Myxofibrosarcoma.
Myxoid mesothelioma, extraskeletal myxoid chondrosarcoma vs., **713**
Myxoid neurofibroma
- acral fibromyxoma vs., **625**
- dermal nerve sheath myxoma vs., **547**
- juxtaarticular myxoma vs., **619**
- superficial angiomyxoma vs., **621**
Myxoinflammatory fibroblastic sarcoma, **202–209**
- differential diagnosis, **204**
- extranodal Rosai-Dorfman disease vs., **312**
- hemosiderotic fibrolipomatous tumor vs., **635**
- molecular genetics, **204**
- myxofibrosarcoma vs., **218**
- pleomorphic hyalinizing angiectatic tumor vs., **627**
- prognosis, **203**
- superficial CD34(+) fibroblastic tumor vs., **211**
Myxoma
- cardiac, **792–795**
  differential diagnosis, **793**
  intimal sarcoma vs., **721**
  molecular genetics, **793**
  prognosis, **793**
- cellular, myxofibrosarcoma vs., **218**
- cutaneous, in Carney complex, dermal nerve sheath myxoma vs., **547**
- dermal nerve sheath, **546–549**
  cellular neurothekeoma vs., **291**
  differential diagnosis of, **547**
  prognosis, **547**
  superficial angiomyxoma vs., **621**
- ganglion cyst vs., **785**
- intramuscular, **614–617**
  differential diagnosis, **615**
  genetic testing, **615**
  juxtaarticular myxoma vs., **619**
  low-grade fibromyxoid sarcoma vs., **224**
  myxofibrosarcoma vs., **218**
  myxoid liposarcoma vs., **102**
  prognosis, **615**
- juxtaarticular, **618–619**
  differential diagnosis, **619**
  genetic testing, **619**
  myxofibrosarcoma vs., **218**
  perineurioma vs., **532**
  prognosis, **619**
- superficial, myxofibrosarcoma vs., **218**

N

Nasal glial heterotopia. *See* Glial heterotopia.
Nasal glioma. *See* Glial heterotopia.
Nasopharyngeal angiofibroma, **800–803**
- differential diagnosis, **802**
- genetics, **801**
- prognosis, **801**
- sinonasal glomangiopericytoma vs., **806**
Necrobiosis lipoidica diabeticorum
- deep granuloma annulare vs., **305**
- rheumatoid nodule vs., **307**
Nerve sheath myxoma, dermal, **546–549**
- cellular neurothekeoma vs., **291**
- differential diagnosis of, **547**
- prognosis, **547**
- superficial angiomyxoma vs., **621**
Nerve sheath tumor
- hybrid, **536–539**
  differential diagnosis, **537**
  gastrointestinal schwannoma vs., **761**
  low-grade fibromyxoid sarcoma vs., **224**
  perineurioma vs., **532**
  prognosis, **537**
- malignant peripheral nerve sheath tumor. *See* Peripheral nerve sheath tumor, malignant.
Neural fibrolipoma. *See* Lipomatosis.
Neural gastrointestinal polyps, benign, **740–743**
- differential diagnosis, **741**
- prognosis, **741**
Neurilemmoma. *See* Schwannoma.
Neuroblastoma
- alveolar rhabdomyosarcoma vs., **388**
- desmoplastic small round cell tumor vs., **702**
- ectomesenchymoma vs., **571**
- embryonal rhabdomyosarcoma vs., **382**
- extraskeletal Ewing sarcoma vs., **708**
- and ganglioneuroblastoma, **832–841**
  differential diagnosis, **834–835**
  favorable vs. unfavorable histology in neuroblastic tumors, **835**
  genetic testing, **834**
  intermixed, **834**

International Neuroblastoma Pathology Committee (INPC) classification, **834**
neuroblastoma staging system, **835**
nodular, **834**
poorly differentiated, **834**
prognosis, **833**
prognosis based on *MYCN* amplification and histology, **835**
undifferentiated, **834**
- melanotic neuroectodermal tumor of infancy vs., **825**
Neuroblastoma-like schwannoma, **510**
Neuroectodermal tumor
- of infancy, melanotic, **824–825**
differential diagnosis, **825**
prognosis, **825**
- malignant gastrointestinal, **776–779**
differential diagnosis, **777–778**
gastrointestinal stromal tumor vs., **747**
immunohistochemistry, **778**
molecular genetics, **777**
Neuroendocrine carcinoma, metastatic, desmoplastic small round cell tumor vs., **702**
Neurofibroma, **522–529**
- atypical, malignant peripheral nerve sheath tumor vs., **560**
- benign neural gastrointestinal polyps vs., **741**
- desmoplastic fibroblastoma vs., **141**
- differential diagnosis, **524**
- diffuse
dermatofibrosarcoma protuberans vs., **176**
lipoma vs., **48**
- ganglion cyst vs., **785**
- ganglioneuroma vs., **551**
- gastrointestinal schwannoma vs., **761**
- glial heterotopia vs., **813**
- hybrid nerve sheath tumor vs., **537**
- myxofibrosarcoma vs., **218**
- myxoid
acral fibromyxoma vs., **625**
dermal nerve sheath myxoma vs., **547**
juxtaarticular myxoma vs., **619**
superficial angiomyxoma vs., **621**
- nodular fasciitis vs., **116**
- perineurioma vs., **532**
- plexiform
plexiform fibromyxoma vs., **773**
solitary circumscribed neuroma vs., **507**
- prognosis, **523**
- schwannoma vs., **510–511**
- spindle cell/pleomorphic lipoma vs., **62**
Neurofibromatosis type 1, lipomatosis of nerve vs., **53**
Neurofibromatosis type 2, **509**
Neurofibrosarcoma. *See* Malignant peripheral nerve sheath tumor.
Neurogenic sarcoma. *See* Malignant peripheral nerve sheath tumor.
Neurolipomatosis. *See* Lipomatosis.
Neuroma
- lipomatosis of nerve vs., **53**
- mucosal
benign neural gastrointestinal polyps vs., **741**
solitary circumscribed neuroma vs., **507**
- solitary circumscribed, **506–507**
differential diagnosis, **507**
prognosis, **507**
- traumatic, solitary circumscribed neuroma vs., **507**
Neuromuscular choristoma, **554–555**
- diagnostic checklist, **555**
- differential diagnosis, **555**
- prognosis, **555**
Neuromuscular hamartoma. *See* Neuromuscular choristoma.
Neurothekeoma
- cellular, **290–293**
differential diagnosis, **291**
ectopic meningioma vs., **811**
plexiform fibrohistiocytic tumor vs., **317**
prognosis, **291**
- cellular neurothekeoma vs., **291**
- dermal nerve sheath myxoma vs., **547**
Nodal metastasis, angiomatoid fibrous histiocytoma vs., **644**
Nodular fasciitis, **114–119**
- aneurysmal bone cyst of soft tissue vs., **631**
- angiomatoid fibrous histiocytoma vs., **644**
- desmoid-type fibromatosis vs., **170**
- desmoplastic fibroblastoma vs., **141**
- differential diagnosis, **116**
- fibroma of tendon sheath vs., **136**
- fibromatosis colli vs., **255**
- inflammatory myofibroblastic tumor vs., **198**
- ischemic fasciitis vs., **125**
- keloid vs., **163**
- molecular genetics, **116**
- myofibroma and myofibromatosis vs., **363**
- myositis ossificans vs., **127**
- prognosis, **115**
- proliferative fasciitis/myositis vs., **121**
Non-Hodgkin lymphoma, histiocytic sarcoma vs., **325**
Noninvoluting congenital hemangioma (NICH). *See* Congenital hemangioma.
Nuchal fibrocartilaginous pseudotumor
- Gardner fibroma vs., **257**
- nuchal-type fibroma vs., **165**
Nuchal fibroma. *See* Nuchal-type fibroma.
Nuchal-type fibroma, **164–165**
- differential diagnosis, **165**
- elastofibromas vs., **143**
- Gardner fibroma vs., **257**
- prognosis, **165**

O

Ormond disease. *See* Idiopathic tumefactive fibroinflammatory lesions.
Ossifying fibromyxoid tumor (OFMT), **650–655**
- differential diagnosis, **652**
- extraskeletal osteosarcoma vs., **498**
- fibroosseous pseudotumor vs., **131**

- malignant, **651**
- molecular genetics, **652**
- myoepithelioma of soft tissue vs., **656**
- myositis ossificans vs., **127**
- prognosis, **651**
- sclerosing epithelioid fibrosarcoma vs., **234**

Osteocartilaginous loose bodies, synovial chondromatosis vs., **493**
Osteochondroma. *See* Soft tissue chondroma.
Osteogenic melanoma, extraskeletal osteosarcoma vs., **498**
Osteosarcoma
- extraskeletal, **496–499**
  - aneurysmal bone cyst of soft tissue vs., **631**
  - diagnostic checklist, **498**
  - differential diagnosis, **498**
  - fibroosseous pseudotumor of digit vs., **131**
  - myositis ossificans vs., **127**
  - ossifying fibromyxoid tumor vs., **652**
  - prognosis, **497**
  - sclerosing epithelioid fibrosarcoma vs., **234**
  - sclerosing rhabdomyosarcoma vs., **397**
  - undifferentiated pleomorphic sarcoma vs., **725**
- extraskeletal mesenchymal chondrosarcoma vs., **502**
- undifferentiated pleomorphic sarcoma vs., **725**

Ovarian serous adenocarcinoma, malignant mesothelioma vs., **600**

P

Palisade myofibroblastoma, intranodal, **152–155**
- differential diagnosis, **153**
- molecular genetics, **153**
- prognosis, **153**

Palisaded encapsulated neuroma. *See* Solitary circumscribed neuroma.
Palisading subcutaneous granuloma. *See* Deep granuloma annulare.
Palmar/plantar fibromatosis, **166–167**
- calcifying aponeurotic fibroma vs., **245**
- differential diagnosis, **167**
- prognosis, **167**

Papillary endothelial hyperplasia (PEH), **408–409**
- angiosarcoma vs., **472**
- diagnostic checklist, **409**
- differential diagnosis, **409**
- prognosis, **409**

Papillary fibroelastoma, cardiac fibroma vs., **797**
Papillary intralymphatic angioendothelioma, **456–457**
- diagnostic checklist, **457**
- differential diagnosis, **457**
- prognosis, **457**
- retiform hemangioendothelioma vs., **459**

Papillary mesothelioma, well-differentiated, **594–597**
- adenomatoid tumor vs., **591**
- differential diagnosis, **595**
- prognosis, **595**

Parachordoma, **657**. *See also* Myoepithelioma, of soft tissue.
Paraganglioma, **814–821**
- adult rhabdomyoma vs., **373**
- alveolar soft part sarcoma vs., **685**
- conventional, gangliocytic paraganglioma vs., **771**
- differential diagnosis, **816**
- gangliocytic, **770–771**
  - differential diagnosis, **771**
- genetic testing, **816**
- genetics, **815**
- glomus tumors vs., **354**
- peripheral hemangioblastoma vs., **823**
- prognosis, **815**

Paraganglioma-like dermal melanocytic tumor, clear cell sarcoma vs., **690**
Parosteal fasciitis. *See* Fibroosseous pseudotumor of digit.
PEComa (perivascular epithelioid cell tumor), **692–699**
- alveolar soft part sarcoma vs., **685**
- angioleiomyoma vs., **367**
- clear cell sarcoma vs., **690**
- deep leiomyoma vs., **339**
- differential diagnosis, **694**
- genetics, **693**
- intranodal palisade myofibroblastoma vs., **153**
- leiomyosarcoma vs., **346**
- peripheral hemangioblastoma vs., **823**
- prognosis, **693**

Penile fibromatosis, **167**
Pericytic (perivascular) tumors
- angioleiomyoma, **366–367**
  - differential diagnosis, **367**
  - prognosis, **367**
- glomus tumors, **352–357**
  - differential diagnosis, **354**
  - prognosis, **353**
- myofibroma and myofibromatosis, **362–365**
  - differential diagnosis, **363**
  - prognosis, **363**
- myopericytoma, **358–361**
  - differential diagnosis, **359**
  - prognosis, **359**

Perineurioma, **530–535**
- acral fibromyxoma vs., **625**
- deep benign fibrous histiocytoma vs., **277**
- dermatofibrosarcoma protuberans vs., **176**
- differential diagnosis, **532**
- hybrid nerve sheath tumor vs., **537**
- inclusion body fibromatosis vs., **251**
- inflammatory fibroid polyp vs., **767**
- intraneural, **531**
- low-grade fibromyxoid sarcoma vs., **224**
- molecular genetics, **531**
- mucosal, gastrointestinal smooth muscle neoplasms vs., **764**
- neurofibroma vs., **524**
- plexiform, **531**
- prognosis, **531**
- reticular, **531**
- sclerosing, **531**

INDEX

Peripheral hemangioblastoma, **822–823**
- differential diagnosis, **823**
- genetics, **823**
- prognosis, **823**

Peripheral nerve sheath tumor
- benign, intramuscular myxoma vs., **615**
- dermal nerve sheath myxoma, **546–549**
  - differential diagnosis of, **547**
  - prognosis, **547**
- ectomesenchymoma, **570–571**
  - differential diagnosis, **571**
  - genetic testing, **571**
  - prognosis, **571**
- ganglioneuroma, **550–553**
  - differential diagnosis, **551**
  - prognosis, **551**
- granular cell tumor, **540–545**
  - differential diagnosis, **542**
  - nonneural, **542**
  - prognosis, **541**
- hybrid nerve sheath tumor, **536–539**
  - differential diagnosis, **537**
  - prognosis, **537**
- malignant, **558–565**
  - adult-type fibrosarcoma vs., **215**
  - atypical fibroxanthoma vs., **638**
  - *BCOR-CCNB3* fusion-positive sarcoma vs., **736**
  - clear cell sarcoma vs., **690**
  - dedifferentiated liposarcoma vs., **96**
  - differential diagnosis, **560**
  - epithelioid, **566–569**. *See also* Epithelioid malignant peripheral nerve sheath tumor.
  - extraskeletal mesenchymal chondrosarcoma vs., **502**
  - extraskeletal osteosarcoma vs., **498**
  - genetic predisposition, **559**
  - hybrid nerve sheath tumor vs., **537**
  - leiomyosarcoma vs., **346**
  - malignant gastrointestinal neuroectodermal tumor vs., **778**
  - metastatic tumors to soft tissue sites vs., **829**
  - myxofibrosarcoma vs., **218**
  - neurofibroma vs., **524**
  - palmar/plantar fibromatosis vs., **167**
  - prognosis, **559**
  - schwannoma vs., **511**
  - spindle cell rhabdomyosarcoma vs., **393**
  - synovial sarcoma vs., **668**
  - undifferentiated pleomorphic sarcoma vs., **725**
  - undifferentiated round cell sarcoma with *CIC-DUX4* translocation vs., **729**
- melanotic schwannoma, **556–557**
  - differential diagnosis, **557**
  - prognosis, **557**
- neurofibroma, **522–529**
  - differential diagnosis, **524**
  - diffuse-type, **523, 524**
  - plexiform, **523, 524**
  - prognosis, **523**
- neuromuscular choristoma, **554–555**
  - diagnostic checklist, **555**
  - differential diagnosis, **555**
  - prognosis, **555**
- perineurioma, **530–535**
  - differential diagnosis, **532**
  - intraneural, **531**
  - molecular genetics, **531**
  - plexiform, **531**
  - prognosis, **531**
  - reticular, **531**
  - sclerosing, **531**
- schwannoma, **508–521**
  - ancient, **510**
  - cellular, **510**
  - differential diagnosis, **510–511**
  - epithelioid, **510**
  - microcystic/reticular, **510**
  - neuroblastoma-like, **510**
  - plexiform, **510**
  - prognosis, **509**
  - pseudoglandular, **510**
- solitary circumscribed neuroma, **506–507**
  - differential diagnosis, **507**
  - prognosis, **507**

Peritoneal mesothelioma, multicystic, **592–593**
- adenomatoid tumor vs., **591**
- differential diagnosis, **593**
- prognosis, **593**

Peritoneal serous carcinoma, well-differentiated papillary mesothelioma vs., **595**

Periungual fibroma, storiform collagenoma vs., **161**

Perivascular epithelioid cell tumor (PEComa), **692–699**
- alveolar soft part sarcoma vs., **685**
- angioleiomyoma vs., **367**
- clear cell sarcoma vs., **690**
- deep leiomyoma vs., **339**
- differential diagnosis, **694**
- genetics, **693**
- intranodal palisade myofibroblastoma vs., **153**
- leiomyosarcoma vs., **346**
- peripheral hemangioblastoma vs., **823**
- prognosis, **693**

Peyronie disease, **167**

PFHT. *See* Plexiform fibrohistiocytic tumor.

PFM. *See* Plexiform fibromyxoma.

Pheochromocytoma, **815**

Phosphaturic mesenchymal tumor (PMT), **664–665**
- differential diagnosis, **665**
- molecular genetics, **665**
- prognosis, **665**
- sinonasal glomangiopericytoma vs., **806**

Pigmented villonodular synovitis, myxoinflammatory fibroblastic sarcoma vs., **204**

PILA. *See* Papillary intralymphatic angioendothelioma.

Pilar leiomyoma
- inclusion body fibromatosis vs., **251**
- smooth muscle hamartoma vs., **333**

Planar xanthoma, **295**

Plantar foot, myxochondroid metaplasia of, soft tissue chondroma vs., **488**

Plaque-like dermal fibromatosis. *See* Dermatomyofibroma.

Plasma cell granuloma. *See* Inflammatory myofibroblastic tumor.

INDEX

Pleomorphic adenoma, ectopic hamartomatous thymoma vs., **633**
Pleomorphic dermal sarcoma
- atypical fibroxanthoma vs., **638**
- superficial CD34(+) fibroblastic tumor vs., **211**
Pleomorphic fibroma, **156–157**
- diagnostic checklist, **157**
- differential diagnosis, **157**
- prognosis, **157**
- storiform collagenoma vs., **161**
Pleomorphic hyalinizing angiectatic tumor, **626–629**
- differential diagnosis, **627**
- hemosiderotic fibrolipomatous tumor vs., **635**
- molecular genetics, **627**
- prognosis, **627**
- schwannoma vs., **511**
Pleomorphic lipoma, **60–65**
- atypical lipomatous tumor/well-differentiated liposarcoma vs., **90**
- differential diagnosis, **62**
- giant cell fibroblastoma vs., **261**
- molecular genetics, **61**
- prognosis, **61**
Pleomorphic liposarcoma (PLPS), **106–111**
- dedifferentiated liposarcoma vs., **96**
- differential diagnosis, **107–108**
- molecular genetics, **107**
- myxofibrosarcoma vs., **218**
- prognosis, **107**
- undifferentiated pleomorphic sarcoma vs., **725**
Pleomorphic melanoma, atypical fibroxanthoma vs., **637–638**
Pleomorphic rhabdomyosarcoma, **400–403**
- differential diagnosis, **401**
- embryonal rhabdomyosarcoma vs., **382**
- epithelioid rhabdomyosarcoma vs., **405**
- prognosis, **401**
- proliferative fasciitis/myositis vs., **121**
Pleomorphic sarcoma
- pleomorphic rhabdomyosarcoma vs., **401**
- undifferentiated, **724–727**
    - adult-type fibrosarcoma vs., **215**
    - angiomatoid fibrous histiocytoma vs., **644**
    - dedifferentiated liposarcoma vs., **96**
    - differential diagnosis, **725**
    - extranodal Rosai-Dorfman disease vs., **312**
    - extraskeletal osteosarcoma vs., **498**
    - with giant cells, giant cell tumor of soft tissue vs., **321**
    - leiomyosarcoma vs., **346**
    - metastatic tumors to soft tissue sites vs., **829**
    - molecular genetics, **725**
    - myxofibrosarcoma vs., **218**
    - nodular fasciitis vs., **116**
    - pleomorphic hyalinizing angiectatic tumor vs., **627**
    - pleomorphic liposarcoma vs., **108**
    - prognosis, **725**
    - proliferative fasciitis/myositis vs., **121**
Pleomorphic spindle cell patterns, **29–30**
Pleuropulmonary blastoma, embryonal rhabdomyosarcoma vs., **382**
Plexiform angiomyxoid myofibroblastic tumor. *See* Plexiform fibromyxoma.
Plexiform angiomyxoid tumor. *See* Plexiform fibromyxoma.
Plexiform fibrohistiocytic tumor, **316–319**
- cellular neurothekeoma vs., **291**
- differential diagnosis, **317**
- ectopic meningioma vs., **811**
- localized-type tenosynovial giant cell tumor vs., **280**
- prognosis, **317**
- xanthomas vs., **296**
Plexiform fibromyxoma, **772–775**
- differential diagnosis, **773**
- gastrointestinal stromal tumor vs., **747**
Plexiform neurofibroma
- plexiform fibromyxoma vs., **773**
- solitary circumscribed neuroma vs., **507**
Plexiform schwannoma, **510**
- xanthomas vs., **296**
Plexiform xanthoma, **295**
Plexiform xanthomatous tumor. *See* Xanthomas.
PMH. *See* Pseudomyogenic hemangioendothelioma.
PMT. *See* Phosphaturic mesenchymal tumor.
Polyp
- antrochoanal, nasopharyngeal angiofibroma vs., **802**
- inflammatory fibroid, **766–769**
    - benign neural gastrointestinal polyps vs., **741**
    - differential diagnosis, **767**
    - gastrointestinal smooth muscle neoplasms vs., **764**
    - gastrointestinal stromal tumor vs., **747**
    - inflammatory myofibroblastic tumor vs., **198**
    - plexiform fibromyxoma vs., **773**
Polyphenotypic small round cell tumor. *See* Desmoplastic small round cell tumor.
Poorly differentiated carcinoma
- epithelioid rhabdomyosarcoma vs., **405**
- gastrointestinal stromal tumor vs., **747**
- myeloid sarcoma vs., **609**
- pleomorphic liposarcoma vs., **108**
Poorly differentiated synovial sarcoma
- *BCOR-CCNB3* fusion-positive sarcoma vs., **736**
- extraskeletal Ewing sarcoma vs., **708**
- lymphoma of soft tissue vs., **611**
- undifferentiated round cell sarcoma with *CIC-DUX4* translocation vs., **730**
PPMS. *See* Primary pulmonary myxoid sarcoma.
Primary carcinoma, paraganglioma vs., **816**
Primary cardiac sarcomas, intimal sarcoma vs., **721**
Primary desmoid fibromatosis, neuromuscular choristoma vs., **555**
Primary extrapulmonary sugar tumor. *See* Perivascular epithelioid cell tumor.
Primary meningioma of CNS, ectopic meningioma vs., **811**
Primary pulmonary myxoid sarcoma (PPMS), **846–849**
- diagnostic checklist, **848**
- differential diagnosis, **847–848**
- immunohistochemistry, **848**
Primary synovial chondromatosis. *See* Synovial chondromatosis.

INDEX

Primitive neuroectodermal tumor. *See* Extraskeletal Ewing sarcoma.
Progonoma, melanotic. *See* Melanotic neuroectodermal tumor of infancy.
Progressive lymphangioma
- atypical vascular lesion vs., **453**
- hobnail hemangioma vs., **435**
- Kaposi sarcoma vs., **478**
- lymphangioma vs., **448**
Proliferative fasciitis/myositis, **120–123**
- desmoid-type fibromatosis vs., **170**
- differential diagnosis, **121**
- ischemic fasciitis vs., **125**
- myxoinflammatory fibroblastic sarcoma vs., **204**
- nodular fasciitis vs., **116**
- prognosis, **121**
Proliferative myositis, focal myositis vs., **371**
Proteinosis, lipoid, hyaline fibromatosis syndrome vs., **253**
Psammomatous melanotic schwannoma. *See* Melanotic schwannoma.
Pseudoglandular schwannoma, **510**
Pseudogout, tophaceous
- soft tissue chondroma vs., **488**
- tumoral calcinosis vs., **787**
Pseudomyogenic hemangioendothelioma (PMH), **462–465**
- differential diagnosis, **463**
- epithelioid hemangioendothelioma vs., **468**
- epithelioid sarcoma vs., **680**
- molecular genetics, **463**
- prognosis, **463**
Pseudorheumatoid nodule. *See* Deep granuloma annulare.
Pseudosarcoma. *See* Massive localized lymphedema.
Pseudosarcoma botryoides. *See* Fibroepithelial stromal polyp.
Pseudosarcomatous fasciitis. *See* Nodular fasciitis.
Pseudosarcomatous myofibroblastic proliferation, nodular fasciitis vs., **116**
Pulmonary adenocarcinoma, malignant mesothelioma vs., **600**
Pyogenic granuloma. *See also* Lobular capillary hemangioma.
- angiofibroma of soft tissue vs., **145**
- antrochoanal, nasopharyngeal angiofibroma vs., **802**
- bacillary angiomatosis vs., **411**
- congenital granular cell epulis vs., **799**
- glomeruloid hemangioma vs., **443**
- infantile hemangioma vs., **418**
- nasopharyngeal angiofibroma vs., **802**
- sinonasal glomangiopericytoma vs., **806**

R

Rapidly involuting congenital hemangioma (RICH). *See* Congenital hemangioma.
RDD. *See* Rosai-Dorfman disease.
Reactive granular cell change, granular cell tumor vs., **542**
Reactive nonlesional fibroblastic proliferation, idiopathic tumefactive fibroinflammatory lesions vs., **790**
Renal cell carcinoma, metastatic, peripheral hemangioblastoma vs., **823**
Resection, soft tissue tumors, **22–25**
- specimens, **23–24**
Reticulohistiocytic granuloma. *See* Reticulohistiocytoma.
Reticulohistiocytoma, **300–303**
- diagnostic checklist, **302**
- differential diagnosis, **301–302**
- prognosis, **301**
- solitary (juvenile) xanthogranuloma vs., **299**
Reticulohistiocytosis
- generalized cutaneous, reticulohistiocytoma vs., **301–302**
- multicentric cutaneous, reticulohistiocytoma vs., **301–302**
Reticulum cell sarcoma, interdigitating dendritic. *See* Interdigitating dendritic cell sarcoma.
Retiform hemangioendothelioma, **458–459**
- angiosarcoma vs., **472**
- composite hemangioendothelioma vs., **461**
- diagnostic checklist, **459**
- differential diagnosis, **459**
- hobnail hemangioma vs., **435**
- papillary intralymphatic angioendothelioma vs., **457**
- prognosis, **459**
Retinal anlage tumor. *See* Melanotic neuroectodermal tumor of infancy.
Retractile mesenteritis. *See* Idiopathic tumefactive fibroinflammatory lesions.
Retroperitoneal fibrosis, idiopathic, **789**
- atypical lipomatous tumor/well-differentiated liposarcoma vs., **90**
- desmoid-type fibromatosis vs., **170**
Retroperitoneum
- anatomic stage/prognostic groups, **9**
- soft tissue sarcoma staging (TNM System), **7**
Rhabdoid tumor
- atypical teratoid, extraskeletal mesenchymal chondrosarcoma vs., **502**
- extrarenal, **716–719**
  - alveolar rhabdomyosarcoma vs., **388**
  - desmoplastic small round cell tumor vs., **702**
  - differential diagnosis, **718**
  - epithelioid rhabdomyosarcoma vs., **405**
  - epithelioid sarcoma vs., **680**
  - molecular genetics, **717–718**
  - prognosis, **717**
Rhabdomyoma
- adult-type, **372–373**
  - cardiac rhabdomyoma vs., **379**
  - congenital granular cell epulis vs., **799**
  - differential diagnosis, **373**
  - embryonal rhabdomyosarcoma vs., **382**
  - granular cell tumor vs., **542**
  - prognosis, **373**
- alveolar soft part sarcoma vs., **685**
- cardiac, **378–379**
  - differential diagnosis, **379**
  - genetics, **379**
  - prognosis, **379**

- crystal-storing histiocytosis vs., **315**
- embryonal rhabdomyosarcoma vs., **382**
- fetal, **374–375**
    differential diagnosis, **375**
    embryonal rhabdomyosarcoma vs., **382**
    genetics, **375**
    genital rhabdomyoma vs., **377**
    prognosis, **375**
    spindle cell rhabdomyosarcoma vs., **394**
- focal myositis vs., **371**
- genital, **376–377**
    botryoid-type embryonal, fibroepithelial stromal polyp vs., **575**
    differential diagnosis, **377**
    embryonal rhabdomyosarcoma vs., **382**
    fetal rhabdomyoma vs., **375**
    prognosis, **377**

Rhabdomyosarcoma
- alveolar, **386–391**
    desmoplastic small round cell tumor vs., **701**
    differential diagnosis, **388**
    embryonal rhabdomyosarcoma vs., **382**
    extraskeletal Ewing sarcoma vs., **708**
    malignant gastrointestinal neuroectodermal tumor vs., **778**
    neuroblastoma and ganglioneuroblastoma vs., **834**
    pleomorphic rhabdomyosarcoma vs., **401**
    prognosis, **387**
    sclerosing epithelioid fibrosarcoma vs., **234**
    sclerosing rhabdomyosarcoma vs., **397**
    undifferentiated round cell sarcoma with *CIC-DUX4* translocation vs., **729**
- angiomatoid fibrous histiocytoma vs., **644**
- botryoid-type embryonal, fibroepithelial stromal polyp vs., **575**
- embryonal, **380–385**
    alveolar rhabdomyosarcoma vs., **388**
    differential diagnosis, **382**
    ectomesenchymoma vs., **571**
    fetal rhabdomyoma vs., **375**
    genital rhabdomyoma vs., **377**
    prognosis, **381**
    spindle cell rhabdomyosarcoma vs., **394**
    undifferentiated embryonal sarcoma of liver vs., **845**
- epithelioid, **404–405**
    differential diagnosis, **405**
    molecular genetics, **405**
    pleomorphic rhabdomyosarcoma vs., **401**
    prognosis, **405**
- extrarenal rhabdoid tumor vs., **718**
- pleomorphic, **400–403**
    differential diagnosis, **401**
    embryonal rhabdomyosarcoma vs., **382**
    epithelioid rhabdomyosarcoma vs., **405**
    prognosis, **401**
    proliferative fasciitis/myositis vs., **121**
- sclerosing, **396–399**
    alveolar rhabdomyosarcoma vs., **388**
    differential diagnosis, **397**
    extraskeletal mesenchymal chondrosarcoma vs., **502**
    prognosis, **397**
    sclerosing epithelioid fibrosarcoma vs., **234**
- spindle cell, **392–395**
    biphenotypic sinonasal sarcoma vs., **851**
    differential diagnosis, **393–394**
    embryonal rhabdomyosarcoma vs., **382**
    fetal rhabdomyoma vs., **375**
    genital rhabdomyoma vs., **377**
    infantile fibrosarcoma vs., **265**
    low-grade myofibroblastic sarcoma vs., **193**
    malignant peripheral nerve sheath tumor vs., **560**
    prognosis, **393**
- undifferentiated pleomorphic sarcoma vs., **725**

RHE. *See* Retiform hemangioendothelioma.
Rheumatoid arthritis, synovial lipomatosis vs., **55**
Rheumatoid nodule, **306–307**
- deep granuloma annulare vs., **305**
- differential diagnosis, **307**
- prognosis, **307**

Rosai-Dorfman disease
- extranodal, **310–313**
    differential diagnosis, **312**
    histiocytic sarcoma vs., **325**
    idiopathic tumefactive fibroinflammatory lesions vs., **790**
    Langerhans cell histiocytosis vs., **309**
    prognosis, **311**
- reticulohistiocytoma vs., **302**
- solitary (juvenile) xanthogranuloma vs., **299**

Round blue cell tumors, various small, myeloid sarcoma vs., **609**
Round cell liposarcoma. *See* Myxoid liposarcoma.

S

Sacrococcygeal ependymoma. *See* Ependymoma, of soft tissue.
Sampling, gross examination, **4**
Sarcoidosis, extranodal Rosai-Dorfman disease vs., **312**
Sarcoma
- alveolar soft part, **684–687**
    adult rhabdomyoma vs., **373**
    alveolar rhabdomyosarcoma vs., **388**
    congenital granular cell epulis vs., **799**
    differential diagnosis, **685**
    granular cell tumor vs., **542**
    molecular genetics, **685**
    paraganglioma vs., **816**
    PEComa vs., **694**
    prognosis, **685**
- atypical fibroxanthoma vs., **638**
- *BCOR-CCNB3* fusion-positive
    diagnostic checklist, **736**
    differential diagnosis, **736**
    prognosis, **735**
    undifferentiated round cell sarcoma with *CIC-DUX4* translocation vs., **729**
- *BCOR-CCNB3* fusion-positive, **734–737**

INDEX

- biphenotypic sinonasal, **850–853**
    - differential diagnosis, **851**
    - prognosis, **851**
- *CIC-FOXO4,* undifferentiated round cell sarcoma with *CIC-DUX4* translocation vs., **729**
- clear cell
    - diagnostic checklist, **690**
    - differential diagnosis, **690**
    - epithelioid malignant peripheral nerve sheath tumor vs., **567**
    - malignant gastrointestinal neuroectodermal tumor vs., **777–778**
    - melanotic schwannoma vs., **557**
    - metastatic tumors to soft tissue sites vs., **829**
    - molecular genetics, **689**
    - PEComa vs., **694**
    - prognosis, **689**
    - of tendon and aponeurosis, **689**
- epithelioid
    - angiosarcoma vs., **472**
    - classic, **679**
    - deep granuloma annulare vs., **305**
    - epithelioid hemangioendothelioma vs., **468**
    - epithelioid rhabdomyosarcoma vs., **405**
    - extrarenal rhabdoid tumor vs., **718**
    - inclusion body fibromatosis vs., **251**
    - ischemic fasciitis vs., **125**
    - molecular genetics, **680**
    - myoepithelioma of soft tissue vs., **656**
    - prognosis, **679**
    - proximal-type, **679–680**
    - pseudomyogenic hemangioendothelioma, **463**
    - rheumatoid nodule vs., **307**
    - solitary extramedullary plasmacytoma vs., **607**
    - superficial CD34(+) fibroblastic tumor vs., **211**
- Ewing
    - alveolar rhabdomyosarcoma vs., **388**
    - *BCOR-CCNB3* fusion-positive sarcoma vs., **736**
    - extrarenal rhabdoid tumor vs., **718**
    - extraskeletal, **706–711**
    - extraskeletal mesenchymal chondrosarcoma vs., **502**
    - low-grade endometrial stromal sarcoma vs., **857**
    - lymphoma of soft tissue vs., **611**
    - myxoid liposarcoma vs., **102**
    - neuroblastoma and ganglioneuroblastoma vs., **834**
    - synovial sarcoma vs., **668**
- follicular dendritic cell, **326–327**
    - angiomatoid fibrous histiocytoma vs., **644**
    - differential diagnosis, **327**
    - extranodal Rosai-Dorfman disease vs., **312**
    - interdigitating dendritic cell sarcoma vs., **329**
    - prognosis, **327**
- histiocytic, **324–325**
    - differential diagnosis, **325**
    - extranodal Rosai-Dorfman disease vs., **312**
    - interdigitating dendritic cell sarcoma vs., **329**
    - Langerhans cell histiocytosis vs., **309**
    - prognosis, **325**
- intimal, **720–721**
    - differential diagnosis, **721**
    - genetic testing, **721**
    - prognosis, **721**
- Kaposi, **476–483**
    - acquired tufted angioma vs., **437**
    - angiolipoma vs., **57**
    - angiomatoid fibrous histiocytoma vs., **644**
    - angiosarcoma vs., **472**
    - bacillary angiomatosis vs., **411**
    - composite hemangioendothelioma vs., **461**
    - dermatofibroma vs., **272**
    - differential diagnosis, **478**
    - glomeruloid hemangioma vs., **443**
    - hobnail hemangioma vs., **435**
    - intranodal palisade myofibroblastoma vs., **153**
    - kaposiform hemangioendothelioma vs., **455**
    - lymphangioma-like, lymphangioma vs., **448**
    - microvenular hemangioma vs., **439**
    - nodular fasciitis vs., **116**
    - papillary intralymphatic angioendothelioma vs., **457**
    - prognosis, **477**
    - retiform hemangioendothelioma vs., **459**
    - spindle cell hemangioma vs., **427**
- Langerhans cell
    - interdigitating dendritic cell sarcoma vs., **329**
    - Langerhans cell histiocytosis vs., **309**
- low-grade endometrial stromal, **856–857**
    - differential diagnosis, **857**
    - prognosis, **857**
- low-grade fibromyxoid, **222–231**
    - angiofibroma of soft tissue vs., **145**
    - desmoid-type fibromatosis vs., **170**
    - desmoplastic fibroblastoma vs., **141**
    - differential diagnosis, **224**
    - intramuscular myxoma vs., **615**
    - juxtaarticular myxoma vs., **619**
    - myxofibrosarcoma vs., **218**
    - myxoid liposarcoma vs., **102**
    - ossifying fibromyxoid tumor vs., **652**
    - perineurioma vs., **532**
    - prognosis, **223**
    - sclerosing epithelioid fibrosarcoma vs., **233**
    - superficial angiomyxoma vs., **621**
- low-grade myofibroblastic
    - adult-type fibrosarcoma vs., **215**
    - desmoid-type fibromatosis vs., **170**
    - differential diagnosis, **193**
    - nodular fasciitis vs., **116**
    - plexiform fibrohistiocytic tumor vs., **317**
    - prognosis, **193**
    - spindle cell rhabdomyosarcoma vs., **394**
- low-grade myofibroblastic, **192–195**
- myeloid, **608–609**
    - differential diagnosis, **609**
    - lymphoma of soft tissue vs., **611**
    - molecular genetics, **609**
    - myelolipoma vs., **79**
    - prognosis, **609**
- myxoinflammatory fibroblastic
    - extranodal Rosai-Dorfman disease vs., **312**
    - pleomorphic hyalinizing angiectatic tumor vs., **627**
    - superficial CD34(+) fibroblastic tumor vs., **211**

INDEX

- pleomorphic, high-grade, undifferentiated pleomorphic sarcoma vs., **725**
- pleomorphic dermal
  - atypical fibroxanthoma vs., **638**
  - superficial CD34(+) fibroblastic tumor vs., **211**
- primary cardiac, intimal sarcoma vs., **721**
- synovial, **666–677**
  - adult-type fibrosarcoma vs., **215**
  - biphasic, **668**
  - biphenotypic sinonasal sarcoma vs., **851**
  - calcifying fibrous tumor vs., **249**
  - differential diagnosis, **668**
  - ectopic hamartomatous thymoma vs., **633**
  - extraskeletal mesenchymal chondrosarcoma vs., **502**
  - extraskeletal osteosarcoma vs., **498**
  - infantile fibrosarcoma vs., **265**
  - leiomyosarcoma vs., **346**
  - low-grade endometrial stromal sarcoma vs., **857**
  - malignant gastrointestinal neuroectodermal tumor vs., **778**
  - malignant mesothelioma vs., **600**
  - molecular genetics, **668**
  - monophasic, **667**
  - monoplastic, calcifying aponeurotic fibroma vs., **245**
  - myxoid liposarcoma vs., **102**
  - prognosis, **667**
  - spindle epithelial tumor with thymus-like differentiation vs., **855**
- undifferentiated pleomorphic, **724–727**
  - adult-type fibrosarcoma vs., **215**
  - angiomatoid fibrous histiocytoma vs., **644**
  - dedifferentiated liposarcoma vs., **96**
  - differential diagnosis, **725**
  - extranodal Rosai-Dorfman disease vs., **312**
  - extraskeletal osteosarcoma vs., **498**
  - with giant cells, giant cell tumor of soft tissue vs., **321**
  - leiomyosarcoma vs., **346**
  - metastatic tumors to soft tissue sites vs., **829**
  - molecular genetics, **725**
  - myxofibrosarcoma vs., **218**
  - nodular fasciitis vs., **116**
  - pleomorphic hyalinizing angiectatic tumor vs., **627**
  - pleomorphic liposarcoma vs., **108**
  - prognosis, **725**
  - proliferative fasciitis/myositis vs., **121**

Sarcomatoid carcinoma
- atypical fibroxanthoma vs., **637**
- ectopic hamartomatous thymoma vs., **633**
- extraskeletal osteosarcoma vs., **498**
- metastatic, follicular dendritic cell sarcoma vs., **327**
- spindle cell rhabdomyosarcoma vs., **394**
- squamous cell, leiomyosarcoma vs., **346**
- undifferentiated embryonal sarcoma of liver vs., **845**

Scar
- early, microvenular hemangioma vs., **439**
- fibrous, desmoid-type fibromatosis vs., **170**
- hypertrophic
  - dermatomyofibroma vs., **159**
  - keloid vs., **163**
- keloidal collagen. *See* Keloid.

SCH. *See* Spindle cell hemangioma.

Schwann cell hamartoma, mucosal, gastrointestinal smooth muscle neoplasms vs., **764**

Schwannian stroma-poor neuroblastic tumor (neuroblastoma), **833**

Schwannian stroma-rich neuroblastic tumor (ganglioneuroblastoma), **833**

Schwannoma, **508–521**
- ancient, **510**
- cellular, **510**
  - deep leiomyoma vs., **339**
  - ganglioneuroma vs., **551**
  - malignant peripheral nerve sheath tumor vs., **560**
  - spindle cell rhabdomyosarcoma vs., **394**
- conventional, melanotic schwannoma vs., **557**
- differential diagnosis, **510–511**
- ependymoma of soft tissue vs., **827**
- epithelioid, **510**
  - epithelioid malignant peripheral nerve sheath tumor vs., **567**
- gastrointestinal, **760–761**
  - differential diagnosis, **761**
  - gastrointestinal smooth muscle neoplasms vs., **764**
  - gastrointestinal stromal tumor vs., **747**
  - melanotic schwannoma vs., **557**
  - prognosis, **761**
- hybrid nerve sheath tumor vs., **537**
- intranodal palisade myofibroblastoma vs., **153**
- melanotic, **556–557**
  - differential diagnosis, **557**
  - prognosis, **557**
- microcystic/reticular, **510**
- myoepithelioma of soft tissue vs., **656**
- neuroblastoma-like, **510**
- neurofibroma vs., **524**
- ossifying fibromyxoid tumor vs., **652**
- perineurioma vs., **532**
- pleomorphic hyalinizing angiectatic tumor vs., **627**
- plexiform, **510**
  - xanthomas vs., **296**
- prognosis, **509**
- pseudoglandular, **510**
- sinonasal glomangiopericytoma vs., **806**
- solitary circumscribed neuroma vs., **507**

Schwannomatosis, **509**

SCL. *See* Spindle cell lipoma.

Sclerosing disease, IgG4-related, inflammatory myofibroblastic tumor vs., **198**

Sclerosing epithelioid fibrosarcoma (SEF), **232–237**
- differential diagnosis, **233–234**
- low-grade fibromyxoid sarcoma vs., **224**
- ossifying fibromyxoid tumor vs., **652**
- prognosis, **233**
- sclerosing rhabdomyosarcoma vs., **397**

Sclerosing mesenteritis. *See* Idiopathic tumefactive fibroinflammatory lesions.

Sclerosing perineurioma, fibroma of tendon sheath vs., **136**

Sclerosing pseudovascular rhabdomyosarcoma. *See* Sclerosing rhabdomyosarcoma.

INDEX

Sclerosing rhabdomyosarcoma, **396–399**
- alveolar rhabdomyosarcoma vs., **388**
- differential diagnosis, **397**
- extraskeletal mesenchymal chondrosarcoma vs., **502**
- prognosis, **397**
- sclerosing epithelioid fibrosarcoma vs., **234**

Sclerotic fibroma. *See also* Storiform collagenoma.
- pleomorphic fibroma vs., **157**

SCN. *See* Solitary circumscribed neuroma.
Secondary lymphangiectasia, lymphangioma vs., **448**
Sectioning, gross examination, **4**
Serous borderline tumor, implants of, well-differentiated papillary mesothelioma vs., **595**
SETTLE. *See* Spindle epithelial tumor with thymus-like differentiation.
Silicone granuloma, pleomorphic liposarcoma vs., **108**
Sinonasal glomangiopericytoma, **804–809**
- diagnostic checklist, **806**
- differential diagnosis, **806**
- genetics, **805**
- nasopharyngeal angiofibroma vs., **802**
- prognosis, **805**

Sinonasal-type hemangiopericytoma. *See* Sinonasal glomangiopericytoma.
Sinus histiocytosis with massive lymphadenopathy. *See* Extranodal Rosai-Dorfman disease; Rosai-Dorfman disease.
Sinusoidal hemangioma, **440–441**
- diagnostic checklist, **441**
- differential diagnosis, **441**
- prognosis, **441**

Skeletal muscle, tumors of
- adult rhabdomyoma, **372–373**
  - differential diagnosis, **373**
  - prognosis, **373**
- alveolar rhabdomyosarcoma, **386–391**
  - differential diagnosis, **388**
  - prognosis, **387**
- cardiac rhabdomyoma, **378–379**
  - differential diagnosis, **379**
  - genetics, **379**
  - prognosis, **379**
- embryonal rhabdomyosarcoma, **380–385**
  - differential diagnosis, **382**
  - prognosis, **381**
- epithelioid rhabdomyosarcoma, **404–405**
  - differential diagnosis, **405**
  - molecular genetics, **405**
  - prognosis, **405**
- fetal rhabdomyoma, **374–375**
  - differential diagnosis, **375**
  - genetics, **375**
  - prognosis, **375**
- focal myositis, **370–371**
  - differential diagnosis, **371**
  - prognosis, **371**
- genital rhabdomyoma, **376–377**
  - differential diagnosis, **377**
  - prognosis, **377**
- pleomorphic rhabdomyosarcoma, **400–403**
  - differential diagnosis, **401**
  - prognosis, **401**
- sclerosing rhabdomyosarcoma, **396–399**
  - differential diagnosis, **397**
  - prognosis, **397**
- spindle cell rhabdomyosarcoma, **392–395**
  - differential diagnosis, **393–394**
  - prognosis, **393**

Skin, normal, from special sites, smooth muscle hamartoma vs., **333**
Small cell carcinoma, extraskeletal Ewing sarcoma vs., **708**
Small cell osteosarcoma, *BCOR-CCNB3* fusion-positive sarcoma vs., **736**
Small round cell tumor, desmoplastic, alveolar rhabdomyosarcoma vs., **388**
Smooth muscle hamartoma, **332–333**
- congenital, superficial leiomyoma vs., **335**
- differential diagnosis, **333**
- prognosis, **333**
- superficial leiomyoma vs., **335**

Smooth muscle neoplasms
- gastrointestinal, **762–765**
  - differential diagnosis, **764**
  - gastrointestinal stromal tumor vs., **747**
  - prognosis, **763**
- low-grade endometrial stromal sarcoma vs., **857**
- sinonasal, sinonasal glomangiopericytoma vs., **806**

Smooth muscle tumors
- deep leiomyoma, **338–341**
  - differential diagnosis, **339**
  - prognosis, **339**
- Epstein-Barr virus-associated smooth muscle tumor, **342–343**
  - differential diagnosis, **343**
  - prognosis, **343**
- leiomyosarcoma, **344–349**
  - differential diagnosis, **346**
  - prognosis, **345**
- smooth muscle hamartoma, **332–333**
  - differential diagnosis, **333**
  - prognosis, **333**
- superficial leiomyoma, **334–337**
  - differential diagnosis, **335**
  - prognosis, **335**

Soft part sarcoma, alveolar, **684–687**
- adult rhabdomyoma vs., **373**
- alveolar rhabdomyosarcoma vs., **388**
- congenital granular cell epulis vs., **799**
- differential diagnosis, **685**
- granular cell tumor vs., **542**
- molecular genetics, **685**
- paraganglioma vs., **816**
- PEComa vs., **694**
- prognosis, **685**

Soft tissue aneurysmal bone cyst, nodular fasciitis vs., **116**
Soft tissue chondroma, **486–491**
- calcified, tumoral calcinosis vs., **787**
- calcifying aponeurotic fibroma vs., **245**
- chondroid lipoma vs., **67**
- diagnostic checklist, **488**
- differential diagnosis, **487–488**
- extraskeletal myxoid chondrosarcoma vs., **713**

- myoepithelioma of soft tissue vs., **656**
- phosphaturic mesenchymal tumor vs., **665**
- prognosis, **487**
- synovial chondromatosis vs., **493**

Soft tissue giant cell tumor of low malignant potential. *See* Giant cell tumor of soft tissue.

Soft tissue immunohistochemistry, **12–17**
- commonly used antibodies in soft tissue pathology, **12**
- epithelioid cell tumors
  - in GI tract, **16**
  - in soft tissue, **15**
- pattern-based diagnostic approach, with prominent CD34 expression, **17**
- pleomorphic soft tissue tumors, **14**
- small round blue cell tumors, **15**
- spindle cell tumors
  - in GI tract, **16**
  - in soft tissue, **14**

Soft tissue metastasis, from axial chordoma, extraaxial soft tissue chordoma vs., **843**

Soft tissue tumors
- diagnostic approach
  - age-based approach, **26**
  - biopsy and resection, **22–25**
  - gastrointestinal mesenchymal tumors, **27**
  - involving lymph nodes, **27**
  - location-based, **27**
- diagnostic molecular and cytogenetic findings, **18**
- feature-based diagnostic approach, **36–43**
  - cytologic features, **36**
  - inflammatory component, **37**
  - multinucleated cells, **37**
  - nuclear features, **37–38**
  - stromal findings, **38**
  - structures, **38**
  - vasculature, **38**
- molecular features, **18–19**
- pattern-based diagnostic approach, **28–35**
  - epithelioid cell patterns, **30**
  - monomorphic spindle cell patterns, **28**
  - pleomorphic spindle cell patterns, **29–30**

Solitary circumscribed neuroma, **506–507**
- differential diagnosis, **507**
- prognosis, **507**

Solitary cutaneous reticulohistiocytoma. *See* Reticulohistiocytoma.

Solitary extramedullary plasmacytoma, **606–607**
- differential diagnosis, **607**
- prognosis, **607**

Solitary extraosseous plasmacytoma. *See* Solitary extramedullary plasmacytoma.

Solitary fibrous tumor, **184–191**
- acral fibromyxoma vs., **625**
- angiofibroma of soft tissue vs., **145**
- *BCOR-CCNB3* fusion-positive sarcoma vs., **736**
- biphenotypic sinonasal sarcoma vs., **851**
- calcifying fibrous tumor vs., **249**
- cellular angiofibroma vs., **581**
- cellular/malignant, extraskeletal mesenchymal chondrosarcoma vs., **502**
- deep benign fibrous histiocytoma vs., **277**
- dermatofibrosarcoma protuberans vs., **176**
- differential diagnosis, **186**
- ectopic hamartomatous thymoma vs., **633**
- gastrointestinal stromal tumor vs., **747**
- low-grade endometrial stromal sarcoma vs., **857**
- malignant mesothelioma vs., **600**
- mammary-type myofibroblastoma vs., **149**
- molecular genetics, **186**
- myopericytoma vs., **359**
- nasopharyngeal angiofibroma vs., **802**
- nuchal-type fibroma vs., **165**
- perineurioma vs., **532**
- peripheral hemangioblastoma vs., **823**
- phosphaturic mesenchymal tumor vs., **665**
- prognosis, **185**
- sinonasal glomangiopericytoma vs., **806**
- spindle cell/pleomorphic lipoma vs., **62**
- spindle epithelial tumor with thymus-like differentiation vs., **855**
- synovial sarcoma vs., **668**

Solitary (juvenile) xanthogranuloma, **298–299**
- differential diagnosis, **299**
- extranodal Rosai-Dorfman disease vs., **312**
- prognosis, **299**
- reticulohistiocytoma vs., **302**
- xanthomas vs., **296**

Specimen inking, **4**

Spindle cell carcinoma, spindle epithelial tumor with thymus-like differentiation vs., **855**

Spindle cell hemangioendothelioma. *See* Spindle cell hemangioma.

Spindle cell hemangioma (SCH), **426–429**
- angiolipoma vs., **57**
- angiomatoid fibrous histiocytoma vs., **644**
- composite hemangioendothelioma vs., **461**
- diagnostic checklist, **427**
- differential diagnosis, **427**
- Kaposi sarcoma vs., **478**
- kaposiform hemangioendothelioma vs., **455**
- prognosis, **427**

Spindle cell lipoma (SCL), **60–65**
- cellular angiofibroma vs., **581**
- differential diagnosis, **62**
- hemosiderotic fibrolipomatous tumor vs., **635**
- lipoma vs., **48**
- mammary-type myofibroblastoma vs., **149**
- molecular genetics, **61**
- myolipoma vs., **71**
- prognosis, **61**
- solitary fibrous tumor vs., **186**

Spindle cell lipomatous tumor, atypical, **84–87**
- differential diagnosis, **85**
- molecular genetics, **85**
- prognosis, **85**
- spindle cell/pleomorphic lipoma vs., **62**

Spindle cell liposarcoma. *See* Atypical spindle cell lipomatous tumor.

Spindle cell melanoma
- atypical fibroxanthoma vs., **637–638**
- desmoplastic, dermatofibrosarcoma protuberans vs., **176**

INDEX

- spindle cell rhabdomyosarcoma vs., **394**

Spindle cell/pleomorphic lipoma, atypical spindle cell lipomatous tumor vs., **85**

Spindle cell rhabdomyosarcoma, **392–395**
- biphenotypic sinonasal sarcoma vs., **851**
- differential diagnosis, **393–394**
- embryonal rhabdomyosarcoma vs., **382**
- genital rhabdomyoma vs., **377**
- infantile fibrosarcoma vs., **265**
- low-grade myofibroblastic sarcoma vs., **193**
- malignant peripheral nerve sheath tumor vs., **560**
- prognosis, **393**

Spindle epithelial tumor with thymus-like differentiation (SETTLE), **854–855**
- differential diagnosis, **855**
- prognosis, **855**

Spitz nevus, cellular neurothekeoma vs., **291**

Spitzoid melanoma, cellular neurothekeoma vs., **291**

Squamous cell carcinoma, epithelioid sarcoma vs., **680**

Stasis changes, microvenular hemangioma vs., **439**

Stasis dermatitis, microvenular hemangioma vs., **439**

Sterno(cleido) mastoid (pseudo)tumor of infancy. *See* Fibromatosis colli.

Storiform collagenoma, **160–161**
- diagnostic checklist, **161**
- differential diagnosis, **161**
- prognosis, **161**

Storiform perineural fibroma. *See* Perineurioma.

Stromal tumor, gastrointestinal, **744–759**
- benign neural gastrointestinal polyps vs., **741**
- calcifying fibrous tumor vs., **249**
- deep leiomyoma vs., **339**
- desmoid-type fibromatosis vs., **170**
- differential diagnosis, **747**
- epithelioid, extraskeletal myxoid chondrosarcoma vs., **713**
- gastrointestinal schwannoma vs., **761**
- gastrointestinal smooth muscle neoplasms vs., **764**
- histiocytic sarcoma vs., **325**
- idiopathic tumefactive fibroinflammatory lesions vs., **790**
- inflammatory fibroid polyp vs., **767**
- inflammatory myofibroblastic tumor vs., **198**
- leiomyosarcoma vs., **346**
- low-grade endometrial stromal sarcoma vs., **857**
- malignant gastrointestinal neuroectodermal tumor vs., **777**
- molecular prognostication, **748**
- paraganglioma vs., **816**
- plexiform fibromyxoma vs., **773**
- prognosis, **745–746**
- risk stratification, **748**
- solitary fibrous tumor vs., **186**
- spindled, gangliocytic paraganglioma vs., **771**

Submucosal leiomyoma, benign neural gastrointestinal polyps vs., **741**

Subungual fibroma, storiform collagenoma vs., **161**

Superficial acral fibromyxoma
- dermal nerve sheath myxoma vs., **547**
- superficial angiomyxoma vs., **621**

Superficial angiomyxoma, **620–623**
- acral fibromyxoma vs., **625**
- deep (aggressive) angiomyxoma vs., **585**
- dermal nerve sheath myxoma vs., **547**
- differential diagnosis, **621**
- juxtaarticular myxoma vs., **619**
- prognosis, **621**

Superficial CD34(+) fibroblastic tumor (SCD34FT), **210–213**
- differential diagnosis, **211**
- prognosis, **211**

Superficial cutaneous lymphangioma. *See* Lymphangioma.

Superficial fibromatosis
- dermatomyofibroma vs., **159**
- fibroma of tendon sheath vs., **136**
- inclusion body fibromatosis vs., **251**

Superficial leiomyoma, **334–337**
- differential diagnosis, **335**
- prognosis, **335**

Superficial leiomyosarcoma, superficial leiomyoma vs., **335**

Synovial cell sarcoma. *See* Synovial sarcoma.

Synovial chondroma. *See* Synovial chondromatosis.

Synovial chondromatosis, **492–495**
- diagnostic checklist, **493**
- differential diagnosis, **493**
- prognosis, **493**
- soft tissue chondroma vs., **487–488**

Synovial chondrometaplasia. *See* Synovial chondromatosis.

Synovial chondrosarcoma, synovial chondromatosis vs., **493**

Synovial lipoma. *See* Synovial lipomatosis.

Synovial lipomatosis, **54–55**
- differential diagnosis, **55**
- prognosis, **55**

Synovial osteochondromatosis. *See* Synovial chondromatosis.

Synovial sarcoma, **666–677**
- adult-type fibrosarcoma vs., **215**
- biphasic, **668**
- biphenotypic sinonasal sarcoma vs., **851**
- calcifying fibrous tumor vs., **249**
- differential diagnosis, **668**
- ectopic hamartomatous thymoma vs., **633**
- extraskeletal mesenchymal chondrosarcoma vs., **502**
- extraskeletal osteosarcoma vs., **498**
- infantile fibrosarcoma vs., **265**
- leiomyosarcoma vs., **346**
- low-grade endometrial stromal sarcoma vs., **857**
- malignant gastrointestinal neuroectodermal tumor vs., **778**
- malignant mesothelioma vs., **600**
- molecular genetics, **668**
- monophasic, **667**
  - clear cell sarcoma vs., **690**
  - malignant peripheral nerve sheath tumor vs., **560**
  - palmar/plantar fibromatosis vs., **167**
  - solitary fibrous tumor vs., **186**
  - spindle cell rhabdomyosarcoma vs., **393**
- monoplastic, calcifying aponeurotic fibroma vs., **245**
- myxoid liposarcoma vs., **102**

- poorly differentiated
  BCOR-CCNB3 fusion-positive sarcoma vs., **736**
  extraskeletal Ewing sarcoma vs., **708**
  lymphoma of soft tissue vs., **611**
  undifferentiated round cell sarcoma with *CIC-DUX4* translocation vs., **730**
- prognosis, **667**
- spindle epithelial tumor with thymus-like differentiation vs., **855**

Systemic angiomatosis. *See* Lymphangioma.

T

Targetoid hemosiderotic hemangioma
- glomeruloid hemangioma vs., **443**
- microvenular hemangioma vs., **439**

Tendinous xanthoma, **295**
Tendon sheath, fibroma, **134–139**
- differential diagnosis, **136**
- prognosis, **135**

Tenosynovial fibroma. *See* Fibroma, tendon sheath.
Tenosynovial giant cell tumor
- diffuse-type, **284–289**
  differential diagnosis, **286**
  localized-type tenosynovial giant cell tumor vs., **280**
  myxoinflammatory fibroblastic sarcoma vs., **204**
  prognosis, **285**
  synovial lipomatosis vs., **55**
- fibroosseous pseudotumor vs., **131**
- giant cell tumor of soft tissue vs., **321**
- localized-type, **278–283**
  deep benign fibrous histiocytoma vs., **277**
  differential diagnosis, **280**
  diffuse-type tenosynovial giant cell tumor vs., **286**
  fibroma of tendon sheath vs., **136**
  prognosis, **279**
  xanthomas vs., **296**
- malignant, diffuse-type tenosynovial giant cell tumor vs., **286**
- soft tissue chondroma vs., **488**

Teratoma, genital rhabdomyoma vs., **377**
Thrombus, organizing, spindle cell hemangioma vs., **427**
Tophaceous gout
- amyloidoma vs., **783**
- tumoral calcinosis vs., **787**

Tophaceous pseudogout
- soft tissue chondroma vs., **488**
- tumoral calcinosis vs., **787**

Translocation-associated undifferentiated sarcomas, neuroblastoma and ganglioneuroblastoma vs., **834**
Traumatic neuroma, solitary circumscribed neuroma vs., **507**
Triton tumor, malignant
- ectomesenchymoma vs., **571**
- embryonal rhabdomyosarcoma vs., **382**

True inflammatory myopathies, focal myositis vs., **371**
Tuberous xanthoma, **295**
Tumoral amyloidosis. *See* Amyloidoma.
Tumoral calcinosis, **786–787**
- amyloidoma vs., **783**
- differential diagnosis, **787**
- prognosis, **787**
- soft tissue chondroma vs., **488**

Tumoral lipocalcinosis. *See* Tumoral calcinosis.
Tumors of uncertain differentiation
- acral fibromyxoma, **624–625**
  differential diagnosis, **625**
  prognosis, **625**
- alveolar soft part sarcoma, **684–687**
  differential diagnosis, **685**
  molecular genetics, **685**
  prognosis, **685**
- aneurysmal bone cyst of soft tissue, **630–631**
  differential diagnosis, **631**
  molecular genetics, **631**
  prognosis, **631**
- angiomatoid fibrous histiocytoma, **642–649**
  differential diagnosis, **644**
  molecular genetics, **644**
  prognosis, **643**
- atypical fibroxanthoma, **636–641**
  differential diagnosis, **637–638**
  immunohistochemistry, **638**
  prognosis, **637**
- clear cell sarcoma, **688–691**
  diagnostic checklist, **690**
  differential diagnosis, **690**
  molecular genetics, **689**
  prognosis, **689**
  of tendon and aponeurosis, **689**
- desmoplastic small round cell tumor, **700–705**
  differential diagnosis, **701–702**
  immunohistochemistry, **702**
  molecular genetics, **701**
  prognosis, **701**
- ectopic hamartomatous thymoma, **632–633**
  differential diagnosis, **633**
  prognosis, **633**
- epithelioid sarcoma, **678–683**
  classic, **679**
  differential diagnosis, **680**
  molecular genetics, **680**
  prognosis, **679**
  proximal-type, **679–680**
- extrarenal rhabdoid tumor, **716–719**
  differential diagnosis, **718**
  genetic factors, **717**
  molecular genetics, **717–718**
  prognosis, **717**
- extraskeletal Ewing sarcoma, **706–711**
  differential diagnosis, **708**
  molecular genetics, **708**
  prognosis, **707**
- extraskeletal myxoid chondrosarcoma, **712–715**
  differential diagnosis, **713**
  genetic testing, **713**
  prognosis, **713**
- hemosiderotic fibrolipomatous tumor, **634–635**
  differential diagnosis, **635**

molecular genetics, **635**
prognosis, **635**
- intimal sarcoma, **720–721**
differential diagnosis, **721**
genetic testing, **721**
prognosis, **721**
- intramuscular myxoma, **614–617**
differential diagnosis, **615**
genetic testing, **615**
prognosis, **615**
- juxtaarticular myxoma, **618–619**
differential diagnosis, **619**
genetic testing, **619**
prognosis, **619**
- myoepithelioma of soft tissue, **656–663**
differential diagnosis, **658**
immunohistochemistry, **658**
molecular genetics, **657**
prognosis, **657**
- ossifying fibromyxoid tumor, **650–655**
differential diagnosis, **652**
malignant, **651**
molecular genetics, **652**
prognosis, **651**
- perivascular epithelioid cell tumor, **692–699**
differential diagnosis, **694**
genetics, **693**
prognosis, **693**
- phosphaturic mesenchymal tumor, **664–665**
differential diagnosis, **665**
molecular genetics, **665**
prognosis, **665**
- pleomorphic hyalinizing angiectatic tumor, **626–629**
differential diagnosis, **627**
molecular genetics, **627**
prognosis, **627**
- superficial angiomyxoma, **620–623**
differential diagnosis, **621**
prognosis, **621**
- synovial sarcoma, **666–677**
biphasic, **668**
differential diagnosis, **668**
molecular genetics, **668**
monophasic, **667**
prognosis, **667**

U

Undifferentiated carcinoma, pleomorphic rhabdomyosarcoma vs., **401**
Undifferentiated embryonal sarcoma of liver (UESL), **844–845**
- differential diagnosis, **845**
- prognosis, **845**
Undifferentiated pleomorphic sarcoma, **724–727**
- adult-type fibrosarcoma vs., **215**
- angiomatoid fibrous histiocytoma vs., **644**
- dedifferentiated liposarcoma vs., **96**
- differential diagnosis, **725**
- extranodal Rosai-Dorfman disease vs., **312**
- extraskeletal osteosarcoma vs., **498**
- with giant cells, giant cell tumor of soft tissue vs., **321**
- leiomyosarcoma vs., **346**
- metastatic tumors to soft tissue sites vs., **829**
- molecular genetics, **725**
- myxofibrosarcoma vs., **218**
- nodular fasciitis vs., **116**
- pleomorphic hyalinizing angiectatic tumor vs., **627**
- pleomorphic liposarcoma vs., **108**
- prognosis, **725**
- proliferative fasciitis/myositis vs., **121**
Undifferentiated round cell sarcoma with *CIC-DUX4* translocation, **728–733**
- diagnostic checklist, **730**
- differential diagnosis, **729–730**
- immunohistochemistry, **730**
- prognosis, **729**
Undifferentiated round or spindle cell sarcomas, *BCOR-CCNB3* fusion-positive sarcoma vs., **736**
Undifferentiated sarcoma with *CIC-DUX4* translocation
- *BCOR-CCNB3* fusion-positive sarcoma vs., **736**
- extraskeletal Ewing sarcoma vs., **708**
Undifferentiated/unclassified sarcomas
- *BCOR-CCNB3* fusion-positive sarcoma
diagnostic checklist, **736**
differential diagnosis, **736**
prognosis, **735**
- *BCOR-CCNB3* fusion-positive sarcoma, **734–737**
- undifferentiated pleomorphic sarcoma, **724–727**
differential diagnosis, **725**
molecular genetics, **725**
prognosis, **725**
- undifferentiated round cell sarcoma with *CIC-DUX4* translocation, **728–733**
diagnostic checklist, **730**
differential diagnosis, **729–730**
immunohistochemistry, **730**
prognosis, **729**

V

Vaginal rhabdomyoma. *See* Genital rhabdomyoma.
Vanek tumor. *See* Inflammatory fibroid polyp.
Vascular leiomyoma. *See* Angioleiomyoma.
Vascular lesion, atypical, **452–453**
- angiosarcoma vs., **472**
- diagnostic checklist, **453**
- differential diagnosis, **453**
- prognosis, **453**
Vascular malformation. *See also* Angiomatosis.
- congenital hemangioma vs., **414**
- infantile hemangioma vs., **418**
Vascular neoplasms, *BCOR-CCNB3* fusion-positive sarcoma vs., **736**
Vascular proliferation, atypical, lymphangioma vs., **448**
Vascular stasis, severe, Kaposi sarcoma vs., **478**

INDEX

Vascular tumors (including lymphatics)
- acquired tufted angioma, **436–437**
  - diagnostic checklist, **437**
  - differential diagnosis, **437**
  - prognosis, **437**
- angiomatosis, **444–445**
  - differential diagnosis, **445**
  - prognosis, **445**
- angiosarcoma
  - differential diagnosis, **472**
  - molecular genetics, **472**
  - prognosis, **471**
- atypical vascular lesion, **452–453**
  - diagnostic checklist, **453**
  - differential diagnosis, **453**
  - prognosis, **453**
- bacillary angiomatosis, **410–411**
  - diagnostic checklist, **411**
  - differential diagnosis, **411**
  - prognosis, **411**
- composite hemangioendothelioma, **460–461**
  - differential diagnosis, **461**
  - prognosis, **461**
- congenital hemangioma, **412–415**
  - differential diagnosis, **414**
  - genetics, **413**
  - prognosis, **413**
- epithelioid hemangioendothelioma
  - differential diagnosis, **468**
  - molecular genetics, **467**
  - prognosis, **467**
- epithelioid hemangioma, **422–425**
  - differential diagnosis, **423**
  - molecular genetics, **423**
  - prognosis, **423**
- glomeruloid hemangioma, **442–443**
  - diagnostic checklist, **443**
  - differential diagnosis, **443**
  - prognosis, **443**
- hobnail hemangioma, **434–435**
  - diagnostic checklist, **435**
  - prognosis, **435**
- infantile hemangioma, **416–419**
  - differential diagnosis, **418**
  - genetics, **417**
  - prognosis, **417**
- intramuscular hemangioma, **430–433**
  - differential diagnosis, **431**
  - prognosis, **431**
- Kaposi sarcoma
  - differential diagnosis, **478**
  - prognosis, **477**
- kaposiform hemangioendothelioma, **454–455**
  - diagnostic checklist, **455**
  - differential diagnosis, **455**
  - prognosis, **455**
- lobular capillary hemangioma, **420–421**
  - differential diagnosis, **421**
  - prognosis, **421**
- lymphangioma, **446–449**
  - diagnostic checklist, **448**
  - differential diagnosis, **448**
  - genetics, **447**
  - prognosis, **447**
- massive localized lymphedema, **450–451**
  - differential diagnosis, **451**
  - prognosis, **451**
- microvenular hemangioma, **438–439**
  - diagnostic checklist, **439**
  - differential diagnosis, **439**
  - hobnail hemangioma vs., **435**
  - Kaposi sarcoma vs., **478**
  - prognosis, **439**
- papillary endothelial hyperplasia, **408–409**
  - diagnostic checklist, **409**
  - differential diagnosis, **409**
  - prognosis, **409**
- pseudomyogenic hemangioendothelioma, **462–465**
  - differential diagnosis, **463**
  - molecular genetics, **463**
  - prognosis, **463**
- retiform hemangioendothelioma, **458–459**
  - diagnostic checklist, **459**
  - differential diagnosis, **459**
  - prognosis, **459**
- sinusoidal hemangioma, **440–441**
  - diagnostic checklist, **441**
  - differential diagnosis, **441**
  - prognosis, **441**
- spindle cell hemangioma, **426–429**
  - diagnostic checklist, **427**
  - differential diagnosis, **427**
  - prognosis, **427**

Venous malformation
- sinusoidal hemangioma vs., **441**
- spindle cell hemangioma vs., **427**

Verruciform xanthoma, xanthomas vs., **296**

Villous lipomatous proliferation of synovial membrane. *See* Synovial lipomatosis.

W

Well-differentiated angiosarcoma, atypical vascular lesion vs., **453**

Well-differentiated liposarcoma, **88–93**
- dedifferentiated liposarcoma vs., **96**
- differential diagnosis, **90**
- elastofibromas vs., **143**
- idiopathic tumefactive fibroinflammatory lesions vs., **790**
- inflammatory myofibroblastic tumor vs., **198**
- ischemic fasciitis vs., **125**
- massive localized lymphedema vs., **451**
- molecular genetics, **90**
- myelolipoma vs., **79**
- peripheral hemangioblastoma vs., **823**
- prognosis, **89**
- synovial lipomatosis vs., **55**

Well-differentiated papillary mesothelioma, **594–597**
- adenomatoid tumor vs., **591**
- differential diagnosis, **595**
- prognosis, **595**

X

Xanthelasma, **295**
Xanthogranuloma, solitary (juvenile), **298–299**
- differential diagnosis, **299**
- extranodal Rosai-Dorfman disease vs., **312**
- prognosis, **299**
- reticulohistiocytoma vs., **302**
- xanthomas vs., **296**
Xanthomas, **294–297**
- clinical forms, **296**
- differential diagnosis, **296**
- eruptive, **295**
- hyperlipoproteinemia (Fredrickson) classification, **296**
- plexiform, **295**
- prognosis, **295**
- solitary (juvenile) xanthogranuloma vs., **299**
- tuberous, **295**
- verruciform, xanthomas vs., **296**
Xanthomatosis, cerebrotendinous, **295**
Xanthomatous tumor, plexiform. *See* Xanthomas.